a LANGE medical book

CURRENT
Diagnosis & Treatment
Pediatrics

TWENTY-FIFTH EDITION

Edited by

William W. Hay Jr., MD
Professor of Pediatrics, University of Colorado, Retired

Myron J. Levin, MD
Professor, Departments of Pediatrics and Medicine
Section of Pediatric Infectious Diseases
University of Colorado School of Medicine
and Children's Hospital Colorado

Mark J. Abzug, MD
Professor and Vice Chair for Academic Affairs,
Department of Pediatrics, Section of Pediatric Infectious
Diseases, University of Colorado School of Medicine and
Children's Hospital Colorado

Maya Bunik, MD, MPH
Professor, Department of Pediatrics, Section of General
Pediatric Academic Medicine, University of Colorado
School of Medicine, Medical Director, Child Health Clinic,
Children's Hospital Colorado

and Associate Authors

The Department of Pediatrics at the University of Colorado School of Medicine
is affiliated with Children's Hospital Colorado.

New York   Chicago   San Francisco   Athens   London   Madrid   Mexico City   Milan
New Delhi   Singapore   Sydney   Toronto

CURRENT Diagnosis & Treatment: Pediatrics, Twenty-Fifth Edition

Previous editions copyright © 2018, 2016, 2014, 2012, 2011, 2009, 2007, 2003, 2001 by McGraw-Hill; © 1999, 1997, 1995, 1991, 1987 by Appleton & Lange.

1 2 3 4 5 6 7 8 9   LCR   25 24 23 22 21 20

ISBN 978-1-260-45782-7
MHID 1-260-45782-6
ISSN 0093-8556

Notice

Medicine is an ever-changing science. As new research and clinical experience broaden our knowledge, changes in treatment and drug therapy are required. The authors and the publisher of this work have checked with sources believed to be reliable in their efforts to provide information that is complete and generally in accord with the standards accepted at the time of publication. However, in view of the possibility of human error or changes in medical sciences, neither the authors nor the publisher nor any other party who has been involved in the preparation or publication of this work warrants that the information contained herein is in every respect accurate or complete, and they disclaim all responsibility for any errors or omissions or for the results obtained from use of the information contained in this work. Readers are encouraged to confirm the information contained herein with other sources. For example and in particular, readers are advised to check the product information sheet included in the package of each drug they plan to administer to be certain that the information contained in this work is accurate and that changes have not been made in the recommended dose or in the contraindications for administration. This recommendation is of particular importance in connection with new or infrequently used drugs.

This book was set in Minion Pro by Cenveo® Publisher Services.
The editors were Andrew Moyer and Peter J. Boyle.
The production supervisor was Catherine H. Saggese.
Project management was provided by Revathi Viswanathan, Cenveo Publisher Services.

This book is printed on acid-free paper.

Contents

17. Oral Medicine & Dentistry 459

Roopa P. Gandhi, BDS, MSD
Chaitanya P. Puranik, BDS, MS, MDentSci, PhD
Anne Wilson, DDS, MS
Katherine L. Chin, DDS, MS

18. Ear, Nose, & Throat 471

Patricia J. Yoon, MD
Melissa A. Scholes, MD
Brian W. Herrmann, MD

19. Respiratory Tract & Mediastinum 499

Monica J. Federico, MD
Christopher D. Baker, MD
Emily M. DeBoer, MD
Oren Kupfer, MD
Stacey L. Martiniano, MD
Paul Stillwell, MD
Stephen Hawkins, MD
Deborah Liptzin, MD

25. Neurologic & Muscular Disorders   740

Ricka Messer, MD, PhD
Teri L. Schreiner, MD, MPH
Diana Walleigh, MD
Michele L. Yang, MD
Jan A. Martin, MD
Scott Demarest, MD

26. Orthopedics   811

Jason T. Rhodes, MD, MS
Alex Tagawa, BS
Cameron Niswander, BA
Wade Coomer, BS
Mark A. Erickson, MD, MMM
Sayan De, MD

37. Genetics & Dysmorphology 1081

Naomi J. L. Meeks, MD
Margarita Saenz, MD
Anne Chun-Hui Tsai, MD, MSc
Ellen R. Elias, MD

38. Allergic Disorders 1112

Ronina A. Covar, MD
David M. Fleischer, MD
Christine Cho, MD
Mark Boguniewicz, MD

39. Antimicrobial Therapy 1152

Sarah K. Parker, MD
Jason Child, PharmD
Christine E. MacBrayne, PharmD, MSC
Andrew Haynes, MD
Justin Searns, MD

Authors

Jordan K. Abbott, MD, MA
Assistant Professor, Department of Pediatrics, Section of Pediatric Allergy and Immunology, University of Colorado School of Medicine and Children's Hospital Colorado
Chapter 33: Immunodeficiency

Daniel R. Ambruso, MD
Professor Emeritus, Department of Pediatrics, Section of Pediatric Hematology, Oncology, and Bone Marrow Transplant, Center for Cancer and Blood Disorders, University of Colorado School of Medicine and Children's Hospital Colorado
Chapter 30: Hematologic Disorders

Abigail S. Angulo, MD, MPH
Assistant Professor, Department of Pediatrics, Section of Developmental Pediatrics, University of Colorado School of Medicine and Children's Hospital Colorado
Chapter 3: Child Development & Behavior

Edwin J. Asturias, MD
Associate Professor, Departments of Pediatrics, Epidemiology and Infectious Diseases, University of Colorado School of Medicine; Associate Director, Center for Global Health, Colorado School of Public Health
Chapter 40: Infections: Viral & Rickettsial

Christopher D. Baker, MD
Associate Professor, Department of Pediatrics, Section of Pediatric Pulmonary Medicine, University of Colorado School of Medicine and Children's Hospital Colorado
Chapter 19: Respiratory Tract & Mediastinum

Peter R. Baker II, MD
Assistant Professor, Department of Pediatrics, Section of Clinical Genetics and Metabolism, University of Colorado School of Medicine and Children's Hospital Colorado
Chapter 36: Inborn Errors of Metabolism

Sarah Bartz, MD
Assistant Professor, Department of Pediatrics, Section of Pediatric Endocrinology, Clinical Lead for Colorado Springs Pediatric Endocrinology, University of Colorado School of Medicine and Children's Hospital Colorado
Chapter 34: Endocrine Disorders

Margret E. Bock, MD, MS
Assistant Professor, Department of Pediatrics, Section of Pediatric Nephrology, Clinic Medical Director, Kidney Transplantation, University of Colorado and Children's Hospital Colorado
Chapter 23: Fluid, Electrolyte, & Acid-Base Disorders & Therapy
Chapter 24: Kidney & Urinary Tract

Mark Boguniewicz, MD
Professor, Department of Pediatrics, Section of Pediatric Allergy and Immunology, University of Colorado School of Medicine and National Jewish Medical and Research Center
Chapter 38: Allergic Disorders

Cortney Braund, MD
Assistant Professor, Department of Pediatrics, Section of Pediatric Emergency Medicine, University of Colorado School of Medicine and Children's Hospital Colorado
Chapter 12: Emergencies & Injuries

David Brumbaugh, MD
Associate Professor, Department of Pediatrics, Section of Pediatric Gastroenterology, Hepatology, and Nutrition, Digestive Health Institute, Associate Chief Medical Officer, University of Colorado School of Medicine and Children's Hospital Colorado
Chapter 21: Gastrointestinal Tract

Dale Burkett, MD
Assistant Professor, Department of Pediatrics, Section of Pediatric Cardiology, University of Colorado School of Medicine and Children's Hospital Colorado
Chapter 20: Cardiovascular Diseases

Adam Burstein, DO
Child, Adolescent & Adult Psychiatrist
Chapter 7: Child & Adolescent Psychiatric Disorders & Psychosocial Aspects of Pediatrics

Todd C. Carpenter, MD
Professor, Department of Pediatrics, Section of Pediatric Critical Care Medicine, University of Colorado School of Medicine and Children's Hospital Colorado
Chapter 14: Critical Care

Jessica R. Cataldi, MD, MSCS
Assistant Professor, Department of Pediatrics, Section of Pediatric Infectious Diseases, University of Colorado School of Medicine and Children's Hospital Colorado
Chapter 10: Immunization

Christina Chambers, MD
Instructor, Department of Pediatrics, Section of Pediatric Endocrinology, University of Colorado School of Medicine and Children's Hospital Colorado
Chapter 34: Endocrine Disorders

Christine M. Chan, MD
Assistant Professor, Department of Pediatrics, Section of
 Pediatric Endocrinology, University of Colorado School of
 Medicine and Children's Hospital Colorado
Chapter 34: Endocrine Disorders

Peter H. Chase, MD
Emeritus Professor of Pediatrics, Department of Pediatrics,
 Clinical Director Emeritus, Barbara Davis Center for
 Childhood Diabetes, University of Colorado School
 of Medicine
Chapter 35: Diabetes Mellitus

Antonia Chiesa, MD
Associate Professor, Department of Pediatrics, University of
 Colorado School of Medicine, Kempe Child Protection
 Team, Kempe Center for the Prevention and Treatment of
 Child Abuse and Neglect, Children's Hospital Colorado
Chapter 8: Child Abuse & Neglect

Jason Child, PharmD
Co-Director, Antimicrobial Stewardship, Department of
 Pharmacy, University of Colorado Skaggs School of
 Pharmacy and Pharmaceutical Sciences
Chapter 39: Antimicrobial Therapy

Katherine L. Chin, DDS, MS
Associate Clinical Professor, Department of Pediatric Dentistry,
 University of Colorado School of Dental Medicine and
 Children's Hospital Colorado
Chapter 17: Oral Medicine & Dentistry

Christine Cho, MD
Assistant Professor, Department of Pediatrics, Section of
 Pediatric Allergy and Clinical Immunology, National
 Jewish Medical and Research Center (primary appointment),
 University Colorado School of Medicine and Children's
 Hospital Colorado
Chapter 38: Allergic Disorders

Gerald H. Clayton, PhD
Senior Instructor (retired), Department of Physical Medicine
 and Rehabilitation Medicine, University of Colorado School
 of Medicine and Children's Hospital Colorado
Chapter 28: Rehabilitation Medicine

Amy C. Clevenger, MD, PhD
Assistant Professor, Department of Pediatrics, Section of
 Pediatric Critical Care Medicine, University of Colorado
 School of Medicine and Children's Hospital Colorado
Chapter 14: Critical Care

Wade Coomer, BS
Research Coordinator, Department of Orthopedic Surgery,
 University of Colorado School of Medicine and Children's
 Hospital Colorado
Chapter 26: Orthopedics

Ronina A. Covar, MD
Associate Professor, Department of Pediatrics, Section of
 Pediatric Allergy and Immunology, University of
 Colorado School of Medicine and National Jewish
 Medical and Research Center
Chapter 38: Allergic Disorders

Melanie Cree-Green, MD, PhD
Associate Professor, Department of Pediatrics, Section of
 Pediatric Endocrinology, Director, Multidisciplinary PCOS
 Clinic, University of Colorado School of Medicine and
 Children's Hospital Colorado
Chapter 34: Endocrine Disorders

Angela S. Czaja, MD, MSc
Associate Professor, Department of Pediatrics, Section of
 Pediatric Critical Care Medicine, University of Colorado
 School of Medicine and Children's Hospital Colorado
Chapter 14: Critical Care

Katherine S. Dahab, MD, FAAP, CAQSM
Assistant Professor, Department of Orthopedic Surgery,
 Director, Pediatric Primary Care Sports Medicine
 Fellowship, University of Colorado School of Medicine
 and Children's Hospital Colorado
Chapter 27: Sports Medicine

Matthew F. Daley, MD
Assistant Professor, Department of Pediatrics, Section of
 General Academic Pediatrics, University of Colorado
 School of Medicine and Children's Hospital Colorado;
 Senior Investigator, Institute for Health Research, Kaiser
 Permanente Colorado
Chapter 10: Immunization

Richard C. Dart, MD, PhD
Professor, Department of Surgery, University of Colorado
 School of Medicine and Children's Hospital Colorado;
 Director, Rocky Mountain Poison and Drug Center, Denver
 Health and Hospital Authority
Chapter 13: Poisoning

Shanlee Davis, MD, MSCS
Assistant Professor, Department of Pediatrics, Section of
 Pediatric Endocrinology, Director of the eXtraOrdinary Kids
 Turner Syndrome Clinic, University of Colorado School of
 Medicine and Children's Hospital Colorado
Chapter 34: Endocrine Disorders

Sayan De, MD
Assistant Professor, Department of Orthopedic Surgery,
 University of Colorado School of Medicine and Children's
 Hospital Colorado
Chapter 26: Orthopedics

Emily M. DeBoer, MD
Assistant Professor, Department of Pediatrics, Section of
Pediatric Pulmonary Medicine, University of Colorado
School of Medicine and Children's Hospital Colorado
Chapter 19: Respiratory Tract & Mediastinum

Scott Demarest, MD
Assistant Professor, Department of Pediatrics, Section of Child
Neurology, University of Colorado School of Medicine and
Children's Hospital Colorado
Chapter 25: Neurologic & Muscular Disorders

Liliane K. Diab, MD
Assistant Professor, Department of Pediatrics, Section of
Pediatric Nutrition, University of Colorado School of
Medicine and Children's Hospital Colorado
Chapter 11: Normal Childhood Nutrition & Its Disorders

Melkon G. DomBourian, MD
Assistant Professor, Department of Pathology, Section of
Pediatric Pathology, University of Colorado School of
Medicine and Children's Hospital Colorado
Chapter 46: Chemistry & Hematology Reference Intervals

Ellen R. Elias, MD
Professor, Departments of Pediatrics and Genetics, Section of
Clinical Genetics and Metabolism, Director, Special Care
Clinic, University of Colorado School of Medicine and
Children's Hospital Colorado
Chapter 37: Genetics & Dysmorphology

Mark A. Erickson, MD
Professor, Department of Orthopedic Surgery, Medical
Director, Spine Center, University of Colorado School of
Medicine and Children's Hospital Colorado
Chapter 26: Orthopedics

Monica J. Federico, MD
Associate Professor, Department of Pediatrics, Section of
Pediatric Pulmonary Medicine, University of Colorado
School of Medicine and Children's Hospital Colorado
Chapter 19: Respiratory Tract & Mediastinum

Amy G. Feldman, MD, MSCS
Assistant Professor, Department of Pediatrics, Section of
Pediatric Gastroenterology, Hepatology and Nutrition,
Digestive Health Institute, University of Colorado School of
Medicine and Children's Hospital Colorado
Chapter 22: Liver & Pancreas

David M. Fleischer, MD
Associate Professor, Department of Pediatrics, Section of
Pediatric Allergy and Immunology, University of Colorado
School of Medicine and Children's Hospital Colorado
Chapter 38: Allergic Disorders

David Fox, MD
Associate Professor, Department of Pediatrics, Section of
General Academic Pediatrics, University of Colorado School
of Medicine and Children's Hospital Colorado
Chapter 9: Ambulatory & Office Pediatrics

Anna R. K. Franklin, MD
Associate Professor, Department of Pediatrics, Section of
Pediatric Hematology, Oncology, and Bone Marrow
Transplant, Center for Cancer and Blood Disorders,
University of Colorado School of Medicine and Children's
Hospital Colorado
Chapter 31: Neoplastic Disease

Brigitte I. Frohnert, MD, PhD
Assistant Professor, Department of Pediatrics, Barbara Davis
Center for Childhood Diabetes, University of Colorado
School of Medicine and Children's Hospital Colorado
Chapter 35: Diabetes Mellitus

Glenn T. Furuta, MD
Professor, Department of Pediatrics, Section of Pediatric
Gastroenterology, Hepatology and Nutrition, Digestive
Health Institute; Director, Gastrointestinal Eosinophil
Disease Program, National Jewish Health, University of
Colorado School of Medicine and Children's Hospital
Colorado
Chapter 21: Gastrointestinal Tract

James Gaensbauer, MD, MScPH
Assistant Professor, Department of Pediatrics, Section of
Pediatric Infectious Diseases, Denver Health, Denver Metro
TB Clinic, University of Colorado School of Medicine and
Children's Hospital Colorado, Center for Global Health,
University of Colorado School of Public Health
Chapter 42: Infections: Bacterial & Spirochetal
Chapter 43: Infections: Parasitic & Mycotic

Jeffrey L. Galinkin, MD
Anesthesiologist, US Anesthesia Partners, Greenwood Village,
Colorado
*Chapter 32: Pain Management & Pediatric Palliative &
End-of-Life Care*

Roopa P. Gandhi, BDS, MSD
Associate Clinical Professor, Residency Program Director,
Department of Pediatric Dentistry, University of Colorado
School of Dental Medicine and Children's Hospital Colorado
Chapter 17: Oral Medicine & Dentistry

Timothy Price Garrington, MD
Associate Professor, Department of Pediatrics, Section of
Pediatric Hematology, Oncology, and Bone Marrow
Transplant, Center for Cancer and Blood Disorders,
University of Colorado School of Medicine and Children's
Hospital Colorado
Chapter 31: Neoplastic Disease

Edward Goldson, MD
Professor Emeritus, Department of Pediatrics, University of Colorado School of Medicine and Children's Hospital Colorado
Chapter 3: Child Development & Behavior

Ryan J. Good, MD
Assistant Professor, Department of Pediatrics, Section of Pediatric Critical Care Medicine, University of Colorado School of Medicine and Children's Hospital Colorado
Chapter 14: Critical Care

Eva N. Grayck, MD
Professor, Department of Pediatrics, Section of Pediatric Critical Care Medicine, University of Colorado School of Medicine and Children's Hospital Colorado
Chapter 14: Critical Care

Brian S. Greffe, MD
Professor, Department of Pediatrics, Section of Pediatric Hematology, Oncology, and Bone Marrow Transplant, Center for Cancer and Blood Disorders, University of Colorado School of Medicine and Children's Hospital Colorado
Chapter 31: Neoplastic Disease
Chapter 32: Pain Management & Pediatric Palliative & End-of-Life Care

Cameron F. Gunville, DO
Associate Professor, Department of Pediatrics, Section of Pediatric Critical Care Medicine, University of Colorado School of Medicine and Children's Hospital Colorado
Chapter 14: Critical Care

Matthew A. Haemer, MD, MPH
Associate Professor, Department of Pediatrics, Section of Pediatric Nutrition, University of Colorado School of Medicine and Children's Hospital Colorado
Chapter 11: Normal Childhood Nutrition & Its Disorders

Melisha G. Hanna, MD, MS
Assistant Professor, Department of Pediatrics, Section of Pediatric Nephrology, Medical Director, Pediatric Dialysis Unit, University of Colorado School of Medicine and Children's Hospital Colorado
Chapter 23: Fluid, Electrolyte, & Acid-Base Disorders & Therapy
Chapter 24: Kidney & Urinary Tract

Pia J. Hauk, MD
Associate Professor, Department of Pediatrics, Section of Pediatric Allergy and Immunology, University of Colorado School of Medicine and National Jewish Medical and Research Center
Chapter 33: Immunodeficiency

Stephen Hawkins, MD, DO
Assistant Professor, Department of Pediatrics, Section of Pediatric Pulmonary Medicine, University of Colorado School of Medicine and Children's Hospital Colorado
Chapter 19: Respiratory Tract & Mediastinum

Andrew Haynes, MD
Fellow, Department of Pediatrics, Section of Pediatric Infectious Diseases, University of Colorado School of Medicine and Children's Hospital Colorado
Chapter 39: Antimicrobial Therapy

Brian W. Herrmann, MD
Associate Professor, Department of Otolaryngology, Head and Neck Surgery, Division of Pediatric Otolaryngology, University of Colorado School of Medicine and Children's Hospital Colorado
Chapter 18: Ear, Nose, & Throat

Edward J. Hoffenberg, MD
Professor, Department of Pediatrics, Section of Pediatric Gastroenterology, Hepatology and Nutrition, Digestive Health Institute, University of Colorado School of Medicine and Children's Hospital Colorado
Chapter 21: Gastrointestinal Tract

Jordana E. Hoppe, MD
Assistant Professor, Department of Pediatrics, Section of Pediatric Pulmonary Medicine, University of Colorado School of Medicine and Children's Hospital Colorado
Chapter 46: Chemistry & Hematology Reference Intervals

Stephanie Hsu, MD, PhD
Associate Professor, Department of Pediatrics, Section of Pediatric Endocrinology, University of Colorado School of Medicine and Children's Hospital Colorado
Chapter 34: Endocrine Disorders

Daniel Hyman, MD
Chief Quality Officer, Children's Hospital Colorado, Department of Pediatrics, Section of Pediatric Administration, University of Colorado School of Medicine and Children's Hospital Colorado
Chapter 1: Advancing the Quality & Safety of Care

Pei-Ni Jone, MD
Associate Professor, Department of Pediatrics, Section of Pediatric Cardiology, University of Colorado School of Medicine and Children's Hospital Colorado
Chapter 20: Cardiovascular Diseases

Jennifer Lee Jung, MD
Assistant Professor, Department of Ophthalmology, University of Colorado School of Medicine and Children's Hospital Colorado
Chapter 16: Eye

Paritosh Kaul, MD
Professor, Department of Pediatrics, Section of Adolescent
    Medicine, University of Colorado School of Medicine,
    Denver Health Medical Center and Children's Hospital
    Colorado
Chapter 5: Adolescent Substance Abuse

Amy K. Keating, MD
Associate Professor, Department of Pediatrics, Section of
    Pediatric Hematology, Oncology, and Bone Marrow
    Transplant, Center for Cancer and Blood Disorders,
    University of Colorado School of Medicine and Children's
    Hospital Colorado
Chapter 31: Neoplastic Disease

Kimberly Kelsay, MD
Associate Professor, Department of Psychiatry, Section of Child
    and Adolescent Psychiatry, University of Colorado School of
    Medicine and Children's Hospital Colorado
*Chapter 7: Child & Adolescent Psychiatric Disorders &
    Psychosocial Aspects of Pediatrics*

John S. Kim, MD
Assistant Professor, Department of Pediatrics, Section of
    Pediatric Cardiology, University of Colorado School of
    Medicine and Children's Hospital Colorado
Chapter 20: Cardiovascular Diseases

Nancy A. King, MSN, RN, CPNP
Senior Instructor, Department of Pediatrics, Section of Pediatric
    Hematology, Oncology, and Bone Marrow Transplant,
    Center for Cancer and Blood Disorders, University of
    Colorado School of Medicine and Children's Hospital
    Colorado
*Chapter 32: Pain Management & Pediatric Palliative &
    End-of-Life Care*

Jessica Knight-Perry, MD, MB
Assistant Professor, Department of Pediatrics, Section of
    Pediatric Hematology, Oncology, and Bone Marrow
    Transplant, Center for Cancer and Blood Disorders,
    University of Colorado School of Medicine and Children's
    Hospital Colorado
Chapter 31: Neoplastic Disease

Gregory E. Kobak, MD
Senior Instructor, Department of Pediatrics, Section of
    Pediatric Gastroenterology, Hepatology and Nutrition,
    Digestive Health Institute, University of Colorado Denver
    and Children's Hospital Colorado
Chapter 21: Gastrointestinal Tract

Robert E. Kramer, MD
Professor, Department of Pediatrics, Section of Pediatric
    Gastroenterology, Hepatology and Nutrition, Digestive
    Health Institute, University of Colorado School of Medicine
    and Children's Hospital Colorado
Chapter 21: Gastrointestinal Tract

Nancy F. Krebs, MD, MS
Professor, Department of Pediatrics, Head, Section of Pediatric
    Nutrition, University of Colorado School of Medicine and
    Children's Hospital Colorado
Chapter 11: Normal Childhood Nutrition & Its Disorders

Oren Kupfer, MD
Assistant Professor, Department of Pediatrics, Section of
    Pediatric Pulmonary Medicine, University of Colorado
    School of Medicine and Children's Hospital Colorado
Chapter 19: Respiratory Tract & Mediastinum

Austin A. Larson, MD
Assistant Professor, Department of Pediatrics, Section of
    Clinical Genetics and Metabolism, University of Colorado
    School of Medicine and Children's Hospital Colorado
Chapter 36: Inborn Errors of Metabolism

Aimee LeDoux, MT (ASCP)
Department of Pathology and Laboratory Medicine
    Children's Hospital Colorado
Chapter 46: Chemistry & Hematology Reference Intervals

Myron J. Levin, MD
Professor, Departments of Pediatrics and Medicine, Section of
    Pediatric Infectious Diseases, University of Colorado School
    of Medicine and Children's Hospital Colorado
Chapter 40: Infections: Viral & Rickettsial
Chapter 43: Infections: Parasitic & Mycotic

Deborah Liptzin, MD
Assistant Professor, Department of Pediatrics, Section of
    Pediatric Pulmonary Medicine, University of Colorado
    School of Medicine and Children's Hospital Colorado
Chapter 19: Respiratory Tract & Mediastinum

Christine E. MacBrayne, PharmD, MSC
Department of Pharmacy, University of Colorado Skaggs
    School of Pharmacy and Pharmaceutical Sciences
Chapter 39: Antimicrobial Therapy

Cara L. Mack, MD
Professor, Department of Pediatrics, Section of Pediatric
    Gastroenterology, Hepatology and Nutrition, Digestive
    Health Institute, University of Colorado School of Medicine
    and Children's Hospital Colorado
Chapter 22: Liver & Pancreas

Kelly Maloney, MD
Professor, Department of Pediatrics, Section of Pediatric
Hematology, Oncology, and Bone Marrow Transplant,
Center for Cancer and Blood Disorders, University of
Colorado School of Medicine and Children's Hospital
Colorado
Chapter 31: Neoplastic Disease

Jacob A. Mark, MD
Assistant Professor, Department of Pediatrics, Section of
Pediatric Gastroenterology, Hepatology and Nutrition,
Digestive Health Institute, University of Colorado School of
Medicine and Children's Hospital Colorado
Chapter 22: Liver & Pancreas

Jan A. Martin, MD
Associate Professor, Department of Pediatrics, Section of Child
Neurology, Associate Program Director, Child Neurology
Residency, University of Colorado School of Medicine and
Children's Hospital Colorado
Chapter 25: Neurologic & Muscular Disorders

Stacey L. Martiniano, MD
Assistant Professor, Department of Pediatrics, Section of
Pediatric Pulmonary Medicine, University of Colorado
School of Medicine and Children's Hospital Colorado
Chapter 19: Respiratory Tract & Mediastinum

Stephanie W. Mayer, MD
Assistant Professor, Department of Orthopedic Surgery,
University of Colorado School of Medicine and Children's
Hospital Colorado
Chapter 27: Sports Medicine

Elizabeth J. McFarland, MD
Professor, Department of Pediatrics, Head, Section of Pediatric
Infectious Diseases, University of Colorado School of
Medicine and Children's Hospital Colorado
Chapter 41: Human Immunodeficiency Virus Infection

Christopher McKinney, MD
Assistant Professor, Department of Pediatrics, Section of
Pediatric Hematology, Oncology, and Bone Marrow
Transplant, Center for Cancer and Blood Disorders,
University of Colorado School of Medicine and Children's
Hospital Colorado
Chapter 30: Hematologic Disorders

Naomi J. L. Meeks, MD
Assistant Professor, Department of Pediatrics, Section of
Clinical Genetics and Metabolism, University of Colorado
School of Medicine and Children's Hospital Colorado
Chapter 37: Genetics & Dysmorphology

Ricka Messer, MD, PhD
Assistant Professor, Department of Pediatrics, Section of Child
Neurology, Director, Pediatric Neurohospitalist Program,
Medical Director of Clinical Informatics for Neurology,
University of Colorado School of Medicine and Children's
Hospital Colorado
Chapter 25: Neurologic & Muscular Disorders

Jean M. Mulcahy Levy, MD
Associate Professor, Department of Pediatrics, Section of
Pediatric Hematology, Oncology, and Bone Marrow
Transplant, Center for Cancer and Blood Disorders, Morgan
Adams Foundation Pediatric Brain Tumor Research
Program, University of Colorado School of Medicine and
Children's Hospital Colorado
Chapter 31: Neoplastic Disease

Kyle B. Nagle, MD, MPH, FAAP, CAQSM
Assistant Professor, Department of Orthopedic Surgery,
University of Colorado School of Medicine, Sports Medicine
for Youth Athletes, Children's Hospital Colorado
Orthopedics Institute
Chapter 27: Sports Medicine

Michael R. Narkewicz, MD, FAASLD
Professor, Department of Pediatrics, Hewitt-Andrews Chair in
Pediatric Liver Disease, Medical Director, The Pediatric Liver
Center and Liver Transplantation Program, Section of
Pediatric Gastroenterology, Hepatology and Nutrition,
Digestive Health Institute, University of Colorado School of
Medicine and Children's Hospital Colorado
Chapter 22: Liver & Pancreas

Daniel Nicklas, MD
Assistant Professor of Pediatrics, Director of Primary Care
Education, Children's Hospital Colorado Residency Program,
University of Colorado and Children's Hospital Colorado
Chapter 9: Ambulatory & Office Pediatrics

Cameron Niswander, BA
Medical Student, University of Colorado School of Medicine
Chapter 26: Orthopedics

Yosuke Nomura, MD
Instructor, Department of Pediatrics, Section of Pediatric
Infectious Diseases, University of Colorado School of
Medicine and Denver Health Medical Center
Chapter 42: Infections: Bacterial & Spirochetal

Rachelle Nuss, MD
Professor, Department of Pediatrics, Section of Pediatric
Hematology, Oncology, and Bone Marrow Transplant, Sickle
Cell Center, University of Colorado School of Medicine and
Children's Hospital Colorado
Chapter 30: Hematologic Disorders

Ann-Christine Nyquist, MD, MSPH
Professor, Department of Pediatrics, Section of Pediatric
  Infectious Diseases, University of Colorado School of
  Medicine and Children's Hospital Colorado
Chapter 10: Immunization
Chapter 44: Sexually Transmitted Infections

John W. Ogle, MD
Professor and Vice Chairman Emeritus, Department of
  Pediatrics, University of Colorado School of Medicine
Chapter 42: Infections: Bacterial & Spirochetal

Sean T. O'Leary, MD, MPH
Associate Professor, Department of Pediatrics, Section of
  Pediatric Infectious Diseases, University of Colorado School
  of Medicine and Children's Hospital Colorado
Chapter 10: Immunization

Daniel Olson, MD
Assistant Professor, Department of Pediatrics, Sections of
  Pediatric Infectious Diseases and Epidemiology, University
  of Colorado School of Public Health, Center for Global
  Health, and Children's Hospital Colorado
Chapter 40: Infections: Viral & Rickettsial

Jonathan Orsborn, MD
Assistant Professor, Department of Pediatrics–Emergency Med/
  Urgent Care/NOC, University of Colorado School of
  Medicine, Director of Quality Improvement, Children's
  Hospital Colorado
Chapter 12: Emergencies & Injuries

Sarah K. Parker, MD
Associate Professor, Department of Pediatrics, Section of
  Pediatric Infectious Diseases, Medical Director of
  Antimicrobial Stewardship, University of Colorado
  School of Medicine and Children's Hospital Colorado
Chapter 39: Antimicrobial Therapy

Laura E. Primak, RD, CNSD, CSP
Coordinator, Professional Research Assistant, Dietitian,
  Department of Pediatrics, Section of Pediatric Nutrition,
  University of Colorado School of Medicine and Children's
  Hospital Colorado
Chapter 11: Normal Childhood Nutrition & Its Disorders

Lori D. Prok, MD
Assistant Professor, Departments of Pediatrics and
  Dermatology, Section of Pediatric Dermatology, University
  of Colorado School of Medicine and Children's Hospital
  Colorado
Chapter 15: Skin

Chaitanya P. Puranik, BDS, MS, MDentSci, PhD
Assistant Clinical Professor, Director of Predoctoral Education
  in Pediatric Dentistry, Department of Pediatric Dentistry,
  University of Colorado School of Dental Medicine and
  Children's Hospital Colorado
Chapter 17: Oral Medicine & Dentistry

Suchitra Rao, MBBS, MSCS
Assistant Professor, Department of Pediatrics, Section of
  Pediatric Infectious Diseases, University of Colorado School
  of Medicine and Children's Hospital Colorado
Chapter 45: Travel Medicine

Dannah M. Raz, MD
Assistant Professor, Department of Pediatrics, Section of
  Developmental Pediatrics, University of Colorado School of
  Medicine and Children's Hospital Colorado
Chapter 3: Child Development & Behavior

Daniel H. Reirden, MD
Associate Professor, Departments of Internal Medicine and
  Pediatrics, Sections of Adolescent Medicine and Pediatric
  Infectious Diseases, University of Colorado School of
  Medicine and Children's Hospital Colorado
Chapter 44: Sexually Transmitted Infections

Marian Rewers, MD, PhD
Professor & Clinical Director, Barbara Davis Center for
  Childhood Diabetes, University of Colorado School of
  Medicine
Chapter 35: Diabetes Mellitus

Ann Reynolds, MD
Associate Professor, Department of Pediatrics, Section of
  Developmental Pediatrics; Director, The Child Development
  Unit, University of Colorado School of Medicine and
  Children's Hospital Colorado
Chapter 3: Child Development & Behavior

Jason T. Rhodes, MD, MS
Associate Professor, Department of Orthopedic Surgery,
  Director, Cerebral Palsy Program, University of Colorado
  School of Medicine and Children's Hospital Colorado,
  Adjunct Associate Professor, Department of Mechanical and
  Materials Engineering, University of Denver
Chapter 26: Orthopedics

Molly J. Richards, MD
Associate Professor, Department of Pediatrics, Section of
  Adolescent Medicine, University of Colorado School of
  Medicine and Children's Hospital Colorado
Chapter 4: Adolescence

Leslie A. Ridall, DO
Assistant Professor, Department of Pediatrics, Section of
Pediatric Critical Care Medicine, University of Colorado
School of Medicine and Children's Hospital Colorado
Chapter 14: Critical Care

Barry H. Rumack, MD
Clinical Professor, Department of Pediatrics, University of
Colorado School of Medicine; Director Emeritus, Rocky
Mountain Poison and Drug Center, Denver Health Authority
Chapter 13: Poisoning

Margarita Saenz, MD
Assistant Professor, Department of Pediatrics, Section of
Clinical Genetics and Metabolism, University of Colorado
School of Medicine and Children's Hospital Colorado
Chapter 37: Genetics & Dysmorphology

Amy E. Sass, MD, MPH
Associate Professor, Department of Pediatrics, Section of
Adolescent Medicine, University of Colorado School of
Medicine and Children's Hospital Colorado
Chapter 4: Adolescence

Carleen Schneiter, MD
Associate Professor, Department of Pediatrics, Section of
Pediatric Critical Care Medicine, University of Colorado
School of Medicine and Children's Hospital Colorado
Chapter 14: Critical Care

Melissa A. Scholes, MD
Associate Professor, Department of Otolaryngology, Head
and Neck Surgery, Section of Pediatric Otolaryngology,
University of Colorado School of Medicine and Children's
Hospital Colorado
Chapter 18: Ear, Nose, & Throat

Teri L. Schreiner, MD, MPH
Associate Professor, Department of Pediatrics, Section of Child
Neurology, Director, Neuroimmunology Center for Kids,
University of Colorado School of Medicine and Children's
Hospital Colorado
Chapter 25: Neurologic & Muscular Disorders

Justin Searns, MD
Pediatric Infectious Disease Fellow, Department of Pediatrics,
Section of Pediatric Infectious Diseases, University of
Colorado School of Medicine and Children's Hospital
Colorado
Chapter 39: Antimicrobial Therapy

Seth Septer, MD
Associate Professor, Department of Pediatrics, Section of
Pediatric Gastroenterology, Hepatology and Nutrition,
Digestive Health Institute, University of Colorado School of
Medicine and Children's Hospital Colorado
Chapter 21: Gastrointestinal Tract

Mary Shull, MD
Assistant Professor, Department of Pediatrics, Section of
Pediatric Gastroenterology, Hepatology and Nutrition,
Digestive Health Institute, Center for Celiac Disease,
University of Colorado School of Medicine and Children's
Hospital Colorado
Chapter 21: Gastrointestinal Tract

Eric J. Sigel, MD
Professor, Department of Pediatrics, Section of Adolescent
Medicine, University of Colorado School of Medicine and
Children's Hospital Colorado
Chapter 6: Eating Disorders

Andrew P. Sirotnak, MD, FAAP
Professor and Vice Chair for Faculty Affairs, Department of
Pediatrics, University of Colorado School of Medicine;
Director, Child Protection Team, Kempe Center for the
Prevention and Treatment of Child Abuse and Neglect,
Children's Hospital Colorado
Chapter 8: Child Abuse & Neglect

Danielle Smith, MD
Assistant Professor, Department of Pediatrics, Section of
Neonatology, University of Colorado School of Medicine and
Children's Hospital Colorado
Chapter 2: The Newborn Infant

Jason Soden, MD
Associate Professor, Department of Pediatrics, Section of
Pediatric Gastroenterology, Hepatology and Nutrition,
Digestive Health Institute, University of Colorado School of
Medicine and Children's Hospital Colorado
Chapter 21: Gastrointestinal Tract

Jennifer B. Soep, MD
Associate Professor, Department of Pediatrics, Section of
Pediatric Rheumatology, University of Colorado School of
Medicine and Children's Hospital Colorado
Chapter 29: Rheumatic Diseases

Ronald J. Sokol, MD
Professor and Vice Chair, Department of Pediatrics, Head,
Section of Pediatric Gastroenterology, Hepatology and
Nutrition; Director, Colorado Clinical Translational Sciences
Institute, University of Colorado School of Medicine and
Children's Hospital Colorado
Chapter 22: Liver & Pancreas

Robert Snyder, MT (ASCP)
Clinical Chemistry Supervisor, Department of Pathology and
Laboratory Medicine, University of Colorado, Children's
Hospital Colorado
Chapter 46: Chemistry & Hematology Reference Intervals

Paul Stillwell, MD
Senior Instructor, Department of Pediatrics, Section of
    Pediatric Pulmonary Medicine, University of Colorado
    School of Medicine and Children's Hospital Colorado
Chapter 19: Respiratory Tract & Mediastinum

Shikha S. Sundaram, MD, MSCI
Associate Professor, Department of Pediatrics, Section of
    Pediatric Gastroenterology, Hepatology and Nutrition,
    Digestive Health Institute, University of Colorado School of
    Medicine and Children's Hospital Colorado
Chapter 22: Liver & Pancreas

Alex Tagawa, BS
Research Coordinator, Department of Orthopedic Surgery,
    University of Colorado School of Medicine and Children's
    Hospital Colorado
Chapter 26: Orthopedics

Ayelet Talmi, PhD
Professor, Departments of Psychiatry and Pediatrics, Section of
    Child Neurology, Director of Integrated Behavioral Health,
    Pediatric Mental Health Institute, Director, Project CLIMB,
    Co-Director, Harris Program in Infant Mental Health,
    University of Colorado School of Medicine and Children's
    Hospital Colorado
*Chapter 7: Child & Adolescent Psychiatric Disorders &
    Psychosocial Aspects of Pediatrics*

Janet A. Thomas, MD
Professor, Department of Pediatrics, Section of Clinical
    Genetics and Metabolism, University of Colorado School of
    Medicine and Children's Hospital Colorado
Chapter 36: Inborn Errors of Metabolism

Carla X. Torres-Zegarra, MD
Assistant Professor, Departments of Dermatology and
    Pediatrics, Section of Pediatric Dermatology, University
    of Colorado School of Medicine and Children's Hospital
    Colorado
Chapter 15: Skin

Meghan Treitz, MD
Assistant Professor, Department of Pediatrics, Section of
    General Academic Pediatrics, University of Colorado School
    of Medicine and Children's Hospital Colorado
Chapter 9: Ambulatory & Office Pediatrics

Anne Chun-Hui Tsai, MD, MSc
Professor, Departments of Pediatrics and Genetics, Section of
    Clinical Genetics and Metabolism, University of Colorado
    School of Medicine and Children's Hospital Colorado
Chapter 37: Genetics & Dysmorphology

Johan L. K. Van Hove, MD, PhD, MBA
Professor, Department of Pediatrics, Section of Clinical
    Genetics and Metabolism, University of Colorado School of
    Medicine and Children's Hospital Colorado
Chapter 36: Inborn Errors of Metabolism

Armando Vidal, MD
Assistant Professor, Department of Orthopedic Surgery, Sports
    Medicine Program, University of Colorado School of
    Medicine and Children's Hospital Colorado
Chapter 27: Sports Medicine

Johannes von Alvensleben, MD
Assistant Professor, Department of Pediatrics, Section of
    Pediatric Cardiology, University of Colorado School of
    Medicine and Children's Hospital Colorado
Chapter 20: Cardiovascular Diseases

Thomas Walker, MD
Professor, Department of Pediatrics, Section of Pediatric
    Gastroenterology, Hepatology and Nutrition, Digestive
    Health Institute, University of Colorado School of Medicine
    and Children's Hospital Colorado
Chapter 21: Gastrointestinal Tract

Diana Walleigh, MD
Assistant Professor, Department of Pediatrics, Section of Child
    Neurology, University of Colorado School of Medicine and
    Children's Hospital Colorado
Chapter 25: Neurologic & Muscular Disorders

George Sam Wang, MD
Associate Professor, Department of Pediatrics, Emergency
    Medicine/Medical Toxicology, University of Colorado School
    of Medicine and Children's Hospital Colorado
Chapter 13: Poisoning

Michael Wang, MD
Professor, Department of Pediatrics, Section of Pediatric
    Hematology, Oncology, and Bone Marrow Transplant,
    Center for Cancer and Blood Disorders, University of
    Colorado School of Medicine and Children's Hospital
    Colorado
Chapter 30: Hematologic Disorders

Anne Wilson, DDS, MS
Professor, Delta Dental of Colorado Endowed Chairperson,
    Department of Pediatric Dentistry, University of Colorado
    School of Dental Medicine and Children's Hospital Colorado
Chapter 17: Oral Medicine & Dentistry

Pamela E. Wilson, MD
Associate Professor, Department of Physical Medicine and
    Rehabilitation, University of Colorado School of Medicine
    and Children's Hospital Colorado
Chapter 28: Rehabilitation Medicine

Michele L. Yang, MD
Assistant Professor, Departments of Pediatrics and Neurology,
    Section of Child Neurology, Director, EMG Laboratory,
    University of Colorado School of Medicine and Children's
    Hospital Colorado
Chapter 25: Neurologic & Muscular Disorders

Patricia J. Yoon, MD
Associate Professor, Department of Otolaryngology, Head
    and Neck Surgery, Section of Pediatric Otolaryngology,
    University of Colorado School of Medicine and Children's
    Hospital Colorado
Chapter 18: Ear, Nose, & Throat

Preface

The 25th edition of *Current Diagnosis & Treatment: Pediatrics (CDTP)* features practical, up-to-date, well-referenced information on the care of children from birth through infancy and adolescence. *CDTP* emphasizes the clinical aspects of pediatric care while also covering important underlying principles. *CDTP* provides a guide to diagnosis, understanding, and treatment of the medical problems of all pediatric patients in an easy-to-use and readable format.

INTENDED AUDIENCE

Like all Lange medical books, *CDTP* provides a concise, yet comprehensive source of current information. Students will find *CDTP* an authoritative introduction to pediatrics and an excellent source for reference and review. *CDTP* provides excellent coverage of The Council on Medical Student Education in Pediatrics (COMSEP) curriculum used in pediatric clerkships. Residents in pediatrics (and other specialties) will appreciate the detailed descriptions of diseases as well as diagnostic and therapeutic procedures. Pediatricians, family practitioners, nurses, nurse practitioners, physician assistants, and other health care providers who work with infants, children, and adolescents will find *CDTP* a useful reference on management of pediatric medicine.

COVERAGE

Forty-six chapters cover a wide range of topics, including neonatal medicine, child development and behavior, emergency and critical care medicine, and diagnosis and treatment of specific disorders according to major problems, etiologies, and organ systems. A wealth of tables and figures provides quick access to important information, such as acute and critical care procedures in the delivery room, the office, the emergency room, and in-hospital critical care units; anti-infective agents; drug dosages; immunization schedules; differential diagnosis; and developmental disorders.

NEW TO THIS EDITION

The 25th edition of *CDTP* has been revised comprehensively by the editors and contributing authors. A major effort involved further streamlining the contents of the book by condensing text into tables, eliminating wordy text, and updating references. New references and up-to-date and useful Web sites have been added, facilitating the reader to consult original material and to go beyond the confines of the textbook. As editors and practicing pediatricians, we have tried to ensure that each chapter reflects the needs and realities of day-to-day practice.

CHAPTERS WITH MAJOR REVISIONS INCLUDE:

3 Child Development & Behavior

5 Adolescent Substance Abuse

7 Child & Adolescent Psychiatric Disorders & Psychosocial Aspects of Pediatrics

9 Ambulatory & Office Pediatrics

10 Immunization

15 Skin

17 Oral Medicine & Dentistry

19 Respiratory Tract & Mediastinum

21 Gastrointestinal Tract

22 Liver & Pancreas

23 Fluid, Electrolyte, & Acid–Base Disorders & Therapy

25 Neurologic & Muscular Disorders

32 Pain Management & Pediatric Palliative & End-of-Life Care

CHAPTER REVISIONS

All chapters have been revised, with new authors added in several cases, reflecting the substantially updated material in each of their areas of pediatric medicine and ensuring conciseness and readability. Especially important are updates to the chapters on immunizations, endocrinology, neurologic and muscular disorders, and adolescent substance abuse. The chapter on HIV includes current guidelines for prevention and treatment of HIV, and updates information on the new antiretroviral therapies. The chapter on immunizations contains the most recently published recommendations, discusses the contraindications and precautions relevant to special populations, and includes the new vaccines licensed since the last edition of this book. All laboratory tables in Chapter 46 Chemistry and Hematology Reference Intervals, including Reference Ranges and Reference Intervals, have been updated. Nineteen new authors have contributed to these revisions.

ACKNOWLEDGMENTS

The editors would like to thank Bonnie Savone for her assistance in helping to manage the flow of manuscripts and materials among the chapter authors, editors, and publishers. The editors also would like to thank Robin Pence, RN, at Children's Hospital Colorado, who produced the cover photograph of Christina Suh, MD, and children.

William W. Hay Jr., MD
Myron J. Levin, MD
Mark J. Abzug, MD
Maya Bunik, MD, MPH

Aurora, Colorado
March 2020

Milestone 25th Silver Anniversary Edition

This tremendously popular book has been written exclusively by faculty and trainees in the Department of Pediatrics and the University of Colorado School of Medicine since its inception in 1970. The book was started as one of the Lange series, now managed by McGraw Hill, by Henry Kempe (then Chair of the Department of Pediatrics), Henry Silver (then Vice Chair of Pediatrics and originator of the Child Health Associate/Physician Assistant Program), and Donough O'Brien (then Head of the first pediatric microchemistry lab in the world). Vincent Fulginiti joined them as the 4th Editor. Bill Hathaway then became the senior editor and recruited colleagues including John Paisley, Jessie Groothuis, and Bill Hay to join as coeditors. Bill Hay assumed the senior editor position with the eighth edition, and recruited Anthony Hayward, Judy Sondheimer, and Myron Levin, followed by Robin Deterding and now Mark Abzug and Maya Bunik, as coeditors. Spinoffs have included CURRENT Essentials Pediatrics that Judy Sondheimer managed, Current Pediatrics Flashcards that Meghan Treitz and Maya Bunik managed, an electronic version through AccessPediatrics.com, and a new Pediatrics Technology version with Robin Deterding as editor. The book is revised and updated every 2 years and continues as an enduring contribution valued the world over, now published in five languages in addition to English. It continues to represent the unique and close collaboration among the exceptional faculty within the Department of Pediatrics at the University of Colorado School of Medicine and Children's Hospital Colorado.

Advancing the Quality & Safety of Care

Daniel Hyman, MD

INTRODUCTION

Hippocrates' famous dictum *primum non nocere* 2500 years ago may have been the earliest reflection of the importance of patient safety, but the Institute of Medicine's (IOM) 1999 landmark report *To Err Is Human* truly galvanized the current focus on eliminating preventable harm from health care. Its most quoted statistic, that between 44,000 and 98,000 Americans die every year because of medical error, was based on studies of hospital mortality in Colorado, Utah, and New York, and extrapolated to an annual estimate for the country. The IOM followed up this report with a second publication, *Crossing the Quality Chasm*, in which they said, "Health care today harms too frequently, and routinely fails to deliver its potential benefits.... Between the health care we have and the care we could have lies not just a gap, but a chasm." These two reports have served as central elements in an advocacy movement that has engaged stakeholders across the continuum of our health care delivery system and changed the nature of how we think about the quality and safety of the care we provide, and receive.

In *Crossing the Quality Chasm*, the IOM included a simple but elegant definition of the word "quality" as it applies to health care. They defined six domains of health care quality: (1) SAFE—free from preventable harm, (2) EFFECTIVE—optimal clinical outcomes; doing what we should do, not what we should not do according to the evidence, (3) EFFICIENT—without waste of resources—human, financial, supplies/equipment, (4) TIMELY—without unnecessary delay, (5) PATIENT/FAMILY CENTERED—according to the wishes and values of patients and their families, and (6) EQUITABLE—eliminating disparities in outcomes between patients of different race, gender, and socioeconomic status.

In the years since these two reports were published, multiple stakeholders who have been concerned about the effectiveness, safety, and cost of health care in the United States and, indeed throughout the world, have accelerated their individual and collective involvement in analyzing and improving care. In the United States, numerous governmental agencies, large employer groups, health insurance plans, consumers/patients, health care providers, and delivery systems are among the key constituencies calling for and working toward better and safer care at lower cost. Similar efforts are occurring internationally. Indeed, the concept of the Triple Aim has been widely accepted as an organizing framework for considering the country's overall health care improvement goals.

Committee on Quality Health Care in America, Institute of Medicine: *Crossing the Quality Chasm: A New Health System for the 21st Century*. Washington, DC: National Academy Press; 2001.
Kohn L, Corrigan JM: *To Err Is Human: Building a Safer Health System*. Washington, DC: National Academy Press; 2000.

CURRENT CONTEXT

The health care industry is in a period of transformation being driven by at least four converging factors: (1) the recognition of serious gaps in the safety and quality of care we provide (and receive), (2) the unsustainable increases in the cost of care as a percent of the national economy, (3) the aging of the population, and (4) the emerging role of health care information technology as a potential tool to improve care. These are impacting health care organizations as well as individual practitioners in numerous ways that can also be traced to expectations regarding transparency and increasing accountability for results. As depicted in Figure 1–1, the Quadruple Aim (advancing the original concept of the Triple Aim) includes the simultaneous goals of achieving better care (outcomes/experience) for individual patients and families, better health status for the population, lower overall cost of care, and enhancing the experience of the health care workforce. Practitioners and trainees (and health care workers in general) must adapt to a new set

*IHI Quadruple Aim

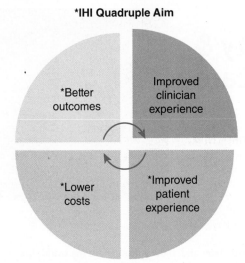

▲ **Figure 1–1.** Quadruple aim.

of priorities that focus attention on new goals to extend our historic focus on the doctor/patient relationship and autonomous physician decision-making. These new imperatives are evidence-based medicine, advancing safety, and reducing unnecessary expense. There is recognition that we need to care for our workforce and understand their challenges if we are to achieve our patient-oriented goals. Staff must be safe, both physically and psychologically, and their resiliency and stress are increasingly a focus of health care systems around the country.

The impact of health care quality improvement will increasingly influence clinical practice and the delivery of pediatric care in the future. This chapter provides a summary of some of the central elements of health care quality improvement and patient safety, and offers resources for the reader to obtain additional information and understanding about these topics.

To understand the external influences driving many of these changes, there are at least six key national organizations central to the transitions occurring:

1. Center for Medicare and Medicaid Services (Department of Health and Human Services)—www.cms.gov
   Center for Medicare and Medicaid Services (CMS) oversees federally funded health care programs of the United States, including Medicare, Medicaid, and other related programs. CMS and the Veterans Affairs Divisions together now provide funding for nearly $1.1 trillion of the total $3.65 trillion the United States spent in 2018 on health care expense (https://www.taxpolicycenter.org/briefing-book/how-much-does-federal-government-spend-health-care). CMS is increasingly promoting payment mechanisms that withhold payment for the costs of

preventable complications of care and giving incentives to providers for achieving better outcomes for their patients, primarily in its Medicare population. The agency has also enabled and advocated for greater transparency of results and makes available on its website comparative measures of performance for its Medicare population. CMS is also increasingly utilizing its standards under which hospitals and other health care provider organizations are licensed to provide care as tools to ensure greater compliance with these regulations. It has instituted a Hospital-Acquired Condition Reduction program (https://www.cms.gov/medicare/medicare-fee-for-service-payment/acuteinpatientpps/HAC-reduction-program.html) which targets a range of conditions, with payment reductions from Medicare based on rates of occurrence. It is worth noting that CMS is able to generate comparative national data only for its Medicare population because it, unlike Medicaid, is a single federal program with a single financial database. Because the Medicaid program functions as 51 state/federal partnership arrangements, patient experience and costs are captured in 51 separate state-based program databases. This segmentation has limited the development of national measures for pediatric care in both inpatient and ambulatory settings. Similarly, while the reporting of hospital-acquired conditions (HACs) is uniform across the United States for Medicare patients, in the Medicaid population it varies by individual state and payment implications are both limited and state based.

2. National Quality Forum—www.qualityforum.org/Home
   National Quality Forum (NQF) is a private, not-for-profit organization whose members include consumer advocacy groups, health care providers, accrediting bodies, employers and other purchasers of care, and research organizations. Its mission is to "drive measurable health improvements" so that "every person experiences high-value care and optimal outcomes." The NQF promotes improvement in the quality of American health care primarily through defining priorities for improvement, approving consensus standards and metrics for performance reporting, and through educational efforts. The NQF, for example, has endorsed a list of 28 "serious reportable events" in health care that include events related to surgical or invasive procedures, products or device failures, patient protection, care management, environmental issues, radiologic events, and potential criminal events (https://www.qualityforum.org/Publications/2007/03/Serious_Reportable_Events_in_Healthcare%E2%80%932006_Update.aspx). This list and the CMS list of HACs are both being used by insurers to reduce payment to hospitals/providers as well as to require reporting to state agencies for public review. In 2012, NQF released a set of 44 measures for the quality of pediatric care, largely representing outpatient preventive

services and management of chronic conditions, and population-based measures applicable to health plans, for example, immunization rates and frequency of well-child care.

3. Leapfrog—www.leapfroggroup.org
Leapfrog is a group of large employers who seek to use their purchasing power to influence the health care community to achieve big "leaps" in health care safety and quality. It promotes transparency and issues public reports of how well individual hospitals meet their recommended standards, including computerized physician-order entry, ICU staffing models, and rates of hospital-acquired infections. There is some evidence that meeting these standards is associated with improved hospital quality and/or mortality outcomes.

4. Agency for Healthcare Research and Quality—www.ahrq.gov
Agency for Healthcare Research and Quality (AHRQ) is currently one of 12 agencies within the US Department of Health and Human Services. AHRQ's primary mission has been to produce evidence to make health care safer and to support health services research initiatives that seek to improve the quality of health care in the United States. Its activities extend well beyond the support of research and now include the development of measurements of quality and patient safety, reports on disparities in performance, measures of patient safety culture in organizations, and promotion of tools to improve care among others. AHRQ also convenes expert panels to assess national efforts to advance quality and patient safety and to recommend strategies to accelerate progress.

5. Specialty Society Boards
Specialty society boards, for example, the American Board of Pediatrics (ABP). The ABP, along with other specialty certification organizations, has responded to the call for greater accountability to consumers by enhancing its maintenance of certification (MOC) programs. All trainees, and an increasing proportion of active practitioners, are now subject to the requirements of the MOC program, including participation in quality improvement activities in the diplomate's clinical practice. The Board's mission is focused on assuring the public that certificate holders have been trained according to their standards and also meet continuous evaluation requirements in six areas of core competency: patient care, medical knowledge, practice-based learning and improvement, interpersonal and communication skills, professionalism, and systems-based practice. These are the same competencies as required of residents in training programs as certified by the Accreditation Council on Graduate Medical Education. Providers need not only to be familiar with the principles of quality improvement and patient safety, but also must demonstrate having implemented quality improvement efforts within their practice settings. The American Board of Medical Specialties is addressing significant concerns with respect to the MOC program and changes are likely to occur in the next few years.

The American Academy of Pediatrics has a number of its own programs to support pediatricians in their pursuit of ongoing certification, and more importantly, ongoing improvement in practice. An example would be the Quality Improvement Innovation Network (QuINN) which is designed to "improve care for children and their families in the outpatient setting." Information on certification can be found at https://www.abp.org/content/maintenance-certification-moc, and information on QuINN can be found at https://www.aap.org/en-us/professional-resources/quality-improvement/Pages/Quality-Improvement-Innovation-Network.aspx.

6. The Joint Commission—www.jointcommission.org
The Joint Commission (JC) is a private, nonprofit agency that is licensed to accredit health care provider organizations, including hospitals, nursing homes, and other health care provider entities in the United States as well as internationally. Its mission is to continuously improve the quality of care through evaluation, education, and enforcement of regulatory standards. Since 2003, JC has annually adopted a set of National Patient Safety Goals designed to help advance the safety of care provided in all health care settings. Examples include the use of two patient identifiers to reduce the risk of care being provided to an unintended patient; the use of time-outs and a universal protocol to improve surgical safety and reduce the risk of wrong site procedures; and adherence to hand hygiene recommendations to reduce the risk of spreading hospital-acquired infections, to name just a few. These goals often become regulatory standards with time and widespread adoption. Failure to meet these standards can result in actions against the licensure of the health care provider, or more commonly, requires corrective action plans, measurement to demonstrate improvement, and resurveying depending on the severity of findings. The JC publishes a monthly journal on quality and safety, available at http://store.jcrinc.com/the-joint-commission-journal-on-quality-and-patient-safety/.

Finally, ongoing governmental impacts on quality and safety will likely be subject to modifications in any future US government changes in the Patient Protection and Affordable Care Act (PPACA) enacted by the US government in 2010. This federal health care legislation sought to provide near-universal access to health care through discounted health care exchanges that supplemented the existing, largely employer-based system. Changes in payment mechanisms for health care will continue irrespective of what happens to the PPACA, and current and future providers' practices will be economically, structurally, and functionally impacted by these emerging trends. Furthermore, changes in the funding and structure of the US health care system may ultimately also result in changes in other countries. Many countries have single-payer systems for providing health care to their citizens and often are leaders in defining new strategies for health care improvement.

Agency for Healthcare Research and Quality: www.ahrq.gov. Accessed April 9, 2019.

American Board of Pediatrics: https://www.abp.org. Accessed April 9, 2019.

Berwick D, Nolan T, Whittington J: The triple aim: care, health, and cost. Health Aff (Millwood) 2008;27(3):759–769. doi:10.1377/hlthaff.27.3.759 [PMID: 18474969].

Center for Medicare and Medicaid Services: Triple Aim.

Center for Medicare and Medicaid Services: www.cms.gov. Accessed April 27, 2019.

CMS list of Hospital-Acquired Conditions: https://www.cms.gov/medicare/medicare-fee-for-service-payment/acuteinpatientpps/HAC-reduction-program.html. Accessed April 9, 2019.

Connors E, Gostin L: Health care reform—a historic moment in US social policy. JAMA 2010;303(24):2521–2522. doi:10.1001/jama.2010.856 [PMID: 20571019].

Hawkins RE, Weiss KB: Commentary: building the evidence base in support of the American Board of Medical Specialties maintenance of certification program. Acad Med 2011;86(1):67. doi:10.1097/ACM.0b013e318201801b [PMID: 21191200]. http://www.nejm.org/doi/full/10.1056/NEJMp0804658. Accessed April 9, 2019.

Jha A, Oray J, Ridgway A, Zheng J, Eptein A: Does the Leapfrog program help identify high-quality hospitals? Jt Comm J Qual Patient Saf 2008;34(6):318–325 [PMID: 18595377].

Leapfrog: www.leapfroggroup.org. Accessed April 9, 2019.

Miller T, Leatherman S: The National Quality Forum: a "me-too" or a breakthrough in quality measurement and reporting? Health Aff (Millwood) 1999;18(6):233–237 [PMID: 10650707].

National Health Expenditure Data: https://www.cms.gov/Research-Statistics-Data-and-Systems/Statistics-Trends-and-Reports/NationalHealthExpendData/index.html. Accessed April 9, 2019.

NQF 29 Serious Reported Events List: http://www.qualityforum.org/Topics/SREs/List_of_SREs.aspx. Accessed April 9, 2019.

Reference on 44 NQF Pediatric measures: http://www.qualityforum.org/Publications/2012/01/Child_Health_Quality_Measures_2010_Final_Report.aspx. Accessed April 29, 2019.

Rosenthal M: Beyond pay for performance—emerging models of provider-payment reform. New Engl J Med 2008;359:1197–1200 [PMID: 18799554].

Shekelle P et al: Advancing the science of patient safety. Ann Intern Med 2011;154(10):693–696 [PMID: 21576538].

Straube B, Blum JD: The policy on paying for treating hospital-acquired conditions: CMS officials respond. Health Aff (Millwood) 2009;28(5):1494–1497 [PMID: 19738268].

The Joint Commission: www.jointcommission.org. Accessed June 21, 2019.

STRATEGIES & MODELS FOR QUALITY IMPROVEMENT (QI)

While there are many approaches to improving the quality of care in health care settings, the following represent three common tools for conducting clinical improvement work. The Model for Improvement (MFI) is primarily emphasized because of its ease of adoption, and because it is the foundation for most improvement efforts included in the Maintenance of Certification program of the ABP. Briefer summaries of Lean and Six-Sigma methods are also included, with listings of resources where the reader can find additional information.

"MODEL FOR IMPROVEMENT"

Widely taught and promoted by the Boston-based educational and advocacy organization the Institute for Healthcare Improvement (IHI), the MFI is grounded in three simple questions that guide the work of the improvement leader and team. The model's framework includes an Aim statement, a measurement strategy, and then the use of "rapid cycle" changes to achieve the aim. The IHI website, www.ihi.org, has an extensive resource library, and hosts an "Open School" that includes a QI/Patient safety modular curriculum for health professional students and their faculty at www.ihi.org/openschool.

AIM STATEMENT

The Aim statement answers the question, "What do we want to accomplish?" The measure question is "How will we know that a change is an improvement?" and the change component is focused on "What changes can we make that will result in improvement?" This model is represented in Figure 1–2.

Aim statements are a *written* description of what the team's improvement goal is, and also include information on who comprises the patient population and a time frame within which the improvement will be achieved. They identify a "stretch" but achievable improvement target goal and,

Model for Improvement

What are we trying to accomplish?

How will we know that a change is an improvement?

What changes can we make that will result in an improvement?

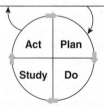

▲ **Figure 1–2.** Model for improvement. (Adapted with permission from Langley G, Moen R, Nolan K, et al: *The Improvement Guide: AIM Model for Improvement.* San Francisco, CA: Jossey-Bass; 2009.)

often, some general statement regarding how the improvement will be achieved. Aim statements are sometimes characterized using the mnemonic SMAART: Specific, Measurable, Achievable, Actionable, Relevant, and Timely. Aim statements should be unambiguous and understandable to the stakeholders and are most likely to be achieved if they are aligned with the strategic goals of the team or organization.

For example, the following statement meets the criteria for a SMAART aim statement: "We will reduce the frequency of emergency department visits and hospitalizations for patients with asthma seen at E Street Pediatrics by 25% by December 31, 2020," whereas this next statement does not: "We will improve the care for patients with asthma by appropriately prescribing indicated medications and better educating families in their use."

The first example provides a specific measurable goal, a time frame, and clarity with respect to who the patients are. A 25% reduction in ED/inpatient asthma visits will require a change in the system for asthma care delivery for the entire population of children with asthma; that extent of level of improvement is a stretch, but it is much more achievable than a goal would be if it was set to "eliminate" such encounters. The second example is unclear in terms of the measure for improvement, the time frame for the goal to be met, and even the population in question. The statement provides some sense of processes that could be utilized to improve asthma care but is missing needed specificity.

MEASURES

Specific measures provide a means to assess whether or not the improvement effort is on track. Three types of measures are useful. *Outcome measures* answer questions concerning the health care impact for the patients, such as how has their health status changed? *Process measures* are related to the health care delivery system itself. They answer questions about how the system is performing. *Balancing measures* seek to identify potential unintended consequences that are related to the improvement effort being undertaken. Examples are helpful to contextualize these conceptual definitions.

Table 1–1 reflects some examples of types of measures that might be employed in an asthma QI initiative.

One might argue that adherence to a treatment plan (third process measure) is an outcome of the work of the practice/practitioner prescribing the medication. It is more consistent, however, to consider the translation of the treatment plan into action as a part of the process of care, and that the health status or outcome measure will be improved by fully improving the measured processes of care, including patient adherence to the treatment plan.

Measures are essential elements of any improvement work. It is a good idea to choose a manageable (4–6) number of measures, all of which can be obtained with limited or no extra effort, and with a mix of outcome, process, and balancing measures. Ideally, the best process measures are those that are directly linked to the outcome goal. The hypothesis in this specific example would be that assessing asthma severity and appropriately using controller medications and action plans would all contribute to reducing the number or frequency of missed school days and the need for ED/hospital utilization.

It is important to note that measurement in the setting of an improvement project is different from measurement in a research study. Improvement projects require "just enough" data to guide the team's continuing efforts. Often, the result seen in a sequence of 10 patients is enough to tell you whether a particular system is functioning consistently or not. For example, considering the first process measure

Table 1–1. Examples of types of measures used in an asthma QI initiative.

Outcome Measures	Process Measures	Balancing Measures
Percent of children with asthma in the practice seen in the ED or hospitalized for asthma in the past 6 months	Proportion of children with an asthma severity assessment in their medical record in the past year	Average difference in the time between the last office patient's scheduled appointment time and the actual office close time
Percent of children with persistent asthma in the practice with fewer than five missed school days due to asthma in the past year	Percent of children with persistent asthma, of any severity, prescribed a controller medication at their most recent visit	Staff satisfaction with their job
	Percent of children prescribed a controller medication who report taking their medicine	
	Percent of children in a practice asthma registry provided with a complete asthma action plan in the past 12 months	

in Table 1–1, if in the last 10 patients seen with asthma, only 2 had their asthma severity documented, how many more charts need be checked to conclude that the system is not functioning as intended and that changes are needed? Other measures may require larger sample sizes, especially when assessing the impact of care changes on a population of patients with a particular condition. See Randolph's excellent summary for a fuller description of measurement for improvement (https://www.pediatric.theclinics.com/article/S0031-3955(09)00066-2/pdf).

CHANGES & IDEAS

Once the team's aim is established and the measures are selected, the third component of the MFI draws from industrial engineering and focuses on what changes in the system must be made that will result in the targeted improvements. To answer the question "What changes will result in improvement?" the improvement team should incorporate "Plan-Do-Study (or check)-Act" cycles, typically referred to as PDSA cycles. The cycles include the following steps.

- *Plan*: What will we do that will likely improve the process measures linked to the outcome target goal? Who will do it? Where? When? How? How will the data be collected?

- *Do*: Implementation of the planned change(s). *TIP!* It is good to make the change cycles as small as possible, for example, trying a new process on the next five patients being seen by one provider as opposed to wide-scale implementation of a new chart documentation form across an entire clinic.

- *Study (or check)*: Once the small test of change is tried, its results are assessed. How many times did the process work as planned for the five patients included in the cycle?

- *Act*: Based on the results of the study of the cycle, recommendations are made as to what the next steps ought to be to achieve the goal. At this point, the cycle then resumes and planning begins for the next cycle.

Over the course of an improvement effort, multiple tests of change might be implemented for any or all of the process measures felt to be likely to impact the outcome measures relevant to the project.

The MFI has been used by improvement teams across numerous health care settings around the world. Further information about the model and examples can be found at www.ihi.org/openschool or in *The Improvement Guide* (Langley et al).

The IHI Open School modules are an excellent online resource for clinicians interested in learning more about the fundamentals of quality improvement and patient safety. These educational lessons are free of charge to health professional students, residents, and university faculty members, and for a modest subscription fee to other clinicians. They are also free to health care practitioners in the developing world. An excellent original resource on implementing this model in clinical practice is in Berwick's summary article from 1998.

Berwick D: The science of improvement. JAMA 2008:299(10): 1182–1184 [PMID: 18334694].

Berwick DM: Developing and testing changes in delivery of care. Ann Intern Med 1998;128:651–656 [PMID: 9537939].

Langley G, Moen R, Nolan K, Nolan T, Norman C, Provost L: *The Improvement Guide: AIM Model for Improvement*. San Francisco, CA: Jossey-Bass; 2009:24.

Randolph G, Esporas M, Provost L, Massie S, Bundy D: Model for improvement—Part Two: measurement and feedback for quality improvement efforts. Pediatr Clin North Am 2009;56(4):779–798 [PMID: 19660627].

"LEAN"

Also grounded in industrial engineering, an increasingly popular method for driving improvement efforts in health care settings is "Lean" or "Lean processing." Early thinking about Lean processes is credited to the Toyota Manufacturing Company in Japan. The crossover to health care from manufacturing is a relatively recent phenomenon, but numerous hospitals and health care delivery settings, including individual clinics, have benefited from the application of these principles to their clinical operations. Lean improvement methods focus on reducing errors and variability in repetitive steps that are part of any process. In health care, examples of repeated processes would include how patients are registered and their information obtained; how medications are ordered, compounded, distributed, and administered; how consent forms are accurately completed in a timely manner prior to surgical procedures; and how antibiotics are reliably and efficiently delivered prior to surgical procedures.

Lean is a philosophy of continuous improvement. It is grounded in recognizing that the way we do things today is merely "current state." With time, effort, focus, and long-term thinking, we can create a "future state" that is better than the status quo. It does so by focusing on identifying the value of all steps in any process and eliminating those steps that do not contribute to the value sought by the customer, or in health care, the patient/family. In doing so, improvements in outcomes, including cost and productivity, and in clinical measures of effectiveness can be realized. See Young for an early critical assessment of the incorporation of Lean into health care settings.

There are four categories that describe the essential elements of Toyota's adoption of "Lean" as a management strategy. These four categories are: (1) *philosophy* (emphasize long-term thinking over short-term gain); (2) *process* (eliminate waste through very defined approaches including an emphasis on process flow and the use of pull systems to reduce overproduction, for example); (3) *people/partners* (respect, challenge, and grow staff); and (4) *problem solving* (create a culture of continuous learning and improvement).

There are a number of hospitals that have fully integrated Lean management as a primary basis for its organizational approach to improvement. Several were featured in a "White Paper" published by the IHI in 2005.

Going Lean in Health Care, Innovation Series White Paper. Institute for Healthcare Improvement: 2005. http://www.ihi. org/knowledge/Pages/IHIWhitePapers/GoingLeaninHealth Care.aspx. Accessed April 9, 2019.

Liker JK: *The Toyota Way*. Madison, WI: McGraw-Hill; 2004.

Young TP, McClean SI: A critical look at Lean Thinking in health-care. BMJ Qual Saf Health Care 2008;17:382–386 [PMID: 18842980].

"SIX SIGMA"

A third quality improvement methodology also arose in the manufacturing industry. Motorola is generally credited with promoting Six Sigma as a management strategy designed to reduce the variability in its processes and thereby reducing the number of defects in its outputs. Organizations adopting Six Sigma as an improvement strategy utilize measurement-based strategies that focus on process improvement and variation reduction to eliminate defects in their work and to reduce cycle times, thereby increasing profitability and enhancing customer satisfaction. Sigma is the statistical measure of standard deviation and Motorola adopted Six Sigma as a performance indicator, promoting consistency of processes in order to have fewer than 3.4 defects per million opportunities. This performance goal has since become the common descriptor for this approach to improvement both in manufacturing and in service industries, including health care. Similar to Lean, the translation of business manufacturing strategies into health care has various challenges, but there are many processes that repeatedly occur in health care that can be routinized and made more consistent. Many health care processes fail far more frequently than 3.4 times per million opportunities. Consider pharmacy dispensing errors, medication ordering or administration errors, and patient-scheduling errors, just to name a few. These are a few of many examples of processes that could potentially benefit from the kind of rigorous analysis that is integral to the Six-Sigma approach.

In a typical Six-Sigma structured improvement project, there are five phases generally referred to as DMAIC: (1) Define (what is the problem, what is the goal?), (2) Measure (quantify the problem and improvement opportunity), (3) Analyze (use of observations and data to identify causes), (4) Improve (implementation of solutions based on data analysis), and finally, (5) Control (sustainable change).

One of the central aspects of Six Sigma as an improvement strategy is its defined focus on understanding the reasons for defects in any process. By understanding these drivers, it is then possible to revise the approach to either the manufacturing process or the service functions in order to reduce these errors and failures.

"Lean-Six Sigma" is a newer entity that draws from both methodologies in order to simplify the improvement work where possible, but retain the rigorous statistical method that is a hallmark of Six-Sigma projects. Lean focuses on where time is lost in any process and can identify opportunities to eliminate steps or reduce time. Six Sigma aims to reduce or eliminate defects in the process, thereby resulting in a higher quality product through a more efficient and lower cost process.

Regardless of the method used, improvement happens because an organization, team, or individual sets a goal to improve a current process through systematic analysis of the way things are done now, and then implement planned changes to see how they impact the outputs or outcomes.

For additional information on Lean and Six Sigma, see www.isixsigma.com (Accessed 04/09/19) or www.asq.org/sixsigma (Accessed 04/09/19).

Pande P, Holpp L: *What Is Six Sigma?* New York, NY: McGraw-Hill; 2002.

PRINCIPLES OF PATIENT SAFETY (INCIDENT REPORTING, JUST CULTURE, DISCLOSURE, FMEA, RCA, RELIABILITY, DATA, & CHECKLISTS)

Safe patient care avoids preventable harm; it is care that does not cause harm as it seeks to cure. The list of adverse events that are considered to be preventable is evolving. As mentioned earlier, both CMS and NQF have endorsed lists of various complications of care as being "never events" or "serious reportable events" for which providers are often now not reimbursed, and which are increasingly reportable to the public through various state transparency programs.

A national network of Children's Hospitals has been active since 2012, collaborating on a shared aim of eliminating serious harm in their now more than 130 organizations. Initially funded as a Hospital Engagement Network by the Center for Medicare and Medicaid Innovation program, Children's Hospitals Solutions for Patient Safety merge approaches to achieving reliability in evidence-based prevention practices ("bundles") with safety practices at both staff and leadership levels to reducing serious safety events (SSEs) and HACs in general. Numerous hospitals have demonstrated dramatic reductions in the occurrence rates of both HACs and SSEs with the following interventions: (1) implementation of structured processes to improve consistency of prevention processes, (2) education and reinforcement of principles of patient safety culture designed to improve communication and reduce error, (3) effective, structured cause analyses after SSEs, and (4) data systems, including both human resources and information technology to support the ongoing focus on improved process reliability and continuous reductions in harm.

Irrespective of one's views about whether various complications are entirely preventable at the current state of science or not, these approaches reflect a changing paradigm that is impacting many aspects of health care delivery. Transparency of results is increasingly expected. Perspectives and data on how these kinds of efforts are impacting actual improvement in outcomes are mixed.

Given these trends, health care providers need to have robust systems for measuring and improving the safety of care provided to patients. The methods for improving quality reviewed earlier are frequently used to reduce harm, just as they can be used to improve effectiveness or efficiency. For example, hospitals attempting to reduce infections have successfully used these types of process improvement approaches to improve antibiotic use prior to surgical procedures or to improve hand hygiene practices.

Common patient safety tools are summarized here.

Incident-reporting systems: Efforts to advance safety in any organization require a clear understanding of the kinds of harm occurring within that organization, as well as the kinds of "near-misses" that are occurring. These reporting systems can range from a simple paper reporting form to a "telephone hotline" to a computerized database that is available to staff (and to potential patients) within the organization. Events are traditionally graded according to the severity of harm that resulted from the incident. One example is the NCC MERP Index, which grades events from A (potential to cause harm) to I (resulting in patient death). Errors that are recognized represent only a fraction of the actual errors and near-misses that are present in the system. Incident-reporting systems depend on people recognizing the error or near-miss, being comfortable reporting it, knowing how and when to report, and then actually doing so. It is no surprise therefore that estimates for how frequently incidents that could or should be reported into incident-reporting systems range from 1.5% to 30% depending on the type of adverse or near-miss event. "Trigger tools" (either manual chart reviews for indications of adverse events, or automated reports from electronic medical records) are increasingly being used to increase the recognition of episodes of harm in health care settings.

"Just culture": The effectiveness of incident-reporting systems is highly dependent on the culture of the organization within which the reporting is occurring. Aviation industry safety-reporting systems are often highlighted for their successes over the past few decades in promoting reporting of aviation events that might have led to accidents. The Aviation Safety Reporting System (ASRS) prioritizes confidentiality in order to encourage reporting and protects reporters from punishment, with certain limitations when they report incidents, even if related to nonadherence to aviation regulations. Although the system is voluntary, more than 880,000 reports have been submitted and used by the Federal Aviation Administration to improve air travel safety.

In health care, the variable recognition of adverse events as well as any fear about reprisal for reporting events both work to reduce the consistent reporting of events. The concept of "just culture" has been promoted as a strategy to increase the comfort of staff members to report the occurrence of errors or near-misses, even if they may have done something incorrectly. See the work of David Marx and the "Just Culture Community" for more information on how to evaluate error so as to support reporting and safer practices in organizations. A great deal of information about "just culture" principles is available at https://www.outcome-eng.com/.

Failure modes and effects analyses (FMEA): An FMEA is a systematic methodology used to proactively identify ways in which any process might fail, and then to prioritize among strategies for reducing the risk or impact of identified potential failures. In conducting an FMEA, which all hospitals are required to do annually, a team will carefully describe and analyze each step in a particular process, consider what and how anything might go wrong, why it would happen, and what the impact would be of such failures. Like Lean and Six Sigma, the FMEA has been adopted into health care from its origins in military and industrial settings. The FMEA is an effective method for identifying strategies to reduce risks in health care settings, thereby protecting patients if interventions are put into place as a result of the analysis. A tool to use in conducting an FMEA is available from the IHI (http://www.ihi.org/resources/Pages/Tools/FailureModesandEffectsAnalysisTool.aspx). Their site includes additional information and resources about the FMEA process.

Root-cause analyses (RCAs) (post-event reviews): As contrasted with the proactive FMEA process, an RCA is a retrospective analysis of an adverse occurrence (or near-miss) that has already happened. It too is a systematic process that in this case allows a team to reach an understanding of why certain things occurred, what systems factors and human factors contributed to the occurrence, and what defects in the system might be changed in order to reduce the likelihood of recurrence. Key to an effective RCA process, and similar to the principles discussed above related to "just culture," RCAs are designed not to ask who was at fault, but rather what system reasons contributed to the event. "Why," not "who," is the essential question to be asked. The answer to the question "why did this occur" almost invariably results in a combination of factors, often illustrated by a series of pieces of Swiss cheese where the holes all line up. Taken from the writings of James Reason, the "Swiss Cheese Model" illustrates the many possible system failures that can contribute to an error, and contributes to identifying potential system changes that reduce the risk of error recurrence. Strategies for approaching retrospective RCA and the causes of human and system error are available at http://www.ncbi.nlm.nih.gov/pmc/articles/pmc1117770. The use of retrospective review processes to learn from adverse events is frequently now referred to as "Safety 1" approach to health care improvement. Increasingly, safety experts are focusing on "Safety 2," which is a complementary strategy oriented to learning from situations "when things go right," and designing systems for reliability using approaches common in the field of human factors engineering. A few selected reading materials for the interested learner are listed as follows.

Communication and team training: Because failures of communication are the most common identified factors in the analysis of reported serious health care events, many health care organizations have incorporated tools from other industries, particularly aviation, in order to enhance patient safety. As a result of the knowledge gained through analysis of tragic aviation accidents, the airline industry implemented methods like crew resource management training to ensure that communication among cockpit team members is effective and clear, thereby reducing risk of air accidents. Similar methods have been used to train teams in operating rooms, delivery rooms, and other team-based settings. Most of these curricula include a few common elements: introductions to be sure all team members know one another's name, promoting the likelihood of speaking up; leader clarity with team members about the expectation that all will speak up if anyone has a concern; and structured language and other tools like verbal read-back of critical information to ensure clarity in interpersonal or interdisciplinary communications. Such training also seeks to flatten the hierarchy, making it more likely that potential risks or problems will be identified and effectively addressed. Common tools used in promoting effective team communication include structured language like SBAR (Situation, Background, Assessment,

and Recommendation), taken from the navy, to promote clarity of communication.

A number of resources exist in the public domain to support better teamwork and communication. One good place to start is the TeamSTEPPS program from the Agency for Healthcare Research and Quality. It can be found at http://teamstepps.ahrq.gov/.

Ashley L, Armitage G, Neary M, Hoolingsworth G: A practical guide to failure mode and effects analysis in health care: making the most of the team and its meetings. Jt Comm J Qual Patient Saf 2010;36(8):351–358 [PMID: 20860241].

Children's Hospitals Solutions for Patient Safety: http://www.solutionsforpatientsafety.org. Accessed April 9, 2019.

Hollnagel E: A Tale of Two Safeties. http://erikhollnagel.com/A%20Tale%20of%20Two%20Safeties.pdf. Accessed April 29, 2019.

http://www.ihi.org/resources/Pages/Tools/FailureModesandEffectsAnalysisTool.aspx. Accessed April 9, 2019.

http://www.wapatientsafety.org/downloads/0610-D-Marx.pdf. Accessed April 29, 2019.

Incident Reporting Systems: http://www.nccmerp.org/. Accessed March 25, 2017.

Marx D: *A Primer for Health Care Executives: Patient Safety and the "Just Culture."* New York, NY: Columbia University; 2011.

Mills R: *Collaborating With Industry to Ensure Regulatory Oversight: The Use of Voluntary Safety Reporting Programs by the Federal Aviation Administration.* Kent State University, College of Arts and Sciences; 2011. [dissertation]. https://etd.ohiolink.edu/!etd.send_file?accession=kent1302102713&disposition=attachment. Accessed April 29, 2019.

Reason J: Human error: models and management. BMJ 2000;320:768–770. doi:10.1136/bmj.320.7237.768:2000 [PMID: 10720363].

Reference on 29 Serious Reportable Events NQF: http://www.qualityforum.org/Topics/SREs/List_of_SREs.aspx. Accessed April 9, 2019.

Shekelle P et al: Advancing the science of patient safety. Ann Intern Med 2011;154(10):693–696 [PMID: 21576538].

Stockwell DC et al: Development of an electronic pediatric all-cause harm measurement tool using a modified Delphi method. J Patient Saf 2014 Aug 26. http://www.ncbi.nlm.nih.gov/pubmed/25162206. Accessed April 9, 2019.

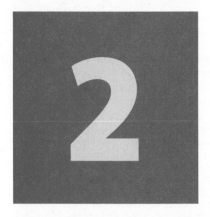

The Newborn Infant

Danielle Smith, MD

INTRODUCTION

The newborn period is defined as the first 28 days of life. In practice, however, sick or very immature infants may require neonatal care for many months. There are four levels of newborn care. Level 1 refers to basic care of well newborns, neonatal resuscitation, and stabilization prior to transport. Level 2 refers to specialty neonatal care of premature infants greater than 1500 g or more than 32 weeks' gestation. Level 3 is subspecialty care of higher complexity neonates without limitations based on newborn size and gestational age. Level 4 includes availability of specialized pediatric surgery, cardiac surgery, and extracorporeal membrane oxygenation (ECMO). Level 4 care is often part of a perinatal center offering critical care and transport to the high-risk mother and fetus as well as the newborn infant.

▼ THE NEONATAL HISTORY

The newborn medical history has three key components:

1. Maternal and paternal medical and genetic history

2. Maternal past obstetric history

3. Current antepartum and intrapartum obstetric history

The mother's medical history includes chronic medical conditions, medications taken during pregnancy, unusual dietary habits, smoking history, substance abuse history, occupational exposure to chemicals or infections of potential risk to the fetus, and any social history that might increase the risk for parenting problems and child abuse. Family illnesses and a history of congenital anomalies with genetic implications should be sought. The past obstetric history includes maternal age, gravidity, parity, blood type, and pregnancy outcomes. The current obstetric history includes the results of procedures during the current pregnancy such as ultrasound, amniocentesis, screening tests (rubella antibody, hepatitis B

surface antigen [HBsAg], serum quadruple screen for genetic disorders, HIV [human immunodeficiency virus]), and antepartum tests of fetal well-being (eg, biophysical profiles, nonstress tests, or Doppler assessment of fetal blood flow patterns). Pregnancy-related maternal complications such as urinary tract infection, pregnancy-induced hypertension, eclampsia, gestational diabetes, vaginal bleeding, and preterm labor should be documented. Significant peripartum events include duration of ruptured membranes, maternal fever, fetal distress, meconium-stained amniotic fluid, type of delivery (vaginal or cesarean section), anesthesia and analgesia used, reason for operative or forceps delivery, infant status at birth, resuscitative measures, and Apgar scores.

▼ ASSESSMENT OF GROWTH & GESTATIONAL AGE

It is important to know the infant's gestational age because normal behavior and possible medical problems can be predicted on this basis. The date of the last menstrual period is the best indicator of gestational age with early fetal ultrasound providing supporting information. Postnatal physical characteristics and neurologic development are also clues to gestational age. Table 2–1 lists the physical and neurologic criteria of maturity used to estimate gestational age by the Ballard method. Adding the scores assigned to each neonatal physical and neuromuscular sign yields a score corresponding to gestational age.

Birth weight and gestational age are plotted on standard grids to determine whether the birth weight is appropriate for gestational age (AGA), small for gestational age (SGA, also known as intrauterine growth restriction [IUGR]), or large for gestational age (LGA). Birth weight for gestational age in normal neonates varies with gender, race, maternal nutrition, access to obstetric care, and environmental factors such as altitude, smoking, and drug and alcohol use. Whenever

Table 2–1. New Ballard score for assessment of fetal maturation of newly born infants.[a]

Neuromuscular Maturity

Neuromuscular Maturity Sign	Score							Record Score Here
	−1	0	1	2	3	4	5	
Posture								
Square window (wrist)	>90°	90°	60°	45°	30°	0°		
Arm recoil		180°	140° to 180°	110° to 140°	90° to 110°	<90°		
Popliteal angle	180°	160°	140°	120°	100°	90°	<90°	
Scarf sign								
Heel to ear								

Total Neuromuscular Maturity Score

Physical Maturity

Physical Maturity Sign	Score							Record Score Here
	−1	0	1	2	3	4	5	
Skin	Sticky, friable, transparent	Gelatinous, red, translucent	Smooth, pink; visible veins	Superficial peeling and/or rash; few veins	Cracking, pale areas; rare veins	Parchment, deep cracking; no vessels	Leathery, cracked, wrinkled	
Lanugo	None	Sparse	Abundant	Thinning	Bald areas	Mostly bald		
Plantar surface	Heel toe 40–50 mm: −1 < 40 mm: −2	50 mm: no crease	Faint red marks	Anterior transverse crease only	Creases anterior 2/3	Creases over entire sole		
Breast	Imperceptible	Barely perceptible	Flat areola; no bud	Stippled areola; 1- to 2-mm bud	Raised areola; 3- to 4-mm bud	Full areola; 5- to 10-mm bud		
Eye/ear	Lids fused loosely: −1 tightly: −2	Lids open; pinna flat; stays folded	Slightly curved pinna; soft; slow recoil	Well-curved pinna; soft but ready recoil	Formed and firm instant recoil	Thick cartilage; ear stiff		
Genitals (male)	Scrotum flat, smooth	Scrotum empty; faint rugae	Testes in upper canal; rare rugae	Testes descending; few rugae	Testes down; good rugae	Testes pendulous; deep rugae		
Genitals (female)	Clitoris prominent and labia flat	Prominent clitoris and small labia minora	Prominent clitoris and enlarging minora	Majora and minora equally prominent	Majora large; minora small	Majora cover clitoris and minora		

Total Physical Maturity Score

Maturity	Score	−10	−5	0	5	10	15	20	25	30	35	40	45	50
Rating	Weeks	20	22	24	26	28	30	32	34	36	38	40	42	44

[a]See text for a description of the clinical gestational age examination.

Reproduced with permission from Ballard JL, Khoury JC, Wedig K, et al: New Ballard Score, expanded to include extremely premature infants. J Pediatr 1991 Sep;119(3):417–423.

possible, standards for newborn weight and gestational age based on local or regional data should be used. Birth weight related to gestational age is a screening tool that should be supplemented by clinical data when entertaining a diagnosis of IUGR or excessive fetal growth. These data include the infant's physical examination and other factors such as parental size and the birth weight–gestational age of siblings.

An important distinction, particularly in SGA infants, is whether a growth disorder is symmetrical (weight, length, and occipitofrontal circumference [OFC] all ≤ 10%) or asymmetrical (only weight ≤ 10%). Asymmetrical growth restriction implies a problem late in pregnancy such as pregnancy-induced hypertension or placental insufficiency. Symmetrical growth restriction implies an event of early pregnancy: chromosomal abnormality, drug or alcohol use, or congenital viral infections. SGA infants, when compared with AGA infants of the same gestational age, have increased morbidity and mortality rates. In general, the outlook for normal growth and development is better in asymmetrically growth-restricted infants whose intrauterine brain growth has been spared.

Knowledge of birth weight in relation to gestational age allows anticipation of some neonatal problems. LGA infants are at risk for birth trauma. LGA infants of diabetic mothers (IDMs) are also at risk for hypoglycemia, polycythemia, congenital anomalies, cardiomyopathy, hyperbilirubinemia, and hypocalcemia. SGA infants are at risk for fetal distress during labor and delivery, polycythemia, hypoglycemia, and hypocalcemia.

▼ EXAMINATION AT BIRTH

The extent of the newborn physical examination depends on the condition of the infant and the setting. Examination in the delivery room consists largely of observation plus auscultation of the chest and inspection for congenital anomalies and birth trauma. Major congenital anomalies occur in 1.5% of live births

and account for 20%–25% of perinatal and neonatal deaths. Because infants are physically stressed during parturition, the delivery room examination should not be extensive. The Apgar score (Table 2–2) should be recorded at 1 and 5 minutes of age. In severely depressed infants, scores can be recorded out to 20 minutes. Although the 1- and 5-minute Apgar scores have almost no predictive value for long-term outcome, serial scores provide a useful description of the severity of perinatal depression and the response to resuscitative efforts.

Skin color is an indicator of cardiac output because of the normal high blood flow to the skin. Stress that triggers a catecholamine response redirects cardiac output away from the skin to preserve oxygen delivery to more critical organs. Cyanosis and pallor are thus two useful signs suggestive of inadequate cardiac output.

Skeletal examination at delivery serves to detect obvious congenital anomalies and to identify birth trauma, particularly in LGA infants or those born after a protracted second stage of labor where a fractured clavicle or humerus might be found.

The placenta and umbilical cord should be examined at delivery. The number of umbilical cord vessels should be determined. Normally, there are two arteries and one vein. In 1% of deliveries (5%–6% of twin deliveries), the cord has only one artery and one vein. This minor anomaly slightly increases the risk of associated defects. The placenta should be examined at delivery. Small placentas are always associated with small infants. The placental examination also includes identification of membranes and vessels (particularly in multiple gestations) as well as placental infarcts or clots (placental abruption) on the maternal side.

▼ EXAMINATION IN THE NURSERY

The purpose of the newborn physical examination is to identify abnormalities or anomalies that might influence the infant's well-being and to evaluate for any acute illness

Table 2–2. Infant evaluation at birth—Apgar score.[a]

		Score	
	0	1	2
Heart rate	Absent	Slow (< 100)	> 100
Respiratory effort	Absent	Slow, irregular	Good, crying
Muscle tone	Limp	Some flexion	Active motion
Response to catheter in nostril[b]	No response	Grimace	Cough or sneeze
Color	Blue or pale	Body pink; extremities blue	Completely pink

[a]One and 5 minutes after complete birth of the infant (disregarding the cord and the placenta), the following objective signs should be observed and recorded.
[b]Tested after the oropharynx is clear.
Data from Apgar V, Holaday DA, James LS, et al: Evaluation of the newborn infant—second report. J Am Med Assoc 1958 Dec 13;168(15):1985–1988.

or difficulty in the transition from intrauterine to extra-uterine life. The examiner should have warm hands and a gentle approach. Start with observation, then auscultation of the chest, and then palpation of the abdomen. Examination of the eyes, ears, throat, and hips should be performed last, as these maneuvers are most disturbing to the infant. The heart rate should range from 120 to 160 beats/min and the respiratory rate from 30 to 60 breaths/min. Systolic blood pressure on day 1 ranges from 50 to 70 mm Hg and increases steadily during the first week of life. An irregularly irregular heart rate, usually caused by premature atrial contractions, is common, benign, and usually resolves in the first days of life.

Approximately 15%–20% of healthy newborns have one minor anomaly (a common variant that would not influence the infant's well-being, eg, a unilateral transverse palmar [simian] crease, or a single umbilical artery). Those with a minor anomaly have a 3% risk of an associated major anomaly. Approximately 0.8% of newborns have two minor anomalies, and 0.5% have three or more, with a risk of 10% and 20%, respectively, of also having a major malformation. Other common minor anomalies requiring no special investigation in healthy infants include preauricular pits, a shallow sacral dimple without other cutaneous abnormality within 2.5 cm of the anus, and three or fewer café au lait spots in a white infant or five or fewer in an African-American infant.

Skin

Observe for bruising, petechiae (common over the presenting part), meconium staining, and jaundice. Visible jaundice in the first 24 hours is never normal, and generally indicates either a hemolytic process or a congenital hepatitis, either of which requires further evaluation. Peripheral cyanosis is commonly present when the extremities are cool or the infant is polycythemic. Generalized cyanosis merits immediate evaluation. Pallor may be caused by acute or chronic blood loss or by acidosis. In dark-skinned infants, pallor and cyanosis should be assessed in the lips, mouth, and nail beds. Plethora suggests polycythemia. Dry skin with cracking and peeling of the superficial layers is common in postterm infants. Edema may be generalized (hydrops) or localized (eg, on the dorsum of the feet in Turner syndrome). Check for birthmarks such as capillary hemangiomas and mongolian spots (bluish-black pigmentation over the back and buttocks). There are many benign skin eruptions such as milia, miliaria, erythema toxicum, and pustular melanosis that are present in the newborn period. See Chapter 15 for a more in-depth description of these conditions.

Head

Check for cephalohematoma (a swelling over one or both parietal bones that is contained within suture lines) and caput succedaneum (edema of the scalp over the presenting part that crosses suture lines). Subgaleal hemorrhages (beneath the scalp) are uncommon but can cause extensive blood loss into this large potential space, resulting in hypovolemic shock. Skull fractures may be linear or depressed and may be associated with cephalohematoma. Check for the presence and size of the fontanelles. The anterior fontanelle varies from 1 to 4 cm in any direction; the posterior fontanelle should be less than 1 cm. A third fontanelle is a bony defect along the sagittal suture in the parietal bones and may be seen in genetic syndromes, such as trisomy 21. Sutures should be freely mobile but are often overriding just after birth. Craniosynostosis, a prematurely fused suture causing an abnormal cranial shape, is more easily diagnosed a few days or more after birth.

Face

Unusual facies may be associated with a specific syndrome. Bruising from birth trauma (especially with face presentation) and forceps application should be identified. Face presentation may cause soft tissue swelling around the nose and mouth and significant facial distortion. Facial nerve palsy is most obvious during crying; the unaffected side of the mouth moves normally, giving an asymmetric grimace.

Eyes

Subconjunctival hemorrhages are a frequent result of birth trauma. Less commonly, a corneal tear (presenting as a clouded cornea), or a hyphema (a layering of blood in the anterior chamber of the eye) may occur. Ophthalmologic consultation is indicated in such cases. Extraocular movements should be assessed. Occasional uncoordinated eye movements are common, but persistent irregular movements are abnormal. The iris should be inspected for abnormalities such as speckling (Brushfield spots seen in trisomy 21) and colobomas. Retinal red reflexes should be present and symmetrical. Dark spots, unilateral blunted red reflex, absent reflex, or a white reflex all require ophthalmologic evaluation. Leukokoria can be caused by glaucoma (cloudy cornea), cataract, or tumor (retinoblastoma). Infants with suspected or known congenital viral infection should have a retinoscopic examination with pupils dilated to look for chorioretinitis.

Nose

Examine the nose for size and shape. In utero compression can cause deformities. Because infants younger than 1 month are obligate nose breathers, any nasal obstruction (eg, bilateral choanal atresia or stenosis) can cause respiratory distress. Unilateral choanal atresia can be diagnosed by occluding each naris, although patency is best checked by holding a cold metal surface or small mirror under the nose, and observing the fog from both nares. Purulent nasal discharge at birth suggests congenital syphilis ("snuffles").

Ears

Malformed or malpositioned (low-set or posteriorly rotated) ears are often associated with other congenital anomalies. Preauricular pits and tags are common minor variants, and may be familial. Any external ear abnormality may be associated with hearing loss.

Mouth

Epithelial (Epstein) pearls are benign retention cysts along the gum margins and at the junction of the hard and soft palates. Natal teeth may be present and sometimes must be removed to prevent their aspiration. Check the integrity and shape of the palate for clefts and other abnormalities. A small mandible and retraction of the tongue with cleft palate is seen with Pierre Robin sequence and can present as respiratory difficulty, as the tongue occludes the airway; prone positioning can be beneficial. A prominent tongue can be seen in trisomy 21 and Beckwith-Wiedemann syndrome. Excessive oral secretions suggest esophageal atresia or a swallowing disorder.

Neck

Redundant neck skin or webbing, with a low posterior hair line, is seen in Turner syndrome. Cervical sinus tracts may be seen as remnants of branchial clefts. Check for masses: midline (thyroglossal duct cysts), anterior to the sternocleidomastoid (branchial cleft cysts), within the sternocleidomastoid (hematoma and torticollis), and posterior to the sternocleidomastoid (cystic hygroma).

Chest & Lungs

Check for fractured clavicles (crepitus, bruising, and tenderness). Check air entry bilaterally and the position of the mediastinum by locating the point of maximum cardiac impulse and assessment of heart tones. Decreased breath sounds with respiratory distress and a shift in the heart tones suggests pneumothorax (tension) or a space-occupying lesion (eg, diaphragmatic hernia). Pneumomediastinum causes muffled heart sounds. Expiratory grunting and decreased air entry are observed in hyaline membrane disease. Rales are not of clinical significance at this age.

Heart

Cardiac murmurs are common in the first hours and are most often benign; conversely, severe congenital heart disease in the newborn infant may be present with no murmur at all. The two most common presentations of heart disease in the newborn infant are (1) cyanosis and (2) congestive heart failure with abnormalities of pulses and perfusion. In hypoplastic left-sided heart and critical aortic stenosis, pulses are diminished at all sites. In aortic coarctation and interrupted aortic arch, pulses are diminished in the lower extremities.

Abdomen

Check for tenderness, distention, and bowel sounds. If polyhydramnios was present or excessive oral secretions are noted, pass a soft catheter into the stomach to rule out esophageal atresia. Most abdominal masses in the newborn infant are associated with kidney disorders (eg, multicystic or dysplastic, and hydronephrosis). When the abdomen is relaxed, normal kidneys may be felt but are not prominent. A markedly scaphoid abdomen plus respiratory distress suggests diaphragmatic hernia. Absence of abdominal musculature (prune belly syndrome) may occur in association with renal abnormalities. The liver and spleen are superficial in the neonate and can be felt with light palpation. A distended bladder may be seen as well as palpated above the pubic symphysis.

Genitalia & Anus

Male and female genitals show characteristics according to gestational age (see Table 2–1). In the female infant during the first few days, a whitish vaginal discharge with or without blood is normal. Check the patency and location of the anus.

Skeleton

Check for obvious anomalies such as absence of a bone, clubfoot, fusion or webbing of digits, and extra digits. Examine for hip dislocation by attempting to dislocate the femur posteriorly and then abducting the legs to relocate the femur noting a clunk as the femoral head relocates. Look for extremity fractures and for palsies (especially brachial plexus injuries) and evidence of spinal deformities (eg, scoliosis, cysts, sinuses, myelomeningocele). Arthrogryposis (multiple joint contractures) results from chronic limitation of movement in utero that may result from lack of amniotic fluid or from congenital neuromuscular disease.

Neurologic Examination

Normal newborns have reflexes that facilitate survival (eg, rooting and sucking reflexes), and sensory abilities (eg, hearing and smell) that allow them to recognize their mother soon after birth. Although the retina is well developed at birth, visual acuity is poor (20/400) because of a relatively immobile lens. Acuity improves rapidly over the first 6 months, with fixation and tracking becoming well developed by 2 months.

Observe the newborn's resting tone. Normal-term newborns should exhibit flexion of the upper and lower extremities and symmetrical spontaneous movements. Extension of the extremities should result in spontaneous recoil to the flexed position. Assess the character of the cry; a high-pitched cry with or without hypotonia may indicate disease of the central nervous system (CNS) such as hemorrhage or infection, a congenital neuromuscular disorder, or systemic disease. Check the following newborn reflexes:

1. *Sucking reflex*: The newborn sucks in response to a nipple in the mouth; observed by 14 weeks' gestation.

2. *Palmar grasp*: Evident with the placement of the examiner's finger in the newborn's palm; develops by 28 weeks' gestation and disappears by age 4 months.

3. *Moro (startle) reflex*: Hold the infant supine while supporting the head. Allow the head to drop 1–2 cm suddenly. The arms will abduct at the shoulder and extend at the elbow with spreading of the fingers. Adduction with flexion will follow. This reflex develops by 28 weeks' gestation (incomplete) and disappears by age 3 months.

▼ CARE OF THE WELL NEONATE

The primary responsibility of the level 1 nursery is care of the well neonate—promoting mother–infant bonding, establishing feeding, and teaching the basics of newborn care. Staff must monitor infants for signs and symptoms of illness, including temperature instability, change in activity, refusal to feed, pallor, cyanosis, early or excessive jaundice, tachypnea, respiratory distress, delayed (beyond 24 hours) first stool or first void, and bilious vomiting.

Several preventive measures are routine in the normal newborn nursery. Prophylactic erythromycin ointment is applied to the eyes within 1 hour of birth to prevent gonococcal ophthalmia. Vitamin K (1 mg) is given intramuscularly or subcutaneously within 4 hours of birth to prevent hemorrhagic disease of the newborn.

All infants should receive hepatitis B vaccine. Both hepatitis B vaccine and hepatitis B immune globulin (HBIG) are administered if the mother is positive for HBsAg. If maternal HBsAg status is unknown, vaccine should be given before 12 hours of age, maternal blood should be tested for HBsAg, and HBIG should be given to the neonate before 7 days of age if the test is positive.

Cord blood is collected from all infants at birth and can be used for blood typing and Coombs testing if the mother is type O or Rh-negative to help assess the risk for development of jaundice.

Bedside glucose testing should be performed in infants at risk for hypoglycemia (IDMs, preterm, SGA, LGA, or stressed infants). Values below 45 mg/dL should be confirmed by laboratory blood glucose testing and treated. Hematocrit should be measured at age 3–6 hours in infants at risk for or those who have symptoms of polycythemia or anemia (see section Hematologic Disorders in the Newborn Infant).

State-sponsored newborn genetic screens (for inborn errors of metabolism such as phenylketonuria [PKU], galactosemia, sickle cell disease, hypothyroidism, congenital adrenal hyperplasia, and cystic fibrosis) are performed prior to discharge, after 24–48 hours of age if possible. In many states, a repeat test is required at 8–14 days of age because the PKU test may be falsely negative when obtained before 48 hours of age. Not all state-mandated screens include the same panel of diseases. Many states now include an expanded screen that tests for other inborn errors of metabolism such as fatty acid oxidation defects and amino or organic acid disorders. Some states also screen for severe combined immunodeficiency syndrome.

Screening for critical congenital heart disease is standard practice in newborn nurseries. The goal of screening is to identify newborn infants with structural heart disease significant enough to require intervention within the first year of life prior to symptoms developing. Newborn infants are screened by pulse oximetry on the second day of life. Infants that screen positive are evaluated by echocardiogram prior to hospital discharge.

Infants should routinely be positioned supine to minimize the risk of sudden infant death syndrome (SIDS). Prone positioning is contraindicated unless there are compelling clinical reasons for that position. Bed sharing with adults and prone positioning are associated with increased risk of SIDS.

FEEDING THE WELL NEONATE

A neonate is ready for feeding if he or she (1) is alert and vigorous, (2) has no abdominal distention, (3) has good bowel sounds, and (4) has a normal hunger cry. These signs usually occur within 6 hours after birth, but fetal distress or traumatic delivery may prolong this period. The healthy full-term infant should be allowed to feed every 2–5 hours on demand. The first breast-feeding should occur within 1 hour from birth if mother and baby are clinically stable. For formula-fed infants, the first feeding usually occurs by 3 hours of life. The feeding volume generally increases from 0.5–1 oz per feeding initially to 1.5–2 oz per feeding on day 3. By day 3, the average full-term newborn takes about 100 mL/kg/day of milk (Table 2–3).

A wide range of infant formulas satisfy the nutritional needs of most neonates. Breast milk is the standard on which formulas are based (see Chapter 11). Despite low concentrations of several vitamins and minerals in breast milk, bioavailability is high. All the necessary nutrients, vitamins, minerals, and water are provided by human milk for the first 6 months of life except vitamin K (1 mg IM is administered at birth), vitamin D (400 IU/day for all infants beginning shortly after birth), and vitamin B_{12} and zinc (if the mother is a strict vegetarian and takes no supplements). Other advantages of breast milk include (1) immunologic, antimicrobial, and anti-inflammatory factors such as immunoglobulin A

Table 2–3. Guidelines for successful breast-feeding.

	First 8 h	First 8–24 h	Day 2	Day 3	Day 4	Day 5	Day 6 Onward
Milk supply	You may be able to express a few drops of milk.		Milk should come in between the second and fourth days.			Milk should be in. Breasts may be firm or leak milk.	Breasts should feel softer after feedings.
Baby's activity	Baby is usually wide-awake in the first hour of life. Put baby to breast within 30 min after birth.	Wake up your baby. Babies may not wake up on their own to feed.	Baby should be more cooperative and less sleepy.	Look for early feeding cues such as rooting, lip smacking, and hands to face.			Baby should appear satisfied after feedings.
Feeding routine	Baby may go into a deep sleep 2–4 h after birth.	Use chart to write down time of each feeding. Feed your baby every 1–4 h or as often as wanted—at least 8–12 times a day.				May go one longer interval (up to 5 h between feeds) in a 24-h period.	
Breast-feeding	Baby will wake up and be alert and responsive for several more hours after initial deep sleep.	As long as the mother is comfortable, nurse at both breasts as long as baby is actively sucking.	Try to nurse both sides each feeding, aiming at 10 min per side. Expect some nipple tenderness.	Consider hand expressing or pumping a few drops of milk to soften the nipple if the breast is too firm for the baby to latch on.	Nurse a minimum of 10–30 min per side every feeding for the first few weeks of life. Once milk supply is well established, allow baby to finish the first breast before offering the second.		Mother's nipple tenderness is improving or is gone.
Baby's urine output		Baby must have a minimum of one wet diaper in the first 24 h.	Baby must have at least one wet diaper every 8–11 h.	You should see an increase in wet diapers (up to four to six) in 24 h.	Baby's urine should be light yellow.	Baby should have six to eight wet diapers per day of colorless or light yellow urine.	
Baby's stool		Baby may have a very dark (meconium) stool.	Baby may have a very dark second (meconium) stool.	Baby's stools should be in transition from black-green to yellow.		Baby should have three or four yellow, seedy stools a day.	The number of stools may decrease gradually after 4–6 wk.

Modified with permission from Gabrielski L: Lactation support services. Childrens Hospital Colorado, 1999.

(IgA) and cellular, protein, and enzymatic components that decrease the incidence of upper respiratory and gastrointestinal (GI) infections; (2) possible decreased frequency and severity of childhood eczema and asthma; (3) improved mother–infant bonding; and (4) improved neurodevelopmental outcome.

Although 85% of mothers in the United States start by breast-feeding, only about 50% continue to do so at 6 months. Hospital practices that facilitate successful initiation of breast-feeding include rooming-in, nursing on demand, and avoiding unnecessary supplemental formula. Nursery staff must be trained to recognize problems associated with breast-feeding and provide help and support for mothers in the hospital. An experienced professional should observe and assist with several feedings to document good latch-on. Good latch-on is important in preventing the common problems of sore nipples, unsatisfied infants, breast engorgement, poor milk supply, and hyperbilirubinemia.

American Academy of Breastfeeding Medicine: www.bfmed.org. Accessed April 2019.
Moon RY: Task Force on Sudden Infant Death Syndrome: SIDS and other sleep-related infant deaths: evidence base for 2016 updated recommendations for a safe infant sleeping environment. Pediatrics 2016;138:1 [PMID: 27940804].

EARLY DISCHARGE OF THE NEWBORN INFANT

Discharge at 24–36 hours of age is safe and appropriate for some newborns if there are no contraindications (Table 2–4) and if a follow-up visit within 48 hours is ensured. Most infants

Table 2–4. Contraindications to early newborn discharge.

Contraindications to early newborn discharge
1. Jaundice ≤ 24 h
2. High risk for infection (eg, maternal chorioamnionitis); discharge allowed after 24 h with a normal transition
3. Known or suspected narcotic addiction or withdrawal
4. Physical defects requiring evaluation
5. Oral defects (clefts, micrognathia)

Relative contraindications to early newborn discharge (infants at high risk for feeding failure, excessive jaundice)
1. Prematurity or early-term infant (< 38 weeks' gestation)
2. Birth weight < 2700 g (6 lb)
3. Infant difficult to arouse for feeding; not demanding regularly in nursery
4. Medical or neurologic problems that interfere with feeding (Down syndrome, hypotonia, cardiac problems)
5. Twins or higher multiples
6. ABO blood group incompatibility or severe jaundice in previous child
7. Mother whose previous breast-fed infant gained weight poorly
8. Mother with breast surgery involving periareolar areas (if attempting to nurse)

Table 2–5. Guidelines for early outpatient follow-up evaluation.

History
Rhythmic sucking and audible swallowing for at least 10 min total per feeding?
Infant wakes and demands to feed every 2–3 h (at least 8–10 feedings per 24 h)?
Do breasts feel full before feedings, and softer after?
Are there at least 6 noticeably wet diapers per 24 h?
Are there yellow bowel movements (no longer meconium)— at least 4 per 24 h?
Is infant still acting hungry after nursing (frequently sucks hands, rooting)?

Physical assessment
Weight, unclothed: should not be more than 8%–10% below birth weight
Extent and severity of jaundice
Assessment of hydration, alertness, general well-being
Cardiovascular examination: murmurs, brachial and femoral pulses, respirations

with cardiac, respiratory, or infectious disorders are identified in the first 12–24 hours of life. The exception may be the infant for whom maternal intrapartum antibiotic prophylaxis for maternal group B streptococcal (GBS) colonization or infection was indicated. The Centers for Disease Control and Prevention (CDC) and the American Academy of Pediatrics (AAP) recommend that such infants be observed in hospital for at least 48 hours if their mothers received no or inadequate intrapartum antibiotic prophylaxis, or cefazolin. Hospital observation beyond 24 hours may not be necessary for well appearing full-term infants whose mothers received adequate intrapartum chemoprophylaxis and for whom ready access to medical care can be ensured if needed. Other problems, such as jaundice and breast-feeding problems, typically occur after 48 hours and can usually be dealt with on an outpatient basis.

The AAP recommends a follow-up visit within 48 hours for all newborns discharged before 72 hours of age. Infants who are small or late preterm—especially if breast-feeding—are at particular risk for inadequate intake; the early visit is especially important for these infants. Suggested guidelines for the follow-up interview and physical examination are presented in Table 2–5. The optimal timing of discharge must be determined in each case based on medical, social, and financial factors.

▶ Circumcision

Circumcision is an elective procedure to be performed only in healthy, stable infants. The procedure has medical benefits, including prevention of urinary tract infections, decreased incidence of penile cancer, and decreased incidence of sexually transmitted diseases (including HIV). Most parental decisions regarding circumcision are religious and social, not medical. The risks of circumcision include local infection, bleeding, removal of too much skin, and urethral injury. The combined incidence of complications is less than 1%. Local anesthesia by dorsal penile nerve block or circumferential ring block using 1% lidocaine without epinephrine, or topical anesthetic cream are safe and effective methods that should always be used. Techniques allowing visualization of the glans throughout the procedure (Plastibell and Gomco clamp) are preferred to blind techniques (Mogen clamp) as occasional amputation of the glans has occurred with the latter technique. Circumcision is contraindicated in infants with genital abnormalities. A coagulation screen should be performed prior to the procedure in infants with a family history of serious bleeding disorders.

HEARING SCREENING

Normal hearing is critical to normal language development. Significant bilateral hearing loss is present in 1–3 per 1000 well neonates and in 2–4 per 100 neonates in the intensive care unit population. Infants should be screened for hearing loss by auditory brainstem evoked responses or evoked otoacoustic emissions as early as possible because up to 40% of hearing loss will be missed by risk analysis alone. Primary care providers and parents should be advised of the possibility of hearing loss and offered immediate referral in suspect cases. With the use of universal screening, the average age at which hearing loss is confirmed has dropped from 24–30 to 2–3 months. If remediation is begun by 6 months, language and social development are commensurate with physical development.

American Academy of Pediatrics Task Force on Circumcision: Male circumcision. Pediatrics 2012;130:e756 [PMID: 22926175]. Prevention of perinatal group B streptococcal disease revised guidelines from CDC, 2010. MMWR 2010;59:132 [PMID: 21088663].

▼ COMMON PROBLEMS IN THE TERM NEWBORN

NEONATAL JAUNDICE

▶ General Considerations

Sixty-five percent of newborns develop visible jaundice with a total serum bilirubin (TSB) level higher than 6 mg/dL during the first week of life. Approximately 8%–10% of newborns develop excessive hyperbilirubinemia (TSB > 17 mg/dL), and 1%–2% have TSB above 20 mg/dL. Extremely high and potentially dangerous TSB levels are rare but can cause kernicterus, characterized by injury to the basal ganglia and brainstem.

Kernicterus caused by hyperbilirubinemia was common in neonates with Rh-isoimmunization until the institution of exchange transfusion for affected infants and postpartum high-titer Rho (D) immune globulin treatment to prevent sensitization of Rh-negative mothers. For several decades after the introduction of exchange transfusion and phototherapy aimed at keeping the neonate's TSB below 20 mg/dL, there were no reported cases of kernicterus in the United States. Since the early 1990s, however, there has been a reappearance of kernicterus. Common factors in recent cases are newborn discharge before 48 hours, breast-feeding, delayed measurement of TSB, unrecognized hemolysis, lack of early post discharge follow-up, and failure to recognize the early symptoms of bilirubin encephalopathy.

Bilirubin is produced by the breakdown of heme (iron protoporphyrin) in the reticuloendothelial system and bone marrow. Heme is cleaved by heme oxygenase to iron, which is conserved; carbon monoxide, which is exhaled; and biliverdin, which is converted to bilirubin by bilirubin reductase. This unconjugated bilirubin is bound to albumin and carried to the liver, where it is taken up by hepatocytes. In the presence of the enzyme uridyl diphosphoglucuronyl transferase (UDPGT; glucuronyl transferase), bilirubin is conjugated to one or two glucuronide molecules. Conjugated bilirubin is then excreted through the bile to the intestine. In the presence of normal gut flora, conjugated bilirubin is metabolized to stercobilins and excreted in the stool. Absence of gut flora and slow GI motility, both characteristics of the newborn, cause stasis of conjugated bilirubin in the intestinal lumen, where mucosal β-glucuronidase removes the glucuronide

molecules and leaves unconjugated bilirubin to be reabsorbed (enterohepatic circulation).

Excess accumulation of bilirubin in blood depends on both the rate of bilirubin production and the rate of excretion. It is best determined by reference to an hour-specific TSB level above the 95th percentile for age in hours (Figure 2–1).

1. Physiologic Jaundice

ESSENTIALS OF DIAGNOSIS & TYPICAL FEATURES

- ▶ Visible jaundice appearing after 24 hours of age.
- ▶ Total bilirubin rises by < 5 mg/dL (86 mmol/L) per day.
- ▶ Peak bilirubin occurs at 3–5 days of age, with a total bilirubin of no more than 15 mg/dL (258 mmol/L).
- ▶ Visible jaundice resolves by 1 week in the full-term infant and by 2 weeks in the preterm infant.

Factors contributing to physiologic jaundice in neonates include low UDPGT activity, relatively high red cell mass, absence of intestinal flora, slow intestinal motility, and increased enterohepatic circulation of bilirubin in the first days of life. Hyperbilirubinemia outside of the ranges noted in Figure 2–1 is not physiologic and requires further evaluation.

2. Pathologic Unconjugated Hyperbilirubinemia

Pathologic unconjugated hyperbilirubinemia can be grouped into two main categories: overproduction of bilirubin or decreased conjugation of bilirubin (Table 2–6). The TSB is a reflection of the balance between these processes. Visible jaundice with a TSB greater than 5 mg/dL before 24 hours of age is most commonly a result of significant hemolysis.

A. Increased Bilirubin Production

1. Antibody-mediated hemolysis (Coombs test–positive)

A. ABO BLOOD GROUP INCOMPATIBILITY—This finding can accompany any pregnancy in a type O mother. Hemolysis is usually mild, but the severity is unpredictable because of variability in the amount of naturally occurring maternal anti-A or anti-B IgG antibodies. Although 15% of pregnancies are "setups" for ABO incompatibility (mother O, infant A or B), only 33% of infants in such cases have a positive direct Coombs test and less than 10% of these infants develop jaundice that requires therapy. Since maternal antibodies may persist for several months after birth, the newborn may

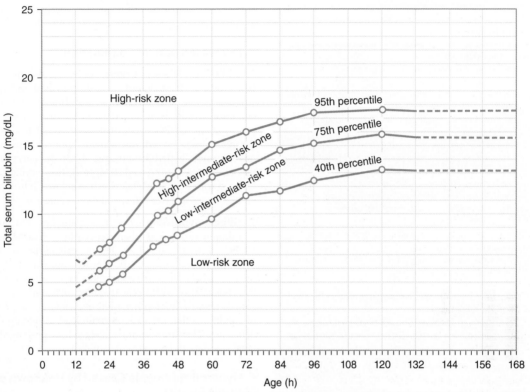

▲ **Figure 2–1.** Risk designation of full-term and near-term newborns based on their hour-specific bilirubin values. (Reproduced with permission from Bhutani VK, Johnson L, Sivieri EM: Predictive ability of a predischarge hour-specific serum bilirubin test for subsequent significant hyperbilirubinemia in healthy term and near-term newborns. Pediatrics 1999 Jan;103(1):6–14.)

become progressively more anemic over the first few weeks of life, occasionally to the point of requiring transfusion.

B. RH-ISOIMMUNIZATION—This hemolytic process is less common, more severe, and more predictable than ABO incompatibility. The severity increases with each immunized pregnancy because of an anamnestic maternal IgG antibody response. Most Rh-disease can be prevented by giving high-titer Rho (D) immune globulin to the Rh-negative woman after invasive procedures during pregnancy or after miscarriage, abortion, or delivery of an Rh-positive infant. Affected neonates are often anemic at birth, and continued hemolysis rapidly causes hyperbilirubinemia and more severe anemia. The most severe form of Rh-isoimmunization, erythroblastosis fetalis, is characterized by life-threatening anemia, generalized edema, and fetal or neonatal heart failure. Without antenatal intervention, fetal or neonatal death often results. The cornerstone of antenatal management is transfusion of the fetus with Rh-negative cells, either directly into the umbilical vein or into the fetal abdominal cavity. Phototherapy is usually started in these

infants upon delivery, with exchange transfusion frequently needed. Intravenous immune globulin (IVIG; 0.5–1 g/kg) given to the infant as soon as the diagnosis is made may decrease the need for exchange transfusion. Ongoing hemolysis occurs until all maternal antibodies are gone; therefore, these infants require monitoring for 2–3 months for recurrent anemia severe enough to require transfusion.

2. Nonimmune hemolysis (Coombs test–negative)

A. HEREDITARY SPHEROCYTOSIS—This condition is the most common of the red cell membrane defects and causes hemolysis by decreasing red cell deformability. Affected infants may have hyperbilirubinemia severe enough to require exchange transfusion. Splenomegaly may be present. Diagnosis is suspected by peripheral blood smear and family history. See Chapter 30 for a more in-depth discussion.

B. G6PD DEFICIENCY—This condition is the most common red cell enzyme defect causing hemolysis, especially in infants of African, Mediterranean, or Asian descent.

Table 2–6. Causes of pathologic unconjugated hyperbilirubinemia.

Overproduction of bilirubin
1. Hemolytic causes of increased bilirubin production (reticulocyte count elevated)
a. Immune-mediated: positive direct antibody (DAT, Coombs) test
• ABO blood group incompatibility, Rh incompatibility, minor blood group antigen incompatibility
b. Nonimmune: negative direct antibody (DAT, Coombs) test
• Abnormal red cell shapes: spherocytosis, elliptocytosis, pyknocytosis, stomatocytosis
• Red cell enzyme abnormalities: glucose-6-phosphate dehydrogenase deficiency, pyruvate kinase deficiency, hexokinase deficiency, other metabolic defects
c. Patients with bacterial or viral sepsis
2. Nonhemolytic causes of increased bilirubin production (reticulocyte count normal)
a. Extravascular hemorrhage: cephalohematoma, extensive bruising, intracranial hemorrhage
b. Polycythemia
c. Exaggerated enterohepatic circulation of bilirubin: bowel obstruction, functional ileus
d. Breast-feeding–associated jaundice (inadequate intake of breast milk causing exaggerated enterohepatic circulation of bilirubin)
Decreased rate of conjugation
1. Crigler-Najjar syndrome (rare, severe)
a. Type I glucuronyl transferase deficiency, autosomal-recessive
b. Type II glucuronyl transferase deficiency, autosomal-dominant
2. Gilbert syndrome (common, milder)
3. Hypothyroidism

Onset of jaundice is often later than in isoimmune hemolytic disease, toward 1 week of age. The role of G6PD deficiency in neonatal jaundice is probably underestimated as up to 10%–13% of African Americans are G6PD-deficient. Although the disorder is X-linked, female heterozygotes are also at increased risk of hyperbilirubinemia due to X-chromosome inactivation. Their increased bilirubin production is further exaggerated by a decreased rate of bilirubin conjugation. Since G6PD enzyme activity is high in reticulocytes, neonates with a large number of reticulocytes may have falsely normal enzyme tests. A low G6PD level should always raise suspicions. Repeat testing in suspect cases with initially normal results is indicated at 2–3 months of age. Please also see Chapter 30 for more details.

3. Nonhemolytic increased bilirubin production—Enclosed hemorrhage, such as cephalohematoma, intracranial hemorrhage, or extensive bruising in the skin, can lead to jaundice. Polycythemia leads to jaundice by increased red cell mass, with increased numbers of cells reaching senescence

daily. Bowel obstruction, functional or mechanical, leads to an increased enterohepatic circulation of bilirubin.

B. Decreased Rate of Conjugation

1. UDPGT deficiency: Crigler-Najjar syndrome type I (complete deficiency, autosomal recessive) and type II (partial deficiency, autosomal dominant)—These rare conditions result from mutations in the exon or encoding region of the UDPGT gene that cause complete or nearly complete absence of enzyme activity. Both can cause severe unconjugated hyperbilirubinemia, bilirubin encephalopathy, and death if untreated. In type II, the enzyme can be induced with phenobarbital, which may lower bilirubin levels by 30%–80%. Liver transplantation is curative.

2. Gilbert syndrome—This is a common mild autosomal dominant disorder characterized by decreased hepatic UDPGT activity caused by genetic polymorphism at the promoter region of the UDPGT gene. Approximately 9% of the population is homozygous, and 42% is heterozygous for this abnormality, with a gene frequency of 0.3. Affected individuals tend to develop hyperbilirubinemia in the presence of conditions that increase bilirubin load, including G6PD deficiency. They are also more likely to have prolonged neonatal jaundice and breast-milk jaundice.

C. Hyperbilirubinemia Caused by Unknown or Multiple Factors

1. Racial differences—Asians (23%) are more likely than whites (10%–13%) or African Americans (4%) to have a peak neonatal TSB greater than 12 mg/dL (206 mmol/L). It is likely that these differences result from racial variations in prevalence of UDPGT gene polymorphisms or associated G6PD deficiency.

2. Prematurity—Premature infants often have poor enteral intake, delayed stooling, and increased enterohepatic circulation, as well as a shorter red cell life. Infants at 35–36 weeks' gestation are 13 times more likely than term infants to be readmitted for hyperbilirubinemia. Even early-term infants (37–38 weeks' gestation) are four times more likely than term neonates to have TSB greater than 13 mg/dL (224 mmol/L).

3. Breast-feeding and jaundice

A. BREAST-MILK JAUNDICE—Unconjugated hyperbilirubinemia lasting until 2–3 months of age is common in breast-fed infants. An increased prevalence of the Gilbert syndrome promoter polymorphism is likely involved. Moderate unconjugated hyperbilirubinemia for 6–12 weeks in a thriving breast-fed infant without evidence of hemolysis, hypothyroidism, or other disease strongly suggests this diagnosis.

B. BREAST-FEEDING–ASSOCIATED JAUNDICE—This common condition has also been called "lack-of-breast-milk" jaundice. Breast-fed infants have a higher incidence (9%) of unconjugated serum bilirubin levels greater than 13 mg/dL (224 mmol/L) than do formula-fed infants (2%). The pathogenesis is probably poor enteral intake and increased enterohepatic circulation. There is no apparent increase in bilirubin production as measured by carbon monoxide exhalation. Although rarely severe enough to cause bilirubin encephalopathy, nearly 100% of the infants with kernicterus reported over the past 20 years were exclusively breast-fed, and in 50%, breast-feeding was the only known risk factor. Excessive jaundice should be considered a possible sign of failure to establish an adequate milk supply, and should prompt specific inquiries. The best way to evaluate successful breast-feeding is to monitor the infant's weight, urine, and stool output (see Table 2–3). If intake is inadequate, the infant should receive supplemental formula and the mother should be instructed to nurse more frequently and to use an electric breast pump every 2 hours to enhance milk production. Consultation with a lactation specialist should be considered. Because hospital discharge of normal newborns occurs before the milk supply is established and before jaundice peaks, a follow-up visit 2 days after discharge is recommended by the AAP to evaluate adequacy of intake and degree of jaundice.

3. Bilirubin Toxicity

Unconjugated bilirubin anion is the agent of bilirubin neurotoxicity. The anion binds to the phospholipids (gangliosides) of neuronal plasma membranes causing injury, which then allows more anion to enter the neuron. Intracellular bilirubin anion binds to the membrane phospholipids of subcellular organelles, causing impaired energy metabolism and cell death. The blood-brain barrier undoubtedly has a role in protecting the infant from brain damage, but its integrity is impossible to measure clinically. The amount of albumin available to bind the unconjugated bilirubin anion and the presence of other anions that may displace bilirubin from albumin-binding sites are also important. It is unknown whether there is a fixed level of bilirubin above which brain damage always occurs. The term *kernicterus* describes the pathologic finding of staining of basal ganglia and brainstem nuclei, as well as the clinical syndrome of chronic brain injury due to hyperbilirubinemia. The term *acute bilirubin encephalopathy* describes the signs and symptoms of evolving brain injury in the newborn.

The risk of bilirubin encephalopathy is small in healthy, term neonates even at bilirubin levels of 25–30 mg/dL (430–516 mmol/L). Risk depends on the duration of hyperbilirubinemia, the concentration of serum albumin, associated illness, acidosis, and the concentrations of competing anions such as sulfisoxazole and ceftriaxone. Premature infants are at greater risk than term infants because of the greater frequency of associated illness affecting the integrity of the blood-brain barrier, reduced albumin levels, and decreased affinity of

albumin-binding sites. For these reasons, the "exchange level" (the level at which bilirubin encephalopathy is thought likely to occur) in premature infants may be lower than that of a term infant.

4. Acute Bilirubin Encephalopathy

 ESSENTIALS OF DIAGNOSIS & TYPICAL FEATURES

- ► Lethargy, poor feeding.
- ► Irritability, high-pitched cry.
- ► Arching of the neck (retrocollis) and trunk (opisthotonos).
- ► Apnea, seizures, coma (late).

Newborn infants with evolving acute bilirubin encephalopathy may be described as "sleepy and not interested in feeding." Although these symptoms are nonspecific, they are also the earliest signs of acute bilirubin encephalopathy and should trigger, in the jaundiced infant, a detailed evaluation of the birth and postnatal history, feeding and elimination history, an urgent assessment for signs of bilirubin-induced neurologic dysfunction (BIND), and a TSB and albumin measurement. Correlation between TSB level and neurotoxicity is poor. Although 65% of recently reported cases of kernicterus had TSB levels above 35 mg/dL, 15% had levels below 30 mg/dL and 8% had TSB levels below 25 mg/dL. Currently the most sensitive means of assessing neurotoxicity may be the auditory brainstem evoked response, which shows predictable, early effects of bilirubin toxicity.

5. Chronic Bilirubin Encephalopathy (Kernicterus)

 ESSENTIALS OF DIAGNOSIS & TYPICAL FEATURES

- ► Extrapyramidal movement disorder (choreoathetoid cerebral palsy).
- ► Gaze abnormality, especially limitation of upward gaze.
- ► Auditory disturbances (deafness, failed auditory brainstem evoked response with normal evoked otoacoustic emissions, auditory neuropathy, auditory dyssynchrony).
- ► Dysplasia of the enamel of the deciduous teeth.

Kernicterus is an irreversible brain injury characterized by choreoathetoid cerebral palsy and hearing impairment.

Intelligence is probably normal but may be difficult to assess because of associated hearing, communication, and coordination problems. The diagnosis is clinical but is strengthened if audiologic testing shows auditory neuropathy and auditory dyssynchrony in which the otoacoustic emission test is normal but the auditory brainstem response is absent. Infants with such findings are usually deaf. Infants with milder kernicterus may have normal audiograms but abnormal auditory processing and subsequent problems with speech comprehension. Magnetic resonance imaging (MRI) scanning of the brain is nearly diagnostic if it shows abnormalities isolated to the globus pallidus, the subthalamic nuclei, or both.

Evaluation of Hyperbilirubinemia

Because most newborns are discharged at 24–48 hours of age, before physiologic jaundice peaks and before maternal milk supply is established, a predischarge TSB or a transcutaneous bilirubin (TcB) measurement is recommended to help predict which infants are at risk for severe hyperbilirubinemia. In all infants, an assessment of risk for severe hyperbilirubinemia should be performed before discharge (Table 2–7).

Table 2–7. Factors affecting the risk of severe hyperbilirubinemia in infants 35 or more weeks' gestation (in approximate order of importance).

Major risk factors
Predischarge TSB or TcB level in the high-risk zone (> 95th percentile; Figure 2–1)
Jaundice observed in the first 24 h
Blood group incompatibility with positive direct Coombs test, other known hemolytic disease (eg, G6PD deficiency), or elevated ETCO
Gestational age 35–36 wk
Previous sibling required phototherapy
Cephalohematoma or significant bruising
Exclusive breast-feeding, particularly if weight loss is excessive
East Asian race[a]

Minor risk factors
Predischarge TSB or TcB level in the high-intermediate-risk zone (75–95th percentile)
Gestational age 37–38 wk
Jaundice observed before discharge
Previous sibling with jaundice
Macrosomic infant of a diabetic mother

Decreased risk (these factors are associated with decreased risk of significant jaundice, listed in order of decreasing importance)
TSB or TcB level in the low-risk zone (Figure 2–1)
Gestational age ≥ 41 wk
Exclusive bottle feeding
Black race[a]
Discharge from hospital after 72 h

ETCO, end-tidal carbon monoxide; G6PD, glucose-6-phosphate dehydrogenase; TcB, transcutaneous bilirubin; TSB, total serum bilirubin.
[a]Race as defined by mother's description.

The greater the number of risk factors, the greater the likelihood of developing severe hyperbilirubinemia. As recommended by the AAP, follow-up within 24–48 hours for all infants discharged before 72 hours of age is imperative. Visual estimation of the bilirubin level is inaccurate. TSB should be measured and interpreted based on the age of the infant in hours at the time of sampling. Term infants with a TSB level greater than the 95th percentile for age in hours have a 40% risk of developing significant hyperbilirubinemia (see Figure 2–1). Serial bilirubin levels should be obtained from a single laboratory whenever possible to make interpretation of serial measurements more meaningful. It is important to remember that these nomograms apply only to infants 36 weeks and older.

Infants with visible jaundice on the first day of life or who develop excessive jaundice require further evaluation. The minimal evaluation consists of the following:

- Feeding and elimination history
- Birth weight and percent weight change since birth
- Examination for sources of excessive heme breakdown
- Assessment of blood type, Coombs testing, complete blood count (CBC) with smear, serum albumin, and TSB
- G6PD test if jaundice is otherwise unexplained, and in African-American infants with severe jaundice
- Fractionated bilirubin level in infants who appear ill, those with prolonged jaundice, acholic stool, hepatosplenomegaly, or dark urine to evaluate for cholestasis

Treatment of Indirect Hyperbilirubinemia

A. Phototherapy

Phototherapy is the most common treatment for indirect hyperbilirubinemia. It is relatively noninvasive and safe. Light of wavelength 425–475 nm (blue-green spectrum) is absorbed by unconjugated bilirubin in the skin converting it to a water-soluble stereoisomer that can be excreted in bile without conjugation. Intensive phototherapy should decrease TSB by 30%–40% in the first 24 hours, most significantly in the first 4–6 hours. The infant's eyes should be shielded to prevent retinal damage.

Phototherapy is started electively when the TSB is approximately 6 mg/dL (102 mmol/L) lower than the predicted exchange level for that infant (eg, at 16–19 mg/dL [272–323 mmol/L] for a full-term infant for whom exchange transfusion would be considered at a TSB of approximately 22–25 mg/dL [374–425 mmol/L]). AAP guidelines for phototherapy and exchange transfusion in infants of 35 or more weeks' gestation are shown in Figures 2–2 and 2–3. Hyperbilirubinemic infants should be fed by mouth if possible to decrease enterohepatic bilirubin circulation. Casein hydrolysate formula to supplement breast milk decreases enterohepatic circulation by inhibiting mucosal β-glucuronidase activity. IVIG (0.5–1.0 g/kg) in severe antibody-mediated

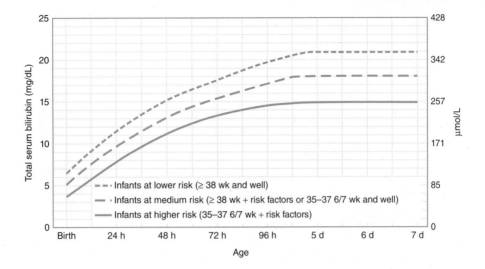

- Use total bilirubin. Do not subtract direct reacting of conjugated bilirubin.
- Risk factors = isoimmune hemolytic disease, G6PD deficiency, asphyxia, significant lethargy, temperature instability, sepsis, acidosis, or albumin < 3.0 g/dL (if measured).
- For well infants 35–37 6/7 wk can adjust TSB levels for intervention around the medium-risk line. It is an option to intervene at lower TSB levels for infants closer to 35 wk and at higher TSB levels for those closer to 37 6/7 wk.
- It is an option to provide conventional phototherapy in hospital or at home at TSB levels 2–3 mg/dL (35–50 mmol/L) below those shown, but home phototherapy should not be used in any infant with risk factors.

▲ **Figure 2–2.** Guidelines for phototherapy in hospitalized infants of 35 or more weeks' gestation. These guidelines are based on limited evidence and levels shown are approximations. (Reproduced with permission from the AAP Subcommittee on Hyperbilirubinemia: management of hyperbilirubinemia in the newborn infant 35 or more weeks of gestation. Pediatrics 2004 Jul;114(1):297–316.)

hemolysis may interrupt the hemolytic process. Although phototherapy has been shown to decrease the need for exchange transfusion, its long-term benefits, if any, in infants with less severe jaundice are unknown.

B. Exchange Transfusion

Although most infants with indirect hyperbilirubinemia can be treated with phototherapy, extreme indirect hyperbilirubinemia is a medical emergency. Infants should be admitted at once to a neonatal intensive care unit where exchange transfusion can be performed before irreversible neurologic damage occurs. Intensive phototherapy should be instituted immediately, during transport to the hospital if possible. As TSB nears the potentially toxic range, serum albumin should be determined. Albumin (1 g/kg) will aid in binding and removal of bilirubin during exchange transfusion, as well as afford some neuroprotection while preparing for the procedure.

Double-volume exchange transfusion (~160–200 mL/kg body weight) is most often required in infants with extreme hyperbilirubinemia secondary to Rh isoimmunization, ABO incompatibility, or hereditary spherocytosis. The procedure decreases serum bilirubin acutely by approximately

50% and removes about 80% of sensitized or abnormal red blood cells and offending antibody so that ongoing hemolysis is decreased. Exchange transfusion is also indicated in any infant with TSB above 30 mg/dL, in infants with signs of encephalopathy, or when intensive phototherapy has not lowered TSB by at least 0.5 mg/dL/h after 4 hours. The decision to perform exchange transfusion should be based on TSB, not on the indirect fraction of bilirubin.

Exchange transfusion is invasive, potentially risky, and infrequently performed. It should therefore be performed at a referral center. Mortality is 1%–5% and is greatest in the smallest, most immature, and unstable infants. Sudden death during the procedure can occur in any infant. There is a 5%–10% risk of serious complications such as necrotizing enterocolitis (NEC), infection, electrolyte disturbances, or thrombocytopenia. Isovolemic exchange (withdrawal through an arterial line with infusion through a venous line) may decrease the risk of some complications.

Bilitool.org. Accessed April 9, 2019.
Lauer BJ, Spector NJ: Hyperbilirubinemia in the newborn. Pediatr Rev 2011;32:341 [PMID: 21807875].

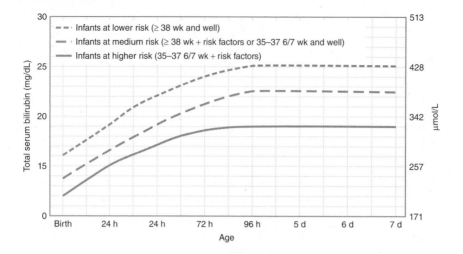

- The dashed lines for the first 24 hours indicate uncertainty due to a wide range of clinical circumstances and a range of responses to phototherapy.
- Immediate exchange transfusion is recommended if infant shows signs of acute bilirubin encephalopathy (hypertonia, arching, retrocolitis, opisthotonos, fever, high-pitched cry) or if TSB is ≥ 5 mg/dL (85 μmol/L) above these lines.
- Risk factors—isoimmune hemolytic disease, G6PD deficiency, asphyxia, significant lethargy, temperature instability, sepsis, acidosis.
- Measure serum albumin and calculate B/A ratio (see legend).
- Use total bilirubin. Do not subtract direct reading or conjugated bilirubin.
- If infant is well and 35–37 6/7 week (median risk), individualize TSB levels for exchange based on actual gestational age.

▲ **Figure 2–3.** Guidelines for exchange transfusion in infants of 35 or more weeks' gestation. These guidelines represent approximations for which an exchange transfusion is indicated in infants treated with intensive phototherapy. (Reproduced with permission from the AAP Subcommittee on Hyperbilirubinemia: Management of hyperbilirubinemia in the newborn infant 35 or more weeks of gestation. Pediatrics 2004 Jul;114(1):297–316.)

HYPOGLYCEMIA

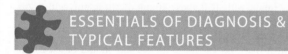

ESSENTIALS OF DIAGNOSIS & TYPICAL FEATURES

▶ Blood glucose < 40 mg/dL at birth to 4 hours, or < 45 mg/dL at 4–24 hours of age.

▶ LGA, SGA, preterm, and stressed infants at risk.

▶ May be asymptomatic.

▶ Infants can present with lethargy, poor feeding, irritability, or seizures.

▶ General Considerations

Blood glucose concentration in the fetus is approximately 15 mg/dL less than maternal glucose concentration. Glucose concentration decreases in the immediate postnatal period, to as low as 30 mg/dL in many healthy infants at 1–2 hours after birth. Concentrations below 40 mg/dL after the first feeding are considered hypoglycemic. By 3 hours, the glucose concentration in normal full-term infants stabilizes at 45 mg/dL or greater. The two groups of full-term newborn infants at highest risk for hypoglycemia are IDMs and growth-restricted infants.

A. Infants of Diabetic Mothers

The IDM has abundant glucose stores in the form of glycogen and fat but develops hypoglycemia because of hyperinsulinemia induced by maternal and fetal hyperglycemia. Increased energy supply to the fetus from the maternal circulation results in a macrosomic infant. The IDM is at increased risk for multiple neonatal problems, including trauma during delivery, cardiomyopathy (asymmetrical septal hypertrophy) which may present with murmur, respiratory distress, or cardiac failure, and microcolon which causes symptoms of low intestinal obstruction similar to Hirschsprung disease. Other neonatal problems include hypercoagulability and polycythemia, a combination that predisposes the infant to large vein thromboses (especially the renal vein). IDMs are often somewhat immature for their gestational age and are at increased risk for surfactant deficiency, hypocalcemia, feeding difficulties, and hyperbilirubinemia.

B. Intrauterine Growth-Restricted Infants

The intrauterine growth-restricted (IUGR) infant has reduced glucose stores in the form of glycogen and body fat and is prone to hypoglycemia. In addition, marked hyperglycemia and a transient diabetes mellitus–like syndrome occasionally develop, particularly in the very premature IUGR infant. These problems usually respond to adjustment in glucose intake, although insulin is sometimes needed transiently. Some IUGR infants have hyperinsulinemia that persists for 1 week or more.

C. Other Causes of Hypoglycemia

Hypoglycemia occurs in disorders with islet cell hyperplasia, including Beckwith-Wiedemann syndrome, nesidioblastosis, and genetic forms of hyperinsulinism. Hypoglycemia also occurs in certain inborn errors of metabolism such as glycogen storage disease and galactosemia. Endocrine causes of hypoglycemia include adrenal insufficiency and hypopituitarism, which should be suspected in the setting of hypoglycemia and micropenis. Hypoglycemia also occurs in infants with birth asphyxia, hypoxia, and bacterial or viral sepsis. Premature infants are at risk for hypoglycemia due to decreased glycogen stores.

▶ Clinical Findings and Monitoring

The signs of hypoglycemia in the newborn infant may be nonspecific and subtle: lethargy, poor feeding, irritability, tremors, jitteriness, apnea, and seizures. Hypoglycemia due to increased insulin is the most severe and most resistant to treatment. Hypoglycemia in hyperinsulinemic states can develop within the first 30–60 minutes of life.

Blood glucose can be measured by heelstick using a bedside glucometer. All infants at risk should be screened, including IDMs, IUGR infants, premature infants, and any infant with suggestive symptoms. All low or borderline values should be confirmed by laboratory measurement of blood glucose concentration. It is important to continue surveillance of glucose concentration until the baby has been on full enteral feedings without intravenous supplementation for 24 hours, with a target of greater than 45 mg/dL before feeding. Relapse of hypoglycemia thereafter is unlikely.

Infants with hypoglycemia requiring IV glucose infusions for more than 5 days should be evaluated for less common disorders, including inborn errors of metabolism, hyperinsulinemic states, and deficiencies of counterregulatory hormones.

▶ Treatment

Therapy is based on the provision of enteral or parenteral glucose. Treatment guidelines are shown in Table 2–8. Enteral glucose is the preferred treatment for an asymptomatic hypoglycemic infant who is vigorous and able to orally feed. Oral dextrose gel can be used to supplement an oral feeding and has been shown to decrease mother-infant separation and promote full breastfeeding at discharge. In hyperinsulinemic states, glucose boluses should be avoided and a higher glucose infusion rate used. After initial correction with a bolus of 10% dextrose in water ($D_{10}W$; 2 mL/kg), glucose infusion should be increased gradually as needed from a starting rate of 6 mg/kg/min, and weaned slowly when normoglycemic. IDMs and IUGR infants with polycythemia are at greatest risk for symptomatic hypoglycemia.

▶ Prognosis

The prognosis of hypoglycemia is good if therapy is prompt. CNS sequelae are more common in infants with hypoglycemic seizures and in neonates with persistent hyperinsulinemic hypoglycemia. Hypoglycemia may also potentiate brain injury after perinatal depression, and should be avoided.

Table 2–8. Hypoglycemia: suggested therapeutic regimens.

Screening Test[a]	Presence of Symptoms	Action
30–45 mg/dL	No symptoms of hypoglycemia	Draw blood glucose[b]; if the infant is alert and vigorous, feed; follow with frequent glucose monitoring. Consider 40% oral glucose gel (0.5 mL/kg) to supplement feeding.
		If the infant continues to have blood glucose < 40 mg/dL or is unable to feed, provide intravenous glucose at 6 mg/kg/min ($D_{10}W$ at 3.6 mL/kg/h).
< 45 mg/dL	Symptoms of hypoglycemia present	Draw blood glucose[b]; provide bolus of $D_{10}W$ (2 mL/kg) followed by an infusion of 6 mg/kg/min (3.6 mL/kg/h).
< 30 mg/dL	With or without symptoms of hypoglycemia	Draw blood glucose[b]; provide bolus of $D_{10}W$ followed by an infusion of 6 mg/kg/min.
		If IV access cannot be obtained immediately, an umbilical vein line should be used.

[a]Rapid bedside determination.
[b]Laboratory confirmation.

Adamkin DH; Committee on Fetus and Newborn: Clinical report—postnatal glucose homeostasis in late preterm and term infants. Pediatrics 2011;127:575 [PMID: 21357346].

Rozance PJ, Hay WW Jr: New approaches to management of neonatal hypoglycemia. Matern Health Neonatol Perinatol 2016 May;10:3 [PMID: 2716842].

RESPIRATORY DISTRESS IN THE TERM NEWBORN INFANT

 ESSENTIALS OF DIAGNOSIS & TYPICAL FEATURES

▶ Tachypnea, respiratory rate > 60 breaths/min.

▶ Intercostal and sternal retractions.

▶ Expiratory grunting.

▶ Cyanosis in room air.

▶ General Considerations

Respiratory distress is one of the most common symptom complexes of the newborn. It may result from cardiopulmonary and noncardiopulmonary causes (Table 2–9). Chest radiography, arterial blood gases, and pulse oximetry are useful in assessing the cause and severity of the distress. It is important to consider the noncardiopulmonary causes, because the natural tendency is to focus on the heart and lungs. Most of the noncardiopulmonary causes can be ruled out by the history, physical examination, and a few simple laboratory tests. The most common pulmonary causes of respiratory distress in the full-term infant are transient tachypnea, aspiration syndromes, congenital pneumonia, and pneumothorax.

A. Transient Tachypnea (Retained Fetal Lung Fluid)

Respiratory distress is typically present at birth, usually associated with a mild-to-moderate oxygen requirement (25%–50% O_2). The infant is usually full term or late preterm, nonasphyxiated, and born following a short labor or cesarean section without labor. The pathogenesis of the disorder is related to delayed clearance of fetal lung fluid via the circulation and pulmonary lymphatics. The chest radiograph shows perihilar streaking and fluid in interlobar fissures. Resolution usually occurs within 12–24 hours. Nasal CPAP can be helpful in the clearance of the fluid.

B. Aspiration Syndromes

Typically occurs in full-term or late preterm infants with fetal distress prior to delivery or depression at delivery. Blood or

Table 2–9. Causes of respiratory distress in the newborn.

Noncardiopulmonary
- Hypothermia or hyperthermia
- Hypoglycemia
- Polycythemia
- Metabolic acidosis
- Drug intoxications or withdrawal
- Insult to the central nervous system
  - Asphyxia
  - Hemorrhage
- Neuromuscular disease
- Phrenic nerve injury
- Skeletal dysplasia

Cardiovascular
- Left-sided outflow tract obstruction
  - Hypoplastic left heart
  - Aortic stenosis
  - Coarctation of the aorta, interrupted aortic arch
- Cyanotic lesions
- Transposition of the great vessels
- Total anomalous pulmonary venous return
- Tricuspid atresia
- Right-sided outflow obstruction

Respiratory tract
- Upper airway obstruction
  - Choanal atresia
  - Vocal cord paralysis
  - Subglottic stenosis
  - Lingual thyroid
- Meconium aspiration
- Clear fluid aspiration
- Transient tachypnea
- Pneumonia
- Pulmonary hypoplasia
- Hyaline membrane disease
- Pneumothorax
- Pleural effusions
- Mass lesions
  - Lobar emphysema
  - Cystic adenomatoid malformation
  - Congenital diaphragmatic hernia

Reproduced with permission from Gabbe SG: *Obstetrics: Normal and Problem Pregnancies.* Philadelphia, PA: Churchill Livingstone, 2007.

meconium may be present in the amniotic fluid. Aspiration of meconium most commonly occurs in utero when the stressed infant gasps. Delivery room management of these infants is discussed in the resuscitation section. Respiratory distress is present from birth, often accompanied by coarse breath sounds. Pneumonitis may cause an increasing oxygen need and may require intubation and ventilation. The chest radiograph shows coarse asymmetric infiltrates, hyperexpansion, and, in the worst cases, lobar consolidation. In some cases, because of secondary surfactant deficiency, the radiograph shows a diffuse homogeneous infiltrate pattern. Infants who aspirate are at risk of pneumothorax because of uneven aeration with segmental overdistention and are at risk for persistent pulmonary hypertension (see section Cardiac Problems in the Newborn Infant).

C. Congenital Pneumonia

The lungs are the most common site of infection in the neonate. Infections usually ascend from the genital tract before or during labor, with the vaginal or rectal flora the most likely agents (group B streptococci and *Escherichia coli*). Infants of any gestational age, with or without a history of prolonged rupture of membranes, chorioamnionitis, or maternal antibiotic administration, may be affected. Respiratory distress may begin at birth or may be delayed for several hours. The chest radiograph may resemble that of retained lung fluid or hyaline membrane disease. Rarely, there may be a lobar infiltrate or pleural effusion. Congenital pneumonia may be complicated by acquired surfactant deficiency or systemic sepsis.

Shock, poor perfusion, absolute neutropenia (< 2000/mL), and elevated C-reactive protein provide supportive evidence for pneumonia. Gram stain of tracheal aspirate may be helpful. Because no signs or laboratory findings can confirm a diagnosis of pneumonia, obtaining a blood culture and treatment with broad spectrum antibiotics should be considered in all term newborn with respiratory distress.

D. Spontaneous Pneumothorax

Spontaneous pneumothorax occurs in 1% of all deliveries. Risk is increased by interventions such as positive-pressure ventilation (PPV) in the delivery room. Respiratory distress (primarily tachypnea) is present from birth and typically is not severe. Breath sounds may be decreased on the affected side; heart tones may be shifted toward the opposite side and may be distant. The chest radiograph shows pneumothorax.

Treatment usually consists of supplemental oxygen and watchful waiting. Drainage by needle thoracentesis or tube thoracostomy is occasionally required. There is a slightly increased risk of renal abnormalities associated with spontaneous pneumothorax. Thus, careful physical examination of the kidneys and monitoring of urine output are indicated. If pulmonary hypoplasia with pneumothorax is suspected, renal ultrasound is indicated.

E. Other Respiratory Tract Causes

Other respiratory tract causes of respiratory distress are rare. Bilateral choanal atresia should be suspected if there is no air movement when the infant breathes through the nose. These infants have good color and heart rate while crying at delivery but become cyanotic and bradycardic when they resume normal nasal breathing. Other causes of upper airway obstruction usually produce some degree of stridor or poor air movement despite good respiratory effort. Pleural effusion is likely in hydropic infants. Space-occupying lesions cause a shift of the mediastinum with asymmetrical breath sounds and are apparent on chest radiographs. Many are associated with severe respiratory distress.

▶ Treatment

Whatever the cause, neonatal respiratory distress is treated with supplemental oxygen sufficient to maintain a Pao_2 of 60–70 mm Hg and an oxygen saturation by pulse oximetry (Spo_2) of 92%–96%. Oxygen should be warmed, humidified, and delivered through an air blender. Concentration should be measured with a calibrated oxygen analyzer. An umbilical or peripheral arterial line should be considered in infants requiring more than 45% fraction of inspired oxygen (Fio_2) by 4–6 hours of life to allow frequent blood gas determinations. Noninvasive monitoring with pulse oximetry should be used.

Supportive treatment includes IV glucose. Unless infection can be ruled out, blood cultures should be obtained, and broad-spectrum antibiotics started. Volume expansion (normal saline) can be given in infusions of 10 mL/kg over 30 minutes for low blood pressure, poor perfusion, and metabolic acidosis. Other specific testing should be done as indicated by the history and physical examination. In most cases, a chest radiograph, blood gas measurements, CBC, and blood glucose determination allow a diagnosis.

Intubation and mechanical ventilation should be undertaken if there is respiratory failure (Pao_2 < 60 mm Hg in > 60% Fio_2, $Paco_2$ > 60 mm Hg, or repeated apnea). Peak pressures should be adequate to produce chest wall expansion and audible breath sounds (usually 18–24 cm H_2O). Positive end-expiratory pressure (4–6 cm H_2O) should be used. Ventilation rates of 20–40 breaths/min are usually required. The goal is to maintain a Pao_2 of 60–70 mm Hg and a $Paco_2$ of 45–55 mm Hg.

▶ Prognosis

Most respiratory conditions of the full-term infant are acute and resolve in the first several days. Meconium aspiration and congenital pneumonia carry a mortality rate of up to 10% and can produce significant long-term pulmonary morbidity. Mortality has been reduced by use of high-frequency oscillatory ventilation and inhaled nitric oxide for treatment of pulmonary hypertension. Only rarely is ECMO needed as rescue therapy.

Edwards MO, Kotecha SJ, Kotecha K: Respiratory distress of the term newborn infant. Paediatr Resp Rev 2013;14(1):2937 [PMID: 23347658].

HEART MURMURS

Heart murmurs are common in the first days of life and do not usually signify structural heart problems (see also Cardiac Problems in the Newborn Infant). If a murmur is present at birth, it should be considered a valvular problem until proved otherwise because the common benign transitional murmurs (eg, patent ductus arteriosus) are not audible until minutes to hours after birth.

If an infant is pink, well-perfused, and in no respiratory distress, with palpable and symmetrical pulses (right brachial pulse no stronger than the femoral pulse), the murmur is most likely transitional. Transitional murmurs are soft (grade 1–3/6), heard at the left upper to midsternal border, and generally loudest during the first 24 hours. If the murmur persists beyond 24 hours of age, blood pressure in the right arm and a leg should be determined. If there is a difference of more than 15 mm Hg (arm > leg) or if the pulses in the lower extremities are difficult to palpate, a cardiologist should evaluate the infant for coarctation of the aorta. If there is no difference, the infant can be discharged home with follow-up in 2–3 days for auscultation and evaluation for signs of congestive failure. If signs of congestive failure or cyanosis are present, the infant should be referred for evaluation without delay. If the murmur persists without these signs, the infant can be referred for elective evaluation at age 2–4 weeks.

BIRTH TRAUMA

Most birth trauma is associated with difficult delivery (eg, large fetus, abnormal presenting position, or fetal distress requiring rapid extraction). The most common injuries are soft tissue bruising, fractures (clavicle, humerus, or femur), and cervical plexus palsies. Skull fracture, intracranial hemorrhage (primarily subdural and subarachnoid), and cervical spinal cord injury can also occur.

Fractures are often diagnosed by the obstetrician, who may feel or hear a snap during delivery. Clavicular fractures may cause decreased spontaneous movement of the arm, with local tenderness and crepitus. Humeral or femoral fractures usually cause tenderness and swelling over the shaft with a diaphyseal fracture, and always cause limitation of movement. Epiphyseal fractures are harder to diagnose radiographically owing to the cartilaginous nature of the epiphysis. After 8–10 days, callus is visible on radiographs. Treatment in all cases is gentle handling, with immobilization for 8–10 days: the humerus against the chest with elbow flexed; the femur with a posterior splint from below the knee to the buttock.

Brachial plexus injuries may result from traction as the head is pulled away from the shoulder during delivery. Injury to the C5–C6 roots is most common (Erb-Duchenne palsy). The arm is limp, adducted, and internally rotated, extended, and pronated at the elbow, and flexed at the wrist (so-called waiter's tip posture). Grasp is present. If the lower nerve roots (C8–T1) are injured (Klumpke's palsy), the hand is flaccid. If the entire plexus is injured, the arm and hand are flaccid, with associated sensory deficit. Early treatment for brachial plexus injury is conservative, because function usually returns over several weeks. Referral should be made to a physical therapist so that parents can be instructed on range-of-motion exercises, splinting, and further evaluation if needed. Return of function begins in the deltoid and biceps, with recovery by 3 months in most cases.

Spinal cord injury can occur at birth, especially in difficult breech extractions with hyperextension of the neck, or in midforceps rotations when the body fails to turn with the head. Infants are flaccid, quadriplegic, and without respiratory effort at birth. Facial movements are preserved. The long-term outlook for such infants is poor.

Facial nerve palsy is sometimes associated with forceps use but more often results from in utero pressure of the baby's head against the mother's sacrum. The infant has asymmetrical mouth movements and eye closure with poor facial movement on the affected side. Most cases resolve spontaneously in a few days to weeks.

Subgaleal hemorrhage into the large potential space under the scalp (Figure 2–4) is associated with difficult

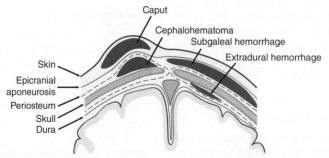

▲ **Figure 2–4.** Sites of extracranial bleeding in the newborn. (Reproduced with permission from Pape KE, Wigglesworth JS: Haemorrhage, ischemia, and the perinatal brain. *Clinics in Developmental Medicine.* Spastics International Medical Publications. William Heinemann Medical Books Limited, London, and JB Lippincott Company, Philadelphia; 1979.)

vaginal deliveries and repeated attempts at vacuum extraction. It can lead to hypovolemic shock and death from blood loss and coagulopathy triggered by consumption of clotting factors. This is an emergency requiring rapid replacement of blood and clotting factors.

INFANTS OF MOTHERS WHO ABUSE DRUGS

Current studies estimate that up to 15% of women use alcohol and 5%–15% use illicit drugs during pregnancy, depending on the population studied and the methods of ascertainment. Drugs most commonly used are tobacco, alcohol, marijuana, cocaine, and methamphetamine. Because mothers may abuse many drugs and give an unreliable history of drug usage, it is difficult to pinpoint which drug is causing the morbidity seen in a newborn infant. Early hospital discharge makes recognition of these infants based on physical findings and abnormal behavior difficult. Except for alcohol, a birth defect syndrome has not been defined for any substance of abuse.

1. Cocaine & Methamphetamine

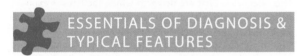
ESSENTIALS OF DIAGNOSIS & TYPICAL FEATURES

▶ Triad of no prenatal care, premature delivery, placental abruption.

▶ Possible IUGR.

▶ Irritability.

Cocaine and methamphetamine are often used in association with other drugs such as tobacco, alcohol, and marijuana. These stimulants can cause maternal hypertension, decreased uterine blood flow, fetal hypoxemia, uterine contractions, and placental abruption. Rates of stillbirth, placental abruption, symmetric IUGR, and preterm delivery are increased in users. In the high-risk setting of no prenatal care, placental abruption, and preterm labor, urine toxicology screens should be performed on the mother and infant; consent from the mother for testing her urine may be required. Meconium or an umbilical cord sample should be sent for drug screening as it enhances diagnosis by indicating cumulative drug exposure from the first trimester forward. Although no specific malformation complex or withdrawal syndrome is described for cocaine and methamphetamine abuse, infants may show irritability, tremors, increased stress response, and poor state regulation.

Children of mothers who use methamphetamines are at particularly high risk for neglect and abuse. Social services evaluation is especially important to assess the home environment for these risks. The risk of SIDS is three to seven times higher in infants of users than in those of nonusers (0.5%–1% of exposed infants). The risk may be lessened by environmental interventions such as avoidance of tobacco smoke and supine infant positioning.

2. Opioids

ESSENTIALS OF DIAGNOSIS & TYPICAL FEATURES

▶ CNS—irritability, hyperactivity, hypertonicity, incessant high-pitched cry, tremors, seizures.

▶ GI—vomiting, diarrhea, weight loss, poor feeding, incessant hunger, excessive salivation.

▶ Metabolic and respiratory—nasal stuffiness, sneezing, yawning, sweating, hyperthermia.

▶ Often IUGR.

▶ Clinical Findings

The withdrawal signs seen in infants born to narcotic-using mothers, whether heroin, prescription narcotics, or methadone, are similar. These symptoms include problems with feeding and sleep, fever, increased tone, tremors, and seizures, and are referred to as neonatal abstinence syndrome (NAS). The symptoms in infants born to methadone-maintained mothers may be delayed in onset, more severe, and more prolonged than those seen with heroin addiction. Symptoms usually begin within 1–3 days of life. The clinical picture is typical enough to suggest a diagnosis even if a maternal history of narcotic abuse has not been obtained. Confirmation should be made with maternal and newborn toxicology screening.

▶ Treatment

If opioid abuse or withdrawal is suspected, the infant is not a candidate for early discharge. A serial scoring system should be used, to objectively diagnose NAS and quantify the severity of symptoms. Supportive treatment includes swaddling the infant and providing a quiet, dimly lit environment, minimizing procedures, and disturbing the infant as little as possible. Specific treatment should be used when the infant has severe symptoms or excessive weight loss. No single drug has been identified as optimally effective. Oral morphine or methadone are the most commonly used first-line agents for NAS. Phenobarbital may be used for increased irritability, particularly in patients who were exposed to multiple drugs. Treatment can be tapered over several days to 2 weeks, as tolerated. It is also important to review maternal tests for HIV, hepatitis B, and hepatitis C, as all are common in intravenous drug users.

Prognosis

These infants often have chronic neurobehavioral handicaps; however, it is difficult to distinguish the effects of in utero drug exposure from those of the environment. Infants of opioid abusers have a four- to fivefold increased risk of SIDS.

3. Alcohol

Alcohol is the only recreational drug of abuse that is clearly teratogenic, and prenatal exposure to alcohol is the most common preventable cause of mental retardation. Prevalence estimates of fetal alcohol syndrome (FAS) in the United States range from 0.5 to 2 per 1000 live births with up to 1 in 100 having lesser effects (fetal alcohol spectrum disorders). The effects of alcohol on the fetus and newborn are determined by the degree and timing of ethanol exposure and by the maternal, fetal, and placental metabolism of ethanol, which is likely genetically determined. Although there is no clear evidence that minimal amounts of alcohol are harmful, there is no established safe dose. Fetal growth and development are adversely affected if drinking continues throughout the pregnancy, and infants can occasionally experience withdrawal similar to that associated with maternal opioid abuse. Clinical features of FAS that may be observed in the newborn period are listed in Table 2–10. This diagnosis is usually easier to recognize in older infants and children.

4. Tobacco Smoking

The fetus is exposed to nicotine concentrations that are 15% higher than in maternal blood. Smoking has a negative effect on fetal growth rate. The more the mother smokes, the greater the degree of IUGR. There is a twofold increase in low birth weight even in light smokers (< 10 cigarettes per day). Infants exposed to nicotine prenatally are also at increased risk for preterm labor and SIDS. Smoking during pregnancy has been associated with irritability, hypertonicity, hyperexcitability, and tremors in the newborn.

5. Marijuana

Marijuana is the most frequently used illegal drug, and now that it is legal in many states, there is concern for increased use among pregnant women. It does not appear to be teratogenic, and although a mild abstinence-type syndrome has been described, infants exposed to marijuana in utero rarely require treatment. Some long-term neurodevelopmental problems, particularly increased impulsivity and hyperactivity and problems in abstract and visual reasoning, have been noted.

6. Other Drugs

Other drugs with potential effects on the newborn fall in two categories. First are drugs to which the fetus is exposed because of therapy for maternal conditions. The human placenta is relatively permeable, particularly to lipophilic solutes. If possible, maternal drug therapy should be postponed until after the first trimester to avoid teratogenic effects. Drugs with potential fetal toxicity include antineoplastics, antithyroid agents, warfarin, lithium, and angiotensin-converting enzyme inhibitors (eg, captopril and enalapril). Anticonvulsants, especially high-dose or multiple-drug therapy, may be associated with craniofacial abnormalities. The use of selective serotonin reuptake inhibitors, benzodiazepines, and antipsychotic medications appears to be generally safe, and risk should be balanced against the risk of untreated psychiatric conditions in the mother. However, up to 33% of infants exposed to SSRI medications in utero experience signs of NAS during the first days of life. Paroxetine seems to have the greatest propensity to cause abstinence symptoms. Phenobarbital may be used for severe irritability in cases of SSRI withdrawal.

In the second category are drugs transmitted to the infant in breast milk. Most drugs taken by the mother achieve some concentration in breast milk, although they usually do not present a problem to the infant. If the drug is one that could have adverse effects on the infant, timing breast-feeding to coincide with trough concentrations in the mother may be useful.

Table 2–10. Features observed in fetal alcohol syndrome in the newborn.

Craniofacial
Short palpebral fissures
Thin vermillion of upper lip
Flattened philtrum
Growth
Prenatal and postnatal growth deficiency (small for gestational age, failure to thrive)
Central nervous system
Microcephaly
Partial or complete agenesis of the corpus callosum
Optic nerve hypoplasia
Hypotonia, poor feeding

McQueen K, Murphy-Oikonen J: Neonatal abstinence syndrome. New Engl J Med 2016;375:2468 [PMID: 28002715].

Oji-Mmuo CN, Corr TE, Doheny KK: Addictive disorders in women: the impact of maternal substance use on the fetus and newborn. NeoReviews 2017;18:e576.

MULTIPLE BIRTHS

ESSENTIALS OF DIAGNOSIS & TYPICAL FEATURES

▶ Monochorial twins
  • Always monozygous (identical twins) and same sex.
  • Can be diamniotic or monoamniotic.
  • Risk for twin-to-twin transfusion and higher risk of congenital anomalies, neurodevelopmental problems, and cerebral palsy.
▶ Dichorial twins
  • Either dizygous (fraternal twins) or monozygous (identical twins); same sex or different sex.
  • Can have growth restriction due to abnormal placental implantation.
  • Not at risk for twin transfusion syndrome; less risk for anomalies and neurodevelopmental problems than monochorial twins.

Historically, twinning occurred at a rate of 1 in 80 pregnancies (1.25%). The incidence of twinning and higher-order multiple births in the United States has increased because of assisted reproductive technologies. In 2017, twins occurred in 3.3% of live births in the United States, a greater than 70% increase since 1980.

A distinction should be made between dizygous (fraternal) and monozygous (identical) twins. Race, maternal parity, and maternal age affect the incidence of dizygous, but not monozygous, twinning. Drugs used to induce ovulation, such as clomiphene citrate and gonadotropins, increase the incidence of dizygotic or polyzygotic twinning. Monozygous twinning also seems to be more common after assisted reproduction. The incidence of malformations is also increased in identical twins and may affect only one of the twins. If a defect is found in one twin, the other should be examined carefully for lesser degrees of the same defect.

Early transvaginal ultrasound and examination of the placenta after birth can help establish the type of twinning. Two amnionic membranes and two chorionic membranes are found in all dizygous twins and in one-third of monozygous twins even when the placental disks appear to be fused into one. A single chorionic membrane always indicates monozygous twins. The rare monochorial, monoamniotic situation (1% of twins) is especially dangerous, with a high risk of antenatal cord entanglement and death of one or both twins. Close fetal surveillance is indicated, and preterm delivery is often elected.

▶ Complications of Multiple Births

A. Intrauterine Growth Restriction

There is some degree of IUGR in most multiple pregnancies, especially after 32 weeks, although it is usually not clinically significant with two exceptions. First, in monochorial twin pregnancy an arteriovenous shunt may develop between the twins (twin-twin transfusion syndrome). The twin on the venous side (recipient) becomes plethoric and larger than the smaller anemic twin (donor), who may ultimately die or be severely growth restricted. The occurrence of poly-hydramnios in the larger twin and severe oligohydramnios in the smaller may be the first sign of this problem. Second, discordance in size (birth weights that are significantly different) can also occur when separate placentas are present if one placenta develops poorly, because of a poor implantation site. In this instance, no fetal exchange of blood takes place but the growth rates of the two infants are different.

B. Preterm Delivery

Length of gestation tends to be inversely related to the number of fetuses. The mean age at delivery for singletons is 38.8 weeks, for twins 35.3 weeks, for triplets 32.2 weeks, and for quadruplets 29.9 weeks. The prematurity rate in multiple gestations is 5–10 times that of singletons, with 50% of twins and 90% of triplets born before 37 weeks. There is an increased incidence of cerebral palsy in multiple births, more so with monochorial than dichorial infants. Prematurity is the main cause of increased mortality and morbidity in twins, although in the case of monochorial twins, intravascular exchange through placental anastomoses, particularly after the death of one twin, also increases the risk substantially.

C. Obstetric Complications

Polyhydramnios, pregnancy-induced hypertension, premature rupture of membranes, abnormal fetal presentations, and prolapsed umbilical cord occur more frequently in women with multiple fetuses. Multiple pregnancies should always be identified prenatally with ultrasound examinations; doing so allows the obstetrician and pediatrician or neonatologist to plan management jointly. Because neonatal complications are usually related to prematurity, prolongation of pregnancy significantly reduces neonatal morbidity.

▼ NEONATAL INTENSIVE CARE

PERINATAL RESUSCITATION

Perinatal resuscitation refers to the steps taken by the obstetrician to support the infant during labor and delivery and the resuscitative steps taken by the pediatrician after delivery.

Intrapartum support includes maintaining maternal blood pressure, maternal oxygen therapy, positioning the mother to improve placental perfusion, readjusting oxytocin infusions or administering a tocolytic if appropriate, minimizing trauma to the infant, obtaining all necessary cord blood samples, and completing an examination of the placenta. The pediatrician or neonatologist focuses on temperature support, initiation and maintenance of effective ventilation, maintenance of perfusion and hydration, and glucose regulation.

A number of conditions associated with pregnancy, labor, and delivery place the infant at risk for birth asphyxia: (1) maternal diseases such as diabetes, pregnancy-induced hypertension, heart and renal disease, and collagen-vascular disease; (2) fetal conditions such as prematurity, multiple births, growth restriction, and fetal anomalies; and (3) labor and delivery conditions, including fetal distress with or without meconium in the amniotic fluid, and administration of anesthetics and opioid analgesics.

Physiology of Birth Asphyxia

Birth asphyxia can be the result of (1) acute interruption of umbilical blood flow (eg, prolapsed cord with cord compression), (2) premature placental separation, (3) maternal hypotension or hypoxia, (4) chronic placental insufficiency, and (5) failure to perform resuscitation properly.

The neonatal response to asphyxia follows a predictable pattern (Figure 2–5). The initial response to hypoxia is an increase in respiratory rate and a rise in heart rate and blood pressure. Respirations then cease (primary apnea) as heart rate and blood pressure begin to fall. The initial period of apnea lasts 30–60 seconds. Gasping respirations (3–6/min) then begin, while heart rate and blood pressure gradually decline. Secondary or terminal apnea then ensues, with further decline in heart rate and blood pressure. The longer the duration of secondary apnea, the greater is the risk for hypoxic organ injury. A cardinal feature of the defense against hypoxia is the underperfusion of certain tissue beds (eg, skin, muscle, kidneys, and GI tract), which allows maintenance of perfusion to core organs (ie, heart, brain, and adrenals).

Response to resuscitation also follows a predictable pattern. During the period of primary apnea, almost any physical stimulus causes the infant to initiate respirations. Infants in secondary apnea require positive pressure ventilation (PPV). The first sign of recovery is an increase in heart rate, followed by an increase in blood pressure with improved perfusion. The time required for rhythmic, spontaneous respirations to occur is related to the duration of the secondary apnea. As a rough rule, for each minute past the last gasp, 2 minutes of PPV is required before gasping begins and 4 minutes is required to reach rhythmic breathing. Not until sometime later do spinal and corneal reflexes return. Muscle tone gradually improves over the course of several hours.

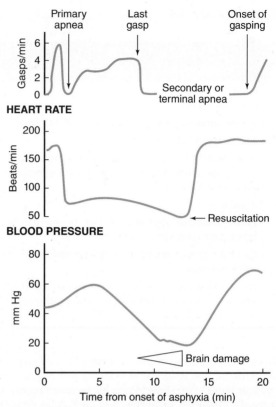

▲ **Figure 2–5.** Schematic depiction of changes in rhesus monkeys during asphyxia and on resuscitation by PPV. (Adapted with permission from Dawes GS: *Fetal and Neonatal Physiology.* Chicago, IL: Year Book Publishing; 1968.)

Delivery Room Management

When asphyxia is anticipated, a resuscitation team of at least two persons should be present: one to manage the airway and one to monitor the heartbeat and provide assistance. The necessary equipment and drugs are listed in Table 2–11.

A. Steps in the Resuscitative Process

1. Dry the infant well and place him or her under a radiant heat source. Do not allow the infant to become hyperthermic.

2. Position the infant to open the airway. Gently suction the mouth, then the nose.

3. Quickly assess the infant's condition. The best criteria are the infant's respiratory effort (apneic, gasping, or regular) and heart rate (> 100 or < 100 beats/min). A depressed heart rate—indicative of hypoxic myocardial depression—is the single most reliable indicator of the need for resuscitation.

Table 2–11. Equipment for neonatal resuscitation.

Clinical Needs	Equipment
Thermoregulation	Radiant heat source with platform, mattress covered with warm sterile blankets, servo control heating, temperature probe, gallon size food-grade plastic bag or plastic wrap and an exothermic blanket (preterm)
Airway management	**Suction:** bulb suction, mechanical suction with sterile catheters (6Fr, 8Fr, 10Fr), meconium aspirator
	Ventilation: manual infant resuscitation bag connected to manometer or with a pressure-release valve, or T-piece resuscitator, capable of delivering 100% oxygen; appropriate masks for term and preterm infants, oral airways, stethoscope, oxygen blender, pulse oximeter
	Intubation: neonatal laryngoscope with No. 0 and 1 blades; endotracheal tubes (2.5, 3.0, 3.5 mm outer diameter with stylet): extra bulbs and batteries for laryngoscope; scissors, adhesive tape, gloves, end-tidal CO_2 detection device
Gastric decompression	Nasogastric tube: 8Fr with 20-mL syringe
Administration of drugs and volume replacement	Sterile umbilical catheterization tray, umbilical catheters (3.5Fr and 5Fr), normal saline, drug box[a] with appropriate neonatal vials and dilutions, sterile syringes, needles, and alcohol sponges
Transport	Warmed transport isolette with oxygen source

[a]Epinephrine 1:10,000; 10% dextrose.
Modified with permission from Gabbe SG: *Obstetrics: Normal and Problem Pregnancies.* Philadelphia, PA: Churchill Livingstone, 2007.

4. Infants who are breathing and have heart rates more than 100 beats/min usually require no further intervention other than supplemental oxygen if persistently cyanotic. Infants with heart rates less than 100 beats/min and apnea or irregular respiratory efforts should be stimulated gently. The infant's back should be rubbed and/or heels flicked.

5. If the infant fails to respond to tactile stimulation within a few seconds, begin bag and mask ventilation, using a soft mask that seals well around the mouth and nose. For the initial inflations, pressures up to 30–40 cm H_2O may be necessary to overcome surface-active forces in the lungs. Adequacy of ventilation is assessed by observing expansion of the infant's chest accompanied by an improvement in heart rate, perfusion, and color. After the first few breaths, lower the peak pressure to 15–20 cm H_2O. The chest movement should resemble that of an easy breath rather than a deep sigh. The rate of bagging should be 40–60 breaths/min. An oximeter probe should be placed on the infant's right hand.

6. Most neonates can be resuscitated effectively with a bag and mask. If the infant does not respond to bag and mask ventilation, reposition the head (slight extension), reapply the mask to achieve a good seal, consider suctioning the mouth and the oropharynx, and try ventilating with the mouth open. An increase in peak pressure should also be attempted, but if the infant does not respond within 30 seconds, intubation is appropriate. Failure to respond to intubation and ventilation can result from (1) mechanical difficulties (Table 2–12), (2) profound asphyxia with myocardial depression, and (3) inadequate circulating blood volume. Quickly rule out the mechanical causes listed in Table 2–12. Check to ensure that the endotracheal tube passes through the vocal cords. A CO_2 detector placed between the endotracheal tube and the bag can be helpful as a rapid confirmation of proper tube position in the airway. Occlusion of the tube should be suspected when there is resistance to bagging and no chest wall movement. Very few neonates (~0.1%) require either cardiac compressions or drugs during resuscitation. Almost all newborns respond to ventilation if done effectively. All resuscitations in term infants should begin using room air. Oxygen concentration can be increased using an oxygen blender during PPV. It is not expected for the preductal (right hand) oxygen saturation to reach 90% until 10 minutes of age. The use of 100% oxygen may increase the risk of postresuscitative oxidative injury without any improvement in efficacy.

Table 2–12. Mechanical causes of failed resuscitation.

Cause	Examples
Equipment failure	Malfunctioning bag, oxygen not connected or running
Endotracheal tube malposition	Esophagus, right main stem bronchus
Occluded endotracheal tube	
Insufficient inflation pressure to expand lungs	
Space-occupying lesions in the thorax	Pneumothorax, pleural effusions, diaphragmatic hernia
Pulmonary hypoplasia	Extreme prematurity, oligohydramnios

Reproduced with permission from Gabbe SG: *Obstetrics: Normal and Problem Pregnancies.* Philadelphia, PA: Churchill Livingstone, 2007.

7. If mechanical causes are ruled out and the heart rate remains less than 60 beats/min after intubation and effective PPV for 30 seconds, cardiac compressions should be initiated. Chest compressions should be synchronized with ventilation at a 3:1 ratio (90 compressions and 30 breaths/min). Electronic cardiac monitoring should be used to monitor the heart rate when chest compressions are administered.

8. If drugs are needed, the drug and dose of choice is epinephrine 1:10,000 solution (0.1–0.3 mL/kg) given via an umbilical venous line. If volume loss is suspected, 10 mL/kg of normal saline should be administered through an umbilical vein line.

B. Continued Resuscitative Measures

The appropriateness of continued resuscitative efforts should be reevaluated in infants who do not respond to initial measures. In current practice, resuscitative efforts are made even in apparent stillbirths (ie, infants whose Apgar score at 1 minute is 0–1). Modern resuscitative techniques have led to improved survival in such infants, with 60% of survivors showing normal development. Although it is clear that resuscitation of these infants should be performed, subsequent continued support depends on the response to resuscitation. If the Apgar score does not improve markedly in the first 10 minutes of life, the mortality rate and the incidence of severe developmental handicaps among survivors are high.

C. Special Considerations

1. Delayed cord clamping—Current recommendations for neonatal resuscitation include that cord clamping should be delayed for at least 30–60 seconds for most vigorous term and preterm newborns. In cases where placental circulation is compromised (placental abruption, umbilical cord compression or avulsion), the umbilical cord should be clamped immediately and the initial steps of resuscitation begun.

2. Preterm infants

A. Minimizing heat loss improves survival. Prewarmed towels should be available. The environmental temperature of the delivery suite should be raised to more than 25°C (especially for infants weighing < 1500 g). An occlusive skin cover such as a gallon-sized food-grade plastic bag with an opening to slip over the infant's head and an exothermic blanket should be used to minimize heat loss in the extremely low-birth-weight (< 1000 g) infant.

B. The lungs of preterm infants are especially prone to injury from PPV due to volutrauma. For this reason, if possible, the infant's respiratory efforts should be supported with nasal continuous positive airway pressure (CPAP) rather than PPV. If PPV is needed, a T-piece resuscitation device should be used to allow precise and consistent regulation of pressure delivery. Resuscitation in the preterm should begin with a blended oxygen concentration of 21%–30% with titration to achieve target oxygen saturations.

C. In the infant of extremely low gestational age (< 26 weeks), immediate intubation for administration of surfactant should be considered.

D. Volume expanders should be infused slowly to minimize rapid swings in blood pressure, especially important in the ELBW infant.

3. Narcotic depression—In the case of opioid administration to the mother within 4 hours of delivery, institute resuscitation as described earlier. The use of naloxone is not recommended for use during neonatal resuscitation due to insufficient evidence of safety and efficacy.

4. Meconium-stained amniotic fluid—Resuscitation of the infant should proceed with the same initial steps as an infant born without meconium-stained amniotic fluid.

5. Universal precautions—In the delivery suite, universal precautions should always be observed.

Treatment of the Asphyxiated Infant

Asphyxia is manifested by multiorgan dysfunction, seizures, neonatal encephalopathy, and metabolic acidemia. The infant with significant perinatal hypoxia and ischemia is at risk for dysfunction of multiple end organs (Table 2–13). The organ of greatest concern is the brain.

The features of neonatal encephalopathy are decreased level of consciousness, poor tone, decreased spontaneous movement, periodic breathing or apnea, and seizures. Brainstem signs (oculomotor and pupillary disturbances, absent gag reflex) may also be present. The severity and duration of clinical signs correlate with the severity of the insult. Other evaluations helpful in assessing severity in the full-term infant include electroencephalogram (EEG) and MRI which, particularly with diffusion-weighted imaging,

Table 2–13. Signs and symptoms caused by asphyxia.

Neonatal encephalopathy, seizures
Respiratory distress due to aspiration or secondary surfactant deficiency, pulmonary hemorrhage
Persistent pulmonary hypertension
Hypotension due to myocardial dysfunction
Transient tricuspid valve insufficiency
Anuria or oliguria due to acute tubular necrosis
Feeding intolerance; necrotizing enterocolitis
Elevated aminotransferases due to liver injury
Adrenal insufficiency due to hemorrhage
Disseminated intravascular coagulation
Hypocalcemia
Hypoglycemia
Persistent metabolic acidemia
Hyperkalemia

is useful in the early evaluation of infants with perinatal asphyxia. A markedly abnormal EEG with voltage suppression and slowing evolving into a burst-suppression pattern is associated with severe clinical symptoms. MRI may show perfusion defects and areas of ischemic injury on diffusion-weighted imaging.

Management is directed at supportive care and treatment of specific abnormalities. Fluids should be restricted initially to 60–80 mL/kg/day; oxygenation should be maintained with mechanical ventilation if necessary; blood pressure should be supported with judicious volume expansion (if hypovolemic) and vasopressor support; and glucose should be in the normal range of 45–100 mg/dL. Hypocalcemia, coagulation abnormalities, and metabolic acidemia should be corrected and seizures treated with IV phenobarbital. Hypothermia, either selective head cooling or whole body cooling, initiated within 6 hours of birth, has been shown to improve outcome at 24 months and 6–7 year follow-up of infants with moderate encephalopathy. Efficacy has not been proved in the most severe cases of neonatal encephalopathy.

Birth Asphyxia: Long-Term Outcome

Fetal heart rate tracings, cord pH, and 1-minute Apgar scores are imprecise predictors of long-term outcome. Apgar scores of 0–3 at 5 minutes in full-term infants are associated with an increased risk of death in the first year of life and an 8% risk of cerebral palsy among survivors. The risks of mortality and morbidity increase with more prolonged depression of the Apgar score. The single best predictor of outcome is the severity of clinical neonatal encephalopathy (severe symptomatology including coma carries a 75% chance of death and a 100% rate of neurologic sequelae among survivors). The major sequela of neonatal encephalopathy is cerebral palsy with or without mental retardation and epilepsy. Other prognostic features are prolonged seizures refractory to therapy, markedly abnormal EEG, and MRI scan with evidence of major ischemic injury.

Papile LA et al: Committee on Fetus and Newborn: hypothermia and neonatal encephalopathy. Pediatrics 2014;133(6):1146 [PMID: 24864176].
Perlman JM: Highlights of the new neonatal resuscitation program guidelines. NeoReviews 2016;17:e435–e446.
Weiner GM: *Textbook of Neonatal Resuscitation*. 7th ed. American Heart Association/American Academy of Pediatrics; 2016.

THE PRETERM INFANT

Premature infants comprise the majority of high-risk newborns. The preterm infant faces a variety of physiologic handicaps:

1. The ability to coordinate sucking, swallowing, and breathing is not achieved until 34–36 weeks' gestation. Therefore, enteral feedings must be provided by gavage.

2. Lack of body fat stores causes decreased ability to maintain body temperature, and may predispose to hypoglycemia.

3. Pulmonary immaturity–surfactant deficiency is associated with structural immaturity in infants younger than 26 weeks' gestation. This condition is exacerbated by the combination of noncompliant lungs and an extremely compliant chest wall, causing inefficient respiratory mechanics.

4. Immature respiratory control leads to apnea and bradycardia.

5. Persistent patency of the ductus arteriosus compromises pulmonary gas exchange because of overperfusion and edema of the lungs.

6. Immature cerebral vasculature and structure predisposes to subependymal and intraventricular hemorrhage, and periventricular leukomalacia (PVL).

7. Impaired substrate absorption by the GI tract compromises nutritional management.

8. Immature renal function (including both filtration and tubular functions) complicates fluid and electrolyte management.

9. Increased susceptibility to infection.

10. Immaturity of metabolic processes predisposes to hypoglycemia and hypocalcemia.

1. Delivery Room Care

See section Perinatal Resuscitation.

2. Care in the Nursery

A. Thermoregulation

Maintaining stable body temperature is a function of heat production and conservation balanced against heat loss. Heat production in response to cold stress occurs through voluntary muscle activity, involuntary muscle activity (shivering), and thermogenesis not caused by shivering. Newborns produce heat mainly through the last of these three mechanisms. This metabolic heat production depends on the quantity of brown fat, which is very limited in the preterm infant. In addition to decreased heat production in preterm infants, heat loss is accelerated because of a high ratio of surface area to body mass, reduced insulation by subcutaneous tissue, and water loss through the immature skin.

The thermal environment of the preterm neonate must be regulated carefully. The infant can be kept warm in an isolette, in which the air is heated and convective heat loss is minimized. The infant can also be kept warm on an open bed with a radiant heat source. Ideally, the infant should be kept in a neutral thermal environment. The neutral thermal environment allows the infant to maintain a stable core body temperature with a minimum of metabolic heat production through oxygen consumption. The neutral thermal environment depends on the infant's size, gestational age, and postnatal age. The neutral thermal environment (for either isolette or radiant warmer care) can be obtained by maintaining an abdominal skin temperature of 36.5°C. Generally, when infants reach 1700–1800 g, they are able to maintain temperature while bundled in an open crib.

B. Monitoring the High-Risk Infant

At a minimum, equipment to monitor heart rate, respirations, and blood pressure should be available. Oxygen saturation is assessed continuously using pulse oximetry, correlated with arterial oxygen tension (Pao_2) as needed. Transcutaneous Po_2 and Pco_2 can also be used to assess oxygenation and ventilation in sicker infants. Arterial blood gases, electrolytes, glucose, calcium, bilirubin, and other chemistries must be measured on small volumes of blood. Early in the care of a sick preterm infant, the most efficient way to sample blood for tests as well as to provide fluids and monitor blood pressure is through an umbilical arterial line. Once the infant is stable and the need for frequent blood samples is reduced (usually 4–7 days), the umbilical line should be removed. All indwelling lines are associated with morbidity from thrombosis, infection, and bleeding.

C. Fluid and Electrolyte Therapy

Fluid requirements in preterm infants are a function of (1) insensible losses (skin and respiratory tract), (2) urine output, (3) stool output (< 5% of total), and (4) other losses, such as nasogastric losses. In most circumstances, the fluid requirement is determined largely by insensible losses plus urine losses. The major contribution to insensible water loss is evaporative skin loss. The rate of water loss is a function of gestational age (body weight, skin thickness, and maturity), environment (losses are greater under a radiant warmer than in an isolette), and the use of phototherapy. Respiratory losses are minimal when humidified oxygen is used. The renal contribution to water requirement is influenced by the limited ability of the preterm neonate either to concentrate the urine and conserve water, or to excrete a water load.

Electrolyte requirements are minimal for the first 24–48 hours until there is significant urinary excretion. Basal requirements thereafter are as follows: sodium, 3 mEq/kg/day; potassium, 2 mEq/kg/day; chloride, 2–3 mEq/kg/day; and bicarbonate, 2–3 mEq/kg/day. In the infant younger than 30 weeks' gestation, sodium and bicarbonate losses in the urine are often elevated, thereby increasing the infant's requirements.

Initial fluid management after birth varies with the infant's size and gestation. Infants of more than 1200 g should start at 80–100 mL/kg/day of $D_{10}W$. Those weighing less should start at 100–120 mL/kg/day of either $D_{10}W$ or D_5W (infants < 800 g and born before 26 weeks' gestation often become

hyperglycemic on $D_{10}W$ at these infusion rates). The most critical issue in fluid management is monitoring. Monitoring body weight, urine output, fluid and electrolyte intake, serum and urine electrolytes, and glucose allows fairly precise determination of the infant's water, glucose, and electrolyte needs. Parenteral nutrition should be started early, preferably on the first day, and continued until an adequate enteral intake is achieved.

D. Nutritional Support

The average caloric requirement for the growing premature infant is 120 kcal/kg/day. Desired weight gain is 15–20 g/kg/day for infants younger than 35 weeks, and 15 g/kg/day for those older than 35 weeks; linear and head circumference growth should average 1 cm/wk. Infants initially require IV glucose infusion to maintain blood glucose concentration in the range of 60–100 mg/dL. Infusions of 5–7 mg/kg/min (~80–100 mL/kg/day of $D_{10}W$) are usually needed. Aggressive nutritional support in the very low-birth-weight infant should be started as soon as possible after birth, with parenteral alimentation solutions containing 3–4 g/kg/day of amino acids (Table 2–14). Small-volume trophic feeds with breast milk or 20 kcal/oz premature formula should be started by gavage at 10% or less of the infant's nutritional intake as soon as possible, generally within the first few days after birth. After several days of trophic feeds the infant can be slowly advanced to full caloric needs over 5–7 days. Even extremely small feedings can enhance intestinal readiness to accept larger feeding volumes. Intermittent bolus feedings are preferred because these appear to stimulate the release of gut-related hormones and may accelerate maturation of the GI tract, although in the extremely low-birth-weight infant (< 1000 g) or the postsurgical neonate, continuous-drip feeds are sometimes better tolerated.

In general, long-term nutritional support for infants of very low birth weight consists either of breast milk supplemented to increase protein, caloric density, and mineral content, or infant formulas modified for preterm infants. In these formulas, protein concentrations and caloric concentrations are relatively high. In addition, premature formulas contain some medium-chain triglycerides—which do not require bile for absorption—as an energy source. Increased calcium and phosphorus are provided to enhance bone mineralization. The infant should gradually be offered feedings of higher caloric density after a substantial volume (100–120 mL/kg/day) of 20 kcal/oz breast milk or formula is tolerated. Success of feedings is assessed by timely passage of feeds out of the stomach without emesis or large residual volumes, an abdominal examination free of distention, and a normal stool pattern.

When the preterm infant approaches term, the nutritional source for the bottle-fed infant can be changed to a transitional formula (22 kcal/oz) until age 6–9 months. Additional iron supplementation (2–4 mg/kg/day) is recommended for premature

Table 2–14. Use of parenteral alimentation solutions.

	Volume (mL/kg/day)	Carbohydrate (g/dL)	Protein (g/kg)	Lipid (g/kg)	Calories (kcal/kg)
Peripheral: short-term (7–10 days)					
Starting solution	100–150	$D_{10}W$	3	1	56–84
Target solution	150	$D_{12.5}W$	3–4	3	80–110
Central: long-term (> 10 days)					
Starting solution	100–150	$D_{10}W$	3	1	56–84
Target solution	130	$D_{12.5}$–$D_{15}W$	3–4	3	80–110

Notes
1. Advance dextrose in central hyperalimentation as tolerated per day as needed to achieve appropriate weight gain, as long as blood glucose remains normal, keeping glucose as 40%–60% of total calories administered.
2. Advance lipids by 0.5–1.0 g/kg/day as long as triglycerides are normal. Use 20% concentration.
3. Total water should be 100–150 mL/kg/day, depending on the child's fluid needs.

Monitoring
1. Blood glucose two or three times a day when changing dextrose concentration, then daily.
2. Electrolytes daily, then twice a week when the child is receiving a stable solution.
3. Every 1–2 weeks: blood urea nitrogen and serum creatinine; total protein and serum albumin; serum calcium, phosphate, magnesium, direct bilirubin, and CBC with platelet counts.
4. Triglyceride level after 24 hours at 2 g/kg/day and 24 hours at 3 g/kg/day, then every other week.

infants, beginning at 2 weeks to 2 months of age, depending on gestational age and number of previous transfusions. Infants who are treated with erythropoietin (epoetin alfa) for anemia of prematurity require a higher dosage of iron (4-6 mg/kg/day). Iron overload is a possibility in multiply transfused sick preterm infants; such infants should be evaluated with serum ferritin levels prior to beginning iron supplementation.

Abrams SA, Committee on Nutrition: Calcium and vitamin D requirements of enterally fed preterm infants. Pediatrics 2013; 131(5):e1676 [PMID: 23629620].
Belfort MB, Ehrenkranz RA: Neurodevelopmental outcomes and nutritional strategies in very low-birth-weight infants. Semin Fetal Neonatal Med 2017 Feb;22:42 [PMID: 27692935].

3. Apnea in the Preterm Infant

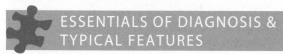

ESSENTIALS OF DIAGNOSIS & TYPICAL FEATURES

▶ Respiratory pause of sufficient duration to result in cyanosis or bradycardia.

▶ Most common in infants born before 34 weeks' gestation; onset before 2 weeks of age.

▶ Methylxanthines (eg, caffeine) provide effective treatment.

▶ General Considerations

Apnea is defined as a respiratory pause lasting more than 20 seconds. Shorter respiratory pauses associated with cyanosis or bradycardia also qualify as significant apnea, whereas periodic breathing, which is common in full-term and preterm infants, is defined as regularly recurring ventilatory cycles interrupted by short pauses *not* associated with bradycardia or color change. By definition, apnea of prematurity is not associated with a predisposing factor, and is a diagnosis of exclusion. A variety of processes may precipitate apnea (Table 2–15) and should be considered before a diagnosis of apnea of prematurity is established.

Apnea of prematurity is the most frequent cause of apnea. Most apnea of prematurity is mixed apnea characterized by a centrally (brainstem) mediated respiratory pause preceded or followed by airway obstruction. Less common is pure central or pure obstructive apnea. Apnea of prematurity is the result of immaturity of both the central respiratory regulatory centers and protective mechanisms that aid in maintaining airway patency.

▶ Clinical Findings

Onset is typically during the first 2 weeks of life. The frequency of spells gradually increases with time. Pathologic apnea should be suspected if spells are sudden in onset, unusually frequent, or very severe. Apnea at birth or on

Table 2–15. Causes of apnea in the preterm infant.

Temperature instability—both cold and heat stress
Response to passage of a feeding tube
Gastroesophageal reflux
Hypoxemia
   Pulmonary parenchymal disease
   Patent ductus arteriosus
   Anemia
Infection
   Sepsis (viral or bacterial)
   Necrotizing enterocolitis
Metabolic causes
   Hypoglycemia
Intracranial hemorrhage
Posthemorrhagic hydrocephalus
Seizures
Drugs (eg, morphine)
Apnea of prematurity

the first day of life is unusual but can occur in the non-ventilated preterm infant. In the full-term or late preterm infant, presentation at birth suggests neuromuscular abnormalities of an acute (asphyxia, birth trauma, or infection) or chronic (eg, congenital hypotonia or structural CNS lesion) nature.

All infants—regardless of the severity and frequency of apnea—require a minimum screening evaluation, including a general assessment of well-being (eg, tolerance of feedings, stable temperature, normal physical examination), a check of the association of spells with feeding, measurement of Pao_2 or Sao_2, blood glucose, hematocrit, and a review of the drug history. Infants with severe apnea of sudden onset require more extensive evaluation for primary causes, especially infection.

► Treatment

Any underlying cause should be treated. If the apnea is due simply to prematurity, symptomatic treatment is dictated by the frequency and severity of apneic spells. Spells frequent enough to interfere with other aspects of care (eg, feeding), or severe enough to cause cyanosis or bradycardia necessitating significant intervention or bag and mask ventilation require treatment. Caffeine citrate is the drug of choice. Side effects of caffeine are generally mild and include tachycardia and occasional feeding intolerance. Nasal CPAP, by treating the obstructive component of apnea, is effective in some infants. Intubation and ventilation can eliminate apneic spells but carry the risks associated with endotracheal intubation. Although many preterm infants are treated medically for possible reflux-associated apnea, there is little evidence to support this intervention. If suspected, a trial of continuous drip gastric or transpyloric feedings can be helpful as a diagnostic and therapeutic intervention.

► Prognosis

In most premature infants, apneic and bradycardiac spells cease by 34–36 weeks postmenstrual age. Spells that require intervention cease prior to self-resolving episodes. In infants born at less than 28 weeks' gestation, episodes may continue past term. Apneic and bradycardiac episodes in the nursery are not predictors of later SIDS, although the incidence of SIDS is slightly increased in preterm infants. Thus, home monitoring in infants who experienced apnea in the nursery is rarely indicated.

4. Hyaline Membrane Disease

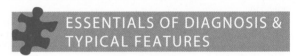

ESSENTIALS OF DIAGNOSIS &
TYPICAL FEATURES

► Tachypnea, cyanosis, and expiratory grunting.
► Poor air movement despite increased work of breathing.
► Chest radiograph showing hypoexpansion and air bronchograms.

► General Considerations

The most common cause of respiratory distress in the preterm infant is hyaline membrane disease. The incidence increases from 5% of infants born at 35–36 weeks' gestation to more than 50% of infants born at 26–28 weeks' gestation. This condition is caused by a deficiency of surfactant production as well as surfactant inactivation by protein leak into airspaces. Surfactant decreases surface tension in the alveolus during expiration, allowing the alveolus to remain partly expanded and maintain a functional residual capacity. The absence or inactivation of surfactant results in poor lung compliance and atelectasis. The infant must expend a great deal of effort to expand the lungs with each breath, and respiratory failure ensues (Figure 2–6).

► Clinical Findings

Infants with hyaline membrane disease show all the clinical signs of respiratory distress. On auscultation, air movement is diminished despite vigorous respiratory effort. The chest radiograph demonstrates diffuse bilateral atelectasis, causing a ground-glass appearance. Major airways are highlighted by the atelectatic air sacs, creating air bronchograms. In the unintubated child, doming of the diaphragm and hypoinflation occur.

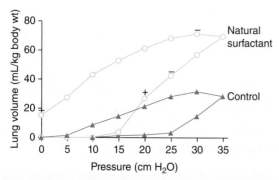

▲ Figure 2–6. Pressure-volume relationships for the inflation and deflation of surfactant-deficient and surfactant-treated preterm rabbit lungs. (Reproduced with permission from Fanaroff AA, Martin RJ: *Neonatal-Perinatal Medicine: Diseases of the Fetus and Infant.* 6th ed. Philadelphia, PA: Mosby; 1997.)

▶ Treatment

Supplemental oxygen, nasal CPAP, early intubation for surfactant administration and ventilation, and placement of umbilical artery and vein lines are the initial interventions required. In stable infants, a trial of nasal CPAP at 5–6 cm H_2O pressure is routinely attempted prior to intubation and surfactant administration. Indications for mechanical ventilation include respiratory acidosis, progressive hypoxia, and apnea. Surfactant replacement can be used both in the delivery room as prophylaxis for infants born before 26 weeks' gestation and with established hyaline membrane disease as rescue, preferably within 2–4 hours of birth. Surfactant therapy decreases both the mortality rate in preterm infants and air leak complications of the disease. During the acute course, ventilator settings and oxygen requirements are significantly lower in surfactant-treated infants than in controls. A total of two to three doses given 8–12 hours apart may be necessary. As the disease evolves, proteins that inhibit surfactant function leak into the air spaces, making surfactant replacement less effective.

For patients requiring mechanical ventilation, a ventilator that can deliver breaths synchronized with the infant's respiratory efforts (synchronized intermittent mandatory ventilation) and accurately deliver a preset tidal volume (5–6 mL/kg) should be used. Alternatively, pressure-limited ventilation with measurement of exhaled tidal volumes can be used. High-frequency ventilators are available for rescue of infants doing poorly on conventional ventilation. For those who require mechanical ventilation, extubation to nasal CPAP should be done as early as possible to minimize lung injury and evolution of chronic lung disease. Nasal intermittent positive-pressure ventilation (NIPPV) is another modality that may be attempted for ventilatory support of the VLBW infant, with potential for less morbidity.

Antenatal administration of corticosteroids to the mother is an important strategy to accelerate lung maturation. Infants whose mothers were given corticosteroids more than 24 hours prior to preterm birth are less likely to have respiratory distress syndrome and have a lower mortality rate.

5. Chronic Lung Disease in the Premature Infant

▶ General Considerations

Chronic lung disease, defined as respiratory symptoms, oxygen requirement, and chest radiograph abnormalities at 36 weeks postconception, occurs in about 20% of preterm infants ventilated for surfactant deficiency. The incidence is higher at lower gestational ages and in infants exposed to chorioamnionitis prior to birth. The development of chronic lung disease is a function of lung immaturity at birth, inflammation, and exposure to high oxygen concentrations and ventilator volutrauma. Surfactant-replacement therapy or early nasal CPAP has diminished the severity of chronic lung disease. The mortality rate from chronic lung disease is very low, but there is still significant morbidity secondary to reactive airway symptoms and hospital readmissions during the first 2 years of life for intercurrent respiratory infection.

▶ Treatment

Long-term supplemental oxygen, mechanical ventilation, and nasal CPAP are the primary therapies for chronic lung disease of the premature infant. Diuretics inhaled β_2-adrenergics, inhaled corticosteroids, and systemic corticosteroids are used as adjunctive therapy. The use of systemic corticosteroids remains controversial. Although a decrease in lung inflammation can aid infants in weaning from ventilator support, there are data associating dexamethasone use in the first week of life with an increased incidence of cerebral palsy. This risk must be balanced against the higher risk of neurodevelopmental handicap in infants with severe chronic lung disease. There is likely a point in the course of these infants at which the benefit of using systemic corticosteroids for the shortest amount of time at the lowest dose possible outweighs the risk of continued mechanical ventilation. After hospital discharge, some of these infants will require oxygen at home. This can be monitored by pulse oximetry with a target Sao_2 of 94%–96%. Some will continue to manifest pulmonary symptomatology into adolescence.

Committee on Fetus and Newborn: Respiratory support in preterm infants at birth. Pediatrics 2014 Jan;133(1):171–174 [PMID: 24379228].

Jobe A: Surfactant for respiratory distress syndrome. NeoReviews 2014;15:e236.

Reuter S, Moser C, Baak M: Respiratory distress in the newborn. Pediatr Rev 2014;35(10):417 [PMID: 25274969].

6. Patent Ductus Arteriosus

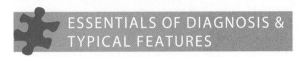

ESSENTIALS OF DIAGNOSIS & TYPICAL FEATURES

▶ Hyperdynamic precordium.

▶ Widened pulse pressure.

▶ Hypotension.

▶ Presence of a systolic heart murmur in many cases.

General Considerations

Clinically significant patent ductus arteriosus usually presents on days 3–7 as the respiratory distress from hyaline membrane disease is improving. Presentation can be as early as days 1 or 2, especially in infants born before 28 weeks' gestation and in those who have received surfactant-replacement therapy. The signs include a hyperdynamic precordium, increased peripheral pulses, and a widened pulse pressure with or without a systolic machinery type heart murmur. Early presentations are sometimes manifested by systemic hypotension without a murmur or hyperdynamic circulation. These signs are often accompanied by an increased need for respiratory support and metabolic acidemia. The presence of patent ductus arteriosus is confirmed by echocardiography.

Treatment

Treatment of patent ductus arteriosus is by medical or surgical ligation. A clinically significant ductus can be closed with indomethacin in about two-thirds of cases. If the ductus reopens or fails to close completely, a second course of drug may be used. For infants that remain symptomatic, the ductus may be closed by cardiac catheterization or surgical ligation. In addition, in the extremely low-birth-weight infant (< 1000 g) who is at very high risk of developing a symptomatic ductus, a prophylactic strategy of indomethacin beginning on the first day of life may be used, with the possible additional benefit of decreasing the incidence of severe IVH, although there is no evidence of an effect on mortality or neurodevelopment. The most common side effect of indomethacin is transient oliguria, which can be managed by fluid restriction until urine output improves. Indomethacin should not be used if the infant is hyperkalemic, if the creatinine is higher than 2 mg/dL, or if the platelet count is less than 50,000/mL. There is an increased incidence of intestinal perforation if indomethacin is used concomitantly with hydrocortisone in extremely low-birth-weight infants (9% vs 2% for either drug alone). Ibuprofen lysine can be used as an alternative to indomethacin. Oliguria is less severe and less frequent than with indomethacin.

Sallmon H, Koehne P, Hansmann G: Recent advances in the treatment of preterm newborn infants with patent ductus arteriosus. Clin Perinatol 2016;43(3):113 [PMID: 26876125].

7. Necrotizing Enterocolitis

ESSENTIALS OF DIAGNOSIS & TYPICAL FEATURES

▶ Feeding intolerance with gastric residuals or vomiting.

▶ Bloody stools.

▶ Abdominal distention and tenderness.

▶ Pneumatosis intestinalis on abdominal radiograph.

General Considerations

NEC is the most common acquired GI emergency in the newborn. It is most common in preterm infants, with an incidence of 10% in infants less than 1500 g. In full-term infants, it occurs in association with polycythemia, congenital heart disease, and birth asphyxia. The pathogenesis of NEC is multifactorial. Ischemia, immaturity, microbial dysbiosis (proliferation of pathogenic bacteria with less colonization with beneficial or commensal bacteria), and genetics are all thought to play a role. In up to 20% of affected infants, the only risk factor is prematurity. IUGR infants with a history of absent or reversed end-diastolic flow in the umbilical artery prior to delivery have abnormalities of splanchnic flow after delivery and have an increased risk of NEC.

Clinical Findings

The most common presenting sign is abdominal distention. Other signs are vomiting, increased gastric residuals, hemepositive stools, abdominal tenderness, temperature instability, increased apnea and bradycardia, decreased urine output, and poor perfusion. There may be an increased white blood cell count with an increased band count or, as the disease progresses, absolute neutropenia. Thrombocytopenia often occurs along with stress-induced hyperglycemia and metabolic acidosis. Diagnosis is confirmed by the presence of pneumatosis intestinalis (air in the bowel wall) or biliary tract air on a plain abdominal radiograph. There is a spectrum of disease, and milder cases may exhibit only distention of bowel loops with bowel wall edema.

Treatment

A. Medical Treatment

NEC is managed by making the infant NPO, nasogastric decompression of the gut, maintenance of oxygenation, mechanical ventilation if necessary, and IV fluids to replace third-space GI losses. Enough fluid should be given to restore good urine output. Other measures include broad-spectrum antibiotics (usually ampicillin, a third-generation cephalosporin or an aminoglycoside, and possibly additional anaerobic coverage), close monitoring of vital signs, and serial physical examinations and laboratory studies (blood gases, white blood cell count, platelet count, and radiographs). Although there are no proven strategies to prevent NEC, use of trophic feedings, breast milk, and cautious advancement of feeds, as well as probiotic agents, may provide some protection.

B. Surgical Treatment

Indications for surgery are evidence of perforation (free air present on a left lateral decubitus or cross-table lateral film), a fixed dilated loop of bowel on serial radiographs, abdominal wall cellulitis, or deterioration despite maximal medical support. All of these signs are indicative of necrotic bowel. In the operating room, necrotic bowel is removed and ostomies are created, although occasionally a primary end-to-end anastomosis may be performed. In extremely low-birth-weight infants, the initial surgical management may simply be the placement of peritoneal drains. Reanastomosis in infants with ostomies is performed after the disease resolves and the infant is bigger (usually > 2 kg and after 4–6 weeks).

Course & Prognosis

Infants treated medically or surgically should not be refed until the disease is resolved (normal abdominal examination and resolution of pneumatosis), usually after 7–10 days. Nutritional support during this time should be provided by total parenteral nutrition.

Death occurs in 10% of cases. Surgery is needed in less than 25% of cases. Long-term prognosis is determined by the amount of intestine lost. Infants with short bowel require long-term support with IV nutrition (see Chapter 21). Late strictures—about 3–6 weeks after initial diagnosis—occur in 8% of patients whether treated medically or surgically, and generally require operative management. Infants with surgically managed NEC have an increased risk of poor neurodevelopmental outcome.

Rich BS, Dolgin SE: Necrotizing enterocolitis. Pediatr Rev 2017 Dec;38(12);552–559 [PMID 29196510].

8. Anemia in the Premature Infant

General Considerations

In the premature infant, the hemoglobin concentration reaches its nadir at about 8–12 weeks and is 2–3 g/dL lower than that of the full-term infant. The lower nadir in premature infants appears to be the result of decreased erythropoietin response to the low red cell mass. Symptoms of anemia include poor feeding, lethargy, increased heart rate, poor weight gain, and perhaps periodic breathing.

Treatment

Transfusion is not indicated in an asymptomatic infant simply because of a low hematocrit. Most infants become symptomatic if the hematocrit drops below 20%. Infants on ventilators and supplemental oxygen are usually maintained with hematocrits above 25%–30%. Alternatively, infants can be treated with erythropoietin. The therapeutic goal is to minimize blood draws and use conservative guidelines for transfusion. Delayed cord clamping 1–2 minutes after birth, if possible, can significantly decrease the need for future transfusion. Use of erythropoietin may increase the rate and severity of retinopathy of prematurity, and should be used judiciously.

Hensch LA, Indrikovs AJ, Shattuck KE: Transfusion in extremely low-birth-weight premature neonates: current practice trends, risks, and early interventions to decrease the need for transfusion. NeoReviews 2015;16:e287.

9. Intraventricular Hemorrhage

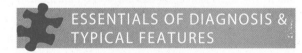

ESSENTIALS OF DIAGNOSIS & TYPICAL FEATURES

► Large bleeds cause hypotension, metabolic acidosis, and altered neurologic status; smaller bleeds can be asymptomatic.

► Routine cranial ultrasound scanning is essential for diagnosis in infants born before 32 weeks' gestation.

General Considerations

Periventricular-intraventricular hemorrhage occurs almost exclusively in premature infants. The incidence is 15%–25% in infants born before 31 weeks' gestation and weighing

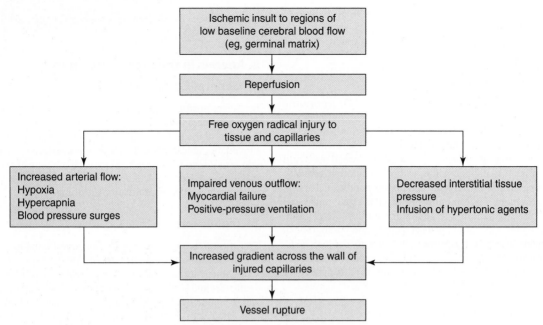

▲ **Figure 2–7.** Pathogenesis of periventricular and intraventricular hemorrhage.

less than 1500 g. The highest incidence occurs in infants of the lowest gestational age (< 26 weeks). Bleeding most commonly occurs in the subependymal germinal matrix (a region of undifferentiated cells adjacent to or lining the lateral ventricles). Bleeding can extend into the ventricular cavity. The proposed pathogenesis of bleeding is presented in Figure 2–7. The critical event is ischemia with reperfusion injury to the capillaries in the germinal matrix in the immediate perinatal period, in the face of immature cerebral pressure autoregulation. The actual amount of bleeding is also influenced by a variety of factors that affect the pressure gradient across the injured capillary wall, such as venous congestion. This pathogenetic scheme applies also to intraparenchymal bleeding (venous infarction in a region rendered ischemic) and to periventricular leukomalacia, also known as PVL (ischemic white matter injury in a water-shed region of arterial supply). CNS complications in preterm infants are more frequent in infants exposed to intrauterine and postnatal infection, implying also the involvement of inflammatory mediators in the pathogenesis of brain injury.

▶ Clinical Findings

Up to 50% of hemorrhages occur before 24 hours of age, and virtually all occur by the fourth day. The clinical syndrome ranges from rapid deterioration (coma, hypoventilation, decerebrate posturing, fixed pupils, bulging anterior fontanelle, hypotension, acidosis, or acute drop in hematocrit) to a more gradual deterioration with more subtle neurologic changes, to absence of any specific physiologic or neurologic signs.

The diagnosis can be confirmed by real-time ultrasound scan. Routine scanning should be done at 10–14 days in all infants born before 29 weeks' gestation. Hemorrhages are graded as follows: grade I, germinal matrix hemorrhage only; grade II, intraventricular bleeding without ventricular enlargement; grade III, intraventricular bleeding with ventricular enlargement; or grade IV, any intraparenchymal bleeding. The amount of bleeding is minor (grade I or II) in 75% of infants who bleed. Follow-up ultrasound examinations are scheduled based on the results of the initial scan. Infants with no bleeding or germinal matrix hemorrhage require only a single follow-up scan at age 4–6 weeks to look for PVL. An infant with blood in the ventricular system is at risk for posthemorrhagic ventriculomegaly. This is usually the result of impaired absorption of cerebrospinal fluid (CSF) but can also occur secondary to obstructive phenomena. An initial follow-up scan should be done 1–2 weeks after the first scan. Infants with intraventricular bleeding and ventricular enlargement should be followed every 7–10 days until ventricular enlargement stabilizes or decreases. Infants born at 29–32 weeks' gestational age need only a single late scan done at 4–6 weeks of age to look for PVL or ventriculomegaly.

Treatment

During acute hemorrhage, supportive treatment (restoration of volume and hematocrit, oxygenation, and ventilation) should be provided to avoid further cerebral ischemia. Progressive posthemorrhagic hydrocephalus is treated initially with a subgaleal shunt. When the infant is large enough, this can be converted to a ventriculoperitoneal shunt.

Although the incidence and severity of intracranial bleeding in premature infants have decreased, strategies to prevent this complication are still needed. Maternal antenatal corticosteroids appear to decrease the risk of intracranial bleeding. Magnesium sulfate administered to the mother appears to reduce the rate of cerebral palsy, although not the rate of IVH per se. The route of delivery may be important as infants delivered by cesarean section have a decreased rate of intracranial bleed. Postnatal strategies are less effective. Early indomethacin administration may have some benefit in minimizing bleeding, especially in males, with unclear influence on long-term outcome.

Prognosis

No deaths occur as a result of grades I and II hemorrhages. Grades III and IV hemorrhages carry a mortality rate of 10%–20%. Posthemorrhagic ventricular enlargement is rarely seen with grade I hemorrhages but is seen in 54%–87% of grades II–IV hemorrhages. Very few of these infants will require a ventriculoperitoneal shunt. Long-term neurologic sequelae are seen slightly more frequently in infants with grades I and II hemorrhages than in preterm infants without bleeding. In infants with grades III and IV hemorrhages, severe sequelae occur in 20%–25% of cases, mild sequelae in 35% of cases, but no sequelae in 40% of cases. Severe PVL, large parenchymal bleeds, especially if bilateral, and progressive hydrocephalus increase the risk of neurologic sequelae. It is important to note that extremely low-birth-weight infants without major ultrasound findings also remain at increased risk for both cerebral palsy and cognitive delays. Recent reports using quantitative MRI scans demonstrate that subtle gray and white matter findings not seen with ultrasound are prevalent in preterm survivors and are predictive of neurodevelopmental handicap. This is especially true in infants born weighing less than 1000 g and before 28 weeks' gestation.

Ballabh P: Pathogenesis and prevention of intraventricular hemorrhage. Clin Perinatol 2014 Mar;41(1):47–67 [PMID:24524446].
Bass WT: Periventricular leukomalacia. NeoReviews 2011; 12:e76.
Whitelaw A: Core concepts: intraventricular hemorrhage. NeoReviews 2011;12:e94.

10. Retinopathy of Prematurity

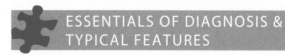

ESSENTIALS OF DIAGNOSIS & TYPICAL FEATURES

► Risk of severe retinopathy is greatest in the most immature infants.

► Diagnosis depends on screening eye examinations in at-risk preterm infants.

► Examination evaluates stage of abnormal retinal vascular development, extent of retinal detachment, and distribution and amount of retina involved.

Retinopathy of prematurity occurs only in the incompletely vascularized premature retina. The incidence of retinopathy in infants weighing less than 1250 g is 66%, but only 6% have retinopathy severe enough to warrant intervention. The incidence is highest in infants of the lowest gestational age. The condition appears to be triggered by an initial injury to the developing retinal vessels and low levels of insulin-like growth factor-1. After the initial injury, normal vessel development may follow or abnormal vascularization may occur due to excessive vascular endothelial growth factor (VEGF), with ridge formation on the retina. Lability in oxygen levels with periods of hypoxia/hyperoxia likely potentiates this progression. The frequency of retinopathy progressing to the need for treatment can be diminished by careful monitoring of the infant's oxygen saturation levels. The process can regress at this point or may continue, with growth of fibrovascular tissue into the vitreous associated with inflammation, scarring, and retinal folds or detachment. The disease is graded by stages of abnormal vascular development and retinal detachment (I–V), by the zone of the eye involved (1–3, with zone 1 being the posterior region around the macula), and by the amount of the retina involved, in "clock hours" (eg, a detachment in the upper, outer quadrant of the left eye would be defined as affecting the left retina from 12 to 3 o'clock).

Initial eye examination should be performed at 31 weeks' postmenstrual age or at 4 weeks of age, whichever is earlier, in infants born at 30 weeks' gestation or less, as well as in infants up to 32 weeks' gestation with an unstable clinical course. Follow-up occurs at 1- to 3-week intervals, depending on the findings, until the retina is fully vascularized. Laser therapy is used in infants with progressive disease at risk for retinal detachment. Although this treatment does not always prevent retinal detachment, it reduces the incidence of poor outcomes based on visual acuity and retinal anatomy. A new form of therapy is intravitreal bevacizumab, an anti-VEGF monoclonal antibody, which may prove to be superior to laser therapy for severe Zone I and II retinopathy of prematurity.

11. Discharge & Follow-up of the Premature Infant

A. Hospital Discharge

Criteria for discharge of the premature infant include maintaining normal temperature in an open crib, adequate oral intake, acceptable weight gain, and absence of apnea and bradycardia spells requiring intervention. Infants going home on supplemental oxygen should not desaturate below 80% in room air or should demonstrate the ability to arouse in response to hypoxia. Factors such as support for the mother at home and the stability of the family situation play a role in the timing of discharge. Home nursing visits and early physician follow-up can be used to hasten discharge. Additionally, the AAP recommends that preterm infants have a period of observation in an infant car seat, preferably their own, before hospital discharge, with careful positioning to mimic optimal restraint as would occur in the car, to see that they do not have obstructive apnea or desaturation for periods up to 90–120 minutes.

B. Follow-up

With advances in obstetric and maternal care, survival of infants born after 28 weeks' gestation or weighing as little as 1000 g at birth is now better than 90%. Seventy to 80% survive at 26–27 weeks' gestation and birth weights of 800–1000 g. Survival at gestational age 25 weeks and birth weight 700–800 g is 50%–70%, with a considerable drop-off below this level.

These high rates of survival come with some morbidity. Major neurologic sequelae, including cerebral palsy, cognitive delay, and hydrocephalus, occur in 10%–25% of survivors of birth weight less than 1500 g. The rate of these sequelae tends to be higher in infants with lower birth weights. Infants with birth weights less than 1000 g also have an increased rate of lesser disabilities, including learning, behavioral, and psychiatric problems. Risk factors for neurologic sequelae include seizures, grade III or IV intracranial hemorrhage, PVL, ventricular dilation, white matter abnormalities on term-equivalent MRI examinations, severe IUGR, poor early head growth, need for mechanical ventilation, chronic lung disease, NEC, and low socioeconomic class. Maternal fever and chorioamnionitis are associated with an increased risk of cerebral palsy. Other morbidities include chronic lung disease and reactive airway disease, resulting in increased severity of respiratory infections and hospital readmissions in the first 2 years; retinopathy of prematurity with associated loss of visual acuity and strabismus; hearing loss; and growth failure. All of these issues require close multidisciplinary outpatient follow-up. Infants with residual lung disease are candidates for monthly palivizumab (Synagis) injections during their first winter after hospital discharge to prevent infection with respiratory syncytial virus. Routine immunizations should be given at the appropriate chronologic age and should not be age-corrected for prematurity.

THE LATE PRETERM INFANT

The rate of preterm births in the United States has increased by more than 30% in the past 30 years, so that preterm infants now comprise 12.8% of all births. Late preterm births, those from 34 0/7 to 36 6/7 weeks' gestation (Figure 2–8), have increased the most, and now account for over 70% of all preterm births. While births less than 34 weeks' gestation have increased by 10% since 1990, late preterm births have increased by 25%. This is in part due to changes in obstetric practice with an increase in inductions of labor (up from 9.5% in 1990 to 22.5% today), and an increase in cesarean

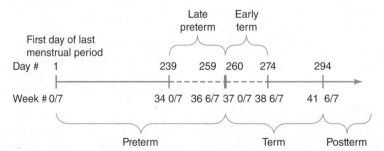

▲ **Figure 2–8.** Definitions of late preterm and early term infant. (Reproduced with permission from Engle WA, Kominiarek MA: Late preterm infants, early term infants, and timing of elective deliveries. Clin Perinatol 2008 Jun;35(2):325–341.)

sections (currently > 30% of all births), as well as a rise in multiple births and an increasing demand for cesarean section "at maternal request."

Compared with term infants, late preterm infants have higher prevalence of acute neonatal problems, including respiratory distress, temperature instability, hypoglycemia, kernicterus, apnea, seizures, feeding problems, and rehospitalization after hospital discharge. The respiratory issues are caused by delayed clearance of lung fluid or surfactant deficiency, or both, and can progress to respiratory failure requiring mechanical ventilation, persistent pulmonary hypertension, and even ECMO support. Feeding issues are caused by immature coordination of suck and swallow, which can interfere with bottle feeding and cause failure to establish successful breast-feeding, putting the infant at risk for excessive weight loss and dehydration. These infants are nearly five times as likely as full-term infants to require either supplemental IV fluids, or gavage feedings. Related both to feeding issues and immaturity, late preterm infants have at least four times the risk of developing a bilirubin level above 20 mg/dL when compared with infants born after 40 completed weeks. As a consequence, late preterm gestation is a major risk factor for excessive hyperbilirubinemia and kernicterus. Rehospitalizations due to jaundice, proven or suspected infection, feeding difficulties, and failure to thrive are much more common than in term infants. Long-term development may also be adversely affected, with some large population-based studies showing a higher incidence of cerebral palsy, developmental delay, and behavioral and emotional disturbances compared with term infants.

Late preterm infants, even if similar in size to their term counterparts, should be considered preterm rather than near term, and require closer in-hospital monitoring after birth for complications. Although they may feed reasonably well for the first day or two, they often fail to increase feeding volume and become sleepier and less interested in feeding as they lose weight and become jaundiced, especially if younger than 36 weeks. Discharge of these newborns should be delayed until they have demonstrated reliable and appropriately increasing intake despite the expected weight loss and jaundice, and absence of other issues such as hypothermia, hypoglycemia, or apnea. If nursing, use of a breast pump to ensure adequate emptying of the breast and milk supply should also be instituted, along with supplementation of the infant's breast-feeding with expressed milk by bottle or gavage. It is better to ensure adequate feeding and mature behaviors for an extra day or two in the hospital than to have a readmission for "lethargy and poor feeding, possible sepsis" after premature discharge. Following nursery discharge, close outpatient follow-up is indicated, generally within 48–72 hours, to ensure continued adequate intake and weight gain.

CARDIAC PROBLEMS IN THE NEWBORN INFANT

STRUCTURAL HEART DISEASE

1. Cyanotic Presentations

ESSENTIALS OF DIAGNOSIS & TYPICAL FEATURES

▶ Cyanosis, initially without associated respiratory distress.

▶ Failure to increase Pa_{O_2} with supplemental oxygen.

▶ Chest radiograph with decreased lung markings suggests right heart obstruction, while increased lung markings suggest transposition or pulmonary venous obstruction.

▶ General Considerations

The causes of cyanotic heart disease in the newborn are transposition of the great vessels, total anomalous pulmonary venous return, truncus arteriosus (some types), tricuspid atresia, and pulmonary atresia or critical pulmonary stenosis. Many are diagnosed antenatally by ultrasound.

▶ Clinical Findings

Infants with these disorders present with early cyanosis. The hallmark of many of these lesions is cyanosis without associated respiratory distress. In most of these infants, tachypnea develops over time either because of increased pulmonary blood flow or secondary to metabolic acidemia from progressive hypoxemia. Diagnostic aids include comparing the blood gas or oxygen saturation in room air to that in 100% F_{IO_2}. Failure of Pa_{O_2} or Sa_{O_2} to increase suggests cyanotic heart disease. *Note:* A Pa_{O_2}, if feasible, is the preferred measure. Saturation in the newborn may be misleadingly high despite pathologically low Pa_{O_2} due to the left-shifted oxyhemoglobin dissociation curve seen with fetal hemoglobin. Other useful aids are chest radiography, electrocardiography, and echocardiography. Routine pulse oximetry screening in the first day of life is recommended for all infants, to detect subtle reductions in Sa_{O_2} that may be the only initial sign of critical congenital heart disease.

Transposition of the great vessels is the most common form of cyanotic heart disease presenting in the newborn. Examination may reveal a systolic murmur and single S_2. Chest radiograph shows cardiomegaly and a narrow mediastinum with normal or increased lung markings. There is little change in Pa_{O_2} or Sa_{O_2} with supplemental oxygen. Total anomalous pulmonary venous return, in which venous return is obstructed, presents early with severe cyanosis and respiratory failure because of severe pulmonary edema. The chest radiograph typically shows a small to normal heart size with marked pulmonary edema. Infants with right-sided heart obstruction (pulmonary and tricuspid atresia, critical pulmonary stenosis, and some forms of truncus arteriosus) have decreased lung markings on chest radiographs and, depending on the severity of hypoxia, may develop metabolic acidemia. Those lesions with an underdeveloped right-sided heart will have left-sided predominance on electrocardiography. Although tetralogy of Fallot is the most common form of cyanotic heart disease, the obstruction at the pulmonary valve is often not severe enough to result in cyanosis in the newborn. In all cases, diagnosis can be confirmed by echocardiography.

2. Acyanotic Presentations

ESSENTIALS OF DIAGNOSIS & TYPICAL FEATURES

▶ Most newborns with symptomatic acyanotic heart disease have left-sided outflow obstruction.

▶ Differentially diminished pulses (coarctation) or decreased pulses throughout (aortic atresia).

▶ Metabolic acidemia.

▶ Chest radiograph showing large heart and pulmonary edema.

▶ General Considerations

Newborn infants who present with serious acyanotic heart disease usually have congestive heart failure secondary to left-sided outflow tract obstruction. Infants with left-to-right shunt lesions (eg, ventricular septal defect) may have murmurs in the newborn period, but clinical symptoms do not occur until pulmonary vascular resistance drops enough to cause significant shunting and subsequent congestive heart failure (usually at 3–4 weeks of age).

▶ Clinical Findings

Infants with left-sided outflow obstruction generally do well in the first days of life until the ductus arteriosus—the source of all or some of the systemic flow—narrows. Tachypnea, tachycardia, congestive heart failure, and metabolic acidosis develop. On examination, these infants have abnormalities of the pulses. In aortic atresia (hypoplastic left-sided heart syndrome) and stenosis, all peripheral pulses are diminished, whereas in aortic coarctation, differential pulses (diminished or absent in the lower extremities) are evident, and Spo_2 and

blood pressure may be lower in the legs than in the right upper extremity. Chest radiographic films in these infants show a large heart and pulmonary edema. Diagnosis is confirmed with echocardiography.

3. Treatment of Cyanotic & Acyanotic Lesions

Early stabilization includes supportive therapy as needed (eg, IV glucose, oxygen, ventilation for respiratory failure, and pressor support). Specific therapy includes infusions of prostaglandin E_1 (0.0125–0.025 mcg/kg/min) to maintain ductal patency. In some cyanotic lesions (eg, pulmonary atresia, tricuspid atresia, and critical pulmonary stenosis) in which lung blood flow is ductus-dependent, this improves pulmonary blood flow and Pao_2 by allowing shunting through the ductus to the pulmonary artery. In left-sided outflow tract obstruction, systemic blood flow is ductus-dependent; prostaglandins improve systemic perfusion and acidosis. Further specific management—including palliative surgical and cardiac catheterization procedures—is discussed in Chapter 20. Neurodevelopmental outcome with congenital heart disease depends on the lesion, associated defects and syndromes, severity of neonatal presentation, and complications related to palliative and corrective surgery.

PERSISTENT PULMONARY HYPERTENSION

ESSENTIALS OF DIAGNOSIS & TYPICAL FEATURES

▶ Onset of symptoms on day 1 of life.

▶ Hypoxia with poor response to high concentrations of inspired oxygen.

▶ Right-to-left shunts through the foramen ovale, ductus arteriosus, or both.

▶ Most often associated with parenchymal lung disease.

▶ General Considerations

Persistent pulmonary hypertension of the newborn (PPHN) results when the normal decrease in pulmonary vascular resistance after birth does not occur. Most affected infants are full term or postterm, and many have experienced perinatal asphyxia. Other clinical associations include meconium aspiration syndrome, hyaline membrane disease, perinatal depression, neonatal sepsis, chronic intrauterine hypoxia, and pulmonary hypoplasia.

There are three underlying pathophysiologic mechanisms of PPHN: (1) vasoconstriction due to perinatal hypoxia related to an acute event such as sepsis or asphyxia;

(2) prenatal increase in pulmonary vascular smooth muscle development, often associated with meconium aspiration syndrome; and (3) decreased cross-sectional area of the pulmonary vascular bed associated with lung hypoplasia (eg, diaphragmatic hernia).

▶ Clinical Findings

Clinically, the syndrome is characterized by onset on the first day of life, usually from birth. Respiratory distress is prominent, and Pao_2 is usually poorly responsive to high concentrations of inspired oxygen. Many infants have associated myocardial depression with systemic hypotension. Echocardiography reveals right-to-left shunting at the level of the ductus arteriosus or foramen ovale, or both. The chest radiograph may show lung infiltrates related to associated pulmonary pathology (eg, meconium aspiration or hyaline membrane disease). If the majority of right-to-left shunting is at the ductal level, pre- and postductal differences in Pao_2 and Sao_2 will be observed.

▶ Treatment

Therapy for PPHN involves treatment of associated multiorgan dysfunction. Specific therapy is aimed at both increasing systemic arterial pressure and decreasing pulmonary arterial pressure to reverse the right-to-left shunting through fetal pathways. First-line therapy includes oxygen and ventilation (to reduce pulmonary vascular resistance) and crystalloid infusions (10–30 mL/kg) to improve systemic pressure. Ideally, systolic pressure should be greater than 50–60 mm Hg. With compromised cardiac function, systemic pressors can be used as second-line therapy (eg, dopamine, 5–20 mcg/kg/min; epinephrine 0.05–0.3 mcg/kg/min; or both). Metabolic acidemia should be corrected because acidemia exacerbates pulmonary vasoconstriction. Pulmonary vasodilation can be enhanced using inhaled nitric oxide, at doses of 5–20 ppm. High-frequency oscillatory ventilation has proved effective in many of these infants, particularly those with severe associated lung disease, by improving lung expansion and recruitment. In cases in which conventional therapy is failing (poor oxygenation despite maximum support), ECMO is used. The lungs are essentially at rest during ECMO, and with resolution of pulmonary hypertension infants are weaned from ECMO back to ventilator therapy. Approximately 10%–15% of survivors of PPHN have significant neurologic sequelae, with cerebral palsy or cognitive delays. Other sequelae such as chronic lung disease, sensorineural hearing loss, and feeding problems have also been reported.

ARRHYTHMIAS

Irregularly irregular heart rates, commonly associated with premature atrial contractions and less commonly with premature ventricular contractions, are common in the first days of life in well newborns. These arrhythmias are typically benign. Clinically significant bradyarrhythmias are seen in association with congenital heart block. Heart block can be seen in an otherwise structurally normal heart (associated with maternal lupus) or with structural cardiac abnormalities. In the absence of fetal hydrops, the bradyarrhythmia is often well tolerated. Cardiac pacing may be required if there are symptoms of inadequate cardiac output.

Tachyarrhythmias can be either wide complex (ventricular tachycardia) or narrow complex (supraventricular tachycardia) on ECG. Supraventricular tachycardia is the most common neonatal tachyarrhythmia and may be a sign of structural heart disease, myocarditis, left atrial enlargement, and aberrant conduction pathways, or may be an isolated event. Acute treatment is ice to the face to induce a vagal response, and if unsuccessful, IV adenosine (50 mcg/kg). If there is no response, the dose can be increased every 2 minutes by 50 mcg/kg to a maximum dose of 250 mcg/kg. Long-term prophylactic antiarrhythmic therapy is generally indicated; cardiology consultation is suggested. Cardioversion is rarely needed for supraventricular tachycardia but is needed acutely for hemodynamically unstable ventricular tachycardia.

Lakshminrusimha S, Keszler M: Persistent pulmonary hypertension of the newborn. NeoReviews 2015;16:e680 [PMID: 26783388].

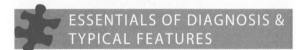

GASTROINTESTINAL & ABDOMINAL SURGICAL CONDITIONS IN THE NEWBORN INFANT

ESOPHAGEAL ATRESIA & TRACHEOESOPHAGEAL FISTULA

ESSENTIALS OF DIAGNOSIS & TYPICAL FEATURES

▶ Polyhydramnios (see also Chapter 21).
▶ Excessive drooling and secretions; choking with attempted feeding.
▶ Unable to pass an orogastric tube to the stomach.

▶ General Considerations

Esophageal atresia is characterized by a blind esophageal pouch with or without a fistulous connection between the proximal or distal esophagus and the trachea. In 85% of infants, the fistula is between the distal esophagus and the airway. Polyhydramnios is common because of high GI obstruction. Incidence is approximately 1 in 3000 births.

Clinical Findings

Infants present in the first hours of life with copious secretions, choking, cyanosis, and respiratory distress. Diagnosis is confirmed with chest radiograph after careful placement of a nasogastric (NG) tube to the point at which resistance is met. The tube will be seen radiographically in the blind pouch. If a tracheoesophageal fistula is present to the distal esophagus, gas will be present in the bowel. In esophageal atresia without tracheoesophageal fistula, no gas is seen in the bowel.

Treatment

The NG tube in the proximal pouch should be placed on low intermittent suction to drain secretions and prevent aspiration. The head of the bed should be elevated to prevent reflux of gastric contents through the distal fistula into the lungs. IV glucose and fluids should be provided and oxygen administered as needed. Definitive treatment is surgical, and the technique used depends on the distance between the segments of esophagus. If the distance is short, the fistula can be ligated and the ends of the esophagus anastomosed. If the ends of the esophagus cannot be brought together, the initial surgery is fistula ligation and a feeding gastrostomy. Echocardiography should be performed prior to surgery to rule out a right-sided aortic arch (for which a left-sided thoracotomy would be preferred).

Prognosis

Prognosis is determined primarily by the presence or absence of associated anomalies, particularly cardiac, and low birth weight. Mortality is highest when the infant is less than 2000 g and has a serious associated cardiac defect. Vertebral, anal, cardiac, renal, and limb anomalies may be observed (VACTERL association). Evaluation for associated anomalies should be initiated early.

Kunisaki SM, Foker JE: Surgical advances in the fetus and neonate: esophageal atresia. Clin Perinatol 2012;39(2):349361 [PMID: 22682384].

INTESTINAL OBSTRUCTION

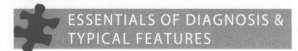

ESSENTIALS OF DIAGNOSIS & TYPICAL FEATURES

▶ Infants with high intestinal obstruction present soon after birth with emesis.

▶ Bilious emesis suggests intestinal malrotation with midgut volvulus until proved otherwise.

▶ Low intestinal obstruction is characterized by abdominal distention and late onset of emesis, often with delayed or absent stooling.

General Considerations

Intestinal obstruction is the most common surgical emergency seen in neonates. A history of polyhydramnios is common, and the fluid, if bile-stained, can easily be confused with thin meconium staining. The higher the location of the obstruction in the intestine, the earlier the infant will develop vomiting and the less prominent the abdominal distention will be. Lower intestinal obstruction presents with abdominal distention and later onset of emesis. Most obstructions are bowel atresias, often caused by an ischemic event during development. Approximately 30% of cases of duodenal atresia are associated with Down syndrome. Meconium ileus is a distal small bowel obstruction caused by viscous meconium produced in utero and may be the presenting symptom of cystic fibrosis. Hirschsprung disease is caused by a failure of neuronal migration to the myenteric plexus of the distal bowel. The distal bowel lacks ganglion cells, causing a lack of peristalsis in that region with a functional obstruction.

Malrotation with midgut volvulus is a surgical emergency that appears in the first days to weeks as bilious vomiting without distention or tenderness. If malrotation is not treated promptly, torsion of the intestine around the superior mesenteric artery will lead to necrosis of the entire small bowel. For this reason, bilious vomiting in the neonate always demands immediate attention and evaluation.

Clinical Findings

Diagnosis of intestinal obstructions depends on plain abdominal radiographs with either upper GI series (high obstruction suspected) or contrast enema (lower obstruction apparent) to define the area of obstruction. Table 2–16 summarizes the findings expected.

Infants with meconium ileus are presumed to have cystic fibrosis, although infants with pancolonic Hirschsprung disease, colon pseudo-obstruction syndrome, or colonic dysgenesis or atresia may also present with meconium impacted in the distal ileum. Definitive testing for cystic fibrosis by the sweat chloride test or genetic testing should be performed. Intestinal perforation in utero results in meconium peritonitis with residual intra-abdominal calcifications. Many perforations are completely healed at birth. If the infant has no signs of obstruction or ongoing perforation, no immediate evaluation is needed. Low intestinal obstruction may present with delayed stooling (> 24 hours in term infants is abnormal) with mild distention. Radiographic findings of gaseous distention should prompt contrast enema to diagnose (and treat) meconium plug syndrome. If no plug is found, the diagnosis may be small left colon syndrome (occurring in IDMs) or Hirschsprung disease. Rectal biopsy is required to clarify these two diagnoses. Imperforate anus is generally apparent on physical examination, although a rectovaginal fistula with a mildly abnormal-appearing anus can occasionally be confused with normal. High imperforate anus in

Table 2–16. Intestinal obstruction.

Site of Obstruction	Clinical Findings	Plain Radiographs	Contrast Study
Duodenal atresia	Down syndrome (30%–50%); early vomiting, sometimes bilious	"Double bubble" (dilated stomach and proximal duodenum, no air distal)	Not needed
Malrotation and volvulus	Bilious vomiting with onset anytime in the first few weeks	Dilated stomach and proximal duodenum; paucity of air distally (may be normal gas pattern)	UGI shows displaced duodenojejunal junction with "corkscrew" deformity of twisted bowel
Jejunoileal atresia, meconium ileus	Bilious gastric contents > 25 mL at birth; progressive distention and bilious vomiting	Multiple dilated loops of bowel; intra-abdominal calcifications if in utero perforation occurred (meconium peritonitis)	Barium or osmotic contrast enema shows microcolon; contrast refluxed into distal ileum may demonstrate and relieve meconium obstruction (successful in about 50% of cases)
Meconium plug syndrome; Hirschsprung disease	Distention, delayed stooling (> 24 h)	Diffuse bowel distention	Barium or osmotic contrast enema outlines and relieves plug; may show transition zone in Hirschsprung disease; delayed emptying (> 24 h) suggests Hirschsprung disease

UGI, upper gastrointestinal contrast study.

males may be associated with rectourethral or rectovesical fistula, with meconium "pearls" seen along the median raphe of the scrotum, and meconium being passed via the urethra.

▶ **Treatment**

OG suction to decompress the bowel, IV glucose, fluid and electrolyte replacement, and respiratory support as necessary should be instituted. Antibiotics are usually indicated in the setting of bowel distention due to risk of bacterial translocation. The definitive treatment for these conditions (with the exception of meconium plug syndrome, small left colon syndrome, and some cases of meconium ileus) is surgical.

▶ **Prognosis**

Up to 10% of infants with meconium plug syndrome are subsequently found to have cystic fibrosis or Hirschsprung disease. For this reason, it is appropriate to consider a sweat chloride test and rectal biopsy in all of these infants before discharge, especially the infant with meconium plug syndrome who is still symptomatic after contrast enema.

In duodenal atresia associated with Down syndrome, the prognosis depends on associated anomalies (eg, heart defects) and the severity of prestenotic duodenal dilation and subsequent duodenal dysmotility. Otherwise, these conditions usually carry an excellent prognosis after surgical repair.

Juang D, Snyder C: Neonatal bowel obstruction. Surg Clin North Am 2012;92(3):685711 [PMID: 22595716].

ABDOMINAL WALL DEFECTS

1. Omphalocele

Omphalocele is a membrane-covered herniation of abdominal contents into the base of the umbilical cord; the incidence is 2 per 10,000 live births. Over 50% of cases have either an abnormal karyotype or an associated syndrome. The sac may contain liver and spleen as well as intestine. Prognosis varies with the size of the lesion, the presence of pulmonary hypoplasia and respiratory insufficiency, and the presence of associated abnormalities.

At delivery, the omphalocele is covered with a sterile dressing soaked with warm saline to prevent fluid loss. NG decompression is performed, and IV fluids, glucose, and antibiotics are given. If the contents of the omphalocele will fit into the abdomen and can be covered with skin, muscle, or both, primary surgical closure is done. If not, staged closure is performed, with placement of a Gore-Tex patch over the exposed contents, and gradual coverage of the patch by skin over days to weeks. A large ventral hernia is left, which is repaired in the future.

2. Gastroschisis

In gastroschisis, the uncovered intestine extrudes through a small abdominal wall defect to the right of the umbilical cord. There is no membrane or sac and no liver or spleen outside the abdomen. Gastroschisis is associated with intestinal atresia in approximately 10%–20% of infants, and with IUGR. The evisceration is thought to be related to abnormal involution of the right umbilical vein or a vascular accident involving the omphalomesenteric artery, although the exact cause is unknown. The prevalence of gastroschisis has been increasing worldwide over the past 20 years, from 0.03% to 0.1%. Environmental factors, including use of illicit drugs such as methamphetamine and cocaine, and cyclooxygenase inhibitors such as aspirin and ibuprofen taken during pregnancy, may be involved. Young maternal age is also strongly linked to the occurrence of gastroschisis.

Therapy initially involves placing the bowel or the lower half of the infant into a Silastic bowel bag to decrease fluid and electrolyte losses as well as to conserve heat. IV fluids, antibiotics, and low intermittent gastric suction are required. The infant is placed right side down to preserve bowel perfusion. Subsequent therapy involves replacement of the bowel into the abdominal cavity. This is done as a single primary procedure if the amount of bowel to be replaced is small. If the amount of bowel is large or if the bowel is much dilated, staged closure with placement of a Silastic silo and gradual reduction of the bowel into the underdeveloped abdominal cavity over several days is preferred. Perioperatively, third-space fluid losses may be extensive; fluid and electrolyte therapy, therefore, must be monitored carefully. Bowel motility may be slow to return if the bowel was dilated, thickened, matted together, and covered with a fibrinous "peel" at delivery. Prolonged intravenous nutrition is often required, but long-term outcome is very good.

Lakshminarayanan B, Lakhoo K: Abdominal wall defects. Early Hum Dev 2014;90(12):917920 [PMID: 25448781].

DIAPHRAGMATIC HERNIA

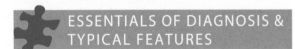

ESSENTIALS OF DIAGNOSIS & TYPICAL FEATURES

▶ Respiratory distress from birth.

▶ Poor breath sounds; flat or scaphoid abdomen.

▶ Bowel loops seen in the chest with mediastinal shift to opposite side on chest radiograph.

This congenital malformation consists of herniation of abdominal organs into the hemithorax (usually left-sided) through a posterolateral defect in the diaphragm. The incidence overall is 1 in 2500 births. It is usually diagnosed antenatally by ultrasound, and, if so, delivery should occur at a perinatal center. If undiagnosed, it should be suspected in any infant with severe respiratory distress, poor breath sounds, and a scaphoid abdomen. The rapidity and severity of presentation depend on several factors: the degree of pulmonary hypoplasia resulting from lung compression by the intrathoracic abdominal contents in utero; degree of associated pulmonary hypertension; and associated anomalies, especially chromosomal abnormalities and congenital cardiac defects. Affected infants are prone to development of pneumothorax during attempts at ventilation of the hypoplastic lungs.

Treatment includes intubation, mechanical ventilation, and decompression of the GI tract with an orogastric (OG) tube. An IV infusion of glucose and fluid should be started. Chest radiograph confirms the diagnosis. Surgery to reduce the abdominal contents from the thorax and close the diaphragmatic defect is delayed until after the infant is stabilized and pulmonary hypertension and lung compliance have improved, usually after 24–48 hours. Both pre- and postoperatively, pulmonary hypertension may require therapy with high-frequency oscillatory ventilation, inhaled nitric oxide, pressors, or ECMO. The survival rate for infants with this condition is improving, and now approaches 70%. Use of a gentle ventilation style and permissive hypercarbia is recommended to avoid barotrauma and further lung injury. Many of these infants have ongoing problems with pulmonary hypertension and severe gastroesophageal reflux, and are at risk for neurodevelopmental problems, behavior problems, hearing loss, and poor growth.

GASTROINTESTINAL BLEEDING

▶ Upper Gastrointestinal Bleeding

Upper GI bleeding sometimes occurs in the newborn nursery but is rarely severe. Old blood ("coffee-grounds" material) in the stomach of the newborn may be either swallowed maternal blood or infant blood from gastritis or stress ulcer. Bright red blood from the stomach is most likely from acute bleeding due to gastritis or iatrogenic from trauma related to a nasogastric tube. Treatment generally consists of gastric lavage to obtain a sample for Apt testing or blood typing to determine if it is mother's or baby's blood, and antacid medication. If the volume of bleeding is large, intensive monitoring, fluid and blood replacement, and endoscopy are indicated. Coagulation studies should also be sent, and vitamin K administration confirmed or repeated.

▶ Lower Gastrointestinal Bleeding

Rectal bleeding in the newborn is less common than upper GI bleeding and is associated with infections (eg, *Salmonella* acquired from the mother perinatally), milk protein intolerance (blood streaks with diarrhea), or, in ill infants, NEC. An abdominal radiograph should be obtained to rule out pneumatosis intestinalis or other abnormalities in gas pattern suggesting inflammation, infection, or obstruction. If the radiograph is negative and the examination is benign, a protein hydrolysate or elemental formula should be tried.

The nursing mother should be instructed to avoid all cow milk protein products in her diet. If the amount of rectal bleeding is large or persistent, endoscopy may be needed.

Boyle JT: Gastrointestinal bleeding in infants and children. Pediatr Rev 2008;29:39 [PMID: 18245300].

GASTROESOPHAGEAL REFLUX

Physiologic regurgitation is common in infants. Reflux is pathologic and should be treated when it results in failure to thrive owing to excessive regurgitation, poor intake due to dysphagia, or chronic respiratory symptoms of wheezing and recurrent pneumonias suggestive of aspiration. Diagnosis is clinical, with confirmation by pH probe or impedance study. Barium radiography is helpful to rule out anatomic abnormalities causing delayed gastric emptying but is not diagnostic of pathologic reflux.

Most antireflux therapies have not been studied systematically in infants, especially in premature infants, and there is little correlation between clinical symptoms and documented gastroesophageal reflux events when studied. Treatment modalities have included thickened feeds for those with frequent regurgitation and poor weight gain, and positioning in a prone or left-side-down position for 1 hour after a feeding, although this may increase risk for SIDS. Gastric-acid suppressants such as ranitidine or lansoprazole can also be used, especially if there is associated irritability; however, these may be associated with an increased incidence of NEC and invasive infections in the young and/or premature infant. Prokinetic agents such as erythromycin or metoclopramide are of little benefit and have significant side effects. Because most infants improve by 12–15 months of age, surgery is reserved for the most severe cases.

Rosen R: Gastroesophageal reflux in infants: more than just a phenomenon. JAMA Pediatr 2014;168(1):83–89 [PMID: 24276411].

▼ INFECTIONS IN THE NEWBORN INFANT

There are three major routes of perinatal infection: (1) blood-borne transplacental infection of the fetus (eg, cytomegalovirus [CMV], rubella, and syphilis); (2) ascending infection with disruption of the barrier provided by the amniotic membranes (eg, bacterial infections after 12–18 hours of ruptured membranes); and (3) infection on passage through an infected birth canal or exposure to infected blood at delivery (eg, herpes simplex, hepatitis B, HIV, and bacterial infections).

Susceptibility of the newborn infant to infection is related to immaturity of the immune system at birth. This feature applies particularly to the preterm neonate. Passive protection against some organisms is provided by transfer of IgG across the placenta, particularly during the third trimester of pregnancy. Preterm infants, especially those born before 30 weeks' gestation, do not have the full amount of passively acquired antibody.

BACTERIAL INFECTIONS

1. Bacterial Sepsis

ESSENTIALS OF DIAGNOSIS & TYPICAL FEATURES

▶ Most infants with early-onset sepsis present at < 24 hours of age.

▶ Respiratory distress is the most common presenting symptom.

▶ Hypotension, acidemia, and neutropenia are associated clinical findings.

▶ The presentation of late-onset sepsis is more subtle.

▶ General Considerations

The incidence of early-onset (< 3 days) neonatal bacterial infection is 1–2 in 1000 live births. If rupture of the membranes occurs more than 24 hours prior to delivery, the infection rate increases to 1 in 100 live births. If early rupture of membranes with chorioamnionitis occurs, the infection rate increases further to 1 in 10 live births. Regardless of membrane rupture, infection rates are five times higher in preterm than in full-term infants.

▶ Clinical Findings

Early-onset bacterial infections appear most commonly on day 1 of life, the majority by 12 hours of age. Respiratory distress due to pneumonia is the most common presenting sign. Other features include unexplained low Apgar scores without fetal distress, poor perfusion, and hypotension. Late-onset bacterial infection (> 3 days of age) presents in a more subtle manner, with poor feeding, lethargy, hypotonia, temperature instability, altered perfusion, new or increased oxygen requirement, and apnea. Late-onset bacterial sepsis is more often associated with meningitis or other localized infections.

Low total white count, absolute neutropenia (< 1000/mL), and elevated ratio of immature to mature neutrophils all suggest neonatal bacterial infection. Thrombocytopenia is another common feature. Other laboratory signs are hypoglycemia or hyperglycemia, unexplained metabolic acidosis, and elevated C-reactive protein and procalcitonin. In early-onset bacterial infection, pneumonia is often present; chest radiography shows infiltrates, but these infiltrates cannot be distinguished from those resulting from other causes of neonatal lung disease. Presence of a pleural effusion makes a diagnosis of pneumonia more likely. Definitive diagnosis is made by positive cultures from blood, CSF, or other body fluids.

Early-onset infection is most often caused by group B β-hemolytic streptococci (GBS) and gram-negative enteric pathogens (most commonly *E coli*). Other organisms to consider are nontypeable *Haemophilus influenzae*, *Enterococcus*, *Staphylococcus aureus*, other streptococci, and *Listeria monocytogenes*. Late-onset sepsis is caused by coagulase-negative staphylococci (most common in infants with indwelling central venous lines), *S aureus*, GBS, *Enterococcus*, and gram-negative organisms, in addition to *Candida* species (see section Fungal Sepsis).

▶ Treatment

A high index of suspicion is important in diagnosis and treatment of neonatal infection. Infants with risk factors (rupture of membranes > 18 hours, maternal chorioamnionitis, prematurity) need to be carefully observed for signs of infection. Evaluation with a CBC and differential, blood and CSF cultures are indicated in infants with clinical signs of early sepsis. Early-onset sepsis is usually caused by GBS or gram-negative enteric organisms; broad-spectrum coverage, therefore, should include ampicillin plus an aminoglycoside or third-generation cephalosporin. Late-onset infections can also be caused by the same organisms, but coverage may

need to be expanded to include staphylococci. In particular, the preterm infant with an indwelling catheter is at risk for infection with coagulase-negative staphylococci, for which vancomycin is the drug of choice. Initial broad-spectrum coverage should also include a third-generation cephalosporin (cefotaxime or ceftazidime, if *Pseudomonas aeruginosa* is strongly suspected) or an aminoglycoside. To prevent the development of vancomycin-resistant organisms, vancomycin should be stopped as soon as cultures and sensitivities indicate that it is not needed. The evaluation for late-onset symptoms should include cultures of blood, urine, and CSF. The duration of treatment for proven sepsis is 10–14 days of IV antibiotics. In sick infants, the essentials of good supportive therapy should be provided: IV glucose and nutritional support, volume expansion and pressors as needed, and oxygen and ventilator support.

▶ Prevention

Prevention of early-onset neonatal GBS infection has been achieved with intrapartum administration of penicillin given more than 4 hours prior to delivery, with overall rates of infection now at 0.3–0.4 cases per 1000 live births. The current guideline (Figure 2–9) is to perform a vaginal and rectal GBS culture at 35–37 weeks' gestation in all pregnant women. Prophylaxis with penicillin or ampicillin is given to GBS-positive women, to those who had GBS bacteriuria during the current pregnancy, to those who had a previous infant with invasive GBS disease, and to those who have unknown GBS status at delivery with risk factors for

Intrapartum GBS prophylaxis indicated	Intrapartum GBS prophylaxis not indicated
• Previous infant with invasive GBS disease	• Colonization with GBS during a previous pregnancy (unless an indication for GBS prophylaxis is present for current pregnancy)
• GBS bacteriuria during any trimester of the current pregnancy[1]	• GBS bacteriuria during previous pregnancy (unless an indication for GBS prophylaxis is present for current pregnancy)
• Positive GBS vaginal-rectal screening culture in late gestation[2] during current pregnancy[1]	• Negative vaginal and rectal GBS screening culture in late gestation[2] during the current pregnancy, regardless of intrapartum risk factors
• Unknown GBS status at the onset of lab or (culture not done, incomplete, or results unknown) and any of the following:	• Cesarean delivery performed before onset of labor on a woman with intact amniotic membranes, regardless of GBS colonization status or gestational age
- Delivery at < 37 weeks' gestation	
- Amniotic membrane rupture ≥ 18 hours	
- Intrapartum temperature ≥ 100.4°F (≥ 38.0°C)[3]	
- Intrapartum NATT[4] positive for GBS	

Abbreviations: GBS, group B streptococcal; NAAT, nucleic acid amplification test.

[1]Intrapartum antibiotic prophylaxis is not indicated in this circumstance if a cesarean delivery is performed before onset of labor on a woman with interact amniotic membranes.
[2]Optimal timing for prenatal GBS screening as at 35–37 weeks' gestation.
[3]If amnionitis is suspected, broad-spectrum antibiotic therapy that includes an agent known to be active against GBS should replace GBS prophylaxis.
[4]NAAT testing for GBS is optional and might not be available in all settings, if intrapartum NAAT is negative for GBS but any other intrapartum risk factor (delivery at ≤ 37 weeks' gestation, amniotic membrane rupture at ≥ 18 hours, or temperature ≥ 100.4°F [≥ 38.0°C]) is present, then intrapartum antibiotic prophylaxis is indicated.

▲ **Figure 2–9.** Indications for intrapartum antimicrobial prophylaxis to prevent early-onset group B streptococcal (GBS) disease using a universal prenatal culture screening strategy at 35–37 weeks' gestation for all pregnant women. (Reproduced with permission from Verani JR, McGee L, Schrag SJ, et al: Prevention of perinatal group B streptococcal disease—revised guidelines from CDC, 2010. MMWR Recomm Rep 2010 Nov 19;59(RR-10):1–36.)

infection. Figure 2–10 presents an algorithm for secondary prevention of early-onset GBS infections in newborns.

2. Meningitis

Any newborn with bacterial sepsis is at risk for meningitis. The incidence is low in infants presenting in the first day of life, and higher in infants with later-onset infection.

The workup for any newborn with possible signs of CNS infection should include a lumbar puncture because blood cultures can be negative in neonates with meningitis. The presence of seizures should increase the suspicion for meningitis. Diagnosis is suggested by a CSF protein level higher than 150 mg/dL, glucose less than 30 mg/dL, leukocytes of more than 20/μL, and a positive Gram stain. The diagnosis is confirmed by culture. The most common organisms are GBS

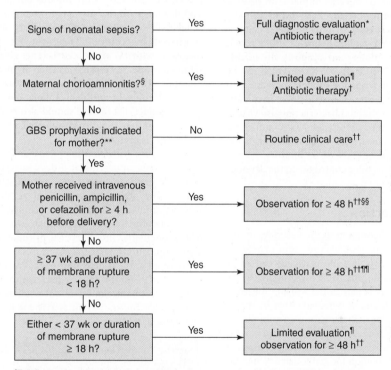

*Full diagnostic evaluation includes a blood culture, a complete blood count (CBC) including white blood cell differential and platelet counts, chest radiograph (if respiratory abnormalities are present), and lumbar puncture (if patient is stable enough to tolerate procedure and sepsis is suspected).

†Antibiotic therapy should be directed toward the most common causes of neonatal sepsis, including intravenous ampicillin for GBS and coverage for other organisms (including Escherichia coli and other gram-negative pathogens) and should take into account local antibiotic resistance patterns.

§Consultation with obstetric providers is important to determine the level of clinical suspicion for chorioamnionitis. Chorioamnionitis is diagnosed clinically and some of the signs are nonspecific.

¶Limited evaluation includes blood culture (at birth) and CBC with differential and platelets (at birth and/or at 6–12 hours of life).

**See Figure 2–13 for indications for intrapartum GBS prophylaxis.

††If signs of sepsis develop, a full diagnostic evaluation should be conducted and antibiotic therapy initiated.

§§If ≥ 37 weeks' gestation, observation may occur at home after 24 hours if other discharge criteria have been met, access to medical care is readily available, and a person who is able to comply fully with instructions for home observation will be present. If any of these conditions is not met, the infant should be observed in the hospital for at least 48 hours and until discharge criteria are achieved.

¶¶Some experts recommend a CBC with differential and platelets at age 6–12 hours.

▲ **Figure 2–10.** Algorithm for secondary prevention of early-onset group B streptococcal (GBS) disease among newborns. (Reproduced with permission from Verani JR, McGee L, Schrag SJ, et al: Prevention of perinatal group B streptococcal disease—revised guidelines from CDC, 2010. MMWR Recomm Rep 2010 Nov 19;59(RR-10):1–36.)

and gram-negative enteric bacteria. Although sepsis can be treated with antibiotics for 10–14 days, meningitis requires 14–21 days. Gram-negative infections, in particular, are difficult to eradicate, and may relapse. The mortality rate of neonatal meningitis is approximately 10%, with significant neurologic morbidity present in one-third of the survivors.

3. Pneumonia

The respiratory system can be infected in utero, on passage through the birth canal, or postnatally. Early-onset neonatal infection is usually associated with pneumonia. Pneumonia should also be suspected in older neonates with a recent onset of tachypnea, retractions, and cyanosis. In infants already receiving respiratory support, an increase in the requirement for oxygen or ventilator support, perhaps with a change in the character of tracheal secretions, may indicate pneumonia. Not only common bacteria but also viruses (CMV, respiratory syncytial virus, adenovirus, influenza, herpes simplex, parainfluenza) and *Chlamydia* can cause pneumonia. In infants with preexisting respiratory disease, intercurrent pulmonary infections contribute to the development of chronic lung disease.

4. Urinary Tract Infection

Infection of the urine is uncommon in the first days of life. Urinary tract infection in the newborn can occur in association with genitourinary anomalies and is usually caused by gram-negative enteric pathogens, or *Enterococcus*. Urine should always be evaluated as part of the workup for later-onset infection. Culture should be obtained either by suprapubic aspiration or bladder catheterization. Antibiotic IV therapy is continued for 3–5 days if the blood culture is negative and clinical signs resolve quickly, and then completed with oral medications. Evaluation for genitourinary anomalies with an ultrasound examination and a voiding cystourethrogram should be done in most cases.

5. Omphalitis

A normal umbilical cord stump atrophies and separates at the skin level. A small amount of purulent material at the base of the cord is common and can be minimized by keeping the cord open to air and dry. The cord can become colonized with streptococci, staphylococci, or gram-negative organisms that can cause local infection. Infections are more common in cords manipulated for venous or arterial lines. Omphalitis is diagnosed when redness and edema develop in the soft tissues around the stump. Local and systemic cultures should be obtained. Treatment is with broad-spectrum IV antibiotics, usually nafcillin or vancomycin, a third-generation cephalosporin, and anaerobic coverage with metronidazole as the infection may be polymicrobial. Complications are determined by the degree of infection of the cord vessels and include septic thrombophlebitis, hepatic abscess, necrotizing fasciitis, and portal vein thrombosis. Surgical consultation should be obtained because of the potential for necrotizing fasciitis.

6. Conjunctivitis

Neisseria gonorrhoeae may colonize an infant during passage through an infected birth canal. Gonococcal ophthalmitis presents at 3–7 days with copious purulent conjunctivitis. The diagnosis can be suspected when gram-negative intracellular diplococci are seen on a Gram-stained smear and confirmed by culture. Treatment for nondisseminated disease is with IV or IM ceftriaxone, given once. For disseminated disease (sepsis, arthritis, or meningitis) cefotaxime for 7–10 days is preferred. Prophylaxis at birth is with 0.5% erythromycin ointment. Infants born to mothers with known gonococcal disease should also receive a single dose of ceftriaxone. If significant hyperbilirubinemia is present, cefotaxime is preferred.

Chlamydia trachomatis is another important cause of conjunctivitis, appearing at 5 days to several weeks of age with conjunctival congestion, edema, and minimal discharge. The organism is acquired at birth after passage through an infected birth canal. Acquisition occurs in 50% of infants born to infected women, with a 25%–50% risk of conjunctivitis. Prevalence in pregnancy is over 10% in some populations. Diagnosis is by isolation of the organism or by rapid antigen detection tests. Treatment is with oral erythromycin for 14 days or oral azithromycin for 3 days. Topical treatment alone will not eradicate nasopharyngeal carriage, leaving the infant at risk for the development of pneumonitis.

Camacho-Gonzalez A et al: Neonatal infectious diseases: evaluation of neonatal sepsis. Pediatr Clin North Am 2013;60:367389 [PMID: 23481106].

Prevention of perinatal group B streptococcal disease revised guidelines from CDC, 2010. MMWR 2010;59:132 [PMID: 21088663].

FUNGAL SEPSIS

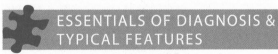

ESSENTIALS OF DIAGNOSIS & TYPICAL FEATURES

▶ Risk factors include low birth weight, indwelling central lines, and multiple antibiotic exposures.

▶ Colonization with *Candida* species is common; systemic infection occurs in 5%–7% of infants.

▶ Presents with often subtle clinical deterioration, thrombocytopenia, and hyperglycemia.

With the survival of smaller, sicker infants, infection with *Candida* species has become more common. Infants of extremely low birth weight with central lines who have had repeated exposures to broad-spectrum antibiotics are at highest risk. For infants of birth weight less than 1500 g, colonization rates of 27%–64% have been demonstrated. Many of these infants develop cutaneous lesions, with the GI tract as the initial site of colonization. A much smaller percentage develops systemic disease. Infection is more common in the smallest and least mature infants; up to 20% in infants 24 weeks' gestation, and 7% overall in those less than 1000 g.

Clinical features of fungal sepsis can be indistinguishable from those of late-onset bacterial sepsis but are often more subtle. Thrombocytopenia or hyperglycemia may be the earliest and only signs. Deep organ involvement (renal, eye, or endocarditis) is commonly associated with systemic candidiasis. Treatment is with intravenous fluconazole or deoxycholate amphotericin B. Prophylaxis for those infants at highest risk, for example, with central venous lines and receiving parenteral nutrition, is recommended. Prophylaxis with fluconazole diminishes intestinal colonization with yeast and decreases the frequency of systemic disease, with an overall reduction in invasive candidal disease of 83%, from 9% to 1.6%, without significant adverse effects, or resistance to fluconazole. Nystatin prophylaxis may also be effective but has been less rigorously tested.

CONGENITAL INFECTIONS

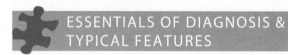

ESSENTIALS OF DIAGNOSIS & TYPICAL FEATURES

▶ Can be acquired in utero, perinatally, and postnatally.

▶ Can be asymptomatic in the newborn period.

▶ Clinical symptom complexes include IUGR, chorioretinitis, cataracts, cholestatic jaundice, thrombocytopenia, skin rash, and brain calcifications.

▶ Diagnosis can be confirmed using polymerase chain reaction (PCR) testing, antigen and antibody studies, and culture.

1. Cytomegalovirus Infection

Cytomegalovirus (CMV) is the most common virus transmitted in utero, affecting approximately 1% of all newborns (see also Chapter 40). Symptomatic disease in the newborn period occurs in 10% of these congenitally infected infants, with a spectrum of findings including hepatosplenomegaly, petechiae and "blueberry muffin" spots, growth restriction, microcephaly, direct hyperbilirubinemia, thrombocytopenia, intracranial calcifications, and chorioretinitis. More

than half of these infants will develop long-term sequelae, including sensorineural deafness in 20%–30%. Sensorineural hearing loss is common even in asymptomatic infants, leading to deafness in another 10%–15%. Transmission of CMV can occur during either primary or reactivated maternal infection; the risk of symptomatic neonatal disease is highest when the mother acquires a primary infection in the first half of pregnancy. Diagnosis in the neonate should be confirmed by culture of the virus from urine. Rapid diagnosis is possible with polymerase chain reaction (PCR) testing of urine or saliva. Diagnosis can also be confirmed in utero from an amniocentesis specimen. Oral valganciclovir therapy for 6 months is recommended for neonates with symptomatic congenital infection, particularly infections affecting the CNS, to prevent progression of hearing loss and neuronal damage. Infection can also be acquired around the time of delivery, and postnatally through blood transfusion or ingestion of CMV-infected breast milk. These infections generally cause no symptoms or sequelae although hepatitis, pneumonia, and neurologic illness may occur in compromised seronegative premature infants. Transfusion risk can be minimized by using frozen, washed red blood cells; leukodepleted blood; or CMV antibody-negative donors.

2. Rubella

Congenital rubella infection occurs as a result of maternal rubella infection during pregnancy (see also Chapter 40). The risk of fetal infection and congenital defects is as high as 80%–85% in mothers infected during the first trimester, but after 12 weeks' gestation, the risk of congenital malformation decreases markedly. Features of congenital rubella syndrome include microcephaly and encephalitis; cardiac defects (patent ductus arteriosus and pulmonary arterial stenosis and arterial hypoplasia); cataracts, retinopathy, and microphthalmia; growth restriction, hepatosplenomegaly, thrombocytopenia, and purpura; and deafness. Affected infants can be asymptomatic at birth but develop clinical sequelae during the first year of life as the viral infection is persistent due to an inadequate immune response. The diagnosis should be suspected in cases of a characteristic clinical illness in the mother (rash, adenopathy, and arthritis) confirmed by an increase in serum rubella-specific IgM or culture of pharyngeal secretions in the infant. Congenital rubella is now rare in industrialized countries because of widespread immunization but is still possible due to the prevalence of unimmunized individuals in the population and widespread travel.

3. Varicella

Congenital varicella syndrome is rare (1%–2% after maternal varicella infection acquired during the first 20 weeks of pregnancy) and may include limb hypoplasia, cutaneous scars, microcephaly, cortical atrophy, chorioretinitis, and cataracts. Perinatal exposure (5 days before to 2 days after delivery) can cause severe to fatal disseminated varicella in the infant. If maternal varicella infection develops within this perinatal risk period, the newborn should receive varicella-zoster immune globulin or IVIG. If this has not been done, subsequent illness can be treated with IV acyclovir.

Hospitalized premature infants of at least 28 weeks' gestation whose mothers have no history of chickenpox—and all infants younger than 28 weeks' gestational age—should receive varicella immune globulin following any postnatal exposure.

4. Toxoplasmosis

Toxoplasmosis is caused by the protozoan *Toxoplasma gondii* (see also Chapter 43). Maternal infection occurs in 0.1%–0.5% of pregnancies and is usually asymptomatic; it is estimated that between 1 in 1000 and 1 in 10,000 infants are infected, 70%–90% are initially asymptomatic. These children may develop mental retardation, visual impairment, and learning disabilities within months to years. The sources of infection include exposure to cat feces and ingestion of raw or undercooked meat. Although the risk of transmission increases to 90% near term, fetal damage is most likely to occur when maternal infection occurs in the second to sixth month of gestation.

Clinical findings may include growth restriction, chorioretinitis, seizures, jaundice, hydrocephalus, microcephaly, intracranial calcifications, hepatosplenomegaly, adenopathy, cataracts, maculopapular rash, thrombocytopenia, and pneumonia. The serologic diagnosis is based on a positive toxoplasma-specific IgA, IgE, or IgM in the first 6 months of life, a rise in serial IgG levels compared to the mother's, or a persistent IgG beyond 12 months. Infants with suspected infection should have eye and auditory examinations and a computed tomographic (CT) scan of the brain. Organism isolation from placenta or cord blood and PCR tests on amniotic fluid or CSF are also available for diagnosis.

Spiramycin (an investigational drug in the United States) treatment of primary maternal infection is used to try to reduce transmission to the fetus. Neonatal treatment using pyrimethamine and sulfadiazine with folinic acid can improve long-term outcome.

5. Parvovirus B19 Infection

Parvovirus B19 is a small, nonenveloped, single-stranded DNA virus that causes erythema infectiosum (fifth disease) in children, with a peak incidence at ages 6–7 years. Transmission to the mother is primarily by respiratory secretions. The virus replicates initially in erythroid progenitor cells and induces cell-cycle arrest, resulting in severe anemia, myocarditis, nonimmune hydrops, or fetal death in approximately 3%–6% of fetuses infected during pregnancy. Resolution of

the hydrops may occur in utero, either spontaneously or after fetal transfusion. Mothers who have been exposed may have specific serologic testing, and serial ultrasound, Doppler examinations, and percutaneous umbilical cord blood sampling of the fetus to assess for anemia. If the fetus survives, the long-term outcome is good with no late effects from the infection.

6. Congenital Syphilis

Active primary and secondary maternal syphilis leads to transplacental passage of *Treponema pallidum* to the fetus in nearly 100% of affected pregnancies while latent maternal infection leads to transplacental infection of the fetus in 40% of cases, and late maternal infection in 10% (see also Chapter 42). Fetal infection is rare before 18 weeks' gestation. Fetal infection can result in stillbirth or prematurity. Findings of early congenital syphilis (presentation before age 2 years) include mucocutaneous lesions, lymphadenopathy, hepatosplenomegaly, bony changes, and hydrops, although newborn infants are often asymptomatic. Late manifestations (after 2 years of age) in untreated infants involve the CNS, bones and joints, teeth, eyes, and skin. An infant should be evaluated for congenital syphilis if he or she has proven or probable congenital syphilis, defined as a suggestive examination, serum quantitative nontreponemal titer more than fourfold the mother's, or positive darkfield or fluorescent antibody test of body fluids, or birth to a mother with positive nontreponemal tests confirmed by a positive treponemal test but without documented adequate treatment (parenteral penicillin G), including the expected fourfold decrease in nontreponemal antibody titer. Infants of mothers treated less than 1 month before delivery also require evaluation. Evaluation should include physical examination, a quantitative nontreponemal serologic test for syphilis, CBC, CSF examination for cell count and protein, Venereal Disease Research Laboratory testing, and long bone radiographs. Treatment in most cases is aqueous penicillin G (50,000 U/kg every 12 hours) or procaine penicillin G (50,000 U/kg IM daily) for 10 days.

7. Congenital Zika Infection

The Zika virus is a mosquito-borne virus that generally causes a mild and self-limited infection. Congenital Zika syndrome is a recently described constellation of congenital anomalies including microcephaly, intracranial calcifications or other brain abnormalities or ocular anomalies associated with maternal Zika infection during pregnancy. The exact risk of complications to the fetus because of congenital infection is unknown, with estimates ranging from a 1% to 13% risk of microcephaly following first-trimester infection. The CDC's current recommendation is to test for Zika infection in infants born to mothers with laboratory evidence of Zika infection during pregnancy and infants who have clinical features of congenital Zika infection and maternal history suggestive of exposure to Zika (travel to areas with high prevalence of infection). Testing should be done directly on the infant's blood (not cord blood) within 2 days of birth, if possible. Both molecular (blood PCR) and immunologic (IgM) testing is recommended. There is no treatment for congenital Zika infection.

American Academy of Pediatrics: In: Pickering LD et al (eds): *Red Book: 2018 Report of the Committee on Infectious Diseases.* 31th ed. American Academy of Pediatrics; 2018.

Centers for Disease Control and Prevention: Zika Virus. www.cdc.gov/zika/. Accessed May, 2019.

Swanson ED, Schleiss MR: Congenital cytomegalovirus infection: new prospects for prevention and therapy. Pediatr Clin North Am 2013;60(2):335349 [PMID: 23481104].

PERINATALLY ACQUIRED INFECTIONS

1. Herpes Simplex

Herpes simplex virus infection is usually acquired at birth during transit through an infected birth canal (see also Chapter 40). The mother may have either primary or reactivated secondary infection. Primary maternal infection, because of the high titer of organisms and the absence of antibodies, poses the greatest risk to the infant. The risk of neonatal infection with vaginal delivery in this setting is 25%–50%. Seventy-five percent of mothers with primary herpes at the time of delivery are asymptomatic. The risk to an infant born to a mother with recurrent herpes simplex is much lower (< 1%). Time of presentation of localized (skin, eye, or mouth) or disseminated disease (pneumonia, shock, or hepatitis) in the infant is usually 5–14 days of age. CNS disease presents later, at 14–28 days with lethargy, fever, and seizures. In rare cases, presentation is as early as day 1 of life, suggesting in utero infection. In about 45% of patients, localized skin, eye, and mouth disease is the first indication of infection. Another 30% present with CNS disease, whereas the remaining 25% have disseminated or multiorgan disease indistinguishable from bacterial sepsis. Herpes infection should be considered in neonates with sepsis syndrome, negative bacteriologic culture results, and liver dysfunction or coagulopathy. Herpes simplex virus also should be considered as a causative agent in neonates with fever, irritability, and abnormal CSF findings, especially in the presence of seizures. PCR testing of vesicles, blood, or CSF is diagnostic but may be falsely negative in the CSF early in the course. If a blood or CSF PCR performed shortly after the onset of symptoms is negative, it should be repeated if herpes simplex virus disease is considered a strong possibility.

Acyclovir is the drug of choice for neonatal herpes infection. Localized disease is treated for 14 days, and a 21-day course is used for disseminated or CNS disease. Prompt initiation of therapy improves survival of neonates with CNS and disseminated disease and prevents the spread of localized disease. Prevention is possible by delivery by cesarean section within 6 hours after rupture of the membranes in the presence of known infection. Given the low incidence of infection in the newborn from recurrent maternal infection, cesarean delivery is not indicated for asymptomatic mothers with a history of recurrent herpes. Cesarean deliveries are performed in mothers with active lesions (either primary or recurrent) at the time of delivery. Infants born to mothers with a history of herpes simplex virus infection but no active lesions can be observed closely after birth, and do not need to be isolated. In infants born to mothers with active lesions—regardless of the route of delivery—cultures of the eye, oropharynx, nasopharynx, and rectum should be performed 24 hours after delivery, and the infant should be in contact isolation. If the infant is colonized (positive cultures) or if symptoms consistent with herpes infection develop, treatment with acyclovir should be started. In cases of primary maternal genital infection at the time of vaginal delivery, infant specimens should be obtained and the infant treated with IV acyclovir for 10 days. The major problem facing perinatologists is the high percentage of asymptomatic primary maternal infection. In these cases, infection in the neonate is not currently preventable. Cultures should be obtained and acyclovir started, pending the results of those cultures, in any infant who presents at the right age with symptoms consistent with neonatal herpes.

The prognosis is good for localized skin and mucosal disease that does not progress, although skin recurrences are common. The mortality rate for disseminated herpes is high (approximately 30%), with significant morbidity among survivors of both disseminated and CNS infections despite treatment. Cutaneous recurrences are common in all types, and examination of the CSF should be considered with skin recurrences. Infants with herpes encephalitis should receive long-term oral acyclovir for 6 months after completion of intravenous treatment.

2. Hepatitis B & C

Infants become infected with hepatitis B at the time of birth; intrauterine transmission is rare. Clinical illness is rare in the neonatal period, but infants born to positive mothers are at risk of becoming chronic HBsAg carriers and developing chronic active hepatitis, and even hepatocellular carcinoma. The presence of HBsAg should be determined in all pregnant women. If the result is positive, the infant should receive HBIG and hepatitis B vaccine as soon as possible after birth, followed by two subsequent vaccine doses at 1 and 6 months of age. If HBsAg has not been tested prior to birth in a mother at risk, the test should be run after delivery and hepatitis B vaccine given within 12 hours after birth. If the mother is subsequently found to be positive, HBIG should be given as soon as possible (preferably within 48 hours, but not later than 1 week after birth). Subsequent vaccine doses should be given at 1 and 6 months of age. In premature infants born to HBsAg-positive mothers, vaccine and HBIG should be given at birth, but a three-vaccine hepatitis B series should be given beginning at 1 month of age.

Perinatal transmission of hepatitis C occurs in about 5% of infants born to mothers who carry the virus; maternal coinfection with HIV increases the risk of transmission. Serum antibody to hepatitis C and hepatitis C RNA have been detected in colostrum, but the risk of hepatitis C transmission is similar in breast-fed and bottle-fed infants. Up to 12 months of age, the only reliable screen for hepatitis C infection is PCR. After that time, the presence of hepatitis C antibodies in the infant strongly suggests that infection has occurred.

3. Enterovirus Infection

Enterovirus infections occur most frequently in the late summer and early fall. Infection is usually acquired in the perinatal period. There is often a history of maternal fever, diarrhea, and/or rash in the week prior to delivery. The illness appears in the infant in the first 2 weeks of life and is most commonly characterized by fever, lethargy, irritability, diarrhea, and/or rash. More severe forms occasionally occur, especially if infection occurs before 1 week of age, including meningoencephalitis, myocarditis, hepatitis, pneumonia, shock, and disseminated intravascular coagulation. Diagnosis is best confirmed by PCR.

Treatment is supportive care. The prognosis is good in most cases, except those with severe hepatitis, myocarditis, or disseminated disease, which carry high mortality rates.

4. HIV Infection

HIV can be acquired in utero or at the time of delivery, or can be transmitted postpartum via breast milk (see also Chapter 41). Testing for HIV should be performed in all pregnant women. Without treatment, transmission of virus occurs in 13%–39% of births to infected mothers, mostly at the time of delivery. The combination of maternal zidovudine treatment during pregnancy and of the infant for the first 6 weeks of life, elective cesarean delivery, and avoidance of breast-feeding can lower transmission to 1%–2%. Current guidelines for antiretroviral drugs in pregnant HIV-infected women are similar to those for nonpregnant patients (eg, highly active antiretroviral combination therapy), and, with maternal virologic suppression, transmission rates of less than 2% are achieved. In cases of unknown HIV status at presentation in labor, rapid HIV testing should be offered, and, if positive, intrapartum maternal treatment and postpartum neonatal treatment should be offered. The risk of transmission is increased in mothers with advanced disease, high viral loads, low CD4 counts, and intrapartum events such as chorioamnionitis and prolonged membrane rupture that increase exposure of the fetus to maternal blood.

Newborns with congenitally acquired HIV are usually asymptomatic. Infants of HIV-infected women should be tested by HIV DNA or RNA PCR at less than 48 hours, at 2 weeks, at 1–2 months, and at 2–4 months. If an infant aged 4 months has a negative PCR result, infection can be reasonably excluded. HIV-positive mothers should be counseled not to breast-feed their infants if safe feeding alternatives are available.

Allen UD, Robinson JL, Canadian Paediatric Society Infectious Diseases and Immunization Committee: Prevention and management of neonatal herpes simplex virus infections. Paediatr Child Health 2014;19(4):201206 [PMID: 24855418].

American Academy of Pediatrics: In: Pickering LD et al (eds): Red Book: 2018 Report of the Committee on Infectious Diseases. 31th ed. American Academy of Pediatrics; 2018.

Chappell CA, Cohn SE: Prevention of perinatal transmission of human immunodeficiency virus. Infect Dis Clin North Am 2014;28(4):529547 [PMID: 25455313].

HEMATOLOGIC DISORDERS IN THE NEWBORN INFANT

BLEEDING DISORDERS

Bleeding in the newborn infant may result from inherited clotting deficiencies (eg, factor VIII deficiency) or acquired disorders—hemorrhagic disease of the newborn (vitamin K deficiency), disseminated intravascular coagulation, liver failure, and isolated thrombocytopenia.

1. Vitamin K Deficiency Bleeding of the Newborn

ESSENTIALS OF DIAGNOSIS & TYPICAL FEATURES

▶ Frequently exclusively breast fed, otherwise clinically well infant.

▶ Bleeding from mucous membranes, GI tract, skin, or internal (intracranial).

▶ Prolonged prothrombin time (PT), relatively normal partial thromboplastin time (PTT), normal fibrinogen and platelet count.

Bleeding is caused by the deficiency of the vitamin K–dependent clotting factors (II, VII, IX, and X). Bleeding occurs in 0.25%–1.7% of newborns who do not receive vitamin K prophylaxis after birth, generally in the first 5 days to 2 weeks in an otherwise well infant. There is an increased risk in infants of mothers receiving therapy with anticonvulsants that interfere with vitamin K metabolism. Early vitamin K deficiency bleeding (0–2 weeks) can be prevented by either parenteral or oral vitamin K administration, whereas late disease (onset 2 weeks to 6 months) is most effectively prevented by administering parenteral vitamin K. Sites of ecchymoses and surface bleeding include the GI tract, umbilical cord, circumcision site, and nose, although devastating intracranial hemorrhage can occur. Bleeding from vitamin K deficiency is more likely to occur in exclusively breast-fed infants because of very low amounts of vitamin K in breast milk and slower and more restricted intestinal bacterial colonization. Differential diagnosis includes disseminated intravascular coagulation and hepatic failure. Coagulation studies reveal a prolonged PT with normal PTT and fibrinogen level.

Treatment consists of 1 mg of vitamin K SC or IV. IM injections should be avoided in infants who are actively bleeding. Such infants may also require factor replacement in addition to vitamin K administration.

2. Thrombocytopenia

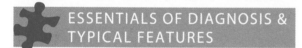

ESSENTIALS OF DIAGNOSIS & TYPICAL FEATURES

▶ Generalized petechiae; oozing at cord or puncture sites.

▶ Thrombocytopenia, often marked (platelets < 10,000–20,000/mL).

▶ In an otherwise well infant, suspect isoimmune thrombocytopenia.

▶ In a sick or asphyxiated infant, suspect disseminated intravascular coagulation.

Infants with thrombocytopenia have generalized petechiae and platelet counts less than 150,000/mL (usually < 50,000/mL; may be < 10,000/mL). Neonatal thrombocytopenia can be isolated in a seemingly well infant or may occur in association with a deficiency of other clotting factors in a sick infant. The differential diagnosis for thrombocytopenia is presented in Table 2–17. Treatment of neonatal thrombocytopenia is transfusion of platelets (10 mL/kg of platelets increases the platelet count by ~70,000/mL). Indications for transfusion in the full-term infant are clinical bleeding or a total platelet count less than 10,000–20,000/mL. In the preterm infant at risk for intraventricular hemorrhage, transfusion is indicated for counts less than 40,000–50,000/mL.

Table 2–17. Differential diagnosis of neonatal thrombocytopenia.

Disorder	Clinical Tips
Immune Passively acquired antibody; idiopathic thrombocytopenic purpura, systemic lupus erythematosus, drug-induced	Proper history, maternal thrombocytopenia
Isoimmune sensitization to HPA-1a antigen	No rise in platelet count from random donor platelet transfusion. Positive antiplatelet antibodies in baby's serum, sustained rise in platelets by transfusion of mother's platelets

Infections
  Bacterial infections
  Congenital viral infections
	Sick infants with other signs consistent with infection

Syndromes
  Absent radii
  Fanconi anemia
	Congenital anomalies, associated pancytopenia

DIC	Sick infants, abnormalities of clotting factors
Giant hemangioma	
Thrombosis	Hyperviscous infants, vascular catheters
High-risk infant with respiratory distress syndrome, pulmonary hypertension, etc	Isolated decrease in platelets is not uncommon in sick infants even in the absence of DIC (localized trapping)

DIC, disseminated intravascular coagulation; HPA, human platelet antigen.

Isoimmune (alloimmune) thrombocytopenia is analogous to Rh-isoimmunization, with a human platelet antigen [HPA]-1a (in 80%)—or HPA-5b (in 15%)—negative mother and an HPA-1a– or HPA-5b–positive fetus. Transplacental passage of IgG antibody leads to platelet destruction. If platelet transfusion is required for acute bleeding, washed maternal platelets may be the most readily available antigen-negative platelet source, because 98% of the general population will also be HPA-1a– or HPA-5b–positive. Treatment with IVIG infusion, 1 g/kg/day for 2–3 days, until the platelet count has doubled or is over 50,000/mL, is potentially beneficial. Twenty to 30% of infants with isoimmune thrombocytopenia will experience intracranial hemorrhage, half of them before birth. Antenatal therapy of the mother with IVIG with or without steroids may reduce this risk.

Infants born to mothers with idiopathic thrombocytopenic purpura are at low risk for serious hemorrhage despite the thrombocytopenia, and treatment is usually unnecessary. If bleeding does occur, IVIG can be used in addition to platelet transfusion.

ANEMIA

ESSENTIALS OF DIAGNOSIS & TYPICAL FEATURES

▶ Hematocrit < 40% at term birth.

▶ Acute blood loss—signs of hypovolemia, normal reticulocyte count.

▶ Chronic blood loss—pallor without hypovolemia, elevated reticulocyte count.

▶ Hemolytic anemia—accompanied by excessive hyperbilirubinemia.

The newborn infant with anemia from acute blood loss presents with signs of hypovolemia (tachycardia, poor perfusion, and hypotension), with an initially normal hematocrit that falls after volume replacement. Anemia from chronic blood loss is evidenced by pallor without signs of hypovolemia, with an initially low hematocrit and reticulocytosis.

Anemia can be caused by hemorrhage, hemolysis, or failure to produce red blood cells. Anemia occurring in the first 24–48 hours of life is the result of hemorrhage or hemolysis. Hemorrhage can occur in utero (fetoplacental, fetomaternal, or twin-to-twin), perinatally (cord rupture, placenta previa, placental abruption, or incision through the placenta at cesarean section), or internally (intracranial hemorrhage, cephalohematoma, or ruptured liver or spleen). Hemolysis is caused by blood group incompatibilities, enzyme or membrane abnormalities, infection, and disseminated intravascular coagulation, and is accompanied by significant hyperbilirubinemia.

Initial evaluation should include a review of the perinatal history, assessment of the infant's volume status, and a complete physical examination. A Kleihauer-Betke test for fetal cells in the mother's circulation should be done. A CBC, blood smear, reticulocyte count, and direct and indirect Coombs tests should be performed. This simple evaluation should suggest a diagnosis in most infants. Most infants tolerate anemia quite well due to the increased oxygen availability in the extrauterine environment; however, treatment with erythropoietin or transfusion might be needed if the infant develops signs of cardiopulmonary compromise. Additionally, if blood loss is the cause of the anemia, early supplementation with iron will be needed. It is important to remember that hemolysis related to blood group incompatibility can

continue for weeks after birth. Serial hematocrits should be followed, because late transfusion may be needed.

POLYCYTHEMIA

ESSENTIALS OF DIAGNOSIS & TYPICAL FEATURES

▶ Hematocrit > 65% (venous) at term.

▶ Plethora, tachypnea, retractions.

▶ Hypoglycemia, irritability, lethargy, poor feeding.

Polycythemia in the newborn is manifested by plethora, cyanosis, respiratory distress with tachypnea and oxygen need, hypoglycemia, poor feeding, emesis, irritability, and lethargy. Hyperbilirubinemia is expected. The consequence of polycythemia is hyperviscosity with decreased perfusion of the capillary beds. Clinical symptomatology can affect several organ systems (Table 2–18). Deep vein or artery thrombosis is a severe complication. Screening can be done by measuring a capillary (heel stick) hematocrit. If the value is greater than 68%, a peripheral venous hematocrit should be measured. Values greater than 65% should be considered consistent with hyperviscosity.

Elevated hematocrits occur in 2%–5% of live births. Delayed cord clamping is the most common cause of benign neonatal polycythemia. Although 50% of polycythemic infants are AGA, the prevalence of polycythemia is greater in the SGA and LGA populations. Other causes of increased hematocrit include (1) twin-twin transfusion, (2) maternal-fetal transfusion, and (3) chronic intrauterine hypoxia (SGA infants, and LGA infants of diabetic mothers).

Treatment should be considered for symptomatic infants. Treatment for asymptomatic infants based strictly on hematocrit is not indicated as there is no proven long-term benefit

Table 2–18. Organ-related symptoms of hyperviscosity.

Central nervous system	Irritability, jitteriness, seizures, lethargy
Cardiopulmonary	Respiratory distress secondary to congestive heart failure, or persistent pulmonary hypertension
Gastrointestinal	Vomiting, heme-positive stools, distention, necrotizing enterocolitis
Renal	Decreased urinary output, renal vein thrombosis
Metabolic	Hypoglycemia
Hematologic	Hyperbilirubinemia, thrombocytopenia

for neurodevelopmental outcome. Treatment for symptomatic infants is isovolemic partial exchange transfusion with normal saline, effectively decreasing the hematocrit. The amount to exchange (in milliliters) is calculated using the following formula:

$$\text{Number of milliliters to exchange} = (PVH - DH)/PVH \times BV(mL/kg) \times Wt(kg)$$

where PVH is the peripheral venous hematocrit, DH is the desired hematocrit, BV is the blood volume in mL/kg, and Wt is the weight in kilograms.

Blood is withdrawn at a steady rate from an umbilical venous line while the replacement solution is infused at the same rate through a peripheral IV line over 15–30 minutes. The desired hematocrit value is 50%–55%; the assumed blood volume is 80 mL/kg.

Watchko JF: Common hematologic problems in the newborn nursery. Pediatr Clin North Am 2015 Apr;62(2):509–524 [PMID: 25836711].

RENAL DISORDERS IN THE NEWBORN INFANT

Renal function and the speed of maturation after birth depend on postmenstrual age (see also Chapter 24). The glomerular filtration rate is 20 mL/min/1.73 m^2 in full-term neonates and 10–13 mL/min/1.73 m^2 in infants born at 28–30 weeks' gestation. Creatinine can be used as a clinical marker of glomerular filtration rate. Values in the first month of life are shown in Table 2–19. Creatinine at birth reflects the maternal level and should decrease slowly over the first 3–4 weeks. An increasing serum creatinine is never normal.

The ability to concentrate urine and retain sodium also depends on gestational age. Infants born before 28–30 weeks' gestation are compromised in this respect and can easily become dehydrated and hyponatremic. Preterm infants also have an increased bicarbonate excretion and are prone to developing metabolic acidosis.

Table 2–19. Normal values of serum creatinine (mg/dL).

Gestational Age at Birth (wk)	Postnatal Age (days)	
	0–2	28
< 28	1.2	0.7
29–32	1.1	0.6
33–36	1.1	0.45
36–42	0.8	0.3

RENAL FAILURE

ESSENTIALS OF DIAGNOSIS & TYPICAL FEATURES

▶ Clinical setting—birth depression, hypovolemia, hypotension, shock.

▶ Low or delayed urine output (< 1 mL/kg/h).

▶ Rising serum creatinine; hyperkalemia; metabolic acidosis; fluid overload.

Renal failure is most commonly seen in the setting of birth asphyxia, hypovolemia, or shock from any cause. The normal rate of urine flow is 1–3 mL/kg/h. After a hypoxic or ischemic insult, acute tubular necrosis may ensue. Typically, 2–3 days of anuria or oliguria is associated with hematuria, proteinuria, and a rise in serum creatinine. The period of anuria or oliguria is followed by a period of polyuria and then gradual recovery. During the polyuric phase, excessive urine sodium and bicarbonate losses may be seen.

The initial management is restoration of the infant's volume status. Thereafter, restriction of fluids to insensible water loss (40–60 mL/kg/day) without added electrolytes, plus milliliter-for-milliliter urine replacement, should be instituted. Serum and urine electrolytes and body weights should be followed frequently. These measures should be continued through the polyuric phase. Hyperkalemia, which may become life-threatening, may occur in this situation despite the lack of added IV potassium. If the serum potassium reaches 7 mEq/L, therapy should be started with glucose and insulin infusion. Nebulized albuterol, IV Lasix, and binding resins per rectum may also be used to quickly decrease serum potassium levels. Calcium chloride (20 mg/kg bolus) and correction of metabolic acidosis with bicarbonate are also helpful in the acute management of arrhythmias resulting from hyperkalemia.

Peritoneal dialysis is occasionally needed for the management of neonatal acute renal failure and for removal of waste products and excess fluid. Hemodialysis, although possible, is difficult due to the small blood volume of the infant and problems with vascular access. Although most acute renal failure in the newborn resolves, ischemic injury severe enough to result in acute cortical necrosis and chronic renal failure can occur. Such infants are also at risk of developing hypertension.

URINARY TRACT ANOMALIES

Abdominal masses in the newborn are most frequently caused by renal enlargement. Most common is a multicystic or dysplastic kidney; congenital hydronephrosis is second in frequency. Chromosomal abnormalities and syndromes with multiple anomalies frequently include renal abnormalities. An ultrasound examination is the first step in diagnosis. In pregnancies complicated by oligohydramnios, renal agenesis or bladder outlet obstruction secondary to posterior urethral valves should be considered.

Only bilateral disease or disease in a solitary kidney is associated with oligohydramnios, significant morbidity, and death. Such infants will generally also have pulmonary hypoplasia, and present with pulmonary rather than renal insufficiency.

Ultrasonography identifies many infants with renal anomalies (most often hydronephrosis) prior to birth. Postnatal evaluation of infants with hydronephrosis should include renal ultrasound at about 1 week of age and, depending on the severity of the antenatal findings, possibly a voiding cystourethrogram. Earlier postnatal ultrasound might underestimate the severity of the hydronephrosis due to low glomerular filtration rates in the first days of life, although cases in which oligohydramnios or severe renal abnormality are suspected will be accurately diagnosed even on the first day of life. Voiding cystourethrogram is indicated to determine the severity of vesicoureteral reflux in the setting of significant hydronephrosis.

RENAL VEIN THROMBOSIS

ESSENTIALS OF DIAGNOSIS & TYPICAL FEATURES

► History of IDM, birth depression, dehydration.

► Hematuria, oliguria.

► Thrombocytopenia, polycythemia.

► Renal enlargement on examination.

Renal vein thrombosis occurs most often in dehydrated polycythemic newborns. At particular risk is the IDM with polycythemia. Thrombosis is unilateral in 70%, usually begins in intrarenal venules, and can extend into larger veins and the vena cava. Hematuria, oliguria, thrombocytopenia, and possibly an enlarged kidney raise suspicion for this diagnosis. With bilateral renal vein thrombosis, anuria ensues. Diagnosis can be confirmed with an ultrasound examination that includes Doppler flow studies of the kidneys. Treatment involves correcting the predisposing condition; systemic heparinization or the use of thrombolytics for this condition is controversial. Prognosis for a full recovery is uncertain. Many infants will develop significant atrophy of the affected kidney, and some develop systemic hypertension. All require careful follow-up.

Mistry K: Renal and urologic diseases of the newborn: neonatal acute kidney injury. Curr Pediatr Rev 2014;10(2):8891 [PMID: 25088261].

Poudel A, Afshan S, Dixit M: Congenital anomalies of the kidney and urinary tract. NeoReviews 2016 Jan;17(1):e18–e27.

NEUROLOGIC PROBLEMS IN THE NEWBORN INFANT

SEIZURES

ESSENTIALS OF DIAGNOSIS & TYPICAL FEATURES

► Usual onset at 12–48 hours.

► Seizure types include subtle (characterized by variable findings), tonic, and multifocal clonic.

► Most common causes include hypoxic-ischemic encephalopathy, intracranial bleeds, and infection.

Newborns rarely have well-organized tonic-clonic seizures because of their incomplete cortical organization and a preponderance of inhibitory synapses. The most common type of seizure is characterized by a constellation of findings, including horizontal deviation of the eyes with or without jerking; eyelid blinking or fluttering; sucking and other oral-buccal movements; swimming or bicycling movements; and desaturation and apneic spells. Strictly tonic or multifocal clonic episodes are also seen.

► Clinical Findings

The differential diagnosis of neonatal seizures is presented in Table 2–20. Most neonatal seizures occur between 12 and 48 hours of age. Later-onset seizures suggest meningitis, benign familial seizures, or hypocalcemia. Information regarding antenatal drug use, the presence of birth asphyxia or trauma, and family history (regarding inherited disorders) should be obtained. Physical examination focuses on neurologic features, other signs of drug withdrawal, concurrent signs of infection, dysmorphic features, and intrauterine growth. Screening workup should include blood glucose, ionized calcium, and electrolytes in all cases. Further workup depends on diagnoses suggested by the history and physical examination. In most cases, a lumbar puncture should be done. Hemorrhages, perinatal stroke, and structural disease of the CNS can be addressed with brain imaging (ultrasound, CT, MRI). Metabolic workup should be pursued when appropriate. EEG should be done; the presence of spike discharges must be noted and the background wave pattern evaluated.

Table 2–20. Differential diagnosis of neonatal seizures.

Diagnosis	Comment
Hypoxic-ischemic encephalopathy	Most common cause (40%), onset in first 24 h
Intracranial hemorrhage	Up to 15% of cases, periventricular/intraventricular hemorrhage, subdural or subarachnoid bleeding
Ischemic stroke	20% of cases
Infection	< 5% of cases
Hypoglycemia	Small for gestational age, IDM
Hypocalcemia, hypomagnesemia	Infant of low birth weight, IDM
Hyponatremia	Rare, seen with SIADH
Disorders of amino and organic acid metabolism, hyperammonemia	Associated acidosis, altered level of consciousness < 5% of cases
Pyridoxine dependency	Seizures refractory to routine therapy; cessation of seizures after administration of pyridoxine
Developmental defects	Congenital brain malformations, chromosomal syndromes
Drug withdrawal	
Genetic causes of neonatal onset epilepsy	Up to 10% of cases
Benign familial neonatal seizures	

IDM, infant of a diabetic mother; SIADH, syndrome of inappropriate secretion of antidiuretic hormone.

Correlation between EEG changes and clinical seizure activity is sometimes absent making a prolonged EEG with video monitoring a useful tool.

Treatment

Adequate ventilation and perfusion should be ensured. Hypoglycemia should be treated immediately with a 2-mL/kg infusion of $D_{10}W$ followed by IV glucose infusion. Other treatments such as calcium or magnesium infusion and antibiotics are indicated to treat hypocalcemia, hypomagnesemia, and suspected infection. Electrolyte abnormalities should be corrected. Intravenous phenobarbital is the first line agent used to stop seizures in neonates. If seizures persist despite maximizing phenobarbital therapy, fosphenytoin or levetiracetam may be indicated. For refractory seizures, a trial of pyridoxine is indicated.

Prognosis

Outcome is related to the underlying cause of the seizure. The outcomes for hypoxic-ischemic encephalopathy and intraventricular hemorrhage have been discussed earlier in this chapter. In these settings, seizures that are difficult to control carry a poor prognosis for normal development. Seizures resulting from hypoglycemia, infection of the CNS, some inborn errors of metabolism, and developmental defects also have a high rate of poor outcome. Seizures caused by hypocalcemia or isolated subarachnoid hemorrhage generally resolve without sequelae.

Hypotonia

One should be alert to the diagnosis of congenital hypotonia when a mother has polyhydramnios and a history of poor fetal movement. The newborn may present with poor respiratory effort and birth asphyxia. For a discussion of causes and evaluation, see Chapter 25.

INTRACRANIAL HEMORRHAGE

1. Primary Subarachnoid Hemorrhage

Primary subarachnoid hemorrhage is the most common type of neonatal intracranial hemorrhage. In the full-term infant, it can be related to trauma of delivery, whereas subarachnoid hemorrhage in the preterm infant can be seen in association with germinal matrix hemorrhage. Clinically, these hemorrhages can be asymptomatic or can present with seizures and irritability on day 2, or rarely, a massive hemorrhage with a rapid downhill course. The seizures associated with subarachnoid hemorrhage are very characteristic—usually brief, with a normal examination interictally. Diagnosis can be suspected on lumbar puncture and confirmed with CT scan or MRI. Long-term follow-up is uniformly good.

2. Subdural Hemorrhage

Subdural hemorrhage is related to birth trauma; the bleeding is caused by tears in the veins that bridge the subdural space. Most commonly, subdural bleeding is from ruptured superficial cerebral veins, with blood over the cerebral convexities. These hemorrhages can be asymptomatic or may cause seizures, with onset on days 2–3 of life, vomiting, irritability, and lethargy. Associated findings include retinal hemorrhages and a full fontanelle. The diagnosis is confirmed by CT scan or MRI.

Specific treatment entailing needle drainage of the subdural space is rarely necessary. Most infants survive; 75% are normal on follow-up.

3. Neonatal Stroke

Focal cerebral ischemic injury can occur in the context of intraventricular hemorrhage in the premature infant and hypoxic-ischemic encephalopathy. Neonatal stroke has also been described in the context of underlying disorders of thrombolysis, maternal drug use (cocaine), a history of infertility, preeclampsia, prolonged membrane rupture, and chorioamnionitis. In some cases, the origin is unclear. The injury often occurs antenatally. The most common clinical presentation of an isolated cerebral infarct is with seizures, and diagnosis can be confirmed acutely with diffusion-weighted MRI scan. The most frequently described distribution is that of the middle cerebral artery.

Treatment is directed at controlling seizures. Use of anticoagulants and thrombolytics is controversial. Long-term outcome is variable, ranging from near normal to hemiplegias and cognitive deficits.

Soul JS: Acute symptomatic seizures in term neonates: etiologies and treatments. Semin Fetal Neonatal Med 2018 Jun;23(3): 183–190 [PMID: 29433814].

van der aA NE et al: Neonatal stroke: a review of the current evidence on epidemiology, pathogenesis, diagnostics, and therapeutic options. Acta Paediatr 2014;103(4):356–364 [PMID: 24428836].

▼ METABOLIC DISORDERS IN THE NEWBORN INFANT

HYPERGLYCEMIA

Hyperglycemia may develop in preterm infants, particularly those of extremely low birth weight who are also SGA. Glucose concentrations may exceed 200–250 mg/dL, particularly in the first few days of life. This transient diabetes-like syndrome usually lasts approximately 1 week.

Management may include simply reducing glucose intake while continuing to supply IV amino acids to prevent protein catabolism with resultant gluconeogenesis and worsened hyperglycemia. Intravenous insulin infusions may be needed in infants who remain hyperglycemic despite glucose infusion rates of less than 5–6 mg/kg/min, but caution should be used as hypoglycemia is a frequent complication.

HYPOCALCEMIA

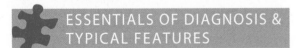

ESSENTIALS OF DIAGNOSIS & TYPICAL FEATURES

▶ Irritability, jitteriness, seizures (see also Chapter 34).

▶ Normal blood glucose.

▶ Possible dysmorphic features, congenital heart disease (DiGeorge syndrome).

Calcium concentration in the immediate newborn period decreases in all infants. The concentration in fetal plasma is higher than that of the neonate or adult. Hypocalcemia is usually defined as a total serum concentration less than 7 mg/dL (equivalent to a calcium activity of 3.5 mEq/L), although the physiologically active fraction, ionized calcium, should be measured whenever possible, and is usually normal even when total calcium is as low as 6–7 mg/dL. An ionized calcium level above 0.9 mmol/L (1.8 mEq/L; 3.6 mg/dL) is not likely to be detrimental.

▶ Clinical Findings

The clinical signs of hypocalcemia and hypocalcemic tetany include a high-pitched cry, jitteriness, tremulousness, and seizures.

Hypocalcemia tends to occur at two different times in the neonatal period. Early-onset hypocalcemia occurs in the first 2 days of life and has been associated with prematurity, maternal diabetes, asphyxia, and rarely, maternal hypoparathyroidism. Late-onset hypocalcemia occurs at approximately 7–10 days and is observed in infants receiving modified cow's milk rather than infant formula (high phosphorus intake), in infants with hypoparathyroidism (DiGeorge syndrome, 22q11 deletion), or in infants born to mothers with severe vitamin D deficiency. Hypomagnesemia should be sought and treated in cases of hypocalcemia that are resistant to treatment.

▶ Treatment

A. Oral Calcium Therapy

The oral administration of calcium salts, often along with vitamin D, is the preferred method of treatment for chronic forms of hypocalcemia resulting from hypoparathyroidism (see Chapter 34).

B. Intravenous Calcium Therapy

IV calcium therapy is usually needed for infants with symptomatic hypocalcemia or an ionized calcium level below 0.9 mmol/L. A number of precautions must be observed when calcium is given intravenously. The infusion must be given slowly so that there is no sudden increase in calcium concentration of blood entering the right atrium, which could cause severe bradycardia and even cardiac arrest. Furthermore, the infusion must be observed carefully, because an IV infiltrate containing calcium can cause full-thickness skin necrosis requiring grafting. For these reasons, IV calcium therapy should be given judiciously and through a central venous line if possible. IV administration of 10% calcium gluconate may be given as a bolus or continuous infusion. Ten percent calcium chloride may result in a larger increment in ionized calcium and greater improvement in mean arterial blood pressure in sick hypocalcemic infants and thus may have a role in the newborn. *Note:* Calcium salts cannot be added to IV solutions that contain sodium bicarbonate because they precipitate as calcium carbonate.

▶ Prognosis

The prognosis is good for neonatal seizures entirely caused by hypocalcemia that is promptly treated.

INBORN ERRORS OF METABOLISM

ESSENTIALS OF DIAGNOSIS & TYPICAL FEATURES

▶ Altered level of consciousness (poor feeding, lethargy, seizures) in a previously well-appearing infant (see also Chapter 36).

▶ Tachypnea without hypoxemia or distress.

▶ Hypoglycemia, respiratory alkalosis, metabolic acidosis.

▶ Recurrent "sepsis" without proven infection.

Each individual inborn error of metabolism is rare, but collectively they have an incidence of 1 in 1000 live births. Expanded newborn genetic screening undoubtedly aids in the diagnosis of these disorders; however, many infants will present prior to these results being available. These diagnoses should be entertained when infants who were initially well present with sepsis-like syndromes, recurrent hypoglycemia, neurologic syndromes (seizures or altered levels of consciousness), or unexplained acidosis (suggestive of organic acidemias).

In the immediate neonatal period, urea cycle disorders present as an altered level of consciousness (coma) secondary to hyperammonemia. A clinical clue that supports this diagnosis is hyperventilation with primary respiratory alkalosis, along with low blood urea nitrogen. The other major diagnostic category to consider consists of infants with severe and unremitting acidemia secondary to organic acidemias.

▼ QUALITY ASSESSMENT & IMPROVEMENT IN THE NEWBORN NURSERY & NICU

Quality improvement initiatives are critical for NICUs to provide the best care possible for patients. This involves recognition that there is a gap between care as it is and care as it could and should be. Clinical units either individually or as part of a consortium need to identify goals for improvement and carry out changes using a plan-do-study-act (PDSA) approach to rapid cycle improvements in care. This involves planning and enacting a change, studying and analyzing the data collected during the change and then acting to assess what changes are to be made for the next PDSA cycle. Individual units can benchmark their care through participation in multicenter databases such as the Vermont Oxford Network or Children's Hospitals Neonatal Consortium, in which many NICUs submit data. These data can form the framework for strategies to improve performance in areas in a unit that are below network standards. Examples of possible initiatives include lowering the incidence of central line-associated bacteremia, decreasing the incidence of ventilator-associated pneumonia or structured feeding protocols to decrease the incidence of NEC.

Garber SJ, Puopolo KM: Prevention of central line-associated bloodstream infections among infants in the neonatal intensive care unit. NeoReviews 2015;16:e211.

Spitzer AR: Has quality improvement really improved outcomes for babies in the neonatal intensive care unit? Clin Perinatol 2017;44:469–483.

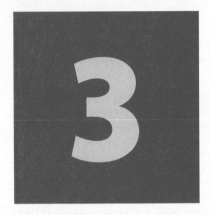

3

Child Development & Behavior

Edward Goldson, MD

Ann Reynolds, MD

Abigail S. Angulo, MD, MPH

Dannah M. Raz, MD

INTRODUCTION

This chapter provides an overview of typical development, identifies developmental variations, and discusses several developmental disorders. The chapter does not cover typical development in the newborn period or adolescence (see Chapters 2 and 4, respectively). It addresses behavioral variations that reflect the spectrum of normal development, along with developmental and behavioral disorders and their treatment. The developmental principle of ongoing change and maturation is integral to the daily practice of pediatrics. It is the basic science of pediatrics. For example, we recognize that a 3-month-old infant is very different from a 3-year-old toddler or a 13-year-old adolescent, not only with respect to what the child can do but also in terms of the kinds of illness he or she might have. From the perspective of the general pediatrician, all these areas should be viewed in the context of a "medical home." The *medical home* is defined as the setting that provides consistent, continuous, culturally competent, comprehensive, and sensitive care to children and their families. It is a setting that advocates for all children, whether they are typical or have developmental challenges or disabilities. By incorporating the principles of child development—the concept that children are constantly changing—the medical home is the optimum setting to understand and enhance typical development and to address variations, delays, and deviations as they may occur in the life trajectory of the child and the family.

▼ NORMAL DEVELOPMENT

Typical children follow a trajectory of increasing physical size (http://www.cdc.gov/growthcharts/clinical_charts.htm) and increasing complexity of function, especially during the first 5 years of life. The child triples his or her birth weight within the first year and achieves two-thirds of his or her adult brain size by age 2½–3 years. The child progresses from a totally dependent infant at birth to a mobile, verbal person who is able to express his or her needs and desires by age 2–3 years. In the ensuing 3 years the child further develops the capacity to interact with peers and adults, achieves considerable verbal and physical prowess, and becomes ready to enter the academic world of learning and socialization.

It is critical for the clinician to identify disturbances in development during these early years as there are windows of opportunity or sensitive periods when appropriate interventions may be instituted to effectively address developmental challenges.

THE FIRST 2 YEARS

From a motor perspective, children develop in a cephalocaudal direction. They can lift their heads with good control at 3 months, sit independently at 6 months, crawl at 9 months, walk at 1 year, and run by 18 months. The child learning to walk has a wide-based gait at first. Next, he or she walks with legs closer together, the arms move medially, a heel-toe gait develops, and the arms swing symmetrically by 18–24 months.

Clinicians often focus on gross motor development, but an appreciation of fine motor development and dexterity, particularly the grasp, can be instructive not only in monitoring normal development but also in identifying deviations in development. The grasp begins as a raking motion involving the ulnar aspect of the hand at age 3–4 months. The thumb is added to this motion at about age 5 months as the focus of the movement shifts to the radial side of the hand. The thumb opposes the fingers for picking up objects just before age 7 months in a radial palmar grasp, and the immature pincer grasp emerges at about age 9 months. The mature pincer grasp is solidified by the first birthday. Most young children have symmetrical movements. Children should not have a significant hand preference before 1 year of age and typically develop handedness between 18 and 30 months.

Language is a critical area to consider as well. Communication is important from birth (Figure 3–1, see Table 3–2), particularly the nonverbal, reciprocal interactions between infant and caregiver. By age 2 months, these interactions begin to include melodic vowel sounds called *cooing* and reciprocal vocal play between parent and child. Babbling, which adds consonants to vowels, begins by age 6–10 months, and the repetition of sounds such as "da-dada-da" is facilitated by the child's increasing oral muscular control. Babbling reaches a peak at age 12 months. The child then moves into a stage of having needs met by using individual words to represent objects or actions. It is common at this age for children to express wants and needs by pointing to objects or using other gestures. Children usually have 5–10 comprehensible words by 12–18 months; by age 2 years they are putting 2–3 words into phrases, 50% of which their caregivers can understand (Tables 3–1 and 3–2; see Figure 3–1), and fluidly use about 50 words for various needs. The acquisition of expressive vocabulary varies greatly between 12 and 24 months of age. As a group, males and children who are bilingual tend to develop expressive language more slowly during that time, though still within the typical time frame. Gender and exposure to two languages should never be used as an excuse for failing to refer a child who has significant delay in the acquisition of speech and language for further evaluation. It is also important to note that most children are not truly bilingual. Most children have one primary language, and any other languages are secondary.

Receptive language usually develops more rapidly than expressive language. Word comprehension begins to increase

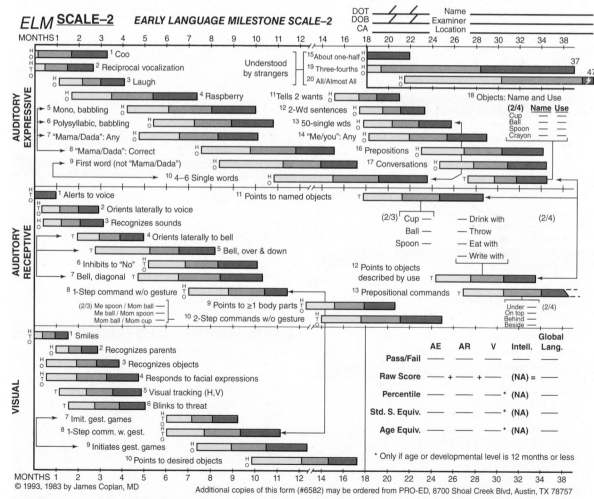

▲ **Figure 3–1.** Early Language Milestone Scale-2. (Reproduced with permission from Coplan J: *Early Language Milestone Scale.* 2nd ed. Austin, TX: Pro Ed; 1993.)

Table 3–1. Developmental charts.

1–2 mo

Activities to be observed:
Holds head erect and lifts head.
Turns from side to back.
Regards faces and follows objects through visual field.
Drops toys.
Becomes alert in response to voice.
Activities related by parent:
Recognizes parents.
Engages in vocalizations.
Smiles spontaneously.

3–5 mo

Activities to be observed:
Grasps cube—first ulnar then later thumb opposition.
Reaches for and brings objects to mouth.
Makes "raspberry" sound.
Sits with support.
Activities related by parent:
Laughs.
Anticipates food on sight.
Turns from back to side.

6–8 mo

Activities to be observed:
Sits alone for a short period.
Reaches with 1 hand.
First scoops up a pellet; then grasps it using thumb opposition.
Imitates "bye-bye."
Passes object from hand to hand in midline.
Babbles.
Activities related by parent:
Rolls from back to stomach.
Is inhibited by the word *no*.

9–11 mo

Activities to be observed:
Stands alone.
Imitates pat-a-cake and peek-a-boo.
Uses thumb and index finger to pick up pellet.
Activities related by parent:
Walks by supporting self on furniture.
Follows 1-step verbal commands, eg, "Come here," "Give it to me."

1 y

Activities to be observed:
Walks independently.
Says "mama" and "dada" with meaning.
Can use a neat pincer grasp to pick up a pellet.
Releases cube into cup after demonstration.
Gives toys on request.
Tries to build a tower of 2 cubes.
Activities related by parent:
Points to desired objects.
Says 1 or 2 other words.

18 mo

Activities to be observed:
Builds tower of 3–4 cubes.
Throws ball.
Seats self in chair.
Dumps pellet from bottle.
Activities related by parent:
Walks up and down stairs with help.
Says 4–20 words.
Understands a 2-step command.
Carries and hugs doll.
Feeds self.

24 mo

Activities to be observed:
Speaks short phrases, 2 words or more.
Kicks ball on request.
Builds tower of 6–7 cubes.
Points to named objects or pictures.
Jumps off floor with both feet.
Stands on either foot alone.
Uses pronouns.
Activities related by parent:
Verbalizes toilet needs.
Pulls on simple garment.
Turns pages of book singly.
Plays with domestic mimicry.

30 mo

Activities to be observed:
Walks backward.
Begins to hop on 1 foot.
Uses prepositions.
Copies a crude circle.
Points to objects described by use.
Refers to self as I.
Holds crayon in fist.
Activities related by parent:
Helps put things away.
Carries on a conversation.

3 y

Activities to be observed:
Holds crayon with fingers.
Builds tower of 9–10 cubes.
Imitates 3-cube bridge.
Copies circle.
Gives first and last name.
Activities related by parent:
Rides tricycle using pedals.
Dresses with supervision.

(Continued)

Table 3–1. Developmental charts. (*Continued*)

3–4 y

Activities to be observed:

Climbs stairs with alternating feet.

Begins to button and unbutton.

"What do you like to do that's fun?" (Answers using plurals, personal pronouns, and verbs.)

Responds to command to place toy *in*, *on*, or *under* table.

Draws a circle when asked to draw a person.

Knows own sex. ("Are you a boy or a girl?")

Gives full name.

Copies a circle already drawn. ("Can you make one like this?")

Activities related by parent:

Feeds self at mealtime.

Takes off shoes and jacket.

4–5 y

Activities to be observed:

Runs and turns without losing balance.

May stand on 1 leg for at least 10 seconds.

Buttons clothes and laces shoes. (Does not tie.)

Counts to 4 by rote. "Give me 2 sticks." (Able to do so from pile of 4 tongue depressors.)

Draws a person. (Head, 2 appendages, and possibly 2 eyes. No torso yet.)

Knows the days of the week. ("What day comes after Tuesday?")

Gives appropriate answers to: "What must you do if you are sleepy? Hungry? Cold?"

Copies + in imitation.

Activities related by parent:

Self-care at toilet. (May need help with wiping.)

Plays outside for at least 30 minutes.

Dresses self except for tying.

5–6 y

Activities to be observed:

Can catch ball.

Skips smoothly.

Copies a + already drawn.

Tells age.

Concept of 10 (eg, counts 10 tongue depressors). May recite to higher number by rote.

Knows right and left hand.

Draws recognizable person with at least 8 details.

Can describe favorite television program in some detail.

Activities related by parent:

Does simple chores at home (eg, taking out garbage, drying silverware).

Goes to school unattended or meets school bus.

Good motor ability but little awareness of dangers.

6–7 y

Activities to be observed:

Copies a Δ.

Defines words by use. ("What is an orange?" "To eat.")

Knows if morning or afternoon.

Draws a person with 12 details.

Reads several 1-syllable printed words. (My, dog, see, boy.)

7–8 y

Activities to be observed:

Counts by 2s and 5s.

Ties shoes.

Copies a ◊.

Knows what day of the week it is. (Not date or year.)

No evidence of sound substitution in speech (eg, *fr* for *thr*).

Draws a man with 16 details.

Reads paragraph #1 Durrell:

Reading:

Muff is a little yellow kitten. She drinks milk. She sleeps on a chair. She does not like to get wet.

Corresponding arithmetic:

7	6	6	8
+4	+7	−4	−3

Adds and subtracts 1-digit numbers.

8–9 y

Activities to be observed:

Defines words better than by use. ("What is an orange?" "A fruit.")

Can give an appropriate answer to the following:

"What is the thing for you to do if …

—you've broken something that belongs to someone else?"

—a playmate hits you without meaning to do so?"

Reads paragraph #2 Durrell:

Reading:

A little black dog ran away from home. He played with two big dogs. They ran away from him. It began to rain. He went under a tree. He wanted to go home, but he did not know the way. He saw a boy he knew. The boy took him home.

Corresponding arithmetic:

	67		
67	16	14	−84
+4	+27	−8	−36

Is learning borrowing and carrying processes in addition and subtraction.

9–10 y

Activities to be observed:

Knows the month, day, and year.

Names the months in order. (15 s, 1 error.)

Makes a sentence with these 3 words in it: (1 or 2. Can use words orally in proper context.)

1. work … money … men

2. boy … river … ball

Reads paragraph #3 Durrell:

Reading:

Six boys put up a tent by the side of a river. They took things to eat with them. When the sun went down, they went into the tent to sleep. In the night, a cow came and began to eat grass around the tent. The boys were afraid. They thought it was a bear.

Should comprehend and answer the question: "What was the cow doing?"

Corresponding arithmetic:

5204	23	837
−530	×3	×7

Learning simple multiplication.

(Continued)

Table 3–1. Developmental charts. (*Continued*)

10–12 y	Reading:
Activities to be observed: Should read and comprehend paragraph #5 Durrell: *Reading:* In 1807, Robert Fulton took the first long trip in a steamboat. He went one hundred and fifty miles up the Hudson River. The boat went five miles an hour. This was faster than a steamboat had ever gone before. Crowds gathered on both banks of the river to see this new kind of boat. They were afraid that its noise and splashing would drive away all the fish. Answer: "What river was the trip made on?" Ask to write the sentence: "The fishermen did not like the boat."	Golf originated in Holland as a game played on ice. The game in its present form first appeared in Scotland. It became unusually popular and kings found it so enjoyable that it was known as "the royal game." James IV, however, thought that people neglected their work to indulge in this fascinating sport so that it was forbidden in 1457. James relented when he found how attractive the game was, and it immediately regained its former popularity. Golf spread gradually to other countries, being introduced in America in 1890. It has grown in favor until there is hardly a town that does not boast of a private or public course. Ask to write a sentence: "Golf originated in Holland as a game played on ice." Answers questions: "Why was golf forbidden by James IV?" "Why did he change his mind?"

Corresponding arithmetic:

$$420 \times 89 \qquad 9\overline{)72} \qquad 31\overline{)62}$$

Should do multiplication and simple division.

Corresponding arithmetic:

$$536\overline{)4762} \qquad \begin{array}{r}\square \\ +\square\end{array} \qquad \begin{array}{r}7\frac{1}{6} \\ -3\frac{1}{6}\end{array}$$

Reduce fractions to lowest forms.
Does long division, adds and subtracts fractions.

12–15 y	
Activities to be observed: Reads paragraph #7 Durrell:	

Modified with permission from Leavitt SR, Goodman H, Harvin D: Use of developmental charts in teaching well child care. Pediatrics 1963 Mar;31:499–508.

at age 9 months, and by age 12 months the child's receptive vocabulary may be as large as 20–100 words. After age 18 months, expressive and receptive vocabularies increase dramatically, and by the end of the second year there is typically a quantum leap in language development. The child begins to put together words and phrases, and begins to use language to represent a new world, the symbolic world. Children begin to put verbs into phrases and focus much of their language on describing their new abilities, for example, "I go out." They begin to incorporate pronouns, such as "I" and "you" into speech and ask "why?" and "what?" questions more frequently. They also begin to appreciate time factors and to understand and use this concept in their speech.

The Early Language Milestone Scale-2 is a simple tool for assessing early language development in the pediatric office setting. Another frequently used screening tool for the ambulatory setting is the Ages and Stages Questionnaire.

One may memorize the developmental milestones that characterize the trajectory of the typical child; however, these milestones become more meaningful and clinically useful if placed in empirical and theoretical contexts. The first 2 years of life have been described as the sensorimotor period, during which infants learn with increasing sophistication how to link sensory input from the environment with a motor response. Infants build on primitive reflex patterns of behavior (termed *schemata*; sucking is an example) and constantly incorporate or assimilate new experiences. The schemata

evolve over time as infants accommodate new experiences and as new levels of cognitive ability unfold in an orderly sequence. This period of behavioral development follows the neurologic development of neural networks through dendritic branching and pruning (apoptosis).

In the first year of life, the infant's perception of reality revolves around their self and what they can see or touch. The infant follows the trajectory of an object through the field of vision, but before age 6 months the object ceases to exist once it leaves the infant's field of vision. At age 9–12 months, the infant gradually develops the concept of object permanence, or the realization that objects exist even when not seen. The development of object permanence correlates with enhanced frontal activity appearing on the electroencephalogram (EEG). The concept attaches first to the image of the primary caregiver because of his or her emotional importance and is a critical part of attachment behavior (see next for further discussion). In the second year, children extend their ability to manipulate objects by using instruments, first by imitation and later by trial and error.

In the first year of life, there is a bidirectional attachment process called *bonding*. The caregivers learn to be aware of and to interpret the infant's cues, which reflect the infant's needs. A more sensitive emotional and social interaction process develops that can be seen in the mirroring of facial expressions by the primary caregiver and infant and in their mutual engagement in cycles of attention and inattention,

Table 3–2. Normal speech and language development.

Age	Speech	Language	Articulation
1 mo	Throaty sounds		Vowels: \ah\, \uh\, \ee\
2 mo	Vowel sounds ("eh"), coos		
2½ mo	Squeals		
3 mo	Babbles, initial vowels		
4 mo	Guttural sounds ("ah," "go")		Consonants: m, p, b
5 mo			Vowels: \o\, \u\
7 mo	Imitates speech sounds		
8 mo			Syllables: da, ba, ka
10 mo		"Dada" or "mama" nonspecifically	Approximates names: baba/bottle
12 mo	Jargon begins (own language)	1 word other than "mama" or "dada"	Understandable: 2–3 words
13 mo		3 words	
16 mo		6 words	Consonants: t, d, w, n, h
18–24 mo		2-word phrases	Understandable 2-word phrases
24–30 mo		3-word phrases	Understandable 3-word phrases
2 y	Vowels uttered correctly	Approximately 270 words; uses pronouns	Approximately 270 words; uses phrases
3 y	Some degree of hesitancy and uncertainty common	Approximately 900 words; intelligible 4-word phrases	Approximately 900 words; intelligible 4-word
4 y		Approximately 1540 words; intelligible 5-word phrases or sentences	Approximately 1540 words; intelligible 5-word phrases
6 y		Approximately 2560 words; intelligible 6- or 7-word sentences	Approximately 2560 words; intelligible 6- or 7-word sentences
7–8 y	Adult proficiency		

Data from Berry MF: *Language Disorders of Children*. New York, NY: Appleton-Century-Crofts; 1969; and from Bzoch K, League R: *Receptive Expressive Emergent Language Scale*. University Park Press; 1970.

which further develop into social play. Basic trust versus mistrust is another way of describing the reciprocal interaction that characterizes this stage. Turn-taking games, which occur between ages 3 and 6 months, are a pleasure for both the parents and the infant and are an extension of mirroring behavior. They also represent an early form of imitative behavior, which is important in later social and cognitive development. More sophisticated games, such as peek-a-boo, become meaningful at approximately age 9 months. The infant's thrill at the reappearance of the face that vanished momentarily demonstrates the emerging understanding of object permanence. Age 8–9 months is also a critical time in the attachment process as this is when separation anxiety and stranger anxiety become marked. The infant at this stage is able to appreciate discrepant events that do not match previously known schemata. These new events cause uncertainty and subsequently, fear and anxiety. The infant must be able to retrieve previous schemata and incorporate new information over an extended time. These abilities are developed by age 8 months and give rise to the fears that may subsequently develop: stranger anxiety and separation anxiety. In stranger anxiety, the infant analyzes the face of a stranger, detects the mismatch with previous schemata or what is familiar, and responds with fear or anxiety, leading to crying. In separation anxiety, the child perceives the difference between the primary caregiver's presence and his or her absence by remembering the schema of the caregiver's presence. Perceiving the inconsistency in the caregiver's absence, the child first becomes uncertain and then anxious and fearful. This begins at age 8 months, reaches a peak at 15 months, and disappears by the end of 2 years in a relatively orderly progression as central nervous system (CNS) maturation facilitates the development of new skills. A parent can put the child's understanding of object permanence to good use by placing a picture of the caregivers near the child or by leaving a comfort object (eg, caregiver's sweater or a special blanket) where the child can see it during the caregiver's absence. A visual substitute for the parent's presence may comfort the child.

Once the child can walk independently, he or she can move away from the parent and explore the environment. Although the child uses the parent as "home base," returning frequently for reassurance, he or she has now taken a major step toward independence. This is the beginning of mastery over the environment and an emerging sense of self. The "terrible twos" and the frequent self-asserting use of "no" are the child's attempt to develop a better idea of what is or might be under his or her control. The child is starting to assert his or her autonomy. As children develop a sense of self, they begin to understand the feelings of others and develop empathy. They hug another child who is in perceived distress or become concerned when one is hurt. They begin to understand how another child feels when he or she is harmed, and this realization helps them to inhibit their own aggressive behavior. Children also begin to understand right and wrong and parental expectations. They recognize that they have done something "bad" and may signify that awareness by saying "uhoh" or with other expressions of distress. They also take pleasure in their accomplishments and become more aware of their bodies.

Also, developing at this age is the important behavior of play. Play is the child's means of learning. Play is a very complex process whose purpose can include the practice and rehearsal of roles, skills, and relationships; a means of revisiting the past; a means of actively mastering a range of experiences; and a way to integrate the child's life experiences into understanding of their environment. Play involves emotional development (affect regulation and gender identification and roles), cognitive development (nonverbal and verbal function and executive functioning and creativity), and social/motor development (motor coordination, frustration tolerance, and social interactions such as turn taking). Of interest is that play has a developmental progression. The typical 6- to 12-month-old engages in the game of peek-a-boo, which is a form of social interaction. During the next several months, although children engage in increasingly complex social interactions and imitation, their play is primarily solitary. However, they do begin to engage in symbolic play such as by drinking from a toy cup and then by giving a doll a drink from a toy cup. By age 2 years, children begin to engage in parallel play (engaging in behaviors that are imitative). This form of play gradually evolves into more interactive or collaborative play by age 3–4 years and is also more thematic in nature. There are of course wide variations in the development of play, reflecting cultural, educational, and socioeconomic variables. Nevertheless, the development of play does follow a sequence that can be assessed and can be very informative in the evaluation of the child.

Brain maturation sets the stage for toilet training. After age 18 months, toddlers have the sensory capacity for awareness of a full rectum or bladder and are physically able to control bowel and urinary tract sphincters. They also take great pleasure in their accomplishments, particularly in appropriate elimination, if it is reinforced positively. Children must be given some control over when elimination occurs. If parents impose severe restrictions, the achievement of this developmental milestone can become a battle between parent and child. The development of bowel control encompasses a more generalized theme of socialized behavior.

AGES 2–4 YEARS

The 2- to 4-year-old stage begins when language has facilitated the creation of mental images in the symbolic sense. The child begins to manipulate the symbolic world; sorts out reality from fantasy imperfectly; and may be terrified of dreams, wishes, and foolish threats. Most of the child's perception of the world is interpreted in reference to his or her needs or influence. Cause-effect relationships are confused with temporal ones or interpreted with respect to themselves. For example, children may focus their understanding of divorce on themselves ("My father left because I was bad" or "My mother left because she didn't love me"). Illness and the need for medical care are also commonly misinterpreted at this age. The child may make a mental connection between a sibling's illness and a recent argument, a negative comment, or a wish for the sibling to be ill. The child may experience significant guilt unless the caregivers are aware of these misperceptions and take time to deal with them.

At this age, children also endow inanimate objects with human feelings. They also assume that humans cause or create all natural events. For instance, when asked why the sun sets, they may say, "The sun goes to his house" or "It is pushed down by someone else." Magical thinking blossoms between ages 3 and 5 years as symbolic thinking incorporates more elaborate fantasy. Fantasy facilitates development of role playing and emotional growth. Children test new experiences in fantasy, both in their imagination and in play. In their play, children often create magical stories and novel situations that reflect issues with which they are dealing, such as aggression, relationships, fears, and control. Children often invent imaginary friends at this time, and nightmares or fears of monsters are common. At this stage, other children become important in facilitating play, such as in a preschool group. Play gradually becomes more cooperative; shared fantasy leads to game playing.

EARLY SCHOOL YEARS: AGES 5–7 YEARS

Attendance at kindergarten at age 5 years marks an acceleration in the separation-individuation theme initiated in the preschool years. The child is ready to relate to peers in a more interactive manner. The brain has reached 90% of its adult weight. Sensorimotor coordination abilities are maturing and facilitating pencil-and-paper tasks and sports, both part of the school experience. Cognitive abilities are still at the preoperational stage, and children focus on one variable in a problem at a time. However, most children have mastered conservation of length by age 5½ years, conservation of mass and weight by 6½ years, and conservation of volume by 8 years.

By first grade, there is more pressure on the child to master academic tasks—recognizing numbers, letters, and words and learning to write. Concrete operations typically begin after age 6 years, when the child is able to perform mental operations concerning concrete objects that involve manipulation of more than one variable. The child is able to order, number, and classify because these activities are related to concrete objects in the environment and because these activities are stressed in early schooling. Magical thinking diminishes greatly at this time, and the reality of cause-effect relationships is better understood. Fantasy and imagination are still strong and are reflected in themes of play.

MIDDLE CHILDHOOD: AGES 7–11 YEARS

From 7 to 11 years of age, children devote most of their energies to school and peer group interactions. For the 7-year-old child, the major developmental tasks are achievement in school and acceptance by peers. Academic expectations intensify, become more abstract, and require the child to concentrate on, attend to, and process increasingly complex auditory and visual information. Children with learning disabilities or problems with attention, organization, and impulsivity may have difficulty with academic tasks. This may subsequently lead to negative reinforcement from teachers, peers, and even parents. Such children may develop a poor self-image manifested as behavioral difficulties. The pediatrician must evaluate potential learning disabilities in any child who is not developing adequately at this stage or who presents with emotional or behavioral problems. The developmental status of school-aged children is not documented as easily as that of younger children because of the complexity of the milestones. In the school-aged child, the quality of the response, the attentional abilities, and the child's emotional approach to the task can make a dramatic difference in success at school. The clinician must consider all of these aspects in the differential diagnosis of learning disabilities and behavioral disorders.

Carey WB, Crocker AC, Elias ER, Feldman HM, Coleman WL: *Developmental-Behavioral Pediatrics.* 4th ed. Philadelphia, PA: Saunders/Elsevier; 2009.

Dixon SD, Stein MT: *Encounters With Children: Pediatric Behavior and Development.* 4th ed. St. Louis, MO: Mosby-Year Book; 2006.

Early Language Milestone Scale. 2nd ed. Austin, Texas: Pro-Ed Incorporated; 1993.

Squires J, Bricker D: *Ages and Stages Questionnaires.* 3rd ed. Baltimore, MD: Brookes Publishing; 2009.

Voigt RG, Macias MM, Myers SM, Tapia CD (eds): *Developmental and Behavioral Pediatrics.* 2nd ed. Itasca, IL: American Academy of Pediatrics; 2018.

▼ BEHAVIORAL & DEVELOPMENTAL VARIATIONS

Variations in children's behavior reflect a blend of intrinsic biological characteristics and the environments with which the children interact. Often identified as complaints by parents, such normal variations in behavior are a reflection of each child's unique, individual biologic and temperament traits and the parents' responses. There are no cures for these behaviors, but management strategies are available that can enhance the parents' understanding of the child and the child's relationship to the environment. These strategies also facilitate the parents' care of the growing infant and child.

The last section of this chapter discusses developmental disorders of cognitive and social competence. Diagnosis and management of these conditions requires a comprehensive and often multidisciplinary approach. The health care provider can play a major role in diagnosis, coordinating the child's evaluation, interpreting the results to the family, and in providing reassurance and support.

Hagan Jr JF, Shaw JS, Duncan PM (eds): *Bright Futures: Guidelines for Health Supervision of Infants, Children, and Adolescents.* 4th ed. Elk Grove Village, IL: American Academy of Pediatrics; 2017.

Medical Home Initiatives for Children With Special Needs Project Advisory Committee; American Academy of Pediatrics: The medical home. Pediatrics 2002;110:184 [PMID: 12093969].

Voigt RG, Macias MM, Myers SM: *American Academy of Pediatrics Developmental and Behavioral Pediatrics.* Elk Grove Village, IL: American Academy of Pediatrics; 2010.

Wolraich ML et al (eds): *Developmental-Behavioral Pediatrics: Evidence and Practice.* Philadelphia, PA: Mosby/Elsevier; 2008.

NORMALITY & TEMPERAMENT

The physician confronted by a disturbance in physiologic function rarely has doubts about what is atypical. Variations in temperament and behavior are not as straightforward. Not infrequently there is an overlap between physiological and behavioral signs requiring other intervention strategies to sort them out. Labeling such variations as disorders is generally not productive in their diagnosis and management.

The behaviors described in this section are part of a continuum of responses by the child to a variety of internal and external experiences. Temperament, for example, is a genetically influenced behavioral disposition that is stable over time. It sometimes is thought of as being the "how" of behavior as distinguished from the "why" (motivation) and the "what" (ability). Temperament is an independent psychological attribute that is expressed as a response to an external stimulus. The influence of temperament is bidirectional: The effect of a particular experience will be influenced by the child's temperament, and the child's temperament will influence the responses of others in the child's environment. Temperament is the style with which the child interacts with the environment.

The perceptions and expectations of parents must be considered when a child's behavior is evaluated. A child whom one parent might describe as hyperactive might not be characterized as such by the other parent. This truism can be expanded to include all the dimensions of temperament. Thus, the concept of "goodness of fit" comes into play. For example, if the parents want and expect their child to be predictable but that is not the child's behavioral style, the parents may perceive the child as being bad or having a behavioral disorder rather than as having a developmental variation. An appreciation of this phenomenon is important because the physician may be able to enhance the parents' understanding of the child and influence their responses to the child's behavior. When there is goodness of fit, there will be more harmony and a greater potential for healthy development not only of the child but also of the family. When goodness of fit is not present, tension and stress can result in parental anger, disappointment, frustration, and conflict with the child.

All models of temperament seek to identify intrinsic behavioral characteristics that lead the child to respond to the world in particular ways. One child may be highly emotional and another less so (ie, calmer) in response to a variety of experiences, stressful or pleasant. The clinician must recognize that each child brings some intrinsic, biologically based traits to its environment and that such characteristics are neither good nor bad, right nor wrong, normal nor abnormal; they are simply part of the child. Thus, as one looks at variations in development, one should abandon the illness model and consider this construct as an aid to understanding the nature of the child's behavior and its influence on the parent-child relationship.

Caring for Your School Age Child: Ages 5 to 12. American Academy of Pediatrics; 2015.

DePauw SSW, Mervield I: Temperament, personality, and developmental psychopathology: a review of the conceptual dimensions underlying childhood traits. Child Psychiatry Hum Dev 2010;41:313–329 [PMID: 20238477].

How to Understand Your Child's Temperament. Healthychildren. org.

Nigg JT: Temperament and developmental psychopathology. J Child Psychol Psychiatry 2006;47:395–422 [PMID: 16492265].

Prior M: Childhood temperament. J Child Psychol Psychiatry 1992;33:249 [PMID: 1737829].

▼ ENURESIS & ENCOPRESIS

ESSENTIALS OF DIAGNOSIS & TYPICAL FEATURES

▶ A child who does not achieve urine and bowel continence by 5–6 years of age and generally has no underlying pathology to which the incontinence can be attributed.

▶ The child does not respond to a full bladder or rectum.

▶ The child is constipated and/or is withholding stools.

Enuresis and encopresis are common childhood problems encountered in the pediatric and family practitioner's office. Bedwetting is particularly common with about 20% of children in the first grade occasionally wetting the bed and 4% wetting the bed two or more times a week. Enuresis is more common in boys than in girls. In a recent large US study, the prevalence of enuresis among boys 7 and 9 years was 9% and 7%, respectively, and among girls at those ages, 6% and 3%, respectively. The data on constipation and encopresis seem less clear with about 1%–3% of children experiencing this problem, but with anywhere from 0.3% to 29% of children worldwide experiencing constipation. Overall, encopresis/constipation accounts for 3% of referrals to pediatricians' offices. What is more striking, however, is that constipation and enuresis often co-occur; in such a case the constipation needs to be dealt with before the enuresis can be addressed.

ENURESIS

Enuresis is defined as repeated urination into the clothing during the day and into the bed at night by a child who is chronologically and developmentally older than 5 years; this pattern of urination must occur at least twice a week for 3 months. Enuresis has been categorized by the International Children's Continence Society as monosymptomatic or non-monosymptomatic. Monosymptomatic enuresis is uncomplicated nocturnal enuresis (NE; must never have been dry at night for over 6 months with no daytime accidents); it is a reflection of a maturational disorder and there is no underlying organic problem. Complicated or non-monosymptomatic enuresis often involves NE and daytime incontinence and often reflects an underlying disorder. The evaluation of both forms needs to take into consideration both the medical and psychological implications of these conditions.

Monosymptomatic enuresis reflects a delay in achieving nighttime continence and reflects a delay in the maturation of the urologic and neurologic systems. Both micturition and anorectal evacuation are dependent on neural connections and communications between the frontal lobes, locus ceruleus, mid pons, sacral voiding center, and the bladder and rectum. With respect to enuresis, most children are continent at night within 2 years of achieving daytime control. However, 15.5% of 7.5-year-old children wet the bed but only about 2.5% meet the criteria for enuresis. With each year of age the frequency of bedwetting decreases: by 15 years only about 1%–2% of children continue to wet. This occurs more commonly among boys than girls.

The causes for NE are varied and probably interact with one another. Genetic factors are strongly implicated, as enuresis tends to run in families. Many children with NE have a higher threshold for arousal and do not awake to the sensation of a full bladder. NE can also be a result of overproduction of urine from decreased production of desmopressin or a resistance to antidiuretic hormone. In such cases, the bladder has decreased functional capacity and empties before it is filled.

The evaluation of a child with NE involves a complete history and physical examination to rule out any anatomical abnormalities, underlying pathology, or the presence of constipation. In addition, every child with NE should undergo a urinalysis including a specific gravity. A urine culture should be obtained, especially in girls.

Treatment involves education and the avoidance of being judgmental and shaming the child. Most children feel ashamed and the goal of treatment is to help the child establish continence and maintain his or her self-esteem. A variety of behavioral strategies have been employed such as limiting liquids before sleep and awakening the child at night so that he/she can go to the toilet. Central to this simple strategy is consistency on the parents' part and the need for the child to be completely awake. If this simple approach is unsuccessful, the use of bedwetting alarms is suggested. Every time the alarm goes off, the child should go to the toilet and void. Therapy needs to be continued for at least 3 months and used every night. Critical to the success of therapy is that parents need to be active participants and get up with the child, as many children will just turn off the alarm and go back to sleep. The alarm system, which is a form of cognitive behavioral therapy, has been found to cure two-thirds of affected children and should be highly recommended to affected children and their parents as a safe, effective treatment for NE. The most common cause of failure of this intervention is that the child does not awaken or the parents do not wake the child.

While behavioral strategies should be the first line of treatment, when these fail one may need to turn to medications. Desmopressin acetate (DDAVP), an antidiuretic hormone analogue, has been used successfully. DDAVP decreases urine production. Imipramine, a tricyclic antidepressant, also has been used successfully to control NE, although the mechanism of action is not understood. However, potential adverse side effects, including the risk of death with an overdose, suggest that imipramine should be used only as a last resort. Unfortunately, when such medications are stopped, there is a very high relapse rate.

Daytime incontinence or non-monosymptomatic enuresis is more complicated than NE. Daytime continence is achieved by 70% of children by 3 years of age and by 90% of children by 6 years. When this is not the case, one needs to consider underlying pathology, including cystitis, diabetes insipidus, diabetes mellitus, seizure disorders, neurogenic bladder, anatomical abnormalities of the urinary tract system such as urethral obstruction, constipation, and psychological stress and child maltreatment. A complete history and physical examination must be obtained, along with a diary that includes daily records of voiding and fecal elimination. Treatment must be directed at the underlying pathology and often requires the input of pediatric subspecialists. Following diagnosis, family support and education are essential.

ENCOPRESIS

Constipation (see Chapter 21) is defined by two or more of the following events for 2 months: (1) fewer than three bowel movements per week, (2) more than one episode of encopresis per week, (3) impaction of the rectum with stool, (4) passage of stool so large that it obstructs the toilet, (5) retentive posturing and fecal withholding, and (6) pain with defecation.

Encopresis is described in the *Diagnostic and Statistical Manual of Mental Disorders*, 5th Edition (DSM-5) as the repeated passage of stool into inappropriate places (such as in the underpants) by child who is chronologically or developmentally older than 4 years. It occurs each month for at least 3 months and is not attributable to the physiologic effects of a substance or another medical condition except to the mechanism involving constipation. Behavioral scientists often divide encopresis into (1) retentive encopresis, (2) continuous encopresis, and (3) discontinuous encopresis. In rare instances children have severe toilet phobia and so do not defecate into the toilet. It is critical to note that more than 90% of the cases of encopresis result from constipation. Thus, in the evaluation of a child with encopresis, one must rule out underlying pathology associated with constipation (see Chapter 21) while at the same time addressing functional and behavioral issues. Conditions associated with constipation include metabolic disorders such as hypothyroidism, neurologic disorders such as cerebral palsy or tethered cord, and anatomical abnormalities of the anus. In addition, children who have been continent can also develop encopresis as a response to stress or child maltreatment.

The prevalence of encopresis is somewhat difficult to precisely ascertain as it is a subject often kept secret by the family and the child. However, some authors report that 1%–3% of children ages 4–11 years of age suffer from encopresis. The highest prevalence is between 5 and 6 years of age.

A complete history and meticulous physical examination must be performed, including a rectal examination, particularly looking for abnormalities around the anus and spine. An abdominal radiograph can be helpful in determining the degree of constipation, the appearance of the bowel, and whether there is obstruction. Assuming no gastrointestinal abnormalities, initial intervention starts with treatment of constipation. Subsequently education, support, and guidance around evacuation are essential, including behavioral strategies such as having the child sit on the toilet after meals to stimulate the gastrocolic reflex. It is most important to avoid punishing the child and making him or her feel guilty and ashamed. Helping the child to clean himself and his clothing in a nonjudgmental, nonpunitive manner is far more productive approach than criticism and reproach. At the same time, if there is an underlying psychiatric disorder such as depression, the child should be treated for the mental health problem along with the treatment of the constipation.

When medical management of constipation is indicated, oral medication or an enema for "bowel cleanout" followed by oral medications should be used. Such treatment can be monitored by abdominal radiographs to be sure that the colon is clean. A bowel regimen needs to be established with the goal of the child achieving continence and defecating in the toilet bowl on a regular basis. The child should be encouraged to have a daily bowel movement, and the use of fiber, some laxatives, and even mineral oil can be helpful. Consultation with a gastroenterologist should be considered in more refractory cases.

Culbert TP, Banez GA: Integrative approaches to childhood constipation and encopresis. Pediatr Clin North Am 2007;54(6): 927–947 [PMID: 18061784].

Nijman, RJM: Diagnosis and management of urinary incontinence and functional fetal incontinence (encopresis) in children. Gastroenterol Clin North Am 2008;37(3):731–748 [PMID: 18794006].

Reiner W: Pharmacotherapy in the management of voiding and storage disorders, including enuresis and encopresis. J Am Acad Child Adolesc Psychiatry 2008;47:491–498 [PMID: 18438186].

Robson WLM: Clinical practice. Evaluation and management of enuresis. N Engl J Med 2009;360:1429–1436 [PMID: 19339722].

Schonwald A, Rappaport LA: Elimination conditions. In: Wolraich ML et al (eds): Developmental-Behavioral Pediatrics: Evidence and Practice. Philadelphia, PA: Mosby/Elsevier; 2008:791–804.

▼ COMMON DEVELOPMENTAL CONCERNS

COLIC

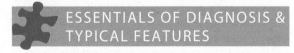

ESSENTIALS OF DIAGNOSIS & TYPICAL FEATURES

▶ An otherwise healthy infant aged 2–3 months seems to be in pain, cries for > 3 hours a day, for > 3 days a week, for > 3 weeks ("rule of threes").

Infant colic is characterized by severe and paroxysmal crying that occurs mainly in the late afternoon. The infant's knees are drawn up and its fists are clenched, flatus is expelled, the facies has a pained appearance, and there is minimal response to attempts at soothing. Studies in the United States have shown that among middle-class infants, crying occupies about 2 hours per day at 2 weeks of age, about 3 hours per day by 6 weeks, and gradually decreases to about 1 hour per day by 3 months. The word "colic" is derived from Greek kolikos ("pertaining to the colon"). Although colic has traditionally been attributed to gastrointestinal disturbances, this has never been proven. Others have suggested that colic reflects a disturbance in the infant's sleep-wake cycling or an infant state regulation disorder. In any case, colic is a behavioral sign or symptom that begins in the first few weeks of life and peaks at age 2–3 months. In about 30%–40% of cases, colic continues into the fourth and fifth months.

A colicky infant is healthy and well fed but cries for more than 3 hours a day, for more than 3 days a week, and for more than 3 weeks—commonly referred to as the "rule of threes." The important word in this definition is "healthy." Thus, before the diagnosis of colic can be made, the pediatrician must rule out diseases that might cause crying. With the exception of the few infants who respond to elimination of cow's milk from its own or the mother's diet, there has been little firm evidence of an association of colic with allergic disorders. Gastroesophageal reflux is often suspected as a cause of colicky crying in young infants. Undetected corneal abrasion, urinary tract infection, and unrecognized traumatic injuries, including child abuse, must be among the physical causes of crying considered in evaluating these infants. Some attempts have been made to eliminate gas with simethicone and to slow gut motility with dicyclomine. Simethicone has not been shown to ameliorate colic. Dicyclomine has been associated with apnea in infants and is contraindicated.

This then leaves characteristics intrinsic to the child (ie, temperament) and parental caretaking patterns as contributing to colic. Behavioral states have three features: (1) They are self-organizing—that is, they are maintained until it is necessary to shift to another one; (2) they are stable over several minutes; and (3) the same stimulus elicits a state-specific response that is different from other states. The behavioral states are (among others) a crying state, a quiet alert state, an active alert state, a transitional state, and a state of deep sleep. The states of importance with respect to colic are the crying state and the transitional state. During transition from one state to another, infant behavior may be more easily influenced. Once an infant is in a stable state (eg, crying), it becomes more difficult to bring about a change (eg, to soothe). How these transitions are accomplished is probably influenced by the infant's temperament and neurologic maturity. Some infants move from one state to another easily and can be diverted easily; other infants sustain a particular state and are resistant to change.

Another factor to be considered in evaluating the colicky infant is the feeding and handling behavior of the caregiver. Colic is a behavioral phenomenon that involves interaction between the infant and the caregiver. Different caregivers perceive and respond to crying behavior differently. If the caregiver perceives the crying infant as being spoiled and demanding and is not sensitive to or knowledgeable about the infant's cues and rhythms—or is hurried and "rough" with the infant—the infant's ability to organize and soothe him- or herself or respond to the caregiver's attempts at soothing may be compromised. Alternatively, if the temperament of an infant with colic is understood and the rhythms and cues deciphered, crying can be anticipated and the caregiver can intervene before the behavior becomes "organized" in the crying state and more difficult to extinguish.

▶ Management

1. Parents need to be educated about the developmental characteristics of crying behavior and made aware that crying increases normally into the second month and abates by the third to fourth month.

2. Parents need reassurance, based on a complete history and physical examination, that the infant is not sick. A discussion of the differential/potential causes and why they have been ruled out can be helpful. Although these behaviors are stressful, they are normal variants and are usually self-limited. This discussion can be facilitated by having the parent keep a diary of crying and weight gain. If there is a diurnal pattern and adequate weight gain, an underlying disease process is less likely to be present. It is important to relieve parental anxiety.

3. For parents to effectively soothe and comfort the infant, they need to understand the infant's cues. The pediatrician (or nurse) can help by observing the infant's behavior and devising interventions aimed at calming both the infant and the parents. One should encourage a quiet environment without excessive handling. Rhythmic stimulation such as gentle swinging or rocking, soft music, drives in the car, or walks in the stroller may be helpful, especially if the parents are able to anticipate the onset of crying. Another approach is to change the feeding habits so that the infant is not rushed, has ample opportunity to burp, adaptive nipple if bottle fed, and, if necessary, can be fed more frequently so as to decrease gastric distention if that seems to be contributing to the problem.

4. Medications such as phenobarbital elixir and dicyclomine should not be used because of the risk of adverse reactions and overdosage. A trial of ranitidine hydrochloride or other proton pump inhibitor might be of help if proven gastroesophageal reflux is contributing to the child's discomfort.

5. For colic that is refractory to behavioral management, a trial of changing the feedings and eliminating cow's milk from the formula or from the mother's diet if she is nursing may be indicated. The use of whey hydrolysate formulas for formula-fed infants has been suggested. There is conflicting evidence regarding the use of probiotics to treat infant colic.

6. There is no conclusive evidence for complementary and alternative interventions to treat colic. While herbal remedies have been suggested, there are no well-designed studies supporting herbal therapies in the treatment of colic. Furthermore, herbal remedies have potential for toxicity and neurologic impairment, compounded by lack of knowledge of appropriate dosing in children. The same holds true for the use of chiropractic interventions and reflexology; there are no well-designed studies to support the use of these interventions, and the risks of adverse events outweigh the possible benefits. However, there are several studies suggesting probiotics—*Lactobacillus reuteri*—may be helpful in the management of colic in breast-fed babies but not in bottle-fed infants.

Bellaïche M, Levy M, Jung C: Treatments for infant colic. J Pediatr Gastroenterol Nutr 2013;57(Suppl 1):S27–S30.

Biagoli E et al: Pain-relieving agents for infantile colic. Cochrane Database Syst Rev 2016 Sep 16;9:CD009999 [PMID: 27631535].

Cohen-Silver J, Ratnapalan S: Management of infantile colic: a review. Clin Pediatr (Phila) 2009;48:14–17 [PMID: 18832537].

Schreck BA et al: Probiotics for the treatment of infantile colic: a systemic review. J Pharm Pract 2017 Jun;30(3):366–374 [PMID: 26940647].

Shamir R et al: Infant crying, colic, and gastrointestinal discomfort in early childhood: a review of the evidence and most plausible mechanisms. J Pediatr Gastroenterol Nutr 2013 Dec;57(Suppl 1): S1–S45 [PMID: 24356023].

FEEDING DISORDERS IN INFANTS & YOUNG CHILDREN

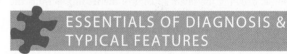

ESSENTIALS OF DIAGNOSIS & TYPICAL FEATURES

▶ Inadequate or disordered intake of food due to any of the following conditions:

- Poor oral-motor coordination.
- Fatigue resulting from a chronic disease.
- Lack of appetite.
- Behavioral issues relating to parent-child interaction.
- Pain associated with feeding.

Feeding problems are common in the general pediatric population. Children can present with feeding problems for various reasons, including fine motor skill deficits, oral-motor dysfunction (gagging, trouble with chewing, and/or swallowing, aspiration), cardiopulmonary disorders leading to fatigue, gastrointestinal disturbances causing pain or discomfort, neuromuscular conditions, social, or emotional issues, and problems with food regulation. Children with medical conditions or developmental disabilities are more likely to experience feeding problems. Infants and young children may refuse to eat if they find eating painful or frightening. The infant or child may refuse to eat if the rhythm of the feeding experience with the caregiver is not harmonious. Food refusal may develop when the infant's cues around feeding are not interpreted correctly by the parent. The infant who needs to burp more frequently or who needs time between bites but instead is rushed may refuse to eat. The child who has had an esophageal atresia repair and has a stricture may find eating uncomfortable. The very young infant with severe oral candidiasis may refuse to eat because of pain. The child who has had a choking experience associated with feeding may be terrified to eat (oral-motor dysfunction or aspiration). The child who is forced to eat by a maltreating parent or an overzealous caregiver may refuse feeds. Children who have required nasogastric feedings or who have required periods of fasting and intravenous nutrition in the first 1–2 months of life are more likely to display food refusal behavior upon introduction of oral feedings. Food refusal can look like a child outright refusing to eat, spitting out the food, or turning their head away. If the child is verbal, they may express that they are not hungry and verbally refuse food offered to them.

The normal developmental and interactive feeding stages through which the child normally progresses are establishment of homeostasis (0–2 months), attachment (2–6 months), and separation and individuation (6 months to 3 years). During the first stage, feeding can be accomplished most easily when the parent allows the infant to determine the timing, amount, pacing, and preference of food intake. During the attachment phase, allowing the infant to control the feeding permits the parent to engage the infant in a positive manner. This paves the way for the separation and individuation phase. When a disturbance occurs in the parent-child relationship at any of these developmental levels, difficulty in feeding may ensue, with both the parent and the child contributing to the dysfunctional interaction. One of the most striking manifestations of food refusal occurs during the stage of separation and individuation. Conflict may arise if the parent seeks to dominate the child by intrusive and controlling feeding behavior at the same time the child is striving to achieve autonomy. The scenario then observed is of the parent forcing food on the child while the child refuses to eat. This often leads to extreme parental frustration and anger, and the child may be inadequately nourished and developmentally and emotionally thwarted.

When the pediatrician is attempting to sort out the factors contributing to food refusal, it is essential first to obtain a complete history, including a social history. This should include information concerning the parents' perception of the child's behavior and their expectations of the child, how often the refusal is happening, if it happens with specific foods or textures, specifics about the environment or setting in which

the child eats, how the family manages the food refusal, when the feeding challenges started, and if any changes or stressors occurred at that time. Other information that is important to include in the history are questions about potential discomfort or pain associated with feeding. This can include asking if the child appears to be uncomfortable when feeding. If the child is having dental pain they may be more likely to refuse foods that require use of dentition such as chewy or crunchy foods. If the child is experiencing gastrointestinal discomfort, they may present with reflux, frequent vomiting, choking or gagging, or difficulty swallowing due to pain or discomfort in their esophagus. Constipation also can impact feeding if the child is uncomfortable and in pain.

Second, a complete physical examination should be performed, with emphasis on oral-motor behavior and other clues suggesting neurologic, anatomic, or physiologic abnormalities that could make feeding difficult. The child's emotional state and developmental level must be determined. This is particularly important if there is concern about depression or a history of developmental delays. Third, the feeding interaction needs to be observed live, if possible. Finally, the physician needs to help the parents understand that infants and children may have different styles of eating and different food preferences, and may refuse foods they do not like. This is not necessarily abnormal but may reflect differences in temperament and variations in the child's way of processing olfactory, gustatory, and tactile stimuli.

When the chief complaint is failure to gain weight, a different approach is required. The differential diagnosis should include not only food refusal but also medical disorders and maltreatment. The most common reason for failure to gain weight is inadequate caloric intake. Excessive weight loss may be due to vomiting or diarrhea, malabsorption, or a combination of these factors. In this situation more extensive diagnostic evaluation may be needed. Laboratory studies may include a complete blood count; erythrocyte sedimentation rate; urinalysis and urine culture; blood urea nitrogen; serum electrolytes and creatinine; and stool examination for fat, occult blood, and ova and parasites. Some practitioners also include liver and thyroid profiles. Occasionally an assessment of swallowing function or evaluation for the presence of gastroesophageal reflux may be indicated. Because of the complexity of the problem, a team approach to the diagnosis and treatment of failure to thrive, or poor weight gain, may be most appropriate.

▶ Management

The goal of intervention is to identify factors contributing to the disturbance and to work to overcome them. The parents may be encouraged to view the child's behavior differently and try not to impose their expectations and desires. Alternatively, the child's behavior may need to be modified so that the parents can provide adequate nurturing. A multidisciplinary approach is recommended in the assessment and treatment of feeding problems in children. The team should include a physician, nurse, and occupational and speech therapists. The team should determine if further workup and referrals would be indicated to provide comprehensive treatment of the concern.

The goals of treatment of the child with feeding challenges are to establish a pattern of eating that is harmonious with the goals of the family or caregivers. Guidelines to accomplishing these goals include the following: (1) Establish a comprehensive diagnosis that considers all factors contributing to poor feeding, (2) monitor the feeding interaction and ensure appropriate weight gain, (3) monitor the developmental progress of the child and the changes in the family dynamics that facilitate optimal weight gain and psychosocial development, and (4) provide support to the family as they seek to help the child.

Aldridge V et al: Identifying clinically relevant feeding problems and disorders. J Child Health Care 2010;14:261–270 [PMID: 20153948].

Bryant-Waugh R et al: Feeding and eating disorders in childhood. Int J Eat Disord 2010;43:98–111 [PMID: 20063374].

Hvelplund K et al: Perinatal risk factors for feeding and eating disorders in children 0-3 years. Pediatrics 2016;137(2):e20152575 [PMID: 26764360].

Lask B, Bryant-Waugh R (eds): *Eating Disorders in Childhood and Adolescence*. 4th ed. East Essex: Routledge; 2013.

Morris N, Knight RM, Bruni T, Sayers L, Drayton A: Feeding disorders. Child Adolesc Psychiatr Clin N Am 2017;26(3): 571–586. doi:10.1016/j.chc.2017.02.011

Williams KE, Field DG, Seiverling L: Food refusal in children: a review of the literature. Res Dev Disabil 2010;31:625–633 [PMID: 20153948].

SLEEP DISORDERS

ESSENTIALS OF DIAGNOSIS & TYPICAL FEATURES

▶ Children aged < 12 years:

- Difficulty initiating or maintaining sleep that is viewed as a problem by the child or caregiver.

- Bedtime resistance or need for caregiver intervention to initiate sleep or to go back to sleep.

- May be characterized by its severity, chronicity, frequency, *and* associated impairment in daytime function in the child *or* family.

- May be due to a primary sleep disorder or occur in association with other sleep, medical, or psychiatric disorders.

▶ Adolescents—difficulty initiating or maintaining sleep, early morning awakening, nonrestorative sleep, or a combination of these problems.

Sleep problems impact quality of life and are considered a public health problem. Poor sleep in children is associated with maladaptive daytime behaviors, poorer developmental outcome, greater parental stress, obesity, insulin resistance, alterations in sympathetic tone, and immune dysfunction. Sleep is a complex physiologic process influenced by intrinsic biologic properties, temperament, cultural norms and expectations, and environmental conditions. Between 20% and 40% of children experience sleep disturbances at some point in the first 4 years of life. The percentage decreases to 10%–12% in school-aged children. The most common sleep disorder encountered by pediatricians is insomnia, or difficulty with initiating and maintaining sleep. Parasomnias refer to abnormalities of arousal, partial arousal, and transitions between stages of sleep. Other sleep disorders include sleep-disordered breathing (covered in greater depth in Chapter 19), restless legs syndrome (RLS)/periodic limb movement disorder (PLMD, narcolepsy, and circadian rhythm disturbances. Narcolepsy, benign neonatal sleep myoclonus, and nocturnal frontal lobe epilepsy will be covered in Chapter 25. DSM-5 no longer differentiates between primary and secondary insomnia in an effort to acknowledge the importance of managing sleep issues no matter what the perceived cause, and to recognize the bidirectional and interactive effects between sleep issues and coexisting conditions.

Sleep is controlled by two mechanisms. One is homeostatic drive, which is the increase in pressure to fall asleep over the course of the day. The second is the circadian rhythm, which is the drive to be alert. This drive for alertness increases over the course of the morning, dips in the early afternoon, and then rises again to the highest levels several hours before bedtime. This increase in alertness prior to bedtime is often called the "forbidden zone," because it may be more difficult to fall asleep during this period. This is very important to take into account when attempting to have a child fall asleep earlier than their current bedtime. If the child typically falls asleep at 10 and the caregiver would like the child to fall asleep at 8:00, they may be asking the child to fall asleep when their body is too alert. The change would need to be made gradually. There also are two different biologic clocks. The first is the circadian rhythm–daily sleep-wake cycle. The second is an ultradian rhythm that occurs several times per night—the stages of sleep. Sleep stages cycle every 50–60 minutes in infants to every 90 minutes in adolescents. The daily circadian clock is longer than 24 hours. Environmental cues entrain the sleep-wake cycle into a 24-hour cycle. The cues include light-dark, ambient temperature, core body temperature, noise, social interaction, hunger, pain, and hormone production. Without the ability to perceive these cues (ie, blindness), a child might have difficulty entraining a 24-hour sleep-wake cycle.

Two major sleep stages have been identified clinically and with the use of polysomnography: rapid eye movement (REM) and nonrapid eye movement (NREM) sleep. In REM sleep, muscle tone is relaxed, the sleeper may twitch and grimace, and the eyes move erratically beneath closed lids. REM sleep occurs throughout the night but is increased during the latter half of the night. NREM sleep is divided into three stages. In the process of falling asleep, the individual enters stage N1, light sleep, characterized by reduced body movements, slow eye rolling, and sometimes opening and closing of the eyelids. Stage N2 sleep is characterized by slowing of eye movements, slowing of respirations and heart rate, and relaxation of the muscles. Most mature individuals spend about half of their sleep time in this stage. Stage N3 is slow-wave sleep, during which the body is relaxed, breathing is slow and shallow, and the heart rate is slow. The deepest NREM sleep occurs during the first 1–3 hours after going to sleep. Most parasomnias occur early in the night during deep NREM sleep. Dreams and nightmares that occur later in the night occur during REM sleep.

Sleep is clearly a developmental phenomenon. Infants are not born with a sleep-wake cycle. REM sleep is more common than NREM sleep in newborns and decreases by 3–6 months of age. Sleep patterns slowly mature throughout infancy, childhood, and adolescence until they become adult like. Newborns sleep 10–19 hours per day in 2- to 5-hour blocks. Over the first year of life, the infant slowly consolidates sleep at night into a 9- to 12-hour block and naps gradually decrease to one per day by about 12 months. Most children stop napping between 3 and 5 years of age. In 2015, the National Sleep Foundation published recommendations for the total number of hours of sleep per day in different age groups: 1- to 2-year-olds—11–14 hours per day; 3- to 5-year-olds—10–13 hours per day; 6- to 13-year-olds—9–11 hours per day. Adolescents need 9–9½ hours per night but often only get 7–7¼ hours per night. This is complicated by an approximate 1- to 3-hour sleep phase delay in adolescence that is due to physiologic changes in hormonal regulation of the circadian system. Often, adolescents are not tired until 2 hours after their typical bedtime but still must get up at the same time in the morning. Some school districts have implemented later start times for high school students because of this phenomenon.

PARASOMNIAS

Parasomnias include both NREM arousal disorders such as confusional arousals, night terrors, sleeptalking (somniloquy), and sleepwalking (somnambulism), and REM-associated sleep disorders which are beyond the scope of this chapter.

▶ Night Terrors & Sleepwalking

Night terrors commonly occur within 2 hours after falling asleep, during the deepest stage of NREM sleep, and are often associated with sleepwalking. They occur in about 3% of children and most cases occur between ages 3 and 8 years.

During a night terror, the child may sit up in bed screaming, thrashing about, and exhibiting rapid breathing, tachycardia, and sweating. The child is often incoherent and unresponsive to comforting. The episode may last up to ½ hour, after which the child goes back to sleep and has no memory of the event the next day. Management of night terrors consists of reassurance of the parents plus measures to avoid stress, irregular sleep schedule, or sleep deprivation, which prolongs deep sleep when night terrors occur. Scheduled awakening (awakening the child 30–45 minutes before the time the night terrors usually occur) has been used in children with nightly or frequent night terrors, but there is little evidence that this is effective.

Sleepwalking also occurs during slow-wave/deep sleep and is common between 4 and 8 years of age. It is often associated with other complex behaviors during sleep. It is typically benign except that injuries can occur while the child is walking around. Steps should be taken to ensure that the environment is free of obstacles and that doors to the outside are locked. Parents may also wish to put a bell on their child's door to alert them that the child is out of bed. As with night terrors, steps should be taken to avoid stress and sleep deprivation.

▶ Nightmares

Nightmares are frightening dreams that occur during REM sleep, typically followed by awakening, which usually occurs in the latter part of the night. The peak occurrence is between ages 3 and 5 years, with an incidence between 25% and 50%. A child who awakens during these episodes is usually alert. He or she can often describe the frightening images, recall the dream, and talk about it during the day. The child seeks and will respond positively to parental reassurance. The child will often have difficulty going back to sleep and will want to stay with their parents. Nightmares are usually self-limited and need little treatment. They can be associated with stress, trauma, anxiety, sleep deprivation that can cause a rebound in REM sleep, and medications that increase REM sleep.

INSOMNIA

Insomnia includes difficulty initiating sleep and nighttime awakenings. Although parasomnias are frightening, insomnia is frustrating. It can result in daytime fatigue for both the parents and the child, parental discord about management, and family disruption.

Several factors contribute to these disturbances. The quantity and timing of feeds in the first year of life will influence nighttime awakening. Most infants beyond age 6 months can go through the night without being fed. Thus, under normal circumstances, night waking for feeds is probably a learned behavior and is a function of the child's arousal and the parents' response to that arousal.

Bedtime habits can influence settling in for the night as well as nighttime awakening. If the child learns that going to sleep is associated with pleasant parental behavior such as rocking, singing, reading, or nursing, going back to sleep after nighttime arousal without these pleasant parental attentions may be difficult. This is called sleep-onset association disorder and usually is the reason for night waking. Every time that the child gets to the light sleep portion of the sleep-wake cycle, he or she may wake up. This is usually brief and not remembered the next morning, but for the child who does not have strategies for getting to sleep independently, getting back to sleep may require the same interventions needed to get to sleep initially. Most of these interventions require a parent. Night waking occurs in 40%–60% of infants and young children.

Parents need to set limits for the child while acknowledging the child's individual biologic rhythms. They should resist the child's attempts to put off bedtime or to engage them during nighttime awakenings. The goal is to establish clear bedtime rituals, to put the child to bed while still awake, and to create a dark, quiet, secure bedtime environment.

The child's temperament is another factor contributing to sleep. It has been reported that children with low sensory thresholds and less rhythmicity (regulatory disorder) are more prone to night waking. Night waking often starts at about 9 months as separation anxiety is beginning. Parents should receive anticipatory guidance prior to that time so that they know to reassure their child without making the interaction prolonged or pleasurable. Finally, psychosocial stressors and changes in routine can play a role in night waking.

Insomnia is common in children with complex medical conditions and neurologic, developmental, and psychiatric disorders.

SLEEP-DISORDERED BREATHING

Sleep-disordered breathing or obstructive sleep apnea is characterized by obstructed breathing during sleep accompanied by loud snoring, chest retractions, morning headaches, dry mouth, and daytime sleepiness. Obstructive sleep apnea occurs in 1%–3% of preschoolers. It has its highest peak in childhood between the ages of 2 and 6 years. It has been associated with daytime behavioral disorders, including attention-deficit/hyperactivity disorder (ADHD) (see Chapter 19).

RESTLESS LEGS SYNDROME & PERIODIC LIMB MOVEMENT DISORDER

RLS and PLMD are common disorders in adults and frequently occur together. The frequency of these disorders in children is about 2%. RLS is associated with an uncomfortable sensation in the lower extremities that occurs at night when trying to fall asleep, is relieved by movement, and is sometimes described by children as "creepy-crawly" or "itchy bones." PLMD is stereotyped, repetitive limb movements often associated with a partial arousal or awakening. These disorders have been associated with iron deficiency. A diagnosis of RLS is generally made by history and a diagnosis of PLMD can be made with

a sleep study. Caffeine, nicotine, antidepressants, and other drugs have been associated with RLS and PLMD. The medical evaluation includes obtaining a serum ferritin and C-reactive protein (CRP) level as ferritin can be falsely elevated during inflammation. If the CRP is normal and the ferritin is less than 30–50 ng/mL, treatment with ferrous sulfate should be considered. Medications have been studied for treatment of RLS and PLMD in adults but not in children.

▶ Management of Sleep Disorders

The **BEARS** is a mnemonic that has been recommended for screening for sleep problems in primary care: **B**edtime resistance, **E**xcessive daytime sleepiness, **A**wakening during the night, **R**egularity and duration of sleep, **S**leep-disordered breathing. Screening for the quality and quantity of sleep at every well-child visit has been recommended by Honaker and Meltzer (2016) due to the impact of sleep problems and evidence that parents will not necessarily bring up sleep issues or be aware of what constitutes poor sleep. Once a problem with sleep is identified, a complete medical and psychosocial history should be obtained, and a physical examination performed. A detailed sleep history and diary should be completed, and both parents should contribute. Assessment for allergies, lateral neck films, and polysomnography may be indicated to complete the evaluation, especially if sleep-disordered breathing is suspected. It is important to consider disorders such as gastroesophageal reflux, which may cause discomfort or pain when recumbent. Dental pain or eczema may cause nighttime awakening. It is also important to make sure that any medications that the child is taking do not interfere with sleep.

The key to treatment of children who have difficulty going to sleep or who awaken during the night and disturb others is for the physician and parents to understand normal sleep patterns, daytime and nighttime habits that promote sleep, responses that inadvertently reinforce undesirable sleep behavior, and the child's individual temperament traits. The **ABCs** of **SLEEPING** were developed by Allen et al (2016) as a mnemonic for typical recommendations offered to improve sleep: **A**ge-appropriate **B**edtimes and wake times with **C**onsistency, **S**chedules and routines, **L**ocation (quiet, dark, cool environment), **E**xercise and diet, no **E**lectronics in the bedroom or before bed, **P**ositivity (positive home environment), **I**ndependence when falling asleep, **N**eeds of child met during the day, equals **G**reat sleep. Good sleep hygiene includes discontinuing any activities that are stimulating in the hour before bedtime. It is also important to dim lights and avoid blue light during the "wind down" time. Television and video games are particularly stimulating. Apps are available to decrease blue light and increase red/orange light at night on computers, phones, and tablets. Exposure to light and physical activity during the day are helpful and it is important to ask about caffeine ingestion. Many recommendations for improving sleep in pediatric patients have limited evidence base. Allen et al reviewed available literature and found moderate to strong evidence to support an association between the following recommendations and good sleep: age-appropriate and consistent nap, bed, and wake times; bedtime by 9 PM; regular schedule; limiting access to electronics during and after bedtime by removing them from the bedroom; need to learn to fall asleep independently; establishing a positive living environment; and supporting emotional needs during the day. The literature does not support limiting exercise in the 1–4 hours prior to bedtime. Other interventions had insufficient, limited, or equivocal evidence. Further study is needed to establish evidence-based practices.

Sleep hygiene education and cognitive behavioral therapy for insomnia are considered first-line treatments for pediatric insomnia.

There is little evidence regarding pharmacologic management of sleep disorders in children. Non-pharmacologic interventions should be tried first. While the role for melatonin in children with typical development is unclear, there is mounting evidence that it can be effective in children with visual impairments, developmental disabilities, and autism spectrum disorders (ASDs). Medications such as clonidine are often used for sleep disorders, especially in children with ADHD and ASD, but there are little data to support its use.

Accardo J (ed): *Sleep in Children With Neurodevelopmental Disabilities.* Chennai, India: Springer Nature; 2018.

Allen SL et al: ABCs of SLEEPING: a review of the evidence behind pediatric sleep practice recommendations. Sleep Med Rev 2016; 29:1–14 [PMID: 26551999].

American Academy of Sleep Medicine: http://sleepeducation. org//.

Badin et al: Insomnia: the sleeping giant of pediatric public health. Curr Psychiatry Rep 2016;18:47 [PMID: 26993792].

Braam W, Smits MG, Didden R, Korzilius H, Van Geijlswijk IM, Curfs LM: Exogenous melatonin for sleep problems in individuals with intellectual disability: a meta-analysis. Dev Med Child Neurol 2009;51(5):340–349 [PMID: 19379289].

Cortese S et al: Assessment and management of sleep problems in youths with attention-deficit/hyperactivity disorder. J Am Acad Child Adolesc Psychiatry 2013;52(8):784–796 [PMID: 23880489].

Economou NT, Ferini-Strambi L, Steiropoulos P: Sleep-related drug therapy in special conditions: children. Sleep Med Clin 2018;13(2):251–262 [PMID: 29759275].

Hirshkowitz M et al: National Sleep Foundation's sleep time duration recommendations: methodology and results summary. Sleep Health 2015;1:40–43.

Honaker SM, Meltzer LJ: Sleep in pediatric primary care: a review of the literature. Sleep Med Rev 2016;25:31–39 [PMID: 26163054].

Jan JE et al: Sleep hygiene for children with neurodevelopmental disabilities. Pediatrics 2008;122(6):1343–1350 [PMID: 19047255].

Meltzer LJ, Crabtree VM: *Pediatric Sleep Problems: A Clinician's Guide to Behavioral Interventions.* American Psychological Association; 2015.

Mindell JA, Owens JA: *A Clinical Guide to Pediatric Sleep: Diagnosis and Management of Sleep Problems.* 3rd ed. Philadelphia, PA: Wolters Kluwer Health, Lippincott Williams & Wilkins; 2015.

National Sleep Foundation: http://www.sleepforkids.org/ http://www.sleepfoundation.org.

Owens J, Midell J (eds): Pediatric sleep medicine update. Pediatr Clin North Am 2011;58.

TEMPER TANTRUMS & BREATH-HOLDING SPELLS

ESSENTIALS OF DIAGNOSIS & TYPICAL FEATURES

▶ Behavioral responses to stress, frustration, and loss of control.

▶ Tantrum—child may throw him- or herself on the ground, kick, scream, or strike out at others.

▶ Breath-holding spell—child engages in a prolonged expiration that is reflexive and may become pale or cyanotic.

▶ Rule out underlying organic disease in children with breath-holding spells (eg, CNS abnormalities, Rett syndrome, seizures).

1. Temper Tantrums

Temper tantrums are common between ages 12 months and 4 years, occurring about once a week in 50%–80% of children in this age group. The child may throw him- or herself down, kick and scream, strike out at people or objects in the room, and hold his or her breath. These behaviors may be considered normal as the young child seeks to achieve autonomy and mastery over the environment. They are often a reflection of immaturity as the child strives to accomplish age-appropriate developmental tasks and meets with difficulty because of inadequate motor and language skills, impulsiveness, or parental restrictions. In the home, these behaviors may be annoying. In public, they are embarrassing.

Some children tolerate frustration well, are able to persevere at tasks, and cope easily with difficulties; others have a much greater problem dealing with experiences beyond their developmental level. Parents can minimize tantrums by understanding the child's temperament and what he or she is trying to communicate. Parents must also be committed to supporting the child's drive to master his or her feelings.

▶ Management

Appropriate intervention can provide an opportunity for enhancing the child's growth. The tantrum is a loss of control on the child's part that may be a frightening event and a blow to the child's self-image. The parents and the physician need to view these behaviors within the child's developmental context rather than from a negative, adversarial, angry perspective.

Several suggestions can be offered to parents and physicians to help manage tantrums:

1. Minimize the need to say "no" by "child-proofing" the environment so that fewer restrictions need to be enforced.

2. Use distraction when frustration increases; direct the child to other, less frustrating activities; and reward the positive response.

3. Present options within the child's capabilities so that he or she can achieve mastery and autonomy.

4. Fight only those battles that need to be won and avoid those that arouse unnecessary conflict.

5. Do not abandon the preschool child when a tantrum occurs. Stay nearby during the episode without intruding. A small child may need to be restrained. An older child can be asked to go to his or her room. Threats serve no purpose and should not be used.

6. Do not use negative terms when the tantrum is occurring. Instead, point out that the child is out of control and give praise when he or she regains control.

7. Never let a child hurt him- or herself or others.

8. Do not "hold a grudge" after the tantrum is over, but do not grant the child's demands that led to the tantrum.

9. Seek to maintain an environment that provides positive reinforcement for desired behavior. Do not overreact to undesired behavior, but set reasonable limits and provide responsible direction for the child.

10. Approximately 5%–20% of young children have severe temper tantrums that are frequent and disruptive. Such tantrums may result from a disturbance in the parent-child interaction, poor parenting skills, lack of limit setting, and permissiveness. They may be part of a larger behavioral or developmental disorder or may emerge under adverse socioeconomic conditions, in circumstances of maternal depression and family dysfunction, or when the child is in poor health. Referral to a psychologist or psychiatrist is appropriate while the pediatrician continues to support and work with the family.

2. Breath-Holding Spells

Whereas temper tantrums can be frustrating to parents, breath-holding spells can be terrifying. The name for this behavior may be a misnomer in that it connotes prolonged inspiration. In fact, breath-holding occurs during expiration and is reflexive—not volitional—in nature. It is a paroxysmal event occurring in 0.1%–5% of healthy children from age 6 months to 6 years. The spells usually start during the first year of life, often in response to anger or a mild injury.

The child is provoked or surprised, starts to cry—briefly or for a considerable time—and then falls silent in the expiratory phase of respiration. This is followed by a color change. Spells have been described as either pallid (acyanotic) or cyanotic, with the latter usually associated with anger and the former with an injury such as a fall. The spell may resolve spontaneously, or the child may lose consciousness. In severe cases, the child may become limp and progress to opisthotonos, body jerks, and urinary incontinence. Only rarely does a spell proceed to asystole or a seizure.

▶ Management

For the child with frequent spells, underlying disorders such as seizures, orthostatic hypotension, obstructive sleep apnea, abnormalities of the CNS, tumors, familial dysautonomia, and Rett syndrome (almost exclusively in girls) need to be considered. An association exists among breath-holding spells, pica, and iron-deficiency anemia. These conditions can be ruled out on the basis of the history, physical examination, and laboratory studies. Once it has been determined that the child is healthy, the focus of treatment is behavioral. Parents should be taught to handle the spells in a matter-of-fact manner and monitor the child for any untoward events. The reality is that parents cannot completely protect the child from upsetting and frustrating experiences and probably should not try to do so. Just as in temper tantrums, parents need to help the child control his or her responses to frustration. Parents need to be careful not to be too permissive and submit to the child's every whim for fear the child might have a spell.

If loss of consciousness occurs, the child should be placed on his or her side to protect against head injury and aspiration. Maintaining a patent oral airway is essential, but cardiopulmonary resuscitation should be avoided. There are no prophylactic medications. Atropine, 0.01 mg/kg given subcutaneously, has been used with some benefit in spells accompanied by bradycardia or asystole.

AAP recommendations for parents: http://www.healthychildren.org/English/family-life/family-dynamics/communication-discipline/pages/Temper-Tantrums.aspx.

Baker J (ed): *No More Meltdowns: Positive Strategies for Managing and Preventing Out-of-Control Behavior*. Arlington, TX: Future Horizons; 2008.

Beers NS, Howard B: Managing temper tantrums. Pediatr Rev 2003;24:70–71.

Bright Futures, 2017: https://www.aap.org/en-us/Documents/periodicity_schedule.pdf.

Daniels et al: Assessment, management and prevention of temper tantrums. J Am Acad Nurse Pract 2012;24(10):569–573 [PMID: 23006014].

Mayo Clinic Staff: *Temper Tantrums in Toddlers: How to Keep the Peace*; 2016.

Temper Tantrums: Am Acad Pediatr 2016. https://patiented.solutions.aap.org/handout.aspx?gbosid=156567.

WELL-CHILD SURVEILLANCE & SCREENING

The American Academy of Pediatrics (AAP) Periodicity Schedule provides guidelines for surveillance and screening at well-child visits. Surveillance is a procedure for recognizing children at risk for a developmental disorder and involves asking parents if they have concerns about their child's development. The PEDS (Pediatric Evaluation of Developmental Status) can be used for this purpose. Screening involves use of a standardized tool to clarify identified risk. An evaluation would be done by a specialist and would involve a more definitive evaluation of a child's development.

Surveillance should occur at all well-child visits. Screening of development should occur at 9, 18, and 30 months. Because a 30-month visit is not part of the standard well-child visit schedule and may not be reimbursed, screening may occur at 24 months instead. It is also recommended that autism-specific screening should occur at the 18-month and 24-month visits. Because children with ASD often experience a regression or plateau in skills between 12 and 24 months of age, some children may be missed by a single screen at 18 months. The Screening Tool for Autism in Toddlers and Young Children (STAT) is a second-line screening tool for children who were found to have concerns for ASD on first-line screener such as the MCHAT-R. The STAT includes direct interaction with the child and was designed to differentiate children with ASD from children with developmental delay. The STAT takes about 20 minutes to complete and is meant to be used by a wide range of community professionals. The measure and training can be found at http://stat.vueinnovations.com/about. Clinicians should keep in mind that if they are administering a screen because they are concerned and the child passes the screen, they should still schedule an early follow-up visit to ensure that appropriate developmental progress has been made and that there are no further concerns.

Implementation of screening requires planning for timing of screening administration during office visits, defining the process for referral, and designing handouts prior to beginning screening. Screening is done to optimize the child's development. However, it also demonstrates to the parent the interest their care provider has not only for the child's physical well-being but also for the child's developmental and psychosocial well-being. Parents of children who receive a developmental assessment express greater satisfaction with their care provider.

Committee on Practice and Ambulatory Medicine; Bright Futures Periodicity Schedule Workgroup: 2016 Recommendations for preventive pediatric health care. Pediatrics 2016;137(1):1–3.

Hagan JF, Shaw JS, Duncan PM (eds): *Bright Futures: Guidelines for Health Supervision of Infants, Children, and Adolescents*, 4th ed. Elk Grove Village, IL: American Academy of Pediatrics; 2017.

http://stat.vueinnovations.com/about.

https://www.aap.org/en-us/Documents/periodicity_schedule.pdf.

Squires J, Bricker D: *Ages and Stages Questionnaires*. 3rd ed. Baltimore, MD: Brookes Publishing; 2009.

DEVELOPMENTAL DISORDERS

Developmental disorders include abnormalities in one or more aspects of development, such as language, motor, visual-spatial, attention, and social abilities. Problems with development are often noted by parents when a child does not meet typical motor and language milestones. Developmental disorders may also include difficulties with behavior or attention. ADHD is the most common neurodevelopmental disorder. ADHD occurs in 2%–10% of school-aged children and may occur in combination with a variety of other learning or developmental issues. Mild developmental disorders are often not noted until the child is of school age.

Many biological and psychosocial factors influence a child's performance on developmental tests. In the assessment of the child, it is important to document adverse psychosocial factors, such as neglect or poverty, which can negatively influence developmental progress. Many of the biological factors that influence development are genetic.

The diagnostic criteria for developmental disorders are found in the DSM-5. The term *mental retardation* has been replaced by *intellectual disability* (ID). The diagnostic criteria for ASDs changed dramatically in DSM-5 with some changes in the criteria for ADHD. There are also subtle changes to communication disorders, specific learning disorder, and motor disorders. These can be found at the following website: https://www.psychiatry.org/psychiatrists/practice/dsm/educational-resources/dsm-5-fact-sheets.

Evaluation

The neurodevelopmental evaluation must focus on (1) defining the child's level of developmental abilities in a variety of domains, including language, motor, visual-spatial, attention, and social abilities; (2) attempting to determine the etiology of the child's developmental delays; and (3) planning a treatment program. These objectives are ideally achieved by a multidisciplinary team that may include a physician, a psychologist, a speech or language therapist, an occupational therapist, and an educational specialist. This type of evaluation is ideal but not always readily available.

Medical & Neurodevelopmental Examination

The medical history should include the pregnancy, labor, and delivery to identify conditions that might compromise the child's CNS function. This includes prenatal exposures to toxins, medications, alcohol, drugs, smoking, and infections;

maternal chronic illness; complications of pregnancy or delivery; and neonatal course. Problems such as poor weight gain, chronic illnesses, hospitalizations, and maltreatment can interfere with typical development. Major illnesses or hospitalizations should be discussed. Any CNS problems, such as trauma, infection, or encephalitis, should be documented. The presence of metabolic diseases and exposure to environmental toxins such as lead should be determined. Chronic diseases such as chronic otitis media, hyper- or hypothyroidism, and chronic renal failure can impact typical development. The presence of motor or vocal tics, seizures, gastrointestinal, or sleep disturbances should be documented. In addition, parents should be questioned about any motor, cognitive, or behavioral regression.

The physician should review and document the child's developmental milestones. The physician should also review temperament, difficulties with sleep or feeding, tantrums, poor attention, impulsivity, hyperactivity, anxiety/fears, and aggression. When asking questions about problematic behaviors, it is important to have the parent describe the behavior including frequency and duration. It is also important to try to determine triggers of the behavior and consequences or potential reinforcers of the behavior (ABC—antecedent/behavior/consequence).

A detailed history of school-related events should be recorded, including previous special education support, evaluations through the school, history of repeating grades, difficulties with specific academic areas, problems with peers, and the teacher's impressions of the child's difficulties, particularly related to problems with attention, impulsivity, or hyperactivity. Input from teachers can be invaluable and should be sought prior to the evaluation.

An important aspect of the medical history is a detailed family history of emotional or behavioral problems, learning disabilities, ASD, ID, or psychiatric disorders. Parental learning strengths and weaknesses, temperament difficulties, or attentional problems may be passed on to the child. For instance, dyslexia is highly heritable.

The neurodevelopmental examination should include a careful assessment of dysmorphic features such as epicanthal folds, palpebral fissure size, shape and length of the philtrum, low-set or posteriorly rotated ears, prominent ear pinnae, unusual dermatoglyphics (eg, a single transverse palmar crease), hyperextensibility of the joints, syndactyly, clinodactyly, or other anomalies. A detailed physical and neurologic examination needs to be carried out with an emphasis on both soft and hard neurologic findings. Soft signs can include motor incoordination, which can be related to handwriting problems and academic delays in written language or drawing. Visual-motor coordination abilities can be assessed by having the child write, copy shapes and designs, or draw a person.

The child's growth parameters, including height, weight, and head circumference, need to be assessed. Normal hearing and visual acuity should be documented or evaluated.

Cranial nerve abnormalities and oral-motor coordination problems need to be noted. The examiner should watch closely for motor or vocal tics. Both fine and gross motor abilities should be assessed. Tandem gait, ability to balance on one foot, and coordinating a skip should be evaluated based on age. Fine motor coordination can be noted when watching a child stack blocks or draw.

The developmental aspects of the examination can include an assessment of auditory processing and perceptual ability with simple tasks, such as two- to fivefold directions, assessing right and left directionality, memory for a series of spoken words or digit span, and comprehension of a graded paragraph. In assessing expressive language abilities, the examiner should look for difficulties with word retrieval, formulation, articulation, and adequacy of vocabulary. Visual-perceptual abilities can be assessed by simple visual memory tasks, puzzles, or object assembly, and evaluating the child's ability to decode words or organize math problems. Visual-motor integration and coordination can be assessed with handwriting, design copying, and drawing a person. Throughout the assessment, the clinician should pay special attention to the child's ability to focus attention and concentrate, and to other aspects of behavior or affect, such as evidence of depression or anxiety.

Additional questionnaires and checklists—such as the Child Behavior Checklist by Achenbach; ADHD scales such as the Conners' Parent/Teacher Rating Scale; Vanderbilt ADHD Diagnostic Parent/Teacher Rating Scales; and the Swanson, Nolan, and Pelham Questionnaire-IV—can be used to help with this assessment.

Referral of family to community resources is critical, as is a medical home (described earlier in this chapter).

American Academy of Pediatrics Council on Children With Disabilities: Care coordination in the medical home: integrating health and related systems of care for children with special health care needs. Pediatrics 2005;116:1238 [PMID: 16264016].
https://www.uptodate.com/contents/children-and-youth-with-special-health-care-needs.
Voigt RG, Macias MM, Myers SM, Tapia CD (eds): *Developmental and Behavioral Pediatrics.* 2nd ed. Itasca, IL: American Academy of Pediatrics; 2018.

ATTENTION-DEFICIT/HYPERACTIVITY DISORDER

ADHD is a common neurodevelopmental disorder that may affect about 7%–8% of children and 2.5% of adults. It is associated with a triad of symptoms: impulsivity, inattention, and hyperactivity. DSM-5 describes three ADHD subtypes: hyperactive-impulsive, inattentive, and combined. To be classified according to one or another of these subtypes, the child must exhibit six or more of the symptoms listed in Table 3–3. DSM-5 include the same 18 symptoms, 2 symptom domains, and require 6 symptoms from each

Table 3–3. Attention-deficit/hyperactivity disorder.

Diagnostic Criteria

A. A persistent pattern of inattention and/or hyperactivity-impulsivity that interferes with functioning or development, as characterized by (1) and/or (2):

1. **Inattention:** Six (or more) of the following symptoms have persisted for at least 6 months to a degree that is inconsistent with developmental level and that negatively impacts directly on social and academic/occupational activities.

   Note: The symptoms are not solely a manifestation of oppositional behavior, defiance, hostility, or failure to understand tasks or instructions. For older adolescents and adults (age ≥ 17), at least five symptoms are required.

   a. Often fails to pay close attention to details or makes careless mistakes in schoolwork, at work, or during other activities (eg, overlooks or misses details, work is inaccurate).

   b. Often has difficulty sustaining attention in tasks or play activities (eg, has difficulty remaining focused during lectures, conversations, or lengthy reading).

   c. Often does not seem to listen when spoken to directly (eg, mind seems elsewhere, even in the absence of any obvious distraction).

   d. Often does not follow through on instructions and fails to finish schoolwork, chores, or duties in the workplace (eg, starts tasks but quickly loses focus and is easily sidetracked).

   e. Often has difficulty organizing tasks and activities (eg, difficulty managing sequential tasks; difficulty keeping materials and belongings in order; messy, disorganized work; has poor time management; fails to meet deadlines).

   f. Often avoids, dislikes, or is reluctant to engage in tasks that require sustained mental effort (eg, schoolwork or homework; for older adolescents and adults, preparing reports, completing forms, reviewing lengthy papers).

   g. Often loses things necessary for tasks or activities (eg, school materials, pencils, books, tools, wallets, keys, paperwork, eyeglasses, mobile telephones).

   h. Is often easily distracted by extraneous stimuli (for older adolescents and adults, may include unrelated thoughts).

   i. Is often forgetful in daily activities (eg, doing chores, running errands; for older adolescents and adults, returning calls, paying bills, keeping appointments).

2. **Hyperactivity and impulsivity:** Six (or more) of the following symptoms have persisted for at least 6 months to a degree that is inconsistent with developmental level and that negatively impacts directly on social and academic/occupational activities:

   Note: The symptoms are not solely a manifestation of oppositional behavior, defiance, hostility, or a failure to understand tasks or instructions. For older adolescents and adults (age ≥ 17), at least five symptoms are required.

   a. Often fidgets with or taps hands or feet or squirms in seat.

   b. Often leaves seat in situations when remaining seated is expected (eg, leaves his or her place in the classroom, in the office or other workplace, or in other situations that require remaining in place).

   c. Often runs about or climbs in situations where it is inappropriate. (**Note:** In adolescents or adults, may be limited to feeling restless.)

   d. Often unable to play or engage in leisure activities quietly.

   e. Is often "on the go," acting as if "driven by a motor" (eg, is unable to be or uncomfortable being still for extended time, as in restaurants, meetings; may be experienced by others as being restless or difficult to keep up with).

   f. Often talks excessively.

   g. Often blurts out an answer before a question has been completed (eg, completes people's sentences; cannot wait for turn in conversation).

   h. Often has difficulty waiting his or her turn (eg, while waiting in line).

   i. Often interrupts or intrudes on others (eg, butts into conversations, games, or activities; may start using other people's things without asking or receiving permission; for adolescents and adults, may intrude into or take over what others are doing).

B. Several inattentive or hyperactive-impulsive symptoms were present prior to age 12 years.

C. Several inattentive or hyperactive-impulsive symptoms are present in two or more settings (eg, at home, school, or work; with friends or relatives; in other activities).

D. There is clear evidence that the symptoms interfere with, or reduce the quality of, social, academic, or occupational functioning.

E. The symptoms do not occur exclusively during the course of schizophrenia or another psychotic disorder and are not better explained by another mental disorder (eg, mood disorder, anxiety disorder, dissociative disorder, personality disorder, substance intoxication or withdrawal).

domain for children younger than 17. DSM-5 includes the following changes: Criteria will address symptoms across the lifespan, symptoms causing the impairment will need to be present prior to age 12 instead of age 7, and some symptoms will need to be present across more than one setting. Overall there are significant challenges in academic functioning and social interactions. A diagnosis will be allowed in children with ASD, and symptom thresholds will be lower in adolescents 17 and older and in adults (only five symptoms required from each category).

The majority of children with ADHD have a combined type with symptoms of inattention as well as hyperactivity and impulsivity. Girls have a higher prevalence of the inattentive subtype; boys have a higher prevalence of the hyperactive subtype. Although symptoms begin in early childhood, they can diminish between ages 10 and 25 years. Hyperactivity declines more quickly, and impulsivity and inattentiveness often persist into adolescence and adulthood. ADHD may be combined with other psychiatric conditions, such as mood disorder in approximately 20% of patients, conduct disorders in 20%, and oppositional defiant disorder in up to 40%. Up to 25% of children with ADHD seen in a referral clinic have tics or Tourette syndrome. Conversely, well over 50% of individuals with Tourette syndrome also have ADHD.

ADHD has a substantial genetic component. Several candidate genes have been identified but only explain a small part of the variance, although there is strong evidence that ADHD is a disorder involving multiple genes. ADHD is also associated with a variety of genetic disorders including fragile X syndrome, Williams syndrome, Angelman syndrome, XXY syndrome (Klinefelter syndrome), and Turner syndrome. Fetal alcohol syndrome (FAS) is also strongly associated with ADHD. CNS trauma, CNS infections, prematurity, and a difficult neonatal course with brain injury can also be associated with later ADHD. Metabolic problems such as hyperthyroidism can sometimes cause ADHD. These organic causes of ADHD should be considered in the evaluation of any child presenting with attentional problems, hyperactivity, or impulsivity. Particularly inattention can occur with obstructive sleep apnea. However, in the majority of children who have ADHD, the cause remains unknown.

▶ Management

The treatment of ADHD varies depending on the complexity of the individual case, including comorbid disorders such as anxiety, sleep disorders, and learning disabilities. It is important to educate the family regarding the symptoms of ADHD and to clarify that it is a neurologic disorder which makes the symptoms difficult for the child to control. Despite that, behavior modification techniques usually help these children and should include structure with consistency in daily routine, positive reinforcement whenever possible, and time-out for negative behaviors. A variety of educational interventions can be helpful, including preferential seating in the classroom, a system of consistent positive behavior reinforcement, consistent structure, the repetition of information when needed, and the use of instruction that incorporates both visual and auditory modalities. Many children with ADHD have significant social difficulties, and social skills training can be helpful. Individual counseling is beneficial in alleviating poor self-esteem, oppositional behavior, and conduct problems.

Stimulant medications (methylphenidate, dextroamphetamine, mixed amphetamine, and lisdexamfetamine) are available in short- and long-acting preparations and in tablet, capsule, liquid, and dermal patch forms. Alternative medications for the treatment of ADHD include extended-release clonidine or guanfacine, which are α_2-adrenergic presynaptic agonists. Atomoxetine, which is a norepinephrine reuptake inhibitor, has also been used as a second-line medication or as an adjunct treatment with the stimulants It should be noted that the stimulants are rapidly acting while atomoxetine takes more time for there to be an effect (ie, 2–4 weeks). It is most important that no matter what medication is used, the diagnosis is correct and the correct dosage is prescribed. A recent study has demonstrated that one of the major factors contributing to treatment failure is inadequate dosing or the failure to recognize the presence of comorbid conditions such as learning disability, anxiety disorders, and depression.

Seventy to 90% of children with normal intellectual abilities respond well to stimulant medications. Stimulants enhance both dopamine and norepinephrine neurotransmission, which seems to improve impulse control, attention, and hyperactivity. The main side effects of methylphenidate and dextroamphetamine include appetite suppression and resulting weight loss, as well as sleep disturbances. Atomoxetine is a selective inhibitor of the presynaptic norepinephrine transporter, which increases norepinephrine and dopamine, and has a similar side-effect profile to the stimulants as well as side effects associated with antidepressants. Some individuals experience increased anxiety, particularly with higher doses of stimulant medications. Children with autism and developmental disabilities may be at increased risk for side effects with stimulants. Stimulants may exacerbate psychotic symptoms. They may also exacerbate motor tics in 30% of patients, but in 10% motor tics may be improved.

Cardiovascular effects of stimulant medications have undergone significant scrutiny over the past several years and do not appear to increase the risk of sudden death over the risk in the general population, especially in children without any underlying risk. Prior to beginning a stimulant medication, it is recommended that clinicians obtain any history of syncope, palpitations, chest pain, and family history of sudden death prior to age 30 that may predispose a child to sudden death. Stimulant products and atomoxetine should generally not be used in patients with serious heart problems or in those for whom an increase in BP or HR would be problematic. Consultation with the child's cardiologist would be indicated prior to making a decision about stimulant use. The US Food and Drug Administration (FDA) includes this statement in the labeling of stimulants: "sudden death has been reported in association with CNS stimulant treatment at usual doses in children and adolescents with structural cardiac abnormalities or other serious heart problems." The FDA has recommended that patients treated with ADHD medications should be monitored for changes in HR or BP.

ADHD CDC website: http://www.cdc.gov/ncbddd/adhd/guidelines.html.

Attention Deficit Disorder Association: http://www.add.org.

Children and Adults With Attention Deficit/Hyperactivity Disorder: http://www.chadd.org.

Diagnostic and Statistical Manual of Mental Disorders. 5th ed. American Psychiatric Association; 2013.

FDA Drug Safety Communication: http://www.fda.gov/Drugs/DrugSafety/ucm277770.htm.

Feldman HM, Reif MI: Attention-deficit hyperactivity disorder in children and adolescents. New Eng J Med 2014;370:838–846.

http://www2.aap.org/pubserv/adhd2/1sted.html.

Questions and Answers: Safety of Pills for Treating ADHD: http://www.aap.org/healthtopics/adhd.cfm.

Reiff MI: *ADHD: What Every Parent Needs to Know.* Elk Grove Village, IL: American Academy of Pediatrics; 2011.

Wolraich M et al: Subcommittee on Attention-Deficit/Hyperactivity Disorder; Steering Committee on Quality Improvement and Management: ADHD: clinical practice guideline for the diagnosis, evaluation, and treatment of attention-deficit/hyperactivity disorder in children and adolescents. Pediatrics 2011;128(5):1007–1022 [PMID: 22003063].

AUTISM SPECTRUM DISORDERS

ESSENTIALS OF DIAGNOSIS & TYPICAL FEATURES

▶ Two core features:

- Persistent deficits in social communication and social interaction across multiple contexts.
- Restricted, repetitive patterns of behavior, interests, or activities.

ASD is a neurologic disorder characterized by (1) persistent deficits in social communication and social interaction across multiple contexts and (2) restricted, repetitive patterns of behavior, interests, or activities. Autism was grouped under the pervasive developmental disorders in the DSM-IV with Asperger disorder, pervasive developmental disorder not otherwise specified, childhood disintegrative disorder (CDD), and Rett syndrome. DSM-5 combines autism, PDD, and Asperger syndrome into ASDs. Table 3–4 lists the DSM-5 criteria for diagnosis of an ASD. DSM-IV stipulated that the typical features or signs should be present prior to 3 years of age. DSM-5 now uses a caveat that the typical features or signs may not be present until social demands become greater and may be difficult to recognize in an individual who has learned compensatory strategies. As with any disorder, the typical features or signs must cause "clinically significant impairment" in function. As ASD and ID may be diagnosed in the same individual, social communication function should be impaired in comparison to the individual's "general developmental level." Severity is now specified as level I: "requiring support," level II: "requiring substantial support," and level III: "requiring very substantial support."

ASDs are relatively common, occurring in approximately 1 in 59 children based on surveillance data from the CDC in 2014. Males are overrepresented by about 4:1. About 31% of children with ASD also have an ID. A rare presumably pathogenic genetic variant can be found in 10%–30% of individuals with ASD, or up to 30%–40% who have had a "thorough clinical genetics evaluation" or have "complex autism" the term used for children with co-occurring microcephaly, seizures, dysmorphic features, or major congenital anomalies. This percentage may increase as newer techniques such as whole-exome sequencing become more widely used. There is a strong familial component. Parents of one child with ASD of unknown etiology have a 7%–23% chance of having a second child with ASD. The prevalence is higher if the second child is male or the affected child is female. The concordance rate among monozygotic twins is high but not absolute, and there is an increased incidence of speech, language, reading, attention, and affective disorders in family members of children with ASD. The genetics of ASD are complex and inheritance patterns appear to be multifactorial. ASD is a heterogeneous disorder for which single-gene disorders are not commonly found. As many as 2500 susceptibility genes have been identified. These genes often have variable penetrance and expression, as well as "pleiotropy" (one genotype associated with different neuropsychiatric or physical phenotypes such as ASD, seizures, or schizophrenia). In addition, epigenetics, gene-gene interactions, and gene-environment interactions may also play a role.

▶ Evaluation & Management

Children with ASD are often not diagnosed until age 3–4 years, when their differences in reciprocal social interaction and communication become more apparent. However, atypical communication and behavior can often be recognized in the first 12–18 months of life. The most common early characteristics are a consistent failure to orient to one's name, regard people directly, use gestures, and to develop speech. Even if one of these skills is present, it is often diminished in frequency, inconsistent, or fleeting. Sharing affect or enjoyment is an important precursor to social interaction. By 16–18 months a child should have "joint attention," which occurs when two people attend to the same thing at the same time. This is usually accomplished by shifting eye gaze, pointing, or saying "look." Toddlers should regularly point to get needs met ("I want that") and to show ("look at that") by 1 year of age. By 18 months a toddler should be able to follow a point, imitate others, and engage in functional play (using toys in the way that they are intended to be used, such as rolling a car, throwing a ball, or feeding a baby doll). Restricted

Table 3–4. Autism spectrum disorder.

Diagnostic Criteria

A. Persistent deficits in social communication and social interaction across multiple contexts, as manifested by the following, currently or by history (examples are illustrative, not exhaustive; see text):

1. Deficits in social-emotional reciprocity, ranging, eg, from abnormal social approach and failure of normal back-and-forth conversation; to reduced sharing of interests, emotions, or affect; to failure to initiate or respond to social interactions.

2. Deficits in nonverbal communicative behaviors used for social interaction, ranging, eg, from poorly integrated verbal and nonverbal communication; to abnormalities in eye contact and body language or deficits in understanding and use of gestures; to a total lack of facial expressions and nonverbal communication.

3. Deficits in developing, maintaining, and understanding relationships, ranging, eg, from difficulties adjusting behavior to suit various social contexts; to difficulties in sharing imaginative play or in making friends; to absence of interest in peers.

Specify current severity:

Severity is based on social communication impairments and restricted, repetitive patterns of behavior.

B. Restricted, repetitive patterns of behavior, interests, or activities, as manifested by at least two of the following, currently or by history (examples are illustrative, not exhaustive; see text):

1. Stereotyped or repetitive motor movements, use of objects, or speech (eg, simple motor stereotypies, lining up toys or flipping objects, echolalia, idiosyncratic phrases).

2. Insistence on sameness, inflexible adherence to routines, or ritualized patterns of verbal or nonverbal behavior (eg, extreme distress at small changes, difficulties with transitions, rigid thinking patterns, greeting rituals, need to take same route or eat same food every day).

3. Highly restricted, fixated interests that are abnormal in intensity or focus (eg, strong attachment to or preoccupation with unusual objects, excessively circumscribed or perseverative interests).

4. Hyper- or hyporeactivity to sensory input or unusual interest in sensory aspects of the environment (eg, apparent indifference to pain/temperature, adverse response to specific sounds or textures, excessive smelling or touching of objects, visual fascination with lights or movement).

Specify current severity:

Severity is based on social communication impairments and restricted, repetitive patterns of behavior.

C. Symptoms must be present in the early developmental period (but may not become fully manifest until social demands exceed limited capacities, or may be masked by learned strategies in later life).

D. Symptoms cause clinically significant impairment in social, occupational, or other important areas of current functioning.

E. These disturbances are not better explained by intellectual disability (intellectual developmental disorder) or global developmental delay Intellectual disability and autism spectrum disorder frequently co-occur; to make comorbid diagnoses of autism spectrum disorder and intellectual disability, social communication should be below that expected for general developmental level.

Reprinted with permission from the *Diagnostic and Statistical Manual of Mental Disorders*, 5th edition. (Copyright ©2013). American Psychiatric Association. All rights reserved.

interests and repetitive behaviors sometimes do not emerge until after age 2, but usually are present before age 2.

There is mounting evidence that a diagnosis of ASD can be made reliably by age 14 to 24 months and is typically stable over time. However, there are a small percentage of children who have been reliably diagnosed with ASD who no longer meet criteria after age 3. Because there is evidence that early intervention is particularly important for children with ASD, the Modified Checklist for Autism in Toddlers—Revised with Follow up (M-CHAT-R/F) was designed for children 16–30 months of age. It is a parent report measure with 20 yes/no questions. There are clinician-administered follow-up questions for those who screen positive. Just under 50% of children who screen positive initially (M-CHAT-R/F score ≥ 3) and after follow-up (M-CHAT-R/F score ≥ 2) will go on to be diagnosed with an ASD; however, 95% will have some type of developmental concern. Fewer children screen positive on the initial parent completed screen with the revised version of the M-CHAT. It can be downloaded

at https://m-chat.org/about.php. The STAT is a second-line screening tool. The STAT includes direct interaction with the child and was designed to differentiate children with ASD from children with developmental delay (See above).

An autism-specific screen is recommended at 18 months and at 24–30 months. The second screen is recommended because some of the symptoms may be more obvious in an older child and because many children with ASD experience a regression or plateau in skills between 12 and 24 months. Screening at 18 months could miss many of these children.

When behaviors raising concern for ASD are noted, the primary care provider should complete a thorough history and examination as discussed in the previous section on developmental disorders and the child should be referred to a team of specialists experienced in the assessment of ASD. At the same time, the child should also be referred to a local early intervention program and to a speech and language pathologist to begin therapy as soon as possible. If the diagnostic features are clearly present, a primary care provider may make a diagnosis of ASD to start autism-specific treatments as soon as possible. All children with ASD should have a formal audiology evaluation. A chromosomal microarray (CMA) and a DNA for fragile X syndrome are currently considered first-tier tests in children with ASD. Second-tier tests such as whole exome sequencing (WES), whole genome sequencing (WGS), and autism gene panels (comprised of up to 2500 genes associated with ASD) are being used more frequently and are used as first tier by some providers. Rare gene variants are considered to play a causal role in 10%–30% of individuals with ASD, and combinations of common gene variants are considered causal in 15%–50%. A more detailed description of genetic workup is beyond the scope of this chapter (see the American College of Medical Genetics and Genomics practice guidelines (2013), review of autism genetics by Vortsman et al (2017), or the review article by Yin and Schaaf (2017) for a more detailed discussion). Metabolic screening, lead level, and thyroid studies may also be done if indicated by findings in the history and physical examination. Although more evidence is needed, routine screening for metabolic disorders has been suggested including screening for mitochondrial disorders if there is evidence of an abnormal neurologic examination or lactic acidosis. An evaluation by a clinical geneticist should be offered to every family. A Wood lamp examination for tuberous sclerosis is also recommended. Neuroimaging is not routinely indicated even in the presence of mild/relative macrocephaly because children with autism often have relatively large heads. Neuroimaging should be done if microcephaly or focal neurologic signs are noted. Retrospective studies have found that approximately 20%–30% of children with ASD have a history of a plateau or loss of skills (usually only language and/or social skills) between 12 and 24 months of age. However, prospective longitudinal studies of high-risk infant siblings who are later diagnosed with ASD have found that up to 80% or more will have a regression/plateau in skills. This is found when the study evaluates skills that are present prior to 12 months of age: eye contact, social interest, and response to name. The loss is often gradual and can co-occur with atypical development. It usually occurs before the child attains a vocabulary of 10 words. If a child presents with regression, he or she may be referred to a child neurologist. Metabolic testing, magnetic resonance imaging (MRI) of the brain, and an overnight EEG to rule out electrical status epilepticus of sleep should be considered when there is a history of regression.

Early, intensive (up to 25 hours per week) behavioral intervention for children with ASD is essential for optimal cognitive and adaptive function. The cost of care and/or supports for an individual with ASD over a lifetime is estimated to be 1.4–2.4 million dollars per person. Intervention prior to 2.5–3.5 years of age can reduce lifetime costs by up to two-thirds. Naturalistic training models for children with ASD implemented before age 3 result in 90% of children attaining functional use of language compared to 20% who begin intervention after age 5. Interventions should include parent training and involvement in treatment; ongoing assessment, program evaluation, and programmatic adjustment as needed. Other interventions focus on communication, social interaction, and play skills that can be generalized in a naturalistic setting. Functional use of language leads to better behavioral and medical outcomes. Early detection and early intervention have a positive impact on children with ASDs. The Early Start Denver Model (ESDM) is one model for early intervention. In a recent study, 48 children 18–30 months of age were randomly assigned to ESDM for 20 h/wk for 2 years or community intervention. The group that received ESDM improved by a mean of 17.6 standard points on developmental testing (Mullen Scales of Early Learning with mean of 100 and standard deviation of 15) versus 7.0 points in the control group. Standard scores for adaptive function were maintained in the ESDM group and decreased in the control group. There are many models for this type of intervention and much variability in what is available in different areas of the country. Families should be encouraged to find a model that best suits the needs of the child and the family.

The primary care provider provides a medical home for children with ASD. This requires coordination of care. One role of the primary care provider is to ensure that medical concerns, such as sleep problems, feeding problems with limited diet, constipation often accompanied by withholding, and seizures, are addressed (see Table 3–5 for co-occurring conditions). Any worsening of behavior in a child with autism may be secondary to unrecognized medical issues such as pain from a dental abscess or esophagitis. Practice pathways for primary care providers for management of multiple co-occurring conditions in children with ASD have been developed through the Autism Speaks-Autism Treatment Network. A practice pathway for the identification, evaluation, and management of insomnia in children with ASDs has been developed. The pathway stresses the importance of screening for sleep

Table 3–5. Co-occurring conditions in children with ASD.

	Prevalence (%)
Sleep problems	50–80
Feeding/limited diet	70–90
Gastrointestinal problems	50–80
Obesity	~23
Seizures	7–38
Anxiety	~22–84
ADHD	~30–50
Irritability, aggression, dysregulation	~20–50
Self-injurious behavior	~30

issues in children with ASD and interviewing around comorbid medical conditions that may impact sleep. Individualizing behavior strategies/sleep hygiene for the child with ASD is also very important, often using creativity and flexibility to adapt strategies used for children with typical development. In addition, psychiatric comorbidities such as anxiety and ADHD are common in children with ASD and should be addressed by the PCP or a specialist. Psychopharmacologic management may be needed to address issues with attention, hyperactivity, anxiety, irritability, aggression, and other behaviors that have a significant impact on daily function. Multiple recent reviews of psychopharmacologic treatments are available. A clinical practice pathway for evaluation and medication choice for ADHD symptoms in children with ASD has also been developed. Children with ASD are less likely to respond to stimulants than children with typical development and are more likely to have side effects. Smaller doses and non-stimulants such as guanfacine should be considered especially in children younger than 5 years, children with IQ less than 50–70, severe anxiety, unstable mood, or low weight/poor appetite. A practice pathway for the management of irritability and problem behavior (aggression toward property, self, or others) in children with ASD was published in 2016. The pathway includes evaluation for conditions that may contribute to irritability and problem behavior: medical (sleep problems, medication side effects, and management of pain or discomfort associated with gastrointestinal, dental, or other medical conditions); impairment in ability to communicate; psychiatric (anxiety, depression); environmental stressors (psychosocial, inadequate educational and behavioral supports, change in routine); and unintentional reinforcement (attention, task avoidance, removal from overwhelming sensory stimuli, or tangible reward such as giving a snack to calm the child). A functional behavioral assessment (FBA) is helpful to characterize the behavior, and to identify the antecedent and consequence of the behavior. Reinforcing positive behavior, providing supports in the environment to assist with tolerance of triggers, providing replacement behaviors for negative behaviors, and avoiding reinforcement are strategies to improve behavior. Risperidone and aripiprazole are the only medications that have an FDA indication for treatment of irritability and aggression in children with ASD. The practice pathway recommended consideration of clonidine and N-acetylcysteine prior to atypical antipsychotics when there were no significant safety concerns necessitating urgent use of the medication that is most likely to improve behavior. These medications have limited evidence for safety and efficacy but appear to have fewer long-term side effects. Anxiety is common in children with ASD with approximately 40% having at least one anxiety disorder. Anxiety can be difficult to diagnose in children with ASD due to difficulty with communication and insight/recognition of feelings and due to some overlap with symptoms of ASD. Anxiety in children with ASD can present with irritability/externalizing behaviors and with dysregulation or symptoms that mimic ADHD. A recent review of diagnosis and management of anxiety in children with ASD recommended using feedback from multiple sources such as the child, parent, clinician, therapists, and school personnel when evaluating for the presence of an anxiety disorder. Randomized controlled trials (RCT) for treating anxiety in children with ASD show moderate efficacy with cognitive behavioral therapy. There have been no RCTs for medications to treat anxiety in children with ASD. Selective serotonin reuptake inhibitors (SSRI) may be used but clinicians should start with low doses and increase slowly while monitoring for behavioral activation. Alpha agonists and propranolol can sometimes be helpful as well. Many complementary and alternative modalities (CAM) treatments for autism have been proposed. As many as 33% of families use special diets and 54% of families use supplements for their child with ASD based on data from the Interactive Autism Network. Most have limited evidence regarding safety and efficacy. The review of CAM prepared by the AAP Task Force on Complementary and Alternative Medicine and the Provisional Section on Complementary, Holistic, and Integrative Medicine is particularly valuable.

AAP Autism Tool Kit: Autism: caring for children with autism spectrum disorders: a resource toolkit for clinicians, 2012. www.aap.org/autism.

Autism Speaks publishes many toolkits for families: http://www.autismspeaks.org.

Baio J et al: Prevalence of autism spectrum disorder among children aged 8 years—Autism and Developmental Disabilities Monitoring Network, 11 Sites, United States, 2014. MMWR Surveill Summ 2018 Apr 27;67(6):1–23 [PMID: 29701730].

Buie T et al: Recommendations for evaluation and treatment of common gastrointestinal problems in children with ASDs. Pediatrics 2010 Jan;125(Suppl 1):S19–S29 [PMID: 20048084].

Diagnostic and Statistical Manual of Mental Disorders. 5th ed. American Psychiatric Association; 2013.

Doyle CA, McDougle CJ: Pharmacotherapy to control behavioral symptoms in children with autism. Expert Opin Pharmacother 2012 Aug;13(11):1615–1629. doi: 10.1517/14656566.2012.674110. [PMID: 22550944].

FDA Center for Safety and Applied Nutrition: http://www.cfsan.fda.gov/%7Edms/ds-warn.html.

First Signs (educational site on autism): http://firstsigns.org.

Golnik A, Scal P, Wey A, Gaillard P: Autism-specific primary care medical home intervention. J Autism Dev Disord 2012; 42(6):1087–1093 [PMID: 21853373].

Hanen Centre (information on family-focused early intervention programs): http://www.hanen.org.

http://www.cdc.gov/ncbddd/autism/data.html.

Kemper KJ, Vohra S, Walls R; Task Force on Complementary and Alternative Medicine; Provisional Section on Complementary, Holistic, and Integrative Medicine: The use of complementary and alternative medicine in pediatrics. Pediatrics 2008;122: 1374–1386 [PMID: 19047261].

Learn the Signs, Act Early (website with resources and free handouts for families): www.cdc.gov/actearly.

Mahajan R et al; Autism Speaks Autism Treatment Network Psychopharmacology Committee: Clinical practice pathways for evaluation and medication choice for attention-deficit/hyperactivity disorder symptoms in autism spectrum disorders. Pediatrics 2012 Nov;130(Suppl 2):S125–S138. doi: 10.1542/peds.2012-0900J [PMID: 23118243].

Malow BA et al; Sleep Committee of the Autism Treatment Network: A practice pathway for the identification, evaluation, and management of insomnia in children and adolescents with autism spectrum disorders. Pediatrics 2012 Nov;130(Suppl 2):S106–S124. doi: 10.1542/peds.2012-0900I [PMID: 23118242].

M-CHAT-RF/Validation: http://pediatrics.aappublications.org/content/early/2013/12/18/peds.2013-1813.full.pdf+html.

McGuire K et al: Irritability and problem behavior in autism spectrum disorder: a practice pathway for pediatric primary care. Pediatrics 2016;137(Suppl 2):A136–S148 [PMID: 26908469].

NCCAM sponsors and conducts research using scientific methods and advanced technologies: http://nccam.nih.gov/. [The National Center for Complementary and Alternative Medicine (NCCAM) was established in 1998.]

Reynolds AM, Malow BA: Sleep and autism spectrum disorders. Pediatr Clin North Am 2011 Jun;58(3):685–698. doi: 10.1016/j.pcl.2011.03.009 [PMID: 21600349].

Schaefer GB, Mendelsohn NJ; Professional Practice and Guidelines Committee: Clinical genetics evaluation in identifying the etiology of autism spectrum disorders: 2013 guideline revisions. Genet Med 2013;15(5):399–407 [PMID: 23519317].

Vasa RA et al: Assessment and treatment of anxiety in youth with autism spectrum disorders. Pediatrics 2016;137(Suppl 2):S115–S123 [PMIID: 26908467].

Vorstman JAS, Parr JR, Moreno-De-Luca D, Anney RJL, Nurnberger JI Jr, Hallmayer JF: Autism genetics: opportunities and challenges for clinical translation. Nat Rev Genet 2017 Jun;18(6):362–376 [PMID: 28260791].

www.dsm5.org.

Yin J, Schaaf C: Autism genetics—an overview. Prenat Diagn 2017;37:14–30 [PMID: 27743394].

INTELLECTUAL DISABILITY

The field of developmental disabilities has been evolving and redefining the constructs of disability and using new terms to reflect that evolution. The term *mental retardation* is considered pejorative, demeaning, and dehumanizing; therefore, the term *intellectual disability* (ID) is used. DSM-5 uses the diagnosis *intellectual disability* (intellectual developmental disorder) and emphasizes the need for evaluation of adaptive function in addition to cognitive testing (IQ). The term *disability* is used by professionals and advocacy groups.

Recently, a rethinking of the construct of disability has emerged that shifts the focus from limitations in intellectual functioning and adaptive capability (a person-centered trait) to a human phenomenon with its source in biologic or social factors and contexts. The current view is a social-ecological conception of disability that articulates the role of disease or disorder leading to impairments in structure and function, limitations in activities, and restriction in participation in personal and environmental interactions. The term *intellectual disability*, which is consistent with this broader view, is increasingly being used and reflects an appreciation of the humanness and potential of the individual. The diagnostic criteria currently remain the same; however, the construct and context has changed.

Having noted this, it is important to acknowledge that significant delays in the development of language, motor skills, attention, abstract reasoning, visual-spatial skills, and academic or vocational achievements are associated with ID. Deficits on standardized testing in cognitive and adaptive functioning greater than two standard deviations below the mean for the population are considered to fall in the range of ID. The most common way of reporting the results of these tests is by using an intelligence quotient. The intelligence quotient is a statistically derived number reflecting the ratio of age-appropriate cognitive function and the child's actual level of cognitive function. A number of accepted standardized measurement tools, such as the *Wechsler Intelligence Scale for Children*, 5th Edition, can be used to assess these capacities. To receive a diagnosis of ID, a child must not only have an intelligence quotient of less than 70 but must also demonstrate adaptive skills more than two standard deviations below the mean. Adaptive function refers to the child's ability to function in his or her environment and can be measured by a parent or teacher interview using an instrument such as the Vineland Adaptive Behavior Scales. Cognitive function tends to predict academic success and adaptive function tends to predict level of independence in daily living skills. Levels of severity are based on adaptive function which determines the level of supports needed.

Global developmental delay (GDD) is the diagnosis used for children with significant delays in at least two developmental domains (cognitive, speech and language, gross and fine motor, social, and daily living skills). This diagnosis is typically used in children younger than 5 years due to poor predictive validity of cognitive testing prior to age 5–6 years. The diagnosis of GDD is also used in children older than 5 who cannot adequately participate in standardized testing.

The prevalence of ID is approximately 1%–3% in the general population and may vary by age. Mild levels of ID are more common and more likely to have a sociocultural cause than are more severe levels. Poverty, deprivation, or a lack of exposure to a stimulating environment can contribute to developmental delays and poor performance on standardized tests.

▶ Evaluation

Children who present with developmental delays should be evaluated by a team of professionals as described at the beginning of this section. For children 0–3½ years of age, the *Bayley Scales of Infant Development*, 3rd Edition, is a well-standardized developmental test. For children older than 3 years, standardized cognitive testing—such as the *Wechsler Preschool and Primary Scale of Intelligence*, 4th Edition; the *Wechsler Intelligence Scale for Children*, 5th Edition; the *Stanford-Binet V*; or the *Differential Abilities Scale*, 2nd Edition—should be administered to assess cognitive function over a broad range of abilities, including verbal and nonverbal scales. For the nonverbal patient, a scale such as the Leiter, 3rd Edition, will assess skills that do not involve language. A full psychological evaluation in school-aged children should include an emotional assessment if psychiatric or emotional problems are suspected. Such problems are common in children with developmental delays or ID.

The evaluation of a child with ID or GDD should include a complete medical and family history; as well as a physical examination, including head circumference, neurologic examination, dysmorphology examination, and skin examination for neurocutaneous stigmata. Clinicians should also screen for co-occurring conditions such as sleep problems, feeding problems, obesity, gastrointestinal disorders, and behavioral and psychiatric conditions. Families should be offered a genetics evaluation. Expert consensus recommends fragile X molecular genetic testing and CMA as the initial workup for ID/GDD unless the child's phenotype suggests more targeted testing, as in the case of Down or Williams syndrome. If there is a family history of multiple miscarriages suggesting a possible balanced translocation, a karyotype is recommended in addition to CMA. In children with ID/GDD, CMA will be positive about 6%–10% of the time and Fragile X testing will be positive in about 2%–3%. Families should be counseled about the possibility of CMA finding a copy number variation of unknown clinical relevance or one with clinical relevance unrelated to ID/GDD. A child with an abnormal result should receive genetic counseling from a medical geneticist or certified genetic counselor. Second-tier testing may include nonsyndromic X-linked ID genes and high-density X-CMA in males, and MECP2 deletion, duplication, and sequencing in females. Whole-exome sequencing may also be considered in patients for whom there is a high index of suspicion that a cytogenetic etiology exists but whose workup has been negative. An audiology evaluation should be completed, even if a child passed a hearing evaluation at birth. An ophthalmology examination should also be considered. An EEG should be considered if there are any concerns for seizures or a regression in skills.

Neuroimaging should be considered in patients with microcephaly, macrocephaly, seizures, loss of psychomotor skills, or specific neurologic signs such as spasticity, dystonia, ataxia, or abnormal reflexes. A lead level should be considered in children who frequently put toys or other nonfood items in their mouth. Thyroid function studies should be carried out in any patient who exhibits clinical features associated with hypothyroidism.

Screening for inborn errors of metabolism (IEM) has a relatively low yield (0%–5%) in children who present with developmental delay or ID. Most patients with IEM will be identified by newborn screening or present with specific indications for more focused testing, such as failure to thrive, recurrent unexplained illnesses, plateauing or loss of developmental skills, coarse facial features, cataracts, recurrent coma, abnormal sexual differentiation, arachnodactyly, hepatosplenomegaly, deafness, structural hair abnormalities, muscle tone changes, and skin abnormalities. However, treatable forms of IEMs may present later or without regression or plateau. There are currently 89 "treatable" types of IEM. Treatments may target improvement in symptoms, slowing progression of the disease, or providing support during an illness. While controversy over cost-benefit of screening for rare diseases exists, van Karnebeek et al proposed a two-tiered approach to screening for treatable IEM, which is based on "availability, affordability, yield, and invasiveness." Tier 1 tests/"nontargeted screening tests" include blood tests for lactate, ammonia, plasma amino acids, total homocysteine, acylcarnitine profile, copper, ceruloplasmin; and urine tests for organic acids, purines and pyrimidines, creatine metabolism, oligosaccharides, and glycosaminoglycans. Testing for 7- and 8-dehydrocholesterol to screen for Smith-Lemli Opitz syndrome and screening for congenital disorders of glycosylation may also be included in first-tier testing. Second-tier testing usually comprises tests that are the only tests for one disease or are more invasive such as tests of cerebrospinal fluid. AAP guidelines for tier 1 tests are somewhat different and include blood tests for plasma amino acids, total homocysteine, acylcarnitine profile; and urine tests for organic acids, purines and pyrimidines, creatine metabolism, oligosaccharides, and mucopolysaccharides. An app has been developed, which is helpful for identifying appropriate tests for treatable etiologies of ID/GDD.

Serial follow-up of patients is important as the physical and behavioral phenotype changes over time and diagnostic testing improves with time. Although cytogenetic testing may have been negative 10 years earlier, advances in high-resolution techniques may now reveal an abnormality that was not identified previously. A stepwise approach to diagnostic testing may also be more cost-effective so that the test most likely to be positive is done first.

► Management

Once a diagnosis of ID is made, treatment should include a combination of individual therapies, such as speech and language therapy, occupational therapy or physical therapy, special education support, behavioral therapy or counseling, and medical intervention, which may include psychopharmacology. To illustrate how these interventions work together, two disorders are described in detail in the next section.

Moeschler JB, Shevell M; Committee on Genetics: Comprehensive evaluation of the child with intellectual disability or global developmental delays. Pediatrics 2014 Sep;134(3):e903–e918 [PMID: 25157020].

Shapiro BK, Accardo PQ: *Neurogenetic Syndromes: Behavioral Issues and Their Treatment*. Baltimore, MD: Paul H Brookes; 2010.

The Arc of the United States (grassroots advocacy organization for people with disabilities): http://www.thearc.org.

van Karnebeek CD, Shevell M, Zschocke J, Moeschler JB, Stockler S: The metabolic evaluation of the child with an intellectual developmental disorder: diagnostic algorithm for identification of treatable causes and new digital resource. Mol Genet Metab 2014 Apr;111(4):428–438 [PMID: 24518794].

www.treatable-id.org.

SPECIFIC FORMS OF INTELLECTUAL DISABILITY & ASSOCIATED TREATMENT ISSUES

1. Fragile X Syndrome

The most common inherited cause of ID is fragile X syndrome, which is caused by a trinucleotide expansion within the fragile X mental retardation I (*FMR1*) gene (see Chapter 37). The full mutation is associated with methylation of the gene, which turns off transcription, resulting in a deficiency in the FMR1 protein. This protein regulates the metabotropic glutamate receptor 5. Fragile X syndrome includes a broad range of symptoms. Children with fragile X syndrome often present with developmental delays, social anxiety, hyperactivity, and difficult behavior in early childhood. Most males will have ID with symptoms such as gaze aversion, perseverative language, hand biting, and significant hypersensitivity to environmental stimuli. About 20% of males with fragile X syndrome meet criteria for an ASD. Girls are usually less affected by the syndrome because they have a second X chromosome that produces FMR1 protein. Approximately 30% of girls with the full mutation have cognitive deficits and a greater proportion have ADHD, anxiety, and shyness. Prominent ears; long, thin face; prominent jaw and forehead; joint hyperextensibility; and macroorchidism (in boys) are common; however, approximately 30% of children with fragile X syndrome may not have these features. The diagnosis should be suspected in any child with behavioral problems and developmental delays. As boys move into puberty, macroorchidism becomes more obvious, and facial features can become more elongated. Medical conditions commonly associated with fragile X syndrome include seizures, strabismus, otitis media, gastroesophageal reflux, mitral valve prolapse, and hip dislocation.

▶ Management

A variety of therapies are helpful for individuals with fragile X syndrome. Speech and language therapy can decrease oral hypersensitivity, improve articulation, enhance verbal output and comprehension, and stimulate abstract reasoning skills. Because approximately 10% of boys with the syndrome will be nonverbal at age 5 years, the use of augmentative communication techniques may be helpful. Occupational therapy can be helpful in providing techniques for calming hyperarousal to stimuli and in improving the child's fine and gross motor coordination and motor planning. If the behavioral problems are severe, it can be helpful to involve a behavioral psychologist who emphasizes positive reinforcement, time-outs, consistency in routine, and the use of both auditory and visual modalities, such as a picture schedule, to help with transitions and new situations.

Psychopharmacology can also be useful to treat ADHD, aggression, anxiety, or severe mood instability. Clonidine or guanfacine may be helpful in low doses to treat hyperarousal, tantrums, or hyperactivity. Stimulant medications such as methylphenidate and dextroamphetamine are usually beneficial by age 5 years and occasionally earlier. Relatively low doses are used because irritability is often a problem with higher doses.

Anxiety may also be a significant problem and the use of a SSRI is often helpful. SSRIs may also decrease aggression or moodiness, although in approximately 25% of cases, an increase in agitation or activation may occur. Aggression may become a significant problem in childhood or adolescence for individuals with fragile X syndrome. In addition to behavioral management, medication may be needed. Clonidine, guanfacine, or an SSRI may decrease aggression, and sometimes an atypical antipsychotic may be needed.

Clinical trials have begun in adults and children with fragile X syndrome to evaluate targeted treatments such as metabotropic glutamate receptor 5 antagonists and γ-aminobutyric acid (GABA) agonists. These medications have shown promising results in mouse models of fragile X syndrome.

An important component of management is genetic counseling. Parents should meet with a genetic counselor after the diagnosis of fragile X syndrome is made because there is a high risk that other family members are carriers or may be affected by the syndrome. A detailed family history is essential. Female carriers have a 50% risk of having a child with the fragile X mutation. Male carriers are at risk for developing FXTAS, a neurodegenerative disorder, as they age.

It is also helpful to refer a newly diagnosed family to a parent support group. Educational materials and parent support information may be obtained on the National Fragile X Foundation website.

Fragile X Research Foundation: http://www.fraxa.org.

Hersh JH, Saul RA; Committee on Genetics: Health supervision for children with fragile X syndrome. Pediatrics 2011;127(5): 994–1006 [PMID: 21518720].

Lozano R, Azarang A, Wilaisakditipakorn T, Hagerman RJ: Fragile X syndrome: a review of clinical management. Intractable Rare Dis Res 2016 Aug;5(3):145–157 [PMID: 27672537].

National Fragile X Foundation: http://www.FragileX.org.

van Karnebeek CD, Bowden K, Berry-Kravis E: Treatment of neurogenetic developmental conditions: from 2016 into the future. Pediatr Neurol 2016 Dec;65:1–13 [PMID: 27697313].

2. Fetal Alcohol Spectrum Disorders

Alcohol exposure in utero is associated with a broad spectrum of developmental problems, ranging from learning disabilities to severe ID. *Fetal alcohol spectrum disorder* (FASD) is an umbrella term describing the range of effects that can occur in an individual exposed to alcohol prenatally. The prevalence of FASD is about 1%–5%. Thus, physicians should always ask about alcohol (and other drug) intake during pregnancy. This is particularly true when evaluating a child presenting with developmental delays. The exact amount of alcohol consumption that leads to teratogenesis remains unclear. Thus, it is best to say that to avoid an FASD, abstention from all alcoholic drinks during pregnancy is essential. Features associated with FASD include facial anomalies, including short palpebral fissures (≤ 10th percentile), thin upper lip, and smooth philtrum (lip/philtrum guide is available for some races/ethniciites); poor prenatal or postnatal growth (height or weight ≤ 10th percentile); CNS abnormalities including poor brain growth (head circumference ≤ 10th percentile), morphogenesis, or neurophysiology (recurrent nonfebrile seizures with no other known etiology); neurobehavioral impairment; and major congenital cardiac, skeletal, renal, ocular, or auditory malformations or dysplasias.

New clinical consensus guidelines for the diagnosis or FASD were published in 2016 by Hoyme et al (Table 3–6). The new guidelines include definitions for prenatal alcohol exposure and neurobehavioral dysfunction, an updated definition of alcohol-related birth defects, a dysmorphology rating system, a lip/philtrum guide for North American white population, and an increase in cutoffs for head circumference, growth, and palpebral fissure percentile cutoffs from less than 3% to 10% or less in an effort to increase sensitivity for identifying children with FASD. The guidelines give criteria for documented prenatal alcohol exposure: six or more drinks per week for 2 weeks or more during the pregnancy; three or more drinks per occasion on two or more occasions during the pregnancy; documented social or legal problems related to alcohol; documented intoxication; positive alcohol-exposure biomarker during pregnancy or at birth such as fatty acid ethyl esters, phosphatidylethanol, or ethyl glucuronide; or increased prenatal risk on a validated screening tool. This does not mean that alcohol use during pregnancy in amounts lower than that guidelines recommend is safe. AAP's position is that no amount of alcohol during pregnancy is considered safe. The guidelines also recommend that a multidisciplinary team make the diagnosis and that

Table 3–6. Fetal alcohol spectrum disorders (FASD).

FASD Diagnoses	Clinical Features Required	Confirmed Prenatal Exposure
Fetal alcohol syndrome	1) At least 2 of 3 specified facial anomalies[a] 2) Poor prenatal or postnatal growth[b] 3) At least 1 CNS abnormality[c] 4) Neurobehavioral impairment	±
Partial fetal alcohol syndrome (with known exposure)	1) At least 2 of 3 specified facial anomalies[a] 2) Neurobehavioral impairment	+
Partial fetal alcohol syndrome (without known exposure)	1) At least 2 of 3 specified facial anomalies[a] 2) Growth deficiency or CNS abnormality[b,c] 3) Neurobehavioral impairment	−
Alcohol-related neurodevelopmental disorder	Neurobehavioral impairment (cannot be made before 3 y of age)	+
Alcohol-related birth defects	One major congenital malformation[d]	+

[a]Facial anomalies: short palpebral fissures (≤ 10th percentile), thin upper lip, and smooth philtrum (lip/philtrum guide is available for some races/ethniciites).

[b]Poor prenatal or postnatal growth (height or weight ≤ 10th percentile).

[c]Central nervous system (CNS) abnormalities: poor brain growth (head circumference ≤ 10th percentile), morphogenesis, or neurophysiology (recurrent nonfebrile seizures with no other known etiology).

[d]Major congenital anomalies, malformations, or dysplasias: cardiac, skeletal, renal, ocular, or auditory.

other disorders be considered or ruled out. Disorders with overlapping features include Cornelia deLange, 22q11.2 deletion syndrome, 15q duplication syndrome, Noonan syndrome, Dubowitz syndrome, and exposure to other teratogens such as valproic acid. The dysmorphology rating system was developed to aid in this process. The DSM-5 also added the diagnosis Neurobehavioral Disorder With Prenatal Alcohol Exposure (ND-PAE) while stipulating that more study is indicated.

▶ Management

Individuals with FASD typically have significant difficulty with complex cognitive tasks and executive function (planning, conceptual set shifting, affective set shifting, response inhibition, and fluency). They process information slowly. They may do well with simple tasks but have difficulty with more complex tasks. They have difficulty with attention and short-term memory. They are also at risk for social difficulties and mood disorders. Functional classroom assessments can be a very helpful part of a complete evaluation. Structure is very important for individuals with FASD. Types of structure that may be helpful are visual structure (color code each content area), environmental structure (keep work area uncluttered, avoid decorations), and task structure (clear beginning, middle, and end). Psychopharmacologic intervention may be needed to address issues such as attention and mood.

FASD: http://www.cdc.gov/ncbddd/fasd/facts.html.

FASD Center for Excellence: http://www.fasdcenter.samhsa.gov/.

Hoyme HE et al: Updated clinical guidelines for diagnosing fetal alcohol spectrum disorders. Pediatrics 2016 Aug;138(2) [PMID: 27464676].

National Organization on Fetal Alcohol Syndrome: http://www.nofas.org.

Petrenko CL, Alto ME: Interventions in fetal alcohol spectrum disorders: an international perspective. Eur J Med Genet 2017 Jan;60(1):79–91 [PMID: 27742482].

Williams JF, Smith VC; Committee on Substance Abuse: Fetal alcohol spectrum disorders, American Academy of Pediatrics Clinical Report. Pediatrics 2015;136(5):e1395–e1406 [PMID: 26482673].

REFERENCES

Print Resources

Carey WB, Crocker AC, Coleman WL, Elias ER, Feldman HM (eds): *Developmental Behavioral Pediatrics.* 4th ed. Philadelphia, PA: Elsevier Saunders; 2009.

Diagnostic and Statistical Manual of Mental Disorders. 5th ed. American Psychiatric Association; 2013.

Dixon SD, Stein MT (eds): *Encounters with Children; Pediatric Behavior and Development.* 4th ed. Philadelphia, PA: Mosby/Elsevier; 2006.

Parker S, Zuckerman B (eds): *Behavioral and Developmental Pediatrics: A Handbook for Primary Care.* Philadelphia, PA; London: Lippincott Williams & Wilkins; 2005.

Voigt RG, Macias MM, Myers SM: *American Academy of Pediatrics Developmental and Behavioral Pediatrics.* Elk Grove Village, IL: American Academy of Pediatrics; 2010.

Wolraich ML: *Disorders of Development and Learning: A Practical Guide to Assessment and Management.* 3rd ed. Ontario, Canada: BC Decker; 2003.

Wolraich ML et al: *Developmental-Behavioral Pediatrics: Evidence and Practice.* Philadelphia, PA: Mosby/Elsevier; 2008.

Web Resources

American With Disabilities Act Information: National Access for Public Schools Project: http://www.adaptenv.org.

Family Voices (website devoted to children and youth with special health care needs): http://www.familyvoices.org.

Hanen Centre (information on family-focused early intervention programs): http://www.hanen.org.

National Association of Developmental Disabilities Councils: http://www.naddc.org.

National Dissemination Center for Children with Disabilities: http://www.nichcy.org.

Parent Training and Information Centers: Alliance Coordinating Office: http://www.taalliance.org.

The American Psychiatric Association (APA) has proposed new diagnostic criteria in the *Diagnostic and Statistical Manual of Mental Disorders*, Fifth Edition (DSM-5) which were released in May 2013: www.psych.org, www.dsm5.org.

The Arc of the United States (grassroots advocacy organization for people with disabilities): http://www.thearc.org.

Title V Program Information: Institute for Child Health Policy: http://www.ichp.edu.s.

Adolescence

Amy E. Sass, MD, MPH

Molly J. Richards, MD

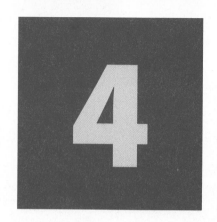

INTRODUCTION

Adolescence is a period of rapid physical, emotional, cognitive, and social development. Generally, adolescence begins at age 11–12 years and ends between ages 18 and 21. Most teenagers complete puberty by age 16–18 years; in Western society, however, for educational and cultural reasons, the adolescent period is prolonged to allow for further psychosocial development before the individual assumes adult status. The developmental passage from childhood to adulthood includes the following steps: (1) completing puberty and somatic growth; (2) developing socially, emotionally, and cognitively, and moving from concrete to abstract thinking; (3) establishing an independent identity and separating from the family; and (4) preparing for a career or vocation.

EPIDEMIOLOGY

Adolescents (ages 10–19) and young adults (ages 20–24) make up 21% of the population of the United States. Adolescence is typically a healthy time of life but several important public health and social problems can greatly affect morbidity and mortality during these years. Environmental factors are critical in challenging or supporting an adolescent's health. The positive development of young people facilitates their adoption of healthy behaviors. The behavioral patterns established during the developmental periods of adolescence help determine young people's current health status and their risk for developing chronic diseases in adulthood.

MORTALITY DATA

In 2017, there were 10,812 deaths among adolescents aged 15–19 years, representing a rate of 51.2 per 100,000. Cultural and environmental rather than organic factors pose the greatest threats to life. The three leading causes of death in adolescents aged 15–19 years were unintentional injury (38.5%), suicide (20.2%), and homicide (15.6%) (Figure 4–1). The primary cause of unintentional injury death was motor vehicle crashes (52%), followed by poisoning (36%), which includes prescription drug overdoses. Since 2000, deaths from opioid overdose have increased by over twofold among 15–24 year olds. Homicide deaths were predominantly attributable to firearms (88%), and firearms were also a leading mechanism of suicide death (47%). The mortality rate of adolescent males aged 15–19 was more than twice that of females (71.4 vs 30 per 100,000, respectively), largely due to higher rates of unintentional injury, homicide, and suicide death among males.

The rate of adolescent mortality has declined significantly since 2000. This decline may be largely attributable to decreases in unintentional injury. Motor vehicle crashes, the leading cause of death among teenagers in the United States, account for more than one-quarter of deaths in this age group. Death rates from motor vehicle accidents have decreased from 26.9/100,000 in 2000 to 16.6/100,000 in 2016.

The most concerning aspect about recent mortality data is the rise in suicide rates. Although the absolute increase has been relatively modest, the mortality rate from suicide in adolescents and young adults 15–24 years has risen steadily: 7.5/100,000 in 2010 to 13.2/100,000 in 2016, and 2013 was the first year in which suicide overtook homicide as the second leading cause of death in adolescents.

MORBIDITY DATA

Demographic and economic changes in the American family have had a profound effect on children and adolescents. In 2014, almost one (18%) in five adolescents was living in families with incomes below the federal poverty line. Adolescents living in poverty have worse academic outcomes

Causes of Death in 2017, ages 15–19 years

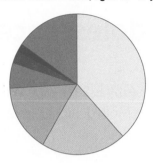

☐ Unintentional injuries (38.5%)

◻ Suicide (20.2%)

◻ Homicide (15.6%)

◼ Malignant neoplasms (5.7%)

◼ Diseases of heart (3.0%)

◼ Congenital malformations, deformations, and chromosomal abnormalities (1.9%)

◼ Other (15.1%)

▲ **Figure 4–1.** Leading causes of death (ages 15–19 years in 2017). (Reproduced with permission from Heron M. Deaths: Leading causes for 2017. National Vital Statistics Reports; vol 68 no 6. Hyattsville, MD: National Center for Health Statistics. 2019.)

and are more likely to suffer from behavioral health problems and engage in high-risk behaviors. Unfortunately, they are less likely to have access to health care. Significant racial and ethnic disparities also exist, with nearly 50% of non-Hispanic American Indian/Alaska Native children, 38.8% of non-Hispanic black children, and 34.3% of Hispanic children living in households with incomes below 100% of the poverty, compared to 12.8% of non-Hispanic white children. Single-parent families are particularly vulnerable to poverty. In 2013, 44.7% of children living in a mother-headed household experienced poverty, as did 21.3% of children living in a father-headed household, compared with 13.2% of children living in two-parent families.

The major causes of morbidity during adolescence are psychosocial and often correlate with poverty: unintended pregnancy, sexually transmitted infection (STI), substance abuse, smoking, dropping out of school, depression, running away from home, physical violence, and juvenile delinquency. High-risk behavior in one area is frequently associated with problems in another (Figure 4–2). For example, teenagers who live in a dysfunctional family (eg, alcoholism or physical or sexual abuse) are much more likely to be depressed than other teenagers. A depressed teenager is at greater risk for drug and alcohol abuse, academic failure, STIs, pregnancy, and suicide.

Early identification of the teenager at risk for these problems is important in preventing immediate complications and future associated morbidities.

D'Angelo LJ et al: Adolescents and driving: a position paper of the Society for Adolescent Health and Medicine. J Adolesc Health 2010;47(2):212214 [PMID: 20638018].

Heron M. Deaths: leading causes for 2017. National Vital Statistics Reports; vol. 68 no. 6. Hyattsville, MD: National Center for Health Statistics; 2019.

Kochanek KD, Murphy SL, Xu JQ, Tejada-Vera B: Deaths: final data for 2014. National vital statistics reports; vol. 65 no. 4. Hyattsville, MD: National Center for Health Statistics; 2016.

Teen Drivers: Fact Sheet: http://www.cdc.gov/motorvehiclesafety/teen_drivers/teendrivers_factsheet.html. Accessed March 15, 2017.

U.S. Census Bureau: Current Population Survey, Annual Social and Economic Supplement; 2014.

U.S. Department of Health and Human Services, Health Resources and Services Administration, Maternal and Child Health Bureau: *Child Health USA 2014*. Rockville, MD: U.S. Department of Health and Human Services; 2015.

Youth Risk Behavior Surveillance System (YRBSS): http://www.cdc.gov/HealthyYouth/yrbs/index.htm. Accessed March 15, 2017.

▼ PROVIDING A MEDICAL HOME FOR ADOLESCENTS

The American Academy of Pediatrics (AAP) developed the primary care medical home (PCMH) as a model of delivering primary care that is accessible, continuous, comprehensive, family-centered, coordinated, compassionate, and culturally effective to every child and adolescent. In addition, a PCMH for pediatric and adolescent patients is a family-centered

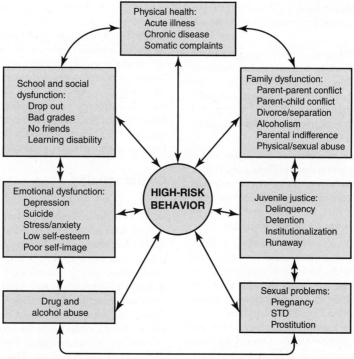

▲ **Figure 4–2.** Interrelation of high-risk adolescent behavior.

partnership within a community-based system that provides uninterrupted care with appropriate payment to support and sustain optimal health outcomes. PCMHs address preventive, acute, and chronic care from birth through transition to adulthood. Adolescent and young adults enrolled in PCMHs are more likely to receive multiple preventive services including immunizations, screening for STI, and contraception. Unfortunately, adolescents and young adults are the most likely age group to be uninsured and have the lowest rates of primary care use of any age group. Furthermore, health care coverage is disproportionately lacking by minority youth. Adolescents, therefore, frequently receive care within a variety of delivery systems with varying access to comprehensive care or specialty care and from a variety of providers with varied levels of training in adolescent care. They are also often seen in pediatric clinics that may not be geared toward teens, making them feel less comfortable and leading them not to access care or to access care in urgent care or emergency room settings. On the other hand, adolescents respond positively to settings and services that communicate sensitivity to their age and progressing autonomy and to age and developmentally appropriate health information pamphlets and educational materials about adolescent health and wellness issues.

Garcia-Huidobro D et al: Effect of patient-centered medical home on preventive services for adolescents and young adults. Pediatrics 2016;137(6) [PMID: 27244851].

Heron M: Deaths: leading causes for 2014. Natl Vital Stat Rep 2016;65(5) [PMID: 27376998].
Medical Home Initiatives for Children With Special Needs Project Advisory Committee: The Medical Home. Pediatrics 2002;110(1) [PMID: 12093969].

▼ RELATING TO THE ADOLESCENT PATIENT

Adolescence is one of the physically healthiest periods in life. The challenge of caring for most adolescents lies not in managing complex organic disease, but in accommodating the cognitive, emotional, and psychosocial changes that influence health behavior. The provider's initial approach to the adolescent may determine the success or failure of the visit. Although providers may have biases, they must learn to put them aside. Adolescents may initially present as closed off, angry, sullen or frustrated but this is often a result of feeling afraid, intimidated or judged. They may be acutely aware of being distrusted, disliked or not listened to as that may have been their experience in other medical settings. The primary care provider should behave simply and honestly, without an authoritarian or excessively professional manner. Because the self-esteem of many young adolescents is fragile, the provider must be careful not to overpower and intimidate the patient. To establish a comfortable and trusting relationship, the provider should strive to present the image of an ordinary person who has special training and skills.

Establishing rapport with an adolescent may not happen during the first visit but is easier to accomplish if the following tips are kept in mind:

1. Remember that the adolescent is your primary patient. Introduce yourself to the adolescent first and address your questions to him/her. This can be a significant change for adolescents and their families from a pediatrics model, where the parent/guardian does most of the talking. It is an important transition and may be initially difficult for both the adolescent and family.

2. Show genuine interest in the adolescent, as a person and as a patient, and point out positive accomplishments. Despite adolescents' reputation as "sullen," they are often very eager to talk about their interests and respond well when the many positive things in their lives are emphasized (instead of focusing on only negative aspects of their behaviors).

3. Treat adolescent concerns seriously and take time to listen. Providers often get frustrated with teenagers' complaints of pain (vague and overstated). Adolescents' reports of severe pain may be attempts to be taken seriously rather than indicating that they are critically ill. Take time listening to adolescents and explain your findings. Many teens just want to be reassured that they are "normal" or that they do not have a serious illness. They may have specific concerns (eg, about an STI or cancer) that they will not disclose unless you ask. Taking time to discuss their concerns and to give reassurance when appropriate often prevents unnecessary testing and multiple repeat visits (especially to emergency rooms).

4. Use a developmentally oriented approach. While it is important to cover areas of sexuality, family, peer group, and drug use, the clinician should keep in mind the developmental stage of the adolescent. For example, it would not be appropriate to ask a 12-year-old prepubertal male the same questions in the same manner as for an 18-year-old fully mature male.

Because the onset and termination of puberty vary from child to child, chronologic age may be a poor indicator of physical, physiologic, and emotional maturity. In communicating with an adolescent, the provider must be sensitive to the adolescent's developmental level, recognizing that outward appearance and chronologic age may not be an accurate reflection of cognitive development.

THE STRUCTURE OF THE VISIT

The Interview

The first few minutes may determine the entire outcome of the interview. Starting the interview with neutral, nonpersonal questions can help the adolescent feel more comfortable and defuse anxiety. Having the adolescent and parent/guardian complete a paper or electronic health history questionnaire prior to the start of the appointment is useful to identify health concerns and collect past medical and surgical historical data, medication use and medication allergies, family history of medical and psychiatric problems, and a review of systems (Figure 4–3). The questionnaire should also contain social history questions that assess healthy behaviors as well as risk behaviors that could be detrimental to health. Adolescents often report health concerns and report behaviors on a questionnaire that they may not articulate verbally. Ideally, the adolescent should complete his/her questionnaire privately without the parent/guardian seeing the responses, particularly about confidential risk behaviors.

Confidentiality

Confidentiality protection is an essential component of health care for adolescents. Assurance of confidential care is needed for adolescents to access health care services. It is also an important part of the provider-patient relationship. Adolescents are more likely to disclose sensitive information, have positive perceptions of care, feel more actively involved in their own healthcare, and return for future care if physicians assure confidentiality. Despite the importance of confidentiality, many teens do not identify their primary care physicians as sources of confidential care.

Families remain crucial to supporting teens' health and psychosocial development. They offer vital information about the home environment, school, medical and family history, and a myriad of other issues that adolescents may not know or may not offer. Beginning in early adolescence, providers should routinely spend at least part of each visit alone with each patient to convey to the young patients and their parents that this is a standard part of adolescent health care and begins the slow transition process into adulthood (independent provider-patient relationships). It is important to discuss with teens and their parents the importance of confidentiality, but that confidentiality does not extend to life-threatening concerns. Although parents hold complex views regarding adolescent confidentiality, studies have shown that parents usually support the idea that adolescents should have the opportunity to openly communicate with their provider alone. At the age of 18 years, it is appropriate to ask adolescents whether or not they want parents involved in their medical visits.

It is important to remind adolescents that sensitive issues are discussed because they are important for health. At the beginning of the interview, it is useful to say, "I am going to ask you some personal questions. This is not because I am trying to pry into your personal business, but because these questions are important to your health. I want to assure you that what we talk about is confidential, just between the two of us, except in certain circumstances. If you tell me that you are hurting yourself or someone else is hurting you or if you intend to hurt someone else, we will have to share this information with your parents (or guardians)."

Revised 04/21/2015

CONFIDENTIAL

ADOLESCENT HEALTH HISTORY CONSULTATION

This information is **CONFIDENTIAL**. Its purpose is to help your doctor give you better care. We request that you fill out the form completely, but you may skip any question that you do not wish to answer.

NAME _____DATE _____

First   Middle Initial   Last

BIRTHDATE _____**AGE** _____ Name you like to be called _____

1. Why did you come to the clinic today? _____
_____

MEDICAL HISTORY

2. Are you allergic to any medicines? .... YES   NO
   If Yes: Name of Medicine _____

3. Are you taking any medicines now? .... YES   NO
   If Yes: Name of Medicine _____
   _____

4. Were you born prematurely or did you have any serious problems as an infant? .... YES   NO
5. Do you have any chronic health conditions? .... YES   NO
   Condition _____
   _____
   _____

6. Have you ever been hospitalized? .... YES   NO
   Have you had any serious or sports related injuries? .... YES   NO
   If YES to any of the above: Describe the reason/problem:
   DATE   **REASON/PROBLEM**
   _____   _____
   _____   _____
   _____   _____

7. Have you ever had any of the following infections, illnesses or problems?
   If Yes: Write down your age when the infection, illness or problem started:

	Yes	No	Age			Yes	No	Age
Chickenpox	___	___	___		Pneumonia	___	___	___
Epilepsy/Seizures	___	___	___		Mononucleosis	___	___	___
Migraines	___	___	___		Tuberculosis	___	___	___
Heart Disease	___	___	___		Arthritis	___	___	___
Asthma	___	___	___		Scoliosis	___	___	___
Acne	___	___	___		Anemia	___	___	___
Stomach Problems	___	___	___		Diabetes	___	___	___
Urine Infections	___	___	___		Thyroid Disease	___	___	___
Hepatitis	___	___	___		Cancer	___	___	___
Sexually Transmitted	___	___	___		Eczema	___	___	___
Diseases					Other_____			___

SCHOOL INFORMATION

8. Are you in school?.. YES   NO
   If Yes: Name of school _____
   a. What grade are you in? (ie, 7th, 8th, 9th, 10th, 11th, 12th, College) _____
   b. What grade do you usually get in English? (ie, A, B, C, D, E, F) _____
   c. What grade do you usually get in math? _____
   d. How many days were you absent from school last semester? _____
   If No: e. Why did you leave? _____
   f. What is the highest grade you completed? _____

9. Have you ever been suspended or expelled? .... YES   NO
10. Have you ever dropped out of school? .... YES   NO

▲ **Figure 4–3.** Adolescent medical history questionnaire. (Reproduced with permission from Kroenke K, Spitzer RL, Williams JB: The PHQ-9: validity of a brief depression severity measure. J Gen Intern Med 2001 Sep;16(9):606–613.)

Revised 04/21/2015

JOB/CAREER INFORMATION

11. Are you working? .... YES   NO

      If yes, what is your job? _____

      How many hours do you work each week? _____

12. What are your future plans or career goals? _____

FAMILY INFORMATION

13. Who do you live with? (Check all that apply)

_____ Both natural parents	_____ Stepmother	_____ Brother(s)/ages: _____
_____ Mother	_____ Stepfather	_____ Sister(s)/ages: _____
_____ Father	_____ Guardian	_____ Foster home: _____
_____ Adoptive parents	_____ Alone	_____ Other: Explain: _____

14. Were you adopted? .... YES   NO

15. Have there been any changes in your family since your last visit here such as:

_____ Marriage	_____ Serious illness	_____ Births
_____ Separation	_____ Loss of job	_____ Deaths
_____ Divorce	_____ Move to a new house	_____ Other

      If Checked: Please explain: _____

16. Father's/stepfather's occupation or job: _____
      Mother's/stepmother's occupation or job: _____

17. How satisfied are you with how well you get along with your family?

     _____ A lot   _____ Somewhat   _____ Not much   _____ Not at all

18. How much tension or conflict is there in your family?

     _____ None   _____ A little   _____ A fair amount   _____ A lot

19. Have you ever lived in foster care or an institution? .... YES   NO

SELF-INFORMATION

20. What do you like about yourself? _____

21. What do you do best? _____

22. If you could, what would you like to change about your life or yourself? _____

_____

_____

23. List any habits you would like to break: _____

24. Have you lost or gained any weight in the last year? .... YES   NO

      If Yes: (circle) Gained **OR** Lost   How much? _____

25. In the past year, have you tried to lose weight or control your weight by vomiting, taking diet pills or laxatives, or starving yourself? .... YES   NO

26. Do you feel you have any friends you can count on? .... YES   NO

27. Have you ever run away from home overnight? .... YES   NO

28. Have you gotten into any trouble because of your anger/temper? .... YES   NO

29. Have you been in a pushing/shoving fight during the past 6 months? .... YES   NO

30. Is there a gun in your house? .... YES   NO

31. Have you ever threatened or been threatened with a knife/gun/or other weapon? .... YES   NO

32. Have you ever seen someone shot or stabbed? .... YES   NO

33. Have you ever been physically or sexually abused? .... YES   NO

▲ **Figure 4–3.** (*Contiuned*)

Revised 04/21/2015

HEALTH CONCERNS

In the past two (2) weeks, how often have you been bothered by the following problems?
Check one:

	Not At All (0)	Several Days (1)	More Than Half the Days (2)	Nearly Every Day (3)
1. Feeling down, depressed, irritable, or hopeless?				
2. Little interest or pleasure in doing things?				
3. Trouble falling asleep, staying asleep, or sleeping too much?				
4. Poor appetite, weight loss, or overeating?				
5. Feeling tired, or having little energy?				
6. Feeling bad about yourself – or feeling that you are a failure, or that you have let yourself or your family down?				
7. Trouble concentrating on things like school work, reading, or watching TV?				
8. Moving or speaking so slowly that other people could have noticed? Or the opposite – being so fidgety or restless that you were moving around a lot more than usual?				
9. Thoughts that you would be better off dead, or of hurting yourself in some way?				

Kroenke K, Spitzer RL. The PHQ-9: a new depression and diagnostic severity measure. Psychiatr Ann 2002;32:509–521.

34. Do you have any questions or concerns about any of the following? (Check all that apply)

_____ Too tall	_____ Wheezing	_____ School problems
_____ Too short	_____ Cough	_____ Future plans/job
_____ Overweight	_____ Breathing problems	_____ Worried about parents
_____ Underweight	_____ Breasts	_____ Family violence/abuse
_____ Blood pressure	_____ Stomach pain	_____ Tobacco, drugs, alcohol
_____ Trouble sleeping	_____ Nausea/vomiting	_____ Feeling down/depression
_____ Tiredness/fatigue	_____ Diarrhea, Constipation	_____ Feeling nervous/anxiety
_____ Dizziness/passing out	_____ Headaches/migraines	_____ Dating
_____ Eyes/vision	_____ Muscles or joints pain	_____ Sexuality
_____ Ears/hearing/earaches	_____ Penis or vagina	_____ Sex
_____ Bloody nose	_____ Period problems	_____ Birth control
_____ Hay fever/allergies	_____ Urination problems	_____ Sexually transmitted disease
_____ Frequent colds	_____ Wetting the bed	_____ Pregnancy/parenting
_____ Mouth/teeth	_____ Acne	_____ Other (explain) _____
_____ Neck/back pain	_____ Rash	
_____ Chest pain	_____ Diet/appetite	
_____ Heart	_____ Eating disorder	

HEALTH BEHAVIOR INFORMATION

35. Do you wear a seatbelt every time you ride in a car? .... YES   NO

36. Have you ever been the driver in an auto accident? .... YES   NO

37. Have you ever driven after drinking alcohol or when high? .... YES   NO

38. Do you ever smoke cigarettes or use chewing tobacco? .... YES   NO

39. Do you ever use marijuana? (inhaled, vaped or edible products)? .... YES   NO

40. In the past month, did you get drunk or very high on beer, wine, or other alcohol? .... YES   NO

▲ **Figure 4–3.** (*Continued*)

Revised 04/21/2015

41. Have you ever used street drugs (speed, cocaine, acid, crack, etc.)? .... YES NO
42. Does anyone in your household smoke? .... YES NO
43. Does anyone in your family have a problem with drugs or alcohol? .... YES NO
44. Have you ever been in trouble with the police or the law? .... YES NO
45. Have you begun dating? .... YES NO
46. Do you currently have a boyfriend or girlfriend? .... YES NO
      If Yes: How old is he/she? _____
47. Do you think you might be gay, lesbian, bisexual or transgender? .... YES NO
48. Have you ever had sex (sexual intercourse)? .... YES NO
      If Yes: Are you (or your partner) using any birth control to prevent pregnancy? .... YES NO
      Have you ever been treated for gonorrhea or chlamydia or other sexually transmitted diseases? .... YES NO
      During your life, with how many people have you had sexual intercourse?... _____
49. Have you been taught how to use a condom correctly? .... YES NO
50. Do you have any other personal problems that you would like to discuss with the doctor but would rather not write down?
.... YES NO

SPORTS
51. Have you ever been diagnosed with a concussion? .... YES NO
52. Do you have severe headaches with exercise? .... YES NO
53. Have you ever passed out or felt light headed or dizzy with exercise? .... YES NO
54. Do you have chest pain with exercise? .... YES NO
55. Have you ever experienced an irregular heart beat with exercise? .... YES NO
56. Do you have a family history of early cardiac death (before age 50) or sudden death with exercise? .... YES NO
57. Have any family members been diagnosed with long QT syndrome or Marfan Syndrome? .... YES NO
58. Have you ever been told that you can't participate in sports due to a medical problem? .... YES NO
For males only
59. If you have had sex, do you use a condom every time? .... YES NO
60. Have you ever fathered a child? .... YES NO
For females only
61. How old were you when your periods began? _____
62. What date did your last period start? _____
63. Are your periods regular (once a month)?... YES NO
64. Do you have painful or excessively heavy periods? .... YES NO
65. Have you ever had a vaginal infection or been treated for a female reproductive health problem? .... YES NO
66. Do you think you might be pregnant? .... YES NO
67. Have you ever been pregnant? .... YES NO
FAMILY HISTORY
68. Have any of your relatives (parents, grandparents, uncles, aunts, brothers or sisters), living or deceased, had any
    of the following problems? If the answer is **YES**, please state their relationship to you.

	YES	RELATIONSHIP		YES	RELATIONSHIP
ADHD			High Blood Pressure		
Alcoholism			High Cholesterol		
Anemia			Kidney Disease		
Anxiety			Mental Retardation		
Asthma			Migraine Headaches		
Bipolar			Obesity		
Blood Clots			Seizure Disorder/Epilepsy		
Cancer			Stomach Disorders		
Depression			Stroke		
Diabetes			Suicide		
Drug Problems			Thyroid Disease		
Eating Disorder			Tuberculosis		
Heart Attack			Other		

▲ **Figure 4–3.** (*Contiued*)

Berlan ED, Bravender T: Confidentiality, consent and caring for the adolescent patient. Curr Opin Pediatr 2009;21:450–456.

SAM Position Statement: Confidential health care for adolescents: position paper of the society for adolescent medicine. J Adolesc Health 2004;35:160–167.

The HEADSS Assessment

Health care providers who see adolescents must be able and willing to take a developmentally appropriate psychosocial history. The HEADSS (Home, Education/employment, Activities, Drugs, Sexuality, and Suicide/depression) assessment acronym is useful for organizing this history (Table 4–1). Ideally the sensitive aspects of the history should be obtained with the adolescent alone. Providers may need to be flexible with history taking to allow for this to happen after the parent/guardian leaves the examination room.

Asking About Abuse & Violence

Using a generalizing scenario to discuss these difficult topics can be helpful. For example, "Some of my patients have told me that their parents may get very angry and hit them. Does anything like this happen in your family?" Questions also should be asked about dating violence and sexual abuse/assault; for example, "Have you ever been pressured or forced to have sex when you didn't want to?" It is also important to ask teens about their personal history of being a victim

Table 4–1. HEADSS assessment.

	Questions	Reasons
Home and environment	Where do you live, and who lives there with you? How do you get along with your parents, siblings? Is there anything you would like to change about your family?	Home life has an important impact on an adolescent's ability to succeed. It is important to know whether they live in a safe and supportive environment.
Education and employment	Are you in school? What are you good at in school? What do you like about school? What is hard for you? What grades do you get? How much school did you miss last year? Why? Have you ever been suspended or expelled? Why? How do you get along with your teachers/peers? Have you been involved with bullying? What are your future plans/goals?	School is likely the primary social activity in the adolescent's life. Problems in school, academically or socially, can be an indicator of other issues (medical and/or psychosocial). Future goals and plans can be important motivators in high-risk behavior change.
Activities	Tell me about your relationships with friends? What do you (or your friends) do for fun? Are you involved in any extracurricular activities or activities in your community? Do you have a job? How many hours a week do you work? Do you play sports or exercise? What activities do you do and how often? How many hours of screen time do you have per day?	Disengagement and withdrawal can be a sign of other problems.
Drugs	Many young people experiment with marijuana, drugs, smoking cigarettes, or drinking alcohol. Have you or your friends ever tried them? What did you try? How often do you use these things? Do you ever operate a vehicle under the influence of drugs or alcohol or ride with an impaired driver?	Positive answers can lead to more in-depth evaluation of use (see Chapter 5).
Sexuality/ Relationships	Are you in a romantic relationship or have you been in one in the past? Tell me about your partner. Do you feel you have a healthy relationship? How do you define a healthy relationship? Have you (or your friends) had sex? How do you feel about it?	It is important to normalize sexual feelings even in the absence of sexual activity. Teens not having sex can still have conversations about sexuality, including masturbation. It is also important to avoid assumptions about patients' sexual orientation and to be nonjudgmental about sexual practices.
Suicide/ depression	Have you had long periods of time where you felt down, depressed, or irritable? Have you ever thought about death, dying or suicide?	Psychosocial history should reveal indicators of depression.

HEADSS, Home, Education/employment, Activities, Drugs, Sexuality, and Suicide/depression.

and/or perpetrator of violence, such as fighting, arrests, and involvement with law enforcement, gang involvement, use of weapons and firearms, violence issues among peers, and the presence and security of weapons/firearms in the home, as these factors may place the adolescent at a higher risk of unintentional injury and death.

Physical Examination

A complete physical examination should be conducted at adolescent annual health supervision visits (Table 4–2). During early adolescence, teenagers may be shy and modest. The examiner should address this concern directly, because it can be allayed by acknowledging the uneasiness verbally and by explaining the purpose of the examination. For example, "Many boys that I see who are your age are embarrassed to have their penis and testes examined. This is an important part of the examination for a couple of reasons. First, I want to make sure that there aren't any physical problems, and second, it helps me determine if your development is proceeding

Table 4–2. Physical examination of adolescents.

A complete physical examination is included as part of every health supervision visit. The following examination components are especially important in the adolescent patient:

Vital signs: Measure and plot height and weight on CDC clinical growth charts (http://www.cdc.gov/growthcharts/clinical_charts.htm). Calculate and plot BMI on CDC clinical growth charts. Measure BP and evaluate elevated BP by age and height percentiles to determine the degree of hypertension per the National Heart, Lung, and Blood Institute BP tables for children and adolescents (http://www.nhlbi.nih.gov/files/docs/guidelines/child_tbl http://www.nhlbi.nih.gov/files/docs/guidelines/child_tbl.pdf).

Skin: Inspect for acne, acanthosis nigricans, atypical nevi, tattoos, piercings, and signs of abuse or self-inflicted injury.

Spine: Examine back for scoliosis with Adam's forward bend test (also assess for leg length discrepancy).

Breast
  Female: Assess SMR. Conduct clinical breast examination for breast disorders if there is a reported concern
  Male: Examine breasts if inspection shows breast hypertrophy and gynecomastia vs other breast pathology is suspected.

Genitalia
  Female: Perform visual inspection of external genitalia to assess SMR, anatomic and skin abnormalities and signs of STIs (warts, vesicles, pathologic vaginal discharge).
  Male: Perform visual inspection for circumcision status, SMR, and signs of STIs (warts, vesicles, penile discharge). Examine testicles for abnormalities (hydroceles, hernias, varicoceles, or masses).

BMI, body mass index (height [cm]/weight [kg²]), BP, blood pressure; CDC, Centers for Disease Control and Prevention; SMR, sexual maturity rating; STI, sexually transmitted infection.

normally." This also introduces the subject of sexual development for discussion. Chaperones may be needed for parts of the physical examination (breast, genitals). The American Academic of Pediatrics recommends chaperones for genital exams but also states the use of a chaperone should be a shared decision between the patient and the physician. Adolescents should be asked if they prefer their parent/guardian is in the room during the physical examination. Attempts should be made to keep the examination as discrete as possible by keeping any parts of the body that are not being examined covered by a sheet, gown, or clothing.

A pictorial chart of sexual development is useful for showing the patient how development is proceeding and what changes to expect. Figure 4–4 shows the relationship between height, penis and testes development, and pubic hair growth in the male, and Figure 4–5 shows the relationship between height, breast development, menstruation, and pubic hair growth in the female. Although teenagers may not admit that they are interested in this subject, they are usually attentive when it is raised. It can be helpful for them to know that puberty progresses in a predictable order, but that the rate of progression is variable. This discussion is particularly useful in counseling teenagers who lag behind their peers in physical development.

▼ GUIDELINES FOR ADOLESCENT PREVENTIVE SERVICES

ADOLESCENT SCREENING

The American Medical Association *Guidelines for Adolescent Preventive Services* (GAPS) and the AAP's *Bright Futures: Guidelines for Health Supervision of Infants, Children, and Adolescents* cover health screening and guidance, immunization, and health care delivery. The goals of these guidelines are to (1) deter adolescents from participating in behaviors that jeopardize health; (2) detect physical, emotional, and behavioral problems early and intervene promptly; (3) reinforce and encourage behaviors that promote healthful living; and (4) provide immunization against infectious diseases. The guidelines recommend that adolescents between ages 11 and 21 years have annual routine health visits. Health services should be developmentally appropriate and culturally sensitive. Confidentiality between patient and provider should be ensured. Table 4–3 lists the current adolescent screening guidelines from the AAP, the U.S. Department of Health and Human Services, and the Centers for Disease Control and Prevention.

CDC Screening Guidelines: 2015 Sexually Transmitted Diseases Treatment Guidelines: https://www.cdc.gov/std/tg2015/special-pops.htm#adol
http://pediatrics.aappublications.org/content/early/2016/03/18/peds.2016-0065

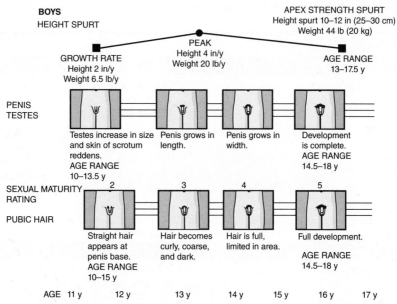

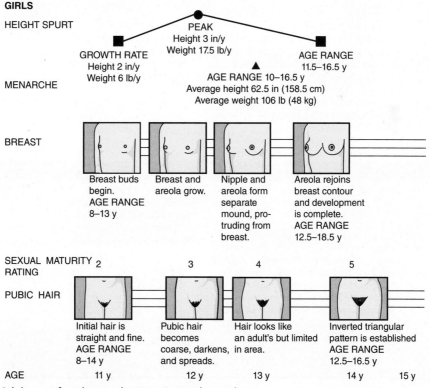

▲ Figure 4–4. Adolescent male sexual maturation and growth.

▲ Figure 4–5. Adolescent female sexual maturation and growth.

Table 4–3. Adolescent Screening Guidelines.

	AAP	USPSTF	CDC
Cancer			
Cervical cancer	Per USPSTF guidelines.	Start cytology screening at age 21 y and screen every 3 y if cytology normal.	Screen women age 21–29 y every 3 y with cytology. Women with HIV should be screened within 1 y of sexual activity or initial HIV diagnosis using conventional or liquid-based cytology; testing should be repeated 6 mo later.
Testicular cancer	AAP Bright Futures recommends testicular examination for hernia, varicocele, or epididymitis.	Screening with physician examination or self-examination is not recommended.	
Cardiovascular (CV)			
Blood pressure	Check annually.	Current evidence is insufficient to assess the balance of benefits and harms of screening for primary hypertension in asymptomatic children and adolescents to prevent subsequent cardiovascular disease in childhood or adulthood.	
Lipid levels	Based on integrated guidelines for CV Health and Risk Reduction in Children and Adolescents https://www.nhlbi.nih.gov/health-pro/guidelines/current/cardiovascular-health-pediatric-guidelines • 9–11 y: Universal lipid screen with nonfasting non-HDL cholesterol or fasting lipid profile. • 12–17 y: Obtain fasting lipid profile if FH newly positive, parent with dyslipidemia, any other RFs or high-risk condition. • 18–21 y: Measuring nonfasting non-HDL cholesterol or fasting lipid profile in all once.	Current evidence is insufficient to assess the balance of benefits and harms of screening for lipid disorders in children and adolescents age ≤ 20 y.	
General Health			
Obesity	Screen BMI annually.	Screen children aged ≥ 6 y for obesity and refer as appropriate for comprehensive, intensive behavioral intervention to promote improvement in weight status.	
Diabetes	Children ≥ 10 y with ≥ 2 RFs should be screened every 2 y. RFs include: BMI > 85 percentile, FH of T2DM, high-risk ethnic group, signs of insulin resistance (dyslipidemia, hypertension, polycystic ovarian syndrome and acanthosis nigricans).		
Scoliosis	Females at age 10 and 12 y. Males once at age 13 or 14 y.	Recommends against the routine screening of asymptomatic adolescents for idiopathic scoliosis.	

(Continued)

Table 4–3. Adolescent Screening Guidelines. (*Continued*)

	AAP	USPSTF	CDC
Anemia	Assess annually for RFs (diet low in iron-rich foods, history of iron deficiency anemia, excessive menstrual bleeding). Screen those with RFs with HgB or HCT at minimum.		Screen all nonpregnant women every 5–10 y, starting in adolescence.
Behavioral Health			
Depression	Screen youth ≥ 12 y using the PHQ2 or other tools available in the GLAD-PC toolkit: http://www.glad-pc.org/	Screen adolescents aged 12–18 y for major depressive disorder. Screening should be implemented with adequate systems in place to ensure accurate diagnosis, effective treatment, and appropriate follow-up.	
Substance use	Screen youth ≥ 11 y with CRAFFT screening tool: http://www.ceasar-boston.org/CRAFFT/index.php	Current evidence is insufficient to assess the balance of benefits and harms of primary care–based behavioral interventions to prevent or reduce illicit drug or nonmedical pharmaceutical use in children and adolescents. This recommendation applies to children and adolescents who have not already been diagnosed with a substance use disorder.	
Tobacco use	Screen youth ≥ 11 y	Clinicians should provide interventions, including education or brief counseling, to prevent initiation of tobacco use among school-aged children and adolescents.	
Sexually Transmitted Diseases			
Chlamydia Trachomatis	Per CDC	Screen sexually active females. Repeat screening if sexual history reveals new or persistent RFs since the last negative test result.	Screen all sexually active women < 25 y annually. Retest ≥ 3 mo after treatment.
Nesseria Gonorrhoeae	Per CDC	Screen sexually active females. Repeat screening if sexual history reveals new or persistent RFs since the last negative test result.	Screen all sexually active women < 25 y annually. Retest approximately 3 mo after treatment. Screen at least annually for sexually active MSM at sites of contact (urethra, rectum, pharynx) regardless of condom use. Screen every 3–6 mo if increased risk.

(Continued)

Table 4–3. Adolescent Screening Guidelines. (*Continued*)

	AAP	USPSTF	CDC
HSV	Per CDC.	Routine serologic screening not recommended.	Consider HSV serology in men and women coming for STD evaluation especially if they have multiple sexual partners.
			Consider HSV serology in MSM if infection status unknown and history of previously undiagnosed genital infection.
HIV	Adolescents should be screened for HIV according to USPSTF recommendations once between the ages of 15 and 18 y, making every effort to preserve confidentiality of the adolescent.	Screen adolescents > 15 y at least once. Repeat screening or screen younger adolescents if RFs for infection present.[a]	Screen all adolescents who seek evaluation and treatment for STD.
			Screen sexually active MSM at least annually if HIV status is unknown or negative and the patient or his sex partner(s) have had more than one sex partner since most recent HIV test.
Syphilis		Screen for syphilis infection in people who are at increased risk for infection (MSM, persons living with HIV, history of incarceration, history of commercial sex work).	Screen sexually active MSM at least annually and every 3–6 mo if at increased risk of infection.[a]

AAP, American Academy of Pediatrics; BMI, body mass index; CDC, Centers for Disease Control and Prevention; FH, family history; HCT, hematocrit; HDL, high-density lipoprotein; HgB, hemoglobin; HIV, human immunodeficiency virus; HSV, herpes simplex virus; MSM, men who have sex with men; RF, risk factor; STD, sexually transmitted disease; T2DM, type 2 diabetes mellitus; USPSTF, US Preventive Services Task Force.
[a]History of STDs, multiple sex partners, inconsistent condom use, sex work, illicit drug use, patients seeking care in high-prevalence settings (eg, clinics located in higher-prevalence geography [prevalence ≥ 1%], STD clinics, correctional facilities, homeless shelters, tuberculosis clinics, clinics serving MSM, adolescent clinics with high STD rates).

Recommendations for Preventive Pediatric Health Care; Bright Futures/American Academy of Pediatrics: https://www.aap.org/en-us/documents/periodicity_schedule.pdf. Accessed date: March 20, 2017.

U.S. Department of Health and Human Services, Health Resources and Services Administration, Maternal and Child Health Bureau: *Child Health USA 2012*. Rockville, MD: U.S. Department of Health and Human Services; 2013.

U.S. Preventive Services Task Force, Published Recommendations. https://www.uspreventiveservicestaskforce.org/BrowseRec/Index?age=Pediatric,Adolescent. Accessed date: March 20, 2017.

Youth Risk Behavior Surveillance System: (YRBSS): http://www.cdc.gov/HealthyYouth/yrbs/index.htm

PROMOTING HEALTHY BEHAVIORS

Motivational Interviewing

The majority of adolescent morbidity and mortality is related to unhealthy behaviors and is preventable. The role of a pediatric provider in adolescent visits is to screen for unhealthy behaviors and promote healthy behaviors. Practitioners may report feeling frustrated with adolescents because they are resistant to change or "do not want help." Primary care in adolescents has historically been delivered as "anticipatory guidance" in a lecture-based format. This model may not be very effective, especially in adolescence. In contrast, motivational interviewing (MI) has been shown to effectively change several health behaviors in adolescents, including tobacco use, substance use, and control of type 1 diabetes.

MI is a counseling style that guides patients toward behavior change by helping to resolve ambivalence. Adolescents may know that certain behaviors are bad for them (smoking, drug use, unprotected sex, binge eating) but also have reasons they do not want to change (enjoy the "high", use with peers, etc) and/or are not confident in their ability to change. MI promotes collaboration between provider and patient, with the patient ultimately deciding what goals he/she would like to achieve and how to achieve them (Table 4–4).

MI starts with a provider assessing a patient's motivation and readiness for change. Some providers do this by asking

Table 4–4. Motivational interviewing skills.

Skill	Description
Evoke Motivations and Commitment to Change	
Ask open-ended questions	*Tell me about…., Describe for me…., Tell me more….*
Explore patients' reason for change	*"Have you ever tried to quit? Why did you try to quit?* *Do you see yourself smoking marijuana in 5 y? Why not?*
Evoke change talk and reflect it back	*"What are the good things about smoking marijuana? What are the not-so-good things about smoking marijuana?"* *When you look at this list of pros and cons, what do you think?"*
Use readiness and confidence "rulers"	*"On a scale from 0 to 10 where 10 is the most and 0 is the least, where would you say you are now?"*
Affirm and accept	Affirmations are statements that provide positive feedback about goal-oriented behaviors or personal characteristics or strengths, reinforcing autonomy and self-efficacy. *"I can see that you are upset about being here, but I'd like to tell you that I am impressed that you chose to come here anyway."*
Listen reflectively	Reflective listening shows that you are listening and understanding. Patient: *"I know it really upsets my parents but it just isn't that big a deal."* Provider: *"You don't think it's such a big deal but you know that your parents are really worried about you and it sounds like you feel badly about that."*
Express empathy	*"You've worked hard on this problem and it's frustrating you that it's not much better yet."*
Develop discrepancies	*"You do not want to quit marijuana because most of your friends smoke and you think it helps you relax, and, at the same time, you know it makes your parents angry and you want to play football and are worried it will get you in trouble with your coach."*
Roll with resistance	Accept patients' statements of resistance rather than confronting them directly: Patient: *"Most of the people I know get high. Why do we even have to talk about it?"* Provider: *"It's hard to figure out why we have to talk about it when it is all around you. Kind of makes you wonder how you could be the only one who is having problems with pot."*
Avoid righting reflex	Avoid the desire to fix things, direct persuasion, and confrontation.
Support self-efficacy	Increase patient perception about his/her skills, resources and abilities that the patient may access to achieve desired goals. *"You say you quit before so you may have good ideas about how to do it again. Tell me what they are."*
Encourage autonomy	Convey that responsibility for making change resides with the patient or parent who must decide if, how, and when change will occur.
Encourage self-direction	Patient: *"I know I made a mistake, but the hoops that they are making me jump through are getting ridiculous."* Provider: *"You don't like what others are asking you to do, but so far you are choosing to follow-through with what they are asking. It takes a lot of fortitude to do that. Tell me what motivates you."*

a patient to indicate on a scale from 0 to 10 how important it is for him/her to change, how ready he/she is to start making a change, and how confident he/she is in his/her ability to make a change. If a patient says he/she feels it is 5/10 important, the provider can then ask why it is so important. Why is it not a 3 or a 4? This provides the patient with the opportunity to tell the provider why it is important to change, rather than telling the provider convincing reasons why it is not important to make changes. This is called "change talk" and is a hallmark of MI. The provider can then ask what it would take to make the number higher. The provider should avoid asking the adolescent why it is *not* important, as that will put the patient in the position of indicating reasons he/she cannot or does not want to change.

Other components of MI are to "roll with resistance" and resist the "righting reflex." Providers often seek to fix problems or challenge patients' stated barriers, causing patients to come up with new reasons they cannot make changes. If the provider is the only one arguing in favor of change, patients and families can become even more entrenched in not changing. They begin arguing against the provider and effectively convincing themselves of reasons that they cannot change. Instead of progressing into this conflictual stance, the provider should focus on the patient's own individual goals and reflect on the patient's challenges.

The guiding principles of MI are to express empathy toward patients and meet them where they are in the process of change, as many patients are ambivalent. The process of MI seeks to progress through stages of change (precontemplative, contemplative, preparation, action), but with the understanding that the provider cannot force a patient into a stage he/she is not ready for. Instead of imposing goals and being disappointed or frustrated when these goals are not accomplished, a patient needs to make his/her own goals if motivated to do so, even if the goals seem insignificant to the provider. It is acceptable to take time to work through this process as long as there is no acute danger. In situations of medical or psychiatric instability, MI is not an appropriate tool.

Developing discrepancies is another MI strategy. This can be done by asking a patient about his/her goals for health and the future and how he/she feels these goals align with current health and/or behaviors (eg, failing school and wanting to go to medical school). Supporting self-efficacy and using the patient's and his/her family's own resources and solutions to break down barriers to change are important, as they will bring longer lasting change. Most essential is for the provider to listen reflectively, avoid confrontation, and roll with resistance. It can be frustrating to see patients putting their health at risk, but it is important, when appropriate, to meet patients where they are in their readiness to change. This allows them to find their internal motivations, encourages autonomy, and establishes collaboration between patients and providers in achieving healthy and attainable goals.

Barnes AJ, Gold MA: Promoting healthy behaviors in pediatrics. Pediatr Rev 2012 Sep;33:9:e57–e68 [PMID: 22942370].

Brief Counseling for Marijuana Dependence—A Manual for Treating Adults http://www.integration.samhsa.gov/clinical-practice/sbirt/brief_counseling_for_marijuana_dependence.pdf. Accessed March 27, 2017.

TRANSITION TO ADULT CARE

It is important for health care providers to have a process for transitioning primary care and subspecialty medical care of adolescents to adult providers. This process should incorporate education, guidance and step-wise planning. Patients should be actively involved in this process to maximize their self efficacy. Even older adolescents and young adults need assistance from providers and their families as they enter the adult health care system.

The AAP clinical report, "Supporting the Health Care Transition From Adolescence to Adulthood in the Medical Home" describes three key components of transition: provider readiness, family readiness, and youth readiness.

- Provider readiness refers to practice policies that allow for a smooth transition. Policies addressing transition should be discussed with patients and families early and regularly and patients should be assessed for transition readiness (often with use of checklists).

- Family readiness: The medical home must understand and address family needs during transition, as the process of transition can be complex and emotional. This includes education and communication with families about the transition process and differences between pediatric and adult models of care.

- Patient readiness: The patient must be the driver in the transition process. It is important to empower and encourage youth to assume increasing responsibility for their own health care. Documenting patient readiness and steps needed to achieve a successful transition are important in this process (eg, ability to schedules one's own medical appointments, obtain medications, know medications and doses).

The final step of transition occurs when the provider implements an adult care model or the patient transfers to an adult medical home provider. Direct communication between pediatric and adult providers is essential for a smooth transition, especially in the case of patients with special needs.

American Academy of Pediatrics, American Academy of Family Physicians, and American College of Physicians, Transitions Clinical Report Authoring Group: Supporting the health care transition from adolescence to adulthood in the medical home. Pediatr 2011;128;182; http://www.gottransition.org/

▼ GROWTH & DEVELOPMENT

PUBERTY

Pubertal growth and physical development are a result of activation of the hypothalamic-pituitary-gonadal axis in late childhood. Before puberty, pituitary and gonadal hormone levels are low. It is estimated that at least 50% of pubertal timing is determined by genetics, and ethnicity is one such factor. Nutrition and general health can also affect the pubertal process. At onset of puberty, the inhibition of gonadotropin-releasing hormone in the hypothalamus is removed, allowing pulsatile production and release of the gonadotropins, luteinizing hormone (LH), and follicle-stimulating hormone (FSH). In early to middle adolescence, pulse frequency and amplitude of LH and FSH secretion increase, stimulating the gonads to produce estrogen or testosterone.

In females, FSH stimulates ovarian maturation, granulosa cell function, and estradiol secretion. LH is important in ovulation and also is involved in corpus luteum formation and progesterone secretion. Initially, estradiol inhibits the release of LH and FSH. Eventually, estradiol becomes stimulatory, and the secretion of LH and FSH becomes cyclic. Estradiol levels progressively increase, resulting in maturation of the female genital tract and breast development.

In males, LH stimulates the interstitial cells of the testes to produce testosterone. FSH stimulates the production of spermatocytes in the presence of testosterone. The testes also produce inhibin, a Sertoli cell protein that inhibits the secretion of FSH. During puberty, circulating testosterone levels increase more than 20-fold. Levels of testosterone correlate with the physical stages of puberty and the degree of skeletal maturation.

PHYSICAL GROWTH

A teenager's weight almost doubles in adolescence, and height increases by 15%–20%. During puberty, major organs double in size, except for lymphoid tissue, which decreases in mass. Before puberty, there is little difference in the muscular strength of boys and girls. Muscle mass and muscle strength both increase during puberty, with maximal strength lagging behind the increase in mass by many months. Boys attain greater mass and strength, and strength continues to increase into late puberty. In boys, the lean body mass increases from 80% to 85% of body weight to approximately 90% at maturity. Muscle mass doubles between 10 and 17 years. By contrast, in girls, the lean body mass decreases from approximately 80% of body weight in early puberty to approximately 75% at maturity. Although motor coordination lags behind growth in stature and musculature, it continues to improve as strength increases.

There is great variability in the timing and onset of puberty and growth, and psychosocial development does not always parallel physical changes. Skeletal maturation correlates well with growth and pubertal development. Chronologic age, therefore, may be a poor indicator of physiologic and psychosocial development. The pubertal growth spurt begins nearly 2 years earlier in girls than in boys. Girls reach peak height velocity between ages 11½ and 12 years, and boys between ages 13½ and 14 years. Linear growth at peak velocity is 9.5 cm/y ± 1.5 cm in boys and 8.3 cm/y ± 1.2 cm in girls. Pubertal growth lasts about 2–4 years and continues longer in boys than in girls. By age 11 years in girls and age 12 years in boys, 83%–89% of ultimate height is attained. An additional 18–23 cm in females and 25–30 cm in males is achieved during late pubertal growth. Following menarche, height rarely increases more than 5–7.5 cm. Males' ability to grow 2 more years prior to peak height velocity and their greater average velocity allows them to leave puberty an average of 13 cm taller than females despite entering puberty at similar heights.

SEXUAL MATURATION

Sexual maturity rating (SMR) is useful for categorizing genital development. SMR staging includes age ranges of normal development and specific descriptions for each stage of pubic hair growth, penis, and testis development in boys, and breast maturation in girls. Figures 4–4 and 4–5 show this chronologic development. SMR 1 is prepuberty and SMR 5 is adult maturity. In SMR 2, the pubic hair is sparse, fine, nonpigmented, and downy; in SMR 3, the hair becomes pigmented and curly and increases in amount; and in SMR 4, the hair is adult in texture but limited in area. The appearance of pubic hair precedes axillary hair by more than 1 year.

Teenagers began entering puberty earlier in the last century because of better nutrition and socioeconomic conditions. Although the first measurable sign of puberty in girls is the beginning of the height spurt, the first conspicuous sign is usually development of breast buds between 8 and 11 years. A large longitudinal study reported a median age of thelarche of 8.8 years for black, 9.3 years for Hispanic, and 9.7 years for Caucasian and Asian girls. Higher BMI was also associated with earlier attainment of SMR 2. Although breast development usually precedes growth of pubic hair, the order may be reversed. Female breast development follows a predictable sequence. Small, raised breast buds appear in SMR 2. In SMR 3, the breast and areolar tissue generally enlarge and become elevated. The areola and nipple form a separate mound from the breast in SMR 4, and in SMR 5 the areola assumes the same contour as the breast. A common concern for girls at this time is whether the breasts will be of the right size and shape, especially because initial breast growth is often asymmetrical.

The growth spurt may precede breast and pubic hair development by approximately one year. Girls gain their peak height velocity of 8.3 cm/year during SMR 2, at an average age of 11.5 years. Girls who mature early will reach peak height velocity sooner and attain their final height earlier. Girls who mature later will attain a greater final height because of the longer period of growth before the growth spurt ends. Final height is related to skeletal age at onset of puberty as well as genetic factors. The height spurt correlates more closely with breast developmental stages than with pubic hair stages.

In the United States, the average age at menarche is 12.53 years but varies by race and ethnicity: 12.57 for non-Hispanic whites; 12.09 years in non-Hispanic blacks, and 12.09 for Mexican-American girls. Menarche usually occurs during SMR 3 or 2 years after breast budding. The range is variable, from 9 to 15 years, and depends on many factors including race and ethnicity as well as nutrition and genetics.

The first sign of puberty in the male (SMR 2), usually between ages 10 and 12 years, is an increase in testicular volume to 4 mL or 2.5 cm in the long axis, accompanied by reddening and thickening of the scrotal skin. Pubic hair development may be the earliest noticeable sign of puberty and may appear anytime between ages 10 and 15 years. The penis begins to grow significantly a year or so after the onset of testicular and pubic hair development. In SMR 3, the penis lengthens, and in SMR 4, the penis enlarges in overall size and the scrotal skin becomes pigmented. The first ejaculation, along with evidence of spermatarche, usually occurs at in SMR 3. The height spurt begins at age 11 years but increases rapidly between ages 12 and 13 years, with the peak height velocity reached at age 13½ years (SMR 3–4). As with girls, there appears to be racial and ethnic differences in pubertal onset. Mean ages for genital development are 10.14 years for non-Hispanic white boys, 9.14 years for black boys and 10.04 years for Hispanic boys. The completion of genital development, similar to girls, is not significantly different. The average length of time is 3 years but can range from 2 to 5 years, and the average age at completion is 15 years. The development of axillary hair, deepening of the voice, and the development of chest hair in boys usually occur in mid-puberty, about 2 years after onset of growth of pubic hair. Facial and body hair begin to increase at age 16–17 years. The duration of pubertal development lasts longer in boys than girls and may not be completed until age 18 years.

Biro FM, et al: Onset of breast development in a longitudinal cohort. Pediatr 2013;132(6):1019–1027 [PMID: 24190685]

Herman-Giddens ME et al: Secondary sexual characteristics in boys: data from the Pediatric Research in Office Settings Network. Pediatr 2012;130(5):e1058e1068 [PMID: 23085608].

Rosenfield RL, Lipton RB, Drum ML: Thelarche, pubarche, and menarche attainment in children with normal and elevated body mass index. Pediatrics 2009;123:84 [PMID: 19117864].

Susman EJ et al: Longitudinal development of secondary sexual characteristics in girls and boys between ages 9½ and 15½ years. Arch Pediatr Adolesc Med 2010;164(2):166173 [PMID: 20124146].

PSYCHOSOCIAL DEVELOPMENT

Adolescence is a period of progressive individuation and separation from the family. Adolescents must learn who they are, decide what they want to do, and identify their personal strengths and weaknesses. Because of the rapidity of physical, emotional, cognitive, and social growth during adolescence, it is useful to divide psychological development into three phases (Table 4–5). Early adolescence is roughly from 10 to 13 years of age; middle adolescence is from 14 to 16 years; and late adolescence is from 17 years and later.

Early Adolescence

Early adolescence is characterized by rapid growth and development of secondary sex characteristics. Body image, self-concept, and self-esteem fluctuate dramatically. Concerns about how personal growth and development deviate from that of peers may be great, especially in boys with short stature or girls with delayed breast development or delayed menarche. Although there is a certain curiosity about sexuality, young adolescents generally feel more comfortable with

Table 4–5. Stages of adolescent development.

Stages of Adolescence	Cognitive Development	Social-Emotional Development
Early adolescence: ~10–13 y	• Growing capacity for abstract thought • Interested in present, limited thought to future • Intellectual interests expand • Deeper moral thinking	• Struggle with sense of identity • Worries about being normal, feels awkward about self and body • Realize parents aren't perfect; increased conflict with parents • Desire for independence • Tendency to return to "childish" behavior especially when stressed • Moodiness • Rule and limit testing • Greater interest in privacy
Middle adolescence: ~14–16 y	• Continued growth of capacity for abstract thought • Greater capacity for setting goals • Interest in moral reasoning • Thinking about meaning of life	• Intense self-involvement • Continued adjustment to changing body and worries about being normal • Distance from parents, drive for independence • Peers gain importance • Feelings of love and passion
Late adolescence: ~ ≥17 y	• Ability to think ideas through • Ability to delay gratification • Examination of inner experiences • Increased concern for future • Continued interest in moral reasoning	• Firmer sense of identity • Increased emotional stability • Increased concern for others • Increased independence and self-reliance • Peer relationships remain important • Development of more serious relationships

Data from American Academy of Child and Adolescent's Facts for Families (2008).

members of the same sex. Peer relationships become increasingly important. Young teenagers still think concretely and cannot easily conceptualize about the future. They may have vague and unrealistic professional goals, such as becoming a movie star or professional athlete.

Middle Adolescence

During middle adolescence, as rapid pubertal development subsides, teenagers become more comfortable with their new bodies. Intense emotions and wide swings in mood are typical. Although some teenagers go through this experience relatively peacefully, others struggle. Cognitively, the middle adolescent moves from concrete thinking to formal operations and abstract thinking. With this new mental power comes a sense of omnipotence and a belief that the world can be changed by merely thinking about it. Sexually active teenagers may believe they do not need to worry about using contraception because they can't get pregnant ("it won't happen to me"). With the onset of abstract thinking, teenagers begin to see themselves as others see them and may become extremely self-centered. Because they are establishing their own identities, relationships with peers and others are narcissistic. Experimenting with different self-images is common. As sexuality increases in importance, adolescents may begin dating and experimenting with sex. Peers determine the standards for identification, behavior, activities, and clothing and provide emotional support, intimacy, empathy, and the sharing of guilt and anxiety during the struggle for autonomy. The struggle for independence and autonomy is often a stressful period for both teenagers and parents.

Late Adolescence

During late adolescence, the young person generally becomes less self-centered and more caring for others. Social relationships shift from the peer group to the individual. Dating becomes much more intimate. By 10th grade, 40.9% of adolescents (41.9% of males and 39.6% of females) have had sexual intercourse, and by 12th grade, this has increased to 62.3% (59.6% of males and 65% of females). Abstract thinking allows older adolescents to think more realistically about their plans for the future. This is a period of idealism; older adolescents have rigid concepts of what is right or wrong.

Sexual Orientation

In addition to rapid physical changes during puberty, adolescence is also characterized by emotional and sexual changes during which sexual discovery, exploration, and experimentation are part of the process of incorporating sexuality into one's identity. Sexual orientation is the preferred term used when referring to an individual's physical and/or emotional attraction to the same and/or opposite gender. Typically,

sexual orientation emerges before or early in adolescence. Gender identity is knowledge of one's self as being male or female and gender expression is the outward expression of being male or female. Gender expression may or may not be congruent with one's sex assigned at birth based on the appearance of external genitalia. Awareness of gender identity happens in early childhood, and by age 3 years, children can identify themselves as a boy or a girl, and by age 4 years, gender identity is stable. It is not uncommon for younger children to experience and display gender role confusion. For some children, interpersonal conflict can develop with awareness that he/she identifies with traits of the opposite gender. This conflict about gender may lead to dysphoria and dislike about the parts of themselves that are different from the gender that they identify with. Many children will resolve their dysphoria by the time they complete adolescence, and others who continue to feel dysphoria may identify as transgender persons, individuals whose gender identity or gender expression differs from their birth sex. The term *transition* refers to the period of time when transgender persons are learning how to cross-live socially as members of the sex category different from their birth-assigned sex. The transition period may include medical treatment with hormones and/or gender affirmation surgery to allow transgender persons to modify their bodies so they may live full time as members of the sex category different from their birth assigned sex.

Individuals who self-identify as heterosexuals are attracted to people of the opposite gender; homosexual individuals self-identify as being attracted to people of the same gender, and bisexual adolescents report attraction to both genders. Generally, self-identified homosexual people are referred to as "gay" if male and "lesbian" if female. Sexuality and identity formation are dynamic processes and adolescents who struggle with their sexual attractions are referred to as "questioning." Sexuality is inherently more complex than these simple definitions; for example, many self-identified heterosexual youth report having sex with same-gendered partners. Many young people also resist definitions and terminology regarding their sexuality. Overall, adolescents who self-identify as lesbian, gay, bisexual, transgender, and/or questioning (LGBTQ) comprise a sexual minority population.

Heterosexism is the societal expectation that heterosexuality is the norm and that LGBTQ youth are "abnormal." Some LGBTQ youth may feel that it is necessary to hide their sexuality from family and friends, and this nondisclosure can be ultimately damaging to a developing self-image. Parents' and other family members' reactions to a young person "coming out" or declaring his/or her self-identified sexuality vary, and parental rejection of sexual minority youth is, unfortunately, common.

Although many LGBTQ youth are resilient, they are a vulnerable population and experience many health disparities that providers should be aware of. Population studies and public health data demonstrate that sexual minority youth are at increased risk of tobacco and substance abuse; being victims of violence including bullying and physical and sexual abuse; increased rates of STI and HIV acquisition; school avoidance and failure; depression and suicide; homelessness; and other crises. As part of providing culturally effective care to reduce health disparities experienced by sexual minority youth, providers should ask their patients what their preferred pronouns are pertaining to their gender identity for the provider to use and encourage adolescents to discuss any questions they have about their sexual orientation and/or sexual behaviors. Providers will optimize opportunities to learn about youths' behaviors by creating an accepting environment and providing nonjudgmental and confidential care. For transgender youth, providers should affirm their feelings of gender dysphoria and provide referrals to qualified mental health and medical professionals for more information about gender transition. Providers can also be sources of support for parents and family members of sexual minority youth. Organizations such as Parents, Families and Friends of Lesbians and Gays (www.pflag.org) or Gay Family Support (www.gayfamilysupport.com) can provide valuable resources. Nonprofit organizations such as the United Way and local LGBTQ and sexual health advocacy organizations are additional resources for sexual minority youth and their families.

Brewster KL, Tillman KH: Sexual orientation and substance use among adolescents and young adults. Am J Public Health 2012;102(6):11681176 [PMID: 22021322].

Gutgesell ME, Payne N: Issues of adolescent psychological development in the 21st century. Pediatr Rev 2004;25:79 [PMID: 14993515].

Institute of Medicine, Committee on Lesbian, Gay, Bisexual, and Transgender Health Issues and Research Gaps and Opportunities: *The Health of Lesbian, Gay, Bisexual, and Transgender People: Building a Foundation for Better Understanding.* Washington, DC: National Academic Press; 2011.

Levine DA et al: Office-based care for lesbian, gay, bisexual, transgender, and questioning youth. Pediatrics 2013;132(1):e297e313 [PMID: 23796737].

Marshal MP et al: Suicidality and depression disparities between sexual minority and heterosexual youth: a meta-analytic review. J Adolesc Health 2011;49(2):115123 [PMID: 21783042].

ADOLESCENT GYNECOLOGY & REPRODUCTIVE HEALTH

BREAST EXAMINATION

The breast examination should be part of the routine physical examination in girls as soon as breast budding occurs. The preadolescent will thus accept breast examination as a routine part of health care, and the procedure can serve as an opportunity to offer reassurance and education. The breast examination begins with inspection of the breasts for symmetry and SMR stage. Asymmetrical breast development is common in young adolescents and is generally transient, although 25% of women may continue to have asymmetry as adults. Organic causes of breast asymmetry include unilateral breast hypoplasia, amastia, absence of the pectoralis major muscle, and unilateral juvenile hypertrophy, in which there is rapid overgrowth of breast tissue usually immediately after thelarche.

The breast examination is performed with the patient supine and the ipsilateral arm placed behind the head. Using flat finger pads, the examiner palpates the breast tissue in concentric circles starting at the outer borders of the breast tissue along the sternum, clavicle, and axilla and then moving in toward the areola. The areola should be compressed gently to check for nipple discharge. Supraclavicular and infraclavicular and axillary regions should be palpated for lymph nodes.

Teaching adolescents to perform breast self-examinations is controversial. Experts have recommended adolescent self-examination as a means of helping them develop comfort with their changing bodies and for future cancer detection. Experts have also questioned whether self-examination might, in fact, result in anxiety, increased physician visits, and unnecessary invasive procedures, since the vast majority of breast masses in adolescents are benign. The U.S. Preventive Services Task Force found little evidence that teaching or performing routine breast self-examination in adolescents reduces breast cancer mortality. Despite the lack of data for or against teaching or performing breast self-examinations during adolescence, there is some consensus that young women at increased risk of breast cancer—adolescents with a history of malignancy, adolescents who are at least 10 years postradiation therapy to the chest, and adolescents 18–21 years of age whose mothers carry the *BRCA1* or *BRCA2* gene should perform monthly breast self-examinations after each menstrual period.

BREAST MASSES

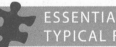

ESSENTIALS OF DIAGNOSIS & TYPICAL FEATURES

▶ Primary breast cancer during adolescence is exceptionally rare.

▶ Fibroadenomas are the most common breast masses.

▶ Typical features of fibroadenomas include 2–3 cm, nontender, rubbery, smooth, well-circumscribed, mobile mass.

The majority of breast masses in adolescents are benign (Tables 4–6 and 4–7). Rare malignancies of adolescent girls include juvenile secretory carcinoma, intraductal carcinoma,

Table 4–6. Breast masses in adolescent females.

Common
   Fibroadenoma
   Fibrocystic changes
   Breast cysts (including subareolar cysts)
   Breast abscess or mastitis
   Fat necrosis (after trauma)
Less common (benign)
   Lymphangioma
   Hemangioma
   Intraductal papilloma
   Juvenile papillomatosis
   Giant fibroadenoma
   Neurofibromatosis
   Nipple adenoma or keratoma
   Mammary duct ectasia
   Intramammary lymph node
   Lipoma
   Hematoma
   Hamartoma
   Galactocele
Rare (malignant or malignant potential)
   Juvenile secretory carcinoma
   Intraductal carcinoma
   Cystosarcoma phylloides
   Sarcomas (fibrosarcoma, malignant fibrous histiocytoma, rhabdomyosarcoma)
   Metastatic cancer (hepatocellular carcinoma, lymphoma, neuroblastoma, rhabdomyosarcoma)

Table 4–7. Characteristics and management of breast lesions in adolescent females.

Fibroadenoma	2- to 3-cm, rubbery, well-circumscribed, mobile, nontender. Commonly found in upper outer quadrant of the breast. Management is observation.
Giant juvenile fibroadenoma	Large, > 5 cm fibroadenoma with overlying skin stretching and dilated superficial veins. Benign but requires excision for confirmation of diagnosis and for cosmetic reasons.
Breast cysts	Usually caused by ductal ectasia or blocked Montgomery tubercles, both of which can have associated nipple discharge. Ultrasound can help differentiate from solid mass. Most resolve spontaneously.
Fibrocystic changes	More common with advancing age after adolescence. Mild swelling and palpable nodularity in upper outer quadrants. Associated with cyclic premenstrual mastalgia.
Abscess	Often associated with overlying mastitis and/or purulent nipple discharge. Culture abscess material and/or nipple discharge before starting antibiotics.
Cystosarcoma phyllodes	Large, rapidly growing tumor associated with overlying skin changes, dilated veins, and skin necrosis. Requires excision. Most often benign but can be malignant.
Intraductal papilloma	Palpable intraductal tumor, which is often subareolar with associated nipple discharge, but may be in the periphery of the breast in adolescents. Requires surgical excision.
Juvenile papillomatosis	Rare breast tumor characterized by a grossly nodular breast mass described as having a "Swiss-cheese" appearance. Requires surgical excision.
Fat necrosis	Localized inflammatory process in the breast; typically follows trauma (sports or seat belt injuries). Subsequent scarring may be confused with changes similar to those associated with malignancy.

rhabdomyosarcoma, malignant cystosarcoma phylloides, and metastatic tumor. Retrospective studies indicate that biopsies of breast masses in adolescents most commonly show fibroadenoma (67%), fibrocystic change (15%), and abscess or mastitis (3%).

1. Fibroadenoma

Fibroadenomas are the most common breast masses of adolescent girls. Fibroadenomas are composed of glandular and fibrous tissue. A fibroadenoma is typically nontender and diagnosed clinically with examination findings of a rubbery, smooth, well-circumscribed, mobile mass most often in the upper outer quadrant of the breast, although fibroadenomas can be found in any quadrant. Ten to 25% of girls will have multiple or bilateral lesions. Fibroadenomas are typically slow growing, with average size 2–3 cm. They may remain static in size for months to years, with 10%–40% completely resolving during adolescence. The dense fibroglandular tissue of the adolescent breast may cause false-positive results on standard mammograms. Thus, ultrasonography is the best imaging modality with which to evaluate a breast mass in an adolescent if further evaluation beyond the clinical

examination is necessary. Fibroadenomas less than 5 cm can be monitored for growth or regression over 3–4 months. Further evaluation will be dictated by the patient's course, with semiannual clinical examinations for a few years followed by annual examinations for a mass that is regressing. Patients with concerning breast masses including fibroadenomas that are larger than 5 cm, undiagnosed breast masses that are enlarging or have overlying skin changes, and any suspicious breast mass in a patient with a history of previous malignancy should be referred to a breast care specialist.

2. Fibrocystic Breast Changes

Fibrocystic breast changes are much more common in adults than adolescents. Symptoms include mild swelling and palpable nodularity, most commonly in the upper outer quadrants. Mastalgia is typically cyclic, usually occurring just before menstruation. Reassuring the young woman about the benign nature of the process may be all that is needed. Nonsteroidal anti-inflammatory drugs (NSAIDs) such as ibuprofen or naproxen sodium help alleviate symptoms. Oral contraceptive pills (OCPs) can also be beneficial. Supportive bras may provide symptomatic relief. Studies have shown no association between methylxanthine and fibrocystic breasts; however, some women report reduced symptoms when they discontinue caffeine.

3. Breast Abscess

ESSENTIALS OF DIAGNOSIS & TYPICAL FEATURES

▶ Common causes of mastitis and breast abscess during adolescence include manipulation of periareolar hair and nipple piercing, with subsequent infection with normal skin flora.

▶ Typical features include breast pain and overlying erythema and warmth.

▶ Breast ultrasound may be helpful to differentiate between mastitis and breast abscess.

Although breast-feeding is the most common cause of mastitis, shaving or plucking periareolar hair, nipple piercing, and trauma occurring during sexual activity are predisposing factors in teenagers. The most common causative organisms are normal skin flora. The female with a breast abscess usually complains of unilateral breast pain, and examination reveals overlying inflammatory changes. The examination may be misleading in that the infection may extend deeper into the breast than suspected. *Staphylococcus aureus* is the most common pathogen. β-Hemolytic streptococci, *Escherichia coli*, and *Pseudomonas aeruginosa* have also been implicated. Fluctuant abscesses should be incised and drained and fluid cultured. Antimicrobial coverage for *S aureus* (including methicillin-resistant strains) should be given initially (generally orally, unless infection is severe), and the patient should be monitored closely for response to therapy until culture and susceptibility test results are available.

Healing time after nipple piercing is 3–6 months. Health risks associated with nipple piercing, in addition to breast abscess, include allergic reactions to jewelry, keloid scar formation, and risk of hepatitis B and C and HIV. Complications associated with abscess formation secondary to nipple piercing include endocarditis, cardiac valve injury, cardiac prosthesis infection, metal foreign-body reaction in the breast tissue, and recurrent infection.

NIPPLE DISCHARGE & GALACTORRHEA

ESSENTIALS OF DIAGNOSIS & TYPICAL FEATURES

▶ Bloody or serosanguineous discharge may indicate a duct problem; milky nipple discharge is typical of galactorrhea.

▶ Galactorrhea is typically benign and caused by chronic nipple stimulation, certain prescription psychiatric drugs, or illicit drug use.

Ductal ectasia is a common cause of nipple discharge in the developing breast and is associated with dilation of the mammary ducts, periductal fibrosis, and inflammation. It can present with bloody, brown, or sticky multicolored nipple discharge and/or a cystic breast mass, which is usually in the subareolar region. Blocked ducts and fluid collections usually resolve spontaneously but can become infected, producing mastitis. Patients should look for erythema, warmth, and tenderness indicating mastitis. Oral antibiotics covering skin flora should be initiated if infection is suspected. Serous or serosanguineous nipple discharge is common and can be associated with fibrocystic breast changes. Montgomery tubercles are small glands located at the outer aspect of the areola that can drain clear or brownish fluid through an ectopic opening on the areola and may be associated with a small subareolar mass. These lesions and discharge typically resolve spontaneously. Intraductal papillomas arising from proliferation of ductal cells projecting into the duct lumen are a rare cause of bloody or serosanguineous nipple discharge and can also present with a subareolar or peripheral mass. These lesions are associated with increased risk of malignancy in adults.

Galactorrhea is distinguishable from other causes of nipple discharge by its milky character and tendency to involve both breasts. It is usually benign. The most common causes include chronic stimulation or irritation of the nipple, medications and illicit drugs (drugs causing galactorrhea are listed in Table 4–8), pregnancy, childbirth, or abortion. Prolactin-secreting tumors (prolactinomas) and hypothyroidism are common pathologic causes of galactorrhea during adolescence. Less common causes of hyperprolactinemia and galactorrhea include diseases in or near the hypothalamus or pituitary that interfere with the secretion of dopamine or its delivery to the hypothalamus. Included are tumors of the hypothalamus and/or pituitary, both benign

Table 4–8. Medications and herbs associated with galactorrhea.

Anticonvulsants (valproic acid)
Antidepressants (selective serotonin reuptake inhibitors, tricyclic antidepressants)
Anxiolytics (alprazolam)
Antihypertensives (atenolol, methyldopa, reserpine, verapamil)
Antipsychotics
Typical (haloperidol, phenothiazine, pimozide)
Atypical (risperidone, olanzapine, molindone)
Antiemetics (prochlorperazine)
Herbs (anise, blessed thistle, fennel, fenugreek seed, nettle)
Hormonal contraceptives
Isoniazid
Illicit drugs (amphetamines, cannabis, opiates)
Motility agents (metoclopramide)
Muscle relaxants (cyclobenzaprine)

(eg, craniopharyngiomas) and malignant (eg, metastatic disease), infiltrative diseases of the hypothalamus (eg, sarcoidosis), and pituitary stalk damage (eg, section due to head trauma or surgery or compression). Stimulation of the intercostal nerves (eg, chest wall surgery or herpes zoster infection), renal failure (decreased prolactin clearance), polycystic ovarian syndrome, and emotional or physical stress can also cause hyperprolactinemia, which can induce galactorrhea.

▶ **Clinical Findings**

Breast ultrasonography can be helpful in determining the cause of nipple discharge and breast masses. Depending on additional findings from the history and examination, evaluation of galactorrhea may include a pregnancy test, prolactin level, and thyroid function studies. If there is a question as to whether the discharge is true galactorrhea, fat staining of the discharge can be confirmatory. Elevated TSH confirms the diagnosis of hypothyroidism. Elevated prolactin and normal TSH, often accompanied by amenorrhea, in the absence of medication known to cause hyperprolactinemia suggests a hypothalamic or pituitary tumor. In such cases, magnetic resonance imaging (MRI) of the brain and consultation with a pediatric endocrinologist are indicated.

▶ **Treatment**

Observation with serial examination is recommended for nipple discharge associated with breast mass unless a papilloma is suspected by the presence of bloody or serosanguineous nipple discharge with or without a subareolar or peripheral mass. The latter entity requires further evaluation and excision by a breast surgeon. For galactorrhea, treating the underlying cause is usually effective. Galactorrhea due to hypothyroidism should be treated with thyroid hormone replacement. An alternative medication can be prescribed

in cases of medication-induced galactorrhea. Adolescents with galactorrhea without a breast mass who have normal prolactin and TSH levels can be followed clinically and counseled about supportive measures such as avoidance of nipple stimulation, stress reduction, and keeping a menstrual calendar to monitor for oligomenorrhea, which might indicate a systemic hormonal problem such as hyperprolactinemia or thyroid disease. In many cases, symptoms resolve spontaneously and no underlying diagnosis is made. Medical management of prolactinomas with dopamine agonists such as bromocriptine is the favored approach.

GYNECOMASTIA

ESSENTIALS OF DIAGNOSIS & TYPICAL FEATURES

▶ Gynecomastia is common in males during puberty and may last 1–3 years.

▶ Typical features include a palpable fibroglandular mass located concentrically beneath the nipple-areolar complex. It may be unilateral or bilateral.

▶ Clinical observation is appropriate; however, further evaluation may be necessary for atypical cases including: prepubertal gynecomastia, eccentric position, rapid breast enlargement, presence of testicular mass, or prolonged persistence.

Gynecomastia, benign subareolar glandular breast enlargement, affects up to 65% of adolescent males. It typically appears at least 6 months after the onset of secondary sex characteristics, with peak incidence during SMR stages 3 and 4. Breast tissue enlargement usually regresses within 1–3 years, and persistence beyond age 17 years is uncommon. Approximately half of young men with gynecomastia have a positive family history of gynecomastia. The pathogenesis of pubertal gynecomastia has long been attributed to a transient imbalance between estrogens that stimulate proliferation of breast tissue and androgens which antagonize this effect. Leptin has recently been implicated in the development of gynecomastia, as levels are higher in healthy nonobese adolescent males with gynecomastia compared to controls. There are several proposed mechanisms in which leptin acts biochemically to alter the estrogen-androgen ratio.

▶ **Clinical Findings**

Palpation of the breasts is necessary to distinguish adipose tissue (pseudogynecomastia) from the glandular tissue found in true gynecomastia, which is palpable as a fibroglandular mass located concentrically beneath the nipple-areolar complex. Gynecomastia is bilateral in almost two-thirds of patients. Findings that indicate more serious disease include hard or firm breast tissue, unilateral breast growth, eccentric masses outside of the nipple-areolar complex, and overlying skin changes. A genitourinary examination is needed to evaluate pubertal SMR, testicular volume and masses, or irregularities of the testes.

In the absence of abnormalities on history or physical examination, clinical monitoring of male gynecomastia for 12–18 months is sufficient. Laboratory evaluation is warranted if the patient with gynecomastia is prepubertal, appears undervirilized, has an eccentric breast mass, has a rapid progression of breast enlargement, has a testicular mass, or has persistence of gynecomastia beyond the usual observation period. The initial laboratory evaluation includes thyroid function tests and testosterone, estradiol, human chorionic gonadotropin (hCG), and LH levels. Additional studies, depending on preliminary findings, include karyotype, liver and renal function studies, and dehydroepiandrosterone sulfate and prolactin levels. Any patient with a testicular mass or laboratory results suggesting possible tumor, such as high serum testosterone, hCG, or estradiol, should have a testicular ultrasound. Further evaluation includes adrenal or brain imaging if a prolactin-secreting pituitary tumor or adrenal tumor is suspected.

Differential Diagnosis

Gynecomastia may be drug induced (Table 4–9). Testicular, adrenal, or pituitary tumors, Klinefelter syndrome, secondary hypogonadism, partial or complete androgen insensitivity syndrome, hyperthyroidism, or chronic diseases (eg, cystic fibrosis, ulcerative colitis, liver disease, renal failure, and AIDS) leading to malnutrition may be associated with gynecomastia. Breast cancer in the adolescent male is extraordinarily rare.

Treatment

If gynecomastia is idiopathic, reassurance about the common and benign nature of the process can be given. Resolution may take up to 2 years. Surgery is reserved for those with persistent severe breast enlargement and/or significant psychological trauma. In cases of drug-induced gynecomastia, the inciting agent should be discontinued if possible. The patient should be referred to an endocrinologist or oncologist if other pathologic etiologies are diagnosed.

De Silva NK: Breast development and disorders in the adolescent female. Best Pract Res Clin Obstet Gynaecol 2018;48:40–50 [PMID: 28935365].
Di Vasta A, Weldon C, Labow BI: The breast: examination and lesions. In: Emans SJ, Laufer MR, Goldstein DP (eds): *Pediatric and Adolescent Gynecology*. 6th ed. Philadelphia, PA: Lippincott Williams & Wilkins; 2012:405–420.

Table 4–9. Drugs associated with gynecomastia.

	Examples
Antiandrogens	Cyproterone, finasteride, flutamide, ketoconazole, nilutamide, spironolactone
Antineoplastic and immunomodulators	Alkylating agents, bleomycin, cisplatin, cyclosporine, imatinib, methotrexate, nitrosurea, vincristine
Antiulcer drugs	Cimetidine, metoclopramide, omeprazole, ranitidine
Cardiovascular drugs	Amiodarone, angiotensin-converting enzyme inhibitors, calcium channel blockers, digitoxin, reserpine, spironolactone
Drugs of abuse	Alcohol, amphetamines, marijuana, opiates
Hormones	Anabolic androgenic steroids, estrogens, testosterone, chorionic gonadotropin
Infectious agents	Antiretrovirals, ketoconazole, isoniazid, metronidazole
Psychoactive medications	Diazepam, tricyclic antidepressants, haloperidol, atypical antipsychotics, phenothiazines

Guss CE, Divasta AD: Adolescent gynecomastia. Pediatri Endocrinol Rev 2017;14(4):371–377 [PMID: 28613047].
Hagan JF, Shaw JS, Duncan PM (eds): *Bright Futures: Guidelines for Health Supervision of Infants, Children, and Adolescents*. 4th ed. Elk Grove Village, IL: American Academy of Pediatrics; 2017.

GYNECOLOGIC CARE & GYNECOLOGIC DISORDERS IN ADOLESCENCE

Physiology of Menstruation

The ovulatory menstrual cycle is divided into three consecutive phases: follicular (days 1–14), ovulatory (midcycle), and luteal (days 16–28). During the follicular phase, pulsatile gonadotropin-releasing hormone from the hypothalamus stimulates anterior pituitary secretion of FSH and LH. Under the influence of FSH and LH, a dominant ovarian follicle emerges by day 5–7 of the menstrual cycle, and the other follicles become atretic. Rising estradiol levels produced by the maturing follicle cause proliferation of the endometrium. By the midfollicular phase, FSH begins to decline secondary to estradiol-mediated negative feedback, while LH continues to rise as a result of estradiol-mediated positive feedback.

Rising LH initiates progesterone secretion and luteinization of the granulosa cells of the follicle. Progesterone in turn further stimulates LH and FSH. This leads to the LH surge, which causes the follicle to rupture and expel the oocyte. During the luteal phase, LH and FSH gradually decline. The corpus luteum secretes progesterone, and the endometrium enters the secretory phase in response to rising levels of estrogen and progesterone, with maturation 8–9 days after ovulation. If pregnancy and placental hCG release do not occur, luteolysis begins; estrogen and progesterone levels decline and the endometrial lining is shed as menstrual flow approximately 14 days after ovulation. In the first 2 years after menarche, the majority of cycles (50%–80%) are anovulatory. Between 10% and 20% of cycles are anovulatory for up to 5 years after menarche.

Pelvic Examination

Indications for a pelvic examination in an adolescent include abdominal or pelvic pain, intra-abdominal or pelvic mass, abnormal vaginal bleeding or other menstrual disorders, pathologic vaginal discharge, or need for cervical cytology screening. The American College of Obstetrics and Gynecology advocates starting Papanicolaou (Pap) cytology screening at age 21 years for both sexually experienced and sexually inexperienced women. Delaying screening until age 21 years is based on the low incidence of cervical cancer in younger women and the potential for adverse effects associated with follow-up of young women with abnormal cytology screening results. Similarly, although reflex testing for high-risk cervical human papillomaviruses (HPV) genotypes for women with an ASC-US (atypical squamous cells of undetermined significance) cytology result can help guide the frequency of follow-up screening, co-testing for HPV is not recommended for women younger than 30 years because of the very high prevalence of high-risk HPV infections, a high rate of spontaneous clearance, and the low incidence of cervical cancer in sexually active women in this age group. Pregnancy during adolescence does not alter screening guidelines. Current guidelines recommend that HIV-positive adolescents should have cervical cytology screening beginning within 1 year of onset of sexual activity or at age 21 years (whichever is earlier). Algorithms for managing abnormal cervical cytology can be found at the American Society for Colposcopy and Cervical Pathology website: http://www.asccp.org/asccp-guidelines. Guidelines for management of abnormal cytology in HIV positive women can be obtained from the CDC and partner organizations at https://aidsinfo.nih.gov/guidelines/html/4/adult-and-adolescent-oi-prevention-and-treatment-guidelines/343/hpv.

The adolescent may be apprehensive about the first pelvic examination. Sensitive counseling and age-appropriate education about the purpose of the examination, pelvic anatomy, and the components of the examination should occur in an unhurried manner. The use of diagrams and models may facilitate discussion. Time should be allotted for the adolescent to ask questions. Ideally, the examination should occur in a controlled and comfortable setting. The adolescent may request to have her mother or family member present during the examination for reassurance; however, in many instances an adolescent will request that the examination occur confidentially. Having another female staff member present to support the adolescent in this setting may be helpful. A female staff chaperone should be present with male examiners.

The pelvic examination begins by placing the patient in the dorsal lithotomy position after equipment and supplies are ready (Table 4–10). Patients with orthopedic or other physical disabilities require accommodation for proper positioning and comfort. The examiner inspects the external genitalia, noting sexually maturity rating; estrogenization of the vaginal mucosa (moist, pink, and more elastic mucosa); shape of the hymen; the size of the clitoris (2–5 mm wide is normal); any unusual rashes or lesions on the vulva such as folliculitis from shaving, warts or other skin lesions; and genital piercing or body art. It can be helpful to ask an adolescent if she has any questions about her body during the inspection as she might have concerns that she was too shy to ask (eg, normalcy of labial hypertrophy). In cases of alleged sexual abuse or assault, the presence of any lesions, including lacerations, bruises, scarring, or synechiae near the hymen, vulva, or anus should be noted.

The patient should be prepared for insertion of the speculum to help her remain relaxed. The speculum should be inserted into the vagina posteriorly with a downward direction to avoid the urethra. A medium Pedersen speculum is most often used in sexually experienced patients; a narrow Huffman is used for virginal patients. In a virginal female prior to the speculum examination, a one-finger examination in the vagina can help the provider identify the position of the cervix and can give the patient an appreciation for the sensation she can expect with placement of the speculum. Warming the speculum with tap water prior to insertion can be more comfortable for the patient and also provide lubrication. Simultaneously

Table 4–10. Items for pelvic examination.

General	Gloves, good light source, appropriate-sized speculums, sterile cotton applicator swabs, large swabs to remove excess bleeding or discharge, patient labels, hand mirror for patient education
Wet prep of vaginal discharge	pH paper, microscope slides and cover slips, NaCl and KOH solutions
Pap smear	Pap smear liquid media or slides with fixative; cervical spatula and endocervical cytologic brush; or broom for collection
STI testing	Gonorrhea and *Chlamydia* test media with specific collection swabs
Bimanual examination	Gloves, water-based lubricant

touching the inner aspect of the patient's thigh or applying gentle pressure to the perineum away from the introitus while inserting the speculum helps distract attention from the placement of the speculum. The vaginal walls and cervix are inspected for anatomical abnormalities, inflammation, and lesions, and the quantity and quality of discharge adherent to the vaginal walls and pooled in the vagina are noted. The presence of a cervical ectropion, extension of the endocervical columnar epithelium outside the cervical os onto the face of the cervix, is commonly observed in adolescents as erythema surrounding the cervical os.

Specimens are obtained in the following order: vaginal pH, saline and KOH wet preparations, cervical cytology (Pap) screening if indicated, and endocervical swabs for gonorrhea and *Chlamydia trachomatis* (Table 4–11). STIs are discussed in further detail in Chapter 44. The speculum is then removed, and bimanual examination is performed with

Table 4–11. Diagnostic tests and procedures performed during speculum vaginal examination.

Vaginal pH	Use applicator swab to sample vaginal discharge adherent to the wall or in the vaginal pool if a speculum is in place; immediately apply it to pH paper for reading.
Saline and KOH wet preparations	Sample discharge as above with different swabs, smear small sample on glass slide, apply small drop of saline or KOH and immediately cover with coverslip, and evaluate under microscope.
Pap smear[a]	Gently remove excessive discharge from surface of cervix. Exocervical cells are sampled with a spatula by applying gentle pressure on the cervix with the spatula while rotating it around the cervical os. Endocervical cells are sampled by gently inserting the cytologic brush into the cervical os and rotating it. Both cell types are collected by the broom when it is centered over the cervical os and rotated.
STI testing[a]	Insert specific test swabs (eg, Dacron for most *Chlamydia* test media) into the cervical os and rotate to obtain endocervical samples for *Chlamydia* and gonorrhea, or if using approved test for vaginal collection, insert the swab into the vagina and rotate, touching the vaginal wall. Vaginal testing for *Trichomonas vaginalis* is also available.

STI, sexually transmitted infection.
[a]Refer to manufacturer instructions for sample collection and processing.

one or two fingers in the vagina and the other hand on the abdomen to palpate the uterus and adnexa for size, position, and tenderness.

▶ Menstrual Disorders

1. Amenorrhea

Primary amenorrhea is defined as having no menstrual periods or secondary sex characteristics by age 13 years or no menses in the presence of secondary sex characteristics by age 15 years. In the adolescent who has achieved menarche, *secondary amenorrhea* is defined as the absence of menses for three consecutive cycles or for 6 months in a patient with irregular cycles.

A. Evaluation of Primary and Secondary Amenorrhea

In evaluating amenorrhea, it is helpful to consider anatomical levels of possible abnormalities from the hypothalamus to the genital tract (Table 4–12).

A stepwise approach, using clinical history, growth charts, physical examination, and appropriate laboratory studies will allow providers to determine the etiology of amenorrhea in most adolescents. Evaluation begins with a thorough developmental and sexual history. Establishing a pubertal timeline including age at thelarche, adrenarche, growth spurt, and menarche is helpful in evaluating pubertal development. Although there can be variations in the onset, degree, and timing of these stages, the progression of stages is predictable. Adrenal androgens are largely responsible for axillary and pubic hair. Estrogen is responsible for breast development; maturation of the external genitalia, vagina, and uterus; and menstruation. Lack of development suggests pituitary or ovarian failure or gonadal dysgenesis. Determining the patient's gynecologic age (time in years and months since menarche) is helpful in assessing the maturity of the hypothalamic-pituitary-ovarian axis. A menstrual history includes date of last menstrual period (LMP), frequency and duration of periods, amount of bleeding, and premenstrual symptoms. Irregular menstrual cycles are common in the first 1–2 years after menarche. Two-thirds of adolescents with a gynecologic age more than 2 years have regular menstrual cycles.

Relevant components of the past medical and surgical histories include the neonatal history, treatment for malignancies, presence of autoimmune disorders or endocrinopathies, and current medications (prescribed and over-the-counter). Family history includes age at menarche of maternal relatives, familial gynecologic or fertility problems, autoimmune diseases, or endocrinopathies. A review of systems should focus on symptoms of hypothalamic-pituitary disease such as weight change, headache, visual disturbance, galactorrhea, polyuria, and/or polydipsia. A history of cyclic abdominal

Table 4–12. Differential diagnosis of amenorrhea by anatomic site of cause.

Hypothalamic-pituitary axis
  Hypothalamic suppression
    Chronic disease
    Stress
    Malnutrition
    Strenuous athletics
    Drugs (haloperidol, phenothiazines, atypical antipsychotics)
  Central nervous system lesion
    Pituitary lesion: adenoma, prolactinoma
    Craniopharyngioma, brainstem, or parasellar tumors
    Head injury with hypothalamic contusion
    Infiltrative process (sarcoidosis)
    Vascular disease (hypothalamic vasculitis)
  Congenital conditions[a]
    Kallmann syndrome (anosmia)
Ovaries
  Gonadal dysgenesis[a]
    Turner syndrome (XO)
    Mosaic (XX/XO)
  Injury to ovary
    Autoimmune disease (oophoritis)
    Infection (mumps)
    Toxins (alkylating chemotherapeutic agents)
    Irradiation
    Trauma, torsion (rare)
  Polycystic ovary syndrome
  Ovarian failure
Uterovaginal outflow tract
  Müllerian dysgenesis[a]
    Congenital deformity or absence of uterus, uterine tubes, or vagina
  Imperforate hymen, transverse vaginal septum, vaginal agenesis, agenesis of the cervix[a]
  Androgen insensitivity syndrome (absent uterus)[a]
  Uterine lining defect
    Asherman syndrome (intrauterine synechiae postcurettage or endometritis)
    Tuberculosis, brucellosis
Defect in hormone synthesis or action (virilization may be present)
  Adrenal hyperplasia[a]
  Cushing disease
  Adrenal tumor
  Ovarian tumor (rare)
  Drugs (steroids, ACTH)

ACTH, adrenocorticotropic hormone.
[a]Indicates condition that usually presents as primary amenorrhea.

Table 4–13. Components of the physical examination for amenorrhea.

General appearance	Syndromic features (eg, Turner syndrome with webbed neck, shield chest, widely spaced nipples, increased carrying angle of the arms)
Anthropometrics	Height, weight, BMI and percentiles for age, vital signs (HR, BP)
Ophthalmologic	Visual field cuts, papilledema
Neck	Thyromegaly
Breast	SMR staging, galactorrhea
Abdomen	Masses
Genital	SMR staging, estrogenization of vaginal mucosa (pink and moist vs thin red mucosa of hypoestrogenization), hymenal patency, clitoromegaly (width > 5 mm)
Pelvic and bimanual	Vaginal depth by insertion of a saline moistened applicator swab into the vagina or by bimanual examination (normal > 2 cm); palpation of the uterus and ovaries by bimanual examination
Skin	Acne, hirsutism, acanthosis nigricans

BMI, body mass index; BP, blood pressure; HR, heart rate; SMR, sexual maturity rating.

problem. A confidential social history should include sexual activity, contraceptive use, the possibility of pregnancy, and use of tobacco, drugs, or alcohol. The patient should also be questioned about major stressors, symptoms of depression and anxiety, dietary habits including any disordered eating or weight-loss behaviors, and athletic participation.

A thorough physical examination should include the components listed in Table 4–13. If a patient cannot tolerate a pelvic or bimanual examination, the presence of the uterus can be assessed by rectoabdominal examination or ultrasonography. Ultrasound provides evaluation of pelvic anatomy and possible genital tract obstruction, measurement of the endometrial stripe as an indicator of estrogen stimulation, and identification of ovarian cysts or masses.

Figure 4–6 illustrates an approach to the laboratory and radiologic evaluation of primary or secondary amenorrhea. Initial studies should include a urine pregnancy test, complete blood count, TSH, prolactin, and FSH. If there is evidence of hyperandrogenemia (acne, hirsutism) and polycystic ovary syndrome (PCOS) is suspected, total and free testosterone and dehydroepiandrosterone sulfate (DHEAS) should be obtained. If systemic illness is suspected, a urinalysis and a chemistry panel (including renal and liver function tests) and erythrocyte sedimentation rate should be obtained. If short stature and delayed puberty are present, a bone age and karyotype should be done.

and/or pelvic pain in a mature adolescent with amenorrhea may indicate an anatomic abnormality such as an imperforate hymen. Acne and hirsutism are clinical markers of androgen excess. Both hypo- and hyperthyroidism can cause menstrual irregularities, and changes in weight, quality of skin and hair, and stooling pattern may indicate a thyroid

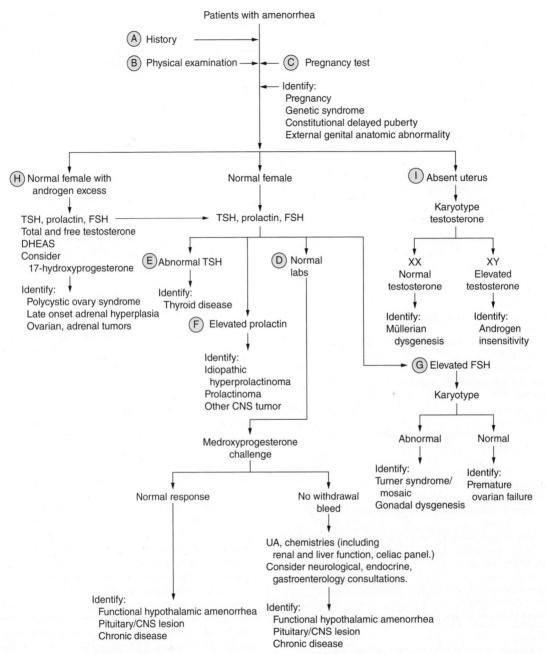

▲ **Figure 4–6.** Evaluation of primary amenorrhea and secondary amenorrhea. CNS, central nervous system; DHEAS, dehydroepiandrosterone sulfate; FSH, follicle-stimulating hormone; TSH, thyroid-stimulating hormone; UA, urine analysis.

If pelvic examination or ultrasonography reveals normal female external genitalia and pelvic organs and the patient is not pregnant, the patient should be given a challenge of oral medroxyprogesterone, 10 mg daily for 10 days. Positive response to the progestin challenge with withdrawal bleeding is suggestive of the presence of a normal, estrogen-primed uterus.

Elevated serum prolactin indicates a possible prolactin secreting tumor. Prolactin testing is sensitive and can be elevated with stress, eating, or sexual intercourse. A mildly elevated test should be repeated prior to MRI of the brain for a prolactinoma. Elevated FSH indicates ovarian insufficiency or gonadal dysgenesis and a karyotype for Turner syndrome or Turner mosaic should be obtained. Autoimmune oophoritis should be assessed by antiovarian antibodies if the chromosome analysis is normal. Normal or low serum gonadotropins indicate hypothalamic suppression and functional amenorrhea if the patient's weight is normal and there is a reasonable explanation such as vigorous exercise. Functional amenorrhea, although relatively common, is a diagnosis of exclusion. Low serum gonadotropin concentration can also be caused by malnutrition as in anorexia nervosa, endocrinopathies, and chronic diseases or by a central nervous system tumor.

If the physical examination or ultrasound reveals an absent uterus, chromosomal analysis and serum testosterone should be obtained to differentiate between Mullerian dysgenesis and androgen insensitivity. Mullerian dysgenesis or Mayer-Rokitansky-Küster-Hauser (MRKH) syndrome is the congenital absence of the vagina with variable uterine development. These women have normal serum testosterone levels. Pelvic MRI is helpful to clarify the nature of the vaginal agenesis and to differentiate it from low-lying transverse vaginal septum, agenesis of the uterus and vagina, and imperforate hymen. Individuals with androgen insensitivity are phenotypically female but have an absent upper vagina, uterus, and fallopian tubes; a male karyotype; and an elevated serum testosterone (normal range for males).

The management of primary or secondary amenorrhea depends on the underlying pathology. Hormonal treatment is used in patients with hypothalamic, pituitary, and ovarian causes. Surgical repair may be required in patients with outflow tract anomalies.

B. Polycystic Ovary Syndrome

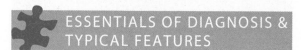

ESSENTIALS OF DIAGNOSIS & TYPICAL FEATURES

▶ Typical features of polycystic ovary syndrome include: menstrual irregularities, clinical signs of hyperandrogenism (eg, hirsutism and moderate to severe acne), and overweight or obesity.

▶ In addition to the laboratory evaluation for secondary amenorrhea, testing for hyperandrogenemia includes total and free testosterone, dehydroepiandrosterone sulfate, and androstenedione.

▶ Obese adolescents with polycystic ovary syndrome should be screened for lipid abnormalities, glucose intolerance and/or type 2 diabetes, fatty liver disease, obstructive sleep apnea and depression and anxiety.

Polycystic ovary syndrome (PCOS) is the most common endocrine disorder of reproductive-aged women. It affects 6%–15% of women of reproductive age. PCOS is characterized by ovarian dysfunction, disordered gonadotropin secretion, and hyperandrogenism, which cause irregular periods, hirsutism, and acne. Many adolescents with PCOS are overweight and the association of PCOS with insulin resistance in adults is well established. Adolescents with PCOS are at increased risk for obesity-related morbidities including type 2 diabetes mellitus; cardiovascular disease including dyslipidemia; fatty liver disease; obstructive sleep apnea; low self-esteem, depression, and anxiety; and adult reproductive health problems including infertility and endometrial cancer.

Hyperandrogenemia occurs during normal puberty and also as a function of prolonged anovulatory cycles as the hypothalamic-pituitary-ovarian axis matures during the first few years of typical pubertal development. The normalcy of this hyperandrogenemia confounds the diagnosis of PCOS in early adolescence if the adult criteria of evidence of chemical hyperandrogenemia are applied. Therefore, many authors recommended avoiding testing androgen levels until 2 years after menarche for symptomatic adolescents. The current diagnostic criteria for PCOS in adolescents include clinical signs and symptoms of androgen excess, increased androgen levels, and exclusion of other causes of hyperandrogenemia in the setting of oligomenorrhea.

Table 4–14 outlines a standard laboratory evaluation for PCOS. If other etiologies of virilization such as late-onset congenital adrenal hyperplasia (history of premature pubarche, high dehydroepiandrosterone sulfate, clitoromegaly) are suspected, a first morning 17-hydroxyprogesterone should be collected to look for 21-hydroxylase deficiency. Urine cortisol or a dexamethasone suppression test is performed if Cushing syndrome is suspected. If the patient is overweight and/or has acanthosis nigricans, a fasting lipid panel and glucose testing are recommended. A 2-hour oral glucose tolerance test (OGTT) to evaluate for impaired glucose tolerance should also be considered as a normal fasting glucose may be falsely reassuring. A hemoglobin A_{1C} test may be considered if a patient is unable or unwilling to complete an OGTT.

Table 4–14. Laboratory evaluation for polycystic ovary syndrome (PCOS).

Pregnancy test	
Testosterone (total and free)	> 200 ng/dL suggests tumor
Sex hormone-binding globulin (SHBG)	
Dehydroepiandrosterone sulfate (DHEAS)	> 700 mcg/dL suggests tumor
Androstenedione	

Additionally, as obstructive sleep apnea, depression and anxiety have been associated with the diagnosis of PCOS, clinicians should screen for patients for these comorbidities. Consultation with a pediatric endocrinologist can assist in further evaluation and management of significantly elevated androgens and possible endocrinopathies.

Encouraging lifestyle changes that will promote weight loss is a primary goal of therapy for PCOS in adolescence. Weight loss is associated with improved menstrual regulation, decreased symptoms of hyperandrogenemia, and improved obesity-related comorbidities. Use of combination hormonal contraceptives will improve menstrual regularity, decrease ovarian and adrenal androgen production, and increase sex hormone–binding globulin (SHBG). There are no current guidelines for the use of insulin-sensitizing medications such as metformin to treat PCOS in adolescents; however, it is prescribed for impaired glucose tolerance or type 2 diabetes. Providers should be aware that metformin will improve the frequency of ovulation, and contraception should also be prescribed for sexually active teens.

2. Dysmenorrhea

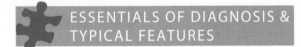

ESSENTIALS OF DIAGNOSIS & TYPICAL FEATURES

▶ The majority of adolescent girls experience primary dysmenorrhea.

▶ Typical features include lower abdominal cramps radiating to the lower back and thighs and nausea and/or vomiting starting a few days before the onset of menses and lasting a few days into the period.

▶ Use of scheduled NSAIDs and contraceptives to suppress ovulation are mainstays of treatment.

Dysmenorrhea or pain with menstrual periods is the most common gynecologic complaint of adolescent girls, with up to 90% of adolescent girls reporting some symptoms. Fifteen percent of adolescent women describe their symptoms as severe. The prevalence of dysmenorrhea increases with gynecologic age due to its association with ovulatory cycles. Dysmenorrhea can be designated as primary or secondary depending on the absence or presence of underlying pelvic pathology (Table 4–15). Potent prostaglandins are the mediators of dysmenorrhea, producing uterine contractions, tissue ischemia, and hypersensitivity of pain fibers in the uterus.

In addition to taking a gynecologic and sexual history, an accurate characterization of the pain (timing with menses, intensity, duration, use of pain medications) is important in determining functional impairment. The pelvic examination

can usually be deferred in nonsexually active adolescents with probable primary dysmenorrhea. Adolescents should be encouraged to keep track of their menstrual cycles using a calendar to predict when a period is imminent, thereby allowing for more proactive use of NSAIDs 1–2 days before the start of the anticipated period or with the first indication of discomfort. NSAIDs are typically continued for an additional 2–3 days after onset of pain. Recommended medications are ibuprofen 400–600 mg every 6 hours or naproxen 500 mg twice a day. If the patient does not respond to NSAIDs, suppression of ovulation with oral contraceptive pills (OCPs) or other combined hormonal contraceptives such as the transdermal patch or intravaginal ring can be effective. OCPs and the intravaginal ring can also be used continuously for extended cycling to decrease the frequency of menstrual periods. This is accomplished by skipping the placebo pill week and immediately starting a new package of birth control pills or skipping the standard 1-week break after removal of the intravaginal ring and immediately placing a new ring. Depot medroxyprogesterone acetate (DMPA) and long-acting reversible contraceptives (LARCs) including the etonogestrel implant and levonorgestrel intrauterine system (IUS) are also effective and may be preferable for patients who may have challenges with compliance. If patients have persistent symptoms despite use of a contraceptive for suppression of ovulation and scheduled NSAIDs, further evaluation for secondary dysmenorrhea is indicated. A pelvic examination, pelvic imaging with ultrasonography or MRI, and diagnostic laparoscopy may be necessary for diagnosis. Secondary dysmenorrhea is more likely to be associated with chronic pelvic pain, midcycle pain, dyspareunia, and metrorrhagia.

3. Abnormal Uterine Bleeding

ESSENTIALS OF DIAGNOSIS & TYPICAL FEATURES

▶ Typical features of abnormal uterine bleeding include heavy menstrual bleeding for longer than 7 days or blood loss that exceeds 80 mL per menses.

▶ The severity of abnormal uterine bleeding is categorized according to hemodynamic status and degree of anemia and classified as mild, moderate, or severe.

▶ Acute management depends on the severity of the problem and its specific etiology and typically consists of hormonal management.

Abnormal uterine bleeding (AUB) describes any aberration of menstrual volume, regulation, frequency, and duration. Examples of AUB include periods that are characterized

Table 4–15. Dysmenorrhea in the adolescent.

	Etiology	Onset and Duration	Symptoms	Pelvic Examination	Treatment
Primary Dysmenorrhea[a]					
Primary	Excessive amount of prostaglandin $F_2\alpha$, which attaches to myometrium, causing uterine contractions, hypoxia, and ischemia. Also, directly sensitizes pain receptors.	Begins just prior to or with the onset of menstrual flow and lasts 1–2 days. Typically does not start until 1–2 y after menarche, when cycles are more regularly ovulatory.	Lower abdominal cramps radiating to lower back and thighs. Associated nausea, vomiting, and diarrhea due to excess prostaglandins.	Normal. May wait to examine if never sexually active and history is consistent with primary dysmenorrhea.	Mild—menstrual calendar, start NSAIDs day before bleeding or at the onset of bleeding or pain if timing of cycle is difficult to predict. Moderate to severe—NSAIDs and OCPs or other birth control product to suppress ovulation.
Secondary Dysmenorrhea[b]					
Infection	Most often due to an STI such as *Chlamydia* or gonorrhea.	Recent onset of pelvic pain. Can also have chronic pain with prolonged untreated infection.	Pelvic pain, excessive or irregular menstrual bleeding, unusual vaginal discharge.	Mucopurulent or purulent discharge from cervical os, cervical friability, cervical motion, uterine or adnexal tenderness, positive wet prep for bacterial vaginosis, positive test for STI.	Appropriate antibiotics.
Endometriosis	Ectopic implants of endometrial tissue in pelvis or abdomen; may result from retrograde menstruation. Definitive diagnosis requires laparoscopy.	Generally starts > 2 y after menarche, is not significantly responsive to standard NSAID and suppression of ovulation therapies, and worsens through time.	Cyclic or acyclic chronic pelvic pain.	Mild to moderate tenderness typically in the posterior vaginal fornix or along the uterosacral ligaments.	Suppression of ovulation with combined hormonal contraceptive methods. Continuous use may provide additional control. If pain persists, refer to a gynecologist for further evaluation of chronic pelvic pain and consideration of gonadotropin-releasing hormone agonists.
Complication of pregnancy	Spontaneous abortion, ectopic pregnancy.	Acute onset.	Pelvic or abdominal pain associated with vaginal bleeding following missed menstrual period.	Positive hCG, enlarged uterus, or adnexal mass.	Pelvic US if hemodynamically stable to evaluate for intrauterine pregnancy. Immediate obstetric or surgical consult with concern for ectopic pregnancy.
Congenital anomalies	Outflow tract anomalies: imperforate hymen, transverse or longitudinal vaginal septum, septate uterus.	Onset at menarche.	Cyclic pelvic or abdominal pain which can become chronic.	Imperforate hymen may be visible on external examination. Pelvic US for general anatomy. Pelvic MRI is most sensitive and specific test for septums.	Gynecology consult for further evaluation and management.
Pelvic adhesions	Previous abdominal surgery or pelvic inflammatory disease.	Delayed onset after surgery or PID.	Abdominal pain, may or may not be associated with menstrual cycles; possible alteration in bowel pattern.	Variable.	Gynecology consult for possible lysis of adhesion.

DMPA, depot medroxyprogesterone acetate; hCG, human chorionic gonadotropin; MRI, magnetic resonance imaging; NSAID, nonsteroidal anti-inflammatory drug; OCP, oral contraceptive pill; PID, pelvic inflammatory disease; STI, sexually transmitted infection; US, ultrasound.
[a]No pelvic pathology.
[b]Underlying pathology present.

Table 4–16. Differential diagnosis of AUB in adolescents.

Condition	Examples
Anovulation	
Sexually transmitted infections	Cervicitis, pelvic inflammatory disease
Pregnancy complications	Ectopic, miscarriage
Bleeding disorders	von Willebrand disease, platelet function abnormalities, thrombocytopenia, coagulopathy
Endocrine disorders	Hypo-/hyperthyroidism, hyperprolactinemia, adrenal insufficiency, PCOS
Anatomic abnormalities	Congenital anomalies, ovarian cysts or tumors, cervical polyps
Trauma	Vaginal laceration
Foreign body	Retained tampon
Chronic illness	Liver, renal, inflammatory bowel, lupus
Malignancy	Leukemia
Drugs	Contraception, anticoagulants

PCOS, polycystic ovary syndrome.

by heavy menstrual bleeding (HMB) such as menorrhagia (prolonged bleeding that occurs at regular intervals) and menometrorrhagia (heavy prolonged bleeding that occurs irregularly and more frequently than normal). The differential diagnosis of common and less common etiologies in adolescence are listed in Table 4–16.

▶ **Evaluation**

In addition to a menstrual and sexual history, the bleeding pattern should be characterized by cycle length, duration, and quantity of bleeding (eg, number of soaked pads or tampons in 24 hours, number of menstrual accidents). Bleeding for longer than 7 days or blood loss that exceeds 80 mL per menses is considered abnormal. The patient should be assessed for symptoms of anemia including fatigue, lightheadedness, syncope, and tachycardia, and for other abnormal bleeding (gingivae, stool, easy bruising). The physical examination includes an assessment of hemodynamic stability with orthostatic heart rate and blood pressure measurements. Mucous membranes and skin should be evaluated for pallor; the heart for tachycardia and murmur; the abdomen for organomegaly; and the external genitalia for signs of trauma or congenital anomalies. If the patient has never been sexually active and the external examination is normal, a pelvic examination is usually unnecessary. In a sexually experienced female, a pelvic and bimanual examination to examine the vagina,

cervix, and adnexa may be helpful to elucidate the diagnosis. Initial laboratory studies should include a pregnancy test, complete blood cell count, prothrombin time, partial thromboplastin time, TSH, fibrinogen level, and iron studies. If the patient has signs of hemodynamic compromise potentially requiring blood transfusion, blood type and cross-match should be obtained. Among adolescents with HMB, up to 20% are reported to have an underlying bleeding disorder. Evaluation for underlying bleeding disorders such as von Willebrand deficiency should be considered for patients who endorse any of the following: insignificant wounds that lead to prolonged bleeding; heavy, prolonged, or recurrent bleeding after surgery or dental procedures; epistaxis greater than 10 minutes in duration or requiring medical attention; unexplained bleeding from the gastrointestinal tract; HMB with iron deficiency; postpartum hemorrhage; and/or a family history of bleeding disorders. Abnormalities in platelet function and/or aggregation can also be considered and consultation with a pediatric hematologist for further evaluation of these potential etiologies can be helpful. For patients suspected of having PCOS, total and free testosterone, dehydroepiandrosterone sulfate and androstenedione should be measured. For sexually experienced females, cervical or vaginal or urine-based testing for *C trachomatis* and gonorrhea should be obtained.

▶ **Treatment**

The goals of treatment include (1) establishment and/or maintenance of hemodynamic stability, (2) correction of acute or chronic anemia, (3) resumption of normal menstrual cycles, (4) prevention of recurrence, and (5) prevention of long-term consequences of anovulation. The severity of AUB is categorized according to hemodynamic status and degree of anemia and classified as mild, moderate, or severe (Table 4–17). Management depends on the severity of the problem and its specific etiology (Table 4–17). Monophasic OCPs containing a potent progestin such as norgestrel 0.3 mg with ethinyl estradiol 30 mcg or levonorgestrel 0.15 mg with ethinyl estradiol 30 mcg are frequently used for patients without medical contraindications to exogenous estrogens (see Table 4–21). The active pills in monophasic formulations contain fixed concentrations of progestins and estrogen and are preferred over multiphasic formulations which contain variable concentrations of estrogen which could potentially increase the risk of breakthrough bleeding. It is important to remind adolescents and their families that compliance with medications to control bleeding and treat anemia is imperative. Adolescents should be treated until the anemia is resolved and often for an additional 6 months or longer if there is an underlying problem such as platelet function abnormality or von Willebrand disease. For patients with contraindications to the use of exogenous estrogens, there are progestin-only methods available for acute management and maintenance treatment of AUB (Table 4–18).

Table 4–17. Management of AUB.

	Mild	Moderate	Severe
HgB value (g/dL)	HgB > 12	HgB 9–12	HgB < 9
Acute treatment	Menstrual calendar; iron supplementation. NSAID with menses may help reduce flow. Consider OCPs if patient is sexually active and desires contraception.	OCP bid until bleeding stops, continue active pill qd for 21 days followed by 1 wk of placebo pills.	Admit to hospital if HgB < 7 g/dL or patient is hemodynamically unstable. Transfusion based on degree of hemodynamic instability and ability to control bleeding. Conjugated estrogens, 25 mg IV every 4 h for up to 48 h. Provide scheduled IV antiemetic. When bleeding stops, step down to 50 mcg OCP PO qid (or tid), then taper as below. If bleeding doesn't stop, gynecology consultation for further evaluation and possible dilation and curettage. Or One 30–35 mcg OCP PO qid until bleeding stops, then decrease to tid for 2 days (and up to 7 days), then bid for 2 days (and up to 7 days), then qd (skipping placebo pills) until Hct > 30%. Antiemetic 2 h prior to OCPs as needed for nausea.
Long-term management	Monitor menstrual calendar and HgB. Follow-up in 2–3 mo.	Iron supplementation. Monitor HgB closely for improvement. May need to revert to bid OCP dosing if bleeding persists. If bleeding controlled, cycle with OCPs (28 days pack) or other combined hormonal contraceptive agent for minimum 3–6 mo.	Iron supplementation. Serial hematocrits. If Hct > 30%, cycle with OCPs (28-day pack) or other combined hormonal contraceptive agent for minimum 3–6 mo. Consider placement of levonorgestrel intrauterine system once anemia improved as alternative to short-acting method.

AUB, abnormal uterine bleeding; bid, twice daily (every 12 hours); Hct, hematocrit; HgB, hemoglobin; IV, intravenous; NSAID, nonsteroidal anti-inflammatory drug; OCP, oral contraceptive pill; PO, by mouth; qd, daily; qid, four times per day (every 6 hours); tid, three times per day (every 8 hours).

4. Mittelschmerz

Mittelschmerz is midcycle discomfort resulting from ovulation. The cause of the pain is unknown but irritation of the peritoneum due to spillage of fluid from the ruptured follicular cyst at the time of ovulation has been suggested. The patient presents with a history of midcycle, unilateral dull or aching abdominal pain lasting a few minutes to as long as 8 hours. Rarely, the pain mimics that of acute appendicitis, torsion or rupture of an ovarian cyst, or ectopic pregnancy. The patient should be reassured and treated symptomatically.

5. Premenstrual Syndrome & Premenstrual Dysphoric Disorder

It is estimated that 51%–86% of adolescent women experience some premenstrual symptoms. Premenstrual syndrome (PMS) is a cluster of physical and psychological symptoms that occur during the luteal phase of the menstrual cycle and resolve with menstruation. Physical symptoms include bloating, breast tenderness, fatigue, headache, myalgia, increased appetite, and food craving. Premenstrual emotional symptoms may include fatigue, mood lability, anxiety, depression, irritability, hostility, sleep dysfunction, and impaired social function. PMS can be diagnosed when at least one disabling physical or psychological symptom is documented prospectively for at least two consecutive menstrual cycles, is restricted to the luteal phase of the menstrual cycle, resolves by the end of menses, results in functional impairment, and is not an exacerbation of another underlying disorder. Severe PMS with functional impairment affects 1.8%–5.8% of women of reproductive age and is classified in the *Diagnostic and Statistical Manual of Mental Disorders*, Fifth Edition, as premenstrual dysphoric disorder (PMDD). The clinical diagnosis of PMDD requires a combination of a minimum of five physical and psychological symptoms in the majority of cycles that must be present in the final week before onset of menses, start to improve within a few days after the onset of menses, and become minimal or absent in the week postmenses.

The pathophysiology of PMS is not well understood; however, there is some evidence of dysregulation of serotonergic

Table 4–18. Progesterone-only hormone regimens for management of AUB.

Hormone	Tapering Regimen
Norethindrone acetate	5–10 mg PO every 4 h until bleeding stops, then qid for 4 days, then tid for 3 days, then bid for 2 days–2 wk, then qd. Once anemia improved, can transition to DMPA 150 mg IM q12 weeks or levonorgestrel intrauterine system placement. Progesterone-only OCPs can also be an alternative, but they require excellent compliance.
Medroxyprogesterone	10 mg PO every 4 h (max 80 mg) until bleeding stops, then qid for 4 days, then tid for 3 days, then bid for 2 days–2 wk, then qd. Once anemia improved, can transition to DMPA 150 mg IM q12 weeks or levonorgestrel intrauterine system placement. Progesterone-only OCPs can also be an alternative, but they require excellent compliance.

bid, twice daily (every 12 hours); DMPA, depot medroxyprogesterone acetate; DUB, dysfunctional uterine bleeding; IM, intramuscular; OCP, oral contraceptive pill; PO, by mouth; qd, daily; qid, four times per day (every 6 hours); tid, three times per day (every 8 hours).

activity and/or of GABAergic receptor functioning during the luteal phase of the menstrual cycle with heightened sensitivity to circulating progesterone metabolites. PMS and PMDD are highly associated with unipolar depressive disorder and anxiety disorders, such as obsessive-compulsive disorder, panic disorder, and generalized anxiety disorder. During adolescence, it may be difficult to determine if the affective symptoms represent a mood or anxiety disorder, a premenstrual exacerbation of a psychiatric disorder, or simple PMS.

Current treatment for PMS in adolescence is based on findings from adult studies and includes lifestyle recommendations and pharmacologic agents that suppress the rise and fall of ovarian steroids or augment serotonin. Proven effective interventions that should be tried include education about pathophysiology, lifestyle changes (eg, increasing physical activity and smoking cessation), stress reduction and cognitive behavioral therapy. If contraception or cycle control is important, a combined hormonal contraceptive pill may be beneficial. The pill containing 20 mcg ethinyl estradiol and 3 mg drospirenone has been shown to be therapeutic in studies of adult women with PMDD. If these interventions do not adequately control symptoms, luteal phase or continuous administration of selective serotonin reuptake inhibitors (SSRIs) can be considered. SSRIs are increasingly used as first-line therapy for PMS and PMDD in adults, and a recent

Cochrane review of SSRIs in severe adult PMS determined that SSRIs administered continuously or during the luteal phase were effective in reducing premenstrual symptoms. Case reports indicate that adolescents with PMDD respond well to luteal phase dosing of fluoxetine at the standard adult dosage of 20 mg/day. SSRIs are not formally approved by the Food and Drug Administration (FDA) for treatment of PMS or PMDD in adolescents.

6. Ovarian Cysts

Functional ovarian cysts account for the majority of benign ovarian tumors in postpubertal adolescents and are a result of the normal process of ovulation. They may be asymptomatic or may cause menstrual irregularities or pelvic pain. Large cysts can cause constipation or urinary frequency. Follicular cysts are the most common functional cysts. They are usually unilateral, less than 3 cm in diameter, and resolve spontaneously in 1–2 months. Cyst pain occurs as the diameter of the cyst increases, stretching the overlying ovarian cortex and capsule. If the patient's discomfort is tolerable, she can be reexamined monthly and observed for resolution. Hormonal contraceptive products that suppress ovulation can be started to prevent additional cysts from forming. Patients with cysts should be counseled about the signs and symptoms of ovarian and/or tubal torsion, which are serious complications. Adnexal torsion presents with the sudden onset of pain, nausea, and vomiting. Low-grade fever, leukocytosis, and the development of peritoneal signs with rebound and guarding can be found. Torsion is a surgical emergency due to the risk of ischemia and death of the ovary. Patients should be referred to a gynecologist for potential laparoscopy if a cyst has a solid component and measures more than 6 cm by ultrasonography, if there are symptoms or signs of hemorrhage or torsion, or if the cyst fails to regress within 2 months. Corpus luteum cysts occur less commonly and may be large, 5–10 cm in diameter. The patient with a corpus luteum cyst may have associated amenorrhea, or as the cyst becomes atretic, heavy vaginal bleeding. There may be bleeding into the cyst or rupture with intraperitoneal hemorrhage. To determine whether the bleeding is self-limited, serial hematocrit measurements and ultrasounds can be used. If the patient is stable, hormonal contraception that suppresses ovulation can be started to prevent additional cyst formation and the patient may be monitored for 3 months for resolution. Laparoscopy may be indicated if the cyst is larger than 6 cm or if there is severe pain or hemorrhage.

ACOG Practice Bulletin No. 168: Cervical cancer screening and prevention. Obstet Gynecol 2016;128(4):e111–e130 [PMID: 27661651].

Braverman PK, Breech L: Committee on Adolescence: Gynecologic examination for adolescents in the pediatric office setting. Pediatrics 2010;126(3):583–590 [PMID: 20805151].

Centers for Disease Control and Prevention: Sexually transmitted diseases treatment guidelines, 2015. MMWR Recomm Rep 2015;64(3):90–93 [PMID: 26042815].

Gordon CM et al: Functional hypothalamic amenorrhea: an Endocrine Society Clinical Practice Guideline. J Clin Endocrinol Metab 2017;102(5):1413–1439 [PMID: 28368518].

Haamid F, Sass AE, Dietrich JE: Heavy menstrual bleeding in adolescents. J Pediatr Gynecol 2017;30(3):335–340 [PMID: 28108214].

Jamieson MA: Disorders of menstruation in adolescent girls. Pediatr Clin North Am 2015;62(4):943–961 [PMID: 26210626].

Massad LS et al: 2012 updated consensus guidelines for the management of abnormal cervical cancer screening tests and cancer precursors. Obstet Gynecol 2013;121(4):829–846 [PMID: 23635684].

Ryan SA: The treatment of dysmenorrhea. Pediatr Clin North Am 2017;64(2):331–342 [PMID: 28292449].

Witchel SF et al: The diagnosis of polycystic ovary syndrome during adolescence. Horm Res Paediatr 2015;83:376–389 [PMID: 25833060].

CONTRACEPTION

According to the CDC 2017 Youth Risk Behavior Survey, 40% of high school students reported having had sexual intercourse and 29% reported being currently sexually active. Fifty-seven percent reported using a condom at their latest intercourse. Most young people have sex for the first time at about the age of 17, but do not marry until their middle or late twenties. This means that young adults are at risk of unwanted pregnancy and STIs for nearly a decade. A sexually active female who does not use contraceptives has almost a 90% chance of becoming pregnant within a year.

Abstinence & Decision Making

Talking with teenagers about sexual intercourse and its implications can help teens make informed decisions regarding engaging in sexual activity. The AAP endorses a comprehensive approach to sexuality education that incorporates encouraging abstinence while providing appropriate risk reduction counseling regarding sexual behaviors. Counseling should include discussions about confidentiality, STI prevention and testing, and contraceptive methods including abstinence and emergency contraception (Table 4–19). Best-practice guidelines recommend that an adolescent sexual history be taken with the adolescent alone in an honest and caring manner with a nonjudgmental attitude and a comfortable, matter-of-fact approach to asking questions. The CDC has a useful *Guide to Taking a Sexual History* for providers, which covers the "five Ps" of sexual health: *p*artners, *p*ractices, *p*rotection from STIs, *p*ast history of STIs, and *p*revention of pregnancy (http://www.cdc.gov/std/treatment/SexualHistory.pdf). Adolescents often delay seeing a clinician for contraceptive services after initiating sexual activity. Concern about lack of confidentiality is an important reason for this delay.

Table 4–19. Contraceptive efficacy.

Method	Percentage of Women Experiencing an Unintended Pregnancy Within the First Year of Use	
	Typical Use	Perfect Use
No method	85	85
Spermicides only	28	18
Withdrawal	22	4
Diaphragm	16	6
Condom		
Female	21	5
Male	18	2
Oral contraceptive pill	9	0.3
Evra Patch	9	0.3
NuvaRing	9	0.3
Depo-Provera	6	0.2
IUD		
ParaGard	0.8	0.6
Mirena	0.2	0.2
Nexplanon	0.05	0.05

IUD, intrauterine device.
Adapted with permission from Hatcher RA: *Contraceptive Technology*, 20th ed (revised). New York, NY: Ardent Media; 2011.

▶ Methods Counseling

The goals of counseling adolescents about contraception include promoting safe and responsible sexual behavior through delaying the initiation of sexual activity, reinforcing consistent condom use for those who are sexually active, and discussing other contraceptive options to provide protection from unwanted pregnancy. Encouraging adolescents to use contraception when they do engage in sexual intercourse does not lead to higher rates of sexual activity. MI can be used to address the ambivalence and discrepancies among adolescents' sexual and contraceptive behaviors, their sexual and relationship values, and future life goals. Providers should familiarize themselves with their state policies regarding the ability of minors to consent for sexual and reproductive health care services. These data are accessible on the Internet from the Guttmacher Institute (http://www.guttmacher.org) and the Center for Adolescent Health and the Law (http://www.adolescenthealthlaw.org).

Providers should consider the adolescent's lifestyle, potential challenges to compliance, need for confidentiality around the use of contraception, previous experiences with contraception and reasons for discontinuation, and any misconceptions regarding contraceptive options. Barriers to health care access including transportation and financial limitations should be identified. Prescribing contraception for other medical reasons (eg, management of dysmenorrhea) can create opportunities for providers and adolescent patients to make parents aware of the use of the medication while maintaining confidentiality around sexual behaviors.

Mechanism of Action

The primary mechanism of action for combined hormonal contraceptives containing estrogen and progestin (OCPs, transdermal patch, intravaginal ring) and the progestin-only methods (pills, DMPA, and the etonogestrel implant) is inhibition of ovulation. Thickening of the cervical mucus also makes sperm penetration more difficult, and atrophy of the endometrium diminishes the chance of implantation. (The mechanisms of action for IUSs and intrauterine devices [IUDs] are discussed later in this chapter in the section Intrauterine Systems & Devices.)

Starting all birth control methods during the menstrual period (either first day of bleeding or first Sunday of bleeding) produces the most reliable suppression of ovulation. Conventional OCPs, transdermal patches, and intravaginal rings typically require that the adolescent wait for her next period to begin before starting. Data show that many women who receive prescriptions or even samples of medication never begin the prescribed method. Furthermore, these women could become pregnant while waiting to start. "Quick start" is an alternative approach to starting contraception that allows the patient to begin contraception on the day of the appointment regardless of menstrual cycle day, following a negative pregnancy test. This approach has been studied in adolescent women and increases adherence with the method of choice. Unfortunately, these studies also highlight the generally poor long-term compliance with contraceptive treatment in this age group.

Medical Considerations

Evaluation of an adolescent female requesting contraception should include a review of current and past medical conditions, current medications and allergies, menstrual history, confidential social history including sexual history, and family medical history. Important components of a sexual history include age at first intercourse, number of partners in lifetime, history of STIs and pelvic inflammatory disease (PID), condom use, current and past use of other contraceptives and reasons for discontinuation, and pregnancy history and outcomes. It is helpful to have a baseline weight, height, BMI, and blood pressure. A pelvic examination is not necessary before initiating contraception. However, if the woman is sexually active and has missed menstrual periods or has symptoms of

pregnancy, a pregnancy test is warranted. Screening for STIs should be offered if a sexually experienced woman is asymptomatic and testing for STIs is indicated if she is symptomatic.

The World Health Organization's (WHO) publication, *Improving Access to Quality Care in Family Planning: Medical Eligibility Criteria for Contraceptive Use* is an evidence-based guide providing criteria for initiating and continuing contraceptive methods based on a risk assessment of an individual's characteristics or known preexisting medical condition. Table 4–20 lists absolute (a condition which represents an unacceptable health risk if the contraceptive method is used) and relative (a condition where the theoretical or proven risks usually outweigh the advantages of using the method) contraindications to using combined hormonal birth control pills. These contraindications can be extended to other combined hormonal products that contain estrogen and progestins, including the transdermal patch and intravaginal ring. The CDC has also published the *US Medical Eligibility Criteria for Contraceptive Use* which was adapted from the WHO

Table 4–20. Contraindications to combined oral contraceptive (COC) pills.

Absolute contraindications
Pregnancy
Breast-feeding (within 6 wk of childbirth)
Hypertension SBP > 160 mm Hg or DBP > 100 mm Hg
History of thrombophlebitis; current thromboembolic disorder, cerebrovascular disease, or ischemic heart disease
Known thrombogenic mutations (factor V Leiden; prothrombin mutation; protein S, protein C, and antithrombin deficiencies)
Systemic lupus erythematosus
Complicated valvular heart disease (with pulmonary hypertension; atrial fibrillation; history of bacterial endocarditis)
Diabetes with nephropathy; retinopathy; neuropathy
Liver disease: active viral hepatitis; severe cirrhosis; tumor (hepatocellular adenoma or hepatoma)
Breast cancer (current)
Migraine headaches with aura
Major surgery with prolonged immobilization
Relative contraindications
Postpartum (first 3 wk)
Breast-feeding (6 wk–6 mo following childbirth)
Hypertension (adequately controlled HTN; any history of HTN where BP cannot be evaluated; SBP 140–159 mm Hg or DPB 90–99 mm Hg)
Migraine headache without aura (for continuation of COC)
Breast cancer history with remission for 5 y
Active gallbladder disease or history of COC-induced cholestasis
Use of drugs that affect liver enzymes (rifampin, phenytoin, carbamazepine, barbiturates, primidone, topiramate, oxcarbazepine, lamotrigine, ritonavir-boosted protease inhibitors)

BP, blood pressure; DBP, diastolic blood pressure; HTN, hypertension; SBP, systolic blood pressure.

publication; this document allows consideration of use of combined hormonal contraceptive products in women who are currently receiving anticoagulation therapy.

It is important to assess patients for possible risk factors for venous thromboembolic events (VTEs) prior to initiating any contraceptive product containing estrogen. The risk of VTE for reproductive-aged women is extremely low (1–5/10,000 woman-years for nonpregnant women not using contraceptive product containing estrogen). The use of estrogen increases the risk of VTE for nonpregnant women (3–15/10,000 woman-years); however, pregnancy itself markedly increases the risk of VTE (5–20/10,000 woman-years in pregnancy and 40–65/10,000 woman-years postpartum). In light of the low population risk of VTE, it is not cost-effective to screen all reproductive-aged women for inherited thrombophilia (factor V Leiden, prothrombin mutation, protein S, protein C, and antithrombin deficiencies). Table 4–21 shows helpful screening questions for personal and family history of VTE. If a close relative had a VTE, determine whether testing for inherited thrombophilia was conducted. If a specific defect was identified, testing the patient for that defect prior to initiating a product containing estrogen is warranted. If testing is unknown but the family history is highly suggested of inherited thrombophilia, testing for all of the inherited thrombophilic disorders prior to initiating estrogen should be considered. Additionally, if testing is indicated but not possible, providers should consider alternative contraceptive products that do not contain estrogen.

▶ Tips for Prescribing & Monitoring Contraceptive Use

It is important to thoroughly review the advantages, disadvantages, potential side effects, and instructions for use of contraceptive methods in a concise and age-appropriate manner with adolescent patients. Written instructions that are clear and at an appropriate educational level can also be helpful (www.youngwomenshealth.org is a useful source for instructions). Some offices utilize consent forms to further ensure that the adolescent has a full understanding of the

Table 4–21. Screening questions for inherited thrombophilia.

Have you or a first-degree relative…	… ever had blood clots in the legs or lungs?
	… ever been hospitalized for blood clots in the legs or lungs?
What were the circumstances in which the blood clot took place?	Cancer, air travel, obesity, immobility, postpartum
Did you or a family member require blood thinning medication?	

chosen contraceptive method. Teens need to be reminded that hormonal contraception will not protect them from STI transmission (including HIV infection), and condoms need to be used consistently. Encouraging teens to be creative about personal reminders such as setting a cell phone alarm to take a pill can help with compliance. Teens often discontinue birth control for nonmedical reasons or minor side effects and should be encouraged to contact their providers if any questions or concerns about the chosen method arise to avoid unintentional pregnancy. Frequent follow-up visits (every few months) with a provider may also improve adherence. These visits also provide opportunities for further reproductive health education and STI screening.

Barrier Methods

Male condoms have been used more widely in the last several decades as a result of educational and marketing efforts driven by the AIDS epidemic. All sexually active adolescents should be counseled to use condoms correctly and consistently with all intimate behaviors (oral, vaginal, and anal intercourse). Condoms offer protection against STIs by providing a mechanical barrier. Polyurethane condoms can be used by adolescents with an allergy to latex. Spermicides containing nonoxynol-9 are no longer recommended, as exposure to spermicide can cause genital irritation which may facilitate the acquisition of STIs including HIV. Patients should be counseled to use water-based lubricants with condoms.

Vaginal barrier methods include the female condom, diaphragm, and cervical cap. The female condom is a polyurethane vaginal pouch that can be used as an alternative to the male condom. Female condoms have lower efficacy in preventing pregnancy and STIs and are more expensive than male condoms. Diaphragms and cervical caps may not be feasible for adolescents as they require prescription, professional fitting, and skill with insertion.

Combined Hormonal Methods

▶ Oral Contraceptive Pills, Transdermal Patch, & Intravaginal Ring

Combined oral contraceptive (COC) pills are the most commonly used contraceptive method in the adolescent age group. COC pills are also utilized for noncontraceptive indications (Table 4–22). All COC pills contain estrogen (ethinyl estradiol). "Low-dose" COC pills contain 20–35 mcg of ethinyl estradiol per pill. There are a variety of progestins used in COC pills, most made from testosterone with differing androgenic profiles. Drospirenone is a progestin derived from spironolactone that possesses antiandrogenic and antimineralocorticoid activity. This formulation has appeal for use with patients who have PCOS, but should not be prescribed for patients with risk of hyperkalemia

Table 4–22. Noncontraceptive health benefits of oral contraceptive pills.

Protection against life-threatening conditions
Ovarian cancer
Endometrial cancer
Pelvic inflammatory disease
Ectopic pregnancy
Morbidity and mortality due to unintended pregnancies
Alleviate conditions affecting quality of life
Iron deficiency anemia
Benign breast disease
Dysmenorrhea
Irregular menstrual cycles
Functional ovarian cysts
Premenstrual syndrome
Acne

(those who have renal, hepatic, or adrenal insufficiency or take certain medications including angiotensin-converting enzyme inhibitors and angiotensin II receptor antagonists). Extended cycle regimens are available which allow women to decrease menstrual frequency from four menstrual cycles per year to formulations that provide hormonal pills daily for the whole year, eliminating menstrual periods altogether. New formulations with fewer placebo pills (4 vs the standard 7) decrease the duration of the menstrual period. There is also a chewable COC for those who cannot swallow pills.

In general, COC side effects are mild and improve or lessen during the first 3 months of use. Table 4–23 shows the more common estrogenic, progestogenic, and combined (estrogenic and progestogenic) effects of COC pills. These symptoms can also be observed with the other combined hormonal methods. If a patient taking contraceptive pills has persistent minor side effects for more than 3 months, a different type of COC can be tried to achieve the hormonal effects desired (eg, decreasing the estrogen content or changing progestin). Breakthrough bleeding is a common side effect in the first few months of COC use and generally resolves without intervention. If breakthrough bleeding is persistent, the provider should rule out other possible etiologies such as missed pills, pregnancy, infection, or interaction with other medications. For women who have spotting or bleeding before completing the active hormonal pills, increasing the progestin content will provide more endometrial support. For those with continued spotting or bleeding after the period, increasing the estrogen content will provide more endometrial support.

▶ Transdermal Patch

The transdermal patch, Ortho Evra, releases 20 mcg of ethinyl estradiol and 150 mcg of norelgestromin daily. One patch is worn for 7 days and changed weekly for 3 consecutive weeks. The patch is an attractive alternative to COC pills for adolescents who have difficulty remembering to take a pill

Table 4–23. Estrogenic, progestenic, and combined effects of COCs by system.

System	Estrogen Effects	Progestin Effects	Estrogen and Progestin Effects
General		Bloating	Cyclic weight gain due to fluid retention
Cardiovascular	Hypertension		Hypertension
Gastrointestinal	Nausea; hepatocellular adenomas	Increased appetite and weight gain; increased LDL cholesterol levels; decreased HDL cholesterol levels; decreased carbohydrate tolerance; increased insulin resistance	
Breast	Increased breast size	Increased breast tenderness or breast size	Breast tenderness
Genitourinary	Leukorrhea; cervical eversion or ectopy		
Hematologic	Thromboembolic complications, including pulmonary emboli (rare), deep venous thrombosis, cerebrovascular accident, or myocardial infarction (rare)		
Neurologic			Headaches
Skin	Telangiectasia, melasma	Acne, oily skin	
Psychological		Depression, fatigue, decreased libido	

COC, combined oral contraceptive (pill); HDL, high-density lipoprotein; LDL, low-density lipoprotein.
Adapted with permission from Hatcher RA: *Contraceptive Technology*, 20th ed (revised). New York, NY: Ardent Media; 2011.

every day; however, the higher bioavailability of estrogens delivered transdermally (60% higher than with 35 mcg COC pills) has raised concern that the patch might increase the risk of VTE over other estrogen-containing contraceptive products. Studies evaluating this risk have shown conflicting results. The FDA updated the safety labeling for Ortho Evra in September 2009 to include its interpretation that these studies show a zero to twofold increase in the risk of thromboembolic events. The FDA maintains that Ortho Evra is a well-tolerated and effective contraceptive for women with low-risk profile for VTE. As with other estrogen-containing contraceptive products, patients should be advised to avoid smoking and consider planned discontinuation of these methods around major surgery and prolonged immobilization. In clinical trials, the most common side effects included breast disorders (pain and swelling), headache, nausea, and skin irritation. The patch may be less effective in women weighing more than 90 kg and those with skin conditions preventing absorption.

▶ Intravaginal Ring

The NuvaRing is a vaginal ring that releases 15 mcg of ethinyl estradiol and 120 mcg of etonogestrel per day. The patient places the ring inside the vagina for 3 weeks and removes it the first day of the fourth week to allow for withdrawal bleeding. A new ring is inserted each month. In clinical trials, the most common side effects included vaginitis and vaginal discharge, headache, weight gain, and nausea.

Progestin-Only Methods

▶ Oral Contraceptive Pills

Progestin-only pills (POPs) do not contain estrogen. They are used in women with contraindications to estrogen-containing products such as the presence of inherited risk factors for thrombophilia or unacceptable estrogen-related side effects with COC pills. The efficacy of POPs in preventing pregnancy is slightly less than COC pills. They require strict compliance and a regular dosing schedule due to the shorter half-life of the progestin; a patient must take POPs daily at the same time (within 3 hours). The primary mechanisms by which pregnancy is prevented include thickening cervical mucous and thinning the endometrial lining. Ovulation is inhibited in approximately 50% of women. The main side effect of POPs is unpredictable menstrual patterns. The need for strict compliance and the possibility of breakthrough bleeding may make POPs a less desirable method for teens.

▶ Injectable Hormonal Contraception

DMPA, or Depo-Provera, is a long-acting injectable progestin contraceptive. It is injected into the gluteal or deltoid muscle every 12 weeks at a dose of 150 mg. The first injection should be given during the first 5 days of the menstrual cycle to ensure immediate contraceptive protection. The quick-start method may also be used with DMPA following a negative pregnancy test. Adolescents who have been sexually active within the previous 2 weeks of administration of DMPA using the quick-start method should be informed of the chance of pregnancy and instructed to return for a repeat pregnancy test 2 weeks after receiving DMPA. With a failure rate of less than 0.3%, long-acting nature reducing compliance issues, reversibility, and lack of estrogen-related side effects, DMPA is an attractive contraceptive option for many adolescents. The hypoestrogenic state that results from DMPA suppression of the hypothalamic-pituitary-ovarian axis reduces the normal effect of estrogen to inhibit bone resorption. The FDA issued a black box warning in 2004 that long-term (> 2 years) use of DMPA was a cause of decreased bone density. This is of particular concern as adolescence is the critical time of peak bone accretion. Current recommendations are that long-term use of DMPA should be limited to situations where other contraceptive methods are inadequate. Although DMPA use is associated with decreased bone density, there are studies showing that bone mineral density recovers after stopping DMPA. There are no studies to date that answer the question of whether decreased bone density from adolescent DMPA use increases the risk of osteoporosis and fractures in adulthood. The consensus of experts at this time is that the advantages of DMPA generally outweigh the theoretical risks of fractures later in life. As with every other contraceptive method, providers need to help their patients weigh the pros and cons of initiating and continuing with this method of contraception. Adolescents using DMPA should be counseled to take adequate dietary calcium (1300 mg/day) and vitamin D (400 IU/day), avoid tobacco smoking and have regular weight-bearing physical activity for overall bone health. Other adverse effects of DMPA include unpredictable menstrual patterns, weight gain (typically 5 lb/y for the first 2 years of use), and mood changes.

▶ Contraceptive Implant

Adolescents most commonly use short-acting hormonal contraceptive methods described previously. Unfortunately, these methods have relatively high failure rates (see Table 4–19) and low continuation rates. Higher failure rates combined with poor continuation rates decrease the efficacy of short-acting contraceptive methods in adolescents. LARCs, which include the contraceptive implants and IUSs and IUDs, have lower rates of failure and discontinuation. In one study comparing 1-year continuation rates for short-acting contraceptives versus LARCs, the continuation rate for short-acting methods was 55% versus 86% for LARCs. The pregnancy rate associated with use of short-acting contraceptives was 22 times higher than the rate of unintended pregnancy associated with the use of LARCs. Adolescents should be encouraged to consider LARCs as the best reversible methods for preventing unintended pregnancy, rapid repeat pregnancy, and abortion.

Nexplanon is a single-rod implant LARC that contains the progestin etonogestrel, a metabolite of desogestrel. Nexplanon also contains barium sulfate which makes it radiopaque. Nexplanon is placed subdermally and provides highly effective contraception for 3 years, with failure rates less than 1%. Nexplanon suppresses ovulation and thickens cervical mucous like DMPA but does not suppress ovarian estradiol production or induce a hypoestrogenic state. The risk of decreased bone density is less than that associated with DMPA. Placement should occur during the first 5 days of the menstrual period or at any time if a woman is correctly using a different hormonal contraceptive method. Proper timing minimizes the likelihood that the implant is placed during an early pregnancy or in a nonpregnant woman too late to inhibit ovulation in the first cycle of use. Irregular menstrual bleeding is the single most common reason for stopping use in clinical trials. On average, the volume of bleeding is similar to the woman's typical menstrual periods but the schedule of bleeding is irregular and unpredictable. Other side effects include headache, weight gain, acne, breast pain, and emotional lability. Return to fertility is rapid following removal. The efficacy of Nexplanon has not been formally defined in women with BMIs greater than 130% ideal and could theoretically be less effective in these women. The etonogestrel implant is not recommended for women who chronically take medications that are potent hepatic enzyme inducers because etonogestrel levels may be substantially reduced.

▶ Intrauterine Systems & Devices

Intrauterine systems (IUSs) and intrauterine devices (IUDs) are LARCs approved for use in nulliparous as well as parous teens and have high efficacy with failure rates of less than 1%. There are four forms of IUS that release the progestin levonorgestrel: Mirena, which releases 20 mcg of levonorgestrel per day and is approved for contraception for up to 5 years; Skyla, which releases an average of 6 mcg/day and is approved for contraception for up to 3 years; Liletta, which releases 18.6 mcg/day initially and declines progressively to 12.6 mcg/day at 3 years after insertion and is approved for contraception for up to 5 years; and Kyleena, which has a release rate of 17.5 mcg/day after 24 days, declining to 7.4 mcg/day after 5 years and is approved for contraception for up to 5 years. The levonorgestrel IUSs have many contraceptive actions including thickening of cervical mucous, inhibiting sperm capacitation and survival, suppressing the endometrium, and suppression of ovulation in some women. Given that the contraceptive effect of levonorgestrel in the IUS devices is mainly due to its local effect versus systemic absorption, ovulation is not always suppressed and cysts related to normal ovulation can occur. Irregular bleeding is common in the first few months following insertion because endometrial suppression takes several months to evolve. Bleeding is then markedly decreased and secondary amenorrhea can occur. Other side effects include abdominal and/or pelvic pain, acne, ovarian cysts, and headache. In addition to pregnancy prevention, women with IUSs report reduced symptoms of dysmenorrhea and reduced pain from endometriosis. Cramping is common during insertion and spontaneous expulsion can occur. Uterine perforation during insertion is an uncommon risk.

The copper T 380A IUD, ParaGard, does not contain hormones and can provide contraception for up to 10 years. Its contraceptive actions include the release of copper ions which inhibit sperm migration and development of a sterile inflammatory reaction which is toxic to sperm and ova and prevents implantation. Menstrual pain and heavy bleeding are the most common reasons for discontinuation.

A common misconception about IUS and IUD use is that they increase the risk of PID. Current research shows that the risk of PID is increased above baseline only for the first 20 days after insertion. IUS and IUD use has also not been shown to increase the risk of tubal infertility or ectopic pregnancy. Contraindications for placement of IUS/IUD include pregnancy, PID, or postabortion sepsis within the past 3 months, current STI, purulent cervicitis, undiagnosed abnormal vaginal bleeding, malignancy of the genital tract, uterine anomalies, or leiomyomata distorting the uterine cavity making insertion incompatible. Allergy to any component of the IUS/IUD is a contraindication. Patients with disorders of copper metabolism (Wilson disease) should not use the copper-containing IUD. Adolescents should be screened for STIs prior to insertion of an IUS or IUD.

Emergency Contraception

Emergency contraception (EC) is the only contraceptive method designed to prevent pregnancy after unprotected or underprotected intercourse (Table 4–24). Indications for EC include unprotected vaginal intercourse, failure of contraceptive methods (broken condoms, missing three or more active COC pills, detached contraceptive patch, removed vaginal ring, or late DMPA injection), and sexual assault. EC medications include products labeled and approved for use as EC by the FDA (levonorgestrel and ulipristal acetate) and the "off-label" use of COC pills (the Yuzpe method).

Levonorgestrel EC, marketed as Plan B One-Step and its generic formulations, Take Action, Next Choice One Dose, and My Way, is a one-pill progesterone-only regimen that contains 1.5 mg of levonorgestrel, taken immediately after unprotected intercourse. The exact mechanism of levonorgestrel EC is unknown but is thought to inhibit ovulation, disrupt follicular development, or interfere with the maturation of the corpus luteum. EC is not teratogenic and does not interrupt a pregnancy that has already implanted in the

Table 4–24. Emergency contraception regimens.

Progestin-Only	Dose: Once
Plan B One-Step, Take Action, Next Choice One Dose, My Way	1 pill
Ulipristal Acetate	**Dose: Once**
Ella	1 pill
Estrogen and Progestin	**Dose: Repeat in 12 h**
Ovral, Ogestrel	2 white pills
Levlen, Nordette	4 orange pills
Lo/Ovral, Low-Ogestrel, Levora, Quasense, Cryselle	4 white pills
Jolessa, Portia, Seasonale, Trivora	4 pink pills
Triphasil, Tri-Levlen	4 yellow pills
Seasonique	4 light blue-green pills
Enpresse	4 orange pills
Alesse, Lessina, Levlite	5 pink pills
Aviane	5 orange pills
Lutera	5 white pills

uterine lining. Therefore, pregnancy testing before use is not required. It is recommended that patients take these products within 72 hours of unprotected intercourse. EC has been studied up to 120 hours following unprotected intercourse; however, its efficacy diminishes with time from the event. EC is 90% effective if used within 24 hours, 75% effective if used within 72 hours, and approximately 60% effective if used within 120 hours. It is therefore important to counsel patients to take the medication as soon as possible following unprotected intercourse or contraception failure. EC could potentially prevent approximately 80% of unintended pregnancies and should be part of anticipatory guidance given to sexually active adolescents of both genders. These products are available without prescription for purchase over the counter by adolescents aged 17 years and older; however, proof of age is not required for purchase. A follow-up appointment should be conducted 10–14 days after administration of EC for pregnancy testing, STI screening, and counseling regarding reproductive health and contraceptive use. A helpful resource for information about EC can be found at http://ec.princeton.edu/index.html.

If an approved EC medication is not available, certain COC pills containing levonorgestrel or norgestrel can also be used for EC in a two-dose regimen separated by 12 hours; this approach is known as the Yuzpe method (see Table 4–24). An antiemetic drug takes 30 minutes prior to pills containing

estrogen may help control nausea. A pregnancy test is not required prior to prescription and administration of EC.

Ulipristal, marketed as Ella, is a single pill containing 30 mg of ulipristal acetate that is available by prescription only and can be used within 120 hours after unprotected intercourse. Ulipristal binds to the human progesterone receptor and prevents binding of progesterone. Unlike levonorgestrel EC, a pregnancy test must be performed to exclude existing pregnancy before taking ulipristal because of the risk of fetal loss if used in the first trimester. Patients should also be counseled that a pregnancy test is indicated if their period is more than 7 days later than expected after taking ulipristal. Patients should be instructed to return for evaluation of the rare occurrence of ectopic pregnancy if severe abdominal pain occurs 3–5 weeks after use.

Providers should be aware that insertion of ParaGard (copper IUD) within 5 days of unprotected intercourse is an additional method of emergency contraception available in the United States.

Committee on Adolescence: Contraception and adolescents. Pediatrics 2014;134:e1257–e1281 [PMID: 17974753].

Committee on Adolescence: Emergency contraception. Pediatrics 2012;130(6):1174–1182 [PMID: 23184108].

Diedrich JT, Klein DA, Peipert JF: Long-acting reversible contraception in adolescents: a systematic review and meta-analysis. Am J Obstet Gynecol 2017;216(4):364.e103642.12 [PMID: 28038902].

Hatcher RA et al: Contraceptive efficacy. In: Hatcher RA et al (eds): *Contraceptive Technology.* 21st ed. New York, NY: Ayer Company Publishers, Inc., 2018.

Kann L et al: Youth risk behavior surveillance—United States, 2017. MMWR Surveill Summ 2018;67(8):1–114 [PMID: 29902162].

Pfeifer S et al: Combined hormonal contraception and the risk of venous thromboembolism: a guideline. Fertil Steril 2017;107(1):43–51 [PMID: 27793376].

World Health Organization: Medical Eligibility Criteria for Contraceptive Use. 5th ed. Geneva: World Health Organization, Reproductive Health and Research, Family and Community Health; 2015 [PMID: 26337268].

PREGNANCY

In the United States, approximately 456,000 women younger than 20 years become pregnant every year. The majority of teen pregnancies are unintended. Approximately 61% of adolescent pregnancies result in live births, 25% end in abortion, and 14% in miscarriage. In the United States, both the teenage pregnancy rate and birth rate have steadily declined over the past two decades, which has been attributed to improved access to contraceptives for youth and increased use of LARCs. In 2018, the birth rate for adolescents, 17.4 births per 1000 women, was the lowest it has ever been for all racial and ethnic groups since the peak rate of 61.8 in 1991. However, despite this trend, racial and ethnic disparities persist, with the pregnancy rate among non-Hispanic white teens less than half that among non-Hispanic blacks and Hispanics. Lower socioeconomic status and lower maternal education are risk factors for teen pregnancy regardless of racial or ethnic group.

Presentation

Pregnancy is the most common cause of secondary amenorrhea and should be considered as a cause of even one missed period. The level of denial about the possibility of pregnancy is high and adolescents with undiagnosed pregnancies may present with abdominal pain, nausea or vomiting, breast tenderness, urinary frequency, dizziness, or other nonspecific symptoms. In addition to denial, difficult social situations can contribute to delays in diagnosis and in seeking prenatal care. Young, newly pregnant adolescents may fear violence from their partner or abandonment by their family. Clinicians should have a low threshold for suspecting pregnancy and obtaining pregnancy tests.

Diagnosis

Enzyme-linked immunosorbent assay test kits specific for the β-hCG subunit and sensitive to less than 50 mIU/mL of serum hCG can be performed on urine (preferably the day's first voided specimen, because it is more concentrated) in less than 5 minutes and are accurate by the expected date of the missed period in almost all patients. Serum radioimmunoassay, also specific for the β-hCG subunit, is accurate within 7 days after fertilization and is helpful in ruling out ectopic pregnancy or threatened abortion, as the quantitative result of this assay can be tracked over time and can be compared to normal ranges for gestational age. Serum hCG doubles approximately every 2 days in the first 6–7 weeks of the pregnancy and a gestational sac is identifiable using transvaginal ultrasonography at hCG levels of 1000–2000 mIU/mL. Pregnancies are dated from the first day of the LMP. The estimated due date can be calculated by adding 7 days to the LMP, subtracting 3 months and adding 1 year. Pregnancy dating calendars are widely available on the Internet. In the absence of an accurate LMP, ultrasonography for confirmation of the presence of an intrauterine pregnancy and accurate dating can be obtained.

A speculum examination is not mandatory at the time of pregnancy diagnosis for an asymptomatic adolescent. If there is vaginal spotting or bleeding, unusual vaginal discharge, symptoms of STI, pelvic pain, or abdominal pain, a speculum examination is required. The differential diagnosis includes infection, miscarriage, ectopic pregnancy, and other disorders of early pregnancy. An 8-week gestational age uterus is about the size of an orange and a 12-week uterus is about the size of a grapefruit on bimanual examination. The uterine fundus is just palpable at the symphysis pubis at 12 weeks' gestational age, midway between the symphysis and umbilicus at 16 weeks and typically at the umbilicus at 20 weeks. If the uterus is smaller than expected for pregnancy dates, possible diagnoses include inaccurate dates, false-positive test, ectopic pregnancy, or incomplete or missed abortion. A uterus that is larger than expected may be caused by inaccurate dates, twin gestation, molar pregnancy, or a corpus luteum cyst of pregnancy.

Management

A. Counseling at the Time of Pregnancy Testing

When an adolescent presents for pregnancy testing, it is helpful, before performing the test, to find out what she hopes the result will be and what she thinks she will do if the test is positive. The diagnosis of pregnancy may be met with shock, fear, anxiety, happiness, or, most likely, a combination of emotions. The clinician should discuss all pregnancy options with the patient including termination or continuing with the pregnancy and either placing the infant for adoption or raising the infant. Patients should be informed of the gestational age and time frames required for the different options. If providers are not comfortable discussing the option of termination, the adolescent should be referred to a provider who is comfortable with comprehensive options counseling. Many teenagers need help in telling and involving their parents. It is also important to ascertain the teen's safety and make appropriate referral to social services if there are legitimate concerns. If the patient knows what she wants to do, she should be referred to the appropriate resources. If a teenager is ambivalent about her plans, it is helpful to follow up in 1 week to be certain that a decision has been made. Avoiding a decision reduces the adolescent's options and may result in poor pregnancy outcomes. Providers can help ensure that the patient obtains prenatal care if she has chosen to continue the pregnancy. In addition, counseling about healthful diet; folic acid supplementation (400 mcg/day); and avoiding alcohol, tobacco, and other drugs is important.

B. Pregnancy Outcomes

Young maternal age, low maternal prepregnancy weight, poor weight gain, delay in prenatal care, maternal depression, exposure to domestic violence, and low socioeconomic status contribute to low birth weight and increased neonatal mortality. The poor nutritional status of some teenagers, substance abuse, and high incidence of STIs also play a role in poor outcomes. Teenagers are at greater risk than adults for preeclampsia, eclampsia, iron deficiency anemia, cephalopelvic disproportion, prolonged labor, premature labor, and maternal death. Good family support, early prenatal care, and good nutrition can positively impact several of these problems.

Psychosocial consequences for the teenage mother and her infant are listed in Table 4–25. Teenagers who are pregnant require additional support from their caregivers.

Table 4–25. Psychosocial consequences of pregnancy for the adolescent mother and her infant.

Mother	Infant
Increased morbidity related to pregnancy	**Greater health risks**
Greater risk of eclampsia, anemia, prolonged labor, premature labor	Increased chance of low birth weight or prematurity
Increased chance of miscarriages, stillbirths	Increased risk of infant death
Increased chance of maternal mortality	Increased risk of injury and hospitalization by age 5 y
Decreased academic achievement	**Decreased educational attainment**
Less likely to get high school diploma, go to college, or graduate	Lower cognitive scores
Delayed education (average 2 y)	Decreased development
Lower occupational attainment and prestige	Greater chance of being behind grade or needing remedial help
Less chance of stable employment (some resolution over time)	Lower chance of advanced academics
Lower job satisfaction	Lower academic aptitude as a teenager and perhaps a higher
Lower income and wages	probability of dropping out of school
Greater dependence on public assistance	**Psychosocial consequences**
Less stable marital relationships	Greater risk of behavior problems
Higher rates of single parenthood	Poverty
Earlier marriage (though less common than in the past)	Higher probability of living in a nonintact home while in high school
Accelerated pace of marriage, separation, divorce, and remarriage	Greater risk of adolescent pregnancy
Faster pace of subsequent childbearing	
High rate of repeat unintended pregnancy	
More births out of marriage	
Closer spacing of births	
Larger families	

Multidisciplinary clinics for young mothers, if available, may be the best providers for pregnant adolescents. Adolescent mothers tend to be more negative and authoritative when disciplining their children. They may have inadequate knowledge of normal behavior and development. Providers can help by educating the adolescent mother during routine visits regarding appropriate discipline and expectations for her child's behavior.

Postpartum contraceptive counseling and follow-up may help prevent additional pregnancies. In untreated girls, the risk of a second unintended pregnancy within the next 2 years is approximately 30%. Combined hormonal contraceptive options can be started 6 weeks after delivery in non–breast-feeding adolescents; progestin-only methods can be started immediately postpartum, even in breast-feeding adolescents.

Ectopic Pregnancy

In the United States, approximately 2% of pregnancies are ectopic. Adolescents have the highest mortality rate from ectopic pregnancy, most likely related to delayed diagnosis. Risk factors include history of PID or STIs. Repeat infections with *C trachomatis* increase risk for ectopic pregnancy, as does cigarette smoking. Conception while on progestin-only methods of contraception also increases the risk of ectopic pregnancy because of the progestin-mediated decrease in tubal motility. The classic presentation is missed menstrual period, abdominal pain, and vaginal bleeding. A urine pregnancy test is usually positive by the time of presentation. The patient may have abdominal or pelvic tenderness, adnexal tenderness, and/or an adnexal mass on examination. The uterus is typically either normal sized or slightly enlarged. Diagnosis is based on serial serum quantitative hCG levels and transvaginal ultrasound. Patients should be referred urgently to an obstetrician gynecologist for management to avoid a ruptured ectopic pregnancy. Ruptured ectopic pregnancy often presents with shock and an acute surgical abdomen and is a surgical emergency.

ACOG Practice Bulletin No. 191: Tubal ectopic pregnancy. Obstet Gynecol 2018;131(2):e65–e77 [PMID: 29232273].

Hornberger LL; Committee on Adolescence: Diagnosis of pregnancy and providing options counseling for the adolescent patient. Pediatrics 2017;140(3):e20172273 [PMID: 28827383].

Kost K, Maddow-Zimet I, Arpaia A: *Pregnancies, Births and Abortions Among Adolescents and Young Women in the United States, 2013: National and State Trends by Age, Race and Ethnicity.* New York, NY: Guttmacher Institute; 2017. http://www.guttmacher.org/report/us-teen-pregnancy-trends-2013#4. Accessed June 25, 2019.

Martin JA et al: Births in the United States, 2018. NCHS Data Brief, no. 346. Hyattsville, MD: National Center for Health Statistics; 2019.

Pinzon JL et al: Care of adolescent parents and their children. Pediatrics 2012;130(6):1743–1756 [PMID: 23184113].

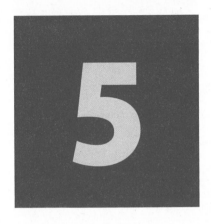

Adolescent Substance Abuse

Paritosh Kaul, MD

Substance abuse tends to be a chronic, progressive disease. Initiation of substance use is becoming such a common feature of an American adult that many authorities call it normative behavior. At this stage, substance use is typically limited to experimentation with tobacco or alcohol (so-called gateway substances). During adolescence, young people are expected to establish an independent, autonomous identity. They try out a variety of behaviors within the safety of families and peer groups. This process often involves experimentation with psychoactive substances, usually in culturally acceptable settings. Continuation of substance abuse, however, is a nonnormative risk behavior with the potential to compromise adolescent development.

The American Psychiatric Association has outlined criteria to judge the severity of substance use disorders (SUD). The most recent version, DSM-5 (*Diagnostic and Statistical Manual of Mental Disorders*, 5th Edition), has moved from the previous terms "substance abuse" and "substance dependency" to mild, moderate, and severe SUD. There are 11 features described in DSM-5. Patients with mild SUD have two or three features, whereas those with moderate have four or five features without loss of control or compulsive features. Patients with severe SUD have more than six features, including loss of control or compulsive features.

Common physiologic effects and symptoms of intoxication (which can occur at any stage of substance use) and withdrawal (a symptom of dependency) for the major classes of substances are shown in Tables 5–1 and 5–2.

American Psychiatric Association: *Diagnostic and Statistical Manual of Mental Disorders*: DSM-5. Washington, DC: American Psychiatric Association; 2013.

SCOPE OF THE PROBLEM

The best current source of information on the prevalence of substance abuse among American adolescents is the Monitoring the Future study (2019), which tracks substance abuse-related behaviors in a sample of 44,500 8th, 10th, and 12th graders in the United States. This study probably understates the magnitude of the problem of substance abuse because it excludes high-risk adolescent groups—school dropouts, runaways, and those in the juvenile justice system. Two other periodic surveys are the Youth Risk Behavior Survey (biannual) of students in grades 9–12 and National Survey of Drug Use and Health that is a home-based computer-assisted interview of individuals 12 years or older. Substance abuse among American youth rose in the 1960s and 1970s, declined in the 1980s, peaked in the 1990s, and has declined in the early 2000s. The most important finding to emerge from the most recent Monitoring the Future survey (2018 data) is the dramatic increase in vaping by adolescents. Vaping of three specific substances, nicotine, marijuana, and flavoring, is a relatively new phenomenon that substantially increased in 2018; the Monitoring the Future study registered some of the largest absolute increases in vaping of all three of these substances that this survey has ever tracked for any substance. Vape devices and electronic cigarettes (e-cigarettes) have rapidly become the most common tobacco products used by youth, driven in large part by marketing and advertising by e-cigarette companies. E-cigarettes are battery-operated devices designed to heat liquid into an aerosol that users inhale. The aerosol can contain nicotine, glycerol, propylene glycol, formaldehyde, cadmium, benzoic acid, lead, cannabis, chromium, nickel, different flavors and other chemicals. Pod-based e-cigarettes that use a salt-based nicotine made popular by Juul Labs have added to the availability of this product. Given that nicotine is involved in most vaping and that nicotine is a highly addictive substance, this presents a serious threat to all of the hard-won progress in adolescent substance abuse that has been made in recent decades.

The Monitoring the Future survey and others show that alcohol is the most frequently abused substance in the United States. Experimentation with alcohol typically begins in or before middle school. It is more common among boys

Table 5–1. Physiologic effects of commonly abused mood-altering substances by organ/system.

Eyes/pupils	
Mydriasis	Amphetamines, MDMA, or other stimulants; cocaine; glutethimide; jimson weed; LSD. Withdrawal from alcohol and opioids
Miosis	Alcohol, barbiturates, benzodiazepines, opioids, PCP
Nystagmus	Alcohol, barbiturates, benzodiazepines, inhalants, PCP
Conjunctival injection	LSD, marijuana
Lacrimation	Inhalants, LSD. Withdrawal from opioids
Cardiovascular	
Tachycardia	Amphetamines, MDMA, or other stimulants; cocaine; LSD; marijuana; PCP. Withdrawal from alcohol, barbiturates, benzodiazepines
Hypertension	Amphetamines, MDMA, or other stimulants; cocaine; LSD; marijuana; PCP. Withdrawal from alcohol, barbiturates, benzodiazepines
Hypotension	Barbiturates, opioids. Orthostatic: marijuana. Withdrawal from depressants
Arrhythmia	Amphetamines, MDMA, or other stimulants; cocaine; inhalants; opioids; PCP
Respiratory	
Depression	Opioids, depressants, GHB
Pulmonary edema	Opioids, stimulants
Core body temperature	
Elevated	Amphetamines, MDMA, or other stimulants; cocaine; PCP. Withdrawal from alcohol, barbiturates, benzodiazepines, opioids
Decreased	Alcohol, barbiturates, benzodiazepines, opioids, GHB
Peripheral nervous system response	
Hyperreflexia	Amphetamines, MDMA, or other stimulants; cocaine; LSD; marijuana; methaqualone; PCP. Withdrawal from alcohol, barbiturates, benzodiazepines
Hyporeflexia	Alcohol, barbiturates, benzodiazepines, inhalants, opioids
Tremor	Amphetamines or other stimulants, cocaine, LSD. Withdrawal from alcohol, barbiturates, benzodiazepines, cocaine
Ataxia	Alcohol, amphetamines, MDMA, or other stimulants; barbiturates; benzodiazepines; inhalants; LSD; PCP; GHB
Central nervous system response	
Hyperalertness	Amphetamines, MDMA, or other stimulants; cocaine
Sedation, somnolence	Alcohol, barbiturates, benzodiazepines, inhalants, marijuana, opioids, GHB
Seizures	Alcohol, amphetamines, MDMA, or other stimulants; cocaine; inhalants; methaqualone; opioids (particularly meperidine, propoxyphene). Withdrawal from alcohol, barbiturates, benzodiazepines
Hallucinations	Amphetamines, MDMA, or other stimulants; cocaine; inhalants; LSD; marijuana; PCP. Withdrawal from alcohol, barbiturates, benzodiazepines
Gastrointestinal	
Nausea, vomiting	Alcohol, amphetamines or other stimulants, cocaine, inhalants, LSD, opioids, peyote, GHB. Withdrawal from alcohol, barbiturates, benzodiazepines, cocaine, opioids

GHB, γ-hydroxybutyrate; LSD, lysergic acid diethylamide; MDMA, methylenedioxymethamphetamine (ecstasy); PCP, phencyclidine hydrochloride. Adapted with permission from Schwartz B, Alderman EM: Substances of abuse. Pediatr Rev 1997 June;18(6):204–215.

Table 5–2. Effects of commonly abused mood-altering substances by agent.

Substance	Pharmacology	Intoxication	Withdrawal	Chronic Use
Alcohol (ethanol)	Depressant; 10 g/drink Drink: 12-oz beer, 4-oz wine, 1½-oz liquor; one drink increases blood level by approximately 0.025 g/dL (varies by weight)	Legal: 0.05–0.1 g/dL (varies by state) Mild (< 0.1 g/dL): disinhibition, euphoria, mild sedation, and impaired coordination Moderate (0.1–0.2 g/dL): impaired mentation and judgment, slurred speech, ataxia Severe: > 0.3 g/dL: confusion, stupor > 0.4 g/dL: coma, depressed respiration	Mild: headache, tremors, nausea and vomiting ("hangover") Severe: fever, sweaty, seizure, agitation, hallucination, hypertension, tachycardia Delirium tremens (chronic use)	Hepatitis, cirrhosis, cardiac disease, Wernicke encephalopathy, Korsakoff syndrome
Marijuana (cannabis)	THC; 4%–6% in marijuana; 20%–30% in hashish	Low: euphoria, relaxation, impaired thinking. High: mood changes, depersonalization, hallucinations Toxic: panic, delusions, paranoia, psychosis	Irritability, disturbed sleep, tremor, nystagmus, anorexia, diarrhea, vomiting	Cough, gynecomastia, low sperm count, infertility, amotivational syndrome, apathy
Cocaine	Stimulant; releases biogenic amines; concentration varies with preparation and route of administration	Hyperalert, increased energy, confident, insomnia, anxiety, paranoia, dilated pupils, tremors, seizures, hypertension, arrhythmia, tachycardia, fever, dry mouth Toxic: coma, psychosis, seizure, myocardial infarction, stroke, hyperthermia, rhabdomyolysis	Drug craving, depression, dysphoria, irritability, lethargy, tremors, nausea, hunger	Nasal septum ulceration, epistaxis, lung damage, intravenous drug use
Opioids (heroin, morphine, codeine, methadone, opium, fentanyl, meperidine, propoxyphene)	Depressant; binds central opioid receptor; variable concentrations with substance	Euphoria, sedation, impaired thinking, low blood pressure, pinpoint pupil, urinary retention Toxic: hypotension, arrhythmia, depressed respiration, stupor, coma, seizure, death	Only after > 3 wk of regular use: drug craving, rhinorrhea, lacrimation, muscle aches, diarrhea, anxiety, tremors, hypertension, tachycardia	Intravenous drug use: cellulitis, endocarditis, embolisms, HIV
Amphetamines	Stimulant; sympathomimetic	Euphoria, hyperalert state, hyperactive, hypertension, arrhythmia, fever, flushing, dilated pupils, tremor, ataxia, dry mouth	Lethargy, fatigue, depression, anxiety, nightmares, muscle cramps, abdominal pain, hunger	Paranoia, psychosis
MDMA (ecstasy)	Stimulant, psychedelic; releases serotonin, dopamine, and norepinephrine; inhibits reuptake of neurotransmitters; increases dopamine synthesis; inhibits MAO	Enhanced empathy, euphoria, increased energy and self-esteem, tachycardia, hypertension, increased psychomotor drive, sensory enhancement, illusions, difficulty concentrating and retaining information, headaches, palpitations, flushing, hyperthermia Toxic: frank psychosis, coma, seizures, intracranial hemorrhage, cerebral infarction, asystole, pulmonary edema, multisystem organ failure, acute renal or hepatic failure, ARDS, DIC, SIADH, death	None	Paranoid psychosis

(Continued)

Table 5–2. Effects of commonly abused mood-altering substances by agent. (*Continued*)

Substance	Pharmacology	Intoxication	Withdrawal	Chronic Use
GHB (liquid ecstasy)	Depressant, endogenous CNS transmitter; influences dopaminergic activity, higher levels of GABA-B activity	10 mg/kg: sleep 30 mg/kg: memory loss 50 mg/kg: general anesthesia Toxic: CNS and respiratory depression, aggressiveness, seizures, bradycardia, apnea	Only after chronic use with dosing every 3 h. Early: mild tremor, tachycardia, hypertension, diaphoresis, moderate anxiety, insomnia, nausea, vomiting Progressive: confusion, delirium, hallucinations, autonomic instability, death	Wernicke-Korsakoff syndrome
Sedative-hypnotics (barbiturates, benzodiazepines, methaqualone)	Depressant	Sedation, lethargy, slurred speech, pinpoint pupils, hypotension, psychosis, seizures Toxic: stupor, coma, cardiac arrest, seizure, pulmonary edema, death	Only after weeks of use: agitation, delirium, psychosis, hallucinations, fever, flushing, hyper-/hypotension, death	Paranoia
Hallucinogens (LSD, peyote, mescaline, mushrooms, nutmeg, jimson weed)	Inhibition of serotonin release	Illusions, depersonalization, hallucination, anxiety, paranoia, ataxia, dilated pupils, hypertension, dry mouth Toxic: coma, terror, panic, "crazy feeling"	None	Flashbacks
Phencyclidine	Dissociative anesthetic	Low dose (< 5 mg): illusions, hallucinations, ataxia, hypertension, flushing Moderate dose (5–10 mg): hyperthermia, salivation, myoclonus High dose (> 10 mg): rigidity, seizure, arrhythmia, coma, death	None	Flashbacks
Inhalants (toluene, benzene, hydrocarbons, and fluorocarbons)	Stimulation progressing to depression	Euphoria, giddiness, impaired judgment, ataxia, rhinorrhea, salivation, hallucination Toxic: respiratory depression, arrhythmia, coma, stupor, delirium, sudden death	None	Permanent damage to nerves, liver, heart, kidney, brain
Nicotine	Releases dopamine, 1 mg nicotine per cigarette	Relaxation, tachycardia, vertigo, anorexia	Drug craving, irritability, anxiety, hunger, impaired concentration	Permanent damage to lung, heart, cardiovascular system
Anabolic steroids[a]	Bind steroid receptor Stacking: use many types simultaneously Pyramiding: increase dosage	Increased muscle bulk, strength, endurance, increased drive, hypogonadism, low sperm count, gynecomastia, decreased libido, virilization, irregular menses, hepatitis, early epiphysial closure, aggressiveness	Drug craving, dysphoria, irritability, depression	Tendon rupture, cardiomyopathy, atherosclerosis, peliosis hepatis (orally active C17 derivatives of testosterone are especially hepatotoxic)

ARDS, acute respiratory distress syndrome; CNS, central nervous system; DIC, disseminated intravascular coagulation; GABA, γ-aminobutyric acid; GHB, γ-hydroxybutyrate; HIV, human immunodeficiency virus; LSD, lysergic acid diethylamide; MAO, monoamine oxidase; MDMA, methylenedioxymethamphetamine; SIADH, syndrome of inappropriate secretion of antidiuretic hormone; THC, δ-9-tetrahydrocannabinol.
[a]Despite conventional assumptions, scientific studies show that anabolic steroids do not improve aerobic athletic performance and improve strength only in athletes trained in weight lifting before they begin using steroids and who continue to train and consume a high-protein diet.

than girls. It is most common among whites, less common among Hispanics and Native Americans, and least common among blacks and Asians. Almost two-thirds (59%) of adolescents consume alcohol before graduating from high school. Approximately one-tenth (9%) of eighth graders and 46% of high school students report being drunk at least once in their life. Marijuana is the most commonly used illicit drug in the United States. First experiences with marijuana and the substances listed in Table 5–2 typically occur during middle or early high school. The lifetime prevalence of marijuana use reported by 12th graders in 2018 was 29.7%. Daily use of marijuana increased until 2011 and has decreased since, with 3% of high school seniors being a daily or near daily user. Synthetic marijuana, often called spice and K-2, was scheduled by the Drug Enforcement Agency in 2011. Despite this intervention, annual synthetic marijuana use remains unchanged at 11.5% making, it the second most widely used class of illicit drug use after marijuana. In the most recent Monitoring the Future survey, there was little change in daily and annual marijuana prevalence rates and annual use of any illicit drug. The annual prevalence of marijuana use has held quite steady for several years, at 36%. In the past decade, lysergic acid diethylamide (LSD), methamphetamine, and cocaine use has decreased. Recently, ecstasy use has increased after a steady decline of several years.

Increasing opioid use has been another important trend in the United States. This issue encompasses a range of behaviors, from opioid misuse (defined as taking a prescription opioid in ways not prescribed by a physician) to use of illicit opioids (such as heroin) or synthetic opioids (such as fentanyl). Initiation of opioid misuse commonly occurs with prescription opioids, and among those with a history of heroin use, most report first opioid exposure having been a prescription opioid. Youth usually acquire opioids from family or friends or they consume opioids prescribed to them for medical indications. Dental visits are a leading source of opioid prescriptions to youth, and use of these prescriptions may be associated with an increased risk for of subsequent opioid use and abuse. In one study, 1 in 10 high school seniors reported nonmedical use of prescription opioids, and almost half (45%) used opioids to "relieve physical symptoms" in the past year. Although Vicodin use decreased among 12th graders to 2.9% in 2016, it remains one of the most widely used illicit drugs.

In the past 10 years, there has also been an increase in the recreational use of other prescription medications and over-the-counter (OTC) cough and cold medications among adolescents. Overall, the psychotherapeutic drugs (amphetamines, sedatives, tranquilizers, and narcotics other than heroin) make up a large part of the overall US drug problem. Medication used in the management of chronic pain, depression, anxiety, and attention-deficit/hyperactivity disorder can all be drugs of abuse.

Studies indicate that variations in the popularity of a substance of abuse are influenced by changes in the perceived risks and benefits of the substance among adolescent users. For example, the use of inhalants was rising until 2006, when both experience and educational efforts resulted in a perception of these substances as being "dangerous." As the perception of danger decreases, old drugs may reappear in common use. This process is called "generational forgetting." Currently, uses of LSD, inhalants, and ecstasy all reflect the effects of generational forgetting. Legalization of marijuana in certain states in the United States may increase the scope and breadth of the substance abuse problem. A recent study has shown an increase in medical marijuana use among adolescents in substance abuse programs. The American Academy of Pediatrics (AAP) has reaffirmed its position against the legalization of marijuana and its opposition to "medical marijuana"; it offers recommendations to protect children and adolescents in states that have legalized marijuana for medical or recreational purposes.

Committee on Substance Abuse, Committee on Adolescence, Committee on Substance Abuse Committee on Adolescence: the impact of marijuana policies on youth: clinical, research, and legal update. Pediatrics 2015 Mar;135(3):584–587 [PMID: 25624383].

Hudgins JD et al: Trends in opioid prescribing for adolescents and young adults in ambulatory care settings. Pediatrics 2019 Jun;143(6) [PMID: 31138669].

Johnston LD et al: Monitoring the Future national survey results on drug use 1975-2018: Overview, key findings on adolescent drug use. Ann Arbor, MI: Institute for Social Research, University of Michigan. http://www.monitoringthefuture.org//pubs/monographs/mtf-overview2018.pdf. Accessed June 22, 2019

Kann L et al: Youth Risk Behavior Surveillance—United States, 2015. MMWR Surveill Summ. 2016 Jun 10;65(6):1–174 [PMID: 27280474].

Peiper NC et al: Overview on prevalence and recent trends in adolescent substance use and abuse. Child Adolesc Psychiatr Clin N Am 2016 Jul;25(3):349–365 [PMID: 27338960].

Schroeder AR, Dehghan M, Newman TB, Bentley JP, Park KT: Association of Opioid Prescriptions From Dental Clinicians for US Adolescents and Young Adults With Subsequent Opioid Use and Abuse. JAMA Intern Med 2019;179(2):145–152 [PMID: 30508022].

Veliz P, Boyd CJ, McCabe SE: Nonmedical use of prescription opioids and heroin use among adolescents involved in competitive sports. J Adolesc Health 2017 Mar;60(3):346–349 [PMID: 27914974].

Supplement Use & Abuse

Use of supplements or special diets to enhance athletic performance dates to antiquity. Today, many elite and casual athletes use ergogenic (performance-enhancing) supplements in an attempt to improve performance. The most popular products used by adolescents are anabolic-androgenic steroids, steroid hormone precursors, creatine, human growth hormone, diuretics, and protein supplements. Anabolic-androgenic steroids increase strength and lean body mass and lessen muscle breakdown. However, they are associated with side effects, including acne, liver tumors, hypertension, premature closure of the epiphysis, ligamentous injury, and precocious puberty. In females, they can cause hirsutism, male pattern baldness, and virilization; in boys, they can cause gynecomastia and testicular atrophy. Creatine increases strength and improves performance in brief, high-intensity exercises but can cause dehydration, muscle cramps, and has potential for renal toxicity. Human growth hormone may increase lean body mass and decrease fat mass but has limited effect on strength and athletic performance. Potential risks include coarsening of facial features and cardiovascular disease. Strength athletes (ie, weight lifters) use protein powders and shakes to enhance muscle repair and mass. The amount of protein consumed often greatly exceeds the recommended daily allowance for weight lifters and other resistance-training athletes (1.6–1.7 g/kg/day). Excess consumption of protein provides no added strength or muscle mass and can provoke renal failure in the presence of underlying renal dysfunction. The AAP cautions against the use of performance-enhancing substances.

As the use of supplements and herbs increases, it is increasingly important for pediatric care providers to be familiar with their common side effects. The Internet has become a source for information about and distribution of these products. The easy accessibility, perceived low risk, and low cost of these products significantly increase the likelihood that they will become substances of abuse by adolescents.

Ali F et al: Energy drinks and their adverse health effects: a systematic review of the current evidence. Postgrad Med 2015 Apr;127(3):308–322 [PMID: 25560302].

Breuner CC: Performance-enhancing substances. Adolesc Med State Art Rev 2014 Apr;25(1):113–125 [PMID: 25022190].

Dandoy C, Gereige RS: Performance-enhancing drugs. Pediatr Rev 2012 Jun;33(6):265–271 [PMID: 22659257].

Das JK et al: Interventions for adolescent substance abuse: an overview of systematic reviews. J Adolesc Health 2016 Oct;59(4S):S61–S75 [PMID: 27664597].

Milicic S et al: The associations between e-cigarettes and binge drinking, marijuana use, and energy drinks mixed with alcohol. J Adolesc Health 2017 Mar;60(3):320–327 [PMID: 28012834].

Scalese M et al: Energy drink and alcohol mixed energy drink use among high school adolescents: association with risk taking behavior, social characteristics. Addict Behav 2017 Mar 27;72:93–99 [PMID: 28388494].

Sepkowitz KA: Energy drinks and caffeine-related adverse effects. JAMA 2013 Jan 16;309(3):243–244 [PMID: 23330171].

MORBIDITY DATA

Use and abuse of alcohol or other mood-altering substances in adolescents in the United States are tightly linked to adolescents' leading causes of death, that is, motor vehicle accidents, unintentional injury, homicide, and suicide. Substance abuse is also associated with physical and sexual abuse. Drug use and abuse contribute to other high-risk behaviors, such as unsafe sexual activity, unintended pregnancy, and sexually transmitted disease. Adolescents may also be involved with selling of drugs.

Risks associated with tobacco, alcohol, and cocaine are listed in Table 5–2. The use of e-cigarettes has been documented to lead to harmful health effects on the heart, lungs, and blood vessels. Nicotine also alters adolescent brain chemistry, making adolescents vulnerable to addiction and other substance use. Use by adolescents can lead to their becoming nicotine dependent, increasing their risk of developing mental health problems. The American Psychological Association notes that nicotine-dependent smokers are up to eight times more likely to develop psychotic disorders, depressive disorders, anxiety, and delirium than smokers who are not dependent on nicotine or those who have never smoked. As e-cigarettes have been used for only a decade, their long-term harms are unknown. Also, less well-known are the long- and short-term adolescent morbidities connected with the currently most popular illicit drugs, marijuana, and synthetic marijuana. The active ingredient in marijuana, δ-9-tetrahydrocannabinol (THC), transiently causes tachycardia, mild hypertension, and bronchodilation. Regular use can cause lung changes similar to those seen in tobacco smokers. Heavy use decreases fertility in both sexes and impairs immunocompetence. It is also associated with abnormalities of cognition, learning, coordination, and memory. It is possible that heavy marijuana use is the cause of the so-called a motivational syndrome, characterized by inattention to environmental stimuli and impaired goal-directed thinking and behavior. Early and frequent use of marijuana during adolescence, compared with occasional use or nonuse, has been associated with development of a higher incidence of psychiatric problems. Analysis of confiscated marijuana recently has shown increasing THC concentration and adulteration with other substances.

Evaluation of the impact of legalization of marijuana on the adolescent and pediatric population has just begun. One observation has been a decrease in perceived harmfulness of marijuana. Adolescents often see nothing wrong with their marijuana use; on contrary; they may believe it has medical and therapeutic use. Additionally, pregnant adolescents tend to use marijuana 1.8 times more often than nonpregnant adolescents. They also use it more compared to pregnant adults. Presence of cannabis products in the home has contributed to an increase in exposure and accidental consumption by younger children. A study in Colorado after marijuana legalization showed an increase in hospitalizations associated with marijuana-related codes from 274 (2010) to 593 (2015) per 100,000 and a fivefold increase in mental health emergency room visits with marijuana-related codes. Calls to emergency rooms related to marijuana exposure increased by 79.7%. As more states legalize marijuana, it will be important to continue to assess potential consequences. Many of the issues related to legalization of marijuana are detailed in the AAP technical report (reference below), and different medical marijuana policies among US states are outlined on the AAP website (reference below).

The popularity and accessibility of ecstasy is again increasing among adolescents. Chronic use is associated with progressive decline of immediate and delayed memory, and with alterations in mood, sleep, and appetite, that may be permanent. Even first-time users may develop frank psychosis indistinguishable from schizophrenia. Irreversible cardiomyopathy, noncardiogenic pulmonary edema, and pulmonary hypertension may occur with long-term use. Acute overdose can cause hyperthermia and multiorgan system failure.

Prenatal and environmental exposure to abused substances also carries health risks. Parental tobacco smoking is associated with low birth weight in newborns, sudden infant death syndrome, bronchiolitis, asthma, otitis media, and fire-related injuries. Maternal use of marijuana during pregnancy is associated with an increased risk of sudden infant death syndrome. In utero exposure to alcohol may produce fetal malformations, intrauterine growth restriction, and brain injury.

American Academy of Pediatrics: https://pediatrics.aappublications.org/content/135/3/584 Accessed June 19, 2019.

Hadland SE et al: Medical comorbidity and complications. Child Adolesc Psychiatr Clin N Am 2016 Jul;25(3):533–548 [PMID: 27338973].

Ryan SA et al: Counseling parents and teens about marijuana use in the era of legalization of marijuana. Pediatrics 2017 Mar;139(3) [PMID: 28242859].

Simpson AK, Magid V: Cannabis use disorder in adolescence. Child Adolesc Psychiatr Clin N Am 2016 Jul;25(3):431–443 [PMID: 27338965].

Storck M et al: Inhalant abuse and dextromethorphan. Child Adolesc Psychiatr Clin N Am 2016 Jul;25(3):497–508 [PMID: 27338970].

Wang GS et al: Impact of marijuana legalization in Colorado on adolescent emergency and urgent care visits. J Adolesc Health 2018;63(2):239–241 [PMID: 29609916].

Yurasek AM et al: Commentary: Adolescent marijuana use and mental health amidst a changing legal climate. J Pediatr Psychol 2016 Apr;41(3):287–289 [PMID: 26883502].

PREDICTING THE PROGRESSION FROM USE TO ABUSE

Initially, most adolescents use mood-altering substances intermittently or experimentally. The challenge to pediatric health care providers is to recognize warning signs, identify potential abusers early, and intervene in an effective fashion before acute or chronic use produces morbidity. The prediction of progression from use to abuse is best viewed within the biopsychosocial model. Substance abuse is a symptom of personal and social maladjustment as often as it is a cause. Because there is a direct relationship between the number of risk factors listed in Table 5–3 and the frequency of substance abuse, a combination of risk factors is the best indicator

of risk. Even so, most teenagers with multiple risk characteristics never progress to substance abuse. It is unclear why only a minority of young people exhibiting the high-risk characteristics listed in Table 5–3 go on to abuse substances, but presumably the protective factors listed in Table 5–3 give most adolescents the resilience to cope with stress in more socially adaptive ways. Being aware of the risk domains in Table 5–3 will help physicians identify youngsters most apt to need counseling about substance abuse.

Simmons S et al: Substance abuse and trauma. Child Adolesc Psychiatr Clin N Am 2016 Oct;25(4):723–734 [PMID: 27613348].

Siqueira LM et al: Nicotine and tobacco as substances of abuse in children and adolescents. Pediatrics 2017 Jan;139(1) [PMID: 27994114].

Yu C et al: Genetics of substance use disorders. Child Adolesc Psychiatr Clin N Am 2016 Jul;25(3):377–385 [PMID: 27338962].

EVALUATION OF SUBSTANCE ABUSE

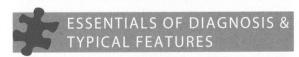

ESSENTIALS OF DIAGNOSIS & TYPICAL FEATURES

► Clues to possible substance abuse include truancy, failing grades, problems with interpersonal relationships, delinquency, depressive affect, chronic fatigue, and unexplained physical complaints.

► Comorbidities, especially psychiatric disorders such as affective disorder, anxiety disorder, and mania, are common among substance-abusing patients.

► When the psychosocial history suggests the possibility of substance use, gather information about extent and circumstances of the problem.

► Pharmacologic screening should be reserved for situations in which the patient's behavioral dysfunction and/or medical condition are of sufficient concern to outweigh practical and ethical drawbacks of testing.

Office Screening

The AAP recommends Screening, Brief Intervention, and Referral to Treatment (SBIRT) as a universal framework for identifying substance use during routine health supervision visits. The three main goals of the integrated, algorithm-based SBIRT screening are to determine whether teens have used any alcohol or drugs; to determine where adolescents are on the substance use spectrum; and finally, for the health care provider to initiate a brief discussion with their teenage patients about substance use and provide them with education, advice, and referrals within a motivational interviewing model.

Table 5–3. Factors that influence the progression from substance use to substance abuse.

Enabling Risk Factors	Potentially Protective Factors
Societal and community	
Experimentation encouraged by media Illicit substances available Extreme economic deprivation Neighborhood disorganization, crowding Tolerance of licit and illicit substance use	Regular involvement in church activities Support for norms and values of society Strict enforcement of laws prohibiting substance use among minors and abuse among adults Neighborhood resources, supportive adults
School	
Lack of commitment to school or education Truancy Academic failure Early, persistent behavior problems	Strong commitment to school or education Future-oriented goals Achievement oriented
Family	
Models of substance abuse and other unconventional behavior Dysfunctional parenting styles; excessive authority or permissiveness High family conflict; low bonding	Models of conventional behavior Attachment to parents Cohesive family Nurturing parenting styles
Peers	
Peer rejection in elementary grades Substance use prevalent among peers Peer attitudes favorable to substance abuse and unconventional behavior	Popular with peers Abstinent friends Peer attitudes favor conventional behavior
Individual	
Genetic predisposition Psychological diagnoses (attention-deficit/hyperactivity disorder; antisocial personality) Depression and low self-esteem Alienation and rebelliousness Sexual or physical abuse Early onset of deviant behavior or delinquency Early onset of sexual behavior Aggressive	Positive self-concept, good self-esteem Intolerance of deviance Internally motivated, takes charge of problems

An important goal of this framework is to identify the range of youth substance use from abstinence to risky substance use to that rising to the level of a SUD. Given the high incidence of substance abuse and the subtlety of its early signs and symptoms, a general psychosocial assessment is the best way to screen for substance abuse among adolescents. In an atmosphere of trust and confidentiality, physicians should ask routine screening questions of all patients and be alert for addictive diseases, recognizing the high level of denial often present in addicted patients. Clues to possible substance abuse include truancy, failing grades, problems with interpersonal relationships, delinquency, depressive affect, chronic fatigue, recurrent abdominal pain, chest pains or palpitations, headache, chronic cough, persistent nasal discharge, and recurrent complaints of sore throat. Substance abuse should be included in the differential diagnosis of all behavioral, family, psychosocial, and medical problems.

A family history of drug addiction or abuse should raise the level of concern about drug abuse in the pediatric patient. Possession of promotional products such as T-shirts and caps with cigarette or alcohol logos should also be a red flag because teenagers who own these items are more likely to use the products they advertise. Pediatricians seeing patients in emergency departments, trauma units, or prison should have an especially high index of suspicion.

In the primary care setting, insufficient time and lack of training are the greatest barriers to screening adolescents for substance abuse. Brief questionnaires can be used if time does not allow for more detailed investigation. A screening instrument that has been rigorously studied in primary care settings is the CAGE questionnaire. CAGE is a mnemonic derived from the first four questions asked of patients regarding their substance use: the need to *c*ut down, *a*nnoyance if asked about it, feeling *g*uilty about the use, and the need of the drug/alcohol as an *eye* opener. A score of 2 or more is highly suggestive of substance abuse. Although constructed as a screening tool for alcohol abuse in adults, the CAGE questionnaire can be adapted to elicit information about use of other mood-altering substances by pediatric patients and their close contacts (eg, parents and older siblings). Clinicians may find it helpful to use such questionnaires to stimulate discussion of the patient's self-perception of his or her substance use. For example, if an adolescent admits to a previous attempt to cut down on drinking, this provides an opportunity to inquire about events that may have led to the attempt. Unfortunately, despite guidance to screen adolescents for substance abuse, recent studies demonstrate that clinicians generally do not regularly ask/advise adolescents about substance use.

Utilizing the SBIRT framework, pediatricians should focus their brief intervention on reducing risks associated with ongoing substance use and motivational interviewing to engage youth in treatment for their SUD. This patient-centered strategy of harm reduction focuses on the risk behaviors identified during intake and aims to meet youth where they are, recognize their inherent strengths and motivation to be well, respect their rights, and create a personalized health promotion strategy in collaboration with the youth. Providers provide education, advice, and referrals within a motivational interviewing model. The Harm Reduction Coalition (https://harmreduction.org) has numerous resources that can be applied in the primary care setting.

Borus J et al: Screening, brief intervention, and referral to treatment. Child Adolesc Psychiatr Clin N Am 2016 Oct;25(4):579–601 [PMID: 27613340].

Levy SJ et al: Substance use screening, brief intervention, and referral to treatment. Pediatrics 2016 Jul;138(1) [PMID: 27325634].

Mitchell SG et al: SBIRT Implementation for adolescents in urban federally qualified health centers. J Subst Abuse Treat 2016;60:81–90 [PMID: 26297321].

Monico LB et al. A comparison of screening practices for adolescents in primary care after implementation of screening, brief intervention, and referral to treatment. J Adolesc Health 2019 Mar 5 [PMID: 30850312].

Roberts E, Martinez J: Harm Reduction Approach, 2016. https://harmreduction.org/wp-content/uploads/2017/07/Webinar-HReduxn_092716.pdf. Accessed June 20, 2019.

Sharma B, Bruner A, Barnett G, Fishman M: Opioid use disorders. Child Adolesc Psychiatr Clin N Am 2016 Jul;25(3):473–487 [PMID: 27338968].

Substance Abuse and Mental Health Services Administration: White paper on Screening, Brief Intervention and Referral to Treatment (SBIRT) in behavioral healthcare. http://www.samhsa.gov/sites/default/files/sbirtwhitepaper_0.pdf. Accessed June 20, 2019.

Diagnosis

When the psychosocial history suggests the possibility of substance use, the primary tasks of the diagnostic interview are the same as for the evaluation of other medical problems (Table 5–4).

Table 5–4. Evaluation of positive psychosocial screens for substance abuse.

I. Define the extent of the problem by determining:
Age at onset of substance use
Which substances are being used
Circumstances of use
  Where?
  When?
  With whom?
To what extent substances are being used
  How frequently?
  How much (quantity)?
  With what associated symptoms (eg, tolerance, withdrawal)?
With what result?
  What does the patient gain from becoming high?
  Does the patient get into risky situations while high?
  Does the patient engage in behaviors while high that
    are later regretted?
II. Define the cause of the problem

First, specific information about the extent and circumstances of the problem is gathered. Eliciting information through multiple-choice questions is a useful technique. For example, "Has anything really good ever happened to you when you are high? Some of my patients like to get high because they feel good; others find it helps them relax and be sociable with friends; and some find it helps them forget their problems. Are any of these things true for you?"

Second, the provider should determine why the patient has progressed from initiation to the continuation or maintenance phase of substance abuse. The cause may be different at different periods of development. Although peer group characteristics are one of the best predictors of substance use among early and middle adolescents, this is not so among older adolescents and young adults.

Although few children and adolescents will have been abusing substances long enough to have developed overt signs and symptoms, it is important to look for them on physical examination. Positive physical findings can be a tool to penetrate a patient's denial and convince him or her of the significance of alcohol or drug use.

Griffin KW et al: Evidence-based interventions for preventing substance use disorders in adolescents. Child Adolesc Psychiatr Clin N Am 2010 Jul;19(3):505–526 [PMID: 20682218].

Harrop E et al: Evidence-based prevention for adolescent substance use. Child Adolesc Psychiatr Clin N Am 2016 Jul;25(3):387–410 [PMID: 27338963].

Margret CP et al: Assessment and treatment of adolescent substance use disorders: alcohol use disorders. Child Adolesc Psychiatr Clin N Am 2016 Jul;25(3):411–430 [PMID: 27338964].

Comorbidity

Comorbidities, especially other psychiatric disorders, are common among substance-abusing patients (Table 5–5).

Table 5–5. Common comorbid conditions associated with adolescent substance abuse.

1. Attention-deficit/hyperactivity disorder
2. Bipolar disorder
3. Depression disorder
4. Anxiety disorders (often with depressive disorders)

Affective disorder, anxiety disorder, and mania are most strongly associated with alcohol and drug dependence. Attention-deficit/hyperactivity has also been closely linked with adolescent substance abuse. Adolescents with depression are likely to use drugs in an attempt to feel pleasure, but this type of self-medication may exacerbate their underlying condition. Although it is often difficult to determine which diagnosis is primary, it is important for pediatric health care providers to recognize the possibility of a comorbid condition and provide appropriate treatment. Finally, in addition to identifying psychiatric comorbidities, it is imperative that providers look for medical conditions that mimic symptoms of drug withdrawal or intoxication.

Burnett-Zeigler I et al: Prevalence and correlates of mental health problems and treatment among adolescents seen in primary care. J Adolesc Health 2012 Jun;50(6):559–564 [PMID: 22626481].

Hanna RC, et al. Cannabis and development of dual diagnoses: a literature review. Am J Drug Alcohol Abuse 2017;43(4); 442–455 [PMID: 27612527].

Harstad E et al: Attention-deficit/hyperactivity disorder and substance abuse. Pediatrics 2014 Jul;134(1):e293–e301 [PMID: 24982106].

Joffe A: Nonmedical use of prescription stimulants by adolescents. Adolesc Med State Art Rev 2014;25(1):89–103 [PMID: 25022188].

Mason MJ et al: Psychiatric comorbidity and complications. Child Adolesc Psychiatr Clin N Am 2016 Jul;25(3):521–532 [PMID: 27338972].

Pharmacologic Screening

The use of urine and blood testing for detecting substance abuse is controversial. The consensus is that pharmacologic screening should be reserved for situations in which behavioral dysfunction is of sufficient concern to outweigh the practical and ethical drawbacks of testing. The AAP recommends testing under certain circumstances (eg, an inexplicably obtunded patient in the emergency department) but discourages routine screening for the following reasons: (1) voluntary screening is rarely truly voluntary owing to the negative consequences for those who decline to participate; (2) infrequent users or individuals who have not used substances recently may be missed; (3) confronting substance-abusing individuals with objective evidence of their use has little or no effect on behavior; and (4) the role of health care providers is

to provide counseling and treatment, not law enforcement, so drug testing should not be done for the purpose of detecting illegal use. If testing is to be performed, the provider should discuss the plan for screening with the patient, explain the reasons for it, and obtain informed consent. The AAP does not consider parental request and permission sufficient justification for involuntary screening of mentally competent minors. It also opposes widespread drug testing in schools because of a lack of solid evidence for its effectiveness.

If testing is to be performed, it is imperative that it be done accurately and that the limitations of testing be understood. Tests range from inexpensive chromatographic spot tests, which can be performed in the office, to gas chromatography and mass spectrometry, which require specialized laboratory equipment and are usually reserved for forensic investigations. Most commercial medical laboratories use the enzyme multiplication immunoassay technique, in which a sample of the fluid to be tested is added to a test reagent containing a known quantity of radiolabeled index drug. If the index drug is present in the patient's urine or serum, it competes with the radiolabeled drug for binding sites on the test kit antibody. The unbound or excess drug can then be quantified with a spectrophotometer. Most of the commonly abused mood-altering substances, with the exception of solvents and inhalants, can be detected by this method.

Interpretation of results is complicated by false positives resulting from antibody cross-reactions with some medications and substances (Table 5–6) or from a patient's passive exposure to illicit substances. The most common cause of false-negative tests is infrequent use. Table 5–7 shows the duration of detectability in the urine after last use by class of substance and duration of use. Detectability ranges from a few hours for alcohol to several weeks for regular marijuana use.

Table 5–6. Causes of false-positive drug screens.

Opioids
  Poppy seeds
  Dextromethorphan
  Chlorpromazine
  Diphenoxylate

Amphetamines
  Ephedrine
  Phenylephrine
  Pseudoephedrine
  N-acetylprocainamide
  Chloroquine
  Procainamide

Phencyclidines
  Dextromethorphan
  Diphenhydramine
  Chlorpromazine
  Doxylamine
  Thioridazine

Table 5–7. Duration of urine positivity for selected drugs.

Drug Class	Detection Time
Amphetamines	< 48 h
Barbiturates	Short acting: 1 days Long acting: 2–3 wk
Benzodiazepines	Single dose: 3 days Habitual use: 4–6 wk
Cocaine metabolites	Acute use: 2–4 days Habitual use: 2 wk
Ethanol	2–14 h
Methadone	Up to 3 days
Opioids	Up to 2 days
Propoxyphene	6–48 h
Cannabinoid	Moderate use: 5 d Habitual use: 10–20 days
Methaqualone	2 wk
Phencyclidine	Acute use: 1 wk Habitual use: 3 wk
Anabolic steroids	Days to weeks

Reproduced with permission from Woolf AD, Shannon MW: Clinical toxicology for the pediatrician. Pediatr Clin North Am 1995 Apr;42(2):317–333.

False-negative results can also occur if the patient alters or adulterates the test specimen. Some of the commercial products used to adulterate samples include glutaraldehyde, nitrite, pyridinium chlorochromate, peroxidase, and peroxide (stealth). Household products such as bleach, vinegar, Visine® eye drops (for marijuana), strong alkali drain cleaners, and detergents are also used. Teenagers should be advised that, despite street lore, ingesting these compounds is an ineffective and potentially dangerous way to prevent drug detection in the urine. Close observation during collection and testing the temperature, specific gravity, and pH of urine samples may detect attempts at deception.

Home drug-testing products are available for parents and can be procured via the Internet; however, these products have limitations and potential risks. The AAP recommends that home (and school-based) drug testing not be implemented until the safety and efficacy of these procedures can be established. It further recommends that parents be encouraged to consult the adolescent's primary care provider rather than relying on home drug-testing products.

Hadland SE et al: Objective testing: urine and other drug tests. Child Adolesc Psychiatr Clin N Am 2016 Jul;25(3):549–565 [PMID: 27338974].

Levy S, Schizer M: Committee on substance abuse: adolescent drug testing policies in schools. Pediatrics 2015 Apr;135(4):782–783 [PMID: 25825537].

Levy S, Siqueira LM: Committee on substance abuse: testing for drugs of abuse in children and adolescents. Pediatrics 2014;133(6):e1798–e1807 [PMID: 24864184].

Terry-McElrath YM, O'Malley PM, Johnston LD: Middle and high school drug testing and student illicit drug use: a national study 1998–2011. J Adolesc Health 2012 Jun;52(6):707–715 [PMID: 23406889].

TREATMENT & REFERRAL

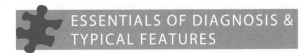

ESSENTIALS OF DIAGNOSIS & TYPICAL FEATURES

▶ Substance-abusing teenagers will generally require repeated discussions about discontinuing substance.

▶ Assessment of the patient's readiness to change is a critical first step in office-based intervention.

▶ Providers should tailor their counseling messages to the patient's stage of readiness to change.

▶ When referral for treatment is indicated, substance-abusing teenagers are best treated in teen-oriented treatment facilities.

▶ Key elements of an effective adolescent drug treatment program include a comprehensive and integrated treatment approach, family involvement, a developmentally appropriate program, and engagement and retention of teens.

Office-Based Treatment

The AAP recommends that all children and adolescents receive counseling about the dangers of substance use and abuse from their primary care providers. By offering confidential health care services and routinely counseling about the risks associated with drug abuse, primary care providers can help most patients avoid the adverse consequences of experimentation with mood-altering substances. However, more intervention is required for youngsters in environments where substance abuse is regarded as acceptable recreational behavior. Counseling strategies appropriate for patients who wish to change their behavior may be ineffective for patients who do not consider use of mood-altering substances to be a problem. It may therefore be preferable to begin discussions about treatment by helping youngsters consider alternative ways of meeting the needs that substance use is currently addressing. The clinician in this way may help the patient devise alternatives that are more attractive than substance use. Brief interventions for adolescents have yielded some improvement among high-risk youth. However, few substance-abusing teenagers will choose to quit because of a single conversation, even with a highly respected health care provider. The message is most effective when offered repeatedly from many sources—family, peers, guidance counselors, and teachers. Motivational interviewing and computer-facilitated screening and brief advice for substance-abusing teens have shown promise.

Assessment of the patient's readiness to change is a critical first step in office-based intervention. Clinicians should consider the construct presented in Table 5–8. In theory, individuals pass through this series of stages in the course of changing problem behaviors. To be maximally effective, providers should tailor their counseling messages to the patient's stage of readiness to change.

Once it has been established that a patient is prepared to act on information about treatment, the next step is to select the program that best fits his or her individual needs. Most drug treatment programs are not designed to recognize and act on the individual vulnerabilities that have predisposed the patient to substance abuse. When programs are individualized, even brief (5- to 10-minutes) counseling sessions may promote reductions in cigarette smoking and drinking. This strategy appears to be most effective when the health care provider's message is part of an office-wide program so that the entire staff reinforces the cessation message with every patient.

Table 5–8. Stages of change and intervention tasks.

Patient Stage	Motivation Tasks
Precontemplation	Create doubt, increase the patient's awareness of risks and problems with current patterns of substance use
Contemplation	Help the patient weigh the relative risks and benefits of changing substance use; evoke reasons to change and risks of not changing; strengthen the patient's self-efficacy for changing current use
Determination	Help the patient determine the best course of action to change substance use from among available alternatives
Action	Help the patient establish a clear plan of action toward changing substance use
Maintenance	Help the patient identify and use strategies to prevent relapse
Relapse	Help the patient renew the process of change starting at contemplation

Reproduced with permission from Werner MJ: Principles of brief intervention for adolescent alcohol, tobacco, and other drug use. Pediatr Clin North Am 1995 Apr;42(2):335–349.

Barclay RP et al: Integrated care for pediatric substance abuse. Child Adolesc Psychiatr Clin N Am 2016 Oct;25(4):769–777 [PMID: 27613351].

Cagande CC, Pradhan BK, Pumariega AJ: Treatment of adolescent substance use disorders. Adolesc Med State Art Rev 2014;25(1):157–171 [PMID: 25022192].

Hammond CJ et al: Pharmacotherapy for substance use disorders in youths. J Child Adolesc Subst Abuse 2016;25(4):292–316 [PMID: 28082828].

Harris SK et al: Computer-facilitated substance use screening and brief advice for teens in primary care: an international trial. Pediatrics 2012 Jun;129(6):1072–1082 [PMID: 22566420].

Horigian VE et al: Family-based treatments for adolescent substance use. Child Adolesc Psychiatr Clin N Am 2016 Oct;25(4):603–628 [PMID: 27613341].

Levy S et al: Medication-assisted treatment of adolescents with opioid use disorders. Pediatrics 2016;138(3):e20161893 [PMID: 27550978].

Stubbs S, Bennett D: Young people and alcohol use: contextualizing and responding to the challenge of problematic drinking. Adolesc Med State Art Rev 2014;25(1):50–69 [PMID: 25022186].

Smoking Cessation in Pediatrics

Although more than half of adolescents who smoke regularly say they want to quit and have tried to quit, only a minority report that they have been advised or helped to do so by a health care provider. Practitioners unfamiliar with approaches to smoking cessation may feel that smoking cessation interventions are time consuming, not reimbursable, and impractical in a busy office. An easy guideline for health care providers is the "five A's" for tobacco cessation (Table 5–9), published by the Public Health Service and endorsed by the AAP.

Smoking cessation is a process that takes time. Relapse must be regarded as a normal part of quitting rather than evidence of personal failure or a reason to forgo further attempts. Patients can actually benefit from relapses if they are helped to identify the circumstances that led to the relapse and to devise strategies to prevent subsequent relapses or respond to predisposing circumstances in a different manner.

Nicotine is a physically and psychologically addictive substance. Providers should be aware that adolescents may not

Table 5–9. "Five A's" for tobacco cessation.

Ask about tobacco use from all patients
Advise all tobacco users to quit
Assess willingness and motivation for tobacco user to make a quit attempt
Assist in the quit attempt
Arrange for follow-up

Adapted with permission from Fiore MC, Bailey WC, Cohen SJ, et al: *Treating Tobacco Use and Dependence. Clinical Practice Guidelines.* U.S. Department of Health and Human Services, Public Health Service; 2000.

exhibit the same symptoms of nicotine dependence as adults and that dependence may be established within as little as 4 weeks. Replacement therapy improves smoking cessation rates and may relieve withdrawal symptoms. Both nicotine gum and transdermal nicotine patch replacement therapies are recommended for teens. Those who are not comfortable prescribing and monitoring nicotine-replacement therapies should limit their involvement with patients who smoke to those who do not exhibit signs of nicotine dependency (eg, patients who smoke less than a pack of cigarettes a day or do not feel a craving to smoke their first cigarette within 30 minutes after waking). Patients who exhibit nicotine dependency can be referred to community smoking cessation programs, including "smoking quit lines." In addition to nicotine-replacement therapies, sustained-release forms of the antidepressants bupropion, clonidine, and nortriptyline have been shown in randomized trials to help smokers quit and to decrease relapse rates fivefold.

The AAP and the World Health Organization recommend against the use of e-cigarettes as a cessation aid or nicotine dependence treatment for adolescents. Public policy recommendations include support for legislation (regulation of all tobacco products and adequate funding of tobacco control), continued education of clinicians, research and evaluation of e-cigarette use, dissemination of effective tobacco-control messaging, increase in taxation on tobacco products, and ban of all flavored products.

Berry KM et al: Association of Electronic Cigarette Use With Subsequent Initiation of Tobacco Cigarettes in US Youths. JAMA Network Open 2019;2(2):e187794 [PMID: 30707232].

Camenga DR et al: Tobacco use disorders. Child Adolesc Psychiatr Clin N Am 2016 Jul;25(3):445–460 [PMID: 27338966].

Gorzkowski JA et al: Pediatrician knowledge, attitudes, and practice related to electronic cigarettes. J Adolesc Health 2016 Jul;59(1):81–86 [PMID: 27338665].

McKelvey K et al: Adolescents' and young adults' use and perceptions of pod-based electronic cigarettes. JAMA Network Open 2018;1(6) [PMID: 30646249].

McMillen R et al: Changes and factors associated with tobacco counseling: results from the AAP Periodic Survey. Acad Pediatr 2017 Jan 17; pii: S1876–2859(17)30004-9 [PMID: 28104489].

Pbert L et al: State-of-the-art office-based interventions to eliminate youth tobacco use: the past decade. Pediatrics 2015;135(4):734–747 [PMID: 25780075].

Spindle T, Eissenberg T. Pod mod electronic cigarettes—an emerging threat to public health. JAMA Network Open 2018;1(6): e183518 [PMID: 30646245].

Stanford Tobacco Prevention Toolkit: https://med.stanford.edu/tobaccopreventiontoolkit.html. Accessed June 20, 2019.

Walley SC et al: A public health crisis: electronic cigarettes, vape, and JUUL. Pediatrics 2019 Jun;143(6) [PMID: 31122947].

Referral

There is no consensus about which substance-abusing patients can be adequately treated in the office, which require referral, and which require hospitalization. Factors to be considered prior to referral are summarized in Table 5–10. When doubt exists about the seriousness of the problem or the advisability of office management, consultation with a specialist should be sought.

Although most primary pediatric providers will not assume responsibility for the treatment of substance-abusing youngsters, clinicians can be instrumental in motivating patients to seek treatment and in guiding them to appropriate treatment resources. Substance-abusing teenagers are best treated in teen-oriented treatment facilities. Despite the similarities between adult and adolescent substance abuse, adult programs are usually developmentally inappropriate and ineffective for adolescents. Many adolescents are concrete thinkers, and their inability to reason deductively, especially about emotionally charged issues, makes it difficult for them to understand the abstract concepts (such as denial) that are an integral component of most adult-oriented programs. This invariably frustrates counselors who misinterpret lack of comprehension as resistance to therapy and concrete responses as evidence of deceit.

Treatment programs range from low-intensity, outpatient, school-based student-assistance programs, which rely heavily on peers and nonprofessionals, to residential, hospital-based programs staffed by psychiatrists and other professionals. Outpatient counseling programs are most appropriate for motivated patients who do not have significant mental health or behavioral problems and are not at risk for withdrawal. Some investigators have raised the concern that in pediatric settings, users who lack significant mental

Table 5–10. Factors to consider prior to referral for substance abuse.

Duration and frequency of substance use
The type of substances being used
Presence of other psychological disorders
Attention-deficit/hyperactivity disorder
Depression
Antisocial personality disorder
Presence of other social morbidities
School failure
Delinquency
Homelessness
Ongoing or past physical or sexual abuse
Program evaluation
View on substance abuse as primary disorder vs symptom
Offers comprehensive evaluation of patient and can manage associated problems identified in initial assessment (eg, comorbid conditions)
Adherence to abstinence philosophy
Patient-staff ratios
Separate adolescent and adult treatment programs
Follow-up and continuing care

health or behavioral comorbidities may actually experience a strengthening of the drug subculture by associating in group therapy with users who have a greater burden of comorbidities. More intensive day treatment programs are available for those who require a structured environment. Inpatient treatment should be considered for patients who need medical care and detoxification in addition to counseling, education, and family therapy.

Finally, special dual-diagnosis facilities are available for substance-abusing patients who also have other psychological conditions. These patients are difficult to diagnose and treat because it is often unclear whether their symptoms are a consequence of substance use or a symptom of a comorbid psychological disorder. Recognition of such disorders is critical because they must be treated in programs that include psychiatric expertise.

Approaches to the treatment of substance abuse in children and adolescents are typically modeled after adult treatment programs. Key elements of an effective adolescent drug treatment program include assessment and treatment matching, a comprehensive and integrated treatment approach, family involvement, a developmentally appropriate program, engagement and retention of teens, qualified staff, gender and cultural competence, continuing care, and satisfactory treatment outcomes. Several studies of adolescent substance abuse treatment programs have shown that many do not adequately address all of the important components of therapy.

Janopaul-Naylor E, Brown JD, Lowenhaupt EA, Tolou-Shams M: Assessment and treatment of substance abuse in the juvenile justice population. Adolesc Med State Art Rev 2014;25(1): 215–229 [PMID: 25022195].

Macgowan MJ et al: Evidence for optimism: behavior therapies and motivational interviewing in adolescent substance abuse treatment. Child Adolesc Psychiatr Clin N Am 2010 Jul;19(3): 527–545 [PMID: 20682219].

Pradhan BK, Cagande CC, Pumariega AJ: Substance abuse among culturally diverse youth. Adolesc Med State Art Rev 2014;25(1):172–183 [PMID: 25022193].

Saloner B, Carson N, Lê Cook B: Explaining racial/ethnic differences in adolescent substance abuse treatment completion in the United States: a decomposition analysis. J Adolesc Health 2014;54(6):646–653 [PMID: 24613095].

Wu SS et al: Cognitive behavioral therapy and motivational enhancement therapy. Child Adolesc Psychiatr Clin N Am 2016 Oct;25(4):629–643 [PMID: 27613342].

PREVENTION

Prevention of substance abuse has been a public health priority since the 1980s. Pediatric health care providers are important advocates and educators of the community and government on developmentally appropriate programs. *Primary-level* programs focus on preventing the initiation of substance use. The Drug Awareness and Resistance Education (DARE) program is a familiar example of a primary prevention program that attempts to educate elementary and middle school students about the adverse consequences of substance abuse and enable them to resist peer pressures.

Secondary-level programs target populations at increased risk for substance use. Their aim is to prevent progression from initiation to continuance and maintenance, relying on individualized intervention to reduce the risk and enhance protective factors listed in Table 5–3. This approach enables the provider to focus scarce resources on those who are most likely to benefit from them. Alateen, which supports the children of alcoholic parents, typifies secondary level prevention.

Tertiary-level prevention programs target young people who have been identified as substance abusers. Their aim is to prevent the morbid consequences of substance use. One example is the identification of adolescents who misuse alcohol and drugs at parties and providing them with a safe ride home. Because prevention is more effective when targeted at reducing the initiation of substance use than at decreasing use or associated morbidity, tertiary prevention is the least effective approach.

Very few population-based programs undergo rigorous scientific evaluation, and few programs have been shown to be effective. Although tertiary prevention programs are the least effective approach, it is the consensus among drug educators that primary prevention programs, such as D.A.R.E., also have limited effect. Parents and others should understand that most adolescents who abuse alcohol and drugs do not do so just for the high. Rather, these behaviors are often purposeful, developmentally appropriate coping strategies. To the extent that these behaviors meet young people's developmental needs, they are not apt to be abandoned unless equally attractive alternatives are available. For example, even though many teenagers cite stress and anxiety as reasons for smoking, teen-oriented smoking cessation programs rarely address the young smoker's need for alternative coping strategies by offering stress management training. Similarly, for the youngster growing up in an impoverished urban environment, the real costs of substance abuse may be too low and the rewards too high to be influenced by talk and knowledge alone. It is unreasonable to expect a talk-based intervention to change attitudes and behaviors in a direction that is opposite to that of the child's own social milieu. The efficacy of the most promising prevention models and interventions is apt to decay over time unless changes in the social environment provide substance-abusing children and adolescents with realistic alternative ways to meet their developmental needs.

Feinstein EC et al: Addressing the critical health problem of adolescent substance use through health care, research, and public policy. J Adolesc Health 2012 May;50(5):431–436 [PMID: 22525104].

REFERENCES

Web Resources

American Lung Association (site for and by teens): http://www
.lungusa.org/smokefreeclass. Monitoring the Future Study
(detailed information and longitudinal data): http://www.moni-
toringthefuture.org. Accessed June 20, 2019.

National Clearinghouse Drug and Alcohol Abuse (information and
resources, including free publications for providers, parents, and
adolescents): http://www.health.org. Accessed June 20, 2019.

National Institute on Drug Abuse: http://www.nida.nih.gov. Accessed
June 20, 2019.

Substance Use and Mental Health Services Administration
(SAMSA; resources for both substance use and mental health
services): http://www.samhsa.gov. Accessed June 20, 2019.

Substance Abuse and Mental Health Services Administration: Key
substance use and mental health indicators in the United States:
results from the 2016 National Survey on Drug Use and Health.
Rockville, MD: Center for Behavioral Health Statistics and
Quality, Substance Abuse and Mental Health Services Administration; 2017. Report No.: HHS, Publication No.: SMA 17-5044,
NSDUH Series H-52.

Tobacco Free Kids: https://www.tobaccofreekids.org. Accessed
June 20, 2019.

Additional References for *AccessPediatrics*

Ammerman S et al: The impact of marijuana policies on
youth: clinical, research, and legal update. Pediatrics 2015
Mar;135(3):e769–e785 [PMID: 25624385].

Biggs JM et al: Abuse and misuse of selected dietary supplements
among adolescents: a look at poison center data. J Pediatr Pharmacol Ther 2017 Nov–Dec;22(6):385–393 [PMID: 29290737].

Callahan ST: Opioids and the urgent need to focus on the health care
of young adults. Pediatrics Jun 2019;143(6) [PMID: 31138665].

Chartier KG et al: Development and vulnerability factors in adolescent alcohol use. Child Adolesc Psychiatr Clin N Am
2010 Jul;19(3):493–504 [PMID: 20682217].

Ewing JA: Detecting alcoholism. The CAGE questionnaire. JAMA
1984 Oct;252(14):1905–1907 [PMID: 6471323].

Grenard JL et al: Exposure to alcohol advertisements and teenage alcohol-related problems. Pediatrics 2013 Feb;131(2):
e369–e379 [PMID: 23359585].

Harris SK, Louis-Jacques J, Knight JR: Screening and brief intervention for alcohol and other abuse. Adolesc Med State Art Rev
2014 Apr;25(1):126–156 [PMID: 25022191].

Jenkins EK et al: Developing harm reduction in the context of
youth substance use: insights from a multi-site qualitative
analysis of young people's harm minimization strategies. Harm
Reduct J 2017;14(1):53 [PMID: 28760146].

Kokotailo B: Alcohol use by youth and adolescents: a pediatric concern. Pediatrics 2010 May;125(5):1078–1087 [PMID:
20385640].

Kuehn BM: Teen perceptions of marijuana risks shift: use of
alcohol, illicit drugs, and tobacco declines. JAMA 2013 Feb 6;
309(5):429–430 [PMID: 23385247].

Meyers JL et al: Genetic and environmental risk factors for adolescent-onset substance use disorders. Child Adolesc Psychiatr
Clin N Am 2010 Jul;19(3):465–477 [PMID: 20682215].

National Institute for Alcohol Abuse and Alcoholism Alcohol
Screening and Brief Intervention for Youth: A Practitioner's
Guide; 2011. http://pubs.niaaa.nih.gov/publications/Practitio-
ner/YouthGuide/YouthGuide.pdf. Accessed June 20, 2019.

Salomonsen-Sautel S et al: Medical marijuana use among adolescents in substance abuse treatment. J Am Acad Child Adolesc
Psychiatry 2012 Jul;51(7):694–702 [PMID: 22721592].

Siqueira L et al: Binge drinking. Pediatrics 2015 Sep;136(3):
e718–e726 [PMID: 26324872].

Strasburger VC: Policy statement—children, adolescents, substance abuse, and the media. Pediatrics 2010 Oct;126(4):
791–799 [PMID: 20876181].

Walton MA et al: Sexual risk behaviors among teens at an urban
emergency department: relationship with violent behaviors
and substance use. J Adolesc Health 2011 Mar;48(3):303–305
[PMID: 21338903].

Wang GS et al: Marijuana and acute health care contacts in
Colorado. Prev Med 2017 Mar 30; pii: S0091-7435(17)30120-2
[PMID: 28365373].

Eating Disorders

Eric J. Sigel, MD

INTRODUCTION

Adolescents as well as younger children engage in disordered eating behavior at an alarming rate, and many develop partial or full-blown eating disorders (EDs). The spectrum of EDs includes anorexia nervosa (AN), bulimia nervosa (BN), binge-eating disorder (BED), atypical anorexia nervosa, and avoidant/restrictive food intake disorder (ARFID). These disorders are best defined in a biopsychosocial context.

ETIOLOGY

There is strong evidence for a genetic basis for EDs. The incidence of AN is 7% in first-degree relatives of anorexic patients compared with 1%–2% in the general population. The concordance rate in monozygotic twins is 55% compared with 7% in dizygotic twins. Twin studies estimate the heritability of AN as 33%–84% and BN as 28%–83%. Most studies also find a higher incidence of EDs among first-degree relatives of bulimic patients.

There is evidence of altered serotonergic and dopaminergic function and alterations in neuropeptides and gut peptides in AN and BN. It remains unclear whether abnormalities of neurotransmitters contribute to the development of EDs or are a consequence of the physiologic changes associated with the disorders. Patients with BN or BED appear to have a blunted serotonin response to eating and satiety. With a decreased satiety response, patients continue to eat, leading to a binge. Treatment with selective serotonin reuptake inhibitors (SSRIs) tends to equilibrate satiety regulation. An alteration in dopamine has also been recognized, although its significance is not clear. Adiponectin is elevated in AN, although it is unclear whether this is merely secondary to the malnourished state. Cholecystokinin is decreased in BN, perhaps contributing to the lack of postingestion satiety that perpetuates a binge. Ghrelin, a gut peptide, is elevated in patients with AN, and it does not decrease normally after a meal in these patients. Obestatin, a gut peptide that inhibits appetite, is elevated in AN as well.

Leptin physiology is deranged in patients with AN. Abnormalities of leptin may mediate energy changes that affect the hypothalamic-pituitary axis and play a role in perpetuating AN. Leptin levels increase excessively as individuals with AN regain weight. The abnormally high levels of leptin may contribute to the difficulty AN patients have when trying to regain weight, as higher leptin levels signal the body to decrease energy intake. Leptin also plays a significant role in some of the sequelae of AN, with low levels signaling the hypothalamus to inhibit reproductive hormone production.

Some experts have hypothesized that the intrauterine hormonal milieu may explain the differences in prevalence of ED between females and males. Procopio and Marriott have studied the risk of developing AN in the same sex and opposite-sex twin pairs when one twin has AN. There was approximately an eightfold risk of developing AN in males with a female twin with AN compared to the risk of developing AN in males who had a male twin with AN. Though the study could not separate environmental influences, evidence from animal models suggests that increased exposure to estrogen and/or decreased exposure to androgens influence brain development and may play a role in determining which individuals are at risk for AN.

Traditional psychological theory has suggested many environmental factors that might promote the development of EDs. Enmeshment of mother with daughter to the point that the teenager cannot develop her own identity (a key developmental marker of adolescence) may be a predisposing factor. The teenager may cope by asserting control over food, as she senses her lack of control in the developmental realm. A second theory involves father-daughter distancing. As puberty progresses and a girl's sexuality blossoms, a father may experience difficulty in dealing with his daughter as a sexual being and may respond by withdrawing emotionally and physically. The teenage girl may intuitively recognize this and subconsciously decrease her food intake in order to become prepubertal again. A third theory is related to puberty itself.

Some teenagers may fear or dislike their changing bodies. By restricting food intake they lose weight, stop menstruating, and effectively reverse pubertal development.

Society has promoted the message that being thin or muscular is necessary for attractiveness and success. The ease of access to diet products—foods and diet pills—as well as Internet instructions (proanorexia sites) makes it simple for adolescents to embark on a quest for thinness or muscularity.

Genetic predisposition, environmental factors, and psychological factors likely combine to create a milieu that promotes development of EDs.

Bulik CM, Slof-Op't Landt MC, van Furth EF, Sullivan PF: The genetics of anorexia nervosa. Annu Rev Nutr 2007a;27:263–275 [PMID: 17430085].

Campbell IC, Mill J, Uher R, Schmidt U: Eating disorders, gene-environment interaction, and epigentics. Neurosci Biobehav Rev 2011;35:784–793 [PMID: 20888360].

Disanto G et al: Season of birth and anorexia nervosa. Brit J Psych 2011;198(5):404–407 [PMID: 21415047].

Grzelak T et al: Neurobiochemical and psychologic factors influencing the eating behaviors and attitudes in anorexia nervosa. J Physiol Biochem 2017;73(2):297–305 [PMID: 27924450].

Procopio M, Marriott P: Intrauterine hormonal environment and risk of developing anorexia nervosa. Arch Gen Psych 2007;64(12):1402 [PMID: 18056548].

Warren MP: Endocrine manifestations of eating disorders. J Clin Endocrin Metabolism 2011;96(2):333 [PMID: 21159848].

INCIDENCE

Anorexia nervosa is the third most common chronic illness of adolescent girls in the United States. The incidence has been increasing steadily in the United States since the 1930s. Although ascertaining exact incidence is difficult, most studies show that 1%–2% of teenagers develop AN and 2%–4% develop BN. Adolescents outnumber adults 5 to 1, although the number of adults with EDs is rising. Incidence is also increasing among younger children. Prepubertal patients often have associated psychiatric diagnoses. Males comprise about 10% of patients with EDs, though this prevalence appears to be increasing as well, associated with the increased media emphasis on muscular, chiseled appearance as the male ideal.

Preadolescents with EDs, in comparison to teenagers with EDs, are more likely to be male and present with rapid weight loss and lower percentile body weight and less likely to engage in bulimic behaviors.

Teenagers' self-reported prevalence of ED behavior is much higher than the official incidence of AN or BN. According to the Youth Risk Behavior Survey of US teenagers (2013), 63% of females and 33% of males had attempted to lose weight during the preceding 30 days. Thirteen percent had fasted for more than 24 hours to lose weight, and 5% had used medications to lose weight (6.6% of girls and 3.4% of boys). Self-induced vomiting or laxative use was reported by 6.6% of females and 2.2% of males. Forty-six percent of females and 30% of males reported at least one binge episode during their lifetime. Although the number of youth with full-spectrum EDs is low, it is alarming that so many youth experiment with unhealthy weight control habits. These behaviors may be precursors to the development of EDs, and clinicians should explore these practices with all adolescent patients.

Halmi KA: Anorexia nervosa: an increasing problem in children and adolescents. Dialogues Clin Neurosci 2009;11(1):100–103 [PMID: 19432392].

Kann L et al: Centers for Disease Control and Prevention (CDC): youth risk behavior surveillance—United States 2013. MMWR Surveill Summ 2014 Jun 13;63(SS-4):39–41 [PMID: 24918634]. http://www.cdc.gov/mmwr/pdf/ss/ss6304.pdf.

Peebles R et al: How do children with eating disorders differ from adolescents with eating disorders at initial evaluation? J Adolesc Health 2006;39:800 [PMID: 17116508].

PREDISPOSING FACTORS & CLINICAL PROFILES

Children involved in gymnastics, figure skating, and ballet—activities that emphasize thin bodies—are at higher risk for AN than are children in sports that do not emphasize body image. Adolescents who believe that being thin represents the ideal frame for a female, those who are dissatisfied with their bodies, and those with a history of dieting are at increased risk for EDs. Sudden changes in dietary habits, such as becoming vegetarian, may be a first sign of anorexia, especially if the change is abrupt and without good reason.

The typical bulimic patient tends to be impulsive and engages in risk-taking behavior such as alcohol use, drug use, and sexual experimentation. Bulimic patients are often an appropriate weight for height or slightly overweight. They have average academic performance. Youth with diabetes have an increased risk of BN. In males, wrestling predisposes to BN, and homosexual orientation is associated with binge eating.

Shaw H et al: Body image and eating disturbances across ethnic groups: more similarities than differences. Psychol Addict Behav 2004;18:8 [PMID: 15008651].

Striegel-Moore RH, Bulik CM: Risk factors for eating disorders. Am Psychol 2007;62:181 [PMID: 17469897].

ANOREXIA NERVOSA

According to the National Eating Disorders Association, the diagnostic criteria for AN, adapted from the *Diagnostic and Statistical Manual of Mental Disorders*, Fifth Edition (DSM-5), are described as follows.

ESSENTIALS OF DIAGNOSIS & TYPICAL FEATURES: ANOREXIA NERVOSA

▶ Restriction of energy intake relative to requirements leading to low body weight in the context of age, sex, physical health, and developmental trajectory.

▶ Strong fear of gaining weight or becoming fat, even though underweight.

▶ Disturbance in the way one's body weight or shape is experienced, undue influence of body weight or shape on self-evaluation, or denial of the seriousness of current low body weight.

https://www.nationaleatingdisorders.org/anorexia-nervosa

Table 6–1. Screening questions to help diagnose anorexia and bulimia nervosa.

How do you feel about your body?
Are there parts of your body you might change?
When you look at yourself in the mirror, do you see yourself as overweight, underweight, or satisfactory?
If overweight, how much do you want to weigh?
If your weight is satisfactory, has there been a time when you were worried about being overweight?
If overweight (underweight), what would you change?
Have you ever been on a diet?
What have you done to help yourself lose weight?
Do you count calories or fat grams?
Do you keep your intake to a certain number of calories?
Have you ever used nutritional supplements, diet pills, or laxatives to help you lose weight?
Have you ever made yourself vomit to get rid of food or lose weight?

There are two major types of AN. In the restricting type, patients do not regularly engage in binge eating or purging. In the binge-purge type, AN is combined with binge eating or purging behavior, or both. Distinguishing between the two is important as they carry different implications for prognosis and treatment. Although patients may not demonstrate all features of AN, they may still exhibit the deleterious symptoms associated with AN. A third form—atypical AN—exists as well, accounting for 18% of all ED diagnoses in one study. These individuals demonstrate typical AN behavior but are within or above normal weight.

▶ Clinical Findings

A. Symptoms and Signs

Clinicians should recognize the early symptoms and signs of AN because early intervention may prevent the full-blown syndrome from developing. Patients may show some typical AN behaviors, such as reduction in dietary fat and intense concern with body image, even before weight loss or amenorrhea occurs.

Making the diagnosis of AN can be challenging because adolescents may try to conceal their illness. Assessing the patient's body image is essential to determining the diagnosis. Table 6–1 lists screening questions that help tease out a teenager's perceptions of body image. Other diagnostic screening tools (eg, EDs Inventory) assess a range of eating and dieting behaviors. Parental observations are critical in determining whether a patient has expressed dissatisfaction over body habitus and which weight loss techniques the child has used. If the teenager is unwilling to share his or her concerns about body image, the clinician may find clues to the diagnosis by carefully considering other presenting symptoms or signs. Weight loss from a baseline of normal body weight is an obvious red flag for the presence of an ED. Additionally, AN

should be considered in any girl with secondary amenorrhea who has lost weight.

Physical symptoms and signs are usually secondary to weight loss and proportional to the degree of malnutrition. The body effectively goes into hibernation, becoming functionally hypothyroid (euthyroid sick) to save energy. Body temperature decreases, and patients report being cold. Bradycardia develops, especially in the supine position. Dizziness, light-headedness, and syncope may occur as a result of orthostasis and hypotension secondary to impaired cardiac function. Left ventricular mass is decreased, stroke volume is compromised, and peripheral resistance is increased, contributing to left ventricular systolic dysfunction. Patients can develop prolonged QTc syndrome and increased QT dispersion (irregular QT intervals), putting them at risk for cardiac arrhythmias. Peripheral circulation is reduced. Hands and feet may be blue and cool. Hair thins, nails become brittle, and skin becomes dry. Lanugo develops as a primitive response to starvation. The gastrointestinal (GI) tract may be affected; inability to take in normal quantities of food, early satiety, and gastroesophageal reflux can develop as the body adapts to reduced intake. The normal gastrocolic reflex may be lost due to lack of stimulation by food, causing bloating and constipation. Delayed gastric emptying may develop. Nutritional rehabilitation improves gastric emptying and dyspeptic symptoms in AN restricting type, but not in those who vomit. Neurologically, patients may experience decreased cognition, inability to concentrate, increased irritability, and depression, which may be related to structural brain changes and decreased cerebral blood flow.

Determining BMI is critical for assessing degree of malnutrition. A gown-only weight after urination is the most accurate way to assess weight. Patients tend to wear bulky clothes and may hide weights in their pockets or drink excessive fluid (water-loading) to trick the practitioner. BMI below the 25th percentile indicates risk for malnutrition and below 5th percentile indicates significant malnutrition. Median body weight (MBW) should be calculated as it serves both as the denominator to determine what percent weight an individual is and to provide a general goal weight during recovery. MBW for height is calculated by using the 50th percentile of BMI for age.

A combination of malnutrition and stress causes hypothalamic hypogonadism. The hypothalamic-pituitary-gonadal axis shuts down as the body struggles to survive, directing finite energy resources to vital functions. This may be mediated by the effect of low serum leptin levels on the hypothalamic-pituitary axis. Pubertal development and skeletal growth may be interrupted, and adolescents may experience decreased libido.

Amenorrhea will continue to be an important clinical sign that the body is malnourished. Amenorrhea occurs for two reasons. The hypothalamic-pituitary-ovarian axis shuts down under stress, causing hypothalamic amenorrhea. In addition, adipose tissue is needed to convert estrogen to its activated form. When weight loss is significant, there is not enough substrate to activate estrogen. Resumption of menses occurs only when both body weight and body fat increase.

Approximately, 73% of postmenarchal girls resume menstruating if they reach 90% of MBW. An adolescent female needs about 17% body fat to restart menses and 22% body fat to initiate menses if she has primary amenorrhea. Some evidence suggests that target weight gain for return of menses is approximately 1 kg higher than the weight at which menses ceased.

B. Laboratory Findings

All organ systems may suffer some degree of damage in the anorexic patient, related to both severity and duration of illness (Table 6-2). Initial screening should include complete blood count with differential; serum levels of electrolytes, blood urea nitrogen, creatinine, phosphorus, calcium, magnesium, and thyroid-stimulating hormone; liver function tests; and urinalysis. Increase in lipids, likely due to abnormal liver function, is seen in 18% of those with AN, with subsequent return to normal once weight is restored. An electrocardiogram (ECG) should be performed, because significant ECG abnormalities may be present, most importantly prolonged QTc syndrome. Bone densitometry should be done if illness persists for 6 months, as patients begin to accumulate risk for osteoporosis.

▶ Differential Diagnosis

If the diagnosis is unclear (ie, the patient has lost a significant amount of weight but does not have typical body image

Table 6–2. Laboratory findings: anorexia nervosa.

Increased blood urea nitrogen and creatinine secondary to renal insufficiency
Decreased white blood cells, platelets, and less commonly red blood cells and hematocrit secondary to bone marrow suppression or fat atrophy of the bone marrow
Increased AST and ALT secondary to malnutrition
Increased cholesterol, thought to be related to altered fatty acid metabolism
Decreased alkaline phosphatase secondary to zinc deficiency
Low- to low-normal thyroid-stimulating hormone and thyroxine
Decreased follicle-stimulating hormone, luteinizing hormone, estradiol, and testosterone secondary to shutdown of hypothalamic pituitary-gonadal axis
Abnormal electrolytes related to hydration status
Decreased phosphorus
Decreased insulin-like growth factor
Increased cortisol
Decreased urine specific gravity in cases of intentional water intoxication

ALT, alanine aminotransferase; AST, aspartate aminotransferase.

distortion or fat phobia), the clinician must consider the differential diagnosis for weight loss in adolescents. This includes inflammatory bowel disease, diabetes, hyperthyroidism, malignancy, depression, and chronic infectious disease such as human immunodeficiency virus (HIV). Less common diagnoses include adrenal insufficiency and malabsorption syndromes such as celiac disease. The history and physical examination should direct specific laboratory and radiologic evaluation.

▶ Complications (Table 6–3)

A. Short-Term Complications

1. Early satiety—Patients may have difficulty tolerating even modest quantities of food when intake increases; this usually resolves after the patients adjust to larger meals. Gastric emptying is poor. Pancreatic and biliary secretion is diminished.

2. Superior mesenteric artery syndrome—As patients become malnourished, the fat pad between the superior mesenteric artery and the duodenum shrinks and compression of the transverse duodenum may cause obstruction and vomiting, especially with solid foods. The upper GI series shows to-and-fro movement of barium in the descending and transverse duodenum proximal to the obstruction. Treatment involves a liquid diet or nasoduodenal feedings until restoration of the fat pad has occurred, coincident with weight gain.

3. Constipation—Patients may be very constipated. Two mechanisms contribute—loss of the gastrocolic reflex and

Table 6–3. Complications of anorexia and bulimia nervosa, by mechanism.

Cardiovascular Bradycardia (WL/MN) Postural hypotension (WL/MN, SIV, LX) Arrhythmia, sudden death (WL/MN, SIV, LX) Congestive heart failure (during refeeding) (WL/MN) Pericardial effusion (WL/MN) Mitral valve prolapse (WL/MN) ECG abnormalities (prolonged QT, low voltage, T-wave abnormalities, conduction defects) (WL/MN) **Endocrine** ↓ LH, FSH (WL/MN) ↓ T_3, ↑ rT_3, ↓ T_4, TSH (WL/MN) Irregular menses (WL/MN, B/P) Amenorrhea (WL/MN) Hypercortisolism (WL/MN) Growth retardation (WL/MN) Delayed puberty (WL/MN) Decreased libido (WL/MN) **Gastrointestinal** Dental erosion (SIV) Parotid swelling (SIV) Esophagitis, esophageal tears (SIV) Delayed gastric emptying (WL/MN, SIV) Gastric dilation (rarely rupture) (SIV) Pancreatitis (WL/MN) Constipation (WL/MN, LXA) Diarrhea (LXA) Superior mesenteric artery syndrome (WL/MN) Hypercholesterolemia (WL/MN) ↑ Liver function tests (fatty infiltration of the liver) (WL/MN)	**Hematologic** Leukopenia (WL/MN) Anemia (WL/MN) Thrombocytopenia (WL/MN) ↓ ESR (WL/MN) Impaired cell-mediated immunity (WL/MN) **Metabolic** Dehydration (WL/MN, SIV, LXA, DU) Acidosis (LXA) Alkalosis (SIV) Hypokalemia (SIV, LXA, DU) Hyponatremia (SIV, LXA, DU, WL/MN) Hypochloremia (SIV) Hypocalcemia (WL/MN, SIV) Hypophosphatemia (WL/MN) Hypomagnesemia (WL/MN) Hypercarotenemia (WL/MN) **Neurologic** Cortical atrophy-white and gray matter (WL/MN) Peripheral neuropathy (WL/MN) Seizures (WL/MN, SIV, LXA) Thermoregulatory abnormalities (WL/MN) ↓ REM and slow-wave sleep (All) **Renal** Hematuria (WL/MN) Proteinuria (WL/MN) ↓ Renal concentrating ability (WL/MN, DU) Enuresis (WL/MN) **Skeletal** Osteopenia (WL/MN) Fractures (WL/MN)

B/P, binge-purge; DU, diuretic abuse; ECG, electrocardiogram; ESR, erythrocyte sedimentation rate; FSH, follicle-stimulating hormone; LH, luteinizing hormone; LXA, laxative abuse; REM, rapid eye movement; rT_3, resin triiodothyronine uptake; SIV, self-induced vomiting; T_3, triiodothyronine; T_4, thyroxine; TSH, thyroid-stimulating hormone; WL/MN, weight loss/malnutrition.

loss of colonic muscle tone. Typically stool softeners are not effective because the colon has decreased peristaltic amplitude. Agents that induce peristalsis, such as bisacodyl, as well as osmotic agents, such as polyethylene glycol-electrolyte solution (MiraLax), are helpful. Constipation can persist for up to 6–8 weeks after refeeding. Occasionally enemas are required.

4. Refeeding syndrome—This syndrome is described in the Treatment section.

5. Pericardial effusion—The degree of malnutrition correlates with increasing prevalence of pericardial effusion. One study demonstrated that 22% of those with AN had silent pericardial effusions, with 88% of effusions resolving after weight restoration.

B. Long-Term Complications

1. Osteoporosis—Approximately 50% of females with AN have reduced bone mass at one or more sites. The lumbar spine has the most rapid turnover and is the area likely to be affected first. Teenagers are particularly at risk as they accrue 40% of their bone mineral during adolescence. Low body weight is most predictive of bone loss. The causes of osteopenia and osteoporosis are multiple. Estrogen and testosterone are essential to potentiate bone development. Bone minerals begin to resorb without estrogen. Elevated cortisol levels and decreased insulin-like growth factor-1 also contribute to bone resorption. Amenorrhea is highly correlated with osteoporosis. Studies show that as few as 6 months of amenorrhea is associated with osteopenia or osteoporosis. Males have similar bone loss related to their degree of malnutrition, likely due to decreased testosterone and elevated cortisol.

The most effective treatment for bone loss in girls with AN has been regaining sufficient weight and body fat to restart the menstrual cycle. Studies do not support the use of hormone replacement therapy delivered orally to improve bone recovery; however, one randomized controlled trial demonstrated that physiologic doses of estrogen, delivered transdermally, over 18 months did improve bone density. Clinicians may consider transdermal estrogen treatment if patients are recalcitrant to intervention and do not restore weight in a timely manner. Bisphosphonates show moderate positive effectiveness for adults with AN, but not for adolescents. Use of dehydroepiandrosterone in combination with oral contraceptive pills is shown to maintain bone mineral density in adolescents with AN compared to controls, though this treatment approach has not been adopted as standard of care.

2. Brain changes—As malnutrition becomes pronounced, brain tissue—both white and gray matter—is lost, with a compensatory increase in cerebrospinal fluid in the sulci and ventricles. Follow-up studies of weight-recovered anorexic patients show a persistent loss of gray matter, although white matter returns to normal. Functionally, there does not seem to be a direct relationship between cognition and brain tissue loss, although studies have shown a decrease in cognitive ability and decreased cerebral blood flow in very malnourished patients. Making patients and family aware that brain tissue can be lost may improve their perception of the seriousness of this disorder.

3. Effects on future children—This area has just recently been studied. Findings suggest that there may be feeding issues for infants who are born to mothers who have a history of either AN or BN. Infants born to mothers with a history of AN have more feeding difficulties at 0 and 6 months and tend to be lower weight (30th percentile on average). Infants born to mothers with current or past BN are more likely to be overweight and have faster growth rates than controls. Pediatricians should ascertain an ED history from mothers of patients who are having feeding issues.

Fazeli PK, Klibanski A: Effects of anorexia nervosa on bone metabolism. Endocr Rev 2018 Dec;39(6):895–910 [PMID: 30165608].

Golden NH et al: Update on the medical management of eating disorders in adolescents. J Adolesc Health 2015;56:370–375 [PMID: 25659201].

Kastner S, Salbach-Andrae H, Renneberg B, Pfeiffer E, Lehmkuhl U, Schmitz L: Echocardiographic findings in adolescents with anorexia nervosa at beginning of treatment and after weight recovery. Eur Child Adolesc Psychiatry 2012 Jan;21(1):15–21 [PMID: 22086424].

Micali N, Simonoff E, Treasure J: Infant feeding and weight in the first year of life in babies of women with eating disorders. J Pediatr 2009;154(1):55–60.e1 [PMID: 18783793].

Misra M et al: Physiologic estrogen replacement increases bone density in adolescent girls with anorexia nervosa. J Bone Miner Res 2011 Oct;26(10):2430–2438 [PMID: 21698665].

Nagata J et al: Assessment of sex differences in bone deficits among adolescents with anorexia nervosa. Int J Eat Disord 2017 Apr;50(4):352–358 [PMID: 27611361].

Sachs KV, Harnke B, Mehler PS, Krantz MJ: Cardiovascular complications of anorexia nervosa: a systematic review. Int J Eat Disord 2016 Mar;49(3):238–248 [PMID: 26710932].

Vo M, Accurso EC, LeGrange D: The impact of DSM-5 on eating disorder diagnoses. Int J Eat Disord 2016 Nov;50(5) [PMID: 27862127].

C. Mortality

Patients with EDs are at a higher risk of death than the general population and those with AN have the highest risk of dying among those with EDs. Meta-analysis estimates the standardized mortality ratio associated with AN to be 5.9. Death in anorexic patients is due to suicide, abnormal electrolytes, and cardiac arrhythmias.

▶ Treatment

A. General Approach

Factors that determine treatment interventions are severity of illness, duration of illness, specific manifestations of disease, previous treatment approaches and outcomes, program availability, financial resources, and insurance coverage. Treatment options include outpatient management, day treatment hospitalization, inpatient medical or psychiatric hospitalization, and residential treatment. The key to determining level of intervention is the degree of malnutrition, the rapidity of weight loss, the degree of medical compromise, and the presence of life-threatening electrolyte abnormalities. No absolute criteria determine level of intervention. The practitioner must examine the degree of medical compromise and consider immediate risks and the potential for an individual to reverse the situation on his or her own. Treatment is costly. Many patients do not have insurance benefits that adequately cover the cost of treatment, leaving parents and practitioners with profound dilemmas as to how to best provide treatment in the face of financial constraints. Legally, however, EDs are now recognized as a parity mental health diagnosis similar to the other biologically based mental health illnesses in many states, which has increased the ease of obtaining insurance coverage.

A multidisciplinary approach is most effective and should include medical monitoring, nutrition therapy, and individual and family psychotherapy by experienced practitioners. Family therapy is an important means of helping families understand the development of the disease and addressing issues that may be barriers to recovery. Both types of psychotherapy are encouraged in most treatment programs, and recovery without psychotherapy is unusual. The average length of psychotherapy is roughly 6–9 months, although some individuals continue therapy for extended periods. Adjunctive modalities include art and horticulture therapy, therapeutic recreation, and massage therapy.

Manualized family therapy, developed in Britain by Maudsley and adapted by Lock and LeGrange, has shifted the therapeutic approach to adolescents with AN. Traditional therapy allowed the adolescent to control his or her eating and the parents to remain uninvolved with the food portion of recovery. The manualized approach gives power and control back to parents.

Treatment is prescribed for 20 weekly sessions. The first 10 weeks are devoted to empowering parents, putting them in control of their child's nutrition and exercise. Parents are educated about the dangers of malnutrition and are instructed to supervise each meal. The next phase, sessions 11–16, returns control over eating to the adolescent once he or she accepts the demands of the parents. The last phase of treatment, sessions 17–20, occurs when the patient is maintaining a healthy weight and shifts the focus away from the ED, examining instead the impact that the ED has had on establishing a healthy adolescent identity. This approach is reported to result in good or intermediate outcomes in 90% of treated adolescents.

Careful instruction in nutrition helps the teenager and family dispel misconceptions about nutrition, identify realistic nutritional goals, and normalize eating. Initially, nutrition education may be the most important intervention as the teenager slowly works through his or her fears of fat-containing foods and weight gain. The teenager begins to trust the nutrition therapist and restore body weight, eventually eating in a well-balanced, healthy manner.

B. Inpatient Treatment

Table 6–4 lists the criteria for hospital admission generally used in the medical community. It is usually quite difficult for a patient who is losing weight rapidly (> 2 lb/wk) to reverse the weight loss because the body is in a catabolic state.

Goals of hospitalization include arresting weight loss and stabilizing hemodynamics. Nutrition is the most vital inpatient medicine. Clinicians can safely begin with a meal plan containing approximately 250 kcal more than the patient has been routinely eating, which can usually be accomplished orally. Studies suggest that meal plans can begin with as high as 1750 kcal regardless of baseline intake. Meal plans should be well balanced with appropriate proportions of carbohydrate, protein, and fat. Oral meals are usually tolerated, although it is important to be supervised by medical staff. If the patient resists, nasogastric or intravenous alimentation can be used. Aside from caloric needs, the clinician needs to

Table 6–4. Criteria for hospitalization for eating disordered patients.

One or more of the following justify hospitalization:
1. Body weight: < 75% median body weight.
2. Dehydration
3. Electrolyte disturbance (hypokalemia, hyponatremia, hypophosphatemia)
4. ECG abnormalities (prolonged QTC, severe bradycardia)
5. Physiologic Instability
   Supine heart rate < 45 beats/min
   Symptomatic hypotension or syncope
   Hypothermia
6. Failure of outpatient management
7. Acute food refusal
8. Uncontrolled bingeing and purging
9. Acute medical complications of malnutrition (syncope, seizures, cardiac failure, pancreatitis)
10. Comorbid psychiatric or medical condition that prohibits or limits appropriate outpatient treatment (severe depression, suicidal ideation, obsessive-compulsive disorder, type 1 diabetes)

consider the patient's hydration and include the appropriate amount of fluid with the meal plan. Dehydration should be corrected slowly. The oral route is usually adequate. Aggressive intravenous fluid administration should be avoided because left ventricular mass is compromised and a rapid increase in volume may not be tolerated. Regulating fluid intake is important, because water intoxication can contribute to abnormal electrolytes and falsified weights.

During the initial introduction of food, the clinician should monitor the patient for refeeding syndrome, a phenomenon that occurs if caloric intake is increased too rapidly. Signs of refeeding syndrome are decreased serum phosphorus (as the body resumes synthesis of adenosine triphosphate), decreased serum potassium (as increased insulin causes K^+ to shift from extracellular fluid into K^+-depleted cells), and, rarely, edema related to fluid shifts or congestive heart failure.

Although specific guidelines do not exist, many practitioners begin phosphorus supplementation if patients are severely malnourished (< 70% MBW) or their intake has been consistently less than 500 kcal/day.

Caloric intake can be increased 250 kcal/day as long as refeeding syndrome does not occur. Weight goals vary depending on programmatic approach. Typically, intake is adjusted to reach a goal of 0.1–0.25 kg/day weight gain.

Overnight monitoring for bradycardia is helpful in assessing degree of metabolic compromise. Usually the more rapid and severe the weight loss, the worse the bradycardia. Improving bradycardia correlates with weight recovery. Orthostatic hypotension is most severe around hospital day 4, improving steadily and correcting by the third week of nutritional rehabilitation. An ECG should be obtained because the patient is at risk for prolonged QTc syndrome and junctional arrhythmias related to the severity of bradycardia.

It usually takes 2–3 weeks to reach the initial goals of hospitalization—steady weight gain, toleration of oral diet without signs of refeeding syndrome, corrected bradycardia (heart rate > 45 beats/min for three consecutive nights), and correction of orthostasis. Specific weight criteria are used by many programs when considering discharge. This depends partly on admission weight. Ideally a patient gains at least 5% of his or her MBW. Some programs set discharge at 80%, 85%, or 90% MBW. Patient outcomes are improved with discharge at a higher body weight. Some evidence exists that patients do better if discharged at 95% MBW. In many practitioners' experience, relapse rates are high if patients are discharged at less than 75% MBW.

C. Pharmacotherapy

Practitioners frequently use psychotropic medications for treatment of AN, despite the lack of evidence supporting efficacy. Several open-label trials suggest that atypical antipsychotics (risperidone, olanzapine, quetiapine) may be helpful. One review found that olanzapine (2.5–15 mg/day) was associated with improved body weight, decreased delusional thinking, improvement in body image, and decreased agitation and premeal anxiety. However, a randomized controlled trial did not show any difference in outcomes between risperidone and placebo.

SSRIs repeatedly have been shown to not be helpful in the initial therapy of AN. A recent study showed that use of SSRIs may decrease bone mineral density when used in malnourished patients. However, once the patient has achieved approximately 85% MBW, SSRIs (fluoxetine, citalopram, or sertraline) may help prevent relapse.

Zinc deficiency is common in AN, and several studies support its use as a supplement during the initial phases of treatment. Because zinc deficiency adversely affects neurotransmitters, administering zinc helps restore neurotransmitter action to baseline. Additionally, zinc may restore appetite and improve depressive mood. Zinc should be administered for approximately 2 months from the beginning of therapy, with at least 14 mg of elemental zinc daily.

Because of global nutritional deficits, a multivitamin with iron is also recommended daily. Symptomatic treatment for constipation and reflux should be used appropriately until symptoms resolve.

D. Outpatient Treatment

Not all patients with AN require inpatient treatment, especially if parents and clinicians recognize the warning signs early. These patients can receive treatment as outpatients, employing the same multidisciplinary team approach.

Manualized family-based treatment is ideal for the outpatient setting if a trained therapist is available. Appropriate nutrition counseling is vital in guiding a patient and family through the initial stages of recovery. As the nutrition therapist is working at increasing the patient's caloric intake, a practitioner needs to monitor the patient's weight and vital signs. Often, activity level needs to be decreased to help reverse the catabolic state. A reasonable weight gain goal may be 0.2–0.5 kg/wk. If weight loss persists, careful monitoring of vital signs, including supine heart rate, is important in determining whether an increased level of care is needed. Concomitantly, the patient should be referred to a psychotherapist and, if indicated, assessed by a psychiatrist.

E. Treatment Goals and Outcomes

Goals of treatment include reaching a healthy body weight, elimination of medical sequelae, and resumption of menses. Symptoms can wax and wane over an extended period for several years. Approximately 50% of adolescents recover in a relatively short period of time. Thirty percent may take several years to get back to a state of health, although symptoms may reappear on occasion. About 20% of adolescents can go on to develop chronic, unremitting AN.

Arcelus J et al: Mortality rates in patients with anorexia nervosa and other eating disorders. A meta-analysis of 36 studies. Arch Gen Psychiatry 2011;68(7):724–731 [PMID: 21727255].

Birmingham CL, Gritzner S: How does zinc supplementation benefit anorexia nervosa? Eat Weight Disord 2006;11:e109 [PMID: 17272939].

Claudino AM et al: Antidepressants for anorexia nervosa. Cochrane Database Syst Rev 2006;(1):CD004365 [PMID: 16437485].

DiVasta AD, Feldman HA, O'Donnell JM: Effect of exercise and antidepressants on skeletal outcomes in adolescent girls with anorexia nervosa. J Adolesc Health 2017 Feb;60(2):229–232 [PMID: 27939877].

Garber AK et al: A systematic review of approaches to refeeding in patients with anorexia nervosa. Int J Eat Disord 2016 Mar;49(3):293–310 [PMID: 26661289].

Hagman J et al: A double-blind, placebo-controlled study of risperidone for the treatment of anorexia nervosa. J Am Acad Child Adolesc Psychiatry 2011;50(9):915–924 [PMID: 21871373].

LeGrange D et al: Manualized family-based treatment for anorexia nervosa: a case series. J Am Acad Child Adolesc Psychiatry 2005;44:41 [PMID: 15608542].

Swenne I: Weight requirements for return of menstruations in teenage girls with eating disorders, weight loss, and secondary amenorrhea. Acta Paediatr 2004;93:1449 [PMID: 08035253].

BULIMIA NERVOSA

The diagnostic criteria for BN are discussed in section Essentials of Diagnosis & Typical Features. Binge eating is either eating excessive amounts of food during a normal mealtime or having a meal that lasts longer than usual. Bulimic individuals feel out of control while eating, unable or unwilling to recognize satiety signals. Any type of food may be eaten in a binge, although typically it includes carbohydrates or junk food. Extreme guilt is often associated with the episode. At some point, either prior to or during a binge, bulimic individuals often decide to purge as a means of preventing weight gain. The most common ways to purge are self-induced vomiting, exercise, and laxative use. Some individuals will vomit multiple times during a purge episode, after using large amounts of water to cleanse their system. This can induce significant electrolyte abnormalities such as hyponatremia and hypokalemia, which may put the patient at acute risk for arrhythmia or seizure. Other methods of purging include diuretics, diet pills, cathartics, and nutritional supplements that promote weight loss, such as Metabolife or Sensa.

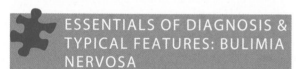

ESSENTIALS OF DIAGNOSIS & TYPICAL FEATURES: BULIMIA NERVOSA

▶ Recurrent episodes of binge eating, characterized by both of the following:

- Eating in a discrete period an amount of food that is larger than most people would eat during a similar period under like circumstances.

- A sense of lack of control during the episode (eg, feeling that one cannot stop eating or control what or how much one is eating).

▶ Recurrent inappropriate compensatory behavior to prevent weight gain (eg, self-induced vomiting; misuse of laxatives, diuretics, or other products; excessive exercise; fasting).

▶ Binge eating and inappropriate compensatory behaviors occur at least once a week for 3 months (on average).

https://www.nationaleatingdisorders.org/bulimia-nervosa

Diagnosing BN can be difficult unless the teenager is forthcoming or parents or caregivers can supply direct observations. Bulimic patients are usually average or slightly above average in body weight and have no physical abnormalities. Screening all teenagers for body image concerns is crucial. If the teenager expresses concern about being overweight, the clinician needs to screen the patient about dieting methods. Asking whether patients have binged, feel out of control while eating, or whether they cannot stop eating can clarify the diagnosis. Parents may report that significant amounts of food are missing or disappearing more quickly than normal. If the physician is suspicious, direct questioning about all the ways to purge should follow. Indicating first

that the behavior is not unusual can make questioning less threatening and more likely to elicit a truthful response. For example, the clinician might say, "Some teenagers who try to lose weight make themselves vomit after eating. Have you ever considered or done that yourself?" (See Table 6–1 for additional screening questions.)

▶ Clinical Findings

A. Symptoms and Signs

Symptoms are related to the mechanism of purging. GI problems are most prominent. Abdominal pain is common. Gastroesophageal reflux occurs as the lower esophageal sphincter becomes compromised due to repetitive vomiting. Frequent vomiting may also cause esophagitis or gastritis, as the mucosa is irritated by acid exposure. Early satiety, involuntary vomiting, and complaints that food is "coming up" on its own are frequent. Hematemesis and esophageal rupture have been reported. Patients may report diarrhea or constipation, especially if laxatives have been used. Sialadenitis (parotid pain and enlargement) may be caused by frequent vomiting. Erosion of dental enamel results from increased oral acid exposure during vomiting. Because comorbid depression is common in BN, patients may report difficulty sleeping, decreased energy, decreased motivation, and headaches. Light-headedness or syncope may develop secondary to dehydration.

It is important to note that most purging methods are ineffective. When patients binge, they may consume thousands of calories. Digestion begins rapidly. Although the patient may be able to vomit some of the food, much is actually digested and absorbed. Laxatives work in the large intestine, leading to fluid and electrolyte loss, but consumed calories are still absorbed from the small intestine. Use of diuretics may result in decreased fluid weight and electrolyte imbalance.

On physical examination, bulimic patients may be dehydrated and have orthostatic hypotension. Sialadenitis, tooth enamel loss, dental caries, and abdominal tenderness are the most common findings. Abrasion of the proximal interphalangeal joints may occur secondary to scraping the fingers against teeth while inducing vomiting. Rarely, a heart murmur is heard which may be due to mitral valve prolapse. Irreversible cardiomyopathy can develop secondary to ipecac use.

B. Laboratory Findings

Electrolyte disturbances are common. The method of purging results in specific abnormalities. Vomiting causes metabolic alkalosis, hypokalemia, and hypochloremia. Laxatives cause metabolic acidosis, hypokalemia, and hypochloremia. Diuretic use may lead to hypokalemia, hyponatremia, hypocalcemia, and metabolic alkalosis. Amylase may be increased secondary to chronic parotid stimulation.

Complications

A. Short-Term Complications

Complications in normal-weight bulimic patients are related to the mechanisms of purging, and many of these complications are listed under Symptoms and Signs. If the bulimic patient is significantly malnourished, complications may be the same as those encountered in the anorexic patient. Other complications of bulimia include esophageal rupture, acute or chronic esophagitis, and, rarely, Barrett esophagitis. Chronic vomiting can lead to metabolic alkalosis, and laxative abuse may cause metabolic acidosis. Diet pill use can cause insomnia, hypertension, tachycardia, palpitations, seizures, and sudden death.

Patients who stop taking laxatives can have severe constipation. Treating constipation can be difficult psychologically, because the practitioner may need to prescribe agents similar to the drugs of abuse used during the ED.

B. Mortality

The mortality rate in bulimic patients is similar to that in anorexic patients. Death usually results from suicide or electrolyte derangements.

Treatment

Treatment of BN depends on the frequency of bingeing and purging and the severity of biochemical and psychiatric derangement. If K^+ is less than 3.0 mEq/L, inpatient medical admission is warranted. Typically, extracellular K^+ is spared at the expense of intracellular K^+, so a patient may become hypokalemic several days after the serum K^+ concentration appears to be corrected. Usually cessation of purging is sufficient to correct K^+ concentration and is the recommended intervention for K^+ above 3.0 mEq/L. If K^+ is 2.5–2.9 mEq/L, oral supplementation is suggested. If K^+ is less than 2.5 mEq/L, intravenous therapy is recommended. Supplements can be stopped once K^+ levels are more than 3.5 mEq/L. Total body K^+ can be assumed to be normal when serum K^+ corrects and remains normal 2 days after supplements are stopped. Continued hospitalization depends on the patient's psychological status.

Some bulimic patients who abuse laxatives may become chronically dehydrated. The renin-angiotensin-aldosterone axis is activated, and the antidiuretic hormone level may be elevated to compensate. These hormones do not normalize immediately when laxatives are stopped, and fluid retention of up to 10 kg/wk may result. This puts patients at risk for congestive heart failure and can scare them as their weight increases dramatically. Diuresis often occurs after 7–10 days.

Hospitalization of bulimic patients is also recommended if there has been failure of outpatient management. The binge-purge cycle is addictive and can be difficult for patients to interrupt on their own. Hospitalization can offer a forced break from the cycle, allowing patients to normalize their eating, interrupt the addictive behavior, and regain the ability to recognize satiety signals.

Outpatient management can be pursued if patients are medically stable. Cognitive-behavioral therapy is crucial to help bulimic patients understand their disease. Nutrition therapy offers patients ways to regulate eating patterns so that they can avoid the need to binge. Medical monitoring should be done to check electrolytes periodically, depending on the purging method used.

SSRIs are generally helpful in treating the binge-purge cycle. Fluoxetine has been studied most extensively; a dose of 60 mg/day is most efficacious in teenagers. Other SSRIs appear to be effective as well and may be used in patients experiencing side effects of fluoxetine. Treatment for gastroesophageal reflux and gastritis should be used when appropriate. The pain and swelling of enlarged parotid glands can be helped by sucking on tart candy and by the application of heat.

Goals of treatment are to interrupt the binge/purge cycle, with the goal of reaching remission as a targeted outcome.

Hail L, LeGrange D: Bulimia nervosa in adolescents: prevalence and treatment challenges. Adolesc Health Med Ther 2018 Jan;9:11–16 [PMID: 29379324].

Mehler PS: Medical complications of bulimia nervosa and their treatments. Int J Eat Disord (0276–3478) 2011 Mar;44(2):95 [PMID: 21312201].

Steinhausen HC, Weber S: The outcome of bulimia nervosa: findings from one-quarter century of research. Am J Psychiatry 2009;166:1331–1341 [PMID: 19884225].

Sysko R, Sha N, Wang W: Early response to antidepressant treatment in bulimia nervosa. Psychol Med 2010;40(6):999 [PMID: 20441691].

BINGE-EATING DISORDER

Binge-eating disorder (BED) is now described in the DSM-5. Studies show that most adults who have BED (a prevalence of 2%–4%) develop symptoms during adolescence. Following are the diagnostic criteria for BED.

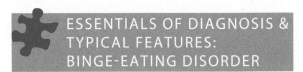

ESSENTIALS OF DIAGNOSIS &
TYPICAL FEATURES:
BINGE-EATING DISORDER

▶ Recurring episodes of binge eating:
  • Eating significantly more food in a short period than most people would eat under similar circumstances.
  • Episodes marked by feelings of lack of control.
▶ Binge eating is associated with marked distress.
▶ Binge eating occurs at least once a week over 3 months (on average).

https://www.nationaleatingdisorders.org/sites/default/files/ResourceHandouts/MultiPageRGB.pdf

► Clinical Findings

A. Symptoms and Signs

BED most often is found in overweight or obese individuals. Eighteen percent of such patients report binging at least once in the past year. Patients with BED have an increased incidence of depression and substance abuse. The possibility of BED should be raised for any significantly overweight patient. Specific questionnaires are available for evaluating patients suspected of BED.

B. Laboratory Findings

The clinician should assess causes and complications of obesity, and laboratory evaluation should include thyroid function tests and measurement of cholesterol and triglyceride levels.

► Treatment

A combination of cognitive-behavioral therapy and antidepressant medication has been helpful in treating BED in adults. Use of SSRIs for BED in adolescents has not been studied, but in adults fluoxetine and citalopram help decrease binge episodes, improve depressive symptoms, and possibly decrease appetite. This evidence suggests that SSRIs in adolescents with BED may be helpful as well. BED has been recognized only recently, and outcomes have not been studied. Little is known regarding long-term prognosis.

Fairburn CG et al: The natural course of bulimia nervosa and binge-eating disorder in young women. Arch Gen Psychiatry 2000;57:659 [PMID: 10891036].

McElroy SL et al: Citalopram in the treatment of binge-eating disorder: a placebo-controlled trial. J Clin Psychiatry 2003;64:807 [PMID: 12934982].

Schneider M: Bulimia nervosa and binge-eating disorder in adolescents. Adolesc Med State Art Rev 2003;14:119 [PMID: 12529196].

AVOIDANT/RESTRICTIVE FOOD INTAKE DISORDER

ARFID was added to the DSM-5 that extends the *Diagnostic and Statistical Manual of Mental Disorders*, 4th Edition (DSM-IV) diagnosis of feeding disorder of infancy or early childhood. The hallmark feature is avoidance or restriction of oral food intake, in the absence of criteria for AN (body image disturbance, fear of weight gain/body fat). For teenagers, food avoidance may be associated with more generalized emotional difficulties that do not meet diagnostic criteria for anxiety or depression. Diagnostic criteria for ARFID are discussed in the following section Essentials of Diagnosis & Typical Features. Similar health effects to AN may be found in youth with ARFID, depending on the degree of malnutrition and how an individual became malnourished.

ESSENTIALS OF DIAGNOSIS & TYPICAL FEATURES: AVOIDANT/RESTRICTIVE FOOD INTAKE DISORDER

► Eating or feeding disturbance (including lack of interest in eating, avoidance due to sensory characteristics of food; concern for aversive consequences of eating) demonstrated by failure to meet appropriate nutritional and/or energy needs and associated with one or more of:

- Weight loss (or failure to achieve expected weight gain or faltering growth).
- Nutritional deficiency.
- Dependence on enteral feeding or oral nutritional supplementation.
- Interference with psychosocial functioning.

► Disturbance not explained by lack of available food or culturally sanctioned practice.

► Eating disturbance does not occur exclusively during AN or BN, and there is no disturbance in experience of one's body weight or shape.

► Eating disturbance not attributable to concurrent medical condition or explained by a different mental disorder, *or*, when eating disturbance occurs in the context of another condition or disorder, severity of eating disturbance exceeds that associated with the other condition or disorder.

PROGNOSIS, QUALITY ASSESSMENT, & OUTCOMES METRICS

Outcome in EDs, especially AN, has been studied extensively. Prior metrics generally defined remission or recovery as being at a healthy body weight and a return of menses. As diagnostic criteria for AN changed, a national collaborative effort that included 14 ED programs defined AN recovery based on reaching at least 90% median BMI, without consideration of return of menses. Most studies have focused on specific inpatient treatment programs, and few have evaluated less ill patients who do not need hospitalization. About 40%–50% of patients receiving treatment recover, 20%–30% have intermittent relapses, and 20% have chronic, unremitting illness. As time from initial onset lengthens, the recovery rate decreases and mortality associated with AN and BN increases. A study from the Swedish registry of EDs revealed that 55% of the participants were in remission and approximately 85% were within a healthy weight range at the end of treatment (15 months on average). The national collaborative showed that 65% of patients demonstrated recovery at 1 year, with higher BMI at baseline the most significant predictor of recovery.

The course of AN often includes significant weight fluctuations over time, and it may be a matter of years until recovery is certain. The course of BN often includes relapses of bingeing and purging, although bulimic patients initially recover faster than do anorexic patients. Up to 50% of anorexic patients may develop bulimia, as well as major psychological complications, including depression, anxiety, and substance abuse disorders. Bulimic patients also develop similar psychological illness but rarely develop anorexia. Long-term medical sequelae, aside from low body weight and amenorrhea, have not been systematically studied, although AN is known to have multiple medical consequences, including osteoporosis and structural brain changes.

It is unclear whether age at onset affects outcome, but shorter length of time between symptom onset and therapy tends to improve outcome. Various treatment modalities can prove effective. Favorable outcomes have been found with brief medical hospitalization and long psychiatric or residential hospitalization. Higher discharge weight, as well as more rapid weight gain during inpatient treatment (> 0.8 kg/wk), seems to improve the initial outcome. It is difficult to compare treatment regimens, because numbers are small and the type of patient and illness varies among studies. No existing studies compare outpatient to inpatient treatment or the effects of day treatment on recovery.

Forman SF et al: Predictors of outcome at 1 year in adolescents with DSM-5 restrictive eating disorders: report of the National Eating Disorders Quality Improvement Collaborative. J Adolescent Health 2014;55(6):750–756 [PMID: 25200345].

Lindstedt K, Kiellin L, Gustafson SA: Adolescents with full or subthreshold anorexia nervosa in a naturalistic sample—characteristics and treatment outcome. J Eat Disord March 2017; 5(1):4 [PMID: 28265410].

Lund BC et al: Rate of inpatient weight restoration predicts outcome in anorexia nervosa. Int J Eat Disord 2009;42(4):301–305 [PMID: 19107835].

Steinhausen HC: Outcome of eating disorders. Child Adolesc Psychiatr Clin N Am 2009;18(1):225–242 [PMID: 19014869].

RESOURCES FOR PRACTITIONERS & FAMILIES

Web Resources

Academy for Eating Disorders: (The Academy for Eating Disorders [AED] is a global, multidisciplinary professional organization that provides cutting-edge professional training and education; inspires new developments in eating disorders research, prevention, and clinical treatments; and is the international source for state-of-the-art information in the field of eating disorders.) www.aedweb.org. Accessed August 13, 2017.

Eating Disorder Hope: Detailed information for patients and families about eating disorders, and treatment centers, and individual providers. https://www.eatingdisorderhope.com.

National Eating Disorders Association: (Information available to help individuals/families locate resources and treatment for eating disorders around the world.) http://www.nationaleatingdisorders.org/. Accessed August 13, 2017.

Child & Adolescent Psychiatric Disorders & Psychosocial Aspects of Pediatrics

7

Kimberly Kelsay, MD

Ayelet Talmi, PhD

Adam Burstein, DO

INTRODUCTION

Pediatric primary care settings are often the first points of identification of mental and behavioral health issues and entry into behavioral health systems for the 14%–20% of children and adolescents affected. Beyond addressing identified and diagnosable mental health conditions, pediatric primary care settings are tasked with (1) screening and surveillance, (2) early identification, (3) triage and initiate treatment for uncomplicated issues, and (4) referral around complex behavioral health issues for the child, their family, and the environments with which the child interacts. Primary care providers see approximately 75% of children with psychiatric disturbances, and half of all pediatric office visits involve behavioral, psychosocial, or educational concerns. Parents and children often prefer discussing these issues with pediatric providers who they already know and trust. As a result, pediatric primary care providers play an important role in the prevention, identification, initiation, management, and coordination of mental health issues, in addition to providing behavioral and development care for children and adolescents. Unfortunately, the shortage of mental health providers, stigma attached to receiving mental health services, chronic underfunding for behavioral/mental health services, institutional barriers within the public mental health system, and disparate insurance benefits contribute to the fact that only 2% of children with diagnosable disorders are seen by mental health specialists.

Despite being strategically positioned as the gatekeepers for identifying mental health and behavioral concerns, primary care providers typically identify fewer than 20% of children with emotional and behavioral problems during routine health supervision visits. In addition, these problems may not be identified when they initially emerge and are most amenable to treatment. This gatekeeper role has become increasingly important over the past decade as advances in mental health awareness and treatment have improved

opportunities for early identification and intervention. The role is especially critical because child psychiatry remains an underserved medical specialty, with only 8300 practicing child and adolescent psychiatrists in the United States. In contrast, more than 50,000 board-certified pediatricians and innumerable midlevel pediatric providers are in a unique position to identify issues affecting the emotional health of children and to initiate treatment or referrals to other providers.

Emotional problems that develop during childhood and adolescence can significantly impact development and may continue into adulthood. In fact, most adult psychiatric disorders involve childhood onset. Many disorders do not present as an all-or-none phenomenon, but rather progress from less severe concerns, such as adjustment problems or perturbations in functioning, to significant disturbances and severe disorders. Pediatricians have the capacity to manage emotional problems and behavioral conditions early on, when improvement can be achieved with less intensive interventions. If pediatricians miss opportunities to appropriately identify mental health problems, provide education about the benefits of intervention, and to encourage and initiate intervention, childhood-onset disorders are more likely to persist, causing worsening impairment and leading to a downward spiral of school and social difficulties, poor employment opportunities, poverty in adulthood, and increased health care utilization and costs as adults. These outcomes are even more pronounced for children and adolescents from underserved, low socioeconomic status backgrounds.

Pediatricians and other pediatric health professionals may be the first, or sometimes only, medical professional to identify a behavioral/mental health problem. Pediatricians working in specialty care settings, hospitalists, and as intensivists will also encounter and need to treat children and adolescents with emotional and behavioral problems. This chapter reviews prevention, surveillance, and screening for mental and behavioral health concerns; situations that may arise in the context of such assessments; psychiatric illnesses that are commonly identified and diagnosed during childhood or adolescence; current treatment recommendations; and indications for referral to mental health professionals.

Costello EJ, Foley DL, Angold A: 10-year research update review: the epidemiology of child and adolescent psychiatric disorders: II. Developmental epidemiology. J Am Acad Child Adolesc Psychiatry 2006;45(1):825 [PMID: 16327577].

Roberts RE, Roberts CR, Xing Y: Prevalence of youth-reported DSM-IV psychiatric disorders among African, European, and Mexican American adolescents. J Am Acad Child Adolesc Psychiatry 2006;45(11):1329–1337 [PMID: 17075355].

MODELS OF CARE ENCOMPASSING BEHAVIORAL HEALTH IN THE PRIMARY CARE SETTING

Mental health, behavior, and development are routinely addressed in the context of pediatric primary care. The continuum of behavioral health services in primary care settings spans from providing anticipatory guidance around development, behavior, and social-emotional well-being plus recommended screening to identification of concerns and making external referrals (routine pediatric care), to utilizing external rapid response consultation (consultation model), and/or providing on-site services to address the identified issues (collocated and integrated model). Table 7–1 describes these models. In addition, practices may utilize a combination of elements from the models described to develop individualized programs and services.

Asarnow JR, Rozenman M, Wiblin J, Zeltzer L: Integrated medical-behavioral care compared with usual primary care for child and adolescent behavioral health: a meta-analysis. JAMA Pediatr 2015;169(10):929–937 [PMID: 26259143].

The American Academy of Child and Adolescent Psychiatry has an excellent resource for pediatric practices interested in integrated care: http://integratedcareforkids.org.

Wissow LS, van Ginneken N, Chandna J, Rahman A: Integrating children's mental health into primary care. Pediatr Clin North Am 2016;63(1):97–113 [PMID: 26613691].

PREVENTION, EARLY IDENTIFICATION, & DEVELOPMENTAL CONTEXT

Developmental contexts and the environments in which children and adolescents grow up play a significant role in their development and well-being. Environments provide access to resources, relationships, and supports in addition to being settings for learning, growth, and development. Longitudinal and retrospective research studies link specific early interventions such as the Perry Preschool Project with health, stable relationships, increased earnings in adulthood, and improved outcomes for the children of participants while adverse experiences in childhood are linked to significant, lifelong health problems. In a study of more than

17,000 adults insured through Kaiser Permanente, researchers found that experiencing adversity in childhood (eg, child abuse, neglect, or household dysfunction) was correlated with poor health outcomes (eg, substance use, heart disease, depression, adolescent pregnancy), lower quality of life, and decreased lifespan. Understanding social determinants of health helps providers attend to the needs of individual children and their families in the context of complex experiences and environments.

However, the major threats to the health of US children increasingly arise from problems that cannot be adequately addressed by the practice model alone. These problems include unacceptably high infant mortality rates in certain communities, extraordinary levels of intentional and unintentional injuries, increasing rates of childhood obesity, substance abuse and dependency, behavioral and developmental consequences of inappropriate care and experience, family dysfunction, sexually transmitted diseases, unplanned pregnancies, and lack of a medical home. The American Academy of Pediatrics (AAP) policy statement, "we must become partners with others, or we will become increasingly irrelevant to the health of children," implies that the work of pediatricians extends to advocacy and community work. Today's community pediatrician seeks to provide a far more realistic and complete clinical picture by taking responsibility for all children in a community, facilitating access to preventive and curative services, and understanding the determinants and consequences of child health and illness, as well as the effectiveness of services provided.

Bright Futures is a national health promotion and disease prevention initiative that addresses children's health needs in the context of family and community. In addition to use in pediatric practice, many states implement Bright Futures principles, guidelines, and tools to strengthen the connections between state and local programs, pediatric primary care, families, and communities. The *Bright Futures Guidelines*, now in its fourth edition, was developed to provide comprehensive health supervision guidelines, including recommendations on immunizations, routine health screenings, and anticipatory guidance. In addition, Bright Futures for Mental Health provides numerous guidelines, tools, and strategies for improving mental health identification, assessment, initiation, management, and coordination.

It is exciting that prevention and early intervention programs are showing promise in helping to reduce risk for patients and their families. Evidenced-based and promising programs and strategies include, but are not limited to:

- Parent–Child Interaction Therapy (PCIT): www.pcit.org
- Triple P (Positive Parenting Program): www.triplep-america.com
- HealthySteps: www.healthysteps.org
- Nurse-Family Partnership: www.nursefamilypartnership.org

Table 7–1. Models of mental health care used in pediatric primary care.

	Routine care	Outside Consultation	Co-location	Collaborative Care
Model description	Surveillance and recommended routine screening Anticipatory guidance Patient referral to specialty mental health and developmental services when needs identified	Various models may include telephone or electronic consultation with option of subsequent 1–2 telepsychiatry or in-person visits with a BH provider	BH provider in same physical space as primary care provider, often with an office on-site BH provider has scheduled appointments to see patients identified with BH needs	BH provider available for in the moment consultation or patient care Operates as a member of the primary care team
Advantages	No change necessary in routine practice No added cost	Rapid response Preferred access to BH providers Consultations may improve provider knowledge and comfort No waitlist	Can care for acute, high needs patients within practice Convenience of being seen for physical and BH in one setting Warm handoffs between primary care and BH providers Patients are more likely to follow through with BH providers to whom they are introduced by their primary care providers Less stigma for patients	No waitlist Ability to address the full continuum of BH needs from prevention and health promotion to early identification, consultation, intervention, and referral Direct communication between providers include shared health records BHC can manage and follow up on referrals Patient sees primary care provider and BHC provide team-based care Provider knowledge and comfort of BH care often improves with co-management of case
Disadvantages	Limited time for providers to discuss anticipatory BH needs Lack of time to address identified issues when screen or surveillance reveals problems Practice must manage referrals and follow-up on referral outcomes Referral follow through ≤ 10% No mechanism to improve provider knowledge and comfort of BH issues Poor communication between BH system and primary care due to regulatory and systemic barriers	Practice responsible for managing referrals to mental health systems as recommended by consultant There must be a structure to pay for system (eg, state funding, pediatric practice fee, grant funding)	BH often becomes "full," and new patients must wait for slots to open Direct communication between providers not built into model, including challenges in documentation and transfer of information about the patient Limited ability to improve provider knowledge and comfort of BH issues	Most severe patients referred to external BH system Costs of hiring BH staff (typically can be covered through billing, institutional support, grant funding, and optimization of health utilization practices)

BH, behavioral health; BHC, behavioral health clinician.

- Hospital-based abusive head trauma prevention approaches (Pennsylvania Abusive Head Trauma Prevention Program)

- Multi-component programs (Child-Parent Centers)

- Incredible Years: www.incredibleyears.com

- Strengthening Families for Parents and Youth: www.extension.iastate.edu/sfp

- Early Head Start: www.ehsnrc.org

- The Safe Environment for Every Kid (SEEK): http://umm.edu/programs/childrens/services/child-protection/seek-project

- Child Parent Psychotherapy (CPP): https://childtrauma.ucsf.edu/child-parent-psychotherapy-resources

- Bright Futures: https://brightfutures.aap.org.

- Centers for Disease Control and Prevention, Injury Prevention & Control: Division of Violence Prevention. http://www.cdc.gov/violenceprevention/acestudy/.

- The Center of Excellence for Infant and Early Childhood Mental Health Consultation: https://www.samhsa.gov/iecmhc.

- Zero to Three: http://www.zerotothree.org.

- The Heckman equation and other resources regarding early intervention return on investments: https://heckmanequation.org/

LIFESTYLE RECOMMENDATIONS

Proper screening, assessment, diagnosis, and treatment of issues are fundamental aspects of practice. In addition, it is equally important that a primary care provider become familiar with factors that can help promote health, both physical and mental. Therefore, activities that support a healthy lifestyle can positively impact health and, in some cases, may help prevent future problems. Many studies demonstrate clear physical and behavioral health benefits from regular exercise, optimal nutrition, meditation, yoga, and participation in prosocial activities. Other contributing factors that directly impact overall health include adequate sleep and use of relaxation techniques. The AAP recommends engaging families in conversations to encourage consumption of fruits and vegetables, avoid sugar-containing drinks, encourage physical activity and to make a family plan around limiting screen time. While these guidelines focus on physical health, successful implementation and adherence to them reside within the relationships and environments in which children live.

American Academy of Pediatrics: Children's Mental Health in Primary Care. http://www.aap.org/mentalhealth/index.html. Accessed September 27, 2015.

Table 7–2. The pediatric primary care provider's role in mental health.

Role	Specific Activities
Prevention	Screen and address social risk factors on intake
	Screen and refer for early socioemotional risk
Identification	Shared family concern
	Surveillance
	Screening
Assessment	Interview and physical
	Assessment tools
	Comorbid conditions
Initiation	Education about condition and treatment options
	Continued collaboration and assessment with family
	Refer to mental health for further evaluation
	Refer for therapy
	Start medication
Management	Monitor condition for improvement
	Monitor for side effects
Coordination	With social work, therapist, psychologist, or psychiatrist
Collaboration	With mental health service providers
	With child protection
	With local schools

U.S. Surgeon General's National Action Agenda: http://www.surgeongeneral.gov/cmh/childreport.htm. Accessed September 27, 2015.

Summary of the Pediatrician's Role

Given these calls for a new pediatric role as the gatekeeper for social-emotional health and well-being, the expanding role of the primary care pediatric provider encompasses the following broad categories: prevention, identification, assessment, initiation, management, coordination, and collaboration (Table 7–2).

IDENTIFICATION & ASSESSMENT DURING HEALTH SUPERVISION VISITS

The possible approaches to identification of problems include surveillance, screening, and assessment. *Surveillance* consists of the following elements: checking in, eliciting concerns, asking open-ended questions, listening for red flags, identifying risk factors, and monitoring closely over time. Like vital signs, which represent an essential

Table 7–3. PSYCH a tool for to open discussion regarding of behavioral health surveillance.

Parent-child interaction	How are things going with you and your parents? Or, in early childhood: What's it like to take care of your baby/toddler?
School	How are things going on in school (or child care); ask about academics, behaviors, and social interactions?
Youth	How are things going on with peer relationships/friendships (how does child get along with same-aged peers)?
Casa	How are things going on at home (including siblings, family stresses, and relationship with parents)?
Happiness	How would you describe your mood? How would you describe your child's mood?

component of the physical evaluation, the essential components of the primary care surveillance for mental health concerns should generally include a review of the youth's general functioning in different aspects of their life. Five questions forming the mnemonic PSYCH provide a helpful tool for opening discussion surveillance topics (Table 7–3).

Many pediatric practices are hampered by lack of continuity and not enough time for in-depth surveillance. Given limited time available for pediatric visits (ie, families spend only a few minutes of in-person time with their pediatric provider during routine health supervision visits), and the fact that only 18% of parents who report elevated behavior problems in children actually tell their providers about it, surveillance should be paired with universal screening for development, mental health, behavior, psychosocial, and environmental risk factors. Surveillance is further hampered by not being a separate and billable service under current Medicaid and insurance reimbursement plans, whereas formal screening is.

Screening involves using standardized instruments to identify areas of risk, delay, or concern. Newborn hearing, vision, and developmental screenings are common in today's pediatric practice. However, the morbidity associated with developmental, emotional, and psychosocial problems requires that social-emotional and psychosocial screening also be performed to identify the presence of symptoms of emotional, behavioral, or relationship disorders and those environmental factors that negatively influence development. Screening tools are brief, easy to use, and can be administered as a questionnaire or using an interview format. While all screenings require review and acknowledgement by the primary care provider that the screening was completed, a positive screen typically warrants referral

for a more thorough assessment. The use of screening tools can facilitate early identification and interrupt the advancement of symptoms. Newer methods of eliciting social-emotional and behavior concerns have been developed (see below for resources and links to access common screening tools). Helpful information can also be obtained from broad screening checklists and symptom-specific questionnaires such as depression or anxiety self-report inventories. Questions can be incorporated into the general pediatric office screening forms or specific questionnaires can be used. Beyond identification, successful screening requires attention to appropriate referrals, referral uptake and completion, and communication back to the referring entity regarding the results of the evaluation. These activities often require additional care coordination resources that could be provided through nonmedical staff such as family navigators and community health workers. Pediatric primary care providers need information about eligibility for services to successfully monitor and address behavioral and developmental issues.

TOOLS FOR MENTAL HEALTH SCREENING IN THE PRIMARY CARE OFFICE SETTING

Given the low rates of identification of psychosocial problems using pediatric surveillance, the use of standardized screening tools has become standard practice. Typically, broad screeners that elicit information regarding multiple domains are employed first and are followed by targeted screens to address symptomatology, severity, impairment, and context of specific psychosocial problems.

Targeted Screening Tools and Assessment Measures

As with broad screening tools, targeted screening or assessment instruments can be very valuable in the clinic since they are standardized and allow for the assessment of current symptoms and severity. They can also be useful for following or reassessing a patient's progress after initiation of treatment. In addition to the Vanderbilt assessment scales for ADHD and the PHQ-9 (Table 7–4), the resources below have other instruments.

Resources for obtaining screening tools:
https://www.mcpap.com/Provider/ScreeningNToolkits.aspx
http://www.brightfutures.org/mentalhealth/pdf/tools.html
http://www.palforkids.org
http://www.schoolpsychiatry.org
http://www.wpic.pitt.edu/research
http://www.theswyc.org
http://www.sdqinfo.com

Table 7–4. Screening tools for primary care settings.

Screening Tool	Area/Domains	Age Range	Notes
Ages and Stages Questionnaire, Third Edition (ASQ-3)	Developmental: Communication, gross motor, fine motor, problem solving, personal-social	1 mo–5.5 y	Parent-completed questionnaire available in Arabic, Chinese, English, French Spanish, and Vietnamese: https://agesandstages.com/
Ages and Stages Questionnaire, Second Edition Socio-Emotional (ASQ: SE-2)	Social-emotional development: Self-regulation, compliance, social communication, adaptive functioning, autonomy, affect, interaction with people	1–72 mo	Parent-completed questionnaire available in English, French, Korean, and Spanish: https://agesandstages.com/
Modified Checklist of Autism in Toddlers (M-CHAT)	Developmental: 20-item screener that detects risk for autism diagnosis	16 and 30 mo	Parent-completed questionnaire available in English, Spanish: https://m-chat.org
Strengths and Difficulties Questionnaires (SDQs)	General behavioral health: Emotional symptoms, conduct problems, hyperactivity/inattention, peer relationship problems, prosocial behavior	2–17 y	Parent-, teacher-, or child-completed questionnaire available in 89 languages: http://www.sdqinfo.com
Pediatric Symptoms Checklist (PSC)	Cognitive, emotional, and behavioral problems	Preschool to 17 y	Parent- or child-completed questionnaire available in English and Spanish: http://www.brightfutures.org/mentalhealth/pdf/professionals/ped_sympton_chklst.pdf
Pediatric Intake Form/Family Psychosocial Screen	Psychosocial: Parental depression, substance use, domestic violence, parental history of abuse, social supports	Adults	Provider-completed screen available in English: https://www.brightfutures.org/mentalhealth/pdf/professionals/ped_intake_form.pdf
WE CARE (Well-child care, Evaluation, Community resources, Advocacy, Referral, Education)	Psychosocial: Parental educational attainment, employment, child care, risk of homelessness, food security, household heat, and electricity	Adults	Parent-completed questionnaire available in English: https://sirenetwork.ucsf.edu/sites/sirenetwork.ucsf.edu/files/HL%20BMC%20Screening%20Tool%20final%20%28English%29.pdf
Patient Health Questionnaire 9 (PHQ-9) modified for teens	Depression and suicide	11–17 y	Child-completed questionnaire available in English and Spanish: http://www.pedpsychiatry.org/pdf/depression/PHQ-9%20Modified%20for%20Teens.pdf
CRAFFT	Substance abuse	12–21 y	Clinician interview and youth-completed questionnaire available in several languages: https://crafft.org/get-the-crafft/
Vanderbilt Assessment Scales	Attention deficit/hyperactivity disorder	6–12 y	Parent- and teacher-completed questionnaire available in English and Spanish: https://www.nichq.org/sites/default/files/resource-file/NICHQ_Vanderbilt_Assessment_Scales.pdf
Center for Epidemiologic Studies Depression Scale for Children (CES-DC)	Depression	6–17 y	Child-completed questionnaire available in English: https://www.brightfutures.org/mentalhealth/pdf/professionals/bridges/ces_dc.pdf
Self-report for Childhood Anxiety-Related Emotional Disorders (SCARED)	Childhood anxiety disorders: General anxiety disorder, separation anxiety disorder, panic disorder, social phobia, school phobia	8–18 y	Parent- and child-completed questionnaire available in 12 languages: https://www.pediatricbipolar.pitt.edu/resources/instruments
Edinburgh Postnatal Depression Scale (EPDS)	Pregnancy-related depression and anxiety	Adult mothers	Self-completed questionnaire: https://www.aap.org/en-us/advocacy-and-policy/aap-health-initiatives/practicing-safety/Documents/Postnatal%20Depression%20Scale.pdf
Bright Futures Toolkit	Numerous guidelines, tools, and other resources for identifying mental health concerns	All ages	Tools for health professionals and families: https://www.brightfutures.org/mentalhealth/pdf/tools.html

Assessment of Behavioral & Emotional Signs & Symptoms

When an emotional/behavioral problem is mentioned by the patient or parents, elicited by an interview, or identified by a screening instrument, the next step should include a more comprehensive assessment and plan for triage. Regardless of access to behavioral health services, the pediatric provider should engage in a meaningful conversation about the findings from screening processes and be integrally involved in follow-up plans. Response to screening results and additional assessment is required to determine appropriate referral resources, safety planning, need for immediate attention or action in the clinic, and follow-up appointments and services.

Situations Requiring Emergent or More Extensive Psychiatric Assessment

If there is any concern about the child's safety, the provider must also evaluate the risk of danger to self (eg, suicidal ideation, plans, or attempts), danger to others (eg, assault, aggression, or homicidal ideation) and screen for other factors that could heighten the risk of danger to self or others such as physical or sexual abuse, substance use or abuse, or unsafe environments. The presence of drug or alcohol abuse in adolescent patients may require referral to community resources specializing in the treatment of these addictive disorders.

The Columbia Lighthouse Project has screens for children of various ages to assess for suicide risk and online training in how to use the tools appropriately.

A. Civil Commitment and Involuntary Mental Health "Holds"

If further assessment indicates a need for inpatient hospitalization, it is optimal if the patient and guardian consent to this care. In a situation in which the guardian is unwilling or unable to give consent for emergency department (ED)–based assessment or inpatient hospitalization of a child or adolescent, an involuntary mental health "hold" may become necessary.

The terms used to describe civil commitment law and involuntary treatment vary by state, as do the criteria for applying these laws. Most states define a process that can be initiated by individuals defined by the state (often providers, police officers, and certified mental health professionals) with reason to believe the patient is at acute risk to seriously harm themselves or others, or is gravely disabled (in the case of children this often means no longer able to eat or perform self-care activities necessary for acute health). The process prevents the individual from leaving the ED or hospital for a brief, defined time (often 72 hours) during which time a formal evaluation to determine safety must be completed. During this allotted time, if an individual is deemed to be safe, they can be discharged prior to 72 hours or the patient or family can also choose to sign in voluntarily. Each state has laws specifying rules and regulations that must be followed as part of this process. Specific forms must be completed and signed by designated professionals, and the patient and family must be informed of their rights. Since mental health holds revoke the civil rights of a patient or their guardian, it is critical to implement the procedure correctly. Providers should familiarize themselves with state's laws regulating this process.

Patients who have a medical condition(s) requiring urgent or emergent treatment do not require a mental health hold. In these cases, the primary team/provider should conduct a capacity evaluation.

B. Mandatory Reporting of Abuse or Neglect or Threat to Others

Mandatory reporting by a provider of suspicion of physical or sexual abuse or neglect to the local human services agency is discussed in greater detail in Chapter 8. The "Tarasoff rule" refers to a California legal case that led to a "duty to warn." Providers are mandated to warn potential victims of harm when plans are disclosed to them about serious threats to harm specific individuals or to perform harmful acts at specific sites. Documentation of a phone call and registered letter to the individual (or site) being threatened are mandated. Under such circumstances, arrangement for the involuntary civil commitment of the potential perpetrator of harm is likely to be in order as well.

Examples of more thorough questions and observations are given in Table 7–5. Targeted assessment screening tools are also useful in determining severity, comorbidity, and context of impairment.

Once it is established that the patient does not need immediate intervention, the provider should determine if the patient's family can return for another visit, or if further assessment can be managed within this visit. Integrated care provides the distinct advantage of immediate further assessment within the primary care setting.

The Mental Status Examination

The Mental Status Examination (MSE) is the mental health provider's equivalent to the physical examination. It includes some standard aspects to help evaluate an individual, including observation of an individual's overall cognitive, emotional, and behavioral presentation. Through observations, interaction, and questions, the MSE identifies current behavioral presentation and areas of clinical concern (eg, suicidal thinking, hallucinations). Depending on the presenting

Table 7–5. Possible topics for discussion and observation when assessing psychosocial problem.

Developmental history
1. Review the landmarks of psychosocial development
2. Summarize the child's temperamental traits
3. Review stressful life events and the child's reactions to them
   a. Separations from primary caregivers or close family members
   b. Losses
   c. Marital conflict, family violence, divorce
   d. Illnesses, injuries, and hospitalizations
   e. Moves, household changes
   f. School transitions
   g. Traumatic events
   h. Financial changes (eg, employment issues) that impact daily living environment
   i. Resource issues including food insecurity, housing instability, and inability to make ends meet
4. Obtain details of past mental health problems and their treatment
Family history
1. Marital/relationship history
   a. Overall satisfaction with the marriage/partnership
   b. Conflicts or disagreements within the relationship
   c. Quantity and quality of time together away from children
   d. Whether the child comes between or is a source of conflict between the parents
   e. Marital history prior to having children
2. Parenting history
   a. Feelings about parenthood
   b. Whether parents feel united in parenting the child
   c. "Division of labor" in parenting
   d. Parental energy or stress level
   e. Sleeping arrangements
   f. Privacy
   g. Attitudes about discipline
   h. Interference with discipline from outside the family (eg, ex-spouses, grandparents)
3. Stresses on the family
   a. Problems with employment
   b. Financial problems
   c. Resource needs
   d. Changes of residence or household composition
   e. Illness, injuries, and deaths
	4. Family history of mental health problems and treatment
	   a. Depression? Who?
	   b. Bipolar Disorder? Who?
	   c. Suicide attempts? Who?
	   d. Psychiatric hospitalizations? Who?
	   e. "Nervous breakdowns"? Who?
	   f. Substance abuse or problems? Who?
	   g. Nervousness or anxiety? Who?
	   h. Other concerns about behavior or mental health problems in family members? Who?
	Observation of the parents
	1. Do they agree on the existence of the problem or concern?
	2. Are they uncooperative or antagonistic about the evaluation?
	3. Do the parents appear depressed or overwhelmed?
	4. Can the parents present a coherent picture of the problem and their family life?
	5. Do the parents accept some responsibility for the child's problems, or do they blame forces outside the family and beyond their control?
	6. Do they appear burdened with guilt about the child's problem?
	Observation of the child
	1. Does the child acknowledge the existence of a problem or concern?
	2. Does the child want help?
	3. Is the child uncooperative or antagonistic about the assessment?
	4. What is the child's predominant mood or attitude?
	5. What does the child wish could be different (eg, "three wishes")?
	6. Does the child display unusual behavior (activity level, mannerisms, fearfulness)?
	7. What is the child's apparent cognitive level?
	Observation of parent-child interaction
	1. Do the parents show concern about the child's feelings?
	2. Does the child control or disrupt the joint interview?
	3. Do the parents set appropriate limits?
	4. Does the child respond to parental limits and control?
	5. Do the parents inappropriately answer questions addressed to the child?
	6. Is there obvious tension between family members?
	Data from other sources
	1. Waiting room observations by office staff
	2. School (teacher, nurse, social worker, counselor, day care provider)
	3. Department of social services
	4. Other caregivers: grandparents, etc

problem, pediatricians may choose to document a complete MSE or a focused MSE. Please refer to standard elements of MSE (Table 7–6).

Diagnostic Formulation & Interpretation of Findings

Diagnosis, the final product of an assessment, starts with a description of the presenting problem, which is then evaluated within the context of the child's age, developmental abilities, the context in which a child exists, including adverse experiences and stressors that impact the child and the family, and the functioning of the family system. In the absence of integrated mental health providers, the primary care provider uses the information gathered to distinguish among possible explanations for the emotional or behavioral problem(s) (Table 7–7).

While it is not necessary to identify a diagnosis in order to refer a patient to a mental health provider, it is important to identify any diagnosis that may be addressed within the community pediatric setting, such as attention-deficit/hyperactivity disorder (ADHD), mild anxiety, mild-moderate depression, and mild adjustment disorders. Diagnoses are made when symptoms cluster to fit criteria for a disorder,

Table 7–6. Standard elements of mental status examination.

Category	Description	Questions to Ask/Observations to Document
General appearance	Physical presentation, attitude and how the child carries themselves (observation, interaction).	Does the child look their stated age? Document physical size compared to peers, dysmorphic features, grooming, cooperation, level of distress, and quality of interaction.
Eye contact	Quality of eye contact in context (observation, interaction).	Observe and document quality of eye contact, eg, good, fair or poor. Is gaze fixed?
Psychomotor activity	Overall energy and physical movement (observation).	Document whether activity level is normal, slowed, or increased.
Musculoskeletal	Gait, range of motion (extremities), abnormal movements (observation and directed tasks).	Document gait and the presence of any rigidity, ataxia, tics, or other abnormal movements.
Speech/language	Rate, volume, tone, articulation, coherence and spontaneity; appropriate naming and word usage (observation).	Observe and document pattern and quality of speech.
Mood/affect	Subjective (child's stated mood); objective (clinician's observation of affect) and how well the two correspond (observation, direct questioning, and optional self-report questionnaire).	Is the child able to identify their mood, happy, sad, angry, anxious? Is the child's affect congruent with mood? What is the observed range of affect?
Thought process; associations	Rate, relevance and reasoning (observation).	Are the child's thoughts goal-directed, logical, tangential, or circumferential? How does the child reason and problem solve? Is thought process concrete or does the child demonstrate abstract reasoning?
Thought content	Content of what the child is actually saying (observation).	Does the child express suicidal or homicidal ideation, and if so, is there intent and a plan? Does the child experience obsessions? Does the child experience perceptual abnormalities such as hallucinations or illusions?
Attention span	Child's ability to stay on task, focus, and concentrate (observation).	Does the child have an age-appropriate attention span? Is the child able to stay on task or are they easily distracted?
Insight; judgment	Child's psychological understanding of his/her situation; ability to make safe and appropriate choices based on situation (observation and response to directed questions).	What is the child's capacity for insight into his/her situation (intact, poor, impaired)?
Orientation	Awareness of oneself, location, date and reason for care (observation and response to directed questions).	Does the child know where he/she is, the date, who he/she is, who the parents are?
Fund of knowledge; memory	Common knowledge, ability to recall long-term events and recent details (observation and response to directed questions).	Response to direct questions about current events and memory.
Cognition	Intelligence	Results of cognitive testing (from outside source), assessment of intellectual capacity based on interaction, and other sources of information (average, below average, above average for age and level of education).

when a child's functioning is impaired in major domains of life, such as learning, peer relationships, family relationships, authority relationships, and recreation, or when substantial deviation from typical developmental trajectories occurs. Providers may need to obtain collateral information to further assess symptoms, such as teacher reports

when assessing symptoms of ADHD. Symptoms can occur across several diagnoses, and children experience a high rate of comorbidity, necessitating providers to consider a differential diagnosis and avoid premature closure.

Identifying and discussing the diagnosis is often the starting point for initiating treatment. The provider's

Table 7–7. Behavior health diagnostic formulation tool.

The behavior falls within the range of normal given the child's developmental level.
The behavior is a temperamental variation.
The behavior is related to central nervous system impairment (eg, prematurity, exposure to toxins in utero, seizure disorder, or genetic disorders).
The behavior is a normal reaction to stressful circumstances (eg, medical illness, change in family structure, or loss of a loved one).
The behavior is related to relationship problems within the family.
The problem is complicated or exacerbated by an underlying medical condition.
The problem reaches threshold for a diagnosis.
Some combination of the above.

Table 7–8. When to consider consultation with a psychotherapist or referral to a child and adolescent psychiatrist.

The diagnosis is not clear
The pediatrician feels that further assessment is needed
The pediatrician believes medication may be needed but will not be prescribing
The pediatrician has started medications and needs further psycho-pharmacologic consultation
Individual, family, or group psychotherapy is needed
Psychotic symptoms (hallucinations, paranoia) are present
Bipolar affective disorder is suspected
Chronic medical regimen nonadherence

interpretation of the presenting problem and diagnosis in the context of current family circumstances and available resources and supports enhances referral uptake, engagement in treatment, and coordinated care. The interpretive process includes the following components:

1. Psychoeducation: An explanation of how the presenting problem or symptom is a reflection of a suspected cause, and typical outcomes both with and without intervention.

2. A discussion of possible interventions, including the following options:

   a. Close monitoring

   b. Counseling provided by the primary care provider or integrated mental health provider

   c. Initiation of medication

   d. Referral to a mental health professional outside of the primary care clinic

   e. Some combination of the above

3. A discussion of the parent's and adolescent's response to the diagnosis and potential interventions.

A joint plan involving the provider, parents, and child is then negotiated to address the child's symptoms and developmental needs in light of the family structure and stresses. If an appropriate plan cannot be developed, or if the provider feels that further diagnostic assessment is required, referral to a mental health practitioner is recommended.

A. Referral of Patients to Mental Health Professionals

Primary care providers often refer patients to a child and adolescent psychiatrist or other qualified child mental health professional when the diagnosis or treatment plan is uncertain, or when medication is indicated and the pediatrician prefers that a specialist initiate or manage treatment of the mental illness (Table 7–8). For academic difficulties not associated with behavioral difficulties, a child educational psychologist or multidisciplinary learning disorder team may be most helpful in assessing patients for learning disorders and potential remediation. For cognitive difficulties associated with head trauma, epilepsy, or brain tumors, a referral to a pediatric neuropsychologist may be indicated.

In many states, patients who are publicly insured or do not have mental health insurance coverage may receive assessment and treatment services at their local mental health care center. Patients with private mental health insurance typically need to contact their insurance company for a list of local mental health professionals trained in the assessment and treatment of children and adolescents who are on their insurance panel. The referring primary care provider or staff should assist the family by providing information to connect with the appropriate resources and services. Personal relationships between staff or providers in the primary care office and community mental health administrators improve the success of referrals. Systems of care in which mental health professionals are co-located in the clinic remove barriers and improve access and care per above. In addition, there are many levels of care between involuntary inpatient psychiatric hospitalization and outpatient treatment including the following: day treatment hospitalization, home-based care, intensive outpatient, and primary care management. The medical home should arrange a follow-up visit after a referral has been made to monitor if the family was able to establish care and to help troubleshoot any barriers to care.

Pediatricians who feel comfortable implementing the recommendations of a mental health professional with whom they have a collaborative relationship should consider remaining involved in the management and coordination of treatment of mental illness in their patients. The local branches of the American Academy of Child and Adolescent Psychiatry and the American Psychological Association and state chapters are often able to provide a list of mental health professionals who are trained in the evaluation and treatment of children and adolescents.

B. Other Resources

The Partnership Access Line (PAL) website (https://www .seattlechildrens.org—Health Care Professionals/Partnership Access Line/Care Guides and Resources) is another useful tool to assist the primary care provider in diagnosis and treatment of the more common psychiatric conditions. The PAL algorithms provide decision trees and guidance for treating specific diagnoses, considering alternative diagnoses in the differential, and reviewing medication treatment tables for specific information regarding psychopharmacologic treatments.

America Academy of Pediatrics mental health initiatives: https:// www.aap.org/en-us/advocacy-and-policy/aap-health-initia- tives/Mental-Health/Pages/implementing_mental_health_ priorities_in_practice.aspx

Dolan MA, Fein JA: Committee on Pediatric Emergency Medicine. Pediatric and adolescent mental health emergencies in the emergency medical services system. Pediatrics 2011;127(5):e13 56–e1366 [Epub 2011 Apr 25] [PMID: 21518712].

Partnership Access Line: http://www.seattlechildrens.org/healthcare- professionals/access-services/partnership-access-line/. Accessed June, 2019.

The Columbia Suicide Screening Rating Scales and training can be assessed through The Columbia Lighthouse Project: http:// cssrs.columbia.edu. Accessed June 25, 2019.

To learn more about state requirements for mental health holds visit the Treatment Advocacy Center: https://www.treatment advocacycenter.org. Accessed June 25, 2019.

▼ PSYCHIATRIC DISORDERS OF CHILDHOOD & ADOLESCENCE

A psychiatric disorder is defined as a characteristic cluster of signs and symptoms (emotions, behaviors, thought patterns, and mood states) that are associated with subjective distress or maladaptive behavior. This definition presumes that the symptoms are of such intensity, persistence, and duration that the ability to adapt to life's challenges is compromised.

The *Diagnostic and Statistical Manual of Mental Disorders*, 5th Edition (DSM-5), the formal reference text for psychiatric disorders, includes the criteria for each of the mental illnesses, including those that begin in childhood and adolescence. Of note, primary care providers frequently see a spectrum of disturbances in their clinical practice, many not achieving full DSM-5 criteria.

Special Considerations in Prescribing Psychotropic Medications

As pediatricians will often manage mental health issues in the primary care setting, such management may include medication treatment. Each primary care provider must establish their comfort level in prescribing psychotropic medications. Table 7–9 includes commonly prescribed

Table 7–9. Psychoactive medications approved by the FDA for use in children and adolescents.

Drug	Indication	Minimum Age for Which Approved (y)
Mixed amphetamine salts (Adderall)	ADHD	≥ 3
Dextroamphetamine (Dexedrine, Dextrostat)	ADHD	≥ 3
Methylphenidate (Concerta, Ritalin, Quillivant XR, and others)	ADHD	≥ 6
Atomoxetine (Strattera)	ADHD	≥ 6
Guanfacine ER (Intuniv)	ADHD	≥ 6
Clomipramine (Anafranil)	OCD	≥ 10
Fluvoxamine (Luvox)	OCD	≥ 8
Sertraline (Zoloft)	OCD	≥ 6
	Aggression and autism	≥ 5
	Schizophrenia and mania	≥ 10
Pimozide (Orap)[a]	Tourette syndrome	≥ 12
Lithium (Eskalith, Lithobid, Lithotabs)	Bipolar disorder	≥ 12
Fluoxetine (Prozac)	Depression	≥ 12
	OCD	≥ 6
Escitalopram (Lexapro)	Depression	≥ 12
Duloxetine	Generalized anxiety disorder	≥ 7
Imipramine (Norpramin)	Enuresis	≥ 6
Aripiprazole (Abilify)	Bipolar disorder	≥ 10
	Schizophrenia	≥ 13
	Aggression and autism	≥ 6
Risperidone (Risperdal)	Bipolar disorder	≥ 10
	Schizophrenia	≥ 13
	Aggression and autism	≥ 6
Quetiapine (Seroquel, XR)	Bipolar disorder	≥ 10
	Schizophrenia	≥ 13
Ziprasidone (Geodon)	Bipolar disorder	≥ 10
	Schizophrenia	≥ 13
Olanzapine (Zyprexa)	Bipolar disorder	≥ 10
	Schizophrenia	≥ 13
Asenapine (Saphris)	Bipolar I disorder	≥ 10
Lurasidone (Latuda)	Schizophrenia	≥ 13
	Bipolar I depression	≥ 10
Paliperidone (Invega)	Schizophrenia	≥ 12
Olanzapine Fluoxetine (Symbyax)	Bipolar I depression	≥ 10

ADHD, attention-deficit/hyperactivity disorder; FDA, Food and Drug Administration; OCD, obsessive-compulsive disorder.
[a]Use of pimozide in the treatment of movement disorders is discussed in Chapter 25.

psychotropic medications and the expected level of comfort of a primary care provider for initiating and managing them. More complete information regarding medication is detailed throughout this chapter. In addition, a list of Food and Drug Administration (FDA)–approved medication for various psychiatric disorders is included in Table 7–9. For a current list of FDA-approved psychotropic medications, refer to the following website: https://www.cms .gov/Medicare-Medicaid-Coordination/Fraud-Prevention/ Medicaid-Integrity-Education/Pharmacy-Education-Materials/pharmacy-ed-materials.html.

ANXIETY DISORDERS

ESSENTIALS OF DIAGNOSIS & TYPICAL FEATURES

▶ Fear or anxiety that is excessive or persisting beyond developmentally appropriate period.

▶ Fear or anxiety is accompanied by behavioral disturbances or physical manifestations.

▶ Symptoms cause functional impairment or significant distress.

Anxiety is described as the anticipation of future threat, and fear is described as the emotional response to real or perceived imminent threat. Both are protective emotions, part of the normal repertoire of children. Distinguishing developmentally appropriate fears and anxiety from those associated with anxiety disorders can be challenging and requires knowledge of normative development. Generally, fears or anxiety that persist beyond the expected developmental period or cause significant distress or impairment suggest an anxiety disorder. Some anxiety disorders are more likely to be precipitated by stress, but many are not. An anxious temperament can be identified as early as infancy, and children with such temperaments are more likely to develop anxiety disorders, especially if they are living with anxious parents. Community-based studies of school-aged children and adolescents suggest that nearly 10% of children have some type of anxiety disorder. According to the CDC, this number has been increasing in the past decade. Anxiety disorders are important to identify and treat early as untreated disorders often persist or evolve into other anxiety disorders.

▶ Identification & Diagnosis

Comorbidity is common with anxiety disorders. Children with one anxiety disorder are likely to have another anxiety disorder and have increased risk for other psychiatric disorders such as depression. It is therefore important to

Table 7–10. Signs and symptoms of anxiety in children.

Psychological
Fears and worries
Increased dependence on home and parents
Avoidance of anxiety-producing stimuli
Decreased school performance
Increased self-doubt and irritability
Frightening themes in play and fantasy
Psychomotor
Motoric restlessness and hyperactivity
Sleep disturbances
Decreased concentration
Ritualistic behaviors (eg, washing, counting)
Psychophysiologic
Autonomic hyperarousal
Dizziness and lightheadedness
Palpitations
Shortness of breath
Flushing, sweating, dry mouth
Nausea and vomiting
Panic
Headaches and stomach aches

carefully screen children with an anxiety disorder to ensure that another disorder is not missed. In addition, children with anxiety, presenting to a pediatrician, are more likely to present with a physical complaint, such as headaches or abdominal pain than with identified anxiety (Table 7–10). While medical causes of anxiety are rare, it is important to not misdiagnose a physical symptom as anxiety, for example, to ascribe the gastrointestinal (GI) upset of inflammatory bowel disease, to anxiety. Screening should also assess for medications and substances that can cause anxiety or present similarly. Such substances include caffeine, marijuana, amphetamines, cocaine, and alcohol during withdrawal. Medications that have been associated with anxiety include steroids, tacrolimus, angiotensin-converting enzyme inhibitors, anticholinergics, dopamine agonists, β-adrenergic agonists, serotonin selective reuptake inhibitors, thyroid medications, and procaine derivatives. Medical illnesses that can lead to symptoms suggestive of anxiety include those associated with hyperthyroid states, hypoglycemia, hypoxia, and, more rarely, pheochromocytoma.

▶ Treatment

Treatment must be tailored to the developmental age of the child. Treatment of younger children focuses on helping parents understand their child's symptoms, developing skills to help their child manage distress, while also helping parents tolerate their child's distress. As soon as children have the developmental capacity to engage in assessing their own anxiety and in learning coping strategies, they are incorporated into therapy.

Cognitive behavioral therapy (CBT) with exposure has the most evidence regarding the successful treatment of anxiety. Exposure refers to planned progressive presentation of low- to midlevel anxiety-provoking stimulus. The aim is to desensitize the child to the stimulus. CBT can be delivered in group settings, or with an individual child and parents. The basic goals include helping children identify and quantify anxiety symptoms, identify maladaptive cognitions, learn cognitive, and behavioral coping strategies to begin exposures to situations or items associated with medium- to low-level anxieties. Parents or caregivers also learn these skills in order to help children or youth practice in settings outside the therapy office. The ultimate goal is to enable the child to face the particular anxiety or set of anxieties that cause distress or dysfunction, experience a decrease in anxiety, and resume normal functioning.

When anxiety symptoms do not remit with cognitive, behavioral, and environmental interventions and continue to significantly affect life functioning, psychopharmacologic agents may be helpful. There is evidence that selective serotonin reuptake inhibitors (SSRIs) are effective in treating anxiety disorders in children as young as 6 years of age, but these medications do not have FDA approval for this indication. The anxiolytic effect of SSRIs can be as rapid as a few days, whereas the effects of benzodiazepines are immediate. Pediatricians are aware of this immediate effect, but the use of benzodiazepines while waiting for the anxiolytic effects of SSRIs is discouraged with youth because the developing brain is at increased risk for dependency and iatrogenic substance abuse. Antihistamines (ie, hydroxyzine), β-blockers, and α-agonists are alternatives that can be used on a scheduled or as-needed based and usually are better tolerated without concern for physiologic dependence. Refer to medication used for treatment of depressive disorders (Table 7–11) as they are commonly used in the treatment for anxiety as well.

Table 7–11. Antidepressant information.

Drug Name and class	Dosage Form	Usual Starting Dose For Adolescent	Increase Increment (After ~4 wk)	RCT Evidence in Kids	FDA Depression Approved for Children?	Editorial Comments
Fluoxetine (Prozac) SSRI	10, 20, 40 mg 20 mg/5 mL	5–10 mg/day (60 mg max)[a]	10– mg[b]	Yes	Yes (over age 8)	Long 1/2 life, no side effect from a missed dose. More potential drug-drug interactions
Sertraline (Zoloft) SSRI	25, 50, 100 mg 20 mg/mL	12.5–25 mg/day (200 mg max)[a]	25–50 mg[b]	Yes	No	May cause more GI upset, more potential side effects when stopping,
Escitalopram (Lexapro) SSRI	5, 10, 20 mg 5 mg/5 mL	2.5–5 mg/day (20 mg max)[a]	5–10 mg[b]	Yes	Yes (for adolescents)	The active isomer of citalopram, less potential for drug-drug interactions.
Citalopram (Celexa) SSRI	10, 20, 40 mg 10 mg/5 mL	5–10 mg/day (40 mg max)[a]	10–20 mg[b]	Yes	No	Few drug interactions for SSRI
Bupropion (Wellbutrin) miscellaneous	75, 100 mg 100, 150, 200 mg SR forms 150, 300 mg XL forms	75 mg/day (later dose this BID) (400 mg max)[a]	75–100 mg[b]	No	No	Also 3rd- or 4th-line treatment for ADHD Potential for increasing seizure risk
Mirtazapine (Remeron) SNRI	15, 30, 45 mg	7.5–15 mg/day (45 mg max)[a]	15 mg[b]	No	No	Sedating, increases appetite
Venlafaxine (Effexor) SNRI	25, 37.5, 50, 75, 100 mg 37.5, 75, 150 mg ER forms	37.5 mg/day (225 mg max)[a]	37.5–75 mg[b]	No (May have higher SI risk than others for children)	No	Only recommended for older adolescents. Withdrawal symptoms can be severe.
Duloxetine (Cymbalta) SNRI	Delayed release (DR) 20, 30, 60 mg	20–30 mg	30 mg after 2 weeks	Yes	Yes	Doses higher than 60 mg daily are rarely more effective.

[a]Recommend low starting dose for young children and children and adolescents with anxiety, to help ease patient or family fears about medication.
[b]If starting at the lowest dose to decrease side effect, may increase again in 1–2 weeks.

Prognosis

Early treatment of anxiety disorders can be very effective and decreases the risk for negative impact on developmental trajectories or the development of other psychiatric disorders. The standard of care is CBT for milder cases and a combination of CBT/antidepressant for more severe cases or cases that do not respond to CBT alone.

Anxiety disorders that present in childhood tend to wax and wane during childhood. Patients who present with more severe anxiety symptoms often develop several anxiety disorders during adolescence and are at risk for depression, substance abuse, and other negative developmental outcomes. Parenting style may contribute to anxiety; specifically, autonomy granting is more likely to result in less anxious children, whereas harsh or rejecting parenting results in more anxious children. Treatment of parental anxiety disorders when present often improves the outcome of the child's anxiety disorder.

As mentioned earlier, the Seattle Children's Hospital website is a great resource for primary care providers. The site includes treatment algorithms and related information for the diagnosis and treatment of commonly encountered mental health disorders.

1. Separation Anxiety

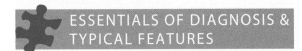

ESSENTIALS OF DIAGNOSIS & TYPICAL FEATURES

▶ Persistent excessive worry about losing or being separated from attachment figures, due to harm, illness, or death befalling either the attachment figure or the patient.

▶ Reluctance or refusal to leave the attachment figure or sleep away from the attachment figure.

▶ Fear of being home without an attachment figure.

▶ Physical complaints when separation occurs or is anticipated.

General Considerations

Very young children may not be symptomatic until the separation is imminent or occurring and may not experience anticipatory fears related to separation. As children get older, they may experience fears in anticipation of separations, particularly around routine separations such as going to preschool/school or at bedtime. Additionally, specific fears such as fears of kidnapping, parents getting into car accidents, and being separated due to natural disasters may emerge. Behaviors associated with separation anxiety also vary by age; young children are more likely to present with difficulties around bedtimes and for older children other

separations, such as school, sleep overs, and camp may be the focus of anxiety. In addition to appearing anxious, children with separation anxiety can appear sad, aggressive, or experience physical symptoms when facing the anxiety-provoking separation. Separation anxiety disorder is more prevalent in younger children (4% 6-month prevalence compared with 1.6% 6-month prevalence in adolescence).

Identification & Diagnosis

Anxiety about separation from attachment figures is typical in early childhood development. Separation anxiety disorder must be distinguished from normal development, occur for more than 4 weeks for children, and lead to impairment or significant distress.

Treatment

Parents and familiar caregivers help alleviate symptoms caused by separation anxiety and can mitigate exacerbations during separation times. Working with caregivers involves developing supportive routines that promote optimal separations. Clinical treatment of separation anxiety includes CBT that is modified to address the developmental level of the child. Children who do not respond to therapy may require medication such as an SSRI. Children younger than school age are generally not treated with medication.

Other Considerations

The differential for separation anxiety is broad and includes other anxiety disorders, mood disorders, oppositional defiant disorder, conduct disorder, psychotic disorder, and personality disorders. Pediatricians are likely to encounter children with school refusal, a common behavioral manifestation of separation anxiety. It is important to recognize and intervene early with school refusal as the longer a child is out of school, the more difficult it is to help the child return to school. Symptoms of school refusal often include physical symptoms and or behavioral outbursts as school time approaches. Parents often notice symptoms abate on the weekend, vacations, or if the child is no longer expected to attend school. Mild cases may be handled with the help of the pediatrician's office, but more severe cases may need the help of a mental health specialist.

School refusal can also be related to other anxiety disorders, learning disorders, mood disorders, psychotic disorders, oppositional defiant disorder, conduct disorder and environmental stressors such as bullying or poor student teacher fit. Identifying the etiology of school refusal helps providers appropriately target the level and type of intervention.

Prognosis

Separation anxiety often abates by adolescence, but adolescents who experienced separation anxiety disorder in childhood are at increased risk to develop other disorders.

2. Selective Mutism Disorder

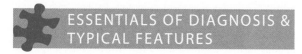

ESSENTIALS OF DIAGNOSIS & TYPICAL FEATURES

▶ Consistent failure to speak in social settings (such as school) where this is expected, despite speaking in other settings.

▶ General Considerations

Selective mutism is more frequent in younger children. Symptoms may be present before 5 but usually do not lead to problems until the child enters school. Children who are new to the country or who initially learned one language and are expected to function in school in a second language may present with selective mutism.

▶ Identification & Diagnosis

Children with selective mutism usually speak with close family members and may also speak with a "best" friend. They may be quite outgoing within a familiar setting but are often shy outside of this setting. They may be comfortable with social roles that do not require verbal communication. Children with selective mutism can become angry and aggressive when facing a demand to speak. Screening for selective mutism is useful as families may not be aware of the problem or may not appreciate how it is interfering with functioning at school. To meet criteria for selective mutism, symptoms must interfere with function in school, work, or social communication, and must last longer than 1 month, not including the first month of school. Symptoms cannot be due to autism, a communication disorder, or psychotic disorders.

▶ Treatment

Selective mutism can be perplexing for parents and teachers as the child's engagement in speaking can vary significantly across settings. Treatment therefore usually begins with psychoeducation. Children with selective mutism can be difficult to engage due to their shyness, so clinicians must be adept at using both verbal and nonverbal methods to form an alliance with the child. CBT with exposure aimed at increasing verbal interactions can be very successful. Patients with more severe symptoms, or symptoms that do not respond to therapy, may benefit from an antidepressant, for example SSRI.

▶ Other Considerations

The differential diagnosis includes other disorders that can interfere with speech, such as autism, communication disorders, and psychotic disorders. Children with selective mutism can have other comorbid anxiety disorders, such as social anxiety disorder, separation anxiety, and specific phobia.

Recognition and treatment of selective mutism is critical as this behavior becomes increasingly entrenched the longer a child avoids verbal communication in settings outside of the family. Children with untreated selective mutism are at risk for depression, social anxiety disorder, and substance abuse as adolescents.

3. Specific Phobias

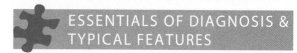

ESSENTIALS OF DIAGNOSIS & TYPICAL FEATURES

▶ Excessive fear or worry about a certain thing, experience, or situation.
▶ The thought about or exposure to this trigger causes excessive anxiety.

▶ General Considerations

Specific phobias are common, impacting 5% of children and 16% of adolescents. Simple phobias often lessen over time while more severe, persistent forms can be debilitating.

▶ Identification & Diagnosis

Specific phobia is an intense fear of a particular object, experience, or situation that persists for at least 6 months. This object or situation is a cause of great distress nearly every time the individual anticipates or is exposed to the stimulus. The perceived harm or threat is well out of proportion to the actual stimulus. To handle the distress, the child avoids the object or situation, therefore reinforcing the anxiety. The distress caused by the stimulus can also present as a panic attack, fainting, or irritability. Young children may present with increased clinginess.

▶ Treatment

The mainstay of treatment for specific phobias is CBT aimed at reducing anxiety or fear of the phobic stimulus.

▶ Other Considerations

Children commonly experience more than one specific phobia and as the number of phobias increases, so does the degree of impairment. The differential diagnosis includes other anxiety disorders, trauma, and stress-related disorders, eating disorders, schizophrenia, and other psychotic disorders.

Significant childhood separation events are associated with later onset of phobia. Addressing specific phobia is important as untreated specific phobias have one of the higher rates of stability over time among childhood anxiety disorders.

4. Panic Disorder

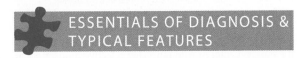

ESSENTIALS OF DIAGNOSIS & TYPICAL FEATURES

► Recurrent, unexpected panic attacks, described as an abrupt onset of intense fear, that crescendos over the course of minutes and is accompanied by physical symptoms.

General Considerations

Panic disorder is more likely to present after the onset of puberty with a prevalence rate of 2%–3% during adolescence. Unlike many other anxiety disorders, there is more likely to be a stressor preceding the onset of panic disorder. Children who experience separation anxiety disorder are at increased risk to develop panic disorder.

Identification & Diagnosis

The physical symptoms of panic disorder are symptoms of a surge in the adrenergic system and include palpitations, sweating, shortness of breath, choking, chest pain or tightness, GI distress, dizziness or associated feelings, chills or heat, numbness, or tingling. Cognitive symptoms can include feelings of unreality and fear of going crazy or of dying. To meet criteria for a panic attack, at least four of the above symptoms must be present. At least one attack much be followed by anticipatory fear of having another attack in the subsequent month. Individuals with panic disorder also experience a fear of or related to future attacks that lead to maladaptive behavior. Youth with panic disorder are most likely to present to the pediatrician with fears related to physical symptoms of autonomic arousal, such as a fear that there is something wrong with their heart. Adolescents are less likely than adults to report panic attacks, and thus specific questions questionnaires should be used when adolescents present with anxiety.

Although over time, individuals with panic disorder can come to expect panic attacks tied to certain cues, they also experience panic attacks randomly.

Treatment

CBT for youth with panic disorder focuses on the cognitions associated with the panic attack as well as the physiologic distressing symptoms. Exposure targets may include situations that trigger panic attacks or some of the physiologic symptoms experienced during an attack. The frequency of treatment can vary depending on the acuity of the patient, with lower levels of care provided during weekly outpatient therapy and higher levels provided several times a week through intensive outpatient treatment programs or daily in psychiatric day treatment programs. Patients who do not respond to therapy alone may benefit from an antidepressant such as an SSRI. Other non-benzodiazepine medication options include antihistamines (eg, hydroxyzine) and occasionally off-label use of β-blockers or low-dose atypical antipsychotics. Benzodiazepines have been used with adults but are discouraged for use with youth in the primary care setting.

Other Considerations

The differential diagnosis of panic attacks includes a physical cause of panic symptoms, which must be ruled out when appropriate. Panic disorder can be debilitating as youth can go to extensive lengths to avoid cues. Youth who avoid going out in public by themselves should be diagnosed with agoraphobia in addition to panic disorder. Although panic disorder increases the risk of developing a substance abuse disorder, withdrawal of some substances can also lead to panic symptoms. For adolescents who are actively using, this can be difficult to distinguish. Panic attacks can present as part of other anxiety disorders, but the panic attacks in other disorders are cued by the underlying fear or anxiety, such as public performance in social anxiety disorder, or anticipation of an event in generalized anxiety disorder. Panic disorder is higher among individuals with other anxiety disorders, depression, and bipolar disorder.

Prognosis

Panic symptoms and panic disorder are both important to recognize and treat. Untreated panic disorder has the highest rate of persistence over time among childhood anxiety disorders. Individuals with panic symptoms that occur in the context of another disorder are at increased risk to develop depression.

5. Agoraphobia

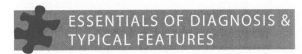

ESSENTIALS OF DIAGNOSIS & TYPICAL FEATURES

► An excessive fear of being in a situation where panic-like symptoms might occur.
► Avoidance of situations that can cause panic attacks.

General Considerations

Agoraphobia can be debilitating. In children and adolescents, it is more likely to present as school refusal than fear of the other situations listed below. Children and adolescents may be reluctant to report symptoms, so a careful screening is warranted for anxious children, or children who are refusing to attend school. In community samples, agoraphobia is more likely to occur in later adolescence; 1.7% of adolescents suffer from agoraphobia, but this may be an underestimate because of the difficulty of assessing youth. Similar to panic disorder, initial symptoms often are triggered by a stressful event.

Identification & Diagnosis

The most well-known fear associated with agoraphobia is fear of open spaces, including the market place. For individuals with agoraphobia, other situations can also trigger intense fear, such as using public transportation, standing in line or being in a crowd, and being in an enclosed space or outside the home alone. Individuals with agoraphobia experience two or more of these fears that last for over 6 months and lead to distress or impairment. Full panic disorder symptoms do not have to be present to meet criteria for agoraphobia.

Treatment

Treatment of individuals with agoraphobia can be very challenging, as treatment typically requires leaving home. Online treatments are available with limited data on efficacy. The current standard remains CBT with exposure, and SSRI for individuals who do not respond to treatment or are severely impacted by agoraphobia.

Other Considerations

The differential diagnosis includes other anxiety disorders, posttraumatic stress disorder (PTSD), depression, and medical conditions. For example, adolescents with postural orthostatic tachycardia syndrome (POTS) may fear leaving the house due to a fear of fainting or individuals with inflammatory bowel disease may fear having an episode of diarrhea.

Prognosis

Individuals with agoraphobia are at risk for comorbid disorders including other anxiety disorders and depression, and males have a high incidence of substance abuse.

6. Generalized Anxiety Disorder (GAD)

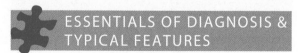

ESSENTIALS OF DIAGNOSIS & TYPICAL FEATURES

▶ Multiple, intense, disproportionate, or irrational worries, often about future events.

▶ Worry is accompanied by other symptoms.

▶ The worry is difficult to control.

General Considerations

Individuals with generalized anxiety disorder often recall a lifetime of anxiety, but community samples find GAD rarely presents before adolescence; the prevalence of GAD in adolescence is 0.9%. Potential reasons for this discrepancy include that the symptoms of anxiety may not meet full criteria for GAD at an earlier age, or symptoms may be underestimated by parents or guardians. Individuals who develop GAD at an early age are more likely to have greater impairment.

GAD is highly heritable, overlapping with the risk for depression and neuroticism. In addition, anxious overprotective parenting increases the risk of GAD, but is not necessary for the development of the disorder.

The differential diagnosis of symptoms of anxiety is presented in Table 7–12.

Identification & Diagnosis

Young children with generalized anxiety often worry about their competence or performance while older youth may worry about additional issues such as family finances or being on time. Worry and anxiety that is not pathologic must be distinguished from the worries or anxieties of GAD. In addition, children with GAD experience at least one symptom of fatigue, restlessness or poor concentration,

Table 7–12. Differential diagnosis of symptoms of anxiety.

- **Normal developmental anxiety**
  A. Stranger anxiety (5 mo–2½ y, with a peak at 6–12 mo)
  B. Separation anxiety (7 mo–4 y, with a peak at 18–36 mo)
  C. The child is fearful or even phobic of the dark and monsters (3–6 y)
- **"Appropriate" anxiety**
  A. Anticipating a painful or frightening experience
  B. Avoidance of a reminder of a painful or frightening experience
  C. Child abuse
- **Anxiety disorder (see Table 7–11), with or without other comorbid psychiatric disorders**
- **Substance abuse**
- **Medications and recreational drugs**
  A. Caffeinism (including colas and chocolate)
  B. Sympathomimetic agents
  C. Idiosyncratic drug reactions
- **Hypermetabolic or hyperarousal states**
  A. Hyperthyroidism
  B. Pheochromocytoma
  C. Anemia
  D. Hypoglycemia
  E. Hypoxemia
- **Cardiac abnormality**
  A. Dysrhythmia
  B. High-output state
  C. Mitral valve prolapsed

irritability, feeling on edge, or sleep disturbance. GAD can also be accompanied by other somatic symptoms, and the pediatrician is more likely to encounter children with GAD who present with symptoms of GI difficulties or headaches. To meet criteria for GAD, the symptoms must cause significant distress or disturbance of function and be present for at least 6 months.

Treatment

As with other anxiety disorders psychotherapy is the first-line treatment, with the possible addition of an SSRI or similar agent (eg. SNRI or Tricyclic) if the response is insufficient.

Other Considerations

It can be challenging to distinguish GAD from other anxiety disorders. Substance-induced anxiety should be considered with adolescents who experience a sudden onset of anxiety. Individuals with GAD are at increased risk to experience depression.

Prognosis

The combination of medication and therapy can be very effective for treating youth with GAD. Individuals with GAD are at increased risk for depression.

7. Social Anxiety Disorder

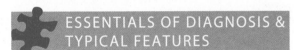

ESSENTIALS OF DIAGNOSIS & TYPICAL FEATURES

▶ Excessive worrying in social settings.
▶ Inability to perform in front of others as expected for age.
▶ Avoidance of events or settings that are social in nature or involve large groups.

General Considerations

Social anxiety disorder is characterized by significant, persistent fear in social settings, or performance situations. The disorder results in overwhelming anxiety and inability to function when exposed to unfamiliar people and/or scrutiny. This is usually a problem of older children and adolescents.

Identification & Diagnosis

Anxiety symptoms in children with social anxiety disorder are related specifically to the social setting and not better explained by another anxiety disorder. Common manifestations of this disorder include consistent avoidance of social functions and persistent somatic complaints that occur in a

social setting and resolve in the absence of social exposure. The symptoms significantly disrupt the child's—and frequently the family's—life, and parents often describe a pattern of overly accommodating their child's avoidance and/or incentivizing their child to attend routine social, extracurricular, or family functions.

Treatment

Like the other anxiety disorders, the mainstay of treatment for social anxiety disorder is CBT. The goal is to modify behavior and diminish the anxiety in social settings through the use of specific cognitive and behavioral techniques. As with other anxiety disorders, if ongoing CBT therapy is not effective at mitigating the anxiety, psychopharmacologic agents may be helpful. SSRIs are the only class of medication to have demonstrated efficacy for children with social anxiety disorder.

Other Considerations

Children with social anxiety disorder are at increased risk for depression and school avoidance. They can also experience panic attacks, and there is high comorbidity between substance use disorders and anxiety disorders, especially social anxiety disorder.

Prognosis

Early age of onset, more severe avoidance, and the presences of panic symptoms are all predictors of persistence over time. Treatment with CBT or a combination of CBT and medication can be very effective for the majority of youth with social anxiety disorder.

Anxiety and Depression Association of America: https://adaa.org/search/.

OBSESSIVE-COMPULSIVE & RELATED DISORDERS

1. Obsessive-Compulsive Disorder

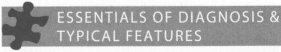

ESSENTIALS OF DIAGNOSIS & TYPICAL FEATURES

▶ Recurrent obsessive thoughts, impulses, or images that are experienced as intrusive at times.
▶ Repetitive compulsive behaviors or mental acts are performed to prevent or reduce distress stemming from obsessive thoughts.
▶ Obsessions and compulsions cause marked distress, are time-consuming, and interfere with normal routines.

General Considerations

Obsessive-compulsive disorder (OCD) is related to anxiety disorders but tends to cluster genetically with other compulsive disorders such as compulsive skin picking, trichotillomania (TTM; hair pulling), and hoarding. Onset often occurs during childhood, and untreated OCD can have a lifelong course. Males have an earlier age of onset, with childhood cases usually occurring before the age of 10 years. OCD often leads to avoidance of situations that trigger obsessions, and for children and adolescents, this can interfere with development.

Identification & Diagnosis

The obsessions that lead to OCD are defined as recurrent, persistent, intrusive thoughts, urges, or images that cause significant distress. The individual tries to avoid, suppress, or ignore the obsessions or to mitigate them through action or thought. The obsessions and compulsions of OCD consume more than 1 hour/day. Obsessions vary by individuals but tend to cluster into the following groups: intrusive "forbidden" images such as sexual, aggressive or religiously taboo images, thoughts of contamination, need for symmetry, fears of harming others, and fears of harm to oneself or loved ones. Individuals often experience more than one cluster and types of obsessions can change over time. In addition to compulsive symptoms, youth who are experiencing obsessions may also experience panic, depressive, irritable, and suicidal symptoms. Sudden onset of symptoms should alert pediatricians to screen for group A streptococcal infections, as pediatric autoimmune disorders associated with these infections have been implicated in the development of OCD for some children.

Caretakers can often identify children who have compulsions, but obsessions can be difficult to recognize because they are experienced internally. Youth who recognize that obsessions and compulsions are strange may not spontaneously reveal symptoms unless specifically asked.

Treatment

Many individuals with OCD feel that their symptoms are "crazy," or alternatively, they do not want to consider giving up their compulsions as they feel these will lead to intense distress. Psychoeducation is an important first step in treatment of OCD to help put symptoms in perspective and outline treatment progression. OCD is best treated with a combination of CBT specific to OCD and with medications in more severe cases. SSRIs are effective in diminishing OCD symptoms, but higher doses—occasionally above maximum recommended daily dose—may be needed than those used to treat anxiety disorders or depression. Fluvoxamine and sertraline have FDA approval for the treatment of pediatric OCD. The tricyclic antidepressant (TCA) clomipramine has

FDA approval for the treatment of OCD in adults. Severe cases have been treated with gamma knife brain surgery interrupting the circuit involved in OCD. Some individuals have benefitted from other nonpharmacologic interventions such as neurofeedback and transcranial magnetic stimulation (TMS); however, they are not FDA approved for this condition.

Other Considerations

OCD often occurs with other compulsive disorders such as TTM (the recurrent pulling out of hair), compulsive skin picking, body dysmorphic disorder, or hoarding. Youth with OCD are at increased risk to have comorbid anxiety, ADHD, depression, and tics. The differential diagnosis includes all of the above as well as eating disorders, psychotic disorders, and obsessive compulsive personality disorder. The perseveration of children with autism spectrum disorders can also be confused with OCD.

Prognosis

The combination of CBT plus medication is most effective for patients who do not respond to either treatment alone. It is important to recognize and treat OCD early, as early age of onset and greater impairment are predictors of poor prognosis. Hoarding is particularly difficult to treat.

International Obsessive Compulsive Foundation: https://iocdf .org/. Accessed June 26, 2019.

2. Excoriation Disorder

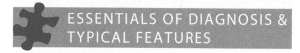

ESSENTIALS OF DIAGNOSIS & TYPICAL FEATURES

▶ Recurrent skin picking resulting in lesions despite efforts to stop.

▶ The skin picking causes significant distress or impairment in school, social settings, or other areas of function.

General Considerations

Excoriation disorder (ED), also known as skin picking disorder, or dermatillomania, is one of the newer diagnoses in the DSM-5. This disorder is a subset of obsessive-compulsive and related disorders. As with other additions to the DSM-5, this disorder has been around for over a century; however, it was not included in previous diagnostic manuals. There are some who believe that ED is closest to OCD in etiology; however, others believe it is better categorized as an "addiction disorder," like alcohol and drug use disorders.

Identification & Diagnosis

The disorder is characterized by repeated skin picking leading to multiple lesions on the skin, despite ongoing efforts to reduce or stop this behavior. ED, like TTM, is not associated with obsessions or preoccupations, as in OCD. Diagnosis of this disorder is characterized by clinically significant distress affecting social, occupational, or other areas of functioning. Distress includes, but is not limited to, experiencing a loss of control, embarrassment, or shame. Symptoms are likely affected by increased stress, anxiety, and boredom. In addition, various substances, namely dopamine agonists (eg, methamphetamines and cocaine) can lead to skin picking.

Treatment

Psychotherapy can be beneficial and should be the first line of treatment in most cases. For severe cases, or cases not responding the therapy, there is mixed evidence supporting the use of SSRIs and evidence for *N*-acetylcysteine (NAC) in adults. Comorbid conditions should be identified and treated. Currently, there are clinical trials looking at treating this disorder by targeting other receptors, such as opioid antagonists and glutaminergic agonists; however, these are still in preliminary phases.

Other Considerations

The differential diagnosis includes TTM, substance use disorder, major depressive disorders, anxiety disorder, OCD, Tourette's or tic disorder, body dysmorphic disorder, substance-induced skin picking, psychosis, and neurodevelopmental disorders, such as Prader-Willi. There is a high comorbidity with OCD and TTM, in addition to major depressive disorder.

Prognosis

The disorder is much more common in females than males, with about a 3:1 ratio. Typical age of onset is teen years, likely associated with picking of acne. The lifetime prevalence for ED in adults is at or above 1.4%. The course is chronic, yet symptoms can wax and wane for months to years at a time.

Posttraumatic Stress Disorder

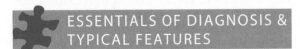

ESSENTIALS OF DIAGNOSIS & TYPICAL FEATURES

► Signs and symptoms of hyperarousal and reactivity.
► Avoidant behaviors.
► Negative changes in thoughts and mood.

► Flashbacks to a traumatic event such as nightmares, intrusive thoughts, or repetitive play.
► Follows traumatic events such as exposure to violence, physical or sexual abuse, natural disasters, car accidents, dog bites, and unexpected personal tragedies.

General Considerations

Factors that predispose individuals to the development of PTSD include proximity to the traumatic event or loss, a history of exposure to trauma, preexisting depression or anxiety disorder, being abused by a caregiver, or witnessing a threat to a caregiver. PTSD can develop in response to natural disasters, terrorism, motor vehicle crashes, and significant personal injury, in addition to physical, sexual, and emotional abuse. Natural disasters, such as hurricanes, fires, flooding, and earthquakes, create situations in which large numbers of affected individuals are at heightened risk for PTSD. Witnessing events through electronic media does not count as exposure to traumatic events. Individuals who have a previous history of trauma or with an unstable social situation are at greatest risk of PTSD.

Long overdue attention is now being paid to the substantial effects of family and community violence on the psychological development of children and adolescents. Abused children are especially likely to develop PTSD and to suffer wide-ranging symptoms and impaired functioning. As many as 25% of young people exposed to violence develop symptoms of PTSD and children with some symptoms of PTSD can suffer significant distress and functional impairment, even when not meeting full criteria for PTSD.

Identification & Diagnosis

Children and adolescents with PTSD typically show persistent fear, anxiety, and hypervigilance. Children may regress developmentally, experience fears of strangers, the dark, and being alone, and avoid reminders of the traumatic event. For young children with magical thinking, this can involve avoiding objects or events that may not be obviously linked to the traumatic event. Children and adolescents with PTSD are often more irritable and can experience detachment and diminished interest in activities. They reexperience elements of the events in the form of nightmares and flashbacks. In the symbolic play of children with PTSD, one can often notice repetition of some aspect of the traumatic event. Children with a history of traumatic experiences or neglect in infancy and early childhood are likely to show signs of reactive attachment disorder and have difficulty forming relationships with caregivers. A subset of children experience dissociative symptoms such as feeling detached or unreal. The criteria for PTSD for children younger than 6 have been adjusted for development, accounting for a more limited repertoire of emotions and behaviors in younger children compared to older youth. Symptoms must be present for at least 1 month to meet criteria for PTSD but can present months after the event.

Treatment

Before considering treatment, it is critical to ensure that the child is living in a safe environment. If there is concern regarding current or past abuse, this must be reported to social services. Treatment of patients with PTSD includes education regarding the nature of the disorder and the many varied symptoms that parents may not recognize as related to PTSD. The child needs support, reassurance, and empathy, and the primary caregiver may also need additional help to provide this. Individual and family psychotherapy are central features of treatment interventions. Treatments differ based on age of child, chronicity of trauma, and access to treatment. Young children may benefit from therapy focused on strengthening the parent child relationship whereas other treatments additionally focus on creating a developmentally appropriate trauma narrative to help the child understand and process their experience. Trauma-focused cognitive behavioral therapy (TF-CBT) has the most evidence for treatment of children and adolescents with PTSD while treatments such as eye movement desensitization and reprocessing therapy (EMDR) have more limited evidence. Pediatricians can help the family establish or maintain daily routines as much as possible, especially after a trauma or disaster that interrupts the family's environment. In the case of media coverage of a disaster or event, children's viewing should be avoided or limited.

For children with more severe and persistent symptoms, assessment for treatment with medication is indicated. Children who have lived for an extended time in abusive environments or have been exposed to multiple traumas are more likely to require treatment with medications. Currently, there are no medications with FDA approval for treating PTSD in children. Child psychiatrists may choose medications to target specific symptoms (eg, anxiety, depression, nightmares, and aggression). Some of the medications used to treat children with PTSD include anti adrenergic agents (clonidine, guanfacine or propranolol), mood stabilizers, antidepressants, and second-generation antipsychotics.

Other Considerations

Growing evidence supports a connection between victimization in childhood and problems in adulthood, including health problems, substance abuse, unstable personality, and mood disorders. It is important to treat PTSD not only to relieve the suffering of youth with PTSD but also to mitigate long-term negative sequelae.

Many of the symptoms of PTSD can be mistaken for other disorders such as depression, anxiety, primary substance abuse, ADHD, learning disorders, ODD, bipolar disorder,

and even psychosis in more severe cases. All behavioral health assessments should include inquiries related to traumatic events. It is important not to miss trauma-related etiology as this may change treatment focus. Traumatic events may not lead to PTSD but may cause grief, an adjustment disorder, depression, or an acute stress disorder (same criteria as PTSD but symptoms last < 1 month). Children with PTSD may have comorbid diagnoses that require treatment. This diagnostic complexity often requires the assistance of the child psychiatrist or other mental health provider.

Prognosis

The best prognostic indicator for children exposed to trauma is a supportive relationship with a caregiving adult. Frequently caregivers exposed to trauma also have PTSD and need referral for treatment so that they can also assist in their child's recovery. Timely access to therapy enhances prognosis. Children with more severe PTSD may require intermittent therapy to identify and treat symptoms that emerge during different stages of development.

For resources and evidence-based interventions: National Child Trauma Stress Network: https://www.nctsn.org. Accessed June 26, 2019.

ATTENTION-DEFICIT/HYPERACTIVITY DISORDER

Inattentive, Hyperactive, & Combined Type

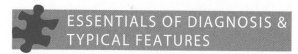

ESSENTIALS OF DIAGNOSIS & TYPICAL FEATURES

- ▶ Significant impairment in attention or concentration.
- ▶ And/or significant hyperactivity and impulsivity in excess of that expected for age.
- ▶ Must be present in two or more settings.

General Considerations

Attention-deficit/hyperactivity disorder (ADHD) is one of the most commonly seen and treated psychiatric conditions in children and adolescents. Although there is no definitive cause or cure for this disorder, with adequate screening and monitoring, it can be identified and effectively treated.

Identification & Diagnosis

Symptoms of ADHD fall into two categories: hyperactive and impulsive or inattentive. If a child has a significant number of symptoms in both categories, a diagnosis of ADHD, combined type is given. Functional impairment is required across at least two settings. Accurate diagnosis includes obtaining information regarding symptoms and functional impairment from two sources: typically parents and teachers. Standardized forms in the public domain such as Vanderbilt parent and teacher evaluation and follow-up forms are helpful in the process. It is important to keep in mind that intermittent symptoms of hyperactivity and/or inattention without functional impairment do not warrant a diagnosis of ADHD.

Not all hyperactivity and/or inattention can be attributed to ADHD. Some of the most common psychiatric conditions that have similar presenting problems to ADHD include mood disorder (ie, bipolar and depression), anxiety disorders, oppositional defiant disorder, adjustment disorder, and PTSD. Learning disorders and other neurodevelopmental disorders can present with symptoms suggestive of ADHD. There are also a number of medical diagnoses with presenting problems similar to ADHD, including head injury, hyperthyroidism, fetal alcohol syndrome, and lead toxicity. Inadequate nutrition and sleep deprivation, including poor quality of sleep, can also cause inattention. It is important to have the correct diagnosis prior to initiating treatment for ADHD.

▶ Treatment

Medication can be very helpful for school age children and adolescents with ADHD. For children diagnosed with ADHD younger than 6, behavioral therapy is the first line of treatment. Stimulants are the most effective and most commonly prescribed medications for ADHD. Approximately 75% of children with ADHD experience symptom improvement when given stimulant medications. Children with ADHD who do not respond favorably to one stimulant may respond to a stimulant from the other class (amphetamines vs methylphenidate stimulants). Children and adolescents with ADHD without prominent hyperactivity (ADHD, predominantly inattentive type) are also likely to be responsive to stimulant medications. When stimulants are not well tolerated or effective, nonstimulants may be used as an alternative. Among nonstimulant medications, atomoxetine, selective noradrenergic reuptake inhibitors, and central α_{2A}-adrenergic receptor agonists (ie, guanfacine and clonidine) have FDA approval for the treatment of ADHD in children.

A device placed on the forehead overnight to stimulate the trigeminal nerve has FDA approval for treatment of children age 7–12 years who are not also being treated with medication. The effect of treatment with the external trigeminal nerve stimulation (ETNS) system is mild and did not separate from placebo until 4 weeks. Side effects include appetite increase, sleep difficulties, teeth clenching, headache, and fatigue.

▶ Other Considerations

ADHD comorbidities are common and include anxiety disorders, mood disorders, oppositional defiant disorder, and conduct disorder. While stimulant medication, the first-line treatment for ADHD, has the potential for abuse, individuals who are treated for ADHD are significantly less likely to abuse substances compared to those who have not been treated. Also, a large majority of children and adolescents with ADHD are not formally diagnosed, and of those who are diagnosed, only 55% receive ongoing treatment.

▶ Special Considerations Regarding the Use of Stimulant Medication

Common adverse events include anorexia, weight loss, abdominal distress, headache, insomnia, dysphoria and tearfulness, irritability, lethargy, mild tachycardia, and mild elevation in blood pressure. Less common side effects include interdose rebound of ADHD symptoms, anxiety tachycardia, hypertension, depression, mania, and psychotic symptoms. Reduced growth velocity can occur, however, for individual patient's ultimate height is not usually compromised. Young children are at increased risk for side effects from stimulant medications. Additive stimulant effects are seen with sympathomimetic amines (ephedrine and pseudoephedrine).

Reports of sudden death and serious cardiovascular adverse events among children taking stimulant medication raised concerns about their safety. The labels for methylphenidate and amphetamine medications note reports of stimulant-related deaths in patients with heart problems and advised against using these products in individuals with known serious structural abnormalities of the heart, cardiomyopathy, or serious heart rhythm abnormalities. Insufficient data continue to confirm whether taking stimulant medication causes cardiac problems or sudden death. The FDA advises providers to conduct a thorough physical examination, paying close attention to the cardiovascular system, and to collect information about the patient's history and any family history of cardiac problems. If this scrutiny suggests a problem, providers should consider a screening electrocardiogram or an echocardiogram. Caution should also be taken if there is a personal or family history of substance abuse or addictive disorders, as these medications can be abused. Formulations such as the methylphenidate transdermal patch or lisdexamfetamine are more difficult to abuse. Students attending college/university may be at increased risk to divert their stimulants to peers. Stimulants should be used with caution in individuals with psychotic disorders, as they can significantly worsen psychotic symptoms. Likewise, stimulants should be used with caution in individuals with bipolar affective disorder as they can worsen mood dysregulation.

Initial medical screening should include observation for involuntary movements and measurement of height, weight, pulse, and blood pressure. (See also Chapter 3.)

Pulse, blood pressure, height, and weight should be recorded every 3–4 months and at times of dosage increases and abnormal movements such as motor tics should be assessed at each visit.

▶ Prognosis

Research indicates that 60%–85% of those diagnosed with ADHD in childhood continue to carry the diagnosis into adolescence and those who don't meet full criteria for ADHD may still have functional impairment. While many have devised ways to cope with their symptoms in a manner that does not require medication, about one-third of adults previously diagnosed with ADHD in childhood require ongoing medication management.

AAP algorithm: Implementing the key action statements: an algorithm and explanation for process of care for the evaluation, diagnosis, treatment, and monitoring of ADHD in children and adolescents. http://pediatrics.aappublications.org/content/suppl/2011/10/11/peds.2011-2654.DC1/zpe611117822p.pdf. Accessed April 29, 2017.

AAP Practice Parameter: http://pediatrics.aappublications.org/content/early/2011/10/14/peds.2011-2654. Accessed April 29, 2017.

FDA press release regarding Trigeminal Nerve Stimulation System: https://www.fda.gov/news-events/press-announcements/fda-permits-marketing-first-medical-device-treatment-adhd.

Medication guide with pictures of medications, drug class, time of action: http://www.adhdmedicationguide.com

MOOD DISORDERS

1. Depression

ESSENTIALS OF DIAGNOSIS & TYPICAL FEATURES

▶ Dysphoric mood, mood lability, irritability, or depressed appearance, persisting for weeks to months at a time.

▶ Characteristic neurovegetative signs and symptoms (eg, changes in sleep, appetite, concentration, and activity levels).

▶ Suicidal ideation, feeling of hopelessness.

▶ General Considerations

The incidence of depression in children increases with age, from 1% to 3% before puberty to around 9% for adolescents, and this is likely even higher in patients seen in primary care. Over the course of adolescence, 20% of individuals will experience depression. The rate of depression in females approaches adult levels by age 15, and the lifetime risk of depression ranges from 10% to 25% for women and 5% to

12% for men. The sex incidence is equal in childhood, but with the onset of puberty, the rates of depression for females begin to exceed those for males. The incidence of depression in children is higher when other family members have been affected by depressive disorders.

▶ Identification & Diagnosis

Clinical depression can be defined as a persistent state of unhappiness or misery that interferes with pleasure or productivity. Children and younger adolescents are more likely to present with an irritable mood state and older adolescents with a sad mood more similar to adults. Typically, a child or adolescent with depression begins to look unhappy and may make comments such as "I have no friends," "life is boring," "there is nothing I can do to make things better," or "I wish I were dead." Behavior patterns change from baseline and can include social isolation, deterioration in schoolwork, loss of interest in usual activities, anger, and irritability. Sleep and appetite patterns commonly change, and the child may complain of tiredness and nonspecific pain such as headaches, stomach aches, or musculoskeletal pains.

Clinical depression is typically identified by asking about the symptoms. Adolescents are often more accurate than their caregivers in describing their own mood state. When several depressive symptoms cluster together over time, are persistent (≥ 2 weeks), and cause impairment, a major depressive disorder may be present. When depressive symptoms are of lesser severity but have persisted for 1 year or more, a diagnosis of dysthymic disorder should be considered. Milder symptoms of short duration in response to some stressful life event may be consistent with a diagnosis of adjustment disorder with depressed mood. Table 7–13

Table 7–13. Clinical manifestations of depression in children and adolescents.

Depressive Symptom	Clinical Manifestations
Anhedonia	Loss of interest and enthusiasm in play, socializing, school, and usual activities; boredom; loss of pleasure
Dysphoric mood	Tearfulness; sad, downturned expression; unhappiness; slumped posture; quick temper; irritability; anger
Fatigability	Lethargy and tiredness; no play after school
Morbid ideation	Self-deprecating thoughts, statements; thoughts of disaster, abandonment, death, suicide, or hopelessness
Somatic symptoms	Changes in sleep or appetite patterns; difficulty in concentrating; bodily complaints, particularly headache, and stomachache

describes some symptoms of depression as they may appear in children and adolescents.

The AAP recommends annual screening for depression in children age 12 and older using a standardized measure. The Center for Epidemiologic Study—Depression Scale for Children (CES-DC), Child Depression Inventory (CDI), Beck Depression Rating Scale, and Reynolds Adolescent Depression Scale and Patient Health Questionnaire-9 modified for teens (PHQ-9) are self-report rating scales that are easily used in primary care to assist in assessment and monitoring response to treatment. Several are available in the public domain.

▶ Treatment

Treatment varies by severity level. Children and adolescents with mild depression should receive close monitoring over several weeks and psychoeducation that includes caregivers. The treatment team (patient, caregiver, and provider) may be able to identify targets for change that may improve depression. See Table 7–14.

Treatment for moderate to severe depression includes developing a comprehensive plan to treat the depressive episode, help the family to respond effectively to the patient's emotional needs, and build supports within the school setting if needed. Referrals should be considered for individual and possibly adjunctive family therapy. CBT and interpersonal therapy (IPT) both have evidence for improving depressive symptoms in children and adolescents. CBT includes a focus on building coping skills to change negative thought patterns that predominate in depressive conditions. It also helps identify, label, and verbalize feelings and misperceptions. In therapy, efforts are also made to resolve conflicts between family members and improve communication skills within the family.

Mild to moderate depressive symptoms often improve with psychotherapy alone. When the symptoms of depression are moderate and persistent, or severe, antidepressant medications may be indicated (see Table 7–11). A positive family history of depression increases the risk of early-onset depression in children and adolescents and the chances of a positive response to antidepressant medication. Depression in toddlers and young children is best approached with parent–child relational therapies.

The carefully conducted Treatment of Adolescent Depression Study (TADS) is a major source of evidence for clinic guidelines regarding the treatment of depression in children and adolescents. This study found that CBT combined with fluoxetine led to the best outcomes in the treatment of pediatric depression during the first 12 weeks of treatment. Although our knowledge is still evolving, these findings suggest that when recommending or prescribing an antidepressant, the provider should consider concurrently recommending CBT or IPT. Providers should discuss the options for medication treatment, including which medications have FDA approval for pediatric indications (see Table 7–6). Target symptoms should be carefully monitored for improvement or worsening, and it is important to ask and document the responses about any suicidal thinking and self-injurious behaviors.

▶ Special Considerations Regarding the Use of Antidepressant Medication

There are some special considerations when prescribing the various classes of antidepressant medication. Table 7–11 outlines the distinct differences between some of the most commonly used antidepressant medications.

A. Selective Serotonin Reuptake Inhibitors (SSRIs)

Each SSRI has different FDA indications. Providers can choose to treat with an SSRI that has not received FDA approval for a specific indication or age group. Typical considerations for using a medication without FDA approval include the side-effect profile and/or whether another family member has responded to a specific medication. In these instances, providers should inform the patient and family that they are using a medication off-label.

The therapeutic response for SSRIs should be expected 4–6 weeks after a therapeutic dose has been reached although many individuals may experience benefit earlier. The starting dose for a child younger than 12 years is generally half the starting dose for an adolescent, but young children may need eventual doses similar to adolescents or adults. Pharmacokinetic studies suggest that SSRIS may be metabolized faster in young children, leading to shorter half-lives. SSRIs are usually given once a day, in the morning with breakfast, but lower doses of sertraline should be administered twice daily. Individuals who experience sedation (1 in 10) or find mornings difficult to remember to take their medication may prefer to take the medication at bedtime. Caution should be used in cases of known liver disease or chronic or severe illness where multiple medications may be prescribed, because SSRIs are metabolized in the liver. In addition, caution should be used when prescribing for an individual with a family history of bipolar disorder, or when the differential diagnosis includes bipolar disorder, because antidepressants can induce manic or hypomanic symptoms.

Adverse effects of SSRIs are often dose related and time limited: GI distress and nausea (can be minimized by taking medication with food), headache, tremulousness, decreased

---

Table 7–14. Targets to improve depression.

Positive lifestyle changes (improve sleep hygiene, exercise, nutrition)
Positive parenting
Increase supports at school
Address stressors
Support positive peer relationships

appetite, weight loss, insomnia, sedation (10%), and sexual dysfunction (25%). Irritability, social disinhibition, restlessness, and emotional excitability can occur in approximately 20% of children taking SSRIs, and activation is more likely to occur with preadolescent children. It is important to systematically monitor for side effects. SSRIs other than fluoxetine should be discontinued slowly to minimize withdrawal symptoms including flu-like symptoms, dizziness, headaches, paresthesias, and emotional lability.

All SSRIs inhibit the hepatic microsomal enzyme system. The order of inhibition is: fluoxetine > fluvoxamine > paroxetine > sertraline > citalopram > escitalopram. This can lead to higher-than-expected blood levels of concomitant medications. Taking tryptophan while on an SSRI may result in a serotonergic syndrome of psychomotor agitation and GI distress. A potentially fatal interaction that clinically resembles neuroleptic malignant syndrome (NMS) may occur when SSRIs are administered concomitantly with monoamine oxidase inhibitors (MAOIs). Fluoxetine has the longest half-life of the SSRIs and should not be initiated within 14 days of the discontinuation of a monoamine oxidase inhibitor, or a monoamine oxidase inhibitor initiated within at least 5 weeks of the discontinuation of fluoxetine. One should be cautious of prescribing SSRIs in conjunction with ibuprofen and other NSAIDs for concerns of GI or other bleeding.

B. Serotonin Norepinephrine Reuptake Inhibitors (SNRI)

Serotonin norepinephrine reuptake inhibitors (SNRIs), which include venlafaxine, duloxetine, desvenlafaxine, and milnacipran, are antidepressants that primarily inhibit reuptake of serotonin and norepinephrine. Desvenlafaxine is the major active metabolite of the antidepressant venlafaxine. It is approved for the treatment of major depression in adults. Contraindications for this class of medication include hypertension, which is typically dose related. SNRIs also can increase heart rate. The most common adverse effects are nausea, nervousness, and sweating. SNRIs should be discontinued slowly to minimize withdrawal symptoms, including flu-like symptoms, dizziness, headaches, paresthesias, and emotional lability. The treatment of resistant depression study in adolescents (TORDIA) compared switching adolescents with depression who had not responded to initial treatment with an SSRI to another SSRI, venlafaxine, or medication plus placebo. Response rates were best for the combination (therapy plus medication) arm but did not differ between the two medications arms. However, the patients treated with venlafaxine experienced more skin problems and elevated blood pressure and heart rate. Duloxetine has been associated with severe skin reactions such as erythema multiforme and Stevens-Johnson syndrome, and venlafaxine has been associated with interstitial lung disease and eosinophilic pneumonia and increased suicidal ideation.

C. Other Antidepressants

Bupropion is an antidepressant that inhibits uptake of norepinephrine and dopamine. It is approved for treatment of major depression in adults. Like the SSRIs, bupropion has very few anticholinergic or cardiotoxic effects. The medication has three different formulations, and consideration for use is based on tolerability and compliance. Bupropion can interfere with sleep, so dosing earlier in the day is paramount to adherence and decreasing side effects. Contraindications of this medication include history of seizure disorder or bulimia nervosa. The most common adverse effects include psychomotor activation (agitation or restlessness), headache, GI distress, nausea, anorexia with weight loss, insomnia, tremulousness, precipitation of mania, and induction of seizures with doses above 450 mg/day.

Mirtazapine is an α_2-antagonist that enhances central noradrenergic and serotonergic activity. It is approved for the treatment of major depression in adults. Mirtazapine should not be given in combination with MAOIs. Very rare side effects are acute liver failure (1 case per 250,000–300,000), neutropenia, and agranulocytosis. More common adverse effects include dry mouth, increased appetite, constipation, weight gain, and increased sedation.

TCAs are an older class of antidepressants, which include imipramine, desipramine, clomipramine, nortriptyline, and amitriptyline. The lack of demonstrated efficacy, high-risk side-effect profile potential, and for lethality with overdose have led steering committees and professional organizations to recommend that primary care providers not prescribe TCAs for depression in children and adolescents. Providers should not be confused by FDA approval of imipramine and desipramine for enuresis in children age 6 years and older.

▶ Other Considerations

The risk of suicide is the most significant side effect associated with depressive episodes. In addition, adolescents with depression are at higher risk for substance abuse and engaging in self-injurious behaviors such as cutting or burning themselves (without suicidal intent). School performance usually suffers during a depressive episode, as children are unable to concentrate or motivate themselves to complete homework or projects. The irritability, isolation, and withdrawal that often result from the depressive episode can lead to loss of peer relationships and tense dynamics within the family. Refer to section on identifying and addressing suicide risk for additional information.

Depression often coexists with other mental illnesses such as ADHD, oppositional defiant disorder, conduct disorder, anxiety disorders, eating disorders, and substance abuse disorders. Medically ill patients also have an increased incidence of depression. Every child and adolescent with a depressed mood state should be asked directly about suicidal ideation and physical and sexual abuse. Depressed adolescents should also be screened for hypothyroidism and substance abuse.

In 2005, the FDA issued a "black box warning" regarding suicidal thinking and behavior for all antidepressants prescribed for children and adolescents. The FDA compiled data from 24 short-term trials of 4–16 weeks that included the use of antidepressants for major depressive disorder and obsessive compulsive disorder. Across these studies, the average risk of suicidal thinking and behavior during the first few months of treatment was 4% or twice the placebo risk of 2%. No suicides occurred in these trials. Subsequent meta-analysis estimated this risk to be lower. Although children face an initial increased risk of suicidal thinking and behaviors during the first few months of treatment, there is now substantial evidence that antidepressant treatment, over time, is protective against suicide. This suggests best practice is to educate the family regarding both the risks and benefits of antidepressant treatment and monitor carefully for any increase in suicidal ideation or self-injurious urges, as well as improvement in target symptoms of depression, especially in the first 4 weeks and subsequent 3 months after beginning their use.

▶ Prognosis

A comprehensive treatment intervention, including psychoeducation for the family, individual and family psychotherapy, medication assessment, and evaluation of school and home environments, often leads to complete remission of depressive symptoms over a 1- to 2-month period. If medications are started and prove effective, they should be continued for 6–12 months after remission of symptoms to prevent relapse. Early-onset depression (before age 15) is associated with increased risk of recurrent episodes and the potential need for longer-term treatment with antidepressants. Education of the family and child/or adolescent will help them identify depressive symptoms sooner and decrease the severity of future episodes with earlier interventions. Some studies suggest that up to 30% of preadolescents with major depression manifest bipolar disorder at 2-year follow-up. Psychotic symptoms during depression, early-onset depression, and family history of bipolar disorder all increase the risk for bipolar disorder. It is important to reassess the child or adolescent with depressive symptoms regularly for at least 6 months and to maintain awareness of the depressive episode in caring for this child in the future.

Guidelines for Adolescent Depression in Primary Care: http://www.gladpc.org. Accessed July 24, 2019.

Depression Resource Center Through American Academy of Child and Adolescent Depression: https://www.aacap.org/AACAP/Families_and_Youth/Resource_Centers/Depression_Resource_Center/Resources_for_Clinicians_Depression.aspx. Accessed June 27, 2019.

2. Bipolar Disorder

ESSENTIALS OF DIAGNOSIS & TYPICAL FEATURES

▶ Periods of abnormally and persistently elevated, expansive, or irritable mood, and heightened levels of energy and activity.

▶ Associated symptoms: grandiosity, diminished need for sleep, pressured speech, racing thoughts, impaired judgment.

▶ Not caused by prescribed or illicit drugs.

▶ The symptoms most commonly reported first are depressive symptoms.

▶ General Considerations

Bipolar illness can be difficult to diagnose and challenging to treat. It is generally recommended that children and adolescents who may have this diagnosis should be evaluated by a child and adolescent psychiatrist for diagnosis and further treatment if indicated.

Recent prospective and family studies have helped differentiate children who were previously diagnosed with bipolar disorder due to chronic irritability, as more likely to develop a mood or anxiety disorder later in adolescence or adulthood. A new disorder was created to help describe the presentation and course of these children: disruptive mood dysregulation disorder (DMDD). Diagnosing bipolar disorder (previously referred to as manic-depressive disorder) relies on meeting full criteria for a current or past manic episode (bipolar I disorder) or current or past hypomanic *and* depressive episode (bipolar II disorder). This change will likely lead to fewer diagnoses of bipolar disorder for children and younger adolescents and decrease the exposure of children to antipsychotic medication. It is still important to be vigilant for bipolar disorder as at least 20% of bipolar adults experience onset of symptoms before age 20 years. Onset of bipolar disorder before puberty is uncommon; however, symptoms often begin to develop and may be initially diagnosed as ADHD or other disruptive behavior disorders. The lifetime prevalence of bipolar disorder in middle to late adolescence is 1%–2%.

▶ Identification & Diagnosis

In about 70% of patients, the first symptoms are primarily those of depression. In the remainder, manic, hypomanic, or mixed states dominate the presentation. Patients with mania display a variable pattern of elevated, expansive, or irritable mood along with rapid speech, high energy levels, increase in goal-directed activity, difficulty in sustaining concentration, and a decreased need for sleep often including lack of fatigue the following day. The child or adolescent may also have hypersexual behavior. It is critical to rule out abuse or be aware of abuse factors contributing to the clinical presentation. Patients often do not acknowledge any problem with their mood or behavior, but the change from baseline is notable to others. The clinical picture can be quite dramatic, with florid psychotic symptoms of delusions and hallucinations accompanying extreme hyperactivity and impulsivity. Hypomanic episodes, characteristic of bipolar II disorder, are lower intensity manic episodes that do not cause social impairment and do not typically last as long as manic episodes. Although common, the co-occurrence of depression with bipolar I disorder is not a diagnostic requirement, while it is for bipolar II disorder. Cyclothymic disorder is diagnosed when the child or adolescent has had 1 year of hypomanic symptoms alternating with depressive symptoms that do not meet criteria for major depressive or hypomanic episode. Symptoms must be interpreted within a developmental context and differentiated from the normal moods and mood changes that occur in childhood and adolescence. Note that other specified bipolar and related disorder criteria describe youth who have hypomania but have not met full criteria for depression, or youth with shorter duration of manic symptoms (2–3 days).

The Mania Rating Scale (Child, CMRS, Youth YMRS, and Parent P-YMRS) can be useful as an additional tool to help patients and families describe moods, but providers should keep in mind that these are not specific. Parent reports of symptoms are typically more diagnostically helpful than patient or teacher reports.

Treatment

It is recommended that primary care providers refer all patients with suspected bipolar mood disorder to a mental health provider for diagnostic clarification and treatment. In situations where bipolar mood disorder is evident, a referral to a psychiatrist is recommended. In cases of severe impairment, hospitalization is required to maintain safety and initiate treatment. Other levels of care that may be appropriate with less severe presentations include day treatment, intensive outpatient therapy (two to three times per week) in home therapy or routine outpatient therapy. Once the goal of stabilization has been attained, it is reasonable for a primary care provider to provide maintenance therapy preferably with ongoing access to child and adolescent psychiatrist if symptoms worsen.

Pediatricians can help reinforce the need for ongoing treatments, provide additional psychoeducation, health maintenance and surveillance for associated problems such as substance abuse, sexually transmitted diseases, and accessing other supports such as a 504 plan or IEP if indicated.

Psychotherapy and medication are the mainstay of treatment. Medications are chosen based on current symptoms, side effects, family preference, and differ by polarity of symptoms (depression vs mania). The best evidence for treatment for mania is with second-generation antipsychotics, followed by lithium. Nonresponders may require a combination of medications. Lithium, risperidone, aripiprazole, quetiapine, asenapine, and olanzapine have been approved by the FDA for the treatment of acute and mixed manic episodes in adolescents. Other mood stabilizers, lamotrigine, carbamazepine, and valproate are less effective. Lithium and aripiprazole are approved for preventing recurrence.

Patients with bipolar disorder experience depressive symptoms that can be challenging to treat. It is generally recommended that patients should be on a mood stabilizer. At least one mood stabilizer is approved for pediatric bipolar depression (lurasidone). Patients with mild depression should receive therapy and other interventions prior to considering adding an antidepressant (refer to depression section) to a second-generation antipsychotic or other mood stabilizer. Choices for additional antidepressants, if the patient fails monotherapy, are similar to depression (refer to that section).

Therapy for children and adolescents with bipolar disorder generally includes psychoeducation, and there is some evidence that psychoeducation alone may have some benefit. More recent studies with youth who met criteria for bipolar I and II disorders found family-focused therapy (FFT) to be effective with outcomes related to bipolar depression and mania. Youth at risk for bipolar disorder, based on parent diagnosis, experienced improved outcomes related to hypomania symptoms. Components of this therapy include (1) psychoeducational activities like monitoring symptoms, recognizing triggers, and the importance of continuing medications, and (2) improving family communication with a focus on problem solving skills, appropriate expression of emotion, and developing and maintaining routines. Other therapies with some evidence include CBT, DBT, interpersonal and social rhythm therapy, and other family therapies.

Once the goal of stabilization has been attained, it is reasonable for a primary care provider to provide maintenance therapy.

Other Considerations

Physical or sexual abuse and exposure to domestic violence can also cause children to be mood labile, hyperactive, and aggressive, and PTSD should be considered by reviewing the history for traumatic life events in children with these symptoms. DMDD, ADHD, oppositional defiant disorder, and conduct disorder can be difficult to differentiate from bipolar and related disorders. The timing of onset of symptoms, severity and chronicity of irritability, and relation of oppositional or conduct behaviors to mood symptoms can help with this differentiation. For adolescents who are abusing substances, it is important to differentiate if mood symptoms of bipolar are "driving" the substance abuse or substance abuse is leading to mood symptoms. Individuals with manic psychosis may resemble those with schizophrenia or schizoaffective disorder. Psychotic symptoms associated with bipolar disorder should clear with resolution of the mood symptoms, which should also be prominent. Patients with mood lability may have a developing personality disorder. Many patients with bipolar disorder experience a worsening of anxiety with mood episodes. Further complicating this diagnostic difficulty is the relatively high likelihood of comorbid disorders for youth with bipolar disorder. Providers should not miss medical causes of symptoms such as hyperthyroidism, head trauma, and rare presentations of tumors. This is especially relevant if the change in personality has been relatively sudden or is accompanied by other neurologic changes.

▶ Prognosis

The chance of recovery from the mood episode of a bipolar illness that results in diagnosis (index episode) is high (80%), but many youth will experience a recurrence (60%) most likely in the same polarity (depression or mania) as the index episode, and are likely to be symptomatic 60% of the time. Early onset, low socioeconomic status, co-morbid illness, and family history of mood disorders all are risk factors for worse outcome. Children and adolescents diagnosed with cyclothymia are at risk to develop bipolar I or II disorder, and youth with bipolar I or II disorder may also change diagnostic categories over time.

Children and adolescents with bipolar illness are at risk for poorer academic, social, legal, and health outcomes. The poor judgment associated with manic episodes predisposes individuals to dangerous, impulsive, and sometimes criminal activity. Legal difficulties can arise from impulsive acts, such as excessive spending and acts of vandalism, theft, or aggression, that are associated with grandiose thoughts. Affective disorders are associated with a 30-fold greater incidence of successful suicide. Substance abuse and risks associated with substance abuse may lead to further poor outcomes.

3. Disruptive Mood Dysregulation Disorder (DMDD)

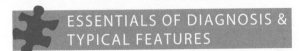

ESSENTIALS OF DIAGNOSIS & TYPICAL FEATURES

▶ Persistent irritability and severe behavioral outbursts at least three times a week for 1 year or more.

▶ The mood in between these symptoms is persistently negative (ie, irritable, angry, or sad), which is observable by others.

▶ The tantrums and negative moods are present in at least two settings.

▶ Onset of illness prior to 10 years old.

▶ Chronological or developmental age of at least 6 years old.

▶ A disruption in functioning in more than one setting (eg, home, school and/or socially).

▶ General Considerations

DMDD is a new diagnosis in the DSM-5. Historically, many of these chronically irritable children would have been diagnosed with some variation of bipolar mood disorder. Studies of the family history, functional brain studies, and developmental progression suggest that these children are different from individuals with bipolar disorder. The prevalence is estimated to be 2%–5% and may decrease from childhood to adolescence. Early studies suggest males are at increased risk for this disorder.

▶ Identification & Diagnosis

Children with DMDD experience severe tantrums in addition to chronic irritability. The tantrums must be inconsistent with the developmental age of the child. Currently, this diagnosis cannot be given to individuals older than 18. In cases where symptoms overlap between DMDD and ODD, DMDD supersedes ODD. Children who have experienced a manic or hypomanic episode cannot be given this diagnosis. Tantrums that occur only in relation to anxiety-provoking situations or when routines are interrupted suggest a diagnosis of anxiety, ASD, or OCD, and do not meet criteria for DMDD.

▶ Treatment

Medication trials for this relatively new diagnosis are few but suggest methylphenidate may be effective in reducing symptoms (open-label trial), and the addition of citalopram to methylphenidate treatment may further reduce temper tantrum severity (randomized placebo-controlled trial). Other recommendations include identifying and treating comorbid conditions and referring patients to therapy that includes a parent component. Therapy is important for children and their families.

▶ Other Considerations

The differential diagnosis for DMDD is similar to that for other mood disorders. In addition, special attention and consideration should include screening for ADHD, anxiety, trauma, and significant interpersonal and relational deficits. Those with DMDD are at a higher risk than the general population to develop major depressive disorder and anxiety disorders as adults.

Children with DMDD have low frustration tolerance and may misread neutral social cues as threatening. They often function poorly in school and have impaired relations with peers and family. The parents or caregivers of these children are often very distressed, and these families tend to seek mental health treatment. Many parents will decrease the demands and limits placed on these children in an attempt to avoid tantrums. This can include withdrawing their children from developmentally appropriate health promoting activities. Children with DMDD often have dangerous behaviors that lead to psychiatric hospitalization.

With the addition of this diagnosis, researchers are now able to collect data to aid with the diagnosis, treatment, and outcome measures.

AACAP Facts for Families Disruptive Mood Dysregulation Disorder: http://www.aacap.org/AACAP/Families_and_Youth/Facts_for_Families/Facts_for_Families_Pages/Disruptive_Mood_Dysregulation_Disorder_DMDD_110.aspx. Accessed September 27, 2015.

SUICIDE IN CHILDREN & ADOLESCENTS

The suicide rate in young people has remained high for several decades. In 2014, suicide became the second leading cause of death among children and adolescents aged 10–24 years in the United States. The suicide rate among adolescents aged 15–24 years has increased dramatically from approximately 2.7 to 14.5 per 100,000 since the 1960s, but there has been no increase from 2015 to 2017. It is estimated that each year, approximately 2 million US adolescents attempt suicide, yet only 700,000 receive medical attention for their attempt. Suicide and homicide rates for children in the United States are two to five times higher than those for the other 25 industrialized countries combined, primarily due to the prevalence of firearms in the United States. For children younger than 10 years, the rate of completed suicide is low but has also increased. Adolescent girls make three to four times as many suicide attempts as boys of the same age, but the number of completed suicides is three to four times greater in boys. Firearms are the most commonly used method in successful suicides, accounting for 40%–60% of cases; hanging, carbon monoxide poisoning, and drug overdoses each account for approximately 10%–15% of cases.

Suicide is almost always associated with a psychiatric disorder and should not be viewed as a philosophic choice about life or death or as a predictable response to overwhelming stress. Most commonly it is associated with a mood disorder and the hopelessness that accompanies a severe depressive episode. Suicide rates are higher for Native American and Native Alaskan populations than for white, black, and Latino/Hispanic populations. Although suicide attempts are more common in individuals with a history of experiencing trauma, behavior problems, and academic difficulties, other suicide victims are high achievers who are temperamentally anxious and perfectionistic and who commit suicide impulsively after a failure or rejection, either real or perceived. Mood disorders (in both sexes, but especially in females), substance abuse disorders (especially in males), a history of trauma, and conduct disorders are commonly diagnosed at psychological autopsy in adolescent suicide victims. Some adolescent suicides reflect an underlying psychotic disorder, with the young person usually committing suicide in response to auditory hallucinations or psychotic delusions.

The vast majority of young people who attempt suicide give some clue to their distress or their tentative plans to commit suicide. Most show signs of dysphoric mood (anger, irritability, anxiety, or depression). For those who are screened, there is often a history of elevated distress reported on a screening instrument. Over 60% make comments such as "I wish I were dead" or "I just can't deal with this any longer" within the 24 hours prior to death. In one study, nearly 70% of subjects experienced a crisis event such as a loss (eg, rejection by a girlfriend or boyfriend), public shaming, a failure, or an arrest prior to completed suicide. With ubiquitous social networking technologies and the presence of digital profiles, posting distress messages electronically and aggression in the form of cyber-bullying are important to identify and discuss when conducting risk assessments and obtaining information about relationships, supports, and sources of stress.

Assessment of Suicide Risk

Routine screening for children 12 and older now includes questions regarding suicide. If a child or adolescent expresses suicidal thinking, the treating provider must ask if he or she has an active plan, intends to complete that plan, and has made previous attempts. **Suicidal ideation accompanied by any plan warrants immediate referral for a psychiatric crisis assessment.** This can usually be accomplished at the nearest emergency room (ER).

Assessment of suicide risk calls for a high index of suspicion and a direct interview with the patient and his or her parents or guardians. The highest risk of suicide is among white, adolescent boys. High-risk factors include previous suicide attempts, self-injurious behavior, a suicide note, and a viable plan for suicide with the availability of lethal means, close personal exposure to suicide, conduct disorder, and substance abuse. Other risk factors are signs and symptoms of major depression or dysthymia, a family history of suicide, a recent death in the family, suicide of student at the patient's school, and a view of death as a relief from the pain in the patient's life.

Intervention

Suicidal ideation and any suicide attempt must be considered a serious matter. The patient should not be left alone, and the treating provider should express concern and convey a desire to help. If a behavioral health clinician (BHC) is embedded in the practice, the BHC can aid in assessing the patient. Either the provider or the BHC should meet with the patient and the family, both alone and together, and listen carefully to their problems and perceptions. It is helpful to explicitly state that with the assistance of mental health professionals, solutions can be found. The practice should err on the side of caution, in deciding whether further referral or an emergency evaluation is indicated. Similar to reporting suspicion of child abuse, although the practice may not have the expertise or time to determine full suicide risk, primary care providers can determine that further evaluation is indicated. A thorough suicide assessment requires some level of expertise, a considerable amount of time, and contact with multiple sources of information. The majority of patients who express suicidal ideation and all who have made a suicide attempt should be referred for psychiatric evaluation and possible hospitalization. Referral for further assessment is always appropriate when there is concern about suicidal thinking and behavior.

Regardless of whether a practice has an embedded BHC, it is useful to have a practice-specific algorithm for suicidal youth. The algorithm should include the steps to be taken for youth who need to be sent to an emergency room, youth who need an urgent or less urgent referral, or youth who will be followed in the practice. The algorithm should specify who in the practice is responsible for each step. This should include who will call for emergency transport, if indicated, and who will flag a patient's record to ensure the patient follows up with care recommendations. Additionally, the primary care practice will need to follow up and document the outcome of the emergency assessment (eg, hospitalization, community referrals) in the patient's record and schedule a follow-up visit in the primary care setting as soon as is feasible given the disposition.

Suicide prevention efforts include heightened awareness in the community and schools to identify at-risk individuals and increased access to services, including hotlines and counseling services. Restricting young people's access to firearms is a critical factor, as firearms are responsible for 85% of deaths due to suicide or homicide in youth in the United States. Other means restriction methods include instructing families to lock up all medications. Many families are not aware that overdoses of over-the-counter medications such as acetaminophen can be lethal. In addition to increasing public awareness of the issue, media depictions of death by suicide, including news reporting and fictionalized accounts, could serve as a conversation starter for discussion of how an adolescent is understanding and thinking about this social issue. It is important to minimize sensationalism of deaths by suicide and have an open dialogue about what happened. This is particularly critical in communities that have recently experienced a death by suicide where there is increased vulnerability to the occurrence of additional incidents.

Finally, the treating provider should be aware of his or her own emotional reactions to dealing with suicidal adolescents and their families. Providers may be reluctant to cause a family stress or go against their will and require an emergency evaluation. Providers may have unfounded fears about precipitating suicide by direct and frank discussions of suicidal risk. Reviewing difficult cases with colleagues, developing formal or informal relationships with psychiatrists, and attending workshops on assessment and management of depression and suicidal ideation can decrease the anxiety and improve competence for primary care providers.

American Foundation for Suicide Prevention: https://afsp.org. Accessed September 15, 2017.

CDC Youth Suicide Prevention: https://www.cdc.gov/violenceprevention/suicide/youth_suicide.html.

Greydanus D, Patel D, Pratt H: Suicide risk in adolescents with chronic illness: implications for primary care and specialty pediatric practice: a review. Dev Med Child Neurol 2010 Dec;52(12):1083–1087 [Epub 2010 Aug 31] [PMID: 20813018].

National Center for the Prevention of Youth Suicide: http://www.suicidology.org/ncpys. Accessed September 15, 2017.

Suicide Awareness Voices of Education: https://www.save.org/. Accessed September 15, 2017.

Suicide Prevention Resource Center: http://www.sprc.org. Accessed September 15, 2017.

The Jed Foundation: https://www.jedfoundation.org/. Accessed September 15, 2017.

DISRUPTIVE, IMPULSE-CONTROL, & CONDUCT DISORDERS

1. Oppositional Defiant Disorder

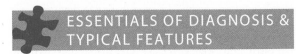

ESSENTIALS OF DIAGNOSIS & TYPICAL FEATURES

► A pattern of negativistic, hostile, and defiant behavior lasting at least 6 months.

► Loses temper, argues with adults, defies rules.

► Blames others for own mistakes and misbehavior.

► Angry, easily annoyed, vindictive.

► Does not meet criteria for conduct disorder.

► General Considerations

Oppositional defiant disorder is more common in families where caregiver dysfunction (eg, substance abuse, parental psychopathology, significant psychosocial stress) is present. It is also more prevalent in children with a history of multiple changes in caregivers, inconsistent, harsh, or neglectful parenting, or serious marital discord.

Identification & Diagnosis

Oppositional defiant disorder usually is evident before 8 years of age and may be an antecedent to the development of conduct disorder. The symptoms usually first emerge at home but then extend to school and peer relationships. The disruptive behaviors of oppositional defiant disorder are generally less severe than those associated with conduct disorder and do not include hurting other individuals or animals, destruction of property, or theft.

Treatment

Interventions include careful assessment of the psychosocial situation and recommendations to support parenting skills and optimal caregiver functioning. Assessment for comorbid psychiatric diagnoses such as learning disabilities, depression, and ADHD should be pursued, and appropriate interventions recommended.

2. Conduct Disorder

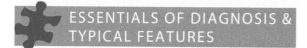

ESSENTIALS OF DIAGNOSIS & TYPICAL FEATURES

▶ A persistent pattern of behavior that includes the following:
- Defiance of authority.
- Violating the rights of others or society's norms.
- Aggressive behavior toward persons, animals, or property.

General Considerations

Disorders of conduct affect approximately 9% of males and 2% of females younger than 18 years. This is a very heterogeneous population, and overlap occurs with ADHD, substance abuse, learning disabilities, neuropsychiatric disorders, mood disorders, and family dysfunction. Many of these individuals come from homes where domestic violence, child abuse, drug abuse, shifting parental figures, and poverty are environmental risk factors. Although social learning partly explains this correlation, the genetic heritability of aggressive conduct and antisocial behaviors is currently under investigation.

Identification & Diagnosis

The typical child with conduct disorder is a boy with a turbulent home life and academic difficulties. Defiance of authority, fighting, tantrums, running away, school failure, and destruction of property are common symptoms. With increasing age, fire-setting, and theft may occur, followed in adolescence by truancy, vandalism, and substance abuse. Sexual promiscuity, sexual perpetration, and other criminal behaviors may develop. Hyperactive, aggressive, and uncooperative behavior patterns in the preschool and early school years tend to predict conduct disorder in adolescence with a high degree of accuracy, especially when ADHD goes untreated. A history of reactive attachment disorder is an additional childhood risk factor. The risk for conduct disorder increases with inconsistent and severe parental disciplinary techniques, parental alcoholism, and parental antisocial behavior.

Treatment

Effective treatment can be complicated by the psychosocial problems often found in the lives of children and adolescents with conduct disorders. These problems may also interfere with achieving compliance with treatment recommendations. Efforts should be made to stabilize the environment and improve functioning within the home, particularly as it relates to parental functioning and disciplinary techniques. Identification of learning disabilities and placement in an optimal school environment is critical. Any associated neurologic and psychiatric disorders should be addressed.

Residential treatment may be necessary for individuals whose symptoms do not respond to lower-level interventions or whose environment is not able to meet their needs for supervision and structure. Juvenile justice system involvement is common in cases where conduct disorder behaviors lead to illegal activities, theft, or assault.

Medications such as mood stabilizers, neuroleptics, stimulants, and antidepressants have all been studied in youth with conduct disorders, yet none has been found to be consistently effective. Each patient suspected of conduct disorder should be screened for other common psychiatric disorders and a history of trauma prior to the initiation of medication. Providers should use caution when prescribing various medications off-label for disruptive behavior. Early involvement in programs, such as Big Brothers, Big Sisters, scouts, and team sports, in which consistent adult mentors and role models interact with youth, decreases the chances that the youth will develop antisocial personality disorder. Multisystemic therapy (MST) is being increasingly used as an intervention for youth with conduct disorders and involvement with the legal system. MST is an intensive home-based model of care that seeks to stabilize and improve the home environment and to strengthen the support system and coping skills of the individual and family.

Other Considerations

Young people with conduct disorders, especially those with more violent histories, have an increased incidence of neurologic signs and symptoms, psychomotor seizures, psychotic symptoms, mood disorders, ADHD, and learning disabilities.

Efforts should be made to identify these associated disorders because they may require specific therapeutic interventions. Conduct disorder is best conceptualized as a final common pathway emerging from a variety of underlying psychosocial, genetic, environmental, and neuropsychiatric conditions.

▶ Prognosis

The prognosis is based on the ability of the child's support system to mount an effective treatment intervention consistently over time. The prognosis is generally worse for children in whom the disorder presents before age 10 years; those who display a diversity of antisocial behaviors across multiple settings; and those who are raised in an environment characterized by parental antisocial behavior, alcoholism or other substance abuse, and conflict. Nearly one-half of individuals with a childhood diagnosis of conduct disorder develop antisocial personality disorder as adults.

HIGH-RISK PATIENTS & HOMICIDE

Aggression & Violent Behavior in Youth

The tragic increase in teenage violence, including school shootings, is of particular concern to health professionals, as well as to society at large. There is strong evidence that screening and initiation of interventions by primary care providers can make a significant difference in violent behavior in youth. Although the prediction of violent behavior remains a difficult and imprecise endeavor, providers can support and encourage several important prevention efforts.

Most of the increase in youth violence, including suicides and homicides, involves the use of firearms. Thus, the presence of firearms in the home, the method of storage and safety measures taken when present, and access to firearms outside the home should be explored regularly with all adolescents as part of their routine medical care.

It is important to note that violent behavior is often associated with suicidal impulses. In the process of screening for violent behavior, suicidal ideation should not be overlooked. Any comment about wishes to be dead, or hopelessness, should be taken seriously and assessed immediately.

Interventions for parents include encouraging parents and guardians to be aware of their child's school attendance and performance. Parents should be encouraged to take an active role and learn about their children's friends, be aware of who they are going out with, where they will be, what they will be doing, and when they will be home. Most students involved in school violence might have been identified earlier and potentially may have benefited from interventions to address problems in social and educational functioning in the school environment. Communities and school districts nationwide have increased their efforts to identify and intervene with students whom teachers, peers, or parents recognize as having difficulty.

Threats & Warning Signs Requiring Immediate Consultation

Any and all threats that children make can be alarming. However, it is important to respond to the more serious and potentially lethal threats. These threats should be taken with the utmost seriousness, and parents/guardians should see a mental health provider immediately. Such threats include threats/warnings about hurting or killing someone or oneself, threats to run away from home, and/or threats to damage or destroy property.

Factors Associated With Increased Risk of Violent and/or Dangerous Behavior

Not all threats signify imminent danger. There are several potential predictors to consider when assessing the dangers and predictors of violent behavior, such as past history of violence or aggressive behavior, including uncontrollable anger outbursts; access to guns or other weapons; history of getting caught with a weapon in school; and family history of violent behaviors. In addition, children who witness abuse and violence at home and/or have a preoccupation with themes and acts of violence (eg, TV shows, movies, music, violent video games) are also at high risk of such behavior. Victims of abuse (ie, physical, sexual, and/or emotional) are more susceptible to feeling shame, loss, and rejection. The difficulty of dealing with abuse can further exacerbate an underlying mood, anxiety, or conduct disorder. Children who have been abused are more likely to be perpetrators of bullying and engage in verbal and physical intimidation toward peers. They also may be much more prone to blame others and are unwilling to accept responsibility for their own actions. Substance use is another major factor frequently associated with violent, aggressive, and/or dangerous behavior, particularly because it impacts judgment and is often associated with decreased inhibition and increased impulsivity. Socially isolated children also carry a high risk for violent and dangerous behavior. These include children with little to no adult supervision, poor connection with peers, and little to no involvement in extracurricular activities. These individuals may be more likely to seek out deviant peer groups for a sense of belonging.

How Adults Can Respond to Concerns of Violence and/or Dangerous Behavior

If a provider, parent, or trusted adult (eg, teacher, coach, clergy) suspects that a child is at risk for violent and/or dangerous behavior, the most important intervention is to talk with the child immediately about alleged threat and/or behavior. One should consider the child's past behavior, personality, and current stressors when evaluating the seriousness and likelihood of them engaging in a destructive or dangerous behavior. If the child already has a mental health provider, he/she should be contacted immediately. If they are not reachable, the parent(s)/guardian(s) should take the child to the closest ED or crisis center to evaluate safety and potential need for hospitalization. It is always acceptable to contact local police for assistance, especially if harm to others or lethal means are suspected. Another indication that warrants a crisis evaluation is if a child refuses to talk, is argumentative, responds defensively, or continues to express violent or dangerous thoughts or plans. Continuous, face-to-face adult supervision is essential while awaiting professional intervention. After evaluation, it is imperative to follow up with recommendations from mental health provider(s) to ensure safety and ongoing management.

Tips for Adults on How to Talk With Children About Violence

Talking about violence and personal safety is a necessary component of child rearing given the rise in violence in public places, including schools and places of worship. The most important factors to consider when discussing such a difficult topic is to be honest, be their source of information, reassure them that they are safe, and try to keep a routine and address *their* concerns at an age-appropriate level. Some reputable national websites that provide guidance on how to talk with children about violence and threats to personal safety include:

- https://www.healthychildren.org/English/family-life/Media/Pages/Talking-To-Children-About-Tragedies-and-Other-News-Events.aspxhttp://www.nea.org/home/72279.htm

- https://www.nctsn.org/sites/default/files/resources//age_related_reactions_to_traumatic_events.pdf

- http://www.pbs.org/parents/talkingwithkids/news/help-kids-feel-safe.html

- https://www.apa.org/topics/violence/school-shooting

- AACAP Facts for Families: http://www.aacap.org/AACAP/Families_and_Youth/Facts_for_Families/Facts_for_Families_Pages/Childrens_Threats_When_Are_They_Serious_65.aspx. Accessed September 27, 2015

SOMATIC SYMPTOM & RELATED DISORDERS

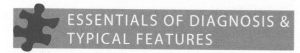

ESSENTIALS OF DIAGNOSIS & TYPICAL FEATURES

▶ Medically unexplained symptoms are no longer required for these disorders other than conversion disorder. Most disorders in this category are characterized by focus on symptoms within a medical setting.

▶ Distress and/or functional impairment are present in somatic symptom disorder while functional impairment is more common in conversion disorder.

▶ General Considerations

The category of somatic symptoms and related disorders includes somatic symptom disorder, illness anxiety disorder, conversion disorder (functional neurologic symptom disorder) psychological factors affecting other medical conditions, factitious disorder, and factitious disorder imposed by another (Table 7–15).

Patients with these disorders are commonly encountered in primary care and can be conceptualized as suffering; differences in presentation are likely related to cultural, contextual factors, individual experiences (such as trauma), and individual differences such as pain sensitivity. Families and cultures that value physical suffering while devaluing or ignoring psychological distress reinforce the development of these disorders. Family members who are ill, physically disabled, or suffer from any of these disorders can serve as models for children. More extreme parental dysfunction can manifest as factitious disorder imposed on another with the child as the victim.

Table 7–15. Somatoform disorders in children and adolescents.

Disorder	Major Clinical Manifestations
Somatic symptom disorder, factitious disorder, other specified somatic symptom and related disorder, unspecified somatic symptom and related disorder	A somatic symptom or symptoms cause significant distress, worry, and concern, and may take up considerable time and energy.
Conversion disorder (functional neurologic symptom disorder)	Symptom onset follows psychologically stressful event; symptoms express unconscious feelings and result in secondary gain.
Illness anxiety disorder	Somatic symptoms if present are mild. Focus is on fear of having or developing an illness leading to maladaptive behaviors.
Psychological factors affecting other medical conditions	Psychological or behavioral factors negatively impact a medical illness.
Factitious disorder or factitious disorder imposed on another	Deliberate false presentation of oneself or another (or causing in oneself or another) signs or symptoms of a physical or psychological problem.

Identification & Diagnosis

Somatic symptom disorder often presents in school age children and adolescents with the somatic symptom of headaches or GI distress. Conversion symptoms by definition involve alterations in voluntary motor or sensory function and are often more transient in pediatric patients than adults. Common symptoms include unusual sensory phenomena, paralysis, and movement or seizure-like disorders. A conversion symptom is thought to be an expression of underlying psychological conflict. The specific symptom may be symbolically determined by the underlying conflict and may resolve the dilemma created by the underlying wish or fear (eg, a seemingly paralyzed child need not fear expressing his or her underlying rage or aggressive retaliatory impulses).

Children with conversion disorder may be surprisingly unconcerned about the substantial disability deriving from their symptoms. Symptoms include unusual sensory phenomena, paralysis, vomiting, abdominal pain, intractable headaches, and movement or seizure-like disorders. For both somatic symptom disorder and conversion disorder, the physical symptoms often begin with a stressful event at school, with peers or within the context of a family experiencing stress, such as serious illness, a death, or family discord.

Treatment

Medical providers are often the first to see the patient and identify these disorders. Many of these patients can be treated within the pediatric primary care setting, utilizing the relationship between the pediatric provider and the family to maximize outcomes. For those who need referral to other settings, ongoing care by the pediatrician can help ensure families engage in other indicated treatments.

In most cases, conversion symptoms resolve quickly when the child and family are reassured that the symptom is a way of reacting to stress. The child is encouraged to continue with normal daily activities, knowing that the symptom will abate when the stress is resolved. Treatment of conversion disorders includes acknowledging the symptom rather than telling the child that the symptom is not medically justified and responding with noninvasive interventions such as physical therapy while continuing to encourage normalization of the symptoms. If the symptom does not resolve with reassurance, further investigation by a mental health professional is indicated. Comorbid diagnoses such as depression and anxiety disorders should be addressed, and treatment with psychopharmacologic agents may be helpful.

Somatic symptom disorder patients may respond to the same treatment. If the family structure or the patient cannot tolerate psychological approaches, somatic symptom patients may respond to regular, short, scheduled medical appointments to address the complaints at hand. In this way they do not need to precipitate emergencies to elicit medical attention. The medical provider should avoid invasive procedures unless clearly indicated and offer sincere concern and reassurance. The provider should also avoid telling the patient "it's all in your head" and should not abandon or avoid the patient, as somatic symptom disorder patients are at great risk of seeking multiple alternative treatment providers and potentially unnecessary treatments. Although not a DSM disorder, many parents worry about their child developing or having a serious illness. These families may also benefit from the above approach, in conjunction with encouragement for the pediatric patient to engage in health promoting activities such as involvement in sports. Parents who do not feel supported are also at risk to seek alternative opinions and procedures for their child.

Treatment for patients who are suffering from psychological factors impacting illness should be targeted to the underlying problem, such as treatment of anxious avoidance, motivational interviewing to target substance abuse, or adherence problems.

Health care providers who suspect factitious disorder imposed on another may need to involve a specialist to confirm the diagnosis. Communication between providers is critical to helping these patients. Child protective services and legal counsel may also need to be alerted. Although parents who are perpetrating factitious disorder imposed on another can appear concerned about the well-being of their child, studies have found child victims' mental health and well-being improved when they were removed from more extreme perpetrating caregivers.

Other Considerations

Somatic symptoms are often associated with anxiety and depressive disorders. Occasionally, psychotic children have somatic preoccupations and even somatic delusions.

Children with conversion disorder may have some secondary gain associated with their symptoms. Several reports have pointed to the increased association of conversion disorder with sexual overstimulation or sexual abuse. As with other emotional and behavioral problems, health care providers should always screen for physical and sexual abuse.

Prognosis

Prognosis is dependent on family factors, age, and disorder. Parents who support the view that symptoms can be related to stress can help patients engage in appropriate treatments. Younger patients with conversion symptoms have better prognosis than older patients with somatic symptom disorder. Patients who have had the disorder for a longer period of time may be less responsive to treatment. Psychiatric consultation can be helpful and for severely incapacitated patients, is indicated.

ADJUSTMENT DISORDERS

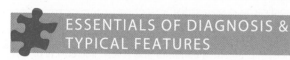

ESSENTIALS OF DIAGNOSIS & TYPICAL FEATURES

▶ The precipitating event or circumstance is identifiable.

▶ The symptoms have appeared within 3 months after the occurrence of the stressful event.

▶ Although the child experiences distress or some functional impairment, the reaction is not severe or disabling.

▶ The reaction does not persist more than 6 months after the stressor has terminated.

▶ General Considerations

The most common and most disturbing stressors in the lives of children and adolescents are the death of a loved one, marital discord, separation and divorce, family illness, a change of residence or school setting, experiencing a traumatic event, and, for adolescents, peer-relationship problems. These stressors naturally have a significant impact on children and adolescents.

▶ Identification & Diagnosis

When faced with stress, children can experience many different symptoms, including changes in mood, changes in behavior, anxiety symptoms, and physical complaints. When the reaction is out of proportion to the stressor and a decline in functioning is noted, a diagnosis of adjustment disorder is highly suspected. The two main categories of adjustment disorders include disturbance in emotions (ie, depression and anxiety) and/or conduct.

▶ Treatment

The mainstay of treatment involves genuine empathy and assurance to the parents and the patient that the emotional or behavioral change is a predictable consequence of the stressful event. This validates the child's reaction and encourages the child to talk about the stressful occurrence and its aftermath. Parents are encouraged to help the child with appropriate expression of feelings, while defining boundaries for behavior that prevent the child from feeling out of control and ensure safety of self and others. Maintaining or reestablishing routines can also alleviate distress and help children and adolescents adjust to changing circumstances by increasing predictability and decreasing distress about the unknown.

▶ Other Considerations

When symptoms emerge in reaction to an identifiable stressor but are severe, persistent, or disabling, mood disorders, anxiety disorders, and conduct disorders should be considered.

▶ Prognosis

The duration of symptoms in adjustment reactions depends on the severity of the stress; the child's personal sensitivity to stress and vulnerability to anxiety, depression, and other psychiatric disorders; and the available support system.

PSYCHOTIC DISORDERS

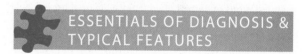

ESSENTIALS OF DIAGNOSIS & TYPICAL FEATURES

▶ Delusional thoughts.

▶ Disorganized speech (rambling or illogical speech patterns).

▶ Disorganized or bizarre behavior.

▶ Hallucinations (auditory, visual, tactile, olfactory).

▶ Paranoia, ideas of reference.

▶ Negative symptoms (ie, flat affect, avolition, alogia).

▶ General Considerations

The incidence of schizophrenia is about 1 per 10,000 per year. The onset of schizophrenia is typically between the middle to late teenage and early 30s. Symptoms usually begin after puberty, although a full "psychotic break" may not occur until the young adult years. Childhood onset (before puberty) of psychotic symptoms due to schizophrenia is uncommon and usually indicates a more severe form of the spectrum of schizophrenic disorders. Childhood-onset schizophrenia is more likely to be found in boys.

Schizophrenia has a strong genetic component. Other psychotic disorders that may be encountered in childhood or adolescence include schizoaffective disorder and unspecified psychosis. Unspecified psychosis may be used as a differential diagnosis when psychotic symptoms are present, but the cluster of symptoms is not consistent with a schizophrenia diagnosis.

Identification & Diagnosis

Children and adolescents display many of the symptoms of adult schizophrenia. Hallucinations or delusions, bizarre and morbid thought content, and rambling and illogical speech are typical. Affected individuals tend to withdraw into an internal world of fantasy and may then equate fantasy with external reality. They generally have difficulty with schoolwork and with family and peer relationships. Adolescents may have a prodromal period of depression prior to the onset of psychotic symptoms. Most individuals with childhood-onset schizophrenia have had nonspecific psychiatric symptoms or symptoms of delayed development for months or years prior to the onset of their overtly psychotic symptoms.

Obtaining a family history of mental illness is critical when assessing children and adolescents with psychotic symptoms. Psychological testing, particularly the use of projective measures, is often helpful in identifying or ruling out psychotic thought processes. Psychotic symptoms in children younger than 8 years must be differentiated from manifestations of normal vivid fantasy life or abuse-related symptoms. Children with psychotic disorders often have learning and attention disabilities, in addition to disorganized thoughts, delusions, and hallucinations. In psychotic adolescents, mania is differentiated by high levels of energy, excitement, and irritability. Any child or adolescent exhibiting new psychotic symptoms requires a medical evaluation that includes physical and neurologic examinations (including consideration of magnetic resonance imaging and electroencephalogram), drug screening, and metabolic screening for endocrinopathies, Wilson disease, and delirium.

Treatment

The treatment of childhood and adolescent schizophrenia focuses on four main areas: (1) decreasing active psychotic symptoms, (2) supporting development of social and cognitive skills, (3) reducing the risk of relapse of psychotic symptoms, and (4) providing support and education to parents and family members. Antipsychotic medications (neuroleptics) are the primary psychopharmacologic intervention. In addition, a supportive, reality-oriented focus in relationships can help to reduce hallucinations, delusions, and frightening thoughts. In situations where psychosis is evident, a referral to a psychiatrist is recommended. In cases of severe impairment, hospitalization is required to maintain safety and initiate treatment. A special school or day treatment environment may be necessary, depending on the child's or adolescent's ability to tolerate the school day and classroom activities. Support for the family emphasizes the importance of clear, focused communication and an emotionally calm climate in preventing recurrences of overtly psychotic symptoms.

Special Considerations Regarding the Use of Antipsychotic Medication

While it is expected that a psychiatrist initiate treatment, primary care providers undoubtedly treat children on antipsychotics and should become familiar with management and potential common and severe side effects of this class of medication. The "atypical or second generation antipsychotics" differ from conventional antipsychotics in their receptor specificity and effect on serotonin receptors. Conventional antipsychotics are associated with a higher incidence of movement disorders and extrapyramidal symptoms due to their wider effect on dopamine receptors. The atypical antipsychotics have a better side-effect profile for most individuals and comparable efficacy for the treatment of psychotic symptoms and aggression. Because of their increased use over conventional antipsychotics, the information that follows primarily focuses on safe use of atypical antipsychotics.

Common adverse effects of the atypical antipsychotics are cognitive slowing, sedation, orthostasis, dystonia, and weight gain. Most side effects tend to be dose related. Less frequent but important side effects are development of type 2 diabetes and change in lipid and cholesterol profile. The risk-benefit ratio of the medication for the identified target symptom should be carefully considered and reviewed with the parent or guardian. Providers should obtain baseline height, weight, and waist circumference; observe and examine for tremors and other abnormal involuntary movements; and establish baseline values for hemoglobin A1c (HbA1c), complete blood count (CBC), liver function tests (LFTs), and lipid profile. Antipsychotics can cause QT prolongation leading to ventricular arrhythmias. Therefore, it is important to obtain an electrocardiogram (ECG) if there is a history of cardiac disease or arrhythmia. Medications that affect the cytochrome P-450 isoenzyme pathway (including SSRIs) may increase the neuroleptic plasma concentration and increase risk of QTc prolongation.

In addition to the above concerns, postmarketing clinical use has demonstrated significant reports of hyperglycemia and diabetes mellitus. Table 7–16 presents the currently recommended monitoring calendar. Baseline and ongoing evaluations of significant markers are considered standard clinical practice. It is important to mention other side effects, which include irregular menses, gynecomastia, and galactorrhea due to increased prolactin, sexual dysfunction, photosensitivity, rashes, lowered seizure threshold, hepatic dysfunction, and blood dyscrasias.

Other troublesome side effects of antipsychotics include dystonia, akathisia (characterized by an urge to be in constant

Table 7–16. Health monitoring and antipsychotics.

Baseline	After Initiation			Thereafter[a]		
	4 wk	8 wk	12 wk	Quarterly	Annually	q5y
Personal/family history					✓	
Weight (BMI)	✓	✓	✓	✓		
Waist circumference					✓	
BP			✓		✓	
Fasting blood sugar			✓		✓	
Fasting lipid profile			✓			✓

[a]More frequent assessments may be warranted based on clinical status.

motion and difficulty sitting still), pseudoparkinsonism, and tardive dyskinesia (TD). These side effects typically occur in a stepwise fashion and are also dose related. The first three are reversible and typically are relieved by anticholinergic agents, such as benztropine (Cogentin) and diphenhydramine, or β-blockers, specifically for akathisia. The risk of TD is small in patients on atypical antipsychotics and those on conventional antipsychotics for less than 6 months. There are two FDA-approved medications for TD (ie, valbenazine and deutetrabenazine); however, the recommendation is to either lower the dose of the offending agent or switch to an alternative. Withdrawal dyskinesias are reversible movement disorders that appear following withdrawal of neuroleptic medications. Dyskinetic movements develop within 1–4 weeks after withdrawal of the drug and may persist for months.

A severe side effect of antipsychotics is NMS. NMS is a very rare medical emergency primarily associated with the conventional antipsychotics, although it has also been reported with atypical antipsychotics. It is manifested by severe muscular rigidity, mental status changes, fever, autonomic lability, and myoglobinemia. NMS can occur without muscle rigidity in patients taking atypical antipsychotics and should be considered in the differential diagnosis of any patient on antipsychotics who presents with high fever and altered mental status. Mortality as high as 30% has been reported. Treatment includes immediate medical assessment and withdrawal of the neuroleptic and may require transfer to an intensive care unit.

The patient should be examined at least every 3 months for side effects, including observation for TD using the Abnormal Involuntary Movement Scale (AIMS), blood pressure, weight gain, abdominal circumference, dietary and exercise habits, and, if indicated, fasting blood glucose and lipid panels. In cases of significant weight gain or abnormal laboratory values, patients should either be switched to an agent with a decreased risk for these adverse events or should receive specific treatments for the adverse events when discontinuation of the offending agent is not possible. In general, a child and adolescent psychiatrist should evaluate children with psychosis, initiate treatment and refer back to the pediatrician once symptoms are adequate control.

▶ **Other Considerations**

Antipsychotics are also used for acute mania and as adjuncts to antidepressants in the treatment of psychotic depression (with delusions or hallucinations). Antipsychotics may also be used cautiously in refractory PTSD, in refractory OCD, and in individuals with markedly aggressive behavioral problems unresponsive to other interventions. In some instances, they may be useful for the body image distortion and irrational fears about food and weight gain associated with anorexia nervosa.

▶ **Prognosis**

Schizophrenia is a chronic disorder with exacerbations and remissions of psychotic symptoms. Generally, earlier onset (prior to age 13 years), poor premorbid functioning (oddness or eccentricity), and predominance of negative symptoms (withdrawal, apathy, or flat affect) over positive symptoms (hallucinations or paranoia) predict more severe disability. Later age of onset, normal social and school functioning prior to onset, and predominance of positive symptoms are associated with better outcomes and life adjustment to the illness.

The American Academy has a practice parameter regarding the use of atypical antipsychotics in youth available at https://www.aacap.org/App_Themes/AACAP/docs/practice_parameters/Atypical_Antipsychotic_Medications_Web.pdf.

OTHER PSYCHIATRIC CONDITIONS

Several psychiatric conditions are covered elsewhere in this book. Refer to the following chapters for detailed discussion:

- ADHD: see Chapter 3.
- Autism and pervasive developmental disorders: see Chapter 3.
- Enuresis and encopresis: see Chapter 3.
- Eating disorders: see Chapter 6.

- Intellectual disability/mental retardation: see Chapter 3.
- Substance abuse: see Chapter 5.
- Sleep disorders: see Chapter 3.
- Tourette syndrome and tic disorders: see Chapter 25.

REFERENCES

Anxiety

Anxiety and Depression Association of America: https://adaa.org/.

Beesdo-Baum K, Knappe S: Developmental epidemiology of anxiety disorder. Child Adolesc Psychiatr Clin N Am 2012;21(3):457–478 doi: 10.1016/j.chc.2012.05.001 [PMID: 22800989].

Gandhi B, Cheek S, Campo JV: Anxiety in the pediatric medical setting. Child Adolesc Psychiatr Clin N Am 2012;21(3):643–653 [PMID: 22800999].

Ginsburg GS, et al: Results From the Child/Adolescent Anxiety Multimodal Extended Long-Term Study (CAMELS): Primary anxiety outcomes. J Am Acad Child Adolesc Psychiatry 2018;57(7):471–480. doi:10.1016/j.jaac.2018.03.017.

Ginsberg GS, et al: Remission after acute treatment in children and adolescents with anxiety disorders: findings from the CAMS. J Consult Clin Psychol 2011;79(6):806–813 [PMID: 22122292].

Mohatt J, Bennett SM, Walkup JT: Treatment of separation, generalized and social anxiety disorders in youths. Am J Psychiatry 2014;171(7):741–748 [PMID: 24874020].

Strawn JR, Sakolsky DJ, Rynn MA: Psychopharmacologic treatment of children and adolescents with anxiety disorders. Child Adolesc Psychiatr Clin N Am 2012;21(3):527–539 [PMID: 22800992].

Walkup JT, et al: Cognitive behavioral therapy, sertraline, or a combination in childhood anxiety. New Engl J Med 2008;359:2753–2766. Epub 2008/11/01. doi: 10.1056/NEJMoa0804633 [PMID: 18974308].

Attention-Deficit/Hyperactivity Disorder

ADHD Medication Guide: Cohen Children's Medical Center. http://www.adhdmedicationguide.com/

American Academy of Pediatrics: Implementing the key action statements: an algorithm and explanation for process of care for the evaluation, diagnosis, treatment, and monitoring of ADHD in children and adolescents. https://pediatrics.aappublications.org/content/suppl/2011/10/11/peds.2011-2654.DC1/zpe611117822p.pdf

Cortese S, et al: Comparative efficacy and tolerability of medications for attention-deficit hyperactivity disorder in children, adolescents, and adults: a systematic review and network meta-analysis. Lancet Psychiatry 2018;5(9):727–738. doi: 10.10/16/S2215-0366(18)30269-4.

Daughton JM, Kratochvil CJ: Review of ADHD pharmacotherapies: advantages, disadvantages, and clinical pearls. J Am Acad Child Adolesc Psychiatry 2009;48(3):240–248 [PMID: 19242289].

"FDA permits marketing of first medical device for treatment of ADHD." (April 19, 2019). U.S. Food & Drug Administration. https://www.fda.gov/news-events/press-announcements/fda-permits-marketing-first-medical-device-treatment-adhd.

Fay TB, Alpert MA: Cardiovascular effects of drugs used to treat attention-deficit/hyperactivity disorder: part 2: impact on cardiovascular events and recommendations for evaluation and monitoring. Cardiol Rev 2019a;27(4):173–178. doi:10.1097/CRD.0000000000000234.

Fay TB, Alpert MA: Cardiovascular effects of drugs used to treat attention-deficit/hyperactivity disorder: part 1: epidemiology, pharmacology, and impact on hemodynamics and ventricular repolarization. Cardiol Rev 2019b;27(3):113–121. doi:10.1097/CRD.0000000000000233.

Goode AP, et al: Nonpharmacologic treatments for attention-deficit/hyperactivity disorder: a systematic review. Pediatrics 2018;141(6). doi:10.1542/peds.2018-0094.

Jensen PS, et al: Findings from the NIMH Multimodal Treatment Study of ADHD (MTA): implications and applications for primary care providers. J Dev Behav Pediatr 2001;22(1):60–73 [PMID: 11265923].

Riddle M: New findings from the preschoolers with attention-deficit/hyperactivity disorder treatment study (PATS). J Child Adolesc Psychopharmacol 2007;17(5):543–546.

Bipolar Disorder

Birmaher B, et al: Four-year longitudinal course of children and adolescents with bipolar spectrum disorders: the Course and Outcome of Bipolar Youth (COBY) study. Am J Psychiatry 2009;166(7):795–804. doi:10.1176/appi.ajp.2009.08101569.

Leibenluft E: Severe mood dysregulation, irritability, and the diagnostic boundaries of bipolar disorder in youths. Am J Psychiatry 2011;168(2):129–142. doi:10.1176/appi.ajp.2010.10050766.

Miklowitz DJ, et al: Family-focused treatment for adolescents with bipolar disorder: results of a 2-year randomized trial. Arch Gen Psychiatry 2008;65(9):1053–1061 [PMID: 18762591].

Miklowitz DJ, Chung B: Family-focused therapy for bipolar disorder: reflections on 30 years of research. Fam Process 2016;55(3):483–499. doi:10.1111/famp.12237.

Shain BN; Committee on Adolescence: Collaborative role of the pediatrician in the diagnosis and management of bipolar disorder in adolescents. Pediatrics 2012;130(6):e1725–e1742. doi:10.1542/peds.2012-2756.

Depression

Brent D, et al: Switching to another SSRI or to venlafaxine with or without cognitive behavioral therapy for adolescents with SSRI-resistant depression: the TORDIA randomized controlled trial. JAMA 2008;299(8):901–913. doi: 299/8/901 [pii]10.1001/jama.299.8.901.

Cheung AH, Zuckerbrot RA, Jensen PS, Laraque D, Stein REK; GLAD-PC Steering Group: Guidelines for Adolescent Depression in Primary Care (GLAD-PC): part II. Treatment and ongoing management. Pediatrics 2018;141(3):e20174082. doi: 10.1542/peds.2017-4082.

Depression Resource Center. American Academy of Child & Adolescent Psychiatry: https://www.aacap.org/AACAP/Families_and_Youth/Resource_Centers/Depression_Resource_Center/Depression%20Resource%20Center.aspx.

Guidelines for Adolescent Depression in Primary Care (GLAD-PC) Toolkit: The REACH Institute. http://www.gladpc.org/.

Kodish I, Richardson L, Schlesinger A: Collaborative and integrated care for adolescent depression. Child Adolesc Psychiatr Clin N Am 2019;28(3):315–325. doi:10.1016/j.chc.2019.02.003.

March J, et al: Treatments for Adolescents with Depression Study (TADS) Team. Fluoxetine, cognitive-behavioral therapy, and their combination for adolescents with depression: Treatment for Adolescents With Depression Study (TADS) randomized controlled trial. JAMA 2004;292(7):807–820. doi:10.1001/jama.292.7.807.

Zuckerbrot RA, et al: Guidelines for Adolescent Depression in Primary Care (GLAD-PC): Part I. Practice preparation, identification, assessment, and initial management. Pediatrics 2018;141(3). doi:10.1542/peds.2017-4081.

Epidemiology of Psychiatric Disorders

Bitsko RH, et al: Health care, family, and community factors associated with mental, behavioral, and developmental disorders in early childhood—United States, 2011–2012. MMWR Morb Mortal Wkly Rep 2016;65(9):221–226 [PMID: 26963052].

Costello EJ, Egger H, Angold A: 10-year research update review: the epidemiology of child and adolescent psychiatric disorders: I. Methods and public health burden. J Am Acad Child Adolesc Psychiatry 2005;44:972–986 [PMID: 16175102].

Costello EJ, Foley DL, Angold A 10-year research update review: the epidemiology of child and adolescent psychiatric disorders: II. Developmental epidemiology. J Am Acad Child Adolesc Psychiatry 2006;45(1):8–25 [PMID: 16327577] doi: 10.1097/01.chi.0000184929.41423.c0.

Excoriation Disorder

Grant JE, et al: N-Acetylcysteine in the treatment of excoriation disorder: a randomized clinical trial. JAMA Psychiatry 2016;73(5):490–496 [PMID: 27007062].

Selles RR, McGuire JF, Small BJ, Storch EA: A systematic review and meta-analysis of psychiatric treatments for excoriation (skin-picking) disorder. Gen Hosp Psychiatry 2016;41:29–37 [PMID: 27143352].

Integrated Collaborative Care

Asarnow JR, Rozenman M, Wiblin J, Zeltzer L: Integrated medical-behavioral care compared with usual primary care for child and adolescent behavioral health: a meta-analysis. JAMA Pediatrics 2015;169(10):929–937. doi: 10.1001/jamapediatrics.2015.1141 [PMID: 26259143].

Kolko DJ, Campo J, Kilbourne AM, Hart J, Sakolsky D, Wisniewski S: Collaborative care outcomes for pediatric behavioral health problems: a cluster randomized trial. Pediatrics 2014;133(4):e981–e982 [PMID: 24664093].

Meadows T, Valleley R, Haack MK, Thorson R, Evans J: Physician "costs" in providing behavioral health in primary care. Clin Pediatr 2011;50(5):447–455 [PMID: 21196418].

Minkovitz CS, et al: A practice-based intervention to enhance quality of care in the first three years of life: results from the Healthy Steps for Young Children Program. JAMA 2003;290(23):3081–3091 [PMID: 14679271].

Pediatric Integrated Care Resource Center; American Academy of Child and Adolescent Psychiatry. http://integratedcareforkids.org.

Talmi A, Stafford B, Buchholz M: Providing perinatal mental health services in pediatric primary care. Zero to Three 2009; 29(5):10–16.

Wissow LS, van Ginneken N, Chandna J, Rahman A: Integrating children's mental health into primary care. Pediatr Clin North Am 2016;63(1):97–113. doi: 10.1016/j.pcl.2015.08.005 [PMID: 26613691].

Miscellaneous

Adverse Childhood Experiences (ACEs). Centers for Disease Control and Prevention. Violence Prevention: http://www.cdc.gov/violenceprevention/acestudy/.

American Psychiatric Association: Diagnostic and Statistical Manual of Mental Disorders. 5th ed. Washington, DC: American Psychiatric Association; 2013.

Bright Futures: https://www.brightfutures.org/.

Correll CU, Kratochvil CJ, March JS: Developments in pediatric psychopharmacology: Focus on stimulants, antidepressants, and antipsychotics. J Clin Psychiatr 2011;72(5):655–670. doi: 10.4088/JCP.11r07064 [PMID: 21658348].

Dolan MA, Fein JA; Committee on Pediatric Emergency Medicine: Pediatric and adolescent mental health emergencies in the emergency medical services system. Pediatrics 2011;127(5):e1356–e1366. doi: 10.1542/peds.2011-0522 [PMID: 21518712].

Roberts RE, Roberts CR, Xing Y: Prevalence of youth-reported DSM-IV psychiatric disorders among African, European, and Mexican American adolescents. J Am Acad Child Adolesc Psychiatry 2006;45(11):1329–1337. doi: 10.1097/01.chi.0000235076.25038.81 [PMID: 17075355].

The Center of Excellence for Infant and Early Childhood Mental Health Consultation (IECMHC). U.S. Department of Health & Human Services. Substance Abuse and Mental Health Services Administration: https://www.samhsa.gov/iecmhc.

Zero to Three: https://www.zerotothree.org/.

Obsessive-Compulsive Disorder

Franklin ME, et al: Cognitive behavior therapy augmentation of pharmacotherapy in pediatric obsessive-compulsive disorder: the Pediatric OCD Treatment Study II (POTS II) randomized controlled trial. JAMA 2011;306(11):1224–1232 [PMID: 21934055].

Practice parameter for the assessment and treatment of children and adolescents with obsessive-compulsive disorder. J Am Acad Child Adolesc Psychiatry 2012;51(1):98–113. doi: 10.1016/ja.jaac.2011.09.019 [PMID: 22176943].

International OCD Foundation: https://iocdf.org/.

Pediatric OCD Treatment Study (POST) Team: Cognitive-behavior therapy, sertraline, and their combination for children and adolescents with obsessive-compulsive disorder: the Pediatric OCD Treatment Study (POTS) randomized controlled trial. JAMA, 2004;292(16):1969–1976. [PMID: 15507582].

Oppositional Defiant Disorder and Conduct Disorder

Byrd AL, Loeber R, Pardini DA: Understanding desisting and persisting forms of delinquency: the unique contributions of disruptive behavior disorders and interpersonal callousness. J Child Psychol Psychiatry 2012;53(4):371–380. doi:10.1111/j.1469-7610.2011.02504.x [PMID: 22176342].

Facts for Families: Disruptive Mood Dysregulation Disorder. American Academy of Child and Adolescent Psychiatry: http://www.aacap.org/App_Themes/AACAP/Docs/facts_for_families/110_disruptive_mood_dysregulation_disorder.pdf.

Viding E, McCrory EJ: Understanding the development of psychopathy: progress and challenges. Psychol Med 2018;48(4):566–577. doi:10.1017/S0033291717002847 [PMID: 29032773].

Posttraumatic Stress Disorder

Cohen JA, et al; AACAP Work Group on Quality Issues: Practice parameter for the assessment and treatment of children and adolescents with posttraumatic stress disorder. J Am Acad Child Adolesc Psychiatry 2010;49(4):414–430 [PMID: 20410735].

Cohen JA, Mannarino AP: Trauma-focused cognitive behavior therapy for traumatized children and families. Child Adolesc Psychiatri Clin N Am 2015;24(3):557–570. doi:10.1016/j.chc.2015.02.005 [PMID: 26092739].

Keeshin BR, Strawn JR: Psychological and pharmacologic treatment of youth with posttraumatic stress disorder: an evidence-based review. Child Adolesc Psychiatr Clin N Am 2014;23(2):399–411, x. doi:10.1016/j.chc.2013.12.002 [PMID: 24656587].

Ross DA, Arbuckle MR, Travis MJ, Dwyer JB, van Schalkwyk GI, Ressler KJ: An integrated neuroscience perspective on formulation and treatment planning for posttraumatic stress disorder: an educational review. JAMA Psychiatry 2017;74(4):407–415. doi:10.1001/jamapsychiatry.2016.3325 [PMID: 28273291].

Schizophrenia

Fusar-Poli P, McGorry PD, Kane JM: Improving outcomes of first-episode psychosis: an overview. World Psychiatry 2017;16(3):251–265. doi: 10.1002/wps.20446 [PMID: 28941089].

Haddad PM, Correll CU: The acute efficacy of antipsychotics in schizophrenia: a review of recent meta-analyses. Ther Adv Psychopharmacol 2018;8(11):303–318. doi:10.1177/2045125318781475 [PMID: 30344997].

McClellan J, Stock S; American Academy of Child and Adolescent Psychiatry Committee on Quality Issues: Practice parameter for the assessment and treatment of children and adolescents with schizophrenia. J Am Acad Child Adolesc Psychiatry 2013;52(9):976–990. doi: 10.1016/j.jaac.2013.02.008 [PMID: 23972700].

Sikich L, et al: Double-blind comparison of first- and second-generation antipsychotics in early-onset schizophrenia and schizo-affective disorder: findings from the treatment of early-onset schizophrenia spectrum disorders (TEOSS) study. Am J Psychiatry 2008;165(11):1420–1431. doi: appi.ajp.2008.08050756 [PMID: 18794207].

Somatic Disorders

Doss JL, Plioplys S: Pediatric psychogenic nonepileptic seizures: a concise review. Child Adolesc Psychiatr Clin N Am 2018;27(1):53–61. doi:10.1016/j.chc.2017.08.007 [PMID: 29157502].

Herzlinger M, Cerezo C: Functional abdominal pain and related syndromes. Child Adolesc Psychiatr Clin N Am 2018;27(1):15–26. doi:10.1016/j.chc.2017.08.006 [PMID: 29157499].

Suicide

American Foundation for Suicide Prevention: https://afsp.org.

Brent DA, et al; The Treatment of Adolescent Suicide Attempters study (TASA): Predictors of suicidal events in an open treatment trial. J Am Acad Child Adolesc Psychiatry 2009;48(10):987–996. doi: 10.1097/CHI.0b013e3181b5dbe4 [PMID: 19730274].

Cha CB, Franz PJ, M Guzman E, Glenn CR, Kleiman EM, Nock MK: Annual research review: suicide among youth—epidemiology, (potential) etiology, and treatment. J Child Psychol Psychiatry 2018;59(4):460–482. doi: 10.1111/jcpp.12831 [PMID: 29090457].

Greydanus D, Patel D, Pratt H: Suicide risk in adolescents with chronic illness: implications for primary care and specialty pediatric practice: a review. Dev Med Child Neurol 2010;52(12):1083–1087. doi: 10.1111/j.1469-8749.2010.03771.x [PMID: 20813018].

Jed Foundation: https://www.jedfoundation.org/.

National Center for the Prevention of Youth Suicide. American Association of Suicidology: https://www.suicidology.org/ncpys.

Suicide Awareness Voices of Education: https://save.org/.

Suicide Prevention Resource Center: http://www.sprc.org.

Suicide Resources: Centers for Disease Control and Prevention. Violence Prevention. https://www.cdc.gov/violenceprevention/suicide/resources.html.

Wilcox HC, Wyman PA: Suicide prevention strategies for improving population health. Child Adolesc Psychiatr Clin N Am 2016;25(2):219–233. doi:10.1016/j.chc.2015.12.003 [PMID: 26980125].

Zalsman G, et al: Suicide prevention strategies revisited: 10-year systematic review. Lancet Psychiatry 2016;3(7):646–659. doi: 10.1016/S2215-0366(16)30030-X. [PMID: 27289303].

Violence

Age-Related Reactions to a Traumatic Event. The National Child Traumatic Stress Network: https://www.nctsn.org/sites/default/files/resources//age_related_reactions_to_traumatic_events.pdf.

How to Help Kids Feel Safe After Tragedy. PBS Parents: http://nunu.pbs.org/parents/talkingwithkids/news/help-kids-feel-safe.html.

Massachusetts Child Psychiatry Access Project: http://www.mcpap .com/.

School Shootings and Other Traumatic Events: How to Talk to Students: http://www.nea.org/home/72279.htm.

Sood AB, Berkowitz SJ: Prevention of youth violence: a public health approach. Child Adolesc Psychiatr Clin N Am 2016;25(2):243–256. doi:10.1016/j.chc.2015.11.004 [PMID: 26980127].

Talking to Children About Tragedies & Other News Events: https:// www.healthychildren.org/English/family-life/Media/Pages/ Talking-To-Children-About-Tragedies-and-Other-News- Events.aspx.

Talking to Your Children About the Recent Spate of School Shootings. American Psychological Association: https://www .apa.org/topics/violence/school-shooting.

Child Abuse & Neglect

Antonia Chiesa, MD

Andrew P. Sirotnak, MD, FAAP

INTRODUCTION

ESSENTIALS OF DIAGNOSIS & TYPICAL FEATURES

▶ Forms of maltreatment:
- Physical abuse
- Sexual abuse
- Emotional abuse and neglect
- Physical neglect
- Medical care neglect
- Medical child abuse (Munchausen syndrome by proxy)

▶ Common historical features in child physical abuse cases:
- Implausible mechanism provided for an injury
- Discrepant, evolving, or absent history
- Delay in seeking care
- Event or behavior by a child that triggers a loss of control by the caregiver
- History of abuse in the caregiver's childhood
- Inappropriate affect of the caregiver
- Pattern of increasing severity or number of injuries if no intervention
- Social or physical isolation of the child or the caregiver
- Stress or crisis in the family or the caregiver
- Unrealistic expectations of caregiver for the child

In 2017, an estimated 4.1 million referrals were made to child protective service agencies, involving the alleged maltreatment of approximately 7.5 million children. Policies about how to screen incoming calls regarding abuse concerns and how to investigate suspicious cases varies among states. Some states investigate every case that is referred, while others may screen out referrals based on certain criteria. More and more states are using an "alternative response" system to handle screened-in reports that are deemed low or moderate risk. While traditional investigative methods focus on identifying whether a child has been maltreated, these alternative response models prioritize service needs of the family over determining victimization. Data collection strategies have been altered to capture both forms of assessment.

Children 3 years of age and younger have the highest rates of maltreatment. The total number of children confirmed as maltreated by child protective services was estimated to be 674,000 in 2017, yielding an abuse victimization rate of 9.1 per 1000 American children. This statistic is referred to as the "unique count" where a child is counted only once regardless of the number of times the child is substantiated as a victim. Sexual abuse rates continue to decline. Rates for physical abuse increased slightly from the immediate past few years; however, all forms of child maltreatment have declined during the preceding decade. Neglect, again the most common form of abuse, was substantiated in 74.9% of cases, while 18.3% of cases involved physical abuse, and 10% involved sexual abuse. Factors such as an overall reduction in crime rates, and improvements in education, reporting, and system responses have also likely played a role in lower rates of child abuse.

There were 1720 victims of fatal child abuse in 2017 from 50 states, resulting in a rate of 2.32 child abuse deaths per 100,000 children, slightly higher than the 2015. Fatalities occur with relatively low frequency, so rates are sensitive to changes in reporting and fluctuations in child population. The topic has garnered national attention, and in 2016 a national commission created by Congress completed a report outlining recommendations to reduce child deaths from abuse.

Substance abuse, poverty and economic strains, parental capacity and skills, and domestic violence are cited as the most common presenting problems in abusive families. Almost a third of substantiated maltreatment cases include domestic violence as a caregiver risk factor. Abuse and neglect of children are best considered in an ecological perspective, which recognizes the individual, family, social, and psychological influences that come together to contribute to the problem. Children whose parents have substance abuse disorders tend to be reported to child protective services at a younger age than other children due to a potential for maltreatment or a harmful home environment. Opioid and prescription drug misuse and the decriminalization of marijuana may adversely impact safe parenting. Kempe and Helfer termed this the *abusive pattern*, in which the child, the crisis, and the caregiver's potential to abuse are components in the event of maltreatment. This chapter focuses on the knowledge necessary for the recognition, intervention, and follow-up of the more common forms of child maltreatment and highlights the role of pediatric professionals in prevention. As childhood adversity, including maltreatment, has been shown to have serious implications for life long health and wellbeing, the delivery of trauma informed behavioral health treatment is now a standard of care.

Ammerman S, Ryan S, Adelman WP; The Committee on Substance Abuse, The Committee on Adolescence: The impact of marijuana policies on youth: clinical, research, and legal update. Pediatrics 2015;135(3):e769–e785 [PMID: 25624385].

Jacob G, van den Heuvel M, Jama N, Moore AM, Ford-Jones L, Wong PD: Adverse childhood experiences: basics for the paediatrician. Paediatr Child Health 2019;24(1):30–37 [PMID: 30792598].

U.S. Department of Health and Human Services: Administration for Children, Youth, and Families. Child Maltreatment 2017. https://www.acf.hhs.gov/cb/resource/child-maltreatment-2015. Accessed June 19, 2019.

PREVENTION

Physical abuse is preventable in many cases. Extensive experience with an evaluation of high-risk families has shown that home visiting services to families at risk can prevent abuse and neglect of children. These services can be provided by public health nurses or trained paraprofessionals, although better outcomes data are available describing public health nurse intervention. Parent education and primary care providers' anticipatory guidance are also helpful, with attention to handling situations that stress parents (eg, colic, crying behavior, and toilet training), age-appropriate discipline, and general education about child developmental issues. Prevention of abusive injuries perpetrated by nonparent caregivers (eg, babysitters, nannies, and unrelated adults in the home) may be addressed by education and counseling of mothers about safe child care arrangements and choosing nonviolent life partners. Hospital-based prevention programs that teach parents about the dangers of shaking an infant and how to respond to a crying infant have demonstrated some positive results; however, no one effort has been shown to be completely effective.

The prevention of sexual abuse is more difficult. Most efforts in this area involve teaching children to protect themselves and their "private parts" from harm or interference. The age of toilet training is a good time to provide anticipatory guidance to encourage parents to begin this discussion. The most rational approach is to place the burden of responsibility of prevention on the adults who supervise the child and the medical providers rather than on the children themselves. Programs such as Stewards of Children® have been designed to train adults on how to prevent and respond to concerns of child sexual abuse and are an important resource for youth-serving organizations. Knowing the parents' own history of any victimization is important, as the ability to engage in this anticipatory guidance discussion with a provider and their child may be affected by that history. Promoting Internet and social media safety and limiting exposure to sexualized materials and media should be part of this anticipatory guidance. Finally, many resources on this topic for parents can be found in the parenting and health sections of most bookstores.

Efforts to prevent emotional abuse of children have been undertaken through extensive media campaigns. No data are available to assess the effectiveness of this approach. The primary care physician can promote positive, nurturing, and nonviolent behavior in parents. The message that they are role models for a child's behavior is important. Screening for domestic violence during discussions on discipline and home safety can be effective in identifying parents and children at risk. Societal factors can influence a family's capacity to parent and care for a child. Issues of crime and safety within a community, the educational system and even the economy may indirectly affect family functioning.

American Academy of Pediatrics. HealthyChildren.org: http://www.healthychildren.org. Accessed June 19, 2017.

Bair-Merritt MH: Intimate partner violence. Pediatr Rev 2010 Apr;31(4):145–150; quiz 150.10.1542/pir.31-4-145 [PMID: 20360408].

Barr RG et al: Eight-year outcome of implementation of abusive head trauma prevention. Child Abuse Negl 2018;84:106–114 [PMID: 30077049].

Dubowitz H, Lane WG, Semiatin JN, Magder LS, Venepally M, Jans M: The safe environment for every kid model: impact on pediatric primary care professionals. Pediatrics 2011;127: e962–e970 [PMID: 21444590].

Duffee JH, Mendelsohn AL, Kuo AA, Legano LA, Earls MF; Council on Community Pediatrics; Council on Early Childhood; Committee on Child Abuse and Neglect: Early childhood home visiting. Pediatrics 2017;140(3):e20172150 [PMID: 28847981].

CLINICAL FINDINGS

Child maltreatment may occur either within or outside the family. The proportion of intrafamilial to extrafamilial cases varies with the type of abuse as well as the gender and age of the child. Each of the following conditions may exist as separate or concurrent diagnoses.

Recognition of any form of abuse and neglect of children can occur only if child abuse is considered in the differential diagnosis of the child's presenting medical condition. The advent of electronic medical records can make documenting concerns and patterns of maltreatment more accessible for all care team members. The approach to the family should be supportive, nonaccusatory, and empathetic. The individual who brings the child in for care may not have any involvement in the abuse. Approximately one-third of child abuse incidents occur in extrafamilial settings. Nevertheless, the assumption that the presenting caregiver is "nice," combined with the failure to consider the possibility of abuse, can be costly and even fatal. Raising the possibility that a child has been abused is not the same as accusing the caregiver of being the abuser. The health professional who is examining the child can explain to the family that several possibilities might explain the child's injuries or abuse-related symptoms. If the family or presenting caregiver is not involved in the child's maltreatment, they may actually welcome an explanation for the child's symptoms and the subsequent necessary report and investigation.

In all cases of abuse and neglect, a detailed psychosocial history is important because psychosocial factors may indicate risk for or confirm child maltreatment. This history should include information on who lives or visits regularly in the home, other caregivers, domestic violence, substance abuse, and prior family history of physical or sexual abuse. Inquiring about any previous involvement with social services or law enforcement can help to determine risk.

Physical Abuse

Physical abuse of children is most often inflicted by a caregiver or family member but occasionally by a stranger. The most common manifestations include bruises, burns, fractures, head trauma, and abdominal injuries. A small but significant number of unexpected pediatric deaths, particularly in infants and very young children (eg, sudden unexpected infant death), are related to physical abuse.

A. History

The medical diagnosis of physical abuse is based on the presence of a discrepant history, in which the history offered by the caregiver is not consistent with the clinical findings. The discrepancy may exist because the history is absent, partial, changing over time, or simply illogical or improbable. A careful past medical, birth, and family history should also be obtained in order to assess for any other medical condition that might affect the clinical presentation. The presence of a discrepant history should prompt a request for consultation with a multidisciplinary child protection team or a report to the child protective services agency. This agency is mandated by state law to investigate reports of suspected child abuse and neglect. Investigation by social services and possibly law enforcement officers, as well as a home visit, may be required to sort out the circumstances of the child's injuries.

B. Physical Findings

The findings on examination of physically abused children may include abrasions, alopecia (from hair pulling), bites, bruises, burns, dental trauma, fractures, lacerations, ligature marks, or scars. Injuries may be in multiple stages of healing. Bruises in physically abused children are sometimes patterned (eg, belt marks, looped cord marks, or grab or pinch marks) and are typically found over the soft tissue areas of the body. Toddlers or older children typically sustain accidental bruises over bony prominences such as shins and elbows. Any unexplained bruise in an infant not developmentally mobile should be viewed with concern. Of note, the dating of bruises is not reliable and should be approached cautiously. (Child abuse emergencies are listed in Table 8–1.) Lacerations of the frenulum or tongue and bruising of the lips may be associated with force feeding or blunt force trauma. Pathognomonic burn patterns include stocking or glove distribution; immersion burns of the buttocks, sometimes with a "doughnut hole" area of sparing; and branding burns such as with cigarettes or hot objects (eg, grill, curling iron, or lighter). The absence of splash marks or a pattern consistent with spillage may be helpful in differentiating accidental from nonaccidental scald burns.

Head and abdominal trauma may present with signs and symptoms consistent with those injuries. Abusive head trauma (eg, shaken baby syndrome) and abdominal injuries may have no visible findings on examination. Symptoms can be subtle and may mimic other conditions such as gastroenteritis. Studies have documented that cases of inflicted head injury will be missed when practitioners fail to

Table 8–1. Potential child abuse medical emergencies.

Any infant with bruises (especially head, facial, or abdominal), burns, or fractures

Any infant or child younger than 2 y with a history of suspected "shaken baby" head trauma or other inflicted head injury

Any child who has sustained suspicious or known inflicted abdominal trauma

Any child with burns in stocking or glove distribution or in other unusual patterns, burns to the genitalia, and any unexplained burn injury

Any child with disclosure or sign of sexual assault within 48–72 h after the alleged event if the possibility of acute injury is present or if forensic evidence exists consider the diagnosis. The finding of retinal hemorrhages in an infant without an appropriate medical condition (eg, leukemia, congenital infection, or clotting disorder) should raise concern about possible inflicted head trauma. Retinal hemorrhages are not commonly seen after cardiopulmonary resuscitation in either infants or children.

C. Radiologic and Laboratory Findings

Certain radiologic findings are strong indicators of physical abuse. Examples are metaphyseal "corner" or "bucket handle" fractures of the long bones in infants, spiral fracture of the extremities in nonambulatory infants, rib fractures, spinous process fractures, and fractures in multiple stages of healing. Skeletal surveys in children aged 3 years or younger should be performed when a suspicious injury is diagnosed. Computed tomography or magnetic resonance imaging findings of subdural hemorrhage in infants—in the absence of a clear accidental history—are highly correlated with abusive head trauma. Abdominal computed tomography is the preferred test in suspected abdominal trauma. Any infant or very young child with suspected abuse-related head or abdominal trauma should be evaluated immediately by an emergency physician or trauma surgeon.

Coagulation studies and a complete blood cell count with platelets are useful in children who present with multiple or severe bruising in different stages of healing. Hepatic transaminases (ALT/alanine aminotransferase and AST/aspartate aminotransferase) should be used to screen for abdominal injury and transaminase levels greater than 80 IU/L should prompt definitive testing for internal injury. Coagulopathy conditions may confuse the diagnostic picture but can be excluded with a careful history, examination, laboratory screens, and hematologic consultation, if necessary.

American Academy of Pediatrics: *Visual Diagnosis of Child Abuse.* 4th ed. American Academy of Pediatrics; 2016 [USB flash drive].

Anderst JD, Carpenter SL, Abshire TC; American Academy of Pediatrics Section on Hematology Oncology, Committee on Child Abuse and Neglect: Evaluation for bleeding disorders for suspected child physical abuse. Pediatrics 2013 Apr;131(4):e1314–e1322. doi: 10.1542 [PMID: 23530182].

Christian CW, Block R; American Academy of Pediatrics Committee on Child Abuse and Neglect: Abusive head trauma in infants and children. Pediatrics 2009;123(5):1409–1411 [PMID: 19403508]. Reaffirmed March, 2013.

Flaherty EG, Perez-Rossello JM, Levine MA, Hennrikus WL; American Academy of Pediatrics Committee on Child Abuse and Neglect; Section on Radiology; Section on Endocrinology; Section on Orthopaedics; Society for Pediatric Radiology: Evaluating children with fractures for child physical abuse. Pediatrics 2013;131:4 [PMID: 24470642].

Hymel KP; American Academy of Pediatrics Committee on Child Abuse and Neglect; National Association of Medical Examiners: Distinguishing sudden infant death syndrome from child abuse fatalities. Pediatrics 2006;118:421 [PMID:16818592]. Reaffirmed March, 2013.

Kempe AM et al: Patterns of skeletal fractures in child abuse: systematic review. BMJ 2008;337:a1518 [PMID: 18832412].

Sheets LK, Leach ME, Koszewski IJ, Lessmeier AM, Nugent M, Simpson P: Sentinel injuries in infants evaluated for child physical abuse. Pediatrics 2013;131(4):701–707 [PMID: 23478861].

Sexual Abuse

Sexual abuse is defined as the engaging of dependent, developmentally immature children in sexual activities that they do not fully comprehend and to which they cannot give consent, or activities that violate the laws and taboos of a society. It includes all forms of incest, sexual assault or rape, and pedophilia. This includes fondling, oral-genital-anal contact, all forms of intercourse or penetration, exhibitionism, voyeurism, exploitation, or prostitution, and the involvement of children in the production of pornography. Over the past decade, there has been a small downward trend nationally in rates of child sexual abuse; however, the exploitation and enticement of children via the Internet and social media and human trafficking cases have gained increases in recognition.

A. History

Sexual abuse may come to the clinician's attention in different ways: (1) The child may be brought in for routine care or for an acute problem, and sexual abuse may be suspected by the medical professional as a result of the history or the physical examination. (2) The parent or caregiver, suspecting that the child may have been sexually abused, may bring the child to the health care provider and request an examination to rule in or rule out abuse. (3) The child may be referred by child protective services or the police for an evidentiary examination following either disclosure of sexual abuse by the child or an allegation of abuse by a parent or third party. Table 8–2 lists the common presentations of child sexual abuse. Certain high-risk behaviors should prompt recognition of possible human trafficking, including substance abuse, runaway activity, multiple sexual partners, law enforcement history, or presenting to care without identification. If suspected, this should be addressed confidentially with the patient. It should be emphasized that with the exception of acute trauma, certain sexually transmitted infections (STIs), or forensic laboratory evidence, none of these presentations is specific. The presentations listed should arouse suspicion of the possibility of sexual abuse and lead the practitioner to ask the appropriate questions—again, in a compassionate and nonaccusatory manner. Asking the young child nonleading, age-appropriate questions is important and is often best handled by the most experienced interviewer after a report is made. Community agency protocols may exist for child advocacy centers that help in the investigation of these reports. Concerns expressed about sexual abuse in the context of divorce and custody disputes should be handled in the same manner, with the same objective, nonjudgmental documentation.

Table 8–2. Presentations of sexual abuse.

General or direct statements about sexual abuse
Sexualized knowledge, play, or behavior in developmentally
    immature children
Sexual abuse of other children by the victim
Behavioral changes
    Sleep disturbances (eg, nightmares and night terrors)
    Appetite disturbances (eg, anorexia, bulimia)
    Depression, social withdrawal, anxiety
    Aggression, temper tantrums, impulsiveness
    Neurotic or conduct disorders, phobias or avoidant behaviors
    Guilt, low self-esteem, mistrust, feelings of helplessness
    Hysterical or conversion reactions
    Suicidal, runaway threats or behavior
    Excessive masturbation
Medical conditions
    Recurrent abdominal pain or frequent somatic complaints
    Genital, anal, or urethral trauma
    Recurrent complaints of genital or anal pain, discharge, bleeding
    Enuresis or encopresis
    Sexually transmitted infections
    Pregnancy
Promiscuity or prostitution, sexual dysfunction, fear of intimacy
School problems or truancy
Substance abuse

The American Academy of Pediatrics has published guidelines for the evaluation of child sexual abuse as well as others relating to child maltreatment.

B. Physical Findings

The genital and anal findings of sexually abused children, as well as the normal developmental changes and variations in prepubertal female hymens, have been described in journal articles and visual diagnosis guides. To maintain a sense of comfort and routine for the patient, the genital examination should be conducted in the context of a full body checkup. For nonsexually active, prepubertal girls, an internal speculum examination is rarely necessary unless there is suspicion of internal injury. The external female genital structures can be well visualized using labial separation and traction with the child in the supine frog leg or knee-chest position. The majority of victims of sexual abuse exhibit no physical findings. The reasons for this include delay in disclosure by the child, abuse that may not cause physical trauma (eg, fondling, oral-genital contact, or exploitation by pornographic photography), or rapid healing of minor injuries such as labial, hymenal, or anal abrasions, contusions, or lacerations. Nonspecific abnormalities of the genital and rectal regions such as erythema, rashes, and irritation may not suggest sexual abuse in the absence of a corroborating history, disclosure, or behavioral changes.

Certain STIs should strongly suggest sexual abuse in prepubertal children. *Neisseria gonorrhoeae* infection or syphilis beyond the perinatal period is diagnostic of sexual abuse.

Chlamydia trachomatis, herpes simplex virus, trichomoniasis, and human papillomavirus are all sexually transmitted, although the course of these potentially perinatally acquired infections may be protracted. Herpes simplex can be transmitted by other means; however, the presence of an infection should prompt a careful assessment for sexual abuse. Risk is higher in children older than five with isolated herpetic genital lesions. In the case of human papillomavirus, an initial appearance of venereal warts beyond the toddler age should prompt a discussion regarding concerns of sexual abuse. Human papillomavirus is a ubiquitous virus and can be spread innocently by caregivers with hand lesions; biopsy and viral typing is rarely indicated and often of limited availability. Finally, sexual abuse must be considered with the diagnosis of *C trachomatis* or human immunodeficiency virus (HIV) infections when other modes of transmission (eg, transfusion or perinatal acquisition) have been ruled out. Postexposure prophylaxis medications for HIV in cases of acute sexual assault should be considered only after assessment of risk of transmission and consultation with an infectious disease expert.

Nucleic acid amplification tests (NAATs) have been used with increasing frequency for screening of STIs in sexual abuse victims, including for children younger than 12 years. For prepubertal children, NAATs can be used for vaginal specimens or urine from girls. If a NAAT is positive, a second confirmatory NAAT test that analyzes an alternate target of the genetic material in the sample or a standard culture is needed. For boys and for extragenital specimens, culture is still the preferred method. Finally, the Centers for Disease Control and Prevention and the AAP Redbook list guidelines for the screening and treatment of STIs in the context of sexual abuse.

C. Examination, Evaluation, and Management

The forensic evaluation of sexually abused children should be performed in a setting that prevents further emotional distress. All the components of a forensic evidence collection kit may not be indicated in the setting of child sexual abuse (as opposed to adult rape cases); the clinical history and exposure risk should guide what specimens are collected. All practitioners should have access to a rape kit, which guides the practitioner through a stepwise collection of evidence and cultures. This should occur in an emergency department or clinic where chain of custody for specimens can be ensured. The most experienced examiner (pediatrician, nurse examiner, or child advocacy center) is preferable. If the history indicates that the adolescent may have had contact with the ejaculate of a perpetrator within 120 hours, a cervical examination to look for semen or its markers (eg, acid phosphatase) should be performed according to established protocols.

Prior to any speculum examination of an assault victim, it is important to consider the child's physiologic and emotional maturation, and whether she has been sexually active or had a speculum examination in the past. A speculum examination in a prepubertal child is rarely indicated unless there is concern for internal injury and in those cases, it is generally advised to perform the examination under anesthesia and with the assistance of gynecology. More important, if there is a history of possible sexual abuse of any child within the past several days, and the child reports a physical complaint or a physical sign is observed (eg, genital or anal bleeding or discharge), the child should be examined for evidence of trauma. Colposcopy may be critical for determining the extent of the trauma and photodocumentation may be helpful in providing documentation for the legal system.

STI screening should include testing for *N gonorrhoeae* and *C trachomatis*, and vaginal secretions evaluated for *Trichomonas*. These infections and bacterial vaginosis are the most frequently diagnosed infections among older girls who have been sexually assaulted. RPR, hepatitis B, and HIV serology should be drawn at baseline and repeated up to 6 months after last contact. Pregnancy testing should be done as indicated.

Acute sexual assault cases that involve trauma or transmission of body fluid should have STI prophylaxis. Using adult doses of ceftriaxone (250 mg IM in a single dose), metronidazole (2 g orally in a single dose), and azithromycin (1 g orally in a single dose) should be offered when older or adolescent patients present for evaluation. (Pediatric treatment and dosing is calculated by weight and can be found in standard references.) Hepatitis B vaccination should be administered to patients if they have not been previously vaccinated and there should be consideration to providing hepatitis B immunoglobulin in certain high-risk cases. No effective prophylaxis is available for hepatitis C. Evaluating the perpetrator for a STI, if possible, can help determine risk exposure and guide prophylaxis. HIV prophylaxis should be considered in certain circumstances (see Chapter 44). For postpubertal girls, contraception should be given if rape abuse occurred within 120 hours.

Although it is often difficult for persons to complete recommended follow-up examinations weeks after an assault, such examinations are essential to detect new infections, complete immunization with hepatitis B vaccination if needed, and continue psychological support.

Centers for Disease Control and Prevention. Sexually Transmitted Diseases Treatment Guidelines 2015: http://www.cdc.gov/std/tg2015. Accessed June 19, 2019.

Chiesa A, Goldson E: Child sexual abuse. Pediatr Rev 2017;38(3):105–118 [PMID: 28250071].

Girardet RG et al: HIV post-exposure prophylaxis in children and adolescents presenting for reported sexual assault. Child Abuse Negl 2009;33:173 [PMID: 19324415].

Greenbaum VJ, Dodd M, McCracken C: A short screening tool to identify victims of child sex trafficking in the health care setting. Pediatr Emerg Care 2018 Jan;34(1):33–37 [PMID: 26599463].

Noll JG, Shenk CE: Teen birth rates in sexually abused and neglected females. Pediatrics 2013;131:e1181–e1187 [PMID: 23530173].

Thackeray et al: Forensic evidence collection and DNA identification in acute child sexual assault. Pediatrics 2011;128:227–232 [PMID: 21788217].

Emotional Abuse & Neglect

Emotional or psychological abuse has been defined as the rejection, ignoring, criticizing, isolation, or terrorizing of children, all of which have the effect of eroding their self-esteem. The most common form is verbal abuse or denigration. Children who witness domestic violence should be considered emotionally abused, as a growing body of literature has shown the negative effects of intimate partner violence on child development.

The most common feature of emotional neglect is the absence of normal parent-child attachment and a subsequent inability to recognize and respond to an infant's or child's needs. A common manifestation of emotional neglect in infancy is nutritional (nonorganic) failure to thrive. Emotionally neglectful parents appear to have an inability to recognize the physical or emotional states of their children. For example, an emotionally neglectful parent may ignore an infant's cry if the cry is perceived incorrectly as an expression of anger. This misinterpretation leads to inadequate nutrition and failure to thrive.

Emotional abuse may cause nonspecific symptoms in children. Loss of self-esteem or self-confidence, sleep disturbances, somatic symptoms (eg, headaches and stomach aches), hypervigilance, or avoidant or phobic behaviors (eg, school refusal or running away) may be presenting complaints. These complaints may also be seen in children who experience domestic violence. Emotional abuse can occur in the home or day care, school, sports team, or other settings.

Physical Neglect & Failure to Thrive

Physical neglect is the failure to provide the necessary food, clothing, and shelter and a safe environment in which children can grow and develop. Although often associated with poverty, physical neglect involves a more serious problem than just lack of resources. There is often a component of emotional neglect and either a failure or an inability, intentionally or otherwise, to recognize and respond to the needs of the child.

A. History

Even though in 2017 neglect was confirmed for over three-quarters of all victims, neglect is not easily documented on history. Given that neglect is the most common form of abuse, providers should be proactive in their approach to recognition and treatment. Physical neglect—which must be differentiated from the deprivations of poverty—will be present even after adequate social services have been provided to families in need. The clinician must evaluate the psychosocial history, family dynamics, and parental mental health, when neglect is a consideration and is in a unique position to intervene when warning signs first emerge. A careful social services evaluation of the home and entire family may be required. The primary care provider must work closely with a social service agency and explain the known medical information to help guide their investigation and decision-making.

The history offered in cases of growth failure (failure to thrive) is often discrepant with the physical findings. Infants who have experienced a significant deceleration in growth may not be receiving adequate amounts or appropriate types of food despite the dietary history provided. Medical conditions causing poor growth in infancy and early childhood can be ruled out with a detailed history and physical examination with minimal laboratory tests. A psychosocial history may reveal maternal depression, family chaos or dysfunction, or other previously unknown social risk factors (eg, substance abuse, violence, poverty, or psychiatric illness). Placement of the child with another caregiver is usually followed by a dramatic weight gain. Hospitalization of the severely malnourished patient is sometimes required, but most cases are managed on an outpatient basis.

B. Physical Findings

Infants and children with nonorganic failure to thrive have a relative absence of subcutaneous fat in the cheeks, buttocks, and extremities. Other conditions associated with poor nutrient and vitamin intake may be present. If the condition has persisted for some time, these patients may also appear and act depressed. Older children who have been chronically emotionally neglected may also have short stature (ie, deprivation dwarfism). The head circumference is usually normal in cases of nonorganic failure to thrive. Microcephaly may indicate a prenatal condition, congenital disease, or chronic nutritional deprivation and increases the likelihood of more serious and possibly permanent developmental delay.

C. Radiologic and Laboratory Findings

Children with failure to thrive or malnutrition may not require an extensive workup. Assessment of the patient's growth curve, as well as careful plotting of subsequent growth parameters after treatment, is critical. Complete blood cell count, urinalysis, electrolyte panel, and thyroid and liver function tests and 25 dihydroxy Vitamin D levels are sufficient screening. Newborn screening should be documented as usual. Other tests should be guided by any aspect of the clinical history that points to a previously undiagnosed condition. A skeletal survey and head computed tomography scan may be helpful if concurrent physical abuse is suspected. The best screening method, however, is placement

in a setting in which the child can be fed and monitored. Hospital or foster care placement may be required. Weight gain may not occur for several days to a week in severe cases.

Medical Care Neglect

Medical care neglect is failure to provide the needed treatment to infants or children with life-threatening illness or other serious or chronic medical conditions. This diagnosis should be considered when caregivers have a clear understanding of the child's condition and the consequences of not providing the recommended treatment, and the provider has made an attempt to address barriers to care. Many states have repealed laws that supported religious exemptions as reason for not seeking medical care for sick children.

Medical Child Abuse

Previously referred to as Munchausen syndrome by proxy, medical child abuse is the preferred term for a relatively unusual clinical scenario in which a caregiver seeks inappropriate and unnecessary medical care for a child. Oftentimes, the caregiver either simulates or creates the symptoms or signs of illness in a child. However, the use of the term medical child abuse emphasizes harm caused to the child as opposed to the psychopathology or motivation of the caregiver. Cases can be complicated, and a detailed review of all medical documentation and a multidisciplinary approach is required. Fatal cases have been reported.

A. History

Children may present with the signs and symptoms of whatever illness is factitiously produced or simulated. The child can present with a long list of medical problems or often bizarre, recurrent complaints. Repetitive visits, persistent doctor shopping, and enforced invalidism (eg, not accepting that the child is healthy and reinforcing that the child is somehow ill) are also described in the original definition of Munchausen syndrome by proxy.

B. Physical Findings

They may be actually ill or, more often, are reported to be ill and have a normal clinical appearance. Among the most common reported presentations are recurrent apnea, dehydration from induced vomiting or diarrhea, sepsis when contaminants are injected into a child, change in mental status, fever, gastrointestinal bleeding, and seizures.

C. Radiologic and Laboratory Findings

Recurrent polymicrobial sepsis (especially in children with indwelling catheters), recurrent apnea, chronic dehydration of unknown cause, or other highly unusual unexplained laboratory findings should raise the suspicion of Munchausen syndrome by proxy. Toxicological testing may also be useful.

Flaherty EG, MacMillan HL; American Academy of Pediatrics; Committee on Child Abuse and Neglect: Caregiver-fabricated illness in a child: a manifestation of child maltreatment. Pediatrics 2013;32:3 [PMID: 23979088].

Hibbard R: Clinical report: psychological maltreatment. Pediatrics 2012 Oct;130(2):372–378.

Hymel KP; American Academy of Pediatrics; Committee on Child Abuse and Neglect: When is lack of supervision neglect? Pediatrics 2006;118:1296 [PMID:16951030].

Larson-Nath C, Biank VF: Clinical review of failure to thrive in pediatric patients. Pediatr Ann 2016;45(2);e46–e49 [PMID 26878182].

Roesler T, Jenny C: *Medical Child Abuse: Beyond Munchausen Syndrome by Proxy.* American Academy of Pediatrics; 2009.

DIFFERENTIAL DIAGNOSIS

The differential diagnosis for abuse and neglect may be straightforward (ie, traumatic vs nontraumatic injury). It can also be more elusive as in the case of multiple injuries that may raise concern for an underlying medical condition or in situations where complex, but nonspecific behavior changes or physical symptoms reflect the emotional impact of maltreatment.

The differential diagnosis of all forms of physical abuse can be considered in the context of a detailed trauma history, family medical history, radiographic findings, and laboratory testing. The diagnosis of osteogenesis imperfecta or other collagen or bone disorders, for example, may be considered in the child with skin and joint findings or multiple fractures with or without the classic radiographic presentation and is best made in consultation with a geneticist, an orthopedic surgeon, and a radiologist. Trauma—accidental or inflicted—leads the differential diagnosis list for subdural hematomas. Coagulopathy; disorders of copper, amino acid, or organic acid metabolism (eg, Menkes syndrome and glutaric acidemia type 1); chronic or previous central nervous system infection; birth trauma; or congenital central nervous system malformation (eg, arteriovenous malformations or cerebrospinal fluid collections) may need to be ruled out in some cases. It should be recognized, however, that children with these rare disorders can also be victims of abuse or neglect.

There are medical conditions that may be misdiagnosed as sexual abuse. When abnormal physical examination findings are noted, knowledge of these conditions is imperative to avoid misinterpretation. The differential diagnosis includes vulvovaginitis, lichen sclerosus, dermatitis, labial adhesions, congenital urethral or vulvar disorders, Crohn disease, and accidental straddle injuries to the labia. In most circumstances, these can be ruled out by careful history and examination.

TREATMENT

A. Management

Physical abuse injuries, STIs, and medical sequelae of neglect should be treated immediately. Children with failure to thrive related to emotional and physical neglect need to be placed in a setting in which they can be fed and cared for. Likewise, the child in danger of recurrent abuse or neglect needs to be placed in a safe environment. Cases can be complicated and psychosocial difficulties are common; therefore, a multidisciplinary approach that works with the family to engage in solving their own problems is helpful. Cooperation and coordination with social work and mental health colleagues are crucial. Given the developmental and emotional implications, prompt referral to mental health resources for any patient with a history of child abuse or neglect is crucial; although not every child with a history of maltreatment will need long-term mental health treatment. There has been significant progress made in identifying, researching, and implementing effective, evidence-based treatment of child maltreatment, especially in the area of treatment for emotional trauma. There are also effective interventions for improving parenting and attachment problems that are common in child maltreatment cases. Pediatricians should be aware of community partners and resources to help families in need of services.

B. Reporting

In the United States, clinicians and many other professionals who come in contact with or care for children are mandated reporters. If abuse or neglect is suspected, a report must be made to the local or state agency designated to investigate such matters. In most cases, this will be the child protective services agency. Law enforcement agencies may also receive such reports. The purpose of the report is to permit professionals to gather the information needed to determine whether the child's environment (eg, home, school, day care setting, or foster home) is safe. Recent studies document physician barriers to reporting, but providers should be mindful that good faith reporting is a legal requirement for any suspicion of abuse. Failure to report concerns may have legal ramifications for the provider or serious health and safety consequences for the patient. Many hospitals and communities make child protection teams or consultants available when there are questions about the diagnosis and management in a child abuse case. A listing of child abuse pediatric consultants is available from the American Academy of Pediatrics.

Finally, communication with social services, case management, and careful follow-up by primary care providers is crucial to ensuring ongoing safety of child.

Flaherty E, Legano L, Idzerda S; Council on Child Abuse and Neglect: Ongoing pediatric health care for the child who has been maltreated. Pediatrics 2019;143(3):e20190284 [PMID: 30886109].

Garner AS et al; Committee on Psychosocial Aspects of Child and Family Health; Committee on Early Childhood, Adoption, and Dependent Care; Section on Developmental and Behavioral Pediatrics: Early childhood adversity, toxic stress, and the role of the pediatrician: translating developmental science into lifelong health. Pediatrics 2012;129;e224–e231 [PMID: 22201148].

National Child Traumatic Stress Network: http://www.nctsn.org/. Accessed June 24, 2019.

Sege R et al: To report or not to report: examination of the initial primary care management of suspicious childhood injuries. Acad Pediatr 2011;11(6):460–466 [PMID: 21996468].

Sege RD, Amaya-Jackson L; American Academy of Pediatrics Committee on Child Abuse and Neglect, Council on Foster Care, Adoption and Kinship Care; American Academy of Child and Adolescent Psychiatry Committee on Child Maltreatment and Violence; National Center for Child Traumatic Stress: Clinical considerations related to the behavioral manifestations of child maltreatment. Pediatrics 2017;139(4):e20170100 [PMID: 28320870].

PROGNOSIS

Depending on the extent of injury resulting from physical or sexual abuse, the prognosis for complete recovery varies. Serious physical abuse that involves head injury, multisystem trauma, severe burns, or abdominal trauma carries significant morbidity and mortality risk. Hospitalized children with a diagnosis of child abuse or neglect have longer stays and are more likely to die. Long-term medical and developmental consequences are common. For example, children who suffer brain damage related to abusive head injury can have significant neurologic impairment, such as cerebral palsy, vision problems, epilepsy, microcephaly, and learning disorders. Other injuries like minor bruises or burns, fractures, and even injuries resulting from penetrating genital trauma can heal well and with no sequelae.

The emotional and psychological outcomes for child victims are often the most detrimental. Research demonstrates that there are clear neurobiologic effects of child maltreatment and other types of early childhood toxic stress. Physiologic changes to the brain can adversely affect the mental and physical health development of children for decades. Adverse childhood experiences (ACEs) have been associated with chronic adult health problems, suicide, alcoholism and drug abuse, anxiety and depression, violence, and early death. The more ACEs in an individual's background, the higher the risk for these negative outcomes. Despite the potential consequences, the effects of maltreatment can be mitigated. There are effective, evidence-based interventions for child maltreatment. Some children may need extra help addressing emotional regulation, coping skills, and rebuilding trust. The primary care provider plays an important role in assuring appropriate medical and mental health care for maltreated children and families, and in advocating for victims across the child and young adult lifespan.

Centers for Disease Control and Prevention: Adverse childhood experiences study. http://www.cdc.gov/violenceprevention/acestudy. Accessed June 24, 2019.

Child Welfare Information Gateway: Long-term consequences of child abuse and neglect. https://www.childwelfare.gov/pubpdfs/long_term_consequences.pdf. Accessed June 24, 2019.

Office of the Administration for Children and Families. Within Our Reach: A National Strategy to Reduce Child Abuse Fatalities. https://www.acf.hhs.gov/cb/resrouce/cecanf-final-report. Accessed June 24, 2019.

Ambulatory & Office Pediatrics

Meghan Treitz, MD

Daniel Nicklas, MD

David Fox, MD

INTRODUCTION

Pediatric ambulatory outpatient services provide children and adolescents with preventive health care and acute and chronic care management services and consultations. In this chapter, special attention is given to the pediatric history and physical examination, normal developmental stages, screening laboratories, and a number of common pediatric issues.

The development of a physician-patient-parent relationship is crucially important if the patient and parent are to effectively confide their concerns. This relationship develops over time, with regular visits, and is facilitated by the continuity of clinicians and other staff members. This clinical relationship is based on trust that develops as a result of several experiences in the context of the office visit. Perhaps the greatest factor facilitating the relationship is for patients or parents to experience advice as valid and effective. Anticipatory guidance should be age-appropriate and timely in order to be most helpful. Important skills include choosing vocabulary that communicates understanding and competence, demonstrating commitment of time and attention to the concern, and showing respect for areas that the patient or parent does not wish to address (assuming that there are no concerns relating to physical or sexual abuse or neglect). Parents and patients expect that their concerns will be managed confidentially and that the clinician understands and sympathizes with those concerns. The effective physician-patient-parent relationship is one of the most satisfying aspects of ambulatory pediatrics.

Tanner JL, Stein MT, Olson LM, Frintner MP, Radecki L: Reflections on well-child care practice: a national study of pediatric clinicians. Pediatrics 2009 Sep;124(3):849–857 [Epub 2009 Aug 10] [PMID: 19706587].

▼ PEDIATRIC HISTORY

A unique feature of pediatrics is that the history represents an amalgam of parents' objective reporting of facts (eg, fever for 4 days), parents' subjective interpretation of their child's symptoms (eg, infant crying interpreted by parents as abdominal pain), and for older children their own history of events. Parents and patients may provide a specific and detailed history, or a vague history that necessitates more focused probing. Parents may or may not be able to distinguish whether symptoms are caused by organic illness or a psychological concern. Understanding the family and its hopes for and concerns about the child can help in the process of distinguishing organic, emotional, and/or behavioral conditions, thus minimizing unnecessary testing and intervention.

Although the parents' concerns need to be understood, it is essential also to obtain as much of the history as possible directly from the patient. Direct histories not only provide firsthand information but also give the child a degree of control over a potentially threatening situation and may reveal important information about the family.

Obtaining a comprehensive pediatric history is time consuming. Many offices provide questionnaires for parents to complete before the clinician sees the child. Data from questionnaires can make an outpatient visit more productive, allowing the physician to address problems in detail while more quickly reviewing areas that are not of concern. Questionnaires may be more productive than face-to-face interviews in revealing sensitive parts of the history. Developmental and mental health screening saves provider time and the results when reviewed with the parent or family member can yield critical information. However, failure to review and assimilate this information prior to the interview may cause a parent or patient to feel that the time and effort have been wasted.

Elements of the history that will be useful over time should be readily accessible in the medical record, including demographic data, a problem list, chronic medications, allergies, and previous hospitalizations. Immunizations, including all data required by the National Childhood Vaccine Injury Act, should also be documented.

The components of a comprehensive pediatric history are listed in Table 9–1. The information should, ideally, be obtained at the first office visit. Items 8 and 9, and a focused review of systems (ROS), are dealt with at each acute or chronic care visit. The entire list should be reviewed and augmented with relevant updates at each health supervision visit.

▼ PEDIATRIC PHYSICAL EXAMINATION

During the pediatric physical examination, time must be taken to allow the patient to become familiar with the examiner. Interactions and instructions help the child understand what is occurring and what is expected. A gentle, friendly manner and a quiet voice help establish a setting that yields a nonthreatening physical examination. The examiner should take into consideration the need for a quiet child, the extent of trust established, and the possibility of an emotional response (crying!) when deciding the order in which the child's organ systems are examined. Unpleasant procedures (eg, otoscopic examination) should be deferred until the end

Table 9–1. Components of the pediatric historical database.[a]

1. Demographic data	Patient's name and nickname, date of birth, social security number, sex, race, parents' names (first and last), siblings' names, and payment mechanism.
2. Problem list	Major or significant problems, including dates of onset and resolution.
3. Allergies	Triggering allergen, nature of the reaction, treatment needed, and date allergy was diagnosed.
4. Chronic medications	Name, concentration, dose, and frequency of chronically used medications.
5. Birth history	Maternal health during pregnancy such as bleeding, infections, smoking, alcohol and any medications, complications of pregnancy; duration of labor; form of delivery; and labor complications. Infant's birth weight, gestational age, Apgar scores, and problems in the neonatal period.
6. Screening procedures	Results of newborn screening, vision and hearing screening, any health screen, or screening laboratory tests. (Developmental screening results are maintained in the development section; see item 14.)
7. Immunizations	Type(s) of vaccine, date administered, vaccine manufacturer and lot number, and name and title of the person administering the vaccine; site, previous reaction and contraindications (eg, immunodeficiency or an evolving neurologic problem), date on vaccine information statement (VIS), and date VIS was provided.
8. Reasons for visit	The patient's or parents' concerns, stated in their own words, serve as the focus for the visit.
9. Present illness	A concise chronologic summary of the problems necessitating a visit, including the duration, progression, exacerbating factors, ameliorating interventions, and associations.
10. Medical history	A statement regarding the child's functionality and general well-being, including a summary record of significant illnesses, injuries, hospitalizations, and procedures.
11. Diet	Eating patterns, likes and dislikes, use of vitamins, and relative amounts of carbohydrates, fat, and protein in the diet, percentage of fat of milk provided. Inquiry about intake of fast food, candy, and sugar drinks.
12. Family history	Information about the illnesses of relatives, preferably in the form of a family tree.
13. Social history	Family constellation, relationships, parents' educational background, religious preference, and the role of the child in the family; socioeconomic profile of the family to identify resources available to the child, access to services that may be needed, and anticipated stressors.
14. Development	(1) Attainment of developmental milestones (including developmental testing results); (2) social habits and milestones (toilet habits, play, major activities, sleep patterns, discipline, peer relationships); (3) school progress and documentation of specific achievements and grades.
15. Sexual history	Family's sexual attitudes, sex education, sexual development, sexual secondary characteristics, activity, sexually transmitted diseases, menstruation onset, and characteristics and birth control measures.
16. ROS, review of systems.	Common symptoms in each major body system.

[a]The components of this table should be included in a child's medical record and structured to allow easy review and modification. The practice name and address should appear on all pages.

of the examination. Whether or not the physician can establish rapport with the child, the process should proceed efficiently and systematically.

Because young children may fear the examination and become fussy, simple inspection is important. For example, the examiner can observe the child's respiratory rate and work of breathing from across the room (often by having a parent lift the child's shirt) before moving near the child for the remainder of the examination. During a health supervision visit, observation will provide the examiner with an opportunity to assess development and parent-child interactions.

Clothing should be removed slowly and gently to avoid threatening the child. A parent or the child is usually the best person to do this. Modesty should always be respected, and gown or drapes should be provided. Examinations of adolescents should be chaperoned whenever a pelvic examination or a stressful or painful procedure is performed.

Examination tables are convenient, but a parent's lap is a comfortable location for a young child. For most purposes, an adequate examination can be conducted on a "table" formed by the parent's and examiner's legs as they sit facing each other.

Although a thorough physical examination is important at every age, certain components of the examination may change based on the age of the patient. An astute clinician can detect signs of important clinical conditions in an asymptomatic child. In infancy, for example, physical examination can reveal the presence of craniosynostosis, congenital heart disease, or developmental dysplasia of the hip. Similarly, examination of a toddler may reveal pallor (possible iron-deficiency anemia) or strabismus. The routine examination of an older child or adolescent may reveal scoliosis or acanthosis nigricans (a finding associated with insulin resistance).

▼ HEALTH SUPERVISION VISITS

One of several timetables for recommended health supervision visits is illustrated in Figure 9–1. (*Note:* A PDF printable format of this figure is available from the American Academy of Pediatrics [AAP].) The federal Maternal and Child Health Bureau has developed comprehensive health supervision guidelines through their Bright Futures program. In areas where evidence-based information is lacking, expert opinion has been used as the basis for these plans. Recently revised *Bright Futures Guidelines* emphasizes working collaboratively with families, recognizing the need for attention toward children with special health care needs, gaining cultural competence, and addressing complementary and alternative care, as well as integrating mental health care into the primary care setting. Practitioners should remember that guidelines are not meant to be rigid; services should be individualized according to the child's needs.

During health supervision visits, the practitioner should review child development and acute and chronic problems, conduct a complete physical examination, order appropriate screening tests, and anticipate future developments. New historical information should be elicited through an interval history. Development should be assessed by parental report and clinician observation. In addition, systematic use of formal parent-directed screening tools, such as the Ages and Stages Questionnaire (ASQ) or the Parents' Evaluation of Developmental Status (PEDS), is recommended. Growth parameters should be carefully recorded, and weight, length, or height, head circumference (up to age 3), and body mass index (BMI) (for > 2 years) should be plotted and evaluated using established growth charts (see Chapter 3). Vision and hearing should be assessed subjectively at each visit, with objective assessments at intervals beginning after the child is old enough to cooperate with the screening test, usually at 3–4 years of age.

Because fewer than 4% of asymptomatic children have physical findings on routine health maintenance visits, a major portion of the health supervision visit is devoted to anticipatory guidance. This portion of the visit enables the health care provider to address behavioral, developmental, injury prevention, nutritional issues, and school problems; and other age-appropriate issues that will arise before the next well-child visit.

Hagan JF, Shaw JS, Duncan PM (eds): *Bright Futures: Guidelines for Health Supervision of Infants, Children, and Adolescents.* 4th ed. Elk Grove Village, IL: American Academy of Pediatrics; 2017.

DEVELOPMENTAL & BEHAVIORAL ASSESSMENT

Addressing developmental and behavioral problems is one of the central features of pediatric primary care. The term *developmental delay* refers to the circumstance in which a child has not demonstrated a developmental skill (such as walking independently) by an age at which the vast majority of normally developing children have accomplished this task. Developmental delays are, in fact, quite common: approximately 18% of children younger than 18 years either have developmental delays or have conditions that place them at risk of developmental delays.

Pediatric practitioners are in a unique position to assess the development of their patients. This developmental assessment should ideally take the form of *developmental surveillance*, in which a skilled individual monitors development in multiple domains (gross motor, fine motor, language, and personal or social) over time as part of providing routine care. Developmental surveillance includes several key elements: listening to parent concerns, obtaining a developmental history, making careful observations during office visits, periodically screening all infants and children for delays using validated screening tools, recognizing conditions and circumstances that place children at increased risk of delays, and referring children who fail screening tests for further evaluation and intervention.

▲ Figure 9-1. 2019 Recommendations for Pediatric Preventive Health care. (Reproduced with permission from Hagan JF, Shaw JS, Duncan PM (eds): *Bright Futures: Guidelines for Health Supervision of Infants, Children, and Adolescents.* 4th ed. Elk Grove Village, IL: American Academy of Pediatrics; 2017. This document has been updated to reflect the 2019 recommendations for Preventive Pediatric Healthcare: *Pediatrics* 2019:143.)

9. Verify results as soon as possible, and follow up, as appropriate.

10. Screen with audiometry including 6,000 and 8,000 Hz high frequencies once between 11 and 14 years, once between 15 and 17 years, and once between 18 and 21 years. See "The Sensitivity of Adolescent Hearing Screens Significantly Improves by Adding High Frequencies" (http://www.jahonline.org/article/S1054-139X(16)00048-3/fulltext).

11. See "Identifying Infants and Young Children With Developmental Disorders in the Medical Home: An Algorithm for Developmental Surveillance and Screening" (http://pediatrics.aappublications.org/content/118/1/405.full).

12. Screening should occur per "Identification and Evaluation of Children With Autism Spectrum Disorders" (http://pediatrics.aappublications.org/content/120/5/1183.full).

13. This assessment should be family centered and may include an assessment of child social-emotional health, caregiver depression, and social determinants of health. See "Promoting Optimal Development: Screening for Behavioral and Emotional Problems" (http://pediatrics.aappublications.org/content/135/2/384) and "Poverty and Child Health in the United States" (http://pediatrics.aappublications.org/content/137/4/e20160339).

14. A recommended assessment tool is available at http://crafft.org.

15. Recommended screening using the Patient Health Questionnaire (PHQ)-2 or other tools available in the GLAD-PC toolkit and at (http://www.aap.org/en-us/advocacy-and-policy/aap-health-initiatives/Mental-Health/Documents/MH_ScreeningChart.pdf.)

16. Screening should occur per "Incorporating Recognition and Management of Perinatal and Postpartum Depression Into Pediatric Practice" (http://pediatrics.aappublications.org/content/126/5/1032).

17. At each visit, age-appropriate physical examination is essential, with infant totally unclothed and older children undressed and suitably draped. See "Use of Chaperones During the Physical Examination of the Pediatric Patient" (http://pediatrics.aappublications.org/content/127/5/991.full).

18. These may be modified, depending on entry point into schedule and individual need.

19. Confirm initial screen was accomplished, verify results, and follow up, as appropriate. The Recommended Uniform Screening Panel (https://www.hrsa.gov/advisory-committees/heritable-disorders/rusp/index.html), as determined by The Secretary's Advisory Committee on Heritable Disorders in Newborns and Children, and state newborn screening laws/regulations (http://genes-r-us.uthscsa.edu/home) establish the criteria for and coverage of newborn screening procedures and programs.

20. Verify results as soon as possible, and follow up, as appropriate.

21. Confirm initial screening was accomplished, verify results, and follow up, as appropriate. See "Hyperbilirubinemia in the Newborn Infant ≥35 Weeks' Gestation: An Update With Clarifications"(http://pediatrics.aappublications.org/content/124/4/1193).

22. Screening for critical congenital heart disease using pulse oximetry should be performed in newborns, after 24 hours of age, before discharge from the hospital, per "Endorsement of Health and Human Services Recommendation for Pulse Oximetry Screening for Critical Congenital Heart Disease" (http://pediatrics.aappublications.org/content/128/1/e1190.full).

23. Schedules, per the AAP Committee on Infectious Diseases, are available at http://redbook.solutions.aap.org/SS/Immunization_Schedules.aspx. Every visit should be an opportunity to update and complete a child's immunizations.

24. Perform risk assessment or screening, as appropriate, per recommendations in the current edition of the AAP Pediatric Nutrition: Policy of the American Academy of Pediatrics (Iron chapter).

25. For children at risk of lead exposure, see "Prevention of Childhood Lead Toxicity" (http://pediatrics.aappublications.org/content/138/1/e20161493) and "Low Level Lead Exposure Harms Children: A Renewed Call for Primary Prevention" (http://www.cdc.gov/nceh/lead/ACCLPP/Final_Document_030712.pdf).

26. Perform risk assessments or screenings as appropriate, based on universal screening requirements for patients with Medicaid or in high prevalence areas.

27. Tuberculosis testing per recommendations of the AAP Committee on Infectious Diseases, published in the current edition of the AAP Red Book: Report of the Committee on Infectious Diseases. Testing should be performed on recognition of high-risk factors.

28. See "Integrated Guidelines for Cardiovascular Health and Risk Reduction in Children and Adolescents" (http://www.nhlbi.nih.gov/guidelines/cvd_ped/index.htm).

29. Adolescents should be screened for sexually transmitted infections (STIs) per recommendations in the current edition of the AAP Red Book: Report of the Committee on Infectious Diseases.

30. Adolescents should be screened for HIV according to the USPSTF recommendations (http://www.uspreventiveservicestaskforce.org/uspstf/uspshivi.htm) once between the ages of 15 and 18, making every effort to preserve confidentiality of the adolescent. Those at increased risk of HIV infection, including those who are sexually active, participate in injection drug use, or are being tested for other STIs, should be tested for HIV and reassessed annually.

31. See USPSTF recommendations (https://www.uspreventiveservicestaskforce.org/Page/Document/UpdateSummaryFinal/cervical-cancer-screening2). Indications for pelvic examinations prior to age 21 are noted in"Gynecologic Examination for Adolescents in the Pediatric Office Setting" (http://pediatrics.aappublications.org/content/126/2/583.full).

32. Assess whether the child has a dental home. If no dental home is identified, perform a risk assessment (https://www.aap.org/en-us/advocacy-and-policy/aap-health-initiatives/Oral-Health/Pages/Oral-Health-Practice-Tools.aspx) and refer to a dental home. Recommend brushing with fluoride toothpaste in the proper dosage for age. See "Maintaining and Improving the Oral Health of Young Children" (http://pediatrics.aappublications.org/content/134/6/1224).

33. Perform a risk assessment (http://www2.aap.org/oralhealth/docs/RiskAssessmentTool.pdf). See "Maintaining and Improving the Oral Health of Young Children" (http://pediatrics.aappublications.org/content/134/6/1224).

34. See USPSTF recommendations (http://www.uspreventiveservicestaskforce.org/uspstf/uspsdnch.htm). Once teeth are present, fluoride varnish may be applied to all children every 3–6 months in the primary care or dental office. Indications for fluoride use are noted in "Fluoride Use in Caries Prevention in the Primary Care Setting" (http://pediatrics.aappublications.org/content/134/3/626).

35. If primary water source is deficient in fluoride, consider oral fluoride supplementation. See "Fluoride Use in Caries Prevention in the Primary Care Setting" (http://pediatrics.aappublications.org/content/134/3/626).

Summary of Changes Made to the
Bright Futures/AAP Recommendations for Preventive Pediatric Health Care
(Periodicity Schedule)

This schedule reflects changes approved in December 2018 and published in March 2019.
For updates and a list of previous changes made, visit www.aap.org/periodicityschedule.

CHANGES MADE IN DECEMBER 2018

BLOOD PRESSURE

- Footnote 6 has been updated to read as follows: "Screening should occur per 'Clinical Practice Guideline for Screening and Management of High Blood Pressure in Children and Adolescents' (http://pediatrics.aappublications.org/content/140/3/e20171904). Blood pressure measurement in infants and children with specific risk conditions should be performed at visits before age 3 years."

ANEMIA

- Footnote 24 has been updated to read as follows: "Perform risk assessment or screening, as appropriate, per recommendations in the current edition of the AAP Pediatric Nutrition: Policy of the American Academy of Pediatrics (Iron chapter)."

LEAD

- Footnote 25 has been updated to read as follows: "For children at risk of lead exposure, see 'Prevention of Childhood Lead Toxicity' (http://pediatrics.aappublications.org/content/138/1/e20161493) and 'Low Level Lead Exposure Harms Children: A Renewed Call for Primary Prevention' (https://www.cdc.gov/nceh/lead/ACCLPP/Final_Document_030712.pdf)."

▲ **Figure 9–1.** (*Continued*)

HRSA

This program is supported by the Health Resources and Services Administration (HRSA) of the U.S. Department of Health and Human Services (HHS) as part of an award totaling $5,000,000 with 10 percent financed with non-governmental sources. The contents are those of the author(s) and do not necessarily represent the official views of, nor an endorsement, by HRSA, HHS, or the U.S. Government. For more information, please visit HRSA.gov.

The prompt recognition of children with developmental delays is important for several reasons. Children with delays can be referred for a wide range of developmental therapies, such as those provided by physical, speech or language, and/or educational therapists. Children with delays, regardless of the cause, make better developmental progress if they receive appropriate developmental therapies than if they do not. Many infants and toddlers younger than 3 years with delays are eligible to receive a range of therapies and other services, often provided in the home, at no cost to families. Children aged 3 years and older with delays are eligible for developmental services through the local school system.

Several parent- and physician-administered developmental screening tools are available and should be utilized in order to more efficiently incorporate this process in the busy well-child care visit. The PEDS, ASQ, and the Child Development Inventories (CDI) are screening tests that rely on parent report. Other screening tools, such as the Denver II screening test, the Early Language Milestone Scale (see Chapter 3, Figure 3–1), and the Bayley Infant Neurodevelopmental Screener, involve the direct observation of a child's skills by a care provider. All developmental screening tests have their strengths and weaknesses. The Denver II is familiar to many pediatric providers and is widely used. However, whereas the Denver II has relatively high sensitivity for detecting possible developmental delays, the specificity is poorer, and this may lead to the over referral of normal children for further developmental testing.

In addition to general developmental screening, autism-specific screens (such as the Modified Checklist for Autism in Toddlers [MCHAT]) should be administered at the 18- and 24-month health supervision visits.

Regardless of the approach taken to developmental screening, there are a number of important considerations: (1) The range of normal childhood development is broad, and therefore a child with a single missing skill in a single developmental area is less likely to have a significant developmental problem than a child showing multiple delays in several developmental areas (eg, gross motor and language delays); (2) continuity of care is important, because development is best assessed over time; (3) it is beneficial to routinely use formal screening tests to assess development; (4) if developmental delays are detected in primary care, these patients need referral and close follow-up to insure evaluation completion for further testing and likely will benefit from receiving developmentally focused therapies and strategies; and (5) parents appreciate when attention is paid to their child's development and generally react positively to referrals for appropriate developmental therapies.

Several developmental charts with age-based expectations for normal development are presented in Chapter 3 (see Tables 3–1, 3–2, 3–3), as well as a discussion of the recommended medical and neurodevelopmental evaluation of a child with a suspected developmental disorder.

In addition to developmental issues, pediatric providers are an important source of information and counseling for parents regarding a broad range of behavioral issues. The nature of the behavioral problems, of course, varies with the child's age. Some common issues raised by parents, discussed in detail in Chapter 3, include colic, feeding disorders, sleep problems, temper tantrums, breath-holding spells, and noncompliance. Behavioral issues in adolescents are discussed in Chapter 4.

American Academy of Pediatrics Council on Children With Disabilities: Identifying infants and young children with developmental disorders in the medical home: an algorithm for developmental surveillance and screening. Pediatrics 2006;118:1808 [PMID: 168118591]. Note: This policy was reaffirmed by the American Academy of Pediatrics in 2014 (Pediatrics 2014;134:e1520).

Godoy L, Carter AS: Identifying and addressing mental health risks and problems in primary care pediatric settings: a model to promote developmental and cultural competence. Am J Orthopsychiatry 2013 Jan;83(1):7388. doi: 10.1111/ajop.12005 [PMID: 23330625].

Talmi A et al: Improving developmental screening documentation and referral completion. Pediatrics 2014 Oct; 134(4):e1181–e1188. doi: 10.1542/peds.2012-1151 [Epub 2014 Sep 1] [PMID: 25180272].

GROWTH PARAMETERS

Monitoring appropriate growth is pivotal in ambulatory pediatric practice.

Height, weight, and head circumference are carefully measured at each well-child examination and plotted on age- and sex-specific growth charts. The Centers for Disease Control and Prevention (CDC) recently recommended use of the World Health Organization (WHO) growth standards to monitor growth for infants and children ages 0–2 in the United States, in lieu of its own growth charts. The WHO standards are based on a sample of 8500 babies (from Brazil, Ghana, India, Norway, Oman, and the United States) who were predominantly breast-fed for at least 4 months, still nursing at 1 year and living in nonsmoking households. The methods used to create the CDC growth charts and the WHO growth charts are similar for children aged 2 years and older.

To ensure accurate weight measurements for longitudinal comparisons, infants should be undressed completely and young children should be wearing underpants only. Recumbent length is plotted on the chart until approximately 2 years of age. When the child is old enough to be measured upright, height should be plotted on the charts for ages 2–20 years. Routine measurements of head circumference may cease if circumferential head growth has been steady for the first 2 years of life. However, if a central nervous system (CNS) problem exists or develops, or if the child has growth deficiency, this measurement continues to be useful. Tracking the growth velocity for each of these parameters allows early recognition of deviations from normal.

It is useful to note that in the first year of life, it is common for height and weight measurements to cross over a percentile line. After approximately 18 months, most healthy children tend to follow the curve within one growth channel.

Determination of whether or not a child's weight falls within a healthy range also relies on growth charts. For children younger than 2 years, the weight-for-length chart is used. For children 2–18 years, a BMI chart is used, which is a measure that correlates well with adiposity- and obesity-related comorbidities. The BMI is calculated as the weight (in kilograms) divided by the squared height (in meters). The BMI is useful for determining obesity (BMI ≥ 95th percentile for age) and overweight (BMI between 85th and 95th percentiles), as well as underweight status (BMI ≤ 5th percentile for age). It must be emphasized that "eyeballing" overweight or underweight is frequently inaccurate and should not substitute for careful evaluation of the data on growth charts.

CDC and WHO growth charts: http://www.cdc.gov/growthcharts/. Accessed June 29, 2019.

Grummer-Strawn LM et al: Use of World Health Organization and CDC growth charts for children aged 0–59 months in the United States. MMWR Recomm Rep 2010;59(RR-9):115 [PMID: 20829749].

US Preventive Services Task Force: Screening for obesity in children and adolescents: US Preventive Services Task Force recommendation statement. Pediatrics 2010;125(2):361–367.

BLOOD PRESSURE

Blood pressure screening at well-child visits starts at age 3 years. There are some conditions that warrant blood pressure monitoring at an earlier age:

- History of prematurity, very low birth weight, or other neonatal complication requiring intensive care
- Congenital heart disease (repaired or nonrepaired)
- Recurrent urinary tract infections, hematuria, or proteinuria
- Known renal disease or urologic malformations
- Family history of congenital renal disease
- Solid organ transplant
- Malignancy or bone marrow transplant
- Treatment with drugs known to raise blood pressure (steroids, oral contraceptives)
- Other conditions associated with hypertension (neurofibromatosis, tuberous sclerosis, etc)
- Evidence of elevated intracranial pressure

Accurate determination of blood pressure requires proper equipment (stethoscope, manometer and inflation cuff, or an automated system) and a cooperative, seated subject in a quiet room. Although automated blood pressure instruments are widely available and easy to use, blood pressure readings from these devices are typically 5 mm Hg higher for diastolic and 10 mm Hg higher for systolic blood pressure compared with auscultatory techniques. Therefore, the diagnosis of hypertension should not be made on the basis of automated readings alone. Additionally, blood pressure varies by the height and weight of the individual. Consequently, hypertension is diagnosed as a systolic or diastolic blood pressure greater than the 95th percentile based on the age and height percentile of the patient using charts from the AAP Clinical Practice Guidelines (see references).

The width of the inflatable portion of the cuff should be 40%–50% of the circumference of the limb. Overweight children need a larger cuff size to avoid a falsely elevated blood pressure reading. Cuffs that are too narrow will overestimate and those that are too wide will underestimate the true blood pressure. Hypertension should not be diagnosed based on readings at one visit, but rather three separate occasions of documented hypertension are required. Repeated measurements at different visits over time should be tracked using flowcharts in an electronic medical record or equivalent in a paper chart. Children with repeated blood pressure readings from the 90th to the 95th percentile may be classified as having elevated blood pressure. Those with greater than between the 95th and 99th percentile plus 12 mm of Hg are classified as Stage 1 hypertension, and those greater than the 99th percentile plus 12 mm of Hg are termed Stage 2 hypertension. National High Blood Pressure Education Program recommends that all children with blood pressure of greater than or equal to 95% should have a complete blood count (CBC), serum nitrogen, creatinine, electrolytes, lipid panel, glucose, urinalysis, and a renal ultrasound in those with abnormal urinalysis or renal function. Nonpharmacologic interventions include diet, exercise, and weight management. Indications for pharmacologic therapy may include the following:

- Symptomatic hypertension
- Stage 2 hypertension without a clearly modifiable factor (eg, obesity)
- Chronic kidney disease
- Diabetes (types 1 and 2)
- Persistent hypertension despite nonpharmacologic measures

Based on a recent systematic review for US Preventive Services Task Force, it is unclear whether screening for hypertension in children and teens reduces adverse outcomes in adults.

Flynn JT et al: Clinical Practice Guideline for Screening and Management of High Blood Pressure in Children and Adolescents. Pediatrics 2017;140(3):e20171904. https://doi.org/10.1542/peds.2017-1904.

National High Blood Pressure Education Program Working Group in High Blood Pressure in Children and Adolescents: The fourth report on diagnosis, evaluation and treatment of high blood pressure in children and adolescents. Pediatrics 2004 Aug;114(2 Suppl 4th Report):555–576 [PMID: 15286277].

Wiesen J et al: Evaluation of pediatric patients with mild to moderate hypertension: yield of diagnostic testing. Pediatrics 2008;122:e988–e993 [PMID: 18977966].

VISION & HEARING SCREENING

Examination of the eyes and an assessment of vision should be performed at every health supervision visit. Eye problems are relatively common in children: refractive errors (including myopia, hyperopia, and astigmatism), amblyopia (loss of visual acuity from cortical suppression of the vision of the eye), and/or strabismus (misalignment of the eyes) occur in 5%–10% of preschoolers. Assessment of vision should include visual inspection of the eyes and eyelids, alignment of eyes, and visual acuity.

Starting at birth, the movement and alignment of the eyes should be assessed and the pupils and red reflexes examined. The red reflex, performed on each pupil individually and then on both eyes simultaneously, is used to detect eye opacities (eg, cataracts or corneal clouding) and retinal abnormalities (eg, retinal detachment or retinoblastoma). By 3 months of age, an infant should be able to track or visually follow a moving object, with both eyes.

Starting after age 3, formal testing of visual acuity should be done if possible. This can be performed in the office with a variety of tests, including the tumbling E chart or picture tests such as Allen cards. In these tests, each eye is tested separately, with the nontested eye completely covered. Credit is given for any line on which the child gets more than 50% correct. Children who are unable to cooperate should be retested, ideally within 6 months, and those who cannot cooperate with repeated attempts should be referred to an ophthalmologist. Because visual acuity improves with age, results of the test are interpreted using the cutoff values in Table 9–2. However, any two-line discrepancy between the two eyes, even within the passing range (eg, 20/20 in one eye, 20/30 in the other in a child aged ≥ 6 years) should be referred to an ophthalmologist.

Throughout childhood, clinicians should screen for undetected strabismus (ocular misalignment). The corneal light reflex test can be used starting at 3 months and the cover test can be used beginning at 6 months to assess for

Table 9–2. Age-appropriate visual acuity.[a]

Age (y)	Minimal Acceptable Acuity
3–5	20/40
≥ 6	20/30

[a]Refer to an ophthalmologist if minimal acuity is not met at a given age or if there is a difference in scores of two or more lines between the eyes.

Table 9–3. Recommended vision screening in the primary care office.

Test	Age for Screening	Indication(s) for Referral
Inspection of eyes and lids	All	
Red reflex	Birth until child can read eye chart	Abnormal red reflex, asymmetry of the red reflexes, or partially obscured red reflex
Assessment of fixation and following	Starting at 2 mo	Poor fixation/following by 3 mo
Corneal light reflex for assessing strabismus	3 mo to 5 y	Asymmetry of light reflex (in relation to iris and pupil)
Cover testing for assessing strabismus	6 mo to 5 y	Presence of refixation movement
Fundoscopic examination	Starting at 3 y	
Preliterate eye chart testing	Starting at 3–4 y	Unable to pass 20/40 for ages 3–5 or 20/30 for 6 and older. Also refer if there is a difference of two or more lines between the eyes.

strabismus. The corneal light reflex test, the cover test, and visual acuity test are described further in Chapter 16.

Recommendations for vision screening and indications for referral are listed in Table 9–3. Referral to an ophthalmologist is also recommended for preterm infants for evaluation of retinopathy of prematurity (ROP), as well as children with a family history of amblyopia, strabismus, retinoblastoma, or retinal degeneration. Children with Down syndrome should be referred to an ophthalmologist at 6 months of age given their increased risk for refractive error, strabismus, and cataracts.

Hearing loss, if undetected, can lead to substantial impairments in speech, language, and cognitive development. Because significant bilateral hearing loss is one of the more common major anomalies found at birth, and early detection and intervention of hearing loss leads to better outcomes for children, universal hearing screening is provided to newborns in most parts of the United States. Hearing in infants is assessed using either evoked otoacoustic emissions or auditory brainstem-evoked responses. Because universal newborn hearing screening is sometimes associated with false-positive test results, confirmatory audiology testing is required for abnormal tests.

Informal behavioral testing of hearing, such as observing an infant's response to a shaken rattle, may be unreliable.

In fact, parental concerns about hearing are of greater predictive value than the results of informal tests, and such concerns should be taken seriously. Prior to age 4, infants should be referred to an audiologist for testing if a concern arises. Conventional screening audiometry, in which a child raises her hand when a sound is heard, can be performed starting at age 4. Each ear should be tested at 500, 1000, 2000, and 4000 Hz and referred at threshold levels of greater than 20 dB at any of these frequencies. Any evidence of hearing loss should be substantiated by repeated testing, and if still abnormal, a referral for a formal hearing evaluation should be made.

The AAP periodicity schedule recommends routine hearing screening at 4, 5, 6, 8, and 10 years of age and several times during adolescence. Children with any risk factors for hearing loss should be closely followed and receive more frequent screening. A number of inherited or acquired conditions increase the risk of hearing loss. Sometimes hearing loss can be mistaken for inattention, and so hearing screening should be part of workup for attention problems. Additional details regarding hearing assessment are provided in Chapter 18.

American Academy of Pediatrics et al: Red reflex examination in neonates, infants, and children. Pediatrics 2008;122:1401 [PMID: 19047263].

Harlor AD, Bower C; American Academy of Pediatrics Committee on Practice and Ambulatory Medicine, Section of Otolaryngology: Hearing assessment in infants and children: recommendations beyond neonatal screening. Pediatrics 2009; 124(4):1252–1263 [PMID: 19786460].

Katbamna B, Crumpton T, Patel DR: Hearing impairment in children. Pediatr Clin North Am 2008;55:1175 [PMID: 18929059].

Loh AR, Chiang MF: Pediatric vision screening. Pediatr Rev 2018 May;225–234 [PMID: 29716965].

Newborn Screening

Newborn screening involves population-wide testing for metabolic and genetic diseases. It has become an essential component in a public health program that screens over 4 million newborns every year. Blood samples are collected by heel stick from newborns before hospital discharge, and results are usually available within 1 week. Some states routinely repeat blood testing between 7 and 14 days of life, while others recommend it if the child is discharged in less than 24 hours. The state-to-state variation seen in newborn screen panels has begun to diminish as a result of national recommendations. In 2010, the Secretary Advisory Committee on Heritable Disorders in Newborns and Children recommended screening for 32 core conditions with another 26 detectable through differential diagnosis. Most states have adopted these guidelines.

Infants with a positive screening result should receive close follow-up, with additional confirmatory studies performed at a center with experience in doing these tests.

Screening tests are usually accurate, but the sensitivity and specificity of a particular screening test must be carefully considered. If symptoms of a disease are present despite a negative result on a screening test, the infant should be tested further. Newborn screening has benefited thousands of infants and their families, preventing and diminishing the morbidity of many diseases. At the same time, the emotional cost of false-positive screening is a continuing challenge. Parents report high levels of stress during the evaluation process. Recommendations for useful resources, given the variability of information on the Internet, and prompt clinical services can help reduce this distress.

Calonge N et al; Advisory Committee on Heritable Disorders in Newborns and Children: Committee report: method for evaluating conditions nominated for population-based screening of newborns and children. Genet Med 2010 Mar;12(3):153–159 [PMID: 20154628].

National Newborn Screening by State: http://genes-r-us.uthscsa.edu/sites/genes-r-us/files/nbsdisorders.pdf. Accessed June 29, 2019.

Lead Screening

The developing infant and child are at risk of lead poisoning or toxicity because of their propensity to place objects in the mouth and their efficient absorption of this metal. Children with lead toxicity are typically asymptomatic. High blood levels (> 70 mcg/dL) can cause severe health problems such as seizures and coma. Numerous neuropsychological deficits have been associated with increased lead levels. Blood lead levels less than 10 mcg/dL have been correlated with lower intelligence quotients. The primary source of lead exposure in this country remains lead-based paint, even though most of its uses have been banned since 1977. Lead levels have declined nationally from a mean of 16 mcg/dL in 1976 to less than 2 mcg/dL in 2008. However, considerable variation in lead levels exists in different regions of the United States, and a majority of children at risk of lead toxicity are not currently screened. Despite the wide variation in the prevalence of lead toxicity, the CDC recommends universal lead screening for children at ages 1 and 2 and targeted screening for older children living in communities with a high percentage of old housing (> 27% of houses built before 1950) or a high percentage of children with elevated blood lead levels (> 12% of children with levels > 10 mcg/dL). Children enrolled in Medicaid are required to be screened at 12 and 24 months.

Communities with inadequate data regarding local blood lead levels should also undergo universal screening. Caregivers of children between 6 months and 6 years of age may be interviewed by questionnaire about environmental risk factors for lead exposure (Table 9–4), although the data to support the use of this screening are inconclusive. If risk factors are present, a blood lead level should be obtained. A venous blood sample is preferred over a capillary specimen.

Table 9–4. Elements of a lead-risk questionnaire.

Recommended questions

1. Does your child live in or regularly visit a house built before 1950? This could include a day care center, preschool, the home of a baby sitter or relative.
2. Does your child live in or regularly visit a house built before 1978 with recent, ongoing, or planned renovation or remodeling?
3. Does your child have a sister or brother, housemate, or playmate being followed for an elevated lead level?

Questions that may be considered by region or locality

1. Does your child live with an adult whose job (eg, at a brass/copper foundry, firing range, automotive or boat repair shop, or furniture refinishing shop) or hobby (eg, electronics, fishing, stained-glass making, pottery making) involves exposure to lead?
2. Does your child live near a work or industrial site (eg, smelter, battery recycling plant) that involves the use of lead?
3. Does your child use pottery or ingest medications that are suspected of having a high lead content?
4. Does your child have exposure to old, nonbrand-type toys or burning lead-painted wood?
5. Does your child play on an athletic field with artificial turf?

An elevated capillary (fingerstick) blood sample should always be confirmed by a venous sample. There is no safe level of lead in a child's blood, but the CDC reference level of 5 mcg/dL should be used to identify children at risk in order to initiate public health actions. The recommended actions can be viewed on the CDC website (see references).

The cognitive development of children with confirmed high blood levels should be evaluated and attempts made to identify the environmental source. Iron deficiency should be treated if present. Chelation of lead is indicated for levels of 45 mcg/dL and higher and is urgently required for levels above 70 mcg/dL. All families should receive education to decrease the risk of lead exposure. With any elevated lead level (> 5 mcg/dL), rescreening should be performed at recommended intervals.

American Academy of Pediatrics Committee on Environmental Health: Lead exposure in children: prevention, detection, and management. Pediatrics 2005;116(4):1036–1046 [PMID: 16199720].

Center for Disease Control Recommended Actions Based on Blood Lead Level: https://www.cdc.gov/nceh/lead/acclpp/actions_blls.html. Accessed June 7, 2019.

Centers for Disease Control and Prevention Lead: http://www.cdc.gov/nceh/lead/ACCLPP/blood_lead_levels.htm. Accessed June 7, 2019.

Lead fact sheet (English and Spanish): http://www.cdc.gov/nceh/lead/acclpp/lead_levels_in_children_fact_sheet.pdf. Accessed June 7, 2019.

Iron Deficiency

Iron deficiency is the most common nutritional deficiency in the United States. Severe iron deficiency causes anemia, behavioral problems, and cognitive effects, but recent evidence suggests that even iron deficiency without anemia may cause behavioral and cognitive difficulties. Some effects, such as the development of abnormal sleep cycles, may persist even if iron deficiency is corrected in infancy.

Risk factors for iron deficiency include preterm or low-birth-weight births, multiple pregnancy, iron deficiency in the mother, use of nonfortified formula or cow's milk before age 12 months, and an infant diet that is low in iron-containing foods. Infants and children with chronic illness, restricted diet, or extensive blood loss (such as gastrointestinal bleeding or injury) are at risk for iron deficiency.

Primary prevention of iron deficiency should be achieved through dietary means, including feeding ground up meats and iron-containing cereals by age 6 months, avoiding low-iron formula during infancy, and limiting cow's milk to 24 oz per day in children aged 1–5 years.

Universal screening for anemia should occur at approximately 12 months of age by obtaining often by obtaining a hemoglobin or hematocrit. Premature and low-birth-weight infants may need testing before 6 months of age.

A full CBC to look at mean corpuscular volume (MCV) can aid in the evaluation. Serum ferritin is a useful test to evaluate iron-deficiency anemia, as it can also pick up iron deficiency in the absence of anemia, and provides more specificity in detecting iron deficiency. Serum ferritin is recommended by the WHO for iron screening. Because ferritin is an acute-phase reactant and can be falsely reassuring in the presence of inflammation, infection, or malignancy, some experts recommend obtaining a concurrent C-reactive protein (CRP) for accurate interpretation of the ferritin level. Elevated lead levels can cause iron-deficiency anemia and should be explored as a cause for at-risk infants and children.

Management of iron deficiency with or without anemia includes treatment doses of 3–6 mg/kg body weight of *elemental* iron.

Baker RD et al; American Academy of Pediatrics; Committee on Nutrition: Diagnosis and prevention and iron-deficiency anemia in infants and young children (0–3 years of age). Pediatrics 2010;126:1040 [PMID: 20923825].

Oatley H, Borkhoff CM et al: Screening for iron deficiency in early childhood using serum ferritin in the primary care setting. Pediatrics 2018 Dec;142(6) [PMID: 30487142].

Hypercholesterolemia & Hyperlipidemia

Cardiovascular disease is the leading cause of death in the United States, and research has documented that the atherosclerotic process begins in childhood. Genetic factors, diet, and physical activity all play a role in the disease process.

Nonfasting lipid screening is recommended universally for children between the ages of 9 and 11. Fasting lipid screening is recommended between the ages of 2 and 8, and ages 12 and 16 if risk factors are present. Diet and weight management strategies are the primary interventions. However, for severe dyslipidemia (LDL ≥ 190 mg/dL), pharmacologic therapy should be considered. However, consideration of pharmacotherapy should be made for severe dyslipidemia (LDL ≥ 190 mg/dL), or at greater than 160 mg/dL if there is a family history of heart disease, and in all patients at greater than 130 mg/dL depending on their level and amount of risk factors.

Daniels SR, Greer FR; Committee on Nutrition: Lipid screening and cardiovascular health in childhood. Pediatrics 2008 Jul; 122(1):198–208 [PMID: 18596007].

Kubo T et al: Usefulness of non-fasting lipid parameters in children. J Pediatr Endocrinol Metab 2017;30(1):77–83.

Tuberculosis

According to the CDC, 9272 cases of tuberculosis (TB) were reported in the United States in 2016. Risk of TB should be assessed at well-child visits, and screening should be based on high-risk status. High risk is defined as contact with a person with known or suspected TB; having symptoms or radiographic findings suggesting TB; birth, residence, or travel to a region with high TB prevalence (Asia, Middle East, Africa, Latin America); contact with a person with AIDS or human immunodeficiency virus (HIV); or contact with a prisoner, migrant farm worker, illicit drug user, or a person who is or has been recently homeless. TB testing can be performed by a skin test or a blood test. The Mantoux test (five tuberculin units of purified protein derivative) is the only recommended skin test. The interferon-gamma release assays (IGRAs) are blood tests that can be useful for patients who have been immunized with bacille Calmette-Guerin (BCG) or for patients who may have difficulty returning for a second appointment to look for skin reaction.

Targeted screening for latent TB for high-risk individuals is the recommended approach based on available evidence. The following screening questions have been validated to determine high-risk status:

1. Was your child born outside the United States? If yes, this question would be followed by: Where was your child born? If the child was born in Africa, Asia, Latin America, or Eastern Europe, a TB testing should be performed.

2. Has your child traveled outside the United States? If yes, this question would be followed by: Where did the child travel, with whom did the child stay, and how long did the child travel? If the child stayed with friends or family members in Africa, Asia, Latin America, or Eastern Europe for more than 1 week cumulatively, TB testing should be performed.

3. Has your child been exposed to anyone with TB disease? If yes, this question should be followed by questions to determine if the person had TB disease or latent TB infection (LTBI), when the exposure occurred, and what the nature of the contact was. If confirmed that the child has been exposed to someone with suspected or known TB disease, TB testing should be performed. If it is determined that a child had contact with a person with TB disease, notify the local health department per local reporting guidelines.

4. Does your child have close contact with a person who has a positive TB test? If yes, go to question 3.

American Academy of Pediatrics: Tuberculosis. In: Pickering LK (ed): *2015 Red Book: Report of the Committee on Infectious Diseases.* 31st ed. American Academy of Pediatrics; 2018.

Pediatric Tuberculosis Collaborative Group: Targeted tuberculin skin testing and treatment of latent tuberculosis infection in children and adolescents. Pediatrics 2004 Oct;114(Suppl 4): 1175–1201 [PMID: 10617723].

Screening of Adolescent Patients

Adolescents may present with chief complaints that are not the true concern for the visit. Repeating the question "Is there anything else you would like to discuss?" should be considered. Since suicide is a leading cause of morbidity and mortality in this age group, screening with the Pediatric Symptom Checklist for Youth is recommended (https://www.brightfutures.org/mentalhealth/pdf/professionals/ped_sympton_chklst.pdf).

Testing adolescents for blood cholesterol, TB, and HIV should be offered based on high-risk criteria outlined in this chapter and in Chapter 41. Females should have a screening hematocrit once after the onset of menses. During routine visits, adolescents should be questioned sensitively about risk factors (eg, multiple partners; early onset of sexual activity, including child sexual abuse) and symptoms (eg, genital discharge, infectious lesions, pelvic pain) of sexually transmitted infections (STIs). An annual dipstick urinalysis for leukocytes is recommended for sexually active adolescents. Because STIs are often not symptomatic, urine polymerase chain reaction (PCR) for gonorrhea and chlamydia and screening tests for trichomoniasis should be considered. Current guidelines recommend that the first Papanicolaou (Pap) test should be performed at age 21 years, regardless of onset of sexual activity. A complete pelvic examination should be performed when evaluating lower abdominal pain in an adolescent.

Please see Chapter 4 for additional details on adolescent preventive services.

American Academy of Pediatrics: Bright Futures: https://brightfutures.aap.org/Bright%20Futures%20Documents/BF4_AdolescenceVisits.pdf. Accessed June 29, 2019.

Centers for Disease Control and Prevention, National Center for HIV, STD and TB Prevention: Tuberculosis Surveillance Reports. http://www.cdc.gov/nchhstp/default.htm. Accessed June 29, 2019.

ANTICIPATORY GUIDANCE

An essential part of the health supervision visit is anticipatory guidance. During this counseling, the clinician directs the parent's or the older child's attention to issues that may arise in the future. Guidance must be appropriate to age, focus on concerns expressed by the parent and patient, and address issues in depth rather than run through a number of issues superficially. Both oral and printed materials are used. When selecting written materials, providers should be sensitive to issues of literacy and primary language spoken by the family members. Areas of concern include diet, injury prevention, developmental and behavioral issues, and health promotion.

Smoking Cessation

Deleterious effects of secondhand smoke (SHS) on children's health are well documented and the AAP has highlighted the importance of tobacco screening and counseling at each pediatric visit. One-third of children live in a home with an adult smoker. The *Ask, Advise,* and *Refer* methodology has been shown to be a feasible approach to smoking cessation. Ask families if there is a smoker at home, advise the family about the benefit of cessation for the child, and refer to a formal cessation program if the family member is ready to quit.

Injury Prevention

For children and adolescents aged 1–19 years, unintentional injuries are the number one cause of death. In every age category, males are at higher risk than females for unintentional injury.

Injury prevention counseling is an important component of each health supervision visit and can be reinforced during all visits. Counseling should focus on problems that are frequent and age appropriate. Passive strategies of prevention should be emphasized, because these are more effective than active strategies; for example, placing chemicals out of reach in high, locked cupboards to prevent poisoning will be more effective than instructing parents to watch their children closely.

Informational handouts about home safety, such as *The Injury Prevention Program* (TIPP; available from the AAP), can be provided in the waiting room. Advice can then be tailored to the specific needs of each family, with reinforcement from age-specific TIPP handouts.

A. Motor Vehicle Injuries

The primary cause of death of children in the United States is motor vehicle injuries. Although the rate of death from this cause is improving, still in 2015, about 35% of children aged 12 years or younger who were killed in motor vehicle accidents were unrestrained.

The type and positioning of safety seats can be confusing. While car seat and booster seat laws differ by state, a recent AAP policy statement describes the best practice recommendations. All infants and toddlers should ride in a rear-facing car safety seat until 2 years of age or until they reach the weight and height limits for convertible car safety seats (usually 35–40 pounds). Infants may ride in infant-only seats (which often have a carrying handle and snap into a base that is secured in the car) until they reach the height and weight limit for that seat, and then transition to a convertible car seat. Once a child reaches 2 years of age (or younger than 2 if outgrown the weight and height limit of a convertible car seat), he or she can be in a forward-facing car safety seat with a harness. The safest scenario is for a child to remain in a car safety seat with a harness as long as possible. Once a child reaches the weight or height limits of a forward-facing seat, he or she may be transitioned to a belt-positioning booster until the vehicle's lap-and-shoulder belt fits properly (child can sit with his back against the vehicle seat, bend his knees at the edge of the seat, have the belt positioned in the center of the shoulder and across the chest, and have the lap belt touching the thighs). These criteria are generally met once a child reaches height of 4 ft 9 in and is between the ages of 8 and 12 years. All children younger than 13 years should be restrained in the rear seats of the vehicle.

Unfortunately, restraint use shows a decreasing trend with advancing age: children from 1 to 8 years of age use restraints over 90% of the time, but those 8–12 years of age use restraints less than 85% of the time. African-American and Hispanic children use child safety seats less often than white children.

A final motor vehicle risk for health involves the use of portable electronic devices. Using a cell phone while driving is associated with a threefold increase in motor vehicle accidents. Texting while driving poses an even greater danger. All should avoid these risks and adults should model safe practices.

B. Bicycle Injuries

Each year, an average of nearly 400 children die from bicycle crashes, and over 450,000 are treated for bicycle-riding injuries. Over 150,000 children are treated annually in emergency departments for head injuries sustained while riding a bicycle. Many observational studies have shown a decreased risk of head injury with the use of bicycle helmets. Community-based interventions, especially those that provide free helmets, have been shown to increase observed bike helmet wearing. Counseling by physicians in various settings has also been shown to increase bike helmet use. While there is no federal law mandating bicycle helmets, some states have passed legislation requiring bicycle helmets.

C. Skiing and Snowboarding Injuries

Recent studies have suggested that the burden of skiing injuries is high among children, and that children have the highest rate of injury of any age group: approximately 3 injuries per 1000 skier days. Traumatic brain injuries are the leading cause of death for pediatric age skiers. Case-control studies have shown a decrease in head injuries associated with helmet use.

D. Firearm Injuries and Violence Prevention

The United States has a higher rate of firearm-related death than any other industrialized country. For children younger than 15, the death rate from firearm-related injuries is nearly 12 times greater than that of 25 other industrialized nations. Some gun deaths may be accidental, but most are the result of homicide or suicide. A gun in the home doubles the likelihood of a lethal suicide attempt. Although handguns are often kept in homes for protection, a gun is more likely to kill a family member or a friend than an intruder. Adolescents with a history of depression or violence are at higher risk with a gun in the home. The most effective way to prevent firearm injuries is to remove guns from the home. Families who keep firearms at home should lock them in a cabinet or drawer and store ammunition in a separate locked location.

E. Drowning and Near Drowning

Drowning is the leading cause of injury-related death in children ages 1–4 years and the third leading cause of injury-related death in children ages 5–19 years. An estimated 8700 children younger than 20 years old were taken to a hospital emergency department for a drowning event in 2017. Children younger than 1 year are most likely to drown in the bathtub. Buckets filled with water also present a risk of drowning to the older infant or toddler. For children aged 1–4 years, drowning or near drowning occurs most often in swimming pools; and for school-aged children and teens, drowning occurs most often in large bodies of water (eg, swimming pools or open water). Parents should be cautioned that inflatable swimming devices are not a substitution for approved live vests or close supervision and can give a false sense of security. All children should be taught to swim, and recreational swimming should always be supervised. Home pools must be fenced securely, and parents should know how to perform cardiopulmonary resuscitation. A phone should be available near the swimming area. Because drowning is a leading cause of death by injury in children, the AAP has produced a Drowning Prevention "toolkit" for pediatric providers and families (see references).

F. Fire and Burn Injuries

Fires and burns are the leading cause of injury-related deaths in the home. Categories of burn injury include smoke inhalation; flame contact; scalding; and electrical, chemical, and ultraviolet burns. Scalding is the most common type of burn in children. Most scalds involve foods and beverages, but nearly one-fourth of scalds are with tap water, and for that reason it is recommended that hot water heaters be set to a maximum of 120°F. Most fire-related deaths result from smoke inhalation. Smoke detectors can prevent 85% of the injuries and deaths caused by fires in the home. Families should discuss a fire plan with children and practice emergency evacuation from the home.

Sunburn is a common thermal injury and often is not recognized because symptoms of excessive sun exposure usually do not begin until after the skin has been damaged. Repeated sunburn and excessive sun exposure are associated with skin cancers. Prevention of sunburn is best achieved by sun avoidance, particularly during the midday hours of 10 AM to 4 PM. A sunscreen with a minimum sun protection factor (SPF) of 30 that protects against both UVA and UVB rays should be used on sunny and cloudy days to help protect against sunburn. Hats, sunglasses, and long-sleeved swim shirts are also important aspects of safe sun exposure. The safety of sunscreen is not established for infants younger than 6 months; thus, sun avoidance, appropriate clothing, and hats are recommended for this age group. In extreme circumstances in which shade is not available, a minimal amount of sunscreen can be applied to small areas, including the face and back of the hands.

G. Choking

Choking is a leading cause of injury and death in young children. Choking hazards include food and small objects. Children younger than 3 are particularly at risk because they do not have fully coordinated chewing and swallowing, and they are more apt to put small objects in their mouths. Foods that are commonly associated with choking include hot dogs, hard candy, nuts, popcorn, raw vegetables, and chunks of meat, fruit, or cheese. Common nonfood items that pose a risk for choking include coins, latex balloons, button batteries, marbles, small toys, and small toy parts. While being mindful of choking hazards is important, accidents can still occur. Again, parents and caregivers should be trained in CPR and choking first aid.

American Academy of Pediatrics: Drowning Prevention Toolkit: https://www.aap.org/en-us/about-the-aap/aap-press-room/campaigns/drowning-prevention/Pages/default.aspx. Accessed June 29, 2019.

American Academy of Pediatrics, Committee on Injury and Poison Prevention: Bicycle helmets. Pediatrics 2001;108:1030 [PMID: 11581464] (reaffirmed Pediatrics 2012;129).

American Academy of Pediatrics, Committee on Injury and Poison Prevention: Firearm-related injuries affecting the pediatric population. Pediatrics 2012;130:5 [PMID: 10742344].

American Academy of Pediatrics, Committee on Injury and Poison Prevention: Reducing the number of deaths and injuries from residential fires. Pediatrics 2000;105:1355 [PMID: 23080412].

American Academy of Pediatrics, Committee on Injury, Violence, and Poison Prevention: Prevention of choking among children. Pediatrics 2010;125:601 [PMID: 20176668].

American Academy of Pediatrics, Committee on Injury, Violence, and Poison Prevention: Child passenger safety. Pediatrics 2011;127:788 [PMID: 21422088].

Bunik M, Cavanaugh KL et al: The ONE step initiative: quality improvement in a pediatric clinic for secondhand smoke reduction. Pediatrics 2013 Aug;132(2):e502–e511 [PMID: 23858424].

Centers for Disease Control and Prevention (CDC). WISQARS (Web-based Injury Statistics Query and Reporting System): www.cdc.gov/injury/wisqars/index.html. Accessed June 29, 2019.

Denny SA; American Academy of Pediatrics, Committee on Injury, Violence, and Poison Prevention: Prevention of drowning. Pediatrics 2019:143e20190850.

Gardner HG; American Academy of Pediatrics Committee on Injury, Violence, and Poison Prevention: Office-based counseling for unintentional injury prevention. Pediatrics 2007 Jan;119(1):202–206 [PMID: 17200289].

NUTRITION COUNSELING

Screening for nutritional problems and guidance for age-appropriate dietary choices should be part of every health supervision visit. Overnutrition, undernutrition, and eating disorders can be detected by a careful analysis of dietary and activity patterns interpreted in the context of a child's growth pattern.

Human milk feeding is species specific and is the preferred method for infant feeding for the first year of life. Pediatricians should assist mother-infant dyads with latch and help manage breast-feeding difficulties in the early newborn period. For exclusively and partially breast-fed infants, vitamin D supplementation should be given. Iron-fortified formula should be used in situations when breast-feeding is contraindicated such as HIV, active untreated TB, galactosemia, and certain medications. As noted in Chapter 11 (Normal Childhood Nutrition & Its Disorders), the positive benefits of continued breast-feeding and breast milk by mothers who have used illicit drugs should be balanced in individual cases against the risk of transmission of such drugs to the infant via the milk. After the first year, breast-feeding may continue or whole cow's milk can be given because of continued rapid growth and high-energy needs. After 2 years of life, milk with 2% fat or lower may be offered. Baby foods and appropriately prepared table foods should be introduced between 4 and 6 months of age and self-feeding with finger foods encouraged by 7–8 months of age.

When obtaining a dietary history, it is helpful to assess the following: who purchases and prepares food, who feeds the child, whether meals and snacks occur at consistent times and in a consistent setting, whether children are allowed to snack or "graze" between meals, the types and portion sizes of food and drinks provided, the frequency of eating meals in restaurants or eating take-out food, and whether the child eats while watching television.

For children 2 years of age and older, a prudent diet consists of diverse food sources, encourages high-fiber foods (eg, fruits, vegetables, grain products), and limits sodium and fat intake. Since obesity is becoming increasingly prevalent, foods to be avoided or limited include processed foods, sugar-sweetened drinks or soda, and candy. Parents should be gently reminded that they are modeling for a lifetime of eating behaviors in their children, both in terms of the types of foods they provide and the structure of meals (eg, the importance of the family eating together). For additional information on nutritional guidelines, undernutrition, and obesity, see Chapter 11; for eating disorders, see Chapter 6; for adolescent obesity, see Chapter 4.

As of 2009, the Women, Infants, and Children (WIC) food packages reflect the recommendations above and include provision of more fruits and vegetables, whole grains, yogurt and soy products, low-fat milk, and limitations on juice. Breast-feeding mothers receive more food as part of their package, less formula supplementation, and breast-fed infants receive baby food meats as a first food (because of more iron and zinc).

American Academy of Pediatrics, Expert Committee Recommendations Regarding the Prevention, Assessment, and Treatment of Child and Adolescent Overweight and Obesity: Summary Report. Pediatrics 2007;120:s164 [PMID: 18055651].

American Academy of Pediatrics Section on Breastfeeding Policy Statement: Breastfeeding and the use of human milk. Pediatrics 2012;129:e841 [PMID: 22371471].

WIC Food Packages. https://www.fns.usda.gov/wic/wic-food-packages. Accessed June 7, 2019.

COUNSELING ABOUT TELEVISION & OTHER MEDIA

Screen time and social media have a significant influence on children and adolescents. The average child in the United States watches approximately 3–5 hours of television per day, and this does not include time spent watching movies, playing video games, playing on computers or tablets, accessing the Internet, or using cell phones. Taking into account these other forms of media, current estimates are around 7.5 hours of media exposure per day for average 8- to 18-year-olds. Figure 9–2 shows a breakdown of media exposure by age group.

Having a television set in the bedroom increases daily media exposure and is also associated with sleep disturbances. According to the Kaiser Family Foundation, over 70% of 8- to 19-year-olds have a television in their bedrooms.

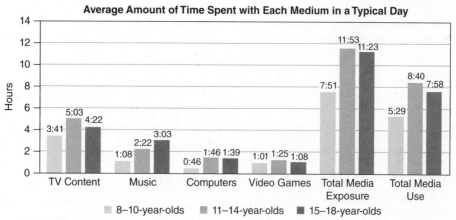

Average Amount of Time Spent with Each Medium in a Typical Day

▲ **Figure 9–2.** Breakdown of media exposure by age showing a significant increase in media use between ages 11 and 14. (Reproduced with permission from Rideout VJ, Foehr UG, Roberts DF; Kaiser Family Foundation Study: *Generation M2: Media in the Lives of 8- to 18-Year-Olds;* January 2010.)

Watching television may have both positive and negative effects. Programs directed toward early childhood may increase knowledge and imaginativeness, and may also teach empathy and acceptance of diversity. However, excessive television viewing of programs with inappropriate content has been shown to have negative effects with respect to violence, sexuality, substance abuse, nutrition, social skills, and body self-image. More recent data suggest that excessive viewing in childhood may have a long-lasting negative effect on cognitive development and academic achievement. Clinicians should assess media exposure in their patients and offer parents concrete advice. Screen time for all media, including television, movies, DVDs, video games, computer activities, computers, tablets, the Internet, and cell phones, should be limited. The AAP recommends that 18- to 24-month-old children should not have any screen time (unless it is video chatting), and that children 2–5 years be limited to 1 hour total screen time each day. The television should not be on during mealtimes, night, or naptimes. Parents should themselves watch sensibly, monitor the program content to which their children are exposed, watch programs and discuss interesting content with children, remove television sets from all bedrooms, and encourage alternative activities. Parents should be advised that research consistently shows that exposure to media violence correlates with childhood aggression.

Social networking sites are becoming increasingly popular, and clinicians need to encourage parents to monitor participation and be aware of potential problems with cyberbullying, "Facebook depression," sexting, and exposure to inappropriate content on sites such as YouTube. Free family media use plans are available through the AAP (www. HealthyChildren.org/MediaUsePlan).

Chassiakos Y, Radesky J, Christakis D, Moreno M, Cross C: Children and adolescents and digital media. Pediatrics 2016; 138(5):e20162593. doi: 10.1542/peds.2016-2593.27940795.

Hill D et al: Media and young minds. Pediatrics 2016;138(5): e20162591.

Radesky J, Christakis D: Increased screen time: implications for early childhood development and behavior. Pediatr Clin North Am 2016;63(5):827–839.

IMMUNIZATIONS

A child's immunization status should be assessed at every visit and every opportunity should be taken to vaccinate. Even though parents may keep an immunization record, it is critical that providers also keep an accurate record of a child's immunizations. This information should be written in a prominent location in the paper or electronic chart or kept in an immunization registry.

Despite high overall national immunization coverage levels, areas of under immunization continue to exist in the United States. An understanding of true contraindications (vs "false contraindications") and a "no missed opportunities" approach to immunization delivery has been shown to successfully increase immunization levels. Therefore, it is important that clinicians screen records and administer required immunizations at all types of visits, not just well child visits, and administer all needed vaccinations simultaneously. Additionally, clinicians should operate reminder or recall systems, in which parents of underimmunized children are prompted by mail, telephone, and text messages (particularly with adolescents) to visit the clinic for immunization. The assessment of clinic-wide immunization levels and feedback of these data to providers have also been shown to increase immunization rates.

Parent refusal of immunizations is an issue in some communities. Because a plethora of incorrect information about vaccine safety and efficacy is on the Internet, it is useful for the provider to direct parents toward reliable sources to help them make an informed decision. A wealth of information for parents and providers about immunizations is available at the National Immunization Program's Web site (www.cdc.gov/vaccines).

Hamborsky J, Kroger A; Center for Disease Control and Prevention. Public Health Foundation. *Epidemiology and Prevention of Vaccine-Preventable Diseases*, E-Book: The Pink Book; 2015. https://www.cdc.gov/vaccines/pubs/pinkbook/index.html. Accessed June 29, 2019.

Kroger A, Sumaya C, Pickering L, Atkinson W; General Recommendations on Immunization: Recommendations of the advisory committee on immunization practices (ACIP). MMWR Recomm Rep 2011;60(RR02):1–60.

Pineda D, Myers MG: Finding reliable information about vaccines. Pediatrics 2011;127:s134–s137 [PMID: 21502244].

Other Types of General Pediatric Service

ACUTE-CARE VISITS

Acute-care visits account for 30% or more of the general pediatrician's office visits. Office personnel should determine the reason for the visit and whether it is an emergent situation, obtain a brief synopsis of the child's symptoms, carefully document vital signs, and list known drug allergies. The clinician should document the events related to the presenting problem and carefully describe them in the medical record. The record should include supporting physical examination data and a diagnosis. Treatments and follow-up instructions must be recorded, including when to return to the office if the problem is not ameliorated. Immunization status should be screened, as previously discussed. Depending on the severity of illness, this may also be an opportunity for age-appropriate health maintenance screenings and anticipatory guidance. This may be particularly true with older school-aged children or adolescents who may be seen more rarely for routine health maintenance visits.

PRENATAL VISITS

Ideally, a couple's first trip to a physician's office should take place before the birth of their baby. A prenatal visit goes a long way toward establishing trust and enables a pediatric provider to learn about a family's expectations, concerns, and fears regarding the anticipated birth. If the infant develops a problem during the newborn period, a provider who has already met the family is in a better position to maintain rapport and communication with the new parents.

In addition to helping establish a relationship between parents and pediatric providers, the prenatal visit can be used to gather information about the parents and the pregnancy, provide information and advice, and identify high-risk situations. A range of information can be provided to parents regarding feeding choices and the benefits of breast-feeding; injury prevention, including sleeping position and the appropriate use of car seats; and techniques for managing colic. Potential high-risk situations that may be identified include mental health issues in the parents, a history of domestic violence, or maternal medical problems that may affect the infant.

Serwint JR: The prenatal pediatric visit. Pediatr Rev 2003;24:31 [PMID: 12509543].

SPORTS PHYSICALS

A preparticipation physical examination (PPE) evaluation is a recommended part of every routine well-child and adolescent care visit. Physicians should be recommending exercise and activity to every child, not just those participating in organized sports.

The goal of the sports physical is to identify medical conditions that would make sports participation unsafe, screen for underlying illness through a traditional history and physical, and recognize preexisting injuries or medical problems that have affected previous sports seasons. As part of the history, the particular sport being played or specific exercise activity should be discussed. Different sports have different potentials for injury, and prevention methods will differ. All patients should be asked about previous cardiac, respiratory, musculoskeletal, or neurologic problems associated with activity. Particular attention should be drawn to any suspicion of cardiac syncope, asthma symptoms, past concussions, or history of unilateral organs, such as kidneys or testicles. Anabolic steroid and nutritional supplement discussion should be explored. Any relevant family history of cardiac death younger than age 50 should be documented.

The physical examination starts with vital signs, including accurate blood pressure screening and examination for obesity. Highlights of the examination include a careful respiratory and cardiac examination, looking for evidence of exercise-induced bronchospasm or anatomic heart disease. Electrocardiogram (ECG) or pulmonary function tests can be considered for suspected abnormalities. The skin examination should look for evidence of potentially contagious skin infections like impetigo or molluscum. The musculoskeletal examination should include all major muscle groups, as well as range of motion and stability testing of the neck, back, shoulder, hips, knees, and ankles. Any pain or limitation should prompt consideration of further investigation or therapy.

A few specific conditions bear mentioning during the counseling phase of the sports participation, including the risks and danger of concussions and performance-enhancing drugs. A list of medical conditions that may affect sports participation can be found in the references. Appropriate protective equipment should be encouraged.

Rice SG: Medical conditions affecting sports participation. *Pediatrics* 2008;*121*(4):841–848. https://doi.org/10.1542/peds.2008-0080

Seto CK: The preparticipation physical examination: an update. Clin Sports Med 2011 Jul;30(3):491–501. doi: 10.1016/j.csm.2011.03.008 [PMID: 21658544].

CHRONIC DISEASE MANAGEMENT

Chronic disease in pediatrics is defined as illness that has been present for more than 3 months. Around 25% children and 35% adolescents have illnesses that meet the definition of a chronic illness. The most common chronic conditions in pediatric practice include asthma, obesity or overweight, attention-deficit/hyperactivity disorder (ADHD), and allergic diseases, but also include congenital anomalies and other conditions. Many patients with chronic conditions are cared for only by a primary care provider. However, when subspecialist care is required, the primary care provider plays an integral part of the care to deal with the complexity of these conditions, which also includes understanding the child's growth and development, routine health promotion and anticipatory guidance, evaluating for social issues, advocating for children and their families, and care coordination.

The goal of chronic disease management is to optimize quality of life while minimizing the side effects of treatment interventions. Problem lists should be used to document chronic diagnoses and monitor associated medications. The child and family's emotional responses to chronic illness should be addressed, and referrals to counselors should be offered if needed. Nutrition and the management of medical devices (eg, catheters, gastrostomy tubes) may need to be addressed, and care coordinated with appropriate specialists.

American Academy of Pediatrics; American Academy of Family Physicians; American College of Physicians, Transitions Clinic Report Authoring Group: Supporting the health care transition from adolescence to adulthood in the medical home. Pediatrics 2011;128:183 [PMID: 21708806].

Ludder-Jackson P, Vessey JA: *Primary Care of the Child with a Chronic Condition.* 5th ed. Mosby-Year Book; 2010.

MEDICAL HOME

The medical home is a concept in which children and their families have an identified, easily accessible primary care provider or group of primary care providers within an office. The AAP has identified seven characteristics of a medical home. The medical home must be (1) accessible, meaning that it must be within the child's community, physically accessible, and all insurances accepted; (2) family centered, with mutual responsibility and decision-making between the patient or family and medical provider, and the family is recognized as an expert of the child; (3) continuous, in that the same medical professionals provide the continuity of care;

(4) comprehensive, with provisions made such that ambulatory and inpatient care are available 24 hours per day, 7 days a week, for 52 weeks of the year; (5) coordinated, with a plan of care developed by the physician and family that is communicated to other providers and agencies as needed; (6) compassionate, meaning that concern is expressed and efforts are made to understand the patient's and family's perspective; and (7) culturally effective, in that the cultural background of the patient and family is respected and incorporated into care, and services are provided in the family's primary language or through a trained medical interpreter.

All children should have a medical home, but it is particularly crucial for children with special health care needs or those with one or more chronic health condition expected to last more than a year. A primary care provider through a medical home should be available for children to assist families with the coordination of consultant recommendations and development of a care plan to implement recommendations.

American Academy of Pediatrics: The medical home. Pediatrics 2002;110:184 [PMID: 12093969].

Medical Home Resources from the American Academy of Pediatrics: https://www.aap.org/en-us/professional-resources/practice-transformation/medicalhome/Pages/home.aspx. Accessed June 20, 2019.

MENTAL & BEHAVIORAL HEALTH

Parents frequently consult their pediatrician on a large variety of parenting and behavioral health issues. Common topics on which the pediatrician must be comfortable counseling include discipline, temper tantrums, toilet training, biting, and sleep problems.

In addition, there are mental health issues that pediatricians will commonly address in the primary care setting, including ADHD, anxiety, depression, school problems, or family stressors (such as separation, divorce, or remarriage). After assessing the situation, the primary care physician must decide whether the child's and family's needs are within his or her area of expertise or whether referral to another professional such as a psychologist or an education specialist would be appropriate.

The pediatrician should know the warning signs of childhood depression and bipolar disorder and have a low threshold for referral of these concerns to the appropriate mental health professional. Ideally, mental health services not provided by the clinician are available in the same setting where physical health services are obtained (see as follows).

Integrated Mental & Behavioral Health in the Primary Care Setting

In the United States, approximately 20% of school-age children suffer from a diagnosable emotional impairment. Prevalence is higher for children living in poor socioeconomic circumstances. About 75% of all children with psychiatric disturbances are seen in primary care settings, and half of all pediatric office visits involve behavioral, psychosocial, or educational concerns.

Child and family concerns routinely manifest in the context of visits with pediatric primary care providers. However, many pediatric providers in community settings do not feel equipped to address the growing mental health and behavioral needs of the populations they serve due to lack of training and perceived lack of support from mental health providers and systems. Parents are most likely to turn to their primary health care provider for information regarding parenting and child development than to another specialist.

Studies have shown that improved detection of mental health conditions is best done when there is a true partnership between clinical providers and families. A small number of clinic settings have moved forward with providing integrated behavior, development, and mental health training for physicians. The HealthySteps for Young Children Program provides an example of training pediatric providers and delivering enhanced developmental services in pediatric primary care settings. Families participating in Healthy Steps received more developmental services, were more satisfied with the quality of care provided, were more likely to attend well-child visits and receive vaccinations on time, and were less likely to use severe discipline techniques with their children. Participation in the program also increased the likelihood that mothers at risk for depression would discuss their symptoms with someone in the pediatric setting.

American Academy of Pediatrics, Committee on Psychosocial Aspects of Child and Family Health and Task Force on Mental Health: The future of pediatrics: mental health competencies for pediatric primary care. Pediatrics 2009 Jul;124:410–421 [PMID: 19564328].

Asarnow J, Rozenman M, Wiblin J, Zeltzer L: Integrated medical-behavioral care compared with usual primary care for child and adolescent behavioral health: a meta-analysis. JAMA Pediatr 2015;169(10):929–937.

TELEPHONE MANAGEMENT & WEB-BASED INFORMATION

Providing appropriate, efficient, and timely clinical advice over the telephone is a critical element of pediatric primary care in the office setting. An estimated 20%–30% of all clinical care delivered by general pediatric offices is provided by telephone. Telephone calls to and from patients occur both during regular office hours and after the office has closed (termed *after-hours*), and the personnel and systems in place to handle office-hours versus before- and after-hours calls may differ. In either circumstance, several principles are important: (1) advice is given only by clinicians or other staff

with formal medical education (eg, nurse, medical assistant), (2) staff is given additional training in providing telephone care, (3) documentation is made of all pertinent information from calls, (4) standardized protocols covering the most common pediatric symptoms are used, and (5) a physician is always available to handle urgent or difficult calls.

During routine office hours, approximately 20%–25% of all telephone calls to pediatric offices involve clinical matters. Many of these calls, however, are routine in nature, and an experienced nurse within the office can screen calls and provide appropriate advice by telephone. Calls from inexperienced or anxious parents about simple concerns should be answered with understanding and respect. Certain types of calls received during office hours should be promptly transferred to a physician: (1) true emergencies, (2) calls regarding hospitalized patients, (3) calls from other medical professionals, and (4) calls from parents who demand to speak with a physician. Nurses should also seek help from a clinician whenever they are uncertain about how to handle a particular call. When in doubt about the diagnosis or necessary treatment, nurses giving telephone advice should err on the side of having the patient seen in the office.

After-hours telephone answering services are available to many clinicians. Pediatric call centers, although not available in all communities, have certain benefits. Calls are managed using standardized protocols, the call centers are typically staffed by nurses with abundant pediatric experience, the calls are well documented, and call centers often perform ongoing quality assurance. Extensive research on pediatric call centers has revealed a high degree of appropriate referrals to emergency departments, safety in terms of outcomes, parent satisfaction with the process, and savings to the health care system.

In general, after-hours pediatric telephone calls tend to be more serious than calls made during regular office hours. Deciding which patients need to be seen, and how urgently, is the most important aspect of these after-hours telephone "encounters." Several factors influence this final patient disposition: (1) the age of the patient, (2) the duration and type of symptom, (3) the presence of any underlying chronic condition, (4) whether the child appears "very sick" to the caller, and (5) the anxiety level of the caller. Once all the pertinent medical information is gathered, a decision is made about whether the child should be seen immediately (by ambulance vs car), seen in the office later (today vs tomorrow), or whether the illness can be safely cared for at home. At the end of the call, it should be confirmed that parents understand and feel comfortable with the plan for their child.

The Internet has become a common tool used in pediatric office settings. Information about the practice and providers, the care of common minor problems, scheduling of appointments, insurance issues, prescription refills, and laboratory test results are often available using the web. Pertinent health information, with appropriate permissions and authority, can often be provided via the electronic medical record to other locations such as hospitals and pharmacies. A well-functioning website is now a crucial service of a pediatric practice.

Bunik M et al: Pediatric telephone call centers—how do they affect health care utilization and costs? Pediatrics 2007;119:e1 [PMID: 17272593].

Kempe A et al: How safe is triage by an after-hours telephone call center? Pediatrics 2006;118:457 [PMID: 16882795].

Liederman EM, Morefield CS: Web messaging: a new tool for patient-physician communication. J Am Med Inform Assoc 2003;10:260 [PMID: 12626378].

▼ ADVOCACY & COMMUNITY PEDIATRICS

Community pediatrics is "a perspective that enlarges the pediatrician's focus from one child to all children in the community." Pediatricians have historically been very involved in supporting and developing services for vulnerable children in their communities. As a group, pediatricians recognize that communities are integral determinants of a child's health and that the synthesis of public health and personal health principles and practices is important in the practice of community pediatrics. As well, pediatricians have long been committed to working with other professionals in the community and advocating for the needs of all children. For example, pediatricians have been instrumental in the passage of laws requiring car seats and bicycle helmets, as well as expanded health care coverage through State Children's Health Insurance Program (SCHIP) working with legislators on both local and federal levels.

Advocacy refers to the act of representing or pleading a cause on behalf of another. Pediatricians and other providers who care for children have a responsibility to be a voice for a population who cannot vote or advocate for themselves very effectively. Advocacy can be broken down into three categories: individual (patient-based), community, and legislative (policy-based).

Pediatricians in practice frequently engage in one-on-one advocacy, which may take the form of writing a letter of medical necessity or referring children and families to valuable services and resources. Pediatricians must be familiar with programs in the community. For example, children with special health care needs may be eligible for services typically funded through state health departments and through programs such as those provided based on the Individuals with Disabilities Education Act (IDEA). A variety of community-based immunization programs can provide access to needed immunizations for eligible children. Food and nutrition programs such as the federally funded WIC program provide sources of food at no cost to eligible families.

Finally, subsidized preschool and child care services such as the federally funded Head Start program provide preschool programs for qualifying children.

Community advocacy goes beyond the walls of the office or hospital. Pediatricians can become involved with local organizations that help children in the community. Pediatricians and other child advocates can work with community partners to address issues that influence child health. Community advocacy might focus on a particular condition (such as obesity) or environmental factors (such as exposure to violence) or improving health prevention (such as promoting programs to incorporate oral health into well-child visits). Finally, pediatricians can learn about issues that affect children and work to affect change at a local, state, or national level. Physician advocates may write or call their legislators, educate the public and disseminate information by writing letters or opinion pieces, provide expert testimony for legislative committees, or even help draft laws.

American Academy of Pediatrics: The pediatrician's role in community pediatrics. Pediatrics 2005;115:1092 [PMID: 15805396].

Duggan A et al: The essential role of research in community pediatrics. Pediatrics 2005;115(Suppl):1195 [PMID: 15821310].

Earnest MA et al: Physician Advocacy: what is it and why do we do it? Acad Med 2010;85:63 [PMID: 20042825].

▼ TOXIC STRESS

Chronic or significant stressors can have a tremendous impact on children, as well as increasing their risk for medical, social, and substance abuse problems later in life. The Adverse Childhood Experiences (ACE) study showed a strongly positive relationship between childhood trauma [abuse (emotional/physical/sexual), household challenges (domestic violence, substance abuse, mental illness, parental separation/divorce, incarcerated family member), and neglect (emotional/physical)] with life-long medical and social problems. When a child experiences chronic stressors, but does not have buffering relationships, toxic stress occurs. Primary care pediatric providers have the opportunity to help families build resiliency by encouraging caregivers to take care of themselves and teaching them how to spend nurturing time with their children. Some families will also benefit from additional supports and resources.

American Academy of Pediatrics Resilience Project: https://www.aap.org/en-us/advocacy-and-policy/aap-health-initiatives/resilience/pages/resilience-project.aspx. Accessed June 29, 2019.

Felitti VJ: Relationship of childhood abuse and household dysfunction to many of the leading causes of death in adults: the adverse childhood experiences (ACE) study. Am J Prev Med 1998:14:245.

▼ COMMON GENERAL PEDIATRIC ISSUES

FEVER

▶ General Considerations

Fever is one of the most common reasons for pediatric office visits, emergency department encounters, and after-hours telephone calls. Several different definitions of fever exist, but most experts define fever as a rectal temperature of 38°C (100.4°F) or above. Temperature in pediatric patients can be measured in a variety of manners: rectal (using a mercury or digital thermometer), oral (mercury or digital), axillary (mercury, digital, or liquid crystal strip), forehead (liquid crystal strip), or tympanic (using a device that measures thermal infrared energy from the tympanic membrane). Tympanic measurement of temperature is quick and requires little patient cooperation. Several cautions apply to the use of this technique: tympanic temperatures have been shown to be less accurate in infants younger than 3 months and are subject to false readings if the instrument is not positioned properly or the external ear canal is occluded by wax.

▶ Causes

Fever occurs when there is a rise in the hypothalamic set point in response to endogenously produced pyrogens. Among the broad range of conditions that cause fever are infections, malignancies, autoimmune diseases, metabolic diseases, chronic inflammatory conditions, medications (including immunizations), CNS abnormalities, and exposure to excessive environmental heat. In most settings, the majority of fevers in pediatric patients are caused by self-limiting viral infections. Meta-analysis has not shown and association between teething and fever.

▶ Evaluation and Clinical Findings

A. Initial Evaluation

When evaluating a child with fever, one should elicit from the parents information about the duration of fever, how the temperature was taken, the maximum height of fever documented at home, all associated symptoms, any chronic medical conditions, any medications taken, medication allergies, fluid intake, urine output, exposures and travel, and any additional features of the illness that concern the parents (Table 9–5). In the office, temperature, heart rate, respiratory rate, and blood pressure should be documented, as well as an oxygen saturation if the child has any increased work of breathing. A complete physical examination, including a neurologic examination, should then be performed, with particular attention paid to the child's degree of toxicity and hydration status. A well-appearing,

Table 9–5. Guidelines for evaluating children with fever.

See immediately if:
1. Child is < age 3 mo with fever > 38°C.
2. Fever is > 40.6°C.
3. Child is crying inconsolably or whimpering.
4. Child is crying when moved or even touched.
5. Child is difficult to awaken.
6. Child's neck is stiff.
7. Purple spots or dots are present on the skin.
8. Child's breathing is difficult and not better after nasal passages are cleared.
9. Child is drooling saliva and is unable to swallow anything.
10. A convulsion has occurred.
11. Child has sickle cell disease, splenectomy, human immunodeficiency virus (HIV), chemotherapy, organ transplant, chronic steroids.
12. Child acts or looks "very sick".

See within 24 h if:
1. Child is 3–6 mo old (unless fever occurs within 48 h after a diphtheria-tetanus-pertussis vaccination and infant has no other serious symptoms).
2. Fever exceeds 40°C (especially if child is < age 3 y).
3. Burning or pain occurs with urination.
4. Fever has been present for > 24 h without an obvious cause or identified site of infection.
5. Fever has subsided for > 24 h and then returned.
6. Fever has been present > 72 h.

well-hydrated child with evidence of a routine viral infection can be safely sent home with symptomatic treatment and careful return precautions.

Depending on patient age, presence of underlying conditions, type of infection, and the provider's assessment of toxicity and hydration, many children with focal bacterial infections can also be treated as outpatients, with appropriate oral antibiotics as discussed in Chapter 42.

B. Fever Without a Focus of Infection

Children who present with fever but without any symptoms or signs of a focal infection are often a diagnostic and management challenge. When assessing a child with fever but no apparent source of infection on examination, the provider needs to carefully consider the likelihood of a serious but "hidden" or occult bacterial infection. With the widespread use of effective vaccines against *Haemophilus influenzae* type b and *Streptococcus pneumoniae*, two of the most common causes of invasive bacterial infections in unimmunized children, the incidence of occult bacterial infections has declined. However, vaccines are not 100% effective, and other organisms cause serious occult infections in children; therefore, febrile children will always demand careful evaluation and observation. Appropriate choices for empiric antibiotic therapy of children with fever without focus are discussed in Chapter 39.

Febrile infants 28 days old or younger, because of their likelihood of serious disease, including sepsis, should always be treated conservatively. Hospitalization and parenteral antibiotics should be strongly considered in all circumstances. An initial diagnostic evaluation should include CBC; blood culture; urinalysis; urine culture; and Gram stain, cerebrospinal fluid protein and glucose tests, as well as culture of the cerebrospinal fluid. Consideration should also be given to the possibility of a perinatal herpes simplex virus infection (neonatal herpes is described in more detail in Chapter 40). A chest radiograph should be obtained for any febrile infant with increased work of breathing.

Infants aged 29–60 days are at risk of developing a variety of invasive bacterial infections. Febrile infants without a focus of infection can be divided into those who appear toxic versus nontoxic, and those at low risk versus higher risk of invasive bacterial disease. As with febrile neonates, toxic children in this age group should be admitted to the hospital for parenteral antibiotics and close observation. Viral illness is the most common cause of fever in this age group; if there is evidence of viral disease (upper respiratory infection, bronchiolitis), further workup may not be necessary. Urinary tract infection is the most common bacterial cause of infection in this age group. Nontoxic low-risk infants in this age group are typically treated as outpatients with close follow-up.

In an era of increasing immunization coverage against the most common invasive pneumococcal serotypes, it is difficult to estimate the risk of occult bacteremia in febrile 3- to 36-month-olds with no focus of infection. Nevertheless, when assessing children aged 3–36 months with temperatures of 39°C or higher, urine cultures should be considered in all male children younger than 6 months and in all females younger than 2 years. Chest radiographs should be performed in any child with increased work of breathing and should also be considered in children with high (20,000/mm³) WBC counts but no respiratory symptoms. Depending on the child's appearance, underlying medical condition, and height of fever, blood cultures should also be obtained. Empiric antibiotic therapy may be considered, particularly for children with temperature of 39°C and WBC count of 15,000/mm³. However, in previously healthy, well-appearing, fully immunized children with reassuring laboratory studies, observation without antibiotics is appropriate.

▶ **Treatment**

Fever phobia is a term that describes parents' anxious response to the fevers that all children experience. In a recent study, 91% of caregivers thought that a fever could cause harmful effects. Around 7% of parents thought that if they did not treat the fever, it would keep going higher. Parents need to be reassured that fevers lower than 41.7°C do not cause brain damage. They should be counseled that, although fevers can occasionally cause seizures—in which case their child needs to be seen—febrile seizures are generally harmless and likewise do not cause brain damage.

Several safe and effective medications are available for the treatment of fever. Acetaminophen is indicated in children older than 2 months who have fever of 39°C or are uncomfortable. Acetaminophen is given in a dosage of 15 mg/kg of body weight per dose and can be given every 4 hours. The other widely used antipyretic is ibuprofen, which can be used in children 6 months and older. Ibuprofen is given in a dosage of 10 mg/kg of body weight per dose and can be given every 6 hours. Ibuprofen and acetaminophen are similar in safety and their ability to reduce fever. Aspirin should not be used for treating fever in any child or adolescent, because of its association with the development of Reye syndrome (particularly during infections with varicella and influenza). With all antipyretics, parents should be counseled to be very careful with dosing and frequency of administration as poisoning can be dangerous. Alternating acetaminophen and ibuprofen is not recommended.

Avner JR: Acute fever. Pediatr Rev 2009;30:5 [PMID: 19118137].

Crocetti M et al: Fever phobia revisited: have parental misconceptions about fever changed in 20 years? Pediatrics 2001;107:1241 [PMID: 11389237].

Sherman JM, Sood SK: Current challenges in the diagnosis and management of fever. Curr Opin Pediatr 2012;24(3):400–406 [PMID: 22525720].

Sullivan JE et al: American Academy of Pediatrics Clinical Report—fever and antipyretic use in children. Pediatrics 2011;127:580 [PMID: 21357332].

GROWTH DEFICIENCY

Growth faltering or growth deficiency—formerly termed *failure to thrive*—is deceleration of growth velocity, resulting in crossing two major percentile lines on the growth chart. The diagnosis also is warranted if a child younger than 6 months has not grown for 2 consecutive months or if a child older than 6 months has not grown for 3 consecutive months. Growth deficiency occurs in about 8% of children.

Patterns of growth deficiency suggest, but are not specific for, different causes. In type I growth deficiency, the head circumference is preserved and the weight is depressed more than the height. This most common type results from inadequate caloric intake, excessive loss of calories, or inability to use calories peripherally. Most cases of type I deficiencies are the result of poverty, lack of caregiver understanding, poor caregiver-child interaction, abnormal feeding patterns, or a combination of factors. Type II growth deficiency, which is associated with genetically determined short stature, endocrinopathies, constitutional growth delay, heart or renal disease, or various forms of skeletal dysplasias, is characterized by normal head circumference and proportionate diminution of height and weight. In type III growth deficiency, all three parameters of growth—head circumference, weight, and height—are lower than normal. This pattern is associated with CNS abnormalities, chromosomal defects, and in utero or perinatal insults.

Just because an infant crosses a growth percentile does not mean an infant necessarily has a problem. Infants can cross growth curves normally, either "lagging down" or "shooting up." This crossing of growth percentiles is usually normal if it meets the following criteria: change in body weight and length are symmetrical, the size of the infant parallels the midparental weight and stature, the development remains normal, and a new growth curve is subsequently established, usually around 15 months of age; this also can be seen in the exclusively breast-fed infants at 4–6 months. WHO growth curves are now the standard and are based on children from various countries who were exclusively or primarily breast-fed in the first 4 months of life.

▶ Clinical Findings

A. Initial Evaluation

The history and physical examination will identify the cause of growth reduction in the vast majority of cases (Table 9–6). The physical examination should focus on signs of organic disease or evidence of abuse or neglect: dysmorphic features, skin lesions, neck masses, adventitial breath sounds, heart murmurs, abdominal masses, and neuromuscular tone and strength. Throughout the evaluation, the physician should observe the caregiver-child interaction and the level of family functioning. Developmental screening and laboratory screening tests (CBC, blood urea nitrogen, creatinine,

Table 9–6. Components of initial evaluation for growth deficiency.

Birth history: newborn screening result; rule out intrauterine growth retardation, anoxia, congenital infections
Feeding and nutrition: difficulty sucking, chewing, swallowing
Feeding patterns: intake of formula, milk, juice, solids
Stooling and voiding of urine: diarrhea, constipation, vomiting, poor urine stream
Growth pattern: several points on the growth chart are crucial
Recurrent infections
Hospitalizations
Human immunodeficiency virus (HIV) risk factors
Developmental history
Social and family factors: family composition, financial status, supports, stresses; heritable diseases, heights and weights of relatives
Review of system

electrolytes, urinalysis, and urine culture) may be useful depending on the history and examination.

B. Further Evaluation

A prospective 3-day diet record should be a standard part of the evaluation. Occasionally, an infant or child may need to be hospitalized to obtain an accurate assessment of intake. This is useful in assessing undernutrition even when organic disease is present. The diet history is evaluated by a dietitian for calories, protein, and micronutrients as well as for the pattern of eating. Additional laboratory tests should be ordered based on the history and physical examination. For example, stool collection for fat determination is indicated if a history of diarrhea suggests malabsorption. Moderate or high amounts of proteinuria should prompt workup for nephrotic syndrome. Vomiting should suggest a gastrointestinal, metabolic, neurologic, infectious, or renal cause. The tempo of evaluation should be based on the severity of symptoms and the magnitude of growth failure.

▶ Treatment

A successful treatment plan addresses the child's diet and eating patterns, the child's development, caregiver skills, and any organic disease. High-calorie diets in the form of higher-calorie formula or liquid supplement are often required and frequent monitoring (every 1 or 2 weeks initially) is essential. Acceptable weight gain varies by age (Table 9–7).

Education in nutrition, child development, and behavioral management as well as psychosocial support of the primary caregiver is essential. If family dysfunction is mild, behavior modification and counseling will be useful. Day care may benefit the child by providing a structured environment for all activities, including eating. If family dysfunction is severe, the local department of social services can help provide structure and assistance to the family. Rarely, the child may need to be temporarily or permanently removed from the home. Hospitalization is reserved for management of dehydration, for cases in which home therapy has failed to result in expected growth, for children who show evidence

Table 9–7. Acceptable weight gain by age.

Age (mo)	Weight Gain (g/day)
Birth to 3	20–30
3–6	15–20
6–9	10–15
9–12	6–11
12–18	5–8
18–24	3–7

of abuse or willful neglect, for management of an illness that compromises a child's ability to eat, or for care pending foster home placement.

Young J: Growth deficiency. In: Bajaj L (ed): *Berman's Pediatric Decision Making*. 5th ed. Mosby-Year Book; 2011.

Web Resources

American Academy of Pediatrics: http://www.aap.org. Accessed June 29, 2019.

Bright Futures National Health Promotion Initiative: http://www.brightfutures.org. Accessed June 29, 2019.

Centers for Disease Control and Prevention (vaccines and immunizations home page): http://www.cdc.gov/vaccines. Accessed June 29, 2019.

National Information Center for Children and Youth With Disabilities: https://www.parentcenterhub.org/. Accessed June 29, 2019.

National Newborn Screening Status Report (2014): http://genes-r-us.uthscsa.edu/sites/genes-r-us/files/nbsdisorders.pdf. Accessed June 29, 2019.

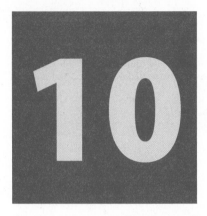

Immunization

Matthew F. Daley, MD

Sean T. O'Leary, MD, MPH

Ann-Christine Nyquist, MD, MSPH

Jessica R. Cataldi, MD, MSCS

Immunization is widely recognized as one of the greatest public health achievements of modern times. Largely due to immunization, the annual incidences of diphtheria, paralytic poliomyelitis, measles, mumps, rubella, and *Haemophilus influenzae* type b (Hib) in the United States have fallen by more than 99% compared with the average annual incidences of these diseases in the 20th century. Invasive pneumococcal disease in children younger than 5 years has declined steeply since routine pneumococcal vaccination began in 2000. Similarly, rotavirus vaccination is associated with substantial declines in hospitalizations and emergency department visits for diarrheal illnesses in young children. Childhood immunization has also led, through herd immunity, to significant decreases in several infectious illnesses in adults, including pneumococcal, rotavirus, and varicella disease.

Every year, approximately 4 million children are born in the United States, and successful immunization of each birth cohort requires the concerted effort of parents, health care providers, public health officials, and vaccine manufacturers. Public perceptions about immunization, particularly routine childhood immunization, are generally positive. However, parent concerns about the safety of vaccines have risen in recent years, in part fueled by unfounded speculation about an association between various vaccines or vaccine components and autism. Modern vaccines have a high degree of safety, serious adverse events following vaccination are rare, and vaccination benefits strongly outweigh these rare risks. Nonetheless, health care providers need to be prepared to discuss the benefits and risks of vaccination with uncertain parents, providing factual information in a clear, empathic, and nonjudgmental manner.

This chapter starts with general principles regarding immunization and the recommended pediatric and adolescent vaccination schedules, followed by a discussion of vaccine safety. Each recommended vaccine is then discussed.

Vaccines only given in special circumstances are discussed in the final section. Several acronyms commonly used in this and other vaccine-related publications are summarized in Table 10–1.

Because the immunization field is rapidly changing, it is important for health care providers to seek the most up-to-date information available. The recommendations outlined are current but will change as technology evolves and our understanding of the epidemiology of vaccine-preventable diseases changes. Several useful sources for regularly updated information about immunization are:

1. The Centers for Disease Control and Prevention (CDC). It maintains a website with extensive vaccine-related resources, including recommendations of the Advisory Committee on Immunization Practices (ACIP), vaccination schedules, Vaccine Information Statements (VISs), and detailed information for the public and providers. Available at: www.cdc.gov/vaccines.

2. CDC Contact Center. The CDC-INFO contact center provides services to the public and health care professionals regarding a variety of health-related issues, including immunizations. Available at: www.cdc.gov/cdc-info, or by phone at 1-800-232-4636 (English and Spanish).

3. *The Red Book: Report of the Committee on Infectious Diseases*. Published at 2- to 3-year intervals by the American Academy of Pediatrics (AAP). A newly revised *Red Book* was published in 2018. Updates are published in the journal *Pediatrics* and can also be accessed at redbook. solutions.aap.org/.

4. Immunization Action Coalition. This nonprofit organization creates and distributes educational materials for the public and health care providers. All materials are provided free of charge and can be accessed at www.vaccineinformation.org (for the public) or www.immunize.org (for health care providers).

Table 10–1. Vaccine-related acronyms.

ACIP	Advisory Committee on Immunization Practices
BCG	Bacillus Calmette-Guérin vaccine against tuberculosis
CDC	Centers for Disease Control and Prevention
CI	Confidence interval
CISA	Clinical Immunization Safety Assessment Network
DT	Pediatric diphtheria and tetanus toxoids
DTaP	Pediatric diphtheria and tetanus toxoids and acellular pertussis vaccine
DTP	Pediatric diphtheria and tetanus toxoids and whole-cell pertussis vaccine
HBIg	Hepatitis B immune globulin
HBsAg	Hepatitis B surface antigen
HepA	Hepatitis A vaccine
HepB	Hepatitis B vaccine
Hib	*Haemophilus influenzae* type b
Hib-MenCY-TT	Hib, meningococcal C and Y, tetanus toxoid vaccine
HIV	Human immunodeficiency virus
HPV	Human papillomavirus
HPV2	HPV vaccine, bivalent
HPV4	HPV vaccine, quadrivalent
HPV9	HPV-vaccine, nine-valent
IIV	Inactivated influenza vaccine
Ig	Immunoglobulin
IPV	Inactivated poliovirus vaccine
LAIV	Live attenuated influenza vaccine
MCV4	Meningococcal conjugate vaccine
MMR	Measles-mumps-rubella vaccine
MMRV	Measles-mumps-rubella-varicella vaccine
MPSV4	Meningococcal polysaccharide vaccine
OPV	Oral poliovirus vaccine
PCV	Pneumococcal conjugate vaccine
PCV7	Pneumococcal conjugate vaccine, 7-valent
PCV13	Pneumococcal conjugate vaccine, 13-valent
PPSV23	Pneumococcal polysaccharide vaccine, 23-valent
PRISM	Post-Licensure Rapid Immunization Safety Monitoring
RV1	Rotavirus vaccine, monovalent
RV5	Rotavirus vaccine, pentavalent
TB	Tuberculosis
Td	Adult tetanus and diphtheria toxoid
Tdap	Tetanus and reduced diphtheria and acellular pertussis vaccine for adolescents and adults
VAERS	Vaccine Adverse Events Reporting System
VariZIG	Varicella-zoster immune globulin
VIS	Vaccine Information Statement
VSD	Vaccine Safety Datalink
VZV	Varicella-zoster virus

5. The Vaccine Education Center at Children's Hospital of Philadelphia. Contains extensive vaccine-related materials, including regarding vaccine safety and vaccine ingredients. Available at: www.chop.edu/centers-programs/vaccine-education-center.

▼ STANDARDS FOR PEDIATRIC IMMUNIZATION PRACTICES

In the United States, every infant requires more than 25 doses of vaccine by age 18 months to be protected against 14 or more childhood diseases. In 2017, immunization coverage rates for children aged 19–35 months were more than 90% for poliovirus, measles-mumps-rubella, varicella, and hepatitis B (HepB) vaccines, and have maintained stable rates around 75% for more recently recommended vaccines such as rotavirus and hepatitis A (HepA) vaccines. CDC recommends the following specific proven strategies to increase vaccination coverage rates: (1) assessing and providing feedback on practice/provider immunization rates; (2) keeping accurate immunization records; (3) recommending vaccination to parents, and reinforcing when to return for vaccination; (4) sending reminder messages to parents; (5) sending reminder messages to providers; (6) reducing missed opportunities to vaccinate; and (7) reducing barriers to immunize within the practice.

The National Childhood Vaccine Injury Act of 1986 requires that for each vaccine covered under the Vaccine Injury Compensation Program, parents should be advised about the risks and benefits of vaccination in a standard manner, using VIS forms produced by CDC. Each time a Vaccine Injury Compensation Program–covered vaccine is administered, the current version of the VIS must be provided to the nonminor patient or legal guardian. Required vaccination documentation in the medical record includes the vaccine manufacturer, lot number, administration date, and expiration date. The VIS version and date and site and route of administration should also be recorded.

Needles used for vaccination should be sterile and disposable to minimize contamination. A 70% solution of alcohol is appropriate for disinfecting the stopper of the vaccine container and the skin at the injection site. A 5% topical emulsion of lidocaine-prilocaine applied to the site of vaccination for 30–60 minutes prior to the injection minimizes pain, especially when multiple vaccines are administered. A separate syringe and needle should be used for each vaccine.

Compliance with the manufacturer's recommendations for route and site of administration of injectable vaccines are critical for safety and efficacy. With few exceptions (Bacillus Calmette-Guérin [BCG] vaccine), all vaccines are given either intramuscularly or subcutaneously. All vaccines containing an adjuvant must be administered intramuscularly to avoid local irritation or granuloma formation. Intramuscular injections are given at a 90-degree angle to the skin, using a needle that is sufficiently long to reach the muscle tissue, but not so long as to injure underlying nerves, blood vessels, or bones. The anterolateral thigh is the preferred site of vaccination in newborns and children up to 2 years of age, and the deltoid muscle is the preferred site for children aged 3–18 years, although the anterolateral thigh is an acceptable site. Needle length and location should be: ⅝ inch in newborn infants (thigh); 1 inch in infants 1- to 12-month-olds (thigh); 1–1¼ inches in 1- to 18-year-olds (thigh), and ⅝–1 inch in 1- to 18-year-olds (deltoid). Subcutaneous injections should be administered at a 45-degree angle into the anterolateral aspect of the thigh (for infants < 12 months) or the upper outer triceps area (for children aged ≥ 12 months) using a 23- or 25-gauge, ⅝-inch needle. Pulling back on the syringe prior to vaccine injection (aspiration) is not recommended.

Many combinations of vaccines can be administered simultaneously without increasing the risk of adverse effects or compromising immune response. Depending on the combination vaccine used, children may receive an "extra" dose of HepB or Hib; these additional doses are not harmful. Inactivated vaccines can be given simultaneously with, or at any time after, a different vaccine. Injectable or intranasal live-virus vaccines (eg, measles-mumps-rubella [MMR], varicella [VAR], or live attenuated influenza [LAIV]), if not administered on the same day, should be given at least 4 weeks apart. If an immunoglobulin (Ig) or blood product has been administered, live-virus vaccination should be delayed 3–11 months to avoid interference with the immune response. The interval depends on the product given (details can be found at: www.cdc.gov/vaccines/hcp/acip-recs/general-recs/timing.html#t-05).

With the large number of vaccine preparations available, interchangeability of vaccines is an issue. All brands of Hib conjugate, HepB, and HepA vaccines are interchangeable. For vaccines containing acellular pertussis antigens, it is recommended that the same brand be used, but when the brand is unknown or the same brand is unavailable, any vaccine with diphtheria and tetanus toxoids and acellular pertussis should be used to continue vaccination. Exceptions to this rule are the serogroup B meningococcal (MenB) vaccines, which are not interchangeable under any circumstance. Extending recommended intervals between vaccinations does not alter final antibody titers, and lapsed schedules do not require restarting the series.

The numerous vaccines and other immunologic products used in routine practice vary in the storage temperatures required. The majority of vaccines should never be subjected to freezing temperatures, except varicella-containing vaccines (MMRV, VAR, and herpes zoster) that should be stored frozen. Product package inserts should be consulted for detailed information on vaccine storage conditions and shelf life.

Vaccines very rarely (about one case per million doses) cause acute anaphylactic-type reactions. All vaccine providers should have the equipment, medications, staff, established protocols, and training to manage emergencies that may occur following vaccination.

CDC: General best practice guidelines for immunization. Best practices guidance of the Advisory Committee on Immunization Practices (ACIP). https://www.cdc.gov/vaccines/hcp/acip-recs/general-recs/index.html.

CDC: Vaccination coverage among children aged 19–35 months-United States, 2017. MMWR Morb Mortal Wkly Rep 2017;67(39):1123–1128 [PMID: 30307907].

McNeil MM et al: Risk of anaphylaxis after vaccination in children and adults. J Allergy Clin Immunol 2016;137:868 [PMID: 26452420].

▼ ROUTINE CHILDHOOD & ADOLESCENT IMMUNIZATION SCHEDULES

Each year, CDC recommends immunization schedules for children and adolescents, which are an important guide for vaccination providers. Vaccines in the schedules are roughly ordered by the age at which the vaccines are first given. Table 10–2 is the 2020 schedule of routine immunizations for normal infants, children, and adolescents from birth through 18 years of age. Table 10–3 is the 2020 schedule for persons aged 4 months through 18 years who start vaccination late or are more than 1 month behind the routine immunization schedule. Annually updated immunization schedules are available at www.cdc.gov/vaccines.

Combination vaccines address the problem of large numbers of injections during a clinic visit. Currently available combination vaccines include MMR, MMRV, and various combinations of Hib, HepB, IPV, and DTaP, including DTaP-HepB-IPV and DTaP-IPV-Hib. There is a newly approved hexavalent (DTaP-IPV-Hib-HepB) vaccine that will likely be available in 2021. Separate vaccines should not be combined into one syringe by the provider unless approved by the Food and Drug Administration (FDA), because this could decrease the efficacy of vaccine components.

VACCINE SAFETY

▶ Vaccine Safety Monitoring

The United States has a sophisticated, multifaceted system to monitor the safety of licensed vaccines. The Vaccine Adverse Event Reporting System (VAERS), the Vaccine Safety Datalink (VSD), the Post-Licensure Rapid Immunization Safety Monitoring (PRISM) system, and the Clinical Immunization Safety Assessment (CISA) system each provide distinct contributions to monitoring vaccine safety. VAERS is a national passive surveillance system administered jointly by the FDA and CDC to accept reports from health care providers and the public about possible vaccine-related adverse events. Reports of adverse events possibly related to vaccination

Table 10–2. Recommended child and adolescent immunization schedule for ages 18 years or younger, United States, 2020.

These recommendations must be read with the notes that follow. For those who fall behind or start late, provide catch-up vaccination at the earliest opportunity as indicated by the green bars. To determine minimum intervals between doses, see the catch-up schedule (Table 2). School entry and adolescent vaccine age groups are shaded in gray.

Vaccine	Birth	1 mo	2 mos	4 mos	6 mos	9 mos	12 mos	15 mos	18 mos	19–23 mos	2–3 yrs	4–6 yrs	7–10 yrs	11–12 yrs	13–15 yrs	16 yrs	17–18 yrs
Hepatitis B (HepB)	1st dose	2nd dose			←———— 3rd dose ————→												
Rotavirus (RV): RV1 (2-dose series), RV5 (3-dose series)			1st dose	2nd dose	See Notes												
Diphtheria, tetanus, acellular pertussis (DTaP <7 yrs)			1st dose	2nd dose	3rd dose		←———— 4th dose ————→					5th dose					
Haemophilus influenzae type b (Hib)			1st dose	2nd dose	See Notes		3rd or 4th dose, See Notes										
Pneumococcal conjugate (PCV13)			1st dose	2nd dose	3rd dose		←——— 4th dose ———→										
Inactivated poliovirus (IPV <18 yrs)			1st dose	2nd dose	←———— 3rd dose ————→							4th dose					
Influenza (IIV)					Annual vaccination 1 or 2 doses						Annual vaccination 1 or 2 doses		Annual vaccination 1 dose only			
Influenza (LAIV)											Annual vaccination 1 or 2 doses		Annual vaccination 1 dose only			
Measles, mumps, rubella (MMR)					See Notes		←——— 1st dose ———→					2nd dose					
Varicella (VAR)					See Notes		←——— 1st dose ———→					2nd dose					
Hepatitis A (HepA)					See Notes		2-dose series, See Notes										
Tetanus, diphtheria, acellular pertussis (Tdap ≥7 yrs)														Tdap			
Human papillomavirus (HPV)													*	See Notes			
Meningococcal (MenACWY-D ≥9 mos, MenACWY-CRM ≥2 mos)														1st dose		2nd dose	
Meningococcal B															See Notes		
Pneumococcal polysaccharide (PPSV23)															See Notes		

Legend	
Range of recommended ages for all children	Range of recommended ages for certain high-risk groups
Range of recommended ages for catch-up immunization	Recommended based on shared clinical decision-making or *can be used in this age group
Range of recommended ages for certain high-risk groups	No recommendation/ not applicable

*can be used in this age group

Reproduced with permission from Centers for Disease Control (CDC) https://www.cdc.gov/vaccines/schedules/hcp/imz/child-adolescent.html.

Table 10–3. Recommended catch-up immunization schedule for children and adolescents who start late or who are more than 1 month behind, United States, 2020.

The table below provides catch-up schedules and minimum intervals between doses for children whose vaccinations have been delayed. A vaccine series does not need to be restarted, regardless of the time that has elapsed between doses. Use the section appropriate for the child's age. **Always use this table in conjunction with Table 1 and the notes that follow.**

Children age 4 months through 6 years

Vaccine	Minimum Age for Dose 1	Minimum Interval Between Doses			
		Dose 1 to Dose 2	Dose 2 to Dose 3	Dose 3 to Dose 4	Dose 4 to Dose 5
Hepatitis B	Birth	**4 weeks**	**8 weeks and at least 16 weeks after first dose.** Minimum age for the final dose is 24 weeks.		
Rotavirus	6 weeks Maximum age for first dose is 14 weeks, 6 days	**4 weeks**	**4 weeks** Maximum age for final dose is 8 months, 0 days.		
Diphtheria, tetanus, and acellular pertussis	6 weeks	**4 weeks**	**4 weeks**	6 months	6 months
Haemophilus influenzae type b	6 weeks	**No further doses needed** if first dose was administered at age 15 months or older. **4 weeks** if first dose was administered before the 1st birthday. **8 weeks (as final dose)** if first dose was administered at age 12 through 14 months.	**No further doses needed** if previous dose was administered at age 15 months or older. **4 weeks** if current age is younger than 12 months **and** first dose was administered at younger than age 7 months **and** at least 1 previous dose was PRP-T (ActHIB, Pentacel, Hiberix) or unknown. **8 weeks and age 12 through 59 months (as final dose)** if current age is younger than 12 months **and** first dose was administered at age 7 through 11 months; OR if current age is 12 through 59 months **and** first dose was administered before the 1st birthday **and** second dose administered at younger than age 15 months; OR if both doses were PRP-OMP (PedvaxHIB, Comvax) **and** were administered before the 1st birthday.	**8 weeks (as final dose)** This dose only necessary for children age 12 through 59 months who received 3 doses before the 1st birthday.	
Pneumococcal conjugate	6 weeks	**No further doses needed** for healthy children if first dose was administered at age 24 months or older. **4 weeks** if first dose was administered before the 1st birthday. **8 weeks (as final dose for healthy children)** if first dose was administered at the 1st birthday or after.	**No further doses needed** for healthy children if previous dose was administered at age 24 months or older. **4 weeks** if current age is younger than 12 months and previous dose was administered at <7 months old. **8 weeks (as final dose for healthy children)** if previous dose was administered between 7–11 months (wait until at least 12 months old); OR if current age is 12 months or older and at least 1 dose was given before age 12 months.	**8 weeks (as final dose)** This dose only necessary for children age 12 through 59 months who received 3 doses before age 12 months or for children at high risk who received 3 doses at any age.	
Inactivated poliovirus	6 weeks	**4 weeks**	**4 weeks** if current age is <4 years. **6 months (as final dose)** if current age is 4 years or older.	**6 months** (minimum age 4 years for final dose).	
Measles, mumps, rubella	12 months	**4 weeks**			
Varicella	12 months	**3 months**			
Hepatitis A	12 months	**6 months**			
Meningococcal ACWY	2 months MenACWY-CRM 9 months MenACWY-D	**8 weeks**	See Notes	See Notes	

Children and adolescents age 7 through 18 years

Vaccine	Minimum Age for Dose 1	Dose 1 to Dose 2	Dose 2 to Dose 3	Dose 3 to Dose 4	
Meningococcal ACWY	Not applicable (N/A)	**8 weeks**			
Tetanus, diphtheria; tetanus, diphtheria, and acellular pertussis	7 years	**4 weeks**	**4 weeks** if first dose of DTaP/DT was administered before the 1st birthday. **6 months (as final dose)** if first dose of DTaP/DT or Tdap/Td was administered at or after the 1st birthday.	**6 months** if first dose of DTaP/DT was administered before the 1st birthday.	
Human papillomavirus	9 years	Routine dosing intervals are recommended.			
Hepatitis A	N/A	**6 months**			
Hepatitis B	N/A	**4 weeks**	**8 weeks and at least 16 weeks after first dose.**		
Inactivated poliovirus	N/A	**4 weeks**	**6 months** A fourth dose is not necessary if the third dose was administered at age 4 years or older and at least 6 months after the previous dose.	A fourth dose of IPV is indicated if all previous doses were administered at <4 years or if the third dose was administered <6 months after the second dose.	
Measles, mumps, rubella	N/A	**4 weeks**			
Varicella	N/A	**3 months** if younger than age 13 years. **4 weeks** if age 13 years and older.			

For vaccine recommendations for persons 19 years of age or older, see the Recommended Adult Immunization Schedule.

Additional information

- Consult relevant ACIP statements for detailed recommendations at www.cdc.gov/vaccines/hcp/acip-recs/index.html.
- For information on contraindications and precautions for the use of a vaccine, consult the General Best Practice Guidelines for Immunization at www.cdc.gov/vaccines/hcp/acip-recs/general-recs/contraindications.html and relevant ACIP statements at www.cdc.gov/vaccines/hcp/acip-recs/index.html.
- For calculating intervals between doses, 4 weeks = 28 days. Intervals of ≥4 months are determined by calendar months.
- Within a number range (e.g., 12–18), a dash (–) should be read as "through."
- Vaccine doses administered ≤4 days before the minimum age or interval are considered valid. Doses of any vaccine administered ≥5 days earlier than the minimum age or minimum interval should not be counted as valid and should be repeated as age-appropriate. The repeat dose should be spaced after the invalid dose by the recommended minimum interval. For further details, see Table 3-1, Recommended and minimum ages and intervals between vaccine doses, in General Best Practice Guidelines for Immunization at www.cdc.gov/vaccines/hcp/acip-recs/general-recs/timing.html.
- Information on travel vaccine requirements and recommendations is available at www.cdc.gov/travel/.
- For vaccination of persons with immunodeficiencies, see Table 8-1, Vaccination of persons with primary and secondary immunodeficiencies, in General Best Practice Guidelines for Immunization at www.cdc.gov/vaccines/hcp/acip-recs/general-recs/immunocompetence.html, and Immunization in Special Clinical Circumstances (In: Kimberlin DW, Brady MT, Jackson MA, Long SS, eds. Red Book: 2018 Report of the Committee on Infectious Diseases. 31st ed. Itasca, IL: American Academy of Pediatrics;2018:67–111).
- For information regarding vaccination in the setting of a vaccine-preventable disease outbreak, contact your state or local health department.

- The National Vaccine Injury Compensation Program (VICP) is a no-fault alternative to the traditional legal system for resolving vaccine injury claims. All routine child and adolescent vaccines are covered by VICP except for pneumococcal polysaccharide vaccine (PPSV23). For more information, see www.hrsa.gov/vaccinecompensation/index.html.

Diphtheria, tetanus, and pertussis (DTaP) vaccination (minimum age: 6 weeks [4 years for Kinrix or Quadracel])

Routine vaccination

- 5-dose series at 2, 4, 6, 15–18 months, 4–6 years
- **Prospectively:** Dose 4 may be administered as early as age 12 months if at least 6 months have elapsed since dose 3.
- **Retrospectively:** A 4th dose that was inadvertently administered as early as 12 months may be counted if at least 4 months have elapsed since dose 3.

Catch-up vaccination

- Dose 5 is not necessary if dose 4 was administered at age 4 years or older and at least 6 months after dose 3.
- For other catch-up guidance, see Table 2.

Haemophilus influenzae type b vaccination (minimum age: 6 weeks)

Routine vaccination

- ActHIB, Hiberix, or Pentacel: 4-dose series at 2, 4, 6, 12–15 months
- PedvaxHIB: 3-dose series at 2, 4, 12–15 months

Catch-up vaccination

- **Dose 1 at 7–11 months:** Administer dose 2 at least 4 weeks later and dose 3 (final dose) at 12–15 months or 8 weeks after dose 2 (whichever is later).
- **Dose 1 at 12–14 months:** Administer dose 2 (final dose) at least 8 weeks after dose 1.
- **Dose 1 before 12 months and dose 2 before 15 months:** Administer dose 3 (final dose) 8 weeks after dose 2.
- **2 doses of PedvaxHIB before 12 months:** Administer dose 3 (final dose) at 12–59 months and at least 8 weeks after dose 2.
- **Unvaccinated at 15–59 months:** 1 dose
- **Previously unvaccinated children age 60 months or older** who are not considered high risk do not require catch-up vaccination.
- For other catch-up guidance, see Table 2.

Special situations

- **Chemotherapy or radiation treatment:**

  <u>12–59 months:</u>
  - Unvaccinated or only 1 dose before age 12 months: 2 doses, 8 weeks apart
  - 2 or more doses before age 12 months: 1 dose at least 8 weeks after previous dose

  Doses administered within 14 days of starting therapy or during therapy should be repeated at least 3 months after therapy completion.

- **Hematopoietic stem cell transplant (HSCT):**
  - 3-dose series 4 weeks apart starting 6 to 12 months after successful transplant, regardless of Hib vaccination history

- **Anatomic or functional asplenia (including sickle cell disease):**

  <u>12–59 months:</u>
  - Unvaccinated or only 1 dose before age 12 months: 2 doses, 8 weeks apart
  - 2 or more doses before age 12 months: 1 dose at least 8 weeks after previous dose

  Unvaccinated persons age 5 years or older*
  - 1 dose

- **Elective splenectomy:**

  Unvaccinated persons age 15 months or older*
  - 1 dose (preferably at least 14 days before procedure)

- **HIV infection:**

  <u>12–59 months:</u>
  - Unvaccinated or only 1 dose before age 12 months: 2 doses, 8 weeks apart
  - 2 or more doses before age 12 months: 1 dose at least 8 weeks after previous dose

  Unvaccinated persons age 5–18 years*
  - 1 dose

- **Immunoglobulin deficiency, early component complement deficiency:**

  <u>12–59 months:</u>
  - Unvaccinated or only 1 dose before age 12 months: 2 doses, 8 weeks apart
  - 2 or more doses before age 12 months: 1 dose at least 8 weeks after previous dose

Unvaccinated = Less than routine series (through 14 months) OR no doses (15 months or older)

(Continued)

Hepatitis A vaccination
(minimum age: 12 months for routine vaccination)

Routine vaccination
- 2-dose series (minimum interval: 6 months) beginning at age 12 months

Catch-up vaccination
- Unvaccinated persons through 18 years should complete a 2-dose series (minimum interval: 6 months).
- Persons who previously received 1 dose at age 12 months or older should receive dose 2 at least 6 months after dose 1.
- Adolescents 18 years and older may receive the combined HepA and HepB vaccine, Twinrix®, as a 3-dose series (0, 1, and 6 months) or 4-dose series (0, 7, and 21-30 days), followed by a dose at 12 months).

International travel
- Persons traveling to or working in countries with high or intermediate endemic hepatitis A (www.cdc.gov/travel/):
- Infants age 6-11 months: 1 dose before departure; revaccinate with 2 doses, separated by at least 6 months, between 12 and 23 months of age.
- Unvaccinated age 12 months and older: Administer dose 1 as soon as travel is considered.

Hepatitis B vaccination
(minimum age: birth)

Birth dose (monovalent HepB vaccine only)
- Mother is HBsAg-negative: 1 dose within 24 hours of birth for all medically stable infants ≥2,000 grams. Infants <2,000 grams: Administer 1 dose at chronological age 1 month or hospital discharge.
- Mother is HBsAg-positive:
  - Administer HepB vaccine and hepatitis B immune globulin (HBIG) (in separate limbs) within 12 hours of birth, regardless of birth weight. For infants <2,000 grams, administer 3 additional doses of vaccine (total of 4 doses) beginning at age 1 month.
  - Test for HBsAg and anti-HBs at age 9-12 months. If HepB series is delayed, test 1-2 months after final dose.
- Mother's HBsAg status is unknown:
  - Administer HepB vaccine within 12 hours of birth, regardless of birth weight.
  - For infants <2,000 grams, administer HBIG in addition to HepB vaccine (in separate limbs) within 12 hours of birth. Administer 3 additional doses of vaccine (total of 4 doses) beginning at age 1 month.
  - Determine mother's HBsAg status as soon as possible. If mother is HBsAg-positive, administer HBIG to infants ≥2,000 grams as soon as possible, but no later than 7 days of age.

Routine series
- 3-dose series at 0, 1-2, 6-18 months (use monovalent HepB vaccine for doses administered before age 6 weeks)
- Infants who did not receive a birth dose should begin the series as soon as feasible (see Table 2).
- Administration of 4 doses is permitted when a combination vaccine containing HepB is used after the birth dose.
- Minimum age for the final (3rd or 4th) dose: 24 weeks
- Minimum intervals: dose 1 to dose 2: 4 weeks / dose 2 to dose 3: 8 weeks / dose 1 to dose 3: 16 weeks (when 4 doses are administered, substitute "dose 4" for "dose 3" in these calculations)

Catch-up vaccination
- Unvaccinated persons should complete a 3-dose series at 0, 1-2, 6 months.
- Adolescents age 11-15 years may use an alternative 2-dose schedule with at least 4 months between doses (adult formulation Recombivax HB only).
- Adolescents 18 years and older may receive a 2-dose series of HepB (Heplisav-B®) at least 4 weeks apart.
- Adolescents 18 years and older may receive the combined HepA and HepB vaccine, Twinrix, as a 3-dose series (0, 1, and 6 months) or 4-dose series (0, 7, and 21-30 days), followed by a dose at 12 months).
- For other catch-up guidance, see Table 2.

Special situations
- Revaccination is not generally recommended for persons with a normal immune status who were vaccinated as infants, children, adolescents, or adults.
- Revaccination may be recommended for certain populations, including:
  - Infants born to HBsAg-positive mothers
  - Hemodialysis patients
  - Other immunocompromised persons
- For detailed revaccination recommendations, see www.cdc.gov/vaccines/hcp/acip-recs/vacc-specific/hepb.html.

Human papillomavirus vaccination
(minimum age: 9 years)

Routine and catch-up vaccination
- HPV vaccination routinely recommended at age 11-12 years (can start at age 9 years) and catch-up HPV vaccination recommended for all persons through age 18 years if not adequately vaccinated
- 2- or 3-dose series depending on age at initial vaccination:
  - Age 9 through 14 years at initial vaccination: 2-dose series at 0, 6-12 months (minimum interval: 5 months; repeat dose if administered too soon)
  - Age 15 years or older at initial vaccination: 3-dose series at 0, 1-2 months, 6 months (minimum intervals: dose 1 to dose 2: 4 weeks / dose 2 to dose 3: 12 weeks / dose 1 to dose 3: 5 months; repeat dose if administered too soon)
- If completed valid vaccination series with any HPV vaccine, no additional doses needed

Special situations
- Immunocompromising conditions, including HIV infection: 3-dose series as above
- History of sexual abuse or assault: Start at age 9 years.
- Pregnancy: HPV vaccination not recommended until after pregnancy; no intervention needed if vaccinated while pregnant; pregnancy testing not needed before vaccination

Influenza vaccination
(minimum age: 6 months [IIV], 2 years [LAIV], 18 years [recombinant influenza vaccine, RIV])

Routine vaccination
- Use any influenza vaccine appropriate for age and health status annually:
  - 2 doses, separated by at least 4 weeks, for children age 6 months-8 years who have received fewer than 2 influenza vaccine doses before July 1, 2019, or whose influenza vaccination history is unknown (administer dose 2 even if the child turns 9 between receipt of dose 1 and dose 2)
  - 1 dose for children age 6 months-8 years who have received at least 2 influenza vaccine doses before July 1, 2019
  - 1 dose for all persons age 9 years and older
- For the 2020-21 season, see the 2020-21 ACIP influenza vaccine recommendations.

Special situations
- Egg allergy, hives only: Any influenza vaccine appropriate for age and health status annually
- Egg allergy with symptoms other than hives (e.g., angioedema, respiratory distress, need for emergency medical services or epinephrine): Any influenza vaccine appropriate for age and health status annually in medical setting under supervision of health care provider who can recognize and manage severe allergic reactions

- **LAIV should not be used** in persons with the following conditions or situations:
  - History of severe allergic reaction to a previous dose of any influenza vaccine or to any vaccine component (excluding egg; see details above)
  - Receiving aspirin or salicylate-containing medications
  - Age 2–4 years with history of asthma or wheezing
  - Immunocompromised due to any cause (including medications and HIV infection)
  - Anatomic or functional asplenia
  - Cochlear implant
  - Cerebrospinal fluid-oropharyngeal communication
  - Close contacts or caregivers of severely immunosuppressed persons who require a protected environment
  - Pregnancy
  - Received influenza antiviral medications within the previous 48 hours

Measles, mumps, and rubella vaccination
(minimum age: 12 months for routine vaccination)
Routine vaccination
- 2-dose series at 12–15 months, 4–6 years
- Dose 2 may be administered as early as 4 weeks after dose 1.

Catch-up vaccination
- Unvaccinated children and adolescents: 2-dose series at least 4 weeks apart
- The maximum age for use of MMRV is 12 years.

Special situations
International travel
- Infants age 6–11 months: 1 dose before departure; revaccinate with 2-dose series with dose 1 at 12–15 months (12 months for children in high-risk areas) and dose 2 as early as 4 weeks later.
- **Unvaccinated children age 12 months and older:** 2-dose series at least 4 weeks apart before departure

Meningococcal serogroup A,C,W,Y vaccination
(minimum age: 2 months [MenACWY-CRM, Menveo], 9 months [MenACWY-D, Menactra])
Routine vaccination
- 2-dose series at 11–12 years, 16 years

Catch-up vaccination
- Age 13–15 years: 1 dose now and booster at age 16–18 years (minimum interval: 8 weeks)
- Age 16–18 years: 1 dose

Special situations
Anatomic or functional asplenia (including sickle cell disease), HIV infection, persistent complement component deficiency, complement inhibitor (e.g., eculizumab, ravulizumab) use:
- **Menveo**
  - Dose 1 at age 8 weeks: 4-dose series at 2, 4, 6, 12 months
  - Dose 1 at age 7–23 months: 2-dose series (dose 2 at least 12 weeks after dose 1 and after age 12 months)
  - Dose 1 at age 24 months or older: 2-dose series at least 8 weeks apart
- **Menactra**
- **Persistent complement component deficiency or complement inhibitor use:**
  - Age 9–23 months: 2-dose series at least 12 weeks apart
  - Age 24 months or older: 2-dose series at least 8 weeks apart
- **Anatomic or functional asplenia, sickle cell disease, or HIV infection:**
  - Age 9–23 months: Not recommended
  - Age 24 months or older: 2-dose series at least 8 weeks apart
  - Menactra must be administered at least 4 weeks after completion of PCV13 series

Travel in countries with hyperendemic or epidemic meningococcal disease, including countries in the African meningitis belt or during the Hajj (www.cdc.gov/travel/):
- **Children less than age 24 months:**
- **Menveo (age 2–23 months):**
  - Dose 1 at 8 weeks: 4-dose series at 2, 4, 6, 12 months
  - Dose 1 at 7–23 months: 2-dose series (dose 2 at least 12 weeks after dose 1 and after age 12 months)
- **Menactra (age 9–23 months):**
  - 2-dose series (dose 2 at least 12 weeks after dose 1; dose 2 may be administered as early as 8 weeks after dose 1 in travelers)
- Children age 2 years or older: 1 dose Menveo or Menactra

First-year college students who live in residential housing (if not previously vaccinated at age 16 years or older) or military recruits:
- 1 dose Menveo or Menactra

Adolescent vaccination of children who received MenACWY prior to age 10 years:
- **Children for whom boosters are recommended** because of an ongoing increased risk of meningococcal disease (e.g., those with complement deficiency, HIV, or asplenia): Follow the booster schedule for persons at increased risk (see below).
- **Children for whom boosters are not recommended** (e.g., those who received a single dose for travel to a country where meningococcal disease is endemic): Administer MenACWY according to the recommended adolescent schedule with dose 1 at age 11–12 years and dose 2 at age 16 years.

Note: Menactra should be administered either before or at the same time as DTaP. For MenACWY booster dose recommendations for groups listed under "Special situations" and in an outbreak setting and for additional meningococcal vaccination information, see www.cdc.gov/vaccines/hcp/acip-recs/vacc-specific/mening.html.

Meningococcal serogroup B vaccination
(minimum age: 10 years [MenB-4C, Bexsero; MenB-FHbp, Trumenba])
Shared clinical decision-making
- Adolescents not at increased risk age 16–23 years (preferred age 16–18 years) based on shared clinical decision-making:
  - Bexsero: 2-dose series at least 1 month apart
  - Trumenba: 2-dose series at least 6 months apart; if dose 2 is administered earlier than 6 months, administer a 3rd dose at least 4 months after dose 2.

Special situations
Anatomic or functional asplenia (including sickle cell disease), persistent complement component deficiency, complement inhibitor (e.g., eculizumab, ravulizumab) use:
- Bexsero: 2-dose series at least 1 month apart
- Trumenba: 3-dose series at 0, 1–2, 6 months

Bexsero and Trumenba are not interchangeable; the same product should be used for all doses in a series. For MenB booster dose recommendations for groups listed under "Special situations" and in an outbreak setting and for additional meningococcal vaccination information, see www.cdc.gov/vaccines/acip/recommendations.html and www.cdc.gov/vaccines/hcp/acip-recs/vacc-specific/mening.html.

(Continued)

Pneumococcal vaccination

(minimum age: 6 weeks [PCV13], 2 years [PPSV23])

Routine vaccination with PCV13

- 4-dose series at 2, 4, 6, 12–15 months

Catch-up vaccination with PCV13

- 1 dose for healthy children age 24–59 months with any incomplete* PCV13 series
- For other catch-up guidance, see Table 2.

Special situations

High-risk conditions below: When both PCV13 and PPSV23 are indicated, administer PCV13 first. PCV13 and PPSV23 should not be administered during the same visit.

Chronic heart disease (particularly cyanotic congenital heart disease and cardiac failure), chronic lung disease (including asthma treated with high-dose, oral corticosteroids), diabetes mellitus:

Age 2–5 years

- Any incomplete* series with:
  - 3 PCV13 doses: 1 dose PCV13 (at least 8 weeks after any prior PCV13 dose)
  - Less than 3 PCV13 doses: 2 doses PCV13 (8 weeks after the most recent dose and administered 8 weeks apart)
- No history of PPSV23: 1 dose PPSV23 (at least 8 weeks after any prior PCV13 dose)

Age 6–18 years

- No history of PPSV23: 1 dose PPSV23 at least 8 weeks after any prior PCV13 dose

Cerebrospinal fluid leak, cochlear implant:

Age 2–5 years

- Any incomplete* series with:
  - 3 PCV13 doses: 1 dose PCV13 (at least 8 weeks after any prior PCV13 dose)
  - Less than 3 PCV13 doses: 2 doses PCV13 (8 weeks after the most recent dose and administered 8 weeks apart)
- No history of PPSV23: 1 dose PPSV23 (at least 8 weeks after any prior PCV13 dose)

Age 6–18 years

- No history of PPSV23: 1 dose PPSV23 (at least 8 weeks after any prior PCV13 dose)

Sickle cell disease and other hemoglobinopathies; anatomic or functional asplenia; congenital or acquired immunodeficiency; HIV infection; chronic renal failure; nephrotic syndrome; malignant neoplasms, leukemias, lymphomas, Hodgkin disease, and other diseases associated with treatment with immunosuppressive drugs or radiation therapy: solid organ transplantation; multiple myeloma:

Age 2–5 years

- Any incomplete* series with:
  - 3 PCV13 doses: 1 dose PCV13 (at least 8 weeks after any prior PCV13 dose)
  - Less than 3 PCV13 doses: 2 doses PCV13 (8 weeks after the most recent dose and administered 8 weeks apart)
- No history of PPSV23: 1 dose PPSV23 (at least 8 weeks after any prior PCV13 dose) and a 2nd dose of PPSV23 5 years later

Age 6–18 years

- No history of either PCV13 or PPSV23: 1 dose PCV13, 2 doses PPSV23 (dose 1 of PPSV23 administered 8 weeks after PCV13 and dose 2 of PPSV23 administered at least 5 years after dose 1 of PPSV23)
- Any PCV13 but no PPSV23: 2 doses PPSV23 (dose 1 of PPSV23 administered 8 weeks after the most recent dose of PCV13 and dose 2 of PPSV23 administered at least 5 years after dose 1 of PPSV23)
- PPSV23 but no PCV13: 1 dose PCV13 at least 8 weeks after the most recent PPSV23 dose and a 2nd dose of PPSV23 administered 5 years after dose 1 of PPSV23 and at least 8 weeks after a dose of PCV13

Chronic liver disease, alcoholism:

Age 6–18 years

- No history of PPSV23: 1 dose PPSV23 (at least 8 weeks after any prior PCV13 dose)

*Incomplete series = Not having received all doses in either the recommended series or an age-appropriate catch-up series See Tables 8, 9, and 11 in the ACIP pneumococcal vaccine recommendations at www.cdc.gov/mmwr/pdf/rr/rr5911.pdf for complete schedule details.

Poliovirus vaccination

(minimum age: 6 weeks)

Routine vaccination

- 4-dose series at ages 2, 4, 6–18 months, 4–6 years; administer the final dose at or after age 4 years and at least 6 months after the previous dose.

- 4 or more doses of IPV can be administered before age 4 years when a combination vaccine containing IPV is used. However, a dose is still recommended at or after age 4 years and at least 6 months after the previous dose.

Catch-up vaccination

- In the first 6 months of life, use minimum ages and intervals only for travel to a polio-endemic region or during an outbreak.
- IPV is not routinely recommended for U.S. residents 18 years and older.

Series containing oral polio vaccine (OPV), either mixed OPV-IPV or OPV-only series:

- Total number of doses needed to complete the series is the same as that recommended for the U.S. IPV schedule. See www.cdc.gov/mmwr/volumes/66/wr/mm6601a6.htm?s_cid=mm6601a6_w.
- Only trivalent OPV (tOPV) counts toward the U.S. vaccination requirements.
  - Doses of OPV administered before April 1, 2016, should be counted (unless specifically noted as administered during a campaign).
  - Doses of OPV administered on or after April 1, 2016, should not be counted.
  - For guidance to assess doses documented as "OPV", see www.cdc.gov/mmwr/volumes/66/wr/mm6606a7.htm?s_cid=mm6606a7_w.
- For other catch-up guidance, see Table 2.

Rotavirus vaccination

(minimum age: 6 weeks)

Routine vaccination

- Rotarix: 2-dose series at 2 and 4 months
- RotaTeq: 3-dose series at 2, 4, and 6 months
- If any dose in the series is either RotaTeq or unknown, default to 3-dose series.

Catch-up vaccination

- Do not start the series on or after age 15 weeks, 0 days.
- The maximum age for the final dose is 8 months, 0 days.
- For other catch-up guidance, see Table 2.

Tetanus, diphtheria, and pertussis (Tdap) vaccination

(minimum age: 11 years for routine vaccination, 7 years for catch-up vaccination)

Routine vaccination

- Adolescents age 11–12 years: 1 dose Tdap
- Pregnancy: 1 dose Tdap during each pregnancy, preferably in early part of gestational weeks 27–36
- Tdap may be administered regardless of the interval since the last tetanus- and diphtheria-toxoid-containing vaccine.

Catch-up vaccination
- Adolescents age 13–18 years who have not received Tdap:
  1 dose Tdap, then Td or Tdap booster every 10 years
- Persons age 7–18 years not fully vaccinated* with DTaP:
  1 dose Tdap as part of the catch-up series (preferably the first dose); if additional doses are needed, use Td or Tdap.
- **Tdap administered at 7–10 years:**
  - Children age 7–9 years who receive Tdap should receive the routine Tdap dose at age 11–12 years.
  - Children age 10 years who receive Tdap do not need to receive the routine Tdap dose at age 11–12 years.

- DTaP inadvertently administered at or after age 7 years:
  - Children age 7–9 years: DTaP may count as part of catch-up series. Routine Tdap dose at age 11–12 years should be administered.
  - Children age 10–18 years: Count dose of DTaP as the adolescent Tdap booster.
- For other catch-up guidance, see Table 2.
- For information on use of Tdap or Td as tetanus prophylaxis in wound management, see www.cdc.gov/mmwr/volumes/67/rr/rr6702a1.htm.

*Fully vaccinated = 5 valid doses of DTaP OR 4 valid doses of DTaP if dose 4 was administered at age 4 years or older

Varicella vaccination
(minimum age: 12 months)
Routine vaccination
- 2-dose series at 12–15 months, 4–6 years
- Dose 2 may be administered as early as 3 months after dose 1 (a dose administered after a 4-week interval may be counted).
Catch-up vaccination
- Ensure persons age 7–18 years without evidence of immunity (see www.cdc.gov/mmwr/pdf/rr/rr5604.pdf) have 2-dose series:
  - **Age 7–12 years:** routine interval: 3 months (a dose administered after a 4-week interval may be counted)
  - **Age 13 years and older:** routine interval: 4–8 weeks (minimum interval: 4 weeks)
  - The maximum age for use of MMRV is 12 years.

can be made via the Internet (vaers.hhs.gov) or by telephone (1-800-822-7967). As a passive surveillance system, VAERS is subject to limitations, including underreporting, overreporting, the reporting of events that are temporally but not causally related to vaccination, the lack of denominator data, and the lack of a comparison group. The VSD and PRISM, in comparison, are active surveillance systems with continuous safety monitoring of vaccines in defined patient populations. The VSD and PRISM can conduct timely investigations of newly licensed vaccines or emerging vaccine safety concerns. The CISA system is designed to develop protocols for the evaluation, diagnosis, and treatment of adverse events following immunization. Patients with rare and serious adverse events following immunization can be referred to CISA for evaluation.

▶ Vaccine Contraindications & Precautions

All vaccines have certain contraindications and precautions that guide their administration. A contraindication indicates that the potential vaccine recipient is at increased risk of a serious adverse event. A vaccine should not be given when a contraindication to that vaccine is present, whereas a precaution indicates a circumstance that might increase the risk of adverse events or diminish vaccine effectiveness. In the setting of precautions, the risks and benefits of vaccination must be carefully weighed prior to a decision regarding vaccination. Precautions are often temporary, in which case vaccination can resume once the precaution no longer applies. Contraindications and precautions are listed with each vaccine in this chapter. Additional, more detailed, information is available from the CDC (www.cdc.gov/vaccines), in the AAP's *Red Book*, and in vaccine package inserts.

DeStefano F, Shimabukuro TT: The MMR vaccine and autism. Annu Rev Virol 2019; Epub ahead of print [PMID: 30986133].

DeStefano F et al: Principal controversies in vaccine safety in the United States. Clin Infect Dis 2019; Epub ahead of print [PMID: 30753348].

Glanz JM et al: White Paper on studying the safety of the childhood immunization schedule in the Vaccine Safety Datalink. Vaccine 2016;34 Suppl 1:A1 [PMID: 26830300].

Moro PL et al: Surveillance systems and methods for monitoring the post-marketing safety of influenza vaccines at the Centers for Disease Control and Prevention. Expert Opin Drug Saf 2016;15:1175 [PMID: 27268157].

VACCINATION IN SPECIAL CIRCUMSTANCES

▶ Minor Acute Illnesses

Minor acute illnesses, with or without low-grade fever, are not contraindications to vaccination, because there is no evidence that vaccination under these conditions increases the rate of adverse effects or decreases efficacy. A moderate to severe febrile illness may be a reason to postpone vaccination. Routine physical examination and temperature assessment are not necessary before vaccinating healthy infants and children.

▶ Children With Chronic Illnesses

Most chronic diseases are not contraindications to vaccination; in fact, children with chronic diseases may be at greater risk of complications from vaccine-preventable diseases, such as influenza and pneumococcal infections. Premature infants are a good example. They should be immunized according to their chronologic, not gestational, age. Vaccine doses should not be reduced for preterm or low-birth-weight infants. One exception is children with progressive central nervous system disorders. Vaccination with DTaP should be deferred until the neurologic condition has been clarified and is stable.

▶ Immunodeficient Children

Congenitally immunodeficient children should not be immunized with live-virus vaccines (oral polio vaccine [OPV, not available in the United States], rotavirus, MMR, VAR, MMRV, yellow fever, or LAIV) or live-bacteria vaccines (BCG or live typhoid fever vaccine). Depending on the nature of the immunodeficiency, other vaccines are safe but may fail to evoke an immune response. Children with cancer and children receiving high-dose corticosteroids or other immunosuppressive agents should not be vaccinated with live-virus or live-bacteria vaccines. This contraindication does not apply if the malignancy is in remission and chemotherapy has not been administered for at least 90 days. Live-virus vaccines may also be administered to previously healthy children receiving low to moderate doses of corticosteroids (defined as up to 2 mg/kg/day of prednisone or prednisone equivalent, with a 20 mg/day maximum) for less than 14 days; children without other immunodeficiency receiving short-acting alternate-day corticosteroids; children being maintained on physiologic corticosteroid therapy; and children receiving only topical, inhaled, or intra-articular corticosteroids.

Contraindication of live-pathogen vaccines also applies to children with HIV infection who are severely immunosuppressed. Those who receive MMR should have at least 15% CD4 cells, a CD4 lymphocyte count equivalent to CDC immunologic class 2, and be asymptomatic from their HIV. MMR for these children is recommended at 12 months of age (after 6 months of age during an epidemic); some experts suggest delaying MMR vaccination in HIV-infected children until they have received antiretroviral therapy for 3 months. For HIV-infected children, a booster MMR dose may be given at least 1 month after the initial dose; in fact, giving this booster dose earlier than at 4–6 years of age is often encouraged. Doses given before 1 year of age should not be considered part of a complete series. VAR vaccination is also recommended for HIV-infected children with CD4 cells preserved or recovered as listed earlier. The ACIP recommends only IPV vaccination for children. Thus, immunodeficient children should no longer be exposed to OPV through household contacts. MMR and VAR are not contraindicated in household contacts of immunocompromised children. HIV-infected children who were vaccinated before their HIV was treated should be reimmunized to ensure adequate protection. The recommended immunization schedule for immunocompromised children is available at https://www.cdc.gov/vaccines/schedules/hcp/imz/child-indications.html.

▶ Allergic or Hypersensitive Children

Severe hypersensitivity reactions are rare following vaccination (1.53 cases per 1 million doses). They are generally attributable to a trace component of the vaccine other than to the antigen; for example, MMR, IPV, and VAR contain microgram quantities of neomycin, and IPV also contains trace amounts of streptomycin and polymyxin B. Children with known anaphylactic responses to these antibiotics should not be given these vaccines. Trace quantities of egg antigens may be present in both inactivated and live influenza and yellow fever vaccines. Guidelines for influenza vaccination in children with egg allergies have recently changed. The trace amounts of egg protein are generally considered below the threshold needed to induce an allergic reaction and there has been no increased risk of anaphylaxis documented in children with severe egg allergies. Therefore, children with severe egg allergy can be vaccinated with influenza vaccine with no special precautions beyond those for any other vaccine. Some vaccines (MMR, MMRV, and VAR) contain gelatin. For any persons with a history of anaphylactic reaction to gelatin or any component contained in a vaccine, the vaccine package insert should be reviewed and additional consultation sought, such as from a pediatric allergist. Some tips and rubber plungers of vaccine syringes contain latex. These vaccines should not be administered to individuals with a history of severe anaphylactic allergy to latex, but may be administered to people with less severe allergies. Thimerosal is an organic mercurial compound used as a preservative in vaccines since the 1930s. While there is no evidence that thimerosal has caused serious allergic reactions or autism, all routinely recommended vaccines for infants have been manufactured without thimerosal since mid-2001. Thimerosal-free formulations of injectable influenza vaccine are available, and LAIV does not contain thimerosal.

▶ Other Special Circumstances

Detailed recommendations for preterm low-birth-weight infants; pediatric transplant recipients; Alaskan Natives/American Indians; children in residential institutions or military communities; or refugees, new immigrants, or travelers are available from the CDC (at http://www.cdc.gov/vaccines) and from the AAP's *Red Book.*

CDC: General recommendations on immunization: recommendations of the Advisory Committee on Immunization Practices (ACIP). MMWR Recomm Rep 2011;60(RR-02):1 [PMID: 21293327].

Kelso JM: Administering influenza vaccine to egg-allergic persons. Expert Rev Vaccines 2014;13:1049 [PMID: 24962036].

COMMUNICATING WITH PARENTS ABOUT VACCINES

Most parents in the United States choose to vaccinate their children. In 2017, 1.1% of young children received no vaccines. However, parental concern about vaccines is on the rise, and an increasing number of parents are choosing to delay or decline vaccination for their children. While there are myriad reasons given for not vaccinating, several themes recur. Some parents do not believe their children are at risk for diseases such as poliomyelitis, measles, and tetanus. Other parents do not believe that certain vaccine-preventable diseases, such as varicella and pertussis, are particularly serious. There are also widespread concerns about the safety of vaccines. Health care providers have a critically important role in discussing the known risks and benefits of vaccination with parents. In this context, it is important that providers recognize that parent decisions are often based on inaccurate information about vaccine risk provided by the media or Internet sources.

AAP, CDC, and others have developed resources to guide providers on how best to communicate with parents about vaccines. A presumptive recommendation ("We have three shots to do today") is likely more effective than a participatory approach ("Have you thought about the shots he is due for today?") for the infant series of vaccines. The presumptive approach has also been shown in a randomized trial to be an effective technique for increasing uptake of HPV vaccine. For parents who resist or have questions about vaccines, some will agree to be vaccinated after simply receiving the necessary knowledge. For many, however, simply correcting misinformation is not enough, and may increase resistance to vaccination. For these parents, it is best to avoid arguments or rebuttals. Motivational interviewing has shown promise as an effective communication technique for both childhood and adolescent vaccines. Other promising techniques include pivoting away from discussions of vaccine side effects to emphasize the importance of the vaccine for disease prevention, personal recommendations ("I vaccinate my own children according to the recommended schedule"), promotion of social norms ("Almost all of our patients are fully vaccinated"), or highlighting circumstances which increase risk ("These infectious diseases are just a plane flight away.").

Parents with questions about vaccine safety may be directed to trusted websites, such as those of the AAP (https://healthychildren.org), CDC (www.cdc.gov/vaccines), and the Immunization Action Coalition (www.immunize.org).

Edwards KM et al: American Academy of Pediatrics: Committee on Infectious Diseases; Committee on Practice and Ambulatory Medicine. Countering vaccine hesitancy. Pediatrics 2016;138 [PMID: 27573088].

HEPATITIS B VACCINATION

Reported cases of acute hepatitis B has declined dramatically in the United States, largely attributable to vaccination. Based on surveillance data from 2015, acute hepatitis B incidence has declined by at least 87% since 1985. The greatest declines are in children younger than 15 years, in whom rates have decreased by 98%.

Success in reducing hepatitis B in the United States is due, in large part, to a comprehensive hepatitis B prevention strategy initiated in 1991. The four central elements of this approach are: (1) immunization of all infants beginning at birth; (2) routine screening of all pregnant women for hepatitis B infection, and provision of hepatitis B immunoglobulin (HBIg) to all infants born to infected mothers; (3) routine vaccination of previously unvaccinated children and adolescents; and (4) vaccination of adults at increased risk of hepatitis B infection.

While high immunization rates have been achieved in young children (> 90% were fully immunized in 2017), there has been less success in identifying hepatitis B–infected mothers and at immunizing high-risk adults. Of the estimated 23,000 mothers who deliver each year who are hepatitis B surface antigen (HBsAg) positive, only 9000 are identified through prenatal screening. While there is an average of 90 cases of perinatally acquired hepatitis B infection reported to the CDC every year, the actual number of perinatal HBV infections is estimated to be 10–20 times higher than the number currently detected and reported. This circumstance represents a significant missed opportunity for prevention in exposed infants, given that administration of HepB vaccine in conjunction with HBIg is 95% effective at preventing mother-to-infant transmission of the virus. Further, many hospitals do not routinely offer HepB to all newborns, despite AAP and ACIP recommendations for universal newborn HepB vaccination. Similarly, while HepB alone is 90%–95% effective at preventing hepatitis B infection, only 45% of high-risk adults have been vaccinated.

All pregnant women should be routinely screened for HBsAg. Infants born to HBsAg-positive mothers should receive both HepB and HBIg immediately after birth. Infants for whom the maternal HBsAg status is unknown should receive vaccine (but not HBIg) within 12 hours of birth. In such circumstances, the mother's HBsAg status should be determined as soon as possible during her hospitalization, and the infant given HBIg if the mother is found to be HBsAg positive. For all infants, the hepatitis B immunization series should be started at birth, with the first dose given prior to 24 hours of age without exception. In 2015, 72% of infants nationally received HepB within 3 days after birth, with wide variation by state (49%–88%).

Routine immunization with three doses of HepB is recommended for all infants and all previously unvaccinated children aged 0–18 years. A two-dose schedule is available for adolescents. Screening for markers of past infection before vaccinating is not indicated for children and adolescents, but may be considered for high-risk adults. Because HepB vaccines consist of an inactivated subunit of the virus, they are not infectious and not contraindicated in immunosuppressed individuals or pregnant women.

▶ **Vaccines Available**

1. HepB vaccine (Recombivax HB, Merck) contains recombinant HepB only.

2. HepB vaccine (Engerix-B, GlaxoSmithKline) contains recombinant HepB only.

3. DTaP-HepB-IPV (Pediarix, GlaxoSmithKline) contains vaccines against diphtheria, tetanus, pertussis, hepatitis B, and poliovirus.

4. HepB vaccine (Heplisav-B, Dynavax Technologies) contains recombinant HepB only, but with a novel adjuvant, and is approved for adults 18 years and older.

5. DTaP-IPV-Hib-HepB (Vaxelis, Merck) contains DTaP, IPV, Hib, and HepB vaccines. Approved for use as a three-dose series at 2, 4, and 6 months of age; not approved for use at 4–6 years of age as the final booster dose of IPV; given intramuscularly (not available until at least 2021).

Only the noncombination vaccines (Recombivax HB and Engerix-B) can be given between birth and 6 weeks of age. Any single or combination vaccine listed above can be used to complete the HepB vaccination series. A combination vaccine against hepatitis A and hepatitis B (Twinrix, GlaxoSmithKline) is available, but is only licensed in the United States for persons 18 years and older.

▶ **Dosage Schedule of Administration**

HepB is recommended for all infants and children in the United States. Table 10–4 presents the vaccination schedule for newborn infants, dependent on maternal HBsAg status. Infants born to mothers with positive or unknown HBsAg status should receive HepB vaccine within 12 hours of birth. Infants born to HBsAg-negative mothers should receive the vaccine prior to 24 hours of age.

For children younger than 11 years not previously immunized, three intramuscular doses of HepB are needed. Adolescents aged 11–15 years have two options: the standard pediatric three-dose schedule or two doses of adult Recombivax HB (1.0 mL dose), with the second dose administered 4–6 months after the first dose. Certain patients may have

Table 10–4. Hepatitis B vaccine schedules for newborn infants, by maternal hepatitis B surface antigen (HBsAg) status.[a]

Maternal HBsAg Status	Single Antigen Vaccine		Single Antigen Followed by Combination Vaccine	
	Dose	Age	Dose	Age
Positive[b]	1[c]	Birth (≤ 12 h)	1[c]	Birth (≤ 12 h)
	HBIg[d]	Birth (≤ 12 h)	HBIg	Birth (≤ 12 h)
	2	1–2 mo	2	2 mo
			3	4 mo
	3[e]	6 mo	4[e]	6 mo (Pediarix)
Unknown[f]	1[c]	Birth (≤ 12 h)	1[c]	Birth (≤ 12 h)
	2	1–2 mo	2	2 mo
			3	4 mo
	3[e]	6 mo	4[e]	6 mo (Pediarix)
Negative	1[c]	Birth (< 24 h)	1[c,g]	Birth (< 24 h)
	2	1–2 mo	2	2 mo
			3	4 mo
	3[e]	6–18 mo	4[e]	6 mo (Pediarix)

[a]See text for vaccination of preterm infants weighing less than 2000 g.
[b]Infants born to HBsAg-positive mothers should be tested at 9–12 months after completion of the immunization series for anti-HBs and HBsAg.
[c]Recombivax HB or Engerix-B should be used for the birth dose. Pediarix cannot be administered at birth or before age 6 weeks.
[d]Hepatitis B immune globulin (HBIg) (0.5 mL) administered intramuscularly in a separate anatomic site from vaccine.
[e]The final dose in the vaccine series should not be administered before age 24 weeks (164 days).
[f]Mothers should have blood drawn and tested for HBsAg as soon as possible after admission for delivery; if the mother is found to be HBsAg-positive, the infant should receive HBIg as soon as possible, but no later than age 7 days.
Adapted with permission from Schillie S, Vellozzi C, Reingold A, et al: Prevention of Hepatitis B Virus Infection in the United States: Recommendations of the Advisory Committee on Immunization Practices, MMWR Recomm Rep. 2018 Jan 12;67(1):1–31.

reduced immune response to HepB vaccination, including preterm infants weighing less than 2000 g at birth, the elderly, immunosuppressed patients, and those receiving dialysis. Preterm infants whose mothers are HBsAg-positive or with unknown HBsAg status should receive both HepB and HBIg within 12 hours of birth. For preterm infants whose mothers are known to be HBsAg-negative, initiation of the vaccination series should be delayed until 30 days of age if the infant is medically stable, or prior to hospital discharge if the infant is discharged before 30 days of age. Pediatric hemodialysis patients and immunocompromised persons may require larger doses or an increased number of doses, with dose amounts and schedules available in the most recent CDC hepatitis B recommendations (see references).

Contraindications & Precautions

HepB should not be given to persons with a serious allergic reaction to yeast or to any vaccine components. Individuals with a history of serious adverse events, such as anaphylaxis, after receiving HepB should not receive additional doses. Vaccination is not contraindicated in persons with a history of Guillain-Barré syndrome, multiple sclerosis, autoimmune disease, other chronic conditions, or in pregnancy.

Adverse Effects

The overall rate of adverse events following vaccination is low. Those reported are minor, including fever (1%–6%) and pain at the injection site (3%–29%). There is no evidence of an association between vaccination and sudden infant death syndrome, multiple sclerosis, autoimmune disease, or chronic fatigue syndrome.

Postexposure Prophylaxis

Postexposure prophylaxis is indicated for unvaccinated persons with perinatal, sexual, household, percutaneous, or mucosal exposure to hepatitis B virus. When prophylaxis is indicated, unvaccinated individuals should receive HBIg (0.06 mL/kg) and the first dose of HepB at a separate anatomic site. Sexual and household contacts of someone with chronic (as opposed to acute) infection should receive HepB only. All vaccinated persons not previously tested for antibody should be tested for anti-HBs after exposure to hepatitis B. If antibody levels are adequate (≥ 10 mIU/mL), no treatment is necessary. If levels are inadequate (< 10 mIU/mL) and the exposure was to HBsAg-positive blood, HBIg and vaccination are required. For non-vaccinated individuals with percutaneous or mucosal exposure to blood, HepB should be given, and HBIg considered depending on the HBsAg status of the person who was the source of the blood exposure.

Antibody Preparations

HBIg is prepared from HIV-negative and hepatitis C virus-negative donors with high titers of hepatitis B surface antibody. The process used to prepare this product inactivates or eliminates any undetected HIV and hepatitis C virus.

American Academy of Pediatrics, Committee on Infectious Diseases: Elimination of perinatal hepatitis B: providing the first vaccine dose within 24 hours of birth. Pediatrics 2017; 140(3):e20171870 [PMID: 28847980].

Schillie S et al: Prevention of hepatitis B virus infection in the United States: recommendations of the Advisory Committee on Immunization Practices. MMWR Recomm Rep 2018;67 (RR-1):1 [PMID: 29939980].

ROTAVIRUS VACCINATION

Rotavirus is the leading cause of hospitalization and death from acute gastroenteritis in young children worldwide. The burden of rotavirus is particularly severe in the developing world, where as many as 215,000 children die each year from rotavirus-associated dehydration and other complications. While deaths from rotavirus were uncommon in the United States (20–60 deaths per year), prior to the introduction of rotavirus vaccine, rotavirus infections caused substantial morbidity annually with an estimated 2.7 million diarrheal illnesses, 410,000 office visits, and 55,000–70,000 hospitalizations.

Rotavirus vaccination has been routinely recommended in the United States since 2006. Two rotavirus vaccines are currently available, a pentavalent rotavirus vaccine (RV5; RotaTeq) and a monovalent rotavirus vaccine (RV1; Rotarix). Hospitalizations and outpatient visits for rotavirus disease have fallen significantly among vaccinated infants in the United States, and disease has also declined among unimmunized older children and adults reflecting herd protection.

Rotavirus vaccination has also reduced morbidity and mortality from rotavirus disease worldwide. While effectiveness of rotavirus vaccines is somewhat lower in developing countries, disease burden is so high that the public health impact of rotavirus vaccination is substantial in developing countries which have introduced these vaccines. Extensive efforts are underway to develop more effective, lower cost, heat-stable (ie, not requiring refrigeration) rotavirus vaccines for use in the developing world.

RV5 and RV1 are known to cause intussusception, although rarely. Intussusception risk has been estimated at 1 excess cases per 20,000 to 100,000 vaccinated infants. At this level of risk, the benefits of vaccination against rotavirus disease continue to greatly outweigh the risks in the United States and globally.

Vaccines Available

1. RV5 (Rotateq, Merck) is a pentavalent, live, oral, human-bovine reassortant rotavirus vaccine. The vaccine is a liquid, does not require any reconstitution, and does not contain any preservatives. The dosing tube is latex-free.
2. RV1 (Rotarix, GlaxoSmithKline) is a monovalent, live, oral, attenuated human rotavirus vaccine. The vaccine needs to be reconstituted with 1 mL of diluent using a prefilled oral applicator. The vaccine does not contain any preservatives. The oral applicator contains latex.

Dosage & Schedule of Administration

Either RV5 or RV1 can be used to prevent rotavirus gastroenteritis. RV5 should be administered orally, as a three-dose series, at 2, 4, and 6 months of age. RV1 should be administered orally, as a two-dose series, at 2 and 4 months of age. For both rotavirus vaccines, the minimum age for dose 1 is 6 weeks, and the maximum age for dose 1 is 14 weeks and 6 days. The vaccination series should not be started at 15 weeks of age or older, because of the lack of safety data around administering dose 1 to older infants. The minimum interval between doses is 4 weeks. All doses should be administered by 8 months and 0 days of age. While the ACIP recommends that the vaccine series be completed with the same product (RV5 or RV1) used for the initial dose, if this is not possible, providers should complete the series with whichever product is available.

Either rotavirus vaccine can be given simultaneously with all other recommended infant vaccines. No restrictions are placed on infant breast or formula feeding before or after receiving rotavirus vaccine. Infants readily swallow the vaccine in most circumstances; however, if an infant spits up or vomits after a dose is administered, the dose should not be readministered; the infant can receive the remaining doses at the normal intervals.

Contraindications & Precautions

Rotavirus vaccine should not be given to infants with a severe hypersensitivity to any components of the vaccine, to infants who had a serious allergic reaction to a previous dose of the vaccine, or to infants with a history of intussusception from any cause. RV1 should not be given to infants with a severe latex allergy. Both vaccines are contraindicated in infants with severe combined immunodeficiency (SCID). RV vaccines should be avoided in infants whose mother received a biologic response modifier (eg, etanercept) during pregnancy. Vaccination should be deferred in infants with acute moderate or severe gastroenteritis. Limited data suggest that rotavirus vaccination is safe and effective in premature infants. Small trials in Africa demonstrated that RV1 and RV5 were well tolerated and immunogenic in HIV-infected children. However, vaccine safety and efficacy in infants with immunocompromising conditions other than SCID, preexisting chronic gastrointestinal conditions (eg, Hirschsprung disease or short-gut syndrome), or a prior episode of intussusception, has not been established. Clinicians should weigh the potential risks and benefits of vaccination in such circumstances. Infants living in households with pregnant women or immunocompromised persons can be vaccinated.

▶ Adverse Effects

In addition to the aforementioned slightly increased risk of intussusception, in prelicensure trials, RV5 was associated with a very small but statistically significant increased risk of vomiting and diarrhea, and RV1 with a similarly small but significant increased risk of cough or runny nose.

Cortese MM, Parashar UD; CDC: Prevention of rotavirus gastroenteritis among infants and children: recommendations of the Advisory Committee on Immunization Practices (ACIP). MMWR Recomm Rep 2009;58(RR-2):1 [PMID: 19194371].

Lo Vecchio A et al: Rotavirus immunization: global coverage and local barriers for implementation. Vaccine 2017;35:1637 [PMID: 28216189].

Tate JE et al: Intussusception rates before and after the introduction of rotavirus vaccine. Pediatrics 2016;138:e20161082 [PMID: 27558938].

DIPHTHERIA-TETANUS-ACELLULAR PERTUSSIS VACCINATION

Diphtheria, tetanus, and pertussis vaccines have been given in a combined vaccine for many decades and have dramatically reduced each of these diseases. The efficacy with antigens in the combined vaccine is similar to that with antigens in single component vaccines. DTP vaccines containing whole-cell pertussis antigens are used widely in the world, but have been entirely replaced in the United States with DTaP vaccines, which contain purified, inactivated components of the pertussis bacterium.

Diphtheria is caused by a gram-positive bacillus, *Corynebacterium diphtheriae*. It is a toxin-mediated disease, with diphtheria toxin causing local tissue destruction, as in pharyngeal and tonsillar diphtheria, as well as systemic disease, particularly myocarditis and neuritis. The overall case fatality rate is between 5% and 10%, with higher death rates in persons younger than 5 years or older than 40 years. Largely because of successful vaccination programs, only two cases of diphtheria have been reported in the United States since 2004. The majority of the rare cases of diphtheria in the United States have been in unimmunized or inadequately immunized persons. The clinical efficacy of diphtheria vaccine is estimated to be greater than 95%.

The anaerobic gram-positive rod *Clostridium tetani* causes tetanus, usually through infection of a contaminated wound. When *C tetani* colonizes devitalized tissue, the exotoxin tetanospasmin is disseminated to inhibitory motor neurons, resulting in generalized rigidity and spasms of skeletal muscles. Tetanus-prone wounds include (1) puncture wounds, including those acquired due to body piercing, tattooing, and intravenous drug abuse; (2) animal bites; (3) lacerations and abrasions; and (4) wounds resulting from nonsterile neonatal delivery and umbilical cord care (neonatal tetanus). In persons who have completed the primary vaccination series and have received a booster dose within the past 10 years, vaccination is virtually 100% protective. In 2014, 29 cases of tetanus and 2 deaths occurred in the United States, almost all in persons who have had inadequate, distant (> 10 years), or no tetanus immunization.

Pertussis is also primarily a toxin-mediated disease caused by *Bordetella pertussis*, which is called "whooping cough" because of the high-pitched inspiratory whoop that can follow intense paroxysms of cough. Pertussis complications include death, often from associated pneumonia, seizures, and encephalopathy. Pertussis incidence in the United States declined dramatically between the 1940s and 1980s, but beginning in the early 1980s, incidence has been slowly increasing, with adolescents and adults accounting for a greater proportion of reported cases. Reasons for increased incidence include improved detection of cases with better laboratory testing methodology (polymerase chain reaction), increased recognition of cases in adolescents and adults, and waning protection from prior infection or with childhood vaccination with only acellular pertussis vaccines. Infants younger than 6 months have the highest rate of pertussis infection (78 cases per 100,000); greater than 90% of pertussis deaths occur in neonates and infants younger than 3 months.

In 2017, 18,975 cases of pertussis were reported in the United States despite widespread underreporting with many localized outbreaks necessitating enhanced vaccination programs. A single booster dose of a different formulation, Tdap, is now recommended for all adolescents and adults, and pregnant women with each pregnancy. Providing a booster dose of pertussis-containing vaccine may prevent adolescent and adult pertussis cases, and also has the potential to reduce the spread of pertussis to infants, who are most susceptible to pertussis complications.

▶ Vaccines Available

A. Diphtheria, Tetanus, and Acellular Pertussis Combinations

1. DTaP (Daptacel, Sanofi; Infanrix, GlaxoSmithKline) contains tetanus toxoid, diphtheria toxoid, and acellular pertussis vaccine. DTaP is licensed for ages 6 weeks through 6 years and can be used for doses 1–5.

2. Tdap (Boostrix, GlaxoSmithKline) is a tetanus-reduced dose diphtheria-acellular pertussis vaccine formulated for persons 10 years of age and older, including adults and the elderly.

3. Tdap (Adacel, Sanofi) is a tetanus-diphtheria-acellular pertussis vaccine approved for persons 11–64 years of age.

B. DTaP Combined With Other Vaccines

1. DTaP-HepB-IPV (Pediarix, GlaxoSmithKline) contains DTaP combined with poliovirus and HepB vaccines. It is approved for the first three doses of the DTaP and IPV series, given at 2, 4, and 6 months of age. Although it is approved for use through age 6 years, it is not licensed for booster doses. It cannot be used, for example, as the fourth dose of DTaP (typically given at 15–18 months of age).

2. DTaP-IPV-Hib (Pentacel, Sanofi) contains DTaP, IPV, and Hib vaccines. The Hib component is Hib capsular polysaccharide bound to tetanus toxoid. This vaccine is approved for use as doses 1–4 of the DTaP series among children 6 weeks to 4 years of age. It is typically given at 2, 4, 6, and 15–18 months of age, and should not be used as the fifth dose in the DTaP series.

3. DTaP-IPV (Kinrix, GlaxoSmithKline, Quadracel, Sanofi) contains DTaP and IPV vaccines. The vaccine is licensed for children 4–6 years of age, for use as the fifth dose of the DTaP vaccine series and the fourth dose of the IPV series. Using this vaccine would reduce by one the number of injections a 4- to 6-year-old child would receive.

4. DTaP-IPV-Hib-HepB (Vaxelis, Merck) contains DTaP, IPV, Hib, and HepB vaccines. Approved for use as a three-dose series at 2, 4, and 6 months of age; not approved for use at 4–6 years of age as the final booster dose of IPV; given intramuscularly (not available until at least 2021).

C. Diphtheria and Tetanus Combinations

1. DT (generic, Sanofi) contains tetanus toxoid and diphtheria toxoid to be used only in children younger than 7 years with a contraindication to pertussis vaccination.

2. Td (Tenivac, Sanofi; generic, Massachusetts Biological Labs) contains tetanus toxoid and a reduced quantity of diphtheria toxoid, which is typically used for adults requiring tetanus prophylaxis.

D. Tetanus Only

TT (generic, Sanofi) contains tetanus toxoid only and can be used for adults or children. However, the use of this single-antigen vaccine is generally not recommended, because of the need for periodic boosting for both diphtheria and tetanus, and is available only on the international market.

▶ Dosage & Schedule of Administration

Although several different vaccines are available, a few general considerations can guide their use in specific circumstances. DTaP (alone or combined with other vaccines) is used for infants and children between 6 weeks and 6 years of age. Children 7–10 years of age not fully immunized against pertussis (meaning those who have not received five prior doses of DTaP, or four doses of DTaP if the fourth dose was given on or after the fourth birthday), who have no contraindications to pertussis immunization, should receive a single dose of Tdap for pertussis protection. For adolescents and adults, a single dose of Tdap is used, followed by booster doses of Td every 10 years; a detailed description of Tdap use is provided later in this chapter.

The primary series of DTaP vaccination should consist of four doses, given at 2, 4, 6, and 15–18 months of age. The fourth dose may be given as early as 12 months of age if 6 months have elapsed since the third dose. Giving the fourth dose between 12 and 15 months of age is indicated if the provider thinks the child is unlikely to return for a clinic visit between 15 and 18 months of age. Children should receive a fifth dose of DTaP at 4–6 years of age. However, a fifth dose of DTaP is not needed if the fourth dose was given after the child's fourth birthday. The same brand of DTaP should be used for all doses if feasible.

▶ Contraindications & Precautions

DTaP vaccines should not be used in individuals who have had an anaphylactic-type reaction to a previous vaccine dose or to a vaccine component. DTaP should not be given to children who developed encephalopathy, not attributable to another identified cause, within 7 days of a previous dose of DTaP or DTP. DTaP vaccination should also be deferred in individuals with progressive neurologic disorders, such as infantile spasms, uncontrolled epilepsy, or progressive encephalopathy, until their neurologic status is clarified and stabilized.

Precautions to DTaP vaccination include high fever ($\geq 40.5°F$), persistent inconsolable crying, or shock-like state within 48 hours of a previous dose of DTP or DTaP; seizures within 3 days of a previous dose of DTP or DTaP; Guillain-Barré syndrome less than 6 weeks after a previous tetanus-containing vaccine; or incident moderate or severe acute illness with or without a fever.

▶ Adverse Effects

Local reactions, fever, and other mild systemic effects occur with acellular pertussis vaccines at one-fourth to two-thirds the frequency noted following whole-cell DTP vaccination. Moderate to severe systemic effects, including fever of 40.5°C, persistent inconsolable crying lasting 3 hours or more, and hypotonic-hyporesponsive episodes, are *much* less frequent than with whole-cell DTP. These are without sequelae. Severe neurologic effects have not been temporally associated with DTaP vaccines in use in the United States. Data are limited regarding differences in reactogenicity among currently licensed DTaP vaccines. More severe local reactions at injection sites appear to occur with increasing dose number (including swelling of the thigh or entire upper arm) after receipt of the fourth and fifth doses for all currently licensed DTaP vaccines.

Diphtheria Antibody Preparations

Diphtheria antitoxin is manufactured in horses. Sensitivity to diphtheria antitoxin must be tested before it is given. Dosage depends on the size and location of the diphtheritic membrane and an estimate of the patient's level of intoxication. Consultation on the use of diphtheria antitoxin is available from the CDC's National Center for Immunization and Respiratory Diseases. Diphtheria antitoxin is not commercially available in the United States and must be obtained from the CDC.

Tetanus Antibody Preparations

Human tetanus immune globulin (TIg) is indicated in the management of tetanus-prone wounds in individuals who have had an uncertain number or fewer than three tetanus immunizations. Persons fully immunized with at least three doses do not require TIg, regardless of the nature of their wounds (Table 10–5). The optimal dose of TIg has not been established, but some experts recommend 500 IU, which appears to be as effective and causing less discomfort, as a single dose of 3000–6000 units with part of the dose infiltrated around the wound.

http://www.cdc.gov/vaccines/pubs/pinkbook/dip.html. Accessed July 18, 2019.

http://www.cdc.gov/vaccines/pubs/pinkbook/pert.html. Accessed July 18, 2019.

http://www.cdc.gov/vaccines/pubs/pinkbook/tetanus.html. Accessed July 18, 2019.

HAEMOPHILUS INFLUENZAE TYPE B VACCINATION

H influenzae type b (Hib) causes a wide spectrum of serious illnesses, particularly in young children, including meningitis, epiglottitis, pneumonia, septic arthritis, and cellulitis. Before the introduction of effective vaccines, Hib was the leading cause of invasive bacterial disease in children younger than 5 years in the United States.

Hib is surrounded by a polysaccharide capsule (polyribosylribitol phosphate [PRP]) that contributes to virulence. Antibodies to this polysaccharide capsule confer immunity to the disease. When Hib polysaccharide is chemically bonded (conjugated) to certain protein carriers, the conjugate vaccine induces T-cell–dependent immune memory that is highly effective in young children. Importantly, polysaccharide-protein conjugate vaccines also prevent carriage of the bacterium, and therefore limit spread from asymptomatic carriers to others in the community. All Hib vaccines are polysaccharide-protein conjugates.

Bacterial serotyping is required to differentiate infections caused by Hib from those caused by other encapsulated and

Table 10–5. Guide to tetanus prophylaxis in routine wound management.

History of Adsorbed Tetanus Toxoid (Doses)	Clean, Minor Wounds		All Other Wounds[a]	
	DTaP, Tdap, or Td[b]	TIG[c]	DTaP, Tdap, or Td[b]	TIG[c]
< 3 or unknown	Yes	No	Yes	Yes
≥ 3	No if < 10 y since last tetanus-containing vaccine dose	No	No[d] if < 5 y since last tetanus-containing vaccine dose	No
	Yes if ≥ 10 y since last tetanus-containing vaccine dose	No	Yes if ≥ 5 y since last tetanus-containing vaccine dose	No

Tdap indicates booster tetanus toxoid, reduced diphtheria toxoid, and acellular pertussis vaccine; DTaP, diphtheria and tetanus toxoids and acellular pertussis vaccine; Td, adult-type diphtheria and tetanus toxoids vaccine; tig, tetanus immune globulin (human).

[a]Such as, but not limited to, wounds contaminated with dirt, feces, soil, and saliva; puncture wounds; avulsions; and wounds resulting from missiles, crushing, burns, and frostbite.

[b]DTaP is used for children younger than 7 years. Tdap is preferred over Td for underimmunized children 7 years and older who have not received Tdap previously.

[c]Immune globulin intravenous should be used when TIG is not available.

[d]More frequent boosters are not needed and can accentuate adverse effects.

Reproduced with permission from Centers for Disease Control and Prevention (CDC).

nonencapsulated *H influenzae* species. In the early 1980s, roughly 20,000 cases of invasive Hib disease occurred each year in the United States. Because of the introduction of protein conjugate Hib vaccines, only about 40 cases of invasive Hib disease occurred in children younger than 5 years in 2017.

Vaccines Available

Four vaccines against Hib disease are available in the United States; three are Hib-only vaccines, and one is a combination vaccines. Each vaccine contains Hib polysaccharide conjugated to a protein carrier, but different protein carriers are used. The Hib conjugate vaccine that uses a meningococcal outer membrane protein carrier is abbreviated PRP-OMP. PRP-T vaccine uses a tetanus toxoid carrier.

Hib-Only Vaccines

1. Hib (PedvaxHIB, Merck, uses PRP-OMP), for use at 2, 4, and 12–15 months of age.
2. Hib (ActHIB, Sanofi, uses PRP-T), for use at 2, 4, 6, and 12–15 months of age.
3. Hib (Hiberix, GlaxoSmithKline, uses PRP-T), for use at 2, 4, 6, and 12–15 months of age.

Hib Combined With Other Vaccines

1. DTaP-IPV-Hib (Pentacel, Sanofi, uses PRP-T) contains DTaP, IPV, and Hib vaccines. This vaccine is approved for use in children 6 weeks to 4 years of age and administered at 2, 4, 6, and 15–18 months of age.

Dosage & Schedule of Administration

Hib vaccination is recommended for all infants in the United States. The vaccine dose is 0.5 mL given intramuscularly. Vaccines containing PRP-OMP (PedvaxHib) are given at 2, 4, and 12–15 months of age; vaccines containing PRP-T (ActHib, Hiberix, Pentacel) are given at 2, 4, 6, and 12–15 months of age. The recommended interval between doses in the primary series is 8 weeks, but a minimal interval of 4 weeks is permitted. For infants who missed the primary vaccination series, a catch-up schedule is used (see Table 10–3). Hib vaccine is not generally recommended for children 5 years of age or older.

Contraindications & Precautions

Hib vaccine should not be given to anyone who has had a severe allergic reaction to a prior Hib vaccine dose or to any vaccine components. Hib vaccine should not be given to infants before 6 weeks of age.

Adverse Effects

Adverse reactions following Hib vaccination are uncommon. Between 5% and 30% of vaccine recipients experience swelling, redness, or pain at the vaccination site. Systemic reactions such as fever and irritability are rare.

Briere EC: Food and Drug Administration approval for use of Hiberix as a 3-dose primary *Haemophilus influenzae* type b (Hib) vaccination series. MMWR Morb Mortal Wkly Rep 2016;65:418–419 [PMID: 27124887].
Briere EC, Rubin L, Moro PL, Cohn A, Clark T, Messonnier N; Division of Bacterial Diseases; National Center for Immunization and Respiratory Diseases; CDC: Prevention and control of *Haemophilus influenzae* type b disease: recommendations of the Advisory Committee on Immunization Practices (ACIP). MMWR Recomm Rep 2014;63(RR-01):1 [PMID: 24572654].

PNEUMOCOCCAL VACCINATION

Before the routine use of pneumococcal conjugate vaccines in infants, *Streptococcus pneumoniae* (pneumococcus) was the leading cause of invasive bacterial disease in children. Pneumococcus remains a leading cause of febrile bacteremia, bacterial sepsis, meningitis, and pneumonia in children and adults in the United States and worldwide. It is also a common cause of otitis media and sinusitis. Over 90 different serotypes of pneumococcus have been identified, and immunity to the capsular polysaccharide antigen of one serotype does not confer immunity to other serotypes.

A conjugate vaccine against a seven-valent pneumococcal conjugate vaccine (PCV7) was first licensed in the United States in 2000. Routine use of PCV7 led to a dramatic decrease in pneumococcal disease overall, however, disease caused by pneumococcal serotypes not included in PCV7 increased. In 2010, a 13-valent pneumococcal conjugate vaccine (PCV13) was licensed for use in the United States. This vaccine contains the serotypes in PCV7 and an additional six pneumococcal serotypes, with the capsular polysaccharide antigens of each serotype individually conjugated to a nontoxic diphtheria cross-reactive material (CRM) carrier protein.

A 23-valent pneumococcal nonconjugated polysaccharide vaccine (PPSV23) is available in the United States, but its use in children is limited to those with certain chronic medical conditions. PPSV23 protects against 23 serotypes and provides protection against the approximately 25% of pneumococcal infections not prevented by PCV13. However, it does not produce a long-lasting immune response and does not reduce nasopharyngeal carriage. While all children and adults are at risk of pneumococcal disease, certain children are at particularly high risk and need enhanced protection against pneumococcal disease including the use of PPSV23 (Table 10–6).

Since the introduction of PCV13, the incidence of invasive pneumococcal disease has decreased dramatically among children younger than 5 years and decreased by more

Table 10–6. Medical conditions or other indications for administration of PCV13[a] and indications for PPSV23[b] administration and revaccination for children aged 6–18 years.[c]

Risk Group	Underlying Medical Condition	PCV13 Recommended	PPSV23 Recommended	PPSV23 Revaccination 5 Years After First Dose
Immunocompetent persons	Chronic heart disease[d]		√	
	Chronic lung disease[e]		√	
	Diabetes mellitus		√	
	Cerebrospinal fluid leaks	√	√	
	Cochlear implants	√	√	
	Alcoholism		√	
	Chronic liver disease		√	
	Cigarette smoking		√	
Persons with functional or anatomic asplenia	Sickle cell disease/other hemoglobinopathies	√	√	√
	Congenital or acquired asplenia	√	√	√
Immunocompromised persons	Congenital or acquired immunodeficiencies[f]	√	√	√
	Human immunodeficiency virus infection	√	√	√
	Chronic renal failure	√	√	√
	Nephrotic syndrome	√	√	√
	Leukemia	√	√	√
	Lymphoma	√	√	√
	Hodgkin disease	√	√	√
	Generalized malignancy	√	√	√
	Iatrogenic immunosuppression[g]	√	√	√
	Solid organ transplant	√	√	√
	Multiple myeloma	√	√	√

[a]13-valent pneumococcal conjugate vaccine.
[b]23-valent pneumococcal polysaccharide vaccine.
[c]Children aged 2–5 years with chronic conditions (eg, heart disease or diabetes), immunocompromising conditions (eg, human immunodeficiency virus), functional or anatomic asplenia (including sickle cell disease), cerebrospinal fluid leaks, or cochlear implants, and who have not previously received PCV13 have been recommended to receive PCV13 since 2010.
[d]Including congestive heart failure and cardiomyopathies.
[e]Including chronic obstructive pulmonary disease, emphysema, and asthma.
[f]Including B- (humoral) or T-lymphocyte deficiency, complement deficiencies (particularly C1, C2, C3, and C4 deficiencies), and phagocytic disorders (excluding chronic granulomatous disease).
[g]Diseases requiring treatment with immunosuppressive drugs, including long-term systemic corticosteroids and radiation therapy.

Reproduced with permission from Centers for Disease Control and Prevention (CDC): Use of 13-valent pneumococcal conjugate vaccine and 23-valent pneumococcal polysaccharide vaccine among children aged 6–18 years with immunocompromising conditions: recommendations of the Advisory Committee on Immunization Practices (ACIP). MMWR Morb Mortal Wkly Rep 2013 Jun 28;62(25):521–524.

than 50% among older adults, largely due to indirect effects of vaccination among children.

▶ Vaccines Available

1. PCV13 (Prevnar13, Pfizer), for use in children 6 weeks of age and older and for adults.
2. PPSV23 (Pneumovax23, Merck), for use in children 2 years of age and older and for adults.

▶ Dosage & Schedule of Administration

PCV13 is given as a 0.5-mL intramuscular dose. PPSV23 is given as a 0.5-mL dose by either the intramuscular or subcutaneous route.

PCV13 is routinely recommended for infants at 2, 4, 6, and 12–15 months of age. For healthy children 24–59 months of age, if they are unvaccinated or did not complete the four-dose PCV13 series, they should receive a single dose of PCV13. Children 24–59 months of age and at high risk of pneumococcal disease (see Table 10–6) should receive two doses of PCV13 (if they previously received fewer than three doses) or one dose of PCV13 (if they previously received three doses). Higher-risk children 24–59 months of age should also receive a dose of PPSV23, at least 8 weeks after their final dose of PCV13. If not previously vaccinated against pneumococcus, higher-risk children 6–18 years of age should receive one dose of PCV13, followed at least 8 weeks later by PPSV23, with PPSV23 repeated 5 years later. Updated and detailed schedule information is available at the CDC (at http://www.cdc.gov/vaccines) and the Immunization Action Coalition (at www.immunize.org).

The rationale for using both PCV13 and PPSV23 in some high-risk children is that while PPSV23 is less immunogenic than PCV13, PPSV23 covers additional serotypes that may cause disease. Table 10–6 also includes the indications for revaccination with PPSV23.

▶ **Contraindications & Precautions**

For both PCV13 and PPSV23, vaccination is contraindicated in individuals who suffered a severe allergic reaction such as anaphylaxis after a previous vaccine dose or to a vaccine component. PCV13 and PPV23 vaccination should be deferred during moderate or severe acute illness, with or without fever.

▶ **Adverse Effects**

The most common adverse effects associated with PCV13 administration are fever, injection site reactions, irritability, and increased or decreased sleep. Although not definitely proven, PCV13 administered simultaneously with inactivated influenza vaccine may lead to a small increased risk of febrile seizures. With PPSV23, 30%–50% of vaccine recipients develop pain and redness at the injection site. Fewer than 1% develop systemic side effects such as fever and myalgia. Anaphylaxis is rare. PPSV23 appears to be safe and immunogenic during pregnancy, although safety data are lacking regarding vaccination during the first trimester of pregnancy.

CDC: Prevention of pneumococcal disease among infants and children—use of 13-valent pneumococcal conjugate vaccine and 23-valent pneumococcal polysaccharide vaccine—recommendations of the Advisory Committee on Immunization Practices (ACIP). MMWR Recomm Rep 2010;59:1 [PMID: 21150868].

CDC: Use of 13-valent pneumococcal conjugate vaccine and 23-valent pneumococcal polysaccharide vaccine among children aged 6–18 years with immunocompromising conditions: recommendations of the Advisory Committee on Immunization Practices (ACIP). MMWR 2013;62:521 [PMID: 23803961].

Yildirim I, Shea KM, Pelton SI: Pneumococcal disease in the era of pneumococcal conjugate vaccine. Infect Dis Clin North Am 2015;29:679 [PMID: 26610421].

POLIOMYELITIS VACCINATION

Polioviruses are highly infectious, spread primarily by fecal-oral and oral-oral routes, and cause acute flaccid paralysis via destruction of motor neurons. There are three polio serotypes; immunity to one serotype does not confer immunity to the others. Poliomyelitis can be prevented by vaccination. Type 2 poliovirus was declared eradicated in 2015, and type 3 poliovirus was last detected in 2012. While the goal of polio eradication has not yet been achieved, the global incidence of polio has decreased from roughly 350,000 cases annually in the prevaccination era, to 33 polio cases detected in 2018. Polio remains endemic in Afghanistan, Nigeria, and Pakistan.

Although extraordinary progress has been made toward the goal of global polio eradication, complex challenges remain. Armed conflict and civil strife continue to impede access to vulnerable populations, and vaccinators have been the target of violence. Also, the attenuated vaccine strains used in trivalent OPV can rarely mutate into pathogenic strains and cause polio disease. To address this issue, while maintaining population immunity to all three poliovirus strains, several steps have been necessary: (1) introduction of IPV into all countries using OPV; (2) switch from trivalent OPV to a more immunogenic bivalent form of OPV; and (3) eventually stopping routine use of OPV altogether. This massive global public health transition occurred during 2015 and 2016 and has largely been successful. However, an IPV vaccine shortage resulted, and strategies are in place to prioritize IPV use and significantly increase vaccine production. Despite setbacks, a polio-free world is achievable. Timely updates on the worldwide polio eradication program can be found at www.polioeradication.org.

IPV, a trivalent inactivated vaccine, is the only vaccine against poliomyelitis available in the United States. IPV cannot cause polio.

▶ **Vaccines Available**

1. IPV (IPOL, Sanofi) is given intramuscularly or subcutaneously.

2. DTaP-HepB-IPV (Pediarix, GlaxoSmithKline) contains DTaP, HepB, and IPV vaccines. Approved for use at 2, 4, and 6 months of age; not approved for use at 4–6 years of age as the final booster dose of IPV; given intramuscularly.

3. DTaP-IPV-Hib (Pentacel, Sanofi) contains DTaP, IPV, and Hib vaccines. Approved for use at 2, 4, 6, and 15–18 months of age; not approved for use at 4–6 years of age as the final booster dose of IPV; given intramuscularly.

4. DTaP-IPV-Hib-HepB (Vaxelis, Merck) contains DTaP, IPV, Hib, and HepB vaccines. Approved for use as a three-dose series at 2, 4, and 6 months of age; not approved for use at 4–6 years of age as the final booster dose of IPV; given intramuscularly (not available until at least 2021).

5. DTaP-IPV (Kinrix, GlaxoSmithKline) contains DTaP and IPV vaccines. Licensed for children 4–6 years of age, for use as a final booster dose of IPV; given intramuscularly.

Dosage & Schedule of Administration

In the United States, all children without contraindications should receive an IPV-containing vaccine at 2, 4, 6–18 months, and 4–6 years of age. A dose of IPV should be given at 4 years of age or older, regardless of the number of prior doses of IPV. Completely immunized adult visitors to areas of continuing wild-type poliovirus circulation should receive a booster dose of IPV. Unimmunized or incompletely immunized adults and children should receive two (preferably three) doses of IPV prior to travel.

Contraindications & Precautions

IPV vaccination is contraindicated in individuals who suffered a severe allergic reaction such as anaphylaxis after a previous vaccine dose or to a vaccine component. IPV vaccination should be deferred during moderate or severe acute illness with or without fever. Pregnancy is also a precaution to IPV vaccination. Receipt of previous doses of OPV is not a contraindication to IPV.

Adverse Effects

Minor local reactions, such as pain or redness at the injection site, may occur following IPV vaccination. No serious adverse reactions following IPV vaccination have been described.

Duintjer Tebbens RJ, Thompson KM: Polio endgame risks and the possibility of restarting the use of oral poliovirus vaccine. Expert Rev Vaccines 2018;17:739 [PMID: 30056767].

Greene SA et al: Progress toward polio eradication, worldwide, January 2017–March 2019. MMWR Morb Mortal Wkly Rep 2019;68:458 [PMID: 31120868].

Shakeel SI et al: Achieving the end game: employing "vaccine diplomacy" to eradicate polio in Pakistan. BMC Public Health 2019;19:79 [PMID: 30654797].

INFLUENZA VACCINATION

Influenza occurs each winter-early spring period, often associated with significant morbidity and mortality in certain high-risk persons. Since 2010, CDC estimates that between 140,000 and 960,000 hospitalizations and up to 36,000 deaths per year in the United States are attributable to influenza, and global epidemics (pandemics) can occur. The recent pandemic H1N1 strain is now incorporated into the seasonal vaccine. Each year, recommendations are formulated in the spring regarding the constituents of influenza vaccine for the coming season. Influenza vaccines contain either three strains (two influenza A strains and one of two influenza B lineages), or all four strains, including two influenza A and two influenza B lineages. It is difficult to predict which influenza B lineages (or both) will predominate in any given influenza season. Children at high risk of seasonal influenza-related complications include those with hemoglobinopathies or with chronic cardiac, pulmonary (including asthma), metabolic, renal, and immunosuppressive diseases (including immunosuppression caused by medications or by HIV); and those with any condition (eg, cognitive dysfunction, spinal cord injuries, seizure disorders, or other neuromuscular disorders) that can compromise respiratory function or the handling of respiratory secretions, or that can increase the risk of aspiration. Children and adolescents receiving long-term aspirin therapy are also at risk of influenza-related Reye syndrome. Healthy children aged 6–23 months are at substantially increased risk of influenza-related hospitalizations, and children aged 24–59 months (ie, 2–4 years) remain at increased risk of influenza-related clinic and emergency department visits and hospitalizations, but less so than younger children.

Annual influenza vaccination is routinely recommended for all persons older than 6 months. Physicians should identify high-risk children in their practices and encourage parents to seek influenza vaccination for their children and themselves as soon as influenza vaccine is available. Influenza prevention will help prevent lower respiratory tract disease or other secondary complications in high-risk groups, thereby decreasing hospitalizations and deaths.

Vaccines Available

Most inactivated influenza vaccine virus is grown in eggs, formalin inactivated, and may contain trace quantities of thimerosal as a preservative. Only split-virus or purified viral antigens are available in the United States. Fluzone (Sanofi), Afluria (Seqirus), Fluarix (GlaxoSmithKline), and FluLaval (Biomedical Corp of Quebec) are approved for children 6 months and older. A cell-culture–based vaccine Flucelvax (Seqirus) is approved for children 4 years and older. There are a number of additional influenza vaccines licensed for adults but not for children, including a high-dose vaccine for older adults, and a recombinant vaccine. Intranasal live attenuated influenza vaccine (LAIV [FluMist, AstraZeneca]) is approved for healthy children and adults aged 2 through 49 years.

Dosage & Schedule of Administration

A. Inactivated Influenza Virus Vaccine (IIV)

Because influenza can circulate from November through early March in the US states, the optimal time to initiate vaccination is as soon as vaccine is available in the early fall. However, providers should continue vaccinating individuals as long as vaccine is available, and there is influenza activity in the community. Children younger than age 6 months should not be immunized. Two doses are recommended for children younger than 9 years who did not receive two vaccine doses in the past. Older children receiving vaccine for the first time require only a single dose. The dose for all children is 0.5 mL given intramuscularly. Pregnancy is not a contraindication to use of inactivated vaccine, which is recommended for all pregnant women and those contemplating pregnancy during the influenza season as complications from influenza infection are greatly increased in the third trimester and up to 2 weeks postpartum. Simultaneous administration with other routine vaccines is acceptable.

B. Live Attenuated Influenza Virus Vaccine (LAIV)

The vaccine is supplied in a prefilled single-use sprayer containing 0.2 mL of the vaccine, approximately half of which is sprayed into each nostril. A dose divider clip is provided to assist in dividing the dose. If the patient sneezes during administration, the dose should not be repeated. It can be administered to children with minor illnesses but should not be given if significant nasal congestion is present. Because it is a live vaccine, it should be administered 48 hours after cessation of therapy in children receiving anti-influenza antiviral drugs, and these should not be given for 2 weeks after vaccination. Two doses are recommended for children younger than 9 years who did not receive two vaccine doses in the past. One dose is recommended for individuals 9–49 years of age.

▶ Contraindications & Precautions

A. Inactivated Influenza Virus Vaccine

Inactivated influenza vaccine is contraindicated in individuals with a severe allergic reaction, such as anaphylaxis, to a previous dose of an inactivated influenza vaccine component. However, guidelines for influenza vaccination in children with egg allergies have recently changed. Children with only urticaria following exposure to egg can be vaccinated. Children with more serious allergic reactions to egg, such as angioedema, respiratory symptoms, or anaphylaxis, may be eligible for inactivated influenza vaccine but should be referred to an allergist for an assessment of vaccination risk and should receive vaccine in an inpatient or outpatient medical setting and by a health care provider who is able to recognize and manage severe allergic conditions.

B. Live Attenuated Influenza Virus Vaccine

LAIV is contraindicated in individuals with a history of severe allergic reaction to any component of the vaccine or to a previous dose of any influenza vaccine, with egg allergy, and in children and adolescents receiving concomitant aspirin or aspirin-containing therapy. LAIV should not be administered to the following persons: (1) children younger than 24 months, because of an increased risk of hospitalization and wheezing that was observed in clinical trials; (2) individuals with asthma or children younger than 5 years with recurrent wheezing unless the potential benefit outweighs the potential risk; (3) pregnant women; (4) and individuals with known or suspected immunodeficiency diseases or immunosuppressed states.

All health care workers, including those with asthma and other underlying health conditions, can administer LAIV. Health care workers who are vaccinated with LAIV can safely provide care to patients within a hospital or clinic, except for severely immunosuppressed patients that require a protected environment (ie, bone marrow transplant patients). In this instance, there should be a 7-day interval between receiving LAIV and care for these patients.

▶ Adverse Effects

A. Inactivated Influenza Virus Vaccine

Injection site reactions are the most common adverse events after inactivated influenza vaccine administration. A small proportion of children will experience some systemic toxicity, consisting of fever, malaise, and myalgias. These symptoms generally begin 6–12 hours after vaccination and may last 24–48 hours. Cases of Guillain-Barré syndrome followed the swine influenza vaccination program in 1976–1977, but careful study by the Institute of Medicine showed no association with that vaccine in children and young adults—nor in any age group that received vaccines in subsequent years.

B. Live Attenuated Influenza Virus Vaccine

The most common adverse reactions include runny nose or nasal congestion in all ages and fever higher than 37.7°C in children 2–6 years of age. These reactions occurred more with the first dose and were self limited.

AAP; Committee on Infectious Diseases: Recommendations for prevention and control of influenza in children, 2019–2020. Pediatrics [PMID: 31477606].

CDC: Prevention and control of seasonal influenza with vaccines: Recommendations of the Advisory Committee on Immunization Practices–United States, 2019–20 Influenza Season. MMWR. 2019;68:1 [PMID: 31441906].

MEASLES, MUMPS, & RUBELLA VACCINATION

Due to an effective vaccination program beginning in 1963, measles was declared eliminated from the United States in 2000. Until 2008, there were sporadic importations of measles from countries with lower vaccination rates, but since then there have been numerous outbreaks of measles, primarily from viral transmission within the United States after initial exposure to imported cases. In 2018–2019, there were numerous outbreaks of measles across the United States, primarily in insular communities, resulting in over 1000 cases in the first half of 2019, the most cases in the United States in any year since 1992. The largest of these outbreaks occurred in New York State in orthodox Jewish communities. In outbreaks such as these, the majority of people who developed measles were unvaccinated.

In the United States, after adding mumps vaccine to the childhood schedule in 1977, there was a 99% decline in mumps to fewer than 300 cases each year between 2001 and 2003. However, since then, there have been several large outbreaks, particularly in 2016–2017 when there were over 9000 cases. University outbreaks accounted for half of all outbreaks and 40% of total mumps cases. Many of these outbreaks were in populations who had a high proportion of individuals fully vaccinated with two doses of MMR vaccine. As a result of these large outbreaks, in 2017 ACIP recommended a third dose of a mumps-containing vaccine in persons previously vaccinated with two doses of a mumps-containing vaccine who are identified by public health as at increased risk for mumps because of an outbreak.

The rubella vaccine is primarily intended to prevent the serious consequences of rubella infection in pregnant women: miscarriage, fetal demise, and congenital rubella syndrome. In the United States and elsewhere, the approach has been to vaccinate young children. Over time, this approach has led to most women being rubella immune by the time they reach child-bearing age; herd immunity also reduces transmission to susceptible women. With the use of rubella vaccines, rubella and congenital rubella syndrome were declared eliminated in the United States in 2004. There are now fewer than 10 rubella cases per year, and all recent cases were infected while living or traveling outside the country. There were only four cases of congenital rubella syndrome in the United States between 2010 and 2015.

Despite many reports in the lay press and on the Internet of a link between MMR and autism, there is overwhelming scientific evidence that there is no causal association between the two. There is also no evidence that separation of MMR into its individual component vaccines lessens the risk of any vaccine adverse event, and such practice is not recommended.

▶ Vaccines Available

1. Measles-mumps-rubella (MMR II, Merck): MMR II is a lyophilized preparation of measles, mumps, and rubella vaccines. The measles and mumps portions are prepared using chick embryo tissue cultures, and rubella is grown in human diploid cells. There is no adjuvant and no preservative. It contains small amounts of gelatin, sorbitol, and neomycin. The individual components of MMR II are no longer available.

2. MMRV: A combined live attenuated measles, mumps, rubella, and varicella vaccine (ProQuad, Merck) is licensed for use in children 1–12 years of age. The measles, mumps,

and rubella components are identical to MMR II. The varicella component has a higher varicella-zoster virus titer than the varicella-only (VAR) vaccine.

▶ Dosage & Schedule of Administration

A. Routine Vaccination

Measles, mumps, and rubella vaccinations should be given as MMR or MMRV at 12–15 months and again at 4–6 years of age. Both MMR and MMRV can cause febrile seizures, although uncommonly. Because febrile seizures following MMRV occur at a rate twice that of MMR at the younger age, the ACIP recommends that after a discussion of the benefits and risks of both vaccination options with the parents or caregivers, either MMR or MMRV may be given at 12–15 months of age. MMRV is the preferred vaccine at 4–6 years of age if available; no excess risk of febrile seizures following MMRV vaccination has been observed at 4–6 years of age. A personal or family history of febrile seizures in an infant is considered a precaution for the use of MMRV, and MMR and VAR given separately are preferred. A dose of 0.5 mL should be given subcutaneously. The second dose of MMR or MMRV is recommended at school entry to help prevent school-based measles and mumps outbreaks. Children not reimmunized at school entry should receive their second dose by age 11–12 years. If an infant receives MMR before 12 months of age (such as for travel), two additional doses are required to complete the series, the first after 12 months of age and the second at least 1 month later. Ig interferes with the immune response to the attenuated vaccine strains of MMR and MMRV. Therefore, MMR and MMRV immunization should be deferred by 3–11 months after Ig administration, depending on the type of Ig product received. Consult the AAP's *Red Book* for specific recommendations.

For measles, mumps, and rubella, most persons can be considered immune if they were fully vaccinated at appropriate intervals, or were born before 1957, or if there is laboratory evidence of serologic immunity or disease. However, special considerations apply to health care workers: for those born before 1957, laboratory confirmation of immunity or disease should be performed, and nonimmune health care workers should be vaccinated. A clinical diagnosis of any of these diseases is not acceptable evidence of immunity. For rubella, susceptible pubertal girls and postpubertal women identified by prenatal screening should be immunized after delivery. Whenever rubella vaccination is offered to a woman of childbearing age, pregnancy should be ruled out and the woman advised to prevent conception for 3 months following vaccination. If a pregnant woman is vaccinated or becomes pregnant within 3 weeks of vaccination, she should be counseled regarding the risk to her fetus, although no cases of rubella-vaccine–related fetal anomalies have been reported. The risk of congenital rubella syndrome after wild-type maternal infection in the first trimester of pregnancy is 20%–85%. All susceptible adults in institutional settings (including colleges), day care center personnel, military personnel, and hospital and health care personnel should be immunized.

B. Vaccination of Travelers

People traveling abroad should be immune to measles, mumps, and rubella. Infants 6–11 months of age traveling to high-risk areas should receive one dose of MMR prior to travel followed by either MMR or MMRV at 12–15 months of age (given at least 4 weeks after the initial dose) and either MMR or MMRV at 4–6 years of age to complete the series. Children over 12 months of age who are traveling to high-risk areas should receive two doses separated by at least 4 weeks. Children traveling internationally to lower-risk areas should be immunized as soon as possible after their first birthday and complete the series at 4–6 years of age in the usual fashion.

C. Revaccination Under Other Circumstances

Persons entering college and other institutions for education beyond high school, medical personnel beginning employment, and persons traveling abroad should have documentation of immunity to measles and mumps, defined as receipt of two doses of measles vaccine after their first birthday, birth before 1957, or a laboratory documented measles or mumps history.

D. Outbreak Control of Measles

A community outbreak is defined as a single documented case of measles. Control depends on immediate protection of all susceptible persons (defined as persons who have no documented immunity to measles in the affected community). In the case of unvaccinated individuals, the following recommendations hold: (1) age 6–11 months, give MMR if cases are occurring in children younger than 1 year, followed by a dose of MMR or MMRV at age 12–15 months and again at age 4–6 years; and (2) age 12 months or older, give MMR or MMRV followed by revaccination at age 4–6 years. A child with an unclear or unknown vaccination history should be reimmunized with MMR or MMRV. Anyone with a known exposure who is not certain of having previously received two doses of MMR should receive an additional dose. Unimmunized persons who are not immunized within 72 hours of exposure, which is the acceptable interval for active postexposure prophylaxis, should be excluded from contact with potentially infected persons until at least 2 weeks after the onset of rash of the last case of measles.

E. Outbreak Control of Mumps

Persons previously vaccinated with two doses of a mumps-containing vaccine who are identified by public health as at increased risk for mumps because of an outbreak should receive a third dose of a mumps-containing vaccine to improve protection against mumps disease and related complications.

▶ Contraindications & Precautions

MMR and MMRV vaccines are contraindicated in pregnant women, women intending to become pregnant within the next 28 days, immunocompromised persons, and persons with an anaphylactic reaction to a prior dose or vaccine component. It is also contraindicated in children receiving high-dose corticosteroid therapy ($\geq$ 2 mg/kg/day, or 20 mg/day total, for longer than 14 days) with the exception of those receiving physiologic replacement doses. In these patients, an interval of 1 month between cessation of steroid therapy and vaccination is sufficient. Leukemic patients who have been in remission and off chemotherapy for at least 3 months can receive MMR and MMRV safely. Persons with HIV infection should receive two doses of MMR vaccine according to the recommended schedule if they do not have evidence of current severe immunosuppression (for persons aged $\leq$ 5 years, they must have CD4 percentages $\geq$ 15% for $\geq$ 6 months; and for persons aged > 5 years, they must have CD4 percentages $\geq$ 15% and CD4 $\geq$ 200 lymphocytes/mm^3 for $\geq$ 6 months). MMRV is contraindicated in HIV-positive individuals. Children with minor acute illnesses (including febrile illnesses), egg allergy, or a history of tuberculosis should be immunized. MMR and MMRV may be safely administered simultaneously with other routine pediatric immunizations.

▶ Adverse Effects

Between 5% and 15% of individuals receiving MMR become febrile to 39.5°C or higher about 6–12 days following vaccination, lasting approximately 1–2 days, and 5% may develop a transient morbilliform rash. MMR and MMRV vaccines can cause febrile seizures, typically 8–14 days after vaccination; these febrile seizures have not been associated with any long-term complications. Other serious adverse events following vaccination are rare and include anaphylaxis, transient thrombocytopenia (1 per 40,000 vaccine recipients), and arthralgias (more common in adults than children).

▶ Antibody Preparations Against Measles

Ig is effective at preventing measles, if given to a nonimmune person within 6 days of exposure to measles. However, the immunity conferred by Ig should be considered temporary. Infants younger than 12 months who have been exposed to measles should receive 0.5 mL/kg of Ig, given intramuscularly. MMR vaccine should also be used, as appropriate, for infants aged 6–11 months. Pregnant women without evidence of measles immunity and severely immune-compromised persons (regardless of evidence of measles immunity) who are exposed to measles should receive 400 mg/kg of Ig given intravenously. Ig given intramuscularly (0.5 mL/kg, maximum dose, 15 mL) may be given to more immune-competent exposed persons without evidence of immunity, with priority for those with the most intense contact with a case.

Albertson JP et al: Mumps outbreak at a university and recommendation for a third dose of measles-mumps-rubella vaccine—Illinois, 2015–2016. MMWR Morb Mortal Wkly Rep 2016;65:731 [PMID: 27467572].

CDC: Prevention of measles, rubella, congenital rubella syndrome, and mumps, 2013: summary recommendations of the Advisory Committee on Immunization Practices (ACIP). MMWR Recomm Rep 2013;62:1 [PMID: 23760231].

Patel M et al: Increase in Measles Cases—United States, January 1–April 26, 2019. MMWR Morb Mortal Wkly Rep 2019; 68(17): 402–404 [PMID: 31048672].

VARICELLA VACCINATION

Prior to the availability of vaccine, about 4 million cases of varicella-zoster virus (VZV) infection occurred as chickenpox annually in the United States, mostly in children younger than 10 years. This resulted in 11,000 hospitalizations and 100 deaths per year due to severe complications such as secondary bacterial infections, pneumonia, encephalitis, hepatitis, and Reye syndrome.

A live, attenuated varicella vaccine (VAR) was licensed in the United States in 1995, and routine immunization of children 12 months of age and older was instituted. The vaccine is almost 100% effective at preventing severe disease. The incidence, morbidity, mortality, and medical costs associated with varicella infection have significantly declined since VAR was licensed. Vaccination prevents an estimated 3.5 million cases of varicella, 9000 hospitalizations, and 100 deaths in the United States each year. Once the routine use of VAR was achieved, it became apparent that there is "breakthrough" (usually very mild) varicella occurring in about 15% of immunized patients. Outbreaks of wild-type infectious VZV were reported in schools with high one-dose VAR vaccination coverage (96%–100%). Varicella attack rates among these children varied between 11% and 17%, and thus it was concluded that a single VAR dose could not prevent endemic varicella.

A second dose of VAR in children, when given 3 months or 4–6 years after the initial dose, greatly increased the magnitude of the anti-VZV antibody response, which is a correlate of vaccine efficacy. A combination MMRV vaccine has also been shown to be immunologically noninferior to the MMR and VAR components administered separately. MMRV is effective as primary immunization or as a booster administered to children age 4–6 years. The two-dose regimen is almost 100% effective against severe varicella, and the risk of breakthrough varicella is threefold less than the risk with a one-dose regimen. Therefore, ACIP and the AAP recommend two doses of VAR for children older than 12 month and for adolescents and adults without evidence of immunity.

The vaccine is also effective in preventing or modifying VZV severity in susceptible individuals exposed to VZV if used within 3 days (and possibly up to 5 days) of exposure, with an efficacy of 95% for preventing any postexposure disease and 100% for preventing moderate or severe disease. There is no evidence that postexposure prophylaxis increases the risk of vaccine-related adverse events or interferes with development of immunity.

▶ Vaccines Available

1. A cell-free preparation of Oka strain VZV is produced and marketed in the United States as Varivax (Merck). Each dose of VAR contains not less than 1350 plaque-forming units of VZV and trace amounts of neomycin, fetal bovine serum, and gelatin. There is no preservative.

2. MMRV (measles-mumps-rubella-varicella, ProQuad, Merck) is licensed for use in children 1–12 years of age. MMRV is well tolerated and provides adequate immune response to all of the antigens it contains. In MMRV, the varicella component is present in higher titer than in VAR. Concomitant administration of MMRV with DTaP, Hib, and HepB vaccines is acceptable.

▶ Dosage & Schedule of Administration

Two doses (0.5 mL) of VAR are recommended for immunization of healthy children aged 12 months and older, and for adolescents and adults without evidence of immunity. For children aged 12 months to 12 years, the immunization interval is at least 3 months, and for persons 13 years or older, it is 4 weeks. MMRV is approved only for healthy children aged 12 months to 12 years. A second dose of catch-up vaccination is required for children, adolescents, and adults who previously received one dose of VAR vaccine. All children should have received two doses of VAR before prekindergarten or school. HIV-infected children (≥ 15% CD4+ cells) should receive two doses of the single-antigen vaccine (with a least a 3-month interval between doses).

VAR may be given simultaneously with MMR at separate sites. If not given simultaneously, the interval between administration of VAR and MMR must be greater than 28 days. Simultaneous VAR administration does not appear to affect the immune response to other childhood vaccines. VAR should be delayed 5 months after receiving intravenous immune globulin, blood, or plasma. In addition, persons who received VAR should not be administered an antibody-containing product for at least 2 weeks or an antiviral medication active against varicella for at least 3 weeks. If this occurs, the individual may need to be tested for immunity or revaccinated. After a discussion of the benefits and risks of both vaccination options with the parents or caregivers (see section "Adverse Effects"), either MMR or MMRV may be given at 12–15 months. MMRV is the preferred vaccine if available at 4–6 years of age.

Contraindications & Precautions

Contraindications to VAR vaccination include a severe allergic reaction after a previous vaccine dose or to a vaccine component. Because VAR and MMRV are live-virus vaccines, they are also contraindicated in children who have acquired treatment-related cellular immunodeficiencies or congenital T-cell abnormalities. The exception to this rule is the recommendation that VAR be administered to HIV-infected children who are not severely immunosuppressed. Household contacts of immunodeficient patients should be immunized. VAR should not be given to pregnant women; however, the presence of a pregnant mother in the household is not a contraindication to immunization of a child within that household. A personal or family history of febrile seizures in an infant is considered a precaution for the use of MMRV; administration of MMR and VAR separately is preferred for the first dose.

Adverse Events

The most commonly recognized adverse reactions, occurring in approximately 20% of vaccines, are minor injection site reactions. Additionally, 3%–5% of patients will develop a rash at the injection site, and an additional 3%–5% will develop a sparse varicelliform rash outside of the injection site. These rashes typically consist of two to five lesions and may appear 5–26 days after immunization. The two-dose vaccine regimen is generally well tolerated with a safety profile comparable to that of the one-dose regimen. The incidence of fever and varicelliform rash is lower after the second dose than the first. Although VAR is contraindicated in pregnancy, there have been hundreds of inadvertent administrations of vaccine to pregnant women tracked by the "Pregnancy Registry for Varivax" with no known cases of congenital varicella syndrome or increases in fetal abnormalities.

Studies comparing MMRV to MMR and VAR administered concomitantly showed more systemic adverse events following MMRV (fever 21.5% vs 14.9% and measles-like rash 3% vs 2.1%, respectively). The risk of febrile seizures in children 12–23 months old with the MMRV preparation is twice that of MMR and VAR given separately, resulting in one additional febrile seizure per 2300–2600 children vaccinated with MMRV.

Transmission of vaccine virus from healthy vaccines to other healthy persons is very rare; has never been documented in the absence of a rash in the index case; and has only resulted in mild disease. Herpes zoster infection occurs in recipients of VAR in immunocompetent and immunocompromised persons within 25–722 days after immunization. Many of these cases were found to be caused by unappreciated latent wild-type virus. Vaccine-strain varicella does cause herpes zoster in children, but the age-specific risk of herpes zoster infection is much lower in children following VAR immunization than after natural infection, and it also tends to be milder.

Antibody Preparations

In the event of an exposure to varicella, there are currently two antibody preparations potentially available in the United States for postexposure prophylaxis, VariZIG (Cangene Corporation) and intravenous Ig. Exposure is defined as a household contact or playmate contact (> 1 h/day), hospital contact (in the same or contiguous room or ward) or intimate contact with a person with herpes zoster deemed contagious. Susceptibility is defined as the absence of a reliable history of varicella or varicella vaccination. Uncertainty in this designation can be resolved with an appropriate test for anti-VZV antibody. Passive postexposure prophylaxis is indicated for neonates, pregnant women, and immunocompromised patients, including those with cancer or taking immunosuppressive therapies.

VariZIG should be administered as soon as possible after exposure, ideally within 96 hours, but may be given within 10 days postexposure. If VariZIG is not available, it is recommended that intravenous Ig be used in its place. The dose is 400 mg/kg administered once. A subsequent exposure does not require additional prophylaxis if this occurs within 3 weeks of intravenous Ig administration.

AAP Committee on Infectious Diseases: Prevention of varicella: recommendations for use of quadrivalent and monovalent varicella vaccines in children. Pediatrics 2011;128:630 [PMID: 21873692].

CDC: Updated recommendations for use of VariZIG—United States, 2013. MMWR Morb Mortal Wkly Rep 2013;62:574 [PMID: 23863705].

Leung J, Harpaz R: Impact of the maturing varicella vaccination program on varicella and related outcomes in the United States, 1994–2012. J Pediatric Infect Dis Soc 2016;5:395 [PMID: 26407276].

HEPATITIS A VACCINATION

The incidence of hepatitis A in the United States had decreased dramatically from an average of 28,000 cases annually in the years prior to availability of a HepA vaccine to 1390 cases reported in 2015. However, more recently hepatitis A incidence has increased to over 11,000 cases reported in 2018 in part related to outbreaks among persons who report drug use or homelessness.

Initial vaccination recommendations for hepatitis A targeted high-risk individuals, primarily adults. However, children, who are more likely than adults to be asymptomatic while infected, usually contribute to the spread of hepatitis A through households and communities. Therefore, since 2006 HepA vaccination has been routinely recommended for children 12–23 months of age. As a consequence of vaccination, the epidemiology of hepatitis A infection has changed such that most cases now occur in adults, often related to travel or contaminated food.

In addition to routine immunization of all children 12–23 months of age, HepA vaccination is indicated for the following groups: (1) travelers to countries with moderate to high rates of hepatitis A, (2) children with chronic liver disease, (3) children with clotting factor disorders, (4) adolescent and adult males who have sex with men, (5) persons with an occupational exposure to hepatitis A, (6) persons reporting drug use, and (7) all previously unvaccinated persons who anticipate close personal contact with an international adoptee from countries with moderate to high rates of hepatitis A. Vaccination should also be considered in previously unimmunized children 2–18 years old, even if none of the above risk factors are present.

HepA vaccines are all inactivated and included two single-antigen vaccines and one combination vaccine.

Vaccines Available

1. HepA (Havrix, GlaxoSmithKline), for use in children 12 months of age and older, and adults.

2. HepA (Vaqta, Merck), for use in children 12 months of age and older, and adults.

3. HepA-HepB (Twinrix, GlaxoSmithKline) contains HepA and HepB vaccines. Approved for use in adults 18 years of age and older.

Dosage & Schedule of Administration

The two HepA vaccines given in childhood (Havrix and Vaqta) are given as a two-dose series. The first dose is recommended at 12–23 months of age; the second dose is recommended 6–18 months later. For individuals 12 months through 18 years of age, these vaccines are administered intramuscularly in a dose of 0.5 mL. Adults 19 years of age and older can receive Havrix (two doses of 1.0 mL each, separated by at least 6 months), Vaqta (two doses of 1.0 mL each, separated by at least 6 months), or Twinrix (for adults 18 years and older, 1.0 mL per dose, in a three-dose series). If needed, such as for imminent travel, Twinrix can be given on an accelerated four-dose schedule, with doses on days 1, 7, and 21–30, with a booster dose given 12 months after the first dose.

Contraindications & Precautions

HepA vaccine should not be given to anyone with a prior severe allergic reaction, such as anaphylaxis, after a previous vaccine dose or to a vaccine component. Precautions to vaccination include pregnancy and moderate or severe acute illness.

Adverse Effects

Adverse reactions, which are uncommon and mild, consist of pain, swelling, and induration at the injection site, headache, and loss of appetite. There have been no reports of serious adverse events attributed definitively to HepA vaccine.

Postexposure Prophylaxis

Postexposure prophylaxis is recommended for household or sexual contacts of persons with serologically confirmed hepatitis A, and for day care staff and attendees in outbreak situations. Postexposure prophylaxis may also be recommended in food-borne outbreaks, depending on the extent and timing of exposure. Postexposure prophylaxis of unimmunized persons should consist of either a single dose of HepA vaccine or Ig (0.1 mL/kg), given as soon as possible after exposure. The efficacy of Ig when given more than 2 weeks after exposure has not been established. For healthy people 12 months through 40 years of age who have not previously completed the two-dose vaccine series, HepA vaccine should be given. For those older than 40 years, Ig may be given in addition to HepA vaccine if there was a high-risk exposure or high risk of complications related to HepA infection. Ig should also be used for children younger than 12 months, immunocompromised persons, those with chronic liver disease, and anyone for whom vaccination is contraindicated. If HepA vaccine and Ig are given at the same time, the vaccine and Ig should be administered at different injection sites.

Preexposure Prophylaxis

Children aged 6–11 months should receive HepA vaccine for preexposure prophylaxis prior to travel and then receive two additional doses on the age-appropriate schedule. Ig is indicated as preexposure prophylaxis in children younger than 6 months at increased risk of hepatitis A infection (eg, those traveling to endemic areas or those with clotting factor disorders) and for travelers > 6 months of age for whom vaccination is contraindicated. Recommended IgIM dosages are 0.1 mL/kg in a single intramuscular dose if the duration of exposure is up to 1 month, 0.2 mL/kg for exposure up to 2 months, and 0.2 mL/kg repeated every 2 months for exposure > 2 months.

CDC: Prevention of hepatitis A through active or passive immunization: recommendations of the Advisory Committee on Immunization Practices (ACIP). MMWR Recomm Rep 2006; 55(RR-7):1 [PMID: 16708058].

Foster MA et al: Increase in hepatitis A virus infections—United States, 2013–2018. MMWR Morb Mortal Wkly Rep 2019;68: 413–415 [PMID: 31071072].

Nelson NP et al: Update: recommendations of the Advisory Committee on Immunization Practices for use of hepatitis A vaccine for postexposure prophylaxis and for preexposure prophylaxis for international travel. MMWR Morb Mortal Wkly Rep 2018;67:1216–1220 [PMID: 30383724].

MENINGOCOCCAL VACCINATION

Infections with *Neisseria meningitidis* cause significant morbidity and mortality, with approximately 350 cases occurring in the United States annually. Even with appropriate treatment, meningococcal disease has an estimated case-fatality rate of 10%–14%, and up to 19% of survivors are left with serious disabilities, including neurologic deficits, hearing loss, and loss of limbs. Six serogroups of meningococcus (A, B, C, W, X, and Y) cause nearly all serious disease worldwide; serogroups B, C, and Y predominate in the United States, while serogroups A and C cause most disease in developing countries. Serogroup B is responsible for more than 50% of cases in children younger than 1 year in the United States; it is also responsible for several recent outbreaks on college campuses.

Five different meningococcal vaccines are available in the United States. Vaccination recommendations are somewhat complex, because disease rates vary substantially by age and depending on whether a chronic condition increasing meningococcal disease risk is present. Updated vaccination recommendations are available at www.cdc.gov/vaccines/vpd/mening/.

Two quadrivalent meningococcal polysaccharide-protein conjugate vaccines are available (MCV4; tradenames Menactra and Menveo), providing protection against serogroups A, C, W, and Y. Menactra is licensed for persons 9 months through 55 years of age; Menveo is licensed for 2 months through 55 years of age. Two doses of either Menactra or Menveo are recommended for all adolescents in the United States, with a first dose at 11–12 years of age and a second dose at 16 years of age.

Two vaccines are available that protect against serogroup B disease (MenB), Bexsero and Trumenba, licensed for use at 10–25 years of age. For healthy young adults who do not have a chronic health condition predisposing to meningococcal disease, Bexsero and Trumenba are not recommended. However, these vaccines may be used with clinical discretion to reduce the risk of serogroup B meningococcal disease. These two vaccines are not interchangeable; the same vaccine product must be used for all doses in the series.

Meningococcal disease risk is significantly higher among children with certain chronic conditions, including anatomic or functional asplenia (including children: with sickle cell disease), with HIV infection, children with complement component deficiencies, being treated with complement inhibitors (eculizumab and possibly ravulizumab). In these circumstances, Menveo may be given as a four-dose series beginning at 2 months of age. Additionally, MenHibrix is a vaccine protecting against Hib as well as meningococcal serogroups C and Y, and can be given as a four-dose series beginning at 6 weeks of age. Alternatively, Menactra may be given to children with anatomic or functional asplenia, or HIV infection, beginning at 2 years of age, or to children with complement deficiencies beginning at 9 months of age.

Children with anatomic or functional asplenia are also at increased risk of meningococcal serogroup B disease and should receive Bexsero or Trumenba starting at 10 years of age. Additionally, individuals traveling abroad to areas with endemic serogroups A, C, and W meningococcal disease should be vaccinated with Menactra or Menveo. Finally, meningococcal disease outbreaks occasionally occur in the United States, and vaccination may be recommended against the serogroups causing the outbreak.

▶ Vaccines Available

1. MCV4 (Menactra, Sanofi): A single 0.5-mL dose contains capsular polysaccharide from serogroups A, C, Y, and W conjugated to diphtheria toxoid.

2. MCV4 (Menveo, Novartis): A single 0.5-mL dose contains serogroups A, C, Y, and W capsular polysaccharide, all of which are conjugated to CRM_{197}, a nontoxic mutant of diphtheria toxoid.

3. Hib-MenCY-TT (MenHibrix, GlaxoSmithKline): A single 0.5-mL dose contains serogroups C and Y capsular polysaccharide conjugated to tetanus toxoid, and Hib capsular polysaccharide conjugated to tetanus toxoid.

4. MenB (Trumenba, Pfizer): A single 0.5-mL dose contains 120 mcg of recombinant lipidated factor H binding protein (fHBP) variants from N meningitidis serogroup B, 0.018 mg of polysorbate 80, and 0.25 mg of aluminum phosphate as an adjuvant.

5. MenB (Bexsero, Novartis): A single 0.5-mL dose contains 50 mcg each of recombinant N meningitidis serogroup B proteins: Neisserial adhesin A (NadA), neisserial heparin-binding antigen (NHBA), factor H–binding protein (fHbp), and 25 mcg of outer membrane vesicles (OMV).

▶ Dosage & Schedule of Administration

MCV4 is given as an intramuscular dose of 0.5 mL. If a dose is inadvertently administered subcutaneously, it does not need to be repeated. Hib-MenCY-TT is given as an intramuscular dose of 0.5 mL; MenB as an intramuscular dose of 0.5 mL in a prefilled syringe. These vaccines can be given at the same time as other vaccines, at a different anatomic site. If a four-dose schedule of Hib-MenCY-TT is given, no additional Hib doses are needed. Protective antibody levels are typically achieved within 10 days of vaccination. The schedule of administration of MCV4 and Hib-MenCY-TT is described previously. Trumenba may be given as a three-dose series (at 0, 1–2, and 6 months) or a two-dose series (at 0 and 6 months). Bexsero is a two-dose series given at least 1 month apart. MenB should be given to persons age 10 years or older at increased risk of meningococcal disease (complement deficiencies, taking complement inhibitors, asplenia, microbiologists, or serogroup B outbreaks). MenB may also be given to healthy adolescents and young adults, but use is discretionary.

▶ Contraindications & Precautions

MCV4 is contraindicated in anyone with a known severe allergic reaction to any component of the vaccine, including diphtheria toxoid (for MCV4) and rubber latex. Although MCV4 vaccination is not contraindicated in someone with a prior history of Guillain-Barré syndrome; providers should discuss the possible risks and benefits of vaccination in anyone with this history. MCV4 can be given to individuals who are immunosuppressed. MCV4 can be given during pregnancy if clinically indicated.

Adverse Effects

MCV4 is generally well tolerated in adolescent patients. Local vaccination reactions (redness, swelling, or induration) occur in 11%–16% of persons 11–18 years old receiving MCV4. The most common solicited complaints among children aged 2–10 years were injection site pain and irritability. More severe systemic reactions (presence of any of the following: fever of ≥ 39.5°C; headache, fatigue, malaise, chills, or arthralgias requiring bed rest; anorexia; multiple episodes of vomiting or diarrhea; rash; or seizures) occur in 4.3% of MCV4 recipients. Although cases of Guillain-Barré syndrome have been reported after MCV4, the current observed rate is above that expected in the absence of vaccination.

Acevedo R et al: The Global Meningococcal Initiative meeting on prevention of meningococcal disease worldwide: epidemiology, surveillance, hypervirulent strains, antibiotic resistance and high-risk populations. Expert Rev Vaccines 2019;18:15 [PMID: 30526162].

CDC: Use of serogroup B meningococcal vaccines in persons aged ≥ 10 years at increased risk for serogroup B meningococcal disease: recommendations of the Advisory Committee on Immunization Practices, 2015. MMWR Morb Mortal Wkly Rep 2015;62:608 [PMID: 26068564].

CDC: Prevention and control of meningococcal disease: recommendations of the Advisory Committee on Immunization Practices (ACIP). MMWR Recomm Rep 2013;62(RR-2):1 [PMID: 23515099].

Myers TR, McNeil MM: Current safety issues with quadrivalent meningococcal conjugate vaccines. Hum Vaccin Immunother 2018;14:1175 [PMID: 28934061].

TETANUS-REDUCED DIPHTHERIA-ACELLULAR PERTUSSIS VACCINATION (ADOLESCENTS & ADULTS)

Pertussis causes disease in all age groups. Although the burden of disease is highest in infants younger than 12 months, pertussis incidence has been rising in children and adolescents, due in part to waning immunity after administration of acellular pertussis vaccines. Routine vaccination with tetanus-reduced dose diphtheria-acellular pertussis (Tdap) has been recommended since 2006. Adolescent, adult, and elderly immunization not only has the capacity to protect vaccine recipients from pertussis but also should limit spread of pertussis from adults to infants and decrease overall pertussis endemicity.

Vaccines Available

1. Tdap (Boostrix, GlaxoSmithKline) contains tetanus toxoid, diphtheria toxoid, and three acellular pertussis antigens (detoxified pertussis toxin [PT], filamentous hemagglutinin [FHA], and pertactin) and is licensed for use in persons aged 10 years and older; this vaccine can be used in adults and the elderly.

2. Tdap (Adacel, Sanofi) contains tetanus toxoid, diphtheria toxoid, and five acellular pertussis antigens (PT, FHA, pertactin, and fimbriae types 2 and 3) and is licensed for use in persons aged 11–64 years.

Dosage & Schedule of Administration

Adolescents 11–18 years of age should receive a 0.5-mL dose of Tdap intramuscularly in the deltoid; the preferred age for Tdap immunization is 11–12 years. Adults 19–64 years of age should receive a single dose of Tdap. Adults 65 years of age and older should receive a single dose of Tdap if they have not previously received Tdap and if they anticipate close contact with an infant younger than 12 months. Women who are pregnant should receive a Tdap booster with each pregnancy, ideally early between 27 and 36 weeks of gestation. Tdap can be administered regardless of the interval since the last tetanus- or diphtheria-toxoid–containing vaccine. Tdap and MCV4 should be administered during the same visit if both vaccines are indicated.

Contraindications & Precautions

Contraindications to Tdap include severe allergic reaction to any vaccine component and encephalopathy (eg, coma, prolonged seizures) not attributable to an identifiable cause within 7 days of administration of a vaccine with pertussis components. Precautions for Tdap administration include Guillain-Barré syndrome occurring within 6 weeks of a previous dose of a tetanus toxoid-containing vaccine, history of Arthus reaction following a previous dose of tetanus or diphtheria toxoid-containing vaccine, a progressive neurologic disorder, uncontrolled epilepsy, or progressive encephalopathy until the condition has stabilized.

Adverse Effects

Pain at the injection site was the most frequently reported local adverse event among adolescents. Headache and fatigue were the most frequently reported systemic adverse events.

Becker-Dreps S et al: Effectiveness of prenatal tetanus, diphtheria, acellular pertussis vaccination in the prevention of infant pertussis in the U.S. Am J Prev Med 2018;55:159 [PMID: 29910115].

CDC: Prevention of pertussis, tetanus, and diphtheria with vaccines in the United States: Recommendations of the Advisory Committee on Immunization Practices (ACIP). MMWR Recomm Rep 2018;67:1 [PMID: 29702631].

Cherry JD: The prevention of severe pertussis and pertussis deaths in young infants. Expert Rev Vaccines 2019;18:205 [PMID: 30736722].
Zerbo O et al: Acellular pertussis vaccine effectiveness over time. Pediatrics 2019;144:e20183466 [PMID: 31182549].

HUMAN PAPILLOMAVIRUS VACCINATION

Genital human papillomavirus (HPV) is the most common sexually transmitted infection in the United States and worldwide. Most of the estimated 14 million persons newly infected every year in the United States have no symptoms. Up to 75% of new infections occur among persons 15–24 years of age. HPV infection is associated with cancers in females (cervical, vulvar, vaginal, oral, and anal) and in males (penile, anal, oral). Other HPV serotypes, distinct from those that cause cancer, cause genital warts in females and males.

A nine-valent HPV vaccine (9vHPV; tradename Gardasil 9) is currently available for use in the United States and is approved for females and males. The vaccine protects against seven cancer-causing HPV types (types 16, 18, 31, 33, 45, 52, and 58), and two genital wart-associated HPV types (types 6 and 11). Two other HPV vaccines licensed in the United States, including a bivalent vaccine (tradename Cervarix) and a quadrivalent vaccine (Gardasil), are no longer distributed in the United States.

Routine HPV vaccination is recommended by ACIP for females and males aged 11–12 years and may be given as early as age 9 years. Because there is some evidence of increased uptake when introduced at a younger age, the AAP recommends starting the series between the ages of 9 and 12, at an age that the provider deems optimal for acceptance and completion of the vaccination series. Catch-up vaccination is recommended for females and males aged 13–26 years who were not previously vaccinated or have not completed the full vaccine series. While not universally recommended, vaccination of adults 27–45 years of age not previously vaccinated can be considered. Females who test positive for a high-risk HPV type, have an abnormal Pap test, or may have been exposed to HPV are still likely to benefit from HPV vaccination through prevention of other HPV types.

More than 10 years has passed since HPV vaccines were licensed. In that time, substantial population-level positive health impacts have been observed, with large reductions in HPV infections, anogenital wart diagnoses, and cervical intraepithelial neoplasia. For example, the prevalence of types 16 and 18, the HPV types most commonly associated with cervical cancer, has fallen by more than 80% in the 5–8 years after vaccination.

▶ Vaccines Available

1. Quadrivalent HPV vaccine (Gardasil, Merck), a nonlive vaccine; a 0.5-mL dose contains HPV-6, 11, 16, and 18 L1 proteins. This vaccine is no longer distributed in the United States.

2. Nine-valent HPV vaccine (Gardasil 9, Merck), a nonlive vaccine; a 0.5-mL dose contains HPV-6, 11, 16, 18, 31, 33, 45, 52, and 58 L1 proteins.

3. Bivalent HPV vaccine (Cervarix, GlaxoSmithKline), a nonlive vaccine is a 0.5-mL dose that contains HPV-16 and HPV-18 L1 protein and the adjuvant AS04. Licensed for use in females only. This vaccine is no longer distributed in the United States.

▶ Dosage & Schedule of Administration

HPV vaccine is administered intramuscularly as two or three separate 0.5-mL doses depending on age at initial vaccination. For healthy adolescents initiating the series prior to their 15th birthday, two doses separated by 6–12 months are recommended (minimum interval 5 months). Three doses are recommended for those initiating vaccination on or after the 15th birthday and for persons with immunocompromising conditions. The second dose should be administered 1–2 months after the first dose and the third dose 6 months after the first dose. The minimum interval between the first and second doses is 4 weeks; the minimum recommended interval between the second and third doses of vaccine is 12 weeks. HPV vaccine may be administered with other vaccines. If the vaccine schedule is interrupted, the series need not be restarted. There is currently no recommendation for repeat vaccination with 9vHPV for persons who have completed a vaccination series with bivalent or quadrivalent HPV vaccine. Additional information on HPV vaccination recommendations can be found at: www.cdc.gov/vaccines/vpd/hpv/hcp/recommendations.html.

▶ Contraindications & Precautions

HPV vaccine is contraindicated in persons with a history of anaphylaxis to any vaccine component. HPV vaccine is not recommended for use in pregnancy. The vaccine can be administered to persons with minor acute illnesses and to immunocompromised persons.

▶ Adverse Effects

Injection site pain (83.9%) and mild to moderate swelling and erythema were the most common adverse events reported by vaccine recipients. Fever (10.3%), nausea (4.2%), and dizziness (2.8%) were reported as systemic adverse events. As with any vaccination, syncope can occur following HPV vaccination; adolescents should be seated or lying down during and for 15 minutes after vaccination, to prevent injuries from falls should syncope occur.

CDC: Human papillomavirus vaccination: recommendations of the Advisory Committee on Immunization Practices (ACIP). MMWR Recomm Rep 2014;63(RR-05):1 [PMID: 25167164].

CDC: Use of a 2-dose schedule for human papillomavirus vaccination—updated recommendations of the Advisory Committee on Immunization Practices. MMWR Morb Mortal Wkly Rep 2016;65:1405 [PMID: 27977643].

CDC: Use of 9-valent human papillomavirus (HPV) vaccine: updated HPV vaccination recommendations of the Advisory Committee on Immunization Practices. MMWR Morb Mortal Wkly Rep 2015;64: 300 [PMID: 25811679].

Drolet M et al: Population-level impact and herd effects following the introduction of human papillomavirus vaccination programmes: updated systematic review and meta-analysis. Lancet 2019; Epub ahead of print [PMID: 31255301].

▼ VACCINATIONS FOR SPECIAL SITUATIONS

RABIES VACCINATION

After symptoms of infection develop, rabies is almost invariably fatal in humans. While sylvan animal and bat rabies in the United States is common, the incidence of human rabies is very low, with fewer than three cases per year. Although dogs represent the most important vector for human rabies worldwide, in the United States because of widespread vaccination of dogs and cats, the most common rabies virus variants responsible for human rabies are bat-related. Rabies is also common in skunks, raccoons, and foxes; it is uncommon in rodents.

Human rabies is preventable with appropriate and timely postexposure prophylaxis. Postexposure care consists of local wound care and both passive and active immunization. Immediately after an animal bite, wounds should be flushed and aggressively cleaned with soap and water. If possible, the wound should not be sutured. Passive immunization after high-risk exposure consists of the injection of human rabies immune globulin (RIg) near the wound. Active immunization is accomplished by completing a schedule of immunization with one of the two available rabies vaccines licensed in the United States. Because bites from bats are often unrecognized, prophylaxis should be considered if a bat is found indoors even if there is no history of contact, especially if found in the same room with a sleeping or unattended child or with an intoxicated or otherwise incapacitated individual.

Local public health officials should be consulted before postexposure rabies prophylaxis is started to avoid unnecessary vaccination and to assist in the proper handling of the animal (if confinement or testing of the animal is appropriate). To facilitate consultation, the health care provider should know the species of animal, its availability for testing or confinement, the nature of the attack (provoked or unprovoked), and the nature of the exposure (bite, scratch, lick, or aerosol of saliva). Rabies immunization should also be considered for some children traveling to countries where rabies is endemic.

▶ Vaccines Available

Rabies vaccines stimulate immunity after 7–10 days, and immunity persists for 2 years or more.

1. HDCV (human diploid cell vaccine; Imovax, Sanofi)
2. PCECV (purified chick embryo cell vaccine; RabAvert, Novartis)

▶ Dosage & Schedule of Administration

These two inactivated rabies vaccines are equally safe and effective for both preexposure and postexposure prophylaxis. For each vaccine, 1 mL is given intramuscularly in the deltoid (for adults and older children) or anterolateral thigh (for infants and young children). The volume of the dose is not reduced for children. Vaccine should not be given in the gluteal region.

▶ Preexposure Vaccination

Preexposure rabies immunization should be considered for individuals at high risk of exposure to rabies (eg, veterinarians, animal handlers, spelunkers, and people moving to or extensively traveling in areas with endemic rabies). Three intramuscular injections of any vaccine are given on days 0, 7, and 21 or 28. Previously vaccinated individuals with potential continued exposure to rabies should have a serum sample tested for rabies antibody every 2 years to assess whether repeat vaccination is indicated.

▶ Postexposure Prophylaxis

After an individual has possibly been exposed to rabies, decisions about whether to initiate postexposure prophylaxis need to be made urgently, in consultation with local public health officials.

1. In previously unvaccinated individuals—After prompt and thorough wound cleansing, an individual exposed to rabies should receive rabies vaccination and RIg. Vaccination is given on the day of exposure (day 0) and on days 3, 7, and 14 following exposure. Immune suppressed individuals should receive an additional dose on day 28. RIg should also be given as soon as possible after exposure, ideally on the day of exposure, in a recommended dose of 20 IU/kg. If anatomically possible, the entire dose of RIg should be infiltrated into and around the wound. Any remaining RIg should be administered intramuscularly at an anatomic site distant from the location used for rabies vaccination. If RIg was not administered when vaccination was begun, it can be administered up to 7 days after the first dose of vaccine. Postexposure failures have occurred only when some deviation from the approved protocol occurred (eg, no cleansing of the wound, less than usual amount of RIg, no RIg at the wound site, or vaccination in the gluteal area).

2. In previously vaccinated individuals—RIg should not be administered, and only two doses of vaccine on days 0 and 3 after exposure are needed.

▶ Adverse Effects

The rabies vaccines are relatively free of serious reactions. Local reactions at the injection site such as pain, swelling, induration, or erythema range in frequency from 11% to 89% of vaccine recipients. Mild systemic reactions, such as headache, nausea, muscle aches, and dizziness, occur in 6%–55% of vaccine recipients. An immune complex-like reaction occurs in about 6% of adults 2–21 days after receiving booster doses of rabies vaccine; symptoms may include generalized urticaria, arthralgias, arthritis, and angioedema.

Travelers to countries where rabies is endemic may need immediate postexposure prophylaxis and may have to use locally available vaccines and RIg. In many developing countries, the only vaccines readily available may be nerve tissue vaccines derived from the brains of adult animals or suckling mice, and the RIg may be of equine origin. Although adverse reactions to RIg are uncommon and typically mild, the nervous tissue vaccines may induce neuroparalytic reactions in 1:200–1:8000 vaccines; this is a significant risk and is another justification for preexposure vaccination prior to travel in areas where exposure to potentially rabid animals is likely.

▶ Antibody Preparations

In the United States, RIg is prepared from the plasma of human volunteers hyperimmunized with rabies vaccine. The recommended dose is 20 IU/kg body weight. The rabies-neutralizing antibody content is 150 IU/mL, supplied in 2- or 10-mL vials.

CDC: Use of a reduced (4-dose) vaccine schedule for postexposure prophylaxis to prevent human rabies: recommendations of the Advisory Committee on Immunization Practices. MMWR Recomm Rep 2010;59(RR-2):1 [PMID: 20300058].

Kessels JA et al: Pre-exposure rabies prophylaxis: a systematic review. Bull World Health Organ 2017;95:210 [PMID: 28250534].

Pierracci EG et al: *Vital Signs:* trends in human rabies deaths and exposures—United States, 1938–2018. MMWR Morb Mortal Wkly Rep 2019;68:524–528 [PMID: 31194721].

TYPHOID FEVER VACCINATION

Typhoid fever causes an estimated 11–21 million illnesses and over 128,000 deaths each year worldwide; in the United States an estimated 5700 cases occur (about 350 cases are reported) each year, predominantly related to international travel.

Two vaccines against *Salmonella enterica typhi*, the bacterium that causes typhoid fever, are available in the United States: a live attenuated vaccine given orally (Ty21a)

and an inactivated vaccine composed of purified capsular polysaccharide (ViCPS) given parenterally. Both vaccines protect 50%–80% of vaccine recipients. The oral vaccine is most commonly used because of its ease of administration. However, noncompliance with the oral vaccine dosing schedule occurs frequently, and correct usage should be stressed or the parenteral ViCPS vaccine used.

Routine typhoid vaccination is recommended only for children who are traveling to typhoid-endemic areas or who reside in households with a documented typhoid carrier. Although typhoid fever occurs throughout the world, areas of highest incidence include southern Asia and sub-Saharan Africa. Travelers should be advised that because the typhoid vaccines are not fully protective, and because of the potential for other food- and waterborne illnesses, careful selection of food and drink and appropriate hygiene remain necessary when traveling internationally.

▶ Vaccines Available

1. Parenteral inactivated ViCPS (Typhim Vi, Sanofi) is for intramuscular use in people 2 years or older.

2. Oral live attenuated Ty21a vaccine (Vivotif Berna Vaccine, Swiss Serum and Vaccine Institute) is supplied as enteric-coated capsules for use in people 6 years or older.

▶ Dosage & Schedule of Administration

ViCPS is administered as a single intramuscular dose (0.5 mL) in the deltoid muscle, with boosters needed every 2 years if exposure continues.

The dose of the oral vaccine (Ty21a) is one capsule every other day for a total of four capsules, taken 1 hour before meals. The capsules should be kept refrigerated and taken with cool liquids. A repeat full course of four capsules is recommended every 5 years if exposure continues. Mefloquine and chloroquine may be given at the same time as the oral vaccine; however, if mefloquine is administered, immunization with Ty21a should be delayed for 24 hours. Proguanil should be administered only if 10 days have lapsed since the last dose of oral vaccine. Oral typhoid vaccine should be given more than 3 days after completing other systemic antibiotics.

▶ Contraindications & Precautions

As with all live attenuated vaccines, Ty21a should not be given to immunocompromised patients.

▶ Adverse Reactions

Both the oral and parenteral vaccines are well tolerated, and adverse reactions are uncommon and usually self-limited. The oral vaccine can cause gastroenteritis-like illness, fatigue, and myalgia, whereas the parenteral vaccine can cause injection site pain, abdominal pain, dizziness, and pruritus.

CDC: Updated recommendations for the use of typhoid vaccine—Advisory Committee on Immunization Practices, United States, 2015. MMWR Morb Mortal Wkly Rep 2015;64:305 [PMID: 25811680].

Martin LB: Vaccines for typhoid fever and other salmonelloses. Curr Opin Infect Dis 2012;25:489 [PMID: 22825288].

World Health Organization: Typhoid vaccines: WHO position paper, March 2018—Recommendations. Vaccine 2019;37(2): 214–216 [PMID: 29661581].

CHOLERA VACCINATION

Cholera is caused by toxigenic *Vibrio cholera* bacteria of serogroup O1 (> 99% of global cases) or O139. The illness manifests as watery diarrhea that can be severe and rapidly fatal without prompt fluid rehydration. Annually in the United States fewer than 25 cases are reported and most occur among travelers to countries where cholera is endemic or epidemic.

A single-dose, live-attenuated monovalent oral vaccine, CVD103-HgR (Vaxchora) is approved by the FDA and available in the United States for use for travelers, age 18–64 years, who are traveling to areas of the world with active cholera transmission. The vaccine has 90% efficacy against severe diarrhea at 10 days after vaccination and 80% efficacy 3 months post-vaccination. CVD103-HgR should not be given to patients who have received antibiotics within the preceding 14 days. CVD103-HgR is an oral live attenuated vaccine that can be shed in the stool and potentially transmitted to close contacts. Additional cholera vaccines are available in countries outside the United States. Vaccinated travelers should continue to utilize careful selection of food and drink and use appropriate hygiene when traveling internationally.

▶ Vaccine Available

1. CVD 103-HgR (Vaxchora, PaxVax, Redwood City, California) is a live-attenuated monovalent oral vaccine that is FDA approved and available in the United States.

CDC: Recommendations of the Advisory Committee on Immunization Practices for use of cholera vaccine. MMWR Morb Mortal Wkly Rep 2017;66:482 [PMID: 28493859].

JAPANESE ENCEPHALITIS VACCINATION

Japanese encephalitis (JE) virus is a mosquito-borne flavivirus. Although most infections are asymptomatic, the disease carries high morbidity and mortality for those with neurologic involvement. It is endemic in parts of Asia, although the risk to most travelers to Asia is low. Travel to rural areas and extended travel in endemic areas may increase the risk. One safe and effective vaccine is available in the United States. Travelers to JE-endemic countries should be advised of risks of JE and the importance of measures to reduce mosquito bites. Vaccination is not recommended for short-term travelers whose visit will be restricted to urban areas or outside of a well-defined JE transmission season, but vaccination is recommended for travelers who plan to spend more than 1 month in endemic areas during the JE transmission season. Vaccination should be *considered* for short-term travelers to endemic areas during the JE transmission season if they will travel outside of an urban area and their activities will increase the risk of JE exposure (time outdoors in rural/agricultural areas, outdoor recreation activities, sleeping in places without mosquito protection) and should also be considered for travelers to an area with an ongoing JE outbreak.

▶ Vaccines Available & Schedule of Administration

JE-VC (Ixiaro, Novartis) is an inactivated Vero cell–derived JE vaccine licensed for use in people ≥2 months of age. It is given intramuscularly in a two-dose series at 0 and 28 days (or 0 and 7–28 days for adults 18–65 years). A booster dose should be given 1 year or more after the primary series if ongoing or repeat exposure to JE virus is expected. For adults and children 3 years or older, each dose is 0.5 mL. For children aged 2–35 months, each dose is 0.25 mL. Adverse reactions include pain at the injection site, headache, myalgias, and fever. JE vaccination is contraindicated for anyone who has had a severe allergic reaction to a previous vaccine dose or component.

CDC: Infectious diseases related to travel: Japanese encephalitis. CDC Health Information for International Travel, 2018. https://wwwnc.cdc.gov/travel/yellowbook/2018/infectious-diseases-related-to-travel/japanese-encephalitis. Accessed July 14, 2019.

CDC: Japanese encephalitis vaccines: recommendations of the Advisory Committee on Immunization Practices (ACIP). MMWR Recomm Rep 2019; 68(RR-1):1 [PMID: 31518342].

CDC: Recommendations for use of a booster dose of inactivated Vero cell culture-derived Japanese encephalitis vaccine: Advisory Committee on Immunization Practices, 2011. MMWR Morb Mortal Wkly Rep 2011;60:661 [PMID: 21617632].

CDC: Use of Japanese encephalitis vaccine in children: recommendations of the ACIP, 2013. MMWR Morb Mortal Wkly Rep 2013;62:898 [PMID: 24226626].

TUBERCULOSIS VACCINATION

Approximately one-fourth of the world's population is infected with *Mycobacterium tuberculosis*, which is a leading cause of death in low- and middle-income nations, killing approximately 1.3 million people annually. It is relatively uncommon in the United States, and most cases occur in persons born abroad or their close contacts. BCG vaccine consists of live attenuated *Mycobacterium bovis*. BCG is the most widely used vaccine in the world, having been administered to over 3 billion people, with a low incidence of adverse events following immunization. BCG vaccine is inexpensive, can be given any time after birth, sensitizes the vaccinated individual for 5–50 years, and stimulates both B-cell and T-cell immune responses. BCG reduces the risk of tuberculous meningitis and disseminated TB in pediatric populations by 50%–100% when administered in the first month of life. Efficacy against pulmonary tuberculosis has been variable (0%–80%) depending on the study setting and other factors.

BCG vaccination should be considered only in children with a negative TB skin test who are not infected with HIV and who are continually exposed to TB without the possibility of being separated from the infected adult. This is essential if the adult is untreated and the child cannot be given preventive treatment. BCG is not recommended for travel.

There is one licensed BCG vaccine in the United States produced by Organon Teknika Corporation (Tice BCG). It is administered intradermally. Adverse effects occur in 1%–10% of healthy individuals, including local ulceration, regional lymph node enlargement, and very rarely lupus vulgaris. The vaccine is contraindicated in pregnant women and in immunocompromised individuals, including those with HIV infection, because it has caused extensive local adenitis and disseminated or fatal infection.

BCG almost invariably causes its recipients to be tuberculin skin test-positive (5–7 mm), but the reaction often becomes negative after 3–5 years. An interferon-γ release assay (IGRA) TB test should be negative. Thus, a positive TST test in a child with a history of BCG vaccination who is being investigated for TB as a case contact should be interpreted as indicating infection with *M tuberculosis*. This is discussed in Chapter 42.

CDC: Updated guidelines for using interferon-gamma release assays to detect Mycobacterium tuberculosis—United States, 2010. MMWR Recomm Rep 2010;59:1 [PMID: 20577159].

CDC (TB information page): https://www.cdc.gov/tb/topic/basics/vaccines.htm. Accessed July 18, 2019.

Perez-Velez CM, Marais BJ: Tuberculosis in children. N Engl J Med 2012;367:348 [PMID: 22830465].

Roy A et al: Effect of BCG vaccination against *Mycobacterium tuberculosis* infection in children: systematic review and meta-analysis. BMJ 2014;349:g4643 doi:10.1136/bmj.g4643 [PMID: 25097193].

YELLOW FEVER VACCINATION

Yellow fever virus is a mosquito-borne flavivirus that is endemic in sub-Saharan Africa and South America. A live, attenuated vaccine against yellow fever is available in the United States but is available only at official yellow fever vaccination locations (typically public health departments) and should only be given after consultation with travel medicine specialists or public health officials. Immunization against yellow fever is indicated for children 9 months or older traveling to endemic areas. Proof of vaccination against yellow fever may be required for travel to certain countries.

▶ Vaccines Available & Schedule of Administration

YF vaccine (YF-VAX, Sanofi) is made from the 17D yellow fever attenuated virus strain grown in chick embryos. When yellow fever vaccine is indicated, a subcutaneous injection of 0.5 mL is administered. Immunity following vaccination is long lasting, and booster doses are no longer recommended for most travelers.

Yellow fever vaccine is contraindicated in infants younger than 6 months (due to an increased risk of vaccine-associated encephalitis), in persons with anaphylactic egg allergy, and in immunocompromised individuals or individuals with a history of thymus disease. In children 6–8 months of age, children with well-controlled HIV, and pregnant women, the vaccine risks and benefits should be weighed on an individual basis. There is no contraindication to giving other live-virus vaccines simultaneously with yellow fever vaccine.

Adverse reactions are generally mild, consisting of low-grade fever, mild headache, and myalgia 5–10 days after vaccination, occurring in fewer than 25% of vaccines. Although very uncommon, several types of severe adverse reactions can occur following vaccination. Serious allergic reactions occur in roughly 1 case per every 55,000 vaccine recipients. The risk of vaccine-associated neurotropic disease within 30 days following vaccination has been estimated to be 1 case per every 125,000 vaccine recipients. The risk of severe multiple organ system failure following vaccination (vaccine-associated viscerotropic disease) has been estimated at 1 case per every 250,000 vaccine recipients. Health care providers should administer yellow fever vaccine only to persons truly at risk of exposure to yellow fever.

CDC: Yellow fever vaccine: recommendations of the Advisory Committee on Immunization Practices (ACIP). MMWR Recomm Rep 2010;59(RR-7):1 [PMID: 20671663].

CDC: Yellow fever vaccine booster doses; recommendations of the Advisory Committee on Immunization Practices, 2015. MMWR Morb Mortal Wkly Rep 2015;64:647 [PMID: 26086636].

Gershman MD et al: Addressing a yellow fever vaccine shortage—United States, 2016–2017. MMWR Morb Mortal Wkly Rep 2017; 66:457–459 [PMID: 28472025].

Monath TP: Review of the risks and benefits of yellow fever vaccination including some new analyses. Expert Rev Vaccines 2012;11:427 [PMID: 22551029].

PASSIVE PROPHYLAXIS

1. Intramuscular & Specific Intravenous Immune Globulin

Ig may prevent or modify infection with hepatitis A virus if administered in a dose of 0.02 mL/kg within 14 days after exposure. Measles infection may be prevented or modified in a susceptible person if Ig is given in a dose of 0.5 mL/kg within 6 days after exposure. Pathogen-specific preparations of Ig include TIg, HBIg, RIg, CMV Ig (IV), botulism Ig (IV), and varicella-zoster Ig (VariZIG). These are obtained from donors known to have high titers of antibody against the organism in question. Ig must be given only by the route (IV or IM) for which it is recommended. The dose varies depending on the clinical indication. Adverse reactions include pain at the injection site, headache, chills, dyspnea, nausea, and anaphylaxis, although all but the first are rare.

Palivizumab (Synagis, MedImmune) is a humanized monoclonal antibody against RSV that is used to prevent RSV infection in high-risk populations with monthly doses during RSV season (Table 10–7). Palivizumab is administered in a dose of 15 mg/kg once a month beginning with the onset of the RSV season and continuing until the end of the season. Prophylaxis should be discontinued in any child who experiences a breakthrough hospitalization.

The maximum number of doses recommended in any one season is five. Palivizumab is packaged in 50- and 100-mg vials. Palivizumab does not interfere with response to routine childhood vaccinations.

2. Intravenous Immune Globulin

The primary indications for IVIg are for replacement therapy in antibody-deficient individuals; for the treatment of Kawasaki disease, immune thrombocytopenic purpura or hemolytic anemia, Guillain-Barré syndrome and other autoimmune diseases; and replacement therapy in chronic B-cell lymphocytic leukemia. IVIg may be beneficial in some children with toxic shock syndrome and for anemia caused by parvovirus B19. It can also be used as postexposure prophylaxis for varicella in at-risk persons when VariZIG is not available.

Table 10–7. Eligibility criteria for palivizumab prophylaxis of high-risk infants and young children based on AAP policy statement.

- Infants born before 29 wk, 0 days, who are aged < 12 mo at the start of RSV season
- Infants aged < 12 mo with chronic lung disease (CLD) of prematurity, defined as gestational age < 32 wk, 0 days, and requiring > 21% oxygen for at least the first 28 days after birth; for the second year of life in children with a history of CLD, consideration of prophylaxis is recommended only for infants who continue to require medical support (chronic corticosteroids, diuretics, or supplemental oxygen) in the 6 mo prior to the start of RSV season
- Certain children aged < 12 mo with significant congenital heart disease (acyanotic heart disease on medication to control heart failure and will require cardiac surgical procedures, infants with moderate to severe pulmonary hypertension)
- Infants with a neuromuscular disease or congenital anomaly that impairs the ability to clear respiratory secretions
- Infants aged < 24 mo who are profoundly immunocompromised at the start of RSV season
- Infants aged < 24 mo with severe cystic fibrosis (respiratory hospitalizations or weight for length < 10th percentile)

AAP: Policy statement—updated guidance for palivizumab prophylaxis among infants and young children at increased risk of hospitalization for respiratory syncytial virus infection. Pediatrics 2014;134(2):415–420 [PMID: 25070315].

Hall CB et al: The burden of respiratory syncytial virus infection in young children. N Engl J Med 2009;360:588 [PMID: 19196675].

Normal Childhood Nutrition & Its Disorders

Matthew A. Haemer, MD, MPH   Laura E. Primak, RD, CNSD, CSP

Liliane K. Diab, MD   Nancy F. Krebs, MD, MS

NUTRITIONAL REQUIREMENTS

NUTRITION & GROWTH

The nutrient requirements of children are influenced by (1) growth rate, (2) body composition, and (3) composition of new growth. These factors vary with age and are especially important during early postnatal life. Growth rates are higher in early infancy than at any other period of life (Table 11–1). Growth rates normally decline rapidly starting in the second month of postnatal life (proportionately later in the preterm infant).

Nutrient requirements also depend on body composition. In the adult, the brain, which accounts for only 2% of body weight, contributes 19% to the total basal energy expenditure. In contrast, in a full-term neonate, the brain accounts for 10% of body weight and for 44% of total energy needs under basal conditions. Thus, in the young infant, total basal energy expenditure and the energy requirement of the brain are relatively high.

Composition of new tissue is a third factor influencing nutrient requirements. For example, fat should account for about 40% of weight gain between birth and 4 months but for only 3% between 24 and 36 months. The corresponding figures for protein are 11% and 21%; for water, 45% and 68%. The high rate of fat deposition in early infancy impacts not only for energy requirements but also for the optimal composition of infant feedings.

Because of the high nutrient requirements for growth and the body composition, the young infant is especially vulnerable to undernutrition. Slowed physical growth is an early and prominent sign of undernutrition in the young infant. The limited fat stores of the very young infant mean that energy reserves are modest. The relatively large size and continued growth of the brain render the central nervous system (CNS) especially vulnerable to the effects of malnutrition in early postnatal life.

ENERGY

The major determinants of energy expenditure are (1) basal metabolism, (2) physical activity, (3) growth, and (4) metabolic response to food. The efficiency of energy use may be a significant factor, and thermoregulation may contribute in extremes of ambient temperature if the body is inadequately clothed. Because adequate data on requirements for physical activity in infants and children are unavailable and because individual growth requirements vary, recommendations have been based on calculations of actual intakes by healthy subjects. Suggested guidelines for energy intake of infants and young children are given in Table 11–2. Also included in this table are calculated energy intakes of infants who are exclusively breast-fed. Weight gain velocity of breast-fed infants during the first 3 months equals and may exceed that of formula-fed infants, but from 6 to 12 months breast-fed infants typically weigh less and lose their body fat more than formula-fed babies and may show a decrease in weight gain velocity. In 2010, the United States adopted the use of the international growth charts developed by The World Health Organization (WHO) for children aged less than 24 months. The WHO charts are growth standards describing the growth of healthy breastfeeding infants under optimal conditions. The use of the WHO charts means that fewer US breastfed infants between the ages of 6 and 18 months will be classified as underweight. (See also section: Pediatric Undernutrition.)

After the first 4 years, energy requirements expressed on a body weight basis decline progressively. The estimated daily energy requirement is about 40 kcal/kg/day at the end of adolescence. Approximate daily energy requirements can be calculated by adding 100 kcal/y to the base of 1000 kcal/day at age 1 year. Appetite and growth are reliable indices of caloric needs in most healthy children, but intake also depends to some extent on the energy density of the food offered. Individual energy requirements of healthy

Table 11–1. Changes in growth rate, energy required for growth, and body composition in infants and young children.

Age (mo)	Growth Rate (g/day)			Energy Requirements for Growth (kcal/kg/day)	Body Composition (%)		
	Male	Both	Female		Water	Protein	Fat
0–0.25		0[a]			75	11.5	11
0.25–1	40		35	50			
1–2	35		30	25			
2–3	28		25	16			
3–6		20		10	60	11.5	26
6–9		15					
9–12		12					
12–18		8					
18–36		6		2	61	16	21

[a]Birth weight is regained by 10 days. Weight loss of more than 10% of birth weight indicates dehydration or malnutrition; this applies to both formula- and breast-fed infants.
Data from Fomon SJ: *Infant Nutrition*, 2nd ed. Philadelphia, PA: WB Saunders; 1974.

infants and children vary considerably, and malnutrition and disease increase the variability. Preterm infant energy requirements can exceed 120 kcal/kg/day, especially during illness or when catch-up growth is desired.

One method of calculating requirements for malnourished patients is to base the calculations on the ideal body weight (ie, 50th percentile weight-for-length, or weight determined from current height and the 50th percentile body mass index [BMI] for age), rather than actual weight.

Scientific Background Papers from the Joint FAO/WHO/UNU Expert Consultation. Oct. 17-24. 2001. Rome, Italy: Human energy requirements. Public Health Nutr 2005 Oct;8(7A): 929–1228 [PMID: 16277811].

PROTEIN

Only amino acids and ammonium compounds are usable as sources of nitrogen in humans. Amino acids are provided through the digestion of dietary protein. Nitrogen is

Table 11–2. Recommendations for energy and protein intake.

Age	Energy (kcal/kg/day)			Protein (g/kg/day)	
	Based on Measurements of Energy Expenditure	Intake From Human Milk	Guidelines for Average Requirements	Intake From Human Milk	Guidelines for Average Requirements
10 d–1 mo	—	105	120	2.05	2.5
1–2 mo	110	110	115	1.75	2.25
2–3 mo	95	105	105	1.36	2.25
3–4 mo	95	75–85	95	1.20	2.0
4–6 mo	95	75–85	95	1.05	1.7
6–12 mo	85	70	90	—	1.5
1–2 y	85	—	90	—	1.2
2–3 y	85	—	90	—	1.1
3–5 y	—	—	90	—	1.1

Data from Krebs NF et al: Growth and intakes of energy and zinc in infants fed human milk. J Pediatr 1994;124–132; Garza C, Butte NF: Energy intakes of human milk-fed infants during the first year. J Pediatr 1990;117:S124.

absorbed from the intestine as amino acids and short peptides. Absorption of nitrogen is more efficient from synthetic diets that contain peptides in addition to amino acids. Some intact proteins are absorbed in early postnatal life, a process that may be important in the development of protein tolerance or allergy.

Because there are no major stores of body protein, a regular dietary supply of protein is essential. In infants and children, optimal growth depends on an adequate dietary protein supply. Relatively subtle effects of protein deficiency are now recognized, especially those affecting tissues with rapid protein turnover rates, such as the immune system and the gastrointestinal (GI) mucosa.

Relative to body weight, rates of protein synthesis and turnover and accretion of body protein are exceptionally high in the infant, especially the preterm infant. Eighty percent of the dietary protein requirement of a preterm infant is used for growth, compared with only 20% in a 1-year-old child. Protein requirements per unit of body weight decline rapidly during infancy as growth velocity decreases. The protein content of human milk decreases from 1.4–1.6 g/100 mL in early lactation to 0.8–1.0 g/100 mL at 3–4 months, then to 0.7–0.8 g/100 mL after 6 months, consistent with the normal decline in growth velocity. Recent research suggests that the higher protein content of typical infant formulas (2–2.5g/100 mL) relative to breast milk is associated with excess weight gain. Regarding the sources of protein in complementary foods, more research is needed to compare the effect of various protein sources such as meat, dairy, and plants on the risk of overweight in infants and children.

The recommendations in Table 11–2 are derived chiefly from the Joint FAO/WHO/UNO Expert Committee and are similar to the Recommended Dietary Allowances (RDAs). They deliver a protein intake above the quantity provided in breast milk. The protein intake required to achieve protein deposition equivalent to the in utero rate in very low-birth-weight infants is 3.7–4.0 g/kg/day simultaneously with adequate energy intake. Protein requirements increase in the presence of skin or gut losses, burns, trauma, and infection. Requirements also increase during times of catch-up growth accompanying recovery from malnutrition (~0.2 g of protein per gram of new tissue deposited). Young infants experiencing rapid recovery may need as much as 1–2 g/kg/day of extra protein. By age 1 year, the extra protein requirement is unlikely to be more than 0.5 g/kg/day.

The quality of protein depends on its amino acid composition. Infants require 43% of protein as essential amino acids, and children require 36%. Adults cannot synthesize nine essential amino acids: histidine, isoleucine, leucine, lysine, methionine, phenylalanine, threonine, tryptophan, and valine. Cysteine and tyrosine are considered partially essential because their rates of synthesis from methionine and phenylalanine, respectively, are limited and may be inadequate in infants, the elderly, and those with malabsorption.

In young infants, synthetic rates for cysteine, tyrosine, and, perhaps, taurine are insufficient for needs. Taurine, an amino acid used to conjugate bile acids, may also be conditionally essential in infancy. Lack of an essential amino acid leads to weight loss within 1–2 weeks. Wheat and rice are low in lysine, and legumes are low in methionine. Appropriate mixtures of vegetable protein are therefore necessary to achieve high protein quality.

Because the mechanisms for removal of excess nitrogen are efficient, moderate excesses of protein are not harmful and may help to ensure an adequate supply of certain micronutrients. Adverse effects of excessive protein intake may include increased calcium losses in urine and, over a life span, increased loss of renal mass. Excessive protein intake of more than 4 g/kg/day in older children and adolescents may also cause elevated blood urea nitrogen, acidosis, and hyperammonemia, and in the preterm infant more than 6 g/kg/day has caused failure to thrive, lethargy, and fever. Impaired capacity to deaminate proteins from liver insufficiency or to excrete excess nitrogen as urea from renal insufficiency can further limit tolerable protein intake.

Arslanoglu S et al. Fortification of human milk for preterm infants: update and recommendations of the European Milk Bank Association (EMBA) Working Group on Human Milk Fortification. Front Pediatr 2019 Mar 22;7:76. doi: 10.3389/fped.2019.00076. eCollection 2019. Review [PMID: 30968003].

LIPIDS

Fats are the main dietary energy source for infants and account for up to 50% of the energy in human milk. Over 98% of breast milk fat is triglyceride (TG), which has an energy density of 9 kcal/g. Fats can be stored efficiently in adipose tissue with a minimal energy cost of storage. This is especially important in the young infant. Fats are required for the absorption of fat-soluble vitamins and for myelination of the CNS. Fat also provides essential fatty acids (EFAs) necessary for brain development, for phospholipids in cell membranes, and for the synthesis of prostaglandins and leukotrienes. The EFAs are polyunsaturated fatty acids, linoleic acid (18:2ω6), and linolenic acid (18:3ω3). Arachidonic acid (20:4ω6) is derived from dietary linoleic acid and is present primarily in membrane phospholipids. Important derivatives of linolenic acid are eicosapentaenoic acid (20:6ω3) and docosahexaenoic acid (DHA, 22:6ω3) found in human milk and brain lipids. Visual acuity and possibly psychomotor development of formula-fed preterm infants is improved in formulas supplemented with DHA (22:6ω3) and ARA (20:4ω6). The benefits of long-chain polyunsaturated fatty acid supplementation in formulas for healthy term infants are unclear (though safety has been established).

Clinical features of EFA omega-6 deficiency include growth failure, erythematous and scaly dermatitis, capillary fragility, increased fragility of erythrocytes, thrombocytopenia, poor wound healing, and susceptibility to infection. The clinical features of deficiency of omega-3 fatty acids are less well defined, but dermatitis and neurologic abnormalities including blurred vision, peripheral neuropathy, and weakness have been reported. Fatty fish are the best dietary source of omega-3 fatty acids. A high intake of fatty fish is associated with decreased platelet adhesiveness and decreased inflammatory response.

Up to 5%–10% of fatty acids in human milk are polyunsaturated, with the specific fatty acid profile reflective of maternal dietary intake. Most of these are omega-6 series with smaller amounts of long-chain omega-3 fatty acids. About 40% of breast milk fatty acids are monounsaturates, primarily oleic acid (18:1), and up to 10% of total fatty acids are medium-chain triglycerides (MCTs) (C_8 and C_{10}) with a calorie density of 7.6 kcal/g. In general, the percentage of calories derived from fat is a little lower in infant formulas than in human milk.

The American Academy of Pediatrics recommends that infants receive at least 30% of calories from fat, with at least 2.7% of total fat as linoleic acid and 1.75% of total fatty acids as linolenic. During at least the first year of life 40%–50% of energy requirements should be provided as fat. Children older than 2 years should be switched gradually to a diet containing approximately 30% of total calories from fat, with no more than 10% of calories from saturated fats.

β-Oxidation of fatty acids occurs in the mitochondria of muscle and liver. Carnitine is necessary for oxidation of the fatty acids, which must cross the mitochondrial membranes as acylcarnitine. Carnitine is synthesized in the human liver and kidneys from lysine and methionine. Carnitine needs of infants are met by breast milk or infant formulas. In the liver, substantial quantities of fatty acids are converted to ketone bodies, which are then released into the circulation as an important fuel for the brain of the young infant.

MCTs are sufficiently soluble that micelle formation is not required for transport across the intestinal mucosa. They are transported directly to the liver via the portal circulation. MCTs are rapidly metabolized in the liver, undergoing β-oxidation or ketogenesis. They do not require carnitine to enter the mitochondria. MCTs are useful for patients with luminal phase defects, absorptive defects, and chronic inflammatory bowel disease. The potential side effects of MCT administration include diarrhea when given in large quantities; high octanoic acid levels in patients with cirrhosis; and, if they are the only source of lipids, deficiency of EFA.

CARBOHYDRATES

The energy density of carbohydrate is 4 kcal/g. Approximately 40% of caloric intake in human milk is in the form of lactose, or milk sugar. Lactose supplies 20% of the total energy in cow's milk. The percent of total energy in infant formulas from carbohydrate is similar to that of human milk.

The rate at which lactase hydrolyzes lactose to glucose and galactose in the intestinal brush border determines how quickly milk carbohydrates are absorbed. Lactase levels are highest in young infants, and decline with age depending on genetic factors. About 20% of nonwhite Hispanic and black children younger than 5 years have lactase deficiency. White children typically do not develop symptoms of lactose intolerance until they are at least 4 or 5 years of age, while nonwhite Hispanic, Asian American, and black children may develop these symptoms by 2 or 3 years of age. Lactose-intolerant children have varying symptoms depending on the specific activity of their intestinal lactase and the amount of lactose consumed. Galactose is preferentially converted to glycogen in the liver prior to conversion to glucose for subsequent oxidation. Infants with galactosemia, an inborn metabolic disease caused by deficient galactose-1-phosphate uridyltransferase, require a lactose-free diet starting in the neonatal period.

After the first 2 years of life, 50%–60% of energy requirements should be derived from carbohydrates, with no more than 10% from simple sugars as recommended by the WHO, or less than 25 g of sugar added to foods per day as recommended by the American Heart Association in 2016. These dietary guidelines are, unfortunately, not reflected in the diets of North American children, who typically derive 25% of their energy intake from sucrose and less than 20% from complex carbohydrates.

Children and adolescents in North America often consume large quantities of sucrose and high-fructose corn syrup in soft drinks and other sweetened beverages, candy, syrups, sweetened breakfast cereals, and a variety of processed foods. A high intake of these sugars, especially in the form of sweetened beverages, may predispose to obesity and insulin resistance, is a major risk factor for dental caries, and may be associated with an overall poorer quality diet, including high intake of saturated fat. Sucrase hydrolyzes sucrose to glucose and fructose in the brush border of the small intestine. Fructose absorption through facilitated diffusion occurs more slowly than glucose absorption through active transport. Fructose does not stimulate insulin secretion or enhance leptin production. Since both insulin and leptin play a role in regulation of food intake, consumption of fructose (eg, as high-fructose corn syrup) may contribute to increased energy intake and weight gain. Fructose is also easily converted to hepatic TGs, which may be undesirable in patients with insulin resistance/metabolic syndrome and cardiovascular disease risk.

Dietary fiber can be classified in two major types: non-digested carbohydrate (β1–4 linkages) and noncarbohydrate (lignin). Insoluble fibers (cellulose, hemicellulose, and lignin) increase stool bulk and water content and decrease gut transit time. Soluble fibers (pectins, mucilages, oat bran) bind bile acids and reduce lipid and cholesterol absorption. Pectins also slow gastric emptying and the rate of nutrient absorption. Few data regarding the fiber needs of children are available. The Dietary Reference Intakes recommend 14 g of fiber per 1000 kcal consumed. The American Academy of Pediatrics recommends that children older than 2 years consume in grams per day an amount of fiber equal to 5 plus the age in years. Fiber intakes are often low in North America. Children who have higher dietary fiber intakes have been found to consume more nutrient-dense diets than children with low-fiber intakes. In general, higher fiber diets are associated with lower risk of chronic diseases such as obesity, cardiovascular disease, and diabetes.

Ruperez AI, Mesana MI, Moreno LA: Dietary sugars, metabolic effects, and child health. Curr Opin Clin Nutr Metab Care 2019 May;22(3):206–216. doi: 10.1097/MCO.0000000000000553 [PMID: 30946053].

Yoshida Y, Simoes EJ: Sugar-sweetened beverage, obesity, and type 2 diabetes in children and adolescents: policies, taxation, and programs. Curr Diab Rep 2018:18(6):31. doi: 10.1007/s11892-018-1004-6. Review [PMID: 29671076].

MAJOR MINERALS

Dietary sources, absorption, metabolism, and deficiency of the major minerals are summarized in Table 11–3. Recommended intakes are provided in Table 11–4.

TRACE ELEMENTS

Trace elements with a recognized role in human nutrition are iron, iodine, zinc, copper, selenium, manganese, molybdenum, chromium, cobalt (as a component of vitamin B_{12}), and fluoride. Information on food sources, functions, and deficiencies of the trace elements is summarized in Table 11–5. Supplemental fluoride recommendations are listed in Table 11–6. Dietary Reference Intakes of trace elements are summarized in Table 11–4. Iron deficiency is discussed in Chapter 30. Recent reviews emphasize the importance of recognizing the risk of iron deficiency without anemia during the first 2 years of life when brain development is rapidly progressing. Testing serum ferritin (and a concurrent marker of inflammation) in older breastfed infants and toddlers with limited dietary iron intake is recommended over checking for anemia (hemoglobin) alone, which identifies severe iron deficiency.

Schwarzenberg SJ et al; AAP Committee on Nutrition: Advocacy for improving nutrition in the first 1000 days to support childhood development and adult health. Pediatrics 2018; 141(2):e20173716 [PMID: 29358479].

VITAMINS

In general, highly restrictive diets (eg, those in which entire food groups are absent) should prompt consideration of vitamin deficiencies. For example, numerous cases of scurvy have been reported in children with autism who have had markedly constrained diets. Untreated fat-malabsorption syndromes (eg, cystic fibrosis, celiac disease, short gut syndrome) are associated with deficiencies of fat-soluble vitamins. See Table 11–7 for other general circumstances that should prompt assessment for vitamin deficiencies.

Fat-Soluble Vitamins

Because they are insoluble in water, the fat-soluble vitamins require digestion and absorption of dietary fat and a carrier system for transport in the blood. Deficiencies of these vitamins develop more slowly than deficiencies of water-soluble vitamins because the body accumulates stores of the fat-soluble vitamins. Prematurity and some childhood conditions (especially those with fat malabsorption) place children at risk (see Table 11–7). Excessive intakes carry potential for toxicity (Table 11–8). A summary of reference intakes is found in Table 11–9. Dietary sources of fat-soluble vitamins, their absorption/metabolism, and causes and clinical features of deficiency are summarized in Table 11–10. Vitamin deficiency and related diagnostic laboratory findings and treatment are detailed in Table 11–11.

Recent recognition of low levels of 25-OH-vitamin D in a relatively large percentage of the population and the broad range of functions beyond calcium absorption have led many experts including the American Academy of Pediatrics to recommend a daily intake of at least 400 IU (10 mcg)/day for all infants, including those who are breast-fed, beginning shortly after birth.

Chang SW, Lee HC: Vitamin D and health—the missing vitamin in humans. Pediatr Neonatol 2019 Jun;60(3):237–244. doi: 10.106/j.pedneo.2019.04.007. Epub 2019 Apr 17. Review [PMID: 31101452].

Water-Soluble Vitamins

Deficiencies of water-soluble vitamins are generally uncommon in the United States because of the abundant food supply and fortification of prepared foods. Cases of deficiencies (eg scurvy) in children with special needs (eg autism) have been reported in the context of sharply restricted diets. Most bread and wheat products are fortified with B vitamins, including the mandatory addition of folic acid to enriched grain products since 1998. Folic acid supplements (400 mcg/day) during the periconceptional period protect against neural tube defects. Dietary intakes of folic acid from natural foods and enriched products are also protective. Biological roles of water-soluble vitamins are listed in Table 11–12. The risk of toxicity from water-soluble vitamins is not as great as that associated with fat-soluble vitamins because excesses are excreted in the urine. However, deficiencies of these vitamins develop more quickly than fat-soluble vitamins because of limited stores, with the

Table 11–3. Summary of major minerals.

Mineral	Absorption/Metabolism	Deficiency	
		Causes	Clinical Features
Calcium *Dietary sources*: dairy products, legumes, broccoli, green leafy vegetables.	20%–30% from diet; 60% from HM. Enhanced by lactose, glucose, protein; impaired by phytate, fiber, oxalate, unabsorbed fat. Absorption is regulated by serum calcitriol, which increases when PTH is secreted in response to low plasma-ionized calcium. PTH also promotes release of calcium from bone. Renal excretion.	Can occur in preterm infants without adequate supplementation and in lactating adolescents with limited calcium intake or in patients with steatorrhea.	Osteopenia or osteoporosis, tetany.
Phosphorus *Dietary sources*: meats, eggs, dairy products, grains, legumes, and nuts; high in processed foods and sodas.	80% from diet. PTH decreases tubular resorption of phosphorus in kidneys; homeostasis is maintained by GI tract and kidneys.	Rare, but can occur in preterm infants fed unfortified HM (results in osteoporosis and rickets, sometimes hypercalcemia). Also seen in patients with protein-energy malnutrition and may occur with refeeding.	Muscle weakness, bone pain, rhabdomyolysis, osteomalacia, and respiratory insufficiency.
Magnesium *Dietary sources*: vegetables, cereals, nuts.	Kidneys regulate homeostasis by decreasing excretion when intake is low.	Occurs as part of refeeding syndrome with protein-energy malnutrition. Renal disease, malabsorption, or magnesium wasting medications may lead to depletion. May cause secondary hypocalcemia.	Neuromuscular excitability, muscle fasciculation, neurologic abnormalities, ECG changes.
Sodium *Dietary sources*: processed foods, table salt.	Hypo- and hypernatremic dehydration are discussed in Chapter 23. Kidneys are primary site of homeostatic regulation.	Results from excess losses associated with diarrhea and vomiting.	Anorexia, vomiting, hypotension, and mental apathy. Severe malnutrition, stress, and hypermetabolism may lead to excess intracellular sodium, affecting cellular metabolism.
Chloride *Dietary sources*: table salt or sea salt, seaweed, many vegetables.	Homeostasis is closely linked to sodium. Plays an important role in physiologic mechanisms of kidneys and gut.	Can occur in infants fed low chloride-containing diets, or in children with cystic fibrosis, vomiting, diarrhea, chronic diuretic therapy, or Bartter syndrome.	Associated with failure to thrive and especially poor head growth; anorexia, lethargy, muscle weakness, vomiting, dehydration, hypovolemia. *Laboratory findings*: may include hypochloremia, hypokalemia, metabolic alkalosis, hyperreninemia.
Potassium *Dietary sources*: nuts, whole grains, meats, fish, beans, fruits and vegetables, especially bananas, orange juice.	Kidneys control potassium homeostasis via the aldosterone renin-angiotensin endocrine system. Amount of total body potassium depends on lean body mass.	Occurs in protein-energy malnutrition (eg, total body depletion + refeeding syndrome) and can cause cardiac failure and sudden death if not treated proactively. With loss of lean body mass, excessive potassium is excreted in urine in any catabolic state. Can also occur during acidosis, from diarrhea, and from diuretic use. Hyperkalemia may result from renal insufficiency.	Muscle weakness, mental confusion, arrhythmias.

ECG, electrocardiogram; GI, gastrointestinal; HM, human milk; PTH, parathyroid hormone.

Table 11–4. Summary of dietary reference intakes for selected major minerals and trace elements.

	0–6 mo	7–12 mo	1–3 y	4–8 y	9–13 y	14–18-y Male	14–18-y Female
Calcium (mg/day)	210[a]	270[a]	500[a]	800[a]	1300[a]	1300[a]	1300[a]
Phosphorus (mg/day)	100[a]	275[a]	460[a]	500	1250	1250	1250
Magnesium (mg/day)	30[a]	75[a]	80	130	240	410	360
Iron (mg/day)	0.27[a]	11	7	10	8	11	15
Zinc (mg/day)	2[a]	3	3	5	8	11	9
Iodine (mcg/day)	110[a]	130	90	90	120	150	150
Copper (mcg/day)	200[a]	220[a]	340	440	700	890	890
Selenium (mcg/day)	15[a]	20[a]	20	30	40	55	55

[a]Adequate Intakes (AI). All other values represent the Recommended Dietary Allowances (RDAs). Both the RDA and AI may be used as goals for individual intakes.

Table 11–5. Summary of trace elements.

Mineral	Deficiency		Treatment
	Causes	Clinical Features	
Zinc *Dietary sources*: meats, shellfish, legumes, nuts, and whole-grain cereals. *Functions*: component of many enzymes and gene transcription factors; plays critical roles in nucleic acid metabolism, protein synthesis, and gene expression; supports membrane structure and function.	Diets low in available zinc (high phytate), unfortified synthetic diets; malabsorptive diseases (enteritis, celiac disease, cystic fibrosis); excessive losses (chronic diarrhea); inborn errors of zinc metabolism (acrodermatitis enteropathica, mammary gland zinc secretion defect). Inadequate intake in breast-fed infants after age 6 mo. Preterm birth and low birth weight are risk factors.	Mild: impaired growth, poor appetite, impaired immunity. Moderate to severe: mood changes, irritability, lethargy, impaired immune function, increased susceptibility to infection; acro-orificial skin rash, diarrhea, alopecia. Response to zinc supplement is gold standard for diagnosis of deficiency; plasma zinc levels are lowered by acute phase response.	1 mg/kg/day of elemental zinc for 2–3 mo (eg, 4.5 mg/kg/day of zinc sulfate salt), given separately from meals and iron supplements. With acrodermatitis enteropathica, 30–50 mg Zn^{2+}/day (or more) sustains remission.
Copper *Dietary sources*: meats, shellfish, legumes, nuts, and whole-grain cereals. *Functions*: vital component of several oxidative enzymes: cytochrome c oxidase (electron transport chain), cytosolic and mitochondrial superoxide dismutase (free radical defense), lysyl oxidase (cross-linking of elastin and collagen), ferroxidase (oxidation of ferrous storage iron prior to transport to bone marrow).	Generalized malnutrition, prolonged PN without supplemental copper, malabsorption, or prolonged diarrhea. Prematurity is a risk factor.	Osteoporosis, enlargement of costochondral cartilages, cupping and flaring of long bone metaphyses, spontaneous rib fractures. Neutropenia and hypochromic anemia resistant to iron therapy. Defect of copper metabolism (Menkes kinky hair syndrome) results in severe CNS disease. Low plasma levels help to confirm deficiency; levels are normally very low in young infants. Age-matched normal data are necessary for comparison. Plasma levels are raised by acute phase response.	1% copper sulfate solution (2 mg of salt) or 500 mcg/day elemental copper for infants.

(Continued)

Table 11–5. Summary of trace elements. (*Continued*)

| Mineral | Deficiency | | |
	Causes	Clinical Features	Treatment
Selenium *Dietary sources*: seafood, meats, garlic (geochemical distribution affects levels in foods). *Function*: essential component of glutathione peroxidase.	Inadequate dietary intake; can occur with selenium-deficient PN. Renal disease. Prematurity	Skeletal muscle pain and tenderness, macrocytosis, loss of hair pigment. Keshan disease, an often fatal cardiomyopathy in infants and children in areas of China with Selenium-poor soil.	Minimum recommended selenium content for full-term infant formulas is 1.5 mcg/100 kcal, and for preterm formulas, 1.8 mcg/100 kcal. PN should be supplemented.
Iodine *Dietary source*: iodized salt. Typical fortification provides 225 mcg/5 g. *Functions*: essential component of thyroid hormones; regulates metabolism, growth, and neural development.	Inadequate dietary intake.	Neurologic endemic cretinism (severe mental retardation, deaf mutism, spastic diplegia, and strabismus) occurs with severe deficiency. Myxedematous endemic cretinism occurs in some central African countries where signs of congenital hypothyroidism are present.	Use of iodized salt is effective in preventing goiter. Injections of iodized oil can also be used for prevention.
Fluoride *Function*: incorporated into the hydroxyapatite matrix of dentin.	Inadequate intake (unfluoridated water supply).	Low intake increases incidence of dental caries.	See Table 11–6 for supplementation guidelines. Excess fluoride intake results in fluorosis.

CNS, central nervous system; PN, parenteral nutrition.

exception of vitamin B_{12}. Major dietary sources of the water-soluble vitamins are listed in Table 11–13. Additional salient details are summarized in Tables 11–7, 11–14, and 11–15.

Carnitine is synthesized in the liver and kidneys from lysine and methionine. In certain circumstances (Table 11–14), synthesis is inadequate, and carnitine can then be considered a vitamin. A dietary supply of other organic compounds, such as inositol, may also be required in certain circumstances.

Table 11–6. Supplemental fluoride recommendations (mg/day).

| Age | Concentration of Fluoride in Drinking Water | | |
	< 0.3 ppm	0.3–0.6 ppm	> 0.6 ppm
6 mo–3 y	0.25	0	0
3–6 y	0.5	0.25	0
6–16 y	1	0.5	0

Adapted with permission from Centers for Disease Control and Prevention: Recommendations for using fluoride to prevent and control dental caries in the United States. Centers for Disease Control and Prevention. MMWR Recomm Rep 2001 Aug 17;50(RR-14):1–42.

Table 11–7. Circumstances associated with risk of vitamin deficiencies.

Circumstance	Possible Deficiency
Preterm birth	All vitamins
Protein-energy malnutrition	B_1, B_2, folate, A
Synthetic diets without adequate fortification (including total parenteral nutrition)	All vitamins
Vitamin-drug interactions	Folate, B_{12}, D, B_6
Fat malabsorption syndromes	Fat-soluble vitamins
Breast-feeding with malnourished mother and/or limited complementary foods	B_1,[a] folate,[b] B_{12},[c] D,[d] K[e]
Periconceptional	Folate
Bariatric surgery (all types)	B vitamins
Highly restrictive diet	Vitamin C, B vitamins

[a]Alcoholic or malnourished mother.
[b]Folate-deficient mother.
[c]Vegan mother or maternal pernicious anemia.
[d]Infant not exposed to sunlight and mother's vitamin D status suboptimal.
[e]Prophylaxis omitted.

Table 11–8. Effects of vitamin toxicity.

Pyridoxine
Sensory neuropathy at doses > 500 mg/day
Niacin
Histamine release → cutaneous vasodilation; cardiac arrhythmias; cholestatic jaundice; gastrointestinal disturbance; hyperuricemia; glucose intolerance
Folic acid
May mask B_{12} deficiency, hypersensitivity
Vitamin C
Diarrhea; increased oxalic acid excretion; renal stones
Vitamin A
(> 20,000 IU/day): Vomiting, increased intracranial pressure (pseudotumor cerebri); irritability; headaches; insomnia; emotional lability; dry, desquamating skin; myalgia and arthralgia; abdominal pain; hepatosplenomegaly; cortical thickening of bones of hands and feet
Vitamin D
(> 50,000 IU/day): Hypercalcemia; vomiting; constipation; nephrocalcinosis
Vitamin E
(> 25–100 mg/kg/day intravenously): Necrotizing enterocolitis and liver toxicity (but probably due to polysorbate 80 used as a solubilizer)
Vitamin K
Lipid-soluble vitamin K: Very low order of toxicity
Water-soluble, synthetic vitamin K: Vomiting; porphyrinuria; albuminuria; hemolytic anemia; hemoglobinuria; hyperbilirubinemia (do not give to neonates)

Diab L, Krebs NF: Vitamin excess and deficiency. Pediatr Rev 2018 Apr;39(4):161–179. doi: 10.1542/pir.2016.0068 [PMID: 29610425].

▼ INFANT FEEDING

BREAST-FEEDING

Breast-feeding provides optimal nutrition for the normal infant during the early months of life. The WHO recommends exclusive breast-feeding for approximately the first 6 months of life, with continued breast-feeding along with appropriate complementary foods through the first 2 years of life. Numerous immunologic factors in breast milk (including secretory immunoglobulin A [IgA], lysozyme, lactoferrin, bifidus factor, oligosaccharides, and macrophages) provide protection against GI and upper respiratory infections.

In developing countries, lack of refrigeration and contaminated water supplies make formula feeding especially hazardous. Although formulas are made to resemble breast milk, they cannot replicate the nutritional or immune composition of human milk. Additional differences of physiologic importance continue to be identified. Furthermore, breastfeeding can foster the maternal-child bond.

Breast-feeding is the predominant *initial* mode of feeding young infants in the United States. Unfortunately, breast-feeding rates remain low among several subpopulations, including low-income, minority, and young mothers. Many mothers face obstacles in maintaining lactation once they return to work, and rates of breast-feeding at 6 months are considerably less than the goal of 50%. Use of an electric breast pump can help to maintain lactation when mothers and infants are separated for extended periods.

Absolute contraindications to breast-feeding are rare. They include active tuberculosis (in the mother) and galactosemia (in the infant). Breast-feeding is associated with maternal-to-child transmission of human immunodeficiency virus (HIV), but the risk is influenced by duration and pattern of breast-feeding and maternal factors, including immunologic status and presence of mastitis. Complete avoidance of breast-feeding by HIV-infected women is presently the only mechanism to prevent maternal-infant transmission. HIV-infected mothers in developed countries are recommended to refrain from breast-feeding if safe alternatives are available. In developing countries, the use of antiretroviral therapy (ART) and exclusive breast-feeding is encouraged; if ART is not available, avoidance of breast-feeding may be considered. The protection of the child against diarrheal illness and malnutrition may outweigh the risk of HIV transmission via breast milk. In such circumstances, HIV-infected women should be encouraged to exclusively breast-feed for 6 months. Mixed feeding should be avoided because of the increased risk of HIV transmission.

In newborns less than 1750 g, human milk should be fortified to increase protein, calcium, phosphorus, micronutrient content, and caloric density. Breast-fed infants with cystic fibrosis can be breast-fed successfully if exogenous pancreatic enzymes are provided. All infants with cystic fibrosis should receive supplemental vitamins A, D, E, K, and sodium chloride. Those with growth faltering should receive caloric supplementation.

Bunik M: The pediatrician's role in encouraging exclusive breast-feeding. Pediatr Rev 2017 Aug;38(8):353–368. doi: 10.154/pir.2016-0109. Review [PMID: 28765198].

Support of Breast-Feeding

In developed countries, health professionals play a significant role in supporting and promoting breast-feeding. Perinatal hospital routines and early pediatric care have a great influence on the successful initiation of breast-feeding by promoting prenatal and postpartum education, frequent mother-baby contact, advice about breast-feeding technique, demand feeding, rooming-in, avoidance of bottle supplements, and early follow-up after delivery. Increasing maternal confidence, family support, adequate maternity leave, and advice about common problems such as sore nipples can foster success. Medical providers can follow best practices and advocate for hospital policies that support breast-feeding.

Table 11–9. Summary of dietary reference intakes for select vitamins.

	0–6 mo	7–12 mo	1–3 y	4–8 y	9–13 y	14–18-y Male	14–18-y Female
Thiamin (mg/day)	0.2[a]	0.3[a]	0.5	0.6	0.9	1.2	1.0
Riboflavin (mg/day)	0.3[a]	0.4[a]	0.5[a]	0.6[a]	0.9[a]	1.3[a]	1.0[a]
Pyridoxine (mg/day)	0.1[a]	0.3[a]	0.5	0.6	1.0	1.3	1.2
Niacin (mg/day)	2[a]	4[a]	6	8	12	16	14
Pantothenic acid (mg/day)	1.7[a]	1.8[a]	2[a]	3[a]	4[a]	5[a]	5[a]
Biotin (mcg/day)	5[a]	6[a]	8[a]	12[a]	20[a]	25[a]	25[a]
Folic acid (mcg/day)	65[a]	80[a]	150	200	300	400	400
Cobalamin (mcg/day)	0.4[a]	0.5[a]	0.9	1.2	1.8	2.4	2.4
Vitamin C (mg/day)	40[a]	50[a]	15	25	45	75	65
Vitamin A (mcg/day)	400[a]	500[a]	300	400	600	900	700
Vitamin D (IU/day)	200[a,b]	200[a,b]	200[a,b]	200[a,b]	200[a,b]	200[a,b]	200[a,b]
Vitamin E (mg/day)	4[a]	5[a]	6	7	11	15	15
Vitamin K (mcg/day)	2[a]	2.5[a]	30[a]	55[a]	60[a]	75[a]	75[a]

[a]Adequate Intakes (AI). All other values represent the Recommended Dietary Allowances (RDAs). Both the RDA and AI may be used as goals for individual intakes.
[b]American Academy of Pediatrics in 2008 recommended 400 IU/day vitamin D for infants, children, and adolescents.
Data from National Academy of Sciences, Food and Nutritional Board, Institute of Medicine: *Dietary Reference Intakes, Applications in Dietary Assessment.* Washington, DC: National Academy Press; 2000:287. http://www.nap.edu.

Table 11–10. Summary of fat-soluble vitamins.

Vitamin	Absorption/Metabolism	Deficiency	
		Causes	Clinical Features
Vitamin A *Dietary sources*: dairy products, eggs, liver, meats, fish oils. Precursor β-carotene is abundant in yellow and green vegetables. *Functions*: has critical role in vision, helping to form photosensitive pigment rhodopsin; modifies differentiation and proliferation of epithelial cells in respiratory tract; and is needed for glycoprotein synthesis.	Retinol is stored in liver and from there is exported, attached to RBP and prealbumin. RBP may be decreased in liver disease or in protein energy malnutrition. Circulating RBP may be increased in renal failure.	Occurs in premature infants, in association with inadequately supplemented PN; protein-energy malnutrition (deficiency worsened by measles); dietary insufficiency and fat malabsorption.	Night blindness, xerosis, xerophthalmia, Bitot spots, keratomalacia, ulceration and perforation of cornea, prolapse of lens and iris, and blindness; follicular hyperkeratosis; pruritus; growth retardation; increased susceptibility to infection.
Vitamin K *Dietary sources*: leafy vegetables, fruits, seeds; synthesized by intestinal bacteria. *Functions*: necessary for the maintenance of normal plasma levels of coagulation factors II, VII, IX, and X; essential for maintenance of normal levels of the anticoagulation protein C; essential for osteoblastic activity.	Absorbed in proximal small intestine in micelles with bile salts; circulates with VLDL.	Occurs in newborns, especially those who are breast-fed and who have not received vitamin K prophylaxis at delivery; in fat malabsorption syndromes; and with use of unabsorbed antibiotics and anticoagulant drugs (warfarin).	Bruising or bleeding in GI tract, genitourinary tract, gingiva, lungs, joints, and brain.

(Continued)

Table 11–10. Summary of fat-soluble vitamins. (*Continued*)

Vitamin	Absorption/Metabolism	Deficiency	
		Causes	Clinical Features
Vitamin E *Dietary sources*: vegetable oils, some cereals, dairy, wheat germ, eggs. *Functions*: free-radical scavenger, stops oxidation reactions. Located at specific sites in cell membrane to protect polyunsaturated fatty acids in membrane from peroxidation and thiol groups and nucleic acids; also acts as cell membrane stabilizer; may function in electron transport chain; may modulate chromosomal expression.	Emulsified in intestinal lumen with bile salts; absorbed via passive diffusion; transported by chylomicrons and VLDL.	May occur with preterm birth, cholestatic liver disease, pancreatic insufficiency, abetalipoproteinemia, and short bowel syndrome. Isolated inborn error of vitamin E metabolism. May result from increased consumption during oxidant stress.	Hemolytic anemia; progressive neurologic disorder with loss of deep tendon reflexes, loss of coordination, vibratory and position sensation, nystagmus, weakness, scoliosis, and retinal degeneration.
Vitamin D *Dietary sources*: fortified milk and formulas, egg yolk, fatty fish. *Functions*: calcitriol, the biologically active form of vitamin D, stimulates intestinal absorption of calcium and phosphate, renal reabsorption of filtered calcium, and mobilization of calcium and phosphorus from bone.	Normally obtained primarily from cholecalciferol (D_3) produced by UV radiation of dehydrocholesterol in skin. Ergocalciferol (D_2) is derived from UV irradiation of ergosterol in skin. Vitamin D is transported from skin to liver, attached to a specific carrier protein.	Results from a combination of inadequate sunlight exposure, dark skin pigmentation, and low dietary intake. Breast-fed infants are at risk because of low vitamin D content of human milk. Cow's milk and infant formulas are routinely supplemented with vitamin D. Deficiency also occurs in fat malabsorption syndromes. Hydroxylated vitamin D may be decreased by CYP-450–stimulating drugs, hepatic or renal disease, and inborn errors of metabolism.	Osteomalacia (adults) or rickets (children), in which osteoid with reduced calcification accumulates in bone. *Clinical findings*: craniotabes, rachitic rosary, pigeon breast, bowed legs, delayed eruption of teeth and enamel defects, Harrison groove, scoliosis, kyphosis, dwarfism, painful bones, fractures, anorexia, and weakness. *Radiographic findings*: cupping, fraying, flaring of metaphyses.

CYP, cytochrome P; GI, gastrointestinal; PN, parenteral nutrition; PTH, parathyroid hormone; RBP, retinol-binding protein; UV, ultraviolet; VLDL, very low-density lipoproteins.

Very few women are physically unable to nurse their babies, but both maternal and/or infant factors can impact successful initiation of nursing and lactogenesis. Mothers with obesity and/or insulin resistance often have delayed lactogenesis, and thus a potential need for additional breastfeeding support to establish successful lactation should be anticipated. The newborn is generally fed ad libitum every 2–3 hours, with longer intervals (4–5 hours) at night. Thus, a newborn infant nurses at least 8–10 times a day, stimulating a generous milk supply. In neonates, a loose stool is often passed with each feeding; later (at age 3–4 months), there may be an interval of several days between stools. Failure to pass several stools a day in the early weeks of breast-feeding suggests inadequate milk intake. Expressing milk using an electric breast pump may be indicated if the mother returns to work or if the infant is preterm, cannot suck adequately, or is hospitalized.

McFadden A et al: Support for healthy breastfeeding mothers with healthy term babies. Cochrane Database Syst Rev 2017 Feb 28;2:CD001141. doi: 10.1002/14651858.CD001141.pub5 [PMID: 28244064].

Technique of Breast-Feeding

Breast-feeding can be started as soon as both mother and baby are stable after delivery, ideally within the first 30–60 minutes. Correct positioning and breast-feeding technique are necessary to ensure effective nipple stimulation and breast emptying with minimal nipple discomfort.

To nurse while the mother is sitting, the infant should be held at the height of the breast and turned to face the mother so that their abdomens touch. The mother's arms supporting the infant should be held tightly at her side, bringing the baby's head in line with her breast. The breast should be supported

Table 11–11. Evaluation and treatment of deficiencies of fat-soluble vitamins.

Vitamin Deficiency	Diagnostic Laboratory Findings and Treatment
Vitamin A	*Laboratory findings*: serum retinol < 20 mcg/dL; molar ratio of retinol:RBP < 0.7 is also diagnostic. *Treatment*: xerophthalmia requires 5000–10,000 IU/kg/day for 5 day PO or IM; with fat malabsorption, standard dose is 2500–5000 IU. Toxicity effects are listed in Table 11–8.
Vitamin K	*Laboratory findings*: assess plasma levels of PIVKA or PT. *Treatment*: Oral: 2.5–5.0 mg/day or IM/IV: 1–2 mg/dose as single dose.
Vitamin E	*Laboratory findings*: normal serum level is 3–15 mg/mL for children. Ratio of serum vitamin E to total serum lipid is normally ≥ 0.8 mg/g. *Treatment*: large oral doses (up to 100 IU/kg/day) correct deficiency from malabsorption; for abetalipoproteinemia, 100–200 IU/kg/day are needed.
Vitamin D	*Laboratory findings*: low serum phosphorus and calcium, high alkaline phosphatase, high serum PTH, low 25-OH-cholecalciferol. American Academy of Pediatrics recommends supplementation, as follows: 400 IU/day for all breast-fed infants, beginning in first 2 mo of life and continuing until infant is receiving ≥ 500 mL/day of vitamin D-fortified formula or cow's milk. *Treatment*: 1600–5000 IU/day of vitamin D_3 for rickets. If poorly absorbed, give 0.05–0.2 mcg/kg/day of calcitriol.

IM, intramuscular; IV, intravenous; PIVKA, protein-induced vitamin K absence; PO, by mouth; PT, prothrombin time; PTH, parathyroid hormone; RBP, retinol-binding protein.

by the lower fingers of her free hand, with the nipple compressed between the thumb and index fingers to make it more protractile. When the infant opens its mouth, the mother should quickly insert as much nipple and areola as possible.

The most common cause of early poor weight gain in breast-fed infants is poorly managed mammary engorgement, which rapidly decreases milk supply. Unrelieved engorgement can result from long intervals between feeding, improper infant suckling, a nondemanding infant, sore nipples, maternal or infant illness, nursing from only one breast, and latching difficulties. Poor technique, maternal dehydration, or excessive fatigue can contribute. Some infants may need waking to feed at night. Primary lactation failure occurs in less than 5% of women.

A sensible guideline for duration of feeding is 5 minutes per breast at each feeding the first day, 10 minutes on each side at

Table 11–12. Summary of biologic roles of water-soluble vitamins.

B vitamins involved in production of energy
  Thiamin (B_1)
    Thiamin pyrophosphate is a coenzyme in oxidative decarboxylation (pyruvate dehydrogenase, α-ketoglutarate dehydrogenase, and transketolase).
  Riboflavin (B_2)
    Coenzyme of several flavoproteins (eg, flavin mononucleotide [FMN] and flavin adenine dinucleotide [FAD]) involved in oxidative/electron transfer enzyme systems.
  Niacin
    Hydrogen-carrying coenzymes: nicotinamide-adenine dinucleotide (NAD), nicotinamide-adenine dinucleotide phosphate (NADP); decisive role in intermediary metabolism.
  Pantothenic acid
    Major component of coenzyme A.
  Biotin
    Component of several carboxylase enzymes involved in fat and carbohydrate metabolism.
Hematopoietic B vitamins
  Folic acid
    Tetrahydrofolate has essential role in one-carbon transfers. Essential role in purine and pyrimidine synthesis; deficiency → arrest of cell division (especially bone marrow and intestine).
  Cobalamin (B_{12})
    Methyl cobalamin (cytoplasm): synthesis of methionine with simultaneous synthesis of tetrahydrofolate (reason for megaloblastic anemia in B_{12} deficiency). Adenosyl cobalamin (mitochondria) is coenzyme for mutases and dehydratases.
Other B vitamins
  Pyridoxine (B_6)
    Prosthetic group of transaminases, etc, involved in amino acid interconversions; prostaglandin and heme synthesis; central nervous system function; carbohydrate metabolism; immune development.
Other water-soluble vitamins
  l-Ascorbic acid (C)
    Strong reducing agent—probably involved in all hydroxylations. Roles include collagen synthesis; phenylalanine → tyrosine; tryptophan → 5-hydroxytryptophan; dopamine → norepinephrine; Fe^{3+}; folic acid → folinic acid; cholesterol → bile acids; leukocyte function; interferon production; carnitine synthesis. Copper metabolism; reduces oxidized vitamin E.

each feeding the second day, and 10–15 minutes per side thereafter. A vigorous infant can obtain most of the available milk in 5–7 minutes, but additional sucking time ensures breast emptying, promotes milk production, and satisfies the infant's sucking urge. The side on which feeding is commenced should be alternated. The mother may break suction gently after nursing by inserting her finger between the baby's gums.

Table 11–13. Major dietary sources of water-soluble vitamins.

Thiamin (B_1)
  Whole and enriched grains, lean pork, legumes
Riboflavin (B_2)
  Dairy products, meat, poultry, wheat germ, leafy vegetables
Niacin (B_3)
  Meats, poultry, fish, legumes, wheat, all foods except fats; synthesized in body from tryptophan
Pyridoxine (B_6)
  Animal products, vegetables, whole grains
Pantothenic acid
  Ubiquitous
Biotin
  Yeast, liver, kidneys, legumes, nuts, egg yolks (synthesized by intestinal bacteria)
Folic acid
  Leafy vegetables (easily destroyed in cooking), fruits, whole grains, wheat germ, beans, nuts
Cobalamin (B_{12})
  Eggs, dairy products, liver, meats; *none in plants*
Vitamin C
  Fruits and vegetables
Carnitine
  Meats, dairy products; *none in plants*

Table 11–14. Causes of deficiencies in water-soluble vitamins.

Thiamin
  Beriberi: in infants breast-fed by mothers with history of alcoholism or poor diet; has been described as complication of parenteral nutrition (PN); protein-energy malnutrition; following bariatric surgery of all types—reported in adults and adolescents; endemic deficiency in mothers and infants reported in Asia where unfortified, refined rice is major food staple
Riboflavin
  General undernutrition; inactivation in total parenteral nutrition (TPN) solutions exposed to light
Niacin
  Maize- or millet-based diets (high-leucine and low-tryptophan intakes); carcinoid tumors
Pyridoxine
  Prematurity (these infants may not convert pyridoxine to pyridoxal-5-P); B_6 dependency syndromes; drugs (isoniazid)
Biotin
  Suppressed intestinal flora and impaired intestinal absorption; regular intake of raw egg whites
Folic acid
  Breast-fed infants whose mothers are folate-deficient; term infants fed unsupplemented processed cow's milk or goat's milk; kwashiorkor; chronic overcooking of food sources; malabsorption of folate because of a congenital defect; celiac disease; drugs (phenytoin)
  Increased requirements: chronic hemolytic anemias, diarrhea, malignancies, extensive skin disease, cirrhosis, pregnancy
Cobalamin (B_{12})
  Breast-fed infants of mothers with latent pernicious anemia or who are on an unsupplemented vegan diet; absence of luminal proteases; short gut syndrome (absence of stomach or ileum); congenital malabsorption of B_{12}
Vitamin C
  Maternal megadoses during pregnancy → deficiency in infants (rebound); diet without fruits or vegetables; seen in infants fed formula based on pasteurized cow's milk (historical)
Carnitine
  Premature infants fed unsupplemented formula or fed intravenously; dialysis; inherited deficits in carnitine synthesis; organic acidemias; infants receiving valproic acid

Follow-up

Assessment before discharge should identify dyads needing additional support. All mother-infant pairs require early follow-up. The second through fourth days postpartum when milk secretion becomes copious is a critical time. Failure to empty the breasts during this time can cause engorgement, which quickly leads to diminished milk production.

Common Problems

Nipple tenderness requires attention to proper positioning of the infant and correct latch-on. Nursing for shorter periods, beginning feedings on the less sore side, air drying the nipples well after nursing, and use of lanolin cream may provide relief. Severe nipple pain and cracking usually indicate improper latch. Temporary pumping may be needed.

Breast-feeding jaundice is exaggerated physiologic jaundice associated with low intake of breast milk, infrequent stooling, and poor weight gain (see Chapter 2). If possible, the jaundice should be managed by increasing the frequency of nursing and, if necessary, augmenting the infant's sucking with regular breast pumping. Supplemental feedings may be necessary, but care should be taken not to decrease breast milk production further.

In a small percentage of breast-fed infants, hyperbilirubinemia with jaundice is caused by an unidentified property of the milk that inhibits conjugation of bilirubin. In severe cases, interruption of breast-feeding for 24–36 hours may be necessary. The mother's breast should be emptied with an electric breast pump during this period.

The symptoms of mastitis include flu-like symptoms with breast tenderness, firmness, and erythema. Antibiotic therapy covering β-lactamase–producing organisms should be given for 10 days. Analgesics may be necessary, but breast-feeding should be continued. Breast pumping may be helpful adjunctive therapy.

Maternal Drug Use

Factors playing a role in the transmission of drugs in breast milk include the route of administration, dosage, molecular weight, pH, and protein binding. Generally, any drug prescribed to a

Table 11–15. Clinical features of deficiencies in water-soluble vitamins.

Thiamin (B$_1$)
   "Dry" Beriberi (paralytic or nervous): peripheral neuropathy, with impairment of sensory, motor, and reflex functions, ophthalmoplegia, vomiting
   "Wet" Beriberi: high output congestive heart failure ± signs of dry beriberi
   Cerebral Beriberi: ophthalmoplegia, ataxia, mental confusion, memory loss
Riboflavin
   Cheilosis; angular stomatitis; glossitis; soreness and burning of lips and mouth; dermatitis of nasolabial fold and genitals; ± ocular signs (photophobia → indistinct vision)
Niacin
   Pellagra (dermatitis, especially on sun-exposed areas; diarrhea; dementia)
Pyridoxine (B$_6$)
   Listlessness; irritability; seizures; anemia; cheilosis; glossitis
Biotin
   Scaly dermatitis; alopecia; irritability; lethargy
Folic acid
   Megaloblastic anemia; neutropenia; growth retardation; delayed maturation of central nervous system in infants; diarrhea (mucosal ulcerations); glossitis; neural tube defects
Cobalamin (B$_{12}$)
   Megaloblastic anemia; hypersegmented neutrophils; neurologic degeneration: paresthesias, gait problems, depression
Ascorbic acid (C)
   Irritability, apathy, pallor; increased susceptibility to infections; hemorrhages under skin, petechiae in mucous membranes, in joints and under periosteum; long bone tenderness; costochondral beading; often presents with refusal to walk secondary to joint pain
Carnitine
   Increased serum triglycerides and free fatty acids; decreased ketones; fatty liver; hypoglycemia; progressive muscle weakness, cardiomyopathy, hypoglycemia

newborn can be consumed by the breast-feeding mother without ill effect. Very few drugs are absolutely contraindicated in breast-feeding mothers; these include radioactive compounds, antimetabolites, lithium, diazepam, chloramphenicol, antithyroid drugs, and tetracycline. For up-to-date information, a regional drug center should be consulted.

Maternal use of illicit or recreational drugs may be a contraindication to breast-feeding, but the risks to the infant should be balanced by the benefits of milk and breastfeeding. Expression of milk for a feeding or two after use of a drug is not an acceptable compromise. The breast-fed infants of mothers taking methadone alone as part of a treatment program have generally not experienced ill effects when the dose is less than 40 mg/day.

United States National Library of Medicine Drugs and Lactation Database (Lactmed): http://toxnet.nlm.nih.gov/newtoxnet/lactmed.htm.

Nutrient Composition

The nutrient composition of human milk is compared to that of cow's milk and formulas in Table 11–16. Outstanding characteristics include (1) lower but highly bioavailable protein content, which is adequate for the normal infant; (2) generous quantity of EFAs; (3) long-chain polyunsaturated fatty acids, of which DHA is thought to be especially important; (4) relatively low sodium and solute load; and (5) lower concentration of highly bioavailable minerals, which are adequate for the needs of normal breast-fed infants for approximately 6 months.

Complementary Feeding

The AAP and the WHO recommend the introduction of solid foods in normal infants at about 6 months of age. Fortified cereals, fruits, vegetables, and meats should complement the breast milk diet. Meats are an important source of iron and zinc, both of which are low in human milk by 6 months. Pureed meats may be introduced as an early complementary food. Single-ingredient complementary foods are introduced one at a time at 3- to 4-day intervals before a new food is given. Fruit juice is not necessary, and if given should be in a cup, not a bottle, and less than 4 oz/day. Whole cow's milk can be introduced after the first year of life. Breast-feeding should ideally continue for at least 12 months.

While breast milk, dairy, soy, legume, and other vegetable sources of protein can provide adequate protein for growth, vegetarian foods are impractical as sources of iron or zinc. A vegetarian diet places older breastfed infants and toddlers at risk for iron and zinc deficiency because of their high requirements during rapid growth and because animal-based foods are best sources of these nutrients. To meet requirements, infants and toddlers consuming vegetarian diets should be offered fortified foods, including cereals and formula or daily supplementation of iron and zinc. A vegan diet that omits all animal protein sources will require supplementation of vitamin B$_{12}$ as well. Guidance from a pediatric registered dietitian is suggested for families seeking for their infant or toddler to follow a vegetarian or vegan diet to ensure adequate protein, calorie, vitamin, and micronutrient intakes.

Results of recent large-scale randomized controlled trials have shifted recommended practice around peanut consumption in infancy by the AAP and National Institute of Allergy and Infectious Diseases (NIAID). For infants with severe eczema or egg allergy but without evidence of active peanut sensitization by skin prick test or specific peanut IgE, introduction of 6–7 g/wk of peanut protein served as a puree is recommended beginning at 4–6 months to reduce the risk of peanut allergy. Infants with less severe eczema are recommended to start consuming peanut purees around 6 months. Furthermore, it was the expert opinion of the NIAID panel that infants without risk factors for food allergy should have

Table 11–16. Composition of human and cow's milk and typical infant formula (per 100 kcal).

Nutrient (unit)	Minimal Level Recommended[a]	Mature Human Milk	Typical Commercial Formula	Cow's Milk (mean)
Protein (g)	1.8[b]	1.3–1.6	2.3	5.1
Fat (g)	3.3[c]	5	5.3	5.7
Carbohydrate (g)	—	10.3	10.8	7.3
Linoleic acid (mg)	300	560	2300	125
Vitamin A (IU)	250	250	300	216
Vitamin D (IU)	40	3	63	3
Vitamin E (IU)	0.7/g linoleic acid	0.3	2	0.1
Vitamin K (mcg)	4	2	9	5
Vitamin C (mg)	8	7.8	8.1	2.3
Thiamin (mcg)	40	25	80	59
Riboflavin (mcg)	60	60	100	252
Niacin (mcg)	250	250	1200	131
Vitamin B_6 (mcg)	15 mcg/g protein intake	15	63	66
Folic acid (mcg)	4	4	10	8
Pantothenic acid (mcg)	300	300	450	489
Vitamin B_{12} (mcg)	0.15	0.15	0.25	0.56
Biotin (mcg)	1.5	1	2.5	3.1
Inositol (mg)	4	20	5.5	20
Choline (mg)	7	13	10	23
Calcium (mg)	5	50	75	186
Phosphorus (mg)	25	25	65	145
Magnesium (mg)	6	6	8	20
Iron (mg)	1	0.1	1.5	0.08
Iodine (mcg)	5	4–9	10	7
Copper (mcg)	60	25–60	80	20
Zinc (mg)	0.5	0.1–0.5	0.65	0.6
Manganese (mcg)	5	1.5	5–160	3
Sodium (mEq)	0.9	1	1.7	3.3
Potassium (mEq)	2.1	2.1	2.7	6
Chloride (mEq)	1.6	1.6	2.3	4.6
Osmolarity (mOsm)	—	11.3	16–18.4	40

[a]Committee on Nutrition, American Academy of Pediatrics.
[b]Protein of nutritional quality equal to casein.
[c]Includes 300 mg of essential fatty acids.

age appropriate peanut-containing products introduced into the diet with other purees and solid foods in a manner consistent with familial and cultural norms.

Greer FR, Sicherer SH, Burks AW; Committee on Nutrition; Section of Allergy and Immunology: The effects of early nutritional interventions on the development of atopic disease in infants and children: the role of maternal dietary restriction, breastfeeding, hydrolyzed formulas, and timing of introduction of allergenic complementary foods. Pediatrics 2019 Apr; 143(4). doi: 10.1542/peds.2019-0281. Epub 2019 Mar 18 [PMID: 30886111].

SPECIAL DIETARY PRODUCTS FOR INFANTS

Soy Protein Formulas

The medical indications for soy formulas are rare: galactosemia and hereditary lactase deficiency. Soy formulas provide an option when a vegetarian diet is preferred. Soy protein formulas are often used in cases of suspected intolerance to cow's milk protein, though cow's milk hydrolysate formulas are preferred because 30%–40% of infants intolerant to cow's milk protein will also react to soy protein. In contrast to this T-cell–mediated protein intolerance, those infants with less commonly documented IgE-mediated allergy to cow's milk protein do not typically cross-react to soy formula. The estrogenic properties of isoflavones from soy had raised concern about potential reproductive system effects, but an Expert Committee of the National Toxicology program found minimal concern for potential harm in their 2011 report.

Semi-elemental & Elemental Formulas

Semi-elemental formulas include protein hydrolysate formulas. The major nitrogen source of most of these products is casein hydrolysate, supplemented with selected amino acids, but partial hydrolysates of whey are also available. These formulas contain an abundance of EFA from vegetable oil; certain brands also provide substantial amounts of MCTs. Elemental formulas are available with free amino acids and varying levels and types of fat components.

Semi-elemental and elemental formulas are invaluable for infants with malabsorption syndromes. They are also effective in infants who cannot tolerate cow's milk and soy protein. Controlled trials suggest that for infants with a family history of atopic disease, partial hydrolysate formulas may delay or prevent atopic disease compared to standard cow milk protein-based formula.

Obbay JE et al: Complementary feeding and food allergy, atopic dermatitis/eczema, asthma, and allergic rhinitis: a systematic review. Am J Clin Nutr 2019 Mar 1;109(Supplement _7): 890S–934S. doi: 10.1093/ajcn/nqy220 [PMID: 30982864].
Vandenplas Y: Prevention and management of cow's milk allergy in non-exclusively breastfed infants. Nutrients 2017 Jul 10;9(7). pii:E731. doi: 10.3390/nu9070731 [PMID: 28698533].

Formula Additives

Occasionally, it may be necessary to increase the caloric density of an infant feeding to provide more calories or to restrict fluid intake. Concentrating formula to 24–26 kcal/oz is usually well tolerated, delivers an acceptable renal solute load, and increases the density of all the nutrients. Beyond this, individual macronutrient additives (Table 11–17) are usually employed to achieve the desired caloric density (up to 30 kcal/oz) based on the infant's needs and underlying condition(s). A pediatric dietitian can provide guidance in formulating calorically dense infant formula feedings. The caloric density of breast milk can be increased by adding infant formula powder or any of the additives used with infant formula. Because of their specialized nutrient composition, human milk fortifiers are generally used only for preterm infants.

Table 11–17. Common infant formula additives.

Additive	Kcal/g	Kcal/Tbsp	Kcal/mL	Comments
Dry rice cereal	3.75	15	—	Thickens formula but not breast milk
Benecalorie (Nestle)	7.3	110	7.3	High-calorie liquid supplement; calcium caseinate, high oleic sunflower oil, mono- and di-glycerides
MCT oil (Mead Johnson)	8.3	116	7.7	Not a source of essential fatty acids
Microlipid (Nestle)	9	68.5	4.5	Safflower oil emulsion with 0.4 g linoleic acid/mL; mixes easily with enteral formulas
Vegetable oil	9	124	8.3	Does not mix well
Beneprotein (Nestle)	3.6	16.7 (4 g protein);	—	Whey protein, soy lecithin (25 kcal/scoop); 1 scoop = 7 g
Duocal (Nutricia)	4.9	42	—	Protein-free mix of hydrolyzed corn starch (60% kcal) and fat (35% MCT)

MCT, medium-chain triglyceride.

Special Formulas

Special formulas are those in which one component, often an amino acid, is reduced in concentration or removed for the dietary management of a specific inborn metabolic disease. Also included under this heading are formulas designed for specific disease states, such as hepatic failure, pulmonary failure with chronic carbon dioxide retention, and renal failure. These condition-specific formulas were formulated primarily for critically ill adults and are used sparingly in those populations; thus, they should be used in pediatrics only with clear indication and caution.

Complete information regarding the composition of formulas can be found in reference texts and in the manufacturers' literature.

American Academy of Pediatrics Committee on Nutrition: In: Kleinman RE, Greer FR (eds): *Pediatric Nutrition*. 7th ed. Elk Grove Village, IL: American Academy of Pediatrics; 2014.

▼ NUTRITION FOR CHILDREN 2 YEARS & OLDER

Because diet impacts the development of chronic diseases such as diabetes, obesity, and cardiovascular disease, learning healthy eating behaviors at a young age is an important preventative measure.

Salient features of the diet for children older than 2 years include the following:

1. Three regular meals per day, and one or two healthful snacks.

2. *A variety of foods*: diet should be nutritionally complete and promote optimal growth and activity.

3. Fat less than 35% of total calories (severe fat restriction < 10% may result in an energy deficit and growth failure). Saturated fats should provide less than 10% of total calories. Monounsaturated fats should provide 10% or more of caloric intake. Trans-fatty acids should provide less than 1% of total calories.

4. Cholesterol intake less than 100 mg/1000 kcal/day, to a maximum of 300 mg/day.

5. Carbohydrates should provide 45%–65% of daily caloric intake, less than 10% in the form of simple sugars. A high-fiber, whole-grain–based diet is recommended.

6. Limitation of grazing behavior, eating while watching television, and the consumption of soft drinks and other sweetened beverages.

7. Limitation of sodium intake by limiting processed foods and added salt.

8. Consumption of lean cuts of meats, poultry, and fish should be encouraged. Skim or low-fat milk, and vegetable oils (especially canola or olive oil) should be used.

Plentiful amounts of fruits and vegetables are recommended. The consumption of processed foods, sugar-sweetened drinks, desserts, and candy should be limited. The American Academy of Pediatrics has endorsed use of low-fat milk in children after 12 months of age.

Lifestyle counseling for children should also include maintenance of a BMI in the healthy range; regular physical activity, limiting sedentary behaviors; avoidance of smoking; and screening for hypertension starting at age 3 years. Current recommendations from the National Heart Lung and Blood Institute are to routinely screen all children for familial hyperlipidemia using a fasting or non-fasting lipid panel once at age 9–11, and to consider screening children at younger ages who have additional risk factors (obesity, diabetes, family history of preterm cardiovascular disease). The preferred time for screening occurs before puberty, a period in which hormonal changes render lipids unreliable in predicting levels in adulthood.

Perak AM, Benuk I: Preserving optimal cardiovascular health in children. Pediatr Ann 2018 Dec 1;47(12):e486. doi: 10.3928/19382359-20181115-01 [PMID: 30543376].
Dietary Guidelines for Americans: https://health.gov/dietary guidelines/2015/guidelines/.

PEDIATRIC UNDERNUTRITION

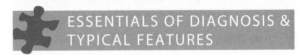

ESSENTIALS OF DIAGNOSIS & TYPICAL FEATURES

▶ Poor weight gain or weight loss.

▶ Loss of subcutaneous fat, temporal wasting.

▶ Most commonly related to inadequate caloric intake.

▶ In toddlers, often associated with low iron and zinc status.

▶ General Considerations

Pediatric undernutrition is usually multifactorial in origin, and successful treatment depends on accurate identification and management of those factors. The terms "organic" and "nonorganic" failure to thrive, though still used by many medical professionals, are not helpful because any systemic illness or chronic condition can cause growth impairment and yet may also be compounded by psychosocial problems.

▶ Clinical Findings

A. Definitions

Failure to thrive is an imprecise term used to describe growth faltering in infants and young children whose weight curve has fallen by two major percentile channels from a previously established rate of growth, or whose weight for length falls below the 5th percentile (see Chapter 9). The WHO growth charts (http://www.who.int/childgrowth/en/) should be used for all infants less than 24 months as these charts reflect the slower velocity of weight gain for healthy breast-fed infants without formula supplementation. Differences in weight gain are particularly notable after 6 months of age. The acute loss of weight, or failure to gain weight at the expected rate, produces a condition of reduced weight for height known as *wasting*. The reduction in height for age, as is seen with more chronic malnutrition, is termed *stunting*.

The typical pattern for mild pediatric undernutrition is decreased weight, with normal height and head circumference. In more chronic malnutrition, linear growth will slow relative to the standard for age, although this should also prompt consideration of nonnutritional etiologies. The term **severe acute malnutrition (SAM)** has generally replaced the term protein energy malnutrition. SAM is used to describe children with severe wasting called *marasmus* (< 3 SD weight for height) and *Kwashiorkor,* also known as edematous malnutrition. Significant protein deprivation, possibly with additional insults such as infection, may produce kwashiorkor.

B. Risk Factors

Multiple medical conditions can cause pediatric undernutrition, and a thorough discussion is beyond the scope of this chapter. However, the most common cause is inadequate dietary intake. In young infants, a weak or uncoordinated suck may be the causative factor. Congenital heart disease, breathing problems (eg, laryngomalacia), and other physical problems that may interfere with normal feeding. Inappropriate formula mixing or a family's dietary beliefs may lead to hypocaloric or unbalanced dietary intakes. Diets restricted because of suspected food allergies or intolerances may result in inadequate intake of calories, protein, or specific micronutrients. Deficiencies of iron or zinc occur in older breast-fed infants whose diets are low in meats or fortified foods, and in toddlers not taking fortified formula or not consuming good dietary sources. Cases of severe malnutrition and kwashiorkor have occurred in infants of parents who substitute milk alternatives (eg, rice, hemp, or almond milk or unfortified soy milk) for infant formula. Such plant source "milks" are hypocaloric, provide an incomplete protein source (ie, low in quality and quantity of protein), and are not adequately fortified with all essential micronutrients to meet infant requirements.

C. Assessment

1. Measurement of weight for age; length/height for age; occipital frontal circumference (OFC) for age (for < 2 years age), weight for length; and calculation of percent ideal body weight (current weight/median weight [50th percentile] for current length). Assess for downward crossing of growth percentiles (acute malnutrition) and for linear growth stunting (chronic malnutrition).

2. History should include details of diet intake and feeding patterns (including restrictive intake, grazing feeding pattern, inappropriate foods for age and development, excessive juice, sugar-sweetened beverages, or water intake); past medical history, including birth and developmental history; family history; social history; and review of systems.

3. Physical examination should include careful examination of skin (for rashes), mouth, eyes, nails, and hair for signs of micronutrient and protein deficiencies, as well as for abnormal neurologic function (eg, loss of deep tendon reflexes, abnormal strength and tone).

4. Laboratory studies are generally of low yield for diagnosis of growth faltering in the absence of other findings, and should be reserved for moderately severe cases of malnutrition. In such cases, risk of and suspicion for nutrient deficiencies and systemic pathology should guide studies ordered. Typical screening laboratories include chemistry panel; complete blood count; and iron panel, including ferritin (and marker of inflammation, eg, CRP or ESR). Thyroid function testing is indicated with linear growth faltering. Serology for celiac disease may also be warranted for toddlers, especially with short stature or linear growth faltering. Guidelines for screening for inborn errors of metabolism are available.

5. Some infants are naturally small and have weight for age percentile values below the 5th percentile and may have length and head circumferences at higher percentiles. Such infants are often called "constitutionally small," as their thinness was present from birth, there was no evidence of intrauterine growth restriction, their mothers had small stature and usually thinness, and the family growth pattern is similar. Mothers of such normally small children should not be discouraged from breast-feeding and should not be counseled to prematurely add food supplements. Workup for failure to thrive is not indicated in these infants and evaluations or referrals for growth failure or child neglect from underfeeding are not warranted.

Refeeding syndrome may occur with nutritional rehabilitation of infants or children with SAM. It is important to monitor for hypophosphatemia, hypokalemia, hypomagnesemia, and hyperglycemia for the first roughly 3–4 days in which caloric intake is advanced to the goal desired for weight gain during nutritional rehabilitation (until stable). Calorie intake should be increased slowly to avoid metabolic instability. More frequent monitoring of electrolytes may be needed if significant amounts of IV dextrose or TPN are used during the initial rehabilitation of a severely malnourished child, and enteral feeding is preferred when possible.

Treatment

Poor eating is often a learned behavior. Families should be counseled regarding choices of foods that are appropriate for the age and developmental level of the child. Increasing the caloric density of foods is associated with increased daily caloric intake and improved weight gain. Food sources should contain both fat and protein to achieve repletion of both lean body mass and fat stores. Micronutrient deficiencies should be corrected. For repletion of iron, 3–6 mg/kg/day, divided BID, can be initiated if acute inflammation has been excluded. Acute inflammation should be allowed to resolve prior to initiating iron supplementation. For zinc, 1 mg/kg/day for 1–2 months, ideally administered several hours apart from iron supplement, is typically adequate. Children should have structured meal times (eg, three meals and two to three snacks during the day), ideally at the same time other family members eat. Consultation with a pediatric dietitian can be helpful for educating the family. Poor feeding may be related to family dysfunction. Children whose households are chaotic and children who are abused, neglected, or exposed to poorly controlled mental illness may be described as poor eaters, and may fail to gain. Careful assessment of the social environment of such children is critical, and disposition options may include support services, close medical follow-up visits, family counseling, and even foster placement while a parent receives therapy.

Bhutta AZ et al: Severe childhood malnutrition. Nat Rev Dis Primers 2017 Sep 21;3:17067. doi: 10.1038/NRDP.2017.67. Review. [PMID: 28933421].

PEDIATRIC OVERWEIGHT & OBESITY

ESSENTIALS OF DIAGNOSIS & TYPICAL FEATURES

► Excessive rate of weight gain; upward change in BMI percentiles (see also Chapter 3 for obesity in adolescents).

► BMI for age between the 85th and 95th percentiles indicates overweight.

► BMI for age greater than 95th percentile indicates obesity and is associated with increased risk of secondary complications.

► BMI for age greater than 99th percentile, or a BMI that exceeds 120% of the 95th percentile, indicates severe obesity and a higher risk of complications.

General Considerations

The prevalence of childhood and adolescent obesity has increased rapidly in the United States and many other parts of the world. Currently in the United States, 18.5% of 2–19-year-olds have obesity, with even higher rates among subpopulations of minority and economically disadvantaged children. The increasing prevalence of childhood obesity is related to a complex combination of socioeconomic, epigenetic, and biologic factors.

Childhood obesity, especially when severe, is associated with significant comorbidities. The probability of obesity persisting into adulthood has been estimated to increase from 20% at 4 years to 80% by adolescence. Rates of persistence from early childhood are much higher when one or both parents have obesity. Obesity is associated with cardiovascular and endocrine abnormalities (eg, dyslipidemia, insulin resistance, and type 2 diabetes), orthopedic problems, pulmonary complications (eg, obstructive sleep apnea), and mental health problems (Table 11–18).

Kumar S et al: Review of childhood obesity: from epidemiology, etiology, and comorbidities to clinical assessment and treatment. Mayo Clin Proc 2017 Feb;92(2):251–265. doi: 10.1016/j.mayocp.2016.09.017 [PMID: 28065514].

Clinical Findings

A. Definitions

BMI is the standard measure of obesity in adults and children. BMI is correlated with more accurate measures of body fatness and is calculated with readily available information: weight and height (kg/m^2). Routine plotting of the BMI on age- and gender-appropriate charts (http://www.cdc.gov/growthcharts) can identify those with excess weight. BMI between the 85th and 95th percentiles for age and sex identifies those who are overweight. Obesity is defined as BMI at or above the 95th percentile and is associated with increased risk of secondary complications. Severe obesity is characterized by BMI for age and sex at or above the 99th percentile and is associated with greatly increased risk of comorbidity. An alternate definition of severe obesity recommended by the American Heart Association numerically approximates the 99th percentile, but provides a framework for clinicians to better gauge progress for children with severe obesity. This standard defines severe obesity class 2 as above 120% of the 95th percentile for a given age and gender, and severe obesity class 3 as above 140% of the 95th percentile. The degree of obesity as a percent of the 95th percentile can be tracked on special growth charts created for this purpose. An upward change in BMI percentiles in any range should prompt evaluation and possible treatment. For children younger than 2 years, weight for length greater than 95th percentile indicates overweight and warrants further assessment, especially of energy intake and feeding behaviors.

B. Risk Factors

There are multiple risk factors for developing obesity, reflecting the complex relationships between genetic and

Table 11–18. Selected complications of childhood obesity.

System	Condition	Note	Review of Systems
Pulmonary	Obstructive sleep apnea	13%–33% of obese youth	Snoring, apnea, poor sleep, nocturnal enuresis, AM headaches, fatigue, poor school performance
	Obesity-hypoventilation syndrome	Severe obesity, restrictive lung disease, may lead to right heart failure	Dyspnea, edema, somnolence
Cardiovascular	Hypertension	3 occasions > 95th percentile on NHLBI tables for gender, age, and height	
	Lipid abnormalities	Total cholesterol 170–199 borderline, > 200 high LDL 110–129 borderline, > 130 high, HDL < 40 low	
		TG > 150 high	Assess for pancreatitis if TG > 400, nausea, vomiting, abdominal pain
GI	NAFLD	10%–25% of obese youth; elevated ALT; rule out other liver disease if ALT highly elevated; steatohepatitis may progress to fibrosis, cirrhosis	Commonly asymptomatic; rarely abdominal pain: vague, recurrent
	GERD	Increased abdominal pressure	Abdominal pain: heartburn
	Gallstones	Associated with rapid weight loss	Abdominal pain: right upper or epigastric
	Constipation	Associated with inactivity, r/o encopresis	Abdominal pain: distension, hard infrequent stools, soiling/incontinence
Endocrine	Impaired glucose metabolism	Elevated fasting glucose = 100–125	Acanthosis nigricans
		Impaired glucose tolerance = 2-h OGTT 140–199	
	Type 2 diabetes (T2DM)	Random glucose > 200 with symptoms; Fasting glucose > 126, 2-h OGTT > 200, HgA_{1c} > 6.5	Polyuria and polydipsia, unintentional weight loss
	Polycystic ovarian syndrome (PCOS)	Diagnoses requires two of three: Hyperandrogenism Oligomenorrhea Polycystic ovaries—ultrasound not used in criteria for adolescents; insulin resistance; risk of infertility and endometrial cancer	Oligomenorrhea (less than 9 menses/y), hyperandrogenism Hyperandrogenism: hirsutism, acne
	Hypothyroid	Associated with poor linear growth	Asymptomatic until uncompensated: linear growth failure, cold intolerance, decline in school performance, coarse features, thin hair
Neurology/ ophthalmology	Pseudotumor cerebri	Papilledema, vision loss possible, consult neuro/ophthalmology	Headaches (severe, recurrent), often worse in AM
Orthopedic	Blount disease	Stress injury to medial tibial growth plate, often painless	Bowed legs, ± knee pain
	SCFE	More likely to progress to bilateral disease in obese	Hip, groin, or knee pain; limp with leg held in external rotation
Dermatology	Acanthosis nigricans	Secondary effect of elevated insulin	Darkening of skin on neck, axillae, groin, ± skin tags
	Intertrigo/furunculosis/panniculitis	Examine skin folds, pannus; bacteria, and/or yeast	Rash/infection in skin folds, inflammatory papules
	Hydradenitis suppurativa	Draining cysts in axillae or groin	Rash/infection in skin folds, blocked glands, recurrent and unrelenting

(Continued)

Table 11–18. Selected complications of childhood obesity. (*Continued*)

System	Condition	Note	Review of Systems
Psychiatric	Depression/anxiety	May lead to worsening obesity if untreated	Full psycho/social review, including mood, school performance, peer and family relationships
	Eating disorder	Assess for binging ± purging behavior	
	History of abuse	Increases risk of severe obesity	

ALT, alanine aminotransferase; GERD, gastroesophageal reflux disease; GI, gastrointestinal; HDL, high-density lipoprotein; HgA$_{1c}$, hemoglobin A$_{1c}$; LDL, low-density lipoprotein; NAFLD, nonalcoholic fatty liver disease; NHLBI, National Heart, Lung, and Blood Institute; OGTT, oral glucose tolerance test; SCFE, slipped capital femoral epiphysis; T2DM, type 2 diabetes mellitus; TG, triglycerides.

environmental factors. Family history is a strong risk factor. Parental obesity, especially in both parents, strongly increases the odds of a child becoming an obese adult.

Risk factors in the home environment offer targets for intervention. Consumption of sugar-sweetened beverages, lack of family meals, large portion sizes, foods prepared outside the home, television viewing, video gaming, poor sleep, and lack of activity are all associated with risk of excessive weight gain.

C. Assessment

Early recognition of rapid weight gain or high-risk behaviors is important. Anticipatory guidance or intervention earlier in childhood and before weight gain becomes severe is more likely to be successful than delayed intervention. Routine evaluation at well-child visits should include the following:

1. Measurement of weight and height, calculation of BMI, and plotting on age- and sex-appropriate growth charts (http://www.cdc.gov/growthcharts). Evaluate for upward crossing of BMI percentile channels.

2. History regarding diet and activity patterns (Table 11–19); family history, and review of systems. Physical examination

Table 11–19. Suggested areas for assessment of diet and activity patterns.

Diet
- Portion sizes: adult portions for young children
- Frequency of meals away from home (restaurants or takeout)
- Frequency/amounts of sugar-sweetened beverages (soda, juice drinks)
- Meal and snack pattern: structured vs grazing, skipping meals
- Frequency of eating fruits and vegetables
- Frequency of family meals
- Television viewing while eating

Activity
- Time spent in sedentary activity: television, video games, computer, or smartphone
- Time spent in vigorous activity: organized sports, physical education, free play
- Activities of daily living: walking to school, chores, yard work
- Sleep duration: risk of obesity is increased with inadequate sleep

should include blood pressure measurement, distribution of adiposity (central vs generalized); markers of comorbidities, such as acanthosis nigricans, hirsutism, hepatomegaly, orthopedic abnormalities; and physical stigmata of genetic syndromes (eg, Prader-Willi syndrome).

3. Laboratory studies are recommended as follows for children beginning by age 10 years or at onset of puberty. Consider testing at younger ages with severe obesity but not younger than 2 years:

- Overweight with personal or family history of heart disease risk factors—fasting lipid profile, fasting glucose and/or hemoglobin A$_{1c}$, alanine aminotransferase (ALT).

- Obese—fasting lipid profile, fasting glucose and/or hemoglobin A$_{1c}$, ALT.

- Other studies should be guided by findings in the history and physical.

▶ Treatment

Treatment should be based on risk factors, including age, severity of obesity, and comorbidities, as well as family history. For children with uncomplicated obesity, the primary goal is to achieve healthy eating and activity patterns, not necessarily to achieve ideal body weight. For children with a secondary complication, improvement of the complication is an important goal. In general, weight goals for children with obesity range from weight maintenance to up to 1 lb/mo weight loss for those younger than 12 years, and up to 2 lb/wk for those older than 12 years. More rapid weight loss should be monitored for pathologic causes that may be associated with nutrient deficiencies and linear growth stunting (Table 11–20).

Treatment focused on behavior changes in the context of family involvement has been associated with sustained weight loss and decreases in BMI. Clinicians should assess the family's readiness to take action. Motivational interviewing is effective in the treatment of excess weight gain in children. This form of counseling uses open-ended questioning

Table 11–20. Weight management goals.

Age (y)	BMI (%)	Weight Change Goal to Achieve BMI < 85%
2–5	85–94	Maintain weight
	95–98	Maintain weight, or if complications lose 1 lb/mo
	99	Lose 1 lb/mo
6–11	85–94	Maintain weight
	95–98	Lose 1 lb/mo
	99	Lose 2 lb/wk
12–18	85–95	Maintain weight
	95–98	Lose 2 lb/wk
	99	Lose 2 lb/wk

BMI, body mass index, % = percentile for age and sex.

and reflective statements to explore and resolve ambivalence toward change, and accepts resistance nonjudgmentally. Providers should engage the family in collaborative decision-making about which behavior change goals will be targeted. Improving dietary habits and activity levels concurrently is desirable for successful weight management. The entire family should adopt healthy eating patterns, with parents modeling healthy food choices, controlling foods brought into the home, and guiding appropriate portion sizes. The American Academy of Pediatrics recommends very limited screen time for children younger than 2 years, a maximum of 2 h/day of television and video games for older children, with lower levels recommended for children during attempts at BMI reduction.

A "staged approach" for treatment has been proposed, with the initial level depending on the severity of overweight, the age of the child, the readiness of the family to implement changes, the preferences of the parents and child, and the skills of the health care provider. The U.S. Preventive Services Task Force has identified that interventions most likely to be successful for childhood obesity treatment are intensive, with 25 or more contact hours.

1. *Prevention plus*: Counseling regarding problem areas identified by screening questions (see Table 11–19); emphasis on lifestyle changes, including healthy eating and physical activity patterns.

2. *Structured weight management*: Provides more specific and structured dietary pattern, such as meal planning, exercise prescription, and behavior change goals. This may be done in the primary care setting. Generally, referral to at least one ancillary health professional will be required: dietitian, behavior specialist, and/or physical therapist. Monitoring is monthly or tailored to patient and family's needs.

3. *Comprehensive multidisciplinary*: This level further increases the structure of therapeutic interventions and support, employs a multidisciplinary team, and may involve weekly group meetings.

4. *Tertiary care intervention*: This level is for patients who have not been successful at the other intervention levels or who have severe obesity. Interventions are prescribed by a multidisciplinary team, and may include intensive behavior therapy, specialized diets, medications, and surgery.

Pharmacotherapy can be an adjunct to dietary, activity, and behavioral treatment. Orlistat, a lipase inhibitor, is approved for patients older than 12 years, but other medications approved for use in adults are used off-label by providers who have expertise in obesity medicine. Bariatric surgery is performed in some centers for adolescents with severe obesity. In carefully selected and closely monitored patients, surgery can result in significant weight loss with a reduction or resolution of comorbidities, including type 2 diabetes, more frequently than in adults undergoing the same surgery.

Inge TH et al; Teen–LABS Consortium: Five-year outcomes of gastric bypass in adolescents as compared with adults. N Engl J Med 2019 May 30;380(22):2136–2145. doi: 10.1056/NEJMoa1813909 [PMID: 31116917].

▼ NUTRITION SUPPORT

ENTERAL

▶ Indications

Enteral nutrition support is indicated when a patient cannot adequately meet nutritional needs by oral intake alone and has a functioning GI tract. This method of support can be used for short- and long-term delivery of nutrition. Even when the gut cannot absorb 100% of nutritional needs, some enteral feedings should be attempted. Enteral nutrition, full or partial, has many benefits:

1. Maintaining gut mucosal integrity

2. Preserving gut-associated lymphoid tissue

3. Stimulating gut hormones and bile flow

▶ Access Devices

Nasogastric feeding tubes can be used for supplemental enteral feedings, but generally are not used for more than 3 months because of the complications of otitis media and sinusitis. Initiation of nasogastric feeding usually requires a brief hospital stay to ensure tolerance to feedings and to allow for parental instruction in tube placement and feeding administration.

Table 11–21. Guidelines for the initiation and advancement of tube feedings.

Age	Drip Feeds		Bolus Feeds	
	Initiation	Advancement	Initiation (mL)	Advancement
Preterm	1–2 mL/kg/h	5–10 mL/kg q8–12 h over 5–7 day as tolerated	10–20 mL/kg	20–30 mL/kg/day as tolerated
Birth–12 mo	5–10 mL/h	5–10 mL q2–8 h	10–60	20–40 mL q3–4 h
1–6 y	10–15 mL/h	10–15 mL q2–8 h	30–90	30–60 mL q feed
6–14 y	15–20 mL/h	10–20 mL q2–8 h	60–120	60–90 mL q feed
> 14 y	20–30 mL/h	20–30 mL q2–8 h	60–120	60–120 mL q feed

If long-term feeding support is anticipated, a more permanent feeding device, such as a gastrostomy tube, may be considered. Referral to a home care company is necessary for equipment and other services such as nursing visits and dietitian follow-up.

Table 11–21 suggests appropriate timing for initiation and advancement of drip and bolus feedings, according to a child's age. Clinical status and tolerance to feedings should ultimately guide their advancement.

▶ **Monitoring**

Monitoring the adequacy of enteral feeding depends on nutritional goals. For critically ill patients in the intensive care unit, provision of enteral nutrition in the first 48 hours is associated with lower mortality. Even when calorie and protein goals cannot be met, provision of more than 60% protein goals enterally is associated with lower odds of mortality in mechanically ventilated children. Evaluating normal growth parameters in critically ill infants and children can be skewed by fluid status changes and loss of muscle mass. While weight and linear growth must still be followed, other measures such as mid-arm muscle circumference may provide another measure to assess nutritional adequacy. Frequent assessment of anthropometrics, medical status changes, biochemical indices, and tolerance to enteral feeds with documentation of delivered nutrition intake versus goal intake is essential in managing this nutritionally challenging population.

For more stable hospitalized young infants and malnourished children, growth data should be regularly obtained and evaluated based on age appropriate growth charts. Hydration status should be assessed carefully at the initiation of enteral feeding and regularly thereafter. Either constipation or diarrhea can be problems, and attention to stool frequency, volume, and consistency can help guide management. When diarrhea occurs, factors such as infection, hypertonic enteral medications, antibiotic use, and alteration in normal gut flora should be addressed.

In medically stable patients, the enteral feeding schedule should be developmentally appropriate (eg, 5–6 small feedings/day for a toddler). When night drip feedings are used in conjunction with daytime feeds, it is suggested that less than 50% of goal calories be delivered at night so as to maintain a daytime sense of hunger and satiety. This will be especially important once a transition to oral intake begins.

Mehta NM et al: Guidelines for the provision and assessment of nutrition support therapy in the pediatric critically ill patient: Society of Critical Care Medicine and American Society for Parenteral and Enteral Nutrition. J Parenter Enteral Nutr 2017 Jul; 41(5):706–742. doi: 10.1177/0148607117711387. Epub 2017 Jun 2. PMID: 286868444.

PARENTERAL NUTRITION

▶ **Indications**

A. Peripheral Parenteral Nutrition

Peripheral parenteral nutrition is indicated when complete enteral feeding is temporarily impossible or undesirable. Short-term partial intravenous (IV) nutrition via a peripheral vein is a preferred alternative to administration of dextrose and electrolyte solutions alone. Because of the osmolality of the solutions required, it is usually impossible to achieve total calorie and protein needs with parenteral nutrition via a peripheral vein.

B. Total Parenteral Nutrition

Total parenteral nutrition (TPN) should be provided only when clearly indicated. Apart from the expense, numerous risks are associated with this method of feeding (see the section Complications). Even when TPN is indicated, every effort should be made to provide at least a minimum of nutrients enterally to help preserve the integrity of the GI mucosa and of GI function.

The primary indication for TPN is the loss of function of the GI tract that prohibits the provision of required nutrients by the enteral route. Important examples include short bowel syndrome, some congenital defects of the GI tract, and prematurity.

In recent years, a number of injectable essential nutrients have been in short supply in the US pharmaceutical market. Shortages have included IV lipids, multivitamins mixtures, and trace minerals. Deficiencies of these micronutrients have led to significant medical morbidity. Nutrition support teams should develop clinical guidelines to ensure injectable micronutrients are available for those patients who have the greatest need, for example, preterm infants and children with long-term dependence upon TPN. Policies to promote use of enteral micronutrient preparations can also help to reduce the reliance on parenteral supplies. National recommendations for the management of IV essential nutrient shortages are available from the American Society for Parenteral and Enteral Nutrition (ASPEN): http://www.nutritioncare.org/News/Product_Shortages/Parenteral_Nutrition_Multivitamin_Product_Shortage_Considerations/.

Fivez T et al: Evidence for the use of parenteral nutrition in the pediatric intensive care unit. Clin Nutr 2017 Feb;36(1):218–223. doi: 10.1016/j.clnu.2015.11.004 [PMID: 26646358].

▶ Catheter Selection & Position

An indwelling central venous catheter is preferred for long-term IV nutrition. For periods of up to 3–4 weeks, a percutaneous central venous catheter threaded into the superior vena cava from a peripheral vein can be used. For the infusion of dextrose concentrations higher than 12.5%, the tip of the catheter should be located in the superior vena cava. Catheter positioning in the right atrium has been associated with complications, including arrhythmias and thrombus. After placement, a chest radiograph must be obtained to check catheter position. If the catheter is to be used for nutrition and medications, a double-lumen catheter is preferred.

▶ Complications

A. Mechanical Complications

1. *Related to catheter insertion or to erosion of catheter through a major blood vessel*: Complications include trauma to adjacent tissues and organs, damage to the brachial plexus, hydrothorax, pericardial effusion with potential cardiac tamponade, pneumothorax, hemothorax, and cerebrospinal fluid penetration. The catheter may slip during dressing or tubing changes, or the patient may manipulate the line.

2. *Clotting of the catheter*: Addition of heparin (1000 U/L) to the solution is an effective means of preventing this complication. If an occluded catheter does not respond to heparin flushing, recombinant tissue plasminogen activator may be effective.

3. *Related to composition of infusate*: Calcium phosphate precipitation may occur if excess amounts of calcium or phosphorus are administered. Factors that increase the risk of calcium phosphate precipitation include increased

pH and decreased concentrations of amino acids. Precipitation of medications incompatible with TPN or lipids can also cause clotting.

B. Septic Complications

Septic complications are the most common cause of nonelective catheter removal, but strict use of aseptic technique and limiting entry into the catheter can reduce the rates of line sepsis. Fever over 38–38.5°C in a patient with a central catheter should be considered a line infection until proved otherwise. Cultures should be obtained and IV antibiotics empirically initiated. Removing the catheter may be necessary with certain infections (eg, fungal), and catheter replacement may be deferred until infection is treated.

C. Metabolic Complications

Many of the metabolic complications of IV nutrition are related to deficiencies or excesses of nutrients in administered fluids, whereas uncommon, specific deficiencies still occur, especially in the preterm infant. Safe and effective IV nourishment requires attention to the nutrient balance, electrolyte composition, and delivery rate of the infusate and careful monitoring, especially when the composition or delivery rate is changed. The most challenging metabolic complication is cholestasis, particularly common in preterm infants of very low birth weight with prolonged feeding intolerance, infants with congenital gut disorders requiring surgery, such as those with gastroschisis, and infants with short gut syndrome following surgical resections for disorders such as necrotizing enterocolitis. See discussion on parenteral nutrition-associated cholestasis (PNAC) in Chapter 22 for details.

Baskin KM et al: Evidence-based strategies and recommendations for preservation of central venous access in children. J Parenter Enteral Nutr 2019 Apr 21. doi: 10.1002/jpen.1591 [PMID: 31006886].

NUTRIENT REQUIREMENTS & DELIVERY

Energy

When patients are fed intravenously, no fat and carbohydrate intakes are unabsorbed, and no energy is used in nutrient absorption. These factors account for at least 7% of energy in the diet of the enterally fed patient. The intravenously fed patient usually expends less energy in physical activity. Average energy requirements may therefore be lower in children fed intravenously, by a total of 10%–15%. Caloric guidelines for the IV feeding of infants and young children are outlined below.

The guidelines are averages, and individuals vary considerably. Factors significantly increasing the energy requirement estimates include exposure to cold environment, fever, sepsis, burns, trauma, cardiac or pulmonary disease, and catch-up growth after malnutrition.

With few exceptions, such as some cases of respiratory insufficiency, at least 50%–60% of energy requirements are provided as glucose. Up to 40% of calories may be provided by IV fat emulsions.

Dextrose

The energy density of IV dextrose (monohydrate) is 3.4 kcal/g. Dextrose is the main energy source provided by total IV feeding. IV dextrose suppresses gluconeogenesis and can be oxidized directly, especially by the brain, red and white blood cells, and wounds. Because of the high osmolality, concentrations of dextrose greater than 10%–12.5% cannot be delivered via a peripheral vein or improperly positioned central line.

Dosing guidelines: The standard initial quantity of dextrose administered will vary by age (Table 11–22). Tolerance to IV dextrose normally increases rapidly due to suppression of hepatic glucose production. Dextrose can be increased by 2.5 g/kg/day, by 2.5%–5%/day, or by 2–3 mg/kg/min/day if there is no glucosuria or hyperglycemia. Standard final infusates for infants via a properly positioned central venous line usually range from 15% to 25% dextrose, though concentrations of up to 30% dextrose may be used at low flow rates. Tolerance to IV dextrose loads is markedly diminished in the preterm neonate and in hypermetabolic states.

Problems associated with IV dextrose administration include hyperglycemia, hyperosmolality, and glucosuria (often with osmotic diuresis and dehydration). Possible causes of hyperglycemia include the following: (1) inadvertent infusion of higher dextrose rates than ordered and achieving higher glucose concentrations than desired, (2) uneven flow rate, (3) sepsis, (4) a stress situation (including administration of catecholamines or corticosteroids), and (5) pancreatitis. If these causes have been addressed and severe hyperglycemia persists, use of insulin may be considered. IV insulin reduces hyperglycemia by suppressing hepatic glucose production and increasing glucose uptake by muscle and fat tissues. It usually increases plasma lactate concentrations, but does not necessarily increase glucose oxidation rates; it may also decrease the oxidation of fatty acids, resulting in less energy for metabolism. Use of IV insulin also increases the risk of hypoglycemia. Furthermore, excessive dextrose infusion paired with insulin infusion can exceed mitochondrial oxidation capacity, produce excess reactive oxidation species leading to cell death and inflammation. Intensive care management strategies that promote enteral feeding and reduce IV dextrose exposure have improved outcomes for critically ill patients. Hence, insulin should be used very cautiously and enteral feeding is strongly preferred. A standard IV dose is 1 U/4 g of carbohydrate, but much smaller quantities may be adequate and, usually, one starts with 0.2–0.3 U/4 g of carbohydrate.

Hypoglycemia may occur after an abrupt decrease in or cessation of IV glucose. When cyclic IV nutrition is provided, the IV glucose load should be decreased steadily for 1–2 hours prior to discontinuing the infusion. If the central line must be removed, the IV dextrose should be tapered gradually over several hours.

Table 11–22. Pediatric macronutrient guidelines for total parenteral nutrition.

	Dextrose		Amino Acids	Lipids
	mg/kg/min	g/kg/day	g/kg/day	g/kg/day
Age	50%–60% kcal		10%–20% kcal	30%–40% kcal
Preterm	Initial 5–8	Initial 7–11	Initial 1.5–2	Initial 0.5–1
	Max 11–12.5	Max 16–18	Max 3–4	Max 2.5–3.5
Birth–12 mo	Initial 6–8	Initial 9–11	Initial 1.5–2	Initial 1
	Max 11–15	Max 16–21.5	Max 3	Max 2.5–3.5
1–6 y	Initial 6–7	Initial 8–10	Initial 1–1.5	Initial 1
	Max 10–12	Max 14–17	Max 2–2.5	Max 2.5–3.5
>6 y	Initial 5–7	Initial 8–10	Initial 1	Initial 1
	Max 9	Max 13	Max 1.5–2	Max 3
>10 y	Initial 4–5	Initial 5–7	Initial 1	Initial 1
	Max 6–7	Max 8–10	Max 1.5–2	Max 2–3
Adolescents	Initial 2–3	Initial 3–4	Initial 1	Initial 0.5–1
	Max 5–6	Max 7–8	Max 1.5–2	Max 2

Oxidation rates for infused dextrose decrease with age. It is important to note that the ranges for dextrose administration provided in Table 11–22 are guidelines and that individual patients may require either less or more dextrose. Quantities of dextrose in excess of maximal glucose oxidation rates are used initially to replace depleted glycogen stores; hepatic lipogenesis occurs thereafter. Excess hepatic lipogenesis may lead to a fatty liver (steatosis). Lipogenesis produces carbon dioxide, as does glucose oxidation. Thus, excess dextrose may elevate the $PaCO_2$ and aggravate respiratory insufficiency or impede weaning from a respirator.

Lipids

The energy density of 20% lipid emulsions is 10 kcal/g of lipid or 2 kcal/mL. Intravenous lipid emulsions can be plant based or fish oil based. Plant-based lipids are derived from either soybean or safflower oil and consist of more than 50% linoleic acid and 4%–9% linolenic acid. This high level of linoleic acid is not ideal due to the proinflammatory potential of omega-6 fatty acids, except when small quantities of lipid are being given to prevent an EFA deficiency. Further disadvantages of soy-based lipid emulsions include phytosterols that contribute to hepatic inflammation and less biologically active Vitamin E. An alternative lipid emulsion recently approved for use in the United States is SMOFlipid, which is composed of 30% **S**oybean oil, 30% **M**edium-chain triglycerides, 25% **O**live oil, and 15% **F**ish oil. The addition of fish oil increases the amount of omega-3 fatty acids and decreases inflammatory potential, as does the addition of Vitamin E. The only available lipid emulsion composed of 100% fish oil is Omegaven. It is not recommended for use as a monotherapy. Recent research indicates favorable outcomes associated with the use of SMOFlipid including a decreased incidence of TPN-induced liver injury. Because 10% and 20% lipid emulsions contain the same concentrations of phospholipids, a 10% solution delivers more phospholipid per gram of lipid than a 20% solution. Twenty percent lipid emulsions are preferred. IV lipid is often used to provide 30%–40% of calorie needs for infants and up to 30% of calorie needs in older children and teens.

Lipoprotein lipase (LPL) activity is the rate-limiting factor in the metabolism and clearance of fat emulsions from the circulation. LPL activity is inhibited or decreased by malnutrition, leukotrienes, immaturity, growth hormone, hypercholesterolemia, hyperphospholipidemia, and theophylline. LPL activity is enhanced by glucose, insulin, lipid, catecholamines, and exercise. Heparin releases LPL from the endothelium into the circulation and enhances the rate of hydrolysis and clearance of TGs. In small preterm infants, low-dose heparin infusions may increase tolerance to IV lipid emulsion.

In general, adverse effects of IV lipid can be avoided by starting with modest quantities and advancing cautiously in light of results of TG monitoring and clinical circumstances.

Monitoring TGs is particularly important in cases of severe sepsis. It should continue periodically with long-term use.

IV lipid dosing guidelines: Check serum TGs before starting and after increasing the dose. Commence with 1 g/kg/day, given over 12–20 hours or 24 hours in small preterm infants. Advance by 0.5–1.0 g/kg/day, every 1–2 days, up to goal (see Table 11–22). As a general rule, do not increase the dose if the serum TG level is above 400 mg/dL during infusion or if the level is greater than 250 mg/dL 6–12 hours after cessation of the lipid infusion.

Serum TG levels above 400–600 mg/dL may precipitate pancreatitis. In patients for whom normal amounts of IV lipid are contraindicated, 4%–8% of calories as IV lipid should be provided to prevent EFA deficiency. Neonates and malnourished pediatric patients receiving lipid-free parenteral nutrition are at high risk for EFA deficiency.

Lapillonne A et al: ESPGHAN/ESPEN/ESPR/CSPEN Guidelines of pediatric parenteral nutrition: lipids. Clin Nutr 2018 Dec;37 (6 Pt. B):2324–2336. doi: 10.1016/j.clin.2018.06.946 Epub 2018 Jun 18 [PMID: 30143306].

Leguina-Ruzzi AA, Ortiz R: Current evidence for the use of Smoflipid emulsion in critical care patients for parenteral nutrition. Crit Care Res Pract 2018 Nov 21;2018:6301293. doi: 10.1155/2018/6301293. eCollection 2018. Review [PMID: 30584476].

Nitrogen

One gram of nitrogen is produced by 6.25 g of protein (1 g of protein contains 16% nitrogen). Caloric density of protein is equal to 4 kcal/g.

A. Protein Requirements

Protein requirements for IV feeding are the same as those for normal oral feeding (see Table 11–2).

B. Intravenous Amino Acid Solutions

Nitrogen requirements can be met by commercially available amino acid solutions. For infants, including preterm infants, accumulating evidence suggests that the use of TrophAmine (McGaw) is associated with a more normal plasma amino acid profile, superior nitrogen retention, and a lower incidence of cholestasis. TrophAmine contains 60% essential amino acids, is relatively high in branched-chain amino acids, contains taurine, and is compatible with the addition of cysteine within 24–48 hours after administration. The dose of added cysteine is 40 mg/g of TrophAmine. The relatively low pH of TrophAmine enhances solubility of calcium and phosphorus.

C. Dosing Guidelines

Amino acids can be started at 1–2 g/kg/day in most patients (see Table 11–22). In severely malnourished infants, the initial amount should be 1 g/kg/day. In infants of very low birth weight, there is evidence that higher initial amounts of amino acids are tolerated with little indication of protein "toxicity." Larger quantities of amino acids in relation to calories can minimize a negative nitrogen balance even when the infusate is hypocaloric. Amino acid intake can be advanced by 0.5–1.0 g/kg/day toward the goal. Normally the final infusate will contain 2%–3% amino acids, depending on the rate of infusion. Concentration should not be advanced beyond 2% in peripheral vein infusates due to osmolality.

Mehta NM et al: Guidelines for the provision and assessment of nutrition support therapy in the pediatric critically ill patient: society of critical care medicine and American Society for Parenteral and Enteral Nutrition. J Parenter Enteral Nutr 2017 Jul; 41(5):706–742. doi: 10.1177/0148607117711387. Epub 2017 Jun 2 [PMID: 286868444].

D. Monitoring

Monitoring for tolerance of the IV amino acid solutions should include blood urea nitrogen. Serum alkaline phosphatase, γ-glutamyltransferase, and bilirubin should be monitored to detect the onset of cholestatic liver disease.

Minerals & Electrolytes

A. Calcium, Phosphorus, and Magnesium

Intravenously fed preterm and full-term infants should be given relatively high amounts of calcium and phosphorus. Current recommendations are as follows: calcium, 500–600 mg/L; phosphorus, 400–450 mg/L; and magnesium, 50–70 mg/L. After 1 year of age, the recommendations are as follows: calcium, 200–400 mg/L; phosphorus, 150–300 mg/L; and magnesium, 20–40 mg/L. The ratio of calcium to phosphorous should be 1.3:1.0 by weight or 1:1 by molar ratio. These recommendations are deliberately presented as milligrams per liter of infusate to avoid inadvertent administration of concentrations of calcium and phosphorus that are high enough to precipitate in the tubing. During periods of fluid restriction, care must be taken not to inadvertently increase the concentration of calcium and phosphorus in the infusate. These recommendations assume an average fluid intake of 120–150 mL/kg/day and an infusate of 25 g of amino acid per liter. With lower amino acid concentrations, the concentrations of calcium and phosphorus should be decreased.

B. Electrolytes

Standard recommendations are given in Table 11–23. After chloride requirements are met, the remainder of the anion required to balance the cation should be given as acetate to avoid the possibility of acidosis resulting from excessive chloride. Electrolyte concentrations should be modified based on the flow rate and if indications dictate for the individual patient. IV sodium should be administered sparingly

Table 11–23. Electrolyte requirements for parenteral nutrition.

Electrolyte	Preterm Infant (mEq/kg)	Full-Term Infant (mEq/kg)	Child (mEq/kg)	Adolescent (mEq/kg)
Sodium	2–5	2–3	2–3	60–150
Chloride	2–5	2–3	2–3	60–150
Potassium	2–3	2–3	2–3	70–180

in the severely malnourished patient because of impaired membrane function and high intracellular sodium levels. Conversely, generous quantities of potassium and phosphorus may be needed.

C. Trace Elements

Recommended IV intakes of trace elements are as follows: zinc 100 mcg/kg, copper 20 mcg/kg, manganese 1 mcg/kg, chromium 0.2 mcg/kg, selenium 2 mcg/kg, and iodide 1 mcg/kg. Of note, IV zinc requirements may be as high as 400 mcg/kg for preterm infants and can be up to 250 mcg/kg for infants with short bowel syndrome and significant GI losses of zinc. When IV nutrition is supplemental or limited to fewer than 2 weeks, and preexisting nutritional deficiencies are absent, only zinc need routinely be added.

IV copper requirements are relatively low in the young infant because of the presence of hepatic copper stores. These are significant even in the 28-week fetus. Circulating levels of copper and manganese should be monitored in the presence of cholestatic liver disease. If monitoring is not feasible, temporary withdrawal of added copper and manganese is advisable in cholestasis.

Copper and manganese are excreted primarily in the bile, but selenium, chromium, and molybdenum are excreted primarily in the urine. These trace elements, therefore, should be administered with caution in the presence of renal failure.

Vitamins

Three vitamin formulations are available for use in pediatric parenteral nutrition: MVI Pediatric (Hospira), Infuvite Pediatric (Baxter), and the adult formulation MVI-12 (AstraZeneca). Detailed content information is available from manufacturers as well as from the Federal Drug Administration (FDA). Recommended MVI dosing is as follows: 5 mL for children weighing more than 3 kg, 3.25 mL for infants 1–3 kg, and 1.5 mL for infants weighing less than 1 kg. Children older than 11 years can receive 10 mL of the adult formulation, MVI-12. It is important to note that MVI-12 contains no vitamin K. For dosing considerations during national shortages, recommendations are available from the American Society for Parenteral and Enteral

Nutrition (ASPEN). It is essential to follow national guidelines in order to prevent deficiencies and use available products appropriately.

IV lipid preparations contain enough tocopherol to affect total blood tocopherol levels. The majority of tocopherol in soybean oil emulsion is γ-tocopherol, which has substantially less biologic activity than the α-tocopherol present in safflower oil emulsions.

A dose of 40 IU/kg/day of vitamin D (maximum 400 IU/day) is adequate for both full-term and preterm infants.

ASPEN. *Appropriate Dosing for Parenteral Nutrition: ASPEN Recommendations.* January 2019. http://www.nutritioncare.org/PNDosing.

Federal Drug Administration data sheet, Infuvite Pediatric: https://www.accessdata.fda.gov/drugsatfda_docs/label/2008/021265s015lbl.pdf.

Federal Drug Administration data sheet, M.V.I Pediatric: https://www.accessdata.fda.gov/drugsatfda_docs/label/2017/018920s036lbl.pdf.

Federal Drug Administration data sheet, MVI-12: https://www.accessdata.fda.gov/drugsatfda_docs/label/2004/08809scf052_mvi-12_lbl.pdf.

Fluid Requirements

The initial fluid volume and subsequent increments in flow rate are determined by basic fluid requirements, the patient's clinical status, and the extent to which additional fluid administration can be tolerated and may be required to achieve adequate nutrient intake. Calculation of initial fluid volumes to be administered should be based on standard pediatric practice. If replacement fluids are required for ongoing abnormal losses, these should be administered via a separate line.

Monitoring

Vital signs should be checked on each shift. With a central catheter in situ, a fever of more than 38.5°C requires peripheral and central-line blood cultures, urine culture, complete physical examination, and examination of the IV entry point. Instability of vital signs, elevated white blood cell count with left shift, and glycosuria suggest sepsis. Removal of the central venous catheter should be considered if the patient is toxic or unresponsive to antibiotics.

Table 11–24. Summary of suggested monitoring for parenteral nutrition.

Variables	Acute Stage	Long-Term[b]
Growth	Daily	Weekly
Weight	Weekly	
Length	Weekly	
Head circumference		
Urine		
Glucose (dipstick)	With each void	With changes in intake or status
Specific gravity	Void	
Volume	Daily	
Blood		
Glucose	4 h after changes,[a] then daily × 2 day	Weekly
Na+, K+, Cl, CO$_2$, blood urea nitrogen	Daily for 2 days after changes,[a] then twice weekly	Weekly
Ca^{2+}, Mg^{2+}, P	Initially, then twice weekly	Weekly
Total protein, albumin, bilirubin, aspartate transaminase, and alkaline phosphatase	Initially, then weekly	Every other week
Zinc and copper	Initially according to clinical indications	Monthly
Triglycerides	Initially, 1 day after changes,[a] then weekly	Weekly
Compete blood count	Initially, then twice weekly; according to clinical indications (see text)	Twice weekly

[a]Changes include alterations in concentration or flow rate.
[b]Long-term monitoring can be tapered to monthly or less often, depending on age, diagnosis, and clinical status of patient.

A. Physical Examination

Monitor especially for hepatomegaly (differential diagnoses include fluid overload, congestive heart failure, steatosis, and hepatitis) and edema (differential diagnoses include fluid overload, congestive heart failure, hypoalbuminemia, and thrombosis of superior vena cava).

B. Intake and Output Record

Calories and volume delivered should be calculated from the previous day's intake and output records (that which was delivered rather than that which was ordered). The following entries should be noted on flow sheets: IV, enteral, and total fluid (mL/kg/day); dextrose (g/kg/day or mg/kg/min); protein (g/kg/day); lipids (g/kg/day); energy (kcal/kg/day); and percent of energy from enteral nutrition.

C. Growth, Urine, and Blood

Routine monitoring guidelines are given in Table 11–24. These are minimum requirements, except in the very long-term stable patient. Individual variables should be monitored more frequently as indicated, as should additional variables or clinical indications. For example, a blood ammonia analysis should be ordered for an infant with lethargy, pallor, poor growth, acidosis, azotemia, or abnormal liver test results.

Emergencies & Injuries

Jonathan Orsborn, MD
Cortney Braund, MD

INTRODUCTION TO PEDIATRIC EMERGENCIES & INJURIES

Of the approximately 140 million annual emergency department (ED) visits in the United States, over 30 million (20%) are children 18 years and younger. Respiratory disorders are the leading cause of all pediatric ED visits (32%), with injuries and poisonings (27%) also accounting for a significant percentage. Though the vast majority (97%) of children presenting for ED evaluation are discharged home, nearly 1 million each year require hospital admission from the ED and, sadly, nearly 3000 children die every year in US EDs.

This chapter begins with the initial approach to the acutely ill pediatric patient, discusses the differentiation and initial management of shock, presents the general approach to the evaluation of pediatric trauma patients, summarizes commonly used emergency drugs, and concludes with the management of a number of common clinical scenarios in pediatric emergency medicine.

INITIAL APPROACH TO THE ACUTELY ILL INFANT OR CHILD

ESSENTIALS OF DIAGNOSIS & TYPICAL FEATURES

▶ Most causes of pediatric cardiac arrest are due to hypoxia from respiratory failure.

▶ Hypotension is a *late* finding in pediatric shock; early signs may include tachycardia, capillary refill > 2 seconds, skin mottling, and decreased mental status.

A pediatric patient in serious distress may present with a known diagnosis or in cardiorespiratory failure of unknown cause. The initial approach must be simple and consistent in order to rapidly identify physiologic derangements and injuries, prioritize management, and reverse life-threatening conditions immediately. Once stabilized following interventions, the provider must then carefully consider the underlying cause, focusing on those that are treatable or reversible. Specific diagnoses can then be made, and targeted therapy initiated.

Pediatric cardiac arrest most commonly results from progressive respiratory deterioration or shock as opposed to a primary cardiac etiology. Unrecognized deterioration may lead to bradycardia, agonal breathing, hypotension, and ultimately asystole. Resulting hypoxic and ischemic insult to the brain and other vital organs make neurologic recovery extremely unlikely, even in the doubtful event that the child survives the arrest. When cardiopulmonary arrest does occur, survival is rare and most often associated with significant neurological impairment. Current data reflect a 6% survival rate for out-of-hospital cardiac arrest, 8% for those who receive prehospital intervention, and 27% survival rate for in-hospital arrest. Children who respond to rapid intervention with ventilation and oxygenation alone or to less than 5 minutes of advanced life support are much more likely to survive neurologically intact. In fact, more than 70% of children with respiratory arrest who receive rapid and effective bystander resuscitation survive with good neurologic outcomes. Therefore, it is essential to recognize the child who is at risk for progressing to cardiopulmonary arrest and to provide aggressive intervention before asystole occurs.

Please see the selected references at the end of this section for more information on the specifics of the American Heart Association's Pediatric Advanced Life Support (PALS) guidelines, most recently updated in 2018. The importance of quality Compressions is emphasized in both pediatric and adult cardiopulmonary resuscitation (CPR), with follow-up close attention paid to Airway and Breathing (acronym "C-A-B"). Please do not confuse this acronym with the "ABCs of resuscitation" approach described later as the following discussion details care of the critically ill pediatric patient who does not require CPR.

Of note, "compressions only" CPR has been touted as a way to encourage bystander CPR and increase survival rates of out-of-hospital cardiac arrests. In the pediatric population, however, conventional CPR (rescue breaths and chest compressions) is still emphasized and should be provided for infants and children in cardiac arrest. This is due to the asphyxial nature of most pediatric cardiac arrests which necessitates ventilation as part of effective CPR, whereas the majority of most adult cardiac arrest is due to a primary cardiac cause which may be more responsive to compressions-only CPR.

THE ABCS OF RESUSCITATION

A severely ill child should be rapidly evaluated in a deliberate sequence known as the *ABCs*: *A*irway patency, *B*reathing adequacy, and *C*irculation integrity. If a potentially life-threatening problem is detected during the evaluation, it must be corrected before proceeding to the next step. Age-appropriate equipment (including laryngoscope blade, endotracheal tubes, nasogastric or orogastric tubes, IV lines, and an indwelling urinary catheter) and monitors (cardio-respiratory monitor, pulse oximeter, and appropriate blood pressure cuff) should be assembled and readily available. Use a length-based emergency tape if available. See Table 12–1 for endotracheal tube and laryngeal mask airways (LMAs) sizes.

Cuffed endotracheal tubes are acceptable for children and infants beyond the newborn period. Cuff inflation pressures must be carefully monitored and maintained below 20 cm H_2O. In certain circumstances, such as poor lung compliance or high airway resistance, the use of cuffed tubes may be preferable in controlled settings.

Airway

In all children, look for evidence of spontaneous breathing. Breath sounds such as stridor, stertor, or gurgling, or increased work of breathing without air movement are suggestive of airway obstruction. Significant airway obstruction often is associated with altered level of consciousness, including agitation or lethargy. During the airway assessment, if the patient is noted to be apneic or producing only gasping (agonal) breaths, chest compressions should be initiated immediately in accordance with PALS guidelines.

If concerned for obstruction, the airway is managed initially by noninvasive means such as oxygen administration, chin lift, jaw thrust, suctioning, or bag-valve mask ventilation (BMV). Invasive maneuvers, such as endotracheal intubation, laryngeal mask insertion, or rarely, cricothyrotomy, are required if the aforementioned maneuvers are unsuccessful. The following discussion assumes that basic life support has been instituted.

Knowledge of pediatric anatomy is important for airway management. Children's tongues are large relative to their

Table 12–1. Equipment sizes and estimated weight by age.

Age (y)	Weight (kg)	Laryngeal Mask Airway (LMA) Size	Endotracheal Tube Size (mm)[a,b]	Laryngoscope Blade Size	Chest Tube (Fr)	Foley (Fr)
Premature	1–2.5	1	2.5 (uncuffed only)	0	8	5
Term newborn	3	1	3.0 (uncuffed only)	0–1	10	8
1	10	1.5	3.5–4.0	1	18	8
2	12	2	4.5	1	18	10
3	14	2	4.5	1	20	10
4	16	2	5.0	2	22	10
5	18	2	5.0–5.5	2	24	10
6	20	2–2.5	5.5	2	26	12
7	22	2.5	5.5–6.0	2	26	12
8	24	3	6.0	2	28	14
10	32	4	6.0–6.5	2–3	30	14
Adolescent	50	4	7.0	3	36	14
Adult	70		8.0	3	40	14

[a]Internal diameter.
[b]Decrease tube size by 0.5 mm if using a cuffed tube.

oral cavities, and the larynx is high and anteriorly located. Infants are obligate nasal breathers; therefore, secretions, blood, or foreign bodies in the nasopharynx can cause significant distress.

1. Place the head in the sniffing position. In the patient without concern for cervical spine injury, the neck should be flexed slightly and the head extended. This position aligns the oral, pharyngeal, and tracheal planes. In infants and children younger than about 8 years, the relatively large occiput causes significant neck flexion and poor airway positioning. This is relieved by placing a towel roll under the shoulders, thus returning the child to a neutral position (Figure 12–1). In an older child, slightly more head extension is necessary. Avoid hyperextension of the neck, especially in infants.

2. Perform the head tilt/chin lift or jaw thrust maneuver (Figure 12–2). Lift the chin upward while avoiding pressure on the submental triangle, or lift the jaw by traction upward on the angle of the jaw. Important: head tilt/chin lift must not be done if cervical spine injury is possible. (See section Approach to the Pediatric Trauma Patient, later.)

3. Assess airway for foreign material. Suction the mouth; use Magill forceps to remove visible foreign bodies. If needed, visualize with a laryngoscope. Do *not* perform blind finger sweeps.

4. If airway obstruction persists, first attempt to reposition the head, then proceed with insertion of an airway adjunct, such as the oropharyngeal or nasopharyngeal airway (Figure 12–3). Such adjuncts relieve upper airway obstruction due to prolapse of the tongue into the

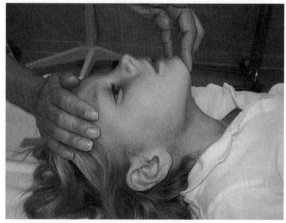

A

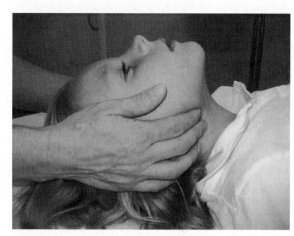

B

▲ **Figure 12–2. A:** Opening the airway with the head tilt and chin lift in patients without concern for spinal trauma: gently lift the chin with one hand and push down on the forehead with the other hand. **B:** Opening the airway with jaw thrust in patients with concern for spinal trauma: lift the angles of the mandible; this moves the jaw and tongue forward and opens the airway without bending the neck.

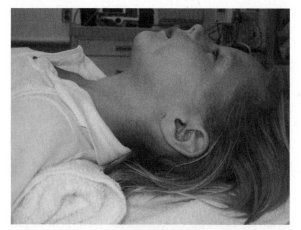

▲ **Figure 12–1.** Correct positioning of the child younger than 8 years for optimal airway alignment: a folded sheet or towel is placed beneath the shoulders to accommodate the occiput and align the oral, pharyngeal, and tracheal airways.

posterior pharynx, the most common cause of airway obstruction in unconscious children. The correct size for an oropharyngeal airway is obtained by measuring from the upper central gumline to the angle of the jaw (Figure 12–4) and should be used only in the unconscious victim. Proper sizing is paramount, as an oropharyngeal airway that is too small will push the tongue further into the airway while one that is too large will obstruct the airway. Nasopharyngeal airways should fit snugly within the nares and should be equal in length to the distance from

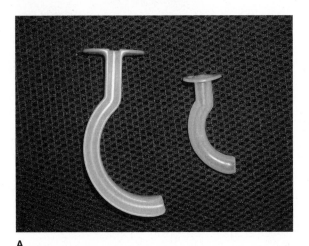

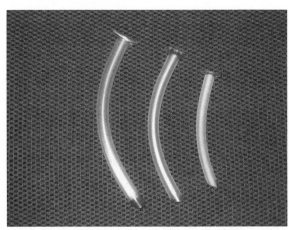

A

B

▲ **Figure 12–3. A:** Oropharyngeal airways of various sizes. **B:** Nasopharyngeal airways of different sizes.

the nares to the tragus (Figure 12–5). This airway adjunct should be avoided in children with significant injuries to the midface due to the risk of intracranial perforation through a damaged cribriform plate.

Breathing

Assessment of respiratory status beings with inspection. *Look* for adequate and symmetric chest rise and fall, rate and work of breathing (eg, accessory muscle use, retractions, flaring, and grunting), skin color, and tracheal deviation. Pulse oximetry measurement and end-tidal CO_2 determination are highly desirable. *Listen* for adventitious breath sounds such

as wheezing. Auscultate for air entry, symmetry of breath sounds, and rales. *Feel* for subcutaneous crepitus.

If spontaneous breathing is inadequate, initiate positive-pressure ventilation with BMV and 100% oxygen. Assisted ventilations should be coordinated with the patient's efforts, if present. Effective BMV is a difficult skill that requires training and practice. To begin, ensure a proper seal by choosing a mask that encompasses the area from the bridge of the nose to the cleft of the chin. Form an E–C clamp around the mask to seal the mask tightly to the child's face. The thumb and index finger form the "C" surrounding the mask, while the middle, ring, and small fingers lift the jaw into the mask (Figure 12–6). Use only enough force and volume to make the

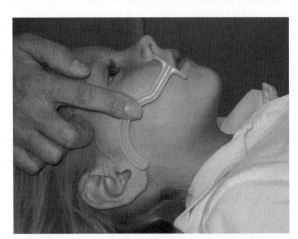

▲ **Figure 12–4.** Size selection for the oropharyngeal airway: hold the airway next to the child's face and estimate proper size by measuring from the upper central gumline to the angle of the jaw.

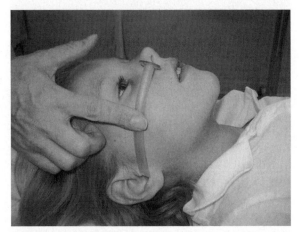

▲ **Figure 12–5.** Size selection for the nasopharyngeal airway: hold the airway next to the child's face and estimate proper size by measuring from the nares to the tragus.

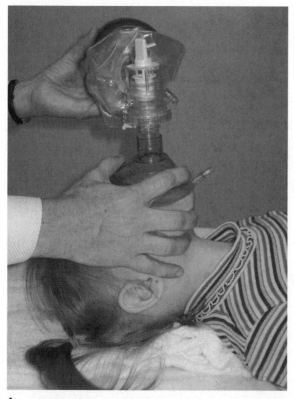

A

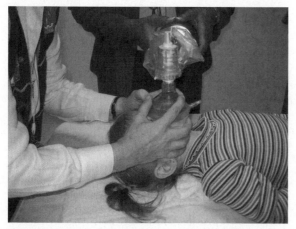

B

▲ **Figure 12–6. A:** Bag-valve-mask ventilation, one-person technique: the thumb and index finger form the "C" surrounding the mask, while the middle, ring, and little fingers lift the jaw into the mask. **B:** Bag-valve-mask ventilation, two-person technique: the first rescuer forms the "C" and "E" clamps with both hands; the second rescuer provides ventilation.

chest rise visibly. In the patient with a pulse, administer one breath every 3–5 seconds (12–20 breaths/min). This may be done using the timing mnemonic "squeeze-release-release" in a normal speaking voice. Two-person ventilation is optimal. When proper technique is used, BMV is effective in the vast majority of cases.

Adequacy of BMV is reflected with appropriate chest rise and auscultation of bilateral air entry. Avoid hyperventilation, as it may lead to barotrauma, increased risk of aspiration, and a decreased likelihood that return of spontaneous circulation will be achieved during cardiac arrest. If the chest does not rise and fall easily with bagging, reposition the airway and assess for foreign material as previously described. The presence of asymmetrical breath sounds in a child in shock or in severe distress suggests pneumothorax and is an indication for needle thoracostomy. In small children, the transmission of breath sounds throughout the chest may impair the ability to auscultate the presence of a pneumothorax. *Note:* Effective oxygenation and ventilation are the keys to successful resuscitation.

Cricoid pressure (Sellick maneuver) during positive-pressure ventilation may decrease gastric inflation; however, it has not been shown to reduce the risk of aspiration and is no longer recommended by the American Heart Association during CPR.

Circulation

The methodical assessment of blood circulation is critical to the diagnosis of shock, defined as the inadequate perfusion of vital organs. Circulation may be assessed in the following ways:

A. Pulses

Check adequacy of peripheral pulses and compare with central pulses. In the infant, central pulses should be checked at the brachial artery.

B. Heart Rate

Compare with age-specific norms. Tachycardia can be a nonspecific sign of distress; bradycardia for age is a sign of imminent arrest and necessitates aggressive resuscitation.

C. Blood Pressure

It is vital to understand that shock may be present even with a normal blood pressure. As intravascular volume falls, peripheral vascular resistance increases. Blood pressure is maintained until there is 35%–40% depletion of blood volume, followed by precipitous and often irreversible deterioration. **Compensated** shock occurs where there is normal blood pressure but signs of decreased organ perfusion. When blood pressure also falls, **decompensated (hypotensive)** shock is present. Blood pressure determination should be performed manually using an appropriately sized cuff, because automated machines can give erroneous readings in children.

D. Extremities

As shock progresses, extremities become cooler from distally to proximal. A child whose extremities are cool distal to the elbows and knees is in severe shock.

E. Capillary Refill Time

When fingertip pressure is applied to a patient's distal extremity and released, blood should refill the area in less than 2 seconds. A prolonged capillary refill time in the setting of other signs of shock indicates a compensated shock state. It is important to recognize that capillary refill time is influenced by ambient temperature, limb position, site, age of the patient, and room lighting.

F. Mental Status

Assess the patient's mental status, as hypoxia, hypercapnia, poor cerebral perfusion, or ischemia will result in altered mental status.

G. Skin Color

Skin that is pale, gray, sallow, mottled, or ashen may indicate compromised circulatory status.

MANAGEMENT OF SHOCK

Intravenous (IV) access is essential but can be difficult to establish in children with shock. Peripheral access, especially via the antecubital veins, should be attempted first. Use short, wide-bore catheters to allow maximal flow rates. Two IVs should be started in severely ill children. Intraosseous (IO) needle placement is an acceptable alternative in any severely ill child when venous access cannot be established rapidly (within 90 seconds) (Figure 12–7). Both manual and automated insertion devices are available for pediatric patients. Increasing evidence suggests that automated devices result in faster, more successful IO placement compared to manual devices. Decisions on more invasive access should be based on individual expertise as well as urgency of obtaining access. Options include percutaneous cannulation of femoral, subclavian, or internal or external jugular veins. Ultrasound guidance could make these attempts safer. In newborns, the umbilical veins may be cannulated. Consider arterial access if beat-to-beat monitoring or frequent laboratory tests will be needed.

Differentiation of Shock States & Initial Therapy

Therapy for inadequate circulation is determined by the cause of circulatory failure.

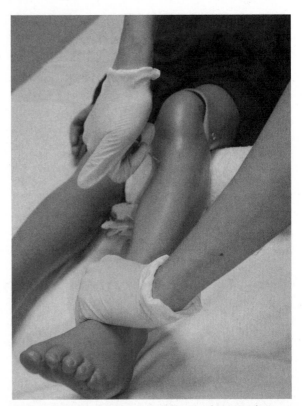

▲ **Figure 12–7.** Interosseous (IO) cannulation technique. The IO line is inserted by grasping the needle hub firmly with the palm of the hand and angling the needle tip perpendicular to the anterior tibial surface approximately two fingerbreadths distal to the tibial plateau. With a firm, twisting motion, advance the needle until a sudden lessening of resistance is felt as the needle enters the marrow space. Aspiration of blood and marrow confirms IO placement.

A. Hypovolemic Shock

The most common type of shock in the pediatric population is hypovolemia. Frequent causes include dehydration, diabetes, heat illness, and hemorrhage. Normal saline or lactated Ringer's solution (isotonic crystalloid) is given as initial therapy in shock and should be initiated even in normotensive patients. There is no advantage to the early administration of colloid (albumin). Give 20 mL/kg body weight (maximum 1 L bolus) and repeat as necessary, until perfusion normalizes, being sure to appropriately monitor and reassess after each intervention. Packed red blood cell transfusion is indicated in trauma patients not responding to initial crystalloid bolus fluid replacement; however, there is insufficient evidence to determine the volume required. Pressors are not typically required in simple hypovolemic shock.

B. Distributive Shock

Distributive shock results from increased vascular capacitance with normal circulating volume. Examples are sepsis, anaphylaxis, and spinal cord injury. Initial therapy is isotonic volume replacement with crystalloid, but pressors may be required if perfusion does not normalize after delivery of two or three 20 mL/kg boluses of crystalloid (total of 40–60 mL/kg). Outcomes improve when threshold heart rates, normalized blood pressure, and a capillary refill in less than 2 seconds are achieved within the first hour of symptom onset. Early identification of septic shock and rapid delivery of goal-directed therapies as fluids, antibiotics, and inotropes within the first hour of presentation to the ED can reduce mortality and neurologic morbidity risks twofold. Recently updated recommendations from the American College of Critical Care Medicine (reference at end of section) stress the importance of aggressively managing hypotension in the pediatric population and recommend no patient be hypotensive for more than 1 hour without starting vasopressor medications. Depending on the clinical scenario, epinephrine, dopamine, norepinephrine, or dobutamine may be used safely in children, though it is important to note that central venous access is preferred for epinephrine and norepinephrine drips. Thus, dopamine may be a preferred agent to be given peripherally until central access can be established.

C. Cardiogenic Shock

Cardiogenic shock can occur as a complication of congenital heart disease, myocarditis, dysrhythmias, ingestions (eg, clonidine, cyclic antidepressants), or as a complication of prolonged shock due to any cause. The diagnosis is suggested by any of the following signs: abnormal cardiac rhythm, distended neck veins, rales, abnormal heart sounds such as an S_3 or S_4, friction rub, narrow pulse pressure, rales, or hepatomegaly. Chest radiographs may show cardiomegaly and pulmonary edema. An initial bolus of crystalloid may be given, but pressors, and possibly afterload reducers, are necessary to improve perfusion. Giving multiple boluses of fluid is deleterious, which is why frequent reassessment and comprehensive monitoring is essential. Bedside ultrasound is useful in rapidly determining if cardiac function is adequate and whether a pericardial effusion is present.

D. Obstructive Shock

Obstructive shock is rare in the pediatric population and involves extracardiac obstruction of blood flow and/or obstruction of adequate diastolic filling. Examples include cardiac tamponade, tension pneumothorax, massive pulmonary embolism, or a critical coarctation of the aorta after closure of the ductus arteriosus. Management is directed toward resolution of the obstruction. In the case of a critical coarctation, management should include emergent prostaglandin initiation to reopen the ductus arteriosus while awaiting surgical repair.

▶ Observation & Further Management

Clinically reassess physiologic response to each fluid bolus to determine additional needs. Serial central venous pressure determinations or a chest radiograph may help determine volume status. Place an indwelling urinary catheter to monitor urine output.

Caution must be exercised with volume replacement if intracranial pressure (ICP) is potentially elevated, as in severe head injury, diabetic ketoacidosis, or meningitis. Even in such situations, however, normal intravascular volume must be restored in order to achieve adequate mean arterial pressure and thus cerebral perfusion pressure.

SUMMARY OF INITIAL APPROACH TO THE ACUTELY ILL INFANT OR CHILD

Assess the ABCs in sequential fashion and, before assessing the next system, immediately intervene if physiologic derangement is detected. It is essential that each system be reassessed after each intervention to ensure improvement and prevent failure to recognize clinical deterioration.

Agency for Healthcare Research and Quality. Welcome to H-CUPnet [home page on internet]. Rockville, MD: AHRQ. http://hcupnet.ahrq.gov/HCUPnet.jsp.

Davis AL et al: American college of critical care medicine clinical practice parameters for hemodynamic support of pediatric and neonatal shock. Critical Care Med 2017;45(6):1061–1093 [PMID: 28509730].

Duff JP, et al: 2018 American Heart Association focused update on pediatric advanced life support: an update to the American Heart Association guidelines for cardiopulmonary resuscitation and emergency cardiovascular care. Circulation 2018;138 [PMID: 30571264].

EMERGENCY PEDIATRIC DRUGS

Although careful attention to airway and breathing remains the mainstay of pediatric resuscitation, medications are often needed. Rapid delivery to the central circulation, which can be via peripheral IV catheter, is essential. Infuse medications close to the catheter's hub and flush with saline to achieve the most rapid systemic effects. In the rare instance that no IV or IO access is achievable, important emergency resuscitation drugs such as epinephrine, atropine, and naloxone may be given endotracheally (see dosing in Table 12–2). However, the dose, absorption, and effectiveness of drugs given via this route are either unknown or controversial. The use of length-based emergency measuring tapes that contain preprinted drug dosages, equipment sizes, and IV fluid amounts (Broselow tapes) or preprinted resuscitation drug charts is much more accurate than estimation formulas and helps minimize dosing errors. Selected emergency drugs used in pediatrics are summarized in Table 12–2.

Table 12-2. Important emergency pediatric drugs.

Drug	Indications	Dosage and Route	Comment
Epinephrine	1. Bradycardia, especially hypoxic-ischemic 2. Hypotension (by infusion) 3. Asystole 4. Fine ventricular fibrillation refractory to initial defibrillation 5. Pulseless electrical activity 6. Anaphylaxis (IM)	*Bradycardia and cardiac arrest*: 0.01 mg/kg of 1:10,000 solution IV/IO: 0.1 mg/kg of 1:1000 solution ET Anaphylaxis: 0.01 mg/kg of 1:1000 solution SC/IM Maximum dose: 0.3 mg. May repeat every 3-5 min. Constant infusion by IV drip: 0.1-1 mcg/kg/min.	Epinephrine is the single most important drug in pediatric resuscitation. Recent pediatric studies have shown no added advantage to high-dose epinephrine in terms of survival to discharge or neurologic outcome. Because other studies have indicated adverse effects, including increased myocardial oxygen consumption during resuscitation and worsened postarrest myocardial dysfunction, high-dose epinephrine is no longer recommended.
Glucose	1. Hypoglycemia 2. Altered mental status (empirical) 3. With insulin, for hyperkalemia	0.5-1 g/kg IV/IO. Continuous infusion may be necessary.	2-4 mL/kg D_{10}W, 1-2 mL/kg D_{25}W.
Naloxone	1. Opioid overdose 2. Altered mental status (empirical)	0.1 mg/kg IV/IO/ET; maximum single dose, 2 mg. May repeat as necessary.	Side effects are few. A dose of 2 mg may be given in children ≥ 5 years or > 20 kg. Repeat as necessary, or give as constant infusion in opioid overdoses.
Sodium bicarbonate	1. Documented metabolic acidosis 2. Hyperkalemia	1 mEq/kg IV or IO; by arterial blood gas: 0.3 × kg × base deficit. May repeat every 5 min.	Infuse slowly. Sodium bicarbonate will be effective only if the patient is adequately oxygenated, ventilated, and perfused. Some adverse side effects.
Calcium chloride 10%	1. Documented hypocalcemia 2. Calcium channel blocker overdose 3. Hyperkalemia, hypermagnesemia	20 mg/kg slowly IV, preferably centrally, or IO with caution. Maximum single dose 2 g.	Calcium is no longer indicated for asystole. Potent tissue necrosis results if infiltration occurs. Use with caution and infuse slowly.

D_5W would be 10 mL/kg; D_{50}W would be 1 mL/kg; D_{10}W/D_{25}W, 10%/25% glucose in water; ET, endotracheally; IO, intraosseously; IV, intravenously; SC, subcutaneously. D_{50}W is not recommended PIV and use caution with D_{25}. D_{10} is preferred for neonates (newborn -1 month of age).

APPROACH TO THE PEDIATRIC TRAUMA PATIENT

Traumatic injuries, including motor vehicle crashes, falls, burns, and immersions, account for the greatest number of deaths among children older than 1 year; injury exceeds all other causes of death combined with motor vehicle accidents accounting for the majority of deaths. Blunt trauma is most common, with penetrating trauma occurring in only 10% of cases. Head and abdominal injuries are particularly common and important.

A coordinated team approach to the severely injured child will optimize outcomes. A calm atmosphere in the receiving area will contribute to thoughtful care. Parents are often anxious, angry, or guilt-ridden, requiring ongoing support from staff, social workers, or child life workers (therapists knowledgeable about child development).

To provide optimal multidisciplinary care, regional pediatric trauma centers provide dedicated teams of pediatric specialists in emergency pediatrics, trauma surgery, orthopedics, neurosurgery, and critical care. However, most children with severe injuries are not seen in these centers. Community providers must often provide initial assessment and stabilization of the child with life-threatening injuries before transport to a verified pediatric trauma center.

MECHANISM OF INJURY

Document the time of occurrence, the type of energy transfer (eg, hit by a car, fall from playground), secondary impacts (if the child was thrown by the initial impact), appearance of the child at the scene, interventions performed, and clinical condition during transport. The report of emergency service personnel is invaluable. Forward all of this information with the patient to the referral facility if secondary transport occurs.

INITIAL ASSESSMENT & MANAGEMENT

The vast majority of children who reach a hospital alive survive to discharge. As most deaths from trauma in children are due to head injuries, cerebral resuscitation must be the foremost consideration when treating children with serious injuries. Strict attention to the ABCs (see the previous section) ensures optimal oxygenation, ventilation, and perfusion, and ultimately, cerebral perfusion.

The primary and secondary survey is a method for evaluating and treating injured patients in a systematic way that provides a rapid assessment and stabilization phase, followed by a head-to-toe examination and definitive care phase.

PRIMARY SURVEY

The primary survey is designed to immediately identify and treat all physiologic derangements resulting from trauma. The mnemonic, *ABCDE*, is a simple way to remember the general steps of the primary survey: *A*irway, with cervical spine control; *B*reathing; *C*irculation, with hemorrhage control; *D*isability (neurologic deficit); *E*xposure (maintain a warm *E*nvironment, undress the patient completely, and *E*xamine)

If the patient is apneic or has agonal breaths, the sequence reverts to the *CABs* of PALS resuscitation (chest compressions, open the *a*irway, provide two rescue *b*reaths). Please refer to PALS guidelines for further information. Refer to preceding discussion regarding details of the ABC assessment. Modifications in the trauma setting are added as follows:

Airway

Failure to manage the airway appropriately is the most common cause of preventable morbidity and death. Administer 100% high-flow oxygen to all patients. Initially, provide cervical spine protection by manual inline immobilization, not traction. A hard cervical spine collar is applied after the primary survey.

Breathing

Most ventilation problems are resolved adequately by the airway maneuvers described earlier and by positive-pressure ventilation. Sources of traumatic pulmonary compromise include pneumothorax, hemothorax, pulmonary contusion, flail chest, and central nervous system (CNS) depression. Asymmetric breath sounds, particularly with concurrent tracheal deviation, cyanosis, or bradycardia, suggest pneumothorax, possibly under tension. To evacuate a tension pneumothorax, insert a large-bore catheter-over-needle assembly attached to a syringe through the second intercostal space in the midclavicular line into the pleural cavity and withdraw air. If a pneumothorax or hemothorax is present (evident by the sound of hissing as the air is evacuated), place a chest tube in the fourth or fifth intercostal space in the anterior axillary line. Connect to water seal. Insertion should be over the rib to avoid the neurovascular bundle that runs below the rib margin. Open pneumothoraces can be treated temporarily by taping petrolatum-impregnated gauze on three sides over the wound, creating a flap valve.

A child with a depressed level of consciousness (Glasgow Coma Scale [GCS] score < 9), a need for prolonged

ventilation, severe head trauma, or an impending operative intervention requires endotracheal intubation after bag-mask preoxygenation. Orotracheal intubation is the route of choice and is possible without cervical spine manipulation. Nasotracheal intubation may be possible in children 12 years of age or older who have spontaneous respirations, if not contraindicated by midfacial injury.

Supraglottic devices, such as the LMA, are being used with increasing frequency, in both the prehospital and hospital settings. The device consists of a flexible tube attached to an inflatable rubber mask (Figure 12–8). The LMA is inserted blindly into the hypopharynx and is seated over the larynx, occluding the esophagus. Advantages to its use include ease of insertion, lower potential for airway trauma, and higher success rates. Patients remain at higher risk for aspiration with LMA use compared with orotracheal intubation; therefore, the LMA should not be used for prolonged, definitive airway management. Rarely, if tracheal intubation cannot be accomplished, particularly in the setting of massive facial trauma, cricothyroidotomy may be necessary. Needle cricothyroidotomy using a large-bore catheter through the cricothyroid membrane is the procedure of choice in patients younger than 12 years.

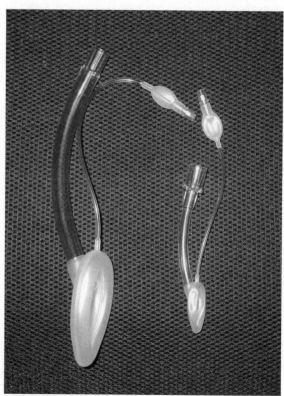

▲ **Figure 12–8.** Laryngeal mask airways of various sizes.

Circulation

Evaluation for ongoing external or internal hemorrhage is important in the trauma evaluation. Large-bore IV access should be obtained early during the assessment, preferably at two sites. If peripheral access is not readily available, an intraosseus line, central line, or cutdown, or IO line is established. Determine hematocrit and urinalysis in all patients. Blood type and cross-match should be obtained in the hypotensive child unresponsive to isotonic fluid boluses or with known hemorrhage. Consider coagulation studies, chemistry panel, liver transaminases, lipase, and toxicologic screening as clinically indicated.

External hemorrhage can be controlled by direct pressure. To avoid damage to adjacent neurovascular structures, avoid placing hemostats on vessels, except in the scalp. Determination of the site of internal hemorrhage can be challenging. Sites include the chest, abdomen, retroperitoneum, pelvis, and thighs. Bleeding into the intracranial vault rarely causes shock in children except in infants. Evaluation by an experienced clinician with adjunctive computed tomography (CT) or ultrasound will localize the site of internal bleeding.

Suspect cardiac tamponade after penetrating or blunt injuries to the chest if shock, pulseless electrical activity, narrowed pulse pressure, distended neck veins, hepatomegaly, or muffled heart sounds are present. Ultrasound may be diagnostic if readily available. Diagnose and treat with pericardiocentesis and rapid volume infusion.

Treat signs of poor perfusion vigorously: A tachycardic child with a capillary refill time of 3 seconds or more, or other evidence of diminished perfusion, is in *shock* and is sustaining vital organ insults. Recall that hypotension is a late finding. Volume replacement is accomplished initially by rapid infusion of normal saline or lactated Ringer solution at 20 mL/kg of body weight. If perfusion does not normalize after two crystalloid bolus infusions, 10 mL/kg of packed red blood cells is infused. Rapid reassessment must follow each bolus. If clinical signs of perfusion have not normalized, repeat the bolus. Lack of response or later or recurring signs of hypovolemia suggest the need for blood transfusion and possible surgical exploration.

A common problem is the brain-injured child who is at risk for intracranial hypertension and who is also hypovolemic. In such cases, circulating volume must be restored to ensure adequate cerebral perfusion; therefore, fluid replacement is required until perfusion normalizes. Thereafter provide maintenance fluids with careful serial reassessments.

Disability-Neurologic Deficit

Assess pupillary size and reaction to light and the level of consciousness. The level of consciousness can be reproducibly characterized by the AVPU (alert, voice, pain, unresponsive) system (Table 12–3). Pediatric GCS assessments can be done as part of the secondary survey (Table 12–4).

Table 12–3. AVPU system for evaluation of level of consciousness.

A Alert
V Responsive to Voice
P Responsive to Pain
U Unresponsive

Exposure & Environment

Significant injuries can be missed unless the child is completely undressed and examined fully, front and back. Any patient transported on a backboard should be removed as soon as possible, as pressure sores may develop on the buttocks and heels of an immobilized patient within hours.

Because of their high ratio of surface area to body mass, infants and children cool rapidly. Hypothermia compromises outcome except with isolated head injuries; therefore, continuously monitor the body temperature and use warming

Table 12–4. Glasgow Coma Scale.[a]

Eye-opening response	
Spontaneous	4
To speech	3
To pain	2
None	1
Verbal response: Child (*Infant modification*)[b]	
Oriented (*Coos, babbles*)	5
Confused conversation (*Irritable cry, consolable*)	4
Inappropriate words (*Cries to pain*)	3
Incomprehensible sounds (*Moans to pain*)	2
None	1
Best upper limb motor response: Child (*Infant modification*)[b]	
Obeys commands (*Normal movements*)	6
Localizes pain (*Withdraws to touch*)	5
Withdraws to pain	4
Flexion to pain	3
Extension to pain	2
None	1

[a]The appropriate number from each section is added to total between 3 and 15. A score less than 8 usually indicates CNS depression requiring positive-pressure ventilation.
[b]If no modification is listed, the same response applies for both infants and children.

techniques as necessary. Hyperthermia can adversely affect outcomes in children with acute brain injuries, so maintain normal body temperatures.

Monitoring

Cardiopulmonary monitors, pulse oximetry, and end-tidal CO_2 monitors should be put in place immediately. At the completion of the primary survey, additional "tubes" may be needed to be placed. See Table 12–1 for age/weight-appropriate equipment sizes.

A. Nasogastric or Orogastric Tube

Children's stomachs should be assumed to be full so a nasogastric tube needs to be placed. Gastric distention from positive-pressure ventilation increases the chance of vomiting and aspiration. Of note, the nasogastric route should be avoided in patients with significant midface trauma.

B. Urinary Catheter

An indwelling urinary bladder catheter should be considered to monitor urine output. Contraindications are based on the risk of urethral transection; signs include blood at the meatus or in the scrotum or a displaced prostate detected on rectal examination. Urine should be tested for blood. After the initial flow of urine with catheter placement, the urine output should exceed 1 mL/kg/h.

SECONDARY SURVEY

After the Primary Survey and resuscitation phase, a focused history and a head-to-toe examination should be performed to reveal all injuries and determine priorities for definitive care.

History

Obtain a rapid, focused history from the patient (if possible), available family members or prehospital personnel. The AMPLE mnemonic is frequently used:

- A—Allergies
- M—Medications
- P—Past medical history/pregnancy
- L—Last meal
- E—Events/environment leading to the injury

Physical Examination

A. Skin

Search for lacerations, hematomas, burns, swelling, and abrasions. Remove superficial foreign material and cleanse as necessary. Cutaneous findings may indicate underlying pathology (eg, a flank hematoma overlying a renal contusion), although surface signs may be absent even with significant internal injury. Do not remove penetrating foreign objects because vital respiratory components, vascular structures, or organs may be involved and require removal in a controlled environment by a surgeon. Make certain that the child's tetanus immunization status is current. Consider tetanus immune globulin for incompletely immunized children.

B. Head

Check for hemotympanum and for clear or bloody cerebrospinal fluid leak from the nares. The "battle sign" (hematoma over the mastoid) and periorbital hematomas ("raccoon eyes") are late signs of basilar skull fracture. Explore wounds, evaluating for foreign bodies and defects in galea or skull. CT scan of the head is an integral part of evaluation for altered level of consciousness, posttraumatic seizure, or focal neurologic findings (see section Head Injury, later). Pneumococcal vaccine may be considered for basilar skull fractures as a preventive measure for meningitis.

C. Spine

Cervical spine injury must be excluded in all children. This can be done clinically in children older than 4 or 5 years with normal neurologic findings on examination who are able to deny midline neck pain or midline tenderness on palpation of the neck and who have no other painful distracting injuries that might obscure the pain of a cervical spine injury. If radiographs are indicated, a cross-table lateral neck view is obtained initially followed by anteroposterior, odontoid, and, in some cases, oblique views. Normal studies do not exclude significant injury, either bony or ligamentous, or involving the spinal cord itself. Therefore, an obtunded child should be maintained in cervical spine immobilization until the child has awakened and an appropriate neurologic examination can be performed. The entire thoracolumbar spine must be palpated and areas of pain or tenderness examined by radiography.

D. Chest

Children may sustain significant internal injury without outward signs of trauma. The most common type of injuries sustained from blunt chest trauma is pulmonary contusions which may lead to hypoxemia. Pneumothoraces are detected and decompressed during the primary survey. Hemothoraces can occur with rib fractures or with injury to intercostal vessels, large pulmonary vessels, or lung parenchyma. Tracheobronchial disruption is suggested by large continued air leak despite chest tube decompression. Myocardial contusions and aortic injuries are unusual in children.

E. Abdomen

Blunt abdominal injury is common in multisystem injuries. Significant injury may exist without cutaneous signs or instability of vital signs. Abdominal pain and tenderness coupled with a linear contusion across the abdomen ("seat belt sign") increases the risk of intra-abdominal injury three-fold. Tenderness, guarding, distention, diminished or absent bowel sounds, or poor perfusion mandate immediate evaluation by a pediatric trauma surgeon. Injury to solid viscera frequently can be managed nonoperatively in stable patients; however, intestinal perforation or hypotension necessitates operative treatment. Intra-abdominal injury is highly likely if the AST is greater than 200 U/L or the ALT greater than 125 U/L; however, elevated levels that are below these thresholds do not exclude significant injury if a significant mechanism has occurred. When measured serially, a hematocrit of less than 30% also may suggest intra-abdominal injury in blunt trauma patients. Coagulation studies are rarely beneficial if no concomitant head injury is present. There is no single test value that can reliably predict intraabdominal injury and therefore laboratory interpretation requires close clinical correlation. Laboratory studies are often most valuable in the nonverbal or obtunded patient, to increase the suspicion for injury and subsequent need for imaging.

Trauma ultrasonography, or the FAST (focused assessment with sonography for trauma), is routinely used in the adult trauma population. The purpose of the four-view examination (Morison pouch, splenorenal pouch, pelvic retrovesical space, and subcostal view of the heart) is to detect free fluid or blood in dependent spaces. In adults, such detection indicates clinically significant injury likely to require surgery. Accuracy and indications in children are much less clear. This examination has a high specificity rate to rule in free abdominal fluid, but low sensitivity to rule out significant intra-abdominal injury. Solid-organ injuries are more frequently missed. Additionally, much of the pediatric trauma management is nonoperative and therefore detection of free fluid by ultrasound in children is less likely to lead to surgery or result in a change in management. At least one recent study showed no change in the rate of pediatric patients eventually undergoing abdominal CT regardless of FAST findings.

F. Pelvis

Pelvic fractures are classically manifested by pain, crepitus, and abnormal motion. Significant blood loss into the pelvis may occur due to vascular injury, thus have a sign index of suspicion in the setting of unexplained tachycardia or hypotension. Pelvic fracture is a relative contraindication to urethral catheter insertion. Many providers perform a rectal examination, noting tone, tenderness, and in boys, prostate position. If this is done, stool should be tested for blood.

G. Genitourinary System

If urethral transection is suspected, perform a retrograde urethrogram before catheter placement. Diagnostic imaging of the child with hematuria less than 50 red blood cells per high-power (hpf) field often includes CT scan or occasionally, IV urograms. Management of kidney injury is largely nonoperative except for renal pedicle injuries.

H. Extremities

Long bone fractures are common but rarely life threatening. Test for pulses, perfusion, and sensation. Neurovascular compromise requires immediate orthopedic consultation. Treatment of open fractures includes antibiotics, tetanus prophylaxis, and orthopedic consultation.

I. Central Nervous System

Most deaths in children with multisystem trauma are from head injuries, so optimal neurointensive care is important. Significant injuries include diffuse axonal injury; cerebral edema; subdural, subarachnoid, and epidural hematomas; and parenchymal hemorrhages. Spinal cord injury occurs less commonly. Level of consciousness should be assessed serially. A full sensorimotor examination should be performed. Deficits require immediate neurosurgical consultation and should be considered for a patient with a GCS less than 12. Extensor or flexor posturing represents intracranial hypertension until proven otherwise. If accompanied by a fixed, dilated pupil, such posturing indicates that a herniation syndrome is present, and mannitol or 3% hypertonic saline should be given if perfusion is normal (see further discussion in next section). Treatment goals include aggressively treating hypotension to optimize cerebral perfusion, providing supplemental oxygen to keep saturations above 90%, achieving eucapnia (end-tidal CO_2 35–40 mm Hg), avoiding hyperthermia, and minimizing painful stimuli. Early rapid sequence intubation, sedation, and paralysis should be considered. Mild prophylactic hyperventilation is no longer recommended, although brief periods of hyperventilation are still indicated in the setting of acute herniation. Seizure activity warrants exclusion of significant intracranial injury. In the trauma setting, seizures are frequently treated with fosphenytoin or levetiracetam. The use of high-dose corticosteroids for suspected spinal cord injury has not been prospectively evaluated in children and is not considered standard of care. Corticosteroids are not indicated for head trauma.

Centers for Disease Control and Prevention, National Center for Injury Prevention and Control, Division of Unintentional Injury Prevention. https://www.cdc.gov/safechild/child_injury_data.html. Accessed June 30, 2019.

Drexel S, Azarow K, Jafri MA: Abdominal trauma evaluation for the pediatric surgeon. Surg Clin North Am 2017 Feb;97(1): 59–74 [PMID: 27894432].

Liang et al: The utility of the focused assessment with sonography in trauma examination in pediatric blunt abdominal trauma: a systematic review and meta-analysis. Pediatr Emerg Care. 2019 Mar 12 [PMID: 30870341].

HEAD INJURY

Closed-head injuries range in severity from minor asymptomatic trauma without sequelae to fatal injuries. Even after minor closed-head injury, long-term disability and neuropsychiatric sequelae can occur.

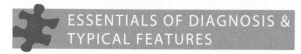

ESSENTIALS OF DIAGNOSIS & TYPICAL FEATURES

▶ Traumatic brain injury (TBI) is the most common injury in children.

▶ Rapid acceleration-deceleration forces (eg, the shaken infant) as well as direct trauma to the head can result in brain injury.

▶ Rapid assessment can be made by evaluating mental status with the GCS score and assessing pupillary light response.

▶ All head injuries require a screening evaluation with symptom inventory and complete neurologic examination.

▶ Prevention

Wearing helmets while riding wheeled recreational devices, playing contact sports, and participating in snow sports is a simple strategy in preventing head injuries. Over 50% of children fail to wear helmets when riding bicycles; rates are lower with other wheeled devices. Adolescents are less likely to use protective equipment and warrant special attention when discussing helmet use. More stringent helmet use while playing contact sports and return to play recommendations are now in place in child and high school sports programs. Toppled televisions, dressers and other unsecured furniture can also result in mild to severe head injuries in young children; anticipatory guidance regarding properly securing furniture should be provided to parents.

▶ Clinical Findings

A. Signs and Symptoms

Head injury symptoms are nonspecific and may include headache, dizziness, nausea/vomiting, disorientation, amnesia, slowed thinking, and perseveration. Loss of consciousness is not necessary to diagnose a concussion (see Chapter 27 for more on concussion). Worsening symptoms in the first 24 hours may indicate more severe TBI. Obtain vital signs and assess the child's level of consciousness by the AVPU system (see Table 12–3) or GCS (see Table 12–4), noting irritability or lethargy and pupillary equality, size, and light reaction. Perform a physical examination, including a

detailed neurologic examination, being mindful of the mechanism of injury. Cerebrospinal fluid or blood from the ears or nose, hemotympanum, or the later appearance of periorbital hematomas ("raccoon eyes") or "battle sign" (bruising over the mastoid process) imply a basilar skull fracture as discussed previously. Evaluate for associated injuries, paying special attention to the cervical spine. Consider child abuse; injuries observed should be consistent with the history, the child's developmental stage, and the injury mechanism.

B. Imaging Studies

CT may be indicated. However, close observation for a period of time may be appropriate management and reduces the use of CT. A 2009 multicenter investigation of head-injured patients presenting to the ED derived and validated a decision rule for identifying those children at very low risk of clinically important traumatic brain injuries (Figure 12–9). Plain films are not generally indicated. In infants, a normal neurologic examination does not exclude significant intracranial hemorrhage. Consider imaging if large scalp hematomas or concerns of nonaccidental trauma are present in younger children.

▶ Differential Diagnosis

CNS infection, toxicological ingestions, or other medical causes of altered mental status may present similarly to head injuries which often have no external signs of injury. In young infants when no history is available, one must also consider sepsis and inborn errors of metabolism.

▶ Complications

A. Central Nervous System Infection

Open-head injuries (fractures with overlying lacerations) pose an infection risk due to direct contamination. Basilar skull fractures that involve the cribriform plate or middle ear cavity may allow a portal of entry for *Streptococcus pneumoniae*. Pneumococcal vaccination is considered for such cases.

B. Acute Intracranial Hypertension

Close observation will detect early signs and symptoms of elevated increased ICP. Early recognition is essential to avoid disastrous outcomes. Symptoms include altered mental status, headache, vision changes, vomiting, gait difficulties, and pupillary abnormalities. Papilledema is a cardinal sign of increased ICP. Other signs may include stiff neck, cranial nerve palsies, and hemiparesis. Cushing triad (bradycardia, hypertension, and irregular respirations) is a late and ominous finding. Consider CT scan before lumbar puncture if there is concern for elevated ICP because of the risk of herniation. Lumbar puncture should be deferred in the unstable patient.

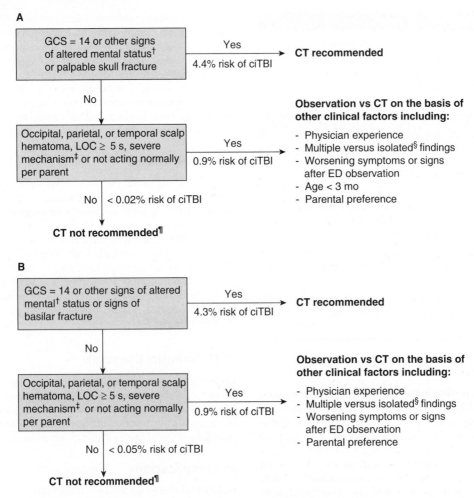

A

GCS = 14 or other signs of altered mental status[†] or palpable skull fracture

Yes → 4.4% risk of ciTBI → **CT recommended**

No ↓

Occipital, parietal, or temporal scalp hematoma, LOC ≥ 5 s, severe mechanism[‡] or not acting normally per parent

Yes → 0.9% risk of ciTBI →

Observation vs CT on the basis of other clinical factors including:

- Physician experience
- Multiple versus isolated[§] findings
- Worsening symptoms or signs after ED observation
- Age < 3 mo
- Parental preference

No | < 0.02% risk of ciTBI ↓

CT not recommended[¶]

B

GCS = 14 or other signs of altered mental[†] status or signs of basilar fracture

Yes → 4.3% risk of ciTBI → **CT recommended**

No ↓

Occipital, parietal, or temporal scalp hematoma, LOC ≥ 5 s, severe mechanism[‡] or not acting normally per parent

Yes → 0.9% risk of ciTBI →

Observation vs CT on the basis of other clinical factors including:

- Physician experience
- Multiple versus isolated[§] findings
- Worsening symptoms or signs after ED observation
- Parental preference

No | < 0.05% risk of ciTBI ↓

CT not recommended[¶]

ciTBI = clinically important traumatic brain injury; GCS = Glasgow Coma Scale; LOC = loss of consciousness.
[†]Other signs of altered mental status: agitation, somnolence repetitive questioning, or slow response to verbal communication.
[‡]Severe mechanism of injury: motor vehicle crash with patient ejection, death of another passenger, or rollover; pedestrian or bicyclist without helmet struck by motorized vehicle; falls of more than 3 ft (or more than 5 ft for panel B); or head struck by a high-impact object.
[§]Patients with certain isolated findings (ie, with no other findings suggestive of traumatic brain injury), such as isolated LOC, isolated headache, isolated vomiting, and certain type of isolated scalp hematomas in infants older than 3 mo, have a risk of ciTBI substantially lower than 1%.
[¶]Risk of ciTBI exceedingly low, generally lower than risk of CT-induced malignancies. Therefore, CT scans are not indicated for most patients in this group.

Adapted from *The Lancet* 374, Kuppermann et al, Identification of children at very low risk of clinically-important brain injuries after head trauma: a prospective cohort study. pp. 1160–1170. © 2009 with permission from Elsevier.

▲ **Figure 12–9.** Suggested CT algorithm for children younger than 2 years (**A**) and for those aged 2 years and older (**B**) with GCS scores 14–15 after head trauma. (Adapted with permission from Kuppermann N et al: Identification of children at very low risk of clinically-important brain injuries after head trauma: a prospective cohort study. Lancet 2009 Oct 3;374(9696):1160–1170.)

Treatment—Therapy for elevated ICP must be swift and aggressive. Maintenance of adequate oxygenation, ventilation, and perfusion is paramount. Rapid sequence intubation is often necessary to protect the airway using a sedative and paralytic to decrease the ICP elevation accompanying intubation. Lidocaine is a controversial adjunct pretreatment medication (administered 2–3 minutes prior to attempt) during RSI and is thought to blunt increases in ICP during intubation by suppressing cough and gag reflexes and protect cerebral perfusion. Avoid hypoperfusion and hypoxemia, as both are associated with increased risk of morbidity and mortality. Hyperventilation (goal PCO_2 30–35 mm Hg) is reserved for acute herniation; otherwise, maintain PCO_2 between 35 and 40 mm Hg. Mannitol (0.5–1 g/kg IV), an osmotic diuretic, will reduce brain water during acute herniation and hypertonic saline (3%; 4–6 mL/kg bolus doses or 1–2 mL/kg/h infusion) also may be used. Adjunctive measures to decreased ICP include elevating the head of the bed 30 degrees, maintaining the head in a midline position and treating hyperpyrexia (fever) and pain. Obtain immediate neurosurgical consultation. Further details about management of intracranial hypertension (cerebral edema) are presented in Chapter 14.

C. Prognosis

Children with concussion should be followed closely, return to sport only when symptom-free at rest and during exercise without medication use and then followed by a graduated return-to-play protocol. All states now have a concussion law and most require a physician's note to return to play. In addition to sport limitations, patients may require a modified academic schedule and additional academic accommodations, including shorter days, longer testing periods, and decreased amounts of homework. Patients should only return to sports after a complete return to other school activities. Most children recover fully within 1–2 weeks. Acute symptoms seen in the ED do not correlate with long-term outcome, and therefore it is crucial for all patients to have follow-up management by their primary care physician. Persistent symptoms indicate the need for rehabilitation and/or neuropsychological referral. The CDC's Heads Up program has accessible concussion and return to play information online and is a good resource for parents, coaches, and health care providers.

The prognosis for children with moderate to severe injuries depends on many factors including severity of initial injury, presence of hypoxia or ischemia, development and subsequent management of intracranial hypertension, and associated injuries.

Centers for Disease Control and Prevention, National Center for Injury Prevention and Control, Division of Unintentional Injury Prevention: https://www.cdc.gov/headsup/index.html. Accessed April, 2019.

Grubenhoff JA et al: Acute concussion symptom severity and delayed symptom resolution. Pediatrics 2014;134(1):54–62 [PMID: 24958583].

Kuppermann N et al: Identification of children at very low risk of clinically-important brain injuries after head trauma: a prospective cohort study. Lancet 2009;374(9696):1160–1170 [PMID: 19758692].

McCrory P et al: Consensus statement on concussion in sport: the 4th International Conference on Concussion in Sport held in Zurich, November 2012. Br J Sports Med 2013;47:250–258 [PMID: 23855362].

Nigrovic LE et al: The effect of observation on cranial computed tomography utilization for children after blunt head trauma. Pediatrics 2011;127(6):1067–1073 [PMID: 21555498].

▼ BURNS

THERMAL BURNS

ESSENTIALS OF DIAGNOSIS & TYPICAL FEATURES

▶ Burn patterns can distinguish accidental burns from inflicted burns.

▶ Burns are categorized into three classes based on skin layer involved: superficial, partial thickness, and full thickness.

▶ Burns of the hands, feet, face, eyes, ears, and perineum are always considered to be major burns.

Burns are a common cause of accidental death and disfigurement in children. Common causes include hot water or food, appliances, flames, grills, vehicle-related burns, and curling irons. Burns occur commonly in toddlers—in boys more frequently than in girls. The association with child abuse and the preventable nature of burns constitute an area of major concern in pediatrics.

▶ Prevention

Hot liquids should be placed as far as possible from counter edges and parents/caregivers should take care when holding a child while drinking a hot beverage. While cooking, panhandles should be turned away from stove edge. Water heater thermostats should be turned to less than 120°F (49°C). Irons and electrical cords should be kept out of reach of children. Barriers around fireplaces are crucial. Infant and young children should wear protective clothing including hats when outdoors. Infant approved sunscreen should be applied, and reapplied frequently, to children 6 months and older, and also in younger infants in long periods of sun exposure outdoors.

▶ Clinical Findings

A. Signs and Symptoms

Superficial-thickness burns are painful, dry, red, and hypersensitive. Sunburn is an example. Partial-thickness burns are sub-grouped as superficial or deep, depending on appearance. Superficial partial-thickness burns are red and often blister. Deep partial-thickness burns are pale, edematous, blanch with pressure, and they display decreased sensitivity to pain. Full-thickness burns affect all epidermal and dermal elements. A full-thickness wound is white or black, dry, depressed, leathery in appearance, and insensate. Deep full-thickness burns are the most severe, extending through all layers of skin as well as into the underlying fascia, muscle, and possibly bone. Singing of nasal or facial hair, carbonaceous material in the nose and mouth, and stridor indicate inhalational burns and may herald critical airway obstruction. Up to 25% of burns in children may be due to child physical abuse. Burn patterns can help distinguish inflicted from accidental causes. If the burn pattern does not fit the mechanism, consider child abuse.

B. Laboratory Findings

Laboratory evaluation is rarely indicated. With extensive partial- and full-thickness burns, baseline complete blood cell count (CBC), basic metabolic panel, and creatinine kinase are helpful for tracking infectious or renal complications. Consider carbon monoxide poisoning after inhalational injury: obtain an arterial blood gas and carboxyhemoglobin levels.

C. Imaging Studies

Imaging studies are rarely indicated. Neck x-rays should not delay intubation when inhalational injury is suspected.

▶ Differential Diagnosis

The differential diagnosis of burns is limited when a history is provided. In the preverbal child when no history is available, the primary alternate consideration is cellulitis.

▶ Complications

Superficial- and superficial partial-thickness burns typically heal well. Deep partial- and full-thickness burns are at risk of scarring. Loss of barrier function predisposes to infection. Damage to deeper tissues in full-thickness burns may result in loss of function, contractures, and in the case of circumferential burns, compartment syndrome. Renal failure secondary to myoglobinuria from rhabdomyolysis is also a concern with more severe burns.

▶ Treatment

Burn extent can be classified as major or minor as determined by calculating the percent of body surface area (BSA) affected by partial- or full-thickness burns. Superficial thickness burns are not counted when assessing % BSA. Minor burns are less than 10% BSA for partial-thickness burns, or less than 2% for full-thickness burns. Partial- or full-thickness burns of the hands, feet, face, eyes, ears, and perineum are considered major.

A. Superficial- and Partial-Thickness Burns

These burns generally can be treated in the outpatient setting. Wounds with a potential to cause disfigurement or functional impairment—especially wounds of the face, hands, feet, digits, or perineum—should be referred promptly to a burn surgeon. Analgesia is paramount. After parenteral narcotic administration, initial treatment of partial-thickness burns with blisters consists of saline irrigation followed by application of clear antibiotic ointment and a non-adherent dressing (eg, petroleum gauze). Digits should be individually dressed to prevent adhesions. Because of the pain associated with aggressive debridement and the ability to provide an infectious barrier, smaller blisters may be left intact under the dressing. Larger bullae may either be drained or left in place. Protect the wound with a bulky dressing, reexamine within 48 hours and serially thereafter. Treatment at home with cool compresses and optimizing pain control with medications.

B. Full-Thickness, Deep or Extensive Partial-Thickness, and Subdermal Burns

Major burns require particular attention to the ABCs of trauma management. Early establishment of an artificial airway is critical with oral or nasal burns because of their association with inhalation injuries and critical airway obstruction. If singeing of the oro- or nasopharynx is noted on initial exam, immediate intubation is recommended.

Perform a primary survey (see earlier discussion). Consider toxicity from carbon monoxide, cyanide, or other combustion products. Place a nasogastric tube and bladder catheter. The secondary survey identifies associated injuries, including those suggestive of abuse.

Fluid losses can be substantial. Initial fluid resuscitation should restore adequate circulating volume. Subsequent fluid administration must account for increased losses. Fluid needs are based on weight and percentage of BSA with partial- and full-thickness burns. Figure 12–10 shows percentages of BSA by region in infants and children. The Parkland formula for fluid therapy is 4 mL/kg/% BSA burned for the first 24 hours, with half administered in the first 8 hours, in addition to maintenance rates. Use of burn tables improves calculation of appropriate fluids. Goal urine output is 1–2 mL/kg/h.

Children with burns greater than 10% BSA in a circumferential pattern, who are suspicious for abuse, or with burns associated with inhalational injury, explosions or fractures,

Infant Less Than 1 Year of Age

Name _____ Age _____ Ward _____

1st-degree erythema not to be included.

2nd-degree   3rd-degree

9½   9½
1½   1½
2   13   2   2   13   2
1½   1½   1½   1½
1¼   1¼   1¼   2   2   1¼
1   2   2
2¾   2¾   2¾   2¾
13   13
2½   2½   2½   2½
1¾   1¾   1¾   1¾

Variations From Adults Distribution in Infants and Children (in Percent).

	New-born	1 Year	5 Years	10 Years
Head	19	17	13	11
Both thighs	11	13	16	17
Both lower legs	10	10	11	12
Neck	2			
Anterior trunk	13			
Posterior trunk	13			
Both upper arms	8	These percentages		
Both lower arms	6	remain constant at		
Both hands	5	all ages		
Both buttocks	5			
Both feet	7			
Genitalia	1			
	100			

▲ **Figure 12–10.** Lund and Browder modification of Berkow scale for estimating extent of burns. (The table under the illustration is compiled from Berkow data.)

should be admitted. Additionally, admission is warranted for adequate pain control in a patient requiring parenteral analgesia. Burns greater than 20% BSA or full-thickness burns greater than 2% BSA should be admitted to a children's hospital or burn center. Children with subdermal burns require immediate hospitalization at a burn center under the care of a burn specialist.

▶ **Prognosis**

Outcome depends on many factors. Healing occurs with minimal damage to epidermis in superficial burns. In contrast, full-thickness burns will be hard, uneven, and fibrotic unless skin grafting is provided. In general, the greater the surface area and depth of burn injury, the greater the risk of long-term morbidity and mortality.

ELECTRICAL BURNS

Electrical injuries vary from exposure to low-voltage, high-voltage, or lightning strike source. Children electrocuted with household current (low-voltage injury) who are awake and alert at the time of medical evaluation are unlikely to have significant injury. An electrocardiogram (ECG) is not necessary but urinalysis should be considered for severe electrical injury as rhabdomyolysis may result. Brief contact with a high-voltage source results in a contact burn and is treated accordingly. Infants and toddlers may bite electric cords, resulting in burns to the commissure of the lips. A late complication is labial artery hemorrhage. If current passes through the body, the pattern of the injury depends on the path of the current. Exposure to high-voltage current often induces a "locking-on" effect due to alternating current causing tetany. Extensive nerve and muscle injury, fractures, and cardiac arrhythmias in addition to dermal burns are possible. Lightning strikes are more likely to induce asystole and blast trauma. These patients often have no obvious physical injuries, but can present in cardiopulmonary arrest.

Arbuthnot MK, Garcia AV: Early resuscitation and management of severe pediatric burns. Semin Pediatr Surg 2019 Feb;28(1): 73–78 [PMID: 30824139].

Lindford AJ, Lim P, Klass B, Mackey S, Dheansa BS, Gilbert PM: Resuscitation tables: a useful tool in calculating pre-burns unit fluid requirements. Emerg Med J 2009;26(4):245–249 [PMID: 19307382].

▼ DISORDERS DUE TO EXTREMES OF ENVIRONMENT

HEAT-RELATED ILLNESSES & HEAT STROKE

ESSENTIALS OF DIAGNOSIS & TYPICAL FEATURES

▶ Heat illness is a spectrum ranging from heat cramps to life-threatening heat stroke.

▶ A high index of suspicion is required to make the diagnosis given the lack of specific symptoms and a usually normal or only slightly elevated temperature.

Prevention

Avoid exposure to extremes of temperature for extended periods. Plan athletic activities for early morning or late afternoon and evening. Acclimatization, adequate water, shade, and rest periods can prevent heat-related illness.

Clinical Findings

Heat cramps are brief, severe cramps of skeletal or abdominal muscles following exertion. Core body temperature is normal or slightly elevated. Electrolyte disturbance is rare and mild: laboratory evaluation is not indicated.

Heat exhaustion includes multiple, vague constitutional symptoms following heat exposure. Patients continue to sweat and have varying degrees of sodium and water depletion. Core temperature should be monitored frequently but is often normal or slightly increased. Symptoms and signs include weakness, fatigue, headache, disorientation, pallor, thirst, nausea with or without vomiting, and occasionally muscle cramps without CNS dysfunction. Shock may be present.

Heat stroke is a life-threatening failure of thermoregulation. Diagnosis is based on a rectal temperature above 40.6°C with associated neurologic dysfunction in a patient with an exposure history. Although typically present, lack of sweating is not a necessary criterion. Symptoms are similar to those of heat exhaustion, but severe CNS dysfunction is a hallmark. Patients may be incoherent or combative. In severe cases, vomiting, shivering, coma, seizures, nuchal rigidity, and posturing may be present. Cellular hypoxia, enzyme dysfunction, and disrupted cell membranes lead to global end-organ derangements and patients may develop rhabdomyolysis, myocardial necrosis, electrolyte abnormalities, acute tubular necrosis and renal failure, hepatic degeneration, acute respiratory distress syndrome (ARDS), and disseminated intravascular coagulation (DIC).

Differential Diagnosis

Viral gastroenteritis, sepsis and other infectious processes, neuroleptic malignant syndrome, malignant hyperthermia, and anticholinergic poisoning may present similarly.

Treatment

Removal from the offending environment and removal of clothing are the first steps in managing any heat-related illness. **Heat cramps** typically respond to rest and rehydration with electrolyte solutions. Severe cramping and **heat exhaustion** should prompt evaluation of electrolytes to guide IV fluid rehydration.

Heat Stroke Management

1. Address the ABCs and administer 100% oxygen.
2. Place monitors, rectal temperature probe, Foley catheter and nasogastric tube.
3. Administer IV fluids: isotonic crystalloid for hypotension; cooled fluids are acceptable. Consider central venous pressure monitoring. Consider providing diazepam for patient comfort.
4. Once resuscitative efforts have begun, initiate active cooling: fanning/misting with cool water; ice application at neck, groin, and axillae. Discontinue active cooling measures once core temperature reaches 38°C to prevent shivering.
5. Order laboratory tests: CBC; electrolytes; glucose; creatinine; prothrombin time and partial thromboplastin time; creatine kinase; liver function tests; arterial blood gases; urinalysis; and serum calcium, magnesium, and phosphate.
6. Admit to the pediatric intensive care unit.

Prognosis

Full recovery is the rule for heat cramps and heat exhaustion. Patients with heat stroke are at risk of end-organ damage. However, even in this critically ill population, most children recover fully with intensive management. Prognostic indicators include initial temperature, duration of elevated temperature, and number of systems involved.

HYPOTHERMIA

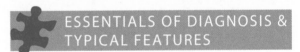

ESSENTIALS OF DIAGNOSIS & TYPICAL FEATURES

▶ Hypothermia is defined as a core temperature of less than 35°C.

▶ Children are at increased risk due to a greater BSA-weight ratio.

▶ In children, hypothermia is most commonly associated with water submersion.

Prevention

Given the high association with submersion injuries, children should be carefully monitored around water. Proper use of life vests is critical.

Clinical Findings

A. Signs and Symptoms

Hypothermia is defined as a core temperature of less than 35°C. In an attempt to maintain core temperature, peripheral vasoconstriction leads to cool, mottled skin. Shivering increases heat production to two to four times basal levels. As temperature falls, heart rate slows and mental status declines. Severe cases (< 28°C) mimic death: patients are pale or cyanotic, pupils may be fixed and dilated, muscles are rigid, and there may be no palpable pulses. Heart rates as low as 4–6 beats/min may provide adequate perfusion due to lowered metabolic needs in severe hypothermia. Besides cold exposure, disorders that cause incidental hypothermia include sepsis, metabolic derangements, ingestions, CNS disorders, and endocrinopathies. Neonates, trauma victims, intoxicated patients, and the chronically disabled are particularly at risk. Because hypothermia may be confused with postmortem changes, death is not pronounced until the patient has been rewarmed and remains unresponsive to resuscitative efforts.

B. Laboratory Findings

Standard evaluation includes CBC, electrolytes, creatinine, coagulation studies, and glucose and blood gas studies. Coagulopathy, hypoglycemia, and acidosis are common. However, correction of derangements is accomplished by rewarming and resuscitating the patient. Also consider toxicology screen depending on the clinical scenario.

C. Imaging Studies

Submersion is the most common cause of hypothermia. Chest x-ray should be performed to assess for pulmonary edema and/or aspiration. Other radiographic studies should be performed according to the history with special attention to potential head or skeletal trauma.

▶ Treatment

A. General Supportive Measures

Management of hypothermia is largely supportive. Administer warmed and humidified 100% oxygen. Continuously monitor core body temperature using a low-reading indwelling rectal thermometer. Handle patients gently as the hypothermic myocardium is exquisitely prone to arrhythmias. Ventricular fibrillation may occur spontaneously or as a result of minor handling or invasive procedures. If asystole or ventricular fibrillation is present on the cardiac monitor, perform chest compressions and use standard pediatric advanced life support techniques as indicated. Defibrillation and pharmacologic therapy (eg, epinephrine) are unlikely to be successful until core rewarming has occurred. Hypoglycemia should be corrected. Spontaneous reversion to sinus rhythm at 28–30°C may take place as rewarming proceeds.

B. Rewarming

Rewarming techniques are categorized as passive external, active external, or active core rewarming. Passive rewarming, such as removing wet clothing, covering with blankets, is appropriate only for mild cases (33–35°C). Active external rewarming methods include warming lights, thermal mattresses or electric warming blanket, and warm bath immersion. Be aware of potential core temperature depression

after rewarming has begun when vasodilation allows cooler peripheral blood to be distributed to the core circulation. This phenomenon is called *afterdrop*.

Active core rewarming techniques supplement active external warming for moderate to severe hypothermia. The techniques include warmed, humidified oxygen, warmed (to 40°C) crystalloid IV fluids, and warm peritoneal and pleural lavage. If available, ECMO is the preferred method for rewarming a severely hypothermic patient, as it stabilizes volume, electrolyte disturbances while being safest for the heart. Bladder and bowel irrigation are not generally effective because of low surface areas for temperature exchange.

▶ Prognosis

Recovery of the hypothermic victim is multifactorial. If associated with submersion injury (see next), CNS anoxic injuries and lung injury play a major role. Mortality rates are high and are related to the presence of underlying disorders and injuries. Children with a core temperature as low as 19°C have survived without neurologic compromise.

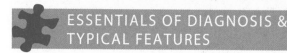

SUBMERSION INJURIES

ESSENTIALS OF DIAGNOSIS & TYPICAL FEATURES

▶ CNS and pulmonary injuries account for major morbidity.

▶ Child may appear well at presentation, but late CNS and pulmonary changes can occur hours later.

▶ Minimum observation period is 12–24 hours.

▶ Prevention

The World Health Organization defines *drowning* as the process of experiencing respiratory impairment from submersion/immersion in liquid. The terms *wet* or *dry drowning*, *near-drowning*, and others are no longer used; nonfatal drowning describes survivors. Water hazards are ubiquitous; even toilets, buckets, and washing machines pose a threat. Risk factors include epilepsy, alcohol, and lack of supervision. Males predominate in submersion deaths. Prevention strategies include protective fencing around public and private pools, use of life vests, avoiding swimming alone, and adequate supervision. Swim lessons may have a role in a comprehensive prevention strategy, even for children 1–4 years of age.

▶ Clinical Findings

A. Signs and Symptoms

Depending on the duration of submersion and any protective hypothermia effects, children may appear clinically dead or completely normal. Major morbidity stems from CNS and pulmonary insult. Cough, nasal flaring, grunting, retractions, wheezes or other lung sounds, and cyanosis are common. A child rewarmed to 33°C but who remains apneic and pulseless is unlikely to survive to discharge or will have severe neurologic deficits. Until a determination of brain death can be made, however, aggressive resuscitation should continue in a patient with return of circulation. Cardiovascular changes include myocardial depression and arrhythmias. Children may develop ARDS.

B. Laboratory Findings

Electrolyte alterations are generally negligible. Unless hemolysis occurs, hemoglobin concentrations change only slightly. Blood gas will show hypoxemia and acidosis.

C. Imaging Studies

Chest radiographs may be normal or may show signs of pulmonary edema. CT of the brain is warranted when the patient is comatose or believed to have suffered prolonged asphyxia or blunt head trauma. Consider cervical spine injury in teens where diving or intoxication may be involved.

▶ Treatment

Care is supportive. Correct hypothermia and treat symptomatically. For children who appear well initially, observe for 12–24 hours for late pulmonary or neurologic compromise. Respiratory distress, an abnormal chest radiograph, abnormal arterial blood gases, or hypoxemia by pulse oximetry require maximal supplemental oxygen, cardiopulmonary monitoring, and frequent reassessment. There is little evidence for use of surfactant following drowning.

▶ Prognosis

Anoxia from laryngospasm or aspiration leads to irreversible CNS damage after only 4–6 minutes. A child must fall through ice or directly into icy water for cerebral metabolism to be slowed sufficiently by hypothermia to provide protection from anoxia. Survival of the drowning victim depends on the duration of anoxia and the degree of lung injury. Children experiencing brief submersion with effective, high-quality resuscitation are likely to recover without sequelae. Children presenting asystolic are unlikely to survive.

AAP: https://www.aap.org/en-us/advocacy-and-policy/aap-health-initiatives/healthy-child-care/Pages/Safety-and-Injury-Prevention.aspx. Accessed June 30, 2019.

Brenner RA et al: Association between swimming lessons and drowning in childhood: a case-control study. Arch Pediatr Adolesc Med 2009;163(3):203–210 [PMID: 19255386].

Safety and Injury Prevention. CDC https://www.cdc.gov/safechild/index.html.

Weiss J: American Academy of Pediatrics Committee on Injury, Violence, and Poison prevention: Technical report—prevention of drowning. Pediatrics 2010;126(1):e253–e262 [PMID: 20498167].

▼ LACERATIONS

ESSENTIALS OF DIAGNOSIS & TYPICAL FEATURES

▶ The basic objectives of wound management are to stop bleeding, prevent infection, and ensure wound healing that achieves optimal functional and cosmetic outcomes.

▶ Options for wound closure include staples, sutures, and tissue adhesives.

Lacerations are a common reason to visit an ED. Lacerations can range from minor cuts that require no repair to complex lacerations that may require surgical consultation for adequate repair. The goals of laceration repair are to stop ongoing bleeding, prevent infection, and ensure wound healing that achieves optimal functional and cosmetic outcomes. Technical instruction of laceration repair is beyond the scope of this text as we present the basics of laceration wound care.

▶ Clinical Findings

A. Signs and Symptoms

Lacerations present in a variety of shapes and sizes and occur over all parts of the body. Patients may present immediately after the injury or several days later. Wounds may contain foreign material, involve muscular, vascular, bony, tendon/ligamentous structures, or extend into joint spaces.

Options for wound repair include staples, suture material (both absorbable and nonabsorbable), and tissue adhesives. Tissue adhesives should *never* be used for highly contaminated wounds (eg, bites).

B. Imaging Studies

Imaging is usually not indicated for simple lacerations; however, plain x-rays may be indicated in certain situations. Lacerations caused by penetrating or crush injury may be associated with fractures. Lacerations across joints require specific evaluation for penetration of the joint space. Foreign bodies may be present in wounds and therefore careful attention must be made to assess complete removal when present.

Treatment

Obtain information regarding mechanism and age of the injury. Assess extent of the wound with identification of foreign bodies, neurovascular compromise, tendon/ligament damage, muscle, or joint involvement. Obtain appropriate surgical consultations as needed.

Provide adequate analgesia or anesthesia, using topical or injectable methods prior to wound care. Irrigate the wound using normal saline (tap water is an appropriate alternative) with high pressure (5–8 psi [pounds per square inch]). Debride devitalized tissue, remove foreign material, and then close wound using staples, sutures, or tissue adhesive. Antibiotic ointment may be applied after wound repair. Consider tetanus prophylaxis depending on immunization status. Patients should return as instructed to have suture material removed if needed (Table 12–5).

Prognosis

Functional and aesthetically pleasing cosmetics is generally achieved with initial repair. Complex lacerations may involve multiple visits with surgical service for wound reconstruction.

Harman S et al: Efficacy of pain control with topical lidocaine-epinephrine-tetracaine during laceration repair with tissue adhesive in children: a randomized controlled trial. CMAJ 2013;185(13):E626–E634 [PMID: 23897942].

Navanandan N, Renna-Rodriguez M, DiStefano M: Pearls in pediatric wound management. Clin Pediatr Emerg Med 2017 March;18(1):53–61.

Trott A: Wounds and lacerations: emergency care and closure. Philadelphia, PA: Mosby INC; 2005.

Weiss EA et al: Water is a safe and effective alternative to sterile normal saline for wound irrigation prior to suturing, a prospective, double-blind, randomized, controlled clinical trial. BMJ Open 2013;16:3(1) [PMID: 23325896].

Table 12–5. Timing of suture removal.

Area of Body	Number of Days
Face	3–4
Neck	5–6
Scalp	6–7
Chest or abdomen	7
Arms and backs of hands	7
Legs and tops of feet	10
Back	10
Palms of hands or soles of feet	14

ANIMAL & HUMAN BITES

Bites account for a large number of visits to the ED. Most fatalities are due to dog bites. Human and cat bites cause the majority of infected bite wounds.

DOG BITES

Prevention

Boys are bitten more often than girls. The dog is known by the victim in most cases. Younger children have a higher incidence of head and neck wounds, whereas school-age children are bitten most often on the upper extremities. Children should be taught to not taunt dogs or approach dogs that are eating, sleeping, or are unknown to them.

Clinical Findings

A. Signs and Symptoms

Dogs may cause abrasions, lacerations, and puncture wounds. Larger dogs may tear skin, subcutaneous tissue, and muscle, or even cause fractures. Other signs and symptoms are related to the structures injured.

B. Imaging Studies

Bites caused by large dogs associated with significant crush injury may be associated with fractures. Dislodged teeth may also be present in the wound. Plain x-rays may be indicated.

Treatment

Provide appropriate analgesia or anesthesia before starting wound care. Debride any devitalized tissue and remove foreign matter. Irrigate using normal saline with high pressure (> 5 psi) and volume (> 1 L). Consider tetanus prophylaxis depending on immunization status. Rabies risk is low among dogs in developed countries; prophylaxis is rarely indicated. Suture wounds only if necessary for cosmesis as closure increases the risk of infection. **Do not use tissue adhesives due to risk of infection.** Prophylactic antibiotics do not decrease infection rates in low-risk dog bites, except those involving the hands and feet. Bites involving a tendon, joint, periosteum, or associated with fracture require prompt orthopedic surgery consultation.

Pasteurella canis and *Pasteurella multocida*, streptococci, staphylococci, and anaerobes may infect dog bites. Broad-spectrum coverage with amoxicillin and clavulanic acid is first-line therapy.

Complications

Complications of dog bites include scarring, skin infections, CNS infections, septic arthritis, osteomyelitis, endocarditis, sepsis, and posttraumatic stress.

CAT BITES

▶ Prevention

Cat-inflicted wounds occur more frequently in girls. The principal complication is infection, and the risk is higher compared to dog bites as cat bites produce a puncture wound. Children should be observed closely when playing with kittens or cats.

▶ Clinical Findings

A. Signs and Symptoms

Cat bites typically result in abrasions and puncture wounds. Within 12 hours, untreated bites may result in cellulitis or, when involving the hand, tenosynovitis and septic arthritis. Other signs and symptoms are related to the structures injured. Cat scratch disease (CSD) can occur after bites or scratches especially from kittens. Local findings include a papule, vesicle, or pustule at the site of inoculation. The hallmark of CSD is regional lymphadenitis. See Chapter 42 for a detailed discussion of CSD.

B. Laboratory Findings

Serologic tests for *Bartonella henselae* are available when cat scratch is suspected. C-reactive protein and erythrocyte sedimentation rate may be useful to monitor treatment response in infected cat bites.

▶ Complications

Cellulitis, tenosynovitis, and septic arthritis are important potential complications of cat bites. Systemic illness is rare.

▶ Treatment

Management is similar to that for dog bites. Provide appropriate analgesia or anesthesia before starting wound care. Debride any devitalized tissue and remove foreign matter. With isolated puncture wounds, high-pressure irrigation is contraindicated as it may force bacteria deeper into the tissue. Although controversial, soaking puncture wounds in an antiseptic solution (eg, dilute povidone-iodine) solution for 15 minutes is an accepted method to cleanse puncture wounds. Some experts recommend the practice to promote wound healing while others report delayed wound healing.

Alternatively, the wound may be soaked in dilute povidone-iodine solution for 15 minutes. Consider tetanus prophylaxis in the under- or unimmunized. As with dogs, rabies risk is low in developed countries and prophylaxis is rarely indicated. Cat bites should *not* be closed except when absolutely necessary for cosmesis.

P multocida is the most common pathogen. Prophylactic antibiotics are recommended. First-line treatment is amoxicillin and clavulanic acid. The dosage of the amoxicillin component should be 80 mg/kg/24 h in three divided doses. The maximum dosage is 2 g/24 h. Strongly consider admission and parenteral antibiotics for infected wounds on the hands and feet.

HUMAN BITES

Most infected human bites occur during fights when a clenched fist strikes bared teeth. Pathogens most commonly include streptococci, staphylococci, anaerobes, and *Eikenella corrodens*. Hand wounds and deep wounds should be treated with antibiotic prophylaxis against *E corrodens* and gram-positive pathogens with a penicillinase-resistant antibiotic (amoxicillin with clavulanic acid). Wound management is the same as for dog bites. Only severe lacerations involving the face should be sutured. Other wounds can be managed by delayed primary closure or healing by secondary intention. A major complication of human bite wounds is infection of the metacarpophalangeal joints. A hand surgeon should evaluate clenched-fist injuries from human bites if extensor tendon injury is identified or joint involvement is suspected.

Halaas GW: Management of foreign bodies in the skin. Am Fam Physician 2007;76(5):683 [PMID: 17894138].

▼ PAIN MANAGEMENT & PROCEDURAL SEDATION

Relief of pain and anxiety is paramount in providing care to pediatric patients and should be assessed and managed at all times. Parenteral agents are effective, safe, and produce few side effects if used judiciously. Intranasal administration of several sedative and narcotic medications is now an accepted route of administration and may omit the need for IV placement. Many agents also have amnestic properties. Refer to Chapter 32 for more information on typical analgesic medications used in pediatric emergency care.

Procedures such as fracture reduction, laceration repair, burn care, sexual assault examinations, abscess incision and drainage, lumbar puncture, and diagnostic procedures such as CT and magnetic resonance imaging may all be performed more effectively and compassionately if effective analgesia, anxiolysis or sedation is used. The clinician should decide whether procedures will require analgesia, anxiolysis, sedation, or a combination of methods.

Safe and effective sedation requires thorough knowledge of the selected agent and its side effects, as well as suitable monitoring devices, resuscitative medications, equipment, and personnel. The decision to perform procedural sedation and analgesia (PSA) must be patient-oriented and tailored to specific procedural needs, while ensuring the child's safety throughout the procedure. In order to successfully complete this task, a thorough preprocedural assessment should be completed, including a directed history and physical examination. Risks, benefits, and limitations of the procedure should be discussed with the parent or guardian and informed; verbal consent must be obtained PSA goals in the ED setting usually involve minimal or moderate sedation. Minimal sedation is a state in which the patient's sensorium is dulled, but he or she is still responsive to verbal stimuli. Moderate sedation is a depression of consciousness in which the child responds to tactile stimuli. In both cases, airway reflexes are preserved. It is important to remember that sedation is a continuum and the child may drift to deeper, unintended levels of sedation. Ensure appropriate resuscitative equipment and personnel are readily available when providing analgesia, anxiolysis, and sedation.

American Academy of Pediatrics; American Academy of Pediatric Dentistry; Coté CJ et al: Guidelines for monitoring and management of pediatric patients during and after sedation for diagnostic and therapeutic procedures: an update. Paediatr Anaesth 2008;18(1):9–10 [PMID: 18095958].

Couloures KG et al: Impact of provider specialty on pediatric procedural sedation complication rates. Pediatrics 2011;127(5): e1154–e1160 [PMID: 21518718].

Gozal D, Gozal Y: Pediatric sedation/anesthesia outside the operating room. Curr Opin Anaesthesiol 2008;21(4):494–498 [PMID: 18660660].

Hartling L et al: What works and what's safe in pediatric emergency procedural sedation: an overview of reviews. Acad Emerg Med 2016 May;23(5):519–530. doi: 10.1111/acem.12938. Epub 2016 Apr 24. Review [PMID: 26858095].

Krauss B, Green SM: Procedural sedation and analgesia in children. Lancet 2006;367:766 [PMID: 16517277].

Ryan PM, Kienstra AJ, Cosgrove P, Vezzetti R, Wilkinson M: Safety and effectiveness of intranasal midazolam and fentanyl use in combination in the pediatric emergency department. Am J Emerg Med 2019 Feb;37(2):237–240. Epub 2018 May 17 [PMID: 30146398].

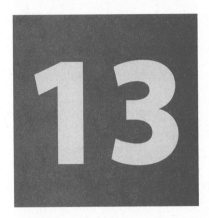

Poisoning

George Sam Wang, MD

Barry H. Rumack, MD

Richard C. Dart, MD, PhD

INTRODUCTION

Accidental and intentional exposures to toxic substances occur in children of all ages. Children younger than 6 years are primarily involved in accidental exposures, with the peak incidence in 2-year-olds. Of the more than 2 million exposures reported by the American Association of Poison Control Centers' National Poison Data System in 2017, almost 60% of exposures occurred in those younger than 20 years: 45% in children aged 5 years and younger, 6% aged 6–12 years, and 8% aged 13–19 years. Fortunately, young children's exposures are typically unintentional and of the low dose or volume type. They can be exposed to intentional poisoning through the actions of parents or caregivers and involvement of child abuse specialists is helpful in these cases (see Chapter 8). Substance abuse and intentional ingestions account for most exposures in the adolescent population. In some locales, small-scale industrial or manufacturing processes may be associated with homes and farms, and exposures to hazardous substances should be considered in the history.

Pediatric patients also have special considerations pertaining to nonpharmaceutical toxicologic exposures. Their shorter stature places them lower to the ground as well as the fact that many are crawling, and some gas and vapor exposures will gather closer to the ground. They may have a greater inhalational exposure due to their higher minute ventilation. They may not be physically mature enough to remove themselves from exposures. They also have a large body surface area to weight ratio making them vulnerable to topical exposures and hypothermia.

Gummin DD et al: 2017 Annual Report of the American Association of Poison Control Centers' National Poison Data System (NPDS): 35th Annual Report. Clin Toxicol (Phila) 2018 Dec;56(13): 1213–1415. doi:10.1080/15563650.2018.1533727 [PMID: 30576252].

PHARMACOLOGIC PRINCIPLES OF TOXICOLOGY

In the evaluation of the poisoned patient, it is important to compare the anticipated pharmacologic or toxic effects with the patient's clinical presentation. If the history is that the patient ingested a sedative 30 minutes ago, but the clinical examination reveals dilated pupils, tachycardia, dry mouth, absent bowel sounds, and active hallucinations—clearly anticholinergic toxicity—diagnosis and therapy should proceed accordingly. In addition, standard pharmacokinetics (absorption, distribution, metabolism, and elimination) often cannot be applied in the setting of a large dose, since these parameters have been extrapolated from healthy volunteers receiving therapeutic doses.

Absorption

Depending on the route, absorption rates can vary in general, intravenous/intra-arterial > inhalation > sublingual > intramuscular > subcutaneous > intranasal > oral > rectal > dermal. Large overdoses, hypotension, and decreased gut mobility are the factors that can delay absorption.

Elimination Half-Life

The $t_{1/2}$ of an agent must be interpreted carefully. Most published $t_{1/2}$ values are for therapeutic dosages. The $t_{1/2}$ may increase as the quantity of the ingested substance increases for many common intoxicants such as salicylates. For example, one cannot rely on the published $t_{1/2}$ for salicylate (2 hours) to assume rapid elimination of the drug. In an acute salicylate overdose (150 mg/kg), the apparent $t_{1/2}$ is prolonged to 24–30 hours. Calculation formula for first-order drugs: $T\ 1/2 = \ln(2)/Ke$ and $Ke = \ln CP1 - \ln CP2/t2 - t1$.

Volume of Distribution

The volume of distribution (Vd) of a drug is determined by dividing the amount of drug absorbed by the blood level. With aspirin for example, the Vd is 150–170 mL/kg body weight, or 10 L in an average adult. In contrast, digoxin distributes well beyond total body water. Because the calculation produces a volume above body weight, this figure is referred to as an "apparent volume of distribution."

Body Burden

Body burden represents the total amount of drug or toxin within the body and may be useful to determine the dose absorbed from an ingestion. For example, a 20-kg child with an acetaminophen blood level of 200 mcg/mL (200 mg/L) would have a body burden of 4000 mg of acetaminophen. This is ascertained by taking the volume of distribution of 1 L times the weight of the child times the blood level in milligram per liter. This would be consistent with an overdose history of having consumed eight extra strength 500-mg tablets but would not be consistent with a history of therapeutic administration of 15 mg/kg for four doses. Such a therapeutic administration would have a maximum administered dose of 1200 mg (20 kg times 15 mg/kg times four doses), which is well under the calculated body burden. Given metabolism of the drug with a normal half-life of 2 hours, it is apparent that much of the first doses would have been metabolized further showing that the dose was not a therapeutic dose. Formula for body burden by patient weight: Dose = Vd*Cp*W, where Vd is the volume of distribution, Cp is the plasma level, and W is the weight in kilograms.

Metabolism & Excretion

The route of excretion or detoxification is important for planning treatment, usually the liver and kidneys. Newborns and toddlers can have low Cytochrome P450 enzyme activity. Methanol, for example, is metabolized to the toxic product, formic acid. This metabolic step may be blocked by the antidote fomepizole or ethanol and patients with renal failure may not eliminate methanol as readily.

Blood Concentrations

Care of the poisoned patient should never be guided solely by laboratory measurements. Concentration results may not return in time to influence acute management. Initial treatment should be directed at symptomatic and supportive care, guided by the clinical presentation, followed by more specific therapy based on laboratory determinations. Clinical information may speed the identification of a toxic agent by the laboratory. CAUTION: Many laboratories report a normal range. When an overdose has occurred several hours earlier than peak times the lab may report a level that is within the normal range such as for aspirin and acetaminophen. It is important to look at the timing as well as signs and symptoms when an overdose is considered.

PREVENTING CHILDHOOD POISONINGS

Inclusion of poison prevention as part of routine well-child care should begin at the 6-month well-baby visit. The poison prevention handout included as Table 13–1 may be copied and distributed to parents. It contains poison prevention information as well as first-aid actions that should be taken in the event of an exposure. All poison control centers in the United States can be reached by dialing 1-800-222-1222; the call will be automatically routed to the correct regional center.

GENERAL TREATMENT OF POISONING

INITIAL TELEPHONE CONTACT

Basic information obtained at the first telephone contact includes the patient's demographics; the agent and amount of agent ingested; location; exposure; the patient's present condition; and the time elapsed since the exposure. Other pertinent information includes the product ingredients, and potential maximum amounts of the drug or chemical involved. An emergency exists if the ingestant is high risk (caustic solutions, hydrogen fluoride, drugs of abuse, or medications such as a calcium channel blocker, opioid, hypoglycemic agent, or antidepressant, supratherapeutic dose) or if the self-poisoning was intentional. If immediate danger does not exist, obtain more details about the suspected toxic agent. If the specific substance is not identified it is important that the surroundings be searched for possible containers or other clues. Poison control centers (1-800-222-1222) are the source of expert telephone advice and have excellent follow-up programs to manage patients in the home as well as provide further poison prevention information.

Obtaining Information About Poisons

Current data on ingredients of commercial products and medications can be obtained from a certified regional poison center. It is important to have the actual container at hand when calling. Safety data sheets (SDSs) can be helpful in providing product ingredient and concentration information. Caution: Antidote information on labels of commercial products or in the *Physicians' Desk Reference* may be incorrect or inappropriate. Many resources found on the Internet are inaccurate.

Table 13-1. Poison prevention and emergency treatment handout.

Poison safety tips
If you or your child has come in contact with poison, call the Poison Center (1-800-222-1222). Poison Information Specialists (typically nurses and pharmacists) will answer your call. In most cases, they can help you take care of the problem right at home. When you need to get to the hospital, they will call ahead with detailed information to help doctors treat you or your child quickly and correctly.

How people get poisoned
People can breathe poison, eat or drink it, or get it on the skin or in the eyes. You probably know that antifreeze, bleach, and bug spray are poisonous. But did you know that vitamins, perfume, and makeup can be dangerous? Eating some plants can be toxic. Some spider bites can be dangerous. Taking medicine that is too old or not prescribed for you can make you sick. Also, mixing different kinds of medicine can be dangerous.

Poison safety "do's" and "don'ts"	
DO:	**DON'T:**
1. Ask for "safety-lock" tops on all prescription drugs.	1. Don't store food and household cleaners together.
2. Keep cleaners, bug sprays, medicines, and other harmful products out of the reach and sight of children. If possible, keep the products locked up.	2. Don't take medicine in front of children; children love to imitate "mommy" and "daddy."
3. Store medicine in original containers.	3. Don't call medicine candy.
4. Read the label before taking medicine; don't take medicine that doesn't have a label.	4. Don't take medicine that is not for you. Never take medicine in the dark.
5. Follow the directions for all products.	5. Don't put gasoline, bug spray, antifreeze, or cleaning supplies in soft-drink bottles, cups, or bowls. Always keep them in their original containers.

Kids can get into things at any age!	
Children aged 0-6 mo	**Children aged 1-3 y**
Learn to roll over and reach for things.	Have the highest accident rate of any group.
Learn about their environment by putting things in their mouths.	Begin to imitate parents and other adults.
Children aged 7-12 mo	Put things in their mouths.
Start to get curious and explore.	Start to climb on things.
Learn to crawl, pull up to stand, and walk holding on.	
Put everything in their mouths.	
Pull things down.	

Different dangers at different times of the year	
Spring and summer dangers	**Fall and winter dangers**
Pesticides	Antifreeze
Fertilizers	Carbon monoxide
Outdoor plants and mushrooms	Black widow spider bites
Snake, spider, and other insect bites	Plants and autumn berries
Bee stings	Holly, mistletoe, and other holiday decorations
Ticks	
Charcoal lighter fluid	

Follow this checklist to make sure your home is safe
Kitchen
—Remove products like detergent, drain cleaner, and dishwashing liquid from under the sink.

(Continued)

Table 13–1. Poison prevention and emergency treatment handout. (*Continued*)

—Remove medicines from counters, tables, refrigerator top, or window sills.

—Put child safety latches on all drawers and cabinets that contain harmful products.

—Store harmful products away from food.

Bathroom

—Regularly clean out your medicine cabinet. **Do not** flush medicines down the toilet. Contact a pharmacy to see if they have a take-back program. If a take-back program is not available, then follow disposal advice recommended by your local health department or the FDA. (https://www.fda.gov/consumers/consumer-updates/where-and-how-dispose-unused-medicines)

—Keep all medicine in original safety-top containers.

—Keep medicine, hair spray, powder, makeup, fingernail polish, hair-care products, and mouthwash out of reach.

Bedroom

—Don't keep medicine in or on dresser or bedside table.

—Keep perfume, makeup, aftershave, and other products out of reach.

Laundry Area

—Keep bleach, soap, fabric softener, starch, and other supplies out of reach.

—Keep all products in their original containers.

Garage/Basement

—Keep bug spray, weed killers, gasoline, oil, paint, and other supplies in locked area.

—Keep all products in their original containers.

General household

—Keep beer, wine, and liquor out of reach.

—Keep ashtrays clean and out of reach.

—Keep plants out of reach.

—Keep paint in good repair.

Emergency action in case your child . . .

Breathes poison

Get child to fresh air right away. Open doors and windows. Always call the Poison Center.

Gets poison on the skin

Remove clothes that have poison on them. Rinse skin with lukewarm water for 10 minutes. Wash gently with soap and water and rinse. Always call the Poison Center.

Gets poison in the eye

Gently pour lukewarm water over the eye from a large glass 2 or 3 inches from the eye or with their face in the shower Repeat for 15 minutes. Have child blink as much as possible while pouring water in the eye. Do not force the eyelid open. Always call the Poison Center. Do not use eye drops without advice from a health care professional.

Swallows poison (Medicines, chemicals, or household products)

Do NOT induce vomiting or administer anything to the child. Call 911 if the child unconscious, seizing, or having difficulty breathing. Otherwise call the Poison Center for further directions.

Pediatrician: _____ (Tel): _____

National Toll Free Number which connects with your local Poison Center: **1-800-222-1222**

Information adapted from, and used, courtesy of the Rocky Mountain Poison Center, Denver Health and Hospital Authority, Denver, CO.

INITIAL EMERGENCY DEPARTMENT CONTACT

Address Initial Resuscitation Evaluation

As in all emergencies, the principles of treatment are attention to Pediatric Advance Life Support algorithms in resuscitation: circulation, airway, and breathing. The most important treatment in toxicological exposures is symptomatic and supportive care.

Treat Burns & Skin Exposures

Burns may occur following exposure to strongly acidic or strongly alkaline agents or petroleum distillates, and should be decontaminated by flooding with sterile saline solution or water. A burn unit should be consulted if more than minimal burn damage has been sustained. Skin decontamination should be performed in a patient with cutaneous exposure. Emergency department personnel in contact with a patient who has been contaminated (eg, with an organophosphate insecticide) should themselves be decontaminated if their skin or clothing becomes contaminated. Ocular exposures can initially be decontaminated at home by placing the child in the shower allowing the water to indirectly flow from the top of the head into the eyes. Otherwise, irrigation with assessment of pH should be performed in the emergency department.

Take a Pertinent History

The history should be taken from the parent/caregiver and all individuals present at the scene. It may be crucial to determine all of the kinds of poisons in the home. These may include drugs used by family members and their medical histories, dietary or herbal supplements, foreign medications, chemicals associated with the hobbies or occupations of family members, or the purity of the water supply.

DEFINITIVE THERAPY OF POISONING

Prevention of Absorption

A. Emesis and Lavage

These measures are rarely used in pediatric patients and have their own associated risk. They should not be used routinely in the management of poisonings and should be performed only in consultation with a poison center or medical toxicologist.

B. Charcoal

The routine use of charcoal has decreased substantially in recent years, especially in unintentional pediatric ingestions where lick, sip, taste ingestions are rarely dangerous. Charcoal can be considered in patients who are awake, alert, and able to drink it voluntarily, but it should not be routinely administered to all poisoned patients. It should never be given to patients with altered sensorium who are unable to protect their airway due to risk of aspiration. It is not recommended in ingestions of heavy metals, hydrocarbons, caustics, and solvent ingestions. The dose of charcoal is 1–2 g/kg (maximum, 100 g) per dose. Repeating the dose of activated charcoal may be useful for those agents that slow passage through the gastrointestinal (GI) tract, but repeated doses of sorbitol or saline cathartics must not be given. Repeated doses of cathartics may cause electrolyte imbalances and fluid loss. Charcoal dosing may be repeated every 4–6 hours until charcoal is passed through the rectum.

C. Catharsis

Cathartics do not improve outcome and should be avoided.

D. Whole Bowel Lavage (or Irrigation)

Whole bowel lavage uses an orally administered, nonabsorbable hypertonic solution such as CoLyte or GoLYTELY. The effectiveness of this procedure in poisoned patients remains controversial. Preliminary recommendations for use of whole bowel irrigation include poisoning with sustained-release preparations, mechanical movement of items through the bowel (eg, drug packets, iron tablets, lead foreign bodies), and poisoning with substances that are poorly absorbed by charcoal (eg, lithium, iron). Underlying bowel pathology and intestinal obstruction are relative contraindications to its use. Consultation with a certified regional poison center is recommended.

American Academy of Clinical Toxicology; European Association of Poisons Centers and Clinical Toxicologists: Position statement and practice guidelines on the use of multi-dose activated charcoal in the treatment of acute poisoning. J Toxicol Clin Toxicol 1999;37:731 [PMID: 10584586].

Benson et al: Poison paper update: gastric lavage. Clin Toxicol 2013 Mar;51(3):140–146 [PMID: 23418938].

Chyka PA et al: Position paper: single-dose activated charcoal. American Academy of Clinical Toxicology; European Association of Poison Centres and Clinical Toxicologists. Clin Toxicol (Phila) 2005;43:61 [PMID: 15822758].

Hojer et al: Position paper update: ipecac syrup for gastrointestinal decontamination. Clin Toxicol 2013 Mar;15(3):134–139 [PMID: 23406298].

Thanacoody R et al: Position paper update: whole bowel irrigation for gastrointestinal decontamination of overdose patients. Clin Toxicol (Phila) Jan 2015;53(1):5–12. doi: 10.3109/15563650.2014.989326 [PMID: 25511637].

Enhancement of Excretion

Excretion of certain substances can be hastened by urinary alkalinization or dialysis and is reserved for special circumstances.

A. Urinary Alkalinization

1. Alkaline diuresis—Urinary alkalinization should be chosen on the basis of the substance's pK_a, so that ionized drug will be trapped in the tubular lumen and not reabsorbed (see Table 13–1). Thus, if the pK_a is less than 7.5, urinary alkalinization is appropriate; if it is over 8.0, this technique is not usually beneficial. The pK_a is sometimes included along with general drug information. Alkaline diuresis is mainly used for salicylate toxicity. Urinary alkalinization is achieved with sodium bicarbonate. It is important to observe for hypokalemia, caused by the shift of potassium intracellularly. If complications such as renal failure or pulmonary edema are present, hemodialysis or hemoperfusion may be required.

B. Dialysis

Hemodialysis is useful in the treatment of some poisons and in the general management of a critically ill patient. Characteristics of drugs amendable to dialysis include low molecular weight, low protein binding, and low volume of distribution. Continuous hemofiltration techniques may be used when hypotensive patients may not tolerate traditional hemodialysis; however, clearance rates will be slower. Dialysis should be considered part of supportive care if the patient satisfies any of the following criteria:

1. Potentially life-threatening toxicity that is caused by a dialyzable drug and cannot be treated by conservative means.

2. Renal failure or insufficiency.

3. Marked hyperosmolality or severe acid–base or electrolyte disturbances not responding to therapy.

▼ MANAGEMENT OF SPECIFIC COMMON POISONINGS

ACETAMINOPHEN (PARACETAMOL)

Overdosage of acetaminophen is common and can produce severe hepatotoxicity. Under than 0.1% of young children develop hepatotoxicity after acetaminophen overdose. In children, toxicity most commonly results from repeated overdosage arising from confusion about the age-appropriate dose, use of multiple products that contain acetaminophen or accidental large volume ingestion.

Acetaminophen is normally metabolized in the liver. A small percentage of the drug goes through a pathway leading to a toxic metabolite. Normally, this electrophilic reactant is removed harmlessly by conjugation with glutathione. In overdosage, the supply of glutathione becomes exhausted, and the metabolite may bind covalently to components of liver cells to produce necrosis.

▶ Treatment

Treatment is to administer acetylcysteine. It may be administered either orally or intravenously. Consultation on difficult cases may be obtained from your regional poison control center. The blood acetaminophen concentration should be obtained 4 hours after a single acute ingestion or as soon as possible thereafter and plotted on Figure 13–1. The nomogram is used only for acute ingestion, not repeated or unknown ingestions. Acetylcysteine is administered to patients whose acetaminophen levels plot in the toxic range on the nomogram. Acetylcysteine is effective even when given more than 24 hours after ingestion, although it is most effective when given within 8 hours post ingestion.

For children weighing 40 kg or more, IV acetylcysteine should be administered as a loading dose of 150 mg/kg administered over 15–60 min; followed by a second infusion of 50 mg/kg over 4 hours, and then a third infusion of 100 mg/kg over 16 hours.

For patients weighing less than 40 kg, IV acetylcysteine must have less dilution to avoid hyponatremia (a dosage calculator is also available at http://www.acetadote.com) (Table 13–2). Patient-tailored therapy is critical when utilizing the IV "20-hour" protocol and those patients who still have acetaminophen measurable and/or elevated aspartate transaminase/alanine transaminase (AST/ALT) may need treatment beyond the 20 hours called for in the product insert. There is now evidence that a 2-bag infusion method of administering acetylcysteine may decrease associated adverse events, including flushing, vomiting and anaphylactoid reactions in addition to decreasing associated medication errors. This is administered as a 200 mg/kg IV bolus over 4 hours, followed by 100 mg/kg over 16 hours.

The oral form of acetylcysteine can also be given and is equally efficacious as intravenous. Consult your regional poison center for dosing recommendations.

AST–serum glutamic oxaloacetic transaminase (AST–SGOT), ALT–serum glutamic pyruvic transaminase (ALT–SGPT), serum bilirubin, and plasma prothrombin time should be followed daily. Significant abnormalities of liver function may not peak until 72–96 hours after ingestion.

Dart RC, Rumack BH: Patient-tailored acetylcysteine administration. Ann Emerg Med 2007;50:280–281 [PMID: 17418449].

Hoyte C, Dart RC: Transition to two-bag intravenous acetylcysteine for acetaminophen overdose: a poison center's experience. Clin Toxicol (Phila) 2019 Jan 28:1–2. doi: 10.1080/15563650.2018.1510127 [PMID: 30689437].

Rumack BH, Bateman DN: Acetaminophen and acetylcysteine dose and duration: past, present and future. Clin Toxicol (Phila) 2012 Feb;50(2):91–98. doi: 10.3109/15563650.2012.659252.22320209 [PMID: 22320209].

Schmidt LE et al: Fewer adverse effects associated with a modified two-bag intravenous acetylcysteine protocol compared to traditional three-bag regimen in paracetamol overdose. Clin Toxicol (Phila) 2018 May 24:1–7. doi: 10.1080/15563650.2018.1475672 [PMID: 29792347].

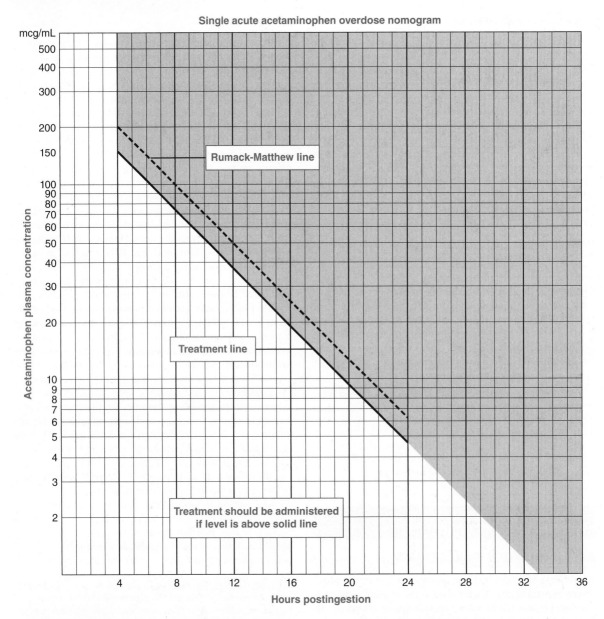

Single acute acetaminophen overdose nomogram

Rumack-Matthew line

Treatment line

Treatment should be administered
if level is above solid line

mcg/mL

Acetaminophen plasma concentration

Hours postingestion

Nomogram: Acetaminophen plasma concentration vs time after acetaminophen ingestion. The nomogram has been developed to estimate the probability of whether a plasma acetaminophen concentration in relation to the interval postingestion will result in hepatotoxicity and, therefore, whether acetylcysteine therapy should be administered.

Cautions for use of this chart:

1. Time coordinates refer to time postingestion.

2. Graph relates only to plasma concentrations following a single, acute overdose ingestion.

3. The Treatment line is plotted 25% below the Rumack-Matthew line to allow for potential errors in plasma acetaminophen assays and estimated time from ingestion of an overdose (Rumack et al. Arch Intern Med 1981;141(suppl):380–385).

▲ **Figure 13–1.** Semilogarithmic plot of plasma acetaminophen levels versus time. (Modified with permission from Rumack BH, Matthew H: Acetaminophen poisoning and toxicity. Pediatrics 1975 Jun;55(6):871–876.)

Table 13–2. Intravenous acetylcysteine administration dosing.

Body Weight		First 150 mg/kg in 5% Dextrose in 60 min		Second 50 mg/kg in 5% Dextrose in 4 h		Third 100 mg/kg in 5% Dextrose in 16 h	
(kg)	(lb)	Acetadote (mL)	Diluent (mL)	Acetadote (mL)	Diluent (mL)	Acetadote (mL)	Diluent (mL)
100	220	75	200	25	500	50	1000
90	198	67.5	200	22.5	500	45	1000
80	176	60	200	20	500	40	1000
70	154	52.5	200	17.5	500	35	1000
60	132	45	200	15	500	30	1000
50	110	37.5	200	12.5	500	25	1000
40	88	30	200	10	500	20	1000
30	66	22.5	100	7.5	250	15	500
25	55	18.75	100	6.25	250	12.5	500
20	44	15	60	5	140	10	280
15	33	11.25	45	3.75	105	7.5	210
10	22	7.5	30	2.5	70	5	140

ALCOHOL, ETHYL (ETHANOL)

Alcoholic beverages, tinctures, cosmetics, perfumes, mouth-washes, food extracts (vanilla, almond, etc), rubbing alcohol, and hand sanitizers are common sources of poisoning in children. Alcohol is even available in powdered form for mixing and consumption. In most states, alcohol levels of 50–80 mg/dL are considered compatible with impaired faculties, and levels of 80–100 mg/dL are considered evidence of intoxication. (Blood levels cited here are for adults; comparable figures for children are not available.)

Recent erroneous information regarding hand sanitizers has indicated that a "lick" following application on the hand could cause toxicity in children. In fact, this is not the case, but because these hand sanitizers contain 62% ethanol, toxicity following ingestion is possible. Potential blood ethanol concentration following consumption of a 62% solution in a 10-kg child is calculated as follows:

$$1 \text{ oz} = 30 \text{ mL} \times 62\% = 18.6 \text{ mL of pure ethanol}$$

$$18.6 \text{ mL} \times 0.79 \text{ (the specific gravity)}$$
$$= 14.7 \text{ g of ethanol, or } 14{,}700 \text{ mg}$$

In a patient weighing 10 kg, the distribution into total body water (Vd) will be 6 L—this is the amount of the body water into which the ethanol will be distributed.

$$14{,}700 \text{ mg} \div 6 \text{ L} = 2450 \text{ mg/L}$$
$$2450 \text{ mg/L} \div 10 = 245 \text{ mg/dL}$$

Based on these calculations, a 10-kg child consuming 0.5 oz would have a concentration of 122.5 mg/dL; a 20-kg child consuming 1 oz would have a concentration of 122.5 mg/dL; a 30-kg child consuming 1 oz would have a concentration of 81.7 mg/dL; and a 70-kg adult consuming 1 oz would have a concentration of 35 mg/dL.

One "pump" from a hand sanitizer bottle dispenses approximately 2.5 mL of the product. If ingested, this amount (containing 62% ethanol) would create a blood ethanol concentration as follows:

1. In a 10-kg child: 23.1 mg/dL.

2. In a 20-kg child: 11.6 mg/dL.

3. In a 30-kg child: 7.7 mg/dL.

Children show a change in sensorium with blood levels as low as 10–20 mg/dL, have higher risk for hypoglycemia than adults, and any child displaying such changes should be seen immediately. Complete absorption of alcohol requires 30 minutes to 6 hours, depending on the volume, the presence of food, and the time spent in consuming the alcohol. The rate of metabolic degradation is constant (about 20 mg/h in an adult). Absolute ethanol, 1 mL/kg, results in a peak blood level of about 100 mg/dL in 1 hour after ingestion.

▶ Treatment

Management of sedation, hypoglycemia and acidosis is usually the only measure required. Start an IV drip of D_5W or $D_{10}W$ if blood glucose is less than 60 mg/dL. Death is usually caused by respiratory failure. In severe cases, cerebral edema may occur and should be appropriately treated. Secondary evaluation for traumatic injury and coingestants should also be performed.

AMPHETAMINES & RELATED DRUGS (STIMULANTS, METHAMPHETAMINE, 3,4-METHYLENEDIOXY-*N*-METHYLAMPHETAMINE)

▶ Clinical Presentation

A. Acute Poisoning

Amphetamine, 3,4-methylenedioxy-*N*-methylamphetamine (MDMA), and methamphetamine poisoning is common because of the widespread availability of "diet pills" and the use of "ecstasy," "speed," "crank," "crystal," and "ice" by adolescents. (Care must be taken in the interpretation of slang terms because they have multiple meanings.) A new cause of stimulant poisoning is drugs for treating attention-deficit/hyperactivity disorder, such as methylphenidate. There are also newer designer drugs, synthetic cannabinoids ("spice, K2") and MPDV or mephedrone ("bath salts, plant food"), which cause effects similar to stimulants.

Symptoms include central nervous system (CNS) stimulation, anxiety, hyperactivity, hyperpyrexia, diaphoresis, hypertension, abdominal cramps, nausea and vomiting, and inability to void urine. MDMA has been associated with hyponatremia and seizures. Severe cases often include rhabdomyolysis and acidosis. A toxic psychosis indistinguishable from paranoid schizophrenia may occur. Methamphetamine laboratories in homes are a potential cause of childhood exposure to a variety of hazardous and toxic substances.

B. Chronic Poisoning

Chronic amphetamine users develop tolerance; more than 1500 mg of IV methamphetamine can be used daily. Hyperactivity, disorganization, and euphoria are followed by exhaustion, depression, and coma lasting 2–3 days. Heavy users, taking more than 100 mg/day, have restlessness, incoordination of thought, insomnia, nervousness, irritability, and visual hallucinations. Psychosis may be precipitated by the chronic administration of high doses. Chronic MDMA use can lead to serotonin depletion, which can manifest as depression, weakness, tremors, GI complaints, and suicidal thoughts.

▶ Treatment

The treatment of choice are benzodiazepines, such as lorazepam, titrated in increments to effect. Very large total doses may be needed. In cases of extreme agitation or hallucinations, droperidol (0.1 mg/kg per dose) or haloperidol (up to 0.1 mg/kg) parenterally has been used. Hyperthermia should be aggressively controlled. Chronic users may be withdrawn rapidly from amphetamines.

Carvalho M et al: Toxicity of amphetamines: an update. Arch Toxicol 2012;86(8):1167–1231 [PMID: 22392347].

Wang GS, Hoyte C: Novel drugs of abuse. Pediatr Rev 2019 Feb;40(2):71–78. doi: 10.1542/pir.2018-0050.

ANESTHETICS, LOCAL

Intoxication from local anesthetics may be associated with CNS stimulation, acidosis, delirium, ataxia, shock, convulsions, and death. Methemoglobinemia has been reported following local mouth or dental analgesia, typically with benzocaine or prilocaine. It has also been reported with use of topical preparations in infants. The maximum recommended dose for subcutaneous (SQ) infiltration of lidocaine is 4.5 mg/kg (Table 13–3). The temptation to exceed this dose in procedures lasting a long time is great and may result in inadvertent overdosage. Oral application of viscous lidocaine may produce toxicity, and the US FDA has published warnings against its use for teething.

Local anesthetics used in obstetrics cross the placental barrier and are not efficiently metabolized by the fetal liver. Mepivacaine, lidocaine, and bupivacaine can cause fetal bradycardia, neonatal depression, and death. Accidental injection of mepivacaine into the head of the fetus during paracervical anesthesia has caused neonatal asphyxia, cyanosis, acidosis, bradycardia, convulsions, and death.

▶ Treatment

If the anesthetic has been ingested, mucous membranes should be cleansed carefully, topical applications should be cleaned and irrigated. Oxygen administration is indicated, with assisted ventilation if necessary. Symptomatic methemoglobinemia is treated with methylene blue, 1%, 0.2 mL/kg (1–2 mg/kg per dose, IV) over 5–10 minutes; this should promptly relieve the cyanosis. Acidosis may be treated with sodium bicarbonate, hypotension with vasopressors, seizures with benzodiazepines, and bradycardia with atropine. In the event of cardiac arrest, 20% lipid (fat) emulsion therapy should be initiated. Initial 1.5 mL/kg bolus over 1 minute, followed by 0.25 mL/kg/min for up to 20–30 minutes until spontaneous circulation returns. Repeat bolus can be considered.

FDA Drug Safety Communication: http://www.fda.gov/Drugs/DrugSafety/ucm402240.htm. Accessed June 1, 2015.

Gosselin S et al: Evidence-based recommendations on the use of intravenous lipid emulsion therapy in poisoning. Clin Toxicol (Phila) 2016 Sep 8;1–25. doi: 10.1080/15563650.2016.1214275 [PMID: 27608281].

Levine M et al: Systematic review of the effect of intravenous lipid emulsion therapy for non-local anesthetics toxicity. Clin Toxicol (Phila) 2016 Mar;54(3):194–221. doi: 10.3109/15563650.2015.1126286 [PMID: 26852931].

Spiller HA et al: Multicenter retrospective evaluation of oral benzocaine exposure in children. Vet Hum Toxicol 2000;42:228 [PMID: 10928690].

Table 13–3. Pharmacologic properties of local anesthetics.

	pK$_a$	Protein Binding (%)	Relative Potency	Duration of Action	Approximate Maximum Allowable Subcutaneous Dose (mg/kg)
Esters					
Chloroprocaine	9.3	Unknown	Intermediate	Short	10
Cocaine	8.7	92	Low	Medium	3
Procaine	9.1	5	Low	Short	10
Tetracaine	8.4	76	High	Long	3
Amides					
Bupivacaine	8.1	95	High	Long	2
Etidocaine	7.9	95	High	Long	4
Lidocaine	7.8	70	Low	Medium	4.5
Mepivacaine	7.9	75	Intermediate	Medium	4.5
Prilocaine	8.0	40	Intermediate	Medium	8
Ropivacaine	8.2	95	Intermediate	Long	3

Reproduced with permission from Nelson LS, Lewin NA, Howland MA, et al: *Goldfrank's Toxicologic Emergencies*, 9th ed. New York, NY: McGraw Hill; 2011.

ANTIHISTAMINES & COUGH & COLD PREPARATIONS

The use of cough and cold preparations in young children has recently been called into question due to potential toxicity. Medications included in this area are antihistamine (brompheniramine, chlorpheniramine, diphenhydramine, doxylamine), antitussive (dextromethorphan), expectorant (guaifenesin), and decongestant (pseudoephedrine, phenylephrine). In 2007, manufacturers voluntarily removed preparations intended for use in children younger than 4 years of age from the market. Most adverse events stem from unintentional ingestions of supratherapeutic doses of antihistamines or dextromethorphan. A high proportion of life threatening cases are associated with child abuse (sedating a child with medication). Considerable controversy remains as to the toxicity of these medications if they are used according to labeled directions and an evaluation of the cases on file at FDA stated, "In the cases judged to be therapeutic intent or unknown intent, several factors appeared to contribute to the administration of an overdosage: administration of two medicines containing the same ingredients, failure to use a measuring device, use of wrong units (mL vs teaspoon), use of an adult product, use of the wrong product because of product misidentification, and two or more caregivers administering the same medication. In the cases of nontherapeutic intent, circumstances involved attempts at sedation and several included apparent attempts of overt child abuse and were under investigation by law enforcement authorities."

Although antihistamines typically cause CNS depression, children often react paradoxically with excitement, hallucinations, delirium, ataxia, tremors, and convulsions followed by CNS depression, respiratory failure, or cardiovascular collapse. A potentially toxic dose is 10–50 mg/kg of the most commonly used antihistamines, but toxic reactions have occurred at much lower doses. Anticholinergic effects such as dry mouth, fixed dilated pupils, flushed face, fever, and hallucinations may be prominent. Dextromethorphan can lead to altered mentation, hallucinations, nystagmus, and serotonin toxicity in large ingestions or when taken with other serotonergic agents. Death may occur with massive overdose.

▶ Treatment

Benzodiazepines, such as lorazepam (0.1 mg/kg IV), can be used to control seizures or agitation. Physostigmine (0.5–2.0 mg IV, slowly administered) dramatically reverses the central and peripheral anticholinergic effects of antihistamines; however, the duration of effect is short. It can also be used only for diagnostic purposes in patients without cardiotoxicity or seizures. Cardiac dysrhythmias and hypotension should be treated with normal saline at a dose of 10–20 mg/kg and a vasopressor if necessary. Sodium bicarbonate may be useful if there is QRS widening at a dose of 1–2 mEq/kg, making certain that the arterial pH does not exceed 7.55. Forced diuresis is not helpful. Exchange transfusion was reported to be effective in one case.

Green JL et al: Safety profile of cough and cold medication use in pediatrics. Pediatrics 2017 Jun;139(6). pii: e20163070. doi: 10.1542/peds.2016-3070 [PMID: 28562262].

Smith MD et al: Out-of-hospital medication errors among young children in the United States, 2002–2012. Pediatrics 2014:124(5):867–879 [PMID: 25332497].

BARBITURATES & BENZODIAZEPINES

Barbiturates are rarely used today, and have mostly been replaced with benzodiazepines for their use in seizures or for sedation. The toxic effects of barbiturates include confusion, poor coordination, coma, miotic or fixed dilated pupils, and respiratory depression. Respiratory acidosis is commonly associated with pulmonary atelectasis, and hypotension. Ingestion of more than 6 mg/kg of long-acting or 3 mg/kg of short-acting barbiturates is usually toxic. Benzodiazepines typically cause CNS depression and lethargy without hemodynamic compromise in unintentional oral ingestions. Large oral overdoses, co-ingestants with other sedative/hypnotics, or iatrogenic IV overdose can cause cardiovascular or respiratory depression.

▶ **Treatment**

Careful, conservative management with emphasis on maintaining a clear airway, adequate ventilation, and control of hypotension is critical. Urinary alkalinization and the use of multiple-dose charcoal may decrease the elimination half-life of phenobarbital but have not been shown to alter the clinical course. Flumazenil can be considered if severe CNS depression or respiratory depression develops after benzodiazepine overdose using a dose of 0.01 mg/kg IV (maximum dose of 0.2 mg).

Bachhuber MA et al: Increasing benzodiazepine prescriptions and overdose mortality in the United States, 1996–2013. Am J Public Health 2016 Apr;106(4):686–688 [PMID: 26890165].

Kreshak AA et al: Flumazenil administration in poisoned pediatric patients. Pediatr Emerg Care 2012;28(5):488 [PMID: 22531190].

BELLADONNA ALKALOIDS (ATROPINE, JIMSONWEED, POTATO LEAVES, SCOPOLAMINE, STRAMONIUM)

The effects of anticholinergic (or antimuscarinic) compounds include dry mouth; thirst; decreased sweating with hot, dry, red skin; high fever; and tachycardia that may be preceded by bradycardia. The pupils are dilated, and vision is blurred. Speech and swallowing may be impaired. Hallucinations, delirium, and coma are common. Leukocytosis may occur, confusing the diagnosis.

Atropinism has been caused by normal doses of atropine or homatropine eye drops. Many common plants and over-the-counter medications (antihistamines and sleep aids) contain belladonna alkaloids or medications with anticholinergic effects.

▶ **Treatment**

Gastric emptying is slowed by anticholinergics, so that gastric decontamination may be useful even if delayed. If the patient is awake and showing no signs or symptoms, administration of activated charcoal can be considered. Benzodiazepines should be administered to control agitation. Bolus dosing should be given in escalating doses, and high doses may be required. Physostigmine (0.5–2.0 mg IV, administered slowly) dramatically reverses the central and peripheral signs of atropinism but should be used only as a diagnostic agent, but clinical improvement is not sustained. Physostigmine infusions have been safely administered. It should not be given in patients with cardiotoxicity or seizures. Hyperthermia should be aggressively controlled. Catheterization may be needed if the patient cannot void.

Arens AM, Kearney T: Adverse effects of physostigmine. J Med Toxicol 2019 Feb 11. doi: 10.1007/s13181-019-00697-z [PMID: 31414401].

Burns MJ et al: A comparison of physostigmine and benzodiazepines for the treatment of anticholinergic poisoning. Ann Emerg Med 2000;35:374 [PMID: 10736125].

Glatstein M et al: Belladonna alkaloid intoxication: the 10-year experience of a large tertiary care pediatric hospital. Am J Ther 2013 Nov; 20 [PMID: 24263161].

β-BLOCKERS & CALCIUM CHANNEL BLOCKERS

β-Blockers and calcium channel blockers primarily cause cardiovascular toxicity; bradycardia, hypotension, and various degrees of heart block; cardiac dysrhythmias may develop. Severe toxicity can cause CNS depression (typically due to hemodynamic collapse). The β-blocker propranolol is associated with seizures and also QRS widening. Hyperglycemia can be seen with calcium channel blocker toxicity.

▶ **Treatment**

Initial stabilization with IV fluid resuscitation with isotonic fluids should be initiated. Atropine can be given for symptomatic bradycardia. Calcium at doses of 20 mg/kg and repeated as needed should be administered. Infusions of calcium chloride 10%, 0.2–0.5 mL/kg/h, can be started after initial bolus dosing. Glucagon can be administered; 50–100 mcg/kg (5–10 mg) IV bolus followed by 2–5 mg/h infusion if patient improves. Vasopressors such as epinephrine or norepinephrine should be started if patient continues to be hypotensive and bradycardic. In patients who are severely poisoned and refractory to these initial measures, hyperinsulinemia euglycemic therapy should be started. Your regional poison control center or medical toxicologist should be contacted for further details on dosing of this therapy.

Dewitt CR, Waksman JC: Pharmacology, pathophysiology and management of calcium channel blocker and beta-blocker toxicity. Toxicol Rev 2004;23(4):223–238 [PMID: 15898828].

Krenz JR, Kaakeh Y: An overview of hyperinsulinemic-euglycemic therapy in calcium channel blocker and β-blocker overdose. Pharmacotherapy 2018 Nov;38(11):1130–1142. doi: 10.1002/phar.2177 [PMID: 30141827].

St-Onge M: Treatment for calcium channel blocker poisoning: a systematic review. Clin Toxicol (Phila) 2014 Nov;52(9):926–944. doi: 10.3109/15563650.2014.965827 [PMID: 25283255].

CARBON MONOXIDE

Carbon monoxide is a colorless, odorless gas produced from burning various fuels. The degree of toxicity correlates well with the carboxyhemoglobin concentration taken soon after acute exposure but not after oxygen has been given or when there has been some time since exposure. Onset of symptoms may be more rapid and more severe if the patient lives at a high altitude, has a high respiratory rate (ie, infants), is pregnant, or has myocardial insufficiency or lung disease. Normal blood may contain up to 5% carboxyhemoglobin (10% in smokers). Neonates may have elevated carboxyhemoglobin levels due to breakdown of bilirubin.

Presenting symptoms can include nonspecific symptoms such as headache or flu-like illness. Other effects include confusion, unsteadiness, and coma. Proteinuria, glycosuria, elevated serum aminotransferase levels, or ECG changes may be present in the acute phase. Other signs may include improvement of symptoms after leaving the exposed environment. Permanent cardiac, liver, renal, or CNS damage occurs occasionally. The outcome of severe poisoning may be complete recovery, vegetative state, or any degree of mental injury between these extremes. The primary delayed mental deficits are neuropsychiatric.

▶ Treatment

The biologic half-life of carbon monoxide on room air is approximately 200–300 minutes; on 100% oxygen, it is 60–90 minutes. Thus, 100% oxygen should be administered immediately. Hyperbaric oxygen therapy at 2.0–2.5 atm of oxygen shortens the half-life to 30 minutes, but is practically difficult to deploy in a timely manner. The use of hyperbaric oxygen therapy for delayed neurologic sequelae can be considered, but remains controversial and the primary focus of care should be acute resuscitation and stabilization. After the level has been reduced to near zero, therapy is aimed at the nonspecific sequelae of anoxia. Evaluation of the source should be performed before the patient returns to the home.

Buckley NA et al: Hyperbaric oxygen for carbon monoxide poisoning. Cochrane Database Syst Rev 2011;13(4):CD002041 [PMID: 21491385].

Macnow TE et al: Carbon monoxide poisoning in children: diagnosis and management in the emergency department. Pediatr Emerg Med Pract 2016 Sep;13(9):1–24 [PMID: 27547917].

CAUSTICS

Both acids and alkalis can burn the skin, mucous membranes, and eyes. Vomiting, dysphagia, airway emergencies, burns, and abdominal pain can occur after ingestion. Respiratory distress may be due to edema of the epiglottis, pulmonary edema resulting from inhalation of fumes, or pneumonia. In severe cases, mediastinitis, intercurrent infections, or shock can occur. Perforation of the esophagus or stomach is rare. Residual lesions include esophageal, gastric, and pyloric strictures as well as scars of the cornea, skin, and oropharynx.

1. Acids (Hydrochloric, Hydrofluoric, Nitric, & Sulfuric Acids; Sodium Bisulfate)

Strong acids are commonly found in metal and toilet bowl cleaners, batteries, and other products, and can lead to coagulative necrosis. Hydrofluoric acid is a particularly dangerous acid. Dermal exposure creates a penetrating burn that can progress for hours or days. Large dermal exposure or small ingestion may produce life-threatening hypocalcemia.

2. Bases (Clinitest Tablets, Clorox, Drano, Liquid-Plumr, Purex, Sani-Clor—Examine the Label or Call a Poison Center to Determine Contents)

Alkalis can produce more severe injuries than acids, resulting in liquefactive necrosis. Some substances, such as Clinitest tablets or Drano, are quite toxic, whereas the chlorinated bleaches (3%–6% solutions of sodium hypochlorite) are usually not toxic. When sodium hypochlorite comes in contact with acid in the stomach, hypochlorous acid, which is very irritating to the mucous membranes and skin, is formed. Chlorinated bleaches, when mixed with a strong acid (toilet bowl cleaners) or ammonia, may produce irritating chlorine or chloramine gas, which can cause serious lung injury if inhaled in a closed space (eg, bathroom).

▶ Treatment

Emetics and lavage are contraindicated. Can be diluted with water, but take care not to induce emesis by excessive fluid administration. Neutralization should not be attempted. Burned areas of the skin, mucous membranes, or eyes should be washed with copious amounts of warm water. The eye should be irrigated for at least 20–30 minutes. Ophthalmologic consultation should be obtained for all alkaline eye burns. An endotracheal tube may be required to alleviate laryngeal edema. The absence of oral lesions does not rule out the possibility of laryngeal or esophageal burns following granular alkali ingestion. Esophagoscopy should be performed if the patient has significant burns or difficulty in swallowing, drooling, vomiting, or stridor. Evidence is not conclusive, but corticosteroids may be helpful in significant esophageal burns. Antibiotics may be needed if mediastinitis develops, but they should not be used prophylactically.

Hydrofluoric acid burns on skin are treated with 10% calcium gluconate gel or calcium gluconate infusion. Severe exposure may require large doses of IV calcium or cardiovascular monitoring. Therapy should be guided by calcium levels, the ECG, and clinical signs.

Chirica M et al: Caustic ingestion. Lancet 2017;389:2014–2052 [PMID: 28045663].

Usta M et al: High doses of methylprednisone in the management of caustic esophageal burns. Pediatrics 2014;133(6):E1518–E1524 [PMID: 24864182].

CENTRAL α₂-ADRENERGIC AGONIST

Central α_2-adrenergic agonists are common over-the-counter and prescribed medication. The imidazolines are found in nasal decongestants and eye drops to relieve redness. Clonidine and guanfacine are used most commonly to treat attention deficit hyperactivity disorder or hypertension. Dexmedetomidine is an IV central α_2-adrenergic agonist used for sedation. These medications exert their effects by stimulating presynaptic α_2-adrenergic receptors in the brain, resulting in decreased norepinephrine release and decreased sympathetic outflow.

▶ Clinical Findings

Most common effects are related to CNS sedation. They can present similar to an opioid toxidrome with miosis, CNS depression, and respiratory depression. Other common effects include bradycardia and hypotension.

▶ Treatment

If the patient becomes obtunded, or has inability to protect their airway, intubation may be indicated. Naloxone has been tried to reverse signs of toxicity with varying success. Symptomatic bradycardia can be treated with IV fluid resuscitation or atropine. Hypotension should be treated initially with IV fluid resuscitation, followed by vasopressors if needed.

Wang et al: Unintentional pediatric exposures to central alpha-2 agonists reported to the National Poison Data System. J Pediatr 2014;164(1):149–152 [PMID: 24094880].

COCAINE

Cocaine is absorbed intranasally, via inhalation or ingestion. Effects are noted almost immediately when the drug is taken intravenously or smoked and are delayed for about an hour when the drug is taken orally or nasally. Cocaine prevents the reuptake of endogenous catecholamines, thereby causing an initial sympathetic discharge, followed by catechol depletion after chronic abuse.

▶ Clinical Findings

A local anesthetic and vasoconstrictor, cocaine is also a potent stimulant to both the CNS and the cardiovascular system. The initial tachycardia, hyperpnea, hypertension, and stimulation of the CNS are often followed by coma, seizures, hypotension, and respiratory depression. In severe cases of overdose, various dysrhythmias may be seen, including sinus tachycardia, atrial arrhythmias, premature ventricular contractions, bigeminy, and ventricular tachycardia and fibrillation. If large doses are taken intravenously, cardiac failure, dysrhythmias, rhabdomyolysis, or hyperthermia may result in death.

In addition to those poisoned through recreational use of cocaine, others are at risk of overdose. A "body stuffer" is one who quickly ingests the drug, usually poorly wrapped, to avoid discovery. A "body packer" wraps the drug carefully for prolonged transport. A stuffer typically manifests toxicity within hours of ingestion; a packer is asymptomatic unless the package ruptures, usually days later. Newborns of cocaine using mothers may continue to have seizures for months after birth. Cocaine can be contaminated with levamisole, which can lead to systemic vasculitis and agranulocytosis.

▶ Treatment

Activated charcoal should be considered in body stuffers, and whole bowel irrigation may be useful in cases of body packers. Testing for cocaine in blood or plasma is generally not clinically useful, but a qualitative analysis of the urine may aid in confirming the diagnosis. Cocaine metabolites can be positive in urine for 3–5 days after exposure. For severe cases, an ECG is indicated. In suspected cases of body packing, radiographs of the GI tract may show multiple packets, but are usually not helpful for identifying stuffers. Seizures are treated with IV benzodiazepines such as lorazepam, titrated to response. Hypotension is treated with standard agents. Because cocaine abuse may deplete norepinephrine, an indirect agent such as dopamine may be less effective than a direct agent such as norepinephrine. Agitation is best treated with a benzodiazepine.

Delaney-Black V: Prenatal cocaine exposure as a risk factor for later developmental outcomes. JAMA 2001;286:46 [PMID: 11434823].

Flach PM et al: "Drug mules" as a radiological challenge: sensitivity and specificity in identifying internal cocaine in body packers, body pushers, and body stuffers by computer tomography, plain radiography and Lodox. Eur J Radiol 2012;81(10): 2518–2526 [PMID: 22178312].

Qureshi AI et al: Cocaine use and the likelihood of nonfatal myocardial infarction and stroke: data from the Third National Health and Nutrition Examination Survey. Circulation 2001; 103:502 [PMID: 11157713].

Vagi SJ: Passive multistate surveillance for neutropenia after use of cocaine or heroin possibly contaminated with levamisole. Ann Emerg Med 2013 Apr;61(4):468–474. doi: 10.1016/j.annemergmed.2012.10.036 [PMID: 23374417].

COSMETICS & RELATED PRODUCTS

Cosmetics and personal care products are the most frequently involved substance in pediatric patients younger than 5 years (14% of all calls reported to NPDS) and second most common in all ages. Luckily, most of them do not cause significant toxicity. The relative toxicities of commonly ingested products in this group are listed in Table 13–4.

CYCLIC ANTIDEPRESSANTS

Cyclic antidepressants (eg, amitriptyline, imipramine) have a very low ratio of toxic to therapeutic doses, and even a moderate overdose can have serious effects. Diphenhydramine toxicity can have similarly symptoms as cyclic antidepressants and is more readily available.

Cyclic antidepressant overdosage can cause a progression of illness beginning with sudden onset coma within 1–2 hours of ingestion, followed by convulsions, hypotension, and dysrhythmias. Usually significant clinical effects occur within hours after the ingestion, may be life-threatening and require rapid intervention. One agent, amoxapine, differs in that it causes fewer cardiovascular complications, but it is associated with a higher incidence of seizures.

▶ Treatment

After a significant ingestion, decontamination should include administration of activated charcoal unless the patient is already symptomatic. Benzodiazepines should be given for seizures.

Table 13–4. Relative toxicities of cosmetics and similar products.

High toxicity	Low toxicity
Permanent wave neutralizers	Perfume
Moderate toxicity	Hair removers
Fingernail polish	Deodorants
Fingernail polish remover	Bath salts
Metallic hair dyes	No toxicity
Home permanent wave lotion	Liquid makeup
Bath oil	Vegetable hair dye
Shaving lotion	Cleansing cream
Hair tonic (alcoholic)	Hair dressing (nonalcoholic)
Cologne, toilet water	Hand lotion or cream
	Lipstick

An ECG should be obtained in all patients. A QRS interval greater than 100 milliseconds specifically identifies patients at risk to develop seizures and dysrhythmias. If dysrhythmias or tachycardia are demonstrated, the patient should be admitted and monitored until free of irregularity for 24 hours. The onset of dysrhythmias is rare beyond 24 hours after ingestion.

Alkalinization with sodium bicarbonate boluses (0.5–1.0 mEq/kg IV) may dramatically reverse ventricular dysrhythmias and narrow the QRS interval. If intubated, hyperventilation may be helpful. Lidocaine may be added for treatment of arrhythmias. Bolus administration of sodium bicarbonate (1–2 mEq/kg) is recommended for all patients with QRS widening to above 120 milliseconds and for those with significant dysrhythmias, to achieve a pH of 7.5–7.6. Lipid-emulsion therapy has been used in the setting of cardiotoxicity.

Cyclic antidepressants block the reuptake of catecholamines, thereby producing initial hypertension followed by hypotension. Vasopressors (such as norepinephrine, 0.1–1 mcg/kg/min, titrated to response) are generally effective. Diuresis and hemodialysis are not effective and physostigmine is contraindicated.

Blaber MS et al: "Lipid rescue" for tricyclic antidepressant cardiotoxicity. J Emerg Med 2012;43(3):465–467 [PMID: 22244291].

Kerr GW et al: Tricyclic antidepressant overdose: a review. Emerg Med J 2001;18:236 [PMID: 11435353].

Woolf AD et al: Tricyclic antidepressant poisoning: an evidence-based consensus guideline for out-of-hospital management. Clin Toxicol (Phila) 2007;45(3):203–333 [PMID: 17453872].

DIGITALIS & OTHER CARDIAC GLYCOSIDES

Acute toxicity with digitalis is typically the result of incorrect dosing, and chronic toxicity is due to unrecognized renal insufficiency. In acute overdosage, hyperkalemia is more common. Hypokalemia is common in chronic toxicity Clinical features include nausea, vomiting, diarrhea, headache, delirium, confusion, and, occasionally, coma. Cardiac dysrhythmias typically involve bradydysrhythmias, but every type of dysrhythmia has been reported in digitalis intoxication, including atrial fibrillation, paroxysmal atrial tachycardia, and atrial flutter. Transplacental intoxication by digitalis has been reported. Cardiac glycosides, such as yellow oleander and foxglove, can cause digitalis toxicity in large ingestions as well.

▶ Treatment

If patient is awake and alert, consider administering activated charcoal. Potassium is contraindicated in acute overdosage unless there is laboratory evidence of hypokalemia. Adequate fluid resuscitation is essential to aid in renal elimination.

The patient must be monitored carefully for ECG changes. Bradycardias have been treated with atropine.

Phenytoin, lidocaine, magnesium salts (but not in renal failure), amiodarone, and bretylium have been used to correct arrhythmias.

Definitive treatment is with digoxin immune Fab (ovine) (Digifab). Indications for its use include hypotension or any dysrhythmia, typically ventricular dysrhythmias and progressive bradydysrhythmias, or hyperkalemia (K > 5) in an acute overdose. Elevated T waves indicate high potassium and may be an indication for digoxin immune Fab (DigiFab) use. Techniques of determining dosage and indications related to levels, when available are described in product literature. High doses of digoxin immune Fab may be needed in cardiac glycoside overdose. Extracorporeal treatment is not indicated for digoxin poisoning.

Botelho AFM et al: A review of cardiac glycosides: Structure, toxicokinetics, clinical signs, diagnosis and antineoplastic potential. Toxicon 2019 Feb;158:63–68 [PMID: 30529380].

Mowry JB: Extracorporeal treatment for digoxin poisoning: systematic review and recommendations from the EXTRIP Workgroup. Clin Toxicol (Phila) 2016;54(2):103–114. doi:10.3109/15563650.2015.1118488 [PMID: 26795743].

Rajapakse S: Management of yellow oleander poisoning. Clin Toxicol (Phila) 2009;47(3):206–212 [PMID: 19306191].

DIPHENOXYLATE WITH ATROPINE (LOMOTIL) & LOPERAMIDE (IMODIUM)

Loperamide (Imodium) has largely replaced Lomotil and does not produce significant toxicity. Ingestions of up to 0.4 mg/kg can safely be managed at home. Both acute and chronic abuse of loperamide has been associated with cardiac dysrhythmias.

Lomotil is still widely available and contains diphenoxylate hydrochloride, a synthetic narcotic, and atropine sulfate. Small amounts are potentially lethal in children; it is contraindicated in children younger than 2 years. Early signs of intoxication with this preparation result from its anticholinergic effect and consist of fever, facial flushing, tachypnea, and lethargy. However, the miotic effect of the narcotic predominates. Later, hypothermia, increasing CNS depression, and loss of the facial flush occur. Seizures are probably secondary to hypoxia. Any ingestion of Lomotil must be observed for 8–12 hours as delayed respiratory arrest may be encountered.

▶ Treatment

Prolonged monitoring (24 hours) with pulse oximetry and careful attention to airway is sufficient in most cases. Naloxone hydrochloride (0.4–2.0 mg IV in children and adults) should be given for signs of respiratory depression. Repeated doses may be required because the duration of action of diphenoxylate is considerably longer than that of naloxone.

Eggleston W: Notes from the field: cardiac dysrhythmias after loperamide abuse–New York, 2008-2016. MMWR Morb Mortal Wkly Rep 2016 Nov 18;65(45):1276–1277. doi: 10.15585/mmwr.mm6545a7 [PMID: 27855148].

Vakkalanka JP, Charlton NP, Holstege CP: Epidemiologic trends in loperamide abuse and misuse. Ann Emerg Med 2016 Nov 4. doi: 10.1016/j.annemergmed.2016.08.444.27823872 [PMID: 27823872].

DISINFECTANTS & DEODORIZERS

1. Naphthalene

Naphthalene is now less commonly found in mothballs, disinfectants, and deodorizers. It is absorbed not only when ingested but also through the skin and lungs. It is potentially hazardous to store baby clothes in naphthalene, because baby oil is an excellent solvent that may increase dermal absorption. Metabolic products of naphthalene may cause severe hemolytic anemia 2–7 days after ingestion. Other physical findings include vomiting, diarrhea, jaundice, oliguria, anuria, coma, and convulsions.

▶ Treatment

If the patient is awake and alert, consideration can be given for administering activated charcoal. Methemoglobinemia and hemolysis may occur 24–48 hours after ingestion. Life-threatening hemolysis and anemia may require blood transfusions.

Moss MJ et al: An algorithm for identifying mothball composition. Clin Toxicol (Phila) 2017 Sep;55(8):919–921 [PMID: 28541143].

2. *p*-Dichlorobenzene, Phenolic Acids, & Others

Disinfectants and deodorizers containing *p*-dichlorobenzene or sodium sulfate are now more commonly found in mothballs and much less toxic than those containing naphthalene. They typically cause mucous membrane irritation and GI upset. Camphor can cause seizures after ingestion.

Disinfectants containing phenolic acids are highly toxic, especially if they contain a borate ion. Phenol precipitates tissue proteins and can also cause systemic toxicity resulting in respiratory alkalosis followed by metabolic acidosis. Some phenols cause methemoglobinemia. Phenol is readily absorbed topically and from the GI tract, causing local injury, diffuse capillary damage and, in some cases, methemoglobinemia. Pentachlorophenol, which has been used in terminal rinsing of diapers, has caused infant fatalities by causing metabolic acidosis.

The toxicity of alkalis, quaternary ammonium compounds, pine oil, and halogenated disinfectants varies with the concentration of active ingredients. Wick deodorizers are usually of moderate toxicity. Iodophor disinfectants are the safest. Spray deodorizers are not usually toxic, because a child is not likely to swallow a very large dose.

Signs and symptoms of acute quaternary ammonium compound ingestion include diaphoresis, strong irritation, thirst, vomiting, diarrhea, cyanosis, hyperactivity, coma, convulsions, hypotension, abdominal pain, and pulmonary edema. Acute liver or renal failure may develop later.

▶ Treatment

Mainstay to phenol toxicity is symptomatic and supportive care. The metabolic acidosis must be managed carefully. Anticonvulsants or measures to treat shock may be needed.

Because phenols are absorbed through the skin, exposed areas should be irrigated copiously with water. Undiluted polyethylene glycol may be a useful solvent as well.

Van Berkel M, de Wolff FA: Survival after acute benzalkonium chloride poisoning. Hum Toxicol 1988;7:191 [PMID: 3378808].
Vearrier D, Jacobs D, Greenberg MI: Phenol toxicity following cutaneous exposure to Creolin®: a case report. J Med Toxicol 2015 Jun;11(2):227–231. doi: 10.1007/s13181-014-0440-1 [PMID: 25326371].

DISK-SHAPED "BUTTON" BATTERIES

Over 60% of batteries that are ingested by children are obtained from manufactured household products. These small, flat, smooth disk-shaped batteries measure between 10 and 25 millimeter in diameter. About 69% of them pass through the GI tract in 48 hours and 85% in 72 hours. Some may become entrapped and lead to caustic injury. Batteries impacted in the esophagus may cause symptoms of refusal to take food, increased salivation, vomiting with or without blood, and pain or discomfort. Fatalities have been reported in association with esophageal perforation or fistula formation.

When a history of disk battery ingestion is obtained, radiographs of the entire respiratory tract and GI tract should be taken immediately so that the battery can be located and the proper therapy determined.

▶ Treatment

Any disk battery ingestion should be referred for evaluation and radiographs. If at home and the patient is greater than 1 year of age, 10 ml of honey every 10 minutes for up to 6 doses is recommended. Upon arrival to an emergency department, sucralfate suspension 10 mL every 10 minutes should be administered until sedation is given for endoscopy. If the disk battery is located in the esophagus, it must be removed immediately. Any prolonged time in the esophagus can cause injury, leading to esophageal perforation, or erosion/ fistula formation into a blood vessel. Consultation with GI or surgical subspecialty is recommended.

Location of the disk battery below the esophagus has been rarely associated with tissue damage. Perforated Meckel diverticulum has been the major complication. It may take as long as 7 days for spontaneous passage to occur, and lack of movement in the GI tract may not require removal in an asymptomatic patient.

Batteries that have opened in the GI tract have been rarely associated with some toxicity due to mercury, but the patients have recovered.

Asymptomatic patients, with known time of ingestion, patients greater than 5 years old, and with disk batteries past the lower esophageal junction may simply be observed and stools examined for passage of the battery. If the battery has not passed within 7 days or if the patient becomes symptomatic, radiographs should be repeated. If the battery has come apart or appears not to be moving, a purgative, enema, or nonabsorbable intestinal lavage solution should be considered. If these methods are unsuccessful, surgical intervention may be required. Levels of heavy metals (mainly mercury) should be measured in patients in whom the battery has opened or symptoms have developed.

Anfang RR et al: pH-neutralizing esophageal irrigations as a novel mitigation strategy for button battery injury. Laryngoscope 2019 Jan;129(1):49–57. doi: 10.1002/lary.27312 [PMID: 30618147].
Centers for Disease Control and Prevention (CDC): Injuries from batteries among children aged < 13 years—United States, 1995–2010. MMWR 2012;61(34):661–666 [PMID: 22932299].
Kramer RE, et al: Management of ingested foreign bodies in children: a clinical report of the NASPGHAN Endoscopy Committee. J Pediatr Gastroenterol Nutr 2015; 60(4):562–74 [PMID: 25611037].
https://www.rmpdc.org/system/user_files/Documents/ Button%20Disc%20Battery%20Guideline%20for%20Management%202018%20Ver%203.pdf.

ETHYLENE GLYCOL & METHANOL

Ethylene glycol and methanol are the toxic alcohols. The primary source of ethylene glycol is antifreeze, whereas methanol is present in windshield wiper fluid and also as an ethanol denaturant. Ethylene glycol causes severe metabolic acidosis and renal failure. Methanol causes metabolic acidosis and blindness. Onset of symptoms with both agents occurs within several hours after ingestion, longer if ethanol was ingested simultaneously. Rarely, glycol ethers can cause acidosis, but only in the setting of large ingestions.

▶ Treatment

The primary treatment is to block the enzyme alcohol dehydrogenase, which converts both agents to their toxic metabolites. This is accomplished with fomepizole (loading dose of 15 mg/kg). Ethanol could be used if fomepizole is unavailable, but can lead to CNS depression and hypoglycemia in children. Hemodialysis is indicated with high concentrations, persistent metabolic acidosis, or end-organ toxicity.

Beauchamp GA, Valento M: Toxic alcohol ingestion: prompt recognition and management in the emergency department. Emerg Med Pract 2016 Sep;18(9):1–20 [PMID: 27538060].

Brent J: Fomepizole for the treatment of pediatric ethylene and diethylene glycol, butoxyethanol, and methanol poisonings. Clin Toxicol (Phila) 2010;48(5):401–406 [PMID: 20586570].

Wang GS et al: Severe poisoning after accidental pediatric ingestion of glycol ethers. Pediatrics 2012;130(4):e1026–e1029 [PMID: 23008459].

γ-HYDROXYBUTYRATE, γ-BUTYROLACTONE, BUTANEDIOL, FLUNITRAZEPAM, & KETAMINE

γ-Hydroxybutyrate (GHB), γ-butyrolactone (GBL), and butanediol have become popular drugs of abuse in adolescents and adults. GHB is a CNS depressant that is structurally similar to the inhibitory neurotransmitter γ-aminobutyric acid. GBL and butanediol are converted in the body to GHB. These drugs cause deep but short-lived coma; the coma often lasts only 1–4 hours. Flunitrazepam (Rohypnol) is a benzodiazepine that can lead to somnolence and CNS depression. Ketamine is a dissociative anesthetic that can also cause rapid onset altered mental status and CNS depression. Although all of these drugs are often referred to as "date rape" drugs, ethanol is the most commonly used substance in drug-facilitated assault.

Treatment consists of supportive care with close attention to airway and endotracheal intubation if respiratory depression or decreased gag reflex complicates the poisoning. Atropine has been used successfully for symptomatic bradycardia.

Withdrawal from GHB, GBL, or butanediol can cause several days of extreme agitation, hallucination, or tachycardia. Treatment with high doses of sedatives such as benzodiazepines or with butyrophenones (eg, haloperidol or droperidol) or secobarbital may be needed for several days.

Schep LJ et al: The clinical toxicology of gamma-hydroxybutyrate, gamma-butyrolactone and 1,4-butanediol. Clin Toxicol (Phila) 2012;50(6):458–470 [PMID: 22746383].

HYDROCARBONS (BENZENE, CHARCOAL LIGHTER FLUID, GASOLINE, KEROSENE, PETROLEUM DISTILLATES, TURPENTINE)

Ingestion of hydrocarbons may cause irritation of mucous membranes, CNS depression, or aspiration pneumonitis. Hydrocarbons with high volatility, low viscosity, and low surface tension have more risk or aspiration pneumonitis. Benzene, kerosene, red seal oil furniture polish, and some of the essential oils are very dangerous. A dose exceeding 1 mL/kg is likely to cause CNS depression. A history of coughing or choking, as well as vomiting, suggests aspiration with resulting hydrocarbon pneumonia. Several weeks may be required for full resolution of hydrocarbon pneumonia. Pulmonary edema and hemorrhage, blebs, cardiac dilation and dysrhythmias, hepatosplenomegaly, proteinuria, and hematuria can occur following large overdoses.

▶ Treatment

Both emetics and lavage should be avoided. Initial supportive care, observing for CNS depression or respiratory distress. Patients who are asymptomatic with a normal chest x-ray (CXR) after 8 hours are unlikely to develop significant illness; however, patients who develop respiratory symptoms, hypoxia, or CXR changes should be observed.

Epinephrine should be avoided with halogenated hydrocarbons because it may affect an already sensitized myocardium. The usefulness of corticosteroids is debated, and antibiotics should be reserved for patients with infections (pneumonitis can cause fevers and infiltrates). Surfactant therapy for severe hydrocarbon-induced lung injury has been used successfully. Extracorporeal membrane oxygenation has been successful in at least two cases of failure with standard therapy.

Makrygianni EA, Palamidou F, Kaditis AG: Respiratory complications following hydrocarbon aspiration in children. Pediatr Pulmonol 2016 Jun;51(6):560–569. doi: 10.1002/ppul.23392 [PMID: 26910771].

Mastropietro SW et al: Early administration of intratracheal surfactant (calfactant) after hydrocarbon aspiration. Pediatrics 2011;127(6):e1600–e1604 [PMID: 21624800].

Tormoehlen LM: Hydrocarbon toxicity: a review. Clin Toxicol (Phila) 2014;52(5):479–489 [PMID: 24911841].

IBUPROFEN

Most exposures in children do not produce symptoms. In one study, for example, children ingesting up to 2.4 g remained asymptomatic. When symptoms occur, the most common are abdominal pain, vomiting, drowsiness, and lethargy. In rare cases, apnea (especially in young children), seizures, metabolic acidosis, and CNS depression leading to coma have occurred.

▶ Treatment

If a child has ingested less than 100 mg/kg, supportive care for GI upset is typically all that is needed. When the ingested amount is more than 400 mg/kg, seizures or CNS depression may occur. There is no specific antidote. Neither alkalization of the urine nor hemodialysis is helpful in elimination of ibuprofen. However, hemodialysis may be needed to correct acid–base abnormalities.

Cuzzolin L et al: NSAID-induced nephrotoxicity from the fetus to the child. Drug Safety 2001;242:9 [PMID: 11219488].

Marciniak KE et al: Massive ibuprofen overdose requiring extracorporeal membrane oxygenation for cardiovascular support. Pediatr Crit Care Med 2007;8:180–182 [PMID: 17273120].

INSECT STINGS (BEE, WASP, & HORNET)

Insect stings are painful but not usually dangerous; however, death from anaphylaxis may occur. Bee venom has hemolytic, neurotoxic, and histamine-like activities that can on rare occasion cause hemoglobinuria and severe anaphylactoid reactions. Massive envenomation from numerous stings may cause hemolysis, rhabdomyolysis, and shock leading to multiple-organ failure.

▶ Treatment

The physician should remove the stinger, taking care not to squeeze the attached venom sac. For allergic reactions, epinephrine 1:1000 solution, 0.01 mL/kg, should be administered IV or SQ above the site of the sting. Albuterol, corticosteroids, and diphenhydramine are useful ancillary drugs but have no immediate effect. Ephedrine or antihistamines may be used for 2 or 3 days to prevent recurrence of symptoms.

For the more usual stings, cold compresses, aspirin, and diphenhydramine (1 mg/kg PO) are sufficient.

Ross RN et al: Effectiveness of specific immunotherapy in the treatment of hymenoptera venom hypersensitivity: a meta-analysis. Clin Ther 2000;22:351 [PMID: 10963289].

Vetter RS et al: Mass envenomations by honey bees and wasps. West J Med 1999;170:223 [PMID: 10344177].

INSECTICIDES

The petroleum distillates or other organic solvents used in these products are often as toxic as the insecticide itself.

1. Chlorinated Hydrocarbons (eg, Aldrin, Carbinol, Chlordane, DDT, Dieldrin, Endrin, Heptachlor, Lindane, Toxaphene)

Signs of intoxication include salivation, GI irritability, abdominal pain, vomiting, diarrhea, CNS depression, and convulsions. Inhalation exposure causes irritation of the eyes, nose, and throat; blurred vision; cough; and pulmonary edema.

Chlorinated hydrocarbons are absorbed through the skin, respiratory tract, and GI tract. Decontamination of skin with soap and evacuation of the stomach contents should be considered in significant ingestions. All contaminated clothing should be removed. Convulsions should be treated with diazepam (0.1–0.3 mg/kg IV). Epinephrine should cautiously be used as it may precipitate cardiac arrhythmias.

2. Organophosphate (Cholinesterase-Inhibiting) Insecticides (eg, Chlorothion, Co-Ral, DFP, Diazinon, Malathion, Paraoxon, Parathion, Phosdrin, TEPP, Thio-TEPP)

Dizziness, headache, blurred vision, miosis, tearing, salivation, nausea, vomiting, diarrhea, hyperglycemia, cyanosis, sense of constriction of the chest, dyspnea, sweating, weakness, muscular twitching, convulsions, loss of reflexes and sphincter control, and coma can occur.

The clinical findings are the result of cholinesterase inhibition, which causes an accumulation of acetylcholine. The onset of symptoms occurs within 12 hours of the exposure. Red cell cholinesterase levels should be measured as soon as possible. (Some normal individuals have a low serum cholinesterase level.) Normal values vary in different laboratories. In general, a decrease of red cell cholinesterase to below 25% of normal indicates significant exposure.

Repeated low-grade exposure may result in sudden, acute toxic reactions. This syndrome usually occurs after repeated household spraying rather than agricultural exposure.

Although all organophosphates act by inhibiting cholinesterase activity, they vary greatly in their toxicity. Parathion, for example, is 100 times more toxic than malathion. Toxicity is influenced by the specific compound, type of formulation (liquid or solid), vehicle, and route of absorption (lungs, skin, or GI tract).

▶ Treatment

Decontamination of skin, nails, hair, and clothing with soapy water is extremely important. Atropine plus a cholinesterase reactivator, pralidoxime, is an antidote for organophosphate insecticide poisoning. After assessment and management of the ABCs, atropine should be given and repeated every few minutes until airway secretions diminish. An appropriate starting dose of atropine is 2–4 mg IV in an adult and 0.05 mg/kg in a child. Severe poisoning may require gram quantities of atropine administered over 24 hours. Glycopyrrolate can also be used if delirium occurs.

Because atropine antagonizes the muscarinic parasympathetic effects of the organophosphates but does not affect the nicotinic receptor, it does not improve muscular weakness. Although the benefits remain controversial, pralidoxime should also be given immediately in more severe cases and repeated every 6–12 hours as needed (25–50 mg/kg diluted to 5% and infused over 5–30 minutes at a rate of no > 500 mg/min). Pralidoxime should be used in addition to—not in place of—atropine if red cell cholinesterase is less than 25% of normal. Pralidoxime is most useful within 48 hours after the exposure but has shown some effects 2–6 days later. Morphine, theophylline, aminophylline, succinylcholine, and tranquilizers of the reserpine and phenothiazine types are contraindicated. Hyperglycemia is common in severe poisonings.

3. Carbamates (eg, Carbaryl, Sevin, Zectran)

Carbamate insecticides are reversible inhibitors of cholinesterase. The signs and symptoms of intoxication are similar to those associated with organophosphate poisoning but are generally less severe. Atropine titrated to effect is sufficient treatment. In combined exposures to organophosphates, give atropine but reserve pralidoxime for cases in which the red cell cholinesterase is depressed below 25% of normal or marked effects of nicotinic receptor stimulation are present.

4. Botanical Insecticides (eg, Black Flag Bug Killer, Black Leaf CPR Insect Killer, Flit Aerosol House & Garden Insect Killer, French's Flea Powder, Raid)

Allergic reactions, asthma-like symptoms, coma, and convulsions have been reported. Pyrethrins, allethrin, and rotenone do not commonly cause significant toxicity. Antihistamines, short-acting benzodiazepines, and atropine are helpful as symptomatic treatment.

Blumberg A et al: Utility of 2-pyridine aldoxime methyl chloride (2-PAM) for acute organophosphate poisoning: a systematic review and meta-analysis. J Med Toxicol 2018 Mar;14(1):91–98. doi: 10.1007/s13181-017-0636-2 [PMID: 29299760].

King AM, Aaron CK: Organophosphate and carbamate poisoning. Emerg Med Clin North Am 2015 Feb;33(1):133–151. doi: 10.1016/j.emc.2014.09.010 [PMID: 25455666].

Roberts JR et al: Pesticide exposure in children. Pediatrics 2012;130(6):e1765–e1788 [PMID: 23184105].

IRON

Iron has many different formulations with varying amounts of elemental iron. Three common formulations include ferrous fumarate (33%), ferrous sulfate (20%), and ferrous gluconate (12%). Typically, doses of more than 20 mg/kg of elemental iron will cause symptoms. Five stages of intoxication may occur in iron poisoning: (1) Hemorrhagic gastroenteritis, which occurs 30–60 minutes after ingestion and may be associated with shock, acidosis, coagulation defects, and coma; this phase usually lasts 4–6 hours; (2) phase of improvement, lasting 2–12 hours, during which patient looks better; (3) delayed shock, which may occur 12–48 hours after ingestion; metabolic acidosis, fever, leukocytosis, and coma may also be present; (4) liver damage with hepatic failure; and (5) residual pyloric stenosis, which may develop about 4 weeks after the ingestion.

▶ Treatment

GI decontamination is based on clinical assessment. The patient should be referred to a health care facility if symptomatic or if the history indicates toxic amounts (typically > 20 mg/kg of elemental iron). Gastric lavage and whole bowel irrigation should be considered in potentially life-threatening overdoses.

Shock is treated in the usual manner. Deferoxamine, a specific chelating agent for iron, is a useful adjunct in the treatment of severe iron poisoning. It forms a soluble complex that is excreted in the urine. It is contraindicated in patients with renal failure unless dialysis can be used. IV deferoxamine chelation therapy should be instituted if the patient has a metabolic acidosis, persistent symptoms, and a serum iron determination cannot be obtained readily, or if the peak serum iron exceeds 500 mcg/dL at 4–5 hours after ingestion.

Deferoxamine should not be delayed until serum iron levels are available in serious cases of poisoning. Intravenous administration is indicated if the patient is in shock, in which case it should be given at a dosage of 10–15 mg/kg/h. Infusion rates up to 35 mg/kg/h have been used in life-threatening poisonings. Rapid IV administration can cause hypotension, facial flushing, urticaria, tachycardia, and shock. Deferoxamine, 90 mg/kg IM every 8 hours (maximum, 1 g), may be given if IV access cannot be established, but the procedure is painful. The indications for discontinuation of deferoxamine have not been clearly delineated. Generally, it can be stopped after 12–24 hours if the acidosis has resolved and the patient is improving. Use of deferoxamine for greater than 24 hours has been associated with acute respiratory distress syndrome (ARDS).

Hemodialysis, peritoneal dialysis, or exchange transfusion can be used to increase the excretion of the dialyzable complex. Urine output should be monitored and urine sediment examined for evidence of renal tubular damage. Initial laboratory studies should include blood typing and cross-matching; total protein; serum iron, sodium, potassium, and chloride; P_{CO_2}; pH; and liver function tests. Serum iron levels fall rapidly even if deferoxamine is not given.

After the acute episode, liver function studies and an upper GI series are indicated to rule out residual damage.

Black J et al: Child abuse by intentional iron poisoning presenting as shock and persistent acidosis. Pediatrics 2003;111:197 [PMID: 12509576].

Chang TP, Rangan C: Iron poisoning: a literature-based review of epidemiology, diagnosis, and management. Pediatr Emerg Care 2011 Oct;27(10):978–985. doi: 10.1097/PEC.0b013e3182302604 [PMID: 21975503].

Juurlink DN et al: Iron poisoning in young children: association with the birth of a sibling. CMAJ 2003;165:1539 [PMID: 12796332].

LEAD

Lead poisoning (plumbism) causes vague symptoms, including weakness, irritability, weight loss, vomiting, personality changes, ataxia, constipation, headache, and colicky abdominal pain. Late manifestations consist of developmental delays, convulsions, and coma associated with increased intracranial pressure, which is a medical emergency.

Plumbism usually occurs insidiously in children younger than age 5 years. The most likely sources of lead include flaking leaded paint, artist's paints, fruit tree sprays, solder, brass alloys, home-glazed pottery, fumes from burning batteries, and foreign country remedies. Only paint containing less than 1% lead is safe for interior use (eg, furniture, toys). Repetitive ingestions of small amounts of lead are far more serious than a single massive exposure. Toxic effects are likely to occur if more than 0.5 mg of lead per day is absorbed. In the United States, lead levels continue to decline and are more common abroad, so particular attention should be paid to immigrant and refugee populations or use of foreign remedies.

Blood lead levels are used to assess the severity of exposure. A complete blood count and serum ferritin concentration should be obtained; iron deficiency increases absorption of lead. Glycosuria, proteinuria, hematuria, and aminoaciduria occur frequently. Abnormal capillary blood lead levels should be repeated with venous sample in asymptomatic patients to rule out laboratory error. Specimens must be meticulously obtained in acid-washed metal-free containers. A normocytic, slightly hypochromic anemia with basophilic stippling of the red cells and reticulocytosis may be present in plumbism. Stippling of red blood cells is absent in cases involving only recent ingestion.

The cerebrospinal fluid (CSF) protein is elevated, and the white cell count usually is less than 100 cells/mL. CSF pressure may be elevated in patients with encephalopathy; lumbar punctures must be performed cautiously to prevent herniation.

▶ Treatment

Refer to the CDC guidelines for the most up-to-date recommendations on lead treatment and evaluation. There is no "safe" concentration of lead. Removing the source of exposure is the most important initial treatment to toxicity. Succimer is an orally administered chelator approved for use in children and reported to be as efficacious as calcium edetate. Succimer should be initiated in asymptomatic children at blood lead levels over 45 mcg/dL. The initial dose is 10 mg/kg (350 mg/m^2) every 8 hours for 5 days. The same dose is then given every 12 hours for 14 days. At least 2 weeks should elapse between courses. Blood lead levels increase somewhat (ie, rebound) after discontinuation of therapy. Courses of dimercaprol/BAL (300–450 mg/m^2/day) and calcium sodium edetate/CaNa2EDTA (1000–1500 mg/m^2/day) should be considered in symptomatic children or levels over 70 mcg/dL.

Encephalopathy associated with cerebral edema needs to be treated with standard measures. Anticonvulsants may be needed. A high-calcium, high-phosphorus diet and large doses of vitamin D may remove lead from the blood by depositing it in the bones. A public health team should evaluate the source of the lead. Necessary corrections should be completed before the child is returned home.

Braun JM et al: Effect of residential lead-hazard interventions on childhood blood lead concentrations and neurobehavioral outcomes: a randomized clinical trial. JAMA Pediatr 2018 Oct 1; 172(10):934–942.doi:10.1001/jamapediatrics.2018.2382[PMID: 30178064].

CDC LEAD: https://www.cdc.gov/nceh/lead/default.htm. Accessed February 20, 2019.

Reuben A et al: Association of childhood blood lead levels with cognitive function and socioeconomic status at age 38 years and with IQ change and socioeconomic mobility between childhood and adulthood. JAMA 2017 Mar 28;317(12):1244–1251. doi: 10.1001/jama.2017.1712 [PMID: 28350927].

Rogan WJ et al: Treatment of lead-exposed children trial group: the effect of chelation therapy with succimer on neuropsychological development in children exposed to lead. N Engl J Med 2001;344:1421 [PMID: 11346806].

MAGNETS

Although not strictly toxic, small magnets have been found to cause bowel obstructions in children. Recent cases have resulted in warnings and a recall by the Consumer Product Safety Commission following intestinal perforation and death in a 20-month-old child. Obstruction may occur following ingestion of as few as two magnets. Radiographs should be obtained and surgical consultation may be indicated.

Alfonzo MJ, Baum CR: Magnetic foreign body ingestions. Pediatr Emerg Care 2016 Oct;32(10):698–702. doi: 10.1097/PEC.0000000000000927 [PMID: 27749667].

Consumer Product Safety Commission: https://www.cpsc.gov/Safety-Education/Safety-Education-Centers/Magnets. Accessed November 20, 2017.

Sola R et al: Magnet foreign body ingestion: rare occurrence but big consequences. J Pediatr Surg 2018 Sep;53(9):1815–1819. doi: 10.1016/j.jpedsurg.2017.08.013 [PMID: 28899548].

MARIJUANA

Marijuana is becoming more readily available as over half of US states have allowed medical marijuana, and several more allowing recreational marijuana. It is also available for use in multiple forms, including high concentrated products (dabs, butters, waxes), vaporizers, and infused edible products that all can have high concentrations of THC (tetrahydrocannabinol), the most psychoactive component.

Young children who ingest edible products can have a range of symptoms. These symptoms can be mild such as sleepiness and ataxia. However, more severe symptoms can develop, including CNS depression, coma, and respiratory depression requiring mechanical ventilation. Symptoms in young children can sometimes last over 24 hours. Inhalational use/abuse of high concentrated products can lead to tachycardia, hypertension, agitation, and acute psychosis. Habitual use has led to significant nausea, vomiting, and abdominal pain relieved by hot showers, often labeled "Cannabinoid Hyperemesis Syndrome (CHS)." Symptomatic and supportive care is mainstay for treatment: supporting cardiorespiratory adverse effects, and treating psychosis and agitation with benzodiazepines or antipsychotics. Capsaicin cream has reported to improve CHS symptoms.

Graham J et al: Capsaicin cream for treatment of cannabinoid hyperemesis syndrome in adolescents: a case series. Pediatrics 2017 Dec;140(6). pii: e20163795. doi: 10.1542/peds.2016-3795 [PMID: 29122973].

Vo KT et al: Cannabis intoxication case series: the dangers of edibles containing tetrahydrocannabinol. Ann Emerg Med 2018 Mar;71(3):306–313. doi: 10.1016/j.annemergmed.2017.09.008 [PMID: 29103798].

Wang GS et al: Unintentional pediatric exposures to marijuana in Colorado, 2009-2015. JAMA Pediatr 2016 Sep 6;170(9):e160971. doi: 10.1001/jamapediatrics.2016.0971 [PMID: 27454910].

MUSHROOMS

Toxic mushrooms are often difficult to distinguish from edible varieties. Contact a poison control center to obtain identification assistance. Symptoms vary with the species ingested, time of year, stage of maturity, quantity eaten, method of preparation, and interval since ingestion. Most mushrooms lead to early GI symptoms and do not lead to significant toxicity; however, some can be fatal and so it is critical to determine from poison center experts what mushroom may have been involved. A mushroom that is toxic to one individual may not be toxic to another. Drinking alcohol and eating certain mushrooms may cause a reaction similar to that seen with disulfiram and alcohol. Cooking destroys some toxins but not the deadly one produced by *Amanita phalloides*, which is responsible for 90% of deaths due to mushroom poisoning. Mushroom toxins are absorbed relatively slowly. Onset of symptoms within 2 hours of ingestion suggests muscarinic toxin, whereas a delay of symptoms for 6–48 hours after ingestion strongly suggests *Amanita* (amanitin) poisoning. Patients who have ingested *A phalloides* may relapse and die of hepatic or renal failure following initial improvement.

► Treatment

Treatment of mushroom poisoning is highly specialized and consultation with a poison center is highly recommended. Supportive care with IV fluid resuscitation may be needed due to emesis and diarrhea. If the patient has muscarinic signs, give atropine, 0.05 mg/kg IM (0.02 mg/kg in toddlers), and repeat as needed (usually every 30 minutes) Atropine, however, is used only when cholinergic effects are present and not for all mushrooms. Hypoglycemia is most likely to occur in patients with delayed onset of symptoms. Try to identify the mushroom if the patient is symptomatic. Local botanical gardens, university departments of botany, and societies of mycologists may be able to help. Supportive care is usually all that is needed; however, in the case of *A phalloides*, silibinin, biliary drainage, and aggressive management of fluids including hemodialysis may be indicated.

Currently, there is clinical trial using intravenous silibinin for amatoxin-induced hepatic failure, protocol available on http://www.clinicaltrials.gov.

Diaz JH: Amatoxin-containing mushroom poisonings: species, toxidromes, treatments, and outcomes. Wilderness Environ Med 2018 Mar;29(1):111–118. doi: 10.1016/j.wem.2017.10.002 [PMID: 29325729].

North American Mycological Association: Mushroom Poisoning Syndromes: http://www.namyco.org/toxicology/poison_syndromes.html. Accessed November 20, 2017.

Silibinin and the full protocol are available from Prevention and Treatment of Amatoxin Induced Hepatic Failure With Intravenous Silibinin (Legalon®SIL): A Nationwide Open Clinical Trial. http://www.clinicaltrials.gov/ct2/show/study/NCT00915681. Accessed February 21, 2019.

White J et al: Mushroom poisoning: a proposed new clinical classification. Toxicon 2019 Jan;157:53–65. doi: 10.1016/j.toxicon.2018.11.007 [PMID: 30682376].

NITRITES, NITRATES, ANILINE, PENTACHLOROPHENOL, & DINITROPHENOL

Nausea, vertigo, vomiting, cyanosis (methemoglobinemia), cramping, abdominal pain, tachycardia, cardiovascular collapse, tachypnea, coma, shock, convulsions, and death are possible manifestations of nitrite or nitrate poisoning.

Nitrite and nitrate compounds found in the home include amyl nitrite, butyl nitrates, isobutyl nitrates, nitroglycerin, pentaerythritol tetranitrate, sodium nitrite, nitrobenzene, and phenazopyridine. Pentachlorophenol and dinitrophenol, which are found in wood preservatives, produce methemoglobinemia and acidosis because of uncoupling of oxidative phosphorylation. Headache, dizziness, and bradycardia have been reported. High concentrations of nitrites in well water or spinach have been the most common cause of nitrite-induced methemoglobinemia. Other common causes of methemoglobinemia include local anesthetics. Symptoms do not usually occur until 15%–50% of the hemoglobin has been converted to methemoglobin. A rapid test is to compare a drop of normal blood with the patient's blood on a dry filter paper. Brown discoloration of the patient's blood indicates a methemoglobin level of more than 15%.

► Treatment

In the setting of a recent ingestion, consider administering activated charcoal if the patient is awake and alert. Decontaminate affected skin with soap and water. Oxygen and artificial respiration may be needed. If the blood methemoglobin level exceeds 30%, or if levels cannot be obtained and the patient is symptomatic, give a 1% solution of methylene blue (0.2 mL/kg IV) over 5–10 minutes. Avoid perivascular infiltration, because it causes necrosis of the skin and subcutaneous tissues. A dramatic change in the degree of cyanosis should occur. Transfusion is occasionally necessary. If reflex bradycardia occurs, atropine should be used.

Cortazzo JA et al: Methemoglobinemia: a review and recommendations for management. J Cardiothorac Vasc Anesth 2014;28(4):1055–1059 [PMID: 23953868].

Grundlingh J, Dargan PI, El-Zanfaly M, Wood DM: 2,4-dinitrophenol (DNP): a weight loss agent with significant acute toxicity and risk of death. J Med Toxicol 2011 Sep;7(3):205–212. doi: 10.1007/s13181-011-0162-6 [PMID: 21739343].

OPIOIDS & OPIATES

Opioid and opiate-related medical problems may include drug addiction, withdrawal in a newborn infant, and accidental overdoses. They can vary in onset of action and duration of action. Many opioids are detected in common urine drug assays, but the substances detected vary by facility. Check with your hospital laboratory to determine which opioids are detected. Use of fentanyl analogs (carfentanyl) and fentanyl contamination in heroin and other drugs of abuse have increased, contributing to local outbreaks and mortality rates.

Opioid-addicted adolescents often have other medical problems, including cellulitis, abscesses, thrombophlebitis, tetanus, infective endocarditis, human immunodeficiency virus (HIV) infection, tuberculosis, hepatitis, malaria, foreign body emboli, thrombosis of pulmonary arterioles, diabetes mellitus, obstetric complications, nephropathy, and peptic ulcer.

▶ **Treatment**

A. Overdose

Opioids and opiates can cause respiratory depression, stridor, coma, increased oropharyngeal secretions, sinus bradycardia, and urinary retention. Pulmonary edema rarely occurs in children but has been reported; deaths usually result from aspiration of gastric contents, respiratory arrest, and cerebral edema.

The indication for the administration of naloxone is respiratory depression. Although suggested doses for naloxone hydrochloride range from 0.01 to 0.1 mg/kg, it is generally unnecessary to calculate the dosage on this basis. This extremely safe antidote should be given in sufficient quantity to reverse opioid-binding sites. Doses as low as 0.04 mg have been affective for reversal. For children younger than 1 year, one ampoule (0.4 mg) should be given initially; if there is no response, five more ampoules (2 mg) should be given rapidly. Older children should be given 0.4–0.8 mg, followed by 2–4 mg if there is no response. An improvement in respiratory status may be followed by respiratory depression, because the antagonist's duration of action is less than 1 hour. Neonates poisoned in utero may require 10–30 mg/kg to reverse the effect. Naloxone infusion can be used for persistent symptoms. Depending on the formulation, some exposures (such as buprenorphine and methadone) may need to be observed for 24 hours due to the duration of effect.

B. Withdrawal in the Addicted Patient

Benzodiazepines such as diazepam (10 mg every 6 hours PO) and antiemetics have been recommended for the treatment of mild narcotic withdrawal in ambulatory adolescents. Management of withdrawal may be accomplished with the administration of clonidine, by substitution with methadone or buprenorphine, or with reintroduction of the original addicting agent, if available through a supervised drug withdrawal program. A tapered course over 3 weeks will accomplish this goal. Death rarely, if ever, occurs. The abrupt discontinuation of narcotics (cold turkey method) is not recommended and may cause severe physical withdrawal signs.

C. Withdrawal in the In-utero Exposed Newborn

A newborn infant in opioid withdrawal is usually small for gestational age and demonstrates yawning, sneezing, decreased Moro reflex, hunger but uncoordinated sucking action, jitteriness, tremor, constant movement, a shrill protracted cry, increased tendon reflexes, convulsions, vomiting, fever, watery diarrhea, cyanosis, dehydration, vasomotor instability, seizure, and collapse.

The onset of symptoms commonly begins in the first 48 hours but may be delayed as long as 8 days, depending on the timing of the mother's last use and her predelivery medication. Several treatment methods, both pharmacologic and nonpharmacologic, have been suggested for narcotic withdrawal in the newborn, including phenobarbital, morphine, methadone, and buprenorphine. The mortality rate of untreated narcotic withdrawal in the newborn may be as high as 45%.

Disher T et al: Pharmacological treatments for neonatal abstinence syndrome: a systematic review and network meta-analysis. JAMA Pediatr 2019 Jan 22. doi: 10.1001/jamapediatrics.2018.5044 [PMID: 30667476].

Gaither JR, Leventhal JM, Ryan SA, Camenga DR: National trends in hospitalizations for opioid poisonings among children and adolescents, 1997 to 2012. JAMA Pediatr 2016 Dec 1; 170(12):1195–1201. doi:10.1001/jamapediatrics.2016.2154 [PMID: 27802492].

Levy S: Youth and the opioid epidemic. Pediatrics 2019 Jan 2. pii: e20182752. doi: 10.1542/peds.2018-2752.

Suzuki J, El-Haddad S: A review: fentanyl and non-pharmaceutical fentanyls. Drug Alcohol Depend 2017 Feb 1;171:107–116. doi: 10.1016/j.drugalcdep.2016.11.033 [PMID: 28068563].

Wachman EM et al: Neonatal abstinence syndrome: advances in diagnosis and treatment. JAMA 2018 Apr 3;319(13):1362–1374. doi: 10.1001/jama.2018.2640 [PMID: 29614184].

ORAL ANTI-DIABETICS (SULFONYLUREAS, METFORMIN)

Noninsulin hypoglycemic and antidiabetic medications include α-glucosidase inhibitors, biguanides (metformin), dipeptidyl peptidase-4 inhibitors (-gliptins), glucagon-like peptides (-glutide), meglitinides (-glinide), sodium glucose transporter inhibitors (-flovzin), sulfonylureas, and thiazolidinediones (-glitazone). They are all used to treat hyperglycemia in diabetics. Sulfonylureas (acetohexamide, glipizide, glyburide) are the only oral hypoglycemic that actively secretes endogenous insulin and can cause hypoglycemia. The meglitinides (nateglinide, repaglinide) have scarce reports of hypoglycemia. Biguanides can rarely cause lactic acidosis in acute large overdose or in renal failure. Hypoglycemic symptoms are variable but can include altered mental status, diaphoresis, seizures, or coma.

▶ **Treatment**

Children with possible exposures to sulfonylureas should be admitted for 12–24 hours. Mainstay of treatment is treating hypoglycemia. If patient is awake and alert, with minimal symptoms, PO glucose can be given. With more severe hypoglycemia or symptomatic, immediate treatment with 0.5–1 g/kg IV dextrose bolus should be administered. With repeated episodes of hypoglycemia, once euglycemia is achieved, octreotide should be considered at 1 mcg/kg SC/IV every 6–8 hours as needed for hypoglycemia. Metformin toxicity should be treated supportively, lactate can be a measure for toxicity, and hemodialysis may be needed for severe acid-base abnormalities or patients with renal failure.

Glatstein M, Scolnik D, Betur Y: Octreotide for the treatment of sulfonylurea poisoning. Clin Toxicol (Phila) 2012;50(9):795–804 [PMID: 23046209].

Llamado R, Czaja A, Stence N, Davidson J: Continuous octreotide infusion for sulfonylurea-induced hypoglycemia in a toddler. J Emerg Med 2013 Dec;45(6):e209–e213. doi: 10.1016/j.jemermed.2013.05.016 [PMID: 23827165].

Wang G, Hoyte C: Review of biguanide (metformin) toxicity. J Intensive Care Med 2018 Aug 21;885066618793385. doi: 10.1177/0885066618793385 [PMID: 30126348].

ANTIPSYCHOTICS (TYPICAL & ATYPICAL)

Typical antipsychotics include butyrophenones (droperidol, haloperidol), and the phenothiazines (promethazine, chlorpromazine, thioridazine). Atypical antipsychotics include benzapines (clozapine, olanzapine, quetiapine) and indoles (risperidone, ziprasidone).

▶ **Clinical Findings**

A. Extrapyramidal Crisis

Episodes characterized by torticollis, stiffening of the body, spasticity, poor speech, catatonia, and inability to communicate although conscious are typical manifestations. Extrapyramidal crises may represent idiosyncratic reactions and are aggravated by dehydration. The signs and symptoms occur most often in children who have received prochlorperazine. They are commonly mistaken for psychotic episodes.

These extrapyramidal symptoms are more common with typical antipsychotics (butyrophenones, phenothiazines).

B. Overdose

Lethargy and deep prolonged coma are the most common symptoms seen in toxicity. Of the typical antipsychotics, promazine, chlorpromazine, and prochlorperazine are the drugs most likely to cause respiratory depression and precipitous drops in blood pressure. Risperidone and quetiapine are atypical antipsychotics that can cause CNS depression. Clozapine, olanzapine, and quetiapine most commonly cause hypotension and also antimuscarinic symptoms. QTc prolongation can occur, most commonly with thioridazine and ziprasidone, however dysrhythmias are rare. Occasionally, paradoxical hyperactivity and extrapyramidal signs as well as hyperglycemia and acetonemia are present. Seizures are uncommon.

C. Neuroleptic Malignant Syndrome

Neuroleptic malignant syndrome is a rare idiosyncratic complication that may be lethal. It is a syndrome involving mental status change (confusion, coma), motor abnormalities (lead pipe rigidity, clonus), and autonomic dysfunction (tachycardia, hyperpyrexia). Typically, it occurs 1–2 weeks after starting therapy, can occur at therapeutic doses, and may last for several days.

▶ **Treatment**

Extrapyramidal signs are alleviated within minutes by the slow IV administration of diphenhydramine, 1–2 mg/kg (maximum, 50 mg), or benztropine mesylate, 1–2 mg IV (1 mg/min). No other treatment is usually indicated. Further doses may be needed.

Patients with overdoses should receive conservative supportive care. Hypotension may be treated with standard agents, starting with isotonic saline administration. Agitation is best treated with benzodiazepines. Neuroleptic malignant syndrome is treated by discontinuing the drug, and treating hyperthermia and agitation aggressively with benzodiazepines and sedation. In refractory cases, bromocriptine can be considered, although the evidence for its use is not clear.

Levine M, Ruha AM: Overdose of atypical antipsychotics: clinical presentation, mechanisms of toxicity and management. CNS Drugs 2012;26(7):601–611 [PMID: 22668123].

Minns AB, Clark RG: Toxicology and overdose of atypical antipsychotics. J Emerg Med 2012;43(5):906–913 [PMID: 22555052].

PLANTS

Many common ornamental, garden, and wild plants are potentially toxic. Only in a few cases will small amounts of a plant cause severe illness or death. Table 13–5 lists the most

Table 13–5. Poisoning due to plants.[a]

	Symptoms and Signs	Treatment
Arum family: *Caladium, Dieffenbachia,* callalily, dumb cane (oxalic acid)	Burning of mucous membranes and airway obstruction secondary to edema caused by calcium oxalate crystals.	Accessible areas should be thoroughly washed. Corticosteroids relieve airway obstruction. Apply cold packs to affected mucous membranes.
Castor bean plant (ricin—a toxalbumin) Jequinty bean (abrin—a toxalbumin)	Mucous membrane irritation, nausea, vomiting, bloody diarrhea, blurred vision, circulatory collapse, acute hemolytic anemia, convulsions, uremia.	Fluid and electrolyte monitoring. Saline cathartic. Forced alkaline diuresis will prevent complications due to hemagglutination and hemolysis.
Foxglove, lily of the valley, and oleander[b]	Nausea, diarrhea, visual disturbances, and -cardiac irregularities (eg, heart block).	See treatment for digitalis drugs in text.
Jimsonweed: See Belladonna Alkaloids section in text	Mydriasis, dry mouth, tachycardia, and -hallucinations.	Benzodiazepines for agitation, physostigmine
Larkspur (ajacine, *Delphinium,* delphinine)	Nausea and vomiting, irritability, muscular paralysis, and central nervous system depression.	Symptomatic. Atropine may be helpful.
Monkshood (aconite)	Numbness of mucous membranes, visual disturbances, tingling, dizziness, tinnitus, hypotension, bradycardia, and convulsions.	Activated charcoal, oxygen. Atropine is probably helpful.
Poison hemlock (coniine)	Mydriasis, trembling, dizziness, bradycardia. Central nervous system depression, muscular paralysis, and convulsions. Death is due to respiratory paralysis.	Symptomatic. Oxygen and cardiac monitoring equipment are desirable. Assisted respiration is often necessary. Give anticonvulsants if needed.
Rhododendron (grayanotoxin)	Abdominal cramps, vomiting, severe diarrhea, muscular paralysis. Central nervous system and circulatory depression. Hypertension with very large doses.	Atropine can prevent bradycardia. Epinephrine is contraindicated. Antihypertensives may be needed.
Yellow jessamine (active ingredient, geisemine, is related to strychnine)	Restlessness, convulsions, muscular paralysis, and respiratory depression	Symptomatic. Because of the relation to strychnine, activated charcoal and diazepam for seizures are worth trying.
Water hemlock (cicutoxin).	Nausea, vomiting, abdominal pain. Followed by seizures. Severe ingestions can result in rhabdomyolysis, metabolic acidosis and renal failure	Symptomatic. Benzodiazepines for seizures.

[a]Many other plants cause minor irritation but are not likely to cause serious problems unless large amounts are ingested. Data from Lampe KF, McCann MA: *AMA Handbook of Poisonous and Injurious Plants.* American Medical Association; 1985.
[b]Done AK: Ornamental and deadly. Emerg Med 1973;5:255.

toxic plants, symptoms and signs of poisoning, and treatment. Contact your poison control center for assistance with identification.

PSYCHOTROPIC DRUGS

Psychotropic drugs consist of four general classes: stimulants (amphetamines, cocaine, nicotine), depressants (eg, narcotics, barbiturates), antidepressants and tranquilizers, and psychoactive drugs (hallucinogens such as lysergic acid diethylamide [LSD], phencyclidine [PCP]).

▶ Clinical Findings

The following clinical findings are commonly seen in patients abusing drugs. See also other entries discussed in alphabetic order in this chapter.

A. Stimulants

Agitation, euphoria, grandiose feelings, tachycardia, fever, abdominal cramps, visual and auditory hallucinations, mydriasis, coma, convulsions, and respiratory depression. Nicotine is associated with vomiting, hypertension and tachycardia, followed by symptoms of cholinergic excess, seizures and weakness.

B. Depressants

Emotional lability, ataxia, diplopia, nystagmus, vertigo, poor accommodation, respiratory depression, coma, apnea, and convulsions. Narcotics cause miotic pupils and, occasionally, pulmonary edema.

C. Antidepressants and Tranquilizers

Hypotension, lethargy, respiratory depression, coma, and extrapyramidal reactions.

D. Hallucinogens and Psychoactive Drugs

Belladonna alkaloids cause anticholinergic toxicity: mydriasis, dry mouth, nausea, vomiting, urinary retention, delirium, agitation, hallucinations, fever, hypotension, convulsions, and coma. Psychoactive drugs such as LSD cause mydriasis, unexplained bizarre behavior, hallucinations, and generalized undifferentiated psychotic behavior. Marijuana can cause tachycardia, anxiety, dysphoria, and vomiting.

▶ Treatment

Only a small percentage of the persons using drugs come to the attention of physicians; those who do are usually experiencing adverse reactions such as panic states, drug psychoses, homicidal or suicidal thoughts, or respiratory depression.

Even with cooperative patients, an accurate history is difficult to obtain. A drug history is most easily obtained in a quiet spot by a gentle, nonthreatening, honest examiner, and without the parents present. Street drugs are often adulterated with one or more other compounds and the exact dose is unknown. Multiple drugs are often taken together. Friends may be a useful source of information.

Hallucinogens are not life-threatening unless the patient is frankly homicidal or suicidal. A specific diagnosis is usually not necessary for management; instead, the presenting signs and symptoms are treated. Does the patient appear intoxicated? In withdrawal? "Flashing back?" Is some illness or injury (eg, head trauma) being masked by a drug effect? (Remember that a known drug user may still have hallucinations from meningoencephalitis.)

The signs and symptoms in a given patient are a function not only of the drug and the dose but also of the level of acquired tolerance, the "setting," the patient's physical condition and personality traits, the potentiating effects of other drugs, and many other factors.

A common drug problem is the "bad trip," which is usually a panic reaction. This is best managed by speaking calmly with the patient and minimizing auditory and visual stimuli. Allowing the patient to sit with a friend while the

drug effect dissipates may be the best treatment. This may take several hours.

Drug therapy is often unnecessary and may complicate the clinical course of a drug-related panic reaction. Although phenothiazines have been commonly used to treat bad trips, they should be avoided if the specific drug is unknown, because they may enhance toxicity or produce unwanted side effects. Benzodiazepines are the drug of choice if a sedative effect is required. Physical restraints are rarely indicated and usually increase the patient's panic reaction. After the acute episode, the physician must decide whether psychiatric referral is indicated.

Wang GS, Hoyte C: Common substances of abuse. Pediatr Rev 2018 Aug;39(8):403–414. doi: 10.1542/pir.2017-0267.

SALICYLATES

The use of childproof containers and publicity regarding accidental poisoning have reduced the incidence of acute salicylate poisoning. Oil of wintergreen ingestion can also lead to salicylate toxicity. Nevertheless, serious intoxication still occurs and must be regarded as an emergency.

Salicylates uncouple oxidative phosphorylation, leading to increased heat production, excessive sweating, and dehydration. They also interfere with glucose metabolism and may cause hypo- or hyperglycemia. Respiratory center stimulation occurs early. The severity of acute intoxication can, in some measure, be judged by serum salicylate levels. High levels are always dangerous irrespective of clinical signs, and low levels may be misleading in chronic cases.

In mild and moderate poisoning, stimulation of the respiratory center produces respiratory alkalosis and may complain of tinnitus or hearing loss. Vomiting is also a common presenting symptom. In severe intoxication (occurring in severe acute ingestion with high salicylate levels and in chronic toxicity with lower levels), respiratory response is unable to overcome the metabolic overdose which may lead to fever, diaphoresis, pulmonary edema, seizures, and death.

Once the urine becomes acidic, less salicylate is excreted. Until this process is reversed, the half-life will remain prolonged, because metabolism contributes little to the removal of salicylate. Chronic severe poisoning may occur as early as 3 days after a regimen of salicylate is begun. Findings usually include vomiting, diarrhea, and dehydration.

▶ Treatment

Charcoal binds salicylates well and should be given for acute ingestions in patients now vomiting with normal mentation. Mild poisoning may require only the administration of oral fluids and confirmation that the salicylate level is falling (< 30 mg/dL). Moderate poisoning involves moderate dehydration and depletion of potassium. Fluids must be administered at a rate of 2–3 mL/kg/h to correct dehydration and produce urine with a pH of greater than 7.0. Initial IV solutions should be isotonic (D5W with 150 mEq sodium bicarbonate). Once the patient is rehydrated, the solution can contain more free water and approximately 40 mEq/L of K^+.

Severe toxicity is marked by major dehydration. Symptoms may be confused with those of Reye syndrome, encephalopathy, and metabolic acidosis. Salicylate levels may even be in the therapeutic range. Major fluid correction of dehydration is required. Once this has been accomplished, hypokalemia must be corrected and sodium bicarbonate given. Usual requirements are sodium bicarbonate, 1–2 mEq/kg/h over the first 6–8 hours, and K^+, 20–40 mEq/L. A urine flow of 2–3 mL/kg/h should be established. Despite this treatment, some patients will develop the paradoxical aciduria of salicylism. This is due to hypokalemia and the saving of K^+ and excretion of H^+ in the renal tubule. Correction of K^+ will allow the urine to become alkaline and ionize the salicylate, resulting in excretion rather than reabsorption of nonionized salicylate in acid urine.

Patients with renal failure, pulmonary edema, mental status changes, seizures, or concentrations of greater than 100 mg/dL should be considered for hemodialysis.

Davis JE: Are one or two dangerous? Methyl salicylate exposure in toddlers. J Emerg Med 2007 Jan;32(1):63–69. doi: 10.1016/j.jemermed.2006.08.009 [PMID: 17239735].

Juurlink DN et al: Extracorporeal treatment for salicylate poisoning: systematic review and recommendations from the EXTRIP workgroup. Ann Emerg Med 2015 Aug;66(2):165–181. doi: 10.1016/j.annemergmed.2015.03.031 [PMID: 25986310].

SCORPION STINGS

Scorpion stings are common in the southwestern United States. Although neurologic manifestations may last a week, most clinical signs subside within 24–48 hours.

The most common scorpions in the United States are *Vejovis*, *Hadrurus*, *Androctonus*, and *Centruroides* species. Stings by the first three produce edema and pain. Stings by *Centruroides* (the Bark scorpion) are most clinically significant and can cause tingling or burning paresthesias that begin at the site of the sting. In small children, hypersalivation, restlessness, muscular fasciculation, abdominal cramps, opisthotonos, convulsions, urinary incontinence, and respiratory failure may occur.

▶ Treatment

Sedation with benzodiazepines is the primary therapy. Antivenom is reserved for severe poisoning, recommended dosing of 1–3 vials. In severe cases, the airway may become compromised by secretions and weakness of respiratory muscles. Endotracheal intubation may be required. Patients may require treatment for seizures, hypertension, or tachycardia. The prognosis is good as long as the patient's airway is managed appropriately and sedation is achieved.

Boyer LV et al: Antivenom for critically ill children with neurotoxicity from scorpion stings. N Engl J Med 2009;360:2090–2098 [PMID: 19439743].

Coorg V, Levitan RD, Gerkin RD, Muenzer J, Ruha AM: Clinical presentation and outcomes associated with different treatment modalities for pediatric bark scorpion envenomation. J Med Toxicol 2016 Aug 3. doi: 10.1007/s13181-016-0575-3 [PMID: 27487782].

Pariury HE et al: A stinging suspicion something was just not right: methamphetamine toxicity in infant mimics scorpion envenomation. Pediatr Emerg Care 2017 Nov;33(11):e124–e125. doi: 10.1097/PEC.0000000000001301 [PMID: 29095780].

SEROTONIN REUPTAKE INHIBITORS

Fluoxetine (Prozac), paroxetine (Paxil), sertraline (Zoloft), and many other agents comprise this class of drugs. Adverse effects in therapeutic dosing include sedation, suicidal thoughts, aggressive behavior, and extrapyramidal effects. In overdose may include vomiting, lethargy, hypertension, tachycardia, hyperthermia, and abdominal pain, but rarely seizures and cardiac dysrhythmias. The findings in overdose are included in the serotonin syndrome due to the action of these drugs, which results in an increase of serotonin (5-hydroxytryptamine [5-HT]). Despite the degree of toxicity these agents generally are not life-threatening and intervention usually is not necessary.

Laboratory measurements of the drugs are not of benefit other than to establish their presence.

Treatment of agitation, hyperthermia with benzodiazepines is most beneficial. Hypotension may be treated with fluids or norepinephrine. Cyproheptadine is an antagonist of serotonin, but evidence for its use is limited. A dose of 0.25 mg/kg/day divided every 6 hours to a maximum of 12 mg/day may be useful in treating the serotonin syndrome. Adults and older adolescents have been treated with 12 mg initially followed by 2 mg every 2 hours to a maximum of 32 mg/day.

Boyer EW, Shannon M: The serotonin syndrome. N Engl J Med 2005;352:1112 [PMID: 15784664].

Kant et al: Recognizing serotonin toxicity in the pediatric emergency department. Pediatr Emerg Care 2012;28(8):817–821 [PMID: 22863827].

SNAKEBITE

Nearly all poisonous snakebites in the United States are caused by pit vipers (rattlesnakes, water moccasins, and copperheads). A few are caused by elapids (coral snakes), and occasional bites occur from cobras and other nonindigenous exotic snakes kept as pets. Snake venom is a complex mixture of enzymes, peptides, and proteins that may have predominantly cytotoxic, neurotoxic, hemotoxic, or cardiotoxic effects but other effects as well. Up to 25% of bites by pit vipers do not result in venom injection. US pit viper venom causes predominantly local injury with pain, discoloration, edema, and thrombocytopenia.

The outcome depends on the size of the child, the site of the bite, the degree of envenomation, the type of snake, and the effectiveness of treatment. Swelling and pain occur soon after rattlesnake bite and are a certain indication that envenomation has occurred. During the first few hours, swelling and ecchymosis extend proximally from the bite. The bite is often obvious as a double puncture mark surrounded by ecchymosis. Hematemesis, melena, hemoptysis, and other manifestations of coagulopathy rarely develop in severe cases. Rarely, respiratory difficulty and shock are the ultimate causes of death.

Coral snake envenomation causes little local pain, swelling, or necrosis, and systemic reactions are often delayed. The signs of coral snake envenomation include bulbar paralysis, dysphagia, and dysphoria; these signs may appear in 5–10 hours and may be followed by total peripheral paralysis and death in 24 hours.

▶ Treatment

A. Emergency (First-Aid) Treatment

The most important first-aid measure is transportation to a medical facility. Splint the affected extremity and minimize the patient's motion. Tourniquets and ice packs are contraindicated. Incision and suction are not useful for either crotalid or elapid snake bite.

B. Definitive Medical Management

Blood should be drawn for hematocrit, clotting time and platelet function, and serum electrolyte determinations. Establish two secure IV sites for the administration of antivenom and other medications.

Specific antivenom is indicated when signs of progressive envenomation are present. For coral snake bites, an eastern coral snake antivenom (Wyeth Laboratories) is sparingly available. Patients with pit viper bites should receive polyvalent crotaline antivenom IV (Fab or Fab$_2$) if progressive local injury, coagulopathy, or systemic signs (eg, hypotension, confusion) are present. See package labeling or call your poison center for details of use. Antivenom will halt progression of symptoms and improve hemorrhage, pain, and shock. For any history of coral snake bites, give three to five vials of antivenom in 250–500 mL of isotonic saline solution if available and observation for at least 24 hours. An additional three to five vials may be required. While generally considered best if administered within the first 6 hours, recent evidence demonstrates that delayed use may be therapeutic.

Administer an opioid or opiate to control pain. Cryotherapy is contraindicated because it commonly causes additional tissue damage. Early physiotherapy minimizes contractures. In rare cases, fasciotomy to relieve pressure within muscular compartments is required; recommend measurements of pressures before fasciotomy. Antihistamines and corticosteroids (hydrocortisone, 1 mg/kg, given PO for a week) are useful in the treatment of serum sickness or anaphylactic shock.

Antibiotics are not needed unless clinical signs of infection occur. Tetanus status should be evaluated and the patient immunized, if needed. Recurrent coagulopathy and thrombocytopenia may occur after discharge, and patients should have follow up examinations and repeat laboratory values within 1 week after hospital discharge.

Gerardo CJ et al: Coagulation parameters in copperhead compared to other Crotalinae envenomation: secondary analysis of the F(ab')2 versus Fab antivenom trial. Clin Toxicol (Phila) 2017 Feb;55(2):109–114. doi: 10.1080/15563650.2016.1250275 [PMID: 27806644].

Goto CS, Feng SY: Crotalidae polyvalent immune Fab for the treatment of pediatric crotaline envenomation. Pediatr Emerg Care 2009 Apr;25(4):273–279; quiz 280-2. doi: 10.1097/PEC.0b013e31819f1f1e [PMID: 19369845].

Lasoff DR et al: A new F(ab')2 antivenom for the treatment of crotaline envenomation in children. Am J Emerg Med 2016 Oct;34(10):2003–2006. doi: 10.1016/j.ajem.2016.07.061 [PMID: 27567423].

Miller AD, Young MC, DeMott MC, Ly BT, Clark RF: Recurrent coagulopathy and thrombocytopenia in children treated with crotalidae polyvalent immune fab: a case series. Pediatr Emerg Care 2010 Aug;26(8):576–582. doi: 10.1097/PEC.0b013e3181ea722b [PMID: 20693856].

SOAPS & DETERGENTS

1. Soaps

Soap is made from salts of fatty acids. Ingestion of soap bars may cause vomiting and diarrhea, but they have a low toxicity.

2. Detergents

Detergents are nonsoap synthetic products used for cleaning purposes because of their surfactant properties. Commercial products include granules, powders, and liquids. Dishwasher detergents are very alkaline and can cause caustic burns. Low concentrations of bleaching and antibacterial agents as well as enzymes are found in many preparations. The pure compounds are moderately toxic, but the concentration used is too small to alter the product's toxicity significantly, although occasional primary or allergic irritative phenomena have been noted in persons who frequently use such products and in employees manufacturing these products. Unit dose detergents, or packets, have become popular and have packaging attractive to young children. They are usually a mix of glycol ethers, ethyl alcohol and surfactant. They typically cause local irritation but can lead to more severe symptoms including corneal injuries, CNS depression and respiratory distress if ingested.

A. Cationic Detergents (Ceepryn, Diaparene Cream, Phemerol, Zephiran)

Cationic detergents in dilute solutions (0.5%) cause mucosal irritation, but higher concentrations (10%–15%) may cause caustic burns to mucosa. Clinical effects include nausea, vomiting, collapse, coma, and convulsions. As little as 2.25 g of some cationic agents have caused death in an adult. In four cases, 100–400 mg/kg of benzalkonium chloride caused death. Cationic detergents are rapidly inactivated by tissues and ordinary soap. Because of the caustic potential and rapid onset of seizures, emesis is not recommended. Anticonvulsants may be needed.

B. Anionic Detergents

Most common household detergents are anionic. Laundry compounds have water softener (sodium phosphate) added, which is a strong irritant and may reduce ionized calcium. Anionic detergents irritate the skin by removing natural oils. Although ingestion causes diarrhea, intestinal distention, and vomiting, no fatalities have been reported. The only treatment usually required is to discontinue use if skin irritation occurs and replace fluids and electrolytes. Induced vomiting is not indicated following ingestion of automatic dishwasher detergent, because of its alkalinity.

C. Nonionic Detergents (Brij Products; Tritons X-45, X-100, X-102, and X-144)

These compounds include lauryl, stearyl, and oleyl alcohols and octyl phenol. They have a minimal irritating effect on the skin and are almost always nontoxic when swallowed.

Perry HE: Pediatric poisonings from household products: hydrofluoric acid and methacrylic acid. Curr Opin Pediatr 2011;13(2):157–161 [PMID: 11317059].

Sjogren PP et al: Upper aerodigestive injuries from detergent ingestion in children. Laryngoscope 2017 Feb;127(2):509–512. doi: 10.1002/lary.26184 [PMID: 27470579].

Yin S et al: Single-use laundry detergent pack exposures in children under 6 years: a prospective study at U.S. Poison Control Centers. J Emerg Med 2018 Sep;55(3):354–365. doi: 10.1016/j.jemermed.2018.05.016 [PMID: 29941372].

SPIDER BITES

Most medically important bites in the United States are caused by the black widow spider (*Latrodectus mactans*) and the North American brown recluse (violin) spider (*Loxosceles reclusa*). Positive identification of the spider is helpful, because many spider bites may mimic those of the brown recluse spider.

1. Black Widow Spider

The black widow spider is endemic to nearly all areas of the United States. The initial bite causes sharp fleeting pain that spreads centripetally. Local and systemic muscular cramping, abdominal pain, periorbital edema, nausea and vomiting, tachycardia, and hypertension are common. Systemic signs of black widow spider bite may be confused with other causes of acute abdomen. Although paresthesias,

nervousness, and transient muscle spasms may persist for weeks in survivors, recovery from the acute phase is generally complete within 2–3 days. In contrast to popular opinion, death is extremely rare.

Initial pain control should be achieved with use of benzodiazepines and opioids or opiates. Antivenom is effective and is recommended in severe cases in which the previously mentioned therapies have failed.

2. Brown Recluse Spider (Violin Spider)

The North American brown recluse spider is most commonly seen in the central and Midwestern areas of the United States. Its bite characteristically produces a localized reaction with progressively severe pain within 24 hours. The initial bleb on an erythematous ischemic base is replaced by a black eschar within 1 week. This eschar separates in 2–5 weeks, leaving an ulcer that heals slowly. Systemic signs (loxoscelism) include cyanosis, morbilliform rash, fever, chills, malaise, weakness, nausea and vomiting, joint pains, hemolytic reactions with hemoglobinuria, jaundice, and delirium and are more common in children. Fatalities are rare. Fatal disseminated intravascular coagulation has been reported.

Although of unproved efficacy, the following therapies have been used: dexamethasone, 4 mg IV four times a day, during the acute phase; polymorphonuclear leukocyte inhibitors, such as dapsone or colchicine. Supportive wound care is recommended, with possible reconstruction/debridement. Plasma exchange has been described for severe hemolysis.

Glatstein M et al: Treatment of pediatric black widow spider envenomation: a national poison center's experience. Am J Emerg Med 2018 Jun;36(6):998–1002. doi: 10.1016/j.ajem.2017.11.011 [PMID: 29133072].

Isbister GK, Fan HW: Spider bite. Lancet Dec 10;2011;378 (9808):2039–2047. doi: 10.1016/S0140-6736(10)62230-1.21762981 [PMID: 21762981].

Said A et al: Successful use of plasma exchange for profound hemolysis in a child with loxoscelism. Pediatrics 2014 Nov;134(5): e1464–e1467. doi: 10.1542/peds.2013-3338 [PMID: 25349320].

VITAMINS

Accidental ingestion of excessive amounts of vitamins rarely causes significant problems. Rare cases of hypervitaminosis A do occur, however, particularly in patients with poor hepatic or renal function. Hypervitaminosis A can result in increased intracranial pressure, ocular toxicity, and hepatotoxicity. However, chronic doses more than 50,000–100,000 IU are required for toxicity. The fluoride contained in many multivitamin preparations is not a realistic hazard, because a 2- or 3-year-old child could eat 100 tablets, containing 1 mg of sodium fluoride per tablet, without experiencing serious symptoms. Iron poisoning has been reported with multivitamin tablets containing iron; most gummy vitamins do not contain iron. Pyridoxine abuse has caused neuropathies; nicotinic acid can result in flushing, and rarely hypotension and hepatotoxicity.

Dean BS, Krenzelok EP: Multiple vitamins and vitamins with iron: accidental poisoning in children. Vet Hum Toxicol 1988;30:23 [PMID: 3354178].

Lab HS et al: Risk of vitamin A toxicity from candy-like chewable vitamin supplements for children. Pediatrics 2006;118(2): 820–824 [PMID: 16882846].

WARFARIN (COUMADIN) & NEWER ORAL ANTICOAGULANTS (NOAC)

Warfarin is used as an anticoagulant and rodenticide. It causes hypoprothrombinemia and capillary injury. A dose of 0.5 mg/kg of warfarin may be toxic in a child. Long-acting anticoagulant rodenticides (brodifacoum, difenacoum, bromadiolone, diphacinone, pinene, valone, and coumatetralyl) can cause a more serious toxicologic problem than warfarin as the anticoagulant activity may persist for periods ranging from 6 weeks to several months. However, most unintentional ingestions can be watched at home without further evaluation. If there are concerns for large ingestions, a prothrombin time at 48 hours can determine extent of toxicity. Treatment with vitamin K_1 at high doses may be needed for weeks for long-acting anticoagulant toxicity.

Refer to published American College of Chest Physicians guidelines on management of bleeding in patient receiving vitamin K antagonists. With evidence for bleeding, give fresh frozen plasma, prothrombin complex concentrated, or activated factor. Without significant bleeding, oral vitamin K is recommended.

Newer oral anticoagulants have been developed that have direct inhibition to specific clotting factors. Examples include direct Xa inhibitors (apixaban, edoxaban, rivaroxaban), and direct thrombin (IIa) inhibitors (dabigatran). Toxic doses have not been established, but accidental ingestions do not typically lead to significant toxicity. If available, chromogenic antifactor Xa assay can quantitate direct Xa inhibition, and ecarin clotting time (ECT) or dilute thrombin time (dTT) is the most the most sensitive coagulation parameter for direct thrombin inhibitors. Activated four-factor prothrombin complex concentrates, activated Factor VII, or fresh frozen plasma should be used to treat potentially life-threatening bleeding. Idaracizumab and andexanet alfa are now available for the reversal of dabigatran and factor Xa inhibitors, respectively. Their availability and clinical experience in overdose is limited.

Gunja N, Coggins A, Bidny S: Management of intentional super warfarin poisoning with long-term vitamin K and brodifacoum levels. Clin Toxicol (Phila) 2011;49(5):385–390 [PMID: 21740137].

Kristiansen A et al: Applying new strategies for the national adaptation, updating, and dissemination of trustworthy guidelines: results from the Norwegian adaptation of the Antithrombotic Therapy and the Prevention of Thrombosis, 9th Ed: American College of Chest Physicians Evidence-Based Clinical Practice Guidelines. Chest 2014 Sep;146(3):735–761. doi: 10.1378/chest.13-2993 [PMID: 25180724].

Lip GYH et al: Antithrombotic therapy for atrial fibrillation: CHEST guideline and expert panel report. Chest 2018 Nov;154(5): 1121-1201. doi: 10.1016/j.chest.2018.07.040 [PMID: 30144419].

Weirthein J et al: Accidental rivaroxaban intoxication in a boy: some lessons in managing new oral anticoagulants in children. Pediatr Emerg Care 2018 Jan 15. doi: 10.1097/PEC.0000000000001392 [PMID: 29337837].

Critical Care

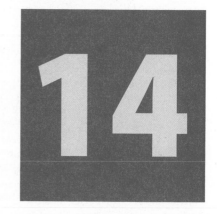

Amy C. Clevenger, MD, PhD

Angela S. Czaja, MD, MSc

Ryan J. Good, MD

Cameron F. Gunville, DO

Leslie A. Ridall, DO

Todd C. Carpenter, MD

Eva N. Grayck, MD

Carleen Schneiter, MD

INTRODUCTION

Critical care medicine is the discipline of caring for patients with acute life-threatening conditions or conditions likely to cause serious harm if not rapidly addressed. This work requires a detailed understanding of human physiology, the pathophysiology of severe illness and injury, the intricate interactions between organ systems and therapies, as well as an understanding of and experience with the rapidly changing technologies available in a modern pediatric intensive care unit (PICU). The science of caring for the critically ill patient continues to advance rapidly as the molecular mediators of illness have become better defined and new therapies are brought into clinical use. Critical care, then, is a highly complex, multidisciplinary field in which optimal patient outcomes require a team-oriented approach, including critical care physicians and nurses; respiratory therapists; pharmacists; consulting specialists; physical, occupational and recreational therapists; and social services specialists.

RESPIRATORY CRITICAL CARE

ACUTE RESPIRATORY FAILURE

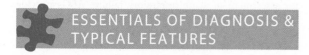

ESSENTIALS OF DIAGNOSIS & TYPICAL FEATURES

► Inability to deliver oxygen or remove carbon dioxide.

► Pao_2 is low while $Paco_2$ is normal in hypoxemic respiratory failure (ventilation/perfusion [V/Q] mismatch, diffusion defects, and intrapulmonary shunt).

► Pao_2 is low and $Paco_2$ is high in hypercapnic respiratory failure (alveolar hypoventilation seen in central nervous system [CNS] dysfunction, oversedation, neuromuscular disorders).

► Noninvasive mechanical ventilation can be an effective treatment for hypercapnic respiratory failure and selected patients with hypoxemic respiratory failure.

► Conventional mechanical ventilation should be accomplished within a strategy of "lung-protective" ventilation.

► Extracorporeal membrane oxygenation (ECMO) is a viable option for patients failing conventional mechanical ventilation.

► Pathogenesis

Acute respiratory failure, defined as the inability of the respiratory system to adequately deliver oxygen or remove carbon dioxide, is a major cause of morbidity and mortality in infants and children. Anatomic and developmental differences place infants and young children at higher risk than older children or adults for respiratory failure. An infant's thoracic cage is more compliant, allowing a greater tendency toward alveolar collapse. The intercostal muscles are poorly developed and unable to achieve the "bucket-handle" motion characteristic of adult breathing, and the diaphragm is shorter and relatively flat with fewer type I muscle fibers, making it less effective and more easily fatigued. The infant's airways are also smaller in caliber resulting in greater resistance to airflow and greater susceptibility to occlusion by mucus plugging and mucosal edema, particularly in the setting of respiratory infections. Alveoli in children are smaller and have less collateral ventilation than adults, again resulting in a greater tendency to collapse and develop atelectasis. Finally, young infants may have a more reactive pulmonary vascular bed, impaired immune system, or residual effects from prematurity, all of which increase the risk of respiratory failure.

Table 14–1. Types of respiratory failure.

Findings	Causes	Examples
Hypoxemic (type I) Pao_2 low $Paco_2$ normal	Ventilation-perfusion (V/Q) defect	Positional (supine in bed), acute respiratory distress syndrome (ARDS), atelectasis, pneumonia, pulmonary embolus, bronchopulmonary dysplasia
	Diffusion impairment	Pulmonary edema, ARDS, interstitial pneumonia
	Shunt	Pulmonary arteriovenous malformation, congenital adenomatoid malformation
Hypercapnic (type II) Pao_2 low $Paco_2$ high	Hypoventilation	Neuromuscular disease (polio, Guillain-Barré syndrome), head trauma, sedation, chest wall dysfunction (burns), kyphoscoliosis, severe reactive airways

Table 14–2. Clinical features of respiratory failure.

Respiratory
  Wheezing
  Expiratory grunting
  Decreased or absent breath sounds
  Flaring of alae nasi
  Retractions of chest wall
  Tachypnea, bradypnea, or apnea
  Cyanosis
Neurologic
  Restlessness
  Irritability
  Headache
  Confusion
  Convulsions
  Coma
Cardiac
  Bradycardia or excessive tachycardia
  Hypotension or hypertension
General
  Fatigue
  Sweating

Respiratory failure can be due to inadequate oxygenation (hypoxemic respiratory failure) or inadequate ventilation (hypercapnic respiratory failure) or both. Hypoxemic respiratory failure occurs in three situations: (1) *Ventilation-perfusion (V/Q) mismatch*, when blood flows to inadequately ventilated lung or when ventilated areas of the lung are inadequately perfused; (2) *diffusion defects*, caused by thickened alveolar membranes or excessive interstitial fluid at the alveolar-capillary junction; and (3) *intrapulmonary shunt*, when structural anomalies in the lung allow blood to flow through the lung without participating in gas exchange. Hypercapnic respiratory failure results from impaired alveolar ventilation, due to conditions such as increased dead space ventilation, reduced respiratory drive due to CNS dysfunction or oversedation, or neuromuscular disorders (Table 14–1).

▶ Clinical Findings

The clinical findings in respiratory failure are the result of hypoxemia, hypercapnia, and arterial pH changes. Common features of respiratory failure are summarized in Table 14–2. These features may not be clinically obvious and many are nonspecific. As a result, a strictly clinical assessment of respiratory failure is not always reliable, and clinical findings of respiratory failure should be supplemented by laboratory data such as blood gas analysis.

▶ Noninvasive Monitoring & Blood Gas Analysis

The adequacy of oxygenation and ventilation can be measured noninvasively and/or through blood gas analysis. *Pulse oximetry* measures *arterial oxygen saturation* (Sao_2) continuously and noninvasively and is an important tool in the assessment and treatment of patients with potential or actual respiratory failure. However, pulse oximetry readings can be much less accurate in patients with saturations below 80%, poor skin perfusion, or significant movement. In addition, pulse oximetry can be dangerously inaccurate in certain clinical settings such as carbon monoxide poisoning or methemoglobinemia. *End-tidal CO_2* ($ETco_2$) *monitoring* measures exhaled carbon dioxide (CO_2) noninvasively, allowing for continuous assessment of ventilation. Normally, the $ETco_2$ level closely approximates the alveolar CO_2 level ($Paco_2$), which should equal arterial CO_2 levels ($Paco_2$) because carbon dioxide diffuses freely across the alveolar-capillary barrier. While most accurate in the intubated patient, this technique can also be used in extubated patients with the proper equipment. However, the $ETco_2$ level may not accurately reflect the $Paco_2$ in patients with increased dead space ventilation or rapid, shallow breathing.

Given the limitations of these noninvasive techniques, *arterial blood gas* (ABG) analysis remains the gold standard for assessment of acute respiratory failure. ABGs provide measurements of the patient's acid-base status (with a measured pH and calculated bicarbonate level) as well as Pao_2 and $Paco_2$ levels. Capillary or venous blood gases may provide some reassurance regarding the adequacy of ventilation and can be useful for following trends; however, they yield virtually no useful information regarding oxygenation and may generate highly misleading information about the ventilatory status of patients who have poor perfusion or who had difficult blood draws. As a result, ABG analysis is important for all patients with suspected respiratory failure, particularly those with abnormal venous or capillary gases.

Knowing the ABG values and the inspired oxygen concentration also enables one to calculate the *alveolar-arterial oxygen difference* ($A-aDO_2$, or A–a gradient). The A–a gradient is less than 15 mm Hg under normal conditions, widening with diffusion impairment, shunts, and V/Q mismatch. The degree of widening has prognostic value in severe hypoxemic respiratory failure, with A–a gradients over 400 mm Hg being strongly associated with mortality. Assessment of intrapulmonary shunting (the percentage of pulmonary blood flow that passes through nonventilated areas of the lung) may also be helpful. Normal individuals have less than a 5% physiologic shunt from bronchial, coronary, and thebesian (cardiac intramural) circulations. Shunt fractions greater than 15% usually indicate the need for aggressive respiratory support. However, calculation of the shunt fraction requires a pulmonary arterial catheter, the use of which has decline significantly over the past decade.

▶ Modes of Respiratory Support

Patients with severe hypoxemia, hypoventilation, or apnea require immediate assistance with bag and mask ventilation. Although assisted ventilation can generally be maintained for some time with a properly sized mask, gastric distention, emesis leading to aspiration of gastric contents, and inadequate tidal volumes leading to atelectasis are possible complications. In patients not requiring immediate intubation, several modalities can be used to provide respiratory support, including supplemental oxygen, heated high-flow nasal cannula (HHFNC), and noninvasive ventilation (NIV).

Supplemental oxygen with a nasal cannula or oxygen mask may be adequate to treat patients with mild respiratory insufficiency (Table 14–3). Patients with hypoventilation and diffusion defects respond better to supplemental oxygen than patients with significant shunts or V/Q mismatch. For patients requiring more support, HHFNC can be considered. *HHFNC* devices deliver heated and humidified oxygen mixtures via nasal cannula at flow rates higher than possible with cooler dry air. Depending on the flow rate and size of patient, HHFNC can also generate some amount of positive pressure and potentially improve work of breathing without further escalation of support. Generally, flow rates of 1–2 L/kg/min are considered high flow in infants and children (up to a maximum of 25 L/min) although some studies have utilized up to 60 L/min in adults. HHFNC use has been studied in children with bronchiolitis and appears to be well tolerated, potentially decreasing the need for noninvasive ventilation or intubation. However, if the patient is not improving on HHFNC after 30–60 minutes, additional escalation of care may be warranted, including initiation of noninvasive ventilation that can deliver positive pressure more consistently.

Noninvasive ventilation (NIV) refers to the administration of positive pressure breathing through various interfaces (mouthpiece or nasal, face, or helmet mask) rather than an invasive artificial airway (endotracheal tube [ETT] or tracheostomy tube). NIV has become an integral tool in the management of both acute and chronic respiratory failure, reducing need for intubation in milder cases of respiratory failure or as a bridge after extubation in patients with marginal lung function and respiratory mechanics. Various modes of support can be used with NIV, such as continuous positive airway pressure (CPAP), bilevel positive airway pressure (BiPAP), or average volume-assured pressure support (AVAPS).

CPAP refers to the constant application of airway pressure, usually in the range of 5–10 cm H_2O. BiPAP cycles between a higher inspiratory positive airway pressure (IPAP) and a lower expiratory positive airway pressure (EPAP). The additional inspiratory support in this mode improves tidal volume and ventilation in patients who are breathing shallowly and can improve oxygenation by

Table 14–3. Supplemental oxygen therapy.

Source	Maximum % O_2 Delivered	Range of Rates (L/min)	Advantages	Disadvantages
Nasal cannula	35%–40%	0.125–4	Easily applied, relatively comfortable	Uncomfortable at higher flow rates, requires open nasal airways, easily dislodged, lower % O_2 delivered, nosebleeds
Simple mask	50%–60%	5–10	Higher % O_2, good for mouth breathers	Unsure of delivered % O_2
Face tent	40%–60%	8–10	Higher % O_2, good for mouth breathers, less restrictive	Unsure of delivered % O_2
Nonrebreathing mask	80%–90%	5–10	Highest O_2 concentration, good for mouth breathers	Unsure of delivered % O_2
Oxyhood	90%–100%	5–10	Stable and accurate O_2 concentration	Difficult to maintain temperature, hard to give airway care

providing a higher mean airway pressure (MAP). Common initial settings would place the IPAP at 12–14 cm H_2O and the EPAP at 6–8 cm H_2O. The IPAP can then be titrated upward to achieve adequate tidal volumes, usually in the range of 5–7 mL/kg, and based on the patient's work of breathing and respiratory rate. EPAP and delivered oxygen concentration can be adjusted upward to achieve adequate oxygenation. AVAPS targets a tidal volume within an allowable inspiratory pressure range. Usually, a tidal volume of approximately 8 mL/kg is set with an IPAP max of 20–30 cm H_2O. EPAP is approached in a similar manner as BiPAP. With any mode of NIV, close respiratory monitoring is essential for assessing response to NIV therapy and guiding further adjustments.

Although NIV is generally well tolerated, successful application of NIV requires careful patient selection and close respiratory monitoring. The best candidates are patients with moderate lung disease, in the recovery phases of their illness, or those with primarily hypercapnic respiratory failure, such as patients with muscular dystrophies or other forms of neuromuscular weakness. These patients should be closely monitored, however, as NIV may mask symptoms of underlying disease progression, making eventual intubation more precarious. Patients suffering from coma, impaired respiratory drive, an inability to protect their airway, or cardiac or respiratory arrest are not candidates for NIV. In patients with severe respiratory failure or those who are not improving with NIV, endotracheal intubation should not be delayed.

For patients with acute respiratory failure, *endotracheal intubation* and the initiation of mechanical ventilation can be life-saving. Safe placement of an ETT in infants and children requires experienced personnel and appropriate equipment at the bedside, including a correctly sized mask, Ambu bag, oral airways, ETTs, and appropriate suction catheters. The patient should first be positioned properly to facilitate air exchange while supplemental oxygen is provided. The sniffing position is used in infants. Head extension with jaw thrust is used in older children without neck injuries. If obstructed by secretions or vomitus, the airway must be cleared by suction. When not obstructed and properly positioned, the airway should be patent and easily visualized, allowing the placement of an oral or nasopharyngeal ETT of the correct size. Patients with normal airway anatomy may be intubated under intravenous (IV) anesthesia by experienced personnel (Table 14–4). Endotracheal intubation of high-risk patients, such as those with significant upper airway obstruction (eg, patients with croup, epiglottitis, foreign bodies, or subglottic stenosis), mediastinal masses, or suspected or known difficult airways should be approached with extreme caution; minimal sedation should be used and paralytic agents should be strictly avoided unless trained airway specialists decide otherwise.

Appropriately sizing the ETT is important for reducing complications and providing adequate respiratory support. An inappropriately large ETT is a risk factor for subglottic pressure necrosis, potentially leading to scarring and stenosis requiring surgical repair. An inappropriately small ETT can

Table 14–4. Drugs commonly used for controlled endotracheal intubation.

Drug	Class of Agent	Dose	Advantages	Disadvantages
Atropine	Anticholinergic	0.02 mg/kg IV, minimum of 0.1 mg	Prevents bradycardia, dries secretions	Tachycardia, fever; seizures and coma with high doses
Fentanyl	Opioid (sedative)	1–3 mcg/kg IV	Rapid onset, hemodynamic stability	Respiratory depression, chest wall rigidity with rapid administration in neonates
Midazolam	Benzodiazepine (sedative)	0.1–0.2 mg/kg IV	Rapid onset, amnestic	Respiratory depression, hypotension
Etomidate	Anesthetic	0.2–0.4 mg/kg IV	Rapid onset, hemodynamic stability, lowers ICP	Suppresses adrenal function, should not be used in sepsis
Ketamine	Dissociative anesthetic	1–2 mg/kg IV 2–4 mg/kg IM	Rapid onset, bronchodilator, hemodynamic stability	Increases oral and airway secretions, may increase ICP and pulmonary artery pressure
Rocuronium	Nondepolarizing muscle relaxant	1 mg/kg	Rapid onset, suitable for rapid sequence intubation, lasts 30 min	Requires refrigeration
Pancuronium	Nondepolarizing muscle relaxant	0.1 mg/kg	Long duration of action (40–60 min)	Tachycardia, slow onset (2–3 min)

ICP, intracranial pressure; IM, intramuscularly; IV, intravenously.

result in excessive air leak around the ETT, making adequate ventilation and oxygenation difficult, or inability to clear secretions effectively. Two useful methods for calculating the correct size of ETT for a child are (1) measuring the child's height with a Broselow tape and then reading the corresponding ETT size on the tape, or (2) in children older than 2 years, choosing a tube size using the formula ETT size = (16 + age in years) ÷ 4. Either cuffed or uncuffed tubes may be used, although a cuffed tube can ensure more effective provision of mechanical ventilation. Assessment of air leakage around the ETT is an important measure of appropriate ETT sizing. An audible leak (with the cuff deflated) noted at pressures of 15–20 cm H_2O generally indicates acceptable ETT size. If there is insufficient leak, the decision to change the ETT needs to be carefully considered, especially in those with severe lung disease. Approximate proper insertion depth (in cm) as measured at the teeth can be estimated by tripling the size of the ETT. Correct placement of the ETT should be confirmed by auscultation for equal bilateral breath sounds and by detecting carbon dioxide using either a colorimetric filter or quantitative capnography. A chest radiograph is necessary for final assessment of ETT placement. A correctly positioned ETT will terminate in the mid-trachea between the thoracic inlet and the carina, at approximately the level of the second thoracic vertebra.

CONVENTIONAL MECHANICAL VENTILATION

▶ Indications

The principal indication for institution of mechanical ventilation is respiratory failure caused either by illness, injury, or treatment with sedating medications. The goals of mechanical ventilation are to facilitate the movement of gas into and out of the lungs (ventilation) and to improve oxygen uptake into the bloodstream (oxygenation). While lifesaving in many situations, positive pressure ventilation can also be harmful. As a result, mechanical ventilation strategies must be adapted to achieve these goals in a way that minimizes further injury to the lung. The overriding principles of this "lung-protective ventilation strategy" are to safely recruit underinflated lung, sustain lung volume, minimize phasic overdistention, and decrease lung inflammation. This strategy requires adjustment of ventilator settings with an understanding of the difference between the gas exchange that is permissible and that which is normal.

▶ Modes of Mechanical Ventilation

The parameters used to control the delivery of mechanical ventilation breaths are known as the trigger, cycle, control, and limit variables. The *trigger variable* describes how breaths are initiated, either by the patient or by the ventilator. The most common triggers are patient effort, sensed as a drop in return pressure or gas flow to the ventilator, and

time. A newer trigger method, neurally adjusted ventilatory assist (NAVA), measures the electrical activity of the diaphragm via an esophageal catheter in order to adjust the ventilator breaths to meet the patient's neural activity. While NAVA holds promise for improving patient-ventilator synchrony and facilitating ventilator weaning, its ideal role in clinical practice remains to be determined. The *cycle variable* describes how the inspiratory phase is terminated, either by the patient or by the ventilator. Most ventilator modes cycle according to a set inspiratory time (I-time) although flow-cycled modes can be used in spontaneously breathing patients. The *control variable* determines whether the ventilator delivers a specific tidal volume (volume-controlled modes) or a specific pressure (pressure-controlled modes). *Limit variables* are parameters whose magnitude is constrained during inspiration in order to prevent excessive pressure or volume from being delivered by the ventilator.

Breathing during mechanical ventilation can be classified as spontaneous or mandatory. The patient controls the timing and size of spontaneous breaths. The ventilator controls the timing and/or size of mandatory breaths, independent of patient activity. In addition, the breathing pattern provided by the ventilator can be set to one of three configurations. In *continuous mandatory ventilation* (CMV), the ventilator determines the size and duration of all breaths. In *intermittent mandatory ventilation* (IMV), the ventilator delivers mandatory breaths, but additional spontaneous breaths between and during mandatory breaths are allowed. In *continuous spontaneous ventilation* (CSV), the patient initiates and controls all breaths, but the ventilator can assist those efforts.

A *ventilator mode* consists of a specific control variable (pressure or volume), a specific pattern of breathing (CMV, IMV, or CSV), and a specific set of phase variables (trigger, limit, and cycle). Initiation of breaths and the length of exhalation are controlled by setting the *respiratory rate*. In time-cycled modes of ventilation, the *inspiratory time* (I-time) determines the length of inspiration and when to allow exhalation. Most modern ventilators can deliver either a pressure-targeted or a volume-targeted breath in several manners. In *synchronized IMV* (SIMV), the ventilator delivers breaths in an IMV pattern, but the machine breaths are synchronized with the patient's efforts. If the patient does not make adequate respiratory efforts to trigger the ventilator, the machine delivers a mandatory breath at a preset time interval. In *pressure-support ventilation*, the patient's own efforts are assisted by the delivery of gas flow to achieve a targeted peak airway pressure. Pressure support ventilation allows the patient to determine the rate and pattern of breaths (CSV breathing pattern), thus improving patient comfort and decreasing the work of breathing. The most commonly used mode of ventilation in many PICUs is *synchronized IMV with pressure support* (SIMV + PS), a mixed mode allowing pressure-supported breaths between the synchronized machine breaths.

In *pressure-controlled ventilation*, air flow begins at the start of the inspiratory cycle and continues until a preset airway pressure is reached. That airway pressure is then maintained until the end of the set I-time, when the exhalation valve on the ventilator opens and gas exits into the machine. With this mode of ventilation, changes in the compliance of the respiratory system will lead to fluctuations in the actual tidal volume delivered to the patient. The advantage of pressure-targeted ventilation lies primarily in the avoidance of high airway pressures that might cause barotrauma or worsen lung injury. The main disadvantage of pressure-controlled ventilation is the possibility of delivering either inadequate or excessive tidal volumes during periods of changing lung compliance. In *volume-controlled ventilation*, the machine delivers a set tidal volume to the patient. Changes in lung compliance will lead to fluctuations in the peak airway pressure generated by the breath. The main advantage of volume ventilation is more reliable delivery of the desired tidal volume and thus better control of ventilation. More reliable tidal volume delivery may also help prevent atelectasis due to hypoventilation. Disadvantages of volume ventilation include the risk of barotrauma from excessive airway pressures and difficulties overcoming leaks in the ventilator circuit. In either pressure- or volume-controlled modes, alarm limits can be set in order to restrict changes in either tidal volume or airway pressure with changing lung compliance; interpreting those alarms and adjusting the ventilator require the ICU clinician to understand the ventilator mode in use.

Finally, in any mode of ventilation, the minimum distending pressure applied to the lung during the respiratory cycle is determined by setting the *positive end-expiratory pressure* (PEEP). PEEP helps prevent the end-expiratory collapse of open lung units, thus preventing atelectasis and shunting. In disease states such as pulmonary edema, pneumonia, or acute respiratory distress syndrome (ARDS), a higher PEEP (10–15 cm H_2O) may increase the patient's functional residual capacity (FRC), helping to keep open previously collapsed alveoli and improve oxygenation. However, high levels of PEEP may also cause complications such as gas trapping and CO_2 retention, barotrauma with resultant air leaks, and decreased central venous return leading to reduced cardiac output or increased intracranial pressure (ICP).

▶ Setting & Adjusting the Ventilator

When initiating either *volume-controlled or pressure-controlled modes* of ventilation, the ICU clinician sets a respiratory rate, an inspiratory time (I-time), and a level of PEEP. The respiratory rate will depend on multiple factors, including patient comfort and blood gas measurements. However, many patients will initially require full support with respiratory rates between 20-30 breaths/min. The minimum PEEP is usually 5 cm H_2O but can be titrated up to maintain adequate oxygenation at acceptable inspired oxygen concentrations

(< 60%–65%), while monitoring for adverse effects of increased intrathoracic pressure. In volume-controlled ventilation, a reasonable initial tidal volume is 8 mL/kg, as long as that volume does not cause excessive airway pressures (> 30 cm H_2O) (see below for open-lung strategies in ARDS). In pressure-controlled ventilation, the amount of peak inspiratory pressure required will depend on the overall respiratory compliance. Patients without lung disease require peak inspiratory pressures of 15–20 cm H_2O, while patients with respiratory illnesses may require 20–30 cm H_2O pressure to provide adequate ventilation. Adequacy of the inspiratory pressure is assessed by observing the patient's chest rise and by measuring the delivered tidal volume and gas exchange.

Ventilated patients require careful *monitoring* for the efficacy of mechanical ventilation, including respiratory rate and activity, chest wall movement, and quality of breath sounds. Gas exchange (oxygenation and ventilation) should be monitored using either noninvasive or invasive methods as described above. Frequent or continuous systemic blood pressure monitoring is also necessary for patients ventilated with high PEEP levels, given the risk of adverse hemodynamic effects.

Ventilator settings can be adjusted to optimize both ventilation ($Paco_2$) and oxygenation (Pao_2). *Ventilation* is most closely associated with the delivered minute volume, or the tidal volume multiplied by the respiratory rate. As a result, abnormal $Paco_2$ values can be most effectively addressed by changes in the respiratory rate or the tidal volume. Increased respiratory rate or tidal volume should increase minute volume and thus decrease $Paco_2$ levels; decreases in respiratory rate or tidal volume should act in the opposite fashion. In some circumstances, additional adjustments may also be necessary. For example, for patients with disease characterized by extensive alveolar collapse, increasing PEEP may improve ventilation by helping to keep open previously collapsed lung units. Also, for patients with disease characterized by significant airway obstruction, decreases in respiratory rate may allow more time for exhalation and improve ventilation despite an apparent decrease in the minute volume provided.

The variables most closely associated with *oxygenation* are the inspired oxygen concentration and the MAP during the respiratory cycle. Increases in inspired oxygen concentration will generally increase arterial oxygenation, unless right-to-left intracardiac or intrapulmonary shunting is a significant component of the patient's illness. Concentrations of inspired oxygen above 60%–65%, however, may lead to hyperoxic lung injury. For patients requiring those levels of oxygen or higher to maintain adequate arterial saturations, increases in MAP should be considered as a means to recruit underinflated lung units. MAP is affected by PEEP, peak inspiratory pressure, and I-time. Increases in any one of those factors will increase MAP and should improve arterial oxygenation. Importantly, increases in MAP may also lead to decreases in cardiac output, primarily by decreasing venous return to the heart. In this circumstance, raising MAP may increase arterial oxygenation but actually compromise oxygen delivery to the tissues. For patients with severe hypoxemic respiratory failure, these tradeoffs highlight the need for careful monitoring by experienced personnel.

Supportive Care of the Mechanically Ventilated Patient

Patients undergoing mechanical ventilation require meticulous supportive care. Mechanical ventilation is often frightening and uncomfortable for critically ill children. In order to reduce dyssynchrony with the ventilator and impaired gas exchange, careful attention must be directed toward optimizing patient comfort and decreasing anxiety. Sedative anxiolytics are typically provided as intermittent doses or continuous infusions. Since oversedation of the ventilated patient may lead to longer durations of ventilation and difficulty weaning from the ventilator, standardized assessments of sedation level and targeting treatment to the minimum sedation level necessary to maintain patient comfort and adequate gas exchange are important.

For patients with severe respiratory illness, even small physical movements can compromise gas exchange. In such cases, muscle paralysis may facilitate oxygenation and ventilation. Nondepolarizing neuromuscular blocking agents are most commonly used for this purpose, given as intermittent doses or as continuous infusions. When muscle relaxants are given, extra care must be taken to ensure that levels of sedation are adequate, as these medications will mask many of the usual signs of patient discomfort. In addition, ventilator support may need to be increased to compensate for the elimination of patient respiratory effort.

Mechanically ventilated patients can usually be fed enterally with the use of temporary or existing feeding tubes. In patients where reflux or emesis is a major concern, transpyloric feeding or parenteral nutrition should be considered. *Ventilator-associated pneumonia* (VAP) is a significant complication of mechanical ventilation, leading to longer ICU stays and increased hospital costs. As a result, many local and national quality improvement initiatives have focused on minimizing the risks of VAP. These preventative measures include proper hand washing, elevation of the head of the bed to 30 degrees to prevent reflux, frequent turning of the patient, proper oral care, the use of closed suction circuits on all ventilated patients and avoidance of breaking the closed suction system, sedation protocols to minimize sedation administration, and daily assessment of extubation readiness.

Mechanical ventilation should be weaned and discontinued as soon as safely possible. Extubation failure rates in mechanically ventilated children have been estimated between 4% and 20%. Considerable effort has been devoted to identifying predictors of extubation readiness and there is literature describing tests used to predict extubation success utilizing trials of spontaneous breathing on pressure support mode. Successful extubation requires adequate gas exchange, adequate respiratory muscle strength, and the ability to protect the airway. To assess extubation readiness, most intensivists will perform a trial of spontaneous breathing in which the patient, while remaining intubated, breathes either without assistance (through a T-piece) or with a low level of pressure support (through the ventilator) for a defined period of time, usually 1–2 hours. The patient is observed carefully for signs of rapid shallow breathing or worsened gas exchange during this trial, and if neither is observed, the patient can generally be safely extubated.

Troubleshooting

Troubleshooting a sudden deterioration in the mechanically ventilated patient should begin with examining the patient. Determine whether the ETT is patent and in the correct position by auscultating for bilateral breath sounds, attempting to pass a suction catheter, assessing for detectable $ETco_2$, and direct laryngoscopy, if necessary. A chest x-ray may also be helpful for ensuring appropriate ETT positioning. If the ETT is patent and correctly positioned, the next step is to determine whether any changes in the physical examination—such as poor or unequal chest rise, or absent or unequal breath sounds—suggest atelectasis, bronchospasm, pneumothorax, or pneumonia. Next, determine whether hemodynamic deterioration could be underlying acute respiratory compromise (shock or sepsis). If the problem cannot be readily identified, take the patient off the ventilator and begin manual ventilation by hand-bagging. Hand-bagging can support the patient while the ventilator is checked for malfunction as well as assess for changes in compliance, informing necessary ventilator adjustments.

OTHER MODES OF RESPIRATORY SUPPORT

High-Frequency Oscillatory Ventilation

High-frequency oscillatory ventilation (HFOV) is an alternative mode of mechanical ventilation in which the ventilator provides very small, very rapid tidal volumes at high rates around a higher MAP. Respiratory rates used during oscillatory ventilation typically range from 5 to 10 Hz (rates of 300–600 breaths/min) in most PICU patients. This mode of ventilation has been used successfully in neonates, older pediatric patients, and adults, although recent work has suggested that HFOV use may be associated with worse outcomes in adults with ARDS. HFOV is most widely used in severe, diffuse lung diseases, such as ARDS, which require high MAP to maintain lung expansion and oxygenation. Diseases characterized by significant heterogeneity or extensive gas trapping often respond too poorly to HFOV, although reports do exist of successful HFOV use in asthma. The advantage of HFOV is that high levels of MAP can be achieved without high peak inspiratory pressures or large tidal volumes, thus theoretically protecting the lung from ventilator-induced lung injury. Disadvantages of HFOV include poor tolerance by patients who are not heavily sedated or paralyzed, the risk of cardiovascular compromise due to high MAP, and the risk of gas-trapping and barotrauma in patients with highly heterogeneous lung disease. Although HFOV can be useful as a rescue mode for selected patients, recent literature suggests that HFOV has a limited role in ARDS compared with carefully managed conventional modes of ventilation.

▶ Extracorporeal Membrane Oxygenation

Extracorporeal membrane oxygenation (ECMO) has been used as a rescue therapy to support pediatric patients with severe respiratory failure who have not improved with mechanical ventilation. ECMO circuits generally consist of a membrane oxygenator, a heater, and a pump. Central venous blood from the patient is directed out of the body, oxygenated, warmed and returned back to the patient. ECMO can be provided in two major modes: venoarterial (VA) and venovenous (VV). VA ECMO bypasses the lungs and the heart, thus supporting both the cardiovascular and respiratory systems, and requires cannulation of a large central artery and vein. VV ECMO utilizes central venous cannulation to provide extracorporeal oxygenation and carbon dioxide removal, thus augmenting the function of the patient's lungs, but the patient's own cardiac output is required to provide systemic oxygen delivery. VV ECMO use has increased over the past 15 years and provides the advantage of a reduced risk of systemic and, particularly, cerebral emboli when compared to VA ECMO. Patients with moderate hemodynamic compromise prior to ECMO initiation can also experience improvements in circulatory status on VV ECMO, likely due to the improvements in acid base status, oxygenation, and decreased intrathoracic pressures achieved with ECMO. ECMO is indicated for patients with *reversible* cardiovascular and/or respiratory failure and is not recommended in patients with severe neurologic compromise or who is in the terminal stages of a lethal condition. Despite an increase in the complexity of patients placed on ECMO, survival has remained acceptable over the past two decades. According to recent registry data, 57% of pediatric respiratory failure patients who are supported with ECMO survive, and survival rates are even better for ECMO patients with a diagnosis of viral pneumonia (especially due to respiratory syncytial virus) and without significant co-morbidities. Of note, in both neonatal and adult randomized controlled trials, patients with severe respiratory failure who were referred to an ECMO center for consideration of ECMO had improved survival, even though not all patients were actually placed on ECMO. These results emphasize the importance of early referral to experienced centers if ECMO is to be considered.

Determining the optimal time to consider ECMO initiation is one of the most challenging aspects of using this technology. Survival appears equally good for most indications with mechanical ventilation for up to 14 days prior to ECMO initiation. Patients placed on ECMO later in the course of their illness or with prolonged ECMO runs (> 14 days) may have worse outcomes. Protocols to improve secretion clearance and lung recruitment have been described and should be considered to hasten lung recovery and shorten the ECMO course, although the optimal mechanical ventilation strategy has yet to be elucidated.

While ECMO remains a viable therapy for selected patients with severe respiratory failure, serious complications such as CNS injury, hemorrhage, renal insufficiency, infection, and complications of immobility do occur, and each patient should be carefully evaluated by experienced personnel in order to choose the optimal timing and mode of ECMO support.

Carroll CL et al: Emergent endotracheal intubations in children: be careful if it's late when you intubate. Pediatr Crit Care Med 2010 May;11(3):343–348 [PMID: 20464775].

Dohna-Schwake C et al: Non-invasive ventilation on a pediatric intensive care unit: feasibility, efficacy, and predictors of success. Pediatr Pulmonol 2011;46(11):1114–1120 [PMID: 21618715].

Faustino EV et al: Accuracy of extubation readiness test in predicting successful extubation in children with acute respiratory failure from lower respiratory tract disease. Crit Care Med 2017;45(1):94–102 [PMID: 27632676].

Fielding-Singh V et al: Beyond low tidal volume ventilation: treatment adjuncts for severe respiratory failure in acute respiratory distress syndrome. Crit Care Med 2018;46(11): 1820–1831 [PMID: 30247273].

Lee JH et al: Use of high flow nasal cannula in critically ill infants, children, and adults: a critical review of the literature. Intensive Care Med 2013;39(2):247–257 [PMID: 23143331].

Nishimura M: High-flow nasal cannula oxygen therapy in adults: physiological benefits, indication, clinical benefits and adverse effects. Respir Care 2016;61(4):529–541 [PMID: 27016353].

Zabrocki LA et al: Extracorporeal membrane oxygenation for pediatric respiratory failure: survival and predictors of mortality. Crit Care Med 2011 Feb;39(2):364–370 [PMID: 20959787].

▼ MAJOR RESPIRATORY DISEASES IN THE PEDIATRIC ICU

ACUTE RESPIRATORY DISTRESS SYNDROME

ESSENTIALS OF DIAGNOSIS & TYPICAL FEATURES

- ▶ ARDS is a severe form of lung injury characterized by hypoxemia and noncardiogenic pulmonary edema.

- ▶ ARDS can arise as a consequence of either direct pulmonary injury or systemic conditions, such as sepsis.

- ▶ Lung protective mechanical ventilation and careful fluid management are crucial to good outcomes in ARDS patients.

ARDS is a syndrome of acute respiratory failure characterized by increased pulmonary capillary permeability resulting in bilateral diffuse alveolar infiltrates on chest radiography, decreased lung compliance, and hypoxemia that is refractory to supplemental oxygen. Mortality rates for pediatric ARDS have fluctuated over time, depending on the diagnostic criteria, the presence of important coexisting conditions, and the quality and consistency of supportive care provided in the ICU. Mortality rates as high as 60%–75% were reported in the 1980s and early 1990s. Since that time there has been a trend toward decreased mortality in pediatric ARDS, ranging from 8% to 40%, though mortality among immunocompromised patients still approaches 60%. Across all subpopulations of pediatric ARDS patients, nonpulmonary organ failure remains an important cause of mortality.

Current consensus diagnostic criteria for ARDS in adult patients include (1) acute onset; (2) bilateral pulmonary infiltrates on chest radiograph; (3) no clinical evidence of left atrial hypertension; and (4) severe hypoxemia in which the ratio of the arterial oxygen level (Pao_2) to inspired oxygen concentration (Fio_2) or P/F ratio is 300 or less while receiving a PEEP of at least 5 cm H_2O via mechanical ventilation. The P/F ratio defines the severity of ARDS, with a P/F ratio between 300 and 200 categorized as mild ARDS; 200–100, moderate ARDS; and less 100, severe ARDS. Pediatric criteria for diagnosing ARDS are similar, but with notable differences including allowing for pulmonary infiltrates to be unilateral, utilizing the oxygenation index (OI) as the marker of ARDS severity in mechanically ventilated patients, and broadening the oxygenation criteria to include measures based on pulse oximetry saturations.

▶ Presentation & Pathophysiology

ARDS may be precipitated by a variety of insults (Table 14–5). Pneumonia and sepsis account for the majority of ARDS cases in children. Despite the diversity of potential causes, the clinical presentation is remarkably similar in most cases. ARDS can be divided roughly into four clinical

phases (Table 14–6). In the earliest phase, the patient may have dyspnea and tachypnea with a relatively normal Pao_2 and hyperventilation-induced respiratory alkalosis. No significant abnormalities are noted on physical or radiologic examination of the chest. Experimental studies suggest that neutrophils accumulate in the lungs at this stage and that their products damage lung endothelium.

Over the next few hours, hypoxemia worsens and respiratory distress becomes clinically apparent, with cyanosis, tachycardia, irritability, and dyspnea. Early radiographic changes include the appearance of increasingly confluent alveolar infiltrates initially appearing in dependent lung fields, in a pattern suggestive of pulmonary edema. Proteinaceous exudates into the alveolar space and direct injury to type II alveolar pneumocytes cause surfactant inactivation and deficiency. As a result, the injured lung requires high inflation pressures to achieve lung opening, and increased PEEP to maintain end-expiratory volume.

Injury to the alveolar type II cell also reduces the capacity for alveolar fluid clearance. Under normal conditions, sodium is taken up from the alveolar space by channels on the apical surface of type II cells and then actively transported across the basolateral cell membrane into the interstitial space. This process creates a gradient for the passive movement of water across the alveolar epithelium and back into the interstitium. In ARDS, this mechanism becomes overwhelmed as direct lung injury depopulates the alveolar epithelium, creating conditions that favor alveolar fluid accumulation. Pulmonary hypertension, reduced lung compliance, and increased airways resistance are also commonly observed in ARDS.

Computed tomography (CT) studies of adult patients in the acute phases of ARDS demonstrate a heterogeneous pattern of lung involvement. The most dependent lung regions remain consolidated throughout the respiratory cycle and can only be recruited using exceedingly high inflation pressures. The most nondependent regions are overinflated throughout the respiratory cycle. Between these two zones lies a region that is either normally inflated or repetitively cycles between inflation and collapse. Attempts to improve oxygenation by recruiting the collapsed dependent lung regions occur at the expense of damaging nondependent regions by hyperinflation. This process, termed *volutrauma*, incites a potent inflammatory response that is capable of worsening non-pulmonary organ dysfunction. Even in normal lungs, ventilation with large tidal volumes and low PEEP levels can produce a lung injury that is indistinguishable from ARDS. This phenomenon is called *ventilator-induced lung injury*. Taken together, these findings suggest that mechanical injury from positive pressure ventilation is superimposed on the initial insult and is an integral part of the pathogenesis of ARDS. Appreciation of this phenomenon has prompted a shift toward ventilating ARDS patients with smaller tidal volumes and a tolerance for the relative

Table 14–5. ARDS risk factors.

Direct Lung Injury	Indirect Lung Injury
Pneumonia	Sepsis
Aspiration of gastric contents	Shock
Inhalation injury (heat or toxin)	Burns
Pulmonary contusion	Trauma
Hydrocarbon ingestion or aspiration	Fat embolism
Near-drowning	Drug overdoses (including aspirin, opioids, barbiturates, tricyclic antidepressants)
	Transfusion of blood products
	Pancreatitis

Table 14–6. Pathophysiologic changes of acute respiratory distress syndrome.

Radiography	Symptoms	Laboratory Findings	Pathophysiology
Phase 1 (early changes)			
Normal radiograph	Dyspnea, tachypnea, normal chest examination	Mild pulmonary hypertension, normoxemic or mild hypoxemia, hypercapnia	Neutrophil sequestration, no clear tissue damage
Phase 2 (onset of parenchymal changes)			
Patchy alveolar infiltrates; normal heart size	Dyspnea, tachypnea, cyanosis, tachycardia, coarse rales	Moderate to severe hypoxemia, increasing shunt, decreased lung compliance, pulmonary hypertension, normal wedge pressure	Neutrophil infiltration, vascular congestion, increased lung permeability, pulmonary edema, fibrin strands, platelet clumps, type I epithelial cell damage
Phase 3 (acute respiratory failure with progression, 2–10 days)			
Diffuse alveolar infiltrates; air bronchograms; decreased lung volume; normal heart size	Tachypnea, tachycardia, sepsis syndrome, signs of consolidation, diffuse rhonchi	Worsening shunt fraction, further decrease in compliance, increased minute ventilation, impaired oxygen extraction	Increased interstitial and alveolar inflammatory exudate with neutrophils and mononuclear cells, type II cell proliferation, beginning fibroblast proliferation, thromboembolic occlusion
Phase 4 (pulmonary fibrosis, pneumonia with progression, > 10 days)			
Persistent diffuse infiltrates; superimposed new pneumonic infiltrates; air leak; normal heart size or enlargement due to cor pulmonale	Symptoms as above, recurrent sepsis, evidence of multiorgan system failure	Phase 3 changes persist; recurrent pneumonia, progressive lung restriction, impaired tissue oxygenation, impaired oxygen extraction; multiorgan system failure	Type II cell hyperplasia, interstitial thickening; infiltration of lymphocytes, macrophages, fibroblasts; loculated pneumonia or interstitial fibrosis; medial thickening and remodeling of arterioles

hypercarbia that typically ensues. Published evidence currently supports using PEEP levels sufficient to stabilize those alveoli with tendency to collapse at end-expiration but below a threshold level that would overdistend nondependent lung regions at end-inspiration. Volutrauma is then mitigated by tidal volume reduction or plateau pressure limitation. This approach is termed the "open-lung strategy" of mechanical ventilation.

The subacute phase of ARDS (2–10 days after lung injury) is characterized by type II pneumocyte and fibroblast proliferation in the interstitium of the lung. This results in decreased lung volumes and signs of consolidation that are noted clinically and radiographically. Worsening of the hypoxemia with an increasing shunt fraction occurs, as well as a further decrease in lung compliance. Some patients develop an accelerated fibrosing alveolitis. The mechanisms responsible for these changes are unclear. Current investigation centers on the role of growth and differentiation factors, such as transforming growth factor-β and platelet-derived growth factor released by resident and nonresident lung cells, such as alveolar macrophages, mast cells, neutrophils, alveolar type II cells, and fibroblasts. During the chronic phase of ARDS (10–14 days after lung injury), fibrosis,

emphysema, and pulmonary vascular obliteration occur. During this phase of the illness, oxygenation defects generally improve, and the lung becomes more fragile and susceptible to barotrauma. Air leak is common among patients ventilated with high airway pressures at this late stage. Also, patients have increased dead space and difficulties with ventilation are common. Airway compliance remains low because of ongoing pulmonary fibrosis and insufficient surfactant production.

Secondary infections are common in the subacute and chronic phases of ARDS and can impact clinical outcomes. The mechanisms responsible for increased host susceptibility to infection during this phase are not well understood. Mortality in the late phase of ARDS can exceed 80%. Death is usually caused by multiorgan failure and systemic hemodynamic instability rather than by hypoxemia.

▶ Treatment

Contemporary *ventilator management* of ARDS is directed at protecting vulnerable lung regions from cyclic alveolar collapse at end expiration and protecting overinflated lung regions from hyperinflation at end inspiration. The actual mode of mechanical ventilation (eg, volume limited vs pressure limited) employed for ARDS is ultimately not as important as limiting phasic alveolar stretch and stabilizing lung units that are prone to repetitive end expiratory collapse. A landmark multicenter trial established that adult ARDS patients who were ventilated using a 6-mL/kg (ideal body weight) tidal volume had a 22% mortality reduction and fewer extrapulmonary organ failures relative to those randomized to receive tidal volumes of 12 mL/kg. Although this trial has never been replicated in pediatric patients, application of these same management principles has gained widespread acceptance among pediatric ICU clinicians.

Given the large body of evidence supporting the benefits of low tidal volume ventilation, we suggest that mechanical ventilation of pediatric ARDS patients be initiated using a tidal volume of 6–8 mL/kg (ideal body weight), combined with PEEP sufficient to produce target arterial saturations ($\geq$ 88%–90%) using an FIO_2 of 0.6 or less. In general, this can be accomplished by incremental increases in PEEP until adequate oxygenation is achieved or until a limiting side effect of the PEEP is reached. Whenever escalating mechanical ventilator settings, clinicians should minimize the ETT cuff leak (if possible), ensure an appropriate plane of patient sedation, and optimize the ventilation to perfusion relationship by verifying that the patient's intravascular volume status is appropriate. Permissive hypercapnia (ie, accepting elevated $Paco_2$) should be used unless a clear contraindication exists (eg, increased ICP). Throughout the course, efforts should be made to limit the alveolar plateau pressure (pressure at end-inspiration) to 25–30 cm H_2O or less.

Fluid management is an important element of the care of patients with ARDS. Given the increased pulmonary capillary permeability in ARDS, further pulmonary edema accumulation is likely with any elevation in pulmonary hydrostatic pressures. Evidence in adults has shown that a "conservative" fluid strategy targeting lower cardiac filling pressures (CVP < 4 mm Hg) is associated with better oxygenation and a shorter duration of mechanical ventilation compared to a "liberal" fluid strategy targeting CVP 10–14 mm Hg. Fluid restriction should only be implemented after hemodynamic variables stabilize and volume resuscitation should not be denied to hemodynamically unstable patients with ARDS.

Patients with ARDS require careful *monitoring*. Given the risks of ventilator-induced lung injury and the inherent limitations of pulse oximetry and capnography, ABG analysis is preferred for accurate assessment of oxygenation and ventilation and careful titration of mechanical ventilation. Indwelling arterial catheters are useful for continuous blood pressure monitoring and frequent laboratory sampling. Since secondary infections are common and contribute to increased mortality rates, surveillance for infection is important by obtaining appropriate cultures and following the temperature curve and white blood cell count. Renal, hepatic, and GI function should be watched closely because of the prognostic implications of multiorgan dysfunction in ARDS.

For patients failing these standard approaches of mechanical ventilation and fluid restriction, several alternative or rescue therapies are available. *Prone positioning* is a technique of changing the patient's position in bed from supine to prone, with the goal of improving ventilation of collapsed dependent lung units via postural drainage and improved V/Q matching. This technique can dramatically improve gas exchange in the short term, particularly for patients early in the course of ARDS, but the gains are often not sustained. Clinical trials examining the role of prone positioning in adults have shown a survival benefit in those with severe disease, but no study in children with ARDS has shown a clear improvement in mortality or in duration of mechanical ventilation. HFOV has been used successfully for many years in pediatric patients with ARDS; however, studies in adults have shown no benefit or an increase in mortality with HFOV. No pediatric studies to date have compared HFOV to a modern lung protective conventional ventilation strategy, and whether HFOV provides any advantage over conventional ventilation for pediatric ARDS remains unclear. In general, HFOV is considered a rescue therapy for patients with severe hypoxemia failing conventional ventilation. Based on the ability of *inhaled nitric oxide* (iNO) to reduce pulmonary artery pressure and to improve the matching of ventilation with perfusion without producing systemic vasodilation, iNO can be used as a therapy for refractory ARDS. Several multicenter trials of iNO in the treatment of ARDS, both in adults and in children, showed acute improvements in oxygenation in subsets of patients, but no significant improvement in overall survival. As a result, iNO cannot be recommended as a standard therapy for ARDS. Finally, *ECMO* has been used to support pediatric patients with severe ARDS. Recent registry data suggest the overall survival rate for children who require ECMO for ARDS is around 50%–60%. To date, the efficacy of ECMO has not been evaluated against lung protective ventilation strategies for pediatric ARDS in a prospective randomized trial. In addition, recent improvements in outcome for pediatric ARDS patients receiving "conventional" therapies have made the role of ECMO less clear and have made further prospective randomized studies of ECMO difficult to complete. For now, ECMO remains a viable rescue therapy for patients with severe ARDS that is unresponsive to other modalities.

Outcomes

Information regarding the long-term outcome of pediatric patients with ARDS remains limited. One report of 10 children followed 1–4 years after severe ARDS showed that three children were still symptomatic and seven had hypoxemia at rest. Until further information is available, all patients with a history of ARDS need close follow-up of pulmonary function.

ARDS Definition Task Force: Acute respiratory distress syndrome: the Berlin definition. JAMA 2012;307(23):2526–2533 [PMID: 22797452].

Khemani RG et al: Pediatric acute respiratory distress syndrome: definition, incidence, and epidemiology. Pediatr Crit Care Med 2015;16:S23–S40 [PMID 26035358].

Fielding-Singh V et al: Beyond low tidal volume ventilation: treatment adjuncts for severe respiratory failure in acute respiratory distress syndrome. Crit Care Med 2018;46:1820–1831 [PMID: 30247273].

STATUS ASTHMATICUS

 ESSENTIALS OF DIAGNOSIS & TYPICAL FEATURES

▶ Status asthmaticus is reversible small airway obstruction refractory to sympathomimetic and anti-inflammatory agents that may progress to respiratory failure without prompt and aggressive intervention.

▶ Dyspnea at rest that interferes with the ability to speak can be an ominous sign.

▶ Absence of wheezing may be misleading because to produce a wheezing sound, the patient must take in sufficient air.

▶ Patients with severe respiratory distress, signs of exhaustion, alterations in consciousness, elevated $Paco_2$, or acidosis should be admitted to the PICU.

▶ Pathogenesis

Life-threatening asthma exacerbations are caused by severe bronchospasm, excessive mucus secretion, inflammation, and edema of the airways (see Chapter 38). Infants and children are at particular risk for respiratory failure from asthma due to several structural and mechanical features of their lungs. They have less elastic recoil than the adult lung, thicker airway walls leading to greater peripheral airway resistance for any degree of bronchoconstriction, increased airway reactivity to bronchoconstrictors, fewer collateral channels of ventilation, and a more compliant chest wall which can lead to increased work of breathing with airway obstruction. Additional risk factors for severe asthma exacerbation include obesity, lower socioeconomic status, non-Caucasian race, and a prior history of previous ICU admissions or intubations.

▶ Clinical Findings

Patients admitted to the PICU with severe asthma exacerbations can have a variety of constitutional and cardiorespiratory findings. They often have tachypnea, increased use of accessory muscles, and variable aeration. Diffuse wheezing is usually present, but absence of wheeze may indicate severe obstruction impeding airflow. Dyspnea at rest that interferes with the ability to speak and cyanosis are also ominous signs of severe airflow obstruction. These children may also display signs of panic or exhaustion and an altered level of consciousness. Agitation, drowsiness, or confusion can be signs of elevated $Paco_2$ levels and impending respiratory failure. Likewise, gasping respirations or frank apnea are indications of respiratory failure and need for intubation.

These patients generally have elevated heart rates (HRs) secondary to stress, dehydration, and β-agonist therapy, and may have systolic and/or diastolic hypotension. Diastolic pressures less than 40 mm Hg in conjunction with extreme tachycardia may impair coronary artery filling and predispose to cardiac ischemia, which can present with chest pain and ST changes on electrocardiogram. Pulsus paradoxus (ie, an exaggerated decrease in systolic blood pressure with inspiration) may be observed and can be used as a marker of disease severity and response to treatment.

▶ Laboratory Findings

In addition to pulse oximetry, blood gas measurements should be considered in critically ill patients with status asthmaticus to evaluate gas exchange and acid-base balance. Although venous blood gas measurements may be acceptable for screening, ABG measurements provide the most accurate and complete information. Patients with severe asthma exacerbations typically have increased minute ventilation and should be expected to have a $Paco_2$ less than 40 mm Hg. Normal to elevated $Paco_2$ levels suggest respiratory failure. Desaturation or reduced Pao_2 on room air may indicate severely impaired gas exchange and impending respiratory failure but also may occur with initiation of β-agonist therapy and associated ventilation/perfusion mismatching. The presence of metabolic acidosis may signify relative dehydration, inadequate cardiac output, or underlying infection.

Other laboratory evaluations may include serum electrolytes, complete blood counts, and other inflammatory markers if clinically indicated. Patients may demonstrate decreased serum potassium, magnesium, and/or phosphate, especially with prolonged β-agonist use. Leukocytosis is commonly observed during asthma exacerbations and may be due to infection or to demargination of polymorphonuclear leukocytes as a result of stress or corticosteroid treatment. Differentiating between these two etiologies of leukocytosis can be difficult, and measurement of other inflammatory markers can be useful if there is concern for infection.

Chest x-rays should be obtained in patients presenting with severe asthma exacerbations to evaluate for treatable conditions such as pneumonia, foreign-body aspiration, air leak, or a chest mass. Pneumothorax and pneumomediastinum are common complications of severe exacerbations and may only be revealed with chest radiography.

Severe wheezing without a prior history of asthma should raise suspicion for alternative diagnoses. Electrocardiograms are not routinely recommended but may be indicated to rule out cardiac ischemia, especially in patients with known cardiac disease, extreme tachycardia and low diastolic blood pressure, or complaints of chest pain.

Although measurements of pulmonary function such as forced expiratory volume in 1 second (FEV_1) or peak expiratory flow (PEF) are recommended in other clinical settings, their use in patients admitted to the PICU with severe asthma exacerbations is limited as those patients are often unable to cooperate with testing. When obtained, values of less than 40% of predicted indicate a severe exacerbation and values less than 25% of predicted indicate imminent respiratory arrest.

▶ Treatment

The key treatment strategy for status asthmaticus is to reverse the underlying process swiftly and aggressively before respiratory failure requiring endotracheal intubation and mechanical ventilation ensues given the complications of providing mechanical ventilation in patients with severe airflow obstruction. Children with status asthmaticus require IV access, continuous pulse oximetry, and cardiorespiratory monitoring, as close monitoring of gas exchange, cardiovascular status, and mental status are crucial to assessing response to therapy and determining appropriate interventions.

Because of inadequate minute ventilation and V/Q mismatching, patients with severe asthma are almost always hypoxemic and should receive supplemental humidified oxygen immediately to maintain saturations more than 90%. The delivery method will depend on the child's age, level of oxygen required, and institutional resources, as described earlier in this chapter. Children with clinical signs of dehydration should receive appropriate fluid resuscitation, while avoiding volume overload. Additionally, the hemodynamic effects of certain asthma therapy (peripheral dilation, diastolic hypotension) may also require further fluid resuscitation to maintain cardiac output and avoid metabolic acidosis. Antibiotics are generally not recommended for treatment of status asthmaticus unless a coexisting infection is identified or suspected.

The first-line treatment for rapidly reversing airflow obstruction is the repetitive or continuous administration of inhaled selective short-acting β_2-*agonist* therapy such as albuterol. The frequency of administration will vary based on the severity of symptoms and the occurrence of adverse side effects. Nebulized albuterol may be given intermittently at a dose of 2.5–5 mg every 10–15 minutes, or it can be administered continuously at a dose of 10 mg/h to a maximum of 20–30 mg/h, usually without serious side effects.

Patients with severe distress and poor inspiratory flow rates may have inadequate delivery of inhaled medications and may require subcutaneous or IV medication. Subcutaneous epinephrine or terbutaline, a relatively specific β_2-agonist,

may be used for initial treatment with an acute exacerbation. Continuous IV therapy with *terbutaline* may also be used with an infusion of 0.5–5 mcg/kg/min after a loading dose of 10 mcg/kg. Because significant tachycardia and other arrhythmias as well as diastolic hypotension are recognized side effects of inhaled and IV β_2-agonist therapy, these children should have close cardiovascular monitoring. An indwelling arterial catheter may be useful for continuous hemodynamic and blood gas monitoring in the most severely ill patients on IV therapy. They may also require additional fluid resuscitation because of hypovolemia from dehydration compounded by the vasodilating effects of β_2-agonist therapies.

In addition to β_2-agonist therapy, immediate administration of systemic *corticosteroids* is critical to the early management of life-threatening status asthmaticus. Because enteral medications may not be tolerated in patients with severe exacerbations, administration of IV or IM steroids should be considered early in these children. Both methylprednisolone and dexamethasone have been used in the treatment of status asthmaticus.

For severe exacerbations unresponsive to the initial treatments listed previously, additional treatments may be considered despite limited clinical pediatric evidence. *Ipratropium bromide*, an inhaled anticholinergic bronchodilator, is commonly used in emergency medicine and is a reasonable intervention in the PICU, despite limited evidence of efficacy. Administration of *magnesium sulfate* may also be considered for patients who are unresponsive to early treatment or who have impending respiratory failure. The bronchodilatory properties of magnesium sulfate are thought to be caused by interference with calcium flux in the bronchial smooth muscle cell. Hypotension and flushing may occur with administration and should be anticipated with adequate fluid resuscitation. *Heliox*-driven albuterol nebulization can also be considered for patients refractory to conventional therapy. Heliox is a mixture of helium and oxygen that has a lower viscosity than ambient air and can improve airway delivery of albuterol and gas exchange. However, a mixture of at least 60%–70% helium is required to be effective, thus limiting its use in patients with severe hypoxia.

Methylxanthines, such as *theophylline and aminophylline*, may also be considered for the management of severe asthma, although their use remains controversial. The theoretical benefit of methylxanthines is relaxation of airway smooth muscle by preventing degradation of cyclic guanosine monophosphate, a mechanism of action distinct from that of β_2-agonists. In addition, mucociliary inflammatory mediators and microvascular permeability are reduced. Unfortunately, the pharmacokinetics of these agents are erratic, and the narrow therapeutic window can be difficult to manage, with serious side effects such as seizures and cardiac arrhythmias occurring with higher drug levels. These concerns, in addition to mixed evidence of benefit, have led to a general recommendation against the routine use of methylxanthines for asthma exacerbations. However, they may still have a role in individual cases of severe refractory asthma as a means to prevent intubation. When a methylxanthine is added to a patient's care, close therapeutic drug monitoring is essential and consultation with a pharmacist recommended.

NIV may be used to support patients with severe asthma exacerbations and help avoid the need for intubation and mechanical ventilation. Positive-pressure ventilation may help avoid airway collapse during exhalation as well as to unload fatigued respiratory muscles by reducing the force required to initiate each breath. Because of its noninvasive interface, spontaneous breathing and upper airway function are preserved, allowing the patient to provide his/her own airway clearance. Data on the effectiveness of NIV for acute severe asthma in children are limited, but some small studies and case series have shown improvements in gas exchange and respiratory effort. Careful titration of inspiratory and expiratory pressures is essential, however, to avoid complications of positive pressure.

If aggressive management fails to result in significant improvement, endotracheal intubation and *mechanical ventilation* may be necessary. Patients who present with apnea or coma should be intubated immediately. If there is steady deterioration despite intensive therapy for asthma, intubation should occur before acute respiratory arrest. The intubation procedure can be dangerous for these patients, given the high risk of barotrauma and cardiovascular collapse, and should be performed by the most experienced provider available.

Mechanical ventilation for patients with asthma is difficult because the severe airflow obstruction often leads to very high airway pressures, air trapping, and resultant barotrauma. Therefore, the goal of mechanical ventilation in this setting is to maintain adequate oxygenation and ventilation with the least amount of barotrauma until other therapies become effective. This approach typically means accepting some degree of hypercarbia in order to avoid complications of aggressive ventilation. Because of the severe inspiratory and expiratory airflow obstruction, these patients will require long inspiratory times to deliver a breath and long expiratory times to avoid air trapping. Either volume- or pressure-targeted modes of ventilation can be used, although volume and pressure limits should be closely monitored and low ($\leq$ 6 cc/kg) tidal volumes used initially. In general, the ventilator rate should be decreased until the expiratory time is long enough to allow emptying prior to the next machine breath. The level of PEEP should be titrated to minimize air trapping from either auto-PEEP or dynamic obstruction. If possible, and when a patient moves toward extubation, a support mode of ventilation is useful, as the patient can set his or her own I-time and flow rate.

These ventilator strategies and the resulting hypercarbia typically are uncomfortable, requiring that patients be heavily sedated. Ketamine is a dissociative anesthetic with bronchodilatory properties that can be used to facilitate intubation and also as a sedative infusion for intubated patients. Ketamine can also increase bronchial secretions, which may limit its use in certain patients or require administration of an anticholinergic agent. Barbiturates and morphine should be avoided, as both can increase histamine release and worsen bronchospasm. Many patients will also require neuromuscular blockade initially to optimize ventilation and minimize airway pressures. In intubated patients not responding to the preceding strategies, inhaled anesthetics, such as isoflurane, should be considered. These agents act not only as anesthetics but also cause airway smooth muscle relaxation. Inhalational anesthetics must be used with caution, however, as they can also cause significant hypotension due to vasodilation and myocardial depression. Finally, use of ECMO has been reported for severe cases of status asthmaticus and could be considered as a rescue therapy.

▶ Prognosis

Status asthmaticus remains among the most common reasons for admission to the PICU, and it is associated with a surprisingly high mortality rate (1%–3%), especially in patients with a previous PICU admission. Careful but expedient management, however, can reduce the associated morbidities and mortality. As many as 75% of patients admitted to the PICU with life-threatening asthma flares will be readmitted with a future exacerbation, emphasizing the need for careful outpatient follow-up of this high-risk population.

Carroll CL et al: Identifying an at-risk population of children with recurrent near-fatal asthma exacerbations. J Asthma 2010 May;47(4):460–464 [PMID: 20528602].

National Asthma Education and Prevention Program: Expert Panel Report 3: Guidelines for the Diagnosis and Management of Asthma—Summary Report 2007, Section 5, Managing Exacerbations of Asthma. http://www.nhlbi.nih.gov/guidelines/asthma/asthgdln.htm.

Ram FS et al: Non-invasive positive pressure ventilation for treatment of respiratory failure due to severe acute exacerbations of asthma. Cochrane Database Syst Rev 2005;(1):CD004360 [PMID: 15674944].

▼ CARDIOVASCULAR CRITICAL CARE

SHOCK

ESSENTIALS OF DIAGNOSIS & TYPICAL FEATURES

▶ Shock is defined as the inadequate delivery of oxygen and nutrients to tissues to meet metabolic needs.

▶ Shock can result from decreased delivery of oxygen, inadequate delivery of oxygen in the face of increased demands, or from impaired utilization of oxygen.

▶ Shock can be categorized as compensated, hypotensive, or irreversible.

▶ Early recognition and intervention are essential to improving patient outcomes from shock.

Pathogenesis

Shock is a syndrome characterized by inadequate oxygen delivery to meet the body's metabolic demands. Shock can complicate multiple different disease processes and can be categorized based on the primary physiologic disturbance (Table 14–7).

Shock, regardless of underlying etiology, can be best understood by examining the factors affecting the balance between delivery of oxygen to the tissues and consumption of oxygen by the tissues. Metabolic failure may occur as a result of reduced oxygen delivery (as in respiratory or cardiac failure or acute hemorrhage), increased tissue demand (as in infection, burns, or other major physiologic stresses), or impaired oxygen utilization (as in severe sepsis), or combinations of all three conditions. These may result in anaerobic cellular metabolism, hypoxia, lactic acidosis, and, ultimately, irreversible cellular damage if not reversed.

Oxygen delivery (DO_2) is defined as the product of the *cardiac output* and the *oxygen content of arterial blood* (Cao_2) delivered by the heart. Cardiac output, in turn, is determined by ventricular stroke volume (SV) and HR. SV is influenced by preload, afterload, contractility, and cardiac rhythm. Numerous conditions can disrupt one or more of these factors, leading to decreased cardiac output. *Preload* can be decreased as a result of hypovolemia due to hemorrhage or dehydration or as a result of vasodilation due to anaphylaxis, medications, or septic shock. Impaired *contractility* can occur with conditions such as cardiomyopathy, myocardial ischemia/reperfusion following a cardiac arrest, postcardiac surgery, and sepsis. Age-dependent differences in myocardial physiology can also affect systolic performance and contractility. For example, in the infant heart, the sarcolemma,

Table 14–7. Categories of shock.

Type of Shock	Examples
Hypovolemic	Dehydration due to vomiting and/or diarrhea Trauma with severe hemorrhage
Cardiogenic	Viral myocarditis Postoperative cardiac patient with poor heart function
Distributive	Septic shock Vasodilation secondary to anaphylaxis
Dissociative	Carbon monoxide poisoning

sarcoplasmic reticulum, and T-tubules are less well developed than in older children, resulting in a greater dependency on extracellular serum calcium concentrations for contraction. *Afterload* can be increased, as seen in late septic shock and cardiac dysfunction, or decreased, as in "warm" septic shock. Cardiac dysrhythmias can also alter cardiac output and contribute to inadequate oxygen delivery. One common example is supraventricular tachycardia, in which reduced time for ventricular filling can lead to reduced SV and cardiac output.

The oxygen content of arterial blood consists of the oxygen *bound* to hemoglobin and the oxygen *dissolved* in the blood. The bound oxygen is determined by the hemoglobin concentration and the percent of the hemoglobin saturated by oxygen. The dissolved oxygen is calculated from the partial pressure of oxygen in the arterial blood (Pao_2). In general, the main determinant of arterial oxygen content is the bound oxygen. Illnesses that affect the oxygen saturation of hemoglobin or alter hemoglobin concentration can impair oxygen delivery. Low hemoglobin oxygen saturations most commonly occur as a result of impaired uptake of oxygen in the lungs. Low hemoglobin concentrations, as in hemorrhage or other causes of anemia, reduce oxygen delivery, as do abnormal hemoglobins such as carboxyhemoglobin (from carbon monoxide poisoning) and methemoglobin.

Clinical Findings

The clinical presentation of shock can be categorized into a series of recognizable stages: compensated, hypotensive or decompensated, and irreversible. Patients in *compensated shock* have relatively normal blood pressures, and compensatory mechanisms preserve oxygen delivery. In infants, a compensatory increase in cardiac output is achieved primarily by increases in HR, given the limited ability of infants to increase SV. In older patients, SV and HR both increase to improve cardiac output. Blood pressure remains normal initially because of peripheral vasoconstriction and increased systemic vascular resistance. Drops in blood pressure occur late, defining *hypotensive shock*. Patients in hypotensive shock are at risk of developing multiorgan system failure (MOSF), which carries a high risk of mortality. In extreme cases, organ damage can progress to the point that restoration of oxygen delivery will not improve organ function, a condition known as *irreversible shock*.

The *symptoms and signs of shock* result from end-organ dysfunction caused by inadequate oxygen delivery. Because this condition can progress rapidly to serious illness or death, rapid assessment of a child in shock is essential to determining the need for resuscitation. In patients with impaired cardiac output and peripheral vasoconstriction, the skin will be cool and pale with delayed capillary refill (> 3 seconds) and thready pulses. Additionally, the skin may appear gray or ashen, particularly in newborns, and mottled or cyanotic in patients with decreased cardiac output. In contrast, patients with "warm" or septic shock can present with warm skin with brisk capillary refill and bounding pulses. The detection of peripheral edema is a worrisome sign and can indicate severe vascular leak due to sepsis or poor cardiac output with fluid and sodium retention. The skin examination can also provide insight into the diagnosis (eg, the presence of rash such as purpura fulminans may indicate an infectious etiology) or reveal the site and extent of traumatic injury. Cracked, parched lips, and dry mucous membranes may indicate severe volume depletion.

Tachycardia is an important and early sign of shock and is typically apparent well before hypotension, which is a late feature in pediatric shock. Not all patients can mount an appropriate increase in HR, however, and the presence of bradycardia in a patient with shock is particularly ominous. Peripheral pulses will weaken first in shock as cardiac output is diverted to the body core. Shock in an infant associated with a discrepancy in pulses between lower extremities and upper extremities may indicate a critical coarctation of the aorta with closure of the ductus arteriosus. A gallop cardiac rhythm can indicate heart failure, while a pathologic murmur suggests the possibility of congenital heart disease or valvular dysfunction. A rub or faint, distant heart sounds may indicate a pericardial effusion. Rales, hypoxia, and increased work of breathing occur in patients with shock from heart failure or acute lung injury, and a patient with severe metabolic acidosis due to shock will have compensatory tachypnea and respiratory alkalosis. Urine output is directly proportionate to renal blood flow and the glomerular filtration rate and, therefore, is a good reflection of cardiac output. Normal urine output is greater than 1 mL/kg/h; output less than 0.5 mL/kg/h is considered significantly decreased. Hepatomegaly may suggest heart failure or fluid overload, while splenomegaly may suggest an oncologic process and abdominal distension may suggest obstruction or perforated viscus as the etiology of shock.

The level of consciousness reflects the adequacy of brain cortical perfusion. When brain perfusion is severely impaired, the infant or child first fails to respond to verbal stimuli, then to light touch, and finally to pain. Lack of motor response and failure to cry in response to venipuncture or lumbar puncture is ominous. In uncompensated shock with hypotension, brainstem perfusion may be decreased. Poor thalamic perfusion can result in loss of sympathetic tone. Finally, poor medullary flow produces irregular respirations followed by gasping, apnea, and respiratory arrest.

▶ Monitoring

Laboratory studies in the patient with suspected shock should be directed at evaluating the etiology of shock, assessing the extent of impaired oxygen delivery, and identifying signs of end-organ dysfunction due to inadequate oxygen delivery

Table 14–8. Laboratory studies in the case of shock.

Evaluation for infectious etiology
Sources include blood, urine, tracheal secretions, CSF, wound, pleural fluid, or stool
Stains, cultures, and other microbiologic tests (PCR, immunofluorescent antibody stains) for bacteria, fungus, viruses
Evaluation of organ function
Pulmonary: ABG (evaluate acid-base status, evaluation of oxygen delivery/consumption)
Cardiac: ABG, mixed venous saturation, lactate
Liver: LFTs, coagulation studies
Renal (and hydration status): BUN, creatinine, bicarbonate, serum sodium
Hematology: WBC count with differential, hemoglobin, hematocrit, platelet count
Evaluation for DIC: PT, PTT, fibrinogen, D-dimer
Extent of inflammatory state: CRP, WBC, ESR, procalcitonin
Additional studies
Electrolytes
Ionized calcium
Magnesium
Phosphate

ABG, arterial blood gas; ACTH, adrenocorticotropic hormone; BUN, blood urea nitrogen; CRP, C-reactive protein; CSF, cerebrospinal fluid; DIC, disseminated intravascular coagulation; ESR, erythrocyte sedimentation rate; LFTs, liver function tests; PCR, polymerase chain reaction; PT, prothrombin time; PTT, partial thromboplastin time; WBC, white blood cell.

(Table 14–8). Assessments of oxygen delivery require measurement of oxygen saturation and hemoglobin concentration. Pulse oximetry is adequate to measure oxygen saturation in patients with low oxygen requirements. ABG analyses provide more accurate oxygen measurements, which are important for optimizing mechanical ventilation in patients with significant hypoxemia, and provide measurements of arterial pH, which can reflect the adequacy of tissue perfusion. Measurements of central venous oxygen saturation can serve as a measure of the adequacy of overall oxygen delivery. If oxygen delivery is inadequate for the needs of the tissues, a greater portion of that oxygen will be consumed and the central venous saturation will be lower than normal (< 70% in a patient without cyanotic heart disease). In contrast, patients with septic shock may have an elevated central venous saturation due to impaired oxygen utilization by the tissues (> 80%).

Additional laboratory signs of organ dysfunction include evidence of anaerobic metabolism such as acidemia and elevated lactate, increased serum creatinine, or abnormal liver function tests such as elevated transaminases or reduced production of clotting factors. Blood chemistry measurements are also essential in patients with shock. Hypo- or hypernatremia are common, as are potentially life-threatening abnormalities in potassium levels, particularly hyperkalemia in patients with impaired renal function due to shock. Patients in shock may have decreased serum ionized calcium levels, which will adversely impact cardiac function, especially in infants. Calcium homeostasis also requires normal magnesium levels, and renal failure may disrupt phosphorus levels. Evaluation of a coagulation panel is required to detect disseminated intravascular coagulation (DIC), particularly in patients with purpura fulminans or petechiae, or in those at risk for thrombosis.

The selection of *imaging studies*, similar to laboratory studies, should be guided by the presumed etiology of shock. For patients presenting with shock secondary to trauma, standard trauma protocols to evaluate organ damage and potential sites of hemorrhage are indicated. Chest x-rays can evaluate the extent of airspace disease and presence of pleural effusions or pneumothorax and evaluate for pulmonary edema and cardiomegaly. CT of the chest or abdomen may be indicated to better evaluate sites of infection in septic shock, and echocardiography can provide important information about cardiac anatomy and function.

Patients with shock often need *invasive hemodynamic monitoring* for diagnostic and therapeutic reasons. *Arterial catheters* provide constant blood pressure readings, and to an experienced interpreter, the shape of the waveform is helpful in evaluating cardiac output. *Central venous catheters* allow monitoring of central venous pressure (CVP) and central venous oxygen saturation. CVP monitoring does not provide information about absolute volume status, but can provide useful information about relative changes in volume status as therapy is given. *Pulmonary artery catheters* can also provide valuable information on cardiac status and vascular resistance and enables calculations of oxygen delivery and consumption (Table 14–9), but these catheters are associated with a higher complication rate than CVP lines and are no longer commonly used in either adult or pediatric critical care. Principles of shock treatment are described in Sepsis section.

SEPSIS

ESSENTIALS OF DIAGNOSIS & TYPICAL FEATURES

▶ Sepsis and septic shock remain major causes of death in children worldwide.

▶ Early recognition and intervention are keys to improving patient outcome.

▶ Organized systematic approaches to the treatment of sepsis within an institution can improve survival.

Sepsis and septic shock require particular consideration because sepsis is one of the major illnesses leading to admission to the PICU. Worldwide, an estimated 18 million patients develop sepsis each year, with 750,000 of those cases in North America. Sepsis is the tenth leading cause of death in the United States and accounts for approximately 40% of intensive care unit (ICU) expenditures in the United States and Europe. Among children, an estimated 42,000 cases of severe sepsis occur annually in the United States, accompanied by a mortality rate of nearly 10%. The incidence of severe sepsis is highest in infancy, remains relatively low from age 1 to mid-life, then rises again in later life.

Published literature regarding sepsis uses a number of overlapping and sometimes confusing terminologies. In earlier definitions, *systemic inflammatory response syndrome* (SIRS) referred to a nonspecific syndrome of systemic inflammation typically associated with fever, tachycardia, tachypnea, and an abnormal white blood cell count. *Sepsis* was defined as documented or suspected infection accompanied by clinical and laboratory signs of systemic inflammation, and *severe sepsis* was defined as sepsis along with evidence

Table 14–9. Hemodynamic parameters.

Parameter	Calculation	Normal Values
Alveolar partial pressure of oxygen	$Pao_2 = (Barometric\ pressure - 47) \times \%$ inspired oxygen concentration	
Alveolar-arterial oxygen difference (mm Hg)	$A-aDO_2 = Pao_2 - (Paco_2/R) - Pao_2$	5–15
Cardiac output (L/min)	$CO = HR \times SV$	
Cardiac index (L/min/m²)	$CI = CO/BSA$	3.0–4.5
Oxygen content of arterial blood (mL/dL)	$Cao_2 = (1.34 \times hemoglobin \times Sao_2) + (0.003 \times Pao_2)$	17–24
Oxygen delivery index (mL/min/m²)	$DO_2 = Cao_2 \times CI \times 10$	550–650
Oxygen content of venous blood (mL/dL)	$Cvo_2 = (1.34 \times hemoglobin \times Svo_2) + (0.003 \times Pvo_2)$	12–17
Oxygen consumption index (mL/min/m²)	$Vo_2 = (Cao_2 - Cvo_2) \times CI \times 10$	120–200

R, respiratory quotient (normally approximates 0.8).

of at least one sepsis-induced major organ dysfunction such as hypotension, hypoxemia, lactic acidosis, oliguria, renal failure, thrombocytopenia, coagulopathy, or hyperbilirubinemia. *Septic shock* was severe sepsis associated with impaired oxygen delivery, typically defined clinically as hypotension requiring either IV fluid boluses or pressor agents and a persistently elevated blood lactate level. A 2016 revision to the definitions effectively eliminated the terms SIRS and severe sepsis, and redefined sepsis as documented or suspected infection with at least one organ failure. Though the criteria used to define sepsis in adults and children differ in published guidelines (Table 14–10), the more specific adult criteria provide a useful framework for thinking about sepsis-related organ dysfunction. Of note, the number of organ systems affected by severe sepsis is an important prognostic factor. The risk of death from sepsis rises with the number of organ failures, with a mortality rate of 7%–10% with single-organ failure and up to 50% mortality with four-organ failures.

In addition to impaired oxygen delivery, sepsis and septic shock are also associated with impaired utilization of delivered oxygen. The etiology of this impaired oxygen utilization is not well understood but is likely multifactorial, including maldistribution of blood flow in the microcirculation as well as mitochondrial dysfunction. Recent work has also brought to light the critical role of the *innate immune system* in sepsis. Infectious agents release *pathogen-associated molecular patterns* (PAMPs) such as lipopolysaccharide or peptidoglycans, and damaged tissues release endogenous proteins and nucleic acids that act as molecular triggers, collectively referred to as *damage-associated molecular patterns* (DAMPs). These molecules are recognized by pattern recognition receptors of the innate immune system, most prominently the *toll-like receptors*, which then trigger inflammatory cascades throughout the body. Derangements of adaptive immunity also contribute to the pathogenesis of sepsis. Toll-like receptor signaling may activate subsets of regulatory T cells in septic patients, leading to either immune paralysis or uncontrolled inflammation depending on the pathophysiologic setting. Cytokine production and leukocyte activation lead to endothelial damage and activation of the clotting system. Microvascular thrombi lead to impaired tissue perfusion, which leads to further tissue damage, which in turn leads to further activation of the immune system. The end result of these processes is impaired oxygen delivery to the tissues, impaired oxygen utilization, and metabolic downregulation, leading to end-organ dysfunction and ultimately to death if the process is not reversed.

▶ Treatment of Shock & Sepsis

Much attention has been directed in recent years to the role of standardized treatment guidelines in improving outcomes from shock and sepsis, and detailed guidelines are now available from several professional organizations, most prominently the American Heart Association Pediatric Advanced

Table 14–10. Diagnostic criteria for sepsis.

Adults
Infection, documented or suspected, and some of the following:
  General signs and symptoms
  - Fever (> 38.3°C)
  - Hypothermia (core temperature < 36°C)
  - Heart rate 90/min or > 2 SD above the normal value for age
  - Tachypnea
  - Altered mental status
  - Significant edema or positive fluid balance (> 20 mL/kg over 24 h)
  - Hyperglycemia (plasma glucose > 140 mg/dL or 7.7 mmol/L) in the absence of diabetes
  Evidence of inflammation
  - Leukocytosis (WBC count > 12,000/μL)
  - Leukopenia (WBC count < 4000/μL)
  - Normal WBC count with > 10% immature forms
  - Plasma CRP > 2 SD above the normal value
  - Plasma procalcitonin > 2 SD above the normal value
  Hemodynamics
  - Arterial hypotension (SBP < 90 mm Hg; MAP < 70 mm Hg; or an SBP decrease 40 mm Hg in adults or > 2 SD below normal for age)
  Organ dysfunction
  - Arterial hypoxemia (Pao_2/Fio_2 < 300)
  - Acute oliguria (urine output < 0.5 mL/kg/h for at least 2 h, despite adequate fluid resuscitation)
  - Creatinine increase > 0.5 mg/dL or 44.2 μmol/L
  - Coagulation abnormalities (INR > 1.5 or a PTT > 60 s)
  - Ileus (absent bowel sounds)
  - Thrombocytopenia (platelet count < 100,000/μL)
  - Hyperbilirubinemia (plasma total bilirubin > 4 mg/dL or 70 μmol/L)
  Tissue perfusion
  - Hyperlactatemia (upper limit of lab normal)
  - Decreased capillary refill or mottling
Children
Signs and symptoms of inflammation plus infection with hyper- or hypothermia (rectal temperature > 38.5°C or < 35°C), tachycardia (may be absent in hypothermic patients), and at least one of the following indications of altered organ function: altered mental status, hypoxemia, increased serum lactate level, or bounding pulses.

aPTT, activated partial thromboplastin time; CRP, C-reactive protein; INR, international normalized ratio; MAP, mean arterial blood pressure; SBP, systolic blood pressure; SD, standard deviation; WBC, white blood cell.

Data from Dellinger RP, Levy MM, Carlet JM, et al: Surviving Sepsis Campaign: international guidelines for management of severe sepsis and septic shock: 2008. Crit Care Med 2008:Jan;36(1):296–327.

Life Support (PALS) guidelines for initial management of shock in children, and the Surviving Sepsis Campaign guidelines for management of sepsis in adults and children. A key principle of both guidelines is that early recognition and treatment of shock and sepsis, preferably stemming from a consistent organized clinical approach, improve outcomes in all age ranges.

Regardless of the etiology, the end result of shock is organ dysfunction, which if untreated can lead to irreversible MOSF. Therefore, early recognition of shock, coupled with early control of underlying cause and supportive care, is necessary to minimize end-organ injury and improve survival. *Airway, breathing, and circulation* should be rapidly assessed, with appropriate stabilization of the airway, support of breathing, and stabilization of circulation. Indications for intubation and mechanical ventilation include altered mental status, significant hemodynamic instability, inability to protect the airway, poor respiratory effort, high work of breathing, poor gas exchange, or need for procedural intervention. Because of low FRC, infants and neonates are more likely to require early initiation of NIV or endotracheal intubation. Use of etomidate for sedation during intubation should be avoided in patients suspected with sepsis due to its association with adrenal suppression and increased mortality. A temporary intraosseous line should be placed if IV access cannot be rapidly obtained for resuscitation fluids and medications. A central venous line should be considered in patients with hemodynamic instability, particularly if they require ongoing resuscitation and infusions of vasoactive medications. While femoral venous lines are simpler and safer to place, subclavian and internal jugular lines are preferred for more accurate and consistent central venous saturation and pressure monitoring, although they do carry the additional risk of pneumothorax. The rapidity and accuracy of placing central venous lines can be improved with the use of ultrasound guidance.

Empiric *antimicrobials* should be delivered promptly, ideally within *1 hour* of presentation in patients with suspected sepsis. Antibiotics should be chosen according to the most likely cause of infection. While it is highly desirable to obtain cultures prior to initiation of antibiotics in order to guide the choice and duration of antibiotic coverage, the acquisition of cultures should never delay antibiotic administration in patients with suspected sepsis. Early and aggressive control of sources of infection is also essential for patients with sepsis and septic shock, including surgical drainage of abscesses or other infected spaces or removal of infected foreign bodies such as vascular catheters.

An important element of the treatment of shock is early aggressive *fluid resuscitation* targeted to measurable physiologic endpoints of organ perfusion, so-called "early goal directed therapy." Fluid resuscitation should begin with 20 mL/kg increments administered over 5–10 minutes and repeated as necessary. Fluid administration should be titrated to reverse hypotension and achieve normal capillary refill, pulses, level of consciousness, and urine output. Trends in serum lactate measurements can also provide a useful marker of reversal of shock to guide fluid administration. If pulmonary edema or hepatomegaly develops, vasoactive medication infusions should be used in place of more fluid, and cardiac function evaluated for evidence of cardiogenic shock. Large volumes of fluid for acute stabilization in children with hypovolemic or septic shock may be necessary to restore adequate oxygen delivery and do not necessarily increase the incidence of ARDS or cerebral edema. Patients who do not respond rapidly to 40–60 mL/kg should be monitored in an intensive care setting and considered for inotropic therapy and invasive hemodynamic monitoring. Initial fluid resuscitation should consist of crystalloid (salt solution), which is readily available and inexpensive. Albumin has been shown to be safe in adults and children with septic shock and should be considered when patients have received large volumes of crystalloid and require ongoing resuscitation. Hydroxyethyl starches (HES) are not recommended as resuscitation fluids in septic shock based on adult studies, which showed no improvement in mortality with HES versus normal saline, but an increased risk of renal failure.

Inotropic and vasopressor agents should be considered for patients with refractory shock despite receiving 60 mL/kg of fluid resuscitation (Table 14–11). Inotropic medications improve cardiac contractility but can increase myocardial oxygen demand and arrhythmia risk; vasopressor medications increase vascular tone and resistance but can increase cardiac afterload. Inotropic or vasopressor therapy should be selected based on the hemodynamic state, that is, cardiac output and systemic vascular resistance, and reassessed with changes in clinical course. These medications can be delivered through an intraosseous or peripheral line until stable central access is secured to prevent a delay in initiation. Although dopamine (α- and β-adrenergic agonist) is no longer recommended for adults with septic shock due to arrhythmogenic effects in this population, *dopamine* remains an acceptable first-line vasopressor in the pediatric population. Either *norepinephrine* (α- and β_1-adrenergic agonist) or *epinephrine* (potent α- and β-adrenergic agonist) may be useful for dopamine-refractory shock; generally, epinephrine has a greater net effect on cardiac output and is preferred for cold shock states, while norepinephrine has a greater net effect on vascular tone and is preferred for warm shock states. *Vasopressin* may be considered for patients failing catecholamine infusions but has not been clearly shown to improve outcomes from severe sepsis in children. In patients with low cardiac output and high systemic vascular resistance, *milrinone*, a type III phosphodiesterase inhibitor with inotropic and vasodilator activity, can be added to other more potent inotropic agents. Alternatively, *dobutamine* (selective β-agonist) may be used to improve myocardial contractility and reduce afterload. As hypocalcemia also may contribute to cardiac dysfunction in shock, *calcium* replacement should be given to normalize ionized calcium levels.

If perfusion is still inadequate despite aggressive fluid and pressor support, the patient can be considered to have *catecholamine-resistant septic shock.* This condition may be related to critical illness-related corticosteroid insufficiency (CIRCI), which is a condition of impaired adrenal responsiveness that may occur in as many as 30%–50% of critically ill patients. Absolute adrenal insufficiency, characterized by

Table 14–11. Pharmacologic support of the patient with shock.

Drug	Dose (mcg/kg/min)	α-Adrenergic Effect[a]	β-Adrenergic Effect[a]	Vasodilator Effect	Actions and Advantages	Disadvantages
Dopamine	1–20	+ to +++ (dose-related)	+ to ++ (dose-related)	None	Moderate inotrope, wide and safe dosage range, short half-life	Neuroendocrine effects; may increase pulmonary artery pressure
Dobutamine	1–10	None	++	+ (via β_2)	Moderate inotrope; less chronotropy, fewer dysrhythmias than epinephrine	Marked variation among patients, tachycardia
Epinephrine	0.05–1	++ to +++ (dose-related)	+++	+ (at lower doses, via β_2)	Strong inotrope and chronotrope; increases SVR	Tachycardia, dysrhythmias; can cause myocardial necrosis at high doses
Norepinephrine	0.05–1	+++	+++	None	Potent vasoconstrictor (systemic and pulmonary), increases SVR	Reduced cardiac output if afterload is too high; renal and splanchnic ischemia
Milrinone	0.25–0.75	None	None	++	Decreases SVR and PVR; increases cardiac contractility but only mild increase in myocardial O_2 consumption	
Nitroprusside	0.05–8	None	None	+++ (arterial and venous vasodilation)	Potent vasodilator, decreases SVR and PVR, very short-acting.	Toxic metabolites (thiocyanates and cyanide); increased intracranial pressure; ventilation-perfusion mismatch; methemoglobinemia

[a]+, small effect; ++, moderate effect; +++, potent effect. PVR, pulmonary vascular resistance; SVR, systemic vascular resistance.

impaired adrenal responsiveness, low-circulating cortisol concentrations, and often associated with adrenal hemorrhage, is less common and occurs in fewer than 25% of children with septic shock. Children with fulminant meningococcemia, congenital adrenal hyperplasia, or recent steroid exposure are at the highest risk of absolute adrenal insufficiency, while CIRCI can occur in any critically ill patient. Pediatric patients with fluid-refractory, catecholamine-resistant septic shock and suspected or proven adrenal insufficiency should receive hydrocortisone. The recommended dose of hydrocortisone is 50 mg/m²/day (up to 200 mg/day) either as a continuous infusion or divided doses; however, some children may require higher doses. Hydrocortisone is generally continued until catecholamine support can be successfully discontinued, and a taper should be considered in those children requiring longer than 7 days of therapy.

Cardiogenic shock is often associated with elevated ventricular filling pressures (> 20 mm Hg). Although increasing preload may augment cardiac output for some patients, volume should be administered cautiously in smaller increments as elevated pulmonary venous pressures from cardiac dysfunction may lead to, or worsen, pulmonary edema.

In this setting, judicious administration of *diuretics* combined with inotropic support can reduce pulmonary edema and improve pulmonary compliance, the work of breathing, and oxygenation.

Blood products can be important supportive therapies in patients with shock. *Red blood cells* can be administered to patients with shock to improve oxygen-carrying capacity. In hemodynamically stable patients, hemoglobin levels are often maintained over 7 g/dL, while the transfusion threshold can be increased to 10 g/dL in unstable patients. DIC is common in shock, particularly septic shock, due to endothelial damage, formation of microvascular emboli, and consumptive coagulopathy. Thus, a process beginning as increased coagulation leads to a bleeding diathesis. *Platelets* are generally transfused when platelet counts are less than 20,000/μL, or less than 40,000–60,000/μL in a patient with bleeding or requiring surgical intervention. For severe coagulopathies associated with bleeding in the setting of shock, the standard treatment is *fresh frozen plasma* (FFP) or, for fibrinogen replacement, *cryoprecipitate*, with close monitoring of prothrombin time (PT), international normalized ratio (INR), and partial thromboplastin time (PTT).

Other supportive therapies for shock and sepsis include mechanical ventilation, sedation and analgesia, renal replacement therapy for renal insufficiency, deep vein thrombosis prophylaxis, stress ulcer prophylaxis, nutrition, and glucose control. Finally, *ECMO* can be considered as a life-saving measure in the treatment of severe shock in patients with recoverable cardiac and pulmonary function who have failed conventional management.

Kleinman ME et al: 2010 American Heart Association Guidelines for Cardiopulmonary Resuscitation and Emergency Cardiovascular Care Science. Part 14: Pediatric Advanced Life Support 2010. Circulation 2010;122:S876–S908 [PMID: 20956230].

Rhodes A et al: Surviving sepsis campaign: international guidelines for management of sepsis and septic shock: 2016. Crit Care Med 2017; 45(3):486–552 [PMID 28098591].

Surviving Sepsis Campaign website (a good source for information on sepsis including protocols and order bundles for the care of patients with sepsis): http://www.survivingsepsis.org/Pages/default.aspx. Accessed January 4, 2018

Wong HR: Genome-wide expression profiling in pediatric septic shock. Pediatr Res 2013 Jan 17 [PMID: 23329198].

▼ NEUROCRITICAL CARE

Pediatric neurocritical care is an emerging multidisciplinary field focused on critically ill pediatric patients with neurologic injury due to conditions such as traumatic brain injury (TBI), stroke, status epilepticus, and hypoxic-ischemic brain injury, as well as brain injury that is secondary to other types of critical illness. Neurointensivists work to better understand the distinct pathophysiological and clinical features of pediatric brain injury, develop and apply new diagnostic and monitoring strategies to better understand brain function and dysfunction in real time, and formulate pediatric-specific management guidelines for common neurocritical care problems. While the field is still relatively young, some basic tenets of support for the injured brain are beginning to emerge.

TRAUMATIC BRAIN INJURY

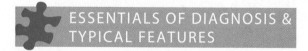

ESSENTIALS OF DIAGNOSIS & TYPICAL FEATURES

► TBI presents in a variety of ways, from alterations in memory or alertness (mild confusion to unresponsiveness), irritability, seizures, and even poor feeding/emesis. TBI should be high on the differential for all patients matching these descriptions.

► Hypotension, hypoxia, hypoglycemia, hyperthermia, and hypermetabolic states can exacerbate brain injury. Timely identification and correction of these factors are essential.

► Early signs and symptoms of intracranial hypertension tend to be nonspecific. The classic Cushing triad of bradycardia, hypertension, and apnea occurs late and is often incomplete.

TBIs can be conceptualized as occurring in two phases. *Primary injury* occurs at the moment that injury disrupts bone, blood vessels, and brain tissue. Prevention through helmets, safety belts, and other injury prevention efforts is the only true means to reduce primary injury. *Secondary injury* is the indirect result of the primary injury and develops minutes to days after the initiating event. Reducing secondary injury is the focus of first responders, emergency medicine doctors, and intensivists. Management of the brain-injured child aims to optimize delivery of oxygen and nutrients (supply) while reducing hypermetabolic states (demand). Therapy, therefore, focuses on avoidance of factors such hypoxia, hypotension, hypoglycemia, hyperthermia, infection, and agitation.

► Pathogenesis

The skull contains a fixed total volume composed of the brain, cerebrospinal fluid (CSF), and cerebral blood. Because of this physical constraint, an increase in volume of one component must be offset by a decrease in one of the other components to maintain a constant ICP (Monro-Kellie doctrine). As a result of a brain injury, the volume of any or all of these components may increase, resulting in increased ICP. *Intracranial hypertension* is defined as an ICP over 20 mm Hg (vs < 15 mm Hg in healthy children) and is associated with increased morbidity and mortality in brain-injured patients. Intracranial hypertension may occur due to other illnesses in addition to TBI (Table 14–12), but in all cases, the pathogenesis of intracranial hypertension can be understood by considering each of the intracranial components.

The uninjured brain occupies about 80% of the volume within the skull, but this volume can increase dramatically after brain injury as a result of cerebral edema. *Vasogenic edema* is frequently associated with trauma, tumors, abscesses, and infarct; breakdown of the tight endothelial junctions that make up the blood-brain barrier (BBB) is a hallmark component. As plasma constituents cross the BBB, extracellular water moves into the brain parenchyma. *Cytotoxic edema* is the most common form of cerebral edema seen in the PICU and is the least easily treated. Cytotoxic edema occurs as a result of direct injury to brain cells, often leading to irreversible cell swelling and death. This form of cerebral edema is typical of TBIs as well as hypoxic-ischemic injuries and metabolic disease. *Hydrostatic edema*, due to transudation of fluid from the capillaries into the parenchyma as a result of elevated cerebral vascular pressures, and *interstitial edema*, which results from obstructed CSF flow and appears in a typical periventricular distribution, are less common. Cerebral edema

Table 14–12. Pediatric illnesses commonly associated with intracranial hypertension.

Diffuse Processes
Hypoxic-ischemic
Near-drowning
Hanging/other strangulation
Cardiorespiratory arrest
Infectious
Encephalitis
Meningitis
Metabolic
Reye syndrome
Liver failure
Inborn errors of metabolism
Toxic
Lead intoxication
Vitamin A overdose
Focal Processes
Trauma
Stroke
Infectious
Abscess
Mass lesions
Tumors
Hematomas

can be diagnosed by characteristic findings on either CT or magnetic resonance imaging (MRI) of the brain.

CSF occupies an estimated 10% of the intracranial space. Intracranial hypertension due primarily to obstructed CSF flow or increased CSF volume (eg, primary or secondary hydrocephalus) is generally easily diagnosed by CT scan and treated with appropriate drainage and shunting. CSF drainage can be of benefit in managing intracranial hypertension even in the absence of overt hydrocephalus.

Cerebral blood volume comprises the final 10% of the intracranial space and is affected by cerebral blood flow. Changes in cerebral blood flow occur by altering cerebral perfusion pressure or vascular resistance. *Cerebral perfusion pressure* (CPP), *defined* as mean systemic arterial pressure minus CVP or ICP, whichever is higher, is the driving pressure across the cerebral circulation. Hypotension, which may occur due to hemorrhage from comorbid injuries or as a part of a systemic inflammatory response following TBI, results in decreased CPP. Changes to vascular resistance generally result from alterations in vascular diameter in response to metabolic demands or vascular pressures, responses termed *autoregulation*. *Metabolic autoregulation* matches cerebral blood flow to tissue demands. High metabolic rates, such as those induced by fever or seizure activity, increase cerebral blood flow by causing vasodilation, which in turn increases cerebral blood volume; lower metabolic rates allow the vessels to constrict, reducing cerebral blood volume. Partial pressure of carbon dioxide is another important determinant,

as elevations in blood $Paco_2$ lead to cerebral vasodilation and decreases in $Paco_2$ lead to vasoconstriction. *Pressure autoregulation*, which works to maintain a constant cerebral blood flow in spite of variable systemic blood pressures, links cerebral blood pressure to cerebral blood flow. Within the autoregulatory range of blood pressure, cerebral vessels dilate with low systemic blood pressures or constrict with high systemic blood pressures to maintain constant cerebral blood flow. Above the autoregulatory range, cerebral vessels are maximally constricted, and further increases in systemic pressure will result in increased cerebral blood flow and volume; the opposite is true below the autoregulatory range, and cerebral blood flow will fall with further decreases in systemic pressure. It is not unusual to see partial or complete loss of cerebral blood flow autoregulation following TBI. Cerebral blood flow then becomes dependent on systemic blood pressure (traditionally termed "pressure passive" blood flow).

In addition to direct damage from elevated ICP and cerebral edema, secondary injury following trauma may also occur due to ischemia and/or excitotoxicity. Ischemia results from decreased cerebral blood flow or hypoxemia. Excitotoxicity occurs via excessive glutamate exposure, sodium-dependent neuronal swelling, and calcium-dependent mitochondrial failure. Depletion of adenosine triphosphate (ATP), oxidative stress, calcium fluxes, hypomagnesemia, and hyponatremia may all contribute to these processes.

▶ Clinical Findings

The clinical presentation of TBI is dependent on the nature, location, and size of affected areas in the brain, as well as the amount of edema and infringement of CSF pathways. Physical deformities such as skull fractures and exposure of the brain parenchyma may or may not be apparent. Clinical presentation can be subtle, such as a headache from a concussion, or more severe, such as manifestations of intracranial hypertension (Table 14–13) or complete unresponsiveness. Often, early signs and symptoms are nonspecific, particularly

Table 14–13. Signs and symptoms of intracranial hypertension in children.

Early
Poor feeding, vomiting
Irritability, lethargy
Seizures
Late
Coma
Decerebrate responses
Cranial nerve palsies
Abnormal respirations
Bradycardia
Hypertension
Apnea

in young children. For these reasons, TBI should be included in the differential diagnosis for a wide range of clinical presentations.

Initial examination of the patient with TBI should include assessment of airway patency, breathing, and cardiovascular function. Mental status should be evaluated, and the Glasgow coma scale (GCS) score calculated. Once stabilized from a cardiac and respiratory standpoint, a more detailed neurologic examination including cranial nerves, spontaneous movement of extremities, strength, sensory perception, and presence or absence of deep tendon reflexes should be performed. Similar considerations apply in patients with suspected intracranial hypertension but no clinical history of trauma. In either setting, repeated neurologic examinations are needed. Head imaging (CT or MRI) is also beneficial to identify specific intracranial injuries, determine the need for surgical intervention, monitor the progression of injuries and cerebral edema, and to monitor for the development of complications.

▶ Treatment

Initial stabilization should begin with support of the airway, breathing, and circulation, but prevention of further neurologic injury should be considered as these steps are completed. Cervical spine immobilization should be strongly considered prior to securing the airway to avoid worsening spinal cord injury. If the GCS is less than 8, or if the patient demonstrates apnea, irregular respirations, significant hypoxia, or other signs concerning for intracranial hypertension, the airway should be secured via endotracheal intubation. Care should be taken during this process to avoid hypercapnia, which will further increase ICP. Similarly, sedative agents used in the process of intubation should be chosen carefully, as adequate sedation is important to blunt further elevations in ICP with airway manipulation. Maintenance of systemic blood pressure is also critically important during this time.

Following intubation and support of systemic blood pressure, treatment strategies for TBI in children are largely focused on optimizing cerebral blood flow and reducing metabolic demand. Minimizing intracranial hypertension is a critical component of management, and current treatment guidelines for children with TBI recommend ICP monitoring for all patients with GCS of 8 or less. Elevated ICP (ICP > 20) can be treated with medical or mechanical interventions.

Medical treatment strategies to reduce ICP rely on *osmotic therapies* such as hypertonic ($\geq 3\%$) saline and mannitol. Hypertonic saline, given in bolus doses of 2–5 mL/kg of 3% saline or as a continuous infusion, encourages intravascular volume expansion and increases serum osmolality, enhancing movement of excess water out of brain cells and interstitium and into blood vessels for removal by the kidneys. Serum sodium and osmolality should be followed closely to avoid severe hypernatremia or severe hypertonicity when this agent is used. Mannitol, given in doses of 0.25–1 g/kg, exerts a rapid rheologic effect, reducing blood viscosity which improves blood flow and subsequent autoregulatory vasoconstriction. Mannitol also exerts a potent osmotic and diuretic effect. While this may further reduce ICP, it can also result in hypovolemia and hypotension, which reduces CPP and exacerbates secondary injury. Volume status and systemic blood pressures should therefore be monitored closely following administration, and treatment should be prompt to reduce these side effects. Renal failure due to intravascular volume depletion and acute tubular necrosis is a rare side effect and is associated with serum osmolality greater than 320 mOsm/L.

Controlled ventilation is another important element of treating intracranial hypertension. Normocapnia, with a goal $Paco_2$ between 35 and 40 mm Hg, is the current standard of care. Hypocapnia (hyperventilation), although acutely effective in causing cerebral vasoconstriction, leads to larger decreases in blood flow than in blood volume, such that hyperventilation may actually compromise CNS perfusion and exacerbate secondary injury. This concept was confirmed by studies showing worse outcomes in head-injured patients consistently hyperventilated to a $Paco_2$ of 25 mm Hg or less. Hyperventilation to $Paco_2$ levels less than 30 mm Hg—in the past a mainstay in the treatment of intracranial hypertension—is no longer recommended although could be considered for short periods in emergent situations in patients with refractory intracranial hypertension while awaiting more definitive therapy.

Mechanical therapies to reduce ICP are aimed at improved drainage of fluids. Midline positioning and head elevation to 30 degrees can aid in cerebral venous drainage. CSF drainage reduces ICP by reducing CSF volume and can be accomplished by placement of an external ventricular drain in the lateral ventricles of the brain. Timely surgical evacuation of hematomas and other pathologic masses is also a mainstay of TBI treatment.

In some cases, intracranial hypertension is refractory to initial medical and mechanical therapies. In these circumstances, 2019 guidelines suggest three additional measures to reduce ICP: decompressive craniectomy (removal of a portion of the skull and opening of the dura), moderate hypothermia (32–33°C), and high-dose *barbiturates*. Of note, barbiturates are potent cardiac depressants and their use often leads to hypotension, necessitating the use of vasopressor medications to maintain adequate cerebral and systemic perfusion pressures. Plasma barbiturate levels correlate poorly with effect on ICP, and monitoring of CNS electrical activity by electroencephalography (EEG) is necessary to accurately titrate their use.

In addition to reducing ICP, *systemic hemodynamic support* is a critical component of optimizing cerebral blood flow. Studies in both adult and pediatric patients with head injury show that even a single episode of hypotension is associated with a marked increase in mortality rates. Maintenance of systemic blood pressure can be accomplished using volume and/or vasopressor medication, and goal systemic pressures are often augmented to maintain CPP in the setting of refractory ICP. Although the ideal CPP in children is not definitively known, 2019 guidelines suggest a goal of 40–50 mmHg, acknowledging that a graded response based on age may be appropriate (eg, 40–55 in infants/toddlers, 50–60 in children, and > 60 in adolescents).

Prevention of ischemia and excitotoxicity are similarly important. Hypoxic episodes (PaO_2 < 60 mm Hg) after TBI are associated with increased morbidity and mortality, and should be prevented. Maintenance of normal ranges for glucose, calcium, magnesium, and phosphorus may be beneficial. Current guidelines also recommend enteral nutrition within 72 hours of injury.

Finally, optimizing oxygen and nutrient delivery to the injured brain should be facilitated by reducing metabolic demands. Aggressive control of fevers (*controlled normothermia*), using antipyretics and surface cooling devices, is warranted, and continuous temperature monitoring helps prevent over- or undercorrection. Induced hypothermia lowers cerebral metabolism, cerebral blood flow, and cerebral blood volume but has not been shown to improve overall outcome in the pediatric population. *Adequate sedation* to reduce episodes of agitation and/or pain can further reduce metabolic demands and ICP, although caution should be used, as bolus administration may contribute to systemic hypotension, and therefore cerebral hypoperfusion. *Neuromuscular blockade* can also be considered as an effective adjunctive therapy. *Seizures* occur in approximately 30% of patients with severe head injury and result in increased metabolic demand and secondary injury. Continuous EEG should be used in patients with persistent altered mental status or in those requiring heavy sedation. A short course (7 days) of empiric antiepileptic medication is suggested, and seizures noted on EEG should be treated rapidly. Corticosteroids may be of use in reducing vasogenic cerebral edema surrounding tumors and other inflammatory CNS lesions, but they are not recommended in the treatment of TBI.

▶ Complications

Complications are frequent in patients with TBIs and should be anticipated. Nosocomial infections are more common in these patients than other critically ill populations and may lead to worse outcomes. Abnormalities of sodium handling such diabetes insipidus, syndrome of inappropriate secretion of antidiuretic hormone (SIADH), or cerebral salt wasting are also relatively common following serious brain injuries and require careful monitoring and intervention. In more severe cases, *cerebral infarctions* may occur as a result of ischemia, thrombosis, and progressive edema compromising blood supply. Finally, *cerebral herniation* presenting with Cushing triad of bradycardia, hypertension, and altered

respirations is an ominous and life-threatening medical emergency, often leading to death or serious disability in brain-injured patients.

▶ Prognosis

Many factors will affect prognosis of patients with TBI, especially the inciting event and severity of injury. Experience has shown that it is difficult to predict overall outcome in the initial stabilization period, but lack of improvement in neurologic examination after 24–72 hours (the peak period for swelling) is associated with worse outcomes. Follow-up studies have also demonstrated that "recovery" occurs over time, even months to years.

▶ Inflicted Traumatic Brain Injury

Inflicted traumatic brain injury (iTBI), also referred to as *nonaccidental trauma* (NAT), accounts for a significant portion of TBIs in infants and young children. Repetitive brain injuries prior to presentation and global hypoxic-ischemic brain damage (as a result of trauma-induced respiratory failure or cardiac arrest) may complicate the pathophysiology. Management of children with iTBI is similar to those with accidental TBI, but additional evaluations should include an ophthalmologic assessment for retinal hemorrhages and a radiologic skeletal survey to identify occult bone fractures. Child advocacy and law enforcement groups should be notified when abuse is suspected. Unfortunately, children with iTBI often have a worse neurologic outcome compared to accidentally injured children.

HYPOXIC-ISCHEMIC ENCEPHALOPATHY

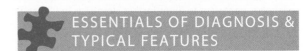

ESSENTIALS OF DIAGNOSIS & TYPICAL FEATURES

▶ Hypoxic-ischemic encephalopathy (HIE) should be suspected when altered mental status persists after prolonged hypoxemia or resuscitation from a cardiorespiratory arrest.

HIE results from global brain hypoxia and ischemia produced by systemic hypoxemia and/or reduced blood flow to the brain. Pediatric HIE is commonly caused by cardiopulmonary arrest due to drowning, hanging or other strangulation, severe respiratory distress, shock, drug overdose/poisoning, lethal arrhythmia, and other insults. Pediatric HIE is associated with poor neurologic outcome. Like TBI, the extent of brain injury in HIE depends on the duration and severity of the initial inciting event and the development of secondary injury over the minutes to days following reestablishment of cerebral blood flow and oxygen delivery.

Clinical Findings

Signs and symptoms of brain injury secondary to hypoxic-ischemic injury are variable and depend on injury severity and affected brain regions. Manifestations of HIE can include cognitive dysfunction, seizures (clinical and subclinical), status epilepticus, stroke, coma, a persistent vegetative state, and irreversible cessation of neurologic function ("brain death").

Treatment

The initial stabilization of a patient with HIE includes airway management, respiratory support, and maintenance of cardiovascular stability. As with TBIs, treatment strategies for victims of HIE are focused on optimizing cerebral blood flow and mitigating neuronal loss. Blood flow to the brain is dependent on cardiac output, which may be impaired following cardiac arrest and/or injury. Optimization of cardiac function and systemic hemodynamics with fluid resuscitation and inotropic and/or vasopressor agents is necessary to ensure adequate delivery of oxygen and nutrients to the injured brain. Cerebral pressure autoregulation may also be impaired in children who develop HIE as a result of cardiac arrest. Several studies in adult victims of cardiac arrest suggest that maintaining a higher mean blood pressure may better support the postischemic brain, but the degree of pressure dysregulation and blood pressure targets to optimize cerebral blood flow in the ischemic pediatric brain remain unclear. Intracranial hypertension may develop as a result of cerebral edema, but the utility of ICP monitoring and titration of therapies to a normal ICP in HIE patients has not been clearly defined. Use of therapies for ICP reduction varies across pediatric referral centers. Seizures should be aggressively treated, and continuous EEG monitoring is useful for identifying subclinical seizure activity. Similar to the case with TBIs, temperature regulation and maintenance of normothermia are also essential, since the risk of severe disability in patients with HIE increases with fevers. *Therapeutic hypothermia* (target body temperature 33–35°C) is a mainstay of treating postcardiac arrest HIE in adults and postanoxic HIE in newborns, but published data in the pediatric population do not demonstrate significant benefit.

Prognosis

Accurately predicting outcome in children with HIE is difficult. Out-of-hospital cardiac arrest and/or prolonged cardiopulmonary resuscitation (> 10–15 minutes) are significant risk factors for poor outcome. Other indicators of likely poor outcome include any of the following, 24 hours or more after the inciting event: (1) GCS score less than 3–5, (2) absent pupillary and motor responses, (3) absent spontaneous respiratory effort, (4) bilateral absence of median nerve somatosensory evoked potential (N20), (5) discontinuous,

nonreactive, or silent EEG (in the absence of confounding drug administration), and (6) MRI demonstrating watershed, basal ganglia, and brainstem injury. Outcome prediction is enhanced when several assessment modalities are combined.

STATUS EPILEPTICUS

ESSENTIALS OF DIAGNOSIS & TYPICAL FEATURES

▶ *Status epilepticus* is defined as a persistent seizure lasting 30 minutes or longer, or several shorter seizures without an intervening return to baseline mental status.

▶ When a patient without epilepsy presents with status epilepticus, multiple etiologies should be considered, including trauma, stroke, infection, tumors, hypertensive encephalopathy, hyponatremia, and hypoglycemia.

▶ Comorbid infections in patients with epilepsy can lower their seizure threshold and result in status epilepticus.

▶ Status epilepticus and its associated treatment can lead to acute cardio-respiratory compromise requiring intervention.

Pathogenesis

Status epilepticus can result from multiple etiologies (Chapter 25). In a patient with a prior diagnosis of epilepsy, common infections such as viral respiratory illnesses can lower the seizure threshold enough to result in prolonged seizure activity, as can nonadherence to antiepileptic medications. In patients without a prior diagnosis of epilepsy, the differential diagnosis is broad. Diagnoses to be considered include complex febrile seizure, CNS tumor, TBI, ischemic or hemorrhagic stroke, CNS infection, hypertensive encephalopathy, electrolyte abnormalities (hyponatremia or hypoglycemia), withdrawal to benzodiazepines or alcohol, acute demyelinating encephalomyelitis, previously unrecognized metabolic disorders, or autoimmune disorders.

Regardless of the etiology, the development of status epilepticus occurs due to an imbalance between excitatory and inhibitory neurotransmission, with rhythmic discharges of multiple neurons in a brain region. Left untreated, these discharges can ultimately result in energy failure and long-lasting changes in neurons, including cell death.

Clinical Findings

While seizures and status epilepticus may be focal in nature (involving only one area of the brain and manifesting in a single body part), classic status epilepticus in considered to be generalized tonic-clonic activity with altered mental status, lasting at least 30 minutes. Loss of bladder or bowel continence may occur. Status epilepticus may be associated with profound respiratory abnormalities, apnea, tachycardia, and/or hypertension or hypotension. Because it is a hypermetabolic state, a long post-ictal period of altered mental status and/or rhabdomyolysis may occur.

Treatment

As with all emergencies, resuscitation begins with attention to airway, breathing, and circulation. If a specific etiology for the seizure can be found (eg, hyponatremia), rapid correction of that abnormality (eg, hypertonic saline) usually results in seizure cessation. In the absence of a clear etiology, treatment generally begins with benzodiazepines, most commonly Ativan 0.1 mg/kg IV, given within the first 5 minutes. This can be repeated, or transition to an alternate agent may be considered. Fosphenytoin 20 mg/kg IV in the general pediatric population or phenobarbital 20 mg/kg IV in the neonatal period are common choices. For refractory status epilepticus that persists after these initial agents, selection of next-line therapies may include infusions of midazolam, propofol, ketamine, or phenobarbital. Close collaboration with neurology and pharmacy experts is encouraged. During treatment of refractory status epilepticus, hypoventilation and apnea may occur, and intubation and initiation of mechanical ventilation are often needed. Similarly, antiepileptic-induced hypotension may occur, and support of systemic blood pressure with volume and/or vasopressor medications is recommended.

Abend NS, Licht DJ: Predicting outcome in children with hypoxic ischemic encephalopathy. Pediatr Crit Care Med 2008;9:32–39 [PMID: 18477911].

Ichord R et al: Neurologic outcomes in pediatric cardiac arrest survivors enrolled in the THAPCA trials. Neurology 2018; 91(2): e123–e131 [PMID: 29884735].

Kochanek P et al: Guidelines for the Management of Pediatric Severe Traumatic Brain Injury, Third Edition: update of the Brain Trauma Foundation Guidelines. Pediatr Crit Care Med 2019; 20(3S):S1–S82 [PMID: 30830016].

Moler FW et al: Therapeutic hypothermia after out-of-hospital cardiac arrest in children. N Engl J Med 2015;372(20):1898–1908 [PMID: 25913022].

ACUTE KIDNEY INJURY & RENAL REPLACEMENT THERAPY

Definitions

The kidney is important in maintaining homeostasis for a number of important physiologic processes, including fluid and electrolyte balance, acid-base status, erythropoiesis, and vascular tone. *Acute kidney injury* (AKI) is a frequent problem in critically ill children, with a range of manifestations from modest reductions in creatinine clearance with preserved urine output to anuria, and even life-threatening

Table 14–14. pRIFLE and KDIGO criteria for diagnosis of acute kidney injury in children.

Stage	Creatinine Criteria	Urine Output Criteria
pRIFLE Criteria		
R (risk)	eCCL down > 25%	< 0.5 cc/kg/h × 8 h
I (injury)	eCCL down > 50%	< 0.5 cc/kg/h × 16 h
F (failure)	eCCL down > 75% or < 20 mL/min/m²	< 0.3 cc/kg/h × 24 h or anuria × 12 h
L (loss)	Meets F criteria for > 4 wk	
E (end stage)	Meets F criteria for > 3 mo	
KDIGO Criteria		
Stage 1	1.5–1.9 times baseline serum creatinine OR ≥ 0.3 mg/dL increase	< 0.5 mL/kg/h for 6–12 h
Stage 2	2.0–2.9 times baseline serum creatinine	< 0.5 mL/kg/h for ≥ 12 h
Stage 3	3.0 times baseline OR increase in serum creatinine to ≥ 4.0 mg/dL OR initiation of renal replacement therapy OR, in patients < 18 y, decrease in eGFR to ≤ 35 mL/min per 1.73 m²	< 0.3 ml/kg/h for ≥ 24 h OR anuria for ≥ 12 h

eCCL, estimated creatinine clearance = 0.413 × height (cm)/serum creatinine.

electrolyte derangements. Several staging systems have been developed, but the most commonly used are the pRIFLE and KDIGO criteria (Table 14–14).

Pathophysiology

The etiology of AKI in critically ill children is most often multifactorial and related to conditions commonly seen in the intensive care unit. Decreased renal perfusion can occur with systemic hypotension from a variety of etiologies or from elevated intra-abdominal pressures reducing local perfusion (eg, abdominal compartment syndrome). In addition to alterating hemodynamics, sepsis can lead to disturbances of the renal microvasculature from inflammatory mediators and activation of the coagulation system. Other conditions associated with AKI, either through direct or indirect mechanisms, include hypoxia, pulmonary-renal and hepatorenal syndromes, and toxic metabolic byproducts as in rhabdomyolysis or tumor lysis syndrome. Finally, nephrotoxic medications contribute to as much as 25% of cases of AKI, most commonly antibiotics (aminoglycosides, vancomycin) and immunosuppressive medications such as cytotoxic cancer chemotherapeutics and calcineurin inhibitors.

Clinical Findings

In general PICU populations, 10%–40% of patients have AKI at some point in their hospital course. Most cases of AKI develop within the first 24–48 hours of hospitalization, and nearly all within the first week. Irrespective of diagnostic criteria, studies consistently show an independent association between AKI and increased ICU length of stay and mortality. Critically ill patients with AKI can have complications such as electrolyte abnormalities, severe metabolic acidosis and fluid overload. Although the mechanisms are unclear and likely complex, fluid overload exceeding 10% of body weight has been shown to be an independent risk factor for worse outcomes, and patients overloaded by 20% of their body weight in fluid may have as much as an eightfold increased risk of death. The causal relationship between fluid overload and poor outcome is uncertain, but based on these findings, some authorities recommend consideration of renal replacement therapies for patients reaching 10%–20% fluid overload.

Treatment

The management of AKI is directed at alleviating potential contributing factors. Methods to *improve renal perfusion* include maintenance of adequate cardiac output and blood pressure with fluids and/or vasopressor medications and relief of excess intrathoracic and intra-abdominal pressures when feasible. For the latter, some experts recommend measurement of intra-abdominal pressures to guide therapy. Prospectively validated thresholds of adequate renal perfusion pressures to prevent or reverse AKI are lacking.

Diuretics are commonly used to address fluid overload associated with AKI, but these agents have not been shown to improve renal recovery in children and have been associated with an increased risk of death in adults with AKI. *Fluid restriction* can be helpful in managing fluid overload and may be of particular benefit in patients with concomitant lung injury.

Renal replacement therapies should be considered for serious electrolyte disturbances, drug or toxin overdoses, refractory acidosis, or when fluid overload associated with AKI is not responsive to fluid restriction and/or diuretic use. Renal replacement modalities include peritoneal dialysis, intermittent hemodialysis, and continuous renal replacement therapy (CRRT), also known as continuous VV hemofiltration with or without dialysis (CVVHF or CVVHD). CRRT involves sending patient venous blood through an extracorporeal filtration circuit and pump to provide slow, continuous fluid removal and/or dialysis. While the ideal renal replacement therapy depends on the individual clinical situation, CRRT is often the preferred modality for managing AKI in PICU patients. CRRT can be performed as ultrafiltration alone if control of intravascular volume is the primary goal, or CRRT can be performed with a dialysate to allow solute control as well. Advantages of CRRT include (1) in hemodynamically labile patients, a slower continuous rate of fluid removal may be better tolerated and can be more precisely controlled than intermittent dialysis; (2) solute and fluid removal can be regulated separately; and (3) CRRT may allow easing of fluid restrictions so that nutrition can be improved. Disadvantages include the technical complexity of the procedure, including anticoagulation of the circuit, and the need for central venous access. No prospective studies have compared CRRT with other modes of renal replacement or demonstrated that early initiation of CRRT improves outcomes in AKI, although retrospective studies have suggested that early initiation of CRRT may be associated with lower mortality. The decision to proceed with CRRT should involve a careful assessment of risks and possible benefits in each individual patient.

Basu RK, Devarajan P, Wong H, Wheeler DS: An update and review of acute kidney injury in pediatrics. Pediatr Crit Care Med 2011;12:339–347 [PMID: 21057358].

Modem V et al: Timing of continuous renal replacement therapy and mortality in critically ill children. Crit Care Med 2014 Apr;42(4):943–953 [PMID: 24231758].

Soler YA et al: Pediatric risk, injury, failure, loss, end-stage renal disease score identifies acute kidney injury and predicts mortality in critically ill children: a prospective study. Pediatr Crit Care Med 2013;14:1–7 [PMID: 23439463].

Acute Kidney Injury Guidelines, Kidney Disease Improving Global Outcomes (KDIGO): https://kdigo.org/guidelines/acute-kidney-injury/.

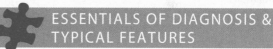

FLUID MANAGEMENT & NUTRITIONAL SUPPORT OF THE CRITICALLY ILL CHILD

ESSENTIALS OF DIAGNOSIS & TYPICAL FEATURES

▶ Fluid overload is an important predictor of poor outcome in critically ill children.

▶ Hyponatremia is also common in the PICU and may be associated with worse outcomes.

▶ Critically ill children are more susceptible to metabolic stress than adults due to lower muscle and fat mass and higher resting energy requirements.

▶ Obese children are more likely to develop complications including sepsis, wound infection, and increased length of stay in the PICU.

▶ Changes in nutritional status can persist for up to 6 months after discharge from a prolonged ICU stay.

▶ Early enteral and parenteral feeding can improve nutrition deficits, and may influence morbidity and mortality in critically ill infants and children.

Fluid Management

The majority of critically ill children are unable to take oral fluids and food, and, as a result, the ICU provider must carefully consider the needs of the individual patient in prescribing a fluid and nutrition regimen. Perhaps the most important issue in prescribing fluids is the patient's overall fluid balance. Standard maintenance IV fluid calculations are based on the assumption of a healthy, normotensive, spontaneously breathing patient. However, the "ideal" amount of fluid in a critically ill patient is variable, depending on the underlying condition, current physiologic state and ongoing fluid losses from urine, hemorrhage, or external drains. Insensible fluid losses may be elevated due to increased work of breathing or fever. In addition to common causes of hypovolemia, inflammatory states can lead to vasodilation and leakage from the vascular space into tissues, producing a "relative hypovolemic" state despite being total body fluid overloaded. Patients may be oliguric due to AKI or have reduced urine output due to excess antidiuretic hormone secretion associated with certain lung diseases and/or positive pressure ventilation. In addition, mechanically ventilated patients generally require less fluid than non-intubated patients because the ventilator delivers humidified gas and the insensible fluid loss that occurs with normal breathing is greatly reduced. Therefore, maintenance fluid requirements for these patients may be as little as two-thirds that of someone who is not mechanically ventilated. Because fluid overload has been associated with worse outcomes, if systemic hemodynamics allow, early consideration of fluid restriction and/or diuretic use may be warranted in these situations.

In addition to rate and volume, the tonicity of IV fluid is another important consideration. Hyponatremia has been associated with significant morbidity and mortality in neurocritical care patients, and even mild to moderate abnormalities in serum sodium are associated with worse outcomes in adult ICU patients. For these reasons, in children with acute brain injury (traumatic or hypoxic-ischemic), isotonic maintenance fluids are generally recommended to avoid worsening the risk of cerebral edema. For other children who are also at high risk for cerebral edema or hyponatremia, such as patients with diabetic ketoacidosis or meningitis, it may also be prudent to use isotonic fluid. When using isotonic fluid, close electrolyte monitoring is warranted to avoid the complications of undesired hypernatremia and hyperchloremic acidosis, particularly given recent literature describing chloride-rich fluids possibly affecting outcomes. No matter the choice of fluid, the critical care practitioner should closely monitor the patient's fluid balance based on physical examination, weight, and laboratory values and modify the fluid management strategy accordingly.

Nutritional Support

When severely ill pediatric patients are admitted to the PICU, provision of adequate nutritional support is often overlooked early in the course of therapy. Malnutrition is, however, a major problem in hospitalized patients, associated with higher rates of infectious and noninfectious complications as well as longer hospital stays and increased hospital costs. In the pediatric ICU, as many as 20% of patients experience either acute or chronic malnutrition, a rate that is largely unchanged over the past 30 years. Malnutrition in PICU patients is typically multifactorial, related to increased demands due to the physiologic and metabolic stresses associated with critical illness (Table 14–15), inaccurate assessments of caloric needs, and/or inadequate delivery of nutrition at the bedside.

Table 14–15. Physiologic and metabolic responses to severe illness.

Physiologic
Cardiovascular
Increased cardiac output
Peripheral vasodilatation and capillary leak
Expansion of vascular compartment
Pulmonary
Increased minute ventilation
Ventilation-perfusion mismatch
Inefficient gas exchange
Increased CO_2 responsiveness
Skeletal muscle
Easier fatigability
Slower relaxation
Altered force-frequency pattern
Renal
Salt and water retention
Impaired concentrating ability
Metabolic
Hormone and biological response modifier levels
Increased insulin
Increased glucocorticoids
Increased catecholamines
Increased interleukin-1
Increased tumor necrosis factor
Carbohydrate metabolism
Increased blood glucose
Increased gluconeogenesis
Increased glucose turnover
Glucose intolerance
Fat metabolism
Increased lipid turnover and utilization
Insuppressible lipolysis
Decreased ketogenesis
Protein metabolism
Increased muscle protein catabolism
Increased muscle branched-chain amino acid oxidation
Increased serum amino acids
Increased nitrogen losses

Nutritional Assessment

Early assessment by a pediatric dietitian or nutritionist can be helpful to establish nutritional requirements and goals in critically ill children and identify factors impeding adequate nutrition intake and tolerance. The initial caloric needs of the critically ill child can be estimated from calculations of the basal metabolic rate (BMR) or the resting energy expenditure (REE), and applying adjustments to those calculations based on the patient's illness and level of support. BMR represents the energy requirements of a healthy, fasting person who recently awoke from sleep, with normal temperature, and no stress, while REE represents the energy requirements of a healthy person at rest, with normal temperature and not fasting (Table 14–16). These closely related parameters are for practical purposes used interchangeably, although the REE tends to be approximately 10% above the BMR. The estimated basal metabolic need can then be multiplied by a stress factor related to the severity of the patient's illness to more accurately estimate overall energy requirements. Unfortunately, because these calculations are based on studies of healthy adults and children, they can be very inaccurate for use in critically ill children and lead to underfeeding or overfeeding. For example, studies have demonstrated significant metabolic instability and alterations in REEs with a predominance of hypometabolism in the PICU population, resulting in a higher risk of overfeeding when using calculations alone.

Indirect calorimetry (IC) is a more accurate means of directly measuring energy expenditure and determining caloric needs, but it is more difficult and expensive to perform and as a result is not always readily available. Identification of patients at highest risk for malnutrition (see Table 14–16) for targeted use of IC assessment has been suggested as one

Table 14–16. Markers of high risk of malnutrition suggested as indications for targeted indirect calorimetry assessment of REE.

- Underweight (< 5th percentile for age) or overweight (> 85th percentile for age)
- > 10% weight gain or loss during ICU stay
- Failure to consistently meet prescribed caloric goals
- Failure to wean from respiratory support
- Need for muscle relaxants for > 7 days
- Neurologic injury with evidence of dysautonomia
- Oncologic diagnoses
- Burns
- Requiring mechanical ventilation for > 7 days
- Suspected hypermetabolic state (eg, status epilepticus, SIRS) or hypometabolic state (eg, hypothermia, induced coma)
- ICU length of stay > 4 wk

ICU, intensive care unit; REE, resting energy expenditure; SIRS; systemic inflammatory response syndrome.

strategy for optimizing the cost-benefit ratio of IC. This technique requires collection of exhaled gases from the patient and can be inaccurate if a significant ETT leak is present, if the F_{IO_2} is more than 60%, and during hemodialysis or CRRT.

Delivery of Nutrition

In adult ICU patients, *enteral nutrition* is associated with fewer infectious complications than parenteral nutrition. No such comparisons in pediatric patients exist, but it is generally accepted that enteral nutrition is preferred in critically ill children as well. Enteral nutrition is generally well tolerated in hemodynamically stable children, with a goal protein intake of 2–3 g/kg/day. Patients with unstable hemodynamics or requiring vasopressor support may not tolerate full-volume enteral feeding, although low-volume continuous "trophic" feeding is generally safe and feasible in all but the most unstable patients and may reduce the incidence of nosocomial infections by protecting GI tract integrity. Use of an enteral feeding protocol and early transpyloric feeding may improve tolerance. Complications of enteral feeding include GI intolerance (vomiting, bleeding, diarrhea, and necrotizing enterocolitis), aspiration events/pneumonia, and mechanical issues (occlusion of tube, errors in tube placement).

Parenteral nutrition should be considered in critically ill children when enteral nutrition cannot be delivered or tolerated within 3–5 days. Although it is common practice to gradually increase the amino acid dose, evidence from preterm neonates shows that it is safe and efficacious to start parenteral amino acids at the target dose. Lipids should be included to decrease carbon dioxide production, minute ventilation, and fat storage, enhance lipid oxidation, augment protein retention, and prevent essential fatty acid deficiency. Hyperglycemia, hypertriglyceridemia, infection, and hepatobiliary abnormalities are all potential complications of parenteral nutrition. Metabolic evaluation (electrolytes, glucose, lipase, and liver function tests) should be performed regularly and the components of parenteral nutrition adjusted as needed.

Regardless of route of nutrition, *monitoring* should include routine physical examination, serial measures of growth (weight, skinfold thickness), serial monitoring of serum electrolyte and mineral concentrations, and repeated measurements of REE when available. Measurements of serum albumin provide limited information about nutritional status given the multiple other influences on albumin concentrations. Prealbumin and CRP measurements may be helpful, however. Prealbumin levels are a good marker of nutritional protein status; they drop during acute illness and return to normal during recovery. CRP levels are a marker of the acute phase response to illness and injury; they rise during acute illness and drop with recovery, typically in association with a return to anabolic metabolism and before increases in prealbumin.

Mehta NM, Duggan CP: Nutritional deficiencies during critical illness. Pediatr Clin North Am 2009 Oct;56(5):1143–1160 [PMID: 19931068].

Mehta NM et al: A.S.P.E.N. clinical guidelines: nutrition support of the critically ill child. J Parent Enteral Nutr 2009;33(3):260–276 [PMID: 19398612].

Valentine SL et al: Fluid balance in critically ill children with acute lung injury. Crit Care Med 2012 Oct;40(10):2883–2889 [PMID: 22824936].

▼ SEDATION & ANALGESIA IN THE PEDIATRIC ICU

ESSENTIALS OF DIAGNOSIS & TYPICAL FEATURES

▶ Pain control and relief of anxiety are standard of care for all patients in the PICU.

▶ Sedation and analgesia must be individualized for each patient and reassessed frequently to avoid inadequate or excessive medication.

▶ Sedative and analgesic medications have unique sets of physiologic effects and side effects, and these agents should only be used with adequate monitoring and support to address potential adverse events.

Children admitted to the PICU often require anxiolytic and analgesic medications to minimize discomfort and keep them safe. Sedation and anxiolysis may also be needed to facilitate mechanical ventilation or the performance of procedures, and analgesia may be needed for postoperative pain or pain related to traumatic injuries. Thus, careful consideration of a patient's sedative and analgesic needs is a vital part of ICU management.

When determining which anxiolytic and analgesic medications to initiate, it is important to distinguish between anxiety and pain, because pharmacologic therapy may be directed at either or both of these symptoms (Table 14–17). Additional considerations in sedative selection are the route of administration and the anticipated duration of treatment. Routes of administration may be limited by the patient's IV access or ability to tolerate oral medications. Children who require more frequent dosing or tighter control of sedation level may benefit from a continuous infusion whereas patients undergoing a bedside procedure may only require a small number of discrete doses. Potential adverse effects in particular clinical circumstances are another important consideration in sedative and analgesic selection.

▶ Sedation

Sedative (anxiolytic) medications may be indicated when the goals of treatment are to reduce anxiety, facilitate treatment or procedures, manage acute confusional states, and

Table 14–17. Commonly used intravenous medications for pain and anxiety control.

Drug	Suggested Starting Dose	Advantages	Disadvantages	Usual Duration of Effect
Morphine	0.1 mg/kg; continuous infusion, 0.05–0.1 mg/kg/h	Excellent pain relief, reversible	Respiratory depression, hypotension, nausea, suppression of GI motility, histamine release	2–4 h
Hydromorphone	0.015 mg/kg; continuous infusion, 1.5–3 mcg/kg/h	Good pain relief, reversible	Respiratory depression, histamine release, nausea, suppression of GI motility	2–4 h
Fentanyl	1–2 mcg/kg; continuous infusion, 0.5–2 mcg/kg/h	Excellent pain relief, reversible, short half-life	Respiratory depression, chest wall rigidity, severe nausea and vomiting	30 min
Midazolam	0.1 mg/kg; continuous infusion 0.05–0.2 mg/kg/h	Short half-life, only benzodiazepine given as continuous infusion	Respiratory depression	20–40 min
Lorazepam	0.1 mg/kg	Longer half-life, sedation and seizure control	Nausea and vomiting, respiratory depression, phlebitis	2–4 h
Diazepam	0.1 mg/kg	Sedation and seizure control	Respiratory depression, jaundice, phlebitis	1–3 h
Dexmedetomidine	0.2–0.7 mcg/kg/h	Sedation, anxiolysis, analgesia without respiratory depression	Bradycardia, hypotension	10 min–2 h

diminish physiologic responses to stress, such as tachycardia, hypertension, or increased ICP. The most commonly used agents in the PICU are the benzodiazepines and the opioids. These should be carefully titrated to effect to avoid oversedation and resultant respiratory depression and/or hemodynamic instability.

A. Benzodiazepines

Benzodiazepines work through the neuroinhibitory transmitter γ-aminobutyric acid (GABA) system, resulting in anxiolysis, sedation, hypnosis, skeletal muscle relaxation, and anticonvulsant effects. Benzodiazepines provide little to no analgesia and thus need to be combined with other medications when pain control is required.

Most benzodiazepines are metabolized in the liver, with their metabolites subsequently excreted in the urine; thus, patients in liver failure are likely to have long elimination times. Benzodiazepines can cause respiratory depression if given rapidly in high doses, an important consideration for the nonintubated patient. They can also cause cardiovascular compromise in critically ill patients, making careful titration of doses essential.

In some children, benzodiazepines can cause a paradoxical effect, producing greater agitation than sedation. In those cases, selection of an alternative agent may be more appropriate than escalation in dose. When overdose is a concern, flumazenil may be used to reverse benzodiazepine effects. Flumazenil must be used with care, however, as its effects generally wear off faster than those of most benzodiazepines. Additionally, in tolerant patients rapid reversal may result in withdrawal symptoms, including seizures.

Commonly used benzodiazepines in the PICU include midazolam, lorazepam, and diazepam. Each has differing half-lives, resulting in varying durations of effect, and multiple possible routes of administration. *Midazolam* has the shortest half-life and produces excellent retrograde amnesia lasting for 20–40 minutes after a single IV dose. Therefore, it can be used for short-term procedural sedation and anxiolysis with single or intermittent doses or for prolonged sedation as a continuous infusion. *Lorazepam* has a longer half-life than midazolam (or diazepam) and can achieve sedation for as long as 6–8 hours. It has less effect on the cardiovascular and respiratory systems than other benzodiazepines and is commonly used for short-term sedation or initial treatment of seizures. Continuous infusions of lorazepam should be avoided because its preservative, polyethylene glycol, can accumulate in patients with renal insufficiency and produce a metabolic acidosis. *Diazepam* has a longer half-life than midazolam and is used most commonly to treat muscle spasticity and seizures. A disadvantage of diazepam in the PICU is the long half-life of its intermediary metabolite, nordazepam, which may accumulate and prolong sedation, making diazepam less ideal for short-term sedation.

B. Other Sedative Medications

Opioids are strong analgesics that also have sedative effects. They are commonly used as adjuncts in combination with other sedatives such as benzodiazepines. Specific medications are described further in the analgesic medication section.

Ketamine is a phencyclidine derivative that produces a trance-like state of immobility and amnesia known as dissociative anesthesia. Ketamine does not cause significant respiratory depression at nonanesthetic doses, an advantage for the nonintubated patient. Ketamine has direct negative inotropic effects, but these are countered by stimulation of the sympathetic nervous system resulting in an increase in HR, blood pressure, and cardiac output for most patients. These effects may make ketamine a good choice for hemodynamically unstable patients unless there is concern that the patient may be catecholamine depleted, such as in the setting of chronic heart failure. Additionally, ketamine has bronchodilatory properties and, thus, may be useful for children with status asthmaticus. Finally, it has strong analgesic effects and therefore may be used as a single agent for sedation for painful procedures. The main side effects seen with ketamine are increased salivary and tracheobronchial secretions and unpleasant dreams or hallucinations. Atropine or glycopyrrolate may be administered ahead of time to reduce secretions, and concurrent administration of benzodiazepines may reduce the hallucinatory effects. Although most frequently used for short-term sedation, low-dose continuous infusions may be used in selected patients.

Dexmedetomidine is a selective α_2-adrenoreceptor agonist that produces sedation, anxiolysis, and some analgesia with minimal respiratory depression. It allows for the ability to rouse the patient easily if necessary. These advantages have resulted in increasing use in critically ill children for procedural sedation as well as sedation to facilitate both invasive and non-invasive mechanical ventilation. The most frequent side effects observed are dose-related bradycardia and hypotension. Dexmedetomidine is primarily used as a short- or long-term continuous infusion. The use of dexmedetomidine may also mitigate the need for increasing doses of opioids and benzodiazepines in patients requiring multiple sedative medications.

Propofol is an anesthetic IV induction agent with strong sedative effects. Its main advantages are a rapid onset and recovery time resulting from its rapid hepatic metabolism. Because propofol has no analgesic properties, an analgesic agent should be concurrently administered for painful procedures. Propofol can cause significant vasodilation, resulting in dose-related hypotension, in addition to dose-dependent respiratory depression. Owing to concerns for propofol infusion syndrome, a sudden-onset, profound, and often fatal acidosis associated with prolonged infusions, propofol is now used in children mostly for procedural or short-term sedation.

Barbiturates (eg, phenobarbital) can cause direct myocardial and respiratory depression and are, in general, poor choices for standard sedation of critically ill patients.

Analgesia

Opioid and nonopioid analgesics are the mainstay of treatment for acute and chronic pain in the PICU. Although several other medications used for sedation also have analgesic properties, they are uncommonly used for primary treatment of pain.

A. Opioid Analgesics

All opioids provide analgesia and have dose-dependent sedative effects. A range of plasma concentrations produce analgesia without sedation; the dose required to produce adequate analgesia varies significantly between patients. Therefore, the best approach to dosing with opioids is to start with a low-end dose but then titrate to effect, monitoring for side effects. The most common side effects of these agents are nausea, pruritus, slowed intestinal motility, miosis, cough suppression, and urinary retention. Opioids can also cause respiratory depression, particularly in infants. Morphine can cause histamine release leading to pruritus and even hypotension; fentanyl generally has few hemodynamic effects in a volume-replete patient. Opioids are metabolized in the liver, with metabolites excreted in the urine. Thus, patients with hepatic or renal impairment may have prolonged responses to their administration.

The choice and mode of delivery of agents within this class depends on the physiologic state of the child and the etiology of pain. In an awake and developmentally capable patient, a patient-controlled analgesia (PCA) approach with an infusion pump may be appropriate. Each of these medications may also be administered intermittently, in which case half-life and tolerability of side effects may be the primary considerations. For many patients in the PICU, a continuous infusion may be the best option. Several IV medications are commonly used as a continuous infusion or by PCA, including fentanyl, morphine, and hydromorphone. For children who have more chronic, less severe pain and who can tolerate oral medications, there are many different options, including hydrocodone, hydromorphone, morphine, methadone, and oxycodone.

Naloxone may be used as an opioid reversal agent for narcotic overdoses. Because of its relatively short half-life compared to many opioids, symptoms may recur and repeat dosing or even a continuous infusion may be necessary. Caution should be used in patients with chronic opioid exposure to avoid precipitating severe withdrawal symptoms.

B. Nonopioid Analgesics

Nonopioid analgesics used to treat mild to moderate pain include acetaminophen, aspirin, and other nonsteroidal anti-inflammatory drugs (NSAIDs). Because the effects of these agents can be additive with opiates, a combination of opiate and nonopiate medications can be a very effective approach to pain management in the ICU.

Acetaminophen is the most commonly used analgesic in pediatrics in the United States and is the drug of choice for mild to moderate pain because of its low toxicity and minimal side-effect profile. With chronic use and higher doses, acetaminophen may cause liver and renal toxicity.

NSAIDs are reasonable alternatives for the treatment of pain, particularly those conditions associated with inflammation. All NSAIDs carry the risk of gastritis, renal compromise, and bleeding due to inhibition of platelet function, limiting their use in patients with thrombocytopenia, bleeding, and kidney disease. *Ketorolac* is the only IV NSAID currently available. It can be very effective for children who cannot take oral medication or require a faster onset of action. Because of the concerns for more serious renal toxicity with longer-term use, ketorolac is primarily used for shorter-term pain control. *Ibuprofen* and *naproxen* are options for patients who can tolerate oral medications. Ibuprofen has a shorter half-life and therefore requires more frequent dosing.

Titration of Sedative & Analgesic Dosing, Delirium, & Withdrawal Syndromes

Sedative analgesic and anxiolytic agents have a number of serious disadvantages, including short- and long-term cognitive deficits, an increased risk of delirium, and withdrawal syndromes. Daily interruption of all continuous sedation with titrated reintroduction as necessary has been shown in adult ICU patients to dramatically reduce the duration of mechanical ventilation and length of stay in the ICU. Similar data are not yet available for pediatric patients. Another proposed intervention to decrease sedation use in children is protocolized, nurse-driven sedation goals. A recent large multicenter, randomized study of this approach in pediatrics demonstrated decreased overall opioid exposure but failed to show a decreased length of mechanical ventilation. The untoward effects of sedation in critically ill children remain a concern and, in general, doses of these agents should be titrated downward daily to the minimum required doses.

Standardized scales have been developed to assist in the titration of sedatives and analgesics in children. In the awake and verbal patient, a pain scale can be used to determine the level of pain and need for treatment. In a nonverbal patient, this assessment can be more difficult, and the medical team may need to depend on changes in physiologic parameters such as HR and blood pressure to indicate pain and the effect of treatment. When using these measures, however, the provider should also exclude or address physiologic causes of agitation, such as hypoxemia, hypercapnia, or cerebral hypoperfusion caused by low cardiac output.

Several scoring systems are available to assess the level of sedation and help guide sedation management decisions. These include the COMFORT score and the State Behavioral Scale (SBS). Utilizing such a measurement tool allows for better communication among team members with regard to the goals of treatment and the effectiveness of any changes in sedation plan.

As with adult patients, critically ill children are at risk for developing *delirium*. Delirium may present with a wide variety of symptoms, commonly grouped as hypoactive, hyperactive or mixed. Hyperactive delirium is associated with restlessness, agitation, emotional lability and combativeness. Hypoactive delirium, on the other hand, may be more difficult to recognize; patients may be quiet, withdrawn, and apathetic with decreased responsiveness. Parents may notice their child's personality is quite different from baseline. PICU delirium scales including the Pediatric Confusion Assessment Method for the ICU (pCAM-ICU) and Cornell Assessment of Pediatric Delirium (CAPD) may help better assess for delirium in the PICU population.

In critically ill children, as in adults, the risk of developing delirium appears to increase with severity of illness, administration of sedative medications such as benzodiazepines, and greater sleep disturbances. Suggested strategies for preventing and treating delirium include reducing sedative exposure, promoting normal circadian rhythms with greater activity during the day and quiet, dark rooms at night, and ensuring the presence of parents and objects familiar to the child. Finally, in more extreme situations, treatment with medications can be considered. Quetiapine is a newer antipsychotic agent that has shown promise in early studies for treating pediatric delirium. Older antipsychotics such as haloperidol are still used at times, but their side-effect profile demands caution. Benzodiazepines may calm the patient but also may induce a paradoxical reaction. Dexmedetomidine may also be an effective medication for treatment of delirium, but this use has not been well studied in the pediatric population.

Withdrawal syndromes are another important aspect of the use of sedative and analgesic agents in the ICU. Long-term administration and high doses of continuous infusions of opioids or benzodiazepines can lead to tolerance and physical dependence. Acute reductions or cessation of these medications can result in withdrawal symptoms such as agitation, tachypnea, tachycardia, sweating, and diarrhea. The risk of withdrawal varies among individuals, but the longer patients receive opiates or benzodiazepines, the more likely they are to have withdrawal symptoms. Gradual tapering of the medication dosage over 7–10 days often effectively prevents withdrawal symptoms. This gradual reduction may be facilitated by transitioning to intermittent dosing of longer half-life agents, such as methadone or lorazepam. While weaning opiates or benzodiazepines, providers should assess daily for symptoms of withdrawal. This assessment can be facilitated by symptom scores such as the Withdrawal Assessment Tool-1 (WAT-1). A higher WAT-1 score suggests greater withdrawal symptoms and may indicate a need to slow the weaning plan. Conversely, if the WAT-1 score is consistently low, the patient is likely to tolerate the current pace or, possibly, an accelerated dose reduction.

Curley MA et al: Protocolized sedation vs usual care in pediatric patients mechanically ventilated for acute respiratory failure: a randomized clinical trial. JAMA 2015 Jan 27;313(4)379–389 [PMID: 25602358].

Harris, J et al: Clinical recommendations for pain, sedation, withdrawal and delirium assessment in critically ill infants and children: an ESPNIC position statement for healthcare professionals. Intensive Care Med 2016;42(6):972–986 [PMID: 27084344].

▼ END-OF-LIFE CARE & DEATH IN THE PICU

ESSENTIALS OF DIAGNOSIS & TYPICAL FEATURES

► End-of-life discussions in the PICU should include the patient, if possible, and family members as well as the medical team.

► PICU providers may assist in defining the limits of care provided, facilitating withdrawal of life support, and providing compassionate palliative care.

► The palliative care and ethics teams, if available, may facilitate end-of-life discussions in the PICU.

► Withdrawal of life-sustaining therapies should include a plan to treat any pain and discomfort in the patient.

► Brain death determination requires a systematic and age-appropriate evaluation consistent with institutional policies.

► Tissue and organ donation must be considered with every death.

► Grief/bereavement support for the family as well as medical team members should be provided following every death in the PICU.

► Death in the PICU

In-hospital pediatric deaths occur infrequently. A large proportion of pediatric deaths occur in the PICU, however, and pediatric intensivists may be called upon to help define the limits to care provided, assist in the withdrawal of life-sustaining medical therapies (LSMTs), and provide compassionate palliative care. End-of-life discussions may have occurred prior to PICU admission for some children with congenital or chronic diseases. For other children, their PICU stay may be the first time a child or family discusses end-of-life decisions. Regardless of the individual patient's situation, the medical team has a responsibility to facilitate discussions regarding the goals of care in an honest and sensitive manner.

Deaths without any limitations on patient care comprise a small minority (10%–12%) of pediatric ICU deaths. In these circumstances, most recent studies have found greater family satisfaction with the care provided if family members are allowed to witness ongoing resuscitative efforts. The remainder of pediatric deaths is divided between brain death declarations (23%) and decisions to limit or withdraw LSMTs (65%).

Brain Death

Patients with severe neurologic injuries may meet the criteria for a diagnosis of brain death. The concept of brain death arose when advances in ICU technologies allowed heart and lung function to be supported even in the absence of any discernible brain activity. Brain death is diagnosed by a clinical examination (Table 14–18) based on published guidelines and is recognized as legally equivalent to somatic (cardiopulmonary) death in all 50 US states. The general approach to the diagnosis of brain death is similar in most medical centers, but subtle institutional variations make it imperative for PICU providers to be familiar with their own institutional policies on brain death declaration. Once a patient is declared legally brain dead, further medical support is no longer indicated, although the timing of discontinuation of mechanical life support should be discussed and agreed upon with the patient's family.

Brain death is determined through a complete clinical assessment of the patient. First and foremost, the provider must be confident that the patient's condition is irreversible and must exclude any potentially reversible conditions that may produce signs similar to brain death. These may include hypotension, hypothermia, or the presence of excessive doses of sedating medications. The brain death examination is a formal clinical examination directed at demonstrating the absence of cortical function (flaccid coma without evidence of response to stimuli) and brainstem function (cranial nerve testing). In order to meet the definition of brain death, guidelines require that qualified physicians document two separate clinical examinations consistent with brain death (ie, no evidence of brain function) separated by a period of observation. If a patient cannot tolerate some portion of the clinical examination (typically apnea testing) or is very young (especially < 1 year of age), an ancillary test such as EEG or cerebral perfusion scan may provide supporting evidence of brain death. Once a child has been declared brain dead, the time of death is noted as occurring at the completion of the second examination even if the child is still receiving cardiopulmonary support.

Limitation or Withdrawal of Medical Care

Most patients who die in the pediatric ICU will do so following a decision to limit or withdraw medical support. The discussions leading to these decisions should include the patient (to the extent possible given their medical condition and developmental age), family members, and members of the medical team. The primary goals of these discussions should be to (1) communicate information regarding the patient's medical status and anticipated prognosis and (2) clarify the goals of ongoing medical care both in regard to the patient's current status and in the event of an acute decompensation. If the opinion of the medical team is that the patient's condition is likely irreversible, the options for care include (1) continuing current support with escalation as deemed medically reasonable by the health care team; (2) continuing current support but not adding any new therapies; (3) withdrawal of life-sustaining therapies such as mechanical ventilation and hemodynamic support. The first two options may include a decision to withhold cardiopulmonary resuscitation in the event of a respiratory or cardiac arrest (do-not-attempt resuscitation [DNAR]). The third option presumes a DNAR but this must be explicitly written in the medical record and communicated to team members.

Discussions with patients and families regarding the decision to limit resuscitation or to withdraw LSMT should be conducted by experienced personnel with the ability to communicate in a clear and compassionate manner and should occur at an appropriate time and place. Cultural needs should be considered prior to major discussions and may include the need for a translator or spiritual guidance. Discussions should begin with a clear statement that the goal is to make decisions in the best interest of the patient and

Table 14–18. Brain death examination.

- Patient must have normal blood pressure, core temperature > 35°C, normal electrolytes and glucose, and not be receiving sedating medications or muscle relaxants.
- 24-h waiting period suggested following CPR or severe brain injury before first brain death exam.
- Flaccid coma with no evidence of cortical function.
- Absence of brain stem reflexes:
  - Apnea ("apnea test": no respirations seen with $Paco_2$ > 60 mm Hg and a change in $Paco_2$ > 20 mm Hg).
  - Fixed dilated pupils with no response to light.
  - Absence of corneal reflexes.
  - Absence of eye movements including spontaneous, oculocephalic (doll's eye), or oculovestibular (cold caloric). Do not perform oculocephalic maneuver if there is potential for cervical spine injury.
  - Absence of gag and cough reflex.
- Examination consistent throughout observation period as documented by two separate clinical examinations by two different attending physicians.
- Recommended observation periods between brain death examinations:
  - Term newborn to 30 d old—24 h
  - 31 d–18 y—12 h
- Ancillary testing (cerebral angiography, radionuclide scanning, electroencephalography, or transcranial Doppler ultrasonography) recommended if unable to perform cranial nerve examination or apnea testing due to patient instability or injuries.

that the health care team will support the patient and family in making reasonable decisions based on that goal. Potential options regarding limitations of care or withdrawal of care should be clearly explained for the decision makers. Withdrawal of LSMT can be considered when the pain and suffering inflicted by prolonging and supporting life outweighs the potential benefit for the individual. If there is no reasonable chance of recovery, the patient has the right to a natural death in a dignified and pain-free manner. The health care team should emphasize that decisions are not irrevocable and that if at any time the family or health care providers wish to reconsider the decision, full medical therapy can be reinstituted until the situation is clarified.

Prior to the withdrawal of LSMT, the patient's family and care team should be prepared for the physiologic process of dying that the child will undergo. Key facets of the process to discuss include the possibility of agonal respirations, which can be disturbing to witness for family members and care providers, as well as the unpredictable length of time that the process may require. Additionally, the fact that the patient will ultimately have a cardiopulmonary arrest and a member of the medical team will declare the time of death should be discussed. The family should also be reassured that the patient will be given appropriate doses of medications to treat signs and symptoms of pain or discomfort and that neither they nor the patient will be abandoned by the medical team during this process.

Palliative Care & Bioethics Consultation

Palliative care teams and ethics consultation services are important resources to help the health care team and families address difficult end-of-life decision making. For families of children with congenital or chronic diseases, the palliative care team may have established relationships with the patient and family outside of the acute illness. For patients with new conditions or whose prognosis has changed, the palliative care team may be newly introduced in the PICU. In either case, the palliative care team can bring invaluable support and resources for families during end-of-life discussions. A more comprehensive discussion of palliative care can be found elsewhere in this book.

If conflict arises surrounding decisions about limiting medical care, an ethics consultation can aid the process by helping to identify, analyze, and resolve ethical problems. Ethics consultation can independently clarify views and allow the health care team, patient, and family to make decisions that respect patient autonomy and promote maximum benefit and minimal harm to the patient.

Tissue & Organ Donation

Organ transplantation is standard therapy for many pediatric conditions and many children die while awaiting a transplant due to short supply of organs. The gift of organ donation can be a positive outcome for a family from the otherwise tragic loss of their child's life. The 1986 U.S. Federal Required Request Law mandates that all donor-eligible families be approached about potential organ donation. The decision to donate must be made free of coercion, with informed consent, and without financial incentive. The state organ-procurement agencies provide support and education to care providers and families to make informed decisions.

To be a solid-organ donor, the patient must be declared dead and have no conditions contraindicating donation. The most frequent type of solid-organ donor in the PICU is a brain-dead donor. The unmet demand for donor organs has, however, led to the emergence of protocols for procuring solid organs from non–heart-beating donors. Although this practice has been described by many terms including Donation after Cardiac Death, the most recent nomenclature is Donation after Circulatory Determination of Death (DCDD). In these cases, the patient does not meet brain death criteria but has an irreversible disease process and the family or patient has decided to withdraw life-sustaining therapy and consented to attempted organ donation. In the DCDD process, LSMT is withdrawn and comfort measures are provided as per usual care. The withdrawal of care may take place in the PICU or the operating room without any surgical staff present, depending on institutional policy. Once the declaring physician has determined cessation of cardiac function, the patient is observed for an additional short time period for auto-resuscitation (the return of cardiac activity without medical intervention). After this waiting period, the patient is declared dead and the organs are immediately harvested for donation. If the patient does not die within a predetermined time limit after discontinuation of LSMT, comfort measures continue but solid-organ donation is abandoned due to unacceptably long ischemic times.

Tissue (heart valves, corneas, skin, and bone) can be donated following a "traditional" cardiac death (no pulse or respirations), brain death, or DCDD.

Bereavement & Grief Support

After any pediatric death, bereavement and grief support for families and health care providers are essential components of comprehensive end-of-life care. Families may need information about care of the body after the death, funeral arrangements, and autopsy decisions as well as about educational, spiritual, and other supportive resources available. Members of the medical team may feel their own grief and sense of loss with the death of a patient. These emotions, if not appropriately addressed, can negatively affect their personal and professional lives. Therefore, similar supportive services should be available to health care workers caring for dying children.

Lee KJ et al: Alterations in end-of-life support in the pediatric intensive care unit. Pediatrics 2010;126(4):e859–e864 [PMID: 20819890].

Nakagawa T et al: Guidelines for the determination of brain death in infants and children: an update of the 1987 task force recommendations. Pediatrics 2011;128(3):e720–e740 [PMID: 21873704].

QUALITY IMPROVEMENT INITIATIVES IN THE PICU

Given the complexity of both the illnesses faced and the care provided in PICUs, these environments are among the most susceptible to medical error. As a result, critical care units also tend to be the areas that are likely to benefit from quality improvement and patient safety initiatives. National and local reporting requirements for a number of hospital-acquired conditions, such as central line-associated bloodstream infections, catheter-associated urinary tract infections, pressure injuries, and venous thromboembolisms, have led to the development of national collaboratives focused on data gathering and sharing of best practices for prevention of those conditions. Improving quality and safety practices relies on creating both a culture of awareness and safe reporting of adverse events and tools or workflows designed to help reduce the likelihood of error. As an example, multipronged efforts to reduce catheter-related bloodstream infections include checklists or tools to ensure strict adherence to sterile procedure during catheter insertion, sterile practice when accessing the catheter during care, reductions in the number of times the catheter is accessed, and removal of catheters at the earliest safe opportunity. More recent efforts have begun to focus on early identification and treatment of sepsis using defined diagnostic triggers and order sets. Most of the data supporting these interventions have been derived from adult ICU populations, and, to date, few large-scale studies have been published documenting efficacy of these measures in the pediatric ICU population. Data that are available suggest that these initiatives are beneficial, although additional studies will likely be needed to refine and optimize these approaches in the pediatric ICU setting.

Skin

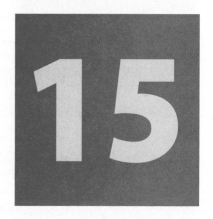

Lori D. Prok, MD

Carla X. Torres-Zegarra, MD

▼ GENERAL PRINCIPLES

DIAGNOSIS OF SKIN DISORDERS

Examination of the skin requires that the entire surface of the body be palpated and inspected in good light. The onset and duration of each symptom should be recorded, together with a description of the primary lesion and any secondary changes, using the terminology in Table 15–1. In practice, characteristics of skin lesions are described in an order opposite to that shown in the table. Begin with distribution, then configuration, color, secondary changes, and primary changes. For example, guttate psoriasis could be described as "generalized, discrete, red, or scaly papules."

TREATMENT OF SKIN DISORDERS

Topical Therapy

Treatment should be simple and aimed at preserving normal skin physiology. Topical therapy is often preferred because medication can be delivered in optimal concentrations to the desired site.

Water is an important therapeutic agent, and optimally hydrated skin is soft and smooth. This occurs at approximately 60% environmental humidity. Because water evaporates readily from the cutaneous surface (epidermal stratum corneum), skin hydration is dependent on the water concentration in the air, and sweating contributes little. However, if sweat is prevented from evaporating (eg, in the axilla, groin), local humidity and hydration of the skin are increased. As humidity falls below 15%–20%, the stratum corneum shrinks and cracks; the epidermal barrier is lost and allows irritants to enter the skin and induce an inflammatory response. Decrease in transepidermal water loss will correct this condition. Therefore, dry and scaly skin is treated by using barriers to prevent evaporation. Oils and ointments prevent

evaporation for 8–12 hours, so they must be applied once or twice a day. In areas already occluded (axilla, diaper area), creams or lotions are preferred, but more frequent application may be necessary.

Overhydration (maceration) can also occur. As environmental humidity increases to 90%–100%, the number of water molecules absorbed by the stratum corneum increases and the tight lipid junctions between the cells of the stratum corneum are gradually replaced by weak hydrogen bonds. The cells eventually become widely separated, and the epidermal barrier falls apart. This occurs in immersion foot, diaper areas, axillae, and the like. It is desirable to enhance evaporation of water in these areas by air drying.

Wet Dressings

By placing the skin in an environment where the humidity is 100% and allowing the moisture to evaporate to 60%, pruritus is relieved. Evaporation of water stimulates cold-dependent nerve fibers in the skin, and this may prevent the transmission of the itching sensation via pain fibers to the central nervous system (CNS). It is also vasoconstrictive, thereby helping to reduce the erythema and also decreasing the inflammatory cellular response.

The simplest form of wet dressing consists of one set of wet underwear (eg, "long johns") worn under dry pajamas. Cotton socks are also useful for hand or foot treatment. The underwear should be soaked in warm (not hot) water and wrung out until no more water can be expressed. Dressings can be worn overnight for a few days up to 1 week. When the condition improves, wet dressings are discontinued.

Topical Glucocorticoids

Twice-daily application of topical corticosteroids is the mainstay of treatment for all forms of dermatitis (Table 15–2). Topical steroids can also be used under wet dressings.

Table 15–1. Examination of the skin.

Clinical Appearance	Description and Examples
Primary lesions (first to appear)	
Macule	Any flat circumscribed color change in the skin < 1 cm. Examples: white (vitiligo), brown (junctional nevus), purple (petechia).
Patch	Any flat circumscribed color change in the skin > 1 cm. Examples: white (nevus depigmentosa), brown (café au lait macule), purple (purpura).
Papule	A solid, elevated area < 1 cm in diameter whose top may be pointed, rounded, or flat. Examples: acne, warts, small lesions of psoriasis.
Plaque	A solid, circumscribed area > 1 cm in diameter, usually flat-topped. Example: psoriasis.
Vesicle	A circumscribed, elevated lesion < 1 cm in diameter and containing clear serous fluid. Example: blisters of herpes simplex.
Bulla	A circumscribed, elevated lesion > 1 cm in diameter and containing clear serous fluid. Example: bullous impetigo.
Pustule	A vesicle containing a purulent exudate. Examples: acne, folliculitis.
Nodule	A deep-seated mass with indistinct borders that elevates the overlying epidermis. Examples: tumors, granuloma annulare. If it moves with the skin on palpation, it is intradermal; if the skin moves over the nodule, it is subcutaneous.
Wheal	A circumscribed, flat-topped, firm elevation of skin resulting from tense edema of the papillary dermis. Example: urticaria.
Secondary changes	
Scales	Dry, thin plates of keratinized epidermal cells (stratum corneum). Examples: psoriasis, ichthyosis.
Lichenification	Induration of skin with exaggerated skin lines and a shiny surface resulting from chronic rubbing of the skin. Example: chronic atopic dermatitis.
Erosion and oozing	A moist, circumscribed, slightly depressed area representing a blister base with the roof of the blister removed. Examples: burns, impetigo. Most oral blisters present as erosions.
Crusts	Dried exudate of plasma on the surface of the skin following disruption of the stratum corneum. Examples: impetigo, contact dermatitis.
Fissures	A linear split in the skin extending through the epidermis into the dermis. Example: angular cheilitis.
Scars	A flat, raised, or depressed area of fibrotic replacement of dermis or subcutaneous tissue. Examples: acne scar, burn scar.
Atrophy	Depression of the skin surface caused by thinning of one or more layers of skin. Example: lichen sclerosus.
Color	
	The lesion should be described as white, red, yellow, brown, tan, or blue. Particular attention should be given to the blanching of red lesions. Failure to blanch suggests bleeding into the dermis (petechiae).
Configuration of lesions	
Annular (circular)	Annular nodules represent granuloma annulare; annular scaly papules are more apt to be caused by dermatophyte infections.
Linear (straight lines)	Linear papules represent lichen striatus; linear vesicles, incontinentia pigmenti; linear papules with burrows, scabies.
Grouped	Grouped vesicles occur in herpes simplex or zoster.
Discrete	Discrete lesions are independent of each other.
Distribution	
	Note whether the eruption is generalized, acral (hands, feet, buttocks, face), or localized to a specific skin region.

Table 15–2. Topical glucocorticoids.

Glucocorticoid	Concentrations
Low potency[a] = 1–9	
Hydrocortisone	0.5%, 1%, 2.5%
Desonide	0.05%
Moderate potency = 10–99	
Mometasone furoate	0.1%
Hydrocortisone valerate	0.2%
Fluocinolone acetonide	0.025%
Triamcinolone acetonide	0.01%
Amcinonide	0.1%
High potency = 100–499	
Desoximetasone	0.25%
Fluocinonide	0.05%
Halcinonide	0.1%
Super potency = 500–7500	
Betamethasone dipropionate	0.05%
Clobetasol propionate	0.05%

[a]1% hydrocortisone is defined as having a potency of 1.

After wet dressings are discontinued, topical steroids should be applied only to areas of active disease. They should not be applied to normal skin to prevent recurrence. Only low-potency steroids (see Table 15–2) are applied to the face or intertriginous areas.

Eichenfield LF et al: Guidelines of care for the management of atopic dermatitis: section 2. Management and treatment of atopic dermatitis with topical therapies. J Am Acad Dermatol 2014 Jul;71(1):116–132 [PMID: 24813302].

Morley KW, Dinulos JG: Update on topical glucocorticoid use in children. Curr Opin Pediatr 2012 Feb;24(1):121–128 [PMID: 22227781].

Schwartz J, Friedman AJ. Exogenous factors in skin barrier repair. J Drugs Dermatol 2016 Nov;1;15(11):1289–1294.

▼ DISORDERS OF THE SKIN IN NEWBORNS

TRANSIENT DISEASES IN NEWBORNS

1. Milia

Milia are tiny epidermal cysts filled with keratinous material. These 1- to 2-mm white papules occur predominantly on the face in 40% of newborns. Their intraoral counterparts are called Epstein pearls and occur in up to 60%–85% of neonates. These cystic structures spontaneously rupture and exfoliate their contents.

2. Sebaceous Gland Hyperplasia

Prominent white to yellow papules at the opening of pilosebaceous follicles without surrounding erythema—especially over the nose—represent overgrowth of sebaceous glands in response to maternal androgens. They occur in more than half of newborns and spontaneously regress in the first few months of life.

3. Neonatal Acne

Inflammatory papules and pustules with occasional comedones predominantly on the face occur in as many as 20% of newborns. Although neonatal acne can be present at birth, it most often occurs between 2 and 4 weeks of age. Spontaneous resolution occurs over a period of 6 months to 1 year. A rare entity that is often confused with neonatal acne is **neonatal cephalic pustulosis**. This is a more monomorphic eruption with red papules and pustules on the head and neck that appears in the first month of life. There is associated neutrophilic inflammation and yeasts of the genus *Malassezia* (*Pityrosporum*). This eruption will resolve spontaneously but responds to topical antiyeast preparations (ie, ketoconazole 2% cream).

4. Harlequin Color Change

A cutaneous vascular phenomenon unique to neonates in the first week of life occurs when the infant (particularly one of low birth weight) is placed on one side. The dependent half develops an erythematous flush with a sharp demarcation at the midline, and the upper half of the body becomes pale. The color change usually subsides within a few seconds after the infant is placed supine but may persist for as long as 20 minutes.

5. Mottling

A lace-like pattern of bluish, reticular discoloration representing dilated cutaneous vessels appears over the extremities and often the trunk of neonates exposed to lowered room temperature. This feature is transient and usually disappears completely on rewarming.

6. Erythema Toxicum

Up to 50% of full-term infants develop erythema toxicum. At 24–48 hours of age, blotchy erythematous macules 2–3 cm in diameter appear, most prominently on the chest but also on the back, face, and extremities. These are occasionally present at birth. Onset after 4–5 days of life is rare. The lesions vary in number from a few up to as many as 100. Incidence is much higher in full-term versus premature infants. The macular erythema may fade within 24–48 hours or may progress to formation of urticarial wheals in the center of the macules or, in 10% of cases, pustules. Examination of a Wright-stained smear of the lesion reveals numerous eosinophils. No organisms are seen on Gram stain. These findings may be accompanied by peripheral blood eosinophilia of up to 20%. The lesions fade and disappear within 5–7 days.

7. Transient Neonatal Pustular Melanosis

Transient neonatal pustular melanosis is a pustular eruption in African-America newborns. The pustules rupture leaving a collarette of scale surrounding a macular hyperpigmentation. Unlike erythema toxicum, the pustules contain mostly neutrophils and often involve the palms and soles.

8. Sucking Blisters

Bullae, either intact or as erosions (representing the blister base) without inflammatory borders, may occur over the forearms, wrists, thumbs, or upper lip. These presumably result from vigorous sucking in utero. They can persist in the newborn period but resolve without complications.

9. Miliaria

Obstruction of the eccrine sweat ducts occurs often in neonates and produces one of two clinical scenarios. Superficial obstruction in the stratum corneum causes miliaria crystallina, characterized by tiny (1- to 2-mm), superficial grouped vesicles without erythema over intertriginous areas and adjacent skin (eg, neck, upper chest). More commonly, obstruction of the eccrine duct deeper in the epidermis results in erythematous grouped papules in the same areas and is called miliaria rubra. Rarely, these may progress to pustules. Heat and high humidity predispose the patient to eccrine duct pore closure. Removal to a cooler environment is the treatment of choice.

10. Subcutaneous Fat Necrosis

This entity presents in the first 7 days of life as reddish or purple, sharply circumscribed, firm nodules occurring over the cheeks, buttocks, arms, and thighs. Cold injury is thought to play an important role, and the clinical manifestations have been observed after iatrogenically induced and therapeutic hypothermia. These lesions resolve spontaneously over a period of weeks, although in some instances they may calcify. Affected infants should be screened for hypercalcemia that can develop up to 28 weeks after these skin changes are noted.

Akcay A et al: Hypercalcemia due to subcutaneous fat necrosis in a newborn after total body cooling. Pediatr Dermatol 2013 Jan–Feb;30(1):120–123 [PMID: 22352980].

Blume-Peytavi U et al: Skin care practices for newborns and infants: review of the clinical evidence for best practices. Pediatr Dermatol 2012 Jan–Feb;29(1):1–14 [PMID: 22011065].

Rayala BZ, Morell DS: Common skin conditions in children: neonatal skin lesions. FP Essent 2017 Feb; 453:11–17 [PMID: 28196316].

PIGMENT CELL BIRTHMARKS, NEVI, & MELANOMA

Birthmarks may involve an overgrowth of one or more of any of the normal components of skin (eg, pigment cells, blood vessels, lymph vessels). A nevus is a hamartoma of highly differentiated cells that retain their normal function.

1. Mongolian Spot

A blue-black macule commonly called a "mongolian spot" is found over the lumbosacral area in 90% of darker-skinned infants. A more descriptive term is "dermal melanocytosis." These spots are occasionally noted over the shoulders and back and may extend over the buttocks. Histologically, they consist of spindle-shaped pigment cells suspended deep in the dermis. The lesions fade somewhat with time as a result of darkening of the overlying skin, but some traces may persist into adult life.

2. Café au Lait Macule

A café au lait macule is a light-brown, oval macule (dark brown on brown or black skin) that may be found anywhere on the body. Café au lait spots over 1.5 cm in greatest diameter are found in 10% of white and 22% of black children. These lesions persist throughout life and may increase in number with age. The presence of six or more such lesions with diameter larger than 0.5 cm in a prepuberal child or 1.5 cm in an adolescent or adult is a major diagnostic criterion for neurofibromatosis type 1 (NF-1). Patients with McCune-Albright syndrome (see Chapter 34) have a large, unilateral café au lait macule.

3. Spitz Nevus

A Spitz nevus presents as a reddish-brown smooth solitary papule appearing on the face or extremities. Histologically, it consists of epithelioid and spindle-shaped nevomelanocytes that may demonstrate nuclear pleomorphism. Although these lesions can look concerning histologically, they follow a benign clinical course in most cases.

MELANOCYTIC NEVI

1. Common Moles

Well-demarcated, brown to brown-black macules represent junctional nevi. They can appear in the first years of life and increase with age. Histologically, single and nested melanocytes are present at the junction of the epidermis and dermis. Approximately 20% may progress to compound nevi—papular lesions with melanocytes both in junctional and intradermal locations. Intradermal nevi are often lighter in color and can be fleshy and pedunculated. Melanocytes in these lesions are located purely within the dermis. Nevi look dark blue (blue nevi) when they contain more deeply situated spindle-shaped melanocytes in the dermis.

2. Melanoma

Melanoma in prepubertal children is very rare. Pigmented lesions with variegated colors (red, white, blue), notched borders, asymmetrical shape, and very irregular or ulcerated surfaces should prompt suspicion of melanoma. Ulceration and bleeding are advanced signs of melanoma. If melanoma is suspected, wide local excision and pathologic examination should be performed.

3. Congenital Melanocytic Nevi

One in 100 infants is born with a congenital nevus. Congenital nevi tend to be larger and darker brown than acquired nevi and may have many terminal hairs. If the pigmented plaque covers more than 5% of the body surface area, it is considered a giant or large congenital nevus; these large nevi occur in 1 in 20,000 infants. Other classification systems characterize lesions over 20 cm as large. Often the lesions are so large they cover the entire trunk (bathing trunk nevi). Histologically, they are compound nevi with melanocytes often tracking around hair follicles and other adnexal structures deep in the dermis. The risk of malignant melanoma in small congenital nevi is controversial in the literature, but most likely very low, and similar to that of acquired nevi. Transformation to malignant melanoma in giant congenital nevi has been estimated between 1% and 7%. Of note, these melanomas often develop early in life (before puberty) and in a dermal location. Two-thirds of melanomas in children with giant congenital nevi develop in areas other than the skin.

Kalani N et al: Pediatric melanoma: characterizing 256 cases from the Colorado Central Cancer Registry. Pediatr Dermatol 2019 Mar;36(2):219–222 [PMID: 30793788]

Kinsler VA: Melanoma in congenital melanocytic naevi. Br J Dermatol 2017 May;176(5):1131–1143 [PMID: 28078671].

LaVigne EA et al: Clinical and dermoscopic changes in common melanocytic nevi in school children: the Framingham school nevus study. Dermatology 2005;211:234 [PMID: 16205068].

Simons EA: Congenital melanocytic nevi in young children: histopathologic features and clinical outcomes. J Am Acad Dermatol 2017 Feb; Epub ahead of print.

VASCULAR BIRTHMARKS

1. Capillary Malformations
▶ Clinical Findings

Capillary malformations are an excess of capillaries in localized areas of skin. The degree of excess is variable. The color of these lesions ranges from light red-pink to dark red.

Nevus simplexes are the light red macules found over the nape of the neck, upper eyelids, and glabella of newborns. Fifty percent of infants have such lesions over their necks. Eyelid and glabellar lesions usually fade completely within the first year of life. Lesions that occupy the total central forehead area usually do not fade. Those on the neck persist into adult life.

Port-wine stains are dark red macules appearing anywhere on the body. A bilateral facial port-wine stain or one covering the entire half of the face may be a clue to Sturge-Weber Syndrome (SWS), which is characterized by seizures, mental retardation, glaucoma, and hemiplegia (see Chapter 25). The overall risk of a facial port-wine stain having the associated abnormalities of the SWS is 8%, but the risk increases to 25% if there is bilateral involvement of V1 or if there is unilateral involvement of all the branches of the trigeminal nerve (V1 to V3). Most infants with smaller, unilateral facial port-wine stains do not have SWS. Similarly, a port-wine stain over an extremity may be associated with hypertrophy of the soft tissue and bone of that extremity (Klippel-Trénaunay syndrome).

▶ Treatment

The pulsed dye laser is the treatment of choice for infants and children with port-wine stains.

Eberson SN et al: A basic introduction to pediatric vascular anomalies. Semin Intervent Radiol 2019 Jun;36(2):149–160 [PMID: 31123389].

Richter GT, Friedman AB: Hemangiomas and vascular malformations: current theory and management. Int J Pediatr 2012;2012:645–678 [PMID: 22611412].

2. Hemangioma
▶ Clinical Findings

A red, rubbery vascular plaque or nodule with a characteristic growth pattern is a hemangioma. The lesion is often not present at birth but is represented by a permanent blanched area on the skin that is supplanted at age 2–4 weeks by red papules. Hemangiomas then undergo a rapid growth or "proliferative" phase within the first 5–7 weeks of life, where growth of the lesion is out of proportion to growth of the child. Growth then slows and, at 9–12 months, growth stabilizes or ceases completely, and the lesion slowly involutes over the next several years. Histologically, hemangiomas are benign tumors of capillary endothelial cells. They may be superficial, deep, or mixed. The terms *strawberry* and *cavernous* are misleading and should not be used. The biologic behavior of a hemangioma is the same despite its location. Fifty percent reach maximal regression by age 5 years, 70% by age 7 years, and 90% by age 9 years, leaving redundant skin, hypopigmentation, and telangiectasia. Local complications include superficial and deep ulcerations particularly for hemangiomas involving the lips and diaper area, leading to pain and scarring.

Disfigurement can result from large facial infantile hemangiomas, or those involving the nasal tip or ears. There is also potential for functional impairment in periorbital hemangiomas which may block vision. Large plaque-like facial hemangiomas may be associated with underlying abnormalities, including intracranial and aortic arch vascular abnormalities accompanying a large facial Infantile hemangioma associated with PHACES syndrome (Posterior fossa malformations, Hemangioma, Arterial anomalies, Cardiac anomalies, Eye anomalies, Supraumbilical raphe or Sternal pit). Similarly, large sacral hemangiomas may be associated with spinal dysraphism and genitourinary abnormalities as seen in LUMBAR syndrome (Lower body hemangioma and other cutaneous defects, Urogenital anomalies, Myelopathy, Bone deformities, Anorectal malformations, arterial anomalies, Renal anomalies). Rare complications include airway obstruction seen with hemangiomas involving lower face in a "beard distribution." Early intervention and referral to a pediatric dermatologist is recommended for certain hemangiomas based on location and associated risk factors to prevent complications.

▶ **Treatment**

Complications that require immediate treatment are (1) visual obstruction (with resulting amblyopia), (2) airway obstruction (hemangiomas of the head and neck ["beard hemangiomas"] may be associated with subglottic hemangiomas), (3) cardiac decompensation (high-output failure), (4) ulceration, and (5) association with underlying anomalies. Historically, the preferred treatment for complicated hemangiomas was systemic prednisolone. Currently, oral propranolol (2 mg/kg/day divided bid) has replaced systemic steroids as the treatment of choice for infantile hemangiomas. Reported side effects are sleep disturbance and acrocyanosis. Hypoglycemia and bradycardia have been described but are rarely seen. Recommendations on pretreatment cardiac evaluation vary between institutions. The topical β-adrenergic receptor antagonist timolol, administered as a gel-forming solution (GFS), is successful in treating small superficial hemangiomas. If the lesion is ulcerated or bleeding, wound care and pulsed dye laser treatment is indicated to initiate ulcer healing and immediately control pain. The Kasabach-Merritt syndrome, characterized by platelet trapping with consumption coagulopathy, does not occur with solitary cutaneous hemangiomas. It is seen only in association with rare vascular tumors such as kaposiform hemangioendotheliomas and tufted angiomas.

Krowchuk DP et al: Clinical practice guideline for the management of infantile hemangiomas. Pediatrics 2019 Jan;143(1). pii: e20183475 [PMID: 30584062].

Raphael MF et al: Is cardiovascular evaluation necessary prior to and during beta-blocker therapy for infantile hemangiomas? A cohort study. J Am Acad Dermatol 2015 Mar;72(3):465–472 [PMID: 25592625].

Semkova K, Kazandjieva J: Rapid complete regression of an early infantile hemangioma with topical timolol gel. Int J Dermatol 2014 Feb;53(2):241–242 [PMID: 24261914].

Smithson SL: Consensus statement for the treatment of infantile haemangiomas with propranolol. Australas J Dermatol 2017 Mar 1; Epub ahead of print.

3. Lymphatic Malformations

Lymphatic malformations may be superficial or deep. Superficial lymphatic malformations present as fluid-filled vesicles often described as resembling "frog spawn." Deep lymphatic malformations are rubbery, skin-colored nodules occurring most commonly in the head and neck. They often result in grotesque enlargement of soft tissues. Histologically, they can be either macrocystic or microcystic.

▶ **Treatment**

Therapy includes compression garments, sclerotherapy with injection of doxycycline, surgical excision, and most recently sirolimus (mToR inhibitor).

EPIDERMAL BIRTHMARKS

1. Epidermal Nevus

▶ **Clinical Findings**

The majority of these birthmarks present in the first year of life. They are hamartomas of the epidermis that are warty to papillomatous plaques, often in a linear array. They range in color from skin-colored to dirty yellow to brown. Histologically they show a thickened epidermis with hyperkeratosis. The condition of widespread epidermal nevi associated with other developmental anomalies (CNS, eye, and skeletal) is called the epidermal nevus syndrome.

▶ **Treatment**

Treatment once or twice daily with topical calcipotriene or keratolytic may flatten some lesions. Fractionated CO_2 laser can be used to remove hyperkeratotic epidermis. The only definitive cure is surgical excision.

2. Nevus Sebaceous

▶ **Clinical Findings**

This is a hamartoma of sebaceous glands and underlying apocrine glands that is diagnosed by the appearance at birth of a yellowish, hairless plaque in the scalp or on the face. The lesions can be contiguous with an epidermal nevus on the face, and widespread lesions can constitute part of the epidermal nevus syndrome.

Histologically, nevus sebaceus represents an overabundance of sebaceous glands without hair follicles. At puberty, with androgenic stimulation, the sebaceous cells in the nevus divide, expand their cellular volume, and synthesize sebum, resulting in a warty mass.

▶ Treatment

Because it has been estimated that approximately 1% of these lesions will develop secondary epithelial tumors, including basal cell carcinomas trichoblastomas, and other benign tumors, surgical excision at puberty is recommended by most experts. The majority of the tumors develop in adulthood, although basal cell carcinomass have been reported in childhood and adolescence.

CONNECTIVE TISSUE BIRTHMARKS (JUVENILE ELASTOMA, COLLAGENOMA)

▶ Clinical Findings

Connective tissue nevi are smooth, skin-colored papules 1–10 mm in diameter that are grouped on the trunk. A solitary, larger (5–10 cm) nodule is called a shagreen patch and is histologically indistinguishable from other connective tissue nevi that show thickened, abundant collagen bundles with or without associated increases of elastic tissue. Although the shagreen patch is a cutaneous clue to tuberous sclerosis (see Chapter 25), the other connective tissue nevi occur as isolated events.

▶ Treatment

These nevi remain throughout life and need no treatment.

HEREDITARY SKIN DISORDERS

1. Ichthyosis

Ichthyosis is a term applied to several diseases characterized by the presence of excessive scales on the skin. These disorders represent a large and heterogeneous group of genetic and acquired defects of cornification of the skin. Classification of these diseases is clinically based, although the underlying genetic causes and pathophysiologic mechanisms responsible continue to be elucidated.

Disorders of keratinization are characterized as syndromic when the phenotype is expressed in the skin and other organs, or nonsyndromic when only the skin is affected. Ichthyoses may be inherited or acquired. Inherited disorders are identified by their underlying gene defect if known. Acquired ichthyosis may be associated with malignancy and medications, or a variety of autoimmune, inflammatory, nutritional, metabolic, infectious, and neurologic diseases. These disorders are diagnosed by clinical examination, with supportive findings on skin biopsy (including electron microscopy) and mutation analysis if available.

▶ Treatment

Treatment consists of controlling scaling with ammonium lactate (Lac-Hydrin or AmLactin) 12% or urea cream 10%–40% applied once or twice daily. Daily lubrication and a good dry skin care regimen are essential.

Oji V et al: Revised nomenclature and classification of inherited ichthyoses: results of the First Ichthyosis Consensus Conference in Sorèze 2009. J Am Acad Dermatol 2010 Oct;63(4):607–641 [PMID: 20643494].
Takeichi T, Akiyama M: Inherited ichthyosis: non-syndromic forms. J Dermatol 2016 Mar;43(3):242–251 [PMID: 26945532].
Yoneda K: Inherited ichthyosis: syndromic forms. J Dermatol 2016 Mar;43(3):252–263 [PMID: 26945533].

2. Epidermolysis Bullosa

This is a group of heritable disorders characterized by skin fragility with blistering. Four major subtypes are recognized, based on the ultrastructural level of skin cleavage (Table 15–3).

For the severely affected, much of the surface area of the skin may have blisters and erosions, requiring daily wound care and dressings. These children are prone to frequent skin infections, anemia, growth problems, mouth erosions and esophageal strictures, and chronic pain issues. They are also at increased risk of squamous cell carcinoma, a common cause of death in affected patients.

▶ Treatment

Treatment consists of protection of the skin with topical emollients as well as nonstick dressings. The other medical needs and potential complications of the severe forms of epidermolysis bullosa require a multidisciplinary approach. For the less severe types, protecting areas of greatest trauma with padding and dressings as well as intermittent topical or oral antibiotics for superinfection are appropriate treatments. If hands and feet are involved, reducing skin friction with 5% glutaraldehyde every 3 days is helpful.

Fine JD et al: The classification of inherited epidermolysis bullosa (EB): report of the Third International Consensus Meeting on Diagnosis and Classification of EB. J Am Acad Dermatol 2008 Jun;58(6):931–950 [PMID: 18374450] [Epub 2008 Apr 18].

▼ COMMON SKIN DISEASES IN INFANTS, CHILDREN, & ADOLESCENTS

ACNE

Acne affects 85% of adolescents. The onset of adolescent acne is between ages 7 and 10 years in 40% of children. The early lesions are usually limited to the face and are primarily closed comedones.

Table 15–3. Major epidermolysis bullosa subtypes.

Cleavage Level	Common Name	Targeted Protein(s)	Inheritance Pattern	Characteristic Clinical Features
Suprabasilar	Epidermolysis bullosa superficialis	Unknown	Autosomal dominant	Superficial erosions at birth; rare to no blistering
Suprabasilar	Plakophilin-deficient EB, Lethal acantholytic EB	Plakophilin, desmoplakin	Autosomal recessive	Similar to above
Basilar	Epidermolysis bullosa simplex	Keratin 5 and 14	Autosomal dominant	Palm and sole blistering presents in early childhood with trauma
Basilar	EB simplex with muscular dystrophy	Plectin	Autosomal recessive	Blisters, muscular dystrophy
Basilar	EB with pyloric atresia	α-6 β-4 integrin	Autosomal recessive	Blisters, pyloric atresia
Junctional (within the basement membrane zone)	Junctional EB—Herlitz or non-Herlitz	Laminin 5, α-6 β-4 integrin, type XVII collagen	Autosomal recessive	Severe generalized blistering, oral involvement
Sub-basilar	Dystrophic EB or "dermolytic" EB	Type VII collagen	Autosomal dominant or recessive	Severe blisters and scarring

▶ Pathogenesis

The primary event in acne formation is obstruction of the sebaceous follicle and subsequent formation of the microcomedo (not evident clinically). This is the precursor to all future acne lesions. This phenomenon is androgen-dependent in adolescent acne. The four primary factors in the pathogenesis of acne are (1) plugging of the sebaceus follicle, (2) increased sebum production, (3) proliferation of *Propionibacterium acnes* in the obstructed follicle, and (4) inflammation. Many of these factors are influenced by androgens.

Drug-induced acne should be suspected in teenagers if all lesions are in the same stage at the same time and if involvement extends to the lower abdomen, lower back, arms, and legs. Drugs responsible for acne include corticotropin (ACTH), glucocorticoids, androgens, hydantoins, and isoniazid, each of which increases plasma testosterone.

▶ Clinical Findings

Open comedones are the predominant clinical lesion in early adolescent acne. The black color is caused by oxidized melanin within the stratum corneum cellular plug. Open comedones do not progress to inflammatory lesions. Closed comedones, or whiteheads, are caused by obstruction just beneath the follicular opening in the neck of the sebaceous follicle, which produces a cystic swelling of the follicular duct directly beneath the epidermis. Most authorities believe that closed comedones are precursors of inflammatory acne lesions (red papules, pustules, nodules, and cysts). In typical adolescent acne, several different types of lesions are present simultaneously. Severe, chronic, inflammatory

lesions may rarely occur as interconnecting, draining sinus tracts. Adolescents with cystic acne require prompt medical attention, because ruptured cysts and sinus tracts result in severe scar formation.

▶ Differential Diagnosis

Consider rosacea, nevus comedonicus, flat warts, miliaria, molluscum contagiosum, and the angiofibromas of tuberous sclerosis.

▶ Treatment

Different treatment options are listed in Table 15–4. Recent data have indicated that combination therapy that targets multiple pathogenic factors increases the efficacy of treatment and rate of improvement.

A. Topical Keratolytic Agents

Topical keratolytic agents address the plugging of the follicular opening with keratinocytes and include retinoids, benzoyl peroxide, and azelaic acid. The first-line treatment for both comedonal and inflammatory acne is a topical retinoid (tretinoin [retinoic acid], adapalene, and tazarotene). These are the most effective keratolytic agents and have been shown to prevent the microcomedone. These topical agents may be used once daily, or the combination of a retinoid applied to acne-bearing areas of the skin in the evening and a benzoyl peroxide gel or azelaic acid applied in the morning may be used. This regimen will control 80%–85% of cases of adolescent acne.

Table 15–4. Acne treatment.

Type of Lesion	Treatment
Comedonal acne	One of the following: Tretinoin, 0.025%, 0.05%, or 0.1% cream; 0.01% or 0.025% gel; 0.4% or 0.1% microgel Adapalene, 0.3% gel, 0.1% gel or solution; 0.05% cream
Papular inflammatory acne	One from first grouping, plus one of the following: Benzoyl peroxide, 2.5%, 4%, 5%, 8%, or 10% gel or lotion; 4% or 8% wash Azelaic acid, 15% or 20% cream Clindamycin, 1% lotion, solution, or gel Combination products include benzoyl peroxide-erythromycin (Benzamycin); benzoyl peroxide-clindamycin (Duac, BenzaClin, Acanya); tretinoin-clindamycin (Ziana, Veltin)
Pustular inflammatory acne	One from first grouping, plus one of the following oral antibiotics: Minocycline or doxycycline, 50–100 mg, bid
Nodulocystic acne	Isotretinoin, 1 mg/kg/day, goal dose 120–150 mg/kg total

B. Topical Antibiotics

Topical antibiotics are less effective than systemic antibiotics and at best are equivalent in potency to 250 mg of tetracycline orally once a day. One percent clindamycin phosphate solution is the most efficacious topical antibiotic. Most *P acnes* strains are now resistant to topical erythromycin solutions. Topical antibiotic therapy alone should never be used. Multiple studies have shown a combination of benzoyl peroxide or a retinoid and a topical antibiotic are more effective than the antibiotic alone. Benzoyl peroxide has been shown to help minimize the development of bacterial resistance at sites of application. The duration of application of topical antimicrobials should be limited unless benzoyl peroxide is used. Several combination products (benzoyl peroxide and clindamycin, tretinoin and clindamycin, adapalene and benzoyl peroxide) are available which may simplify the treatment regimen and increase patient compliance.

C. Systemic Antibiotics

Antibiotics that are concentrated in sebum, such as tetracycline, minocycline, and doxycycline, should be reserved for moderate to severe inflammatory acne. The usual dose of tetracycline is 0.5–1.0 g divided twice a day on an empty stomach; minocycline and doxycycline 50–100 mg taken once or twice daily can be taken with food. Oral antibiotics should never be used alone without concurrent retinoid and/or benzoyl peroxide. Recent recommendations are that oral antibiotics should be used for a finite time period, and then discontinued as soon as there is improvement in the inflammatory lesions. The tetracycline antibiotics should not be given to children younger than 8 years of age due to the effect on dentition (staining of teeth). Doxycycline may induce significant photosensitivity, and minocycline can cause bluish-gray dyspigmentation of the skin, vertigo, headaches, and drug-induced lupus. These antibiotics have anti-inflammatory effects in addition to decreasing *P acnes* in the follicle.

D. Oral Retinoids

An oral retinoid, 13-*cis*-retinoic acid (isotretinoin), is the most effective treatment for severe cystic acne. The precise mechanism of its action is unknown, but apoptosis of sebocytes, decreased sebaceous gland size, decreased sebum production, decreased follicular obstruction, decreased skin bacteria, and general anti-inflammatory activities have been described. The initial dosage is 0.5–1 mg/kg/day. This therapy is reserved for severe nodulocystic acne, or acne recalcitrant to aggressive standard therapy. Side effects include dryness and scaling of the skin, dry lips, and, occasionally, dry eyes and dry nose. Fifteen percent of patients may experience some mild achiness with athletic activities. Up to 10% of patients experience mild, reversible hair loss. Elevated liver enzymes and blood lipids have rarely been described. Acute depression and mood changes have been reported, but no definitive relationship to the drug has been proven. Most importantly, isotretinoin is teratogenic. Because of this and other potential side effects, it is not recommended unless strict adherence to the Food and Drug Administration (FDA) guidelines is ensured. The FDA has implemented a strict registration program (iPLEDGE) that must be used to obtain and/or prescribe isotretinoin.

E. Other Acne Treatments

Hormonal therapy (oral contraceptives) is often an effective option for girls who have perimenstrual flares of acne or have not responded adequately to conventional therapy. Adolescents with endocrine disorders such as polycystic ovary syndrome also see improvement of their acne with hormonal therapy and spironolactone 50 mg–100 mg PO bid. Oral contraceptives can be added to a conventional therapeutic regimen and should always be used in female patients who are prescribed oral isotretinoin unless absolute contraindications exist. There is growing data regarding the use of light, laser, and photodynamic therapy in acne. However, existing studies are of variable quality, and although there is evidence to suggest that these therapies offer benefit in acne, the evidence is not sufficient to recommend any device as monotherapy in acne.

F. Patient Education and Follow-up Visits

The multifactorial pathogenesis of acne and its role in the treatment plan must be explained to adolescent patients. Good general skin care includes washing the face consistently and using only oil-free, noncomedogenic cosmetics, face creams, and hair sprays. Acne therapy takes 8–12 weeks to produce improvement, and this delay must be stressed to the patient. Realistic expectations should be encouraged in the adolescent patient because no therapy will eradicate all future acne lesions. A written education sheet is useful. Follow-up visits should be made every 3–4 months. An objective method to chart improvement, including photographs, should be documented by the provider, because patients' assessment of improvement can be inaccurate.

Bhate K, Williams HC: Epidemiology of acne vulgaris. Br J Dermatol 2013 Mar;168(3):474–485 [PMID: 23210645].

Bienenfeld A: Oral antibiotic therapy for acne vulgaris: an evidence-based review. Am J Clin Dermatol 2017 Mar 2; Epub ahead of print.

Eichenfield LF et al: Evidence-based recommendations for the diagnosis and treatment of pediatric acne. Pediatrics 2013 May;131 Suppl 3:S163–S186 [PMID: 23637225].

BACTERIAL INFECTIONS OF THE SKIN

1. Impetigo

Erosions covered by honey-colored crusts are diagnostic of impetigo. Staphylococci and group A streptococci in combination are the pathogens in this disease, which histologically consists of superficial invasion of bacteria into the upper epidermis, forming a subcorneal pustule.

▶ Treatment

Impetigo should be treated with an antimicrobial agent effective against *Staphylococcus aureus* and group A streptococci (β-lactamase–resistant penicillins or cephalosporins, clindamycin, amoxicillin–clavulanate) for 7–10 days. Topical mupirocin, polymyxin, gentamycin, and erythromycin are also effective but not recommended in children because of the need to eradicate nasopharyngeal carriage. In severe and recalcitrant cases, skin swab for bacterial culture should be performed prior to initiation of empiric antibiotic therapy.

2. Bullous Impetigo

In bullous impetigo there is, in addition to the usual erosion covered by a honey-colored crust, a border filled with clear fluid. Staphylococci may be isolated from these lesions, and systemic signs of circulating exfoliatin are absent. Bullous impetigo lesions can be found anywhere on the skin, but a common location is the diaper area.

▶ Treatment

Treatment with oral antibiotic for 7–10 days is effective. Application of cool compresses to debride crusts is a helpful symptomatic measure.

3. Ecthyma

Ecthyma is a firm, dry crust, surrounded by erythema that exudes purulent material. It represents invasion by group A β-hemolytic streptococci through the epidermis to the superficial dermis, therefore it is often referred as a deeper form of impetigo. This should not be confused with ecthyma gangrenosum. Lesions of ecthyma gangrenosum may be similar in appearance, but they are seen in a severely ill or immunocompromised patient and are due to systemic dissemination of bacteria, usually *Pseudomonas aeruginosa*, through the bloodstream.

▶ Treatment

Treatment is with systemic penicillin.

4. Cellulitis

Cellulitis is characterized by erythematous, hot, tender, ill-defined, edematous plaques accompanied by regional lymphadenopathy. Histologically, this disorder represents invasion of microorganisms into the lower dermis and sometimes beyond, with obstruction of local lymphatics. Group A β-hemolytic streptococci and coagulase-positive staphylococci are the most common causes; pneumococci and *Haemophilus influenzae* (in younger unvaccinated children) are rare causes. Staphylococcal infections are usually more localized and more likely to have a purulent center; streptococcal infections spread more rapidly, but these characteristics cannot be used to specify the infecting agent. An entry site of prior trauma or infection (eg, varicella, dermatophyte) is often present. Septicemia is a potential complication.

▶ Treatment

Treatment is with an appropriate systemic antibiotic.

5. Folliculitis

A pustule at a follicular opening represents folliculitis. Deeper follicular infections are called furuncles (single follicle) and carbuncles (multiple follicles). Staphylococci and streptococci are the most frequent pathogens. Lesions are painless and tend to occur in crops, usually on the buttocks and extremities in children. Methicillin-resistant *S aureus* (MRSA) is now an increasing cause of folliculitis and skin abscesses. Cultures of persistent or recurrent folliculitis for MRSA are advisable.

Treatment

Treatment consists of measures to remove follicular obstruction—either warm, wet compresses for 24 hours or keratolytics such as those used for acne. Topical or oral anti-staphylococcal antibiotics may be required.

6. Abscess

An abscess occurs deep in the skin, at the bottom of a follicle or an apocrine gland, and is diagnosed as an erythematous, firm, acutely tender nodule with ill-defined borders. Staphylococci are the most common organisms.

Treatment

Recent studies have suggested that incision and drainage alone may be adequate for uncomplicated MRSA skin abscesses in otherwise healthy patients. In more extensive cases adjuvant systemic antibiotics may be required.

7. Scalded Skin Syndrome

This entity consists of the sudden onset of bright red, acutely painful skin, most obvious periorally, periorbitally, and in the flexural areas of the neck, the axillae, the popliteal and antecubital areas, and the groin. The slightest pressure on the skin results in severe pain and separation of the epidermis (positive Nikolsky sign). The disease is caused by a circulating toxin (exfoliatin) elaborated by phage group II staphylococci. Exfoliatin binds to desmoglein-1 resulting in a separation of cells in the granular layer. The causative staphylococci may be isolated from the nasopharynx, an abscess, sinus, blood culture, joint fluid, or other focus of infection, but not from the skin.

Treatment

Treatment is with systemic antistaphylococcal drugs.

McNeil JC, Fritz SA: Prevention strategies for recurrent community-associated *Staphylococcus aureus* skin and soft tissue infections. Curr Infect Dis Rep 2019 Mar 11;21(4):12 [PMID: 30859379].

Yamamoto LG: Treatment of skin and soft tissue infections. Pediatr Emerg Care 2017 Jan;33(1):49–55 [PMID: 28045842].

Zabielinski M et al: Trends and antibiotic susceptibility patterns of methicillin-resistant and methicillin-sensitive *Staphylococcus aureus* in an outpatient dermatology facility. JAMA Dermatol 2013 Apr;4(149):427–432 [PMID: 23325388].

FUNGAL INFECTIONS OF THE SKIN

1. Dermatophyte Infections

Dermatophytes become attached to the superficial layer of the epidermis, nails, and hair, where they proliferate. Fungal infection should be suspected with any red and scaly lesion.

Classification & Clinical Findings

A. Tinea Capitis

Thickened, broken-off hairs with erythema and scaling of underlying scalp are the distinguishing features (Table 15–5). Hairs are broken off at the surface of the scalp, leaving a "black dot" appearance. Diffuse scaling of the scalp and pustules are also seen. A boggy, fluctuant mass on the scalp called a kerion, represents an exaggerated host response to the organism. *Microsporum canis* and *Trichophyton tonsurans* are the cause. Fungal culture should be performed in all cases of suspected tinea capitis.

B. Tinea Corporis

Tinea corporis presents either as annular marginated plaques with a thin scale at the periphery and clear center or as an annular confluent dermatitis. The most common organisms are *Trichophyton mentagrophytes*, *Trichophyton rubrum*, and *M canis*. The diagnosis is made by scraping thin scales from the border of the lesion, dissolving them in 20% potassium hydroxide (KOH), and examining for hyphae.

C. Tinea Cruris

Symmetrical, sharply marginated lesions in inguinal areas occur with tinea cruris. The most common organisms are *T rubrum*, *T mentagrophytes*, and *Epidermophyton floccosum*.

D. Tinea Pedis

Tinea pedis presents with red scaly soles, blisters on the instep of the foot, or fissuring between the toes. *T rubrum* and *T mentagrophytes* are the cause.

E. Tinea Unguium (Onychomycosis)

Loosening of the nail plate from the nail bed (onycholysis), giving a yellow discoloration, is the first sign of fungal invasion of the nails. Thickening of the distal nail plate then occurs, followed by scaling and a crumbly appearance of the

Table 15–5. Clinical features of tinea capitis.

Most Common Organisms	Clinical Appearance	Microscopic Appearance in KOH
Trichophyton tonsurans (90%)	Hairs broken off 2–3 mm from follicle; "black dot"; diffuse pustule; seborrheic dermatitis-like; no fluorescence	Hyphae and spores within hair
Microsporum canis (10%)	Thickened broken-off hairs that fluoresce yellow-green with Wood lamp	Small spores outside of hair; hyphae within hair

entire nail plate surface. *T rubrum* is the most common cause. The diagnosis is confirmed by KOH examination and fungal culture. Usually only one or two nails are involved. If every nail is involved, psoriasis, lichen planus, or idiopathic trachyonychia is a more likely diagnosis than fungal infection.

Treatment

The treatment of dermatophytosis is quite simple: If hair is involved (ie, scalp infections), systemic therapy is necessary. Griseofulvin and terbinafine are both effective. Terbinafine does not work for *M canis*. Topical antifungal agents do not enter hair or nails in sufficient concentration to clear the infection. The absorption of griseofulvin from the gastrointestinal tract is enhanced by a fatty meal; thus, whole milk or ice cream taken with the medication increases absorption. The dosage of griseofulvin is 20 mg/kg/day divided bid (maximum 500 mg/dose). With hair infections, cultures should be done every 4 weeks, and treatment should be continued for 4 weeks following a negative culture result. The side effects are few, and the drug has been used successfully in the newborn period. Terbinafine dosing is weight dependent: 62.5 mg/day, < 20 kg; 125 mg/day, 20–40 kg; 250 mg/day, > 40 kg. For nails, daily administration of topical ciclopirox 8% (Penlac nail lacquer) can be considered; however, success rates are lower than 20%, terbinafine can be used for 6–12 weeks or pulsed-dose itraconazole (50 mg/twice a day < 20 kg; 100 mg/twice a day, 20–40 kg; 200 mg/twice a day, > 40 kg) given in three 1-week pulses separated by 3 weeks.

Tinea corporis, tinea pedis, and tinea cruris can be treated effectively with topical medication after careful inspection to make certain that the hair and nails are not involved. Treatment with any of the imidazoles, allylamines, benzylamines, or ciclopirox applied twice daily for 3–4 weeks is recommended.

Chen X et al: Systemic antifungal therapy for tinea capitis in children. Cochrane Database Syst Rev 2016 May 12;(5):CD004685 [PMID: 27169520].

Kelly BP: Superficial fungal infections. Pediatr Rev 2012;33:e22–e37 [PMID: 22474120].

2. Tinea Versicolor

Tinea versicolor is a superficial infection caused by *Malassezia globosa*, a yeast-like fungus. It characteristically causes polycyclic connected hypopigmented macules and very fine scales in areas of sun-induced pigmentation. In winter, the polycyclic macules appear reddish brown. Recurrent infection is common.

Treatment

Treatment consists of application of selenium sulfide (Selsun), 2.5% suspension, zinc pyrithione shampoo, or topical antifungals. Selenium sulfide and zinc pyrithione shampoo should be applied to the whole body and left on overnight. Treatment can be repeated again in 1 week and then monthly thereafter. It tends to be somewhat irritating, and the patient should be warned about this difficulty. Topical antifungals are applied twice a day for 1–2 weeks. Fluconazole 400 mg single dose may also be used.

3. *Candida albicans* Infections

Clinical Findings

Candida albicans causes diaper dermatitis; thick, white patches on the oral mucosa (thrush); fissures at the angles of the mouth (perleche); and periungual erythema and nail plate abnormalities (chronic paronychia) (see also Chapter 43). Candida dermatitis is characterized by sharply defined erythematous patches, sometimes with eroded areas. Pustules, vesicles, or papules may be present as satellite lesions. Similar infections may be found in other moist areas, such as the axillae and neck folds. This infection is more common in children who have recently received antibiotics.

Treatment

A topical imidazole cream is the drug of first choice for *C albicans* infections. In diaper dermatitis, the cream form can be applied twice a day. In oral thrush, nystatin suspension should be applied directly to the mucosa with the parent's finger or a cotton-tipped applicator. In candidal paronychia, the antifungal agent is applied over the area, covered with occlusive plastic wrapping, and left on overnight after the application is made airtight. Refractory candidiasis will respond to a brief course of oral fluconazole.

VIRAL INFECTIONS OF THE SKIN

1. Herpes Simplex Infection

Clinical Findings

Painful, grouped vesicles or erosions on a red base suggest herpes simplex (see also Chapter 40). Rapid immunofluorescent tests for herpes simplex virus (HSV) and varicella-zoster virus (VZV) are available. A Tzanck smear is done by scraping a vesicle base with a No. 15 blade, smearing on a glass slide, and staining the epithelial cells with Wright stain. The smear is positive if epidermal multinucleated giant cells are visualized. A positive Tzanck smear indicates herpesvirus infection (HSV or VZV). In infants and children, lesions resulting from herpes simplex type 1 are seen most commonly on the gingiva, lips, and face. Involvement of a digit (herpes whitlow) will occur if the child sucks the thumb or fingers. Herpes simplex type 2 lesions are seen on the genitalia and in the mouth in adolescents. Cutaneous dissemination of herpes simplex occurs in patients with atopic dermatitis (eczema herpeticum) and appears clinically as very tender, monomorphic punched-out erosions among the eczematous skin changes. Herpes gladiatorum occurs on the face, lateral neck, and medial arms and is commonly seen in wrestlers and rugby players.

Treatment

The treatment of HSV infections is discussed in Chapter 40.

2. Varicella-Zoster Infection

Clinical Findings

Grouped vesicles in a dermatome, usually on the trunk or face, suggest varicella-zoster reactivation. Zoster in children may not be painful and usually has a mild course. In patients with compromised host resistance, the appearance of an erythematous border around the vesicles is a good prognostic sign. Conversely, large bullae without a tendency to crusting and systemic illness imply a poor host response to the virus. Varicella-zoster and herpes simplex lesions undergo the same series of changes: papule, vesicle, pustule, crust, slightly depressed scar. Lesions of primary varicella appear in crops, and many different stages of lesions are present at the same time (eg, papules), eccentrically placed vesicles on an erythematous base ("dew dropon a rose petal"), erosions, and crusts.

Treatment

The treatment of VZV infections is discussed in Chapter 41.

3. Human Immunodeficiency Virus Infection

Clinical Findings

The average time of onset of skin lesions after perinatally acquired HIV infection is 4 months; after transfusion-acquired infection, it is 11 months (see also Chapter 41). Persistent oral candidiasis and recalcitrant candidal diaper rash are the most frequent cutaneous features of infantile HIV infection. Severe or recurrent herpetic gingivostomatitis, varicella zoster infection, and molluscum contagiosum infection occur. Recurrent staphylococcal pyodermas, tinea of the face, and onychomycosis are also observed. A generalized dermatitis with features of seborrhea (severe cradle cap) is extremely common. In general, persistent, recurrent, or extensive skin infections should make one suspicious of HIV infection.

Treatment

The treatment of HIV infections is discussed in Chapter 46.

VIRUS-INDUCED TUMORS

1. Molluscum Contagiosum

Molluscum contagiosum is a poxvirus that induces the epidermis to proliferate, forming a pale papule. Molluscum contagiosum consists of umbilicated, flesh-colored papules in

groups anywhere on the body. They are common in infants and preschool children, as well as sexually active adolescents.

Treatment

Treatment for molluscum is usually observational. Other treatments are either immunological (topical imiquimod, oral cimetidine, intralesional candida antigen injection) or cytodestructive (topical cantharidin, cryotherapy with liquid nitrogen, and curettage). Destructive therapies can be painful and potentially scarring. Choosing not to treat is an appropriate alternative, depending on patient symptoms. Left untreated, the lesions resolve over months to years.

2. Warts

Warts are skin-colored papules with rough (verrucous) surfaces caused by infection with human papillomavirus (HPV). There are over 200 types of this DNA virus, which induces the epidermal cells to proliferate, thus resulting in the warty growth. Flat warts are smoother and smaller than common warts and are often seen on the face and other sun-exposed areas. Certain types of HPV are associated with certain types of warts (eg, flat warts) or location of warts (eg, genital warts).

Treatment

Thirty percent of warts will clear in 6 months. As with molluscum, the treatment of warts is also immunological (topical imiquimod, oral cimetidine, intralesional candida antigen injection, and squaric acid contact therapy) or cytodestructive. Liquid nitrogen is painful, user dependent, and can lead to blistering and scarring. Topical salicylic acid may also be used. Large mosaic plantar warts are treated most effectively by applying 40% salicylic acid plaster cut with a scissors to fit the lesion. The adhesive side of the plaster is placed against the lesion and taped securely in place with duct or athletic tape. The plaster and tape should be placed on Monday through Friday. Over the weekend, the patient should soak the skin in warm water for 30 minutes to soften it. Then the white, macerated tissue should be pared with a pumice stone, cuticle scissors, or a nail file. This procedure is repeated every week, and the patient is seen every 4 weeks. Most plantar warts resolve in 6–8 weeks when treated in this way. Vascular pulsed dye lasers are a useful adjunct therapy for the treatment of warts.

For flat warts, a good response to 0.025% tretinoin gel or topical imiquimod cream, applied once daily for 3–4 weeks, has been reported. Candida albicans antigen, 0.3 mL injected every 4–6 weeks intradermally into the lesion for has been effective. 5-fluoruracil applied directly to warts under occlusion for 12 weeks has been approved to be use in children with a success rate of over 80%.

Surgical excision, electrosurgery, and nonspecific burning laser surgery should be avoided; these modalities do not have higher cure rates and result in scarring.

Cantharidin may cause small warts to become larger and should not be used.

Venereal warts (condylomata acuminata) (see Chapter 44) may be treated with imiquimod, 25% podophyllum resin (podophyllin) in alcohol, or podofilox, a lower concentration of purified podophyllin, which is applied at home. Podophyllin should be painted on the lesions in the practitioner's office and then washed off after 4 hours. Retreatment in 2–3 weeks may be necessary. Podofilox is applied by the patient once daily, Monday through Thursday, whereas imiquimod is used three times a week on alternating days. Lesions not on the vulvar mucous membrane but on the adjacent skin should be treated as a common wart and frozen.

No wart therapy is immediately and definitively successful. Realistic expectations should be set and appropriate follow-up treatments scheduled.

Gladsio JA et al: 5% 5-Fluorouracil cream for treatment of verruca vulgaris in children. Pediatr Dermatol 2009 May–Jun;26(3): 279–285 [PMID: 19706088].

Park IU, Introcaso C, Dunne EF: Human papillomavirus and genital warts: a review of the evidence for the 2015 Centers for Disease Control and Prevention Sexually Transmitted Diseases Treatment Guidelines. Clin Infect Dis 2015 Dec 15;61 Suppl 8: S849–S855 [PMID: 26602622].

INSECT INFESTATIONS

1. Scabies

▶ Clinical Findings

Scabies is suggested by linear burrows about the wrists, ankles, finger webs, areolas, anterior axillary folds, genitalia, or face (in infants). Often there are excoriations, honey-colored crusts, and pustules from secondary infection. Identification of the female mite or her eggs and feces is necessary to confirm the diagnosis. Apply mineral oil to a No. 15 blade and scrape an unscratched papule or burrow and examine microscopically to confirm the diagnosis. In a child who is often scratching, scrape under the fingernails. Examine the parents for unscratched burrows.

▶ Treatment

Permethrin 5% is the treatment of choice for scabies. It should be applied as a single overnight application and repeated in 7 days to patient and household contacts. Oral ivermectin 200 mcg/dose × 1 and repeated in 7 days may be used in resistant cases.

2. Pediculoses (Louse Infestations)

▶ Clinical Findings

The presence of excoriated papules and pustules and a history of severe itching at night suggest infestation with the human body louse. This louse may be discovered in the seams of underwear but not on the body. In the scalp hair, the gelatinous nits of the head louse adhere tightly to the hair shaft. The pubic louse may be found crawling among pubic hairs, or blue-black macules may be found dispersed through the pubic region (maculae ceruleae). The pubic louse is often seen on the eyelashes of newborns.

▶ Treatment

Initial treatment of head lice is often instituted by parents with an over-the-counter pyrethrin or permethrin product. These products are not ovicidal, and are more effective if nits are removed manually, by hand or with a lice comb. If head lice are not eradicated after two applications 7 days apart with these products, malathion 0.5% is ovicidal and highly effective but is toxic, if ingested, and flammable. A second application 7–9 days after initial treatment may be necessary. Other ovicidal products include topical ivermectin and spinosad (oral ivermectin is also effective but is not FDA approved for this indication). These ovicidal products do not require manual nit removal. Treatment of pubic lice is similar. Treatment of body lice is clean clothing and washing the infested clothing at high temperature.

3. Papular Urticaria

▶ Clinical Findings

Papular urticaria is characterized by grouped erythematous papules surrounded by an urticarial flare and distributed over the shoulders, upper arms, legs, and buttocks in infants. Although not a true infestation, these lesions represent delayed hypersensitivity reactions to stinging or biting insects. Fleas from dogs and cats are the usual offenders. Less commonly, mosquitoes, lice, scabies, and bird and grass mites are involved. The sensitivity is transient, lasting 4–6 months. Usually, no other family members are affected. It is often difficult for the parents to understand why no one else is affected.

▶ Treatment

The logical therapy is to remove the offending insect, although in most cases it is very difficult to identify the exact cause. Topical corticosteroids and oral antihistamines will control symptoms.

DERMATITIS (ECZEMA)

The terms *dermatitis* and *eczema* are currently used interchangeably in dermatology, although the term *eczema* truly denotes an acute weeping dermatosis. All forms of dermatitis, regardless of cause, may present with acute edema, erythema, and oozing with crusting, mild erythema alone, or lichenification. Lichenification is diagnosed by thickening of the skin with a shiny surface and exaggerated, deepened skin markings. It is the response of the skin to chronic rubbing or scratching.

Although the lesions of the various dermatoses are histologically indistinguishable, clinicians have nonetheless divided the disease group called dermatitis into several categories based on known causes in some cases and differing natural histories in others.

1. Atopic Dermatitis

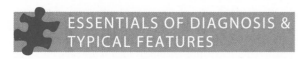

ESSENTIALS OF DIAGNOSIS & TYPICAL FEATURES

Clinical features of atopic dermatitis:

▶ Essential feature: Pruritus (or parental reporting of itching or rubbing) in the past 12 months, plus at least three of the following:

- History of generalized dry skin in the past 12 months
- Personal history of allergic rhinitis or asthma (or history in first-degree family member if patient is < 4 years old)
- Onset before 2 years of age
- History of skin crease involvement (antecubital or popliteal fossae, front of ankles, neck, periorbital)
- Visible flexural dermatitis (if child is < 4 years, include cheeks or forehead, and extensor surface of limbs)

▶ Pathogenesis

Atopic dermatitis is a polygenic disease with positive and negative modifiers. Atopic dermatitis results from an interaction among susceptibility genes, the host environment, skin barrier defects, pharmacologic abnormalities, and immunologic response. The case for food and inhalant allergens as specific causes of atopic dermatitis is not strong. There is significant evidence that a primary defect in atopic dermatitis is an abnormality in the skin barrier formation due to defects in the filaggrin gene. Not all people with filaggrin abnormalities have atopic dermatitis and not all people with atopic dermatitis have filaggrin abnormalities.

▶ Clinical findings

A. Symptoms & Signs

Many (not all) patients go through three clinical phases. In the first, infantile eczema, the dermatitis begins on the cheeks and scalp and frequently expresses itself as oval patches on the trunk, later involving the extensor surfaces of the extremities. The usual age at onset is 2–3 months, and this phase ends at age 18 months to 2 years. Only one-third of all infants with infantile eczema progress to phase 2 childhood

or flexural eczema in which the predominant involvement is in the antecubital and popliteal fossae, the neck, the wrists, and sometimes the hands or feet. This phase lasts from age 2 years to adolescence. Only one-third of children with typical flexural eczema progress to adolescent eczema, which is usually manifested by the continuation of chronic flexural eczema along with hand and/or foot dermatitis. Atopic dermatitis is quite unusual after age 30 years.

▶ Differential Diagnosis

All other types of dermatitis must be considered.

A few patients with atopic dermatitis have immunodeficiency with recurrent pyodermas, unusual susceptibility to HSVs, hyperimmunoglobulinemia E, defective neutrophil and monocyte chemotaxis, and impaired T-lymphocyte function (see Chapter 33).

▶ Complications

A faulty epidermal barrier predisposes the patient with atopic dermatitis to dry, itchy skin. Inability to hold water within the stratum corneum results in rapid evaporation of water, shrinking of the stratum corneum, and cracks in the epidermal barrier. Such skin forms an ineffective barrier to the entry of various irritants. Chronic atopic dermatitis is frequently infected secondarily with *S aureus* or *Streptococcus pyogenes*. HSV virus may also superinfect atopic dermatitis and severe widespread disease is known as Kaposi's varicelliform eruption or eczema herpeticum. Patients with atopic dermatitis have a deficiency of antimicrobial peptides in their skin, which may account for the susceptibility to recurrent skin infection.

▶ Treatment

A. Acute Stages

Application of wet dressings and medium-potency topical corticosteroids is the treatment of choice for acute, weeping atopic eczema. The use of wet dressings is outlined at the beginning of this chapter. Superinfection with *S aureus*, *S pyogenes*, and HSV may occur, and appropriate systemic therapy may be necessary. If the expected improvement is not seen, bacterial and HSV cultures should be obtained to identify the possibility of a superinfection.

B. Chronic Stages

Treatment is aimed at avoiding irritants and restoring moisture to the skin. No soaps or harsh shampoos should be used, and the patient should avoid woolen or any rough clothing. Bathing is minimized to every second or third day. Twice-daily lubrication of the skin is very important.

Nonperfumed creams or lotions are suitable lubricants. Plain petrolatum is an acceptable lubricant, but some people find it too greasy and during hot weather it may also cause considerable sweat retention. Liberal use of a thick moisturizer four to five times daily as a substitute for soap is also satisfactory as a means of lubrication. A bedroom humidifier is often helpful. Topical corticosteroids should be limited to medium strength (see Table 15–2). There is seldom a reason to use super or high-potency corticosteroids in atopic dermatitis. In superinfected atopic dermatitis, systemic antibiotics for 10–14 days are necessary.

Tacrolimus and pimecrolimus ointments are topical immunosuppressive agents that are effective in atopic dermatitis. Because of concerns about the development of malignancies, tacrolimus and pimecrolimus should be reserved for children older than 2 years with atopic dermatitis unresponsive to medium-potency topical steroids. It has been argued that an increased risk of malignancy has not been seen in immunologically normal individuals using these products. Recommendations for usage likely will change with time. Narrow-band UV-B is recommended for extensive disease, starting with twice-weekly sessions in addition to topical steroids. Numerous immunosuppressive have been successful in controlling severe generalized eczema, including methotrexate, mycophenolate mofetil, azathioprine, or cyclosporine. Dipilumab (Dupixent®) is the first biological therapy approved to treat atopic dermatitis in patients 12 years and older. This antibody blocks IL-4 and IL-13, inhibiting immune system and subsequent inflammation. Leukotriene antagonists (used in asthma) are not effective.

Treatment failures in chronic atopic dermatitis are most often the result of noncompliance or nonadherence to a consistent therapy plan. This is a frustrating disease for parent and child. Return to a normal lifestyle for the parent and child is the ultimate goal of therapy.

Barrett M, Luu M: Differential diagnosis of atopic dermatitis. Immunol Allergy Clin North Am 2017 Feb;37(1):11–34 [PMID: 27886900].

Kalamaha K et al: Atopic dermatitis: a review of evolving targeted therapies. Expert Rev Clin Immunol 2019 Mar;15(3):275–288. doi: 10.1080/1744666X.2019.1560267. Epub 2019 Jan 14 [PMID: 30577713].

Yang EJ et al: Recent developments in atopic dermatitis. Pediatrics 2018 Oct;142(4). pii: e20181102 [PMID: 30266868].

2. Nummular Eczema

Nummular eczema is characterized by numerous symmetrically distributed coin-shaped patches of dermatitis, principally on the extremities. These may be acute, oozing, and crusted or dry and scaling. The differential diagnosis should include tinea corporis, impetigo, and atopic dermatitis.

▶ Treatment

The same topical measures should be used as for atopic dermatitis, although more potent topical steroids may be necessary.

3. Primary Irritant Contact Dermatitis (Diaper Dermatitis)

Contact dermatitis is of two types: primary irritant and allergic. Primary irritant dermatitis develops within a few hours, reaches peak severity at 24 hours, and then disappears. Allergic contact dermatitis (described in the next section) has a delayed onset of 18 hours, peaks at 48–72 hours, and often lasts as long as 2–3 weeks even if exposure to the offending antigen is discontinued.

Diaper dermatitis, the most common form of primary irritant contact dermatitis seen in pediatric practice, is caused by prolonged contact of the skin with urine and feces, which contain irritating chemicals such as urea and intestinal enzymes.

▶ Clinical Findings

The diagnosis of diaper dermatitis is based erythema and scaling of the skin in the perineal area and the history of prolonged skin contact with urine or feces, with sparing of inguinal folds. This is frequently seen in the "good baby" who sleeps many hours through the night without waking. In 80% of cases of diaper dermatitis lasting more than 3 days, the affected area is colonized with *C albicans* even before appearance of the classic signs of a beefy red, sharply marginated dermatitis with satellite lesions. Streptococcal perianal cellulitis and infantile psoriasis should be included in the differential diagnosis.

▶ Treatment

Treatment consists of changing diapers frequently. The area should only be washed with clean cloth and water following a bowel movement. Because rubber or plastic pants prevent evaporation of the contactant and enhance its penetration into the skin, they should be avoided as much as possible. Air drying is useful. Treatment of long-standing diaper dermatitis should include application of a barrier cream such as zinc oxide with each diaper change and an imidazole cream twice a day.

4. Allergic Contact Dermatitis

▶ Clinical Findings

Plants such as poison ivy, poison sumac, and poison oak cause most cases of allergic contact dermatitis in children. Allergic contact dermatitis has all the features of delayed type (T-lymphocyte–mediated) hypersensitivity. Many substances may cause such a reaction; other than plants, nickel sulfate, potassium dichromate, and neomycin are the most common causes. Nickel is found to some degree in all metals. Nickel allergy is commonly seen on the ears secondary to the wearing of earrings, and near the umbilicus from pants snaps and belt buckles. The true incidence of allergic contact dermatitis in children is unknown. Children often present with acute dermatitis with blister formation, oozing, and crusting. Blisters are often linear and of acute onset.

▶ Treatment

Treatment of contact dermatitis in localized areas is with potent topical corticosteroids. In severe generalized involvement, prednisone, 1–2 mg/kg/day orally for 10–14 days, can be used.

> Bonitisis NG et al: Allergens responsible for allergic contact dermatitis among children: a systematic review and meta-analysis. Contact Dermatitis 2011;64:245 [PMID: 21480911].

5. Seborrheic Dermatitis

▶ Clinical Findings

Seborrheic dermatitis is an erythematous scaly dermatitis accompanied by overproduction of sebum occurring in areas rich in sebaceous glands (ie, the face, scalp, and perineum). This common condition occurs predominantly in the newborn and at puberty, the ages at which hormonal stimulation of sebum production is maximal. Although it is tempting to speculate that overproduction of sebum causes the dermatitis, the exact relationship is unclear.

Seborrheic dermatitis on the scalp in infancy is clinically similar to atopic dermatitis, and the distinction may become clear only after other areas are involved. Psoriasis also occurs in seborrheic areas in older children and should be considered in the differential diagnosis.

▶ Treatment

Seborrheic dermatitis responds well to low-potency topical corticosteroids, antifungal shampoos (ketoconazole 1% or 2%), and antidandruff shampoos. For severe recalcitrant cases, pulse courses of oral itraconazole have been shown to be effective.

6. Dandruff

Dandruff is physiologic scaling or mild seborrhea, in the form of greasy scalp scales. The cause is unknown. Treatment is with medicated dandruff shampoos.

7. Dry Skin Dermatitis (Asteatotic Eczema, Xerosis)

Children who live in arid climates are susceptible to dry skin, characterized by large cracked scales with erythematous borders. The stratum corneum is dependent on environmental humidity for its water, and below 30% environmental humidity the stratum corneum loses water, shrinks, and cracks. These cracks in the epidermal barrier allow irritating substances to enter the skin, predisposing the patient to dermatitis.

▶ Treatment

Treatment consists of increasing the water content of the skin in the immediate external environment. House humidifiers are very useful. Minimize bathing to every second or third day.

Frequent soaping of the skin impairs its water-holding capacity and serves as an irritating alkali, and all soaps should therefore be avoided. Frequent use of emollients (eg, Cetaphil, Eucerin, Vaseline, Vanicream) should be a major part of therapy.

8. Keratosis Pilaris

Follicular papules containing a white inspissated scale characterize keratosis pilaris. Individual lesions are discrete and may be red. They are prominent on the extensor surfaces of the upper arms and thighs and on the buttocks and cheeks. In severe cases, the lesions may be generalized.

▶ Treatment

Treatment is with keratolytics such as urea cream or lactic acid, followed by skin hydration.

9. Pityriasis Alba

White, scaly macular areas with indistinct borders are seen over extensor surfaces of extremities and on the cheeks in children with pityriasis alba. Sun tanning exaggerates these lesions. Histologic examination reveals a mild dermatitis. These lesions may be confused with tinea versicolor.

▶ Treatment

Low-potency topical corticosteroids may help decrease any inflammatory component and may lead to faster return of normal pigmentation. Strict sun avoidance and sun protection is also recommended.

COMMON SKIN TUMORS

If the skin moves with the nodule on lateral palpation, the tumor is located within the dermis; if the skin moves over the nodule, it is subcutaneous. Seventy-five percent of lumps in childhood will be either epidermoid cysts (60%) or pilomatricomas (15%).

1. Epidermoid Cysts

▶ Clinical Findings

Epidermoid cysts are the most common type of cutaneous cyst. Other names for epidermoid cysts are epidermal cysts, epidermal inclusion cysts, and "sebaceous" cysts. This last term is a misnomer since they contain neither sebum nor sebaceous glands. Epidermoid cysts can occur anywhere, but are most common on the face and upper trunk. They usually arise from and are lined by the stratified squamous epithelium of the follicular infundibulum. Clinically, epidermoid cysts are dermal nodules with a central punctum, representing the follicle associated with the cyst. They can reach several centimeters in diameter. **Dermoid cysts** are areas of sequestration of skin along embryonic fusion lines. They are present at birth and occur most commonly on the lateral eyebrow. When present in the midline nasal dorsum, they develop a superficial pit. Imaging prior to any intervention is recommended in this case to evaluate for intracranial connection.

▶ Treatment

Epidermoid cysts can rupture, causing a foreign-body inflammatory reaction, or become infected. Infectious complications should be treated with antibiotics. Definitive treatment of epidermoid and dermoid cysts is surgical excision.

2. Pilomatricomas

These are benign tumors of the hair matrix. They are most commonly seen on the face and upper trunk. They are firm and may be irregular. Their color varies, flesh colored or blue. The firmness is secondary to calcification of the tumor.

▶ Treatment

Treatment is by surgical excision.

3. Granuloma Annulare

Violaceous circles or semicircles of nontender intradermal nodules found over the lower legs and ankles, the dorsum of the hands and wrists, and the trunk suggest granuloma annulare. Histologically, the disease appears as a central area of tissue death (necrobiosis) surrounded by macrophages and lymphocytes.

▶ Treatment

No treatment is necessary. Lesions resolve spontaneously within 1–2 years in most children.

4. Pyogenic Granuloma

These lesions appear over 1–2 weeks at times following skin trauma as a dark red papule with an ulcerated and crusted surface that may bleed easily with minor trauma. Histologically, this represents excessive new vessel formation with or without inflammation (granulation tissue). It should be regarded as an abnormal healing response.

▶ Treatment

Pulsed dye laser, Imiquimod 5% cream and Timolol 0.05% GFS daily have been successful in treating very small lesions. Curerettage followed by electrocautery is the treatment of choice for larger or recurrent lesions.

5. Keloids

Keloids are scars of delayed onset that continue to grow for up to several years and to progress beyond the initial wound margins. The tendency to develop keloids is inherited. They are often found on the face, earlobes, neck, chest, and back.

▶ Treatment

Treatment includes intralesional injection with triamcinolone acetonide, 20–40 mg/mL, or excision and injection with corticosteroids. For larger keloids, excision followed by postoperative radiotherapy may be indicated.

PAPULOSQUAMOUS ERUPTIONS

Papulosquamous eruptions (Table 15–6) comprise papules or plaques with varying degrees of scale.

1. Pityriasis Rosea

▶ Pathogenesis & Clinical Findings

Pink to red, oval plaques with fine scales that tend to align with their long axis parallel to skin tension lines (eg, "Christmas tree pattern" on the back) are characteristic lesions of pityriasis rosea. The generalized eruption is usually preceded for up to 30 days by a solitary, larger, scaling plaque with central clearing and a scaly border (the herald patch). The herald patch is clinically similar to ringworm and can be confused. In whites, the lesions are primarily on the trunk; in blacks, lesions are primarily on the extremities and may be accentuated in the axillary and inguinal areas (inverse pityriasis rosea).

This disease is common in school-aged children and adolescents and is presumed to be viral in origin. The role of human herpesvirus 7 in the pathogenesis of pityriasis rosea is debated. The condition lasts 6–12 weeks and may be pruritic.

▶ Differential Diagnosis

The major differential diagnosis is secondary syphilis, and a VDRL (Venereal Disease Research Laboratories) test should be done if syphilis is suspected, especially in high-risk patients with palm or sole involvement. Fever and

Table 15–6. Papulosquamous eruptions in children.

Psoriasis
Pityriasis rosea
Tinea corporis
Lichen planus
Pityriasis lichenoides (acute or chronic)
Dermatomyositis
Lupus erythematosus
Pityriasis rubra pilaris
Secondary syphilis

widespread lymphadenopathy is often found in secondary syphilis. "Pityriasis rosea" lasting more than 12 weeks is likely to be pityriasis lichenoides.

▶ Treatment

Exposure to natural sunlight may help hasten the resolution of lesions. Oral antihistamines and topical steroids can be used for pruritus. Often, no treatment is necessary. Pityriasis rosea that lasts more than 12 weeks should be referred to a dermatologist for evaluation.

2. Psoriasis

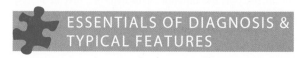

ESSENTIALS OF DIAGNOSIS & TYPICAL FEATURES

▶ Erythematous papules and plaques with thick, white scales.

▶ Elbows, knees, and scalp often affected.

▶ Nail pitting and distal onycholysis.

▶ Pathogenesis

The pathogenesis of psoriasis is complex and incompletely understood. It has immune-mediated inflammation, is a familial condition, and multiple psoriasis susceptibility genes have been identified. There is increased epidermal turnover; psoriatic epidermis has a turnover time of 3–4 days versus 28 days for normal skin. These rapidly proliferating epidermal cells produce excessive stratum corneum, giving rise to thick, opaque scales.

▶ Clinical Findings

Psoriasis is characterized by erythematous papules covered by thick white scales. Guttate (droplike) psoriasis is a common form in children that often follows by 2–3 weeks an episode of streptococcal pharyngitis. The sudden onset of small papules (3–8 mm), seen predominantly over the trunk and quickly covered with thick white scales, is characteristic of guttate psoriasis. Chronic psoriasis is marked by thick, large scaly plaques (5–10 cm) over the elbows, knees, scalp, and other sites of trauma. Pinpoint pits in the nail plate are seen, as well as yellow discoloration of the nail plate resulting from onycholysis. Psoriasis occurs frequently on the scalp, elbows, knees, periumbilical area, ears, sacral area, and genitalia.

▶ Differential Diagnosis

Papulosquamous eruptions that present problems of differential diagnosis are listed in Table 15–6.

▶ Treatment

Topical corticosteroids are the initial treatment of choice. Penetration of topical steroids through the enlarged epidermal barrier in psoriasis requires that more potent preparations be used, for example, fluocinonide 0.05% (Lidex) or clobetasol 0.05% (Temovate) ointment twice daily.

The second line of therapy is topical vitamin D_3 medications such as calcipotriene (Dovonex) or, calcitriol (Vectical), applied twice daily or the combination of a superpotent topical steroid twice daily on weekends and calcipotriene or calcitriol twice daily on weekdays.

Topical retinoids such as tazarotene (0.1%, 0.5% cream, gel) can be used in combination with topical corticosteroids to help restore normal epidermal differentiation and turnover time.

Anthralin therapy is also useful. Anthralin is applied to the skin for a short contact time (eg, 20 minutes once daily) and then washed off with a neutral soap (eg, Dove). This can be used in combination with topical corticosteroids.

Crude coal tar therapy is messy and stains bedclothes. The newer tar gels (Estar, PsoriGel) and one foam product (Scytera) cause less staining and are most efficacious. They are applied twice daily. These preparations are sold over the counter and are not usually covered by insurance plans.

Scalp care using a tar shampoo requires leaving the shampoo on for 5 minutes, washing it off, and then shampooing with commercial shampoo to remove scales. It may be necessary to shampoo daily until scaling is reduced.

More severe cases of psoriasis are best treated by a dermatologist. Narrow band UVB phototherapy and multiple systemic medications and new biologic agents (antibodies, fusion proteins, and recombinant cytokines) are effective in more widespread, severe cases.

Bronkers et al: Psoriasis in children and adolescents: diagnosis, management and comorbidities. Paediatr Drugs 2015 Oct;17(5): 373–384 [PMID: 26072040].

Relvas M, Torres T: Pediatric psoriasis. Am J Clin Dermatol 2017 Dec;18(6):797–811 [PMID: 28540590].

HAIR LOSS (ALOPECIA)

Hair loss in children (Table 15–7) imposes great emotional stress on the patient and the parent. A 60% hair loss in a single area is necessary before hair loss can be detected clinically. Examination should begin with the scalp to determine whether inflammation, scale, or infiltrative changes are present. The hair should be gently pulled to see if it is easily removable. Hairs should be examined microscopically for breaking and structural defects and to see whether growing or resting hairs are being shed. Placing removed hairs in mounting fluid (Permount) on a glass microscope slide makes them easy to examine.

Table 15–7. Other causes of hair loss in children.

Hair loss with scalp changes
Atrophy:
Lichen planus
Lupus erythematosus
Birthmarks:
Epidermal nevus
Nevus sebaceous
Aplasia cutis congenita
Hair loss with hair shaft defects (hair fails to grow out enough to require haircuts)
Monilethrix—alternating bands of thin and thick areas
Pili annulati—alternating bands of light and dark pigmentation
Pili torti—hair twisted 180 degrees, brittle
Trichorrhexis invaginata (bamboo hair)—intussusception of one hair into another
Trichorrhexis nodosa—nodules with fragmented hair

Three diseases account for most cases of hair loss in children: alopecia areata, tinea capitis (described earlier in this chapter), and hair pulling.

1. Alopecia Areata

▶ Clinical Findings

Complete hair loss in a localized area is called alopecia areata. This is the most common cause of hair loss in children. An immunologic pathogenic mechanism is suspected because dense infiltration of lymphocytes precedes hair loss. Fifty percent of children with alopecia areata completely regrow their hair within 12 months, although as many may have a relapse in the future.

A rare and unusual form of alopecia areata begins at the occiput and proceeds along the hair margins to the frontal scalp. This variety, called ophiasis, often eventuates in total scalp hair loss (alopecia totalis). The prognosis for regrowth in ophiasis is poor.

▶ Treatment

Superpotent topical steroids, minoxidil (Rogaine), contact therapy, and anthralin are topical treatment options. Systemic corticosteroids given to suppress the inflammatory response will result in hair growth, but the hair may fall out again when the drug is discontinued. Systemic corticosteroids should never be used for a prolonged time period. In children with alopecia totalis, a wig is most helpful. Treatment induced hair growth does not alter risk of recurrence. New therapies including topical and systemic JAK inhibitors (Tofacitinib) are currently being studied, but are not yet approved for the treatment of alopecia areata in the pediatric population,

Craiglow BG et al: Tofacitinib for the treatment of alopecia areata in preadolescent children. J Am Acad Dermatol 2019 Feb;80(2):568–570 [PMID: 30195571].

Strazzulla LC et al: Alopecia areata: an appraisal of new treatment approaches and overview of current therapies. J Am Acad Dermatol 2018 Jan;78(1):15–24 [PMID: 29241773].

2. Hair Pulling

▶ Clinical Findings

Traumatic hair pulling causes the hair shafts to be broken off at different lengths, with an ill-defined area of hair loss, petechiae around follicular openings, and a wrinkled hair shaft on microscopic examination. This behavior may be merely habit, an acute reaction to severe stress, trichotillomania, or a sign of another psychiatric disorder. Eyelashes and eyebrows rather than scalp hair may be pulled out.

▶ Treatment

If the behavior has a long history, psychiatric evaluation may be helpful. Cutting or oiling the hair to make it slippery is an aid to behavior modification.

REACTIVE ERYTHEMAS

1. Erythema Multiforme

▶ Clinical Findings

Erythema multiforme begins with papules that later develop a dark center and then evolve into lesions with central bluish discoloration or blisters and the characteristic target lesions (iris lesions) that have three concentric circles of color change. Erythema multiforme has sometimes been diagnosed in patients with severe mucous membrane involvement, but Stevens-Johnson syndrome is the diagnosis when severe involvement of conjunctiva, oral cavity, and genital mucosa also occur.

Many causes are suspected, particularly concomitant HSV; drugs, especially sulfonamides; and *Mycoplasma* infections. Recurrent erythema multiforme is usually associated with reactivation of HSV. In erythema multiforme, spontaneous healing occurs in 10–14 days, but Stevens-Johnson syndrome may last 6–8 weeks.

▶ Treatment

Treatment is symptomatic in uncomplicated erythema multiforme. Removal of offending drugs is an obvious measure. Oral antihistamines such as cetirizine 5–10 mg every morning and hydroxyzine 1 mg/kg/day at bedtime are useful. Cool compresses and wet dressings will relieve pruritus. Steroids have not been demonstrated to be effective. Chronic acyclovir therapy has been successful in decreasing attacks in patients with herpes-associated recurrent erythema multiforme.

Table 15–8. Common drug reactions.

Urticaria
Barbiturates
Opioids
Penicillins
Sulfonamides
Morbilliform eruption
Anticonvulsants
Cephalosporins
Penicillins
Sulfonamides
Fixed drug eruption, erythema multiforme, toxic epidermal necrolysis, Stevens-Johnson syndrome
Anticonvulsants
Nonsteroidal anti-inflammatory drugs
Sulfonamides
DRESS syndrome
Anticonvulsants
Photodermatitis
Psoralens
Sulfonamides
Tetracyclines
Thiazides

DRESS syndrome, drug eruptions with fever, eosinophilia, and systemic symptoms.

2. Drug Eruptions

Drugs may produce urticarial, morbilliform, scarlatiniform, pustular, bullous, or fixed skin eruptions. Urticaria may appear within minutes after drug administration, but most reactions begin 7–14 days after the drug is first administered. These eruptions may occur in patients who have received these drugs for long periods, and eruptions continue for days after the drug has been discontinued. Drug eruptions with fever, eosinophilia, and systemic symptoms (DRESS syndrome) is most commonly seen with anticonvulsants but may be seen with other drugs. Drugs commonly implicated in skin reactions are listed in Table 15–8.

Heinze A et al: Characteristics of pediatric recurrent erythema multiforme. Pediatr Dermatol 2018 Jan;35(1):97–103 [PMID: 29231254].

MISCELLANEOUS SKIN DISORDERS SEEN IN PEDIATRIC PRACTICE

1. Aphthous Stomatitis

Recurrent erosions on the gums, lips, tongue, palate, and buccal mucosa are often confused with herpes simplex. A smear of the base of such a lesion stained with Wright stain will aid in ruling out herpes simplex by the absence of epithelial multinucleate giant cells. A culture for herpes simplex is also useful in differential diagnostics. The cause remains unknown, but T-cell–mediated cytotoxicity to various viral antigens has been postulated.

▶ **Treatment**

There is no specific therapy for this condition. Rinsing the mouth with liquid antacids provides relief in most patients. Topical corticosteroids in a gel base may provide some relief. In severe cases that interfere with eating, prednisone, 1 mg/kg/day orally for 3–5 days, will suffice to abort an episode. Colchicine, 0.2–0.5 mg/day, sometimes reduces the frequency of attacks.

2. Vitiligo

Vitiligo is characterized clinically by the development of areas of depigmentation. These are often symmetrical and occur mainly on extensor surfaces. The depigmentation results from a destruction of melanocytes. The basis for this destruction is unknown, but immunologically mediated damage is likely and vitiligo sometimes occurs in individuals with autoimmune endocrinopathies.

▶ **Treatment**

Treatment is with potent topical steroids or tacrolimus. Topical calcipotriene has also been used. Narrow-band ultraviolet B radiation (UVB 311 nm) may be used in severe cases. Response to treatment is slow often requiring many months to years.

Tamesis ME, Morellij JG: Vitiligo in childhood: a state of the art review. Pediatr Dermatol 2010;27:437 [PMID: 20553403].

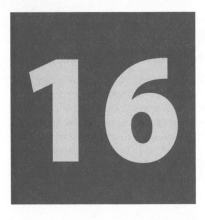

Eye

Jennifer Lee Jung, MD

INTRODUCTION

Normal vision is a sense that develops during infancy and childhood. Pediatric ophthalmology emphasizes early diagnosis and treatment of pediatric eye diseases in order to obtain the best possible visual outcome. Eye disease can also be a manifestation of systemic disease.

COMMON NONSPECIFIC SIGNS & SYMPTOMS

Nonspecific signs and symptoms commonly occur as the chief complaint or as an element of the history of a child with eye disease. Five of these findings are described here, along with a sixth—abnormal red reflex. Do not hesitate to seek the help of a pediatric ophthalmologist when you believe the diagnosis and treatment of these signs and symptoms require in-depth clinical experience.

RED EYE

Redness (injection) of the bulbar conjunctiva or deeper vessels is a common presenting complaint. It may be localized or diffuse. Causes include infection, inflammation (ocular or systemic, like Kawasaki disease or Stevens-Johnson syndrome [SJS]), allergy, irritation from noxious agents (acidic or alkali exposure), and trauma. Subconjunctival hemorrhage may be traumatic, spontaneous, or associated with hematopoietic disease, vascular anomalies, or inflammatory processes.

TEARING

Tearing in infants is usually due to nasolacrimal obstruction but may also be associated with congenital glaucoma, in which case photophobia and blepharospasm may also be present. Any irritation in the eye can cause tearing including infections, allergy, and dryness.

DISCHARGE

Purulent discharge is usually associated with bacterial conjunctivitis. *Watery discharge* occurs with viral conjunctivitis/keratitis, iritis, and corneal abrasions/foreign bodies. *Mucoid discharge* may be a sign of allergic conjunctivitis or nasolacrimal obstruction. Infants with nasolacrimal duct obstruction commonly have tearing associated with yellow crusts, but their eye remains white and quiet. A mucoid discharge due to allergy typically contains eosinophils, whereas a purulent bacterial discharge contains polymorphonuclear leukocytes.

PAIN & FOREIGN-BODY SENSATION

Pain in or around the eye may be due to foreign bodies, corneal abrasions, lacerations, acute infections of the globe or ocular adnexa, iritis, and elevated eye pressure. Large refractive errors or poor accommodative ability may manifest as headaches and eye strain. Trichiasis (inturned lashes) and contact lens problems also cause ocular discomfort.

PHOTOPHOBIA

Acute aversion to light may occur with corneal abrasions, foreign bodies, and uveitis. Squinting of one eye in bright light is a common sign of intermittent exotropia (eye drifting). Photophobia is present in infants with glaucoma, albinism, aniridia, and retinal dystrophies such as achromatopsia. Photophobia is common after ocular surgery and after pharmacologic dilation of the pupil.

ABNORMAL RED REFLEX

Checking for an abnormal red reflex is a crucial part of every pediatric exam starting from the newborn period. Abnormal red reflex can be unilateral or bilateral. Any abnormality altering the penetration of light into the retina can result

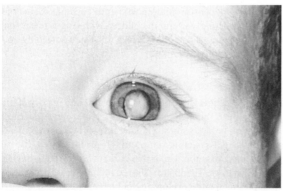

▲ **Figure 16–1.** Leukocoria of the left eye caused by retrolental membrane (persistent hyperplastic primary vitreous or persistent fetal vasculature).

in abnormal red reflex. This includes cloudy corneas, cloudy lens (cataracts), abnormality in the retina itself, and significant refractive errors (nearsightedness, farsightedness, astigmatism). Causes of cloudy corneas include congenital glaucoma, Peter anomaly, infections, and anterior segment dysgenesis. Leukocoria (white pupil) can be caused by cataracts or retinal problems like retinoblastoma (RB), retinal detachment, *Toxocara* infection, and Coat disease (nonhereditary retinal vascular disorder) (Figure 16–1).

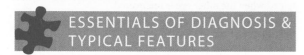

ESSENTIALS OF DIAGNOSIS & TYPICAL FEATURES

▶ Significant refractive errors (myopia, hyperopia, astigmatism, or anisometropia) may cause decreased visual acuity (VA), amblyopia, and strabismus.

▶ Symptoms and signs of uncorrected refractive error include blurred vision, squinting, headaches, fatigue with visual tasks, and failed vision screening.

▶ **Pathogenesis**

Refractive error refers to the optical state of the eye (Figure 16–2). The shape of the cornea and, to a lesser extent, the shape of the lens and length of the eye play a role in the refractive state of the eye. Children at particular risk for refractive errors requiring correction with glasses include those who are born prematurely; have Down syndrome; have parents with refractive errors; or have certain systemic conditions such as Stickler, Marfan, or Ehlers-Danlos syndrome.

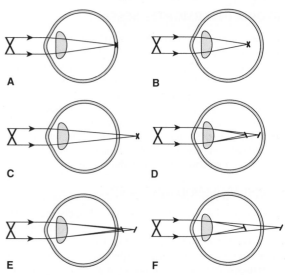

▲ **Figure 16–2.** Different refractive states of the eye. **A:** Emmetropia. Image plane from parallel rays of light falls on retina. **B:** Myopia. Image plane focuses anterior to retina. **C:** Hyperopia. Image plane focuses posterior to retina. **D:** Astigmatism, myopic type. Images in horizontal and vertical planes focus anterior to retina. **E:** Astigmatism, hyperopic type. Images in horizontal and vertical planes focus posterior to retina. **F:** Astigmatism, mixed type. Images in horizontal and vertical planes focus on either side of retina.

▶ **Diagnosis**

There are three common refractive errors: myopia, hyperopia, and astigmatism. High refractive errors or inequality of the refractive state between the two eyes (anisometropia) can cause amblyopia (reduced vision caused by conditions affecting normal vision development). The refractive state can be determined by instrument-based screening or by an eye care professional. Use of the autorefractor in children can overestimate the amount of nearsightedness. Cycloplegia is used to fully relax their accommodation, and the process of retinoscopy is used to determine the accurate refractive error in children.

▶ **Treatment**

Refractive errors in children are most commonly treated with glasses. An eye care professional can determine if the refractive error requires treatment. Contact lenses are prescribed for children with very high or asymmetrical refractive errors and adolescents who do not want to wear glasses. Laser refractive surgery is not indicated for most children.

MYOPIA (NEARSIGHTEDNESS)

For the myopic individual, objects nearby are in focus; those at a distance are blurred. There is a global rise in prevalence of myopia. Onset is typically in elementary school age and often progresses throughout adolescence and young adulthood. A myopic person may squint to produce a pinhole effect, which improves distance vision. Treatment requires glasses or contact lenses. Daily use of low-dose atropine 0.01% eye drops has been shown to slow myopia progression by approximately 50%. Side effects include minimal pupil dilation and loss of accommodation without reduction in VA.

HYPEROPIA (FARSIGHTEDNESS)

A hyperopic child is able to see clearly both at distance and at near because the child can focus on near objects through the process of accommodation if the hyperopia is not excessive. Large amounts of uncorrected hyperopia can cause esotropia (crossed eyes) as accommodation and convergence are closely linked. Most young children have hyperopic refraction that diminishes with age and does not require glasses.

ASTIGMATISM

When either the cornea or the crystalline lens is not perfectly spherical, an image will not be sharply focused in one plane. Schematically, there will be two planes of focus. This refractive state is described as *astigmatism*. Large amounts of astigmatism can cause amblyopia, and it is treated with glasses or toric contact lenses. Keratoconus is a corneal disorder that results in progressive corneal thinning and irregular astigmatism and requires special attention. It is more commonly seen in children with Down syndrome, atopy, and connective tissue disorders.

▼ OPHTHALMIC EXAMINATION

The ophthalmic examination should be a part of every well-child assessment. A history of poor vision, misalignment of the eyes, failed vision screening, eyelid malposition, abnormal pupil reactivity or shape, and an asymmetric/abnormal red reflex requires referral to an ophthalmologist. Prompt detection and treatment of ocular conditions can prevent a lifetime of visual disability.

From birth to 3 years of age, the ophthalmic examination should include taking a history for ocular problems, vision assessment, inspection of the eyelids and eyes, pupil examination, ocular motility assessment, and red reflex check. Instrument-based screening may be attempted at this age.

The ophthalmic examination of children older than 3 years should include all of the previously mentioned tests and VA testing with eye charts such as HOTV, Snellen, or LEA. Testing of binocular vision, or use of both eyes at the same time, can be accomplished by various stereoacuity tests. Instrument-based screening can identify children with amblyogenic risk factors and are particularly useful in children with language barriers or cognitive delays. See AAPOS.org for vision screening and referral recommendations.

HISTORY

Evaluation begins with the chief complaint and history of the present illness. Elements of the ocular history include onset of the complaint, its duration, laterality, previous treatment, and associated systemic symptoms. If an infectious disease is suspected, ask about possible contact with others having similar findings. The history should include prior ocular disease, perinatal and developmental history, history of allergy, and history of familial ocular disorders.

VISUAL ACUITY

Visual acuity (VA) testing is the most important test of visual function and should be part of every well-child check. Acuity should be tested in each eye individually using an adhesive eye patch to prevent peeking. Glasses should be worn during vision screening.

In the sleeping newborn, the presence of lid squeezing to bright light is an adequate response. At age 6 weeks, eye-to-eye contact with slow, following movements is usually present. By age 3 months, the infant should demonstrate fixing and following ocular movements for objects at a distance of 2–3 ft. At age 6 months, interest in movement across the room is the norm. Vision can be recorded for the presence or absence of fixing and following behavior, and whether vision is steady (unsteady when nystagmus is present) and maintained when the other eye is uncovered.

Children who can identify or match objects on a chart can provide direct measurements of their VA. This may be possible in children as young as 3 years. Vision is tested first with both eyes open on large optotypes to ensure that the child understands the test. Then, vision should be tested monocularly, preferably with one eye patched (with tape or occlusive patch) to prevent peeking.

Currently preferred optotypes are LEA and HOTV symbols. For those who can identify letters, Snellen or Sloan charts are recommended. Most accurate assessment is obtained when using charts with lines of optotypes or single optotype with crowding bars around it. Using single optotypes without crowding bars can overestimate VA. Crowding bars surrounding an optotype make individual letters more difficult to identify by an amblyopic eye, thus increasing the sensitivity to detect amblyopia.

"Threshold" acuity testing is a time-honored method where children start at the top of an eye chart and read down each line until they can identify the smallest line discernable with each eye tested separately. This method helps identify the best level of VA in each eye and allows the detection of mild difference in acuity between each eye. However,

Table 16–1. "Critical line" vision screening evaluation.

Age (mo)	Critical Line For Vision
36–47	20/50
48–59	20/40
≥ 60	20/30 or 20/32 in some charts

threshold evaluation can be time-consuming and may result in loss of attention in young children.

"Critical line" screening is an effective alternative for identifying children with potentially serious vision problems and can be administered more quickly. The "critical line" is the age-dependent line a child is expected to see and pass. This critical line to pass becomes smaller in size as age increases. Most eye charts have 4–6 optotypes per line. Passing the screening requires the child to correctly answer the majority of the optotypes present on the critical line appropriate for his or her age (Table 16–1).

Children with nystagmus (eye shaking) require special considerations during vision testing. They may have a compensatory head position (head turn or tilt) to achieve their null point (where shakiness is dampened). Because VA can decrease when forced to face straight ahead, these children should be tested in their compensatory head positions. In addition, children with nystagmus often also have "latent nystagmus," which results in worsened shakiness when one eye is covered. For this reason, testing both eyes simultaneously without occlusion gives a better VA measurement than when either eye is tested individually.

Instrument-based screening modalities including photo screeners and autorefractors are used by various volunteer programs, schools, daycare facilities, and physician offices. Photo screening does not screen directly for amblyopia but for amblyogenic factors that include strabismus, media opacities, eyelid ptosis, and refractive errors. Autorefractors can determine if there is a significant refractive error present in either eye or if there is a significant difference between the two eyes. Some instruments also detect strabismus, media opacities, pupil abnormalities, and eyelid ptosis. If the screening results suggest an amblyogenic factor, children are referred to an eye care professional for a complete eye examination. Problems exist with sensitivity and specificity of the instruments and poor follow-up for referrals to eye care professionals. If available, instrument-based screening can be initiated beginning at age 12 months. Once children can read, optotype-based acuity should supplement instrument-based testing.

American Academy of Ophthalmology: Visual system assessment in infants, children, and young adults by pediatricians: policy statement—2016. January 1, 2016. https://www.aao.org/clinical-statement/visual-system-assessment-in-infants-children-young.

Donahue SP, Baker CN: Procedures for the evaluation of the visual system by pediatricians. Pediatrics 2016 Jan;137(1). doi: 10.1542/peds.2015-3597 [PMID: 26644488].

Pineles SL et al: Atropine for the prevention of myopia progression in children: a report by the American Academy of Ophthalmology. Ophthalmology 2017 Dec;124(12):1857–1866. doi: 10.1016/j.ophtha.2017.05.032 [PMID: 28669492].

ESSENTIALS OF DIAGNOSIS & TYPICAL FEATURES

▶ The handheld ophthalmoscope is the tool necessary to check the red reflex of the eye.

▶ Simultaneous examination of both pupils at the same time is called the *Brückner test*.

Red Reflex Test

An ophthalmoscope is used to check the red reflex of both eyes. The examiner should use the largest diameter of light and have the setting at zero. The room should be darkened for maximal pupil dilation. Both pupils are evaluated with the ophthalmoscope at arm's length from the child with the child looking straight at the light. If the child is looking off to the side, the reflex can be asymmetric. The observed red reflexes should be a light orange-yellow in color in lightly pigmented eyes or a dark red in darkly pigmented brown eyes. A difference in quality of the red reflexes between the two eyes constitutes a positive Brückner test and requires referral to an ophthalmologist. The American Academy of Pediatrics (AAP), American Association for Pediatric Ophthalmology and Strabismus (AAPOS), and the American Academy of Ophthalmology (AAO) policy statements for red reflex testing can be accessed at https://www.aao.org/clinical-statement/procedures-evaluation-of-visual-system-by-pediatri.

EXTERNAL EXAMINATION

A penlight provides good illumination for inspection of the anterior segment of the globe and its adnexa. A slit lamp provides optimal illumination and magnification for an ocular examination.

In cases of suspected foreign body, pulling down on the lower lid provides excellent visualization of the inferior cul-de-sac (palpebral conjunctiva). Visualizing the upper cul-de-sac and superior bulbar conjunctiva is possible by having the patient look down, while the upper lid is lifted up. The upper lid should be everted to evaluate the superior tarsal conjunctiva (Figure 16–3).

When indicated for further evaluation of the cornea, a small amount of fluorescein solution should be instilled into the lower cul-de-sac. A Wood lamp or a blue filter cap

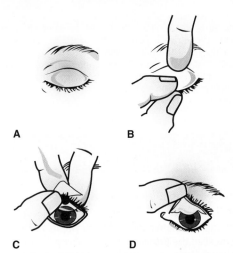

▲ **Figure 16–3.** Eversion of the upper lid. **A:** The patient looks downward. **B:** The fingers pull the lid down, and an index finger or cotton tip is placed on the upper tarsal border. **C:** The lid is pulled up over the finger. **D:** The lid is everted.

placed over a penlight will illuminate the epithelial defects as yellow-green. Disease-specific staining patterns may be observed. For example, herpes simplex lesions of the corneal epithelium produce a dendrite or branchlike pattern. A foreign body lodged beneath the upper lid shows one or more vertical lines of stain on the cornea due to the constant movement of the foreign body over the cornea. Contact lens overwear produces a central staining pattern. A fine, scattered punctate pattern may be a sign of medication toxicity. Punctate erosions of the inferior third of the cornea can be seen with staphylococcal blepharitis or exposure keratitis secondary to incomplete lid closure.

PUPILS

The pupils should be evaluated for reaction to light, regularity of shape, and equality of size as well as for the presence of afferent pupillary defect (APD). This defect, which occurs in optic nerve disease, is evaluated by the swinging flashlight test (see section Diseases of the Optic Nerve). Irregular pupils are associated with iritis, trauma, pupillary membranes, and structural defects such as iris coloboma (see section Iris Coloboma).

Pupils vary in size due to lighting conditions and age. In general, infants have miotic (constricted) pupils. Children have larger pupils than either infants or adults, whereas the elderly have miotic pupils.

Anisocoria, a size difference between the two pupils, may be physiologic if the size difference is within 1 mm. Anisocoria can result when the abnormal pupil is smaller

Table 16–2. Function and innervation of each of the extraocular muscles.

Muscle	Function	Innervation
Medial rectus	Adductor	Oculomotor (third)
Lateral rectus	Abductor	Abducens (sixth)
Inferior rectus	Depressor, adductor, extorter	Oculomotor
Superior rectus	Elevator, adductor, intorter	Oculomotor
Inferior oblique	Elevator, abductor, extorter	Oculomotor
Superior oblique	Depressor, abductor, intorter	Trochlear (fourth)

(Horner syndrome) or when it is bigger (third nerve palsy, Adie tonic pupil, trauma, medication). Systemic antihistamines and scopolamine patches can dilate the pupils and interfere with accommodation (focusing).

ALIGNMENT & MOTILITY EVALUATION

Alignment and motility should be tested because amblyopia is associated with strabismus. Ocular rotations should be evaluated in the six cardinal positions of gaze (Table 16–2; Figure 16–4). A small toy is an interesting target for testing ocular rotations in infants; a penlight works well in older children.

Alignment can be assessed in several ways. In order of increasing accuracy, these methods are observation, the corneal light reflex test, and cover testing. Observation is an educated guess about whether the eyes are properly aligned. Corneal light reflex evaluation (Hirschberg test) is performed by shining a penlight at the patient's eyes, observing the reflections of each cornea, and estimating whether these "reflexes"

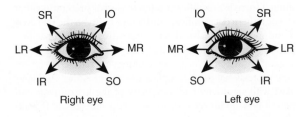

MR = medial rectus	LR = lateral rectus
SR = superior rectus	IR = inferior rectus
SO = superior oblique	IO = inferior oblique

▲ **Figure 16–4.** Cardinal positions of gaze and muscles primarily tested in those fields of gaze. Arrow indicates position in which each muscle is tested.

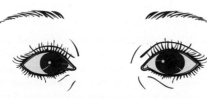

▲ **Figure 16–5.** Temporal displacement of light reflection showing esotropia (inward deviation) of the right eye. Nasal displacement of the reflection would show exotropia (outward deviation) of the left eye.

appear to be positioned symmetrically. If the reflection of light is noted temporally on the cornea, esotropia (crossed eyes) is suspected (Figure 16–5). Nasal reflection of the light suggests exotropia (outward deviation). Pseudostrabismus is the appearance of crossed eyes due to wide nasal bridge and/or prominent epicanthal skin folds that cover the medial portion of the sclera. Despite the false impression of esotropia, they will have symmetric corneal light reflexes.

Another way of evaluating alignment is with the cover test. As the child attends to the target, each eye is alternately covered. A shift in an eye's alignment as it assumes fixation onto the target is a possible indication of strabismus (Figure 16–6). A deviated eye that is blind or has very poor vision will not fixate on a target. Consequently, spurious results to cover testing may occur, which can happen with disinterest on the part of the patient, small-angle strabismus, and inexperience in administering cover tests.

Intermittent strabismus is a normal finding in infancy. However, if this persists beyond 4 months of age, referral to ophthalmology is necessary.

OPHTHALMOSCOPIC EXAMINATION

A handheld ophthalmoscope allows visualization of the ocular fundus. As the patient's pupil becomes more constricted, viewing the fundus becomes more difficult. Although pupillary dilation can precipitate an attack of closed-angle glaucoma in the predisposed adult, children are very rarely predisposed to angle closure. Exceptions include those with a dislocated lens, past surgery, or an eye previously compromised by a retrolental membrane, such as in ROP. Therefore, if an adequate view of the fundus is precluded by a miotic pupil, use of a dilating agent (eg, one drop in each eye of 2.5% phenylephrine or 0.5% or 1% tropicamide) can provide adequate mydriasis (dilation). In infants younger than 1 year, one drop of a combination of 1% phenylephrine with 0.2% cyclopentolate (Cyclomydril) is safer. Structures to be observed during ophthalmoscopy include the optic disc, blood vessels, the macular reflex, and retina, as well as the clarity of the vitreous media. By increasing the amount of plus lens dialed into the instrument, the point of focus moves anteriorly from the retina to the lens and finally to the cornea.

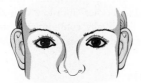

Eyes straight (maintained in position by fusion).

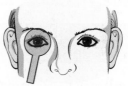

Position of eye under cover in orthophoria (fusion-free position). The right eye under cover has not moved.

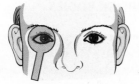

Position of eye under cover in esophoria (fusion-free position). Under cover, the right eye has deviated inward. Upon removal of cover, the right eye will immediately resume its straight-ahead position.

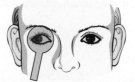

Position of eye under cover in exophoria (fusion-free position). Under cover, the right eye has deviated outward. Upon removal of the cover, the right eye will immediately resume its straight-ahead position.

▲ **Figure 16–6.** Cover testing. The patient is instructed to look at a target at eye level 20 ft away. Note that in the presence of constant strabismus (ie, a tropia rather than a phoria), the deviation will remain when the cover is removed. (Reproduced with permission from Riordan-Eva P, Cunningham ET: *Vaughan & Asbury's General Ophthalmology*, 18th ed. New York, NY: McGraw Hill; 2011.)

OCULAR TRAUMA

ESSENTIALS OF DIAGNOSIS & TYPICAL FEATURES

▶ A careful history of the events that led to the ocular injury is crucial in the diagnosis and treatment of ocular trauma.

▶ If the extent of the eye injury is difficult to determine or if it is sight threatening, it is best to cover the eye with a shield and refer to ophthalmology urgently.

PREVENTION OF OCULAR INJURIES

Air rifles, paintballs, bungee cords, and fireworks are responsible for many serious eye injuries in children. Golf, baseball/softball, and lacrosse injuries are common and can be very severe. Safety/sport goggles or prescription glasses should be used while in laboratories and industrial arts classes, when operating power tools, hammers, nails, and while participating in organized sports. The one-eyed individual should be specifically advised to always wear polycarbonate eyeglasses at all times and goggles for all sports. High-risk activities such as boxing and the martial arts should be avoided by one-eyed children.

CORNEAL ABRASION

ESSENTIALS OF DIAGNOSIS & TYPICAL FEATURES

▶ The cornea is one of the most sensitive parts of the body. Corneal abrasion can cause severe ocular pain, tearing, and blepharospasm.

▶ Corneal abrasion is most commonly associated with trauma.

▶ Pathogenesis

Children often suffer corneal abrasions accidentally while playing with siblings or pets and participating in sports. Contact lens users may develop abrasions due to poorly fitting lenses, overnight wear, and use of torn or damaged lenses.

▶ Prevention

Proper contact lens care and parental supervision can prevent activities that can lead to a corneal abrasion.

▶ Clinical Findings

Symptom of a corneal abrasion is sudden and severe eye pain, usually after an inciting event. Decreased vision secondary to pain and tearing are common complaints. Eyelid edema, tearing, injection of the conjunctiva, and poor cooperation with the ocular examination due to pain are common signs of a corneal abrasion. Pain improves with instillation of ophthalmic anesthetic drops and can aid in examination. Fluorescein dye will stain the abrasion with bright yellow-green when illuminated with Wood lamp. Both upper and lower eyelids should be everted to evaluate for foreign bodies.

▶ Differential Diagnosis

Ocular or adnexal foreign bodies, corneal ulcer, and corneal laceration.

▶ Complications

Possible vision loss from corneal infection and scarring.

▶ Treatment

Topical anesthetic should never be given to patients as they can lead to corneal melting. Ophthalmic ointment, such as erythromycin ointment, lubricates the surface of the cornea and also helps prevent infections. Patching the affected eye when a large abrasion is present may provide comfort, but it is not advised for corneal abrasions caused by contact lens wear or other potentially contaminated sources. Frequent follow-up is required until healing is complete.

▶ Prognosis

Excellent if corneal infection and scarring do not occur.

OCULAR FOREIGN BODIES

ESSENTIALS OF DIAGNOSIS & TYPICAL FEATURES

▶ Vertical corneal abrasion can be a sign of foreign body under the eyelid so lid eversion should be performed.

▶ Prevention

Protective goggles or prescription glasses can help prevent ocular injuries and should be encouraged while participating in sports and activities at risk for eye injuries.

Clinical Findings

Foreign bodies on the surface of the globe and palpebral conjunctiva usually cause discomfort, tearing, and a red eye. Pain with blinking suggests that the foreign body may be trapped under the eyelid or on the corneal surface.

Magnification with a slit lamp may be needed for inspection. Foreign bodies that lodge on the upper palpebral conjunctiva are best viewed by everting the lid on itself and removing the foreign body with a cotton applicator.

Differential Diagnosis

Corneal abrasion, corneal ulcer, and globe rupture/laceration.

Complications

Pain, infection, and potential vision loss from scarring.

Treatment

When foreign bodies are noted on the bulbar conjunctiva or cornea (Figure 16–7), removal of the foreign body with irrigation or with a cotton applicator after instillation of a topical anesthetic can be attempted. Referral to an ophthalmologist may be necessary if the aforementioned measures fail to remove the foreign body or if a corneal rust ring secondary to a metallic foreign body is present. Patients should be warned that foreign-body sensation may persist for 1–2 days even after removal due to the epithelial defect that occurs after removal. An ophthalmic antibiotic ointment is typically prescribed for several days after foreign-body removal.

Prognosis

Usually excellent with prompt treatment.

INTRAOCULAR FOREIGN BODIES & PERFORATING OCULAR INJURIES

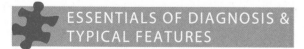

ESSENTIALS OF DIAGNOSIS & TYPICAL FEATURES

► Signs of perforating ocular injuries include irregularly shaped pupil, shallow anterior chamber, hyphema (blood in the anterior chamber), or dark tissue showing through the white sclera (Figure 16–8).

Pathogenesis

Intraocular foreign bodies and penetrating injuries/corneal/scleral laceration (ruptured globes) are most often caused by being in close proximity to high-velocity projectiles such as

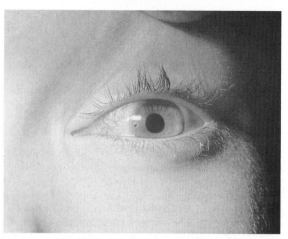

A

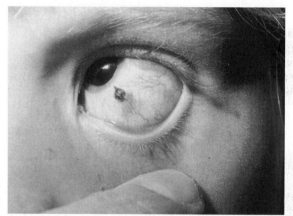

B

▲ **Figure 16–7. A:** Corneal foreign body at the nasal edge of the cornea. **B:** Subconjunctival foreign body of graphite.

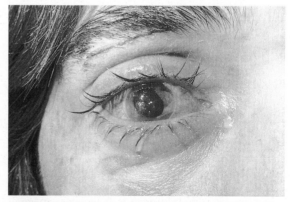

▲ **Figure 16–8.** Corneal laceration with irregular pupil and vitreous loss.

windshield glass broken during a motor vehicle accident, metal grinding without use of protective safety goggles, BB gun injury, and sports-related injuries.

Prevention

Use protective eyewear when engaging in activities that may be a risk for ocular injury.

Clinical Findings

Sudden ocular pain with vision loss occurs after an inciting event. Diagnosis may be difficult if obvious signs of globe rupture as stated above are not present.

Computed tomographic (CT) scan is useful in evaluating ocular trauma, including bony injury and intraocular foreign bodies. Nonradiopaque materials such as glass will not be seen on imaging. Magnetic resonance imaging (MRI) must be avoided if a magnetic foreign body is suspected. B scan ultrasound should not be performed on suspected globe injury.

Differential Diagnosis

Corneal abrasion and superficial foreign body of the eye or eyelids.

Complications

Traumatic cataract, retinal detachment, intraocular infection, loss of vision or eye.

Treatment

In cases of suspected intraocular foreign body or perforation of the globe, it may be best to keep the child at rest, gently shield the eye with a metal shield or cut-down paper cup, and keep the extent of examination to a minimum to prevent expulsion of intraocular contents. In this setting, the child should be given nothing by mouth in case eye examination under anesthesia or surgical repair is required. Emergent consultation with ophthalmologist is warranted.

Prognosis

Prognosis depends on the extent of the trauma.

BLUNT ORBITAL TRAUMA

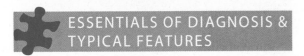

ESSENTIALS OF DIAGNOSIS & TYPICAL FEATURES

▶ In "White-eyed blowout fracture," injury to the eye and lids may appear minimal except for restriction of eye movements, especially upgaze. It requires emergent surgery.

Pathogenesis

Blunt trauma to the orbit can lead to orbital fractures. Retrobulbar hemorrhage (bleeding behind the globe within the orbit) can lead to orbital compartment syndrome, which can lead to permanent vision loss.

Prevention

Protective eyewear during athletic activities and adequate supervision of children at home and school.

Clinical Findings

The orbital floor is a common location for a fracture (called a *blowout fracture*). Patients can have double vision, pain with eye movements, and restriction of extraocular movements. *White-eyed blowout fracture* is a greenstick fracture with entrapment of orbital contents within the fracture. It is called "white-eyed" because the only abnormality on examination may be restricted eye movements, especially upward. Entrapment of orbital contents often stimulates the oculo-cardiac reflex resulting in bradycardia and emesis. CT scan is helpful in diagnosing the extent of injuries. Consultation with an ophthalmologist is necessary to determine the full spectrum of the injuries.

Orbital compartment syndrome is also an emergency requiring immediate treatment. Patients present with severe eyelid edema and proptosis. With true orbital compartment syndrome, eyelids will be too tight to open even with fingers or instruments because of the pressure from behind the orbit. Neuroimaging will show retrobulbar hemorrhage and proptosis.

Treatment

Orbital compartment syndrome requires emergent lateral eyelid canthotomy and cantholysis to decompress the orbit. Treatment should not be delayed in order to image the orbits. Prompt treatment can prevent permanent vision loss.

Patients with clinical signs of muscle entrapment require urgent surgical repair to avoid permanent ischemic injury to the involved extraocular muscle. Large fractures may need nonurgent repair to prevent enophthalmos (sunken appearance to the orbit). Patients with any orbital fracture must be warned not to blow their nose as it can cause orbital emphysema and worsening proptosis.

Cold compresses or ice packs for brief periods in the first 24 hours after injury may help reduce hemorrhage and swelling.

Prognosis

The prognosis depends on the severity of the blunt trauma, associated ocular injuries, and extent of the orbit fractures.

LACERATIONS

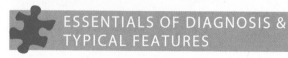

ESSENTIALS OF DIAGNOSIS & TYPICAL FEATURES

▶ Lacerations of the nasal third of the eyelid are at risk for lacrimal system injury.

▶ Pathogenesis

Lacerations of the eyelids and lacrimal system often result from dog bites, car accidents, falls, and fights.

▶ Prevention

Supervision of children at home and at school.

▶ Clinical Findings

Eyelid lacerations may be partial or full thickness in depth. Foreign bodies, such as glass or gravel, may be present depending on the mechanism of the injury.

▶ Differential Diagnosis

Globe injury may be associated with eyelid lacerations as well.

▶ Complications

Poor surgical repair of lacerations of the eyelid margin can result in eyelid malposition, which causes chronic ocular surface irritation and possible corneal scarring.

▶ Treatment

Superficial lacerations away from the lid margins can be repaired by nonophthalmologists. Lacerations involving the lid margin or canaliculus (Figure 16–9) and those associated

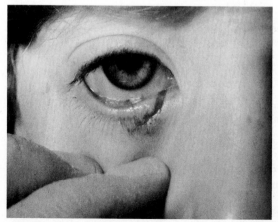

▲ **Figure 16–9.** Laceration involving right lower lid and canaliculus.

with significant tissue loss are best repaired by an ophthalmologist and may require intubation of the nasolacrimal system with silicone tubes.

▶ Prognosis

Prognosis depends on severity of the injury, tissue loss, and adequacy of surgical repair.

BURNS

ESSENTIALS OF DIAGNOSIS & TYPICAL FEATURES

▶ For all chemical burns, pH should be checked and eyes irrigated until pH is close to 7.

▶ In severe burns, the eye may not look red due to perilimbal ischemia.

▶ Alkalis tend to penetrate deeper than acids into ocular tissue and often cause severe injury.

▶ Pathogenesis

Burns of the conjunctiva and cornea may be thermal, radiant, or chemical. Chemical burns with strong acidic and alkaline agents can be blinding and constitute a true ocular emergency. Examples are burns caused by splash injury with cleaning supplies, spilled drain cleaner, and bleach. Radiant energy causes ultraviolet keratitis. Typical examples are welder's burn and burns associated with skiing without goggles in bright sunlight. In addition to thermal and blunt trauma, chemical eye injury can occur from airbag deployment as a result of alkaline burn due to the chemical components of the inflation reaction.

▶ Prevention

Protective eyewear when engaging in activities that pose a potential risk for exposure to hazardous chemicals, radiant energy, or when explosive conditions is possible.

▶ Clinical Findings

Superficial thermal burns cause pain, tearing, and injection. Corneal epithelial defects can be diagnosed using fluorescein dye, which will stain areas of the cornea bright yellows green where the epithelium is absent. Conjunctiva may be injected diffusely. In severe burns, there is relative lack of redness around the cornea indicative of perilimbal ischemia. Eyelashes may be singed due to thermal burns. The fluorescein dye pattern will show a uniformly stippled appearance of the corneal epithelium in ultraviolet keratitis. It is important to check the pH after any suspected chemical burn injury including airbag deployment.

Differential Diagnosis

Corneal abrasion, foreign body, and traumatic iritis.

Complications

Significant corneal injury, especially if associated with an alkali burn, may lead to scarring and vision loss. Eyelid scarring can result in chronic exposure, dry eye, and entropion or ectropion.

Treatment

Immediate treatment consists of copious irrigation and removal of precipitates as soon as possible after the injury. Irrigation should be continued until the pH is close to 7. Initial stabilization of the injury is initiated by using topical antibiotics. A cycloplegic agent such as cyclopentolate 1% may be added to reduce ciliary spasm that contributes to pain. Topical steroids may also be necessary but should be guided by an ophthalmologist. Ultraviolet keratitis can be extremely painful, and patients often need opioids for pain control. Patients should be referred to an ophthalmologist after immediate first aid has been given.

Prognosis

Prognosis depends on the severity of the injury.

HYPHEMA

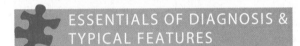

ESSENTIALS OF DIAGNOSIS & TYPICAL FEATURES

- ▶ Slit-lamp examination or penlight examination may reveal a layer of blood within the anterior chamber.
- ▶ A hyphema may be microscopic or may fill the entire anterior chamber (Figure 16–10).

Pathogenesis

Blunt trauma to the globe may cause a hyphema, which is bleeding within the anterior chamber from a ruptured vessel from the iris or in the anterior chamber angle (see Figure 16–10).

Prevention

Protective eyewear and appropriate supervision at home and at school.

Clinical Findings

Blunt trauma severe enough to cause a hyphema may be associated with additional ocular injury, including lens subluxation, cataract, retinal edema or detachment, and

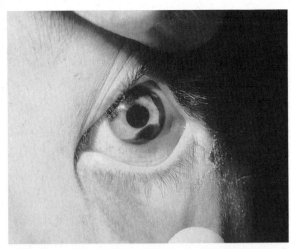

▲ **Figure 16–10.** Hyphema filling approximately 20% of the anterior chamber.

ruptured globe. It is important to note the height and color of the hyphema. Most will be layered inferiorly unless patient has been lying down for a long time, in which case it will be dispersed and have a hazy appearance. Sometimes, it can be seen as a clot over the iris. Total hyphema (100%) may appear black or red. A black total hyphema is referred to as "eight-ball hyphema." The black color is suggestive of impaired aqueous circulation and decreased oxygen concentration. This distinction is important because an eight-ball hyphema is more likely to cause pupillary block and secondary angle closure. In patients with sickle cell anemia or trait, even a small amount of hyphema can lead to significantly elevated intraocular pressure that can result in permanent vision loss. Therefore, all African Americans should have their sickle cell status determined if hyphema is observed. These patients require extra vigilance in diagnosing and treating hyphema.

Differential Diagnosis

Nontraumatic causes of hyphema include juvenile xanthogranuloma and blood dyscrasias.

Complications

Increased intraocular pressure, glaucoma, permanent corneal staining, and vision loss.

Treatment

A shield should be placed over the eye, the head elevated, and arrangements made for ophthalmologic referral.

Prognosis

Majority of children with isolated traumatic hyphema do well with outpatient treatment, activity restriction, and close follow-up with an ophthalmologist. Prognosis is worse if intraocular pressure is elevated, the patient has sickle cell disease, or if other associated ocular injuries are present.

ABUSIVE HEAD TRAUMA & NONACCIDENTAL TRAUMA

ESSENTIALS OF DIAGNOSIS & TYPICAL FEATURES

▶ Abusive head trauma (AHT), formerly known as *shaken baby syndrome*, is a form of nonaccidental trauma characterized by a constellation of examination findings, including intracranial injury, retinal hemorrhages, and fractures of long bones or ribs.

▶ The history leading to the diagnosis of AHT is often vague and poorly correlated with the extent of injury.

▶ Pathogenesis

AHT includes shaking as a mechanism of injury, shaking with impact, or impact alone. The most widely accepted theory is that retinal hemorrhages occur due to the vitreoretinal traction from accelerating-decelerating forces from shaking alone or combined with impact. Additional injury may result from spinal cord injuries and hypoxia.

▶ Clinical Findings

Victims often have multiple-organ system involvement that includes, but is not limited to, traumatic brain injury, bone fractures, and retinal hemorrhages. The presentation can include irritability, change in mental status, or cardiopulmonary arrest.

Ophthalmic consultation with dilated retinal examination is necessary to document retinal hemorrhages. Hemorrhages may be unilateral or bilateral and may be located in the posterior pole or periphery. Often, retinal hemorrhages are multilayered (intraretinal, preretinal, and subretinal), too numerous to count, and diffuse. Intraretinal hemorrhages may resolve rapidly within days, whereas preretinal or vitreous hemorrhages can take time. If a blood clot lies over the macula, deprivation amblyopia may occur and may require intraocular surgery by a retinal specialist. Other ocular findings associated with AHT include lid ecchymosis, subconjunctival hemorrhage, hyphema, retinal folds, retinoschisis (traumatic separation of the retinal layers), and optic nerve edema.

▶ Differential Diagnosis

The differential diagnosis of retinal hemorrhages includes birth trauma (in < 1 month old), sepsis, blood dyscrasia, and severe crush injuries or high-velocity trauma. A team effort between the primary treating physician, neurosurgery, orthopedics, ophthalmology, social services, and law enforcement is crucial in determining the true cause of a patient's injuries.

▶ Complications

The severity of injuries dictates the long-term outcome. Persistent hemorrhages involving the macula can lead to amblyopia. Often, poor vision results from cortical visual impairment in patients with severe neurologic injuries. Children with history of AHT are at higher risk of strabismus and significant refractive error, requiring glasses correction.

▶ Treatment

Management of any systemic injuries is required. Observation by an ophthalmologist for resolution of retinal hemorrhages is the usual management. Vitreous hemorrhages or large preretinal hemorrhages that do not resolve within several weeks may need surgical treatment by a retinal specialist.

▶ Prognosis

Prognosis depends on the severity of ocular and brain injuries.

Binenbaum G, Chen W, Huang J, Ying GS, Forbes BJ: The natural history of retinal hemorrhage in pediatric head trauma. J AAPOS 2016 Apr;20(2):131–135. doi: 10.1016/j.jaapos .2015.12.008 [PMID: 27079593].

Levin AV, Cordovez JA, Leiby BE, Pequignot E, Tandon A: Retinal hemorrhage in abusive head trauma: finding a common language. Trans Am Ophthalmol Soc 2014;112:1–10 [PMID: 25075150].

▼ DISORDERS OF THE OCULAR STRUCTURES

DISEASES OF THE EYELIDS

The eyelids can be affected by various dermatologic, infectious, or inflammatory conditions.

Blepharitis/Blepharokeratoconjunctivitis

ESSENTIALS OF DIAGNOSIS & TYPICAL FEATURES

▶ Blepharokeratoconjunctivitis (BKC) is a chronic inflammatory disorder of the eyelid and ocular surface that can be sight-threatening.

▶ Patients with BKC often have chronic, recurrent "pink eye" and frequent chalazia, leading to delay in diagnosis and proper treatment.

Pathogenesis

Blepharitis is caused by inflammation of the eyelid margin, meibomian gland obstruction, and tear film imbalance. The term *BKC* is used when the conjunctiva and cornea are affected in addition to the lids. Meibomian glands, located in the eyelids, secrete the lipid layer of tear film. Bacterial flora on lid margins secrete enzymes that can further destabilize the tear film. Higher numbers of *Staphylococcus aureus* and *Staphylococcus epidermis* have been cultured in patients with BKC. Refractory cases of BKC can be caused by ocular rosacea or *Demodex* (mite) infestation.

Prevention

Eyelid hygiene is essential to prevent or control blepharitis. Eyelid scrubs with baby shampoo help decrease the bacterial load on the eyelid margins and lashes. Warm compresses help loosen the secretions of the meibomian glands.

Clinical Findings

Patients commonly present with concerns of redness, tearing, photophobia, and foreign-body sensation. They may have decreased vision. Diagnosis is clinical with examination findings of the lid margin (thickening, telangiectasia, stye, crusting, collarettes), meibomian gland inspissation, follicular conjunctivitis, and corneal changes (punctate keratitis, corneal opacities, peripheral pannus and vascularization, ulceration, thinning, and scarring). Findings are often bilateral but can be asymmetric. Corneal scarring, if present, is usually peripheral and inferior but can be diffuse and central in severe cases. Vision loss can be from corneal scarring and also from induced astigmatism, leading to amblyopia.

Differential Diagnosis

Allergic or viral conjunctivitis. Herpes keratitis is the most frequent misdiagnosis. Contrary to BKC, HSV will be unilateral with decreased corneal sensation.

Complications

Permanent corneal and eyelid margin scarring in severe cases. Amblyopia with vision loss.

Treatment

It should be emphasized that BKC is a chronic condition with exacerbations and remissions. Treatment is targeted to opening the plugged meibomian glands to clear them of excess bacteria and oily secretions. Hot compresses of the lids with microwavable heat packs and eye masks is essential in melting the glandular debris followed by lid massage to express the glands. Lids should also be scrubbed with baby shampoo

daily. When suspecting Demodex, addition of tea tree oil shampoo is helpful. Topical and oral antibiotics can be used to decrease the bacterial burden. These include erythromycin ointment, azithromycin drops, and oral azithromycin. Topical steroids may be required to treat the inflammation and requires close follow up with an ophthalmologist.

Prognosis

Generally good with early diagnosis and treatment.

O'Gallagher M, Banteka M, Bunce C, Larkin F, Tuft S, Dahlmann-Noor A: Systemic treatment for blepharokeratoconjunctivitis in children. Cochrane Database Syst Rev 2016 May;30(5):CD011750. doi: 10.1002/14651858.CD011750.pub2 [PMID: 27236587].

O'Gallagher M, Bunce C, Hingorani M, Larkin F, Tuft S, Dahlmann-Noor A: Topical treatments for blepharokeratoconjunctivitis in children. Cochrane Database Syst Rev 2017 Feb 7;2:CD011965. doi: 10.1002/14651858.CD011965.pub2 [PMID: 28170093].

Rousta ST: Pediatric blepharokeratoconjunctivitis: is there a 'right' treatment? Curr Opin Ophthalmol 2017 Sep;28(5):449–453. doi: 10.1097/ICU.0000000000000399 [PMID: 28696955].

Chalazion

ESSENTIALS OF DIAGNOSIS & TYPICAL FEATURES

► A chalazion is an aseptic, nontender eyelid nodule.
► Patients report slowly enlarging lump with variability in size from day to day.

Pathogenesis

Obstruction of the eyelid meibomian glands with resultant inflammation, fibrosis, and lipogranuloma formation.

Prevention

See section Blepharitis.

Clinical Findings

Eyelid nodule of variable size and localized erythema of the corresponding palpebral conjunctiva that may be associated with a yellow lipogranuloma (Figure 16–11). It is a nontender, painless lesion.

Differential Diagnosis

Clinical presentation of acute chalazion and internal hordeolum can be difficult to distinguish, but management is the same.

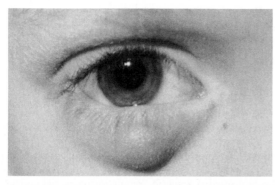

A

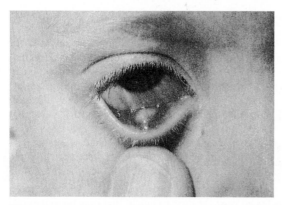

B

▲ **Figure 16–11.** Chalazion. **A:** Right lower lid, external view. **B:** Right lower lid conjunctival surface.

Treatment

See section Blepharitis. Since chalazia are inflammatory and not infectious, antibiotics are not necessary. If incision and curettage are needed because the lesion is slow to resolve, the child will often require a general anesthetic.

Prognosis

Generally good.

Hordeolum

ESSENTIALS OF DIAGNOSIS & TYPICAL FEATURES

▶ Hordeolum is a painful red bump on the eyelid caused by an acute bacterial infection of eyelash hair follicle or Meibomian glands.

▶ It is a self-limiting condition lasting 1–2 weeks.

Pathogenesis

Hordeolum is usually caused by *Staphylococcus* infection occurring from stasis of eyelid glands, which normally produce antiseptic secretions. External hordeolum (stye) occurs from blockage of the sebaceous (Zeis) and sweat (Moll) glands, resulting in painful red swollen bump that develops into a pustule. Internal hordeolum is due to blockage of Meibomian glands and pustules form on the inner side of the eyelids.

Prevention

See section Blepharitis.

Clinical Findings

It presents as painful, red bump on the eyelid with localized erythema. Pustule can be seen on the eyelid margin for external hordeolum or on the palpebral conjunctiva for internal hordeolum (Figure 16–12).

Differential Diagnosis

Periorbital cellulitis, chalazion

Treatment

Hordeolum generally drain spontaneously without any treatment. Treatments used for chalazia can be helpful (warm compresses, lid massage, lid scrubs). Erythromycin ointment can provide lubrication. Oral antibiotic is rarely indicated unless infection leads to periorbital cellulitis, when systemic antibiotic is necessary. Incision and draining of a persistent lesion can be performed by ophthalmologists.

Prognosis

Generally good.

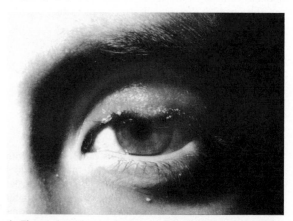

▲ **Figure 16–12.** Hordeolum and blepharitis, left upper lid.

VIRAL EYELID DISEASE

Pathogenesis

HSV may involve the conjunctiva and lids at the time of primary herpes simplex infection resulting in blepharoconjunctivitis. Vesicular lesions with an erythematous base occur. Herpes zoster causes vesicular disease in association with a skin eruption in the dermatome of the ophthalmic branch of the trigeminal nerve.

Prevention

Avoid contact with individuals with active HSV infection.

Clinical Findings

A vesicular rash is the most common sign of herpes viral eyelid infection. Fluorescein dye should be administered topically to the affected eye followed by examination with a cobalt blue light to assess for the presence of dendrites. When vesicles are present on the tip of the nose with herpes zoster (Hutchinson sign), ocular involvement, including iritis, is more likely. Eyelid edema in herpes zoster ophthalmicus (HZO) can be severe and mistaken for preseptal cellulitis. Herpes simplex or herpes zoster can be diagnosed by polymerase chain reaction or viral culture. Molluscum contagiosum lesions are typically umbilicated papules, which may or may not be inflamed. It can cause acute or chronic follicular conjunctivitis.

Differential Diagnosis

Impetigo.

Complications

Conjunctivitis and keratitis (corneal infection).

Treatment

Herpes simplex blepharoconjunctivitis can be treated with systemic acyclovir or valacyclovir. An alternative includes topical ganciclovir 0.15%. Treatment of ophthalmic herpes zoster with systemic nucleoside analogues within 3 days after onset may reduce the morbidity. Molluscum contagiosum lesions may be treated with observation, cautery, or excision.

Prognosis

Generally good unless corneal involvement is present.

MISCELLANEOUS EYELID INFECTIONS

Pediculosis

Pediculosis of the lids (phthiriasis palpebrarum) is caused by *Phthirus pubis*. Nits and adult lice can be seen on the eyelashes when viewed with appropriate magnification. Mechanical removal as well as medical treatment is effective (see Chapter 15). Other bodily areas of involvement must also be treated if involved. Family members and contacts may also be infected.

Papillomavirus

Papillomavirus may infect the lid and conjunctiva. Warts may be recurrent, multiple, and difficult to treat. Treatment modalities include cryotherapy, cautery, carbon dioxide laser, and surgery.

EYELID PTOSIS

Pathogenesis

Eyelid ptosis—a droopy upper lid (Figure 16–13)—may be congenital or acquired but is usually congenital in children owing to a defective levator muscle. Other causes of ptosis are myasthenia gravis, lid injuries, third nerve palsy, and

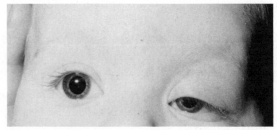

▲ **Figure 16–13.** Congenital ptosis of severe degree, left upper lid.

Horner syndrome (see section Horner Syndrome). Marcus Gunn jaw-winking phenomenon is a congenital ptosis associated with synkinetic movements of the upper eyelid and muscles of mastication. It is due to an aberrant connection between the motor branches of trigeminal nerve innervating the external pterygoid muscle and the superior branches of oculomotor nerve supplying the levator palpebrae superioris.

▶ Clinical Findings

The upper eyelid is lower than normal, which narrows the vertical dimension of the palpebral fissure. In congenital ptosis, the upper lid crease is poorly defined or absent with poor elevation of lid when looking up due to fibrotic levator muscle. This may be compensated by use of forehead muscles to lift the brow. It is important to note the extraocular motility and check for anisocoria in any child with ptosis.

▶ Differential Diagnosis

Congenital ptosis, traumatic ptosis, neurogenic ptosis (oculomotor nerve palsy), Horner syndrome.

▶ Complications

Amblyopia

▶ Treatment

Children with ptosis should be monitored for development of amblyopia. They may require correction of refractive error. Surgical correction is indicated for moderate to severe ptosis. Generally, surgery is delayed until preschool age when most of the facial growth has occurred, but it can be considered earlier in the presence of amblyopia or severe chin-up position.

▶ Prognosis

The prognosis depends on the presence of amblyopia and whether it is adequately treated.

HORNER SYNDROME

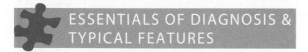

ESSENTIALS OF DIAGNOSIS & TYPICAL FEATURES

▶ Horner syndrome, which may be congenital or acquired, presents with signs of unequal pupils (anisocoria), eyelid ptosis, and anhidrosis.

▶ Pathogenesis

The syndrome is caused by an abnormality or lesion to the sympathetic chain. Most cases of pediatric Horner syndrome are idiopathic or caused by trauma. Acquired cases may occur in children who have had cardiothoracic surgery, trauma, neoplasm, or brainstem vascular malformation. Most worrisome is a Horner syndrome caused by neuroblastoma of the sympathetic chain in the apical lung region.

▶ Clinical Findings

Parents may notice unequal pupils or different colored eyes. Penlight examination of the eyes may reveal anisocoria and eyelid ptosis of the affected eye.

The affected pupil is smaller in size and the difference is most pronounced in the dark as the problems lies in poor dilation due to sympathetic dysfunction. Ptosis is usually mild with a well-defined upper lid crease. The whole eye may appear smaller due the smaller palpebral fissure from upper lid ptosis and lower lid elevation (lower lid also has sympathetic innervation). A key finding of *congenital* Horner syndrome is iris heterochromia, with the lighter colored iris on the affected side (Figure 16–14). Anhidrosis can occur in congenital and acquired cases. Of note, not all of the three signs must be present to make the diagnosis.

Pharmacologic assessment of the pupils with topical cocaine and hydroxyamphetamine will help determine whether Horner syndrome is due to a preganglionic or postganglionic lesion of the sympathetic chain, but these drugs are difficult to obtain in a clinical setting. Use of apraclonidine may be more practical, but its use is limited in pediatric population as it can lead to lethargy and bradycardia. Physical examination, including palpation of the neck and abdomen for masses, should be performed. The need for an extensive evaluation for neuroblastoma (urinary catecholamine test, MRI of the brain, neck, chest, abdomen, and abdominal ultrasound) in children with isolated Horner syndrome remains controversial as many studies show that isolated Horner syndrome is an unlikely sign of "occult" neuroblastoma, and sedation and gadolinium involved in MRI are not without risk. Further evaluation of children with Horner syndrome is recommended for suspicious cases without a history of trauma, surgery, or pneumonia, in the presence of other signs or symptoms of neuroblastoma.

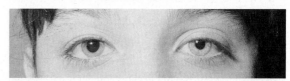

▲ **Figure 16–14.** Congenital Horner syndrome. Ptosis, miosis, and heterochromia. Lighter colored iris is on the affected left side.

Differential Diagnosis

Congenital or neurogenic ptosis and physiologic anisocoria.

Complications

Prognosis depends on the etiology. Ptosis associated with Horner syndrome is usually mild and rarely results in amblyopia.

Treatment

Management of any underlying disease is required. The ptosis and vision should be monitored by an ophthalmologist.

Prognosis

Prognosis depends on the etiology. The vision is usually normal.

Ben SA, Ash S, Luckman J, Toledano H, Goldeberg-Cohen N: Likelihood of diagnosing neuroblastoma in isolated Horner syndrome. J Neuroophthalmol 2019;39(3):308–312. doi: 10. 1097/WNO.0000000000000764 [PMID: 30801444].

EYELID TICS

Eyelid tics may occur as a transient phenomenon lasting several days to months. Although a tic may be an isolated finding in an otherwise healthy child, it may also occur in children with multiple tics, attention-deficit/hyperactivity disorder, or Tourette syndrome. Caffeine consumption may cause or exacerbate eyelid tics. If the disorder is a short-lived annoyance, no treatment is needed.

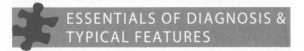

▼ DISORDERS OF THE NASOLACRIMAL SYSTEM

NASOLACRIMAL DUCT OBSTRUCTION

> ### 🧩 ESSENTIALS OF DIAGNOSIS & TYPICAL FEATURES
>
> ▶ Nasolacrimal duct obstruction (NLDO) occurs in up to 20% of infants < 1 year.
>
> ▶ Most cases (> 90%) clear spontaneously during the first year.

Pathogenesis

Congenital NLDO occurs from mechanical obstruction located distally at the valve of Hasner. Nasolacrimal obstruction is more commonly seen in individuals with craniofacial abnormalities or Down syndrome.

Prevention

Not applicable.

Clinical Findings

Nasolacrimal duct obstruction can be unilateral, bilateral, and asymmetric in severity. Signs and symptoms include tearing (epiphora) or mucoid discharge from the affected eye(s), especially in the morning (Figure 16–15). The conjunctiva is usually white and quiet, distinguishing it from infectious conjunctivitis. The eyelid skin can become irritated from constant wetness or dabbing. Fluorescein dye disappearance test can evaluate the clearance of dye from the tear meniscus in both eyes over a 5-minute period.

Differential Diagnosis

The differential diagnosis of tearing includes congenital glaucoma, foreign bodies, nasal disorders, and, in older children, allergies. Light sensitivity and blepharospasm suggest possible congenital glaucoma and warrant an urgent ophthalmic referral.

Complications

Dacryocystitis, orbital cellulitis, higher prevalence of anisometropic amblyopia has been demonstrated in children with congenital NLDO.

Treatment

Massage over the nasolacrimal sac may empty debris from the nasolacrimal sac and clear the obstruction, although the efficacy of massage in clearing nasolacrimal obstruction is debated. Use of topical antibiotics should be reserved only

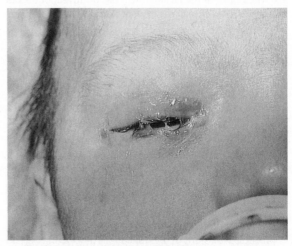

▲ **Figure 16–15.** Nasolacrimal obstruction, right eye. Mattering on upper and lower lids.

for concurrent signs of conjunctivitis or dacryocystitis as there is no evidence that it affects resolution of NLDO and can also promote overgrowth of resistant flora that can cause chronic NLD infection.

The mainstay of surgical treatment is probing, which has 75%–80% success rate. In general, probing is recommended for children older than 12 months and under general anesthesia. Other surgical procedures include infraction of the inferior nasal turbinate and balloon dilation. Silicone tube intubation may be necessary if probing fails in older children or those with craniofacial abnormalities or Down syndrome. Much less often, dacryocystorhinostomy is required.

► Prognosis

Generally good with surgical treatment.

Vagge A et al: Congenital nasolacrimal duct obstruction (CNLDO): a review. Diseases 2018 Dec;6(4):96. doi: 10.3390/diseases6040096 [PMID: 30360371].

CONGENITAL DACRYOCYSTOCELE

ESSENTIALS OF DIAGNOSIS & TYPICAL FEATURES

► Congenital dacryocystocele (CDC) presents as a bluish mass located below the medial canthus.

► This entity is different from regular congenital NLD obstruction and is associated with high rates of acute dacryocystitis and intranasal cysts, and warrants urgent ophthalmology and ENT referral.

► Pathogenesis

CDC is thought to result from obstructions proximal and distal to the nasolacrimal sac.

► Clinical Findings

CDC presents in the neonatal period with the majority within the first 10 days of life. It is most often a unilateral (80%) bluish mass lesion, which may or may not be compressible, and can displace the medial canthus superiorly (Figure 16–16). Not all patients have associated epiphora/discharge. More than one-half can be associated with intranasal cysts that can cause respiratory distress and feeding difficulties. Therefore, nasal endoscopic examination should be performed in all cases of CDC. Infection (dacryocystitis) can develop in up to 85%, usually in the first 1–2 weeks of life, and can progress to orbital cellulitis and sepsis. Typically, CDCs are not associated with any syndromes or congenital anomalies.

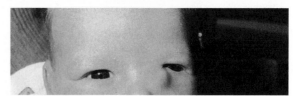

▲ **Figure 16–16.** Congenital dacryocystocele on the left side. Raised, bluish discolored mass of enlarged nasolacrimal sac. Note superiorly displaced medial canthus.

► Differential Diagnosis

Eyelid hemangioma, encephalocele, and meningoencephalocele (these are usually located above the medial canthus).

► Complications

Dacryocystitis, orbital cellulitis, sepsis, respiratory distress, feeding difficulties.

► Treatment

All patients with CDC should be referred to an ophthalmologist urgently due to the high risk of infection and possible need for surgical intervention. In the meantime, parents can perform massage as long as there are no signs of respiratory distress. Nasolacrimal duct probing and endoscopic marsupialization of the intranasal cyst under general anesthesia are often required. For treatment of dacryocystitis, hospital admission and use of systemic antibiotics are advised prior to probing in order to monitor respiratory status and reduce the rate of probing-induced bacteremia. Consultation with an ENT specialist is recommended to aid in the diagnosis and treatment of an associated intranasal cyst.

► Prognosis

Generally good.

Singh S, Ali MJ: Congenital dacryocystocele: a major review. Ophthalmic Plast Reconstr Surg 2019;35:309–317. doi: 10.1097/IOP.0000000000001297 [PMID: 30601463].

DACRYOCYSTITIS

ESSENTIALS OF DIAGNOSIS & TYPICAL FEATURES

► Dacryocystitis is an infection of the nasolacrimal sac that causes erythema and edema over the nasolacrimal sac.

Pathogenesis

Acute dacryocystitis is most commonly caused by *S aureus* followed by *Streptococcus pneumoniae*, and *Haemophilus* species. Rare causes of fungal or viral infections have been reported. Pediatric acute dacryocystitis can be categorized into four groups that are managed differently: acute dacryocystitis in neonates with dacryocystocele, dacryocystitis with periorbital cellulitis, dacryocystitis post facial trauma, and dacryocystitis associated with orbital abscess.

Prevention

Treatment of nasolacrimal duct obstruction.

Clinical Findings

Acute dacryocystitis presents with inflammation, swelling, tenderness, and pain over the lacrimal sac (located inferior to the medial canthal tendon). Fever may be present. The infection may point externally (Figure 16–17). A purulent discharge within the lacrimal sac may reflux with sac pressure.

Chronic dacryocystitis and recurrent episodes of low-grade dacryocystitis are caused by nasolacrimal obstruction.

Differential Diagnosis

Dacryocystocele and preseptal cellulitis.

Complications

Preseptal cellulitis, orbital cellulitis, and sepsis.

Treatment

Management of acute dacryocystitis depends on the category. All acute types will require systemic antibiotics. Dacryocystitis associated with dacryocystocele in neonates are managed by probing with or without marsupialization of intranasal cysts. Dacryocystitis with periorbital cellulitis is treated with probing after the acute episode. Those that occur from facial trauma often require dacryocystorhinostomy (DCR) with stents. Those complicated by orbital

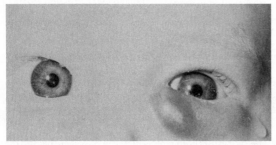

▲ **Figure 16–17.** Acute dacryocystitis in an 11-week-old infant.

abscess require simultaneous abscess drainage with probing and stent placement.

Warm compresses are beneficial to help express discharge from the lacrimal sac.

Prognosis

Generally good.

Ali MJ: Pediatric acute dacryocystitis. Ophthal Plast Reconstr Surg 2015 Sep–Oct;31(5):341–347. doi: 10.1097/IOP.0000000000000472 [PMID: 25856337].

▼ DISEASES OF THE CONJUNCTIVA

Conjunctivitis may be infectious, allergic, or associated with systemic disease. In conjunctivitis, the eye becomes red as a result of dilation of blood vessels. Edema can accumulate leading to *chemosis*, a boggy appearance of conjunctiva. When eyelids are everted, there can be a papillary or follicular reaction of the palpebral conjunctiva. In *papillary* reaction, the palpebral conjunctiva has a cobblestoning appearance with large nodules with central vessel core. *Follicular* reaction causes dome-shaped, gel-like nodules surrounding surrounded at its base by vessels.

Trauma and intraocular inflammation can cause injection of conjunctival vessels that can be confused with conjunctivitis.

OPHTHALMIA NEONATORUM

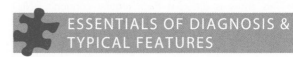

ESSENTIALS OF DIAGNOSIS & TYPICAL FEATURES

▶ Ophthalmia neonatorum (conjunctivitis in the newborn) occurs during the first month of life.

Pathogenesis

Pathogenesis may be due to bacterial infection (gonococcal, staphylococcal, pneumococcal, or chlamydial) or viral infection. In developed countries, *Chlamydia* is the most common cause. Neonatal conjunctivitis may lead to rapid corneal perforation if caused by *Neisseria gonorrhoeae*. Herpes simplex is a rare but serious cause of neonatal conjunctivitis.

Prevention

Treatment of maternal infections prior to delivery can prevent ophthalmia neonatorum. Although no single prophylactic medication can eliminate all cases of neonatal conjunctivitis, povidone-iodine may provide broader coverage against the organisms causing this disease. Silver nitrate is not effective against *Chlamydia* and can cause chemical

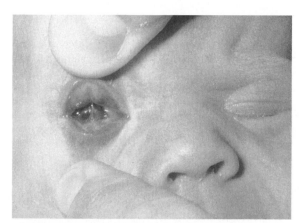

▲ **Figure 16–18.** Ophthalmia neonatorum due to *Chlamydia trachomatis* infection in a 2-week-old infant. Note marked lid and conjunctival inflammation.

conjunctivitis. The choice of prophylactic agent is often dictated by local epidemiology and cost considerations, but erythromycin ophthalmic ointment is most often routinely administered immediately after birth to help prevent ophthalmia neonatorum.

▶ Clinical Findings

Ophthalmia neonatorum is characterized by redness, discharge, and swelling of the lids and conjunctiva (Figure 16–18). *N gonorrhoeae* causes severe purulence with pseudomembrane formation and can rapidly lead to corneal perforation. Gram staining with cultures and PCR amplification for *Chlamydia trachomatis*, *N gonorrhoeae*, and HSV aid in making an etiologic diagnosis. Neonates may have systemic manifestations of disease.

▶ Differential Diagnosis

Chemical/toxic conjunctivitis, viral conjunctivitis, bacterial conjunctivitis.

▶ Complications

Chlamydia can cause a delayed-onset pneumonitis. Gonococcal infections can cause blindness through corneal perforation and can cause sepsis.

▶ Treatment

Treatment for ophthalmia neonatorum is shown in Table 16–3. Parents should be examined and receive treatment when a sexually associated pathogen is present. They need close monitoring by an ophthalmologist due to the risk of corneal involvement that can lead to permanent vision loss.

▶ Prognosis

Prognosis depends on the infectious agent as well as the rapidity of treatment.

BACTERIAL CONJUNCTIVITIS

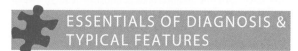

ESSENTIALS OF DIAGNOSIS & TYPICAL FEATURES

▶ In general, bacterial conjunctivitis is accompanied by a significant purulent discharge.

▶ Pathogenesis

Common bacterial causes of conjunctivitis in children include *Haemophilus* species, *S pneumoniae*, *Moraxella catarrhalis*, and *S aureus*.

▶ Prevention

Hand-washing and contact precautions.

▶ Clinical Findings

Presence of significant discharge helps distinguish bacterial from viral conjunctivitis. Regional lymphadenopathy is not

Table 16–3. Features and treatment of ophthalmia neonatorum.

Cause	Typical Onset	Features	Topical Treatment	Systemic Treatment
Chlamydia	5–14 days after birth	Mucoid discharge	Erythromycin 4 times daily × 14 days	Erythromycin or azithromycin
Gonorrhea	2–4 days after birth	Hyperpurulent discharge, corneal perforation	Saline lavage, erythromycin	Ceftriaxone or cefotaxime
HSV	4–21 days after birth	Mucoid discharge, corneal involvement	Ganciclovir gel	Acyclovir
Chemical	1 day after birth	Redness, lid swelling	Lubricants	

a common finding in bacterial conjunctivitis except in cases of oculoglandular syndrome due to *S aureus*, group A β-hemolytic streptococci, *Mycobacterium tuberculosis* or atypical mycobacteria, *Francisella tularensis*, and *Bartonella henselae*. Chlamydia serotypes A and C cause trachoma with severe follicular reaction of tarsal conjunctiva that can lead to scarring (Arlt's line), limbal follicles (Herbert pits), and eventual cicatrization of cornea. Chlamydial D through K causes inclusion conjunctivitis, a unilateral chronic follicular form seen in sexually active adolescents.

▶ Differential Diagnosis

Viral, allergic, traumatic, or chemical/toxic conjunctivitis.

▶ Complications

Bacterial conjunctivitis is usually self-limited unless caused by *C trachomatis*, *N gonorrhoeae*, and *N meningitidis*, which may have systemic manifestations and can lead to ocular complications without treatment.

▶ Treatment

If conjunctivitis is not associated with systemic illness, topical antibiotics such as polymyxin/trimethoprim sulfate or fluoroquinolones may be helpful in hastening the resolution of symptoms. Using a delayed treatment strategy (waiting 3 days for spontaneous improvement) before use of antibiotics may prevent unnecessary medication. Systemic therapy in addition to topical treatment is recommended for conjunctivitis associated with *C trachomatis*, *N gonorrhoeae*, and *N meningitidis*.

▶ Prognosis

Generally good.

Alfonso SA, Fawley JD, Alexa Lu X: Conjunctivitis. Prim Care 2015 Sep;42(3):325–345. doi: 10.1016/j.pop.2015.05.001 [PMID: 26319341].
Chen FV, Chang TC, Cavuoto KM: Patient demographic and microbiology trends in bacterial conjunctivitis in children. J AAPOS 2018;22:66–67 [PMID: 29247795].

VIRAL CONJUNCTIVITIS

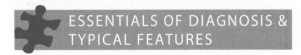

ESSENTIALS OF DIAGNOSIS & TYPICAL FEATURES

▶ Children with viral conjunctivitis usually present with injection of the conjunctiva of one or both eyes and watery ocular discharge.

▶ Pathogenesis

Adenovirus infection is often associated with pharyngitis, a follicular reaction of the palpebral conjunctiva, and preauricular adenopathy (pharyngoconjunctival fever). Epidemics of adenoviral keratoconjunctivitis occur. Less commonly, acute hemorrhagic conjunctivitis due to Coxsackievirus or enterovirus can present with extensive subconjunctival hemorrhage and injection. Other causes include measles, Zika virus, HSV, and varicella-zoster virus (VZV).

▶ Prevention

Hand-washing and contact precautions.

▶ Clinical Findings

Watery discharge associated with conjunctival injection of one or both eyes. Significant eyelid edema can occur. Enlarged preauricular lymph nodes can be present. A vesicular rash involving the eyelids or face suggests HSV or herpes zoster (unilateral).

▶ Differential Diagnosis

Bacterial, allergic, traumatic, or chemical/toxic conjunctivitis.

▶ Complications

Generally, viral conjunctivitis is self-limited. Cornea involvement in epidemic keratoconjunctivitis may prolong the course of disease. Herpes conjunctivitis may be associated with keratitis or retinal involvement.

▶ Treatment

Treatment of adenovirus conjunctivitis is supportive. Children with presumed adenoviral keratoconjunctivitis are considered contagious 10–21 days from the day of onset or as long as the eyes are red. They should stay out of school and group activities until redness and tearing resolve. Strict hand-washing precautions are recommended. In severe cases with cornea involvement, a short course of topical steroids can improve the symptoms. However, steroids can also prolong the duration of disease. Steroids should only be used when it is certain that HSV is not the cause.

Herpes conjunctivitis can be treated with topical or oral antivirals (see section Viral Keratitis).

▶ Prognosis

Generally good.

ALLERGIC CONJUNCTIVITIS

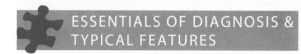

ESSENTIALS OF DIAGNOSIS & TYPICAL FEATURES

► Allergic conjunctivitis causes itching associated with redness, tearing, and papillary reaction of palpebral conjunctiva.

► It is commonly seen with allergic rhinitis and asthma

▶ Prevention

Decrease exposure to allergens.

▶ Clinical Findings

The history of itchy, watery, and red eyes is essential in making the diagnosis of allergic conjunctivitis. Allergic "shiners" or dark circles under eyes can be present. Atopic keratoconjunctivitis (AKC) can cause year-round symptoms. Vernal keratoconjunctivitis (VKC), which is similar to AKC but occurs more often in the spring and summer (75%), is associated with intense tearing, itching, and a stringy discharge. VKC is more common in males, usually in the first decade of life, and may present with giant cobblestone papillae (Figure 16–19) on the tarsal conjunctiva, Horner-Trantas dots (white accumulation of degenerated eosinophils and epithelial cells at corneal limbus), phlyctenules (nodular inflammation on conjunctiva or cornea), and even sterile corneal ulcers (shield ulcers) due to rubbing of the giant papillae against the corneal surface. Contact lens wear may induce a giant papillary conjunctivitis that appears similar to the palpebral form of vernal conjunctivitis.

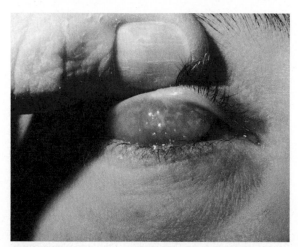

▲ **Figure 16–19.** Vernal conjunctivitis. Cobblestone papillae in superior tarsal conjunctiva.

▶ Treatment

Topical ophthalmic solutions that combine both an antihistamine and mast cell stabilizer are very effective at treating allergic conjunctivitis. Table 16–4 lists the various combinations available for treatment of allergic conjunctivitis. Corticosteroids should be used with caution because their extended use causes glaucoma or cataracts and requires close follow-up with an ophthalmologist. Topical antibiotics are used to prevent secondary infections in those with shield ulcers. Systemic antihistamines and limitation of exposure to allergens may help reduce symptoms and are important part of the treatment, especially for AKC.

▶ Prognosis

Generally good but inadequate treatment and poor follow-up can result in corneal scarring and permanently decreased vision.

MUCOCUTANEOUS DISEASES

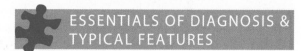

ESSENTIALS OF DIAGNOSIS & TYPICAL FEATURES

► Stevens-Johnson syndrome (SJS) and toxic epidermal necrolysis (TEN) are systemic conditions that often affect the eyes, as well as the skin, oral, and genitourinary mucosa.

► Ocular involvement may result in permanent conjunctival scarring, eyelid malposition, severe dry eye syndrome, and permanent vision loss. Early intervention is key to preventing ocular complications.

▶ Pathogenesis

SJS/TEN is a spectrum of serious delayed-type hypersensitivity reaction to drugs. Recently, a separate pattern of mucocutaneous eruptions associated with *Mycoplasma pneumoniae* infection, called mycoplasma-induced rash and mucositis (MIRM), has been described. These mucocutaneous conditions can have ocular involvement with potential permanent and serious ocular complications.

▶ Clinical Findings

Eye involvement can vary in severity from self-limited mild conjunctivitis to sloughing of the entire mucosal surface. Intense inflammation can lead to formation of pseudomembrane, frank membrane, and corneal ulceration. Conjunctival ulceration can result in fusion of bulbar and forniceal surfaces leading to permanent symblepharon (adhesions

Table 16–4. Common ocular allergy medications.

Generic Name	Brand Name	Side Effects	Dosage
Mast cell stabilizer			
Lodoxamide tromethamine 0.1%	Alomide	Transient burning or stinging	1 drop 4 times daily—taper
Cromolyn Na 4%	Crolom, Opticrom	Transient burning or stinging	1 drop 1–4 times daily
Nedocromil	Alocril	Bitter tasting, nasal congestion (10%)	1 drop 1–2 times daily
Pemirolast potassium	Alamast	Burning, nasal congestion (10%)	
Antihistamines			
Emedastine difumarate	Emadine	Headache	1 drop 1–4 times daily
Levocabastine HCL 0.05%	Livostin	Headache, burning	1 drop 1–4 times daily
H1–Antihistamines/Mast cell stabilizer combination			
Olopatadine	Patanol, Pataday	Headache, burning or stinging	1 drop 1–2 times daily
Ketotifen	Zyrtec Eye, Claritin Eye	Redness, rhinitis	1 drop 3 times daily
Azelastine	Optivar	Burning, bitter taste	1 drop 2 times daily
Bepostastine	Bepreve	Bitter taste, headache	1 drop 2 times daily
Epinastine	Elestat	Cold symptoms	1 drop 2 times daily
Alcaftadine	Lastacaft	Burning, stinging	1–2 drops daily
Nonsteroidal anti-inflammatory			
Ketorolac tromethamine 0.5%	Acular	Transient burning or stinging	1 drop 4 times daily
Vasoconstrictor			
Naphazoline HCl 0.1%	AK-Con, Naphcon, Opcon, Vasocon	Mydriasis, increased redness, irritation, discomfort, punctate keratitis, increased intraocular pressure, dizziness, headache, nausea, nervousness, hypertension, weakness, cardiac effects, hyperglycemia, rebound redness	Varies by preparation

between conjunctiva), ankyloblepharon (adhesions between eyelids), and lid malposition. The extent of epithelial cell loss of ocular surface is visualized with fluorescein staining. Patients require daily examinations by ophthalmologists. The severity of ocular involvement may not correlate with systemic skin and mucocutaneous manifestations.

▶ **Differential Diagnosis**

Viral or bacterial conjunctivitis until the diagnosis of SJS/TEN is apparent.

▶ **Complications**

Severe ocular involvement can result in permanent scarring of the conjunctiva leading to eyelid malposition, trichiasis (misdirected eyelashes), and vision loss and blindness from chronic ocular irritation and extreme tear film deficiency.

▶ **Treatment**

Management of acute ocular SJS/TEN/MIRM involves controlling the intense ocular surface inflammation. Treatment of the underlying disease includes discontinuation of offending medications and use of appropriate antimicrobials as necessary. Aggressive ophthalmic treatment should be initiated as soon as possible, including use of lubrication, topical corticosteroids, topical cyclosporine, and topical antibiotics. Extensive sloughing requires urgent amniotic membrane transplants to the lid margins and conjunctiva within the first weeks of illness in order to prevent chronic ocular complications.

▶ **Prognosis**

Prognosis depends on the severity of the underlying condition. Visual prognosis can be excellent with early medical and surgical treatment.

Gregory DG: New grading system and treatment guidelines for the acute ocular manifestations of Stevens-Johnson syndrome. Ophthalmology 2016 Aug;123(8):1653–1658. doi: 10.1016/j .ophtha.2016.04.041 [PMID: 27297404].

▼ DISORDERS OF THE IRIS

IRIS COLOBOMA

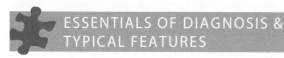

ESSENTIALS OF DIAGNOSIS & TYPICAL FEATURES

▶ Iris coloboma is a developmental defect due to incomplete closure of the anterior embryonal fissure.

▶ Iris coloboma may occur as an isolated defect or in association with various chromosomal abnormalities and syndromes.

▶ Clinical Findings

Penlight examination of the pupils reveals a keyhole shape to the pupil rather than the normal round configuration (Figure 16–20). A dilated examination by an ophthalmologist is necessary to determine if the coloboma involves additional structures of the eye including the optic nerve, retina, and choroid, in which case vision can be affected. A genetic evaluation is usually recommended due to the high rate of associated genetic syndromes.

▶ Differential Diagnosis

Anterior segment dysgenesis, aniridia, and previous iris trauma.

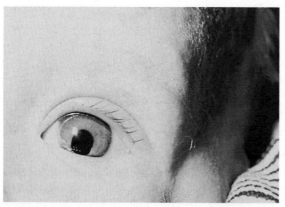

▲ **Figure 16–20.** Iris coloboma located inferiorly.

▶ Complications

Low vision and rarely a secondary retinal detachment from chorioretinal coloboma.

▶ Treatment

Patients with coloboma should be monitored by an ophthalmologist for signs of amblyopia, significant refractive errors, and strabismus.

▶ Prognosis

The prognosis depends on whether there are other ocular structures involved. VA is guarded if a large retinal coloboma is present.

ANIRIDIA

ESSENTIALS OF DIAGNOSIS & TYPICAL FEATURES

▶ Aniridia is a bilateral congenital disorder that affects all ocular tissue but most notably results in iris hypoplasia (Figure 16–21).

▶ Pathogenesis

Aniridia can occur in isolation without systemic involvement, due to PAX6 gene mutation, or as part of the Wilms tumor-aniridia-genitourinary anomalies-retardation (WAGR) syndrome, which is caused by deletion of 11p13, including PAX6 and adjacent WT1 locus. Two-thirds of cases are familial (autosomal dominant), and one-third are known to be sporadic. Sporadic cases are due to "de novo" mutations that subsequently are inherited in an autosomal dominant manner with variable expressivity. One-third of the sporadic cases are associated with WAGR syndrome.

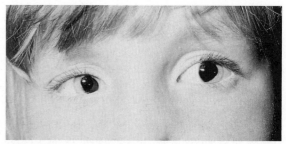

▲ **Figure 16–21.** Bilateral aniridia. Iris remnants present temporally in each eye.

Clinical Findings

Aniridia involves all ocular tissue and can manifest as iris hypoplasia, keratopathy, glaucoma, cataract, optic nerve hypoplasia (ONH), and foveal hypoplasia. If foveal hypoplasia is present, nystagmus is usually apparent by 6 weeks of age due to poor vision. Slit-lamp or penlight examinations reveal little to no visible iris (see Figure 16–21). Photophobia may be present. Glaucoma, cataracts, and keratopathy usually develop with time in teenage years or adulthood.

Differential Diagnosis

Microphthalmia, iris coloboma, and previous iris trauma.

Complications

Low vision, cataracts, glaucoma, keratopathy.

Treatment

An ophthalmologist should evaluate and treat refractive error as well as monitor for signs of cataracts and glaucoma. Abdominal ultrasonography is indicated in the sporadic form of aniridia to diagnose Wilms tumor. Referral to genetics is recommended unless there is clear family history of autosomal dominant aniridia.

Prognosis

Patients tend to have low vision.

ALBINISM

ESSENTIALS OF DIAGNOSIS & TYPICAL FEATURES

▶ Oculocutaneous albinism (OCA) is a heterogenous group of autosomal recessive disorders causing reduced or absent pigmentation of hair, skin, and eyes. Ocular albinism (OA) is an X-linked recessive disorder where hypopigmentation is limited to eyes only.

Pathogenesis

OCA is most often due to a defect in tyrosine conversion affecting pigment production. There are at least four types of OCA for which the clinical spectrum can vary from complete lack of pigmentation in OCA1A to milder forms where pigments can accumulate over time. OA, which represents 10% of all albinism, is due to a mutation in the *GPR143* gene whose protein product controls the number and size of melanosomes.

Clinical Findings

Iris, skin, and hair color vary with the type of albinism. Iris transillumination is abnormal transmission of light through an iris with decreased pigment. The iris can appear to be pink in color as the red fundus shows through the hypopigmented iris. This may be obvious or may require slit-lamp examination with retroillumination to detect focal areas of transillumination. Affected individuals usually have poor vision and nystagmus due to foveal hypoplasia. Other ocular abnormalities include abnormal optic pathway projections, strabismus, and poor stereoacuity.

Differential Diagnosis

Albinism may be associated with other systemic manifestations. Bleeding problems occur in individuals with Hermansky-Pudlak syndrome (chromosome 10q23 or 5q13), in which OCA is associated with a platelet abnormality. Chédiak-Higashi syndrome (chromosome 1q42–44) is characterized by neutrophil defects, recurrent infections, and OCA. Other conditions associated with albinism are Waardenburg, Prader-Willi, and Angelman syndromes.

Complications

Low vision, strabismus, high refractive errors, and visual field (VF) abnormalities.

Treatment

Children with albinism should be evaluated by a pediatric ophthalmologist in order to optimize their visual function. Vision teachers in schools and ophthalmic specialists trained in treating low-vision patients can improve the patient's ability to perform activities of daily living and function within society. Affected individuals should use sunscreen and protective clothing to prevent skin cancer.

Prognosis

Vision is subnormal in most individuals.

MISCELLANEOUS IRIS CONDITIONS

Heterochromia, or a difference in iris color, can occur in congenital Horner syndrome, after iritis, or with tumors and nevi of the iris. Lisch nodules, which occur in type 1 neurofibromatosis, usually become apparent by age 8 years. When seen on slit-lamp examination, Lisch nodules are 1–2 mm in diameter and often beige in color. Iris xanthogranuloma occurring with juvenile xanthogranuloma can cause hyphema and glaucoma. Patients with juvenile xanthogranuloma should be evaluated by an ophthalmologist for ocular involvement.

GLAUCOMA

ESSENTIALS OF DIAGNOSIS & TYPICAL FEATURES

▶ Pediatric glaucoma can be congenital or acquired, unilateral or bilateral.

▶ The classic triad of symptoms in primary congenital glaucoma (PCG) includes epiphora, photophobia, and blepharospasm.

Clinical Findings

Primary signs of PCG are buphthalmos and corneal clouding. Buphthalmos occurs from elevated eye pressure that lends to enlargement of the globe due to low scleral rigidity of an infant eye. Horizontal breaks in Descemet's membrane called Haab's striae can be visible in the cornea. Unlike in adults, optic nerve cupping may be reversible in children with lowering of eye pressure. In general, a red, inflamed eye is not typical of PCG.

Sudden eye pain, redness, corneal clouding, and vision loss suggest possible pupillary block or angle-closure glaucoma. Urgent referral to an ophthalmologist is indicated. Genetic evaluation should be completed if other systemic abnormalities are noted.

Glaucoma also occurs with ocular and systemic syndromes such as aniridia, anterior segment dysgenesis, Sturge-Weber syndrome, the oculocerebrorenal syndrome of Lowe, Weill-Marchesani syndrome, and the Pierre Robin syndrome. Glaucoma can be secondary to trauma, uveitis, lens dislocation, intraocular tumor, and retinal disorders.

Differential Diagnosis

Buphthalmos is glaucoma until proven otherwise. Nasolacrimal duct obstruction can cause tearing, but other signs of blepharospasm and photophobia are absent.

Treatment

Treatment depends on the cause, but surgery is often indicated. Topical medications have limited success in pediatric glaucoma but can be used as temporizing measures until the time of surgery. Treatment of refractive error and amblyopia is essential.

Prognosis

In general, the prognosis is guarded although excellent results can be seen. Patients may require multiple surgeries to achieve adequate eye pressure control.

Yu Chan JY, Choy BN, Ng AL, Shum JW: Review on the management of primary congenital glaucoma. J Curr Glaucoma Pract 2015 Sep–Dec;9(3):92–99. doi: 10.5005/jp-journals-10008-1192 [PMID: 26997844].

UVEITIS

Inflammation of the uveal tract can be subdivided according to the uveal tissue primarily involved (iris, choroid, or retina) or by location (anterior, intermediate, or posterior uveitis). The most commonly diagnosed form of uveitis in childhood is traumatic iridocyclitis or iritis.

ANTERIOR UVEITIS/IRIDOCYCLITIS/IRITIS

ESSENTIALS OF DIAGNOSIS & TYPICAL FEATURES

▶ Anterior uveitis (iritis or iridocyclitis) can present with redness, photophobia, and blurred vision.

▶ These symptoms may be absent despite severe ocular inflammation in children with juvenile idiopathic arthritis (JIA).

Pathogenesis

Approximately 10%–20% of children with JIA are at risk for uveitis. Those with positive antinuclear antibodies are young at arthritis diagnosis (6 years old or younger), and early in their disease course (≤ 4 years), they are considered at highest risk and are recommended to be screened by an ophthalmologist every 3 months. Uveitis is also a common extra-articular manifestation of ankylosing spondylitis (10%–15%). It is less common in association with inflammatory bowel disease (IBD) or psoriatic arthritis (2%–7%). Other causes of anterior uveitis in children include trauma and infection. A substantial percentage of cases are of unknown origin.

Clinical Findings

Injection, photophobia, pain, and blurred vision usually accompany anterior uveitis. An exception to this is iritis associated with JIA (see Chapter 29). The eye in such cases is quiet and asymptomatic, but slit-lamp examination reveals anterior chamber inflammation with inflammatory cells and protein flare. JIA-associated uveitis is often bilateral but can be asymmetric. HLA-B27–associated uveitis is usually unilateral and recurrent. Uveitis associated with IBD tends to be bilateral and also have vitritis. Children with JIA should be screened according to a schedule recommended by the AAP (http://www.aap.org).

Other findings include band keratopathy (calcium deposits on the cornea as a result of chronic inflammation), keratic precipitates (seen on the endothelium of cornea), posterior synechiae (iris adhesions to the lens often causing irregular shaped pupil), and iris nodules. Severe anterior uveitis can also result in vitritis and panuveitis.

Posterior subcapsular cataracts can develop in patients with ocular inflammation. Many of these patients have been taking corticosteroids as part of the long-term treatment of their autoimmune disease, which can contribute to cataract formation.

▶ Differential Diagnosis

Trauma, infection, autoimmune disorders, medications, and masquerade syndromes such as RB and juvenile xanthogranuloma. Tubulointerstitial nephritis and uveitis (TINU) is a rare cause of bilateral anterior uveitis seen in children. Early-onset sarcoidosis and Blau syndrome are also rare causes of uveitis in children.

▶ Complications

Cataract and glaucoma can develop due to severe inflammation but also due to corticosteroid treatment. Other complications include band keratopathy, cyclitic membranes, optic nerve and retinal edema, and permanent decreased vision.

▶ Treatment

Topical or periocular corticosteroids are used to control the inflammation. Cycloplegic agents help release and prevent iris adhesion to the lens and also reduce ciliary muscle spasm that causes photophobia and eye pain. Depending on the etiology, systemic immunosuppressive agents may be needed. Methotrexate is the most commonly used systemic therapy for children. Other options include anti-TNFα agents and T-cell inhibitors for refractory cases.

▶ Prognosis

Prognosis depends on the severity of ocular inflammation, development of cataracts, and secondary glaucoma.

Angeles-Han ST, Rabinovich CE: Uveitis in children. Curr Opin Rheumatol 2016 Sep;28(5):544–549. doi: 10.1097/BOR.0000000000000316 [PMID: 27328333].

Ozdal PC, Berker N, Tugal-Tutkun I: Pars Planitis: epidemiology, clinical characteristics, management and visual prognosis. J Ophthalmic Vis Res 2015 Oct–Dec;10(4):469–480. doi: 10.4103/2008-322X.176897 [PMID: 27051493].

Rosenbaum JT: Uveitis in spondyloarthritis including psoriatic arthritis, ankylosing spondylitis, and inflammatory bowel disease. Clin Rheumatol 2015 Jun;34(6):999–1002. doi: 10.1007/s10067-015-2960-8 [PMID: 25953065].

POSTERIOR UVEITIS

ESSENTIALS OF DIAGNOSIS & TYPICAL FEATURES

▶ The terms *choroiditis*, *retinitis*, and *retinochoroiditis* denote the tissue layers primarily involved in posterior uveitis. Infectious agents are the most common cause of posterior uveitis in the pediatric population.

▶ Clinical Findings

Children with posterior uveitis may have both acute inflammation and chronic chorioretinal changes. Fundus examination by an ophthalmologist and serologic testing are used to identify or rule out the causes of posterior uveitis.

A granular "salt and pepper" retinopathy can be seen in congenital chorioretinitis due to TORCH complex (toxoplasmosis, rubella, CMV, HSV, syphilis). With congenital infections, they often have systemic manifestations including deafness, skin and bony lesions, CNS disease with developmental delay, and cardiac abnormalities.

Ocular toxoplasmosis (see Chapter 43) is the most common cause of pediatric posterior uveitis. Active toxoplasmosis produces a white lesion appearing as a "headlight in the fog" owing to the overlying vitritis. Inactive lesions have a hyperpigmented border. Classically, reactivation of the infection is characterized by new white lesions (satellite lesions) adjacent to an old atrophic scar with hyperpigmentation.

Although rare, acute retinal necrosis is a serious vaso-occlusive necrotizing retinitis that can be caused by HSV-1 and 2, VZV, and rarely by CMV. It is seen in immunocompetent patients and characterized by circumferentially advancing peripheral white necrotic lesions, vitritis, and vasculitis. Necrosis leads to retinal atrophy that can result in rhegmatogenous and tractional retinal detachment in up to 75% of cases. Patients may present with vision loss or a red and painful eye.

CMV infection is the most common cause of retinitis in immune compromised children, especially those with hematopoietic stem cell transplantation or human immunodeficiency virus (HIV) infection. CMV retinitis appears as a white retinal lesion, typically but not always associated with hemorrhage, or as a granular, indolent-appearing lesion with hemorrhage and a white periphery.

Ocular candidiasis/endogenous endophthalmitis typically occurs in an immunocompromised host or a low-birth-weight premature infant in the intensive care nursery receiving hyperalimentation. Candidal chorioretinitis appears as multifocal, whitish yellow, fluffy retinal lesions that may spread into the vitreous and produce a so-called cotton or fungus ball vitritis.

In toddlers and young children, *Toxocara canis* or *Toxocara cati* infections (ocular larva migrans; see Chapter 43) occur from ingesting soil contaminated with parasite eggs. The disease is usually unilateral. Presenting features include unilateral blurriness, strabismus, leukocoria, and photophobia. The anterior segment is usually white and quiet. Posterior segment may show localized granulomas that are seen as a white, hazy mass that may be peripheral or in the posterior pole. Peripheral lesions may have inflammatory vitreous membranes that extend from the granuloma to the optic nerve, forming characteristic retinal folds and traction. Vitritis and nematode endophthalmitis can be present. Diagnosis is based on the appearance of the lesion and serologic testing using ELISA for *T canis* and *T cati* (see Chapter 43).

▶ Differential Diagnosis

Posterior uveitis due to autoimmune disorder, trauma, infection, malignancy, or idiopathic etiology.

▶ Complications

Permanent vision loss due to retinal scarring and detachment.

▶ Treatment

Treatment of acute retinal necrosis includes antiviral medication, corticosteroids, and prophylactic laser. The goal is rapid recovery of disease and prevention of fellow eye involvement as well as complication. Congenital toxoplasmosis infections must be treated with systemic antimicrobials (see Chapter 43). Ophthalmic and neurologic outcomes are improved with prolonged treatment. Treatment of toxocariasis includes periocular corticosteroid injections and vitrectomy. The benefit of anthelminthic medications, such as albendazole, thiabendazole, and mebendazole, is not well established, as they can worsen the inflammatory response as the larvae die.

▶ Prognosis

The prognosis for vision depends on the severity of retinal and systemic involvement.

INTERMEDIATE UVEITIS

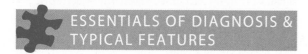

ESSENTIALS OF DIAGNOSIS & TYPICAL FEATURES

▶ Intermediate uveitis or pars planitis is inflammation located in the far anterior periphery of the retina and vitreous base.

▶ Clinical Findings

The term "intermediate uveitis" describes inflammation of the anterior vitreous, ciliary body, and peripheral retina which may or may not be associated with infection or systemic disease. The term "pars planitis" is a particular subset (85%–95%) of intermediate uveitis associated with characteristic snowbank and snowball formation in the absence of an infectious or systemic disease. Intermediate uveitis accounts for 5%–27% of pediatric uveitis.

Pars planitis has a bimodal age distribution and affects both children (5–15 years) and adults (20–40 years). It is most commonly bilateral and can be asymmetric. Patients can follow three clinical courses: 10% self-limiting, benign course; 31% smoldering course with few episodes of exacerbation; or prolonged course without exacerbations. Pars planitis may "burn out" after 5–15 years.

Most common clinical symptoms are blurry vision and floaters. Less commonly, patients can have red eye, photophobia, or pain. Some are asymptomatic and are diagnosed incidentally on routine eye examination. A dilated examination is crucial to identifying vitritis and inflammation along the pars plana (snowballs and snowbanking).

▶ Differential Diagnosis

Intermediate uveitis is most often idiopathic. It is important to rule out infectious causes. Noninfectious etiologies such as JIA, sarcoidosis, Blau syndrome, and neoplasms should be considered. Intermediated uveitis can be associated with multiple sclerosis (MS).

▶ Complications

Although it is most often a benign entity, it can potentially be a blinding disease due to complications including macula edema, optic nerve edema, cataract and vitreous opacities, or hemorrhage. The most common cause of decreased vision is from macular edema.

▶ Treatment

Treatment is topical or periocular steroid injections, systemic steroids, and systemic immunosuppression. Vitrectomy by a retinal surgeon may be needed in refractory cases.

▶ Prognosis

Prognosis depends on the severity of the disease and secondary complications. Younger children often have worse prognosis due to delayed detection and development of amblyopia.

DISORDERS OF THE CORNEA

CLOUDY CORNEA

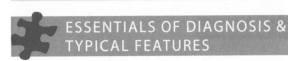

ESSENTIALS OF DIAGNOSIS & TYPICAL FEATURES

► Corneal clouding can be caused by developmental abnormalities, metabolic disorders, trauma, and infection.

Clinical Findings

The cornea may have a white, hazy appearance on penlight examination. Findings can be unilateral or bilateral. The red reflex may be decreased or absent.

Differential Diagnosis

Corneal clouding, tearing, blepharospasm, and photophobia in a newborn are signs of congenital glaucoma until proven otherwise. Peter anomaly and sclerocornea are congenital malformations of the anterior segment of the eye that can be unilateral or bilateral. Direct trauma to the cornea during a forceps delivery can result in corneal haze, scarring, and significant amblyopia. Systemic abnormalities, such as developmental delay and liver or kidney failure, associated with cloudy cornea, suggest metabolic disorders such as mucopolysaccharidoses, Wilson disease, and cystinosis. Corneal infiltrates occur with viral infections, staphylococcal lid disease, and corneal dystrophies. Interstitial keratitis is a manifestation of congenital syphilis.

A complete ocular evaluation by an ophthalmologist is required and should be completed urgently when congenital glaucoma is suspected.

Complications

Amblyopia.

Treatment

Treatment depends on the underlying condition. Surgical treatment of glaucoma and possible corneal transplantation or keratoprosthesis may be required.

Prognosis

Prognosis depends on the amount of corneal involvement and response to surgical treatment. Corneal transplants have a very high frequency of rejection and subsequently a poor prognosis in children.

Fecarotta CM, Huang WW: Pediatric genetic disease of the cornea. J Pediatr Genet Dec 2014;3(4):195–207. doi: 10.3233/PGE-14102 [PMID: 27625877].

VIRAL KERATITIS

ESSENTIALS OF DIAGNOSIS & TYPICAL FEATURES

► A dendritic or branch-like pattern can be seen with fluorescein staining in herpetic keratitis.
► Children with HSV keratitis may not complain of eye pain due to decreased corneal sensation.

Clinical Findings

In the anterior segment, HSV can present as blepharoconjunctivitis, keratitis (epithelial, stromal or endothelial), and keratouveitis. Most often, children present with recurrent unilateral red eye with tearing, photophobia, and decreased vision. In epithelial keratitis, fluorescein administration will reveal areas of staining when viewed with a blue light. The pattern of epithelium staining may be dendritic or irregular and round if a geographic ulcer is present. In stromal keratitis, there is corneal haze, scarring, and neovascularization, usually without epithelial fluorescein staining. Stromal keratitis is more commonly seen in children than in adults due to increased inflammatory response. Recurrence is more common in children, especially with stromal keratitis. Up to 75% of children with herpes keratitis develop damage to corneal nerves leading to decreased corneal sensation and complications associated with neurotrophic cornea. Bilateral disease in adults has been associated with atopy and immune suppression, but this relationship remains unclear in children.

HZO is more commonly seen in adults but can present in children. It occurs with reactivation of VZV involving the ophthalmic branch of the trigeminal nerve and can affect the ocular structures anywhere from the conjunctiva to the optic nerve. In the cornea, punctate keratitis and pseudodendrites represent swollen, poorly adherent epithelial cells having a "stuck on" appearance. In contrast to HSV dendrites, these pseudodendrites lack terminal bulbs and dichotomous branching and stain poorly with fluorescein.

Adenovirus can cause bilateral epidemic keratoconjunctivitis with corneal subepithelial infiltrates (see section Viral Conjunctivitis). Adenovirus conjunctivitis may progress to keratitis 1–2 weeks after onset. Vision may be decreased.

Differential Diagnosis

BKC, allergic conjunctivitis.

Treatment

Oral acyclovir is a well-tolerated and effective treatment for children with herpes simplex infection. Topical treatment can also be helpful in refractory cases of acyclovir-resistant strains of HSV. For acute HZO, oral antiviral medication can be helpful when started within 72 hours of onset of disease. Topical antivirals for HZO are controversial. Topical steroids are used for the treatment of stromal keratitis with close monitoring by an ophthalmologist. Long-term prophylactic oral acyclovir is frequently employed in children with stromal keratitis or those with recurrence and continued for at least 1 year after the last recurrence.

In adenovirus keratoconjunctivitis, no treatment is necessary as it is most often self-limiting. However, judicious use of topical steroids can help decrease the symptoms (see section Viral Conjunctivitis).

▶ **Prognosis**

Recurrence of herpetic keratitis is common in children. Permanent vision loss due to scarring and amblyopia is common in children with HSV keratitis, occurring in more than 50% of affected children.

CORNEAL ULCERS

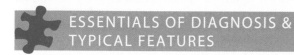

ESSENTIALS OF DIAGNOSIS & TYPICAL FEATURES

▶ Acute pain, decreased vision, injection, a white corneal infiltrate or ulcer (Figure 16–22), and hypopyon (pus in the anterior chamber) may be present.

▶ **Pathogenesis**

Most common risk of infectious keratitis and corneal ulcer is contact lens use, especially with extended wear, overnight use, orthokeratology, and using tap water for cleaning.

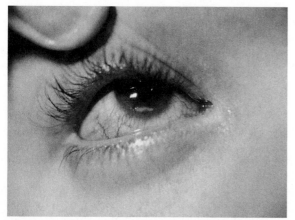

▲ **Figure 16–22.** Corneal ulcer. Note white infiltrate located on inferior cornea.

Common pathogens causing infectious keratitis are *Pseudomonas aeruginosa*, **staphylococci,** and *Acanthamoeba*. In children younger than 3 years, ocular trauma is a common cause of infectious corneal ulcers.

▶ **Clinical Findings**

Patients present with acute pain, photophobia, redness, and decreased vision. On examination, they have a white spot on the cornea with overlying epithelial defect that stains with fluorescein (see Figure 16–22). Other examination findings include corneal thinning, anterior chamber inflammation, and hypopyon. *Acanthamoeba* keratitis can cause unilateral or bilateral rapidly progressing ulcers with pain that seems out of proportion to exam findings.

▶ **Differential Diagnosis**

Viral keratitis, corneal abrasion, and penetrating foreign body.

▶ **Complications**

Corneal perforation and corneal scarring.

▶ **Treatment**

Treatment of corneal ulcers requires special expertise, and urgent referral to an ophthalmologist is necessary. It is helpful for patients to bring their contact lens and case, which can be used for culture.

▶ **Prognosis**

Prognosis depends on how large the ulcer is and whether the central cornea is involved.

▼ DISORDERS OF THE LENS

Lens disorders involve abnormality of clarity or position. Lens opacification (Figure 16–23) can affect vision depending on its density, size, and position. Visual potential is also influenced by age at onset and the success of amblyopia treatment.

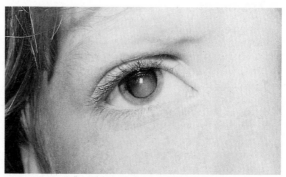

▲ **Figure 16–23.** Cataract causing leukocoria.

CATARACTS

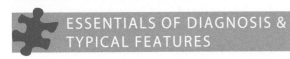

ESSENTIALS OF DIAGNOSIS & TYPICAL FEATURES

▶ Cataracts in children may be unilateral or bilateral, may exist as isolated defects, or may be accompanied by other ocular disorders or systemic disease (see Figure 16–23).

▶ Clinical Findings

Leukocoria, poor fixation, and strabismus or nystagmus may be the presenting complaints. Absence or asymmetry of a red reflex in the newborn may be due to a cataract, which requires an urgent referral to an ophthalmologist.

Bilateral congenital cataracts can be inherited in an autosomal dominant manner. If there is no family history of bilateral cataracts, laboratory investigation for infectious, genetic and metabolic causes of bilateral congenital cataracts is indicated. Such investigation would include serologic tests for TORCH infections, as well as evaluation for inborn metabolic errors, such as galactosemia or Lowe syndrome. Unilateral cataracts can be associated with other structural ocular abnormalities (persistent fetal vasculature), isolated and developmental (posterior or anterior polar cataracts) or secondary to tumor, uveitis, or trauma.

▶ Differential Diagnosis

Cloudy cornea, intraocular tumor, and retinal detachment.

▶ Complications

Pediatric cataracts are frequently associated with deprivation amblyopia.

▶ Treatment

Early diagnosis and treatment are necessary to prevent deprivation amblyopia in children younger than 9 years. Cataracts that are visually significant require removal. Visually significant unilateral cataracts in infants are removed prior to 6 weeks of age and bilateral cataracts within 8 weeks of age to reduce the risk of deprivation amblyopia. Rehabilitation of the vision will require the correction of refractive errors and amblyopia treatment. Contact lenses, glasses, bifocals, and artificial intraocular lenses are used to correct refractive errors after cataract extraction. Concomitant treatment of associated amblyopia, glaucoma, and the underlying systemic disease is indicated.

▶ Prognosis

The ultimate VA depends on the age when the cataract developed and was removed, whether it was unilateral or bilateral, whether it was associated with glaucoma, and compliance with amblyopia treatment.

DISLOCATED LENSES/ECTOPIA LENTIS

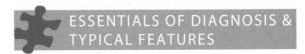

ESSENTIALS OF DIAGNOSIS & TYPICAL FEATURES

▶ Nontraumatic lens dislocation is usually bilateral.
▶ Subluxation causes refractive errors of large magnitude that are difficult to correct.

▶ Pathogenesis

Marfan syndrome, homocystinuria, Weill-Marchesani syndrome, sulfite oxidase deficiency, hyperlysinemia, syphilis, Ehlers-Danlos syndrome, and trauma.

▶ Clinical Findings

Slit-lamp examination reveals malposition of the intraocular lens. Refraction often reveals significant astigmatism. A complete ophthalmic evaluation, as well as genetic and metabolic evaluation, may be warranted.

▶ Differential Diagnosis

Ectopia lentis due to systemic disease versus trauma.

▶ Complications

Ectopia lentis can cause decreased vision and amblyopia due to induced refractive errors. Another ophthalmologic concern is pupillary block glaucoma, in which a malpositioned unstable lens interferes with the normal flow of aqueous humor from the ciliary body (posterior to the pupil), where it is produced, into the trabecular meshwork (anterior to the pupil).

▶ Treatment

Surgical lensectomy may be required if the VA is not improved significantly with glasses or contact lenses. Underlying metabolic and/or genetic disorders require a multidisciplinary approach.

▶ Prognosis

Prognosis depends on the severity of the lens dislocation and need for lensectomy.

▼ DISORDERS OF THE RETINA

RETINAL HEMORRHAGES IN THE NEWBORN

ESSENTIALS OF DIAGNOSIS & TYPICAL FEATURES

▶ Retinal hemorrhages associated with birth most often resolves by 6 weeks of life.

▶ Clinical Findings

Birth-related retinal hemorrhages can occur in approximately 25% of newborns. Retinal hemorrhages are more commonly seen after spontaneous vaginal delivery with higher rates up to 50% after vacuum- or forceps-assisted deliveries. Retinal hemorrhages are less common after cesarean sections but still occur (5%). Most retinal hemorrhages from birth resolve by 2–4 weeks. Small, isolated deeper hemorrhages may persist to 6 weeks. Examination of the retina of an otherwise healthy newborn infant is not indicated.

▶ Differential Diagnosis

See section Abusive Head Trauma & Nonaccidental Trauma.

▶ Treatment

Observation is indicated since retinal hemorrhages of the newborn usually disappear by 6 weeks of life.

▶ Prognosis

Excellent.

RETINOPATHY OF PREMATURITY (ROP)

ESSENTIALS OF DIAGNOSIS & TYPICAL FEATURES

▶ ROP screening examinations are recommended for infants with:

• Birth weight ≤ 1500 g or

• Gestational age ≤ 30 weeks or

• Select infants with an unstable clinical course who may not meet criteria above

▶ Pathogenesis

Premature infants have incomplete retinal vascularization and are at risk for developing abnormal peripheral retinal vascularization, which may lead to retinal detachment and blindness. Recent studies suggest that insulin-like growth factor I (IGF-I) and vascular endothelial growth factor (VEGF) may play key roles in ROP development. Other associations for severe ROP are bronchopulmonary dysplasia, intraventricular hemorrhage, sepsis, apnea and bradycardia, and mutations of the Norrie disease gene. Very low birth weight and gestational age have a higher risk of developing severe ROP that requires treatment.

▶ Prevention

The risk of vision loss from ROP can be reduced by timely screening of premature infants by an ophthalmologist.

▶ Clinical Findings

The Cryotherapy for Retinopathy of Prematurity (CRYOROP) study outlined a standard nomenclature to describe the progression and severity of ROP (Table 16–5). Since retinal blood vessels emanate from the optic nerve and do not fully cover the developing retina until term, the optic nerve is used as the central landmark. The most immature zone of the retina, zone I, is the most posterior concentric imaginary circle around the optic nerve. The next peripheral area is zone II, and peripheral to that is zone III. Zone I disease by definition is higher risk than disease in more anterior/peripheral zones. Similarly, the stages of the abnormal vessels are numbered from zero (simply incomplete vascularization) through stages 1–5.

Initial examinations are performed 4 weeks after delivery or at 31 weeks for those with GA 26 weeks or less. The frequency of follow-up examinations depends on the findings and the risk factors for developing ROP. Most infants are evaluated every 1–2 weeks. ROP may persist beyond 40 weeks post menstrual age. Examinations can be discontinued when the retinas are fully vascularized. Complete retinal vascularization may be prolonged in infants with moderate to severe ROP.

▶ Complications

Low vision and retinal detachment.

Table 16–5. Stages of retinopathy of prematurity.

Stage	
Stage I	Demarcation line or border dividing the vascular from the avascular retina.
Stage II	Ridge. Line of stage I acquires volume and rises above the surface retina to become a ridge.
Stage III	Ridge with extraretinal fibrovascular proliferation.
Stage IV	Subtotal retinal detachment.
Stage V	Total retinal detachment.

Treatment

Treatment of ROP is indicated when there is type I ROP [zone I ROP with any stage and plus disease (severe vessel dilation and tortuosity), zone I ROP stage III without plus disease, zone II ROP with stage II or III and plus disease] as defined by the Early Treatment Retinopathy of Prematurity (ETROP) study. Treatment includes laser photocoagulation and, in certain cases, anti-VEGF intravitreal injections. Surgical treatment for a retinal detachment involves scleral buckling or a lens-sparing vitrectomy by a vitreoretinal specialist.

Prognosis

Most cases of ROP do not progress to retinal detachment and require no treatment. However, ROP remains a leading cause of blindness in children. Premature infants, especially those who had ROP, are at a higher risk of developing strabismus, amblyopia, and refractive error than the average child.

Fierson WM; American Academy of Pediatrics Section on Ophthalmology; American Academy of Ophthalmology; American Association for Pediatric Ophthalmology and Strabismus; American Association of Certified Orthoptists: Screening examination of premature infants for retinopathy of prematurity. Pediatrics 2018;142(6). pii: e20183061. doi: 10.1542/peds.2018-3061 [PMID: 30824604].

Liegl R, Lofqvist C, Hellström A, Smith LE: IGF-1 in retinopathy of prematurity, a CNS neurovascular disease. Early Hum Dev 2016 Nov;102:13–19. doi: 10.1016/j.earlhumdev.2016.09.008 [PMID: 27650433].

Owen LA, Morrison MA, Hoffman RO, Yoder BA, DeAngelis MM: Retinopathy of prematurity: a comprehensive risk analysis for prevention and prediction of disease. PLoS One 2017 Feb 14;12(2):e0171467. doi: 10.1371/journal.pone.0171467 [PMID: 28196114].

RETINOBLASTOMA

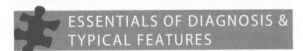

ESSENTIALS OF DIAGNOSIS & TYPICAL FEATURES

▶ Retinoblastoma (RB) is the most common primary intraocular malignancy of childhood, with an incidence estimated between 1 in 14,000–18,000 live births, and 8000 new cases each year globally.

▶ Most patients present before age 3 years.

Pathogenesis

RB is a tumor that arises from the retina due to mutation of both copies of the RB1 tumor suppressor gene (13q14). From the retina, it can grow under the retina or into the vitreous. It can directly invade the choroid and sclera into the orbit, spread via optic nerve to CNS, or metastasize hematogenously.

The two forms of RB are heritable (germline) and non-heritable. Heritable RB accounts for 45% of all cases, of which 85% are bilateral, 10% unilateral, and 5% trilateral (bilateral RB with pineal midline neuroectodermal tumor). The "two-hit hypothesis" states that biallelic inactivation of the *RB1* gene, a tumor-suppressor gene, results in RB development. In heritable cases, a germline mutation is present in all cells, and the second "hit" occurs in somatic retinal cell development. In sporadic RB, both mutations are somatic. Children of a parent with heritable RB have a 45% chance of being affected by RB (50% risk of inheritance and 90% penetrance). However, most heritable RBs arise de novo and often are proband with the disease.

Children with germline RB1 mutation are at increased risk of developing second primary malignancies, especially osteosarcomas, soft tissue sarcomas, and melanomas. Those who received radiation therapy are at an additional higher risk.

Clinical Findings

The most common presenting sign in a child with previously undiagnosed RB is leukocoria (see Figure 16–1). Evaluation of the pupillary red reflex is important, although a normal red reflex does not rule out RB. Other presentations include strabismus, red eye, glaucoma, or pseudohypopyon (appearance of pus-like material in the anterior chamber). Children with heritable RB are usually diagnosed earlier and present with bilateral, multifocal tumors.

Genetic testing and counseling is important in the management of RB. Once the causative mutation is found in an affected individual, unaffected members of the family should be tested to determine their personal and reproductive risk.

Differential Diagnosis

Coats disease, cataracts, uveitis, *Toxocara* infection, persistent fetal vasculature, and medulloepithelioma.

Complications

This disease can be fatal. Decreased vision depends on the location of tumor. Loss of vision and loss of eye.

Treatment

The primary goal is to save the child's life through early tumor detection and prevention of metastasis. Secondary goals are to preserve the eye and maximize visual potential. Management begins with staging exam under anesthesia and MRI. Treatment depends on laterality and extent of RB. Multimodal therapeutic options include chemotherapy (systemic, intra-arterial, or intravitreal) combined with focal treatment (laser, cryotherapy), radiotherapy (brachytherapy, stereotactic, external beam), or surgery.

Prognosis

Survival exceeds 95% in developed countries. Patients with germline mutations need lifelong monitoring for secondary neoplasms.

Abramson DH, Shields CL, Munier FL, Chantada GL: Treatment of retinoblastoma in 2015: agreement and disagreement. JAMA Ophthalmol 2015 Nov;133(11):1341–1347. doi: 10.1001/jamaophthalmol.2015.3108 [PMID: 26378747].

AlAli A, Kletke S, Gallie B, Lam WC: Retinoblastoma for pediatric ophthalmologists. Asia Pac J Ophthalmol (Phila) 2018 May–June;7(3):160–168 [PMID: 29737052].

Shields CL et al: Targeted retinoblastoma management: when to use intravenous, intra-arterial, periocular, and intravitreal chemotherapy. Curr Opin Ophthalmol 2014 Sep;25(5):374–385 [PMID: 25014750].

RETINAL DETACHMENT

ESSENTIALS OF DIAGNOSIS & TYPICAL FEATURES

▶ A retinal detachment may present as an abnormal or absent red reflex.

▶ Older children may complain of decreased vision, flashes, floaters, or VF defects.

Pathogenesis

Common causes are trauma, ocular anomalies, and history of ocular surgery. The most common inherited cause of childhood retinal detachment is Stickler syndrome, a genetic connective tissue disorder. Other risk factors include high myopia, ROP, and Marfan syndrome.

Clinical Findings

Symptoms of detachment are floaters, flashing lights lasting seconds, and loss of VF; however, children often cannot appreciate or verbalize their symptoms. Self-injurious behavior is associated with high rates of retinal detachment and traumatic cataracts.

Differential Diagnosis

Intraocular tumor.

Complications

Vision loss, strabismus.

Treatment

Treatment of retinal detachment is surgical. Examination under anesthesia with prophylactic cryotherapy or laser photocoagulation is recommended for all patients with Stickler syndrome.

Prognosis

Prognosis depends on the location and duration of the detachment.

DIABETIC RETINOPATHY

ESSENTIALS OF DIAGNOSIS & TYPICAL FEATURES

▶ Diabetic retinopathy (DR) is a specific microvascular complication of diabetes mellitus. Patients with type 1 diabetes are at higher risk of developing severe proliferative retinopathy leading to visual loss than are those with type 2 diabetes.

Prevention & Detection

Control of diabetes is the best way to prevent ocular complications. Risk factors for developing DR include longer duration of disease and poor glycemic control. The screening guidelines differ among different medical societies. The AAP recommends that children older than 9 years should be examined by an ophthalmologist within 3–5 years after the onset of type 1 diabetes. Based on research in adults with type 2 diabetes, screening examination is recommended at initial diagnosis and annually thereafter for children with type 2 diabetes.

Clinical Findings

Acute onset of diabetes may be accompanied by sudden blurred vision due to shift in refractive error and/or cataract formation. DR can range in severity from mild, moderate, or severe nonproliferative retinopathy to proliferative retinopathy that can lead to tractional retinal detachment. Macula edema may occur with any retinopathy. Vision-threatening DR is less common in children.

Complications

Vision loss due to vitreous hemorrhage, macular edema, neovascular glaucoma, cataracts, and/or retinal detachment.

Treatment

Good glycemic control is essential to decrease the risk and severity of DR. Severe proliferative DR requires pan-retinal laser photocoagulation or vitreoretinal surgery (or both). Most children with DR do not require treatment until adulthood.

▶ Prognosis

Prognosis depends on the severity of the retinopathy and associated complications.

Geloneck MM, Forbes BJ, Shaffer J, Ying GS, Binenbaum G: Ocular complications in children with diabetes mellitus. Ophthalmology 2015 Dec;122(12):2457–2464. doi: 10.1016/j .ophtha.2015.07.010 [PMID: 26341461].

Wang SY, Andrews CA, Herman WH, Gardner TW, Stein JD: Incidence and risk factors for developing diabetic retinopathy among youths with type 1 or type 2 diabetes throughout the United States. Ophthalmology 2016 Nov 30. doi: 10.1016/j .ophtha.2016.10.031 [PMID: 27914837].

▼ DISEASES OF THE OPTIC NERVE

OPTIC NEUROPATHY

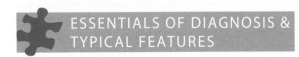

ESSENTIALS OF DIAGNOSIS & TYPICAL FEATURES

▶ Poor optic nerve function may result in decreased central or peripheral vision, decreased color vision, strabismus, and nystagmus.

▶ Clinical Findings

Optic nerve disorders can be due to congenital malformation, malignancy, inflammation, infection, infiltration, medication toxicity, metabolic or genetic disorders, ischemia, and trauma. Optic nerve function is evaluated by checking VA, color vision, pupillary response, and VFs.

The swinging flashlight test is used to assess the relative function of each optic nerve. It is performed by shining a light alternately in front of each pupil to check for an afferent pupillary defect (APD). Normal pupil should constrict when the light is shined directly and also when the light is shined into the fellow eye (consensual pupil constriction). An abnormal response in the affected eye is pupillary dilation when the light is directed into that eye after having been shown in the other eye with its healthy optic nerve. Hippus—rhythmic dilating and constricting movements of the pupil—can be confused with an APD. Patients with bilateral optic nerve dysfunction may not show an APD but have bilaterally sluggishly reactive pupils.

The optic nerve is evaluated as to size, shape, color, and vascularity. Occasionally, myelinization past the entrance of the optic nerve head occurs. It appears white, with a feathered edge (Figure 16–24). Myelinization onto the retina is

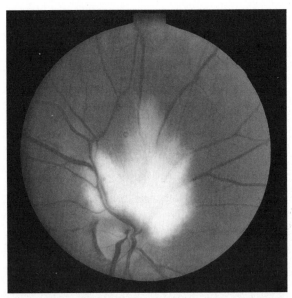

▲ **Figure 16–24.** Myelinization of the optic nerve.

congenital and nonprogressive but can be associated with myopia, anisometropia, and amblyopia. Anatomic anomalies of the optic nerve include colobomatous defects, optic nerve pits, and ONH.

▶ Treatment

Management of the underlying condition resulting in the optic neuropathy is necessary.

▶ Prognosis

Prognosis depends on the severity of optic neuropathy and the underlying disease.

OPTIC NERVE HYPOPLASIA

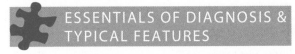

ESSENTIALS OF DIAGNOSIS & TYPICAL FEATURES

▶ Optic nerve hypoplasia (ONH), regardless of laterality or neuroanatomic abnormalities, is an independent risk factor for hypothalamic-pituitary dysfunction, which occurs in 60%–80%.

▶ Neuroimaging of the brain and endocrine consultation should be performed in all patients with ONH.

Pathogenesis

ONH is a complex congenital disorder, involving a spectrum of anatomic malformations and clinical manifestations ranging from isolated hypoplasia of one or both optic nerves to extensive brain malformations, hypothalamic-pituitary dysfunction, and neurocognitive disability. In the past, ONH has been considered as part of the septo-optic dysplasia or de Morsier syndrome due to the co-occurrence of hypothalamic-pituitary dysfunction and absent septum pellucidum. Absent septum pellucidum has no prognostic significance. Growth hormone abnormality is the most common endocrine dysfunction in children with ONH. Most cases of ONH are nonhereditary.

To date, the most consistently found risk factors for ONH are young maternal age and primiparity although the mechanism by which these lead to ONH development still needs to be elucidated.

Clinical Findings

Visual function with ONH ranges from functional vision to complete blindness. Vision impairment is nonprogressive. If only one eye is involved, the child usually presents with strabismus (usually esotropia). If both eyes are affected, nystagmus is usually the presenting sign. Visual signs often may not develop until children are at least 3 months of age. Systemic signs of congenital hypopituitarism may present earlier with signs, including prolonged hyperbilirubinemia, transient or permanent hypoglycemia, or poor linear growth.

Ophthalmoscopy is performed to directly visualize the optic nerves and to determine the severity of the hypoplasia. In ONH, optic nerves can be smaller than average to nearly absent. Vessels are often abnormal in caliber. Classic "double-ring sign" refers to the circular hypo- or hyperpigmented ring (scleral canal) seen around the small optic nerve.

Treatment

ONH is an incurable congenital disorder. Research in stem cell therapy has not shown benefits with unknown long-term risks. Sensory amblyopia and significant refractive errors should be treated by an ophthalmologist. Strabismus surgery may be necessary in certain patients. Endocrine abnormalities should be managed as necessary. A referral to a teacher for the visually impaired is a beneficial adjunct to children with ONH at any age to help optimize vision.

Prognosis

Severe bilateral ONH may result in blindness.

PAPILLEDEMA

ESSENTIALS OF DIAGNOSIS & TYPICAL FEATURES

▶ Optic nerve edema is abnormal swelling of the optic nerves. Causes include elevated intracranial pressure (ICP), infection, inflammation, ischemia, and infiltrative causes.

▶ Papilledema is a specific term used for optic nerve edema caused by elevated intracranial pressure.

Pathogenesis

In papilledema, ICP can be elevated primarily (idiopathic intracranial hypertension [IIH]/pseudotumor cerebri) or secondarily as a direct result of an identifiable condition. Secondary causes include intracranial mass, structural abnormalities (Chiari malformation, obstructive hydrocephalus), vascular causes (cerebral venous sinus thrombosis, hypertensive emergency), or medication-induced. Most common medications associated with papilledema are the tetracycline class, vitamin A derivatives, growth hormone supplementation, and corticosteroid use or withdrawal.

IIH, formerly known as pseudotumor cerebri, is a poorly understood primary cause of intracranial hypertension in the presence of normal brain parenchyma and cerebrospinal constituents. In children, IIH is often divided into prepubertal and pubertal groups. In the pubertal group, female gender and obesity are associated with IIH, similar to adults.

Not every patient with elevated ICP develops papilledema. It is speculated that transmission of ICP to the optic nerve sheath results in axoplasmic flow stasis leading to papilledema. There may be anatomic variations in the optic canal that provide protective effects in some individuals. In addition, optic nerves with atrophy may not swell even in the setting of severely elevated ICP.

Clinical Findings

Acute rise in ICP can result in headaches, tinnitus, nausea, vomiting, and vision changes (transient visual obscurations). Patients can develop diplopia from sixth nerve (CN VI) palsy that occurs when elevated ICP leads to a downward displacement of the brainstem that stretches CN VI as it crosses over the petrous ridge and enters Dorello's canal. CN VI palsy associated with elevated ICP is more commonly seen in children compared to adults. Photophobia is also a unique symptom of elevated ICP seen in children. Gradual rise in ICP may not cause obvious symptoms. For IIH, clinical symptoms vary with age with symptoms being less obvious in younger patients. Optic nerve edema may be an incidental finding in a routine eye examination in young children.

Direct visualization of the optic nerve by ophthalmoscopy reveals an elevated disc with indistinct margins, dilated and tortuous vessels that may be obscured by the edema around the disc margin, and central hyperemia of the nerve head. Hemorrhages may be present in more severe cases. Optic nerve changes are often bilateral but can be asymmetric.

When optic nerve edema is noted, it is important to search for the cause. MRI of the brain with and without contrast is the preferred method of neuroimaging. MRV is recommended in atypical cases to rule out venous sinus thrombosis. In secondary causes, abnormalities will be evident on MRI. In IIH, characteristic MRI findings are empty sella turcica, decreased pituitary gland size, optic nerve tortuosity, perioptic subarachnoid space enlargement, posterior globe flattening, and intraocular protrusion of the optic nerve head. These findings are not direct causes of elevated ICP but associated findings that may be seen in IIH patients. When a mass or structural abnormality is ruled out with neuroimaging, obtaining a lumbar puncture (LP) for opening pressure and CSF analysis may be necessary. Elevated ICP in children 18 years and younger is greater than 25 cm H_2O in nonobese, nonsedated children, and greater than 28 cm H_2O for the all others.

Other ancillary modalities for evaluation include optic coherence tomography, which may show thickened retinal nerve fiber layer, and VF tests, which most commonly show an enlarged blind spot.

▶ Differential Diagnosis

Pseudopapilledema is a normal variant of the optic disc in which the disc appears elevated, with indistinct margins and a normal vascular pattern. Pseudopapilledema sometimes occurs in hyperopic individuals. Optic disc drusen, which are acellular deposits that calcify over time, is commonly misdiagnosed as papilledema. Optic nerve edema can also be caused by infections and inflammation.

▶ Treatment

Treatment of papilledema depends on the cause. Cessation of inciting agents may be adequate in medication-related papilledema. Anticoagulation and antibiotics may be needed for cerebral venous sinus thrombosis. For IIH, medications that are commonly used include acetazolamide, topiramate, and furosemide. For obese individuals with IIH, weight loss and healthy diet can be significantly helpful. When conservative treatment fails, or with concerns for optic nerve compression, surgery may be necessary. Surgical options are ventriculoperitoneal or lumboperitoneal shunts and optic nerve sheath fenestration.

▶ Complications

Optic atrophy and vision loss.

▶ Prognosis

Prognosis depends on the underlying etiology, duration, and control of the increased ICP.

Aylward SC, Reem RE: Pediatric intracranial hypertension. Pediatr Neurol Jan 2017;66:32–43. doi: 10.1016/j.pediatrneurol.2016.08.010 [PMID: 27940011].

Aylward SC, Waslo CS, Au JN, Tanne E: Manifestations of pediatric intracranial hypertension from the intracranial hypertension registry. Pediatr Neurol 2016 Aug;61:76–82 doi: 10.1016/j.pediatrneurol.2016.04.007 [PMID: 27255412].

Gilbert AL, Heidary G: Update on the evaluation of pediatric idiopathic intracranial hypertension. Curr Opin Ophthalmol 2016 Nov;27(6):493–497. doi: 10.1097/ICU.0000000000000317 [PMID: 27585209].

Phillipis PH, Sheldon CA: Pediatric pseudotumor cerebri syndrome. J Neuroophthalmol 2017 Sep;37 Suppl 1: S33–S40 [PMID: 28806347].

Sheldon CA: Pediatric idiopathic intracranial hypertension: age, gender, and anthropometric features at diagnosis in a large, retrospective, multisite cohort. Ophthalmology 2016 Nov;123(11):2424–2431. doi: 10.1016/j.ophtha.2016.08.004 [PMID: 27692528].

OPTIC NEURITIS

ESSENTIALS OF DIAGNOSIS & TYPICAL FEATURES

▶ Compared to adults, optic neuritis (ON) in children is more often bilateral, more often associated with papillitis (up to 69% vs 33% in adults), more often present after a preceding viral illness, less often associated with painful eye movements, but with more severe visual deficit.

▶ Pathogenesis

ON in children is a heterogenous disorder that may occur as an isolated event (ie, postinfectious, idiopathic) or as a component of a generalized inflammatory CNS disease or an underlying rheumatologic condition such as systemic lupus erythematosus. Inflammatory CNS diseases that can present with ON include acute disseminated encephalomyelitis (ADEM), MS, and neuromyelitis optica (NMO).

▶ Clinical Findings

Cardinal features of ON are decreased VA, abnormal color vision (notably red color desaturation), pain with eye movements, and VF deficits. APD will be present in unilateral cases. Symptoms may present over hours to days. Anterior ON results in optic nerve edema (papillitis). Patients with posterior ON may have normal appearing nerves on examination despite signs of optic nerve dysfunction and abnormal MRI findings.

Diagnostic workup includes LP, MRI, serum autoimmune and rheumatologic studies, and complete ophthalmic examination. MRI of the brain/orbits with and without contrast may show thickening of the optic nerves on T1-weighted imaging, bright T2 signal along the optic nerve or chiasm, and postgadolinium enhancement. Up to 36% of children who present with ON are eventually diagnosed with MS clinically or radiologically. Likelihood is higher in children with white matter lesions in MRI of the brain and cerebrospinal fluid (CSF) oligoclonal bands (present in 80% of children with MS vs 15% in monophasic ON). Normal MRI at the time of ON conveys a low likelihood of MS.

Severe bilateral ON with severe vision loss, poor response to steroids, signs of hypothalamic/brainstem symptoms, or the presence of longitudinally extensive lesions of the optic nerve and spinal cord should prompt evaluation of aquaporin-4 (AQP4) IgG (NMO IgG). Clinical manifestations with AQP4-IgG positivity are supportive of NMO.

Serum myelin oligodendrocyte glycoprotein (MOG) antibodies are associated with non-MS subgroup of CNS demyelination and frequently found in patients with ADEM with ON. ADEM is most commonly seen in younger children and manifests as encephalopathy with polyfocal neurologic deficits.

▶ Differential Diagnosis

Papilledema, infection, neoplasm.

▶ Complications

Decreased VA, color vision, peripheral vision, and contrast sensitivity. ON may be the first manifestation of relapsing disease that can result in ocular and systemic disability.

▶ Treatment

No clinical trials have been performed for pediatric ON. Clinical practice follows evidence from the optic neuritis treatment trial (ONTT) where recovery after IV steroids followed by oral steroids was more rapid than after placebo or oral steroids alone. Although treatment may not change the medical outcome, recovery of visual symptoms can be shortened from 7 to 2 weeks, which may prevent psychosocial challenges faced by children including the need to make up school work and other sequelae from visual limitations. Plasmapheresis or intravenous immunoglobulin therapy may be considered for refractory cases.

▶ Prognosis

Prognosis depends on the underlying disease process. Despite the severe vision deficit at presentation, the majority have good visual recovery.

Lehman SS, Lavrich JB: Pediatric optic neuritis. Curr Opin Ophthalmol 2018 Sep; 29(5):419–422 [PMID: 30096089].

OPTIC ATROPHY

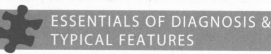

ESSENTIALS OF DIAGNOSIS & TYPICAL FEATURES

▶ Optic atrophy is the pathologic endpoint of numerous diseases that result in intrinsic and extrinsic insults to optic nerves.

▶ Clinical Findings

Most common causes of optic atrophy are tumors, warranting a timely evaluation and diagnosis. More recently, perinatal events (insults in gestation, at birth or in immediate postnatal period) are emerging as a common cause of optic atrophy. An example is optic atrophy resulting from intraventricular hemorrhage or periventricular white matter changes in premature infants. Other causes include structural intracranial abnormalities (craniosynostosis, hydrocephalus), post-papilledema or papillitis, toxins, ischemia, and inherited causes (autosomal dominant, autosomal recessive, X-linked, and mitochondrial). Neuroimaging is helpful for delineating CNS abnormalities.

Direct examination of the optic nerve by ophthalmoscopy reveals an optic nerve head with a cream or white color and possibly cupping. Vessels may appear attenuated. Patients may not complain of decreased vision but often have low vision on exam. Nystagmus can be present if optic atrophy was acquired as an infant.

▶ Complications

Vision loss, decreased peripheral vision or central scotoma, and contrast sensitivity.

▶ Treatment

There is no treatment to reverse optic atrophy.

▶ Prognosis

Prognosis depends on the severity of the optic nerve atrophy and associated neurologic deficits.

▼ DISEASES OF THE ORBIT

PERIORBITAL & ORBITAL CELLULITIS

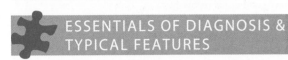

ESSENTIALS OF DIAGNOSIS & TYPICAL FEATURES

▶ Decreased vision, restricted eye movements, and an APD suggest orbital cellulitis.

▶ Pathogenesis

The fascia of the eyelids joins with the fibrous orbital septum to isolate the orbit from the lids. The orbital septum helps decrease the risk of an eyelid infection extending into the orbit. Infections arising anterior to the orbital septum are termed *preseptal*. Orbital cellulitis denotes infection posterior to the orbital septum and may cause serious complications, such as a cavernous sinus thrombosis, cerebral abscess, meningitis, septicemia, and optic neuropathy.

Preseptal (periorbital) cellulitis usually arises from a local exogenous source such as an abrasion or insect bite of the eyelid or from other infections (hordeolum, dacryocystitis). *S aureus* and *S pyogenes* are the most common pathogens cultured from these sources. Preseptal cellulitis can progress to orbital cellulitis.

Orbital cellulitis most commonly arises from paranasal sinus infection (most commonly ethmoid sinusitis) because the walls of three sinuses make up portions of the orbital walls, and infection can breach these walls or extend by way of a richly anastomosing venous system. The pathogenic agents are those of acute or chronic sinusitis—respiratory flora and anaerobes, In addition to the normal culprits of preseptal cellulitis, *Streptococcus anginosis* is an emerging cause of orbital cellulitis and often causes a more serious infection with increased frequency of intracranial or spinal abscesses that may require neurosurgical intervention.

Rhino-orbital-cerebral mucormycosis is an uncommon but devastating infection that can lead to blindness and death in children with immunosuppression and poorly controlled diabetes.

▶ Clinical Findings

Children with preseptal cellulitis present with red and swollen eyelids, pain, and mild fever. The vision, eye movements, and eye itself are normal.

Orbital cellulitis presents with orbital signs, which are proptosis, eye movement restriction, decreased vision, and may have an APD. The eye often appears red and chemotic. CT with contrast helps establish the extent of the infection within the orbit and sinuses.

▶ Differential Diagnosis

Severe conjunctivitis can cause (often bilateral) eyelid swelling and redness that can mimic preseptal/orbital cellulitis. Other confusing diseases are primary or metastatic neoplasm of the orbit, orbital pseudotumor (idiopathic orbital inflammation), and orbital foreign body with secondary infection.

▶ Complications

Orbital cellulitis can result in permanent vision loss due to compressive optic neuropathy. Proptosis can cause corneal exposure, dryness, and scarring. Cavernous sinus thrombosis, intracranial extension, blindness, and death can result from severe orbital cellulitis.

▶ Treatment

Initial therapy for preseptal and orbital cellulitis infection is with broad-spectrum systemic antibiotics, which may be later narrowed based on culture findings and clinical improvement. Treatment may require surgical drainage for subperiosteal abscess in addition to drainage of infected sinuses, which is a crucial part of the therapy. Surgery is indicated for decreased VA attributable to orbital cellulitis, failure to improve clinically after 24–48 hours of IV antibiotics, or demonstration of worsened abscess on repeat CT. Patients with proptosis, eye movement restriction, elevated eye pressure, and age greater than 9 years are significantly more likely to require surgical intervention.

▶ Prognosis

Most patients do well with timely treatment.

Smith JM, Bratton EM, DeWitt P, Davies BW, Hink EM, Durairaj VD: Predicting the need for surgical intervention in pediatric orbital cellulitis. Am J Ophthalmol 2014 Aug;158(2):387–394 [PMID: 24794092].

CRANIOFACIAL ANOMALIES

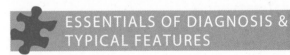

ESSENTIALS OF DIAGNOSIS & TYPICAL FEATURES

▶ Children with craniosynostosis and craniofacial abnormalities often have strabismus and abnormal eye versions.

▶ Clinical Findings

Ocular abnormalities associated with craniofacial abnormalities involving the orbits include visual impairment, proptosis, corneal exposure, hypertelorism (widely spaced orbits), strabismus, amblyopia, lid coloboma, papilledema, refractive errors, and optic atrophy.

Treatment

Orbital and ocular abnormalities associated with craniofacial anomalies often require a multispecialty approach. Management may require orbital and strabismus surgery. Ophthalmologists also treat amblyopia, refractive errors, and corneal exposure when present.

Taub PJ, Lampert JA: Pediatric craniofacial surgery: a review for the multidisciplinary team. Cleft Palate Craniofac J 2011;48(6):670–683 [PMID: 21740182].

ORBITAL TUMORS

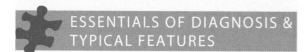

ESSENTIALS OF DIAGNOSIS & TYPICAL FEATURES

▶ The most common benign tumor of infancy is capillary hemangioma, arising in the first few weeks of life and exhibiting a characteristic sequence of growth and spontaneous involution (Figure 16–25).

▶ The most common primary malignant tumor of the orbit is rhabdomyosarcoma.

Clinical Findings

Capillary hemangiomas may be located superficially in the lid or deep in the orbit and can cause ptosis (see Figure 16–25), refractive errors, and amblyopia. Deeper lesions may cause proptosis.

Orbital dermoid cysts are benign congenital orbital choristomas that vary in size and are usually found temporally at the brow and orbital rim or supranasally. These lesions are firm, well encapsulated, and mobile. Rupture of the cyst causes a severe inflammatory reaction.

Lymphangioma occurring in the orbit is typically poorly encapsulated, increases in size with upper respiratory infection,

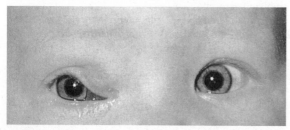

▲ **Figure 16–25.** Right upper-lid hemangioma causing ptosis.

and is susceptible to hemorrhage. Other benign tumors of the orbit are varix, plexiform neurofibroma, teratoma, and tumors arising from bone, connective tissue, and neural tissue.

Orbital rhabdomyosarcoma (see Chapter 31) grows rapidly and displaces the globe. The average age at onset is 6–7 years. The tumor is often initially mistaken for orbital swelling due to insignificant trauma or can mimic orbital cellulitis.

Tumors metastatic to the orbit also occur; neuroblastoma is most common. The patient may exhibit proptosis, orbital ecchymosis (raccoon eyes), Horner syndrome, or opsoclonus (dancing eyes). Ewing sarcoma, leukemia, Burkitt lymphoma, and Langerhans cell histiocytosis may involve the orbit.

Examination of vision, eye movements, eyelids, and orbits often reveals amblyopia, eyelid malposition, strabismus, and proptosis. Neuroimaging with CT or MRI is required to delineate the location and size of orbital tumors.

Differential Diagnosis

Orbital pseudotumor (idiopathic orbital inflammation) and orbital cellulitis.

Treatment

Most capillary hemangiomas do not require treatment. Topical and systemic β-blockers have shown success in treating capillary hemangiomas. Treatment is indicated if the lesion is large enough to cause amblyopia. Induced astigmatism or amblyopia (or both) are treated with glasses and patching, respectively. Treatment of orbital dermoids is by excision.

Treatment modalities for rhabdomyosarcoma include radiation, chemotherapy, and surgery. With expeditious diagnosis and proper treatment, the survival rate of patients with orbital rhabdomyosarcoma confined to the orbit approaches 90%.

Treatment of metastatic disease requires management by an oncologist and may require chemotherapy and radiation therapy.

Prognosis

Prognosis depends on the underlying disease.

NYSTAGMUS

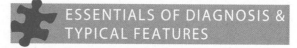

ESSENTIALS OF DIAGNOSIS & TYPICAL FEATURES

▶ Nystagmus is an involuntary rhythmic oscillation of eyes. It may be unilateral or bilateral or be gaze dependent.

▶ Nystagmus can be caused by poor vision. Reduced VA can also occur from nystagmus due to excessive motion of images on the retina.

Pathogenesis

Nystagmus can be grouped into infantile nystagmus, which usually appears in the first 3–6 months of life, and acquired nystagmus, which appears later in life. Infantile nystagmus can be idiopathic, associated with retinal diseases (ie. retinal dystrophy), due to low vision (ie, ONH, foveal hypoplasia), or due to visual deprivation early in life (ie, cataracts). Foveal hypoplasia can be isolated or be associated with aniridia, albinism, and achromatopsia.

Nystagmus can also occur with normal ocular structures and seemingly normal CNS development. Infantile nystagmus syndrome, also known as congenital motor nystagmus, is an ocular disorder of unknown etiology that presents at birth or early infancy. Positive family history may be present. Latent nystagmus occurs when one eye is occluded and can be seen in patients with strabismus. Acquired nystagmus can result from neurologic disorders, vestibular dysfunction, and drug toxicity.

Clinical Findings

When characterizing nystagmus, the examiner can note the laterality (unilateral, bilateral, asymmetric), plane (horizontal, vertical, torsional), conjugacy, amplitude, and frequency of nystagmus.

Nystagmus due to low vision or foveal hypoplasia may exhibit a slow "roving" nystagmus. Infantile nystagmus syndrome is characterized by horizontal, uniplanar nystagmus that increases in intensity with fixation and decreases in intensity with convergence and at a null point (gaze where shakiness is the least). Children may have an abnormal head posture in order to hold their gaze at the null point. They may have crossing (esotropia) due to nystagmus blockage syndrome since nystagmus is dampened by convergence. Children with infantile nystagmus do not complain of oscillopsia (perception of oscillations in vision). See-saw nystagmus is associated with a suprasellar mass (ie, craniopharyngioma).

Spasmus nutans, in which a rapid, shimmering, asymmetric nystagmus occurs often with head bobbing and torticollis, is a benign disorder that resolves with time. Clinically, nystagmus of spasmus nutans is indistinguishable from nystagmus due to optic pathway glioma. MRI of brain/orbits, with and without contrast, is necessary to determine if the cause of the nystagmus is due to a CNS disease.

Neurologic disease should be suspected and neuroimaging performed in acquired nystagmus and also when nystagmus is unilateral or asymmetrical. An electroretinogram may be required to rule out retinal pathology as the cause of nystagmus if neuroimaging is normal.

Differential Diagnosis

Opsoclonus (chaotic bilateral eye movements), voluntary eye movements (cannot be prolonged).

Treatment

Therapy is directed at managing the underlying ocular or CNS disease. An ophthalmologist can optimize vision by correcting significant refractive errors and strabismus. The range of vision varies depending on the cause of the nystagmus. Some patients may benefit from extraocular muscle surgery and contact lenses.

Prognosis

Most affected individuals have subnormal vision, but spasmus nutans usually improves with time.

AMBLYOPIA

ESSENTIALS OF DIAGNOSIS & TYPICAL FEATURES

▶ Amblyopia is a unilateral or bilateral reduction in VA resulting from abnormal or inadequate stimulation of the visual system during the critical early period of visual development.

▶ Amblyopia is defined as a difference of best-corrected VA of two lines or more on an acuity chart between the two eyes.

Pathogenesis

Amblyopia is classified according to its cause. Unilateral amblyopia has two main causes: strabismus (misalignment of the eyes resulting in abnormal binocular interaction and amblyopia of the nondominant eye) and anisometropia (difference in refractive error between two eyes resulting in poor visual input in one eye). Bilateral amblyopia can result from high refractive errors (high hyperopia, myopia, or astigmatism). Less commonly, amblyopia can occur due to organic causes such as cataracts, corneal opacities, lid ptosis, or vitreous hemorrhages. This type is called deprivation amblyopia and is least common but most difficult to treat. Children can have combined or mixed mechanism amblyopia as well.

Normal binocular development leads to progressive refinement of monocular VA, stereoacuity (3D vision), and fusion of images from both eyes. The critical early period for vision development is thought to end around 8 years of age. Individuals with amblyopia may have not only decreased VA but also decreased contrast sensitivity, stereoacuity, and fixation stability, and increased vulnerability to "crowding," difficulty identifying shapes surrounded by visual "clutter."

▶ Prevention

Vision screening and referral to an eye care professional if amblyopia is suspected.

▶ Clinical Findings

Screening for amblyopia should be a component of periodic well-child examinations. The single best screening technique to discover amblyopia is obtaining VA in each eye. In preverbal children unable to respond to VA assessment, amblyogenic factors are sought, including strabismus, media opacities, unequal Brückner reflexes (pupillary red reflexes), and a family history suggestive of strabismus, amblyopia, or ocular disease occurring in childhood (see section Ophthalmic Examination).

▶ Treatment

The earlier treatment is begun, the better will be the chance of improving VA. Treatment is continued until amblyopia resolves or until at least 8–9 years of age. Amblyogenic factors such as refractive errors are addressed. Because of the extreme sensitivity of the visual nervous system in infants, congenital cataracts and media opacities must be diagnosed and treated within the first few weeks of life. Visual rehabilitation and amblyopia treatment must then be started to foster visual development.

After eradicating amblyogenic factors, the mainstay of treatment is to increase stimulation of the amblyopic eye by part-time occlusion (patching) of the amblyopic eye. Other treatment modalities include "fogging" the sound eye with cycloplegic drops (atropine), lenses, and filters.

▶ Prognosis

Prognosis depends on the compliance with treatment and the cause of amblyopia.

STRABISMUS

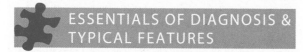

ESSENTIALS OF DIAGNOSIS & TYPICAL FEATURES

- ▶ Strabismus is misalignment of the eyes.
- ▶ Its prevalence in childhood is about 2%–3%.
- ▶ Strabismus is categorized by the direction of the deviation (esotropia, exotropia, hypertropia, hypotropia) and its frequency (constant or intermittent).
- ▶ Strabismus may cause or be due to amblyopia.

▼ ESOTROPIA (CROSSED EYES)

ESSENTIALS OF DIAGNOSIS & TYPICAL FEATURES

- ▶ Pseudoesotropia can result from prominent epicanthal folds and wide nose bridges that give the appearance of crossed eyes when they are actually straight.
- ▶ Esotropia is deviation of the eyes toward the nose and may involve one or both eyes.

▶ Pathogenesis

Primary infantile esotropia (also known as congenital esotropia) has its onset in the first year of life. The deviation of the eyes toward the nose is large and obvious. The most frequent type of acquired esotropia is the accommodative type (Figure 16–26). Onset is usually between ages 2 and 5 years. The deviation is variable in magnitude and constancy and is often accompanied by amblyopia. Refractive accommodative esotropia is associated with a high hyperopic refraction. In another type, the deviation is worse with near than with distant vision (high AC/A accommodative esotropia). This type of esodeviation is usually associated with lower refractive errors.

Esotropia can be associated with certain syndromes. In Möbius syndrome (congenital facial diplegia), a sixth nerve palsy causing esotropia is associated with palsies of the 7th and 12th cranial nerves and limb deformities. Duane syndrome can affect the medial or lateral rectus muscles (or both). It may be an isolated defect or may be associated with a multitude of systemic defects (eg, Goldenhar syndrome). Duane syndrome is often misdiagnosed as a sixth (abducens) nerve palsy. The left eye is involved more commonly, but both eyes can be involved. Girls are affected more frequently.

After age 5 years, any esotropia of recent onset should arouse suspicion of CNS disease. Intracranial masses, hydrocephalus, demyelinating diseases, and IIH are causes of abducens palsy, where patients may present with esotropia and diplopia. Papilledema is often, but not invariably, present with increased ICP.

Besides the vulnerability of the abducens nerve to increased ICP, it is susceptible to infection and inflammation. Otitis media and Gradenigo syndrome (inflammatory disease of the petrous bone) can cause sixth nerve palsy. Less commonly, migraine and diabetes mellitus are considerations in children with sixth nerve palsy.

▶ Clinical Findings

Observation of the reflection of a penlight on the cornea, the corneal light reflex, is an accurate means of determining if

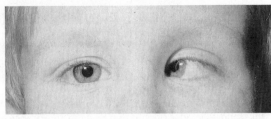

A

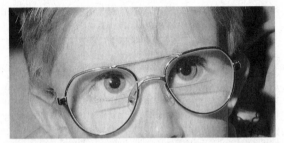

B

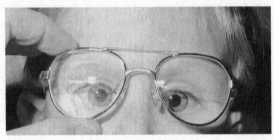

C

▲ **Figure 16–26.** Accommodative esotropia. **A:** Without glasses, esotropic; **B:** With glasses, well aligned at distance; **C:** At near with bifocal correction.

the eyes are straight. This is a good way to differentiate true esotropia from pseudostrabismus. If strabismus is present, the corneal light reflex will not be centered in one or both eyes. Observation of eye movements may reveal restriction of eye movements in certain positions of gaze. Children with unilateral paretic or restrictive causes of esotropia may develop face turns toward the affected eye to maintain binocularity. The face turn is an attempt to maintain binocularity away from the field of action of the paretic muscle. Alternate cover testing of the eyes while the child is fixating on a near and/or distant target will reveal refixation movements in the opposite direction of the deviation. Motility, cycloplegic refraction, and a dilated funduscopic examination by an ophthalmologist are necessary to determine the etiology of esotropia. Some children require imaging studies and neurologic consultation.

▶ **Complications**

Amblyopia and poor stereoacuity/depth perception.

▶ **Treatment**

Surgery is the mainstay of treatment for primary infantile esotropia. Surgery is typically performed between 6 months and 2 years of age in order to obtain optimal results.

Management of accommodative esotropia includes glasses with or without bifocals, amblyopia treatment, and, in some cases, surgery.

Underlying neurologic disease should be referred to the appropriate specialists for further management.

▶ **Prognosis**

Usually good.

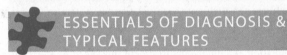

EXOTROPIA (WALL-EYED, DRIFTING OF EYES)

ESSENTIALS OF DIAGNOSIS & TYPICAL FEATURES

- ▶ Exotropia is a type of strabismus in which the eyes are divergent (Figure 16–27).
- ▶ Exotropia may be intermittent or constant and involve one or both eyes.

▶ **Clinical Findings**

The deviation of the eyes toward the ears most often begins intermittently and occurs after age 2 years (see Figure 16–27). Congenital (infantile) exotropia is extremely rare in an otherwise healthy infant. Early-onset exotropia may occur in infants and children with severe neurologic problems. All children with constant, congenital exotropia require CNS neuroimaging. Referral to an ophthalmologist is indicated.

Evaluation of the corneal light reflex reveals the penlight's reflection in the deviated eye is displaced nasally. Cover uncover test or alternate cover test will reveal refixation eye movements inward (toward the nose) when exotropia is present.

Convergence insufficiency is a special type of exotropia where the deviation is larger at near compared to distance. They have poor convergence (ability to converge or cross their eyes when looking at a near target). Common symptoms include asthenopia, binocular diplopia, or visual blur with near visual tasks.

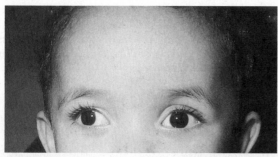

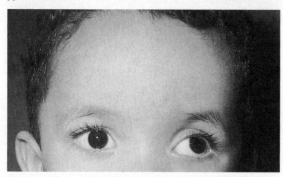

A

B

▲ **Figure 16–27.** Exotropia. **A:** Fixation with left eye. **B:** Fixation with right eye.

▶ Complications

Poor stereoacuity/depth perception. Amblyopia is less commonly seen in exotropia compared to esotropia but can occur in monocular or poorly controlled exotropia.

▶ Treatment

Treatment of exotropia includes observation, glasses, and/ or surgery. Indications for surgery of intermittent exotropia include poor control of deviation, large angle deviation, and worsening stereoacuity. There is strong evidence that orthoptic exercises can improve the symptoms and signs of convergence insufficiency. Classic exercise is pencil push-ups, which can be performed at home or in the office. There are other computer-based exercises that can help reduce the symptoms of convergence insufficiency. Vision exercises or therapy for all other types of strabismus are not endorsed by pediatric ophthalmologists due to the lack of scientific evidence.

▶ Prognosis

Generally good.

UNEXPLAINED DECREASED VISION IN INFANTS & CHILDREN

ESSENTIALS OF DIAGNOSIS & TYPICAL FEATURES

▶ Blindness in infants and children is commonly caused by retinal dystrophies, optic nerve disorders, or cortical visual impairment due to significant CNS disease.

▶ Pathogenesis

Occult causes of poor vision and blindness in children may be due to hereditary retinal dystrophies such as Leber congenital amaurosis and optic nerve abnormalities, including ONH and atrophy.

Cerebral visual impairment is visual impairment that is not fully explainable by their eye exam findings and deemed to be due to neurologic injury. The term *cortical visual impairment* was first applied as an umbrella term to describe impairments of visual processes like VA, contrast sensitivity, and VFs. But since injuries can involve more than the outer cortex of the brain, the term *cerebral visual impairment* was later adopted. Cerebral visual impairment can occur from generalized cerebral damage or from insults in the dorsal and ventral pathways of vision (higher processes of vision). Perinatal hypoxia, trauma, intracranial hemorrhage, and periventricular leukomalacia are some of the causes of cortical visual impairment.

▶ Clinical Findings

Affected infants will have poor eye contact, fail to fixate and follow a visual target, and be unresponsive to visual threat. Wandering or roving eye movements and nystagmus are common. Eye poking can be seen in some infants with low vision.

Referral to an ophthalmologist is indicated to determine the etiology of the low vision. Diagnostic tests such as an electroretinogram and visual evoked response may be required. Imaging studies of the brain, genetics, and neurology consultations may be useful.

▶ Differential Diagnosis

Delayed visual maturation, vision loss due to an ocular versus neurologic disease.

▶ Treatment

Low-vision aids enhance remaining vision. Devices used include magnifiers for both distance and near vision, closed-circuit television, and large-print reading materials. Vision rehabilitation specialists and support groups can help teach the affected child and their family how to best use these devices. Clinical trials are underway for treatment of Leber congenital amaurosis with gene therapy.

▶ Prognosis

Generally poor for vision.

LEARNING DISABILITIES & DYSLEXIA

ESSENTIALS OF DIAGNOSIS & TYPICAL FEATURES

▶ Learning disabilities and dyslexia result in poor reading comprehension and writing.

▶ Children often have vague complaints of ocular fatigue, headaches, and difficulty reading.

▶ Clinical Findings

Evaluation of the child with learning disabilities and dyslexia should include ophthalmologic examination to identify any ocular disorders that could cause or contribute to poor school performance. Most children with learning difficulties have no demonstrable problems on ophthalmic examination.

▶ Treatment

A multidisciplinary approach is recommended by the AAP, the AAPOS, and the AAO for evaluating and treating children with learning disabilities. According to the joint AAP report, there is no scientific evidence to support the claims that visual training, muscle exercises, ocular pursuit-and-tracking exercises, behavioral/perceptual vision therapy, "training"

glasses, prisms, and colored lenses and filters are effective treatments for learning disabilities, dyslexia, and strabismus. There is no evidence that children who participate in vision therapy are more responsive to educational instruction than children who do not participate.

Handler SM, Fierson WM; Section on Ophthalmology; Council on Children With Disabilities; American Academy of Ophthalmology; American Association for Pediatric Ophthalmology and Strabismus; American Association of Certified Orthoptists: Learning disabilities, dyslexia, and vision. Pediatrics 2011; 127(3):e818–e856 [PMID: 21357342].

Rucker JC, Phillips PH: Efferent vision therapy. J Neuroophthalmol 2017 Jan 4;1–7. doi: 10.1097/WNO.0000000000000480 [PMID: 28059865].

Web Resources

Ali MJ: Pediatric acute dacryocystitis. Ophthal Plast Reconstr Surg 2015 Sep–Oct;31(5):341–347. doi: 10.1097/IOP.0000000000000472 [PMID: 25856337].

American Academy of Ophthalmology: www.aao.org. Accessed November 27, 2017.

American Association of Pediatric Ophthalmology and Strabismus: www.aapos.org. Accessed November 27, 2017.

Hammersmith KM: Blepharokeratoconjunctivitis in children. Curr Opin Ophthalmol 2015 Jul;26(4):301–305 [PMID: 26058029].

O'Gallagher M, Banteka M, Bunce C, Larkin F, Tuft S, Dahlmann-Noor A: Systemic treatment for blepharokeratoconjunctivitis in children. Cochrane Database Syst Rev 2016 May;30(5):CD011750. doi: 10.1002/14651858.CD011750.pub2 [PMID: 27236587].

O'Gallagher M, Bunce C, Hingorani M, Larkin F, Tuft S, Dahlmann-Noor A: Topical treatments for blepharokeratoconjunctivitis in children. Cochrane Database Syst Rev 2017 Feb 7;2:CD011965. doi: 10.1002/14651858.CD011965.pub2 [PMID: 28170093].

Oral Medicine & Dentistry

Roopa P. Gandhi, BDS, MSD
Chaitanya P. Puranik, BDS, MS, MDentSci, PhD
Anne Wilson, DDS, MS
Katherine L. Chin, DDS, MS

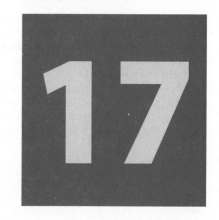

PEDIATRIC ORAL HEALTH

Concept of the Dental Home

Establishment of a dental home during the infant phase provides a vital foundation for oral health promotion and prevention of oral disease, such as early childhood caries. Analogous to the American Academy of Pediatrics concept of a medical home, the dental home has been defined by the American Academy of Pediatric Dentistry as "the ongoing relationship between the dentist and the patient, inclusive of all aspects of oral health care delivered in a comprehensive, continuously accessible, coordinated, and family-centered way." The dental home encompasses all aspects of oral health that result from the interaction of the patient, parents, dentists, dental professionals, and nondental professionals. A dental home is initiated by the determination of involved individuals and their collaborative interaction to establish awareness of factors influencing the patient's oral health.

Achieving optimal oral health care as part of a dental home requires a dentist who is knowledgeable about pediatric oral health or a pediatric dentist (a specialist in care for children and those with more complex oral health needs), in partnership with the child's primary caregiver. Together, the dentist and primary caregiver can develop a comprehensive preventive program based on an assessment of disease susceptibility. Similar to preventive care guidelines as part of a medical home, the preventive oral health plan for children provides anticipatory guidance for caregivers on age-appropriate preventive measures. These include oral hygiene practices, the importance of fluoride, dietary guidance, dental trauma, and the value of a dental home.

Addressing risk factors for early childhood caries is a central component of anticipatory guidance during routine visits to medical and dental providers. Beyond the focus on preventive oral health, the dental home provides access to comprehensive, routine, and urgent dental care, and facilitates referral to other dental and medical providers as indicated. By providing continuously accessible dental care, the time and cost of urgent or emergent dental treatment may be reduced for the family and society.

Prenatal and Perinatal Factors and Infant Oral Health Care

Oral health promotion by health care providers during the prenatal and perinatal periods provides preventive information to mothers and other family members. Mothers may be unaware of the potential consequences of their own oral health, which can impact their systemic health, pregnancies, and the well-being of their children. Also, a mother's and/or primary caregiver's oral health knowledge, behaviors, and attitudes have an influence on the oral health trajectory of children. Infant oral health care is the foundation for preventive dental care. The infant oral health program should (1) establish with caregivers the goals of oral health, (2) inform caregivers of their role in reaching these goals, (3) motivate caregivers to learn and practice optimal preventive oral health behaviors, and (4) initiate a long-term dental care relationship with caregivers. These goals are enhanced through anticipatory guidance on topics such as teething, oral hygiene, diet, fluoride, injury prevention, nonnutritive sucking habits, and regular dental health supervision. This approach advances dental care from monitoring for disease to oral health promotion.

Typically, pediatricians encounter newborns and infants at an earlier age than dental providers, providing them an opportunity to address risk factors associated with early childhood caries. Pediatricians are encouraged to incorporate caries-risk assessment and anticipatory guidance focused on oral health into their routine practice. Caries-risk assessment estimates the likelihood of developing carious lesions based on the complex interaction of risk factors at multiple levels (individual, family, community, and social environment). Risk indicators for the age group 0 to 3 years of age that predict development of dental caries are listed in caries-risk assessment forms that are available for physicians and other nondental health care providers through the American Academy of Pediatric Dentistry and American Academy of Pediatrics. By 6 months of age, every infant should have a caries-risk assessment performed by a pediatric health care provider. Since the risk of caries increases with age, anticipatory guidance by pediatricians and nondental health care providers is recommended beyond age 3 years as part of routine pediatric care.

Ladrillo TE, Hobdell MH, Caviness AC: Increasing prevalence of emergency department visits for pediatric dental care, 1997–2001. J Am Dent Assoc 2006 Mar;137(3):379–385 [PMID: 16570472].

Mouradian WE et al: Addressing disparities in children's oral health: a dental-medical partnership to train family practice residents. Dent Educ 2003 Aug;67(8):886–895 [PMID: 12959162].

Rozier RG, Sutton BK, Bawden JW, Haupt K, Slade GD, King RS: Prevention of early childhood caries in North Carolina medical practices: implications for research and practice. J Dent Educ 2003 Aug;67(8):876–885 [PMID: 12959161].

Salone LR, Vann WF, Dee DL: Breastfeeding: an overview of oral and general health benefits. J Am Den Assoc 2013 Feb, 28;144(2):143–151 [PMID: 23372130].

Sanchez OM, Childers NK: Anticipatory guidance in infant oral health: rationale and recommendations. Am Fam Physician. 2000 Jan 1;61(1):115–120, 123–124 [PMID: 10643953].

Watt RG: From victim blaming to upstream action: tackling the social determinants of oral health inequalities. Community Dent Oral Epidemiol 2007;35(1):1–11 [PMID: 17244132].

ORAL EXAMINATION OF CHILDREN

Exam Positioning

For children under age 3, a knee-to-knee position allows the provider to complete the oral examination in a safe and comfortable way (Figure 17–1). The parent is instructed to

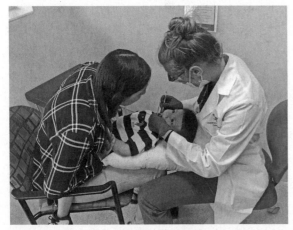

▲ **Figure 17–1.** Knee-to-knee position.

sit facing the provider with the knees of both the parent and provider touching or interlocking to create a table. The infant is then positioned on the parent's lap facing the parent, with each leg wrapped around the parent's waist. The child's head is lowered onto a pillow on the provider's lap for the examination, with the parent being instructed to stabilize the child's arms and legs with their hands and elbows, respectively. Crying during the examination is a normal response in healthy children and will allow for better visualization of the oral cavity. For older, more cooperative children, the oral examination can be performed on the dental chair. With the chair reclined and the patient in a supine position, a pillow can be added for support for the legs depending on the size of the patient.

During the examination, the clinician assesses the extra-oral tissues, intra-oral hard and soft tissues, and overall oral hygiene maintenance.

Extra-Oral Examination

Extra-oral examination includes assessing the overall symmetry of the face. This can easily be done by holding a piece of floss across the patient's facial midline. Evaluation of the face can be done by dividing the face in equal thirds. The facial upper third extends from the hair line to the glabella, the middle third spans from the glabella to the base of the nose (subnasale), and the lower third extends from subnasale to the chin. The length of each facial thirds is usually equal or similar. Extraoral findings such as muscle strain over the chin can also point to a skeletal or orthodontic problem. The submandibular glands and lymph nodes should be palpated to identify any enlargement or pain. A temperomandibular joint (TMJ) examination should determine the range of motion and any deviation while opening or closing the jaw. The preauricular area is palpated to determine the presence of any TMJ crepitations or clicking indicative of underlying joint pathology.

Intra-Oral Soft Tissue Examination

The mouth of the normal newborn is lined with an intact, smooth, moist, shiny mucosa (Figure 17–2). The alveolar ridges are continuous and relatively smooth. Within the alveolar bone are numerous tooth buds, which at birth are mostly primary teeth. The sagittal and vertical maxillo-mandibular relationships are different at birth, with an anterior open bite being considered physiologic before the onset of tooth eruption. The mouth is more triangularly shaped and the oral cavity is small and filled by the tongue due to a small and slightly retrognathic lower jaw. This pseudo micrognathia is due to ventral positioning of the fetus to facilitate its passage through the birth canal and will generally correct after birth.

Frena

Small maxillary and mandibular frena can be found in the anterior midline region (Figure 17–3), and small accessory

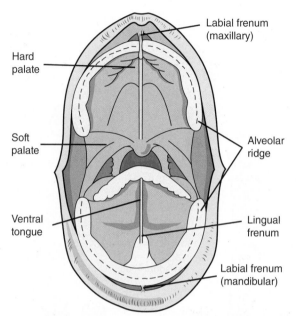

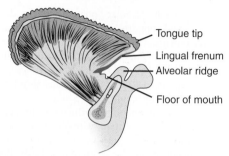

▲ **Figure 17–4.** Normal position of lingual frenum.

▲ **Figure 17–2.** Normal anatomy of the newborn mouth.

frena are often present posteriorly. A more prominent midline maxillary labial frenum, which is observed in 25% of children, tends to diminish in size and recede apically with normal development and the eruption of teeth.

The tongue is connected to the floor of the mouth by the lingual frenum (Figures 17–4 and 17–5), whereas the upper lip is connected to gingiva above the upper central incisors by the maxillary frenum. With ankyloglossia, the attachment

is tight, closer to the tip of the tongue or high up on the alveolar ridge (see Figure 17–5) and may restrict movement. Ankyloglossia typically does not inhibit normal growth and development; however, it can cause feeding problems, such as difficulty latching or pain during nursing. These concerns can be addressed with frenotomy of the lingual frenum shortly after birth. In most cases breastfeeding will be improved. In contrast, frenotomy of the maxillary frenum is rarely indicated as there is no evidence that this reduces breastfeeding difficulties.

Soft Tissue Variations

The most common soft tissue pathology in newborns are neonatal cysts, including Bohn's nodules, Epstein pearls, and dental lamina cysts. Bohn's nodules are remnants of mucous gland tissue that occur on the buccal and lingual aspects of the alveolar ridges. Epstein pearls are remnants of epithelial tissue trapped at the time of palatal fusion during early fetal development and are found along the mid-palatal raphe. Dental lamina cysts are remnants of the dental lamina and are typically located on the alveolar mucosa. These cysts are 1–3 mm round, smooth, nontender white, gray, or yellow nodules that are self-limiting in nature and typically resolve by 3 months of age.

Intra-Oral Hard Tissue

The development of alveolar bone is evident with development of tooth buds and later eruption of the primary teeth

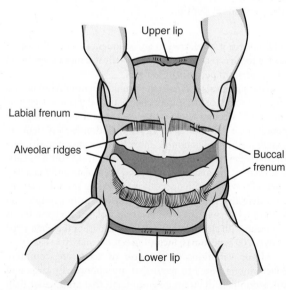

▲ **Figure 17–3.** The frena.

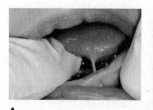

A   B

▲ **Figure 17–5.** Ankyloglossia (tongue-tie) in a 6-week-old, before (**A**) and after (**B**) lingual frenectomy.

and permanent teeth. Alveolar bone encases the developing tooth buds and supports the teeth through periodontal ligament attachments. Alveolar ridges are usually horseshoe-shaped at birth and the mandibular and maxillary alveolar ridges contact each other at their most posterior aspects at birth. With eruption of teeth during further development, these ridges will no longer contact each other.

Hard tissue formation of the primary teeth begins at approximately 14 weeks in utero, with all 20 primary teeth being calcified to varying degrees, with traces of the enamel of first permanent molars being present at birth. Primary teeth generally begin to erupt around 7 months of age but may appear as early as 3–4 months or as late as 12–16 months of age. A complete set of primary teeth (20 teeth) is usually erupted between 30 and 36 months. Although there are variations, usually anterior teeth erupt before posterior teeth, and mandibular teeth before their maxillary counterparts.

Between 6 and 7 years of age, the first permanent molars erupt distal to the existing primary second molars. This phase of development, when both primary and permanent teeth simultaneously exist, is known as the mixed dentition. Following eruption of the first permanent molars, mandibular permanent central incisors erupt, replacing existing primary central incisors and resulting in the exfoliation of the first primary tooth. Children continue to exfoliate primary teeth as their permanent successors erupt until approximately the age of 12, with the maxillary canines typically being the final primary tooth to be shed. Around the same time, the second permanent molars erupt, followed later in adolescence by the development of the permanent third molars, colloquially referred to as wisdom teeth. Once the patient has erupted a complete set of permanent teeth (with the exception of third molars), they are considered to have adolescent dentition.

Tooth Numbering Systems

Tooth numbering systems enable clinicians to more effectively communicate unequivocally about a patient's teeth. In the United States, the Universal Numbering System (Figure 17–6) is used, which assigns the uppercase letters A–T for primary teeth and the numbers 1–32 for permanent teeth. The initial designation begins on the upper right, most posterior tooth and continues along the upper teeth to the left side. The count then drops to the lower, most posterior tooth on the left side and continues along the bottom teeth to end on the lower right side.

Hard Tissue Variations

Potential variations in dental hard tissues involve the number and size of primary and permanent teeth. When an extra tooth or teeth are present they are referred to as supernumerary tooth/teeth and the condition is known as hyperdontia. If a supernumerary tooth occurs in the maxillary incisor

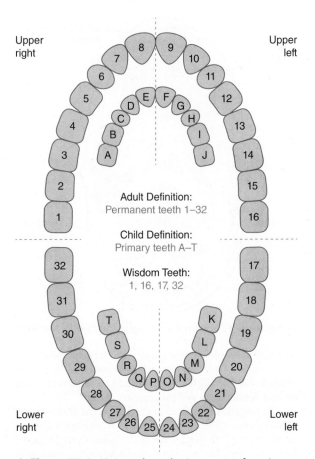

▲ **Figure 17–6.** Universal numbering system for primary and permanent dentition.

midline area it is referred to as mesiodentes. The removal of such a tooth is recommended especially if it hinders eruption of the adjacent permanent incisors.

Tooth agenesis is rare in the primary dentition but occurs with an incidence of 5% in the permanent dentition. Depending on the number of teeth that are congenitally missing, the condition is referred to as either hypodontia (less than six absent teeth) or oligodontia (more than six absent teeth). The most frequently missing permanent teeth are the third molars, followed by the mandibular second premolars and maxillary lateral incisors. Tooth agenesis is caused by several independent defective genes, which can act alone or in combination with other genes. It can occur as an isolated problem but is common with cleft lip/cleft palate or as part of the phenotype of over 200 syndromes, including ectodermal dyplasias.

Minor variations in the size of teeth are common. Macrodontia refers to teeth that are abnormally large and microdontia is the term given to teeth that are smaller than the usually expected size. Apart from the number and shape of the teeth, there may also be abnormalities in the overall formation of the hard tissue structures such as enamel and dentin (amelogenesis imperfecta or dentinogenesis imperfecta, respectively).

Eruption Symptoms

Many symptoms are ascribed to the process of tooth eruption or teething. However, any temporal association with fever, upper respiratory infection, or systemic illness is coincidental rather than related to the eruption process. Attributing fever to teething without a thorough diagnostic evaluation for other sources has resulted in missing serious organic disease.

Common therapies for teething pain include the application of over the counter teething gels or liquids. For teething children, their main ingredient, benzocaine, can rarely cause methemoglobinemia. While "natural" benzocaine-free formulations are available, systemic analgesics such as acetaminophen or ibuprofen are safer and more effective. Chewing on a teething object can be beneficial, if only for distraction purposes.

Occasionally, swelling of the alveolar mucosa overlying an erupting tooth can be seen. This usually asymptomatic condition appears as localized red to purple, round, raised, and smooth lesion. Treatment is rarely needed as these eruption cysts/hematomas resolve with tooth eruption.

Pathologies of Tooth Eruption

▶ Natal Teeth

On rare occasions (1:3000), natal teeth are present at birth and neonatal teeth erupt into the oral cavity within the first month of life. These are most commonly (85%) primary mandibular incisors. A radiograph should be taken to determine whether they are regular or supernumerary teeth (10%). Although the preferred approach is to leave the tooth in place, natal teeth that are supernumerary, hypermobile, or of inferior structural quality should be extracted. Other indications for removal of natal teeth include nursing difficulties and when their sharp incisal edges cause laceration of the ventral surface of the infant's tongue (Riga-Fede disease).

▶ Delayed Eruption

Premature loss of a primary tooth can either delay or accelerate eruption of the underlying permanent tooth. Accelerated eruption occurs when the primary tooth is removed within 6–9 months of its normal exfoliation, but loss of the primary tooth more than 1 year before its expected exfoliation typically delays eruption of its successor. The loss of a primary tooth often causes adjacent teeth to tip or drift into the resulting space, leading to space loss for the underlying permanent tooth. Placement of a space maintainer can prevent such space loss.

Other local factors delaying or preventing tooth eruption include supernumerary teeth, cysts, odontogenic tumors, over-retained or ankylosed primary teeth, and impacted teeth. A generalized delay in eruption may be associated with global developmental delays, endocrinopathies, and other systemic conditions.

▶ Ectopic Eruption

Insufficient space in the dental arch may cause permanent teeth to erupt ectopically and cause a usually painless root resorption of the adjacent primary tooth. This phenomenon is observed most commonly with the maxillary first permanent molars.

Occasionally, mandibular incisors erupt lingually and lead to over-retention of the primary predecessor, resulting in a "double row of teeth." If the primary tooth is still firmly in place, the dentist should remove it to allow its successor to drift into proper position.

▶ Impaction

Impaction occurs when a permanent tooth is prevented from erupting. Although crowding is a frequent reason, over-retained primary or supernumerary teeth are other causes. The teeth most often affected in the developing dentition are the maxillary incisors and canines. Often, they are brought into correct alignment by early extraction of the preceding or adjacent primary teeth. If this approach is ineffective, surgical exposure of the impacted tooth and orthodontic treatment are indicated.

Casamassimo PS, Fields HW, McTigue DJ, Nowak AJ: *Pediatric Dentistry: Infancy Through Adolescence.* 5th ed. St. Louis, MO: Mosby Elsevier.

Dean JA, Avery DR, McDonald RE: *McDonald and Avery's Dentistry for the Child and Adolescent.* 9th ed. Maryland Heights, MO: Mosby Elsevier.

DENTAL CARIES

Dental caries is the most common chronic disease of childhood and the most prevalent unmet health need of US children. Largely a disease of poverty, dental caries primarily affects almost 80% of children and adolescents living in low-income families.

Early Childhood Caries

Formerly termed "baby bottle tooth decay" or "nursing bottle caries," early childhood caries (ECC) is a particularly virulent and rapidly progressive form of caries that begins on the smooth surfaces of the teeth soon after eruption. According to the American Academy of Pediatric Dentistry (AAPD), ECC is defined as one or more decayed (d), missing (m), or filled (f) tooth surfaces (s) in any primary tooth in a child under 6 years of age. The disease typically involves the maxillary incisors, but any other teeth may be affected. A lack of adequate preventive care and poor feeding habits can place children at high risk for ECC.

Any sign of smooth-surface caries in a child less than 3 years is termed severe ECC (S-ECC). From 3 to 5 years, a *dmfs* score of 1 or more in maxillary front teeth or a total *dmfs* score of 4 or higher must be present to make a diagnosis of S-ECC. Children with S-ECC are at higher risk for new carious lesions. They are also likely to experience frequent hospitalizations, emergency department visits, and school absences due to the severity of existing carious lesions. The presence of S-ECC can also result in below-normal height and weight gain and diminished oral health-related quality of life for the affected child. Although S-ECC can affect all children, it is 32 times more likely in children who consume sugary foods and whose mothers are of low socioeconomic status and education level.

Pathogenesis

Development of caries requires the interaction of four factors: (1) a host (tooth in the oral environment); (2) a suitable dietary substrate (fermentable carbohydrates); (3) cariogenic microorganisms that adhere to the tooth; and (4) time, measured as the frequency of exposure to fermentable carbohydrates and the duration of acid exposure. The main organisms implicated in the initiation of caries are *Streptococcus mutans* (MS) and *Streptococcus sobrinus*. *Lactobacillus acidophilus* and *Lactobacillus casei* are also linked to the progression of caries. MS organisms are most commonly passed from mother to child. A "window of infectivity" between ages 19 and 30 months has been described, but MS colonization of the oral cavity can occur as early as 3 months of age. Earlier colonization increases the risk of caries.

Dental plaque is an adherent biofilm on the tooth surface that harbors acidogenic bacteria in close proximity to the enamel. As bacteria metabolize sucrose, they produce lactic acid that solubilizes calcium phosphate in tooth enamel. Demineralization of the dental enamel occurs below pH 5.5 and is the first step in cariogenesis. The flow rate of saliva and its buffering capacity are important modifiers of demineralization. Demineralization of enamel and dentin can be halted

or even reversed by redeposition of calcium, phosphate, and fluoride from saliva.

If caries progresses it penetrates the enamel, advancing through the dentin toward the pulp of the tooth. In response, blood vessels in the pulp dilate and inflammatory cells begin to infiltrate (pulpitis), resulting in tooth pain. When the carious lesion is still untreated, pulp invasion will occur, triggering invasion of more inflammatory cells and the eventual formation of a small pulpal abscess. Once the pulp in the root of the tooth becomes necrotic, a periapical abscess develops (Figure 17–7), which usually causes severe pain, fever, and swelling.

Caries Prevention

Since caregivers are more likely to establish a medical home for well-child visits at birth and prior to initiating a dental home, medical offices have opportunities to provide preventive dental services that includes dental screening, caries risk assessment, caregiver counseling about their child's oral health, and referrals to dentists for establishment of a dental home or follow-up for concerns.

Prevention of dental caries necessitates restoration of the delicate balance between pathologic factors and protective influences. Pathologic factors include a susceptible host, cariogenic bacteria, deficient fluoride exposure, and fermentable carbohydrates. The most studied protective influences include fluoride, sugar substitutes (xylitol), and frequency of brushing. Among these, only fluoride from topical and systemic sources (food, beverages, drinking water, and oral care products) has demonstrated a consistent protective effect.

Dietary Guidelines

Since dental caries requires frequent exposure to fermentable carbohydrates, poor feeding habits increase the risk for caries development. Dietary practices that can reduce caries risk in nursing infants include giving only water in the bottle at bedtime. Infants should also be weaned from the bottle between 12 and 18 months of age and encouraged to drink from an uncovered cup (rather than a no-spill training cup). Soda, 100% juice, and powdered beverages should be avoided.

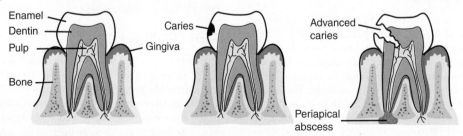

▲ **Figure 17–7.** Tooth anatomy and progression of caries.

Dietary counseling should be based on maintaining a diet in accordance with the World Health Organization (WHO) recommendations in which free-sugar consumption is less than 10% of total daily energy intake and preferably below 5% of the total energy intake. Foods considered to be protective against caries are high in fat, protein, and minerals such as milk and cheese, which contain calcium and phosphate.

▶ Oral Hygiene

Soon after birth, caregivers should clean intra-oral surfaces on a daily basis using a moist, soft cloth. Once the teeth erupt, oral hygiene must be practiced in earnest, particularly in high-risk children as caries formation has been associated with biofilm accumulation on tooth surfaces. Due to a lack of manual dexterity in children younger than 8 years of age, caregivers should be brushing, as well as flossing for their children's teeth if there is no spacing between the teeth. With respect to caries, mechanical removal of biofilm from tooth surfaces without concomitant use of fluoridated toothpaste has a weaker association with caries reduction. Thus, as part of oral hygiene practices, fluoridated toothpaste is recommended to reduce risk of caries in the primary and permanent dentition. Caregivers should be instructed regarding the appropriate amount of fluoridated toothpaste at each brushing; "smear or rice-sized amount" (under age 3 years) or "pea-sized" amount (ages 3–6 years) of toothpaste. The beneficial effect of fluoride-containing toothpaste can be maximized by brushing teeth twice daily and either avoiding or rinsing minimally after brushing. Supplemental fluoride use is based on the individual's caries risk.

▶ Fluoride

Fluoride is a one of the most effective means of caries prevention through the topical and systemic mechanisms of action. By both routes of administration, fluoride can affect the dentin and enamel of erupted and unerupted teeth. Topical application inhibits bacterial metabolism by interfering with enzyme activity, inhibiting demineralization, and enhancing remineralization.

Systemic benefits are achieved by oral ingestion from sources such as fluoridated drinking water, beverages, infant formulas, and prepared food. The U.S. Department of Health and Human Services has specified a level of 0.7 ppm fluoride in community water supplies to balance the benefits of preventing dental caries while minimizing the risk for enamel fluorosis. Infants receiving concentrated infant formula as the main source of nutrition are at increased risk for enamel fluorosis in the permanent dentition if fluoride-containing formulas are reconstituted with fluoridated drinking water.

Fluoride supplements also help reduce dental caries prevalence and are a consideration for children at high caries risk and without access to fluoridated community water, depending on their age and existing fluoride exposure from other sources. A child's true exposure to all sources of fluoride must be thoroughly evaluated before supplements are prescribed so as to avoid enamel fluorosis.

A. Fluoride Varnish for High-Risk Populations

Applications of fluoride varnish during well-child visits with physicians is successful in reducing dental caries among vulnerable children (ICD-10-CM Diagnosis Code Z29.3: Encounter for Prophylactic Fluoride Administration). The sticky nature of the varnish's resin base allows for extended contact time of its fluoride content with the tooth surface.

The varnish in single-dose packages (0.3–0.5 mL) should be stirred before application and the contents of larger tubes (5 mL) massaged to dissolve any precipitated fluoride. The former are preferable because consistent availability of fluoride cannot be guaranteed with multidose packages. The average amount of varnish needed depends on the number of teeth present and ranges from 0.1 mL for infants to 0.3 mL for preschool children. Teeth should be dried with gauze before the varnish is applied with a small brush. It will set quickly to a dull yellow film upon contact with saliva. Caregivers should be instructed not to brush or floss and to give their children only soft foods until the next morning to provide enough time for absorption of the fluoride into enamel.

B. Other Adjunctive Measures

Xylitol containing products are marketed in many forms (eg, gums, mints, lollipops, chewable tablets, toothpastes, mouthwashes) as an adjunctive measure in caries prevention. Xylitol is considered a noncariogenic substitute due to the inability of oral bacteria to metabolize this five-carbon sugar alcohol. However, recent systematic reviews suggest that there is limited evidence for caries reduction from xylitol-containing products.

▶ Treatment of Caries

Caries is usually diagnosed by visual and tactile oral examination supplemented by radiographs to detect caries on the surfaces between teeth. The initial defect observed on enamel beneath dental plaque is the so-called "white-spot lesion," a white, chalky, decalcified area along the gingival margin or on approximated tooth surfaces. Frank carious lesions are light to dark brown spots or cavities of varying size on the tooth. A light shade of brown indicates rampant decay, while arrested caries is almost black in color.

In the early stages of decay, the tooth may be sensitive to temperature changes or sweets. Removing the carious tooth structure and filling the early defect with a restorative material can repair the tooth. As decay progresses deeper into the pulp, inflammation and pain increase. Eventually, the entire pulp becomes necrotic, and a choice must be made between root canal therapy (pulpectomy) and removal of the tooth. In the presence of cellulitis, extraction and antibiotic therapy are the treatments of choice.

When restorative materials are used to repair a tooth, the primary choices include dental amalgam, composite resin, or glass ionomer cement. For primary molars with extensive caries and/or pulpal involvement, full coverage crowns are the restorations of choice and these are available as preformed stainless steel crowns and in various cosmetic iterations.

Silver diamine fluoride has been utilized to slow or arrest caries progression in select patients. Its use may be considered in circumstances where the risk of morbidity or mortality under sedation or general anesthesia outweighs the benefit of definitive restorations. Once applied, the medicament produces a gray-black discoloration of carious defects of treated teeth and may be interpreted as caries.

Achembong LN, Kranz AM, Rozier RG: Office-based preventive dental program and statewide trends in dental caries. Pediatrics 2014 Apr;133(4):e827–e834 [PMID: 24685954].

Guideline: Sugars Intake for Adults and Children. Geneva: World Health Organization; 2015. Available from: https://www.ncbi .nlm.nih.gov/books/NBK285537/.

Policy on early childhood caries (ECC): classifications, consequences, and preventive strategies. Pediatr Dent 2016;38(6): 52–54 [PMID: 29179321].

Policy on early childhood caries (ECC): unique challenges and treatment Options. Pediatr Dent 2016;38(6):55–56 [PMID: 27931421].

Rozier RG et al: Evidence-based clinical recommendations on the prescription of dietary fluoride supplements for caries prevention: a report of the American Dental Association Council on Scientific Affairs. J Am Dent Assoc. 2010 Dec;141(12): 1480–1489 [PMID: 21158195].

PERIODONTAL DISEASE

Periodontal diseases are a group of conditions affecting a tooth's supporting structures: bone, gingiva, and periodontal ligament (Figure 17–8). Plaque and bacterial accumulation in the gingival sulcus cause a localized inflammation of the gingival tissue adjacent to a tooth. This initial phase, called dental plaque-induced gingivitis, is found almost universally in children and adolescents. This affects about half of the population by 5 years of age and reaches a prevalence of nearly 100% at puberty. Gingivitis is considered reversible,

and generally responds well to removal of dental plaque and improved oral hygiene.

Periodontitis, the subsequent phase, is characterized by irreversible loss of the periodontal attachment and destruction of bone. Abnormalities in neutrophil function such as chemotaxis, phagocytosis, and antibacterial activity increase the risk of periodontitis. Actinobacillus actinomycetemcomitans in combination with *bacteroides* species are implicated in this disease process. If oral hygiene does not improve and local contributing factors are not removed, chronic periodontitis can become more severe, resulting in generalized loss of the periodontal attachment. Chronic periodontitis is most easily arrested in its early stages before deep pockets develop with gradual loss of attachment. Aggressive periodontitis, previously labeled as early-onset periodontitis, is defined by rapid attachment loss and alveolar bone destruction. Treatment consists of combined surgical and nonsurgical mechanical debridement, and antibiotic therapy.

Concomitant medical conditions, hormonal alterations associated with the onset of puberty, certain medications, and malnutrition can intensify the inflammatory response to plaque. Periodontitis as a manifestation of systemic disease is associated with hematological (acquired neutropenia, leukemias) or genetic disorders, such as Down, Papillon-Lefèvre, Chediak-Higashi, hypophosphatasia, and leukocyte adhesion deficiency syndromes. The incidence of necrotizing periodontal diseases is lower (1%) in North America than in developing countries (2%–5%). These diseases are characterized by interproximal ulceration and necrosis of the dental papillae, rapid onset of dental pain, and often fever. Predisposing factors include viral infections, malnutrition, emotional stress, and systemic disease. The condition usually responds well to mechanical debridement, improved oral hygiene, and antibiotic therapy for febrile patients.

Armitage GC: Development of a classification system for periodontal diseases and conditions. Ann Periodontol 1999 Dec, 1;4(1): 1–6 [PMID: 10863370].

Periodontal diseases of children and adolescents. Pediatr Dent 2016;38(6):388–396 [PMID: 27931482].

Treatment of plaque-induced gingivitis, chronic periodontitis, and other clinical conditions. Pediatr Dent 2016;38(6): 403–411 [PMID: 27931484].

DENTAL EMERGENCIES

▶ Orofacial Trauma

Orofacial trauma consists mainly of abrasion or laceration of the lips, gingiva, tongue, or oral mucosa (including the frena), without damage to the teeth. Lacerations should be cleansed, inspected for foreign bodies, and sutured if necessary. Radiographs of lacerations of the tongue, lips, or cheeks should be taken to detect missing tooth fragments or other foreign bodies as palpation alone may not be adequate.

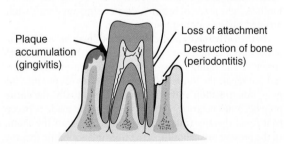

Plaque accumulation (gingivitis)

Loss of attachment

Destruction of bone (periodontitis)

▲ **Figure 17–8.** Periodontal disease.

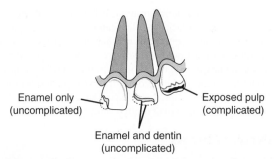

Enamel only
(uncomplicated)

Exposed pulp
(complicated)

Enamel and dentin
(uncomplicated)

▲ **Figure 17–9.** Patterns of crown fractures.

All patients with facial trauma should be evaluated for jaw fractures. Blows to the chin are among the most common childhood orofacial traumas. They are also a leading cause of condylar fracture in the pediatric population. Condylar fracture should be suspected if significant pain or deviation occurs when the mouth is opened.

Tooth-related trauma affects the dental hard tissues and pulp, the alveolar process, and the periodontal tissues. The range of dental injuries includes root, crown, and alveolar fractures; concussion, subluxation, intrusive, extrusive, and lateral luxations; and avulsion. Figure 17–9 demonstrates different degrees of tooth fractures, and Figure 17–10 shows the types of luxation injuries.

Primary Teeth

The most common injuries in the primary dentition are luxation injuries, with the greatest incidence of trauma occurring between 2 and 3 years of age. Treatment recommendations are primarily guided by assessing the risk of damage to the

developing permanent tooth which is in close proximity to the apex of the root of the primary tooth. Parents should be advised of any permanent tooth complications such as enamel hypocalcification, dilacerations (severe angular distortions of the crown or root of a tooth), ectopic eruption, or impaction caused by intrusion injuries of the primary maxillary anterior teeth. An intrusive luxation is usually observed for a period to discern whether the tooth will spontaneously re-erupt (see Figure 17–10) unless the root of the primary tooth is impinging on the crown of the permanent tooth bud as diagnosed with an occlusal radiograph. Severe luxation in any direction is treated with extraction. Avulsed primary teeth are rarely replanted because the risk of ankylosis and damage to the permanent tooth successor outweigh the esthetic benefit of having the primary tooth in place for a few years. In a root fracture, the crown and apical fragment are generally extracted, but the latter should be left for physiologic resorption if its retrieval would result in potential damage to the permanent tooth.

When planning treatment, other important factors such as the child's maturity and level of cooperation should be considered along with the time to exfoliation of the injured tooth. Complex procedures such as root canal treatment, crown placement, and splinting require high levels of cooperation when compared to extraction and must be carefully discussed with parents if advanced behavior guidance modalities such as sedation or general anesthesia are required.

Permanent Teeth

The most common injury in the permanent dentition is crown fracture occurring secondary to falls, motor vehicle accidents, violence, and sports. Treatment is aimed at preserving the health of the pulp. Intrusions of permanent teeth are corrected with repositioning unless the tooth is immature and has incomplete root formation, the intrusion is minor (less than 3 mm), or there is no re-eruption after a few weeks. Lateral and extrusive luxations are generally repositioned and splinted for up to 2 weeks. Splints should stabilize the tooth in correct position while allowing physiologic movement of the tooth, good oral hygiene, and nontraumatic removal.

Because the prognosis for viability worsens rapidly as time outside the mouth increases, an avulsed permanent tooth should be replanted into its socket as soon as possible at or near the accident scene after gentle rinsing with clean water. The patient must seek emergency dental care immediately thereafter. Hank's balanced salt solution (HBSS) is the best storage and transport medium for avulsed teeth that are to be replanted at a distant site. The next best storage mediums in decreasing order are milk, saline, saliva (buccal vestibule), or water. The commercially available FDA-approved Save-a-Tooth kit which contains HBSS should be part of first-aid kits in school and sports facilities. Root canal treatment is necessary in the majority of cases to prevent inflammatory

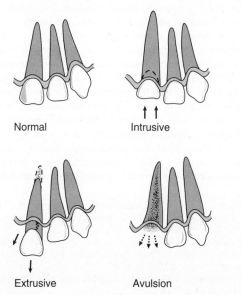

Normal

Intrusive

Extrusive

Avulsion

▲ **Figure 17–10.** Patterns of luxation injuries.

root resorption and needs to be initiated within 10 days from time of the initial injury.

Alveolar Fracture

Severe injuries can result in a fractured alveolus. The alveolar ridge and teeth within the fractured segment often move together when palpated and result in a disturbance in occlusion. Fractures should be evaluated with radiographs to determine their extent and involvement with the remaining teeth. The entire fractured segment should be repositioned and splinted with the teeth in place for 4 weeks after gingival lacerations are sutured. Removal of teeth which are firmly positioned in the alveolar segment is not indicated.

Home Care, Follow-Up, and Prevention

Healing outcomes are improved when home care instructions are observed and follow-up visits to the dentist are made. Excellent oral hygiene and rinsing with 0.12% chlorhexidine gluconate for 1–2 weeks reduces the presence of bacteria in the affected areas. A soft diet for 1–2 weeks and prevention of further injury is critical to healing and parents should be advised to keep children out of contact sports and rough play during this sensitive time of healing. Additionally, infants should be restricted from using a pacifier. During dental follow-up visits, the vitality of the teeth will be assessed through temperature, percussion, palpation, and radiographic testing.

Following healing of the injury, prevention of future injuries should be encouraged through the use of mouthguards for sports prone to injury.

Antibiotic Usage

There is limited evidence for the use of systemic antibiotics for dental injuries; however, antibiotic use remains at the discretion of the clinician as traumatic dental injuries frequently occur in unclean environments and are often accompanied by soft tissue lacerations, maxillofacial trauma, and affect medically compromised patients. For avulsion injuries, tetracycline is the antibiotic of choice for the first week after replantation of an avulsed tooth. While one of the significant side effects of tetracyclines is permanent tooth discoloration, such a risk is more likely to occur with longer courses (> 21 days) that are generally not given to children who are younger than 8 years of age. Per the International Association for Dental Traumatology (IADT), penicillin or amoxicillin can also be prescribed as an effective alternative to tetracycline for children under 12 years of age for whom the risk for discoloration of permanent teeth may be considered a significant concern.

▶ Odontogenic Infections

Odontogenic infections can result from carious lesions, restorations approximating the pulp tissue, periodontal complications, and dental trauma. If left untreated, pain, a dental abscess, and facial cellulitis can result. These sequelae can lead to serious complications such as dehydration from difficulties with eating or drinking, cavernous sinus thrombosis, and Ludwig's angina. While acetaminophen or ibuprofen can help relieve pain, prompt intervention and removal of the source of infection is needed to avoid adverse sequelae. Topical medications are of limited value for pain relief.

Alveolar Abscess

When left untreated, the infection that causes necrosis of the pulp tissue can spread outward from the apical foramen of the root of the tooth through bone and periosteum to produce an alveolar abscess. In its acute form, the abscess presents as a painful and diffuse infection of the gingival soft tissues that requires immediate attention. Treatment includes root canal therapy or extraction for the drainage of pus from the site of infection and for pain relief. A chronic alveolar abscess (or parulis) is a localized smaller swelling confined to the gingival tissue associated with the infected tooth. A parulis does not represent an urgent situation and antibiotic therapy is not warranted as the pus is draining through a fistula tract. Definitive treatment includes root canal therapy or extraction of the offending tooth.

Facial Cellulitis

Facial cellulitis results if the odontogenic infection invades the facial spaces. Elevated temperature (> 38.8°C), lethargy, difficulty swallowing, and difficulty breathing are signs of serious infections. Swelling of the midface—especially the bridge of the nose and the lower eyelid—should be urgently evaluated as a potential dental infection. Depending on the clinical situation and the patient's overall health, treatment choices range from treating or extracting the offending tooth/teeth, with antibiotic coverage, to achieve drainage and eliminate the source of infection. Occasionally, treatment is delayed for several days while antibiotics are administered orally or IV (for hospitalized patients) so that the infection can be properly drained. The first-line antibiotic of choice is penicillin and secondarily clindamycin or ampicillin-sulbactam (Unasyn). Hospitalization is a prudent choice for younger children with severe facial cellulitis especially if other systemic signs and symptoms are present—fever, dehydration, airway compromise, or possible noncompliance.

Andersson LA, et al: Guidelines for the management of traumatic dental injuries: 2. Avulsion of permanent teeth. Pediatr Dent 2012;28: 88–96 [PMID: 29179383].

DiAngelis AJ, et al: Guidelines for the management of traumatic dental injuries: 1. Fractures and luxations of permanent teeth. Dent Traumatol 2012;28:2–12.

Guideline on use of antibiotic therapy for pediatric dental patients. Pediatr Dent 2018–19;40(6):383–385.

Malmgren B, et al: Guidelines for the management of traumatic dental injuries: 3. Injuries in the primary dentition. Dent Traumatol 2012;28(3):174–182.

SPECIAL PATIENT POPULATIONS

▶ Oral Conditions

Children with special health care needs (C-SHCN) may have anomalies affecting their teeth and/or oral soft tissues as a primary manifestation of a systemic condition or secondary to medical interventions. For children with Trisomy 21 for example, conditions such as hypodontia and delayed eruption are considered primary oral manifestations of the syndrome. Rare systemic conditions such as osteogenesis imperfecta can be associated with dentinogenesis imperfecta—a defect affecting the dentin of primary and permanent dentition resulting in early loss of teeth if left unrecognized and untreated.

Medical interventions such as chemotherapy and radiation therapy can have immediate and long-term oral effects. Most immediate are xerostomia, particularly where the salivary glands are in the path of the radiation beam, mucositis due to atrophy of the oral mucosa, and severe oral pain from mucositis. Long-term effects include microdontia, hypocalcification, short and blunted roots, and delayed tooth eruption. Patients undergoing hematopoietic stem cell transplantation are at risk for oral fungal and herpes simplex virus infections during the initial engraftment and reconstitution period. Allogeneic transplants further predispose a child to oral graft-versus-host disease, which can cause ulcerations, erosive lesions, or whitish reticulations affecting various oral soft tissues.

▶ Preventive Measures

Dental caries affects C-SHCN for reasons that are uniquely related to their medical condition. The long-term use of many medications is associated with increased caries risk as some of these contain sucrose as a sweetener. Likewise, the frequent consumption of supplemental nutrition drinks that are typically high in carbohydrates significantly increases the risk for dental caries. Simple preventive steps such as rinsing with fluoridated water or a fluoridated mouth rinse, and/or tooth brushing with fluoridated toothpaste after each medication or supplemental nutrition intake lowers caries risk in such patients. The prescription of sugar-free alternatives for medications is recommended as a preventive measure.

The susceptibility of C-SHCN to periodontal diseases increases with difficulty performing oral hygiene due to a child's oral aversions, limited mouth opening, or erratic body movements. Parents may also wrongly choose not to brush their child's teeth believing it to be unnecessary since the child takes no foods my mouth. G-tube fed children typically exhibit increased calculus build-up due to the lack of mechanical stimulation associated with oral feedings, increasing their risk for periodontal disease.

Preventive Measures for the Oncology Patient

It is imperative that a dentist knowledgeable about pediatric oncology evaluate children with cancer soon after diagnosis. The aims are to (1) develop a dental treatment plan in collaboration with the oncologist prior to cancer therapy, (2) educate the patient and caregivers about the importance of good oral hygiene, and (3) remove all existing and potential sources of dental infection (eg, abscessed teeth, extensive caries) before the child becomes neutropenic from chemotherapy.

Preventive strategies aimed at reducing oral complications from cancer therapy include reduction of refined sugars, fluoride therapy, mucositis prevention, and patient education. Meticulous oral hygiene reduces the risk for severe mucositis. In children receiving radiation therapy, customized fluoride applicators and artificial saliva are used in combination with regular follow-up visits to minimize rapid and extensive destruction of teeth due to xerostomia.

▶ Dental Treatment Considerations

Indications for Antibiotic Prophylaxis

All dental procedures (even tooth brushing) often result in transient bacteremia. Patients with certain medical conditions are at increased risk for bacteremia-induced infections and require prophylactic antibiotic coverage prior to invasive dental procedures. These include children with cardiac conditions such as heart valves, previous infective endocarditis, repaired congenital heart disease with residual defects related to a prosthetic patch, and unrepaired cyanotic congenital heart disease. For nonvalvular devices such as indwelling vascular catheters and cardiovascular implantable electronic devices, antibiotic coverage is only indicated at the time of placement and possibly 3–6 months afterward. Hydrocephalus shunts with vascular access (ie, ventriculoatrial, ventriculocardiac, ventriculovenous) require antibiotic prophylaxis to minimize risk for infection from dental procedures, whereas the nonvascular type (ventriculoperitoneal) does not.

Antibiotic prophylaxis is generally not indicated for dental patients with pins, plates, screws, or other orthopedic hardware that is not within a synovial joint. Likewise, most patients with total joint replacements do not routinely require antibiotic prophylaxis except for the early postsurgical period (6 months).

For immunocompromised patients, the absolute neutrophil count (ANC) is important for the dentist because of the risk for systemic sepsis from dental procedures. The AAPD guideline indicates for neutrophil levels above 2000/mm^3 antibiotic prophylaxis is not indicated. Between 1000 and 2000/mm^3, prophylaxis is subject to the clinical judgment of the dentist, the patient's health status, and the planned procedures. Both the dentist and physician should discuss and plan the need for antibiotic prophylaxis in these unique circumstances.

Management of Bleeding Disorders

Oral surgical procedures on any child with a bleeding disorder should be planned in a coordinated approach between the child's hematologist and dentist. Patients with mild bleeding disorders (eg, mild von Willebrand's disease) can be treated in the ambulatory dental setting with local hemostatic measures such as topical hemostatic agents (eg, Gelfoam, thrombin). Patients with severe coagulation disorders (eg, severe hemophilia A and/or Factor VIII antibodies) requiring dental surgery should be admitted to a hospital. Preoperative planning includes prescription of antifibrinolytic medications such as ε-aminocaproic or tranexamic acid to minimize postoperative oral bleeding. Intra-operatively, the placement of topical hemostatic agents within tooth sockets and additional sutures immediately following extractions improves clot formation.

For patients receiving anticoagulation therapy, dosage reduction before dental surgery is generally not recommended as the risk of embolism outweighs the risk for bleeding complications. In these instances, the dentist should consult with the hematologist to obtain the most recent INR and discuss the most appropriate anticoagulation level at which a dental procedure can occur. Also, the administration of a "bridging agent" such as enoxaparin in preparation for the planned dental procedure reduces postoperative bleeding concerns while minimizing embolic complications.

Patients undergoing chemotherapy and/or hematopoietic stem cell transplantation are also at risk for intra-oral bleeding. They can experience spontaneous oral hemorrhage, particularly when the platelet count is less than 20,000/μL. Typically, platelet counts greater than 75,000/μL do not require additional measures for dental procedures, while lower levels require pre- and postoperative platelet transfusions.

Guideline on antibiotic prophylaxis for dental patients at risk for infection. Pediatr Dent 2016;38(6):328–333.

Guideline on dental management of pediatric patients receiving chemotherapy, hematopoieticcell transplantation, and/or radiation therapy. Pediatr Dent 2016. October;38(6):334–342.

Guideline on management of dental patients with special health care needs. Pediatr Dent 2016;38(6):171–176.

Moursi AM, Fernandez JB, Daronch M, Zee L, Jones CL: Nutrition and oral health considerations in children with special health care needs: implications for oral health care providers. Pediatr Dent 2010 Aug, 15;32(4):333–342 [PMID: 20836954].

Norwood KW, Slayton RL: Oral health care for children with developmental disabilities. Pediatrics 2013;131(3):614–619 [PMID: 23439896].

ORTHODONTIC REFERRAL

The pediatric dentist is involved in the timely detection of orthodontic concerns in the mixed or permanent dentition and facilitates appropriate referral to an orthodontist for correction of the malocclusion to promote normal growth development of jaws and teeth. For any child with a cleft palate or other craniofacial growth disorder, referral is indicated when maxillary permanent incisors are starting to erupt and an alveolar bone graft is contemplated.

The orthodontic evaluation to detect a malocclusion usually involves detailed examination of the craniofacial and intra-oral structures. The extra-oral analysis includes assessment of head shape, facial form, and mandibular growth pattern. The intra-oral analysis includes assessment of the sagittal relationship between the permanent first molars, canines, and incisors of the maxilla and mandible. Discrepencies between these teeth in the coronal and sagittal planes can result in crossbites involving the anterior and posterior dentition. The clinical assessment is typically coupled with a radiographic evaluation utilizing panoramic or cephalometric radiographs. The radiographic assessment provides supplemental detailed information regarding the malocclusion by assessing the relative position of the jaws with respect to the cranial base and teeth, as well as the growth pattern of the mandible.

Franco FCM, Araujo TM, Vogel CJ, Quintão CCA: Brachycephalic, dolichocephalic and mesocephalic: Is it appropriate to describe the face using skull patterns? Dental Press J Orthod 2013;18(3):159–163 [PMID: 24094027].

Proffit WR, Sarver DM, Ackerman JL: Orthodontic diagnosis: the problem-oriented approach. In: Proffit WR, Fields HW, Sarver DM (eds): *Contemporary Orthodontics*. 5th ed. St. Louis, MO: Mosby; 2012:150–219.

Ear, Nose, & Throat

Patricia J. Yoon, MD

Melissa A. Scholes, MD

Brian W. Herrmann, MD

INFECTIONS OF THE EAR

1. Acute Otitis Externa

ESSENTIALS OF DIAGNOSIS & TYPICAL FEATURES

▶ Rapid onset of symptoms within the past 3 weeks.

▶ **Symptoms** of ear canal inflammation, including otalgia, itching, or fullness, with or without hearing loss or jaw pain.

▶ **Signs** of ear canal inflammation, including tenderness of the tragus and/or pinna, ear canal edema and/or erythema, otorrhea, regional lymphadenitis, tympanic membrane (TM) erythema, or cellulitis of the pinna and adjacent skin.

▶ Differential Diagnosis

Acute or chronic otitis media with eardrum rupture, furunculosis of the ear canal, herpes zoster oticus, mastoiditis, referred temporomandibular joint pain, and chronic otitis externa.

▶ Pathogenesis

Otitis externa (OE) is a cellulitis of the soft tissues of the external auditory canal (EAC), which can extend to surrounding structures such as the pinna, tragus, and lymph nodes. Humidity, heat, and moisture in the ear are known to contribute to the development of OE, thus it is more common in the summer months and in humid climates. Cerumen serves as a hydrophobic protective barrier to the underlying skin and its acidic pH inhibits bacterial and fungal growth. Trauma to the ear canal skin can break this skin-cerumen barrier, which is the first step in developing OE. Sources of trauma can include cotton swab use, earbuds, digital manipulation (scratching), and ear plugs. Dermatologic conditions such as atopic dermatitis can also predispose one to OE. The most common organisms causing OE are *Staphylococcus aureus*, *Staphylococcus epidermidis*, and *Pseudomonas aeruginosa*. However, anaerobic bacteria are also seen. Fungal infection occurs in 2%–10% of patients, usually following treatment for a bacterial OE.

▶ Clinical Findings

Symptoms include acute onset of pain, aural fullness, decreased hearing, and itching in the ear. Symptoms tend to peak within 3 days. Manipulation of the pinna or tragus causes considerable pain. Discharge may be clear or purulent and may also cause secondary eczema of the auricle. The EAC is typically swollen and narrowed, and the patient may resist any attempt to insert an otoscope. Debris is often present in the canal, and it may be difficult to visualize the TM. However, it is important to determine the status of the eardrum to rule out secondary OE caused by middle ear drainage that may need to be managed differently.

▶ Complications

If untreated, cellulitis of neck and face may result. Immunocompromised individuals can develop malignant OE, which is a spread of the infection to the skull base with resultant osteomyelitis. This is a life-threatening condition and should be evaluated emergently if suspected.

CHAPTER 18

Treatment

Management of OE includes pain control, removal of debris from the canal, topical antimicrobial therapy, and avoidance of causative factors. Cultures are not routinely sent on initial presentation as most cases will resolve with these primary interventions. Fluoroquinolone eardrops alone are first-line therapy for OE in the absence of systemic symptoms. The topical therapy chosen must be nonototoxic because a perforation or patent tube may be present; if the TM cannot be visualized, a perforation should be presumed to exist. If the ear canal is too edematous to allow entry of the eardrops, a Pope ear wick (expandable sponge) should be placed to ensure antibiotic delivery. Oral antibiotics are indicated for any signs of invasive infection, such as fever, cellulitis of the face or auricle, or tender periauricular or cervical lymphadenopathy. In such cases, in addition to ototopical therapy, cultures of the ear canal discharge should be sent, and an antistaphylococcal antibiotic prescribed while awaiting culture results. The ear should be kept dry until the infection has cleared. If drainage persists despite therapy, cultures should be sent. Patients can have difficulty applying drops to the affected ear canal, which may cause prolonged symptoms and treatment failures. If this is suspected, thoroughly explain and demonstrate the application of the topical therapy as outlined in the Clinical Practice Guideline on Acute Otitis Externa. A new formulation of ciprofloxacin suspension has recently become available; it is liquid at cooler temperatures and thickens into a gel at body temperature. This allows a single application to work for multiple days and may be useful when there are compliance problems.

Rosenfeld RM et al: Clinical practice guideline: acute otitis externa executive summary. Otolaryngol Head Neck Surg 2014 Nov;150(2):161–168 [PMID: 24492208].

Web Resources

Goguen LA. External Otitis: Pathogenesis, Clinical Features and Diagnosis. https://www.uptodate.com/contents/external-otitis-pathogenesis-clinical-features-and-diagnosis?search=external%20otitis&source=search_result&selectedTitle=2~30&usage_type=default&display_rank=2. Accessed June 2, 2019.

Waitzman AA et al. Otitis Externa. http://emedicine.medscape.com/article/994550-overview. Accessed June 2, 2019.

2. Acute Otitis Media

Acute otitis media (AOM) is the most common reason antibiotics are prescribed for children in the United States. It is an acute infection of the middle ear space associated with inflammation, effusion, or, if a patent tympanostomy tube or perforation is present, otorrhea (ear drainage).

ESSENTIALS OF DIAGNOSIS & TYPICAL FEATURES

▶ Moderate to severe bulging of the TM or new otorrhea not associated with OE.

▶ Mild bulging of the TM and less than 48 hours of otalgia (ear-holding, tugging, or rubbing in a nonverbal child) or intense erythema of the TM.

▶ Middle ear effusion (MEE), proven by pneumatic otoscopy or tympanometry, must be present.

▶ Differential Diagnosis

Otitis media with effusion (OME), bullous myringitis, acute mastoiditis, and middle ear mass.

▶ Clinical Findings

Two findings are critical in establishing a diagnosis of AOM: a bulging TM and a MEE. The presence of MEE is best determined by visual examination and either pneumatic otoscopy or tympanometry (Figure 18–1). To distinguish AOM from OME, signs and symptoms of middle ear inflammation and acute infection must be present. Otoscopic findings specific for AOM include a bulging TM, impaired visibility of ossicular landmarks, yellow or white effusion (pus), an opacified and inflamed eardrum, and occasionally squamous exudate or bullae on the eardrum.

A. Pathophysiology and Predisposing Factors

1. Eustachian tube dysfunction (ETD)—The Eustachian tube regulates middle ear pressure and allows for drainage of the middle ear. The ciliated respiratory epithelium of the Eustachian tube also defends against pathogens by producing lysozyme and mucus, which helps rid the ear of microorganisms. It must periodically open to prevent the development of negative pressure and effusion in the middle ear space. If the Eustachian tube does not work properly, negative pressure leads to transudation of cellular fluid into the middle ear, as well as influx of fluids and pathogens from the nasopharynx and adenoids. Middle ear fluid may then become infected, resulting in AOM. The Eustachian tube of infants and young children is more prone to dysfunction because it is shorter, more compliant, and more horizontal than in adults. The Eustachian tube reaches its adult configuration by the age of 7 years. Children with craniofacial differences, such as those with Trisomy 21 or cleft palate, may be particularly susceptible to ETD because of abnormal anatomy of the Eustachian tube.

2. Bacterial colonization—Nasopharyngeal colonization with *S pneumoniae*, *Haemophilus influenzae*, or *Moraxella catarrhalis* increases the risk of AOM, whereas colonization

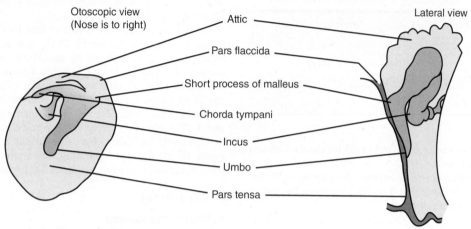

▲ **Figure 18–1.** Tympanic membrane.

with normal flora such as viridans streptococci may prevent AOM by inhibiting growth of these pathogens.

3. Viral upper respiratory infections—Upper respiratory infections (URIs) impair Eustachian tube function by causing adenoid hypertrophy and edema of the Eustachian tube itself. Viral infections also inhibit the antibacterial properties of mucus and mucociliary clearance.

4. Smoke exposure—Passive smoke increases the risk of persistent MEE by enhancing colonization, prolonging the inflammatory response, and impeding drainage of the middle ear through the Eustachian tube. For infants aged 12–18 months, cigarette exposure is associated with an 11% per pack increase in the duration of MEE.

5. Impaired host immune defenses—Immunocompromised children such as those with selective IgA deficiency usually experience recurrent AOM, rhinosinusitis, and pneumonia. However, most children who experience recurrent or persistent otitis only have selective impairments of immune defenses against specific otitis pathogens.

6. Bottle feeding—Bottle feeding especially with bottle propping in the crib or carseat increases the risk of AOM because of aspiration of contaminated secretions into the middle ear space. Breastfeeding reduces the incidence of acute respiratory infections and provides immunoglobulin A (IgA) antibodies that reduce colonization with otitis pathogens.

7. Season—The incidence of AOM correlates with the activity of respiratory viruses, accounting for the annual surge in otitis media cases during the winter months in temperate climates.

8. Daycare attendance—Children exposed to large groups of children have more respiratory infections and OM. The increased number of children in day care over the past three

decades has undoubtedly played a major role in the increase in AOM.

9. Genetic susceptibility—Genetics is thought to play a role in 40%–70% of ear infections. Most of the genes responsible regulate immunity. However, environmental and pathogen-related causes also play a role. The role of genetics in AOM is an area of active research.

10. Age—Children ages 1–3 years are at greatest risk for AOM.

B. Microbiology of Acute Otitis Media

Bacterial or viral pathogens can be detected in up to 96% of middle ear fluid samples from patients with AOM. Peak activity of respiratory syncytial virus, metapneumovirus, and influenza A corresponds with increased visits for AOM and 71% of middle ear aspirates from children undergoing ear tube surgery for recurrent OM contain viruses. Polybacterial infections are seen in up to 55% of cases, with bacterial and viral coinfections occurring in up to 70%. S pneumoniae and H influenzae account for 35%–40% and 30%–35% of isolates, respectively. With widespread use of the pneumococcal conjugate vaccine starting in 2000, the incidence of AOM caused by H influenzae rose while that of the S pneumoniae vaccine serotypes declined. However, there has been an increase in disease caused by S pneumoniae serotypes not covered by the vaccine, as well as S aureus. The third most common pathogen cited is M catarrhalis, which causes 15%–25% of AOM cases in the United States (Table 18–1). The fourth most common organism in AOM is Streptococcus pyogenes, which is found more frequently in school-aged children than in infants. S pyogenes and S pneumoniae are the predominant causes of mastoiditis.

Drug-resistant S pneumoniae is a common pathogen in AOM and strains may be resistant to only one drug class

Table 18–1. Microbiology of acute otitis media (AOM).

Organism	Percentage of AOM Cases
S pneumoniae	35–40
H influenzae	30–35
M catarrhalis	15–25
S pyogenes	4

(eg, penicillins or macrolides) or to multiple classes. Children with resistant strains tend to be younger and to have had more unresponsive infections. History of antibiotic treatment in the preceding 3 months increases the risk of harboring resistant pathogens.

C. Examination Techniques and Procedures

1. Pneumatic otoscopy—AOM is overdiagnosed, leading to inappropriate antibiotic therapy, unnecessary surgical referrals, and significant associated costs. Contributing to errors in diagnosis is the temptation to accept the diagnosis without removing enough cerumen to adequately visualize the TM, and the mistaken belief that a red TM establishes the diagnosis. Redness of the TM is often a vascular flush caused by fever or crying.

A pneumatic otoscope with a rubber suction bulb and tube is used to assess TM mobility. When used correctly, pneumatic otoscopy can improve diagnostic ability by 15%–25%. The largest possible speculum should be used to provide an airtight seal and maximize the field of view. When the rubber bulb is gently squeezed, the TM should move freely with a snapping motion; if fluid is present in the middle ear space, the mobility of the TM will be absent or resemble a fluid wave. The ability to assess mobility is compromised by failure to achieve an adequate seal with the otoscope and poor visualization of the TM.

2. Cerumen removal—In order to adequately visualize the TM, cerumen (ear wax) removal is an essential skill for anyone who cares for children. Please refer to section on cerumen impaction below.

3. Tympanometry—Tympanometry can be helpful in assessing middle ear status, particularly when pneumatic otoscopy is inconclusive or difficult to perform. Tympanometry can reveal the presence or absence of a MEE but cannot differentiate between acutely infected fluid (AOM) and a chronic effusion (also referred to as OME).

Tympanometry measures TM compliance and displays it in graphic form. It also measures the volume of the ear canal, which can help differentiate between an intact and perforated TM.

Standard 226-Hz tympanometry is not reliable in infants younger than 6 months. A high-frequency (1000 Hz) probe is used in this age group.

Tympanograms can be classified into four major patterns, as shown in Figure 18–2. The pattern shown in Figure 18–2A, characterized by maximum compliance at normal atmospheric pressure, indicates a normal TM, good Eustachian tube function, and absence of effusion. Figure 18–2B identifies a nonmobile TM with normal volume, which indicates MEE. Figure 18–2C indicates an intact, mobile TM with excessively negative middle ear pressure (> –150 daPa), indicative of poor Eustachian tube function. Figure 18–2D shows a flat tracing with a large middle ear volume, indicative of a patent tube or TM perforation.

▶ Treatment

A. Pain Management

Pain is the primary symptom of AOM, and the 2013 clinical practice guidelines emphasize the importance of addressing this symptom. As it may take 1–3 days before antibiotic therapy leads to a reduction in pain, ibuprofen or acetaminophen should be administered as needed to relieve discomfort. Topical analgesics have a very short duration and studies do not support efficacy in children younger than 5 years.

B. The Observation Option

The choice to observe an episode of AOM and not treat with antibiotics is an option in otherwise healthy children with mild to moderate otitis media without other underlying conditions such as cleft palate, craniofacial abnormalities, immune deficiencies, cochlear implants, or tympanostomy tubes. The decision should be made in conjunction with the parents, and a mechanism must be in place to provide antibiotic therapy if there is worsening of symptoms or lack of improvement within 48–72 hours. A Safety-Net Antibiotic Prescription (SNAP) given to parents with instructions to be filled only if symptoms do not resolve lowered overall antibiotic use in a large pediatric practice-based research network. The American Academy of Pediatrics clinical practice guidelines include age, presence of otorrhea, severity of symptoms, and laterality as criteria for antibiotic treatment versus observation (Table 18–2).

C. Antibiotic Therapy

Antibiotics have been shown to shorten the duration of AOM. Therefore, high-dose amoxicillin remains the first-line antibiotic for treating AOM, even with a high prevalence of drug-resistant S pneumoniae, because data show that isolates of the bacteria remain susceptible to the drug 83%–87% of the time.

Amoxicillin-clavulanate enhanced strength (ES), with 90 mg/kg/day of amoxicillin dosing (14:1 ratio of

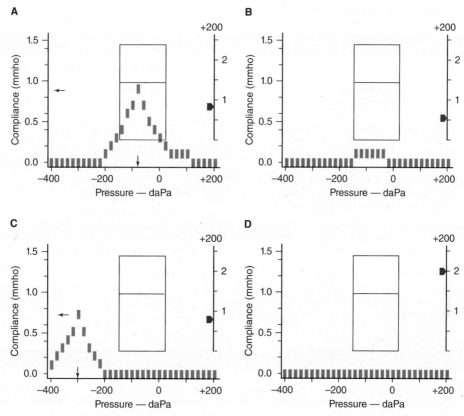

▲ **Figure 18–2.** Four types of tympanograms obtained with Welch-Allyn MicroTymp 2. **A:** Normal middle ear. **B:** Otitis media with effusion or AOM. **C:** Negative middle ear pressure due to ETD. **D:** Patent tympanostomy tube or perforation in the TM. Same as B except for a very large middle ear volume.

amoxicillin:clavulanate), is an appropriate choice when a child has had amoxicillin in the last 30 days, or is clinically failing after 48–72 hours on amoxicillin (Table 18–3) or has concomitant conjunctivitis. Purulent conjunctivitis is often caused by nontypeable *H influenzae*. The regular strength formulations of amoxicillin-clavulanate (7:1 ratio) should not be doubled in dosage to achieve 90 mg/kg/day of amoxicillin, because the increased amount of clavulanate will cause diarrhea.

Table 18–2. Recommendations for initial management of uncomplicated AOM. [a]

Age	Otorrhea With AOM[a]	Unilateral or Bilateral AOM[a] With Severe Symptoms[b]	Bilateral AOM[a] Without Otorrhea	Unilateral AOM[a] Without Otorrhea
6 mo to 2 y	Antibiotic therapy	Antibiotic therapy	Antibiotic therapy	Antibiotic therapy or additional observation
≥ 2 y	Antibiotic therapy	Antibiotic therapy	Antibiotic therapy or additional observation	Antibiotic therapy or additional observation[c]

[a]Applies only to children with well-documented AOM and a high certainty of diagnosis.
[b]A toxic-appearing child, persistent otalgia for more than 48 hours, temperature > 39°C (102.2°F) in the past 48 hours, or if there is uncertain access to follow-up after the visit.
[c]This plan of initial management provides an opportunity for shared decision-making with the child's family for those categories appropriate for initial observation. If observation is offered, a mechanism must be in place to ensure follow-up and begin antibiotics if the child worsens or fails to improve within 48–72 hours of AOM onset.

Table 18–3. Antibiotic therapies for AOM.

A. Initial Immediate or Delayed Antibiotic Treatment	
First-Line Treatment	**Alternative Treatments (if Penicillin-Allergic)**
Amoxicillin (80–90 mg/kg/day in two divided doses) • For children aged < 2 y or children of all ages with severe symptoms, treat for 10 days. • Age 2–6 y with mild-moderate symptoms, treat for 7 days. • Age > 6 y with mild-moderate symptoms, treat for 5 days. or Amoxicillin-clavulanate (90 mg/kg/day or amoxicillin, with 6.4 mg/kg/day of clavulanate in two divided doses) • For patients who have received amoxicillin in the previous 30 days or who have otitis-conjunctivitis syndrome	Cefdinir (14/mg/kg/day in 1 or 2 doses) Cefuroxime (30 mg/kg/day divided BID) Cefpodoxime (10 mg/kg/day in two divided doses) Ceftriaxone (50 mg IM or IV per day for 1 or 3 days) • If unable to take oral medications For children with severe penicillin allergies (IgE-mediated events) or known cephalosporin allergy: • Trimethoprim-sulfamethoxazole • Macrolides • Clindamycin (30–40 mg/kg/day, divided TID)
B. Antibiotic Treatment After 48–72 h of Failure of Initial Antibiotic	
First-Line Treatment	**Alternative Treatment**
Amoxicillin-clavulanate (90 mg/kg/day or amoxicillin, with 6.4 mg/kg/day of clavulanate in two divided doses) • For patients who have received amoxicillin in the previous 30 days or who have otitis-conjunctivitis syndrome. or Ceftriaxone (50 mg IM or IV per day for 3 days)	Ceftriaxone (50 mg IM or IV per day for 3 days) Clindamycin (30–40 mg/kg/day, divided TID) with or without a third-generation cephalosporin Consider tympanocentesis Consult specialist
C. Recurrence > 4 wk After Initial Episode	
1. A new pathogen is likely, so restart first-line therapy. 2. Be sure diagnosis is not OME, which may be observed for 3–6 mo without treatment.	

Three oral cephalosporins (cefuroxime, cefpodoxime, and cefdinir) are more β-lactamase–stable and are alternative choices in children who develop a papular rash with amoxicillin (see Table 18–3). Of these, cefdinir suspension is most palatable; the other two have a bitter aftertaste which is difficult to conceal.

A second-line antibiotic is indicated when a child experiences symptomatic infection within 1 month of finishing amoxicillin; however, repeated use of high-dose amoxicillin is indicated if more than 4 weeks have passed without symptoms. Macrolides are not recommended as second-line agents because *S pneumoniae* is resistant in approximately 30% of respiratory isolates, and because virtually all strains of *H influenzae* have an intrinsic macrolide efflux pump, which pumps the antibiotic out of the bacterial cell. However, if there is a history of type 1 hypersensitivity reaction, macrolides may be used.

Reasons for failure to eradicate a sensitive pathogen include drug noncompliance, poor drug absorption, or vomiting of the drug. If a child remains symptomatic for longer than 3 days while taking a second-line agent, a tympanocentesis is useful to identify the causative pathogen. If a highly resistant pneumococcus is found or if tympanocentesis is not feasible, intramuscular ceftriaxone at 50 mg/kg/dose for 3 consecutive days is recommended. If a child has experienced a severe reaction, such as anaphylaxis, to amoxicillin, cephalosporins should not be substituted. Otherwise, the risk of cross-sensitivity is less than 0.1%. Multidrug-resistant *S pneumoniae* poses a treatment dilemma and newer antibiotics, such as fluoroquinolones or linezolid, may need to be employed. However, these drugs are not approved by the U.S. Food and Drug Administration (FDA) for the treatment of AOM in children.

In patients with tympanostomy tubes with uncomplicated acute otorrhea, ototopical antibiotics (fluoroquinolone eardrops) are first-line therapy. The eardrops serve two purposes: (1) They treat the infection and (2) they physically "rinse" drainage from the tube which helps prevent plugging of the tube. Oral antibiotics are not indicated in the absence of systemic symptoms.

If a TM perforation has occurred with otorrhea then topical antibiotics are recommended as first-line agents due to the ability to provide high concentrations of antibiotic directly to the middle ear. Topical fluoroquinolone otic drops (ofloxacin and ciprofloxacin) with or without steroids are considered safe for administration into the middle ear. If there is a large amount of debris or drainage in the ear canal, the canal may need to be suctioned first to allow drops to gain access to the middle ear.

D. Tympanocentesis

Tympanocentesis is performed by placing a needle through the TM and aspirating the middle ear fluid. The fluid is sent for culture and sensitivity. Indications for tympanocentesis are (1) AOM in an immunocompromised patient, (2) research studies, (3) evaluation for presumed sepsis or meningitis, such as in a neonate, (4) unresponsive otitis media despite courses of two appropriate antibiotics, and (5) acute mastoiditis or other suppurative complications.

E. Prevention of Acute Otitis Media

1. Antibiotic prophylaxis—Strongly discouraged due to poor efficacy and concern for antibiotic resistance.

2. Possible lifestyle modifications—Parental education plays a major role in decreasing AOM.

- Smoking is a risk factor both for URI and AOM. Primary care physicians should provide information on smoking cessation programs and measures.

- Breastfeeding protects children from AOM. Clinicians should encourage exclusive breastfeeding for 6 months.

- Bottle-propping in the crib should be avoided. It increases AOM risk due to the reflux of milk into the Eustachian tubes.

- Pacifiers are controversial. There may be a protective effect of pacifiers against SIDS but they may increase risk of AOM. Currently, the recommendation from the American Academy of Family Physicians is to wean pacifiers after 6 months of age to reduce the risk of AOM.

- Day care is a risk factor for AOM, but working parents may have few alternatives. Possible alternatives include care by relatives or child care in a setting with fewer children.

3. Surgery—Tympanostomy tubes are effective in the treatment of recurrent AOM as well as OME.

4. Immunologic evaluation and allergy testing—While immunoglobulin subclass deficiencies may be more common in children with recurrent AOM, there is no practical immune therapy available. More serious immunodeficiencies, such as selective IgA deficiency, should be considered in children who suffer from a combination of recurrent AOM, rhinosinusitis, and pneumonia. In the school-aged child or preschooler with an atopic background, skin testing may be beneficial in identifying allergens that can predispose to AOM.

5. Vaccines—The pneumococcal conjugate and influenza vaccines are recommended. The seven-valent pneumococcal conjugate vaccine (PCV7) was introduced in the United States in 2000, and the 13-valent pneumococcal conjugate vaccine (PCV13) in 2010. The transition from PCV7 to PCV13 has resulted in a decline of otitis media among children younger

than 2 years due to decreased risk of both the first and subsequent episodes of otitis media.

Barenkamp SJ et al: Panel 4: Report of the microbiology panel. Otolaryngol Head Neck Surg 2017 April; 156(4 Suppl):S51–S62 [PMID: 28372529].

Lieberthal AS et al: The diagnosis and management of acute otitis media. Pediatrics 2013;131:e964–e999 [PMID: 23439909].

Schilder AG et al: Panel 7: Otitis media and complications. Otolaryngol Head Neck Surg 2017;156(4s):S88–S105 [PMID: 28372534].

Siegel RM et al: Treatment of otitis media with observation and a safety-net antibiotic prescription. Pediatrics 2003 Sep;112(3 Pt 1):527–531 [PMID: 12949278].

Wiese AD et al: Changes in otitis media episodes and pressure equalization tube insertions among young children following introduction of the 13-valent pneumococcal conjugate vaccine: A birth-cohort based study. Clin Infect Dis 2019 Nov 27;69(12):2162–2169. doi: 10.1093/cid/ciz142 [PMID: 30770533].

3. Otitis Media With Effusion

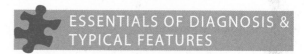

ESSENTIALS OF DIAGNOSIS & TYPICAL FEATURES

► MEE with decreased TM mobility as diagnosed on pneumatic otoscopy.

► No signs or symptoms of acute inflammation.

► OME should not be treated with antibiotics.

► Clinical Findings

OME is the presence of fluid in the middle ear space without signs or symptoms of acute inflammation. This is common, with 90% of children having one episode of OME by age 5. On examination, the TM may be opacified and thickened and the middle ear fluid can be clear, amber-colored, or opaque. Pneumatic otoscopy can confirm the presence of a MEE. If the pneumatic otoscopy examination is uncertain, then tympanometry should be performed to confirm presence of middle ear fluid.

Children with OME can develop AOM if the middle ear fluid should become infected. After AOM, fluid can remain in the ear for several weeks, with 60%–70% of children still having MEE 2 weeks after successful treatment. This drops to 40% at 1 month and 10%–25% at 3 months after treatment. It is important to distinguish OME from AOM because the former does not benefit from treatment with antibiotics.

► Management

An audiology evaluation should be performed after approximately 3 months of continuous bilateral effusion in most children. However, children who are at risk of language delay due to socioeconomic circumstances, craniofacial anomalies, or other risk factors should undergo a hearing evaluation at the time that OME is diagnosed. Children with hearing loss or speech delay should be referred to an otolaryngologist for possible tympanostomy tube placement. Antibiotics, antihistamines, and steroids have not been shown to be useful in the treatment of OME.

In uncomplicated cases, OME is observed for 3 months prior to consideration for tympanostomy tube placement. Longer periods of observation may be acceptable in children with normal or very mild hearing loss on audiogram, no risk factors for speech and language issues, and no structural changes to the TM. These children should be followed every 3–6 months until the effusions clear or problems develop. Indications for tympanostomy tubes include hearing loss greater than 40 dB, TM retraction pockets, ossicular erosion, adhesive atelectasis, and cholesteatoma. In children older than age 4, adenoidectomy may be recommended with ear tubes as studies show this can reduce failure rate and need for additional surgeries.

▶ Prognosis & Sequelae

Prognosis is variable based on age of presentation. Infants who are very young at the time of first otitis media are more likely to need surgical intervention. Other factors that decrease the likelihood of resolution are onset of OME in the summer or fall, history of prior tympanostomy tubes, presence of adenoids, and hearing loss greater than 30 dB.

Rosenfeld RM et al: Clinical practice guideline: tympanostomy tubes in children. Otolaryngol Head Neck Surg 2013 July;149(1Suppl):S1–S35 [PMID: 23818543].

Rosenfeld RM et al: Clinical Practice Guideline: otitis media with effusion executive summary (update). Otolaryngol Head Neck Surg 2016 Feb;154(2):201–214. doi: 10.1177/0194599815624407.26833645 [PMID: 26833645].

4. Complications of Otitis Media

A. Changes of the Tympanic Membrane

Tympanosclerosis is an acquired disorder of calcification and scarring of the TM and middle ear structures secondary to inflammation. If tympanosclerosis involves the ossicles, a conductive hearing loss may result. The term *myringosclerosis* applies to calcification of the TM only and is a fairly common sequela of OME and AOM. Myringosclerosis may also develop at the site of a previous tympanostomy tube; tympanosclerosis is not a common sequela of tube placement. Myringosclerosis rarely causes hearing loss, unless the entire TM is involved ("porcelain eardrum").

The appearance of a small defect or invagination of the pars tensa or pars flaccida of the TM suggests a retraction pocket. Retraction pockets occur when chronic inflammation and negative pressure in the middle ear space produce atrophy and atelectasis of the TM.

Continued inflammation can cause adhesions to form between the retracted TM and the ossicles. This condition, referred to as *adhesive otitis*, predisposes one to formation of a cholesteatoma or fixation and erosion of the ossicles.

B. Cholesteatoma

A greasy-looking or pearly white mass seen in a retraction pocket or perforation behind the eardrum suggests a cholesteatoma (Figure 18–3). If infection is superimposed, serous or purulent drainage will be seen, and the middle ear cavity may contain granulation tissue or even polyps. Persistent, recurrent, or foul-smelling otorrhea following appropriate medical management should make one suspect a cholesteatoma and prompt an ENT (Ear-Nose-Throat/Otolaryngology) referral.

C. Tympanic Membrane Perforation

Occasionally, an episode of AOM may result in rupture of the TM. Discharge from the ear is seen, and often there is rapid relief of pain. Perforations due to AOM usually heal spontaneously within a couple of weeks. Ototopical antibiotics are recommended for a 10- to 14-day course and patients should be referred to an otolaryngologist 2–3 weeks after the rupture for examination and hearing evaluation.

When perforations fail to heal, surgical repair may be needed. TM repair is generally delayed until the child is older and Eustachian tube function has improved. Repair of the

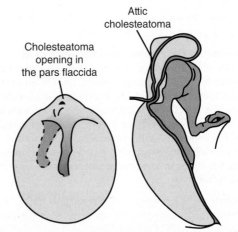

▲ **Figure 18–3.** Attic cholesteatoma, formed from an indrawing of an attic retraction pocket.

eardrum (tympanoplasty) is generally deferred until around 7 years of age, which is approximately when the Eustachian tube reaches adult orientation.

In the presence of a perforation, water activities should be limited to surface swimming, preferably with the use of an ear plug.

D. Facial Nerve Paralysis

The facial nerve traverses the middle ear as it courses through the temporal bone to its exit at the stylomastoid foramen. Normally, the facial nerve is completely encased in bone, but occasionally bony dehiscence in the middle ear is present, exposing the nerve to infection and making it susceptible to inflammation during an episode of AOM. The acute onset of a facial nerve paralysis should not be deemed idiopathic Bell palsy until all other causes have been excluded. If middle ear fluid is present, prompt myringotomy and tube placement are indicated. CT is indicated if a cholesteatoma or mastoiditis is suspected.

E. Chronic Suppurative Otitis Media

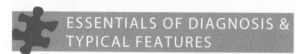

ESSENTIALS OF DIAGNOSIS & TYPICAL FEATURES

▶ Ongoing purulent ear drainage.

▶ Nonintact TM: perforation or tympanostomy tubes.

▶ May be associated with cholesteatoma.

Chronic suppurative otitis media (CSOM) is present when persistent otorrhea occurs in a child with tympanostomy tubes or TM perforation for greater than 6–12 weeks. It starts with an acute infection that becomes chronic with mucosal edema, ulceration, granulation tissue, and eventual polyp formation. Risk factors include a history of, multiple episodes of otitis media, living in crowded conditions, day care attendance, and being a member of a large family. The most common associated bacteria include *P aeruginosa*, *S aureus*, *Proteus* species, *Klebsiella pneumoniae*, and diphtheroids.

Visualization of the TM, meticulous cleaning with culture of the drainage, and appropriate antimicrobial therapy, usually topical, are the keys to management.

Occasionally, CSOM may be a sign of cholesteatoma or other disease process such as foreign body, neoplasm, Langerhans cell histiocytosis, tuberculosis, granulomatosis, fungal infection, or petrositis. If CSOM is not responsive to culture-directed treatment, imaging and biopsy may be needed to rule out other possibilities. Patients with facial palsy, vertigo, or other CNS signs should be referred immediately to an otolaryngologist.

Web Resources

Roland PS et al. Chronic Suppurative Otitis Media. http://emedicine.medscape.com/article/859501-overview. Updated March 13, 2019. Accessed June 2, 2019.

F. Labyrinthitis

Suppurative infections of the middle ear can spread into the membranous labyrinth of the inner ear. Symptoms include vertigo, hearing loss, and fevers. The child often appears extremely toxic. Intravenous antibiotic therapy is used, and intravenous steroids may also be used to help decrease inflammation. Sequelae can be serious, including a condition known as *labyrinthitis ossificans*, or bony obliteration of the inner ear, including the cochlea, leading to profound hearing loss.

G. Mastoiditis

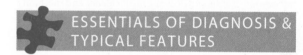

ESSENTIALS OF DIAGNOSIS & TYPICAL FEATURES

▶ AOM is almost always present.

▶ Postauricular pain and erythema.

▶ Ear protrusion (late finding).

▶ Pathogenesis

Mastoiditis occurs when infection spreads from the middle ear space to the mastoid portion of the temporal bone, which lies just behind the ear and contains air-filled spaces. Mastoiditis can range in severity from inflammation of the mastoid periosteum to bony destruction of the mastoid air cells (coalescent mastoiditis) with abscess development. Mastoiditis can occur in any age group, but more than 60% of the patients are younger than 2 years. Many children do not have a prior history of recurrent AOM.

▶ Clinical Findings

A. Symptoms and Signs

Patients with mastoiditis usually have postauricular pain, fever, and an outwardly displaced pinna. On examination, the mastoid area often appears indurated and red and with disease progression, it may become swollen and fluctuant. The earliest finding is severe tenderness on mastoid palpation. AOM is almost always present. Late findings include a pinna that is pushed forward by postauricular swelling and an ear canal that is narrowed due to pressure on the posterosuperior wall from the mastoid abscess. In infants younger than 1 year, the swelling occurs superior to the ear and pushes the pinna downward rather than outward.

B. Imaging Studies

The best way to determine the extent of disease is by CT scan. Early mastoiditis is radiographically indistinguishable from AOM, with both showing opacification but no destruction of the mastoid air cells. With progression of mastoiditis, coalescence of the mastoid air cells is seen with bone destruction. Mastoiditis is a clinical diagnosis, based on pain as well as physical exam findings.

C. Microbiology

The most common pathogens are *S pneumoniae* followed by *H influenzae* and *S pyogenes*. Rarely, gram-negative bacilli and anaerobes are isolated. In the preantibiotic era, up to 20% of patients with AOM developed mastoiditis requiring mastoidectomy. Antibiotics decrease the incidence and morbidity of acute mastoiditis. However, acute mastoiditis still occurs in children who are treated with antibiotics for an acute ear infection. In the Netherlands, where only 31% of AOM patients receive antibiotics, the incidence of acute mastoiditis is 4.2 per 100,000 person-years. In the United States, where more than 96% of patients with AOM receive antibiotics, the incidence of acute mastoiditis is 2 per 100,000 person-years. Despite the routine use of antibiotics, the incidence of acute mastoiditis has been rising in some cities. The pattern change may be secondary to the emergence of resistant *S pneumoniae*.

▶ Differential Diagnosis

Lymphadenitis, parotitis, trauma, tumor, histiocytosis, OE, and furuncle.

▶ Complications

Meningitis can be a complication of acute mastoiditis and should be suspected when a child has associated high fever, stiff neck, severe headache, or other meningeal signs. Lumbar puncture should be performed for diagnosis after imaging. Brain abscess occurs in 2% of mastoiditis patients and may be associated with persistent headaches, recurring fever, or changes in sensorium. Facial palsy, sigmoid sinus thrombosis, epidural abscess, cavernous sinus thrombosis, and thrombophlebitis may also be encountered.

▶ Treatment

Intravenous antibiotic treatment alone may be successful if there is no evidence of coalescence or abscess on CT. However, if there is no improvement within 24–48 hours, surgical intervention should be undertaken. Minimal surgical management starts with tympanostomy tube insertion,

during which cultures are taken. If a subperiosteal abscess is present, incision and drainage is also performed, with or without a cortical mastoidectomy. Intracranial extension requires complete mastoidectomy with decompression of the involved area.

Antibiotic therapy (intravenous and topical ear drops) is instituted along with surgical management and relies on culture-directed antibiotic therapy for 2–3 weeks. An antibiotic regimen should be chosen which is able to cross the blood-brain barrier. After significant clinical improvement is achieved with parenteral therapy, oral antibiotics are begun and should be continued for 2–3 weeks. A patent tympanostomy tube must also be maintained with continued use of otic drops until drainage abates.

▶ Prognosis

Prognosis for full recovery is good. Children that develop acute mastoiditis with abscess as their first ear infection are not necessarily prone to recurrent otitis media.

Anne S et al: Medical versus surgical treatment of pediatric acute mastoiditis: a systematic review. Laryngoscope 2019 Mar;129(3):754–760 [PMID: 30284265].

Chesney J et al: What is the best practice for acute mastoiditis in children? Laryngoscope 2014 May;124(5):1057–1058 [PMID: 23852990].

ACUTE TRAUMA TO THE MIDDLE EAR

Head injuries, a blow to the ear canal, sudden impact with water, blast injuries, or the insertion of pointed objects into the ear canal can lead to perforation of the TM, ossicular chain disruption, facial nerve injury, hearing loss, vertigo, and hematoma of the middle ear. One study reports that 50% of serious penetrating wounds of the TM are due to parental use of a cotton swab.

If there is facial paralysis, severe vertigo or subjective hearing loss after ear trauma, urgent otolaryngology consultation is warranted. Middle ear trauma can lead to a perilymphatic fistula which is a breach of the inner ear that causes sensorineural (nerve) hearing loss and vertigo. This hearing loss can be prevented or reversed with emergent surgery. Facial nerve injury in the setting of middle ear trauma also often needs to be addressed emergently with possible facial nerve decompression. Other sequelae of middle ear trauma may be treated with observation. Blood collecting in the middle ear space may cause a conductive hearing loss that will resolve with time. Antibiotics are not necessary unless signs of infection appear. The patient needs to be followed with audiometry or by an otolaryngologist until hearing has returned to normal, which is expected within 6–8 weeks. If the conductive hearing loss does not resolve, there may be injuries to the ossicular chain. A CT scan may be needed to evaluate the middle ear structures in this case.

Traumatic TM perforations should be referred to an otolaryngologist for examination and hearing evaluation. Spontaneous healing may occur within 6 months of the perforation. In the acute setting, antibiotic eardrops are often recommended to provide a moist environment which is thought to speed healing.

EAR CANAL FOREIGN BODY & CERUMEN IMPACTION

Foreign bodies of the ear canal, both intentional (placement by patient or other person) or accidental (eg, insect, playground mulch), are common in childhood. Cerumen can also be obstructive, acting like a foreign body. These objects can be removed if they are easy to visualize and there is appropriate instrumentation. Factors that may make them difficult to remove include size of foreign body, particularly when large enough to obscure the TM, rounded or globular objects, and objects deep in the ear canal adjacent to the TM. If these conditions exist or you are unable to remove the object on the first attempt, an ENT referral is often necessary for resolution. Vegetable matter should never be irrigated as it can swell and become more difficult to remove. An emergency condition exists if the foreign body is a disk-type battery. An electric current is generated in the moist canal, and a severe burn can occur in less than 4 hours. If the TM cannot be visualized, assume a perforation and avoid irrigation or ototoxic medications.

Cerumen impaction is common in children and using cotton swabs or other devices in the ear canal predisposes to the problem. Not only do these objects block the natural outflow of cerumen, they can also increase cerumen production from irritation. Cerumen impaction should be removed if it is symptomatic or obstructs visualization of the TM. Education on the proper techniques of ear cleaning (such as only cleaning the external meatus) is important to avoid impactions. Explaining to parents that cerumen production is normal and cerumen protects the ear canal skin can help reinforce proper ear care.

Oyama LC: Foreign bodies of the ear, nose and throat. Emerg Med Clin North Am 2019 Feb;37(1):121–130 [PMID: 30454775].

Schwartz SR: Clinical practice guideline (update). Otolaryngol Head Neck Surg 2017 Jan;156(1 suppl):S1–S29. doi: 10.1177/0194599816671491.28045591 [PMID: 28045632].

Sharpe SJ, Rochette LM, Smith GA: Pediatric battery-related emergency department visits in the United States, 1990–2009. Pediatrics 2012 Jun;129(6):1111–1117 [PMID: 22585763].

AURICULAR HEMATOMA

Trauma to the outer ear can result in formation of a hematoma between the perichondrium and cartilage of the pinna. This is different from a bruise, which does not change the ear shape and where the blood is in the soft tissue outside of the perichondral layer. A hematoma appears as a boggy purple swelling of the cartilaginous auricle, and the normal folds of the ear are obscured. If untreated, neocartilage is deposited after 7–10 days resulting in "cauliflower ear." To prevent this cosmetic deformity, physicians should urgently refer patients to an otolaryngologist for drainage and application of a pressure dressing.

CONGENITAL EAR MALFORMATIONS

The external ear and EAC start to develop at 3 weeks gestation. Variable anomalies can present depending on timing of abnormal development. **Atresia** is failure of the ear canal to form. This results in conductive hearing loss and should be evaluated within the first 3 months of life by an audiologist and otolaryngologist. **Microtia** is the term used for an external ear that is small, collapsed, or only has an earlobe present. Usually there is a deficiency of cartilage and tissue. **Anotia** refers to an absent external ear. Often, there is an associated atresia with microtia and anotia. Reconstruction of the auricle usually occurs around ages 6–8 years and requires introduction of additional tissue or implants.

Malformations of the auricle can occur that are not due to a deficiency of tissue. This can range from ears that lack the proper folds and therefore protrude from the skull (**prominotia**) to ears that are folded over due to lack of cartilage stiffness or in utero positioning. Taping of the ears into correct anatomic position is very effective if performed in the first 72–96 hours of life. Tape is applied over a molding of wax or plastic and continued for at least 2 weeks. If this window of opportunity is missed or taping is unsuccessful, surgical correction, called an "otoplasty," can be performed at school age.

An ear is considered "low-set" if the upper pole is below eyebrow level. This condition is often associated with other congenital anomalies, and in these patients a genetics evaluation should be considered.

Preauricular tags, ectopic cartilage, fistulas, and cysts require surgical correction primarily for cosmetic reasons. Since the inner ear forms in conjunction with the outer ear children with ear malformations should have their hearing tested. Renal ultrasound should be considered, as external ear anomalies can also be associated with renal anomalies, as both structures form during the same period of embryogenesis. Most preauricular pits are asymptomatic but may become infected and require antibiotic treatment and possible surgical management.

Anstadt EE et al: Neonatal ear molding: timing and technique. Pediatrics 2016 Mar;137(3): e20152831 [PMID: 26908661].

Bly et al: Microtia reconstruction. Facial Plast Surg Clin North Am 2016 Nov;24(4):577–591 [PMID: 27712823].

IDENTIFICATION & MANAGEMENT OF HEARING LOSS

Hearing loss is classified as being conductive, sensorineural, or mixed in nature. Conductive hearing loss occurs when sound transmission is blocked somewhere between the opening of the external ear and the cochlear receptor cells. The most common cause of conductive hearing loss in children is fluid in the middle ear. Sensorineural hearing loss (SNHL) is due to a defect in the neural transmission of sound, arising from a defect in the cochlear hair cells or the auditory nerve. Mixed hearing loss is characterized by elements of both conductive and sensorineural loss.

Hearing is measured in decibels (dB). The threshold, or 0 dB, refers to the level at which a sound is perceived in normal subjects 50% of the time. Hearing is considered normal if an individual's thresholds are within 20 dB of normal. In children, severity of hearing loss is commonly graded as follows: 20–40 dB mild, 41–55 dB moderate, 56–70 dB moderately severe, 71–90 dB severe, and 91+ dB profound.

Hearing loss can significantly impair a child's ability to communicate and hinder academic, social, and emotional development. Studies suggest that periods of auditory deprivation may have enduring effects on auditory processing, even after normal hearing is restored. Even a unilateral loss may be associated with difficulties in school and behavioral issues. Early identification and management of any hearing loss is therefore critical.

Conductive Hearing Loss

The most common cause of childhood conductive hearing loss is otitis media and related conditions such as MEE and ETD. Other causes may include EAC atresia or stenosis, TM perforation, cerumen impaction, cholesteatoma, and middle ear abnormalities, such as ossicular fixation or discontinuity. Often, a conductive loss may be corrected with surgery.

MEE may be serous, mucoid, or purulent, as in AOM. Effusions are generally associated with a mild conductive hearing loss that normalizes once the effusion is gone. The American Academy of Pediatrics recommends that hearing and language skills be assessed in children who have recurrent AOM or MEE lasting longer than 3 months.

Sensorineural Hearing Loss

SNHL arises due to a defect in the cochlear receptor cells or the auditory nerve (cranial nerve VIII). The loss may be congenital (present at birth) or acquired. In both the congenital and acquired categories, the hearing loss may be either hereditary (due to a genetic mutation) or nonhereditary. It is estimated that SNHL affects 2–3 out of every 1000 live births, making this the most common congenital sensory impairment. The incidence is thought to be considerably higher among the neonatal intensive care unit population. Well-recognized risk factors for SNHL in neonates include positive family history of childhood SNHL, birthweight less than 1500 g, low Apgar scores (0–4 at 1 minute or 0–6 at 5 minutes), craniofacial anomalies, hypoxia, in-utero infections (eg, TORCH syndrome), hyperbilirubinemia requiring exchange transfusion, and mechanical ventilation for more than 5 days.

A. Congenital Hearing Loss

Approximately 50% of congenital hearing loss is nonhereditary. Examples include loss due to infection, teratogenic drugs, and perinatal injuries. The other 50% is attributed to genetic factors. Among children with hereditary hearing loss, approximately one-third of cases are thought to be due to a known syndrome, while the other two-thirds are considered nonsyndromic.

Syndromic hearing loss is associated with malformations of the external ear or other organs, or with medical problems involving other organ systems. Over 400 genetic syndromes that include hearing loss have been described. All patients being evaluated for hearing loss should be also evaluated for features commonly associated with these syndromes. These include branchial cleft cysts or sinuses, preauricular pits, ocular abnormalities, white forelock, café au lait spots, and craniofacial anomalies. Some of the more frequently mentioned syndromes associated with congenital hearing loss include the following: Waardenburg, branchio-oto-renal, Usher, Pendred, Jervell and Lange-Nielsen, and Alport.

Over 70% of hereditary hearing loss is not related to a syndrome (ie, there are no associated visible abnormalities or related medical problems). The most common known mutation associated with nonsyndromic hearing loss is in the *GJB2* gene, which encodes the protein Connexin 26. The *GJB2* mutation has a carrier rate of about 3% in the general population. Most nonsyndromic hearing loss, including that due to the *GJB2* mutation, is autosomal recessive.

B. Acquired Hearing Loss

Hereditary hearing loss may be delayed in onset, as in Alport syndrome and most types of autosomal dominant nonsyndromic hearing loss. Vulnerability to aminoglycoside-induced hearing loss has also been linked to a mitochondrial gene defect.

Nongenetic etiologies for delayed-onset SNHL include exposure to ototoxic medications, meningitis, autoimmune or neoplastic conditions, noise exposure, and trauma. Infections such as syphilis or Lyme disease have been associated with hearing loss. Hearing loss associated with congenital cytomegalovirus (CMV) infection may be present at birth, or may have a delayed onset. The loss is progressive in approximately half of all patients with congenital CMV-associated hearing loss. Other risk factors for delayed-onset, progressive loss include a history of persistent pulmonary hypertension and extracorporeal membrane oxygenation therapy.

C. Congenital CMV Infection and Hearing Loss

Congenital CMV (cCMV) associated hearing loss can be congenital, but is more often acquired. It deserves special mention as it is believed to be the most common cause of nongenetic hearing loss in the US pediatric population, and it can present at birth or have a delayed onset as long as several years. Congenital CMV is the most common in utero infection in the United States today, and an estimated 0.5%–1% of all newborns are infected in the prenatal period. While some manifest severe symptoms at birth such as petechiae, hyperbilirubinemia, hepatosplenomegaly, seizures, neurologic deficits and retinitis, 90%–95% of newborns with cCMV infection are completely asymptomatic. Thirty to fifty percent of symptomatic and 8%–12% of asymptomatic infants will go on to develop SNHL in early childhood. Congenital CMV infection can only be confirmed in the newborn period, so given that most newborns are asymptomatic during this period, it has been very difficult to accurately determine the percentage of SNHL attributable to cCMV. There is currently no universal screening for cCMV, but with the increased awareness of this problem, some centers are now performing targeted screening on newborns who fail newborn hearing screening. There is no consensus on the management of cCMV but trials of valganciclovir have shown promise in the treatment of cCMV hearing loss.

Identification of Hearing Loss

A. Newborn Hearing Screening

Prior to the institution of universal newborn screening programs, the average age at identification of hearing loss was 30 months. Recognizing the importance of early detection, in 1993, a National Institutes of Health Consensus Panel recommended that all newborns be screened for hearing impairment prior to hospital discharge. Today, all 50 states and the District of Columbia have Early Hearing Detection and Intervention (EHDI) laws or screening programs, and as of 2014, 97% of newborns in the United States were screened for hearing loss. The EHDI goal is loss identification and confirmation of hearing loss by 3 months of age, and appropriate intervention by the age of 6 months. Subjective testing is not reliable in infants, and therefore objective, physiologic methods are used for screening. Auditory brainstem response and otoacoustic emission testing are the two commonly employed screening modalities.

B. Audiologic Evaluation of Infants and Children

A parent's report of his or her infant's behavior cannot be relied upon for identification of hearing loss. A deaf infant's behavior can appear normal and mislead parents and professionals. Deaf infants are often visually alert and able to actively scan the environment which may be mistaken for an appropriate response to sound. In children, signs of hearing loss include inconsistent response to sounds, not following directions, speech and language delays, and turning the volume up on televisions or radios. Any child who fails a hearing screening or is suspected to have hearing loss should be referred for formal audiometric testing by an audiologist who is knowledgeable about testing the pediatric population.

Audiometry subjectively evaluates hearing. There are several different methods used, based on patient age:

- Behavioral observational audiometry (birth to 6 months): Sounds are presented at various intensity levels, and the audiologist watches closely for a reaction, such as change in respiratory rate, starting or stopping of activity, startle, head turn, or muscle tensing. This method is highly tester-dependent and error-prone.

- Visual reinforcement audiometry (6 months to 2.5 years): Auditory stimulus is paired with positive reinforcement. For example, when a child reacts appropriately by turning toward a sound source, the behavior is rewarded by activation of a toy that lights up. After a brief conditioning period, the child localizes toward the tone, if audible, in anticipation of the lighted toy.

- Conditioned play audiometry (2.5–5 years): The child responds to sound stimulus by performing an activity, such as putting a peg into a board.

- Conventional audiometry (5 years and up): The child indicates when he or she hears a sound.

Objective methods such as auditory brainstem response and otoacoustic emission testing may be used if a child cannot be reliably tested using the above methods.

In addition to infants who fall into the high-risk categories for SNHL as outlined earlier, hearing should be tested in children with a history of developmental delay, bacterial meningitis, ototoxic medication exposure, neurodegenerative disorders, or a history of infection such as mumps or measles. Children with bacterial meningitis should be referred immediately to an otolaryngologist, as cochlear ossification can necessitate urgent cochlear implantation. Even if a newborn screening was passed, all infants who fall into a high-risk category for progressive or delayed-onset hearing loss, such as in utero CMV exposure, should be referred for regular audiologic monitoring for the first 3 years and at appropriate intervals thereafter to avoid a missed diagnosis.

Management of Hearing Loss

While identification of hearing loss is the critical first step, it is largely meaningless without appropriate follow-up and management. Prompt and appropriate intervention can minimize the potential lifelong detrimental effects that hearing loss can have on language, academic, emotional and social development, and hearing-related quality of life. Optimal management requires a multidisciplinary approach. The team may include audiologists, otolaryngologists, speech-language pathologists, early intervention specialists, deaf-hard of hearing educational specialists and family counselors.

Any child with confirmed hearing loss should be referred to an otolaryngologist for further evaluation and possible medical and/or surgical management. Etiologic workup can include radiographic imaging and/or laboratory tests and should be tailored to each individual patient's history, examination, and audiometric results. Within the past decade, major advances have made comprehensive genetic testing for syndromic and nonsyndromic hearing loss using next-generation sequencing technology available to the public.

The medical management of hearing loss depends upon the type and severity. Conductive hearing loss is sometimes fixable if the point at which sound transmission is compromised can be corrected. For example, hearing loss due to chronic effusions usually normalizes once the fluid has cleared, whether by natural means or by the placement of tympanostomy tubes. As of yet, SNHL is not reversible. Most sensorineural loss is managed with amplification. Cochlear implantation is an option for some children when benefit is no longer achieved with amplification. It is FDA approved down to the age of 12 months. Unlike hearing aids, cochlear implants do not amplify sound, but directly stimulate the cochlea with electrical impulses.

When a hearing loss is diagnosed, it is not known whether it will remain stable, or if it will fluctuate or worsen. Therefore, children with hearing loss should receive ongoing audiologic monitoring, as well as periodic assessments of global development and functional performance.

The Individuals with Disabilities Education Act 2004 (IDEA 2004) is a United States law mandating free access to individualized educational opportunities with qualified instructors for children with disabilities, including hearing loss. Part C provides early intervention for children up to age 3 years. Audiologists play an important role in the transition from diagnosis to intervention, as they are required to initiate a referral to their state's Part C program within 7 days of a new confirmed permanent hearing loss diagnosis. An Individualized Family Service Plan (IFSP) is developed and may enlist the services of audiologists, speech-language pathologists, and other related professionals. The IFSP is family-centered, and family support services are often available. Between the ages of 3 and 21 years, children are covered under Part B of IDEA 2004. Part B is managed through the local school systems' special education programs. Under Part B, an Individualized Education Plan (IEP) is developed with a goal of maximizing a child's academic success.

Prevention

Appropriate care may treat or prevent certain conditions causing hearing deficits. Aminoglycosides and diuretics, particularly in combination, are potentially ototoxic and should be used judiciously and monitored carefully. Given the association of a mitochondrial gene defect with aminoglycoside ototoxicity, use should be avoided when possible, in patients with a family history of aminoglycoside-related hearing loss. Reduction of repeated exposure to loud noises may prevent high-frequency hearing loss associated with acoustic trauma. Any patient with sudden-onset SNHL should be seen by an otolaryngologist immediately, as in some cases, steroid therapy may reverse the loss if initiated right away.

Web Resources

Congenital CMV and Hearing Loss. Updated September 27, 2018: https://www.cdc.gov/cmv/hearing-loss.html?CDC_AA_refVal=https%3A%2F%2Fwww.cdc.gov%2Fcmv%2Ffact-sheets%2Fhearing-loss.html. Accessed June 2, 2019.

NCHAM: Newborn Hearing & Infant Hearing—Early Hearing Detection and Intervention Resources and Information: http://www.infanthearing.org/screening/. Accessed June 2, 2019.

OtoSCOPE Genetic Testing: https://morl.lab.uiowa.edu/otoscope-genetic-testing. Accessed June 2, 2019.

Smith RJH, Shearer AE, Hildebrand MS, Van Camp G: Deafness and hereditary hearing loss overview. Last update July 27, 2017. http://www.ncbi.nlm.nih.gov/books/NBK1434/. Accessed June 2, 2019.

▼ THE NOSE & PARANASAL SINUSES

ACUTE VIRAL RHINITIS

The common cold (viral URI) is the most common pediatric infectious disease, and the incidence is higher in early childhood than in any other period of life (Common Cold; See also Chapter 40). Children younger than 5 years typically have 6–12 colds per year. Approximately 30%–40% are caused by rhinoviruses, of which there are over 100 subtypes. Other culprits include adenoviruses, coronaviruses, enteroviruses, influenza and parainfluenza viruses, and respiratory syncytial virus. Since so many viruses can cause a cold, development of a vaccine has not been possible.

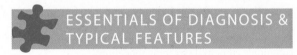

ESSENTIALS OF DIAGNOSIS & TYPICAL FEATURES

► Clear or mucoid rhinorrhea, nasal congestion, sore throat.

► Possible fever, particularly in younger children (under 5–6 years).

► Possible hoarseness and/or cough.

► Symptoms resolve by 7–10 days, but cough and hoarseness can linger for several weeks afterward.

Differential Diagnosis

Rhinosinusitis (acute or chronic), allergic rhinitis, nonallergic rhinitis, influenza, pneumonia, gastroesophageal reflux disease, asthma, and bronchitis.

Clinical Findings

The patient usually experiences a sudden onset of sore throat followed by clear or mucoid rhinorrhea, nasal congestion, and sneezing. Cough or fever may develop. Although fever is not a prominent feature in older children and adults, in the first 5 or 6 years of life it can be as high as 40.6°C without superinfection. The nose, throat, and TMs may appear red and inflamed. The average duration of symptoms is about 1 week. Nasal secretions tend to become thicker and more purulent after day 2 of infection due to shedding of epithelial cells and influx of neutrophils. This discoloration should not be assumed to be a sign of bacterial rhinosinusitis, unless it persists beyond 10–14 days, by which time the patient should be experiencing significant symptomatic improvement. A mild cough may persist for several weeks following resolution of other symptoms.

Treatment

Treatment for the common cold is symptomatic (Figure 18–4). Because colds are viral infections, antibiotics are not helpful. Acetaminophen or ibuprofen can relieve fever and pain. Humidification may provide relief for congestion and cough. Nasal saline drops and bulb suctioning may be used for an infant or child unable to blow his or her nose.

Available scientific data suggest that over-the-counter cold and cough medications are not effective in children and may be associated with serious adverse effects. Use in children younger than 4 years is not recommended. Antihistamines have not proven effective in relieving cold symptoms in children; in rhinoviral colds, increased levels of histamine are not observed. Oral decongestants may provide symptomatic relief in adults but have not been well studied in children. Studies have shown that most cough medicines are no better than placebo and use of narcotic antitussives is discouraged, as these may be associated with respiratory depression. There is no convincing evidence that naturopathic or alternative therapies are effective in children.

Only time cures the common cold. Education and reassurance may be the most important "therapy" for parents.

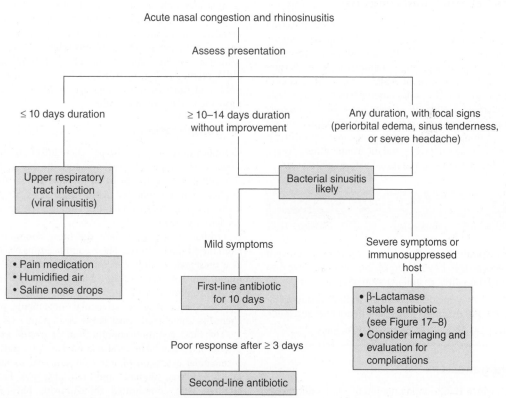

▲ **Figure 18–4.** Algorithm for acute nasal congestion and rhinosinusitis.

They should be informed about the expected nature and duration of symptoms, efficacy and potential side effects of medications, and the signs and symptoms of complications of the common cold, such as bacterial rhinosinusitis, bronchiolitis, or pneumonia.

Kenealy T, Arroll B: Antibiotics for the common cold and acute purulent rhinitis. Cochrane Database Syst Rev 2013 Jun 4;6:CD000247. doi: 10.1002/14651858.CD000247.pub3 [PMID: 23733381].

Web Resources

U.S. Food and Drug Administration: Using over-the-counter cough and cold products in children. Last updated February 8, 201: https://www.fda.gov/drugs/special-features/use-caution-when-giving-cough-and-cold-products-kids. Accessed June 2, 2019.

RHINOSINUSITIS

The use of the term *rhinosinusitis* has replaced sinusitis. Rhinosinusitis acknowledges that the nasal and sinus mucosa are involved in similar and concurrent inflammatory processes.

1. Acute Bacterial Rhinosinusitis

Acute bacterial rhinosinusitis (ABRS) is a bacterial infection of the paranasal sinuses which lasts less than 30 days and the symptoms resolve completely. It is almost always preceded by a cold. Other predisposing conditions include allergies and trauma. The diagnosis of ABRS is made when a cold does not improve by 10–14 days or worsens after 5–7 days. The maxillary and ethmoid sinuses are most commonly involved and these sinuses are present at birth. Other sinuses are involved in older children as the sphenoid sinuses typically form by the age of 5 years, and the frontal sinuses by age 7–8 years. Frontal sinusitis is unusual before age 10 years.

ESSENTIALS OF DIAGNOSIS & TYPICAL FEATURES

▶ Upper respiratory infection (URI) symptoms are present 10 or more days beyond onset, or symptoms worsen within 10 days after an initial period of improvement.

▶ Symptoms may include nasal congestion, nasal drainage, postnasal drainage, facial pain, headache, and fever.

▶ Symptoms resolve completely within 30 days.

▶ Pathogenesis

Situations which lead to inflammation of sinonasal mucosa and obstruction of sinus drainage underlie the development of rhinosinusitis. A combination of anatomic, mucosal, microbial, and immune factors are involved. Both viral and bacterial infections play integral roles in the pathogenesis. Viral URIs may cause sinus mucosal injury and swelling, resulting in sinus outflow obstruction, loss of ciliary activity, and mucous hypersecretion. The bacterial pathogens that commonly cause acute rhinosinusitis are *S pneumoniae*, *H influenzae* (nontypeable), *M catarrhalis*, and β-hemolytic streptococci.

▶ Clinical Findings

The onset of symptoms in ABRS may be gradual or sudden and commonly include nasal drainage, nasal congestion, facial pressure or pain, postnasal drainage, hyposmia or anosmia, fever, cough, fatigue, maxillary dental pain, and ear pressure or fullness. The physical examination is rarely helpful in making the diagnosis, as the findings are essentially the same as those in a child with an uncomplicated cold.

In complicated or immunocompromised patients, sinus aspiration and culture by an otolaryngologist should be considered for diagnostic purposes and to facilitate culture-directed antibiotic therapy. Gram stain or culture of nasal discharge does not necessarily correlate with cultures of sinus aspirates. If the patient is hospitalized because of rhinosinusitis-related complications, blood cultures should also be obtained.

Imaging of the sinuses during acute illness is not recommended unless evaluating for possible complications, or for patients with persistent symptoms which do not respond to medical therapy. As with the physical examination, the radiographic findings of ABRS, such as sinus opacification, fluid, and mucosal thickening, are indistinguishable from those seen in the common cold.

▶ Complications

Complications of ABRS occur when infection spreads to adjacent structures like the eye and the brain. *S aureus* (including methicillin-resistant *S aureus*) is frequently implicated in complicated ABRS, as well as *Streptococcus anginosus* (*milleri*), which has been found to be a particularly virulent organism.

Orbital complications are the most common, arising from the ethmoid sinuses. These complications usually begin as a preseptal cellulitis, but can progress to postseptal cellulitis, subperiosteal abscess, orbital abscess, and cavernous sinus thrombosis. Associated signs and symptoms include eyelid edema, restricted extraocular movements, proptosis, chemosis, and altered visual acuity (see Chapter 16).

The most common complication of frontal sinusitis is osteitis of the frontal bone, also known as Pott's puffy tumor. Intracranial extension of infection can lead to meningitis and to epidural, subdural, and brain abscesses. Frequently, children with complicated rhinosinusitis have no prior history of sinus infection.

▶ Treatment

For children with cold symptoms that are not improving by 10 days, observation for up to 3 more days or antibiotic therapy may be chosen, depending upon individual circumstances, such as ability to follow-up and treat with antibiotics if needed. For children with uncomplicated ABRS who have worsening or severe symptoms (fever of at least 39°C and purulent nasal drainage for at least 3 consecutive days), antibiotic therapy is recommended. Antibiotics are generally thought to decrease duration and severity of symptoms.

First-line antibiotic therapy should be amoxicillin or amoxicillin-clavulanate. Cefuroxime, cefpodoxime, and cefdinir are recommended for patients with a non–type I hypersensitivity to penicillin, and in most cases may be safely used in patients with an anaphylactoid reaction, as recent studies seem to indicate almost no risk of a serious reaction to second- and third-generation cephalosporins among these patients. Other agents which may be used, particularly in more severe cases where resistant *S pneumoniae* and *H influenzae* are suspected, include clindamycin, linezolid, and quinolone antibiotics. Due to high resistance of *S pneumoniae* and *H influenzae*, the use of trimethoprim-sulfamethoxazole and azithromycin is not advised.

Duration of therapy should be for 7 days after symptoms have resolved.

Failure to improve after 48–72 hours of antibiotic therapy suggests a resistant organism or potential complication. Second-line therapies should be initiated at this point, or, if the patient is already on amoxicillin-clavulanate or a cephalosporin, intravenous antibiotic therapy should be considered. Imaging and referral for sinus aspiration should be strongly considered as well.

Patients who are toxic, or who have evidence of invasive infection or CNS complications, should be hospitalized immediately. Intravenous therapy with nafcillin or clindamycin plus a third-generation cephalosporin such as ceftriaxone should be initiated until culture results become available.

Decongestants, antihistamines, and nasal saline irrigations are frequently used in acute rhinosinusitis to promote drainage. To date, there are no methodologically sound studies supporting their efficacy in children. If used, topical nasal decongestants, such as oxymetazoline or phenylephrine sprays, should not be used for more than 3 days due to risk of rebound edema. Patients with underlying allergic rhinitis may benefit from intranasal cromolyn or corticosteroid nasal spray.

Shaikh N, Wald ER: Decongestants, antihistamines and nasal irrigation for acute sinusitis in children. Cochrane Database Syst Rev 2014 Oct 27;(10):CD007909 [PMID: 25347280].

Wald ER et al: Clinical practice guideline for the diagnosis and management of acute bacterial sinusitis in children aged 1 to 18 years. Pediatrics 2013;134:e262–e280 [PMID: 23796742].

2. Recurrent or Chronic Rhinosinusitis

Recurrent rhinosinusitis occurs when episodes of ABRS clear for at least 10 days but recur at least four times per year. Chronic rhinosinusitis (CRS) is diagnosed when the child has not cleared the infection in 90 days, but has not developed acute complications. Both symptoms and physical findings are required to support the diagnosis, and CT scan may be a useful in making the diagnosis. Although recent meta-analysis evaluations have resulted in recommendations for ABRS, there is a paucity of data for the treatment of recurrent or CRS. Important factors to consider include allergies, anatomic variations, and disorders in host immunity. Mucosal inflammation leading to obstruction is most commonly caused by allergic rhinitis and occasionally by nonallergic rhinitis. There is a great deal of evidence that allergic rhinitis, rhinosinusitis, and asthma are all manifestations of a systemic inflammatory response. Gastroesophageal reflux has also been implicated in CRS. Less commonly, CRS is caused by anatomic variations, such as septal deviation, polyp, or foreign body.

Allergic nasal polyps are unusual in children younger than 10 years and should prompt a workup for cystic fibrosis. In cases of chronic or recurrent pyogenic pansinusitis, poor host resistance (eg, an immune defect, primary ciliary dyskinesia, or cystic fibrosis)—though rare—must be ruled out by immunoglobulin studies, electron microscopy studies of respiratory cilia, nasal nitric oxide measurements if available, a sweat chloride test, and genetic testing (see Chapter 19). Anaerobic and staphylococcal organisms are often responsible for CRS. Evaluation by an allergist and an otolaryngologist may be useful in determining the underlying causes.

▶ Treatment

A. Medical Therapy

Antibiotic therapy is similar to that used for ABRS, but the duration is longer, typically 3–4 weeks. Antimicrobial choice should include drugs effective against staphylococcal organisms. Nasal saline irrigations and intranasal steroid sprays have been shown to be helpful in the reduction of symptoms of CRS.

B. Surgical Therapy

The mainstay of treatment for pediatric CRS is medical management, with appropriate antibiotic therapy and treatment of comorbid conditions such as allergic rhinitis and asthma. Only a small percentage of children will warrant surgical management.

1. Antral lavage—Antral lavage, generally regarded as a diagnostic procedure, may have some therapeutic value. An aspirate or a sample from the maxillary sinus is retrieved under anesthesia. The maxillary sinus is then irrigated. In the very young child, this may be the only procedure performed.

2. Adenoidectomy—Adenoidectomy is thought to be effective in 50%–75% of children with CRS, up to the age of 12 years. The adenoids serve as a reservoir of pathogenic bacteria and may also interfere with mucociliary clearance and drainage. Biofilms have been reported in the adenoids of children with CRS and may explain the resistance of these infections to standard antibiotic therapy.

3. Endoscopic sinus surgery—Endoscopic sinus surgery in children was controversial because of concerns regarding facial growth. However, recent studies have not supported this concern. Endoscopic sinus surgery is reported to be effective in over 80% of cases, and may be indicated if adenoidectomy or balloon dilation is not effective.

4. External drainage—External drainage procedures are reserved for complications arising from ethmoid and frontal sinusitis.

Brietzke SE et al: Clinical consensus statement: pediatric chronic rhinosinusitis. Otolaryngol Head Neck Surg 2014;151(4): 542–553 [PMID: 25274375].

Orlandi RR et al: International consensus statement on allergy and rhinology: rhinosinusitis. Int Forum Allergy Rhinol 2016 Feb 6; Suppl 1:S22–S209 [PMID: 26889651].

CHOANAL ATRESIA

Choanal atresia occurs in approximately 1 in 7000 live births. The female-male ratio is 2:1, as is the unilateral-bilateral ratio. Bilateral atresia results in severe respiratory distress at birth and requires immediate placement of an oral airway or intubation, and otolaryngology consultation for surgical treatment. Unilateral atresia usually appears later as a unilateral chronic nasal discharge that may be mistaken for CRS. Diagnosis may be suspected if a 6F catheter cannot be passed through the nose and is confirmed by axial CT scan. Approximately 50% of patients with bilateral choanal atresia have CHARGE association (**C**oloboma, **H**eart disease, **A**tresia of the choanae, **R**etarded growth and retarded development or CNS anomalies, **G**enital hypoplasia, and **E**ar anomalies or deafness) (see Chapter 37) or other congenital anomalies.

RECURRENT RHINITIS

Recurrent rhinitis is frequently seen in pediatrics. The child is brought in with the chief complaint of having "one cold after another," "constant colds," or "always being sick." Approximately, two-thirds of these children have recurrent colds; the rest have either allergic rhinitis or recurrent rhinosinusitis.

1. Allergic Rhinitis

Allergic rhinitis is a chronic disorder of the upper airway which is induced by IgE-mediated inflammation secondary to allergen exposure. It is more common in children than in adults and affects up to 40% of children in the United States.

It significantly affects quality of life, interfering with physical and social activities, concentration, school performance, and sleep. Allergic rhinitis can contribute to the development of rhinosinusitis, otitis media, and asthma. Symptoms may include nasal congestion, sneezing, rhinorrhea, and itchy nose, palate, throat, and eyes. On physical examination, the nasal turbinates are swollen and may be red or pale pink-purple. Several classes of medications have proven effective in treating allergic rhinitis, including intranasal corticosteroids, oral and intranasal antihistamines, leukotriene antagonists, and decongestants. Ipratropium nasal spray may also be used as an adjunctive therapy. Nasal saline rinses are helpful to wash away allergens. Recent studies have indicated that use of intranasal steroid sprays may not only decrease the impairment caused by allergic rhinitis symptoms, but also help prevent progression to more severe disease and decrease the risk of related comorbidities such as asthma and sleep-disordered breathing. These intranasal steroids can be used in children as young as 2 years of age.

2. Nonallergic Rhinitis

Nonallergic rhinitis also causes rhinorrhea and nasal congestion, but does not seem to involve an immunologic reaction. Its mechanism is not well understood. Triggers can include sudden changes in environmental temperature, air pollution, and other irritants such as tobacco smoke. Medications can also be associated with nonallergic rhinitis. Nasal decongestant sprays, when used for long periods of time, can cause *rhinitis medicamentosa*, which is a rebound nasal congestion and can be very difficult to treat. Oral decongestants, nasal corticosteroids, antihistamines, and ipratropium spray have all been shown to offer symptomatic relief.

Rachelefsky G, Farrar JR: A control model to evaluate pharmacotherapy for allergic rhinitis in children. JAMA Pediatr 2013;167(4):380–386 [PMID: 23440263].

Web Resources

American Academy of Allergy, Asthma, and Immunology: Rhinitis (Hay Fever): https://www.aaaai.org/conditions-and-treatments/library/allergy-library/rhinitis. Accessed June 2, 2019.

Becker JM: Pediatric Allergic Rhinitis. Medscape: https://www.fda.gov/drugs/special-features/use-caution-when-giving-cough-and-cold-products-kids. Updated July 17, 2018. Accessed June 2, 2019.

EPISTAXIS

The nose is a highly vascular structure. In most cases, epistaxis (nosebleed) arises from the anterior portion of the nasal septum (Kiesselbach area). It is often due to dryness, nose rubbing, nose blowing, or nose picking. Examination of the anterior septum usually reveals a red, raw surface with fresh clots or old crusts. Presence of telangiectasias, hemangiomas, or varicosities should also be noted. If a patient has been using a nasal corticosteroid spray, check the patient's technique to make sure he or she is not directing the spray toward the septum. If proper technique does not reduce the nosebleeds, the spray should be discontinued.

In fewer than 5% of cases, epistaxis is caused by a bleeding disorder such as von Willebrand disease. A hematologic workup is warranted if any of the following is present: family history of a bleeding disorder; medical history of easy bleeding, particularly with circumcision or dental work; spontaneous bleeding at any site; bleeding that lasts for more than 30 minutes or blood that will not clot with direct pressure by the physician; onset before age 2 years; or a drop in hematocrit due to epistaxis. High blood pressure may rarely predispose to prolonged nosebleeds in children.

Juvenile nasopharyngeal angiofibroma (JNA) is a benign, but often aggressive, tumor that tends to bleed and may present as recurrent epistaxis (45%–60%). JNA is only seen in males; females with JNA should undergo karyotyping. CT and MRI are diagnostic.

▶ Treatment

The patient should sit up and lean forward so as not to swallow the blood. Swallowed blood may cause nausea and hematemesis. The nasal cavity should be cleared of clots by gentle blowing. The soft part of the nose below the nasal bones is pinched and held firmly enough to prevent arterial blood flow, with pressure over the bleeding site (anterior septum) being maintained for 5 minutes. For persistent bleeding, a one-time only application of oxymetazoline into the nasal cavity may be helpful. If bleeding continues, the bleeding site needs to be visualized. A small piece of gelatin sponge (Gelfoam) or collagen sponge (Surgicel) can be inserted over the bleeding site and held in place.

Friability of the nasal vessels is often due to dryness and can be decreased by increasing nasal moisture. This can be accomplished by daily application of a water-based ointment to the nose. A pea-sized amount of ointment is placed just inside the nose and spread by gently squeezing the nostrils. Twice-daily nasal saline irrigation and humidifier use may also be helpful. Aspirin and ibuprofen should be avoided, as should nose picking and vigorous nose blowing. Otolaryngology referral is indicated for refractory cases. Cautery of the nasal vessels is reserved for treatment failures.

NASAL INFECTION

A nasal furuncle is an infection of a hair follicle in the anterior nares. Hair plucking or nose picking can provide a route of entry. The most common organism is S aureus. A furuncle presents as an exquisitely tender, firm, red lump in the anterior nares. Treatment includes dicloxacillin or cephalexin orally for 5 days to prevent spread. The lesion should be gently incised and drained as soon as it points with a

sterile needle. Topical antibiotic ointment may be of additional value. Because this lesion is in the drainage area of the cavernous sinus, the patient should be followed closely until healing is complete. Parents should be advised never to pick or squeeze a furuncle in this location—and neither should the physician. Associated cellulitis or spread requires hospitalization for administration of intravenous antibiotics.

A nasal septal abscess is usually the result of nasal trauma or a nasal furuncle. Examination reveals fluctuant gray septal swelling, which is usually bilateral. The possible complications are the same as for nasal septal hematoma (see following discussion). In addition, spread of the infection to the CNS is possible. Treatment consists of immediate hospitalization, incision and drainage by an otolaryngologist, and antibiotic therapy.

NASAL TRAUMA

Newborn infants rarely present with subluxation of the quadrangular cartilage of the septum. In this disorder, the top of the nose deviates to one side, the inferior septal border deviates to the other side, the columella leans, and the nasal tip is unstable. This disorder must be distinguished from the more common transient flattening of the nose caused by the birth process. In the past, physicians were encouraged to reduce all subluxations in the nursery. Otolaryngologists are more likely to perform the reduction under anesthesia for more difficult cases.

After nasal trauma, it is essential to examine the inside of the nose in order to rule out hematoma of the nasal septum, as this can quickly lead to septal necrosis, causing permanent nasal deformity. This diagnosis is confirmed by the abrupt onset of nasal obstruction following trauma and the presence of a boggy, widened nasal septum. The normal nasal septum is only 2–4 mm thick. A cotton swab can be used to palpate the septum. Treatment consists of immediate referral to an otolaryngologist for drainage and packing of the nose.

Most blows to the nose result in epistaxis without fracture. A persistent nosebleed after trauma, crepitus, instability of the nasal bones, and external deformity of the nose indicate fracture. Septal injury cannot be ruled out by radiography, and can only be ruled out by careful intranasal examination. Patients with suspected nasal fractures should be referred to an otolaryngologist for definitive therapy. Since the nasal bones begin healing immediately, the child must be seen by an otolaryngologist within 48–72 hours of the injury to allow time to arrange for fracture reduction before the bones become immobile.

FOREIGN BODIES IN THE NOSE

If this diagnosis is delayed, unilateral foul-smelling rhinorrhea, halitosis, bleeding, or nasal obstruction often result.

There are many ways to remove nasal foreign bodies. The obvious first maneuver is vigorous nose blowing if the child is old enough. The next step in removal requires nasal decongestion, good lighting, correct instrumentation, and physical restraint. Topical tetracaine or lidocaine may be used for anesthesia in young children. Nasal decongestion can be achieved by topical phenylephrine or oxymetazoline. When the child is properly restrained, most nasal foreign bodies can be removed using a pair of alligator forceps or right-angle instrument through an operating head otoscope. If the object seems unlikely to be removed on the first attempt, is wedged in, or is quite large, the patient should be referred to an otolaryngologist rather than worsening the situation through futile attempts.

Because the nose is a moist cavity, the electrical current generated by disk-type batteries—such as those used in clocks, watches, and hearing aids—can cause necrosis of mucosa and cartilage destruction in less than 4 hours. Batteries constitute a true foreign body emergency.

▼ THE THROAT & ORAL CAVITY

ACUTE STOMATITIS

Stomatitis is inflammation in the oral cavity, and can arise from infection, autoimmune disorders, drug reactions, and chemoradiation. Acute episodes are often painful, and limit oral intake.

1. Recurrent Aphthous Stomatitis

Aphthous ulcers, or canker sores, are small painful ulcers (3–10 mm) usually found on the inner aspect of the lips, gingiva, or tongue. Typically lasting 1–2 weeks, there is usually no associated fever or cervical adenopathy. These may reoccur throughout life, with infectious or autoimmune cause suspected. Treatment is symptomatic with acetaminophen or ibuprofen and temporary choice of a bland diet. A topical corticosteroid, such as triamcinolone dental paste, may also reduce symptomatic duration and intensity. A Cochrane review was unable to promote a single systemic treatment for those unresponsive to local therapy.

Less common causes of recurrent oral ulcers include Behçet disease, familial Mediterranean fever, and PFAPA syndrome (**P**eriodic **F**ever, **A**phthous stomatitis, **P**haryngitis, and cervical **A**denopathy). Behçet disease requires two of the following: genital ulcers, uveitis, and erythema nodosum–like lesions. Patients with Mediterranean fever usually have a positive family history, serosal involvement, and recurrent fever. PFAPA typically begins before the age of 5 years, continues through adolescence, and then spontaneously resolves. Fever and other symptoms recur at regular intervals. Episodes last approximately 5 days and are not associated with other URI symptoms or illnesses. Steroids may shorten episodes but do not prevent recurrence. PFAPA has been shown to resolve with prolonged cimetidine use and adenotonsillectomy.

Brocklehurst P et al: Systemic interventions for recurrent aphthous stomatitis (mouth ulcers). Cochrane Database Syst Rev 2012 Sep 12;(9):CD005411 [PMID: 22972085].

Manthiram K et al: Physician's perspectives on the diagnosis and management of periodic fever, aphthous stomatitis, pharyngitis, and cervical adenitis (PFAPA) syndrome. Rheumatol Int 2017 Jun;37(6):883–889. doi: 10.1007/s00296-017-3688-3 [PMID 28271158].

2. Herpes Simplex Gingivostomatitis (See Chapter 40 Infections: Viral & Rickettsial)

HSV-1 is more often associated with oral ulcerations than HSV-2. HSV transmission is almost always through direct contact, and the virus migrates to reside in the trigeminal ganglion. Reactivation from a dormant state can arise from a variety of stimuli, leading to symptomatic ulcerated lesions of the lips and oral cavity.

3. Thrush (See Chapter 43 Infections: Parasitic & Mycotic)

Candida is normally found in the oral flora of 60% of the population. In infants it presents as white plaques with an erythematous base that typically involves the buccal mucosa and dorsal tongue. Spread to the pharynx and larynx causes odynophagia and can be seen in older children using inhaled steroids and those with compromised immune systems. The breast-feeding mother-infant dyad require simultaneous treatment—the mother with oral diflucan and the infant with a one-time application of Gentian Violet or a course of Nystatin suspension.

4. Traumatic Oral Ulcers

Mechanical trauma most commonly occurs on the buccal mucosa secondary to biting by the molars. Thermal trauma, from very hot foods, can also cause ulcerative lesions. Chemical ulcers can be produced by mucosal contact with aspirin or other caustic agents. Oral ulcers can occur with leukemia or on a recurrent basis with cyclic neutropenia.

PHARYNGITIS

Figure 18–5 is an algorithm for the management of a sore throat.

1. Acute Viral Pharyngitis

Over 90% of sore throats and fever in children are due to viral infections. The findings seldom point toward any particular viral agent, but four types of viral pharyngitis are sufficiently distinctive to warrant discussion below.

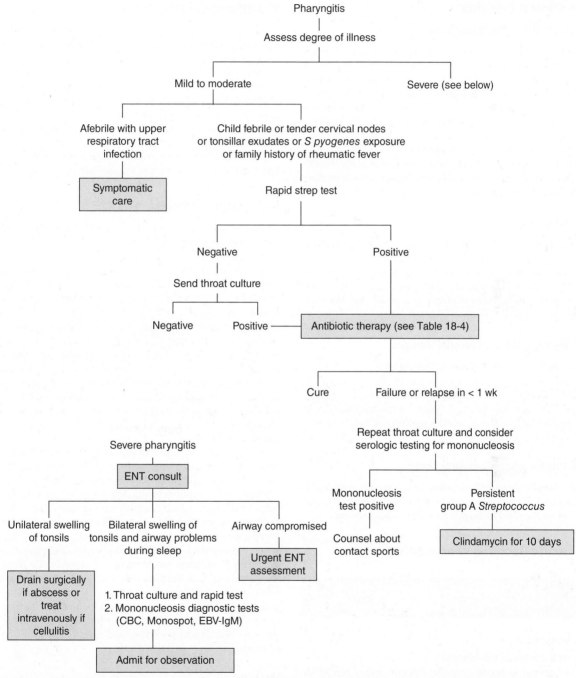

▲ **Figure 18–5.** Algorithm for pharyngitis. CBC, complete blood count; EBV, Epstein-Barr virus; ENT, ear, nose, and throat.

Clinical Findings

A. Infectious Mononucleosis

Findings include exudative tonsillitis, generalized cervical adenitis and fever, usually in patients older than 5 years. A palpable spleen or axillary adenopathy increases the likelihood of the diagnosis. The presence of more than 10% atypical lymphocytes on a peripheral blood smear or a positive mononucleosis spot test supports the diagnosis, although these tests are often falsely negative in children younger than 5 years. Epstein-Barr virus serology showing an elevated IgM-capsid antibody is definitive. Amoxicillin is contraindicated in patients suspected of having mononucleosis because the drug often precipitates a rash.

B. Herpangina

Herpangina ulcers are classically 3 mm in size, surrounded by a halo and are found on the anterior tonsillar pillars, soft palate, and uvula; the anterior mouth and tonsils are spared. Herpangina is caused by the Coxsackie A group of viruses. Polymerase chain reaction testing is available, but not typically indicated, as this is a self-limited illness.

C. Hand, Foot, and Mouth Disease

This entity is caused by several enteroviruses, one of which (enterovirus 71) can rarely cause encephalitis. Ulcers occur anywhere in the mouth. Vesicles, pustules, or papules may be found on the palms, soles, interdigital areas, and buttocks. In younger children lesions may be seen on the distal extremities and even the face.

D. Pharyngoconjunctival Fever

This disorder is caused by an adenovirus and often is epidemic. Exudative tonsillitis, conjunctivitis, lymphadenopathy, and fever are the main findings. Treatment is symptomatic.

2. Acute Bacterial Pharyngitis

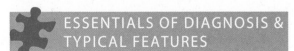

ESSENTIALS OF DIAGNOSIS & TYPICAL FEATURES

▶ Sore throat
▶ At least one of the following:
  • Cervical lymphadenopathy (lymph nodes tender or > 2 cm)
  • Tonsillar exudates
  • Positive group A β-hemolytic *Streptococcus* culture
  • Fever > 38.3°C

Differential Diagnosis

Viral pharyngitis, infectious mononucleosis, bacterial pharyngitis other than streptococcal, diphtheria, and peritonsillar abscess.

Approximately 20%–30% of children with pharyngitis have a group A streptococcal (GAS) infection. It is most common in children between 5 and 15 years in the winter or early spring. Less common causes of bacterial pharyngitis include *Mycoplasma pneumoniae*, *Chlamydia pneumoniae*, groups C and G streptococci, and *Arcanobacterium hemolyticum*. Of the five, *M pneumoniae* is by far the most common and may cause over one-third of all pharyngitis cases in adolescents and adults.

Clinical Findings

Sudden onset of sore throat, fever, tender cervical adenopathy, palatal petechiae, a beefy-red uvula, and a tonsillar exudate suggest streptococcal infection. Other symptoms may include headache, stomachache, nausea, and vomiting. The only way to make a definitive diagnosis is by throat culture or rapid antigen test. Rapid antigen tests are very specific, but have a sensitivity of only 85%–95%. Therefore, a positive test indicates *S pyogenes* infection, but a negative result requires confirmation by performing a culture. Diagnosis is important because untreated streptococcal pharyngitis can result in acute rheumatic fever, glomerulonephritis, and suppurative complications (eg, cervical adenitis, peritonsillar abscess, otitis media, cellulitis, and septicemia). The presence of conjunctivitis, cough, hoarseness, symptoms of URI, anterior stomatitis, ulcerative lesions, viral rash, and diarrhea should raise suspicion of a viral etiology.

Occasionally, a child with group A streptococcal infection develops scarlet fever within 24–48 hours after the onset of symptoms. Scarlet fever is a diffuse, finely papular, erythematous eruption producing a bright red discoloration of the skin, which blanches on pressure. The rash is more intense in the skin creases. The tongue has a strawberry appearance.

A controversial but possible complication of streptococcal infections is pediatric autoimmune neuropsychiatric disorders associated with *Streptococcus* (PANDAS). PANDAS is a relatively newly recognized condition. It describes a subset of pediatric patients who experience a sudden onset of obsessive-compulsive disorder and/or tics, or worsening of such symptoms in children who previously had these, following a strep infection.

Web Resources

National Institute of Mental Health: Information About PANS/PANDAS: https://www.nimh.nih.gov/research/research-conducted-at-nimh/research-areas/clinics-and-labs/sbp/information-about-pans-pandas.shtml. Accessed June 2, 2019.

Table 18–4. Treatment of group A streptococcal pharyngitis.*

Treatment of acute group A strep pharyngitis		
Antibiotic	**Dose**	**Notes**
Penicillin	**Penicillin V** 250 mg 2–3 times per day for 10 days if less than 27 kg; 500 mg 2–3 times per day for 10 days if greater than 27 kg **Benzathine Penicillin** 600,000 units IM single dose if less than 27 kg; 1.2 million units IM single dose if greater than 27 kg	Resistance to penicillin, amoxicillin, and first-generation cephalosporins has not been reported. Each is equally effective if compliance is assured.
Amoxicillin	50 mg/kg/day once daily for 10 days (max 1200 mg)	
Cephalexin	25–50 mg/kg/day in 2 divided doses for 10 days	
Clindamycin	20 mg/kg/day in 3 divided doses for 10 days	Rare resistance reported in the United States.
Azithromycin	12 mg/kg once daily for 5 days (max 500 mg/day)	Some resistance reported in the United States.
Eradication of carrier state		
Clindamycin	20 mg/kg/day in 3 divided doses for 10 days	Most effective
Cephalexin	25–50 mg/kg/day in 2 divided doses for 10 days	Also effective
Penicillin + Rifampin	See above penicillin doses; Rifampin 20 mg/kg/day twice daily for final 4 days	

*Tetracyclines, sulfonamides (including trimethoprim-sulfamethoxazole), and quinolones should not be used for treating GAS infections.

▶ Treatment

Suspected or proven group A streptococcal infection should be treated with penicillin (oral or intramuscular) or amoxicillin as outlined in Table 18–4. For patients allergic to penicillin, alternative treatments include cephalexin, azithromycin, and clindamycin. Tetracyclines, sulfonamides (including trimethoprim-sulfamethoxazole) and quinolones should not be used for treating GAS infections.

Repeat culture after treatment is not recommended and is indicated only for those who remain symptomatic, have a recurrence of symptoms, or have had rheumatic fever. Of note, children who have had rheumatic fever are at a high risk of recurrence if future GAS infections are inadequately treated. In this group of patients, long-term antibiotic prophylaxis is recommended, sometimes life-long in patients with residual rheumatic heart disease (see Chapter 20).

In general, the carrier state is harmless, self-limited (2–6 months), and not contagious. An attempt to eradicate the carrier state is warranted only if the patient or another family member has frequent streptococcal infections, or if a family member or patient has a history of rheumatic fever or glomerulonephritis. If eradication is chosen, a course of clindamycin for 10 days or rifampin for 5 days should be used.

In the past, daily penicillin prophylaxis was occasionally recommended; however, because of concerns about the development of drug resistance, tonsillectomy is now preferred for patients with recurrent streptococcal tonsillitis.

Wessels MR: Clinical practice. Streptococcal pharyngitis. N Engl J Med 2011;364(7):648–655 [PMID: 21323542].

PERITONSILLAR CELLULITIS OR ABSCESS (QUINSY)

ESSENTIALS OF DIAGNOSIS & TYPICAL FEATURES

▶ Severe sore throat.

▶ Unilateral tonsillar swelling.

▶ Deviation of the uvula.

▶ Trismus (limited mouth opening).

Tonsillar infection extending to the surrounding tissues is called peritonsillar cellulitis. If untreated, necrosis occurs, with peritonsillar abscess formation. The most common pathogen is β-hemolytic *Streptococcus*, but others include group D *Streptococcus*, *S pneumoniae*, and anaerobes. A severe sore throat and high fever is usually present, and the process is almost always unilateral. The tonsil bulges medially, and the anterior tonsillar pillar is prominent. The soft palate and uvula on the involved side are edematous and displaced toward the uninvolved side. As the infection progresses, trismus, ear pain, dysphagia, and drooling may occur. The most serious complication of untreated peritonsillar abscess is a lateral pharyngeal abscess.

While peritonsillar cellulitis will often respond to parenteral antibiotics (penicillin, cephalosporin, or clindamycin), an abscess within the peritonsillar space will typically require drainage. Failure to respond to therapy during the first 12–24 hours indicates a high probability of abscess formation and need for otolaryngology consultation. A peritonsillar abscess may be needle aspirated or formally incised and drained. The risk of bilateral and/or recurrent peritonsillar abscess is low (7%–10%), so tonsillectomy is not usually indicated for a single incident.

RETROPHARYNGEAL ABSCESS

Retropharyngeal lymph nodes drain the oropharynx, nasopharynx, and paranasal sinuses. Infections of these nodes are most often due to β-hemolytic streptococci and S aureus. The diagnosis of retropharyngeal abscess should be suspected in a child with fever, respiratory symptoms, and neck hyperextension. Dysphagia, drooling, dyspnea, and gurgling respirations may also be present. This occurs most commonly during the first 2 years of life. After this age, the most common cause of retropharyngeal abscess is penetrating injury of the posterior pharyngeal wall.

Prominent swelling on one side of the posterior pharyngeal wall is characteristic. Swelling usually stops at the midline because a medial raphe divides the prevertebral space. Although nonspecific, lateral neck x-ray may demonstrate retropharyngeal tissues wider than the C4 vertebral body; CT scan with contrast can distinguish between soft tissue swelling versus abscess.

Although a retropharyngeal abscess is a surgical emergency, frequently it cannot be distinguished from retropharyngeal adenitis. Immediate hospitalization and intravenous antimicrobial therapy with a semisynthetic penicillin or clindamycin is the first step for most cases. In most instances, a period of 12–24 hours of antimicrobial therapy will help differentiate the two entities. In the child with adenitis, fever will decrease and oral intake will improve. A child with retropharyngeal abscess will typically not improve. A surgeon should incise and drain the abscess under general anesthesia to prevent its extension. Immediate surgical drainage is indicated if there is concern for airway compromise.

LUDWIG ANGINA

Ludwig angina is a rapidly progressive cellulitis of both submandibular spaces that pushes the tongue posteriorly against the pharyngeal wall, causing life threatening airway obstruction. Symptoms include fever and tender swelling of the tongue and floor of the mouth. Most often arising from an odontogenic source, this infection is unusual in infants and children. Group A strep is the most common culprit.

Treatment consists of high-dose intravenous clindamycin or ampicillin plus nafcillin until culture and sensitivities are available. Treatment for airway obstruction in patients with Ludwig angina has transitioned through the years from tracheotomy to intensive care unit monitoring and intubation. An otolaryngologist should be consulted for airway evaluation and management, and to perform a drainage procedure if needed.

ACUTE CERVICAL ADENITIS

Local infections of the ear, nose, and throat can involve a regional lymph node and cause abscess formation. The typical case involves a unilateral, solitary, anterior cervical node. About 70% of these cases are due to β-hemolytic streptococcal infection, 20% to staphylococci (including MRSA), and the remainder to viruses, atypical mycobacteria, and Bartonella henselae.

The initial evaluation of cervical adenitis should generally include a rapid group A streptococcal test, and a complete blood count with differential looking for atypical lymphocytes. A purified protein derivative skin test, looking for nontuberculous mycobacteria, should also be considered. If multiple enlarged nodes are found, a rapid mononucleosis test is useful. Early treatment with antibiotics prevents many cases of adenitis from progressing to suppuration. However, once abscess formation occurs, antibiotic therapy alone is often insufficient and a drainage procedure may be necessary. Because of the increase in community-acquired MRSA, it is a prudent to send a specimen for culture and sensitivity.

Cat-scratch disease, caused by B henselae, causes indolent ("cold") adenopathy. The diagnosis is supported if a primary papule is found at the scratch site on the face. In over 90% of patients, there is a history of contact with kittens. The node is usually only mildly tender but may, over a month or more, suppurate and drain. About one-third of children have fever and malaise; rarely neurologic sequelae and prolonged fever occur. Cat-scratch disease can be diagnosed by serologic testing, but testing is not always confirmatory. If blood is to be drawn, one should wait 2–8 weeks after onset of symptoms. Because most enlarged lymph nodes infected with B henselae spontaneously regress within 1–3 months, the benefit of antibiotics is controversial. In a placebo-controlled trial, azithromycin for 5 days caused a more rapid decrease in node size. Other drugs likely to be effective include rifampin, trimethoprim-sulfamethoxazole, erythromycin, clarithromycin, doxycycline*, ciprofloxacin*, and gentamicin (*be aware of age restrictions).

Cervical lymphadenitis can also be caused by nontuberculous mycobacterial species or Mycobacterium avium complex. Mycobacterial disease is unilateral and may involve several matted nodes. A characteristic violaceous appearance may develop over a prolonged period of time without systemic signs or much local pain. Atypical mycobacterial infections are often associated with positive purified protein derivative skin test reactions less than 10 mm in diameter, and a second-strength (250-test-unit) purified protein derivative skin test is virtually always positive.

Lawrence R, Bateman N: Controversies in the management of deep neck space infection in children: an evidence-based review. Clin Otolaryngol 2017 Feb;42(1):156–163. doi: 10.1111/coa.12692. Epub 2016 Jun 30 [PMID: 27288654].

▶ Differential Diagnosis

A. Neoplasms and Cervical Nodes

Malignant tumors usually are not suspected until adenopathy persists despite antibiotic treatment. Classically, malignant lymph nodes are painless, nontender, and of firm consistency. They may be fixed to underlying tissues. They may occur as a single node, as unilateral nodes in a chain, bilateral cervical nodes, or as generalized adenopathy. Common malignancies that may manifest in the neck include lymphoma, rhabdomyosarcoma, and thyroid carcinoma.

B. Imitators of Adenitis

Several structures in the neck can become infected and resemble a lymph node. The first three masses are of congenital origin.

1. Thyroglossal duct cyst—These are midline, usually near the level of the hyoid bone. Thyroglossal duct cysts move upward when the tongue is protruded or with swallowing. Occasionally, a thyroglossal duct cyst may have a sinus tract with an opening just lateral to the midline. When infected, these can become acutely swollen and inflamed.

2. Branchial cleft cyst—These masses are found along the anterior border of the sternocleidomastoid muscle and are smooth and fluctuant. Sometimes a branchial cleft cyst may be attached to the overlying skin by a small dimple or a draining sinus tract. When infected, they can become a tender mass 3–5 cm in diameter.

3. Lymphatic malformation—Most lymphatic cysts are located in the posterior triangle just above the clavicle. These are soft and compressible and can be transilluminated. Over 60% are noted at birth; the remaining malformations usually become apparent by the age of 2 years. If large enough, they can compromise the patient's ability to swallow and breathe.

4. Parotitis—Parotitis is commonly mistaken for cervical adenitis. The parotid salivary gland crosses the angle of the jaw. Parotitis may be bacterial or viral and may occur unilaterally or bilaterally. Mumps was once the most common cause of viral parotitis, but because of routine vaccinations, parainfluenza is the primary viral cause in the United States. An amylase level will be elevated in parotitis.

5. Ranula—A ranula is a saliva filled cyst in the floor of mouth caused by obstruction of the sublingual salivary gland. A "plunging" ranula extends down through the mylohyoid muscle and can present as a neck mass.

6. Sternocleidomastoid muscle hematoma—Also known as *fibromatosis colli*, these are noted at age 2–4 weeks. On examination, the mass is found to be part of the muscle body and not movable. An associated torticollis usually confirms the diagnosis. A neck ultrasound can help confirm the diagnosis. Treatment involves physical therapy, with range of motion exercises.

TONSILLECTOMY & ADENOIDECTOMY

Tonsillectomy

A tonsillectomy, with or without adenoidectomy, is most often performed for either hypertrophy or recurrent infections. The most common indication for adenotonsillectomy is adenotonsillar hypertrophy associated with an obstructive breathing pattern during sleep (see Chapter 19). Adenotonsillar hypertrophy may also cause other problems such as dysphagia or dental malocclusion.

Recurrent tonsillitis is the second most common reason for tonsillectomy. Tonsillitis is considered "recurrent" when a child has seven or more documented infections in 1 year, five per year for 2 years, or three per year for 3 years. For an infection to be considered clinically significant, there must be a sore throat and at least one of the following clinical features: cervical lymphadenopathy (tender lymph nodes or > 2 cm), OR tonsillar exudate, OR positive culture for group A β-hemolytic *Streptococcus*, OR temperature greater than 38.3°C.

Tonsillectomy is reasonable with fewer infections if the child has missed multiple school days due to infection, has a complicated course, or under other circumstances such as recurrent peritonsillar abscess, persistent streptococcal carrier state, or multiple antibiotic allergies. Unless neoplasm is suspected, tonsil asymmetry is not an indication.

A new indication for tonsillectomy is PFAPA syndrome (see earlier section on Recurrent Aphthous Stomatitis), in which fever recurs predictably, typically every 4–8 weeks. Tonsillectomy has been shown to be an effective treatment.

Ingram DG, Friedman NR: Toward adenotonsillectomy in children: a review for the general pediatrician. JAMA Pediatr 2015 Dec;169(12):1155–1161. doi: 10.1001/jamapediatrics.2015 .2016. Review [PMID: 26436644].
Mitchell RB et al: Clinical practice guideline: tonsillectomy in children (update). Otolaryngol Head Neck Surg 2019 Feb;160(1_suppl): S1–S42. doi: 10.1177/0194599818801757 [PMID: 30798778].

Web Resources

American Academy of Otolaryngology/Head and Neck Surgery–sponsored site dedicated to children: http://www.entnet.org/content/pediatric-sleep-disordered-breathingobstructive-sleep-apnea. Accessed June 2, 2019.

Adenoidectomy

The adenoid is composed of lymphoid tissue in the nasopharynx and is a part of the Waldeyer ring of lymphoid tissue, which also includes the palatine and lingual tonsils. Enlarged adenoids, with or without infection, can obstruct the nose, alter normal orofacial growth, and interfere with speech, swallowing, and Eustachian tube function. Children who are persistent mouth breathers can develop dental malocclusion and "adenoid facies," where the face appears "pinched" and the maxilla narrowed because the molding pressures of the orbicularis oris and buccinator muscles are unopposed by the tongue. The adenoid can also harbor biofilms, which have been associated with CRS and otitis media.

Indications for adenoidectomy with or without tonsillectomy include upper airway obstruction, orofacial conditions such as mandibular growth abnormalities and dental malocclusion, speech abnormalities, persistent MEE, recurrent otitis media, and CRS.

Complications of Tonsillectomy & Adenoidectomy

The mortality rate associated with tonsillectomy and adenoidectomy is reported to approximate that of general anesthesia alone. The rate of hemorrhage varies between 0.1% and 8.1%, depending on the definition of hemorrhage; the rate of postoperative transfusion is 0.04%. Other potential complications include permanently hypernasal speech (< 0.01%) and, more rarely, nasopharyngeal stenosis, atlantoaxial subluxation, mandibular condyle fracture, and psychological trauma.

Contraindications to Tonsillectomy & Adenoidectomy

A. Palatal Abnormalities

Adenoid tissue should not be removed completely in a child with a cleft palate or submucous cleft palate because of the risk of velopharyngeal incompetence which may cause hypernasal speech and nasal regurgitation. If needed, a partial adenoidectomy can be performed in at-risk children. A bifid uvula can be a sign of a palatal abnormality.

B. Bleeding Disorder

When suspected, bleeding disorders must be diagnosed and treated prior to surgery.

C. Acute Tonsillitis

An elective tonsillectomy and adenoidectomy can usually be postponed until acute tonsillitis is resolved. Urgent tonsillectomy may occasionally be required for tonsillitis unresponsive to medical therapy.

DISORDERS OF THE LIPS

1. Labial Sucking Tubercle

A young infant may present with a small callus in the mid-upper lip. The cause is likely strong sucking in utero but can persist into early infancy. It usually is asymptomatic and disappears after cup feeding is initiated.

2. Cheilitis

Dry, cracked, scaling lips are usually caused by sun or wind exposure. Contact dermatitis from mouthpieces or various woodwind or brass instruments has also been reported. Licking the lips exacerbates cheilitis. Liberal use of lip balm gives excellent results.

3. Inclusion Cyst

Inclusion or mucous retention cysts are due to obstruction of mucous glands or other mucous membrane structures, such as minor salivary glands. In the newborn, they occur on the hard palate or gums and are called *Epstein pearls*. These resolve spontaneously in 1–2 months. In older children, inclusion cysts usually occur on the palate, uvula, or tonsillar pillars. They appear as taut yellow sacs varying in size from 2 to 10 mm. Inclusion cysts that do not resolve spontaneously may undergo incision and drainage. Occasionally, a mucous cyst on the lower lip (mucocele) will require excision for cosmetic reasons.

DISORDERS OF THE TONGUE

1. Geographic Tongue (Benign Migratory Glossitis)

This condition of unknown etiology occurs in 1%–2% of the population with no age, sex, or racial predilection. It is characterized by irregularly shaped patches on the tongue that are devoid of papillae and surrounded by parakeratotic reddish borders. The pattern changes as alternating regeneration and desquamation occurs. The lesions are generally asymptomatic and require no treatment.

2. Fissured Tongue (Scrotal Tongue)

This condition is marked by numerous irregular fissures on the dorsum of the tongue. It occurs in approximately 1% of the population and is usually a dominant trait. It is also frequently seen in children with trisomy 21.

3. Coated Tongue (Furry Tongue)

The tongue becomes coated if mastication is impaired and the patient is limited to a liquid or soft diet. Mouth breathing, fever, or dehydration can accentuate the process.

4. Macroglossia

Tongue hypertrophy and protrusion may be due to trisomy 21, Beckwith-Wiedemann syndrome, glycogen storage diseases, cretinism, mucopolysaccharidoses, lymphangioma, or hemangioma. Tongue reduction procedures should be considered in otherwise healthy subjects if macroglossia affects airway patency.

HALITOSIS

Bad breath is usually due to acute stomatitis, pharyngitis, rhinosinusitis, nasal foreign body, or dental hygiene problems. In older children and adolescents, halitosis can be a manifestation of CRS, gastric bezoar, bronchiectasis, or lung abscess. The presence of orthodontic devices or dentures can cause halitosis if good dental hygiene is not maintained. Halitosis can also be caused by decaying food particles embedded in cryptic tonsils. Mouthwashes and chewable breath fresheners give limited improvement. Treatment of the underlying cause is indicated, and a dental referral may be in order.

SALIVARY GLAND DISORDERS

1. Parotitis

A first episode of parotitis may safely be considered to be of viral origin, unless fluctuance is present. Mumps was the leading cause until adoption of vaccination; now the leading viruses are parainfluenza and Epstein-Barr virus. HIV infection should be considered if the child is known to be at risk.

2. Suppurative Parotitis

Suppurative parotitis occurs chiefly in newborns and debilitated elderly patients. The parotid gland is swollen, tender, and often erythematous, usually unilaterally. The diagnosis is made by expression of purulent material from Stensen duct. The material should be cultured. Fever and leukocytosis may be present. Treatment includes intravenous antibiotic therapy. *S aureus* is the most common causative organism.

3. Juvenile Recurrent Parotitis

Some children experience recurrent nonsuppurative parotid inflammation with swelling or pain and fever. Juvenile recurrent parotitis (JRP) is most prevalent between the ages of 3 and 6 years, and it generally decreases by adolescence. The cause is unknown, but possible etiologic factors include ductal anomaly, autoimmune, allergy, and genetic. It usually occurs unilaterally. Treatment includes analgesics and some recommend an antistaphylococcal antibiotic for prophylaxis of bacterial infection and quicker resolution. Endoscopy and irrigation of Stensen duct is being performed more frequently, not only to confirm diagnosis but also to provide treatment.

4. Tumors of the Parotid Gland

Mixed tumors, hemangiomas, sarcoidosis, and leukemia can manifest in the parotid gland as a hard or persistent mass. A cystic mass or multiple cystic masses may represent an HIV infection. Workup may require consultation with oncology, infectious disease, hematology, and otolaryngology.

5. Ranula

A ranula is a retention cyst of a sublingual salivary gland. It occurs on the floor of the mouth to one side of the lingual frenulum. It is thin walled and can appear bluish. Referral is indicated to an otolaryngologist for surgical management.

CONGENITAL ORAL MALFORMATIONS

1. Tongue-Tie (Ankyloglossia)

A short lingual frenulum can hinder protrusion and elevation of the tongue. Dimpling of the midline tongue tip is noted with tongue movement. Ankyloglossia can cause feeding difficulties in the neonate, speech problems, and dental problems. If the tongue cannot protrude past the teeth or alveolar ridge or move between the gums and cheek, referral to an otolaryngologist is indicated. A frenulectomy should be performed in the neonatal period if the infant is having difficulty breast-feeding, specifically inefficient milk transfer or persistent pain in the mother. Early treatment is favored because it can easily be performed in clinic. When an infant is even a few months old, general anesthesia is required for the procedure to be performed safely. Lip tie concerns have become more common as breast-feeding initiation is increasing but there is little evidence that this has any effect on nursing.

O'Shea JE et al: Frenotomy for tongue-tie in newborn infants. Cochrane Database Syst Rev 2017 Mar 11;3:CD011065. doi: 10.1002/14651858.CD011065.pub2 [PMID: 28284020].

2. Torus Palatini

Torus palatini are hard, midline, palate masses which form at suture lines of the bone. They are usually asymptomatic and require no therapy, but they can be surgically reduced if necessary.

3. Cleft Lip & Cleft Palate

A. Submucous Cleft Palate

A bifid uvula is present in 3% of healthy children (see Chapter 37). However, a close association exists between bifid uvula and submucous cleft palate. A submucous cleft can be diagnosed by noting a translucent zone in the middle of the soft palate (zona pellucida). Palpation of the hard palate reveals absence of the posterior bony protrusion. Affected children have a 40% risk of developing persistent MEE. They are at risk for velopharyngeal incompetence, or an inability to close the palate against the posterior pharyngeal wall, resulting in hypernasal speech and nasal regurgitation of food. Children with submucous cleft palate causing abnormal speech or significant nasal regurgitation of food should be referred for possible surgical repair.

B. High-Arched Palate

A high-arched palate is usually a genetic trait of no consequence. It also occurs in children who are chronic mouth breathers and in premature infants who undergo prolonged oral intubation. Some rare causes of high-arched palate are congenital disorders such as Marfan syndrome, Treacher Collins syndrome, and Ehlers-Danlos syndrome. Orthodontic treatment of a high arched palate can be an effective treatment for childhood OSA.

C. Pierre Robin Sequence

This group of congenital malformations is characterized by the triad of micrognathia, cleft palate, and glossoptosis. Affected children often present as emergencies in the newborn period because of infringement on the airway by the tongue and also because of feeding difficulties. The main objective of treatment is to prevent asphyxia until the mandible becomes large enough to accommodate the tongue. In some cases, this can be achieved by leaving the child in a prone position when unattended. Other airway manipulations such as a nasal trumpet may be necessary. Distraction osteogenesis has been used to avoid tracheostomy. In severe cases, a tracheostomy is required. The child requires close observation and careful feeding until the problem is outgrown.

Gómez OJ et al: Pierre robin sequence: an evidence-based treatment proposal. J Craniofac Surg 2018 Mar;29(2):332–338. doi: 10.1097/SCS.0000000000004178 [PMID: 29215441].

Respiratory Tract & Mediastinum

19

Monica J. Federico, MD

Christopher D. Baker, MD

Emily M. DeBoer, MD

Oren Kupfer, MD

Stacey L. Martiniano, MD

Paul Stillwell, MD

Stephen Hawkins, MD

Deborah Liptzin, MD

▼ RESPIRATORY TRACT

Pediatric pulmonary diseases account for almost 50% of deaths in children younger than 1 year and about 20% of all hospitalizations of children younger than 15 years. Approximately 7% of children have a chronic disorder of the lower respiratory system. Understanding the pathophysiology of many pediatric pulmonary diseases requires an appreciation of the normal growth and development of the lung.

▼ GROWTH & DEVELOPMENT

Normal fetal lung development progresses through five stages with considerable overlap in the timing of each stage (Table 19–1). Interruption of the sequence leads to significant neonatal pulmonary difficulties that may extend lifelong. The normal human term newborn infant does not have a full complement of alveoli at birth, usually 100–150 million; this will increase with normal growth to the adult number of 300–600 alveoli. Infants who miss even the last few weeks of gestation may be challenged to meet the demands of transition from fetal life to air breathing due to incomplete alveolarization, and this may be accentuated by additional stress such as higher altitude or infection

Stocks J, Hislop A, Sonnappa S: Early lung development: lifelong effect on respiratory health and disease. Lancet Respir Med 2013;1:728–742 [PMID: 24429276].

▼ DIAGNOSTIC AIDS

PHYSICAL EXAMINATION OF THE RESPIRATORY TRACT

The complete pulmonary examination includes inspection, palpation, auscultation, and percussion. *Inspection* of respiratory rate and work of breathing is critical to the detection of pulmonary disease. Tachypnea, abnormalities of attentiveness, inconsolability, increased respiratory effort, color, and movement are reliable signs of hypoxemia. *Palpation* of tracheal position, symmetry of chest wall movement, and vibration with vocalization can help in identifying intrathoracic abnormalities. For example, a shift in tracheal position from midline can suggest pneumothorax or significant unilateral atelectasis. Tactile fremitus may change with consolidation or air in the pleural space. *Auscultation* should assess the intensity and symmetry of breath sounds and the presence of abnormal sounds such as fine or coarse crackles, wheezing, or rhonchi. Wheezing or prolonged expiratory compared to inspiratory time suggests intrathoracic airways obstruction. Tachypnea with an equal inspiratory and expiratory time suggests decreased lung compliance. It is important to know the lung anatomy in order to identify the location of abnormal findings (Figure 19–1). In older patients, unilateral crackles are the most valuable examination finding in pneumonia. *Percussion* may identify tympanic or dull sounds that can help define an effusion or pneumothorax. This component of the examination can prove challenging in young children.

Extrapulmonary manifestations of pulmonary disease include acute findings such as cyanosis and altered mental status; and signs of chronic respiratory insufficiency including growth failure, clubbing, and osteoarthropathy. Evidence of cor pulmonale (loud pulmonic component of the second heart sound, hepatomegaly, elevated neck veins, and rarely, peripheral edema) signifies pulmonary hypertension and may accompany advanced lung disease.

Respiratory disorders can be secondary to disease in other systems. It is therefore important to look for other conditions such as fever, metabolic acidosis, congenital heart disease, neuromuscular disease, immunodeficiency, autoimmune disease, and occult malignancy. Children with an elevated body mass index are more likely to present with sleep or respiratory symptoms and need to be evaluated for pulmonary pathology versus deconditioning or dyspnea.

Table 19–1. Sequence of fetal lung development.

Stage of Development	Weeks of Gestation	Transitions	Pathology
Embryonic	4–6	Mainstem bronchi form from foregut outpouching. Main PAs develop.	Lung aplasia Tracheaesophageal fistula Diaphragmatic hernia
Pseudoglandular	6–16	Major bronchi form to terminal bronchioles. Conducting airways branching complete at 16 wk.	Foregut malformations: CPAM, sequestration, bronchogenic cyst
Canalicular	16–26	Growth extends to respiratory bronchioles. Extensive angiogenesis.	Nonviable fetus below 22–23 wk gestation
Saccular	26–36	Primitive air sacs and alveolar ducts form off respiratory bronchioles. Surfactant production begins.	Respiratory distress syndrome of the newborn
Alveolar	36+	Increased number and complexity of alveoli.	Incomplete alveolarization

CPAM, congenital pulmonary airway malformation.

Advanced Physical Diagnosis Learning and Teaching at the Bedside: Skill Modules: Pulmonary Examination. https://depts.washington.edu/physdx/pulmonary/tech.html. Accessed May 30, 2017.

Bohadana A, Izbicki G, Kraman SS: Fundamentals of lung auscultation. N Engl J Med 2014;370:744–751 [PMID: 24552321].

Sly PD, Collins RA: Physiologic basis of respiratory signs and symptoms. Paediatr Respir Rev 2006;7:84–88.

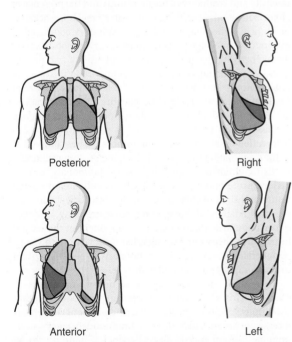

Posterior

Right

Anterior

Left

▲ **Figure 19–1.** Projections of the pulmonary lobes on the chest surface. The upper lobes are white, the right-middle lobe is the darker color, and the lower lobes are the lighter color.

PULMONARY FUNCTION TESTS

Pulmonary function tests (PFTs) are objective measures of pulmonary physiology that can differentiate obstructive from restrictive lung diseases, measure disease progression, and evaluate response to therapy. Because the normal values change with growth, serial determinations of lung function are often more informative than a single determination. Patient cooperation and consistent effort is essential for almost all standard PFTs. Most children aged 5 and older can perform pulmonary function testing. Younger children may be able to produce reliable results with coaching and visual incentives. Children with cystic fibrosis (CF) and asthma should perform pulmonary function testing routinely as early as they can cooperate. The values measured include forced vital capacity (FVC), which is the total volume of air that is exhaled; forced expiratory volume in the first second of the exhalation (FEV_1); the ratio of the FEV_1/FVC; forced expiratory flow at the middle of the vital capacity (FEF_{25-75}); and peak expiratory flow rate (PEFR). With a more robust sample of normal subjects, reference equations are now available from age 4 to 80, and the lower limit of normal is defined by a Z-score of 1.64. Commonly seen obstructive lung processes include asthma, bronchopulmonary dysplasia (BPD), and (CF). Common restrictive lung diseases include chest wall deformities, muscle weakness, and interstitial lung diseases (ILDs). Confirmation of restrictive lung physiology requires lung volume measurements (eg, total lung capacity, residual volume, and functional residual capacity) with special equipment. (For examples of PFTs, see Figures 19–2 to 19–4.)

PEFR, the maximal flow recorded during an FVC maneuver, can be assessed by handheld devices. These devices are not as well calibrated as spirometers, and the PEFR measurement can vary greatly with patient effort, so they are not good substitutes for actual spirometry. However, peak flow

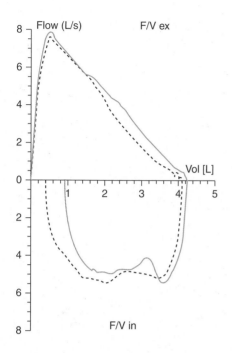

		Pred	Pre	%Pred	Post	%Pred	%Change
FVC	[L]	4.19	4.09	98	4.24	101	4
FEV$_1$	[L]	3.58	3.42	95	3.74	104	9
FEV$_1$ %FVC	[%]		83.46		88.07		6
FEF 25/75	[L/s]	3.89	3.47	89	4.08	105	18
PEF	[L/s]	7.38	7.59	103	7.84	106	3
V back extrapol. %FVC	[%]		2.56		2.29		−11

▲ **Figure 19–2.** Normal flow volume loop pre- and post-bronchodilator.

monitoring can be helpful in a patient with asthma that is difficult to control or for patients with poor perception of their airflow obstruction.

Coates AL: Using reference values to interpret pulmonary function tests. Paediatr Respir Rev 2011;12:206–207 [PMID: 21722850].
Stanojevic S et al. Reference ranges for spirometry across all ages: a new approach. Am J Respir Crit Care Med 2008;177:253–260 [PMID: 18006882].

ASSESSMENT OF OXYGENATION & VENTILATION

Arterial blood gas measurements define the acid-base balance between respiration in the tissue and in the lungs. Blood gas measurements evaluate hypoxemia, acidosis, and hypercarbia and can be used to categorize acid-base disturbances as respiratory, metabolic, or mixed. Blood gas measurements are affected by abnormalities of ventilation/perfusion ($\dot{V}/\dot{Q}$) matching, respiratory control, ventilation, and respiratory mechanics. In pediatrics, hypoxemia (low partial pressure of arterial oxygen [Pa_{O_2}]) most commonly results from ventilation ($\dot{V}$) and perfusion ($\dot{Q}$) mismatch. Common pediatric diseases associated with hypoxemia due to $\dot{V}/\dot{Q}$ mismatch include acute asthma, CF, pneumonia, bronchiolitis, and BPD. Other causes of hypoxemia include hypoventilation, shunts (physiologic and anatomic), and diffusion barrier for oxygen. Hypercapnia (elevated partial pressure of arterial carbon dioxide [Pa_{CO_2}]) results from hypoventilation (ie, inability to clear the CO_2 produced). Causes include decreased central respiratory drive, respiratory muscle weakness, and low-tidal-volume breathing as seen in restrictive lung or chest wall diseases. Hypercapnea can also occur when severe $\dot{V}/\dot{Q}$ mismatch is present, which may occur with severe CF or BPD. Table 19–2 gives normal values for arterial pH, Pa_{O_2}, and Pa_{CO_2} at sea level and at 5000 ft.

Venous blood gas analysis or capillary blood gas analysis can be useful for the assessment of P_{CO_2} and pH, but not P_{O_2} or saturation. Noninvasive assessment of oxygenation can be

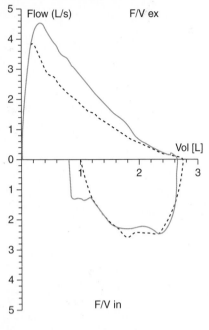

		Pred	Pre	%Pred	Post	%Pred	%Change
FVC	[L]	2.11	2.74	130	2.62	125	−4
FEV$_1$	[L]	1.85	1.77	96	2.03	110	15
FEV$_1$ %FVC	[%]		64.74		77.46		20
FEF 25/75	[L/s]	2.21	1.09	49	1.66	75	53
PEF	[L/s]	3.89	3.85	99	4.50	116	17
V back extrapol. %FVC	[%]		1.39		2.20		59

▲ **Figure 19–3.** Flow volume loops from a child with asthma (obstructive pattern with bronchodilator response).

achieved with pulse oximetry (Spo$_2$). Values of Spo$_2$ are reliable as low as 80%. Reliability is reduced with poor arterial pulsation (eg, with hypothermia, hypotension, or infusion of vasoconstriction). Carbon monoxide bound to hemoglobin results in falsely high Spo$_2$ readings. Exhaled or end-tidal CO$_2$ monitoring can be used to noninvasively estimate arterial CO$_2$ content. It is used to monitor alveolar ventilation and is most accurate in patients without significant lung disease, particularly those good $\dot{V}/\dot{Q}$ matching and without airway obstruction. Monitoring of exhaled or end-tidal CO$_2$ is commonly used during polysomnogram (PSG) and anesthesia. Transcutaneous Pco$_2$ monitoring is also feasible but may be less reliable than transcutaneous Po$_2$ monitoring and should be used with caution.

Ammaddeo A, Faroux B: Oxygen and carbon dioxide monitoring during sleep. Paediatr Respir Rev 2016;20:42–44. doi: 10.1016/j.prrv.2015.11.009. Epub 2015 Dec 4 [PMID: 26724141].

Berend K, de Vries APJ, Gans ROB: Physiological approach to assessment of acid-base disturbances. N Engl J Med 2014; 371:1434–1445 [PMID: 25295502].

Fouzas S, Priftis KN, Anthracopoulos MB: Pulse oximetry in pediatric practice. Pediatrics 2011;128:740 [PMID: 21930554].

DIAGNOSIS OF RESPIRATORY TRACT INFECTIONS

Respiratory tract infections may be caused by bacteria, viruses, atypical bacteria (eg, *Mycoplasma pneumoniae* and *Chlamydia pneumoniae*), *Mycobacterium tuberculosis*, nontuberculous mycobacterium, or fungi (eg, *Aspergillus* and *Pneumocystis jiroveci*). The type of infection suspected and appropriate diagnostic tests vary depending on factors such as underlying lung disease, immune function, and geographic region. Sources of respiratory tract secretions for diagnostic testing include nasopharyngeal and oropharyngeal swabs; expectorated and induced sputum; tracheal aspirates; direct lung or pleural fluid sampling; bronchoalveolar

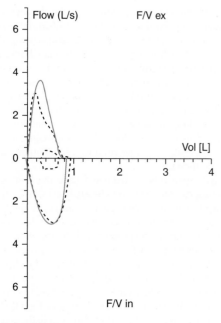

Spirometry							
		Pred	**Pre**	**%Pred**	**Post**	**%Pred**	**%Change**
FVC	L	1.89	0.91	48	0.83	44	−9
FEV$_1$	L	1.77	0.78	44	0.74	42	−5
FEV$_1$ %FVC	%		85.90		89.61		4
FEF 25/75	L/s	2.37	1.18	50	1.23	52	5
PEF	L/s	4.43	3.10	70	3.66	83	18

▲ **Figure 19–4.** Flow volume loops from a child with scoliosis (restrictive pattern), which restricts vital capacity due to changes in the configuration of the thorax. Lung volume studies are needed to confirm restriction.

lavage (BAL) fluid; and gastric aspirates, specifically for *M tuberculosis*. Spontaneously expectorated sputum is the least invasive way to collect a sample for diagnostics, though it is rarely available from patients younger than 6 years. Sputum induction, performed by inhaling aerosolized hypertonic saline, is a relatively safe, noninvasive means of obtaining lower airway secretions. Sputum induction has been used in patients with CF and may be useful in patients with suspected *M tuberculosis*, *P jiroveci* pneumonia, or complicated community-acquired pneumonia (CAP). Tracheal aspirates can be obtained easily from patients with endotracheal or tracheostomy tubes. Culture of respiratory tract samples is the most commonly used approach to detect and identify airway pathogens. Molecular diagnostic tests, based on polymerase chain reaction (PCR) amplification and detection of nucleic acid from microbes, are often more rapid and sensitive, and may be used for detection of typical bacterial pathogens (eg, *Streptococcus pneumoniae*, methicillin-resistant *Staphylococcus aureus*), as well as detection of *M tuberculosis*, *P jiroveci*, and fastidious bacteria such as anaerobes. Blood and urine samples also may be used for serologic and antigen testing.

Table 19–2. Normal arterial blood gas values on room air.

	pH	Pao$_2$ (mm Hg)	Paco$_2$ (mm Hg)
Sea level	7.38–7.42	85–95	36–42
5000 ft	7.36–7.40	65–75	35–40

Paco$_2$, partial pressure of arterial carbon dioxide; Pao$_2$, partial pressure of arterial oxygen; Sao$_2$, percent hemoglobin saturation.

Hammitt LL et al: Specimen collection for the diagnosis of pediatric pneumonia. Clin Infect Dis 2012;54(S2):S132–S139 [PMID: 22403227].

Waterer GW: Diagnosing viral and atypical pathogens in the setting of community-acquired pneumonia. Clin Chest Med 2017;38:21–28 [PMID: 28159158].

Zumla A et al: Tuberculosis. N Engl J Med 2013;368(8):745–755 [PMID: 23425167].

IMAGING OF THE RESPIRATORY TRACT

The plain chest radiograph remains the foundation for investigating the pediatric thorax. Both frontal (posterior-anterior) and lateral views should be obtained if feasible. The radiograph is useful for evaluating chest wall abnormalities, heart size and shape, mediastinum, diaphragm, airways, and lung parenchyma. When pleural fluid is suspected, lateral decubitus radiographs may be helpful in determining the extent and mobility of the fluid. When a foreign body is suspected, forced expiratory radiographs may show focal air trapping and shift of the mediastinum to the contralateral side. Lateral neck radiographs can be useful in assessing the size of adenoids and tonsils and also in differentiating croup from epiglottitis, the latter being associated with the "thumbprint" sign.

Fluoroscopic studies including upper gastrointestinal (UGI) series, esophagram, or videofluoroscopic swallow studies (VFSS) are indicated for detection of swallowing dysfunction in patients with suspected aspiration, tracheo-esophageal fistula, vascular rings and slings, and achalasia. Fluoroscopy or ultrasound of the diaphragm can detect paralysis by demonstrating paradoxic movement of the involved hemidiaphragm.

Volumetric chest CT is recommended for evaluation of congenital lung lesions, pleural disease (eg, effusion or recurrent pneumothorax), complicated pneumonia, mediastinal disorders (eg, lymphadenopathy), interstitial lung disease (ILD) and bronchiectasis. The addition of contrast may be needed to evaluate masses and nodules and CT angiography to delineate vasculature. Magnetic resonance imaging (MRI) is also useful for defining vascular or bronchial anatomical abnormalities. Concerns about radiation exposure in children led to the *Image Gently* campaign, an initiative of The Alliance for Radiation Safety in Pediatric Imaging, dedicated to increasing awareness of the need for radiation protection for children. Identified challenges include the need for continued education particularly at adult-focused hospitals, increased emphasis on appropriateness of pediatric imaging and research to validate CT outcomes, and establishing ranges of optimal CT technique when imaging children.

Don S et al: Image gently campaign back to basics initiative: ten steps to help manage radiation dose in pediatric digital radiography. AJR Am J Roentgenol 2013;200(5):W431–W436 [PMID: 23617510].
Image Gently Campaign website: http://www.imagegently.org/.
Schneebaum et al: Use and yield of chest computed tomography in the diagnostic evaluation of pediatric lung disease. Pediatrics 2009;124:472–479 [PMID: 19620200].

LARYNGOSCOPY & BRONCHOSCOPY

Direct visualization of the airways may be necessary for diagnosis despite an extensive history and physical and sophisticated imaging. This can be achieved with rigid or flexible instrumentation. Indications for laryngoscopy include hoarseness, stridor, symptoms of obstructive sleep apnea (OSA), and laryngeal wheezing. Indications for bronchoscopy include wheezing, suspected foreign body, suspected tracheoesophageal fistula, recurrent pneumonia, persistent atelectasis, chronic cough, and hemoptysis. A flexible bronchoscope can also be used to assess placement and patency of an endotracheal tube. In general, the more specific the indication, the higher the diagnostic yield. Rigid and flexible bronchoscopes have individual advantages, and for some patients, both should be employed sequentially under the same anesthesia.

The rigid, open tube instruments have the best optics and allow surgical intervention to be easily achieved, such as removal of a foreign body. Flexible laryngoscopes and bronchoscopes are of a smaller caliber, and therefore do not stent the airway open during the procedure. Dynamic airway collapse is better evaluated by flexible bronchoscopy, and more distal airways can be evaluated better with the flexible scope than with the rigid scope. In fiberoptic endoscopic evaluation of swallowing (FEES), a laryngoscope is used to visualize the larynx while the patient swallows liquids or food that has been dyed blue or green. BAL is useful to sample the alveolar space for infection, inflammation, or hemorrhage. Although removal of foreign bodies has been achieved with the flexible bronchoscope in larger children, the standard of care in most institutions is to remove foreign bodies via the rigid bronchoscope. Rigid bronchoscopy is done with general anesthesia. Flexible laryngoscopy may be performed awake. Flexible bronchoscopy is typically performed in children with general anesthesia, although can be performed with less sedation, especially through a tracheostomy tube.

Transbronchial biopsy in children is limited to evaluation of infection and rejection in lung transplant patients. There is low diagnostic yield in most other conditions. Transbronchial biopsy may have a role in sarcoidosis. Video-assisted thoracoscopic lung surgery (VATS) provides a more substantial specimen for pathologic assessment.

Giraldo-Cadavid LF et al: Accuracy of endoscopic and videofluoroscopic evaluations of swallowing for oropharyngeal dysphagia. Laryngoscope 2017 Sep; 127(9):2002–2010 [PMID: 27859291].
Nicholai T: The role of rigid and flexible bronchoscopy in children. Paediatr Respir Rev 2011;12:190–195 [PMID: 21722848].

▼ GENERAL THERAPY FOR PEDIATRIC LUNG DISEASES

OXYGEN THERAPY

Oxygenation can be measured by the arterial oxygen tension or pulse oximetry (SpO_2). The advantages of the latter noninvasive method include obtaining continuous measurements during normal activities and avoiding artifacts caused by crying or breath-holding during arterial or venous puncture. For children with cardiopulmonary disorders that require chronic supplemental oxygen therapy (eg, BPD or CF), frequent noninvasive assessments are essential to ensure the safety and adequacy of oxygenation.

Supplemental oxygen (O_2) therapy is used to relieve hypoxemia, and the benefits may include reducing the work of breathing, reducing respiratory symptoms, relaxing the pulmonary vasculature, and improving feeding tolerance. Patients breathing spontaneously can receive supplemental O_2 via nasal cannula, head hood, or mask (including simple, rebreathing, nonrebreathing, or Venturi masks). The goal of O_2 therapy is to achieve an arterial oxygen tension of 65–90 mm Hg or SpO_2 above 90%. Lower PaO_2 or SpO_2 levels may be acceptable in certain situations, particularly cyanotic congenital heart disease. The actual O_2 concentration achieved by nasal cannula or mask depends on the flow rate, the type of mask used, and the patient's age. Small changes in flow rate during O_2 administration by nasal cannula can lead to substantial changes in inspired oxygen concentration in young infants. The amount of oxygen required to correct hypoxemia may vary with activity; for example, an infant with chronic lung disease who uses 0.25 L/min while awake may need 0.5 L/min while asleep or feeding.

Head hood O_2 delivery is not often used if the patient can use a nasal cannula, which allows more mobility. Even at high flow rates, O_2 by nasal cannula rarely delivers inspired oxygen concentrations greater than 40%–45%. In contrast, partial rebreathing and nonrebreathing masks or head hoods can achieve inspired oxygen concentrations as high as 90%–100%. Heated humidified high-flow nasal cannula delivery allows a much higher high flow rate and is used with increasing frequency when standard low flow supplemental O_2 is not meeting SpO_2 goals.

Fedor KL: Noninvasive respiratory support in infants and children. Resp Care 2017;62(6):699–717. doi: 10.4187/respcare.05244 [PMID: 28546373].

Franklin S et al: A randomized trial of high-flow oxygen therapy in infants with bronchiolitis. N Engl J Med 2018;378:1121–1131 [PMID: 29562151].

Levy SD et al: High-flow oxygen therapy and other inhaled therapies in intensive care units. Lancet 2016;387:1867–1878 [PMID: 27203510].

INHALATION OF MEDICATIONS

Inhalation of medications is a mainstay of therapy for pediatric respiratory conditions and are routinely used CF, BPD, and asthma, as well as in acute illnesses such as infectious laryngotracheobronchitis and bronchiolitis (Table 19–3). Short-acting β-agonists and anticholinergics provide acute bronchodilitation (relievers), whereas inhaled corticosteroids and cromones provide anti-inflammatory effects (controllers). Nebulized antibiotics have documented benefit in CF and nebulized mucolytic medications (eg, rhDNAse and hypertonic saline) are used in CF and other conditions with impaired secretion control such as non-CF bronchiectasis.

The medications can be delivered by pressurized metered dose inhaler (pMDI), dry powder inhaler (DPI), or compressed air-driven wet nebulization. Careful attention to delivery technique is critical to optimize medication delivery to the airways. A valved holding chamber or similar spacer should be used with pMDI use, and this technique has been shown to be effective in infants as young as 4 months of age. A face-mask interface is recommended for both pMDI and wet nebulization in infants and toddlers; a simple mouth piece suffices for older children who can form a seal around the mouthpiece. Delivery technique should be assessed and reviewed at each clinical visit.

Table 19–3. Common uses for inhaled medications in pediatric respiratory illness.

Disease Process	Short-Acting Bronchodilator	Anticholinergic Bronchodilator	Inhaled Steroid	Other
Asthma	Acute relief and prior to exercise to prevent exercise induced bronchospasm	Acute relief	Chronic use for control of inflammation	Inhaled corticosteroid + long-acting bronchodilator for control
Bronchopulmonary dysplasia	Acute relief	Acute relief	Chronic use for control of inflammation if bronchial reactivity is present	
Cystic fibrosis	Prior to airway clearance	Limited data	Chronic use for control of inflammation if bronchial reactivity is present	Mucolytics and inhaled antibiotics
Infectious laryngotracheo-bronchitis (croup)	Acute relief (racemic epinephrine)		Acute relief (nebulized steroid)	
Bronchiolitis (acute infectious)	Acute relief. May have limited benefit.		Ongoing investigation of inhaled epinephrine and hypertonic saline	Recent interest in inhaled epinephrine and hypertonic saline

Restreppo MI, Keyt H, Reyes LF: Aerosolized antibiotics. Respir Care 2015;60:762–773 [PMID: 26070573].

Rottier BL, Rubin BK: Asthma medication delivery: mists and myths. Paediatr Respir Rev 2013;14:112–118 [PMID: 23522986].

AIRWAY CLEARANCE THERAPY

Airway clearance is the mobilization and expulsion of airway secretions or debris. Innate airway clearance comprises mucociliary clearance and cough. Airway clearance therapies intend to reproduce or augment these functions. Currently available airway clearance techniques include: manual percussion or chest physiotherapy, postural drainage, forced expiratory technique (huff cough), autogenic drainage, positive expiratory pressure with handheld devices, intermittent positive pressure breathing, high-frequency chest wall oscillation or compression, intrapulmonary percussive ventilation, and manual or mechanical insufflation-exsufflation. All the above except insufflation-exsufflation techniques have been used in CF, bronchiectasis, and tracheobronchomalacia due to impaired mucociliary function. Often, therapies are combined (eg, high-frequency chest wall compression plus huff cough) to maximize the effect. Insufflation-exsufflation (commonly called cough assist) is used when cough force is weakened as in neuromuscular diseases, neurologic injury, or prolonged immobility. The decision about which technique to use should be based on the patient's underlying airway clearance impairment, age, preference, and ability to participate. Bronchodilators or mucolytic medications may be given prior to or during airway clearance therapy. If prescribed, inhaled corticosteroids and inhaled antibiotics should be given after airway clearance therapy so that the airways are first cleared of secretions, allowing the medications to maximally penetrate the lung. Airway clearance has not been shown to be beneficial for patients with acute respiratory illnesses such as pneumonia, bronchiolitis, and asthma. Contraindications to airway clearance therapy include retained foreign body, hemoptysis, untreated pneumothorax, chest trauma, recent airway or open chest surgery, and concerns for increased intracranial pressure. Daily exercise is an important adjunctive therapy for airway clearance and overall lung health.

Kravitz RM: Airway clearance in Duchenne muscular dystrophy. Pediatrics 2009;123:S231–S235 [PMID: 19420150].

McIlwaine M et al: Personalizing airway clearance in chronic lung disease. Eur Respir Rev 2017;26:143 [PMID: 28223396].

AVOIDANCE OF ENVIRONMENTAL HAZARDS

Environmental insults can aggravate existing lung diseases, impair pulmonary function, and cause lung disease in children. Outdoor air pollution (ozone and particulates), indoor pollution, diesel exhaust, and household fungi are examples. Environmental tobacco smoke dramatically increases childhood pulmonary morbidity. The impact of other tobacco products such as e-cigarettes and marijuana smoke is unclear but being studied. Smoking family members should be counseled to quit smoking and do everything possible to minimize environmental smoke exposure to the people around them. Homes with mold should have remediation, particularly if children with lung disease are in residence. Ozone exposure can be limited by avoiding outdoor activities during the height of daily ozone levels. Recent data show that improvements in air quality reduce lung function impairments in children.

Pet exposure and infestations such as cockroaches or mice may be a significant trigger in children who have asthma and allergies to the pets or pests. Despite the known risk, many families are reluctant to eliminate the risk of exposure to the pet and smoke exposure of any kind. Limiting exposure to outdoor pollutants may be impossible for many families and children.

Breysse PN et al: Indoor air pollution and asthma in children. Proce Am Thorac Soc 2010;7:102–106 [PMID: 20427579].

Guarnieri M, Balmes JR: Outdoor air pollution and asthma. Lancet 2014;383:1581–1592 [PMID: 24792855].

State of the Air Report 2017: Report by the American Lung Association: http://www.stateoftheair.org/. Accessed June 19, 2019.

DISORDERS OF THE CONDUCTING AIRWAYS

The conducting airways include the nose, mouth, pharynx, larynx, trachea, bronchi, and terminal bronchioles. These airways direct inspired air to the gas-exchange units of the lung but do not participate in gas exchange. Airflow obstruction in the conducting airways can occur at extrathoracic sites (eg, above the thoracic inlet) or at intrathoracic sites (eg, below the thoracic inlet). Extrathoracic or upper airway obstruction disrupts the inspiratory phase of respiration and is often manifest by stridor or "noisy breathing." Intrathoracic obstruction disrupts the expiratory phase of respiration and is often manifest by wheezing and prolongation of the expiratory phase. After assessing whether the obstruction is extrathoracic or intrathoracic the next challenge is to determine if the obstruction is fixed or variable. Fixed obstructions disrupt each breath and the abnormal sounds are consistently heard. Fixed obstructions can be intrinsic to the airway or due to airway compression (extrinsic). They are often associated with anatomic abnormalities that may be amenable to surgical correction (Table 19–4).

Variable obstruction leads to abnormal sounds with breathing that are softer or absent with normal quiet breathing and may sound different with every breath. Variable obstructions are often due to dynamic changes in airway caliber that occurs with laryngomalacia, tracheomalacia, or bronchomalacia. The onset and progression of the

Table 19–4. Classification and causes of upper airway obstruction.

Fixed, Extrathoracic, Not Acute	Fixed, Extrathoracic, Acute	Fixed Intrathoracic, Intrinsic	Fixed, Intrathoracic, Extrinsic
Vocal cord paralysis	Infectious laryngotracheobronchitis	Tracheal stenosis	Tumor (compressing the airways)
Laryngeal atresia/web	Epiglottitis	Complete tracheal rings	Vascular ring or sling
Laryngocele/cyst	Bacterial tracheitis	Foreign body aspiration	Bronchogenic cyst
Laryngeal papillomas	Anaphylaxis	Endobronchial tumor	Congenital pulmonary airway malformation
Subglottic hemangioma	Angioneurotic edema		Esophageal duplication
Tracheal web	Foreign body aspiration		Congenital lobar overdistention

obstruction can provide important clues as to the etiology and help determine the urgency of evaluation and management. Obstructions due to dynamic airway collapse often improve with age, whereas fixed obstructions typically progress or fail to improve with age. Acute-onset extrathoracic obstruction is often infectious. Clinical indications that the obstruction is severe include high-pitched stridor or wheezing, biphasic stridor, drooling or dysphagia, poor-intensity breath sounds, severe retractions, and poor color or cyanosis.

Helpful diagnostic studies in the evaluation of extrathoracic obstruction include chest and lateral neck radiographs and bronchoscopy. Patients who have symptoms of severe chronic obstruction should have an electrocardiogram and/or ECHO to evaluate for right ventricular hypertrophy and pulmonary hypertension. Patients suspected to have OSA should have a PSG (see section Sleep-Disordered Breathing). Diagnostic studies for intrathoracic obstruction may include chest radiographs, CT, sweat test, PFTs, and bronchoscopy. In older children, PFTs can differentiate fixed from variable airflow obstruction and may identify the site of obstruction. Other diagnostic studies are dictated by the history and physical findings. If asthma is suspected, a trial of bronchodilators and/or anti-inflammatories should be considered. Treatment should be directed at relieving airway obstruction and correcting the underlying condition if possible.

LARYNGOMALACIA & CONGENITAL DISORDERS OF THE EXTRATHORACIC AIRWAY

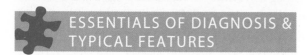

ESSENTIALS OF DIAGNOSIS & TYPICAL FEATURES

▶ Presentation from birth or within the first few weeks of life.

▶ Intermittent, high-pitched, inspiratory stridor.

▶ Moderate to severe symptoms require visualization of the airway.

LARYNGOMALACIA

Laryngomalacia is a congenital disorder in which the cartilaginous support for the supraglottic structures is underdeveloped. It is the most common cause of variable extrathoracic airway obstruction and manifests as **intermittent stridor** in infants, usually within the first 6 weeks of life. Stridor is generally worse in the supine position, with increased activity, with upper respiratory infections, and during feeding. The diagnosis is established by laryngoscopy, which shows inspiratory collapse of an omega-shaped epiglottis (with or without long, redundant arytenoids). Typically the condition is benign and resolves by the time the child is 2 years old, but occasionally signs can be more severe or persist beyond 2 years of age. In mildly affected patients with no stridor at rest and no retractions, treatment is not usually needed. Surgical epiglottoplasty may be recommended in patients with either severe symptoms of airway obstruction such as stridor with each breath, retractions, OSA, and increased work of breathing or more chronic signs such as feeding difficulties or failure to thrive.

Thompson DM et al: Laryngomalacia: factors that influence disease severity and outcomes of management. Curr Opin Otolaryngol Head Neck Surg 2010;18(6):564 [PMID: 20962644].

Thorne MC, Garetz SL: Laryngomalacia: review and summary of current clinical practice in 2015. Paediatr Respir Rev 2016; 17:3–8 [PMID: 25802018].

OTHER CAUSES OF CONGENITAL EXTRATHORACIC OBSTRUCTION

Other congenital lesions of the larynx such as laryngeal atresia, laryngeal web, laryngocele and cyst of the larynx, subglottic hemangioma, laryngeal cleft, and subglottic stenosis usually present as fixed extrathoracic obstruction and are best evaluated by direct laryngoscopy.

• Laryngeal atresia, also known as complete high airway obstruction syndrome (CHAOS), presents at birth with severe respiratory distress and is often fatal or requires a fetal EXIT procedure (ex utero intrapartum treatment) with immediate tracheostomy.

- Laryngeal web, representing fusion of the anterior portion of the true vocal cords, is associated with hoarseness, aphonia, and stridor at birth and severe cases require immediate intervention.

- Laryngeal cysts and laryngocoeles present with stridor and significant airway obstruction. Laryngeal cysts are superficial and are generally fluid filled. Laryngocoeles communicate with the interior of the larynx and may be either air- or fluid-filled. Both require surgery or laser therapy.

- Subglottic hemangiomas are a rare cause of upper airway obstruction in infants and are associated with cutaneous vascular lesions of the skin in 50%–60% of patients. Although vascular malformations regress spontaneously, airway obstruction requires intervention. Medical management options include propranolol, systemic steroids, or intralesional steroids. Surgical intervention with laser ablation is usually successful. Tracheostomy is rarely required.

- Laryngeal cleft is an uncommon condition resulting from failure of posterior cricoid fusion. Patients present with dysphagia or silent aspiration. A type 1 laryngeal cleft (at the level of the vocal cords) may not show aspiration on a VFSS while more severe types 2 and 3 laryngeal clefts almost always do. All types of clefts may result in recurrent or chronic pneumonia and failure to thrive. The diagnosis is made by rigid laryngoscopy/bronchoscopy with attention to spreading the posterior glottic structures apart and assessing for the absence of tissue above the vocal folds. The decision to correct type 1 clefts should be made after multidisciplinary consideration of the pulmonary complications and other comorbidities. Repair of type 1 clefts may be addressed surgically or with an injection laryngoplasty. More severe clefts require surgical repair and may require tracheostomy. Normal swallow function without aspiration may not return for months, even after repair.

- Subglottic stenosis can be congenital or acquired (see acquired disorders of the extrathoracic airway).

Ahmad SM, Soliman AM: Congenital anomalies of the larynx. Otolaryngol Clin North Am 2007;40(1):177–191 [PMID: 17346567].
Huoh KC, Rosbe KW: Infantile hemangiomas of the head and neck. Pediatr Clin North Am 2013;60(4):937–949 [PMID: 23905829].

▼ ACQUIRED DISORDERS OF THE EXTRATHORACIC AIRWAY

Acquired disorders of the extrathoracic airway can present acutely or with recurrent symptoms of upper airway obstruction. Children with acquired disorders of the extrathoracic airway present with inspiratory sounds consistent with stridor. The pitch of the sound varies depending on the diagnosis. Upper airway obstruction can progress quickly and may be life threatening, requiring close observation. The differential for acquired disorders includes aspiration, infection, and injury or trauma leading to vocal cord paralysis or subglottic stenosis.

FOREIGN-BODY ASPIRATION IN THE EXTRATHORACIC AIRWAY

ESSENTIALS OF DIAGNOSIS & TYPICAL FEATURES

▶ Sudden onset of coughing or respiratory distress.
▶ History of choking.
▶ Difficulty vocalizing.

Aspiration of a foreign body into the respiratory tract is a significant cause of accidental death each year. The foreign body can lodge anywhere along the respiratory tract. Foreign bodies that lodge in the esophagus may compress the airway and cause respiratory distress. More typically, the foreign body lodges in the supraglottic airway, triggering protective reflexes that result in laryngospasm. Small objects such as coins may pass through the glottis and obstruct the trachea. Objects that pass into the lower airway cause coughing and more variable respiratory distress (see section Acquired Causes of Intrathoracic Airway Obstruction).

Foreign-body aspiration is commonly seen with small, round foods such as nuts and seeds, berries, corn/popcorn, hot dogs, and beans. Children 6 months to 3 years are at the highest risk. Homes and child care centers in which an older sibling or child feeds age-inappropriate foods (eg, peanuts, hard candy, or carrot slices) to the younger child are typical in the history. Without treatment, progressive cyanosis, loss of consciousness, seizures, bradycardia, and cardiopulmonary arrest can follow.

▶ Clinical Findings

Signs at the time of aspiration can include coughing, choking, or wheezing. Onset is generally abrupt, with a history of the child running with food in the mouth or playing with seeds, small coins, or toys.

The diagnosis is established by acute onset of choking along with *inability* to vocalize or cough and cyanosis with marked distress (complete obstruction), or with drooling, stridor, and *ability* to vocalize (partial obstruction). Chest x-rays and other imaging studies have been used to evaluate for foreign-body ingestion; however, rigid bronchoscopy is the gold standard for diagnosis.

▶ Treatment

Prevention is paramount. Pediatricians should counsel caregivers regarding age-specific safe foods. Small toys and latex balloons should have age-appropriate choking warnings on their labels. In the event of acute upper airway obstruction due to foreign-body aspiration, emergency treatment depends on the amount of obstruction. If partial obstruction is present, the choking subject should be allowed to use his or her own cough reflex to remove the foreign body. If the obstruction increases or the airway is *completely obstructed*, acute intervention is required and Red Cross recommendations for choking in a child should be followed. https://www.redcross.org/take-a-class/first-aid/performing-first-aid/child-baby-first-aid.

Blind finger sweeps *should not* be performed in infants or children because the finger may push the foreign body further into the airway. The airway should be opened by jaw thrust, and if the foreign body can be directly visualized, careful removal with the fingers or instruments should be attempted. Patients with persistent apnea and inability to achieve adequate ventilation may require emergency intubation, tracheotomy, or needle cricothyrotomy, depending on the setting and the rescuer's skills. If the child of any age becomes unresponsive, cardiopulmonary resuscitation (CPR) is recommended. Chest compressions may help to dislodge the foreign body. If the foreign body moves into the lower airway, foreign-body removal is most successfully performed using rigid bronchoscope under general anesthesia.

Green SS: Ingested and aspirated foreign bodies. Pediatr Rev 2015;6(10):430–436 [PMID: 26330203].
https://www.redcross.org/take-a-class/first-aid/performing-first-aid/child-baby-first-aid.

CROUP SYNDROMES

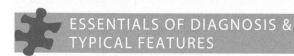

ESSENTIALS OF DIAGNOSIS & TYPICAL FEATURES

▶ New-onset stridor in the setting of an upper respiratory illness or fever.

Croup describes acute inflammatory diseases of the larynx, including viral croup (laryngotracheobronchitis), epiglottitis (supraglottitis), and bacterial tracheitis. These are the main entities in the differential diagnosis for patients presenting with acute stridor, although spasmodic croup, angioedema, laryngeal or esophageal foreign body, and retropharyngeal or peritonsillar abscess should be considered as well.

1. Viral croup

Viral croup generally affects young children 6 months to 5 years of age in the fall and early winter and is most often caused by *parainfluenza virus* serotypes. However, many other viral organisms as well as *M pneumoniae* can cause croup. Edema in the subglottic space accounts for the predominant signs of upper airway obstruction although inflammation of the entire airway is often present.

▶ Clinical Findings

A. Symptoms and Signs

Usually, a prodrome of upper respiratory tract symptoms is followed by a barking cough and stridor. Fever is usually absent. Patients with mild disease may have stridor when agitated. As obstruction worsens, stridor occurs at rest, accompanied in severe cases by retractions, air hunger, and cyanosis. On examination, the presence of cough and the absence of drooling favor the diagnosis of viral croup over epiglottitis.

B. Imaging

Anteroposterior and lateral neck radiographs are not routinely indicated for patients with classic presentation of croup. For atypical presentation, x-ray shows subglottic narrowing (the steeple sign) without the irregularities seen in tracheitis and a normal epiglottis. A severely ill patient should never be left unattended in the imaging suite.

▶ Treatment

Treatment of viral croup is based on the symptoms. Mild croup, signified by a barking cough and no stridor at rest, requires supportive therapy with oral hydration and minimal handling. Mist therapy has historically been used, but clinical studies do not demonstrate effectiveness. Conversely, patients with stridor at rest require active intervention. Oxygen should be administered to patients with oxygen desaturation. Nebulized racemic epinephrine (0.5 mL of 2.25% solution diluted in sterile saline) is commonly used because it has a rapid onset of action within 10–30 minutes. Both racemic epinephrine and epinephrine hydrochloride (L-epinephrine, an isomer) are effective in alleviating symptoms and decreasing the need for intubation.

The efficacy of glucocorticoids in croup is firmly established. Dexamethasone, 0.6 mg/kg intramuscularly as one dose, improves symptoms, reduces the duration of hospitalizations and frequency of intubations, and permits earlier discharge from the emergency department. Oral dexamethasone (0.15 mg/kg) may be equally effective for mild to moderate croup. Dexamethasone has been shown to be more effective than prednisolone in equivalent doses, but inhaled budesonide (2–4 mg) can improve symptoms and decrease hospital stay and may be as effective as dexamethasone. The use of heliox, a mixture of helium and oxygen, improves turbulent airflow but is not superior to nebulized medication. Its use is limited in hypoxic children because of its low fractional concentration of inspired oxygen.

If symptoms resolve within 3–4 hours of glucocorticoids and nebulized epinephrine, patients can safely be discharged without fear of a sudden rebound in symptoms. If, however, recurrent nebulized epinephrine treatments are required or if respiratory distress persists, patients require hospitalization for close observation, supportive care, and nebulization treatments as needed. In patients with impending respiratory failure, an airway must be established. Intubation with an endotracheal tube of slightly smaller diameter than would ordinarily be used is reasonably safe. Extubation should be accomplished within 2–3 days to minimize the risk of laryngeal injury. Other underlying causes should be considered in hospitalized patients with persistent symptoms over 3–4 days despite treatment.

Prognosis

Most children with viral croup have an uneventful course and improve within a few days. Some evidence suggests that patients with a history of croup associated with wheezing may have airway hyperreactivity. It is not always clear if the hyperreactivity was present prior to the croup episode or if the viral infection causing croup altered airway function.

Petrocheilou A et al: Viral croup: diagnosis and a treatment algorithm. Ped Pulm 2014;49(5):421 [PMID: 24596395].
Tyler A et al: Variation in inpatient croup management and outcomes. Pediatrics 2017;139(4):e20163582. doi: 10.1542/peds.2016-3582.

2. Epiglottitis

With the introduction of the *Haemophilus influenzae* conjugate vaccine, the incidence of epiglottitis is rare in countries with immunization programs. If disease occurs, it is likely to be associated with *H influenzae* in unimmunized children, or another organism such as nontypeable *H influenzae*, *Neisseria meningitidis*, or *Streptococcus* species in immunized populations.

Clinical Findings

A. Symptoms and Signs

The classic presentation is a sudden onset of high fever, dysphagia, drooling, muffled voice, inspiratory retractions, cyanosis, and soft stridor. Patients often sit in the so-called sniffing dog position, with the neck hyperextended and the chin stretched forward, which gives them the best airway possible under the circumstances. Progression to total airway obstruction may occur and result in respiratory arrest. The definitive diagnosis is made by direct inspection of the epiglottis, a procedure that should be done by an experienced airway specialist under controlled conditions (typically in the operating room during intubation). The typical findings are a cherry-red and swollen epiglottis and swollen arytenoids.

B. Imaging

Diagnostically, lateral neck radiographs may be helpful in demonstrating a classic "thumbprint" sign caused by the swollen epiglottis. Obtaining radiographs, however, may delay important airway intervention.

Treatment

Once the diagnosis of epiglottitis is made, endotracheal intubation must be performed immediately in children but not necessarily in adults. Most anesthesiologists prefer general anesthesia (but not muscle relaxants) to facilitate intubation. After an airway is established, cultures of the blood and epiglottis should be obtained, and the patient should be started on appropriate intravenous antibiotics to cover *H influenzae* and *Streptococcus* species (ceftriaxone sodium or an equivalent cephalosporin). Extubation can usually be accomplished in 24–48 hours, when direct inspection shows a significant reduction in the size of the epiglottis. Intravenous antibiotics should be continued for 2–3 days, followed by oral antibiotics to complete a 10-day course.

Prognosis

Prompt recognition and appropriate treatment usually results in rapid resolution of swelling and inflammation. Recurrence is unusual.

Guardiani E et al: Supraglottitis in the era following widespread immunization against *Haemophilus influenzae* type B: evolving principles in diagnosis and management. Laryngoscope 2010;120(11):2183 [PMID: 20925091].
Tibballs J et al: Symptoms and signs differentiating croup and epiglottitis. J Paediatr Child Health 2011;47(3):77 [PMID: 21091577].

3. Bacterial Tracheitis

Bacterial tracheitis (pseudomembranous croup) is a severe life-threatening form of laryngotracheobronchitis. As the management of severe viral croup has been improved with the use of dexamethasone, and vaccination has decreased the incidence of epiglottitis, tracheitis is relatively more common as a cause of a pediatric airway emergency requiring admission to the pediatric intensive care unit. This diagnosis must be high in the differential when a patient presents with severe upper airway obstruction and fever. The organism most often isolated is *S aureus*, but organisms such as *H influenzae*, group A *Streptococcus pyogenes*, *Neisseria* species, *Moraxella catarrhalis*, and others have been reported. A viral prodrome is common. Viral coinfections are described and influenza should be treated. The disease probably represents localized mucosal invasion of bacteria in patients with primary viral croup, resulting in inflammatory edema, purulent secretions, and pseudomembranes. Although cultures of the tracheal secretions are frequently positive, blood cultures are almost always negative.

Clinical Findings

A. Symptoms and Signs

The early clinical picture is similar to that of viral croup. However, instead of gradual improvement, patients develop higher fever, toxicity, and progressive or intermittent severe upper airway obstruction that is unresponsive to standard croup therapy. The incidence of sudden respiratory arrest or progressive respiratory failure is high, requiring airway intervention. Findings of toxic shock and the acute respiratory distress syndrome may also be seen. Aggressive medical treatment and debridement is indicated.

B. Laboratory Findings and Imaging

The white cell count is usually elevated with a left shift. Cultures of tracheal secretions usually demonstrate one of the causative organisms. Lateral neck radiographs show a normal epiglottis but severe subglottic and tracheal narrowing. Irregularity of the contour of the proximal tracheal mucosa can frequently be seen radiographically and should elicit concern for tracheitis. Bronchoscopy showing a normal epiglottis and the presence of copious purulent tracheal secretions and membranes confirms the diagnosis.

▶ Treatment

Patients with suspected bacterial tracheitis may require direct visualization of the airway in a controlled environment and debridement of the airway. Most patients will be intubated because the incidence of respiratory arrest or progressive respiratory failure is high. Patients may also require further debridement, humidification, frequent suctioning, and intensive care monitoring to prevent endotracheal tube obstruction by purulent tracheal secretions. Intravenous antibiotics to cover *S aureus, H influenzae,* and the other organisms are indicated. Thick secretions persist for several days, usually resulting in longer periods of intubation for bacterial tracheitis than for epiglottitis or croup. Despite the severity of this illness, the reported mortality rate is very low if it is recognized and treated promptly.

Dawood FS et al: Complications and associated bacterial coinfections among children hospitalized with seasonal or pandemic influenza, United States, 2003–2010. J Infect Dis 2014;209(5):686 [PMID: 23986545].
Tebruegge M et al: Bacterial tracheitis: a multi-centre perspective. Scand J Infect Dis 2009;41(8):548–557 [PMID: 19401934].

VOCAL FOLD IMMOBILITY

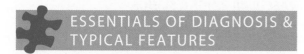

ESSENTIALS OF DIAGNOSIS & TYPICAL FEATURES

▶ Hoarseness or stridor.

▶ May present with difficulty swallowing.

Unilateral or bilateral vocal fold (cord) paresis and paralysis may be congenital, or more commonly may result from injury

to the recurrent laryngeal nerves. Patients may present with varying degrees of hoarseness, dysphagia, or high-pitched stridor. If partial function is preserved (paresis), the adductor muscles tend to move better than the abductors, with a resultant high-pitched inspiratory stridor and normal voice. Risk factors for acquired paresis/paralysis include difficult delivery (especially face presentation), neck and thoracic surgery (eg, ductal ligation or repair of tracheoesophageal fistula), trauma, mediastinal masses, and central nervous system disease (eg, Arnold-Chiari malformation). Unilateral cord paralysis is more likely to occur on the left because of the longer course of the left recurrent laryngeal nerve and its proximity to major thoracic structures. With bilateral cord paralysis, the closer to midline the cords are positioned, the greater the airway obstruction; the more lateral the cords are positioned, the greater the tendency to aspirate and experience hoarseness or aphonia.

Airway intervention (tracheostomy) is rarely indicated in unilateral paralysis but is often necessary for bilateral paralysis. Clinically, paralysis can be assessed by direct visualization of vocal fold function with laryngoscopy or more invasively by recording the electrical activity of the muscles (electromyography). Electromyogram recordings can differentiate vocal fold paralysis from arytenoid dislocation, which has prognostic value. Recovery is related to the severity of nerve injury and the potential for healing.

King EF, Blumin JH: Vocal cord paralysis in children. Curr Opin Otolaryngol Head Neck Surg 2009;17(6):483 [PMID: 19730263].

SUBGLOTTIC STENOSIS

ESSENTIALS OF DIAGNOSIS & TYPICAL FEATURES

▶ Chronic or recurrent stridor.

▶ History of airway trauma is common in acquired subglottic stenosis.

Subglottic stenosis may be congenital, or more commonly may result from endotracheal intubation. Neonates and infants are particularly vulnerable to subglottic injury from intubation. The subglottis is the narrowest part of an infant's airway, and the cricoid cartilage, which supports the subglottis, is the only cartilage that completely encircles the airway. This area is therefore susceptible to injury when an endotracheal tube is inserted. The clinical presentation may vary from asymptomatic to severe upper airway obstruction. Subglottic stenosis should be suspected in children who repeatedly fail extubation or children with multiple, prolonged, or severe episodes of croup. Diagnosis is made by direct visualization of the subglottic space with bronchoscopy and maneuvers to size the airway. Tracheostomy is often required when airway compromise is severe. Laryngotracheal reconstruction, in which a cartilage graft from another source (eg, rib) is used to expand the airway, has become the standard procedure for severe subglottic stenosis in children. In mild cases, balloon dilation of the subglottis is a less invasive alternative.

Jefferson ND, Cohen AP, Rutter MJ: Subglottic stenosis. Semin Pediatr Surg Jun 2016;25(3):138–143 [PMID: 27301599].

▼ CONGENITAL CAUSES OF INTRATHORACIC AIRWAY OBSTRUCTION

Congenital disorders of intrathoracic airway obstruction can present acutely or with recurrent symptoms of lower airway obstruction. Children with disorders of the intrathoracic airway often present with expiratory sounds such as wheeze, recurrent cough, and/or recurrent pneumonia due to retained secretions. The differential for intrathoracic airway obstruction includes airway malacia, extrinsic compression (eg, vascular ring), and congenital anomalies such as bronchogenic cysts.

MALACIA OF AIRWAYS

ESSENTIALS OF DIAGNOSIS & TYPICAL FEATURES

▶ Chronic monophonic wheeze with or without a barking cough.
▶ Respiratory symptoms do not respond to bronchodilators.

▶ Pathogenesis

Tracheomalacia or bronchomalacia exists when the cartilaginous framework of the airway is inadequate to maintain airway patency. Airway collapse is dynamic and can lead to partial or complete airway obstruction. Because infant airway cartilage is normally soft, infants have some degree of dynamic collapse of the central airway during the phases of respiration. Tracheomalacia and bronchomalacia can be congenital or acquired, although comorbidities associated with congenital tracheomalacia overlap with acquired causes. Congenital or innate abnormalities of the trachealis or tracheal cartilage are associated with developmental syndromes and other congenital abnormalities such as tracheoesophageal fistula and vascular ring. Congenital tracheomalacia may be localized or diffuse and may extend through to the remainder of the conducting airways (bronchomalacia). Acquired tracheomalacia has been associated with long-term ventilation of preterm infants due to delayed cartilaginous development with or without direct positive pressure. Other acquired causes include severe tracheobronchitis, surgical repair of airways anomalies such as tracheoesophageal fistula and complete tracheal rings, extrinsic airway compression due to tumors, abscess or cysts, and compression as seen in congenital heart disease with associated ventricular hypertrophy or vascular anomalies.

▶ Clinical Findings

Coarse and recurrent wheezing, cough, or stridor that do not respond to bronchodilators are common findings. Preterm infants with trachea or bronchomalacia may have hypoxemia that requires continuous nasal cannula or positive pressure ventilation. Symptoms classically present insidiously over the first few months of life and can increase with agitation, excitement, activity, or upper respiratory tract infections. Diagnosis can be made by bronchoscopy or combined inspiratory/expiratory imaging modalities like CT or MRI.

▶ Treatment

Observation is usually indicated for mild symptoms, which generally improve over time with growth. Coexisting lesions such as tracheoesophageal fistulas and vascular rings need primary repair. In severe cases of tracheomalacia, non-invasive or invasive ventilation may be necessary. Unfortunately, tracheostomy alone is seldom satisfactory because airway collapse continues to exist below the tip of the artificial airway. Surgical intervention (posterior tracheopexy, aortopexy, or stents) may be considered for the most challenging situations.

▶ Prognosis

The resolution of symptoms due to airway malacia depends on the severity and extent of the airway malacia and any underlying illness in the child. Children with mild malacia without other underlying lung disease or neuromuscular disease will most likely have at least partial resolution by the time they are 3–4 years old.

Fraga JC, Jennings RW, Kim PC: Pediatric trachomalacia. Semin Pediatr Surg 2016;25(3):156–164 [PMID: 27301602].
Goyal V, Masters IB, Chang AB: Interventions for primary (intrinsic) tracheomalacia in children. Cochrane Database Syst Rev 2012;CD005304 [PMID: 23076914].

VASCULAR RINGS & SLINGS

ESSENTIALS OF DIAGNOSIS & TYPICAL FEATURES

▶ Chronic barking cough, wheeze.
▶ A UGI fluoroscopy series showing esophageal compression is the mainstay of diagnosis.

The most common vascular anomaly to compress the trachea or esophagus is a vascular ring. A vascular ring can be formed by a double aortic arch or a right aortic arch with left ligamentum arteriosum or a patent ductus arteriosus. The pulmonary sling is created when the left pulmonary artery branches off the right pulmonary artery. Other common vascular anomalies include an anomalous innominate artery, a left carotid artery, and an aberrant right subclavian artery. All but the right subclavian artery can cause tracheal compression. The pulmonary sling may compress the trachea but can also compress the right upper lobe bronchus or the right mainstem takeoff. A pulmonary sling is associated with long segment tracheal stenosis 50% of the time.

▶ Clinical Findings

A. Symptoms and Signs

Symptoms of chronic airway obstruction (stridor, coarse wheezing, and croupy cough) are often worse in the supine position. Respiratory compromise is most severe with double aortic arch and may lead to apnea, respiratory arrest, or even death. Esophageal compression may result in feeding difficulties. UGI fluoroscopy series showing esophageal compression is the mainstay of diagnosis in all but anomalous innominate or carotid artery. Chest radiographs and echocardiograms may miss abnormalities. Anatomy can be further defined by angiography, chest CT with contrast, MRI or magnetic resonance angiography, or bronchoscopy.

▶ Treatment

Patients with significant symptoms require surgical correction, especially those with double aortic arch. Patients usually improve following correction but may have persistent but milder symptoms of airway obstruction due to associated tracheomalacia.

Backer CL et al: Vascular rings. Semin Pediatr Surg 2016; 25(3):165–175 [PMID: 27301603].

McLaren CA, Elliott MJ, Roebuck DJ: Vascular compression of the airway in children. Paediatr Respir Rev 2008;9(2):85–94 [PMID: 18513668].

BRONCHOGENIC CYSTS

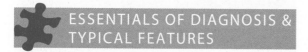

ESSENTIALS OF DIAGNOSIS & TYPICAL FEATURES

- ▶ Can present with symptoms of airway compression, infection, or chest pain.
- ▶ Chest radiograph may show a spherical lesion along the airway.

Bronchogenic cysts generally occur in the middle mediastinum (see section Mediastinal Masses) near the carina and adjacent to the major bronchi but can be found elsewhere in the lung. They range in size from 2 to 10 cm. Cyst walls are thin and may contain air, pus, mucus, or blood. Cysts develop from abnormal lung budding of the primitive foregut and can occur in conjunction with other congenital pulmonary malformations such as pulmonary sequestration or lobar emphysema.

▶ Clinical Findings

Bronchogenic cysts can present acutely with respiratory distress in early childhood due to airway compression or with symptoms of infection. Other patients present with chronic symptoms such as chest pain, chronic wheezing, cough, intermittent tachypnea, recurrent pneumonia, or recurrent stridor, depending on the location and size of the cysts and the degree of airway compression. Still other patients remain asymptomatic until adulthood. However, all asymptomatic cysts will eventually become symptomatic; chest pain is the most common presenting complaint. The physical examination is often normal.

A. Laboratory Findings and Imaging Studies

The choice of diagnostic studies for bronchogenic cysts is controversial. Chest radiographs can show air trapping and hyperinflation of the affected lobes or may show a spherical lesion with or without an air-fluid level. However, smaller lesions may not be seen on chest radiographs. CT scan is the preferred imaging study and can differentiate solid versus cystic mediastinal masses and define the cyst's relationship to the airways and the rest of the lung. Fluoroscopy can help determine whether the lesion communicates with the gastrointestinal tract. MRI and ultrasound are other imaging modalities used.

▶ Treatment

Treatment is surgical resection. Resection should be performed as soon as the cyst is detected to avoid future complications including infection. Postoperatively, vigorous pulmonary physiotherapy is required to prevent complications (atelectasis or infection of the lung distal to the site of resection of the cyst).

Chowdhury MM, Chakraboty S: Imaging of congenital lung malformations. Semin Pediatr Surg 2015;24(4):168–175 [PMID: 26051049].

Durell J, Lajhoo K: Congenital cystic lesions of the lung. Early Human Dev 2014;90(12):935–939 [PMID: 25448785].

ACQUIRED CAUSES OF INTRATHORACIC AIRWAY OBSTRUCTION

Acquired disorders of intrathoracic airway obstruction airway can present acutely or with recurrent symptoms of lower airway obstruction. Children with disorders of the intrathoracic airway often present with expiratory sounds such as wheeze, recurrent cough, and/or recurrent pneumonia due to retained secretions. The differential for intrathoracic airway obstruction includes foreign-body aspiration, infection, extrinsic compression not present at birth (eg, lymphadenopathy), and chronic lung diseases causing airway swelling such as disorders of mucociliary clearance, recurrent aspiration, and asthma.

FOREIGN-BODY ASPIRATION IN THE INTRATHORACIC AIRWAY

ESSENTIALS OF DIAGNOSIS & TYPICAL FEATURES

▶ Sudden onset of coughing, wheezing, or respiratory distress.

▶ History of choking.

▶ Asymmetrical physical findings of decreased breath sounds or localized wheezing.

▶ Asymmetrical radiographic findings, especially with forced expiratory view.

▶ Clinical Findings

A. Symptoms and Signs

Respiratory symptoms and signs vary depending on the site of obstruction and the duration following the acute episode. (See section Foreign-Body Aspiration in the Extrathoracic Airway.) The acute cough or wheezing caused by a foreign body in the lower respiratory tract may diminish over time only to recur later as chronic cough or persistent wheezing, monophonic wheezing, asymmetrical breath sounds on chest examination, or recurrent pneumonia in one location. Foreign-body aspiration should be suspected in children with chronic cough, persistent wheezing, or recurrent pneumonia. Asymmetrical breath sounds or localized wheezing also suggests a foreign body.

B. Laboratory Findings and Imaging Studies

Inspiratory and forced expiratory (obtained by manually compressing the abdomen during expiration) chest radiographs should be obtained if foreign-body aspiration is suspected. Chest radiographs may be normal up to 17% of the time. A positive forced expiratory study shows unilateral hyperinflation. There also may be a mediastinal shift away from the affected side. If obstruction of a distal airway is complete, atelectasis and related volume loss will be the major radiologic findings. Virtual bronchoscopy and CT are alternative approaches for detecting a foreign body.

C. Treatment

When a foreign body is highly suspected, a normal chest radiograph is not sufficient to rule out the possibility of an airway foreign body. If clinical suspicion persists based on two of three findings—history of possible aspiration, focal abnormal lung examination, or an abnormal chest radiograph—then a bronchoscopy is indicated. Rigid bronchoscopy under general anesthesia is recommended. Flexible bronchoscopy may be helpful for follow-up evaluations (after the foreign object has been removed).

Children with suspected acute foreign-body aspiration should be admitted to the hospital for evaluation and treatment. Chest postural drainage is no longer recommended because the foreign body may become dislodged and obstruct a major central airway. Bronchoscopy should not be delayed in children with respiratory distress but should be performed as soon as the diagnosis is made—even in children with more chronic symptoms. Following the removal of the foreign body, β-adrenergic nebulization treatments followed by chest physiotherapy are recommended to help clear related mucus or treat bronchospasm. Failure to identify a foreign body in the lower respiratory tract can result in bronchiectasis or lung abscess. This risk justifies an aggressive approach to suspected foreign bodies in suspicious cases.

Green SS: Ingested and aspirated foreign bodies. Pediatr Rev 2015;36(10):430–436 [PMID: 26430203].

▼ DISORDERS OF MUCOCILIARY CLEARANCE

Mucociliary clearance is the primary defense mechanism for the lung. Inhaled particles including microbial pathogens are also entrapped in mucus on the airway surface, then cleared by the coordinated action of cilia. The volume and composition of airway surface liquid influence the efficiency of ciliary function and mucus clearance. Mucus that cannot be cleared normally can obstruct the airways. If mucociliary clearance is not normal, bacteria that are not cleared can cause a vicious cycle of infection and inflammation and increased mucus production. The two main genetic diseases of mucociliary clearance involve disorders of ion transport (cystic fibrosis [CF]) and disorders in ciliary function (primary ciliary dyskinesia [PCD]).

CYSTIC FIBROSIS

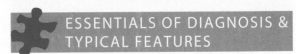

ESSENTIALS OF DIAGNOSIS & TYPICAL FEATURES

▶ Greasy, bulky, malodorous stools; failure to thrive.

▶ Recurrent respiratory infections.

▶ Digital clubbing.

► Bronchiectasis on chest imaging.

► Sweat chloride greater than 60 mmol/L.

Pathogenesis

Cystic fibrosis (CF), an autosomal recessive disease, results in a syndrome of chronic sinopulmonary infections, malabsorption, and nutritional abnormalities. It is one of the most common lethal genetic diseases in the United States, with an incidence of approximately 1:3000 among Caucasians and 1:9200 in the US Hispanic population. Although abnormalities occur in the hepatic, gastrointestinal, and male reproductive systems, lung disease is the major cause of morbidity and mortality. Most individuals with CF develop obstructive lung disease associated with chronic infection that leads to progressive loss of pulmonary function.

The cause of CF is a defect in a single gene on chromosome 7 that encodes an epithelial chloride channel called the CF transmembrane conductance regulator (CFTR) protein. The most common mutation is F508del, although approximately 1800 other disease-causing mutations been identified. Gene mutations lead to absence or defects in CFTR, altering salt and water movement across cell membranes, resulting in abnormally thick secretions in various organs and critically altering host defense in the lung.

Clinical Findings

A. Symptoms and Signs

All states in the United States and many other countries now perform newborn screening for CF by measuring immunoreactive trypsin (IRT), a pancreatic enzyme, in blood with or without concurrent DNA testing. Most infants with CF have elevated IRT in the newborn period, although false-negative results are possible. In newborns with positive newborn screen, the diagnosis of CF must be confirmed by sweat testing, mutation analysis, or both (http://www.cff.org/AboutCF/Testing/NewbornScreening/).

Approximately 15% of newborns with CF are born with meconium ileus, a severe intestinal obstruction resulting from inspissation of tenacious meconium in the terminal ileum. Meconium ileus is virtually diagnostic of CF, so the infant should be treated presumptively as having CF until a sweat test or genotyping can be obtained.

During infancy and beyond, a common presentation of CF is failure to thrive due to malabsorption from exocrine pancreatic insufficiency, failure of the pancreas to produce sufficient enzymes to digest fats and protein. Children with pancreatic insufficiency fail to gain weight despite good appetite and typically have frequent, bulky, foul-smelling, oily stools. Pancreatic insufficiency occurs in about 85% of persons with CF. (Chapter 22 describes gastrointestinal and hepatobiliary manifestations of CF; see also Table 22–12.)

Infants with undiagnosed CF may also present with hypoproteinemia, anemia, and deficiency of the fat-soluble vitamins A, D, E, and K, because of ongoing steatorrhea.

CF should also be considered in children who present with severe dehydration and hypochloremic alkalosis, bronchiectasis, nasal polyps, chronic sinusitis, rectal prolapse, or unexplained pancreatitis or cirrhosis. Respiratory symptoms can include productive cough, wheezing, recurrent pneumonia, progressive obstructive airways disease, exercise intolerance, dyspnea, or hemoptysis. Chronic airway infection with bacteria, including *Staphylococcus aureus* and *H influenzae*, often begins in the first few months of life, even in asymptomatic infants. Eventually, *Pseudomonas aeruginosa* and other gram-negative opportunistic bacteria become the predominant pathogens. Chronic infection leads to airflow obstruction and progressive airway and lung destruction resulting in bronchiectasis.

Episodic increases in respiratory symptoms are generically termed pulmonary exacerbations. Clinically, an exacerbation manifests by increased cough and sputum production, decreased exercise tolerance, malaise, and weight loss, and decrease in measures of lung function. Treatment for pulmonary exacerbations generally consists of antibiotics and augmented airway clearance.

B. Laboratory Findings and Imaging Studies

The diagnosis of CF is made by a sweat chloride concentration greater than 60 mmol/L following an abnormal newborn screen or when obtained for clinical signs or family history of CF. Sweat testing should be performed at a Cystic Fibrosis Foundation–accredited laboratory. A diagnosis can also be confirmed by genotyping that reveals two disease-causing CFTR mutations (www.cftr2.org).

Intermediate sweat chloride values of 30–60 may be associated with "mild" CFTR mutations that result in residual functioning CFTR protein. Patients with residual CFTR function typically have adequate pancreatic exocrine function, but may develop severe lung disease. CFTR-related metabolic syndrome, diagnosed based on elevated IRT on newborn screen but sweat test less than 60 mmol/L and up to two CFTR mutations, at least one of which is not considered disease-causing, appears to have an even milder disease phenotype. The natural history of this condition is still being defined.

Treatment

Individuals with CF should be followed at a Cystic Fibrosis Foundation–accredited CF care center (http://www.cff.org) in addition to a primary care provider. Care is provided by a multidisciplinary team that includes pulmonologists and advanced practice providers trained in CF care, nurses, respiratory therapists, dietitians, social workers, and psychologists. Recently a large study highlighted the importance of screening for depression and anxiety in patients with CF, as these are prevalent and negatively impact quality of life and adherence to treatment.

The cornerstone of gastrointestinal treatment is pancreatic enzyme supplementation combined with a high-calorie, high-protein, and high-fat diet. Persons with CF are required to take pancreatic enzyme immediately prior to each meal and with snacks and should also take daily multivitamins that contain vitamins A, D, E, and K. Caloric supplements are often added to the diet to optimize growth. Daily salt supplementation also is required to prevent hyponatremia, especially during hot weather.

Airway clearance therapy and aggressive antibiotic use form the mainstays of treatment for CF lung disease. Antibiotic therapy appears to be one of the primary reasons for the increased life expectancy of persons with CF. Respiratory treatments typically include recombinant human dornase alpha, inhaled hypertonic saline, and for those with chronic *Pseudomonas* infection, anti-pseudomonal antibiotics (tobramycin or aztreonam), and oral azithromycin. These therapies have been shown to maintain lung function and reduce the need for hospitalizations and intravenous antibiotics. Early detection of *P aeruginosa* and treatment with inhaled tobramycin can often eradicate the bacteria and delay chronic infection. Bronchodilators and anti-inflammatory therapies are also frequently used.

Recent development of protein-rescue therapies that directly target the underlying defects in CFTR (termed CFTR modulators) have made significant impacts on the lives of patients with CF. The first treatment that directly works to correct the function of the defective CF protein was approved in 2012, and currently there are three CFTR modulators that are FDA approved for people with certain CFTR mutations: ivacaftor, lumacaftor/ivacaftor, and tezacaftor/ivacaftor. These medications are currently available to about 50% of the CF population based on genotype. Addition of these modulators to treatment regimens significantly improves lung function and body mass index and reduces exacerbations. Recently, there have been promising results from clinical trials of "triple" combination CFTR modulators that would extend CFTR modulator access to approximately 90% of the CF population.

Prognosis

A few decades ago, CF was fatal in early childhood. Now the median life expectancy is 70 years of age. The rate of lung disease progression usually determines survival. Lung transplantation may be performed in those with end-stage lung disease. In addition, new treatments, including gene therapy and gene editing trials and improved CFTR modulators, are in development to improve life expectancy and quality of life.

Ramsey BW et al: A CFTR potentiator in patients with cystic fibrosis and the G551D mutation. N Engl J Med 2011;365(18): 1663–1672 [PMID: 22047557].

Rosenfeld M, Sontag MK, Ren CL: Cystic fibrosis diagnosis and newborn screening. Pediatr Clin North Am 2016;63(4):599–615 [PMID: 27469178].

Taylor-Cousar JL et al: Tezacaftor-Ivacaftor in patients with cystic fibrosis homozygous for Phe508del. N Engl J Med 2017 Nov 23;377(21):2013–2023 [PMID: 29099344].

PRIMARY CILIARY DYSKINESIA

ESSENTIALS OF DIAGNOSIS & TYPICAL FEATURES

▶ Unexplained neonatal respiratory distress in a term infant.

▶ Daily year-round cough and nasal congestion.

▶ Recurrent otitis media with effusions and conductive hearing loss.

▶ Situs inversus in approximately 50% of cases.

▶ Diagnosis confirmed by low nasal nitric oxide, presence of mutations in primary ciliary dyskinesia (PCD) genes, and/or a ciliary ultrastructure abnormality on electron microscopy (EM).

PCD is a rare, genetic disorder (usually inherited in an autosomal recessive fashion) of impaired mucociliary clearance leading to chronic otosinopulmonary disease. It is believed to occur in approximately 1 in 15,000 births. Approximately half of patients with PCD have situs abnormalities, and men are usually infertile. The triad of situs inversus totalis, bronchiectasis, and chronic sinusitis is known as Kartagener syndrome.

▶ Clinical Findings

A. Symptoms and Signs

Upper and lower respiratory tract manifestations are cardinal features of PCD. The majority of children with PCD present in the immediate newborn period with respiratory distress (commonly diagnosed as neonatal pneumonia or transient tachypnea of the newborn) and often require supplemental oxygen. Upper respiratory tract problems include chronic year-round nasal drainage that may begin in the first weeks of life, chronic sinusitis, nasal polyps, and chronic serous otitis media. Conductive hearing loss with chronic middle ear effusion is common. If myringotomy tubes are placed, chronic otorrhea often ensues. Lower respiratory tract features include chronic year-round productive cough, chronic and recurrent bronchitis, and recurrent pneumonia. They are at risk to develop obstructive lung disease and bronchiectasis. Situs inversus totalis occurs in approximately 50% of patients with PCD.

Nonrespiratory ciliopathies that have been associated with PCD include heterotaxy, with congenital heart disease, asplenia, polysplenia, autosomal dominant polycystic kidney disease, retinitis pigmentosa, and biliary atresia.

B. Laboratory Findings and Imaging Studies

The diagnosis of PCD currently requires a compatible clinical phenotype with at least two of four key clinical features: (1) unexplained neonatal respiratory distress in term infant, (2) year-round daily cough, (3) year-round daily nasal congestion, and (4) organ laterality defect. Additionally, identification of low nasal nitric oxide, biallelic pathogenic mutations in PCD-associated genes, and/or ultrastructural defects of the cilia by EM is also required. In patients with a compatible clinical history, nasal nitric oxide at a PCD specialty center is the preferable diagnostic test in cooperative children ages 5 and older. Extended genetic testing (> 12 genes) has emerged as the test of choice if nasal nitric oxide testing is not available. Cilia samples may be obtained from either the upper airways (nasal passage) or lower airways (trachea) for EM testing. Significant expertise is required to produce high-quality EM of cilia, and to distinguish primary (genetic) defects from secondary (acquired) defects in ciliary ultrastructure. Multiple different defects in EM include abnormalities in the outer dynein arms, inner dynein arms, radial spokes, and the central apparatus. Some patients with PCD can also have normal EM ultrastructure. Ciliary beat frequency and motion analysis analyzed via high speed videomicroscopy are also used for diagnosis in some settings.

▶ Treatment

At present, no specific therapies are available to correct the ciliary dysfunction in PCD. Treatment is not evidence-based and recommendations are largely extrapolated from CF and other suppurative lung diseases. Respiratory management includes routine pulmonary monitoring (lung function testing, respiratory cultures, chest imaging), airway clearance by combinations of physiotherapy and physical exercise, and aggressive treatment of upper and lower airways infections.

▶ Prognosis

The progression of lung disease in PCD is quite variable. Importantly, persons with PCD are at risk for chronic obstructive lung disease with bronchiectasis. With monitoring and aggressive treatment during times of illness, most individuals with PCD should experience a normal or near-normal life span.

Davis SD et al: Primary ciliary dyskinesia: longitudinal study of lung disease by ultrastructure defect and genotype. Am J Respir Crit Care Med 2019 Jan 15;199(2):190–198 [PMID: 30067075].
Shapiro AJ et al: Diagnosis of primary ciliary dyskinesia: an official American Thoracic Society clinical practice guideline. Am J Respir Crit Care Med 2018 Jun 15;197(12):e24–e39 [PMID: 29905515].

BRONCHIECTASIS

ESSENTIALS OF DIAGNOSIS & TYPICAL FEATURES

▶ Chronic cough with sputum production.

▶ Rhonchi or wheezes (or both) on chest auscultation.

▶ Diagnosis is confirmed by volumetric chest CT scan.

▶ Pathogenesis

Bronchiectasis is the permanent dilation of bronchi resulting from airway obstruction by retained mucus secretions or inflammation in response to chronic or repeated infection. It occurs either as a consequence of a preceding illness (severe pneumonia or foreign-body aspiration) or as a manifestation of an underlying systemic disorder leading to chronic airway inflammation and injury (CF, PCD, chronic aspiration, or immunodeficiency).

▶ Clinical Findings

A. Symptoms and Signs

Persons with bronchiectasis will typically have chronic cough, purulent sputum, fever, and weight loss. Recurrent respiratory infections and dyspnea on exertion are also common. Hemoptysis occurs less frequently in children than in adults with bronchiectasis. On physical examination, digital clubbing may be seen. Rales, rhonchi, and decreased air entry are often noted over the bronchiectatic areas.

B. Laboratory Findings and Imaging Studies

The most common bacteria detected in cultures from the lower respiratory tract include *Streptococcus pneumoniae*, *Staphylococcus aureus*, nontypeable *H influenzae*, and *Pseudomonas aeruginosa*. Nontuberculous mycobacterial species may also be detected in patients with bronchiectasis.

Chest radiographs may be mildly abnormal with slightly increased bronchovascular markings or areas of atelectasis, or they may demonstrate cystic changes in one or more areas of the lung. The extent of bronchiectasis is best defined by volumetric chest CT, which often reveals far wider involvement of lung than expected from the chest radiograph. Airflow obstruction and air trapping often is seen on pulmonary function testing. Evaluation of lung function after use of a bronchodilator is helpful in assessing the benefit from bronchodilators. Serial assessments of lung function help define the progression or resolution of the disease.

Differential Diagnosis

Bronchiectasis is the hallmark finding in patients with disorders of mucociliary; thus, CF and PCD must be considered in all children with bronchiectasis. Bronchiectasis has numerous other causes to consider. It can occur following severe respiratory tract infections by bacteria (eg, *Bordetella pertussis*), viruses (eg, adenovirus), or other atypical organisms (eg, mycobacteria). Bronchiectasis can also be due to persistent inflammation and is commonly seen in persons with recurrent aspiration pneumonia, CF, PCD, immunodeficiency, surfactant deficiencies, and collagen-vascular conditions. Other diagnostic considerations include foreign-body aspiration and allergic bronchopulmonary aspergillosis.

Treatment

Aggressive antibiotic therapy during pulmonary exacerbations and routine airway clearance are mainstays of treatment. Chronic antibiotic use, anti-inflammatory therapy, hyperosmolar agents (hypertonic saline), and bronchodilators have not proven effective in non-CF bronchiectasis, although individual patients may benefit. However, a large study in adults with idiopathic bronchiectasis concluded that those who received dornase alpha twice a day had more frequent exacerbations, hospitalizations, and lower lung function compared to placebo; thus, dornase alpha is not indicated in adult idiopathic bronchiectasis. Chronic azithromycin was recently shown to reduce exacerbations in adults with non-CF bronchiectasis. Whether these results translate to children with idiopathic bronchiectasis is not known.

Surgical removal of an area of lung affected with severe bronchiectasis is considered when the response to medical therapy is poor. Other indications for operation include severe localized disease, repeated hemoptysis, and recurrent pneumonia in one area. If bronchiectasis is widespread, surgical resection offers little advantage.

Prognosis

The prognosis depends on the underlying cause and severity of bronchiectasis, the extent of lung involvement, and the response to medical management. Good pulmonary hygiene and avoidance of infectious complications in the involved areas of lung may reverse cylindrical bronchiectasis.

Goyal V et al: Pediatric bronchiectasis: no longer an orphan disease. Pediatr Pulmonol 2016;51(5):450–469 [PMID: 26840008].

Wong C et al: Azithromycin for prevention of exacerbations in non-cystic fibrosis bronchiectasis (EMBRACE): a randomised, double-blind, placebo-controlled trial. Lancet 2012 Aug 18;380(9842):660–667 [PMID: 22901887].

CONGENITAL MALFORMATIONS OF THE LUNG PARENCHYMA

PULMONARY AGENESIS & HYPOPLASIA

ESSENTIALS OF DIAGNOSIS & TYPICAL FEATURES

▶ Pulmonary aplasia is not compatible with life.

▶ Pulmonary hypoplasia is due to incomplete development.

▶ Pulmonary hypoplasia often leads to prolonged oxygen requirement and increased oxygen need with illness and activity. Other symptoms vary by degree of hypoplasia.

In unilateral pulmonary agenesis (complete absence of one lung), the trachea continues into a main bronchus and often has complete tracheal rings. With compensatory postnatal growth, the remaining lung often herniates into the contralateral chest. Chest radiographs show a mediastinal shift toward the affected side. Absent or incomplete lung development may be associated with vertebral and other congenital abnormalities, such as absence of one or both kidneys or fusion of ribs, and the outcome is primarily related to the severity of associated lesions. About 37% of patients with pulmonary agenesis survive; the mortality rate is higher with agenesis of the right lung than of the left lung.

Pulmonary hypoplasia is incomplete development of one or both lungs, characterized by a reduction in alveolar number and a reduction in airway branches and surface area for gas exchange. Pulmonary hypoplasia results from premature disruption of lung development. Causes include decreased amniotic fluid production (such as with renal agenesis), premature loss of amniotic fluid through prolonged premature rupture of membranes, decreased blood flow to the early fetal developing lungs, chromosomal abnormalities, or possibly a primary mesodermal defect affecting multiple organ systems leading to structural immaturity. Chest cage abnormalities, intrathoracic masses, diaphragmatic hernia or elevation, fetal hydrops, severe musculoskeletal disorders, and cardiac lesions may also result in hypoplastic lungs. Postnatal factors may play important roles. For example, infants with advanced BPD can have pulmonary hypoplasia.

Clinical Findings

A. Symptoms and Signs

The clinical presentation is highly variable and related to the severity of hypoplasia as well as associated abnormalities. Lung hypoplasia is often associated with pneumothorax in newborns. Some newborns present with perinatal stress, severe acute respiratory distress, and persistent pulmonary hypertension secondary to primary pulmonary hypoplasia (without associated anomalies). Children with lesser degrees of hypoplasia may present with chronic cough, tachypnea, wheezing, and recurrent pneumonia.

B. Laboratory Findings and Imaging Studies

Chest radiographic findings include variable degrees of volume loss in a small hemithorax with mediastinal shift. Pulmonary agenesis should be suspected if tracheal deviation is evident on the chest radiograph. The chest CT scan is the optimal diagnostic procedure if the chest radiograph is not definitive, though ultrasound or fetal MRI are also used for prenatal diagnosis. Ventilation-perfusion scans, angiography, and bronchoscopy are often helpful in the evaluation, demonstrating decreased pulmonary vascularity or premature blunting of airways associated with the maldeveloped lung tissue. The degree of respiratory impairment is defined by analysis of arterial blood gases.

▶ Treatment & Prognosis

Treatment is supportive. The outcome is determined by the severity of underlying medical problems, the extent of the hypoplasia, and the degree of pulmonary hypertension.

Cotton CM: Pulmonary hypoplasia. Semin Fetal Neonatal Med 2017;22(4):250–255 [PMID: 28709949].

PULMONARY SEQUESTRATION

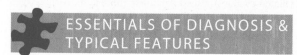

ESSENTIALS OF DIAGNOSIS & TYPICAL FEATURES

▶ Congenital lung malformation with a blood supply from systemic arteries usually found in a lower lobe.

▶ Often presents with recurrent pneumonia or chronic cough.

▶ Diagnosed postnatally by chest CT.

Pulmonary sequestration is the second most common congenital lung abnormality, is characterized by nonfunctional pulmonary tissue that does not communicate with the tracheobronchial tree, and receives its blood supply from one or more anomalous systemic arteries. This abnormality originates during the embryonic period of lung development. It is classified as either extralobar or intralobar.

Extralobar sequestration is a mass of pulmonary parenchyma anatomically separate from the normal lung, with a distinct pleural investment. Its blood supply derives from

the systemic circulation (more typical), from pulmonary vessels, or from both. In contrast to intralobar sequestrations, venous drainage is usually through the systemic or portal venous system. Pathologically, extralobar sequestration appears as a solitary thoracic lesion near the diaphragm. Abdominal sites are rare. Size varies from 0.5 to 12 cm. The left side is involved in more than 65% of cases. Other congenital anomalies are seen in 50% of patients with extralobar sequestration.

Intralobar sequestration is an isolated segment of lung within the normal pleural investment that often receives blood from one or more arteries arising from the aorta or its branches. Intralobar sequestration is usually found within the lower lobes (98%), 55% are found on the left side, and it is rarely associated with other congenital anomalies (< 2%).

▶ Clinical Findings, Imaging, & Treatment

Pulmonary sequestrations have been detected by prenatal ultrasound. Doppler imaging may allow for distinction between intralobar and extralobar malformations. Postnatal clinical presentation includes chronic cough, wheezing, and/or recurrent pneumonias. Rarely, patients with sequestration present with hemoptysis. Diagnosis is often suggested by CT imaging postnatally, though it can be diagnosed via prenatal ultrasound. CT angiography or magnetic resonance angiography have proved useful in identifying anomalous systemic arterial supply to the lung. Treatment is surgical resection.

Baird R, Puligandla PS, LaBerge JM: Congenital lung malformations: informing best practice. Semin Pediatr Surg 2014;23(5):270–277 [PMID 25459011]
Wall J, Coates A: Prenatal imaging and postnatal presentation, diagnosis, and management of congenital lung malformations. Curr Opin Pediatr 2014;26(3):315–319 [PMID: 24739492].

CONGENITAL LOBAR OVERINFLATION

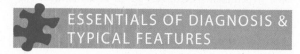

ESSENTIALS OF DIAGNOSIS & TYPICAL FEATURES

▶ Presents in the first year of life and may be diagnosed prenatally.

▶ Chest imaging shows overinflation of the affected lobe (usually right upper or middle).

Patients with congenital lobar overinflation (CLO)—also known as congenital lobar emphysema—present most commonly with neonatal respiratory distress or progressive respiratory impairment during the first year of life. Rarely the mild or intermittent nature of the symptoms in older children or young adults results in delayed diagnosis. Most patients are white males. Although the cause of congenital lobar emphysema is not well understood, some lesions show bronchial cartilaginous dysplasia due to abnormal orientation or distribution of the bronchial cartilage or other cause of bronchial obstruction, leading to a partial ball-valve effect and resultant air trapping. This leads to expiratory collapse, producing obstruction, and air trapping.

▶ Clinical Findings

A. Symptoms and Signs

Clinical features include respiratory distress, tachypnea, wheezing, and cough. Breath sounds are reduced on the affected side, perhaps with hyperresonance to percussion, mediastinal displacement, and bulging of the chest wall.

B. Imaging Studies

Radiologic findings include overdistention of the affected lobe (usually an upper or middle lobe; > 99%), with wide separation of bronchovascular markings, collapse of adjacent lung, shift of the mediastinum away from the affected side, and a depressed diaphragm on the affected side. The radiographic diagnosis may be confusing in the newborn because of retention of alveolar fluid in the affected lobe causing the appearance of a homogeneous density. The most commonly used diagnostic studies are chest CT and bronchoscopy.

▶ Differential Diagnosis

The differential diagnosis of CLO includes pneumothorax, pneumatocele, atelectasis with compensatory hyperinflation, diaphragmatic hernia, and congenital cystic adenomatoid malformation. The most common site of involvement is the left upper lobe (42%) or right middle lobe (35%). Evaluation must differentiate regional obstructive emphysema from lobar hyperinflation secondary to an uncomplicated ball-valve mechanism due to extrinsic compression (ie, bronchogenic cyst, tumor, lymphadenopathy, vascular compression) or intrinsic obstruction from a mucus plug due to infection and inflammation from various causes.

▶ Treatment

When respiratory distress is marked, a segmental or complete lobectomy is usually required. Less symptomatic and older children may do equally well with or without lobectomy.

Seear M et al: A review of congenital lung malformations with a simplified classification system for clinical and research use. Pediatr Surg Int 2017;33(6):657–664 [PMID: 2820492].

Wall J, Coates A: Prenatal imaging and postnatal presentation, diagnosis, and management of congenital lung malformations. Curr Opin Pediatr 2014;26(3):315–319 [PMID: 24739492].

CONGENITAL PULMONARY AIRWAY MALFORMATION (PREVIOUSLY NAMED CYSTIC ADENOMATOID MALFORMATION)

ESSENTIALS OF DIAGNOSIS & TYPICAL FEATURES

▶ May be diagnosed prenatally by ultrasound.

▶ Newborns generally present with respiratory distress and evidence of a space occupying density on chest x-ray.

Congenital pulmonary airway malformations (CPAMs; previously known as congenital cystic adenomatoid malformations) are unilateral hamartomatous lesions that generally present with marked respiratory distress within the first days of life. This disorder accounts for 95% of cases of congenital cystic lung disease.

Right and left lungs are involved with equal frequency. These lesions originate in the first 5–22 weeks of gestation during the embryonic period of lung development. They are space-occupying masses that can appear to be solid or cystic. Histopathology varies based on type of CPAM and may show an increase in terminal respiratory structures, forming intercommunicating cysts of various sizes, lined by cuboidal or ciliated pseudostratified columnar epithelium. Air passages appear malformed and tend to lack cartilage.

There are five types of such malformations (Table 19–5).

▶ Clinical Findings

A. Symptoms and Signs

CPAMs are most commonly identified on routine prenatal ultrasound. In children, 86% are identified by age five. Presenting symptoms include respiratory distress with focal findings of decreased breath sounds, and recurrent pulmonary infection. With type 3 lesions, dullness to percussion may be present. Older patients can present with a spontaneous pneumothorax or with pneumonia-like symptoms.

B. Laboratory Findings and Imaging Studies

Chest radiographic findings differ by the type of lesion. Placement of a radiopaque feeding tube into the stomach helps in the differentiation from diaphragmatic hernia. Differentiation from sequestration is not difficult because congenital CPAMs have no systemic blood supply.

Table 19–5. Types of congenital pulmonary airway malformations.

CPAM Type	Epidemiology	Pathologic Characteristics	Presentation	Prognosis and Treatment
Type 0	1%–3%	Firm with small cysts and made of irregular bronchial tissue. Often involving entire lung.	Not compatible with life.	Not compatible with life.
Type 1	60%–70% of cases	Single or multiple large cysts; rarely bilateral.	Prenatal diagnosis may occur when cysts are large. In the newborn period, respiratory distress will be seen if large cysts expand causing compression of the adjacent lung or mediastinal shift. Smaller cysts may present with recurrent pneumonia later.	Resection leads to symptom resolution.
Type 2	15%–20%	Bulky, firm masses with small cysts isolated to one lobe.	Often first present with associated nonpulmonary anomalies.	Resection.
Type 3	5%–10%	Bulky, solid appearance. Small cysts. This CPAM is often large involving one whole lobe or multiple lobes. Frequent mediastinal shift.	Infants present in the newborn period with severe respiratory distress.	50% survival due to the association with cardiac compression and fetal hydrops in large, type 3 CPAMs. Infants may be stillborn. Treatment includes pre- and postnatal resection.
Type 4	< 10%	Large, thin-walled cysts in the periphery of a whole lung or isolated to one lobe.	Newborns present with severe respiratory distress.	Resection.

CPAM, congenital pulmonary airway malformation.

▶ Treatment

Postnatal treatment of types 1 and 3 lesions involves surgical removal of the affected lobe. Attention must be paid to complications of these lesions such as hydrops and cardiac compression. Resection is often indicated because of the risk of infection and air trapping, since the malformation communicates with the tracheobronchial tree but mucus clearance is compromised. Segmental resection is not feasible because smaller cysts may expand after removal of the more obviously affected area. Of note, some CPAMs have been shown to spontaneously resolve. However, CPAMs have been reported to have malignant potential; therefore, expectant management with observation alone should proceed with caution. Recent development of intrauterine surgery for congenital malformations has led to promising results.

Baird R, Puligandla PS, Laberge JM: Congenital lung malformations: informing best practice. Semin Pediatr Surg 2014;23(5):270–277 [PMID: 25459011].

David M, Lamas-Pinheiro R, Henriques-Coelho T: Prenatal and postnatal management of congenital pulmonary airway malformation. Neonatology 2016;110(2):101–115 [PMID: 27070354].

Wall J, Coates A: Prenatal imaging and postnatal presentation, diagnosis, and management of congenital lung malformations. Curr Opin Pediatr 2014;26(3): 315–319 [PMID: 24739492].

▼ ACQUIRED ABNORMALITIES OF THE LUNG PARENCHYMA

BRONCHOPULMONARY DYSPLASIA

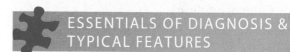

ESSENTIALS OF DIAGNOSIS & TYPICAL FEATURES

▶ Respiratory distress after preterm birth.

▶ Required oxygen therapy or positive pressure ventilation at 36 weeks' gestational age or 28 days of life.

▶ Persistent respiratory abnormalities, including physical signs and radiographic findings.

BPD remains one of the most significant sequelae of acute respiratory distress in the neonatal intensive care unit, with an incidence as high as 68% for infants born at 22–28 weeks' gestation. This disease was first characterized in 1967 when Northway reported the clinical, radiologic, and pathologic findings in a group of preterm newborns who required prolonged mechanical ventilation and oxygen therapy.

The pathologic findings and clinical course of BPD have changed over time due to technological advances (artificial surfactant, antenatal steroids) and protective/noninvasive ventilatory strategies. Improvements in care have also increased survival of infants born at earlier gestational ages. Extremely preterm infants born at less than 28 weeks' gestation are at risk to develop "new" BPD and arrest of lung development, which is characterized by alveolar simplification and vascular hypoplasia that can lead to sequelae, such as impaired gas exchange, exercise intolerance, and pulmonary hypertension.

The mechanisms that cause BPD are unclear. Current studies suggest that structural immaturity of the alveolar-capillary network, surfactant deficiency, atelectasis, and pulmonary edema cause impaired gas exchange and, potentially, respiratory failure. Mechanical ventilation and supplemental oxygen, though necessary to sustain life, may result in barotrauma and oxidative stress. Excessive fluid administration, patent ductus arteriosus, pulmonary interstitial emphysema, pneumothorax, infection, pulmonary hypertension, and inflammatory stimuli secondary to lung injury or infection also play important roles in the pathogenesis of the disease. Infants can develop aggressive, fibroproliferative pathologic lesions as well as physiologic abnormalities (increased airway resistance) and biochemical markers of lung injury that may predict BPD during the first weeks of life. Ongoing injuries may further contribute to ventilator and oxygen dependence. The lungs of extremely preterm newborns with BPD show simplified histology with fewer alveoli, early inflammation, and hypercellularity followed by healing with fibrosis.

▶ Clinical Findings

The clinical definition of BPD includes the need for postnatal oxygen for at least 28 days. The severity of BPD is determined by a physiologic assessment of oxygen status at 36 weeks' gestation or on day of life for infants born after 32 weeks' gestation. Full-term newborns with disorders such as meconium aspiration, congenital diaphragmatic hernia, and persistent pulmonary hypertension also can develop BPD.

The clinical course of infants with BPD ranges from an oxygen requirement that gradually resolves over a few months to more severe disease requiring tracheostomy for chronic mechanical ventilation during early childhood. In general, patients show slow, steady improvements in oxygen or ventilator requirements. Sufficient respiratory support should be provided to ensure that the preterm infant breathes comfortably without distress. Clinical management also includes paying careful attention to growth and nutrition (infants with oxygen dependence have high caloric requirements) and partnering with developmental therapists to ensure the optimal neurocognitive outcomes.

▶ Treatment

A. Medical Therapy

Early use of surfactant therapy with adequate lung recruitment increases the chance for survival without BPD, reduces the need for mechanical ventilation, and can decrease mortality. Short courses of postnatal glucocorticoid therapy have been helpful in increasing the success of weaning from the ventilator. Longer courses of postnatal glucocorticoids have been linked to an increased incidence of cerebral palsy. Routine use of inhaled corticosteroids and β-adrenergic agonists do not decrease the incidence of BOD, but there may be some benefit to infants who have airway hyper-reactivity.

Salt and water retention secondary to chronic hypoxemia, hypercapnia, or other stimuli may be present. Chronic or intermittent diuretic therapy is commonly used if pulmonary edema is present. Clinical studies show acute improvement in lung function with this therapy, but their impact on long-term outcomes is unclear. Unfortunately, diuretics often have adverse effects, including volume contraction, hypokalemia, alkalosis, hyponatremia, and nephrocalcinosis. Potassium and arginine chloride supplements may be required.

B. Airway Evaluation

Children with significant stridor, sleep apnea, chronic wheezing, or excessive respiratory distress require diagnostic bronchoscopy to evaluate for structural lesions (eg, subglottic stenosis, vocal cord paralysis, tracheal or bronchial stenosis, tracheobronchomalacia, or airway granulomas). The contribution of gastroesophageal reflux and aspiration should be considered in the face of worsening chronic lung disease.

C. Management of Pulmonary Hypertension

Infants with BPD are at risk of developing pulmonary hypertension. In many of these children even mild hypoxemia can cause significant elevations of pulmonary arterial pressure. To minimize the harmful effects of hypoxemia, the arterial oxygen saturation should be kept above 93% in children with pulmonary hypertension, with care to avoid hyperoxia during retinal vascular development. Echocardiograms should be performed to monitor for the development of right ventricular hypertrophy. Management of neonatal pulmonary hypertension should involve expert consultation with a pulmonary hypertension specialist. Cardiac catheterization may be necessary to diagnose unsuspected cardiac or pulmonary lesions and to measure the response of the pulmonary vasculature to vasodilators such as inhaled nitric oxide before chronic therapy, such as oral sildenafil, is initiated. A barium esophagram, esophageal pH/impedence studies, video fluoroscopic swallow study, PSG or overnight pulse oximetry, and bronchoscopy may aid in diagnosing gastroesophageal reflux, aspiration, OSA, and airway abnormalities that contribute to the underlying pathophysiology. Long-term care should include monitoring for systemic hypertension and the development of left ventricular hypertrophy.

D. Nutrition and Immunizations

Nutritional problems in infants with BPD may be due to increased oxygen consumption, feeding difficulties, gastroesophageal reflux, and chronic hypoxemia. Hypercaloric formulas and gastrostomy tubes are often required to ensure adequate intake while avoiding overhydration. Routine vaccinations including the influenza vaccine are recommended. Immune prophylaxis of RSV reduces the severity morbidity of bronchiolitis in infants with BPD. In children older than 2 years with severe BPD, pneumococcal polysaccharide 23-valent vaccine should be considered in addition to standard pneumococcal vaccination.

E. Ventilation

For children with established severe BPD and persistent positive pressure dependence, a supportive approach to ventilation is warranted. The lungs of infants with severe BPD demonstrate very heterogeneous disease with regions of both atelectasis and extreme hyperinflation. In this context, an effective ventilation strategy involves delivery of larger tidal volumes (10–12 mL/kg) given more slowly (inspiratory time ≥ 0.6 seconds) with slower rates (10–14 breaths/min) to permit adequate exhalation. Sufficient peak end-expiratory pressure (PEEP) should be provided to overcome dynamic collapse of the airways. Counterintuitively, increasing PEEP may effectively decrease hyperinflation in infants with severe tracheobronchomalacia. This approach to ventilation can reduce air hunger, prevent hypoxemic spells, and decrease the infant's work of breathing.

▶ Differential Diagnosis

The differential diagnosis of BPD includes meconium aspiration syndrome, congenital infection (eg, with cytomegalovirus or *Ureaplasma*), cystic adenomatoid malformation, recurrent aspiration, pulmonary lymphangiectasia, total anomalous pulmonary venous return, overhydration, childhood ILD, and idiopathic pulmonary fibrosis.

▶ Prognosis

Surfactant replacement therapy has had a markedly beneficial effect on reducing morbidity and mortality from BPD. The incidence of BPD and chronic lung disease due to prematurity is increasing due to increased survival or early and extremely preterm infants. The long-term outlook for most survivors is favorable, although follow-up studies suggest that lung function may be altered for life. As smaller, more immature infants survive, abnormal neurodevelopmental outcomes become more likely. The incidence of cerebral palsy, hearing/visual impairment, and developmental delays

is increased. Feeding abnormalities, behavior difficulties, and increased irritability have also been reported. A focus on alleviating respiratory distress, optimal nutrition, prophylaxis against respiratory infection, developmental therapies (physical, occupational, and speech), attention to neurocognitive function, and family support provide the best outcomes.

Baraldi E, Filippone M: Chronic lung disease after premature birth. N Engl J Med 2007;357:1946 [PMID: 17989387].

Higgins RD et al: Executive summary of the workshop on oxygen in neonatal therapies: controversies and opportunities for research. Pediatrics 2007;119:790 [PMID: 17403851].

Islam JY et al: Understanding the short- and long-term respiratory outcomes of prematurity and bronchopulmonary dysplasia. Am J Respir Crit Care Med 2015;(192)2:134–156 [PMID: 26038806]

COMMUNITY-ACQUIRED BACTERIAL PNEUMONIA

ESSENTIALS OF DIAGNOSIS & TYPICAL FEATURES

- ▶ Fever, cough, dyspnea.
- ▶ Abnormal chest examination (focal crackles or decreased breath sounds).
- ▶ Abnormal chest radiograph (opacities, hilar adenopathy, pleural effusion).

Community-acquired pneumonia (CAP) is the most common cause of childhood mortality worldwide. Infectious etiologies vary widely by geographic region and by the age of the child. In developed countries the majority of pneumonias are caused by viral infections. Physical examination, white blood cell count and differential, and chest radiograph do not reliably distinguish between viral and bacterial pathogens. Children with CAP complicated by parapneumonic effusions are more likely to have a prolonged illness and are at higher risk for long term complications of CAP. Empyema is covered in the next section of this chapter.

The most common cause of bacterial pneumonia in children of all ages is *S pneumoniae*, but the spectrum of potential pathogens to be considered also includes aerobic, anaerobic, and acid-fast bacteria as well as other atypical bacteria and respiratory viruses. Bacterial pneumonia usually follows a viral lower respiratory tract infection. Compromised pulmonary defense systems increase the risk of pneumonia in children. For example, abnormal mucociliary clearance, impaired cough function, immunocompromised status, aspiration of oral secretions or oral intake, and malnutrition, increase the risk for bacterial pneumonia. Certain immunocompromised patients, such as those who have undergone splenectomy or who have hemoglobin SS or SC disease or thalassemia, are especially prone to overwhelming sepsis associated with bacterial pneumonia.

Clinical Findings

A. Symptoms and Signs

The pathogen, severity of the infection, and age of the patient may cause substantial variations in the presentation of CAP. Fever (> 39°C), tachypnea, and cough are hallmarks of CAP. Respiratory distress and hypoxemia are signs of more severe disease. Chest auscultation may reveal focal crackles or decreased breath sounds in the setting of consolidation or an associated pleural effusion. Some patients may have additional extrapulmonary findings, such as abdominal pain, due to pneumonia itself. Others may have evidence of infection at other sites due to the same organism causing their pneumonia such as otitis media, sinusitis, or meningitis.

B. Laboratory Findings and Imaging Studies

Chest x-rays may be helpful diagnostic tool in CAP but are not specific to bacterial pneumonia. Chest radiographs are indicated in children ill enough to be in the hospital for CAP to evaluate for complicated CAP. Laboratory studies may also impact the management of children hospitalized for CAP, but they are not indicated for the outpatient management of children with CAP. Blood cultures should be obtained in children admitted to the hospital with severe distress or complicated pneumonia. Inflammatory markers such as erythrocyte sedimentation rate, C-reactive protein (CRP), and procalcitonin may inform clinical decision making, especially in complicated CAP. Complete blood counts can help evaluate for complications of pneumonia such as thrombocytopenia, anemia, or hemolytic uremic syndrome. Sputum cultures may be helpful in older children capable of providing a satisfactory sample. Invasive diagnostic procedures should be undertaken in critically ill patients when other means do not adequately identify the cause (see section Diagnosis of Respiratory Tract Infections).

If a pleural effusion is suspected, radiographs should be taken in the lateral decubitus position. Chest ultrasonography may also be useful to confirm the clinical suspicion and to localize the effusion. A diagnostic (and possibly therapeutic) thoracentesis should also be performed in a child with a pleural effusion. For further recommendations, see section Parapneumonic Effusions & Empyema.

Differential Diagnosis

Noninfectious pulmonary disease (including gastric aspiration, foreign-body aspiration, atelectasis, congenital malformations, congestive heart failure, tumors such as plasma cell granulomas, chronic ILD, and pulmonary hemosiderosis) should be considered in the differential diagnosis of localized or diffuse infiltrates. When effusions are present, additional noninfectious disorders such as collagen vascular diseases, neoplasm, and pulmonary infarction should also be considered.

Treatment

If a bacterial pneumonia is suspected, empiric antibiotic therapy should be considered. Children younger than 4 weeks should be treated with ampicillin and an aminoglycoside. Infants 4–12 weeks of age should be admitted to the hospital and treated with intravenous ampicillin for 7–10 days. Admission to the hospital should also be considered in any child from 3 to 6 months of age with bacterial pneumonia. All children older than 6 months who do not have significant respiratory distress should be treated with oral amoxicillin (50–90 mg/kg/dose) in doses given three times per day for 7–10 days. Macrolide antibiotics should be used if an atypical infection such as *M pneumoniae* is suspected, although the utility of treating *Mycoplasma* infections is questionable. (See Chapter 39). When possible, therapy can be guided by the antibiotic sensitivity pattern of the organisms isolated. (For further discussion, see Chapter 39.) Whether older children should be hospitalized depends on age, the severity of illness, the suspected organism, and the anticipated reliability of adherence to the treatment regimen at home. Moderate to severe respiratory distress, apnea, hypoxemia, poor feeding, clinical deterioration on oral antibiotic treatment, or associated complications (large effusions, empyema, or abscess) indicate the need for immediate hospitalization. Careful outpatient follow-up within 12 hours to 5 days is indicated in those not admitted.

Additional therapeutic considerations include oxygen, humidification of inspired gases, hydration and electrolyte supplementation, and nutrition. Removal of pleural fluid for diagnostic purposes is indicated to guide antimicrobial therapy and may be required for therapeutic purposes.

Prognosis

Immunocompetent children who live in developed countries in whom bacterial pneumonia is adequately recognized and treated have a high survival rate. For example, the mortality rate from uncomplicated pneumococcal pneumonia is less than 1%. If the patient survives the initial illness, persistently abnormal pulmonary function following even complicated CAP is surprisingly uncommon, even when treatment has been delayed or inappropriate.

Messinger AI, Kupfer O, Hurst A, Parker S: Management of pediatric community-acquired bacterial pneumonia. Pediatr Rev 2017;38(9):394–409 [PMID 28864731].

PARAPNEUMONIC EFFUSION & EMPYEMA

ESSENTIALS OF DIAGNOSIS & TYPICAL FEATURES

▶ Respiratory distress and chest pain.

▶ Fever.

▶ Chest x-ray showing a meniscus or layering fluid on a lateral decubitus film.

Parapneumonic effusions can be associated with pneumonia, autoimmune disease, trauma, malignancy, hypoalbuminemia due to liver or kidney disease, hypothyroidism, autoimmune disease, and pancreatitis. Some parapneumonic effusions associated with pneumonia harbor infection. Others are inflammatory reactions to the infection. The nomenclature in this area is somewhat confusing. Some authors use the term *empyema* for grossly purulent fluid and *parapneumonic effusion* for nonpurulent fluid. It is clear, however, that some nonpurulent effusions will also contain organisms and represent either partially treated or early empyema. It is probably best to refer to all effusions associated with pneumonia as parapneumonic effusions, some of which are infected and some not.

The most common organism associated with empyema is *S pneumoniae*. Other common organisms include *H influenzae*, and *S aureus*. Less common causes are group A *Streptococcus*, gram-negative organisms, anaerobic organisms, and *M pneumoniae*. Effusions associated with tuberculosis are almost always sterile and constitute an inflammatory reaction.

▶ Clinical Findings

A. Symptoms and Signs

Patients usually present with typical signs of pneumonia, including fever, tachypnea, and cough. Patients with complicated pneumonia may have chest pain, decreased breath sounds, and dullness to percussion on the affected side and may prefer to lie on the affected side. With large effusions, there may be tracheal deviation to the contralateral side. Empyema is more likely to occur in children younger than 5 years and in immunocompromised hosts.

B. Diagnostic Studies

The presence of pleural fluid is suggested by a homogeneous density that obscures the underlying lung on chest radiograph. Large effusions may cause a shift of the mediastinum to the contralateral side. Small effusions may only blunt the costophrenic angle. Lateral decubitus radiographs may help to detect freely movable fluid by demonstrating a layering-out effect, unless the fluid is loculated. Chest ultrasound is preferred to chest CT for identifying septations or loculations. Chest CT scan can help determine the presence of a parenchymal abscess in cases of pneumonia that does not respond as expected.

Blood cultures may be positive up to 18% of the time in complicated pneumonia. The tuberculin skin test is positive in most cases of tuberculosis. Gram stain, cultures, and antigen detection sent from a diagnostic or therapeutic thoracocentesis may help establish the etiology of the pneumonia. Cells in the pleural fluid are usually neutrophils in bacterial disease and lymphocytes in tuberculous effusions. Although in adults the presence of low pH and glucose indicates the need for aggressive and thorough drainage procedures, the prognostic significance of these findings in children is unknown. When the sitology of the effusion is unknown, Light's criteria should be used to determine if the fluid obtained by thoracocentesis is an exudate or a transudate. Light's criteria indicate an exudate if one of the following is positive: pleural fluid protein/Serum protein greater than 0.5, pleural fluid lactate dehydrogenase (LDH)/serum LDH greater than 0.6, or pleural fluid LDH greater than 2/3 serum upper limit of normal (mdcalc.com.).

▶ Treatment

After initial thoracentesis and identification of the organism, appropriate intravenous antibiotics and adequate drainage of the fluid are the mainstay of therapy. Although there is a trend toward managing smaller pneumococcal empyemas without a chest tube, larger effusions require chest tube drainage. Early use of fibrinolytics is becoming standard of care in pediatrics. Surgical interventions including video-assisted thoracoscopic surgery (VATS) done by an experienced surgeon may reduce morbidity and shorten the length of hospital stay. The therapeutic choice will vary depending on the resources available and the preferences of the clinician.

▶ Prognosis

The prognosis is related to the severity of disease but is generally excellent, with complete or nearly complete recovery in most instances.

Langle JM et al: Empyema associated with community acquired pneumonia: a Pediatric Investigator's Collaborative Network on Infections in Canada (PICNIC) study. BMC Infect Dis 2008;8:129 [PMID: 18816409].

Messinger AI, Kupfer O, Hurst A, Parker S: Management of pediatric community-acquired bacterial pneumonia. Pediatr Rev 2017;38(9):394–409 [PMID: 28864731].

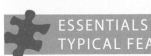

ATYPICAL PNEUMONIAS

VIRAL PNEUMONIA

> ## ESSENTIALS OF DIAGNOSIS & TYPICAL FEATURES

► Upper respiratory infection prodrome (fever, coryza, cough, hoarseness).

► Wheezing or rales.

► Myalgia, malaise, headache (older children).

Viral infection is a common cause of CAP in children. Viral pneumonia is most common in children younger than 2 years. Respiratory syncytial virus (RSV), human rhinovirus, adenovirus, parainfluenza (types 1–3), influenza (A and B) viruses, coronavirus, and human metapneumovirus are responsible for the large majority of cases. Severity of disease, severity of fever, radiographic findings, and the characteristics of cough or lung sounds do not reliably differentiate viral from bacterial pneumonias. Furthermore, viral infections may predispose to bacterial pneumonia. However, substantial pleural effusions, pneumatoceles, abscesses, lobar consolidation with lobar volume expansion, and "round" pneumonias are generally inconsistent with viral disease.

► Clinical Findings

A. Symptoms and Signs

An upper respiratory infection frequently precedes the onset of lower respiratory disease due to viruses. Although wheezing or stridor may be prominent in viral disease, other findings, such as cough, signs of respiratory distress (tachypnea, retractions, grunting, and nasal flaring), and physical findings (rales and decreased breath sounds), are similar to those in bacterial pneumonia.

B. Laboratory Findings

Rapid viral diagnostic methods such as fluorescent antibody tests, enzyme-linked immunosorbent assay, and/or PCR should only be performed on nasopharyngeal secretions if the result will change management, is necessary a viral etiology in high-risk patients, or is required for epidemiology or infection control. The peripheral white blood cell count is not useful in distinguishing viral from bacterial disease.

C. Imaging Studies

Chest radiographs frequently show perihilar streaking, increased interstitial markings, peribronchial cuffing, or patchy bronchopneumonia. Lobar consolidation or atelectasis may occur, however. Hyperinflation of the lungs may occur when involvement of the small airways is prominent.

► Differential Diagnosis

The differential diagnosis of viral pneumonia is the same as for bacterial pneumonia. Patients with prominent wheezing may have asthma, airway obstruction caused by foreign-body aspiration, and acute bacterial or viral tracheitis.

► Complications

Viral pneumonia or laryngotracheobronchitis may predispose the patient to subsequent bacterial tracheitis or pneumonia as immediate sequelae. Bronchiolitis obliterans or severe chronic respiratory failure may follow adenovirus pneumonia. The results of studies evaluating the development of asthma after a viral pneumonia are variable. Bronchiectasis, chronic hypersensitivity pneumonia and unilateral hyperlucent lung (Sawyer-James syndrome) may follow measles, adenovirus, and influenza pneumonias.

► Treatment

General supportive care for viral pneumonia does not differ from that for bacterial pneumonia. Patients can be quite ill and should be hospitalized according to the level of their illness. Because bacterial disease often cannot be definitively excluded, antibiotics may be indicated.

Patients at risk for life-threatening RSV infections (eg, those with BPD or other severe pulmonary conditions, congenital heart disease, or significant immunocompromise) should be hospitalized and ribavirin should be considered. Rapid viral diagnostic tests may be a useful guide for such therapy.

All children with influenza should be treated with the appropriate therapy for the specific type of influenza (A, B, H1N1). When available epidemiologic data indicate an active influenza infection in the community, antiviral therapy should be considered early for high-risk infants and children who appear to be infected. For dosing recommendations, refer to the American Academy of Pediatrics (AAP) 2018 *Redbook*. Children with suspected viral pneumonia should be placed in respiratory isolation.

► Prognosis

Although most children with viral pneumonia recover uneventfully, worsening asthma, abnormal pulmonary function or chest radiographs, persistent respiratory insufficiency, and even death may occur in high-risk patients such as newborns or those with underlying lung, cardiac, or immunodeficiency disease. Patients with coinfections, virus-virus coinfections, or virus-bacterium co-infections have worse outcomes.

Jain S: Epidemiology of viral pneumonia. Clin Chest Med 2017;38:1–9 [PMID: 28159152].

Nolan VG et al: Etiology and impact of coinfections in children hospitalized with community-acquired pneumonia. J Infect Dis 2018; 218(2):179–188 [PMID: 29228381].

BRONCHIOLITIS

ESSENTIALS OF DIAGNOSIS & TYPICAL FEATURES

▶ Clinical syndrome characterized by one or more of the following findings: coughing, tachypnea, labored breathing, and hypoxia.

▶ Irritability, poor feeding, vomiting.

▶ Wheezing and crackles on chest auscultation.

Bronchiolitis is the most common serious acute respiratory illness in infants and young children. The diagnosis of bronchiolitis is based on clinical findings including an upper respiratory infection that has progressed to cough, tachypnea, respiratory distress, and crackles or wheeze by physical examination. In most literature from the United States, this definition of bronchiolitis specifically applies to children younger than 2 years. One to 3% of infants with bronchiolitis will require hospitalization, especially during the winter months. Respiratory syncytial virus (RSV) is by far the most common viral cause of acute bronchiolitis. Parainfluenza, human metapneumovirus, influenza, and adenovirus are less common causes of bronchiolitis during early infancy.

▶ Prevention

The most effective preventions against RSV infection are proper handwashing techniques and reducing exposure to potential environmental risk factors. Prophylaxis with a monoclonal antibody (palivizumab) is effective at reducing the rate of hospitalization and associated morbidity in high-risk premature infants and those with chronic cardiopulmonary conditions. Dosing recommendations in the United States are available in the AAP 2018 *Redbook*.

▶ Clinical Findings

A. Symptoms and Signs

The usual course of RSV bronchiolitis is 1–2 days of fever, rhinorrhea, and cough, followed by wheezing, tachypnea, and respiratory distress. Typically, the breathing pattern is shallow, with rapid respirations. Nasal flaring, cyanosis, retractions, and rales may be present, along with prolongation of the expiratory phase and wheezing, depending on the severity of illness. Some young infants present with apnea and few findings on auscultation but may subsequently develop rales, rhonchi, and expiratory wheezing.

B. Laboratory Findings and Imaging Studies

A nasal wash can be used to identify the causative pathogen but is not necessary to make the diagnosis of bronchiolitis. The peripheral white blood cell count may be normal or show a mild lymphocytosis. Chest radiographs are not indicated in children who have bilateral, symmetrical findings on examination, who are not in significant respiratory distress, and who do not have elevated temperature. Chest radiograph findings are generally nonspecific and typically include hyperinflation, peribronchial cuffing, increased interstitial markings, and subsegmental atelectasis.

▶ Complications

Bacterial superinfection is a rare complication of viral pneumonia. The results of studies investigating the risk for the subsequent development of chronic airway hyperreactivity (asthma) are variable. Bronchiolitis due to RSV infection contributes substantially to morbidity and mortality in children with underlying medical disorders, including chronic lung disease of prematurity, CF, congenital heart disease, and immunodeficiency.

▶ Treatment

Although most children with RSV bronchiolitis are readily treated as outpatients, hospitalization is required in infected children with hypoxemia on room air, a history of apnea, moderate tachypnea with feeding difficulties, and marked respiratory distress with retractions. Children at high risk for hospitalization include infants (aged < 6 months), especially with any history of prematurity, and those with underlying chronic cardiopulmonary disorders. While in the hospital, treatment should include supportive strategies such as frequent suctioning and providing adequate fluids to maintain hydration. If hypoxemia is present, supplemental oxygen should be administered. There is no evidence to support the use of antibiotics in children with bronchiolitis unless there is evidence of an associated bacterial pneumonia. Bronchodilators and corticosteroids have not been shown to change the severity or the length of the illness in bronchiolitis and therefore are not recommended. Studies evaluating the effectiveness of hypertonic saline and heated high-flow oxygen therapy are ongoing.

Patients at risk for life-threatening RSV infections (eg, children born at < 35 weeks, children with other severe pulmonary conditions, congenital heart disease, neuromuscular disease, or significant immunocompromise) should be considered for RSV prophylaxis therapy. For more detail, refer to the AAP 2018 *Redbook*. High-risk patients with RSV bronchiolitis may need to be hospitalized and treated with ribavirin.

Prognosis

The prognosis for most infants with acute bronchiolitis is very good. With improved supportive care and prophylaxis with palivizumab, the mortality rate among high-risk infants has decreased substantially.

Meissner HC: Viral bronchiolitis in children. New Engl J Med 2016;374(1):62–72 [PMID: 26735994].

Ralston SL et al: Clinical practice guideline: the diagnosis, management, and prevention of bronchiolitis. Pediatrics 2014; 134(5):e1474–e1502 [PMID: 25349312].

MYCOPLASMA PNEUMONIA

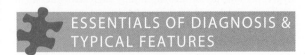

ESSENTIALS OF DIAGNOSIS & TYPICAL FEATURES

► Fever and cough.
► Most common in children older than 5 years.

M pneumoniae is a common cause of symptomatic pneumonia in older children although it may be seen in children younger than 5 years. Endemic and epidemic infection can occur. The incubation period is long (2–3 weeks), and the onset of symptoms is slow. Although the lung is the primary infection site, extrapulmonary complications sometimes occur. Extrapulmonary complications in CAP suggest the diagnosis of M. pneumoniae.

Clinical Findings

A. Symptoms and Signs

Fever, cough, headache, and malaise are common symptoms as the illness evolves. Although cough is usually dry at the onset, sputum production may develop as the illness progresses. Sore throat, otitis media, otitis externa, and bullous myringitis may occur. Rales and chest pain are frequently present on chest examination; decreased breath sounds or dullness to percussion over the involved area may be present.

B. Laboratory Findings and Imaging Studies

PCR is the gold standard for diagnosis. However, like other respiratory pathogens, Mycoplasma can be carried in the upper respiratory tract after resolution of active infection. Enzyme immunoassay (EIA) and complement fixation are sensitive and specific for M pneumoniae but may also be positive in asymptomatic children. Serologic (IgG) testing collected over 2 weeks showing a fourfold or greater rise in specific antibodies confirms the diagnosis of active respiratory disease due to M pneumoniae. The total and differential white blood cell counts are usually normal.

Chest radiographs usually demonstrate interstitial or bronchopneumonic infiltrates, frequently in the middle or lower lobes. Pleural effusions are extremely uncommon.

Complications

Extrapulmonary involvement of the blood, central nervous system, skin, heart, or joints can occur. Direct Coombs–positive autoimmune hemolytic anemia, occasionally a life-threatening disorder, is the most common hematologic abnormality that can accompany M pneumoniae infection. Coagulation defects and thrombocytopenia can also occur. Cerebral infarction, meningoencephalitis, Guillain-Barré syndrome, cranial nerve involvement, and psychosis all have been described. A wide variety of skin rashes, including erythema multiforme and Stevens-Johnson syndrome, can occur. Bronchiolitis obliterans due to Stephens-Johnson syndrome associated with M pneumoniae also has been reported.

Treatment

Antibiotic therapy with a macrolide for 7–10 days may shorten the course of illness. Ciprofloxacin is a possible alternative. Supportive measures, including hydration, antipyretics, and bed rest, are helpful.

Prognosis

In the absence of the less common extrapulmonary complications, the outlook for recovery is excellent.

Atkinson TP, Waites KB: Mycoplasma pneumoniae infections in childhood. Pediatr Infect Dis 2014;33(1):92–94 [PMID: 24346598].

Meyer Sauteur PM, Unger WWJ, van Rossum AMC, Berger C: The art and science of diagnosing Mycoplasma infection. Pediatr Infect Dis J 2018;37(11):1192–1195 [PMID: 30169485].

ASPIRATION PNEUMONIA

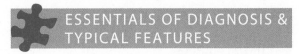

ESSENTIALS OF DIAGNOSIS & TYPICAL FEATURES

► History of recurrent aspiration or an aspiration event.
► New-onset respiratory distress, oxygen requirement, or fever, after the aspiration.
► Any new-onset respiratory distress or increase in oxygen requirement in a child with known aspiration.
► Focal findings on physical examination.

Table 19–6. Risk factors for aspiration pneumonia.

Anatomic abnormalities (laryngeal cleft, tracheoesophageal fistula, vocal cord paralysis)
Delayed maturation (Down syndrome or prematurity)
Static encephalopathy
CNS malformation, mass, or traumatic brain injury
Neuromuscular disorders
Seizures
Depressed sensorium (medications)
Near-drowning
Iatrogenic (anesthesia, nasogastric or tracheostomy tubes)
Gastrointestinal disease (reflux, achalasia, or obstruction)

CNS, central nervous system.

Patients whose anatomic defense mechanisms are impaired are at risk of aspiration pneumonia (Table 19–6). Aspiration pneumonia may be acute or chronic but is more common in children with other underlying medical conditions (see Table 19–6). An acute aspiration event may lead to a typical pneumonia syndrome with fever, asymmetrical auscultation findings, and asymmetric imaging findings. Chronic aspiration pneumonitis is more indolent and can cause chronic respiratory symptoms of "rattling," cough or wheezing, chronic chest infiltrates, bronchiectasis, or failure to thrive. Pneumonitis is worsened by gram-negative anaerobes and other bacteria present in the mouth.

▶ Clinical Findings

A. Symptoms and Signs

Acute onset of fever, cough, respiratory distress, or hypoxemia in a patient at risk suggests acute aspiration pneumonia. Chest physical findings, such as rales, rhonchi, or decreased breath sounds, may initially be limited to the lung region into which aspiration occurred. Although any region may be affected, the right side—especially the right upper lobe in the supine patient—is commonly affected. In patients with chronic aspiration "chest rattling" is often described by parents. Generalized rales and wheezing may also be present.

B. Laboratory Findings and Imaging Studies

Chest radiograph abnormalities can vary widely. They may reveal lobar consolidation or atelectasis and focal or generalized alveolar or interstitial infiltrates. Complications such as empyema or lung abscess may complicate acute aspiration pneumonia. In some patients with chronic aspiration, perihilar infiltrates with or without bronchiectasis may be seen. If there is clinical concern, chest CT can better delineate these complications.

In patients with chronic aspiration pneumonitis, attempts should be made to evaluate dysphagia. VFSS is typically performed to evaluate the swallow. Fiberoptic endoscopic examination of swallowing (FEES) is done at specialty centers to directly visualize the larynx during swallowing via laryngoscope. Radionuclide studies have low sensitivity to diagnosis aspiration. Although biomarkers such as lipid-laden macrophages obtained from BAL samples have low sensitivity and specificity, BAL may be considered to diagnose bacterial infection (see section Diagnosis of Respiratory Tract Infections). Anatomic abnormalities such as laryngeal cleft can be evaluated by rigid laryngoscopy/bronchoscopy. Tracheoesophageal fistula is rare and can be difficult to diagnose: UGI fluoroscopy series, rigid or flexible bronchoscopy, or esophageal endoscopy may aid in diagnosis. The role of esophageal disease, gastroesophageal reflux, and impaired esophageal motility in chronic aspiration may warrant evaluation by a gastroenterologist or multidisciplinary aerodigestive team.

▶ Differential Diagnosis

In the acutely ill patient, bacterial and viral pneumonias should be considered. In the chronically ill patient, the differential diagnosis may include disorders causing recurrent pneumonia (eg, immunodeficiencies, ciliary dysfunction, or foreign body), chronic wheezing, or interstitial lung disorders (see the next section), depending on the presentation.

▶ Treatment

Aspiration pneumonia leads to a chemical pneumonitis, and supportive treatment is recommended. Antimicrobial therapy for patients who are acutely ill from aspiration pneumonia includes coverage for anaerobic organisms. In general, clindamycin is appropriate initial coverage.

Treatment of chronic aspiration pneumonitis may include the following: surgical correction of anatomic abnormalities; paced swallowing systems/bottles, thickening of liquids taken by mouth, swallowing therapy, improved oral hygiene, inhaled corticosteroids, and chest physiotherapy. In patients with compromise of the central nervous system, exclusive feeding by gastrostomy may be required. Because of the widespread causes and consequences of chronic aspiration, multidisciplinary aerodigestive management is often recommended.

Durvasula VS, O'Neill AC, Richter GT: Oropharyngeal dysphagia in children: mechanism, source, and management. Otolaryngol Clin North Am 2014;47(5):691 [PMID: 25213278].

PNEUMONIA IN THE IMMUNOCOMPROMISED HOST

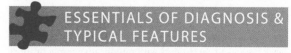
ESSENTIALS OF DIAGNOSIS & TYPICAL FEATURES

▶ The nature of the immunocompromised state may help predict etiology of pulmonary infection.

Compromised immune function occurs following solid organ or hematopoietic stem cell transplantation, in patients with congenital immune deficits, and in patients receiving cancer chemotherapy or other immunosuppressant therapy, including chronic corticosteroids.

Pulmonary infection, which is the most common infection in these patients, can present as focal pneumonia, pulmonary nodules, disseminated disease, or diffuse ILD. The underlying cause of the immunocompromised state often determines the spectrum of infectious agents responsible for disease (see also Chapter 33). Pneumonia in an immunocompromised host may be due to any common community-acquired bacteria or less common pathogens such as opportunistic fungi, *Toxoplasma gondii*, *P jiroveci*, anaerobic bacteria, *Nocardia* species, *Legionella pneumophila*, mycobacteria, and viruses. Multiple organisms are commonly isolated in culture.

▶ Clinical Findings

A. Symptoms and Signs

Patients often present with subtle signs such as mild cough, tachypnea, or low-grade fever that can rapidly progress to high fever, respiratory distress, and hypoxemia or Children's Interstitial and diffuse Lung Disease (chILD) syndrome. An obvious portal of infection, such as an intravascular catheter, may predispose to bacterial or fungal infection via hematogenous spread.

B. Laboratory Findings and Imaging Studies

Fungal, parasitic, or bacterial infection, especially with antibiotic-resistant bacteria, should be suspected in the neutropenic child. Cultures of peripheral blood and through intravascular catheters, sputum, tracheobronchial secretions, nasopharynx or sinuses, pleural fluid, biopsied lymph nodes, bone marrow, or skin lesions should be considered and obtained as soon as infection is suspected. Serum $(1, 3)$-β-d-glucan assays and serum and BAL galactomannan assays for invasive pulmonary fungal disease are being used in some centers. Urine can be tested for typical pathogens and *Legionella* urinary antigens.

Invasive methods are commonly required to make a diagnosis. Appropriate samples should be obtained soon after a patient with pneumonia fails to respond to initial treatment. The results of these procedures usually lead to important changes in empiric therapy. Sputum is often unavailable in the young child. BAL frequently detects one or more organisms and should be done early in evaluation. The combined use of a wash, brushing, endobronchial biopsy, and lavage has a high yield. In patients with rapidly advancing, or more peripheral disease, lung biopsy becomes more urgent. The morbidity and mortality of this procedure can be reduced by VATS techniques.

Because of the multiplicity of organisms that may cause disease, a comprehensive set of studies should be done on lavage and biopsy material. These consist of rapid diagnostic studies including culture, PCR, and antigen detection for viruses and rapid fluorescent antibody studies for *P jiroveci* and *Legionella*; Gram, acid-fast, and fungal stains; cytologic examination for viral inclusions; and cultures for anaerobic and aerobic bacteria, fungi, mycobacteria, and *Legionella*.

Chest radiographs and volumetric CT scans may be useful in identifying the pattern and extent of disease. In early *P jiroveci* pneumonia, dyspnea and hypoxemia may be marked despite minimal radiographic abnormalities. Distinctive radiographic findings such as the halo sign can be seen in aspergillosis.

▶ Differential Diagnosis

The organisms causing disease vary with the type of immunocompromise present. For example, the splenectomized or sickle cell disease patient may be overwhelmed by infection with encapsulated bacteria. The child with HIV/AIDS or receiving immunosuppressant therapy or chemotherapy is more likely to have *P jiroveci* infection. The febrile neutropenic child who has been receiving adequate doses of intravenous broad-spectrum antibiotics or systemic steroid therapy may have fungal disease. The key to diagnosis is to consider all possibilities of infection.

Depending on the form of immunocompromise, perhaps only one-half to two-thirds of new pulmonary infiltrates in such patients represent infection. The remaining infiltrates are caused by pulmonary toxicity of radiation, chemotherapy, or other drugs; pulmonary disorders, including hemorrhage, embolism, atelectasis, or aspiration; idiopathic pneumonia syndrome or acute respiratory distress syndrome in bone marrow transplant patients; recurrence or extension of primary malignant growths or immunologic disorders; transfusion reactions, leukostasis, or tumor cell lysis; or ILD, such as lymphocytic interstitial pneumonitis with HIV infection.

▶ Complications

Necrotizing pneumonia, lung abscess, and parapneumonic effusions can develop. Progressive respiratory failure, shock, multiple organ damage, disseminated infection, and death commonly occur in the infected immunocompromised host.

▶ Treatment

Early use of broad-spectrum intravenous antibiotics is indicated in febrile, neutropenic, or immunocompromised children. Trimethoprim-sulfamethoxazole (for *P jiroveci*), macrolides (for *Legionella*) are/or antifungals may also be indicated early in the treatment of immunocompromised children before an organism is identified. Targeted therapy should be based on studies of specimens obtained from BAL or lung biopsy. Recent data suggest that use of noninvasive ventilation strategies early in the course of pulmonary insufficiency or respiratory failure may decrease mortality.

Prognosis

Prognosis is based on the severity of the underlying immunocompromise, appropriate early diagnosis and treatment, and the infecting organisms. Intubation and mechanical ventilation have been associated with high mortality, especially in hematopoietic stem cell transplant patients.

Collaco JM, Gower WA, Mogayzel PJ Jr: Pulmonary dysfunction in pediatric hematopoietic stem cell transplant patients: overview, diagnostic considerations, and infectious complications. Pediatr Blood Cancer 2007;49(2):117 [PMID: 17029246].

Nouér Simone A et al: Earlier response assessment in invasive aspergillosis based on the kinetics of serum Aspergillus galactomannan: proposal for a new definition. Clin Infect Dis 2011;53(7):671 [PMID: 21846834].

LUNG ABSCESS

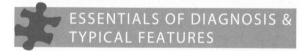

ESSENTIALS OF DIAGNOSIS & TYPICAL FEATURES

► High fever, malaise, and weight loss in the setting of pneumonia.

► Chest radiographs and CT scans usually reveal lung cavities, often with air-fluid levels.

Pathogenesis

Lung abscesses are thick-walled cavities that form from inflammation and central necrosis following an initial pulmonary infection. A lung abscess can occur in a previously well child, a child prone to aspiration, or in children with immunosuppression or underlying lung or systemic disease. Lung abscesses may also occur via embolic spread. Organisms such as staphylococci and streptococci more commonly affect the healthy host, while anaerobic and gram-negative organisms as well as *Nocardia*, mycobacteria, *Legionella* species, fungi (*Candida* and *Aspergillus*), and drug-resistant pathogens should be considered in the immunocompromised host or in patients not responding to typical antibiotic treatment.

Clinical Findings

A. Symptoms and Signs

Symptoms and signs referable to the chest may or may not be present. High fever, malaise, and weight loss are often present. In infants, evidence of respiratory distress can be present.

B. Laboratory Findings and Imaging Studies

Elevated peripheral white blood cell count with a neutrophil predominance or an elevated erythrocyte sedimentation rate or CRP may be present. Blood cultures are rarely positive except in the immunocompromised patient.

Chest radiographs usually reveal single or multiple thick-walled lung cavities, often with air-fluid levels. Local compressive atelectasis, pleural thickening, or adenopathy may also occur. Chest CT scan may provide better localization and understanding of the lesions.

In patients producing sputum, stains, and cultures may provide the diagnosis. Direct percutaneous aspiration of material for stains and cultures should be considered although complications can occur.

Differential Diagnosis

Loculated pyopneumothorax, neoplasms, plasma cell granuloma, and infected congenital cysts and sequestrations should be considered. Pneumatoceles, non–fluid-filled cysts, are common in children with empyema and usually resolve over time.

Complications

Although complications due to abscesses are now rare, mediastinal shift, tension pneumothorax, and spontaneous rupture can occur. Diagnostic maneuvers such as radiology-guided lung puncture to drain and culture the abscess may also cause pneumothorax or a bronchopulmonary fistula.

Treatment

Because of the risks of lung puncture, uncomplicated abscesses are frequently conservatively treated in the immune competent host with appropriate broad-spectrum intravenous antibiotics. Additional coverage for anaerobic gram-negative organisms and fungi should be provided for others. Prolonged therapy with 2–3 weeks of intravenous antibiotics followed by oral therapy may be required. Attempts to drain abscesses via bronchoscopy have caused life-threatening airway compromise. Surgical drainage or lobectomy is occasionally required, primarily in immunocompromised patients. However, such procedures may themselves cause life-threatening complications.

Prognosis

Although radiographic resolution may be very slow (6 weeks–5 years), resolution occurs in most patients without risk factors for lower respiratory tract infections or loss of pulmonary function. In the immunocompromised or medically complex host, the outlook depends on the underlying disorder.

Chan PC et al: Clinical management and outcome of childhood lung abscess: a 16-year experience. J Microbiol Immunol Infect 2005;38:183 [PMID: 15986068].

Patradoon-HoP et al: Lung abscess in children. Paediatr Respir Rev 2007;8(1):77–84 [PMID: 17419981].

▼ BRONCHIOLITIS OBLITERANS

 ESSENTIALS OF DIAGNOSIS & TYPICAL FEATURES

▶ Persistent symptoms of airway obstruction 8 weeks after the resolution of a lower respiratory tract infection.

▶ Chest CT shows a mosaic pattern of hyperinflation and vascular attenuation.

Bronchiolitis obliterans is a rare chronic obstructive lung disease characterized by complete obliteration of the small airways following a severe insult. The most common etiology in children is post-infectious, following a lower airway tract infection with adenovirus, although influenza, rubeola, *Bordetella*, and *Mycoplasma* are also implicated. Other causes include connective tissue diseases, chronic aspiration, Stevens-Johnson syndrome, posttransplantation (lung or bone marrow), and inhalational injury. Many cases of bronchiolitis obliterans are idiopathic. Mechanical ventilation for severe adenoviral respiratory infection is a strong risk factor for development of bronchiolitis obliterans.

▶ Clinical Findings

A. Symptoms and Signs

Persons with bronchiolitis obliterans usually experience dyspnea, coughing, and exercise intolerance. This diagnosis should be considered in children with persistent cough, wheezing, crackles, or hypoxemia lasting longer than 60 days following a lower respiratory tract infection.

B. Laboratory Findings and Imaging Studies

Chest radiograph abnormalities include evidence of heterogeneous air trapping and airway wall thickening. Traction bronchiectasis can occur as the disease progresses. Classic findings on chest CT include a mosaic perfusion pattern, vascular attenuation, and central bronchiectasis. After hematopoietic stem cell transplantation, bronchiectasis may not be present. This finding along with pulmonary function testing showing airway obstruction unresponsive to bronchodilators may be diagnostic in patients with the appropriate clinical history. Although not typically required for diagnosis, ventilation-perfusion scans may show a pattern of ventilation and perfusion mismatch. Pulmonary angiograms reveal decreased vasculature in involved lung, and bronchograms show marked pruning of the bronchial tree. Lung biopsy is necessary typically only in cases where clinical history and/or CT scan are not classic. Pathologic findings include airway scarring (eg, with fibrin) with partial or complete obstruction of bronchioles.

▶ Differential Diagnosis

Poorly treated asthma with remodeling, CF, and BPD must be considered in children with persistent airway obstruction. A trial of medications (including bronchodilators and corticosteroids) may help determine the reversibility of the process when the primary differential is between asthma and bronchiolitis obliterans. Others without classic findings on CT scan and lung function testing may require a lung biopsy.

▶ Complications

Sequelae of bronchiolitis obliterans include persistent airway obstruction, recurrent wheezing, bronchiectasis, chronic atelectasis, recurrent pneumonia, and unilateral hyperlucent lung syndrome.

▶ Treatment

Supportive care, including supplemental oxygen for hypoxemia, routine vaccination, avoidance of environmental irritant exposure, exercise, and nutritional support should be provided. Ongoing airway damage due to problems such as aspiration should be prevented. Inhaled bronchodilators (β-agonists and anticholinergic) may reverse airway obstruction if the disease has a reactive component. Systemic corticosteroids may help reverse the obstruction or prevent ongoing damage; these can be given orally or with monthly intravenous doses (intravenous doses may decrease systemic side effects). Azithromycin is beneficial in bronchiolitis obliterans syndrome after lung transplantation and in patients with bronchiectasis. Fluticasone, azithromycin, and montelukast have been used to treat bronchiolitis obliterans after hematopoietic stem cell transplantation. There are concerns for disease recurrence (ie, leukemia) with prophylactic use of azithromycin. Lung transplant may be an option for patients with severe, progressive disease. If bronchiectasis is present, airway clearance and early antibiotics with respiratory illnesses (ie, to treat endobronchitis) are helpful.

▶ Prognosis

Prognosis depends in part on the underlying cause as well as the age of onset. Postinfectious bronchiolitis obliterans tends to be nonprogressive with low mortality and the possibility of slow improvement. Conversely, posttransplantation or Stevens-Johnson syndrome–related bronchiolitis obliterans may have a rapidly progressive course leading to death or need for lung transplantation.

Colom AJ et al: Pulmonary function of a paediatric cohort of patients with postinfectious bronchiolitis obliterans. A long term follow-up. Thorax 2015 Feb;70(2):169–174 [PMID: 25388479].

Kutzke JL et al: Relapse rates in patients receiving azithromycin for the treatment of bronchiolitis obliterans after allogeneic hematopoietic stem cell transplant. Biol Blood Marrow Transplant 2019; Mar 1;25(3):S286.

Li YN et al: Post-infectious bronchiolitis obliterans in children: a review of 42 cases. BMC Pediatr Sep 25, 2014;14:238 [PMID: 25252824].

Teixeira MFC, Rodrigues JC, Leone C, Adde FV: Acute bronchodilator responsiveness to tiotropium in postinfectious bronchiolitis obliterans in children. Chest 2013;144(30):974–980 [PMID: 23558666].

Tomikawa SO et al: Follow-up on pediatric patients with bronchiolitis obliterans treated with corticosteroid pulse therapy. Orphanet J Rare Dis 2014 Aug 15;9:128 [PMID: 25124141].

Williams KM et al: Fluticasone, azithromycin, and montelukast treatment for new-onset bronchiolitis obliterans syndrome after hematopoietic cell transplantation. Biol Blood Marrow Transplant 22.4 (2016):710–716 [PMID: 26475726].

CHILDREN'S INTERSTITIAL LUNG DISEASE SYNDROME

ESSENTIALS OF DIAGNOSIS & TYPICAL FEATURES

▶ Diverse group of rare pulmonary disorders: somewhat more unique in children younger than 2 years but can occur at any age.

▶ Can involve the airways, alveoli, and/or interstitium.

▶ Diagnosis: First exclude more common pulmonary diseases that can have similar presentations: CF, PCD, BPD, aspiration, etc. Patients present with at least three of the following:

- Respiratory symptoms such as tachypnea, retractions, cough, wheeze, dyspnea

- Respiratory signs such as crackles, wheezing, decreased breath sounds, clubbing, weight loss

- Hypoxemia breathing ambient room air

- Abnormality on chest imaging: chest CT scan or plain CXR

▶ May need a lung biopsy for precise diagnosis.

Children's Interstitial and diffuse Lung Disease (chILD) syndrome describes a constellation of signs and symptoms and not a specific diagnosis (Table 19–7). Once recognized, chILD syndrome should elicit a search for a more specific

Table 19–7. Classification of diffuse lung diseases in infancy and childhood.

Developmental disorders	Acinar dysplasia
	Congenital alveolar dysplasia
	Alveolar capillary dysplasia with misaligned pulmonary veins
Growth abnormalities	Pulmonary hypoplasia
	Chronic neonatal lung disease/bronchopulmonary dysplasia (BPD)
	Related to chromosomal defects (eg, Down syndrome)
	Related to congenital heart disease with normal chromosomes
Specific conditions with undefined etiology	Pulmonary interstitial glycogenosis (PIG)
	Neuroendocrine cell hyperplasia of infancy (NEHI)
Disorders of surfactant metabolism (Genetic disorders of surfactant protein B, surfactant protein C, ABCA3, and TTF1 or NKX2.1)	Pulmonary alveolar proteinosis (PAP)
	Chronic pneumonitis of infancy (CPI)
	Desquamative interstitial pneumonia (DIP)
	Nonspecific interstitial pneumonitis (NSIP)
Disorders in a normal host	Infectious and postinfectious processes (eg, bronchiolitis obliterans [BO])
	Hypersensitivity pneumonitis (HP)
	Chronic aspiration syndromes
	Eosinophilic pneumonia
	Toxic inhalations
Associated with systemic diseases	Rheumatologic diseases
	Storage diseases
	Sarcoidosis
	Langerhans cell histiocytosis
	Malignant Infiltrates
	Alveolar hemorrhage syndromes and vasculitis
	Tuberous sclerosis with lymphangioleiomyomatosis
Immunocompromised host	Opportunistic infections
	Drug toxicities
	Idiopathic diffuse alveolar damage (DAH)
	Lymphoid hyperplasia and lymphoid interstitial pneumonitis (LIP)
	Lymphoproliferative disease
Lymphatic disorders	Lymphangiectasis
	Lymphangiomatosis

Data Kurland G, Deterding RR, Hagood JS, et al: An official American Thoracic Society clinical practice guideline: classification, evaluation, and management of childhood interstitial lung disease in infancy. Am J Respir Crit Care Med. 2013 Aug 1;188(3):376–94; Dishop MK: Diagnostic Pathology of Diffuse Lung Disease in Children. Pediatr Allergy Immunol Pulmonol. 2010 Mar;23(1):69–85.

diagnosis. More common pulmonary diseases that can present similarly to chILD should be evaluated and excluded first, including CF, cardiac disease, asthma, acute infection, immunodeficiency, neuromuscular disease, thoracic cage abnormality, chronic lung disease of prematurity, and aspiration.

Clinical Findings

A. Symptoms and Signs

chILD presents acutely in infants and young children with respiratory failure and inability to wean supplemental O_2 or alternatively insidiously with cough, exercise intolerance, clubbing, dyspnea, tachypnea, retractions, hypoxemia, barrel chest, and failure to thrive. Crackles are common on chest auscultation.

B. Laboratory Findings

After a comprehensive history and examination, initial evaluation may include PFTs, allergy skin tests, complete blood count with WBC differential, CRP and erythrocyte sedimentation rate (ESR), and comprehensive metabolic panel. Cardiac evaluation including an electrocardiogram and echocardiogram should be obtained. Immunologic assessment includes serum immunoglobulins and markers of collagen vascular disease. DNA analysis for surfactant protein dysfunction syndromes is done commonly in young children.

C. Imaging Studies

Chest radiographs are normal in up to 10%–15% of patients, but volumetric CT scans are always abnormal. Certain specific chILD disorders such as bronchiolitis obliterans and neuroendocrine cell hyperplasia of infancy can be diagnosed by characteristic CT findings alone.

D. Special Tests

Pulmonary function testing is typically abnormal in chILD. Depending on the specific type of chILD, PFTs may show (1) a restrictive pattern of decreased lung volumes, compliance, and carbon monoxide diffusing capacity, (2) an obstructive pattern with hyperinflation, or (3) a mixed obstructive-restrictive pattern. Six-minute walk test often demonstrates SpO_2 desaturation and reduced distance capacity. Exercise-induced or nocturnal hypoxemia may be the earliest physiologic abnormality in chILD.

Bronchoscopy can exclude anatomic abnormalities and obtain BAL for microbiologic and cytologic testing but is seldom diagnostic alone. Commercial genetic testing is available for surfactant dysfunction mutations (*SFTPB*, *SFTPC*, *ABCA3*, and *NKX2*.1), alveolar capillary dysplasia (*FOXF1*), pulmonary alveolar proteinosis (GMCSF receptor mutations or autoantibodies), and pulmonary hemorrhage (COPA). Lung biopsy is often required for a definitive diagnosis, and video-assisted thoracoscopically lung biopsies are preferred.

Differential Diagnosis

Many disorders have similar presentations: CF cardiac disease, asthma, acute infection, immunodeficiency, neuromuscular disease, scoliosis, thoracic cage abnormality, chronic lung disease of prematurity, and aspiration.

Complications

Complications from chILD include being behind in school, failure to thrive, respiratory insufficiency, respiratory failure, and pulmonary hypertension. Mortality and morbidity can be significant and varies by specific diagnosis.

Treatment

The mainstays of treatment include support with supplemental O_2 and nutritional support. Corticosteroids are used for many of the specific chILD diagnoses as well as other disease specific medications. Patients with severe disease may need noninvasive respiratory support. All patients should be evaluated for comorbidities such as pulmonary hypertension, aspiration, failure to thrive, sleep apnea and hypoxemia. All vaccines should be provided, including annual influenza vaccine, palivizumab in infancy, and pneumococcal polysaccharide vaccine. Nutritional and respiratory support should be provided as appropriate to encourage optimal growth and development. Environmental irritant exposure (recreational and occupational) should be avoided. Most treatment for chILD is disease specific and based on expert opinion, case reports, and small case series. Children with chILD should be evaluated and cared for by an experienced multidisciplinary team. Lung transplantation may be an option for patients with progressive respiratory failure. The chILD Family Foundation can provide further supportive resources for families (http://www.childfoundation.us).

Prognosis

Prognosis varies by chILD diagnosis from mild disease to progressive respiratory failure and death.

Spagnolo P, Bush A: Interstitial lung disease in children younger than 2 years. Pediatrics 2016;137:e20152725 [PMID: 27245831].

Thacker PG, Vargas SO, Fishman MP, Casey AM, Lee EY: Current update on interstitial lung disease in infancy: new classification system, diagnostic evaluation, imaging algorithms, imaging findings, and prognosis. Radiol Clin N Am 2016;54:1065–1076 [PMID: 27719976].

Vece TJ, Young LR: Update on diffuse lung disease in children. Chest 2016;149:836–845 [PMID: 26502226].

HYPERSENSITIVITY PNEUMONITIS

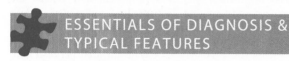

ESSENTIALS OF DIAGNOSIS & TYPICAL FEATURES

▶ Recurrent respiratory symptoms, especially exercise intolerance, cough, weight loss, and fever.

▶ History of exposure to an inhaled organic particle (birds) or low molecular weight chemicals.

Hypersensitivity pneumonitis (HP), or extrinsic allergic alveolitis, is a T-cell–mediated disease involving the peripheral airways, interstitium, and alveoli. The disease is triggered by the host response to an environmental exposure. Both acute and chronic forms may occur. In children, the most common antigen(s) are birds or bird droppings (eg, pigeons, parakeets, parrots, or doves); this is also known as "bird fancier's lung." However, a multitude of antigens have been documented to cause HP, including moldy hay, compost, logs or tree bark, sawdust, or aerosols from humidifiers or hot tubs. Methotrexate-induced hypersensitivity has also been described in a child with juvenile rheumatoid arthritis. Hot tub lung can be caused by exposure to aerosolized *Mycobacterium avium* complex. A high level of suspicion and a thorough environmental exposure history are required for diagnosis.

▶ Clinical Findings

A. Symptoms and Signs

Episodic cough and fever can occur following acute exposures. Chronic exposure results in weight loss, fatigue, hypoxemia, and dyspnea. Physical examination findings include crackles, loud cardiac P2, and clubbing.

B. Laboratory Findings and Imaging Studies

Acute exposure may cause polymorphonuclear leukocytosis with eosinophilia and airway obstruction or restriction on lung function testing. Chronic HP results in a restrictive pattern.

Serum precipitins (precipitating IgG antibodies) to the triggering antigen may be detected, but perhaps only if the identical antigen is used. The cell counts on BAL typically show lymphocytosis. Chest radiograph findings are variable and may include normal lung fields, air-space consolidation, and linear nodular or reticulonodular opacities. Chest CT often shows small centrilobular nodules, ground-glass opacities, and air-trapping. Chronic HP may progress to pulmonary fibrosis.

Lung biopsy reveals bronchiolocentric interstitial lymphocytic inflammation interstitial nonnecrotizing, poorly formed granulomas, and intraalveolar foci of organizing pneumonia.

▶ Differential Diagnosis

Patients with acute symptoms must be differentiated from acute asthma exacerbations. Patients with chronic symptoms must be distinguished from chILD due to collagen-vascular, immunologic dysfunction, or other forms of chILD.

▶ Complications

Prolonged exposure to offending antigens may result in pulmonary hypertension due to chronic hypoxemia, irreversible restrictive lung disease, and pulmonary fibrosis.

▶ Treatment & Prognosis

The primary goal is complete elimination of exposure to the offending antigen. Corticosteroids treatment is controversial. With early diagnosis and avoidance of offending antigens, the prognosis is excellent.

Vasakova M, Morell F, Walsh S, Leslie K, Raghu G: Hypersensitivity pneumonitis: perspectives in diagnosis and management. Am Rev Respir Crit Care Med 2017;196:680–689 [PMID: 28598197].

▼ DISEASES OF THE PULMONARY CIRCULATION

PULMONARY HEMORRHAGE

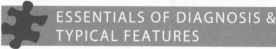

ESSENTIALS OF DIAGNOSIS & TYPICAL FEATURES

▶ History of hemoptysis.

▶ New-onset respiratory distress, oxygen requirement, or fatigue with evidence of infiltrate by chest imaging and blood in the tracheal aspirate.

Pulmonary hemorrhage can be caused by a spectrum of disorders affecting the large and small airways and alveoli. It can occur as an acute or chronic process. If pulmonary hemorrhage is subacute or chronic, hemosiderin-laden macrophages can be found in tracheal aspirates 48–72 hours after the bleeding begins. Many cases are secondary to bacterial, mycobacterial, parasitic, viral, or fungal infections (such as the toxigenic mold *Stachybotrys chartarum*). Lung abscess, bronchiectasis (from CF or other causes), foreign body, coagulopathy (often with overwhelming sepsis), or elevated pulmonary venous pressure (secondary to congestive heart failure, anatomic heart lesions, or ascent to high altitude) may also cause pulmonary hemorrhage. Other causes include lung contusion from trauma, pulmonary embolus with infarction, arteriovenous fistula or telangiectasias, autoimmune vasculitis, HP pulmonary sequestration, agenesis of a single pulmonary artery, and esophageal duplication or bronchogenic cyst. In children, pulmonary hemorrhage due to airway tumors (eg, bronchial adenoma) is very rare.

Hemorrhage involving the alveoli is termed diffuse alveolar hemorrhage. This may be idiopathic, drug-related, or may occur in Goodpasture syndrome, rapidly progressive glomerulonephritis, and systemic vasculitides (often associated with such collagen-vascular diseases as systemic lupus erythematosus, rheumatoid arthritis, Wegener granulomatosis, polyarteritis nodosa, Henoch-Schönlein purpura, and Behçet disease). Idiopathic pulmonary hemosiderosis refers to the accumulation of hemosiderin in the lung, especially in alveolar macrophages, as a result of chronic or recurrent hemorrhage (usually from pulmonary capillaries) that is not associated with the previously listed causes. Children and young adults are mainly affected, with the age at onset ranging from 6 months to 20 years.

▶ Clinical Findings

A. Symptoms and Signs

Large airway hemorrhage presents with hemoptysis and symptoms of the underlying cause, such as infection, foreign body, or bronchiectasis in CF. Hemoptysis from larger airways is often bright red or contains clots. Children with diffuse alveolar hemorrhage may present with massive hemoptysis, marked respiratory distress, stridor, or a pneumonia-like syndrome. However, most patients with diffuse alveolar hemorrhage and idiopathic pulmonary hemosiderosis present with nonspecific respiratory symptoms (cough, tachypnea, and retractions) with or without hemoptysis, poor growth, and fatigue. Fever, abdominal pain, and chest pain may also be reported. Jaundice and hepatosplenomegaly may be present with chronic bleeding. Physical examination often reveals decreased breath sounds, rales, rhonchi, or wheezing and digital clubbing.

B. Laboratory Findings and Imaging Studies

Laboratory studies depend on the cause of hemorrhage. When gross hemoptysis is present, large airway bronchiectasis, epistaxis, foreign body, and arteriovenous malformations should be considered. Flexible bronchoscopy and imaging (MRI or CT-assisted angiography) can be used to localize the site of bleeding. Alveolar bleeding with hemoptysis is often frothy and pink. Long-standing idiopathic pulmonary hemorrhage may cause iron deficiency anemia and heme-positive sputum. Nonspecific findings may include lymphocytosis and an elevated erythrocyte sedimentation rate. Peripheral eosinophilia is present in up to 25% of patients. Chest radiographs may demonstrate perihilar infiltrates, fluffy alveolar infiltrates with or without atelectasis, and mediastinal adenopathy. Pulmonary function testing generally reveals restrictive impairment, with low lung volumes, poor compliance, and an increased diffusion capacity. Hemosiderin-laden macrophages are found in the BAL fluid and tracheal aspirates. The diagnostic usefulness of lung biopsy is controversial.

Patients with diffuse alveolar hemorrhage with an underlying systemic disease may need a lung biopsy. In patients with systemic lupus erythematosus, granulomatosis and polyangiitis (formerly called Wegener granulomatosis), and occasionally Goodpasture syndrome diffuse alveolar hemorrhage can occur in the setting of necrotizing pulmonary capillaritis. Lung biopsy reveals alveolar septa infiltrated with neutrophils, edema, or necrosis in addition to alveolar hemorrhage. Idiopathic pulmonary hemosiderosis is a mild form of capillaritis associated with focal or diffuse alveolar hemorrhage. Other causes of pulmonary hemosiderosis include collagen-vascular disease, immune-mediated vasculitis, and pulmonary fibrosis must be ruled out to diagnose idiopathic pulmonary hemosiderosis. Lung biopsy often shows immune-mediated capillaritis in the absence of an identifiable serologic marker. Serologic studies such as circulating antineutrophilic cytoplasmic autoantibodies for Wegener granulomatosis, perinuclear antineutrophilic cytoplasmic autoantibodies for microscopic polyangiitis, antinuclear antibodies for systemic lupus erythematosus, and anti–basement membrane antibodies for Goodpasture syndrome should be obtained. α_1-Antitrypsin deficiency should also be considered.

Cow's milk-induced pulmonary hemosiderosis (Heiner syndrome) can be confirmed by high titers of serum precipitins to multiple constituents of cow's milk and positive intradermal skin tests to cow's milk proteins. Improvement after eliminating cow's milk supports the diagnosis.

▶ Differential Diagnosis

Bleeding from the nose or mouth can present as hemoptysis. Therefore, a complete examination of the nose and mouth is required before confirming the diagnosis of intrapulmonary bleeding. Hematemesis can also be confused with hemoptysis; confirming that the blood was produced after coughing and not with emesis should also be part of the initial evaluations. A complete past medical history including underlying systemic illness and cardiovascular anomalies may direct the search for the site of respiratory bleeding.

▶ **Treatment**

Therapy should be aimed at direct treatment of the underlying disease. In severe bleeding, intubation with application of positive pressure during mechanical ventilation and/or endotracheal administration of epinephrine may help attenuate bleeding. Patients with CF or bronchiectasis from other causes who develop massive (> 240 mL) or recurrent hemoptysis may require bronchial artery embolization. Although its use requires anticoagulation, extracorporeal life support has resulted in the survival of children with severe pulmonary hemorrhage. For chronic bleeding, supportive measures, including iron therapy, supplemental oxygen, and blood transfusions, may be needed. A diet free of cow's milk should be tried in infants. Systemic corticosteroids have been used for various causes of diffuse alveolar hemorrhage and have been particularly successful in those secondary to collagen-vascular disorders and vasculitis. Case reports have been published describing the variable effectiveness of steroids, chloroquine, cyclophosphamide, and azathioprine for idiopathic pulmonary hemosiderosis.

▶ **Prognosis**

The outcome of pulmonary hemorrhage depends on the cause of the bleeding and how much blood has been lost. The course of idiopathic pulmonary hemosiderosis is variable, characterized by a waxing and waning course of intermittent intrapulmonary bleeds and the gradual development of pulmonary fibrosis. The severity of the underlying renal disease influences mortality associated with Goodpasture syndrome and Wegener granulomatosis. Diffuse alveolar hemorrhage is considered a lethal pulmonary complication of systemic lupus erythematosus.

Bull TM et al: Pulmonary vascular manifestations of mixed connective tissue disease. Rheum Dis Clin North Am 2005;31:451 [PMID: 16084318].

Flume PA et al: Cystic Fibrosis Pulmonary Guidelines–Pulmonary Complications: Hemoptysis and Pneumothorax. Am J Respir Crit Care Med 2010;182(3):298 [PMID: 20675678].

Godfrey S: Pulmonary hemorrhage/hemoptysis in children. Pediatr Pulmonol 2004;37:476 [PMID: 15114547].

PULMONARY EMBOLISM

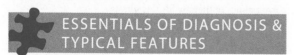

ESSENTIALS OF DIAGNOSIS & TYPICAL FEATURES

▶ Acute-onset dyspnea and tachypnea.

▶ Evidence of embolism on chest imaging.

Pulmonary embolism is a rare, but severe cause of respiratory distress in children. Etiologies include sickle cell anemia (as part of the acute chest syndrome), malignancy, rheumatic fever, infective endocarditis, bone fracture, dehydration, polycythemia, nephrotic syndrome, atrial fibrillation, and other conditions. Many children with pulmonary emboli referred for hematology evaluation have coagulation regulatory protein abnormalities and antiphospholipid antibodies. Emboli result in clinical signs and symptoms in proportion to the severity of pulmonary vascular obstruction. In children, tumor emboli are a more common cause of massive pulmonary embolism than embolization from a lower extremity deep venous thrombosis.

▶ **Clinical Findings**

A. Symptoms and Signs

Pulmonary embolism usually presents as an acute onset of dyspnea and tachypnea. Heart palpitations, pleuritic chest pain, and a sense of impending doom may be reported.

Hemoptysis is rare but may occur along with splinting, cyanosis, and tachycardia. Massive emboli may be present with syncope and cardiac arrhythmias. Physical examination is usually normal (except for tachycardia and tachypnea) unless the embolism is associated with an underlying disorder. Mild hypoxemia, rales, focal wheezing, or a pleural friction rub may be found.

B. Laboratory Findings and Imaging Studies

Radiographic findings may be normal, but a peripheral infiltrate, small pleural effusion, or elevated hemidiaphragm can be present. If the emboli are massive, differential blood flow and pulmonary artery enlargement may be appreciated. The electrocardiogram is usually normal unless the pulmonary embolus is massive. Echocardiography is useful in detecting the presence of a large embolus in the great vessels. A negative D-dimer has a more than 95% negative predictive value for an embolus, but has poor specificity. Ventilation-perfusion scans show localized areas of ventilation without perfusion.

Spiral CT with contrast may be helpful, but pulmonary angiography is the gold standard. A recent case series suggests that bedside chest ultrasound may aid in diagnosing pulmonary emboli, particularly in critically ill children. Further evaluation may include Doppler ultrasound studies of the legs to search for deep venous thrombosis. Coagulation studies, including assessments of antithrombin III, fibrinogen, antiphospholipid antibodies, homocysteine, coagulation regulatory proteins (proteins C and S, and factor V Leiden), and the prothrombin G20210A mutation are abnormal in up to 70% of pediatric patients with pulmonary embolism.

Treatment

Acute treatment includes supplemental oxygen, and anti-coagulation. Current recommendations include heparin therapy to maintain an activated partial thromboplastin time of greater than 1.5 times the control value for the first 24 hours. Urokinase or tissue plasminogen activator can be used to help dissolve the embolus. These therapies should be followed by warfarin therapy for at least 6 weeks with an international normalized ratio (INR) greater than 2.

Baird JS et al: Massive pulmonary embolism in children. J Pediatr 2010;156:148 [PMID: 20006766].

Konstantinides S et al: Heparin plus alteplase compared with heparin alone in patients with submassive pulmonary embolism. N Engl J Med 2002;347:1143 [PMID: 12374874].

Thacker PG, Lee EY: Pulmonary embolism in children. Am J Roentgenol 2015;204(6):1278–1288 [PMID: 26001239].

PULMONARY EDEMA

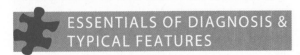

ESSENTIALS OF DIAGNOSIS & TYPICAL FEATURES

▶ Dyspnea and oxygen requirement.

▶ Evidence of pulmonary edema on chest imaging.

Pathogenesis

Pulmonary edema is excessive accumulation of extravascular fluid in the lung. This occurs when fluid is filtered into the lungs faster than it can be removed, leading to changes in lung mechanics such as decreased lung compliance, worsening hypoxemia from ventilation-perfusion mismatch, bronchial compression, and if advanced, decreased surfactant function. There are two basic types of pulmonary edema: increased pressure (cardiogenic or hydrostatic) and increased permeability (noncardiogenic or primary). Hydrostatic pulmonary edema is usually due to excessive increases in pulmonary venous pressure, in the setting of congestive heart failure. Postobstructive pulmonary edema occurs when airway occlusion (or its sudden relief) causes a sudden drop in airway pressure that leads to increased venous return and decreased left heart blood flow. These changes result in elevated hydrostatic pressures and transudation of fluid from the pulmonary capillaries to the alveolar space.

In contrast, many lung diseases, especially acute respiratory distress syndrome, are characterized by the development of pulmonary edema secondary to changes in permeability due to injury at the alveolar-capillary interface.

In this setting, pulmonary edema occurs independently of the elevations of pulmonary venous pressure.

Clinical Findings

A. Symptoms and Signs

Cyanosis, tachypnea, tachycardia, and respiratory distress are commonly present. Physical findings include rales, diminished breath sounds, and (in young infants) expiratory wheezing. More severe disease is characterized by progressive respiratory distress with marked retractions, dyspnea, and severe hypoxemia.

B. Imaging Studies

Chest radiographic findings depend on the cause of the edema. Pulmonary vessels are prominent, often with diffuse interstitial or alveolar infiltrates. Heart size is usually normal in permeability edema but enlarged in hydrostatic edema.

Treatment

Although specific therapy depends on the underlying cause, supplemental oxygen therapy and ventilator support may be indicated. Diuretics, digoxin, and vasodilators may be indicated for congestive heart failure along with restriction of salt and water. Loop diuretics, such as furosemide, are primarily beneficial because they increase systemic venous capacitance, not because they induce diuresis. Improvement can even be seen in anuric patients. Recommended interventions for pulmonary edema include reduction of vascular volume and maintenance of the lowest central venous or pulmonary arterial wedge pressure possible without sacrificing cardiac output or causing hypotension (see following discussion). β-Adrenergic agonists such as terbutaline have been shown to increase alveolar clearance of lung water, perhaps through the action of a sodium-potassium channel pump. Maintaining normal albumin levels and a hematocrit concentration above 30 maintains the filtration of lung liquid toward the capillaries.

High-altitude pulmonary edema (HAPE) occurs when susceptible individuals develop noncardiogenic edema after rapid ascent to altitudes above 3000 m. HAPE in children may be variable. Oxygen therapy and prompt descent are the cornerstones of therapy for this illness.

Bartsch P et al: Physiologic aspects of high-altitude pulmonary edema. J Appl Physiol 2005;98:1101 [PMID: 15703168].

O'Brodovich H: Pulmonary edema in infants and children. Curr Opin Pediatr 2005;17:381 [PMID: 15891430].

Udeshi A et al: Postobstructive pulmonary edema. J Crit Care 2010;25:508 [PMID: 20413250].

CONGENITAL PULMONARY LYMPHANGIECTASIA

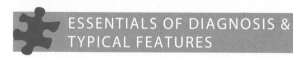

ESSENTIALS OF DIAGNOSIS & TYPICAL FEATURES

▶ Respiratory distress and oxygen requirement at birth.

▶ Diagnosed by chest CT shows dilated lymphatic suggested by interstitial prominence.

Congenital pulmonary lymphangiectasia consists of dilated subpleural and interlobular lymphatic channels, often as part of a generalized lymphangiectasis (in association with obstructive cardiovascular lesions—especially total anomalous pulmonary venous return) or as an isolated idiopathic lesion. Pathologically, the lung appears firm, bulky, and noncompressible, with prominent cystic lymphatics visible beneath the pleura. On cut section, dilated lymphatics are present near the hilum, along interlobular septa, around bronchovascular bundles, and beneath the pleura. Histologically, dilated lymphatics have a thin endothelial cell lining overlying a delicate network of elastin and collagen.

▶ Clinical Findings

Congenital pulmonary lymphangiectasia is a rare, usually fatal, disease that generally presents as acute, severe, or persistent respiratory distress at birth. There are reports of children developing symptoms in the first few months of life and others report diagnosis later in childhood. Chylothorax has been reported. Chest radiographic findings include a ground-glass appearance, prominent interstitial markings suggesting lymphatic distention, diffuse hyperlucency of the pulmonary parenchyma, and hyperinflation with depression of the diaphragm.

Congenital pulmonary lymphangiectasia may be associated with Noonan syndrome, asplenia, total anomalous pulmonary venous return, septal defects, atrioventricular canal, hypoplastic left heart, aortic arch malformations, and renal malformations. Patients with generalized lymphangiectasia have less severe pulmonary disease.

▶ Prognosis

The outcomes for children with congenital pulmonary lymphangiectasia are improving due to improvements in perinatal respiratory support and care. Most deaths occur within weeks after birth and thereafter respiratory symptoms improve after the first year of life suggesting that maximal medical treatment remains warranted. In those with the most severe disease, rapid diagnosis is essential in order to expedite the option of lung transplantation.

Reiterer F et al: Congenital pulmonary lymphangiectasia. Pediatr Resp Rev 2014;15(3):275–280 [PMID: 24997116].

▼ DISORDERS OF THE CHEST WALL

SCOLIOSIS

ESSENTIALS OF DIAGNOSIS & TYPICAL FEATURES

▶ Scoliosis is a lateral curve of the spine. Pectus carinatum is a protrusion of the sternum while pectus excavatum is an anterior depression of the chest wall.

▶ Scoliosis is a common cause of restrictive lung disease in children.

Scoliosis is defined as lateral curvature of the spine and is categorized as idiopathic, congenital, or neuromuscular. No pulmonary impairment is typically seen with a Cobb angle showing thoracic curvature of less than 35 degrees. Most cases of idiopathic scoliosis occur in adolescent girls and are corrected before significant pulmonary impairment occurs. Congenital scoliosis of severe degree or with other major abnormalities carries a more guarded prognosis. Patients with progressive neuromuscular disease, such as Duchenne muscular dystrophy, can be at risk for respiratory failure due to severe scoliosis and restrictive lung disease. Severe scoliosis can also lead to impaired lung function and, if uncorrected, possible death from cor pulmonale. (See also Chapter 26.) Small studies indicate that surgical correction of neuromuscular scoliosis should lead to improved quality of life, although pulmonary function may not improve.

Gill I: Correction of neuromuscular scoliosis in patients with preexisting respiratory failure. Spine 2006;31(21):2478–2483 [PMID: 17023858].

Johnston CE et al: Correlation of preoperative deformity magnitude and pulmonary function tests in adolescent idiopathic scoliosis. Spine 2011;36:1096–1102 [PMID: 21270699].

PECTUS CARINATUM

Pectus carinatum is a protrusion of the upper or lower (more common) portion of the sternum, more commonly seen in males. Impairment of cardiopulmonary function due to pectus carinatum is debated. The decision to repair this deformity is often based on cosmetic concerns. Patients with reduced endurance or dyspnea with mild exercise experienced marked improvement within 6 months following repair, suggesting possible physiologic indications. Pectus carinatum may be associated with systemic diseases such as the mucopolysaccharidoses and congenital heart disease.

Lawson ML et al: Impact of pectus excavatum on pulmonary function before and after repair with the Nuss procedure. J Pediatr Surg 2005;40:174 [PMID: 15868581].

Obermeyer RJ, Goretsky MJ: Chest wall deformities in pediatric surgery. Surg Clin North Am 2012;92(3):669–684 [PMID: 22595715].

PECTUS EXCAVATUM

Pectus excavatum is anterior depression of the chest wall that may be symmetrical or asymmetrical with respect to the midline. The effect of pectus excavatum on cardiopulmonary function is controversial. While subjective exertional dyspnea can be reported and may improve with repair, objective cardiopulmonary function may not change postoperatively. Therefore, the decision to repair the deformity may be based on cosmetic or physiologic considerations. Timing of repair is critical and based on growth plate maturation. Pectus excavatum may be associated with congenital heart disease, PCD, and neuromuscular disorders.

Obermeyer RJ, Goretsky MJ: Chest wall deformities in pediatric surgery. Surg Clin North Am 2012;92(3):669–684 [PMID: 22595715].

Williams AM, Crabbe DC: Pectus deformities of the anterior chest wall. Paediatr Respir Rev 2003;4:237 [PMID: 12880759].

NEUROMUSCULAR DISORDERS & LUNG DISEASE

ESSENTIALS OF DIAGNOSIS & TYPICAL FEATURES

▶ Neuromuscular disease is associated with impaired cough, sleep-disordered breathing (SDB), and restrictive lung disease in children.

Neuromuscular disorders are discussed in detail in Chapter 25. Weakness of the diaphragm, intercostal muscles, and pharyngeal muscles leads to chronic or recurrent pneumonia secondary to weak cough and poor mucus clearance, aspiration and infection, persistent atelectasis, hypoventilation, and respiratory failure in severe cases. Scoliosis, which frequently accompanies neuromuscular disorders, may further compromise respiratory function. Children born with significant neuromuscular weakness may present with signs and symptoms of respiratory distress or failure early in life. The time to presentation for children with progressive or acquired neuromuscular disease depends on the underlying neuromuscular defect. Typical examination findings in children at increased risk for pulmonary disease are a weak cough, decreased air exchange, crackles, and dullness to percussion. The child also may have symptoms of sleep-related hypoventilation or OSA.

Positional changes in chest movement and paradoxical thoracoabdominal movement during quiet breathing are indications of respiratory insufficiency. Signs of cor pulmonale may be evident in advanced cases. Chest radiographs generally show small lung volumes. Other radiographic findings include abnormal rib orientation and generalized osteopenia of disuse. If chronic aspiration is present, increased interstitial infiltrates and areas of atelectasis or consolidation may be present. Arterial blood gases demonstrate hypoxemia in the early stages and compensated respiratory acidosis in the late stages. Typical pulmonary function abnormalities include decreased vital capacity, decreased inspiratory and/or expiratory pressure, and decreased peak cough flow.

▶ Treatment & Prognosis

Treatment is supportive and includes vigorous airway clearance with a focus on assisted cough maneuvers, noninvasive ventilation, and antibiotics with infection. Supplemental oxygen may correct hypoxemia but does not correct the mechanical defect leading to hypoxemia. Depending on the diagnosis, routine PSG may be indicated to identify hypoventilation before it becomes clinically apparent. Consideration of bilevel positive airway pressure and mechanical airway clearance support, like mechanical in-exsufflation, should be introduced before respiratory failure is present. Due to risk of malignant hyperthermia and difficulty extubating, expert consultation prior to any anesthesia is required.

Many neuromuscular conditions progress to respiratory failure and death. The decision to intubate and ventilate is a difficult one; it should be made only when there is real hope that deterioration, though acute, is potentially reversible or when chronic ventilation is desired. Chronic mechanical ventilation using either noninvasive or invasive techniques is being used more frequently in patients with chronic respiratory insufficiency. New therapies in spinal muscular atrophy, including gene replacement and antisense oligonucleotide, are changing the landscape of this disease.

Finkel RS et al; SMA Care group: Diagnosis and management of spinal muscular atrophy: Part 2: pulmonary and acute care; medications, supplements and immunizations; other organ systems; and ethics. Neuromuscul Disord 2018 Mar;28(3):197–207 [PMID: 29305137].

Sheehan DW et al: Respiratory management of the patient with Duchenne muscular dystrophy. Pediatrics 2018 Oct;142(Suppl 2): S62–S71 [PMID: 30275250].

DISORDERS OF THE PLEURA & PLEURAL CAVITY

The *parietal* pleura covers the inner surface of the chest wall. The *visceral* pleura covers the outer surface of the lungs. Disease processes can lead to accumulation of air or fluid or both in the pleural space. Pleural effusions are classified as transudates or exudates. Transudates occur when there is imbalance between hydrostatic and oncotic pressure, so that fluid filtration exceeds reabsorption (eg, congestive heart failure). Exudates form because of inflammation of the pleural surface leading to increased capillary permeability (eg, parapneumonic effusions). Other pleural effusions include chylothorax and hemothorax.

Thoracentesis is helpful in characterizing the fluid and providing definitive diagnosis. Recovered fluid is considered an exudate when Light's criteria are present (pleural fluid–serum protein ratio > 0.5, a pleural fluid–serum LDH ratio > 0.6, or a pleural fluid LDH level greater than two-thirds the upper limit for normal serum LDH). Important additional studies on pleural fluid include cell count; pH and glucose; Gram stain, acid-fast and fungal stains; aerobic and anaerobic cultures; and counterimmunoelectrophoresis for specific organisms. Cytologic examination of pleural fluid should be performed to rule out leukemia or other neoplasm.

Wilcox M et al: Does this patient have an exudative pleural effusion? The rational clinical examination systematic review. JAMA 2014;311(23):2422–2431 [PMID: 24938565].

HEMOTHORAX

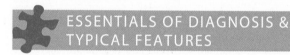

ESSENTIALS OF DIAGNOSIS & TYPICAL FEATURES

▶ Sudden-onset shortness of breath.
▶ Thoracocentesis reveals blood in the pleural space.

Accumulation of blood in the pleural space can be caused by surgical or accidental trauma, coagulation defects, and pleural or pulmonary tumors. A hemothorax is defined as a parapneumonic effusion when the hematocrit of the fluid is more than 50% of the peripheral blood. Hemopneumothorax may be caused by trauma. Symptoms are related to blood loss and compression of underlying lung parenchyma. There is some risk of secondary infection, resulting in empyema.

▶ Treatment

Drainage of a hemothorax is required when significant compromise of pulmonary function is present, as with hemopneumothorax. In uncomplicated cases, observation is indicated because blood is readily absorbed spontaneously from the pleural space.

VATS has been used successfully in the management of hemothorax. Chest CT scan is helpful to select patients who may require surgery, as identification of blood and the volume of blood may be more predictive by this method than by chest radiograph.

Muzumdar H, Arens R: Pleural fluid. Pediatr Rev 2007;28(12):462–464 [PMID: 18055645].

CHYLOTHORAX

ESSENTIALS OF DIAGNOSIS & TYPICAL FEATURES

▶ Respiratory distress with evidence of fluid in the pleural space on chest imaging.
▶ Thoracocentesis reveals milky fluid that is high in triglycerides and lymphocytes.

Accumulation of chyle, fluid of intestinal origin containing fat digestion products (mostly lipids), in the pleural space usually results from accidental or surgical trauma to the thoracic duct. The most common cause of a pleural effusion in the first few days of life is a chylothorax. In a newborn, chylothorax can be due to congenital abnormalities of the lymph vessels or secondary to birth trauma. Abnormalities of lymph vessels are seen in several congenital syndromes such as Down syndrome and Noonan syndrome. In an older child, a chylothorax can be due to laceration or obstruction of the thoracic duct due to trauma or any surgery involving the chest wall (cardiac surgery, scoliosis repair, etc); obstruction of the vessels due to a benign or malignant mass or lymphadenopathy; a granulomatous infection such as tuberculosis; or increased venous pressure due to obstruction or left ventricular failure. Symptoms of chylothorax are related to the amount of fluid accumulation and the degree of compromise of underlying pulmonary parenchyma. Thoracentesis reveals typical milky fluid (unless the patient has been fasting) containing chiefly T lymphocytes.

▶ Treatment

Treatment should be conservative because many chylothoraces resolve spontaneously. Oral feedings with medium-chain triglycerides reduce lymphatic flow through the thoracic duct. Somatostatin or the long-acting somatostatin analogue, octreotide, are viable therapeutic options. Drainage of chylous effusions should be performed only for respiratory compromised because the fluid often rapidly reaccumulates. Repeated or continuous drainage may lead to protein malnutrition and T-cell depletion, rendering the patient relatively immunocompromised. If reaccumulation of fluid persists, surgical ligation of the thoracic duct or sclerosis of the pleural space can be attempted, although the results may be less than satisfactory.

Tutor JD: Chylothorax in infants and children. Pediatrics 2014;133(4):722–733 [PMID: 24685960].

PNEUMOTHORAX & RELATED AIR LEAK SYNDROMES

ESSENTIALS OF DIAGNOSIS & TYPICAL FEATURES

- ▶ Sudden-onset shortness of breath.
- ▶ Focal area of absent breath sounds on chest auscultation.
- ▶ Shift of the trachea away from the area with absent breath sounds.

Pneumothorax can occur spontaneously in newborns and in older children or, more commonly, as a result of birth trauma, positive pressure ventilation, underlying obstructive or restrictive lung disease, or rupture of a congenital or acquired lung cyst. Pneumothorax can also occur as an acute complication of tracheostomy. Air usually dissects from the alveolar spaces into the interstitial spaces of the lung. Migration to the visceral pleura ultimately leads to rupture into the pleural space. Associated conditions include pneumomediastinum, pneumopericardium, pneumoperitoneum, and subcutaneous emphysema. These conditions are more commonly associated with dissection of air into the interstitial spaces of the lung with retrograde dissection along the bronchovascular bundles toward the hilum.

▶ Clinical Findings

A. Symptoms and Signs

The clinical spectrum can vary from asymptomatic to severe respiratory distress. Associated symptoms include cyanosis, chest pain, and dyspnea. Physical examination may reveal decreased breath sounds and hyperresonance to percussion on the affected side with tracheal deviation. When pneumothorax is under tension, cardiac function may be compromised, resulting in hypotension or narrowing of the pulse pressure. Pneumopericardium is a life-threatening condition that presents with muffled heart tones and shock. Pneumomediastinum rarely causes complications other than chest pain.

B. Laboratory Findings and Imaging Studies

Chest radiographs demonstrate the presence of free air in the pleural space. When the pneumothorax is large and under tension, compressive atelectasis of the underlying lung and shift of the mediastinum to the contralateral side may be observed. Cross-table lateral and lateral decubitus radiographs can aid in the diagnosis of free air. Pneumopericardium is identified by the presence of air entirely surrounding the heart, whereas in patients with pneumomediastinum, the

heart and mediastinal structures may be outlined with air, but the air does not involve the diaphragmatic cardiac border. Chest CT may identify subtle pleural disease (eg, blebs) in recurrent pneumothoraces.

▶ Differential Diagnosis

Acute deterioration of a patient on a ventilator can be caused by tension pneumothorax, obstruction or dislodgment of the endotracheal tube, or ventilator failure. Radiographically, pneumothorax must be distinguished from diaphragmatic hernia, lung cysts, congenital lobar emphysema, and CPAM.

▶ Treatment

Small (< 15%) or asymptomatic pneumothoraces usually do not require treatment and can be managed with close observation. Larger or symptomatic pneumothoraces require drainage, although inhalation of 100% oxygen to wash out blood nitrogen can be tried. Needle aspiration should be used to relieve tension acutely, followed by chest tube or pigtail catheter placement. Pneumopericardium requires immediate identification, and if clinically symptomatic, needle aspiration to prevent death, followed by pericardial tube placement.

▶ Prognosis

In older patients with spontaneous pneumothorax, recurrences are common; sclerosing and surgical procedures are often required.

Dotson K, Johnson LH: Pediatric spontaneous pneumothorax. Pediatr Emerg Care 2012;28(7):715–720 [PMID: 22766594].

Johnson NN, Toledo A, Endom EE: Pneumothorax, pneumomediastinum, and pulmonary embolism. Pediatr Clin North Am 2010;57(6):1357–1383 [PMID: 21111122].

▼ MEDIASTINUM

MEDIASTINAL MASSES

ESSENTIALS OF DIAGNOSIS & TYPICAL FEATURES

- ▶ Presentation varies depending on the location of the mass.
- ▶ Most mediastinal masses are discovered on routine chest x-rays.

Children with mediastinal masses may present because of symptoms produced by pressure on the esophagus, airways, nerves, or vessels within the mediastinum, or the masses may be discovered incidentally on chest radiograph. Once the mass is identified, localization to one of four mediastinal compartments aids in the differential diagnosis. The superior mediastinum is the area above the pericardium that is bordered inferiorly by an imaginary line from the manubrium to the fourth thoracic vertebra. The anterior mediastinum is bordered by the sternum anteriorly and the pericardium posteriorly, and the posterior mediastinum is defined by the pericardium and diaphragm anteriorly and the lower eight thoracic vertebrae posteriorly. The middle mediastinum is surrounded by these three compartments.

Clinical Findings

A. Symptoms and Signs

Respiratory symptoms, when present, are due to pressure on an airway (cough or wheezing) or an infection (unresolving pneumonia in one area of lung). Hemoptysis can also occur but is an unusual presenting symptom. Dysphagia may be due to compression of the esophagus. Pressure on the recurrent laryngeal nerve can cause vocal cord paralysis and hoarse voice. Superior vena caval syndrome presents with dilation of neck vessels and other signs and symptoms of venous obstruction; superior mediastinal syndrome presents similarly but includes tracheal compression.

B. Laboratory Findings and Imaging Studies

The mass is initially defined by frontal and lateral chest radiographs together with chest CT scans or MRI. A barium esophagram may help define the extent of a mass. Other studies that may be required include angiography (to define the blood supply to large tumors), electrocardiography, echocardiography, ultrasound of the chest, fungal and mycobacterial skin tests, and urinary catecholamine assays. MRI or myelography may be necessary in children suspected of having a neurogenic tumor in the posterior mediastinum. Mediastinal masses, particularly anterior masses, can cause life-threatening airway compromise in the supine position and during sedation even in patients with mild symptoms; thus, any sedation or anesthesia should be avoided if possible and performed cautiously.

Differential Diagnosis

The differential diagnosis of mediastinal masses is determined by their location. Superior mediastinal masses include cystic hygromas, vascular or neurogenic tumors, thymic masses, teratomas, intrathoracic thyroid tissue, mediastinal abscess, and esophageal lesions. Anterior mediastinal masses include thymic tissue (thymomas, hyperplasia, and cysts), intrathoracic thyroid, teratomas, vascular tumors, reactive lymphadenopathy, leukemia, and lymphoma. Middle mediastinum masses include lymphomas, hypertrophic lymph nodes, granulomas, bronchogenic or enteric cysts, metastases, and pericardial cysts. Abnormalities of the great vessels and aortic aneurysms may also present as masses in this compartment. Posterior mediastinal masses include neurogenic tumors, enterogenous cysts, thoracic meningoceles, and aortic aneurysms.

In some series, more than 50% of mediastinal tumors occur in the posterior mediastinum and are mainly neurogenic tumors or enterogenous cysts. Most neurogenic tumors in children younger than 4 years are malignant (neuroblastoma or neuroganglioblastoma), whereas a benign ganglioneuroma is the most common histologic type in older children. In the middle and anterior mediastinum, lymphoma and leukemia are the primary concern. Definitive diagnosis in most instances relies on surgical excision or biopsy for histologic examination.

Treatment & Prognosis

The appropriate therapy and the response to therapy depend on the cause of the mediastinal mass.

Garey CL et al: Management of anterior mediastinal masses in children. Eur J Pediatr Surg 2011;21(5):310–313 [PMID: 21751123].

SLEEP-DISORDERED BREATHING

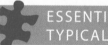

ESSENTIALS OF DIAGNOSIS & TYPICAL FEATURES

► Nighttime symptoms of habitual snoring, apnea, or labored respirations are characteristic of OSA, where central sleep apnea or periodic breathing may be more subtle.

► Sleep studies are used to diagnose sleep apnea and guide treatment.

Sleep apnea is recognized as a major public health problem in adults, due to its associated impact on health and the risks of excessive daytime sleepiness, impairment while driving, and poor work performance. Pediatric sleep-related breathing disorders are less commonly recognized because the risk factors, presentations, management, and outcomes differ from those in adults, although the adverse impact on health is similar in scope and perhaps severity. SDB in children has been associated with problems in a multitude of realms, including social, behavioral, and neurocognitive. It has been shown to significantly impact quality of life and has been associated with growth impairment and cardiovascular complications. Recent studies also indicate that sleep-disordered breathing (SDB) is associated with systemic inflammation.

SDB is any abnormal respiratory pattern during sleep, which may include noisy breathing, mouth breathing, and/or pauses in breathing that may be obstructive, central, or mixed in etiology. SDB encompasses a spectrum of obstructive disorders from primary snoring to OSA, but also includes periodic breathing, central sleep apnea, hypoventilation syndromes, etc. SDB is a presumptive clinical diagnosis where PSG is necessary to more specifically characterize the disorder.

▼ PRIMARY SNORING & OBSTRUCTIVE SLEEP APNEA

▶ Clinical Findings

A. Symptoms and Signs

Obstructive sleep apnea (OSA) occurs in normal children with an incidence of about 2%, increasing in children with medical conditions such as craniofacial abnormalities or neuromuscular diseases, or use of medications, such as hypnotics, sedatives, or anticonvulsants. OSA should be suspected whenever a child presents with symptoms of loud or habitual snoring (snoring 3 or more nights per week), witnessed apnea, labored breathing, mouth breathing, or frequent nighttime arousals, especially in the setting of failure to thrive or obesity, nocturnal oxygen desaturations, life-threatening events, craniofacial abnormalities, poor school performance, or behavioral problems such as hyperactivity. In children, airway obstruction is often associated with nasal congestion, atopy, and adenotonsillar hypertrophy, where tonsillar hypertrophy is most common between the ages of 2 and 7 years. Obesity is widely recognized as an etiologic component in adult OSA and is increasingly cited in pediatric OSA.

B. Diagnostic Studies: Polysomnography & Airway Evaluation

In 2012, the AAP updated their clinical practice guideline for the diagnosis and management of uncomplicated childhood OSA syndrome. The guideline emphasizes that pediatricians should screen all children for snoring. If the child exhibits additional signs and symptoms of SDB, referral for a sleep study is recommended, but referral to an otolaryngologist or sleep specialist is also an option. The American Academy of Sleep Medicine (AASM) has similar recommendations.

A patient's history and clinical examination cannot predict the presence or severity of OSA. Similarly, an overnight oximetry study is a poor screening test for OSA, as obstructive respiratory events can occur without oxygen desaturations. Therefore, the gold standard for diagnosis of OSA is a PSG, commonly called a "sleep study." This test measures sleep state with electroencephalogram leads and electromyography, oronasal airflow, chest and abdominal effort, heart rate and rhythm, gas exchange (O_2 and CO_2), and leg movements, along with body position, vibrations representing snoring, and audiovisual recording. PSG is utilized not only for characterizing SDB but also for diagnosing periodic limb movements. Sleep apnea is defined as cessation of breathing and can be classified as obstructive (airflow stops despite persistence of respiratory effort) or central (the lack of effort to breathe). A hypopnea is counted when airflow and respiratory effort decrease for at least two respiratory cycles with an associated oxygen desaturation or arousal. The criteria for diagnosing OSA differ between children and adults, and normative values for children are still being established. The AASM states that for children, the occurrence of more than one apnea-plus-hypopnea per hour of sleep (the apnea-hypopnea index, or AHI) is abnormal. However, the AASM has qualified its recommendation, stating that the criteria may be modified once more comprehensive data become available. One study of children aged 6–11 years found that an AHI of between one and five events per hour (mild OSA) was associated with daytime sleepiness and learning problems when associated with 3% oxygen desaturation, whereas an AHI of five events per hour or more (moderate to severe OSA) was associated with clinical symptoms even in the absence of desaturation. Notably, many studies have shown little correlation between the severity of OSA by PSG and morbidity. Furthermore, even primary snoring, which is habitual snoring without gas exchange abnormalities or arousals, has been associated with neurobehavioral consequences.

A PSG is generally recommended for children with suspected sleep apnea if they have any of the following comorbid conditions: obesity, Down syndrome, craniofacial abnormalities, neuromuscular disorders, sickle cell disease, or mucopolysaccharidoses. PSG also is recommended for children without the above comorbidities if the need for surgery is uncertain, or if there is discordance between tonsillar size on physical examination and the reported severity of symptoms, no adenotonsillar hypertrophy or nasal obstruction, but significant symptoms of SDB for example. Other conditions, especially a periodic limb movement disorder, may mimic the daytime symptoms of SDB.

If a PSG indicates OSA in a child without tonsillar hypertrophy, a complete evaluation of the upper airway by awake flexible laryngoscopy should be performed to look for other possible sites of obstruction, including the nose (turbinate hypertrophy), nasopharynx (adenoid), hypopharynx (base of tongue or lingual tonsils), and larynx (laryngomalacia). The adenoid can also be assessed with a lateral neck x-ray. Alternative methods to evaluate a child for anatomical sites of obstruction include sedated cine MRI of the upper airway or drug-induced sleep endoscopy (DISE).

▶ Clinical Evaluation & Management

Most pediatric otolaryngologists perform adenotonsillectomy (AT) in healthy patients with obstructive SDB without obtaining a PSG. AT without PSG may be considered in a healthy child if the following are present:

1. Nighttime symptoms: habitual snoring along with gasping, pauses, or labored breathing. Other symptoms that may be related to SDB include night terrors, sleep walking, secondary enuresis, or morning headaches.

2. Daytime symptoms: unrefreshed sleep, attention deficit, hyperactivity, emotional lability, temperamental behavior, poor weight gain, and daytime fatigue. Other signs include daytime mouth breathing or dysphagia.

3. Enlarged tonsils.

If the three findings cannot be confirmed, but the child has other indications for an AT—that is, recurrent tonsillitis or markedly enlarged (4+) tonsils with dysphagia—referral to a pediatric otolaryngologist to consider surgery is warranted. See Chapter 18 for a thorough discussion of AT.

Figure 19–5 is an algorithm for management of SDB complaints in an otherwise healthy child. The pathway relies on clinical symptoms and tonsil size. The most commonly used grading scale for tonsil size ranges from 0 to 4. With grade 1 the tonsils are small and contained within the tonsillar fossa; in grade 4 the tonsils are so large they may touch ("kissing"); grade 0 describes prior tonsillectomy. As mentioned, tonsil size alone does not predict the presence of significant SDB, as children without significant tonsil hypertrophy may still have OSA due to factors such as low muscle tone, atopy, etc. Clinical suspicion of SDB should be heightened if a child has enlarged tonsils, especially if the parents cannot provide a reliable history. Although the pathway states that an asymptomatic child with markedly enlarged tonsils (4+) should undergo PSG, a period of observation or trial of conservative management is reasonable. If the child has no clinical symptoms and the tonsils are only moderately enlarged (3+), observation is appropriate. Educating the parents about the risks of SDB and what to look for is paramount.

A landmark randomized prospective study on AT outcomes (CHAT Study) demonstrated overall success at 79%. Success was defined as AHI reduced to less than 2 and obstructive apnea index to less than one event an hour. Obesity, black ethnicity, and an AHI more than 4.7 events an hour were associated with lower cure rates. Interestingly, 47% of the children in the watchful waiting group had spontaneous resolution of their OSA at 7 months. Children who had mild OSA or normal weight were more likely to improve spontaneously.

As for postoperative PSG, the AASM and AAP agree that a child with mild OSA (AHI fewer than five events an hour) does not require a follow-up study. However, those with persistent symptoms, more severe OSA, obesity, or other comorbidities should routinely have a postoperative study. When OSA persists or AT is

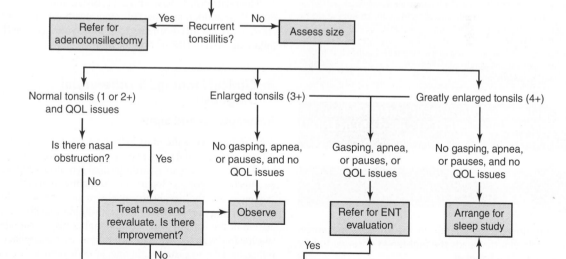

▲ **Figure 19–5.** Algorithm for evaluation of snoring in a healthy child.

contraindicated/refused/delayed for whatever reason, treatment with continuous or bilevel positive airway pressure (CPAP or BiPAP) may be considered.

Regardless of the underlying etiology of SDB, maintaining a healthy weight, addressing abnormal dentition (with the use of orthodontics, such as oral appliances or rapid maxillary expanders) and optimizing airway health (by treating nasal obstruction, atopy, and asthma with topical intranasal steroids and leukotriene modifiers, for example) are cornerstones of OSA management.

PERIODIC BREATHING & CENTRAL SLEEP APNEA

Pediatric sleep-related breathing disorders of central etiology, including periodic breathing and central sleep apnea, are less well understood. Central apneas are common in infants and children, particularly at increased elevation. These are pauses in breathing without concomitant effort and may occur in a pattern of alternating apnea and tachypnea known as periodic breathing. Clinical significance is uncertain, as healthy children have been shown to have central apneas lasting 25 seconds without clear consequences. These central respiratory events may be relevant if they occur frequently or are associated with gas exchange abnormalities or sleep fragmentation, and should then prompt a thorough evaluation by a pediatric sleep specialist. Though no intervention is needed in most cases of periodic breathing and central sleep apnea, supplemental oxygen may be used to reduce oxygen desaturation and stabilize the respiratory pattern.

Marcus CL et al: Childhood Adenotonsillectomy Trial (CHAT). A randomized trial of adenotonsillectomy for childhood sleep apnea. N Engl J Med 2013 Jun 20;368(25):2366–2376 [PMID: 22926173].
Marcus CL et al: Diagnosis and management of childhood obstructive sleep apnea syndrome. Pediatrics 2012;130(3):576–584 [PMID: 22926173].

BRIEF RESOLVED UNEXPLAINED EVENTS (FORMERLY APPARENT LIFE-THREATENING EVENTS)

ESSENTIALS OF DIAGNOSIS & TYPICAL FEATURES

▶ Acute, unexpected change in breathing, appearance, and behavior that leads the frightened observer to fear that the infant has died.

▶ Infants are characterized as low versus high risk to facilitate evaluation and management.

In 2016, the AAP suggested renaming apparent life-threatening events (ALTE) to brief resolved unexplained events (BRUE), just as ALTE previously replaced "near-miss sudden infant death syndrome" (SIDS). The BRUE nomenclature serves to clarify clinical care and research, while also providing a framework for evaluation of lower- versus higher-risk infants following a BRUE. BRUEs are defined in infants younger than 1 year who are observed to have apnea or irregular breathing, cyanosis or pallor (not redness), marked change in muscle tone (either hypotonia/limpness or hypertonia), or decreased responsiveness that lasts less than 1 minute (more often < 20–30 seconds) and returns to baseline with subsequent reassuring history and physical examination by a clinician. This definition highlights that the event remains unexplained, whereas the ALTE label overlaps with events such as fever, upper airway congestion, or labored respirations attributable to acute viral illness, or gagging/choking with gastroesophageal reflux, as examples.

Once a clinician has made the BRUE diagnosis, the infant is determined to be either low or high risk, which will determine what, if any, evaluation is needed. Infants with a BRUE are considered high risk if they are younger than 60 days, were born less than 32 weeks' gestation, received CPR at the time of the event, or have had a prior BRUE.

Immaturity likely plays a major role in the pathogenesis of BRUEs. Classic studies on the nervous system, reflexes, or responses to apnea or gastroesophageal reflux during sleep in infants and immature animals show profound cardiovascular changes during stimulation of the vagus nerve, whereas adults are not affected.

The relationship between ALTE/BRUE and future risk of SIDS or sudden unexpected infant death (SUID) is not clear, as ALTE/BRUE infants tend to be younger. See the following SUID/SIDS section for more detail.

▶ Clinical Findings & Differential Diagnosis

A. Symptoms and Signs

A careful history is the most helpful part of the evaluation. A history of several days of poor feeding, temperature instability, or respiratory or gastrointestinal symptoms suggests an infectious process. Reports of "struggling to breathe" or "trying to breathe" imply airway obstruction. Episodes following crying may be related to breath-holding spells. Association of the episode with feeding implies dis-coordinated swallowing with or without aspiration, gastroesophageal reflux, or delayed gastric emptying, or may imply an airway abnormality. Episodes occurring while awake are associated with very different diagnoses than episodes occurring during sleep. Association of episodes with sleep may suggest

Table 19–8. Potential causes of brief resolved unexplained events (formerly apparent life-threatening events).

Infectious	Viral: respiratory syncytial virus and other respiratory *viruses*
	Bacterial: sepsis, pertussis, *Chlamydia*
Gastrointestinal	Gastroesophageal reflux with or without obstructive apnea
Respiratory	Airway abnormality; vascular rings, pulmonary slings, tracheomalacia
	Pneumonia
Neurologic	Seizure disorder
	Central nervous system infection: meningitis, encephalitis
	Vasovagal response
	Leigh encephalopathy
	Brain tumor
Cardiovascular	Congenital malformation
	Dysrhythmias
	Cardiomyopathy
Nonaccidental trauma	Battering
	Drug overdose
	Munchausen syndrome by proxy
No definable cause	Apnea of infancy

seizure, gastroesophageal reflux, apnea of infancy, or SDB. It is helpful to role-play the episode with the family and then use the event characteristic (such as cyanosis, hypotonia, unresponsiveness, etc) to describe the event, as opposed to the vaguer term "ALTE." Details regarding the measures taken to resuscitate the infant and the infant's recovery from the episode may be useful in determining severity. Table 19–8 classifies disorders that may present as higher-risk BRUEs.

The physical examination provides further direction in pursuing the diagnosis. Fever or hypothermia suggests infection. An altered state of consciousness implies a postictal state or drug overdose, or central nervous system anomaly or infection. Respiratory distress implies cardiac or pulmonary lesions.

Apneic episodes have been linked to child abuse in several ways. Head injury following nonaccidental trauma may be first brought to medical attention because of apnea. Other signs of abuse are usually immediately apparent in such cases. Drug overdose, either accidental or intentional, may also present with apnea. Several studies document that apneic episodes may be falsely reported by parents who are seeking attention (ie, Munchausen syndrome by proxy, now referred to as medical child abuse). Parents may physically interfere with a child's respiratory efforts, in which case pinch marks on the nares are sometimes found.

B. Laboratory Findings

Patients with low-risk BRUEs may not need inpatient observation or further testing. One may consider pertussis testing, electrocardiogram, brief pulse oximetry, and/or serial observations based on history, examination, or suspicion, but other blood work, lumbar puncture, imaging, acid-suppression therapy, hospitalization, etc are generally discouraged as they provoke unwarranted worry and stress in both patients and caregivers.

Those at high risk, however, should undergo more thorough evaluation for potential underlying etiologies, as referenced in Table 19–8, where clinical suspicion prioritizes the appropriate workup. In these cases, patients may be hospitalized for observation in order to reduce stress on the family and allow prompt completion of the evaluation. Diagnostic testing should be based primarily on the history and physical examination. Laboratory evaluation might include a complete blood count, blood culture with urinalysis, and urine culture for evidence of infection, especially in the face of fever, hypothermia, or an abnormal physical examination. Serum electrolytes may reveal electrolyte disturbances from metabolic disorders, dehydration, or ingestions. An elevation in serum bicarbonate indicates chronic hypoventilation, whereas decreases indicate acute acidosis, perhaps due to hypoxia during the episode. Chronic acidosis suggests an inherited metabolic disorder. Arterial blood gas studies provide an initial assessment of oxygenation and acid-base status. Low Pa_{O_2}, elevated Pa_{CO_2}, or both indicate cardiorespiratory disease. A significant base deficit suggests that the episode was accompanied by hypoxia or circulatory impairment. Oxygen saturation measurements in the hospital assess oxygenation status during different activities and are more comprehensive than a single blood gas sample. Because apnea has been associated with respiratory infections, diagnostic studies for RSV and other viruses, *Bordetella pertussis*, and *Chlamydophila pneumoniae* may help with diagnosis. Apnea occurring with infection often precedes other physical findings.

C. Imaging Studies

The chest radiograph is examined for infiltrates indicating acute infection or chronic aspiration and for cardiac size as a clue to intrinsic cardiac disease. Electrocardiogram is helpful to rule out cardiac dysrhythmias, and echocardiogram may be indicated if there is suspicion of congenital heart disease based on history and physical examination. If the episode might have involved airway obstruction, the airway should be examined either directly by fiberoptic bronchoscopy or radiographically by CT. VFSS or FEES can be done to evaluate for dysphagia and aspiration, and UGI fluoroscopy series is a useful tool to rule out the possibility of anatomic abnormalities such as vascular ring and tracheoesophageal fistula.

Gastroesophageal reflux is common in infants; however, it may be a marker of autonomic immaturity as opposed to a cause of the event. Infants with reflux and apnea can be given medical antireflux treatment. Infants with reflux and repeated episodes of apnea may benefit from evaluation by a multidisciplinary aerodigestive team.

D. Special Tests: Polysomnography and Other Studies

Depending on the discretion of the clinician, PSG can be useful in detecting abnormalities of cardiorespiratory function, sleep state, oxygen saturation, carbon dioxide retention, and seizure activity. Sleep studies can be used in conjunction with pH monitoring to determine the contribution of reflux to apnea. Esophageal pressure manometry can be useful to detect subtle changes in espiratory effort related to partial obstructive breathing (hypopnea). Due to their immature nervous system, infants are more likely to experience adverse events from sleep disordered breathing than adults.

Among the neurologic causes of BRUEs, seizure disorder has been found to be a cause of BRUE in a significant number of cases. Apnea as the sole manifestation of a seizure disorder is unusual but may occur. In cases of repeated episodes, 24-hour electroencephalographic monitoring may be helpful in detecting a seizure disorder.

▶ Treatment

Therapy is directed at the underlying cause, if one is found. After blood cultures are taken, antibiotics should be given to infants who appear toxic. Seizure disorders are treated with anticonvulsants. Gastroesophageal reflux should be treated if symptomatic, though this may not prevent future episodes. Cardiovascular anomalies, such as vascular rings and pulmonary slings, require cardiovascular surgical evaluation considering the potential for severe morbidity and mortality.

For both low- and high-risk BRUEs caregivers should be provided with education to reduce modifiable risk factors and taught CPR. Home monitoring has been used in the past as treatment, but the efficacy of monitoring has not been demonstrated in controlled trials. After more than 30 years of home monitoring, the sudden infant death rate has not changed. Although monitors can detect central apnea or bradycardia, they do not predict which children will have future events or SUID. Apnea monitors are prone to frequent false alarms, and it must be noted that many parents cannot handle the stress associated with having a monitor in the home.

Supplemental oxygen has been used as therapy for BRUEs for several reasons. Oxygen reduces periodic breathing of infancy, an immature pattern of breathing that can cause some degree of oxygen desaturation. Second, infants have small chest capacities with increased chest wall compliance that reduces lung volume. Supplemental oxygen can increase the baseline saturation, reducing the severity of desaturation with short apneas. Respiratory stimulants such as caffeine and aminophylline have been used in specific cases of central apnea or periodic breathing.

▶ Prevention

All infants younger than 1 year should be evaluated for the presence of modifiable SUID risk factors. Parents should be educated on how to avoid these risk factors, especially in infants at increased risk such as former preterm infants, children exposed to cigarette smoke environmentally or prior to birth, African American or Native American infants, and infants in poor socioeconomic areas. Recommendations from the AAP Task Force on SIDS include:

- Always place a baby on its back to sleep (this includes a baby with reflux).
- Infants should sleep in the parents' room, close to the parents' bed but on a separate surface designed for infants, ideally for the first year of life but at least for the first 6 months.
- Soft objects and loose bedding, including blankets, nonfitted sheets, stuffed animals, or wedge positioners, should be kept away from the infant's sleep area to reduce the risk of SIDS, suffocation, entrapment, and strangulation.
  - Wearable blankets are preferred to blankets and other coverings to keep the infant warm while reducing the chance of head covering. There is no evidence to recommend swaddling as a strategy to reduce the risk of SIDS.
  - Avoid overheating, overwrapping, and covering the face and head.
- Breast-feeding is recommended.
- Consider offering a pacifier at naptime and bedtime.
- Avoid exposure to cigarette smoke during pregnancy and after birth.
- Car seats, swings, and baby slings should not be used for sleep as the infant's head tends to fall forward or to the side, compromising the airway.
- Avoid the use of adult beds, bed rails, etc, which increase the risk of suffocation and entrapment.
  - There are no studies supporting the safety of bedside or in-bed sleepers, and therefore these products cannot be recommended.
- Health care professionals, hospital staff, and childcare providers should endorse and model infant safe sleep recommendations from birth.

- Pediatricians and other primary care providers should actively participate in the "Safe to Sleep" campaign, focusing on ways to reduce the risk of all sleep-related infant deaths, including SIDS, suffocation, and other unintentional deaths.

SUDDEN UNEXPECTED INFANT DEATH & SUDDEN INFANT DEATH SYNDROME

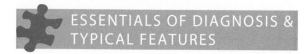

ESSENTIALS OF DIAGNOSIS & TYPICAL FEATURES

► Sudden, unexpected death of an infant or child, including accidental suffocation.

SIDS is defined as the sudden death of an infant younger than 1 year that remains unexplained after a thorough case investigation, including performance of a complete autopsy, examination of the death scene, and review of the clinical history. The postmortem examination is an important feature of the definition because approximately 20% of cases of sudden death can be explained by autopsy findings. After the "Back to Sleep" campaign began in the United States in 1994, the incidence of SIDS declined from approximately 2 per 1000 to 0.5 per 1000 live births. However, the incidence of SIDS has leveled off since 1999.

SUID, defined as any sudden and unexpected infant death, whether explained (such as accidental suffocation or strangulation) or unexplained (such as SIDS) has gained favor as the preferred term to refer to infant deaths that were previously classified as SIDS. SIDS is neither a true diagnosis nor a syndrome, and labeling an infant death as SIDS tends to give parents a false sense that the cause of their child's death is known and understood. SUID also includes deaths due to infection, ingestions, metabolic diseases, cardiac arrhythmias, and trauma. Recent evidence shows that the incidence of accidental suffocation and strangulation in bed is increasing due to unsafe sleep surfaces and environments.

► Epidemiology & Pathogenesis

Epidemiologic and pathologic data constitute most of what is known about SUID. Like SIDS, SUID deaths peak between ages 2 and 4 months. Most deaths occur at night, while the infant and the caregiver are sleeping. In fact, the only unifying features of all cases are age and sleep. SUID is more common among ethnic and racial minorities and socioeconomically disadvantaged populations. Racial disparity in the prevalence of prone positioning and especially in bed-sharing may be contributing to the continued disparity in SUID rates between black and white infants. There is a 3:2 male

predominance in most series. Other risk factors include preterm birth, low birth weight, recent infection, young maternal age, high maternal parity, maternal tobacco or drug use, and crowded living conditions. Most of these risk factors are associated with a two- to threefold increased incidence but are not specific enough to be useful in predicting which infants will die unexpectedly. **Recent immunization is not a risk factor.**

The most consistent pathologic findings in SUID deaths from unknown cause (previously classified as SIDS) are intrathoracic petechiae and mild inflammation and congestion of the respiratory tract. More subtle pathologic findings include brainstem gliosis, extramedullary hematopoiesis, and increases in periadrenal brown fat. These latter findings suggest that infants who succumb to SUID have had intermittent or chronic hypoxia before death.

In cases where a distinct cause cannot be identified, the mechanism or mechanisms of death in SUID are unknown. For example, it is unknown whether the initiating event at the time of death is cessation of breathing, cardiac arrhythmia, or asystole. Hypotheses have included upper airway obstruction, catecholamine excess, and increased fetal hemoglobin. However, maldevelopment or delayed maturation of the brainstem, which is responsible for arousal from sleep, remains the predominant theory. A history of mild symptoms of upper respiratory infection before death is not uncommon, and SUID victims are sometimes seen by physicians a day or so before death. The postmortem examination is essential and may help the family by excluding other possible causes of death. A death scene investigation is also important in determining the cause of sudden unexpected deaths in infancy.

Families must be supported following the death of an infant. The National SIDS Resource Center (http://www.sidscenter.org) provides information about psychosocial support groups and counseling for families of SIDS victims.

► Prevention

Since 1990, SIDS rates have declined more than 60% worldwide. Population studies in New Zealand and Europe identified risk factors, which when changed had a significant effect on the incidence of SIDS. Since 1994 the AAP's "Back to Sleep" campaign has promoted education about the risk of prone positioning.

AAP Task Force on Sudden Infant Death Syndrome: SIDS and other sleep-related infant deaths: updated 2016 recommendations for a safe infant sleeping environment. Pediatrics 2016;138(5):e20162938 [PMID: 27940804].

Tieder JS et al: Brief resolved unexplained events (formerly apparent life-threatening events) and evaluation of lower-risk infants. Pediatrics 2016 May;137(5) [PMID: 27244835].

QUALITY ASSESSMENT & OUTCOMES METRICS

Pediatric pulmonary medicine is constantly adjusting to improve the outcomes for children with respiratory illness. The foundation of the work in quality improvement is in the many clinical care guidelines that inform the care of patients and in the data that indicate the success of the care. For example, as mentioned (and referenced) earlier, the Cystic Fibrosis Foundation works with providers and centers of care to create and implement guidelines for the diagnosis and management of children with CF. This foundation also maintains a registry of children with CF and reports on outcomes including lung function, body mass index, and mortality data. The ChILD foundation mentioned earlier has also created guidelines for diagnosis and management and follows patient outcomes including those mentioned above. The National Heart, Lung, and Blood Institute has updated the asthma guidelines three times. International and United States based organizations have studied adherence to those guidelines. The Centers for Disease Control and Prevention in the United States reports asthma outcomes including utilization, mortality, and cost of care. AAP, as mentioned earlier, has published guidelines for SIDS and SUID prevention. There are ongoing studies of the impact of those guidelines and the data demonstrates clearly that these guidelines are saving lives. Finally, respiratory disease requires a multidisciplinary team to care for patients in and out of the hospital. The American Academy of Respiratory Care publishes guidelines on oxygen use, aerosolized device use, and ventilation (acute and chronic) for pediatric patients.

Cardiovascular Diseases

Pei-Ni Jone, MD

John S. Kim, MD

Johannes von Alvensleben, MD

Dale Burkett, MD

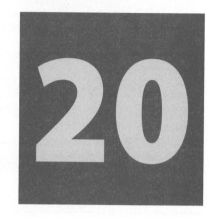

20

INTRODUCTION

Eight in 1000 infants are born with a congenital heart defect. Advances in medical and surgical care allow more than 90% of such children to enter adulthood. Pediatric cardiac care includes not only the diagnosis and treatment of congenital heart disease but also the prevention of risk factors for adult cardiovascular disease—obesity, smoking, and hyperlipidemia. Acquired and familial heart diseases such as Kawasaki disease (KD), viral myocarditis, cardiomyopathies, and rheumatic heart disease are also a significant cause of morbidity and mortality in children.

DIAGNOSTIC EVALUATION

HISTORY

Symptoms related to congenital heart defects primarily vary according to the alteration in pulmonary blood flow (Table 20–1). The presence of other cardiovascular symptoms such as palpitations and chest pain should be determined by history in the older child, paying particular attention to the timing (at rest or activity-related), onset, and termination (gradual vs sudden), as well as precipitating and relieving factors.

PHYSICAL EXAMINATION

General

The examination begins with a visual assessment of mental status, signs of distress, perfusion, and skin color. Documentation of heart rate, respiratory rate, blood pressure (in all four extremities), and oxygen saturation is essential. Many congenital cardiac defects occur as part of a genetic syndrome (Table 20–2), and complete assessment includes evaluation of dysmorphic features that may be clues to the associated cardiac defect.

Cardiovascular Examination

A. Inspection and Palpation

Chest conformation should be noted in the supine position. A precordial bulge indicates cardiomegaly. Palpation may reveal increased precordial activity, right ventricular (RV) lift, or left-sided heave; a diffuse point of maximal impulse; or a precordial thrill caused by a grade IV/VI or greater murmur. The thrill of aortic stenosis is found in the suprasternal notch. In patients with severe pulmonary hypertension (PH), a palpable pulmonary closure (P_2) is frequently noted at the upper left sternal border.

B. Auscultation

1. Heart sounds—The first heart sound (S_1) is the sound of atrioventricular (AV) valve closure. It is best heard at the lower left sternal border and is usually medium pitched. Although S_1 has multiple components, only one of these (M_1—closure of the mitral valve) is usually audible.

The second heart sound (S_2) is the sound of semilunar valve closure. It is best heard at the upper left sternal border. S_2 has two component sounds, A_2 and P_2 (aortic and pulmonic valve closure). Splitting of S_2 varies with respiration, widening with inspiration and narrowing with expiration. Abnormal splitting of S_2 may be an indication of cardiac disease (Table 20–3). A prominent or loud P_2 is associated with PH.

The third heart sound (S_3) is the sound of rapid left ventricular (LV) filling. It occurs in early diastole, after S_2, and is medium- to low-pitched. In healthy children, S_3 diminishes or disappears when going from supine to sitting or standing. A pathologic S_3 is often heard in the presence of poor cardiac function or a large left-to-right shunt. The fourth heart sound (S_4) is associated with atrial contraction and increased atrial pressure and has a low pitch similar to that of S_3. It occurs just prior to S_1 and is not normally audible. It is heard

Table 20–1. Symptoms of increased and decreased pulmonary blood flow.

Decreased Pulmonary Blood Flow	Increased Pulmonary Blood Flow
Infant/toddler	
Cyanosis	Tachypnea with activity/feeds
Squatting	Diaphoresis
Loss of consciousness	Poor weight gain
Older child	
Dizziness	Exercise intolerance
Syncope	Dyspnea on exertion, diaphoresis

Table 20–2. Cardiac defects in common syndromes.

Genetic Syndrome	Commonly Associated Cardiac Defect
Down syndrome	AVSD
Turner syndrome	Bicuspid aortic valve, coarctation, dilated aortic root, hypertension
Noonan syndrome	Dysplastic pulmonic valve, HCM
Williams-Beuren syndrome	Supravalvular aortic stenosis, PPS, coronary ostial stenosis
Marfan syndrome	MVP, MR, dilated aortic root
Fetal alcohol syndrome	VSD, ASD
Maternal rubella	PDA, PPS
Loeys-Dietz syndrome	Aneurysmal PDA, dilated aortic root, tortuous arteries throughout the body

ASD, atrial septal defect; AVSD, atrioventricular septal defect; HCM, hypertrophic cardiomyopathy; MR, mitral regurgitation; MVP, mitral valve prolapse; PDA, patent ductus arteriosus; PPS, peripheral pulmonary stenosis; VSD, ventricular septal defect.

Table 20–3. Abnormal splitting of S_2.

Causes of wide split S_2
RV volume overload: ASD, anomalous pulmonary venous return, PI
RV pressure overload: Pulmonary valve stenosis
Delayed RV conduction: RBBB
Causes of narrow split S_2
Pulmonary hypertension
Single semilunar valve (aortic atresia, pulmonary atresia, truncus arteriosus)

ASD, atrial septal defect; PI, pulmonic insufficiency; RBBB, right bundle branch block; RV, right ventricle.

in the presence of atrial contraction into a noncompliant ventricle as in hypertrophic or restrictive cardiomyopathy or from other causes of diastolic dysfunction.

Ejection clicks are usually related to dilate great vessels or valve abnormalities. They are heard during ventricular systole and are classified as early, mid, or late. Early ejection clicks at the mid-left sternal border are from the pulmonic valve. Aortic clicks are typically best heard at the apex. In contrast to aortic clicks, pulmonic clicks vary with respiration, becoming louder during inspiration. A mid to late ejection click at the apex is most typically caused by mitral valve prolapse (MVP).

2. Murmurs—A heart murmur is the most common cardiovascular finding leading to a cardiology referral. Innocent or functional heart murmurs are common, and 40%–45% of children have an innocent murmur at some time during childhood.

A. CHARACTERISTICS—All murmurs should be described based on the following characteristics:

(1) Location and radiation—Where the murmur is best heard and where the sound extends.

(2) Relationship to cardiac cycle and duration—Systolic ejection (immediately following S_1 with a crescendo/decrescendo change in intensity), pansystolic (occurring throughout most of systole and of constant intensity), diastolic, or continuous. The timing of the murmur provides valuable clues as to the underlying pathology (Table 20–4).

(3) Intensity—Grade I describes a soft murmur heard with difficulty; grade II, soft but easily heard; grade III, loud but without a thrill; grade IV, loud and associated with a precordial thrill; grade V, loud, with a thrill, and audible with the edge of the stethoscope; grade VI, very loud and audible with the stethoscope off the chest.

(4) Quality—Harsh, musical, or rough; high, medium, or low in pitch.

(5) Variation with position—Audible changes in murmur when the patient is supine, sitting, standing, or squatting.

B. INNOCENT MURMURS—The six most common innocent murmurs of childhood are as follows:

(1) Newborn murmur—Heard in the first few days of life, this murmur is at the lower left sternal border, without significant radiation. It has a soft, short, vibratory grade I–II/VI quality that often subsides when mild pressure is applied to the abdomen. It usually disappears by age 2–3 weeks.

(2) Peripheral pulmonary artery stenosis (PPS)—This murmur, often heard in newborns, is caused by the normal branching of the pulmonary artery. It is heard with equal intensity at the upper left sternal border, at the back, and in one or both axillae. It is a soft, short, high-pitched, grade I–II/VI systolic ejection murmur and usually disappears by age 2. This murmur must be differentiated from true peripheral pulmonary stenosis (Williams syndrome,

Table 20–4. Pathologic murmurs.

Systolic Ejection	Pansystolic	Diastolic	Continuous
Semilunar valve stenosis (AS/PS/truncal stenosis)	VSD	Semilunar valve regurgitation	Runoff lesions
ASD	AVVR (MR/TR)	AI/PI/truncal insufficiency	PDA/AVM/aortopulmonary collaterals
Coarctation		AV valve stenosis (MS/TS)	

AI/PI, aortic insufficiency/pulmonic insufficiency; AS/PS, aortic stenosis/pulmonic stenosis; ASD, atrial septal defect; AV, atrioventricular; AVVR, atrioventricular valve regurgitation; MR/TR, mitral regurgitation/tricuspid regurgitation; PDA/AVM, patent ductus arteriosus/arteriovenous malformation; VSD, ventricular septal defect.

Alagille syndrome, or rubella syndrome), coarctation of the aorta, and valvular pulmonary stenosis. Characteristic facial features, extracardiac physical examination findings, history, and laboratory abnormalities suggestive of the syndromes listed above are the best way to differentiate true peripheral pulmonary stenosis from benign PPS of infancy as the murmurs can be similar.

(3) Still murmur—This is the most common innocent murmur of early childhood. It is typically heard between 2 and 7 years of age. It is the loudest midway between the apex and the lower left sternal border. Still murmur is a musical or vibratory, short, high-pitched, grade I–III early systolic murmur. It is loudest when the patient is supine. It diminishes or disappears with inspiration or when the patient is sitting. The still murmur is louder in patients with fever, anemia, or sinus tachycardia from any reason.

(4) Pulmonary ejection murmur—This is the most common innocent murmur in older children and adults. It is heard from age 3 years onward. It is usually a soft systolic ejection murmur, grade I–II in intensity at the upper left sternal border. The murmur is louder when the patient is supine or when cardiac output is increased.

(5) Venous hum—A venous hum is usually heard after age 2 years. It is located in the infraclavicular area on the right. It is a continuous musical hum of grade I–III intensity and may be accentuated in diastole and with inspiration. It is best heard in the sitting position. Turning the child's neck, placing the child supine, and compressing the jugular vein obliterates the venous hum. Venous hum is caused by turbulence at the confluence of the subclavian and jugular veins.

(6) Innominate or carotid bruit—This murmur is more common in the older child and adolescents. It is heard in the right supraclavicular area. It is a long systolic ejection murmur, somewhat harsh and of grade II–III intensity. The bruit can be accentuated by light pressure on the carotid artery and must be differentiated from all types of aortic stenosis. The characteristic findings of aortic stenosis are outlined in more detail later in this chapter.

When innocent murmurs are found in a child, the physician should assure the parents that these are normal heart sounds of the developing child and that they do not represent heart disease.

Extracardiac Examination

A. Arterial Pulse Rate and Rhythm

Cardiac rate and rhythm vary greatly during infancy and childhood, so multiple determinations should be made. This is particularly important for infants (Table 20–5) whose heart rates vary with activity. The rhythm may be regular, or there may be a normal phasic variation with respiration (sinus arrhythmia).

B. Arterial Pulse Quality and Amplitude

A bounding pulse is characteristic of runoff lesions, including patent ductus arteriosus (PDA), aortic regurgitation, arteriovenous malformation, or any condition with a low diastolic pressure (fever, anemia, or septic shock). Narrow or thready pulses occur in patients with conditions reducing cardiac output such as decompensated heart failure (HF) pericardial tamponade, or severe aortic stenosis. A reduction in pulse amplitude or blood pressure (> 10 mm Hg) with inspiration is referred to as pulsus paradoxus and is a sign of pericardial tamponade. The pulses of the upper and lower extremities should be compared. The femoral pulse should be palpable and equal in amplitude and simultaneous with the brachial pulse. A femoral pulse that is absent or weak, or

Table 20–5. Resting heart rates.

Age	Low	High
< 1 mo	80	160
1–3 mo	80	200
2–24 mo	70	120
2–10 y	60	90
11–18 y	40	90

that is delayed in comparison with the brachial pulse, suggests coarctation of the aorta.

C. Arterial Blood Pressure

Blood pressures should be obtained in the upper and lower extremities. Systolic pressure in the lower extremities should be greater than or equal to that in the upper extremities. The cuff must cover the same relative area of the arm and leg. Measurements should be repeated several times. A lower blood pressure in the lower extremities suggests coarctation of the aorta.

D. Cyanosis of the Extremities

Cyanosis results from an increased concentration (> 4–5 g/dL) of reduced hemoglobin in the blood. Bluish skin color is usually, but not always, a sign. Visible cyanosis also accompanies low cardiac output, hypothermia, and systemic venous congestion, even in the presence of adequate oxygenation. Cyanosis should be judged by the color of the mucous membranes (lips). Bluish discoloration around the mouth (acrocyanosis) does not correlate with cyanosis.

E. Clubbing of the Fingers and Toes

Clubbing is often associated with severe cyanotic congenital heart disease. It usually appears after age 1 year. Hypoxemia with cyanosis is the most common cause, but clubbing also occurs in patients with endocarditis, chronic liver disease, inflammatory bowel diseases, chronic pulmonary disease, and lung abscess. Digital clubbing may be a benign genetic variant.

F. Edema

Edema of dependent areas (lower extremities in the older child and the face and sacrum in the younger child) is characteristic of elevated right heart pressure, which may be seen with tricuspid valve pathology or HF.

G. Abdomen

Hepatomegaly is the cardinal sign of right HF in the infant and child. Left HF can ultimately lead to right HF, and therefore hepatomegaly may also be seen in the child with pulmonary edema from lesions causing left-to-right shunting (pulmonary overcirculation) or LV failure. Splenomegaly may be present in patients with long-standing HF, and is also a characteristic of infective endocarditis (IE). Ascites is a feature of chronic right HF. Examination of the abdomen may reveal shifting dullness or a fluid wave.

Etoom Y, Ratnapalan S: Evaluation of children with heart murmurs. Clin Pediatr (Phila) 2014 Feb;53(2):111–117 [PMID: 23671266].

Kostopoulou E, Dimitriou G, Karatza A: Cardiac murmurs in children: a challenge for the primary care physician. Curr Pediatr Rev 2019 Mar 20 [PMID: 30907325].

ELECTROCARDIOGRAPHY

The electrocardiogram (ECG) is essential for the evaluation of the cardiovascular system. The heart rate should first be determined, then the cardiac rhythm (Is the patient in a normal sinus rhythm or other rhythm as evidenced by a P wave with a consistent PR interval before every QRS complex?), and then the axis (Are the P and QRS axes normal for patient age?). Finally, assessment of chamber enlargement, cardiac intervals, and ST segments should be performed.

Age-Related Variations

The ECG evolves with age. The heart rate decreases and intervals increase with age. Right ventricle (RV) dominance in the newborn changes to left ventricle (LV) dominance in the older infant, child, and adult. The normal ECG of the 1-week-old infant is abnormal for a 1-year-old child, and the ECG of a 5-year-old child is abnormal for an adult.

Electrocardiographic Interpretation

Figure 20–1 defines the events recorded by the ECG.

A. Rate

The heart rate varies markedly with age, activity, and state of emotional and physical well-being (see Table 20–5).

B. Rhythm

Sinus rhythm should always be present in healthy children. Extra heartbeats representing premature atrial and ventricular contractions (PAC and PVC) are common during childhood, with atrial ectopy predominating in infants and ventricular ectopy during adolescence. Isolated premature beats in patients with normal heart structure and function are usually benign.

C. Axis

1. P-wave axis—The P wave is generated from atrial contraction beginning in the high right atrium at the site of the sinus node. The impulse proceeds leftward and inferiorly, thus leading to a positive deflection in all left-sided and inferior leads (II, III, and aVF) and negative in lead aVR.

2. QRS axis—The net voltage should be positive in leads I and aVF in children with a normal axis. In infants and young children, RV dominance may persist, leading to a negative deflection in lead I. Several congenital cardiac lesions are associated with alterations in the normal QRS axis (Table 20–6).

D. P Wave

In the pediatric patient, the amplitude of the P wave is normally no greater than 3 mm and the duration no more than 0.08 second. The P wave is best seen in leads II and V_1.

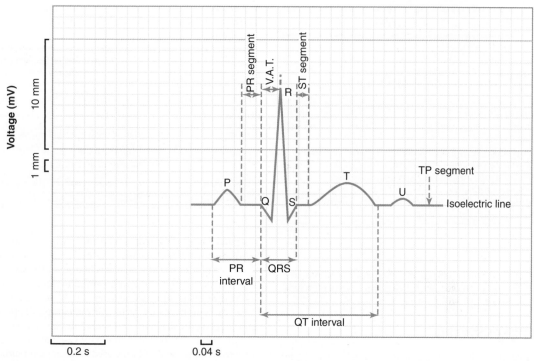

▲ **Figure 20–1.** Complexes and intervals of the electrocardiogram.

E. PR Interval

The PR is measured from the beginning of the P wave to the beginning of the QRS complex. It increases with age and with slower rates. The PR interval ranges from a minimum of 0.10 second in infants to a maximum of 0.18 second in older children with slow rates. Rheumatic heart disease, digitalis, β-blockers, and calcium channel blockers can prolong the PR interval.

F. QRS Complex

This represents ventricular depolarization, and its amplitude and direction of force (axis) reveal the relative ventricular mass in hypertrophy, hypoplasia, and infarction. Abnormal

Table 20–6. QRS axis deviation.

Right-Axis Deviation	Left-Axis Deviation
Tetralogy of Fallot	Atrioventricular septal defect
Transposition of the great arteries	Pulmonary atresia with intact ventricular septum
Total anomalous pulmonary venous return	Tricuspid atresia
Atrial septal defect	

ventricular conduction (eg, right bundle-branch block [RBBB] or left bundle-branch block [LBBB]) is also revealed.

G. QT Interval

This interval is measured from the beginning of the QRS complex to the end of the T wave. The QT duration may be prolonged as a primary condition or secondarily due to drugs or electrolyte imbalances (Table 20–7). The normal QT duration is rate-related and must be corrected using the Bazett formula:

$$QTc = \frac{QT\ interval\,(s)}{\sqrt{R-R}\ interval\,(s)}$$

The normal QTc is less than or equal to 0.44 second.

H. ST Segment

This segment, lying between the end of the QRS complex and the beginning of the T wave, is affected by drugs, electrolyte imbalances, or myocardial injury.

I. T Wave

The T wave represents myocardial repolarization and is altered by electrolytes, myocardial hypertrophy, and ischemia.

Table 20–7. Causes of QT prolongation.[a]

Cardiac medications
   Antiarrhythmics: class IA (quinidine, procainamide, disopyramide) class III (amiodarone, sotalol)
   Inotropic agents: dobutamine, dopamine, epinephrine, isoproterenol
Noncardiac medications
   Antibiotics/antivirals: azithromycin, clarithromycin, levofloxacin, amantadine
   Antipsychotics: risperidone, thioridazine, lithium, haloperidol
   Sedatives: chloral hydrate, methadone
   Other: albuterol, levalbuterol, ondansetron, phenytoin, pseudoephedrine
   Electrolyte disturbances: hypokalemia, hypomagnesemia, hypocalcemia

[a]Partial list only.

O'Connor M, McDaniel N, Brady WJ: The pediatric electrocardiogram. Part I: age-related interpretation. Am J Emerg Med 2008 May;26(4):506–512 [PMID: 18416018].

CHEST RADIOGRAPH

Evaluation of the chest radiograph for cardiac disease should focus on (1) position of the heart, (2) position of the abdominal viscera, (3) cardiac size, (4) cardiac configuration, and (5) character of the pulmonary vasculature. The standard posteroanterior and left lateral chest radiographs are used (Figure 20–2).

Cardiac position is either levocardia (heart predominantly in the left chest), dextrocardia (heart predominantly in the right chest), or mesocardia (midline heart). The position of the liver and stomach bubble is either in the normal position (abdominal situs solitus), inverted with the stomach bubble on the right (abdominal situs inversus), or variable with midline liver (abdominal situs ambiguous). The heart appears

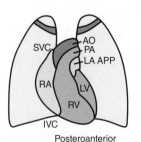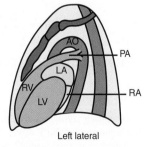

▲ **Figure 20–2.** Position of cardiovascular structures in principal radiograph views. AO, aorta; IVC, inferior vena cava; LA, left atrium; LA APP, left atrial appendage; LV, left ventricle; PA, pulmonary artery; RA, right atrium; RV, right ventricle; SVC, superior vena cava.

Table 20–8. Radiographic changes with cardiac chamber enlargement.

Chamber Enlarged	Change in Cardiac Silhouette on Anteroposterior Film
Right ventricle	Apex of the heart is tipped upward
Left ventricle	Apex of the heart is tipped downward
Left atrium	Double shadow behind cardiac silhouette
	Increase in subcarinal angle
Right atrium	Prominence of right atrial border of the heart

relatively large in normal newborns at least in part due to a prominent thymic shadow. The heart size should be less than 50% of the chest diameter in children older than 1 year. The cardiac configuration on chest radiograph may provide useful diagnostic information (Table 20–8). Some congenital cardiac lesions have a characteristic radiographic appearance that suggests the diagnosis but should not be viewed as conclusive (Table 20–9). The pulmonary vasculature should be assessed. The presence of increased or decreased pulmonary blood flow suggests a possible congenital cardiac diagnosis, particularly in the cyanotic infant (Table 20–10).

Laya BF et al: The accuracy of chest radiographs in the detection of congenital heart disease and in the diagnosis of specific congenital cardiac lesions. Pediatr Radiol 2006;36:677–681 [PMID: 16547698].

Dextrocardia

Dextrocardia is a radiographic term used when the heart is on the right side of the chest. When dextrocardia occurs with reversal of position of the other important organs of the chest and abdomen (eg, liver, lungs, and spleen), the condition is

Table 20–9. Lesion-specific chest radiographic findings.

Diagnosis	Chest Radiograph Appearance
D-transposition of the great arteries	Egg on a string
Tetralogy of Fallot	Boot-shaped heart
Unobstructed total anomalous pulmonary venous drainage	Snowman
Obstructed total anomalous pulmonary venous drainage	Small heart with congested lungs
Coarctation	Figure 3 sign + rib notching

Table 20–10. Alterations in pulmonary blood flow in cyanotic cardiac lesions.

Increased Pulmonary Blood Flow	Decreased Pulmonary Blood Flow
Total anomalous pulmonary venous return	Pulmonic stenosis
Tricuspid atresia with large ventricular septal defect	Tricuspid atresia/restrictive ventricular septal defect
Transposition of the great arteries	Tetralogy of Fallot
Truncus arteriosus	Pulmonary atresia with intact ventricular septum

called situs inversus totalis, and the heart is usually normal. When dextrocardia occurs with the other organs normally located (situs solitus), the heart usually has severe defects.

Other situs abnormalities include situs ambiguous with the liver central and anterior in the upper abdomen and the stomach pushed posteriorly, bilateral right-sidedness (asplenia syndrome), and bilateral left-sidedness (polysplenia syndrome). In virtually all cases of situs ambiguous, congenital heart disease is present.

ECHOCARDIOGRAPHY

Echocardiography is a fundamental tool of pediatric cardiology. Using multiple ultrasound modalities (two-dimensional imaging, Doppler, and M-mode), cardiac anatomy, blood flow, intracardiac pressures, and ventricular function can be assessed. Echocardiography is based on the physical principles of sound waves. The ultrasound frequencies utilized in cardiac imaging range from 2 to 10 million cycles/s.

M-mode echocardiography uses short bursts of ultrasound sent from a transducer. At acoustic interfaces, sound waves are reflected back to the transducer. The time it takes for the sound wave to return to the transducer is measured, and the distance to the interface is calculated. That calculated distance is displayed against time, and a one-dimensional image is constructed that demonstrates cardiac motion. **Two-dimensional imaging** extends this technique by sending a rapid series of ultrasound bursts across a 90-degree sector, which allows construction of a two-dimensional image of the heart. **Doppler ultrasound** measures blood flow. The ultrasound transducer sends out a known frequency of sound that reflects off moving red blood cells. The transducer receives the reflected frequency and compares it with the transmitted frequency. The blood flow velocity can be calculated from the measured frequency shift. This information is used to estimate pressure gradients by the simplified Bernoulli equation, in which the pressure gradient is equal to four times the calculated velocity (pressure gradient = $4(V^2)$).

A transthoracic echocardiogram is obtained by placing the transducer on areas of the chest where there is minimal lung interference. At each transducer position, the beam is swept through the heart and a two-dimensional image appears on the screen. Complex intracardiac anatomy and spatial relationships can be described, making possible the accurate diagnosis of congenital heart disease. In addition to structural details, Doppler gives information about intracardiac blood flow and pressure gradients. Commonly used Doppler techniques include color-flow imaging, pulsed-wave, and continuous-wave Doppler. Color-flow imaging gives general information on the direction and velocity of flow. Pulsed- and continuous-wave Doppler imaging give more precise measurements of blood velocity. The role of M-mode in the ultrasound examination has decreased as other ultrasound modalities have been developed. M-mode is still used to measure LV end-diastolic and end-systolic dimensions and permits calculation of the LV-shortening fraction, a standard estimate of LV function (SF = LV end-diastolic volume – LV systolic volume/LV end-diastolic volume). Three-dimensional echocardiography, tissue Doppler, strain, and strain rate imaging are newer modalities that provide more sophisticated assessment of systolic and diastolic function and can detect early changes in myocardial function.

A typical transthoracic echocardiogram performed by a skilled sonographer takes about 30 minutes, and patients must be still for the examination. Frequently infants and children cannot cooperate for the examination and sedation is required. Transesophageal echocardiography requires general anesthesia in infants and children and is primarily used to guide interventional procedures and surgical repair of congenital heart disease. In cases of difficult imaging windows due to patient size, air interference or when looking for evidence of vegetations on cardiac valves, transesophageal echocardiography may be necessary.

It is important to note that fetal echocardiography plays an important role in the prenatal diagnosis of congenital heart disease. A fetal echocardiogram is recommended if the fetus is considered high risk for the development of congenital heart disease or if there is suspicion for structural heart disease or fetal arrhythmias based on the obstetric fetal ultrasound. In utero management of fetal arrhythmias and postdelivery planning for the fetus with complex heart disease have resulted in improved outcomes for this challenging group of patients.

Donofrio MT et al: Diagnosis and treatment of fetal cardiac disease: a scientific statement from the American Heart Association. Circulation 2014 May 27;129(21):2183–2242 [PMID: 24763516].

Elkiran O, Karakurt C, Kokac G, Karadaq A: Tissue Doppler, strain, and strain rate measurements assessed by two-dimensional speckle-tracking echocardiography in healthy newborns and infants. Cardiol Young 2014 Apr;24(2):201–211 [PMID: 23388082].

Simpson J et al: Three-dimensional echocardiography in congenital heart disease: an expert consensus document from the European Association of Cardiovascular Imaging and the American Society of Echocardiography. J Am Soc Echocardiogr 2017 Jan;30(1):1–27 [PMID: 27838227].

MAGNETIC RESONANCE IMAGING

Magnetic resonance imaging (MRI) of the heart is valuable for evaluation and noninvasive follow-up of many congenital heart defects. It is particularly useful in imaging the thoracic vessels, which are difficult to image by transthoracic echocardiogram. Cardiac gated imaging allows dynamic evaluation of structure and blood flow of the heart and great vessels. Cardiac MRI provides unique and precise imaging in patients with newly diagnosed or repaired aortic coarctation and defines the aortic dilation in Marfan, Turner, and Loeys-Dietz syndromes. Cardiac MRI can quantify regurgitant lesions such as pulmonary insufficiency (PI) after repair of tetralogy of Fallot (ToF) and can define ventricular function, chamber size, and wall thickness in patients with inadequate echocardiographic images or cardiomyopathies. MRI is especially useful to characterize RV size and function as this chamber is often difficult to image comprehensively by echocardiogram. Because it allows computer manipulation of images of the heart and great vessels, three-dimensional MRI is an ideal noninvasive way of obtaining accurate reconstructions of the heart. General anesthesia is often required to facilitate cardiac MRI performance in children younger than 8 years.

Van der Hulst AE et al: Cardiac MRI in postoperative congenital heart disease patients. J Magn Reson Imaging 2012;36(3):511–528 [PMID: 2290365].

CARDIOPULMONARY STRESS TESTING

Cardiopulmonary stress testing provides objective measurements in children with congenital cardiac lesions to ascertain limitations, develop exercise programs, assess effects of medical or surgical therapies, and determine need for cardiac transplantation. Most children with heart disease are capable of normal activity. Bicycle ergometers or treadmills can be used in children as young as 5 years. The addition of a metabolic cart enables one to assess whether exercise impairment is secondary to cardiac limitation, pulmonary limitation, deconditioning, or lack of effort. Exercise variables include the ECG, blood pressure response to exercise, oxygen saturation, ventilation, maximal oxygen consumption, and peak workload attained. Stress testing is also employed in children with structurally normal hearts who have complaints of exercise-induced symptoms to rule out cardiac or pulmonary pathology. Significant stress ischemia or dysrhythmias warrant physical restrictions or appropriate therapy. Children with poor performance due to suboptimal conditioning benefit from a planned exercise program.

Miliaresis C et al: Cardiopulmonary stress testing in children and adults with congenital heart disease. Cardiol Rev 2014 Nov–Dec; 22(6):275–280 [PMID: 25162333].

ARTERIAL BLOOD GASES & PULSE OXIMETRY

Quantitating the partial arterial oxygen pressure (Pao_2) or O_2 saturation (Sao_2) during the administration of 100% oxygen is the most useful method of distinguishing hypoxemia produced primarily by heart disease or by lung disease—the so-called hyperoxia test. In cyanotic heart disease, hypoxemia is caused by shunting of de-oxygenated blood to the systemic circulation and, thus, when compared to values obtained while breathing room air, the Sao_2 and Pao_2 increase very little when 100% oxygen is administered. However, in a patient with hypoxemia caused by lung disease, the Sao_2 and Pao_2 usually increase significantly when oxygen is administered. Table 20–11 illustrates the respective responses seen in patients during the hyperoxia test.

In 2010, the US Department of Health and Human Services (HHS) recommended newborn screening for critical congenital heart disease with pulse oximetry screening at 24–48 hours of age. Both the American Academy of Pediatrics (AAP) and American Heart Association (AHA) endorsed this recommendation in 2012.

Hoffman JI: Is pulse oximetry useful for screening neonates for critical congenital heart disease at high altitudes? Pediatr Cardiol 2016 Jun;37(5):812–817. doi: 10.1007/s00246-016-1371-1 [PMID: 27090652].

Kemper AR et al: Strategies for implementing screening for critical congenital heart disease. Pediatrics 2011 Nov;128(5):e1259–e1267 [PMID: 21987707].

Mahle WT et al: Endorsement of health and human services recommendation for pulse oximetry screening for critical congenital heart disease. Pediatrics 2012 Jan;129(1):190–192 [PMID: 22201143].

Table 20–11. Examples of responses to 10 minutes of 100% oxygen in lung disease and heart disease.

	Lung Disease		Heart Disease	
	Room Air	100% Fio$_2$	Room Air	100% Fio$_2$
Color	Blue → Pink		Blue → Blue	
Oximetry (Sao$_2$)	60% → 99%		60% → 62%	
Pao$_2$ (mm Hg)	35 → 120		35 → 38	

Fio$_2$, fraction of inspired oxygen; Pao$_2$, partial arterial oxygen pressure; Sao$_2$, oxygen saturation.
Data from Mahle WT, Newburger JW, Matherne GP, et al: Role of pulse oximetry in examining newborns for congenital heart disease: a scientific statement from the AHA and AAP. Pediatrics 2009 Aug;124(2):823–836.

CARDIAC CATHETERIZATION & ANGIOCARDIOGRAPHY

Cardiac catheterization is an invasive method to evaluate anatomic and physiologic conditions in congenital or acquired heart disease. Management decisions may be made based on oximetric, hemodynamic, or angiographic data obtained through a catheterization. In an increasing number of cases, intervention may be performed during a catheterization that may palliate, or even cure, a congenital heart defect without open heart surgery.

Cardiac Catheterization Data

Figure 20–3 shows oxygen saturation (in percent) and pressure (in millimeters of mercury) values obtained at cardiac catheterization from the chambers and great arteries of the heart. These values represent the normal range for a school age child.

A. Oximetry, Shunts, and Cardiac Output

Measurement of oxygen levels throughout the heart and surrounding blood vessels can provide a wealth of information about a patient's physiology. The difference between systemic saturation (in the aorta) and mixed venous saturation

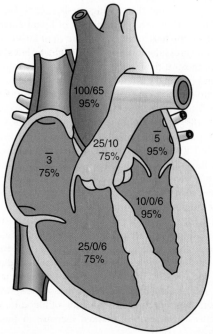

▲ **Figure 20–3.** Pressures (mm Hg) and oxygen saturation (%) obtained by cardiac catheterization in a healthy child. 3, mean pressure of 3 mm Hg in the right atrium; 5, mean pressure of 5 mm Hg in the left atrium.

(usually in the superior vena cava [SVC]) is usually inversely proportional to the overall cardiac output. Cardiac output is determined by saturation difference across a vascular bed, taking into account oxygen consumption and hemoglobin. This is known as the Fick principle. Cardiac output in a healthy heart varies directly with the body's oxygen consumption and is inversely proportional to hemoglobin. The circulatory system of patients who are anemic usually tries to generate a higher cardiac output to maintain oxygen delivery to the cells of the body.

An *increase* in saturation across the *right* side of the heart (anywhere between SVC and pulmonary arteries) represents a left-to-right shunt. If oxygenated blood can mix with venous blood, the saturation rises—the degree of which correlates with the size of the shunt. Conversely, a *fall* in saturation across the *left* heart, between the pulmonary veins and the aorta, is abnormal. This represents the addition of deoxygenated blood to oxygenated blood—a right-to-left shunt.

A commonly referenced ratio in pediatric cardiology is the Qp:Qs. In a normal heart, systemic cardiac output (Qs) and pulmonary blood flow (Qp) are equal, or Qp:Qs = 1. If a step-up in saturation is noted across the right heart, suggesting a left-to-right shunt, pulmonary blood flow will exceed systemic blood flow. This can result, in cases of large shunts, in a Qp:Qs of as high as 3:1 or more. This level of shunt is usually poorly tolerated, but small shunts (such as 1.5:1) may be well tolerated for months or years. In cases of right-to-left shunts, Qs will exceed Qp. In these cyanotic patients, the Qp:Qs may be 0.7 or 0.8.

B. Pressures

Pressures should be determined in all chambers and major vessels entered. Systolic pressure in the RV should be equal to the systolic pressure in the pulmonary artery. Likewise, the systolic pressure in the LV should be equal to the systolic pressure of the aorta. The mean pressure in the atria should be nearly equal to (or a point or two lower than) the end-diastolic pressure of the ventricles. If a gradient in pressure exists, an obstruction is present, and the severity of the gradient is one criterion for the necessity of intervention.

For example, an LV systolic pressure in a small child of 140 mm Hg and an aortic systolic pressure of 80 mm Hg, a gradient of 60 mm Hg, would classify as severe aortic valve stenosis. Balloon aortic valvuloplasty would be indicated at the time of the catheterization.

C. Vascular Resistance

In addition to pressure and flow, resistance completes the "concept triad" of congenital heart physiology. Resistance is related to pressure and flow as described in the below equation:

$$\text{Resistance} = \frac{\text{Pressure}}{\text{Flow}}$$

The resistance across a vascular bed can be concretely calculated. Patients with congenital heart disease or pulmonary vascular disease may have elevation in pulmonary vascular resistance (PVR), which can adversely impact circulation and heart function. To calculate PVR, the pressure drop from the pulmonary arteries to the left atrium is divided by pulmonary blood flow (Qp) to obtain a value in units. For example, a patient with a mean pulmonary artery pressure (PAP) of 15 mm Hg and a left atrial pressure of 9 mm Hg, with a Qp of 3 L/min/m^2, has a PVR of 2 U/m^2.

Normal PVR is less than 3 U/m^2. Systemic vascular resistance normally covers a wider range, usually from 10 to 30 U/m^2. The ratio of pulmonary to systemic vascular resistance is usually less than 0.3. High pulmonary resistance, or a high ratio of resistance, denotes abnormal pulmonary vasculature. It often represents increased risk in patients with congenital heart disease or PH and results in higher risk of death in severely affected patients.

Cardiac catheterization can be performed to evaluate the effects of pharmaceutical therapy. An example of this use of catheterization is monitoring changes in PVR during the administration of nitric oxide or prostacyclin in a child with primary PH.

Angiography

In the past, angiography was a mainstay of the initial diagnostic methods for congenital heart disease. It is still used for diagnostic purposes in selected cases but currently is used more frequently to plan interventions or evaluate postsurgical anatomy that is poorly seen by noninvasive methods. Injection of contrast liquid via a well-positioned catheter can illuminate detailed intracardiac and intravascular anatomy more clearly than any other method. Cardiac function can be observed, and anatomic abnormalities may be easily identified. In a growing number of centers, three-dimensional reconstruction of angiograms can provide exquisite delineation of cardiac and vascular structures.

Interventional Cardiac Catheterization

Interventional cardiac catheterization procedures are performed to occlude lesions such as a PDA, atrial septal defect (ASD), or ventricular septal defect (VSD). Obstruction of heart valves can be addressed through balloon valvuloplasty. Intervention may also be performed on vascular obstruction through angioplasty or stent placement in pulmonary arteries or the aorta. Systemic and pulmonary veins can be modified in a similar fashion, unfortunately with often minimal success in the latter. Devices are now available to allow patients to undergo replacement of failing heart valves without open heart surgery, and an increasing armamentarium of devices are becoming available for treatment of other defects and abnormal vasculature.

With the progression of improved noninvasive imaging, fewer diagnostic cardiac catheterization studies are performed today. The number of interventional procedures, however, is on the rise. Although the risks of cardiac catheterization are very low for elective studies in older children (< 1%), the risk of major complications in distressed or small patients is higher. Interventional procedures, particularly in unstable babies and children, increase these risks further. Increased use of registries is currently being employed to better understand efficacy rates and risks of these procedures, with the hope of optimizing the care of infants and children in the catheterization laboratory.

Backes CH et al: Low weight as an independent risk factor for adverse events during cardiac catheterization of infants. Catheter Cardiovasc Interv 2013 Nov 1;82(5):786–794 [PMID: 23436647].

PERINATAL & NEONATAL CIRCULATION

At birth, two events affect the cardiovascular and pulmonary system: (1) the umbilical cord is clamped, removing the placenta from the maternal circulation and (2) breathing commences. As a result, marked changes in the circulation occur. During fetal life, the placenta offers low resistance to blood flow. In contrast, the pulmonary arterioles are markedly constricted and there is high resistance to blood flow in the lungs. Therefore, the majority of blood entering the right side of the heart travels from the right atrium into the left atrium across the foramen ovale (right-to-left shunt). In addition, most of the blood that makes its way into the RV and then pulmonary arteries will flow from the pulmonary artery into the aorta through the ductus arteriosus (right-to-left shunt). Subsequently, pulmonary blood flow accounts for only 7%–10% of the combined in utero ventricular output. At birth, pulmonary blood flow dramatically increases with the fall in PVR and pressure. The causes of prolonged high PVR include physical factors (lack of an adequate air-liquid interface or ventilation), low oxygen tension, and vasoactive mediators such as elevated endothelin peptide levels or leukotrienes. Clamping the umbilical cord produces an immediate increase in resistance to flow in the systemic circuit.

As breathing commences, the Po$_2$ of the small pulmonary arterioles increases, resulting in a decrease in PVR. Increased oxygen tension, rhythmic lung distention, and production of nitric oxide as well as prostacyclin play major roles in the fall in PVR at birth. The PVR falls below that of the systemic circuit, resulting in a reversal in direction of blood flow across the ductus arteriosus and marked increase in pulmonary blood flow.

Functional closure of the ductus arteriosus begins shortly after birth. The ductus arteriosus usually remains patent for 1–5 days. During the first hour after birth, a small right-to-left shunt is present (as in the fetus). However, after 1 hour, bidirectional shunting occurs, with the left-to-right direction predominating. In most cases, right-to-left shunting disappears completely by 8 hours. In patients with severe hypoxia (eg, in the syndrome of persistent PH of the newborn), PVR remains high, resulting in a continued right-to-left shunt. Although flow through the ductus arteriosus usually is gone by 5 days of life, the vessel does not close anatomically for 7–14 days.

In fetal life, the foramen ovale serves as a one-way valve shunting blood from the inferior vena cava (IVC) through the right atrium into the left atrium. At birth, because of the changes in the pulmonary and systemic vascular resistance and the increase in the quantity of blood returning from the pulmonary veins to the left atrium, the left atrial pressure rises above that of the right atrium. This functionally closes the flap of the foramen ovale, preventing flow of blood across the septum. The foramen ovale remains probe patent in 10%–15% of adults.

Persistent PH is a clinical syndrome of full-term infants. The neonate develops tachypnea, cyanosis, and PH during the first 8 hours after delivery. These infants have massive right-to-left ductal and/or foramen shunting for 3–7 days because of high PVR. Progressive hypoxia and acidosis will cause early death unless the pulmonary resistance can be lowered. Postmortem findings include increased thickness of the pulmonary arteriolar media. Increased alveolar Po_2 with hyperventilation, alkalosis, paralysis, surfactant administration, high-frequency ventilation, and cardiac inotropes can usually reverse this process. Inhaled nitric oxide selectively dilates pulmonary vasculature, produces a sustained improvement in oxygenation, and has resulted in improved outcomes.

In the normal newborn, PVR and pulmonary arterial pressure continue to fall during the first weeks of life as a result of demuscularization of the pulmonary arterioles. Adult levels of pulmonary resistance and pressure are normally achieved by 4–6 weeks of age. It is at this time typically that signs of pulmonary overcirculation associated with left-to-right shunt lesions VSD or atrioventricular septal defect [AVSD]) appear.

Rudolph AM: The fetal circulation and congenital heart disease. Arch Dis Child Fetal Neonatal Ed 2010;95(2):F132–F136 [PMID: 19321508].

▼ HEART FAILURE

Heart failure (HF) is the clinical condition in which the heart fails to meet the circulatory and metabolic needs of the body. Right and left HF can result from volume or pressure overload of the respective ventricle or an intrinsic abnormality of the ventricular myocardium. Causes of RV volume overload include an ASD, pulmonary valve insufficiency, or anomalous pulmonary venous return. LV volume overload occurs with any left-to-right shunting lesion (eg, VSD, PDA), aortic valve insufficiency, or a systemic arteriovenous malformation. Causes of RV failure as a result of pressure overload include PH, valvar pulmonary stenosis, or severe branch PPS. LV pressure overload results from left heart obstructive lesions such as aortic stenosis (subvalvar, valvar, or supravalvar) or coarctation of the aorta. Abnormalities of the RV myocardium that can result in right HF include Ebstein anomaly (atrialization of the RV) and arrhythmogenic RV dysplasia (a genetic disorder where the RV myocardium is replaced by fat). Abnormalities of the LV myocardium are more common and include dilated cardiomyopathy (DCM), myocarditis, or hypertrophic cardiomyopathy (HCM). As a result of elevated left atrial pressure and impaired relaxation of the LV, left HF can lead to right HF. Other causes of HF in infants include AVSD, coronary artery anomalies, and chronic atrial tachyarrhythmias. Metabolic, mitochondrial, and neuromuscular disorders with associated cardiomyopathy present at various ages depending on the etiology. HF due to acquired conditions such as myocarditis can occur at any age. Children with HF may present with irritability, diaphoresis with feeds, fatigue, exercise intolerance, or evidence of pulmonary congestion (see Table 20–1).

Treatment of Heart Failure

The therapy of HF should be directed toward the underlying cause as well as the symptoms. Regardless of the etiology, neurohormonal activation occurs early when ventricular systolic dysfunction is present. Plasma catecholamine levels (eg, norepinephrine) increase causing tachycardia, diaphoresis, and activation of the renin-angiotensin system (which, in turn, results in peripheral vasoconstriction and salt and water retention). Although an evidence basis for treatment of pediatric HF is lacking, therapies should be aimed at improving cardiac performance by targeting the three determinants of cardiac performance: (1) preload, (2) afterload, and (3) contractility.

Inpatient Management of Heart Failure

Patients with cardiac decompensation may require hospitalization for initiation or augmentation of HF therapy. Table 20–12 demonstrates intravenous inotropic agents used to augment cardiac output and their relative effect on heart rate, systemic vascular resistance, and cardiac index. The drug used will depend in part on the cause of the HF. Of the drugs listed in Table 20–12, norepinephrine would not be utilized alone due to its mild effect on contractility and cardiac index and more profound effect of increasing systemic vascular resistance, and thus afterload.

Table 20–12. Intravenous inotropic agents.

Drug	Dose	Renal Perfusion	Heart Rate	Cardiac Index	SVR
Dopamine	2–5 mcg/kg/min	↑ via vasodilatation	0	0	0
	5–15	↑/↓ depending on balance of ↑ cardiac index and ↑ SVR	↑	↑	↑↓
	15–20	↓ via vasoconstriction	↑	↑	↑
Dobutamine	2–20 mcg/kg/min	↑ via ↑ cardiac index	Mild ↑	↑	↓
Epinephrine	0.05–2 mcg/kg/min	↑ at low dose via vasodilatation ↓ at high dose via vasoconstriction	↑	↑	↓ at low dose ↑ at high dose
Norepinephrine	0.05–2 mcg/kg/min	↓	0	Very mild ↑	↑↑
Isoproterenol	0.05–5 mcg/kg/min	0	↑↑	↑	↓↓

SVR, systemic vascular resistance.

A. Inotropic and Mechanical Support

1. Afterload reduction and systemic vasodilatation

A. MILRINONE—This phosphodiesterase-3 inhibitor potentiates calcium delivery to the myocardium, thereby improving the inotropic state of the heart. Milrinone is an inodilator with systemic and pulmonary vasodilatory effects, in addition to a dose-dependent increase in cardiac contractility. Thus, milrinone is an effective agent in both right and left HF. Milrinone also reduces the incidence of low cardiac output syndrome following open-heart surgery. The usual intravenous infusion dosage range is 0.25–0.75 mcg/kg/min.

B. NITRATES—Nitroprusside is a nitric oxide donor that induces arterial and venous vasodilatation. Venous vasodilatation allows for increased capacitance, reduction of venous preload, and reduction of right atrial pressure. Arterial vasodilatation reduces LV afterload but can also cause hypotension. A common adverse effect is reflex tachycardia. Nitroglycerin exerts similar effects with increased venous selectivity and is also used to improve coronary blood flow in settings of myocardial infarction or coronary underperfusion following congenital heart surgery. The usual intravenous infusion dosages for nitroprusside and nitroglycerin range are 0.25–3 mcg/kg/min.

2. Enhancement of contractility

A. EPINEPHRINE—Also known as adrenaline, this catecholamine is a potent stimulator of α_1-, β_1-, and β_2-adrenergic receptors resulting in bronchodilatation, cardiac stimulation, and systemic vasodilatation. Epinephrine demonstrates dose-dependent effects on the vasculature with vasodilatation at low doses via β_2 receptors and vasoconstriction at high doses via α_1-receptor activation. The β_1 effects induce both increased inotropy and chronotropy (heart rate). The usual intravenous infusion dosage range is 0.05–2 mcg/kg/min. Other non-HF indications for epinephrine include anaphylaxis, bronchoconstriction, shock, and bradycardia or pulseless cardiac arrest.

B. DOPAMINE—This naturally occurring catecholamine increases myocardial contractility primarily via stimulation of adrenergic and dopaminergic receptors. Renal dopamine receptor activation improves renal perfusion. The usual dose range for HF is 2–10 mcg/kg/min.

C. DOBUTAMINE—This synthetic catecholamine increases myocardial contractility secondary to cardiospecific β-adrenergic activation and produces little peripheral vasoconstriction. Dobutamine does not usually cause marked tachycardia, which is a distinct advantage. However, the drug does not selectively improve renal perfusion as does dopamine. The usual intravenous infusion dose range is 2–10 mcg/kg/min.

3. Mechanical circulatory support—Mechanical support is indicated in children with severe, refractory myocardial failure secondary to cardiomyopathy, myocarditis, or following cardiac surgery. Mechanical support is used for a limited time while cardiac function improves or as a bridge to cardiac transplantation.

A. EXTRACORPOREAL MEMBRANE OXYGENATION (ECMO)—ECMO is a temporary means of providing gas exchange and hemodynamic support to patients with cardiac or pulmonary failure refractory to conventional therapy. Blood is withdrawn from the patient by a pump via a cannula positioned at the SVC or right atrium and passes through a membrane oxygenator (to exchange both O_2 and CO_2). This oxygenated blood is then delivered back to the patient through a cannula in the aorta (via the common carotid artery). Systemic anticoagulation is needed to prevent clot formation in the circuit. The patient is monitored closely while awaiting improvement in cardiac function. Risks are significant and include severe bleeding, infection, end organ injury (kidneys, in particular), stroke, and patient or circuit thrombosis.

B. Ventricular assist devices—Use of ventricular assist devices is increasing in children as device development has progressed. These devices allow for less invasive hemodynamic support than ECMO. In this case, a cannula is usually positioned in the apex of the ventricle and blood is withdrawn from the ventricle using a battery-operated pump. Blood is then returned to the patient through a separate cannula positioned in the aorta or pulmonary artery, depending on the ventricle being supported. One or both ventricles can be supported, if necessary. Ventricular assist carries lower risk of circuit thrombosis than ECMO, but the risk of infection, patient thrombosis, and bleeding complications remains.

Outpatient Management of Heart Failure

A. Medications

1. Afterload-reducing agents—Oral afterload-reducing agents improve cardiac output by decreasing systemic vascular resistance. Angiotensin-converting enzyme (ACE) inhibitors (captopril, enalapril, and lisinopril) are first-line therapy in children with HF requiring long-term treatment. These agents block angiotensin II–mediated systemic vasoconstriction and are particularly useful in children with reduced LV myocardial function (eg, myocarditis or DCMs).

2. β-Blockade—Although clearly beneficial in adults with HF, β-blocker therapy in children with HF did not demonstrate any significant improvement compared to placebo. However, β-blockers may still be useful adjunctive therapy in some children who are already taking ACE inhibitors and have refractory HF requiring additional afterload reduction. The neurohumoral response to HF includes excessive circulating catecholamines due to activation of the sympathetic nervous system. Although beneficial acutely, this compensatory response over time produces myocardial fibrosis, myocyte hypertrophy, and myocyte apoptosis that contribute to the progression of HF. β-Blockers (eg, carvedilol and metoprolol) antagonize this sympathetic activation and may offset these deleterious effects. Side effects of β-blockers include bradycardia, hypotension, and worsening HF in some patients.

3. Diuretics—Diuretic therapy is often necessary in HF to maintain the euvolemic state and control symptoms related to pulmonary or hepatic congestion caused by sodium and water retention as a consequence of renin-angiotensin system activation.

A. Furosemide—This loop diuretic inhibits sodium-chloride-potassium cotransport and reabsorption at the loop of Henle. When used chronically, loop diuretics induce potassium and chloride excretion, producing hypochloremic metabolic alkalosis and hypokalemia for which electrolytes should be monitored.

B. Thiazides—Thiazides inhibit sodium chloride reabsorption at the distal convoluted tubule and are used to complement furosemide in severe cases of HF.

C. Spironolactone—Spironolactone is an aldosterone inhibitor used frequently in conjunction with other diuretics for its potassium sparing effect (often helps avoid the need for potassium supplementation). Though not proven in children, the aldosterone inhibitory effect of spironolactone has benefit in adults with HF, separate from its diuretic effect, as aldosterone is associated with the development of fibrosis, sodium retention, and vascular dysfunction.

4. Digitalis—Digitalis is a cardiac glycoside with a positive inotropic effect on the heart and an associated decrease in systemic vascular resistance. The preparation of digitalis used in clinical practice is digoxin. Large studies in adult patients with HF have not demonstrated decreased mortality of HF with digoxin use, but treatment is associated with reduced hospitalization rates for HF exacerbations. No controlled studies exist in children,

A. Digitalis toxicity—Any dysrhythmia that occurs during digoxin therapy should be attributed to the drug until proven otherwise. Ventricular dysrhythmia and first-, second-, or third-degree AV block are characteristic of digoxin toxicity. A trough level should be obtained if digoxin toxicity is suspected.

B. Digitalis poisoning—This acute emergency must be treated without delay. Digoxin poisoning most commonly occurs in toddlers who have taken their parents' or grandparents' medications. The child's stomach should be emptied immediately by gastric lavage, and activated charcoal may be indicated in severe poisonings. Toxicity may induce high grade heart block, for which atropine or temporary ventricular pacing may be needed. Antiarrhythmic agents may also be needed. Digoxin immune Fab can be used to reverse potentially life-threatening intoxication.

Kirk R et al: The International Society of Heart and Lung Transplantation Guidelines for the management of pediatric heart failure: executive summary. J Heart Lung Transplant 2014 Sep; 33(9):888–909 [PMID: 25110323].

Morales DL et al: Use of ventricular assist devices in children across the United States: analysis of 7.5 million pediatric hospitalizations. Ann Thorac Surg 2010 Oct;90(4):1313–1318; discussion 1318–1319 [PMID: 20868835].

GENETIC BASIS OF CONGENITAL HEART DISEASE

Environmental factors such as maternal diabetes, alcohol consumption, progesterone use, viral infection, and other maternal teratogen exposure are associated with an increased incidence of cardiac malformations. However, the importance of genetics as a cause of congenital heart disease is becoming more evident as advances in the field occur. Microdeletion in the long arm of chromosome 22 (22q11) is associated with DiGeorge syndrome. These children often have conotruncal abnormalities such as truncus arteriosus, ToF, double-outlet RV, or interrupted aortic arch. Alagille, Noonan, Holt-Oram, and Williams syndromes and the trisomies 13, 18, and 21 are all commonly associated with congenital heart lesions. Understanding these associations as well as further targeted study investigating the genetic basis of other cardiac lesions will offer opportunities for early diagnosis, gene therapy, and recurrence risk counseling for families.

Pierpont ME et al: Genetic basis for congenital heart defects: current knowledge: a scientific statement from the American Heart Association Congenital Cardiac Defects Committee, Council on Cardiovascular Disease in the Young: endorsed by the American Academy of Pediatrics. Circulation 2007;115:3015–3038 [PMID: 17519398].

▼ ACYANOTIC CONGENITAL HEART DISEASE

DEFECTS IN SEPTATION

1. Atrial Septal Defect

ESSENTIALS OF DIAGNOSIS & TYPICAL FEATURES

▶ Fixed, widely split S_2, RV heave.

▶ Grade I–III/VI systolic ejection murmur at the pulmonary area.

▶ Large shunts cause a diastolic flow murmur at the lower left sternal border (increased flow across the tricuspid valve).

▶ ECG shows rsR′ in lead V_1.

▶ Frequently asymptomatic.

▶ General Considerations

Atrial septal defect (ASD) is an opening in the atrial septum permitting the shunting of blood between the atria. There are three major types: ostium secundum, ostium primum, and sinus venosus. Ostium secundum is the most common type and represents an embryologic deficiency in the septum secundum or too large of a central hole in the septum primum. Ostium primum defect is associated with AVSDs. The sinus venosus defect is frequently associated with abnormal pulmonary venous return, as the location of the sinus venosus is intimately related to the right upper pulmonary vein.

Ostium secundum ASD occurs in 10% of patients with congenital heart disease and is two times more common in females than in males. The defect is most often sporadic but may be familial or have a genetic basis (Holt-Oram syndrome). After the third decade, atrial arrhythmias or pulmonary vascular disease may develop. Irreversible PH resulting in cyanosis as atrial level shunting becomes right-to-left and ultimately right HF can occur and is a life-limiting process (Eisenmenger syndrome).

▶ Clinical Findings

A. Symptoms and Signs

Most infants and children with an ASD have no cardiovascular symptoms. Older children and adults can present with exercise intolerance, easy fatigability, or, rarely, HF. The direction of flow across the ASD is determined by the compliance of the ventricles. Because the RV is normally more compliant, shunting across the ASD is left-to-right as blood follows the path of least resistance. Therefore, cyanosis does not occur unless RV dysfunction occurs, usually as a result of PH, leading to reversal of the shunt across the defect.

Peripheral pulses are normal and equal. The heart is usually hyperactive, with an RV heave felt best at the mid to lower left sternal border. S_2 at the pulmonary area is widely split and often fixed. In the absence of associated PH, the pulmonary component is normal in intensity. A grade I–III/VI ejection-type systolic murmur is heard best at the left sternal border in the second intercostal space. This murmur is caused by increased flow across the pulmonic valve, not flow across the ASD. A mid-diastolic murmur is often heard in the fourth intercostal space at the left sternal border. This murmur is caused by increased flow across the tricuspid valve during diastole. The presence of this murmur suggests high flow with a pulmonary-to-systemic blood flow ratio greater than 2:1.

B. Imaging

Radiographs may show cardiac enlargement. The main pulmonary artery may be dilated and pulmonary vascular markings increased in large defects owing to the increased pulmonary blood flow.

C. Electrocardiography

The usual ECG shows right-axis deviation. In the right precordial leads, an rsR′ pattern is usually present. A mutation in the cardiac homeobox gene (*NKX2-5*) is associated with an ASD, and AV block would be seen on the ECG.

D. Echocardiography

Echocardiography shows a dilated right atrium and RV. Direct visualization of the exact anatomic location of the ASD by two-dimensional echocardiography, and demonstration of a left-to-right shunt through the defect by color-flow Doppler, confirms the diagnosis and has eliminated the need for cardiac catheterization prior to surgical or catheter closure of the defect. Assessment of all pulmonary veins should be made to rule out associated anomalous pulmonary venous return.

E. Cardiac Catheterization

Although cardiac catheterization is rarely needed for diagnostic purposes, transcatheter closure of an ostium secundum ASD is now the preferred method of treatment.

If a catheterization is performed, oximetry shows a significant step-up in oxygen saturation from the SVC to the right atrium. The PAP and PVR are usually normal. The Qp:Qs may vary from 1.5:1 to 4:1.

▶ Treatment

Surgical or catheterization closure is generally recommended for symptomatic children with a large atrial level defect and associated right heart dilation. In the asymptomatic child with a large hemodynamically significant defect, closure is performed electively at age 1–3 years. Most defects are amenable to nonoperative device closure during cardiac catheterization, but the defect must have adequate tissue rims on all sides on which to anchor the device. The mortality for surgical closure is less than 1%. When closure is performed by age 3 years, late complications of RV dysfunction and dysrhythmias are avoided.

▶ Course & Prognosis

Patients usually tolerate an ASD well in the first two decades of life, and the defect often goes unnoticed until middle or late adulthood. PH and reversal of the shunt are rare late complications. Infective endocarditis (IE) is uncommon. Spontaneous closure occurs, most frequently in children with a defect less than 4 mm in diameter; therefore, outpatient follow-up is recommended. Exercise tolerance and oxygen consumption in surgically corrected children are generally normal, and restriction of physical activity is unnecessary.

Moore J et al: Transcatheter device closure of atrial septal defects: a safety review. JACC Cardiovasc Interv 2013 May;6(5):433–442 [PMID: 23702008].

Silvestry FE et al: Guidelines for the echocardiographic assessment of atrial septal defect and patent foramen ovale: from the American Society of Echocardiography and Society for Cardiac Angiography and Interventions. J Am Soc Echocardiogr 2015 Aug;28(8): 910–958. doi: 10.1016/j.echo.2015.05.015 [PMID: 26239900].

2. Ventricular Septal Defect

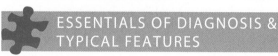

ESSENTIALS OF DIAGNOSIS & TYPICAL FEATURES

▶ Holosystolic murmur at lower left sternal border with RV heave.

▶ Presentation and course depend on size of defect and the PVR.

▶ Clinical features are failure to thrive, tachypnea, and diaphoresis with feeds.

▶ Left-to-right shunt with normal PVR.

▶ Large defects may cause Eisenmenger syndrome if not repaired early.

▶ General Considerations

VSD is the most common congenital heart malformation, accounting for about 30% of all congenital heart disease. Defects in the ventricular septum occur both in the membranous portion of the septum (most common) and the muscular portion. VSDs follow one of four courses:

A. Small, Hemodynamically Insignificant Ventricular Septal Defects

Between 80% and 85% of VSDs are small (< 3 mm in diameter) at birth and will close spontaneously. In general, small defects in the muscular interventricular septum will close sooner than those in the membranous septum. In most cases, a small VSD never requires surgical closure. Fifty percent of small VSDs will close by age 2 years, and 90% by age 6 years, with most of the remaining closing during the school years.

B. Moderate-Sized Ventricular Septal Defects

Asymptomatic patients with moderate-sized VSDs (3–5 mm in diameter) account for 3%–5% of children with VSDs. In general, these children do not have clear indicators for surgical closure. Historically, in those who had cardiac catheterization, the ratio of pulmonary to systemic blood flow is usually less than 2:1, and serial cardiac catheterizations demonstrate that the shunts get progressively smaller. If the patient is asymptomatic and without evidence of PH, these defects can be followed serially as some close spontaneously over time.

C. Large Ventricular Septal Defects With Normal Pulmonary Vascular Resistance

These defects are usually 6–10 mm in diameter. Unless they become markedly smaller within a few months after birth, they often require surgery. The timing of surgery depends on the clinical situation. Many infants with large VSDs and normal PVR develop symptoms of failure to thrive, tachypnea, diaphoresis with feeds by age 3–6 months, and require correction at that time. Surgery before age 2 years in patients with large VSDs essentially eliminates the risk of pulmonary vascular disease.

D. Large Ventricular Septal Defects With Pulmonary Vascular Obstructive Disease

The direction of flow across a VSD is determined by the resistance in the systemic and pulmonary vasculature, explaining why flow is usually left-to-right. In large VSDs, ventricular pressures are equalized, resulting in increased PAP. In addition, shear stress caused by increased volume in the pulmonary circuit causes increased resistance over time. The vast majority of patients with inoperable PH develop the condition progressively. The combined data of the multicenter National History Study indicate that almost all cases of irreversible PH can be prevented by surgical repair of a large VSD before age 2 years.

▶ Clinical Findings

A. Symptoms and Signs

Patients with small or moderate left-to-right shunts usually have no cardiovascular symptoms. Patients with large left-to-right shunts are usually ill early in infancy. These infants have frequent respiratory infections and gain weight slowly. Dyspnea, diaphoresis, and fatigue are common. These symptoms can develop as early as 1–6 months of age. Older children may experience exercise intolerance. Over time, in children and adolescents with persistent large left-to-right shunt, the pulmonary vascular bed undergoes structural changes, leading to increased PVR and reversal of the shunt from left-to-right to right-to-left (Eisenmenger syndrome). Cyanosis will then be present.

1. Small left-to-right shunt—No lifts, heaves, or thrills are present. The first sound at the apex is normal, and the second sound at the pulmonary area is split physiologically. A grade II–IV/VI, medium- to high-pitched, harsh pansystolic murmur is heard best at the left sternal border in the third and fourth intercostal spaces. The murmur radiates over the entire precordium. No diastolic murmurs are heard.

2. Moderate left-to-right shunt—Slight prominence of the precordium with moderate LV heave is evident. A systolic thrill may be palpable at the lower left sternal border between the third and fourth intercostal spaces. The second sound at the pulmonary area is most often split but may be single. A grade III–IV/VI, harsh pansystolic murmur is heard best at the lower left sternal border in the fourth intercostal space. A mitral diastolic flow murmur indicates that pulmonary blood flow and subsequently the pulmonary venous return are significantly increased by the large shunt.

3. Large ventricular septal defects with pulmonary hypertension—The precordium is prominent, and the sternum bulges. Both LV and RV heaves are palpable. S_2 is palpable in the pulmonary area. A thrill may be present at the lower left sternal border. S_2 is usually single or narrowly split, with accentuation of the pulmonary component. The murmur ranges from grade I to IV/VI and is usually harsh and pansystolic. Occasionally, when the defect is large or ventricular pressures approach equivalency, a murmur is difficult to hear. A diastolic flow murmur may be heard, depending on the size of the shunt.

B. Imaging

In patients with small shunts, the chest radiograph may be normal. Patients with large shunts have significant cardiac enlargement involving both the LV and RV and the left atrium. The main pulmonary artery segment may be dilated. The pulmonary vascular markings are increased.

C. Electrocardiography

The ECG is normal in small left-to-right shunts. Left ventricular hypertrophy (LVH) usually occurs in patients with large left-to-right shunts and normal PVR. Combined ventricular enlargement occurs in patients with PH caused by increased flow, increased resistance, or both. Pure right ventricular hypertrophy (RVH) occurs in patients with PH secondary to pulmonary vascular obstruction induced by long-standing left-to-right shunt (Eisenmenger syndrome).

D. Echocardiography

Two-dimensional echocardiography can reveal the size of a VSD and identify its anatomic location. Multiple defects can be detected by combining two-dimensional and color-flow imaging. Doppler can further evaluate the VSD by estimating the pressure difference between the LV and RV. A pressure difference greater than 50 mm Hg in the LV compared to the RV confirms the absence of severe PH.

E. Cardiac Catheterization and Angiocardiography

The ability to describe the VSD anatomy and estimate the PAPs on the basis of the gradient across the VSD allows for the vast majority of isolated defects to be repaired without cardiac catheterization and angiocardiography. Catheterization is indicated in those patients with increased PVR. Angiocardiographic examination defines the number, size, and location of the defects.

▶ Treatment

A. Medical Management

Patients who develop symptoms can be managed with anticongestive treatment, particularly diuretics and systemic afterload reduction, prior to surgery or if it is expected that the defect will close over time.

B. Surgical Treatment

Patients with cardiomegaly, poor growth, poor exercise tolerance, or other clinical abnormalities who have a significant shunt (> 2:1) typically undergo surgical repair at age 3–6 months. A synthetic or pericardial patch is used for primary closure. In most centers, these children have surgery before age 1 year. As a result, Eisenmenger syndrome has been virtually eliminated. The surgical mortality rate for VSD closure is below 2%.

Transcatheter closure of muscular VSDs is also a possibility. Perimembranous VSDs have also been closed in children during catheterization, but a high incidence of complete heart block after placement of the occluding device has slowed the acceptance of this approach.

▶ Course & Prognosis

Significant late dysrhythmias are uncommon. Functional exercise capacity and oxygen consumption are usually normal, and physical restrictions are unnecessary. Adults with corrected defects have normal quality of life.

Jortveit J et al: Mortality and complications in 3495 children with isolated ventricular septal defects. Arch Dis Child 2016 Sep; 101(9):808–813. doi: 10.1136/archdischild-2015-310154 [PMID: 27091847].

Sondheimer HM, Rahimi-Alangi K: Current management of ventricular septal defect. Cardiol Young 2006;16(Suppl 3):131–135 [PMID: 17378052].

3. Atrioventricular Septal Defect

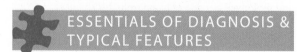

ESSENTIALS OF DIAGNOSIS & TYPICAL FEATURES

- ▶ Murmur often inaudible in neonates.
- ▶ Loud pulmonary component of S_2.
- ▶ Common in infants with Down syndrome.
- ▶ ECG with extreme left-axis deviation.

▶ General Considerations

Atrioventricular septal defect (AVSD) results from incomplete fusion of the embryonic endocardial cushions. The endocardial cushions help to form the "crux" of the heart, which includes the lower portion of the atrial septum, the membranous portion of the ventricular septum, and the septal leaflets of the tricuspid and mitral valves. AVSD accounts for about 4% of all congenital heart disease. Sixty percent of

children with Down syndrome have congenital heart disease, and of these, 35%–40% have an AVSD.

AVSDs are defined as partial or complete. The physiology of the defect is determined by the location of the AV valves. If the valves are located in the midportion of the defect (complete AVSD), both atrial and ventricular components of the septal defect are present and the left- and right-sided AV valves share a common ring or orifice. In the partial form, there is a low insertion of the AV valves, resulting in a primum ASD without a ventricular defect component. In partial AVSD, there are two separate AV valve orifices and usually a cleft in the left-sided valve.

Partial AVSD behaves like an isolated ASD with variable amounts of regurgitation through the cleft in the left AV valve. The complete form causes large left-to-right shunts at both the ventricular and atrial levels with variable degrees of AV valve regurgitation. If there is increased PVR, the shunts may be bidirectional. Bidirectional shunting is more common in Down syndrome or in older children who have not undergone repair.

▶ Clinical Findings

A. Symptoms and Signs

The partial form may produce symptoms similar to ostium secundum ASD. Patients with complete AVSD usually have symptoms such as failure to thrive, tachypnea, diaphoresis with feeding, or recurrent bouts of pneumonia.

In the neonate with the complete form, the murmur may be inaudible due to relatively equal systemic and pulmonary vascular resistance (PVR). After 4–6 weeks, as PVR drops, a nonspecific systolic murmur develops. The murmur is usually not as harsh as that of an isolated VSD. There is both right- and left-sided cardiac enlargement. S_2 is loud, and a pronounced diastolic flow murmur may be heard at the apex and the lower left sternal border.

If severe pulmonary vascular obstructive disease is present, there is usually dominant RV enlargement. S_2 is palpable at the pulmonary area, and no thrill is felt. A nonspecific short systolic murmur is heard at the lower left sternal border. No diastolic flow murmurs are heard. If a right-to-left shunt is present, cyanosis will be evident.

B. Imaging

Cardiac enlargement is always present in the complete form and pulmonary vascular markings are increased. Often, only the right heart size may be increased in the partial form, although a severe mitral valve cleft can rarely lead to left heart enlargement as well.

C. Electrocardiography

In all forms of AVSD, there is extreme left-axis deviation with a counterclockwise loop in the frontal plane. The ECG is an important diagnostic tool. Only 5% of isolated VSDs have this ECG abnormality. First-degree heart block occurs in over 50% of patients. Right, left, or combined ventricular hypertrophy is present depending on the particular defect and the presence or absence of PH.

D. Echocardiography

Echocardiography is the diagnostic test of choice. The anatomy can be well visualized by two-dimensional echocardiography. Both AV valves are at the same level, compared with the normal heart in which the tricuspid valve is more apically positioned. The size of the atrial and ventricular components of the defect can be measured. AV valve regurgitation can be detected. The LV outflow tract is elongated (gooseneck appearance), which produces systemic outflow obstruction in some patients.

E. Cardiac Catheterization and Angiocardiography

Cardiac catheterization is not routinely used to evaluate AVSD but may be used to assess PAPs and resistance in the older infant with Down syndrome, as this patient group is predisposed to early-onset PH. Increased oxygen saturation in the RV or the right atrium identifies the level of the shunt. Angiocardiography reveals the characteristic gooseneck deformity of the LV outflow tract in the complete form.

▶ Treatment

Spontaneous closure of this type of defect does not occur, and therefore surgery is required. In the partial form, surgery carries a low mortality rate (1%–2%), but patients require follow-up because of late-occurring LV outflow tract obstruction and mitral valve dysfunction. The complete form carries a higher mortality rate. Complete correction in the first year of life, prior to the onset of irreversible PH, is obligatory.

Colen T, Smallhorn JF: Three-dimensional echocardiography for the assessment of atrioventricular valves in congenital heart disease: past, present and future. Semin Thorac Cardiovasc Surg Pediatr Card Surg Annu 2015;18(1):62–71. doi: 10.1053/j.pcsu.2015.01.003 [PMID: 25939845].

Craig B: Atrioventricular septal defect: from fetus to adult. Heart 2006;92:1879–1885 [PMID: 17105897].

PATENT (PERSISTENT) DUCTUS ARTERIOSUS

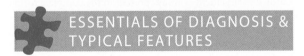

ESSENTIALS OF DIAGNOSIS & TYPICAL FEATURES

▶ Continuous machinery-type murmur.

▶ Bounding peripheral pulses if large ductus present.

▶ Presentation and course depends on size of the ductus and the PVR.

▶ Clinical features of a large ductus are failure to thrive, tachypnea, and diaphoresis with feeds.

▶ Left-to-right shunt with normal PVR.

▶ General Considerations

Patent ductus arteriosus (PDA) is the persistence of the normal fetal vessel joining the pulmonary artery to the aorta. It closes spontaneously in normal-term infants at 1–5 days of age. PDA accounts for 10% of all congenital heart disease. The incidence of PDA is higher in infants born at altitudes over 10,000 ft. It is twice as common in females as in males. The frequency of PDA in preterm infants weighing less than 1500 g ranges from 20% to 60%. The defect may occur as an isolated abnormality or with associated lesions, commonly coarctation of the aorta and VSD. Patency of the ductus arteriosus may be necessary in some patients with complex forms of congenital heart disease (eg, hypoplastic left heart syndrome [HLHS], pulmonary atresia [PA]). Prostaglandin E$_2$ (PGE$_2$) is a product of arachidonic acid metabolism and continuous intravenous infusion maintains ductal patency.

▶ Clinical Findings

A. Symptoms and Signs

The clinical findings and course depend on the size of the shunt and the degree of PH.

1. Moderate to large patent ductus arteriosus—Pulses are bounding, and pulse pressure is widened due to diastolic runoff through the ductus. S$_1$ is normal and S$_2$ is usually narrowly split. In large shunts, S$_2$ may have a paradoxical split (eg, S$_2$ narrows on inspiration and widens on expiration). Paradoxical splitting is caused by volume overload of the LV and prolonged ejection of blood from this chamber.

The murmur is characteristic. It is a rough machinery murmur maximal at the second left intercostal space. It begins shortly after S$_1$, rises to a peak at S$_2$, and passes through the S$_2$ into diastole, where it becomes a decrescendo murmur and fades before the S$_1$. The murmur tends to radiate well to the anterior lung fields but relatively poorly to the posterior lung fields. A diastolic flow murmur is often heard at the apex.

2. Patent ductus arteriosus with increased pulmonary vascular resistance—Flow across the ductus is diminished. S$_2$ is single and accentuated, and no significant heart murmur is present. The pulses are normal rather than bounding.

B. Imaging

In an isolated PDA, the appearance of the chest radiograph depends on the size of the shunt. If the shunt is small, the heart is not enlarged. If the shunt is large, both left atrial and LV enlargement may be seen. The aorta and the main pulmonary artery segment may also be prominent.

C. Electrocardiography

The ECG may be normal or may show LVH, depending on the size of the shunt. In patients with PH caused by increased blood flow, biventricular hypertrophy usually occurs. In pulmonary vascular obstructive disease, pure RVH occurs.

D. Echocardiography

Echocardiography provides direct visualization of the ductus and confirms the direction and degree of shunting. High-velocity left-to-right flow argues against abnormally elevated PVR, and as PVR drops during the neonatal period, higher velocity left-to-right shunting is usually seen. If suprasystemic PVR is present, flow across the ductus will be seen from right to left. Associated cardiac lesions and ductal-dependent pulmonary or systemic blood flow must be recognized by echocardiography, as closure of a PDA in this setting would be contraindicated.

E. Cardiac Catheterization and Angiocardiography

PDA closure in the catheterization laboratory with a vascular plug or coils is now routine in all but the smallest of neonates and infants.

▶ Treatment

Surgical closure is indicated when the PDA is large and the patient is small. Caution must be given to closing a PDA in patients with pulmonary vascular obstructive disease and right-to-left shunting across the ductus as this could result in RV failure. Patients with large left-to-right shunts require repair by age 1 year to prevent the development of progressive pulmonary vascular obstructive disease. Symptomatic PDA with normal PAP can be safely coil or device-occluded in the catheterization laboratory, ideally after the child has reached 5 kg.

Patients with nonreactive pulmonary vascular obstruction, PVR greater than 10 Wood units (normal, < 3), and a ratio of pulmonary to systemic resistance greater than 0.7 (normal, < 0.3) despite vasodilator therapy (eg, nitric oxide) should not undergo PDA closure. These patients are made worse by PDA closure because the flow through the ductus allows preserved RV function and maintains cardiac output to the systemic circulation. These patients can be managed with pulmonary vasodilator therapy but eventually may require heart-lung transplant in severe cases.

Presence of a symptomatic PDA is common in preterm infants. Indomethacin, a prostaglandin synthesis inhibitor, is often used to close the PDA in premature infants. Indomethacin does not close the PDA of full-term infants or children. The success of indomethacin therapy is as high as 80%–90% in premature infants with a birth weight greater than 1200 g, but it is less successful in smaller infants. Indomethacin (0.1–0.3 mg/kg orally every 8–24 hours or 0.1–0.3 mg/kg parenterally every 12 hours) can be used if there is adequate renal, hematologic, and hepatic function. Because indomethacin may impair renal function, urine output, BUN, and creatinine should be monitored during therapy. If indomethacin is not effective and the ductus remains hemodynamically significant, surgical ligation should be performed. If the ductus partially closes so that the shunt is no longer hemodynamically significant, a second course of indomethacin may be tried.

▶ Course & Prognosis

Patients with an isolated PDA and small to moderate shunts usually do well without surgery. However, in the third or fourth decade of life, symptoms of easy fatigability, dyspnea on exertion, and exercise intolerance appear in those patients who develop PH and/or HF. Percutaneous closure can be done later in life if there has not been development of severe pulmonary vascular disease. For those with severe and irreversible PH prognosis is not good and heart-lung transplant may be needed.

Spontaneous closure of a PDA may occur up to age 1 year, especially in preterm infants. After age 1 year, spontaneous closure is rare. Because endocarditis is a potential complication, some cardiologists recommend closure if the defect persists beyond age 1 year, even if it is small. Most of these patients undergo percutaneous occlusion as opposed to surgical ligation.

Lam JY, Lopushinsky SR, MaI W, Dicke F, Brindle ME: Treatment options for pediatric patent ductus arteriosus: systematic review and meta-analysis. Chest 2015 Sep;148(3):784–793. doi: 10.1378/chest.14-2997 [PMID: 25835756].

Takata H et al: Long-term outcome of coil occlusion in patients with patent ductus arteriosus. Circ J 2011 Feb;75(2):407–412 [PMID: 21173496].

RIGHT-SIDED OBSTRUCTIVE LESIONS

1. Pulmonary Valve Stenosis

ESSENTIALS OF DIAGNOSIS & TYPICAL FEATURES

▶ No symptoms in mild or moderate stenosis.

▶ Cyanosis and a high incidence of right-sided HF in ductal-dependent lesions.

▶ RV lift with systolic ejection click heard at the third left intercostal space.

▶ S_2 widely split with soft to inaudible P_2; grade I–VI/VI systolic ejection murmur, maximal at the pulmonary area.

▶ Dilated pulmonary artery on chest radiograph.

General Considerations

Pulmonic valve stenosis accounts for 10% of all congenital heart disease. The pulmonary valve annulus is usually small with moderate to marked poststenotic dilation of the main pulmonary artery. Obstruction to blood flow across the pulmonary valve causes an increase in RV pressure. Pressures greater than systemic are potentially life threatening and are associated with critical obstruction. Because of the increased RV strain, severe RVH and eventual RV failure can occur.

When obstruction is severe and the ventricular septum is intact, a right-to-left shunt will often occur at the atrial level through a patent foramen ovale (PFO). In neonates with severe obstruction and minimal antegrade pulmonary blood flow (critical PS), left-to-right flow through the ductus is essential, making prostaglandin a necessary intervention at the time of birth. These infants are cyanotic at presentation.

Clinical Findings

A. Symptoms and Signs

Patients with mild or even moderate valvular pulmonary stenosis are acyanotic and asymptomatic. Patients with severe valvular obstruction may develop cyanosis early. Patients with mild to moderate obstruction are usually well developed and well nourished. They are not prone to pulmonary infections. The pulses are normal. The precordium may be prominent, often with palpable RV heave. A systolic thrill is often present in the pulmonary area. In patients with mild to moderate stenosis, a prominent ejection click of pulmonary origin is heard at the third left intercostal space. The click varies with respiration, being more prominent during expiration than inspiration. In severe stenosis, the click tends to merge with S_1. S_2 varies with the degree of stenosis. In mild pulmonic stenosis, S_2 is normal. In moderate pulmonic stenosis, S_2 is more widely split and the pulmonary component is softer. In severe pulmonary stenosis, S_2 is single because the pulmonary component cannot be heard. A rough systolic ejection murmur is best heard at the second left interspace. It radiates well to the back. With severe pulmonary valve obstruction, the murmur is usually short. No diastolic murmurs are audible.

B. Imaging

The heart size is normal. Poststenotic dilation of the main pulmonary artery and the left pulmonary artery often occurs.

C. Electrocardiography

The ECG is usually normal with mild obstruction. In severe obstruction, RV hypertrophy with an RV strain pattern (deep inversion of the T wave) occurs in the right precordial leads (V_{3R}, V_1, V_2). Right atrial enlargement may be present. Right-axis deviation occurs in moderate to severe stenosis.

D. Echocardiography

The diagnosis often is made by physical examination, but the echocardiogram confirms the diagnosis, defines the anatomy, and can identify any associated lesions. The pulmonary valve has thickened leaflets with reduced valve leaflet excursion. The transvalvular pressure gradient can be estimated accurately by Doppler, which provides an estimate of RV pressure and can assist in determining the appropriate time to intervene.

E. Cardiac Catheterization and Angiocardiography

Catheterization is reserved for therapeutic balloon valvuloplasty. In severe cases with associated RV dysfunction, a right-to-left shunt at the atrial level is indicated by a lower left atrial saturation than pulmonary vein saturation. PAP is normal. The gradient across the pulmonary valve varies from 10 to 200 mm Hg. In severe cases, the right atrial pressure is elevated, with a predominant "a" wave. Angiocardiography in the RV shows a thick pulmonary valve with a narrow opening producing a jet of contrast into the pulmonary artery. Infundibular (RV outflow tract) hypertrophy may be present and may contribute to obstruction to pulmonary blood flow.

Treatment

Treatment of pulmonic stenosis is recommended for children with RV systolic pressure greater than two-thirds of systemic pressure. Immediate correction is indicated for patients with systemic or suprasystemic RV pressure. Percutaneous balloon valvuloplasty is the procedure of choice. It is as effective as surgery in relieving obstruction and causes less valve insufficiency. Surgery is needed to treat pulmonic valve stenosis when balloon pulmonic valvuloplasty is unsuccessful.

Course & Prognosis

Patients with mild pulmonary stenosis live normal lives. Even those with moderate stenosis are rarely symptomatic. Those with severe valvular obstruction may develop cyanosis in infancy as described earlier.

After balloon pulmonary valvuloplasty or surgery, most patients have good maximum exercise capacity unless they have significant PI. Limitation of physical activity is unwarranted. The quality of life of adults with successfully treated pulmonary stenosis and minimal PI is normal. Patients with PI, a frequent side effect of intervention, may be significantly limited in exercise performance. Severe PI leads to progressive RV dilation and dysfunction, which may precipitate ventricular arrhythmias or right HF in adulthood. Patients with severe PI may benefit from replacement of the pulmonic valve.

Harrild DM et al: Long-term pulmonary regurgitation following balloon valvuloplasty for pulmonary stenosis risk factors and relationship to exercise capacity and ventricular volume and function. J Am Coll Cardiol 2010 Mar 9;55(10):1041–1047 [PMID: 20202522].

Van Hare GF: Eligibility and disqualification recommendations for competitive athletes with cardiovascular abnormalities: Task Force 4: congenital heart disease: a scientific statement from the American Heart Association and American College of Cardiology. Circulation 2015 Dec 1;132(22):e281–e291. doi: 10.1161/CIR.0000000000000240 [PMID: 26621645].

2. Subvalvular Pulmonary Stenosis

Isolated infundibular (subvalvular) pulmonary stenosis is rare. More commonly it is found in combination with other lesions, such as in ToF. Infundibular hypertrophy that is associated with a small perimembranous VSD may lead to a "double-chambered RV" characterized by obstruction between the inflow and outflow portion of the RV. One should suspect such an abnormality if there is a prominent precordial thrill, no audible pulmonary ejection click, and a murmur maximal in the third and fourth inter-costal spaces rather than in the second intercostal space. The clinical picture is otherwise identical to that of pulmonic valve stenosis. Intervention, if indicated, is always surgical because this condition does not improve with balloon catheter dilation.

3. Supravalvular Pulmonary Stenosis

Supravalvular pulmonary stenosis is a relatively rare condition defined by narrowing of the main pulmonary artery. The clinical picture may be identical to valvular pulmonary stenosis, although the murmur is maximal in the first inter-costal space at the left sternal border and in the suprasternal notch. No ejection click is audible, as the valve itself is not involved. The murmur radiates toward the neck and over the lung fields. Children with Williams syndrome can have supravalvular and PPS as well as supravalvular aortic stenosis.

4. Peripheral (Branch) Pulmonary Artery Stenosis

In PPS, there are multiple narrowings of the branches of the pulmonary arteries, sometimes extending into the vessels in the periphery of the lungs. Systolic murmurs may be heard over both lung fields, anteriorly and posteriorly, radiating to the axilla. Mild, nonpathologic pulmonary branch stenosis produces a murmur in infancy that resolves by 6 months of age. Williams syndrome, Alagille syndrome, and congenital rubella are commonly associated with severe forms of peripheral PAS. Surgery is often unsuccessful, as areas of stenoses near and beyond the hilum of the lungs are not accessible to the surgeons. Transcatheter balloon angioplasty and even stent placement are used to treat this condition, with moderate success. In some instances, the stenoses improve spontaneously with age.

5. Ebstein Malformation of the Tricuspid Valve

In Ebstein malformation of the tricuspid valve, the septal leaflet of the tricuspid valve is displaced toward the apex of the heart and is attached to the endocardium of the RV rather than at the tricuspid annulus. As a result, a large portion of the RV functions physiologically as part of the right atrium. This "atrialized" portion of the RV is thin-walled and does not contribute to RV output. The portion of the ventricle below the displaced tricuspid valve is diminished in volume and represents the functioning RV.

▶ Clinical Findings

A. Symptoms and Signs

The clinical picture of Ebstein malformation varies with the degree of displacement of the tricuspid valve. In the most extreme form, the septal leaflet is markedly displaced into the RV outflow tract, causing obstruction of antegrade flow into the pulmonary artery, and there is very little functioning RV as the majority of the ventricle is "atrialized." The degree of tricuspid insufficiency may be so severe that forward (antegrade) flow out the RV outflow tract is further diminished leading to a right-to-left atrial level shunt and cyanosis. At the opposite extreme when antegrade pulmonary blood flow is adequate, symptoms may not develop until adulthood when tachyarrhythmias associated with right atrial dilation or reentrant electrical pathways occur. These older patients typically have less displacement of the septal leaflet of the tricuspid valve and therefore more functional RV tissue.

B. Imaging

The chest radiograph shows cardiomegaly with prominence of the right heart border. The extent of cardiomegaly depends on the degree of tricuspid valve insufficiency and the presence and size of the atrial level shunt. Massive cardiomegaly with a "wall-to-wall heart" (the heart shadow extends across the entire chest cavity from right to left) occurs with severe tricuspid valve displacement and/or a restrictive atrial level defect.

C. Electrocardiography

ECG may be normal but usually shows right atrial enlargement and RBBB. There is an association between Ebstein anomaly and Wolff-Parkinson-White (WPW) syndrome, in which case a delta wave is present (short PR with a slurred upstroke of the QRS).

D. Echocardiography

Echocardiography is necessary to confirm the diagnosis and may aid in predicting outcome. Degree of tricuspid valve displacement, size of the right atrium, and presence of associated atrial level shunt all affect outcome.

▶ Course & Prognosis

In cyanotic neonates, PGE$_2$ is used to maintain pulmonary blood flow via the ductus arteriosus until PVR decreases, facilitating antegrade pulmonary artery flow. If the neonate remains significantly cyanotic, surgical intervention is required.

The type of surgical repair varies and depends on the severity of the disease. For example, in order to decrease the amount of tricuspid regurgitation surgery may involve atrial plication and tricuspid valve repair. The success of the procedure is highly variable. Late arrhythmias are common due to the preexisting atrial dilation. If a significant Ebstein malformation is not treated, atrial tachyarrhythmias frequently begin during adolescence and the enlarged atrialized RV could impede LV function. Postoperative exercise tolerance improves but remains lower than age-related norms.

Dearani JA, Mora BN, Nelson TJ, Haile DT, O'Leary PW: Ebstein anomaly review: what's now, what's next? Expert Rev Cardiovasc Ther 2015 Oct;13(10):1101–1109. doi: 10.1586/14779072. 2015.1087849 [PMID: 26357983].

LEFT-SIDED LESIONS

1. Coarctation of the Aorta

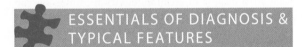

ESSENTIALS OF DIAGNOSIS & TYPICAL FEATURES

▶ Absent or diminished femoral pulses.

▶ Upper to lower extremity systolic blood pressure gradient.

▶ Blowing systolic murmur in the back or left axilla.

▶ General Considerations

Coarctation of the aorta is a narrowing in the aortic arch, usually in the proximal descending aorta at the insertion of the ductus arteriosus, near the takeoff of the left subclavian artery (which is usually proximal to the obstruction). Coarctation accounts for 7% of all congenital heart disease and has a male predominance (1.5:1); many affected females have Turner syndrome (45, XO). Coarctation is associated with bicuspid aortic valve in up to 85% of cases and intracerebral (berry) aneurysms in 10% of cases.

▶ Clinical Findings

A. Symptoms and Signs

The cardinal physical findings are decreased/absent femoral pulses and blood pressure gradient between the arms and legs. Normally, blood pressure in the legs is at least that of the arms, and typically higher. This is reversed in coarctation, with upper extremity blood pressure often greater than 15 mm Hg above that of lower extremities; the gradient may be diminished in the setting of significant LV dysfunction or collateralization. Blood pressure should be measured in all four extremities; the left subclavian artery may be distal to the coarctation, with decreased blood pressure and pulses in the left upper extremity. Lower extremity pulses may be normal until the PDA closes (ductal patency ensures flow to the descending aorta distal to the coarctation).

Approximately 40% of children with coarctation present as neonates, often with acute LV dysfunction, low cardiac output, shock and systemic acidosis from impaired tissue perfusion when the PDA closes. The remaining 60% of children with coarctation often have no symptoms in infancy, presenting insidiously with systemic hypertension, claudication, or failure to thrive. A systolic or continuous murmur may be present in the left back or left axilla, in addition to possible findings associated with a bicuspid aortic valve, if present.

B. Imaging

Infants with coarctation and associated cardiac dysfunction often have marked cardiac enlargement and pulmonary venous congestion on chest radiograph. Older children may have normal LV size but demonstrate a "figure 3" sign (prominent aorta proximal to the coarctation, an indentation at the level of the coarctation, and postcoarctation dilation) or inferior notching of the ribs due to significant collateralization of intercostal arteries bypassing the obstruction. CT and MRI are occasionally utilized to provide three-dimensional imaging of the aorta, especially with complex coarctation and extensive aortic hypoplasia.

C. Electrocardiography

The ECG in infants is often normal, with dominant RV forces, as the RV serves as the systemic ventricle during fetal life. ECGs in older children often demonstrate LVH.

D. Echocardiography

Two-dimensional echocardiography can directly visualize the coarctation, ventricular size and function. Color-flow and spectral Doppler demonstrate turbulent flow at the coarctation and estimate velocity across the obstruction; diastolic runoff flow is present with significant obstruction. In neonates with a PDA, future development of a coarctation cannot be excluded, as PDA closure can constrict aortic tissue, causing coarctation. Other left heart obstructive lesions, such as bicuspid aortic valve or mitral abnormalities, may be present.

E. Cardiac Catheterization and Angiocardiography

Cardiac catheterization and angiocardiography are rarely performed for diagnosis in infants or children with coarctation but are used if transcatheter intervention is planned.

▶ Treatment

Infants with coarctation of the aorta may present in extremis, and the primary resuscitative measure is PGE_1 infusion (0.05–0.1 mcg/kg/min) to reopen the ductus arteriosus and relax ductal tissue in the aorta. End-organ damage distal to the coarctation is not uncommon, and inotropic support is frequently needed.

Once stabilized, the infant should undergo corrective repair. Neonatal repair of native coarctation is typically addressed with surgery (extended end-to-end anastomosis); surgery may also address other associated lesions at that time. Palliative neonatal balloon angioplasty of native coarctation is rarely performed in those with substantial cardiac dysfunction. In older children, balloon angioplasty of the coarctation can be the definitive treatment; stenting (including covered stent placement) may be appropriate if the stent implanted can be expanded to an adult size.

Recurrent coarctation, the primary complication of both baseline surgery and balloon angioplasty, is more common after initial angioplasty intervention. Recurrent coarctation is typically treatable in the catheterization laboratory with angioplasty and possible stent placement.

▶ Course & Prognosis

Children who survive the neonatal period without HF do well through childhood and adolescence. Systemic hypertension is common, even after successful coarctation repair, especially in those repaired after age 5 years. Fatal complications (eg, hypertensive encephalopathy or intracranial bleeding) are uncommon in childhood. Infective endarteritis is rare before adolescence but can occur in both repaired and unrepaired coarctation. Exercise testing is mandatory prior to participation in competitive athletic activities.

Feltes TF et al: Indications for cardiac catheterization and intervention in pediatric cardiac disease: a scientific statement from the American Heart Association. Circulation 2011 Jun 7; 123(22):2607–2652. doi: 10.1161/CIR.0b013e31821b1f10 [PMID: 21536996].

Meadows J, Minahan M, McElhinney DB, McEnaney K, Ringel R: Intermediate outcomes in the prospective, multicenter coarctation of the Aorta Stent Trial (COAST). Circulation 2015 May 12;131(19):1656–1664. doi: 10.1161/CIRCULATIONAHA.114.013937 [PMID: 25869198].

2. Aortic Stenosis

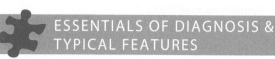

ESSENTIALS OF DIAGNOSIS & TYPICAL FEATURES

- ▶ Harsh systolic ejection murmur at the upper right sternal border with radiation to the neck.
- ▶ Thrill in suprasternal notch and carotid arteries.
- ▶ Systolic click at the apex.
- ▶ Dilation of the ascending aorta on chest radiograph.

▶ General Considerations

Aortic stenosis, accounting for 3%–8% of congenital heart disease, is defined as obstruction to outflow from the LV at/near the aortic valve, producing a systolic pressure gradient greater than 10 mm Hg. Three isolated anatomic variants of aortic stenosis exist (at, below, or above the valve), though multiple levels of obstruction commonly occur.

A. Valvular Aortic Stenosis (60%–75%)

Valvular aortic stenosis has a male predominance (3–5:1) and is typically associated with a bicuspid or unicuspid aortic valve. Bicuspid aortic valve is present in 1.3% of the population, making it the most common congenital heart lesion; the valve is composed of only two leaflets or three leaflets with complete or partial fusion of two of the leaflets. A unicuspid aortic valve has fusion of the three leaflets. Leaflet fusion typically results in reduced leaflet mobility and potential obstruction to flow.

B. Subvalvular Aortic Stenosis (10%–20%)

Subvalvular aortic stenosis, also with a male predominance (2–3:1), is associated with a discrete membrane or muscular narrowing in the LV outflow tract. The aortic valve may be normal or malformed, and membranes are often attached to the anterior leaflet of the mitral valve. Membranes typically develop postnatally, often associated with other left heart obstructive lesions and perimembranous VSDs, and they are typically progressive.

C. Supravalvular Aortic Stenosis (8%–14%)

Supravalvular aortic stenosis involves narrowing of the ascending aorta, typically at the aortic sinotubular junction. This is typically associated with an elastin defect, such as in Williams syndrome (with supravalvular pulmonary stenosis, abnormal facies, and developmental delays).

► Clinical Findings

A. Symptoms and Signs

Isolated valvular aortic stenosis seldom causes symptoms in infancy, though severe congenital stenosis can be associated with severe LV dysfunction and cardiogenic shock and require a PDA to supply systemic cardiac output ("critical" aortic stenosis). Physical findings vary depending on the level of obstruction:

1. Valvular aortic stenosis—If the stenosis is severe, pulses are diminished with a slow upstroke. Palpation reveals an LV thrust at the apex and, possibly, a systolic thrill at the suprasternal notch and over the carotid arteries with moderate or severe stenosis.

An aortic ejection click, associated with valve opening, may be heard at the apex, distinct from S_1 and without respiratory variation. A loud, harsh, medium-to-high-pitched ejection-type systolic murmur is present at the right upper sternal border, radiating to the suprasternal notch and carotids; the frequency of the murmur correlates with stenosis severity.

2. Discrete membranous subvalvular aortic stenosis—The findings are the same as those of valvular aortic stenosis, though an ejection click is absent. The murmur is located lower on the left sternal border, in the third and fourth intercostal spaces. Associated aortic insufficiency, a common sequela of subaortic stenosis, may have a high-pitch diastolic decrescendo murmur.

3. Supravalvular aortic stenosis—The harsh systolic murmur is best heard in the suprasternal notch (with possible thrill) and carotids but is well transmitted over the aortic area. There may be a difference in pulses and blood pressure between the right and left arms, with more prominent pulse and higher pressure in the right arm (the Coanda effect).

Most patients with aortic stenosis who do not present in infancy have no cardiovascular symptoms. Except in the most severe cases, patients do well until the third to fifth decades of life. Some patients have mild exercise intolerance and fatigability. Infrequently, significant symptoms (eg, exertional chest pain, dizziness, syncope) manifest in the first decade. Sudden death is uncommon but may occur in all forms of aortic stenosis, with the greatest risk in patients with subvalvular obstruction.

B. Imaging

In most cases, the heart is not enlarged. The LV, however, may be slightly prominent. In valvular aortic stenosis, post-stenotic dilation of the ascending aorta is common.

C. Electrocardiography

Patients with mild aortic stenosis have normal ECGs. LVH and LV strain may be present with more severe obstruction, but even those with severe stenosis may have a normal ECG in up 30%. Progressive LVH on serial ECGs indicates a significant obstruction. LV strain is one indication for intervention.

D. Echocardiography

This reliable noninvasive technique can be used to diagnose and follow all forms of aortic stenosis. Two-dimensional images and color Doppler can visualize the affected area, and the mean gradient estimated by spectral Doppler approximates the transvalvular gradient by cardiac catheterization.

E. Cardiac Catheterization and Angiocardiography

Left heart catheterization demonstrates the pressure gradient from LV to aorta and the anatomic level at which the gradient exists. Catheterization should be considered for severe valvular aortic stenosis (mean gradient > 40 mm Hg, peak gradient > 70 mm Hg by echocardiography), and those with critical aortic stenosis or decreased LV function regardless of gradient.

► Treatment

PGE_1 infusion is necessary in critical aortic stenosis patients until surgical or percutaneous therapy can be performed. Percutaneous balloon valvuloplasty is usually the standard initial treatment for patients with valvular aortic stenosis, though it is typically ineffective for significant annular hypoplasia or subvalvular and supravalvular stenosis. Surgery should be considered in patients with a high residual resting gradient despite balloon angioplasty or coexisting aortic insufficiency. In many cases, the gradient cannot be significantly diminished by valvuloplasty without producing aortic insufficiency. Patients who develop significant aortic insufficiency require surgical intervention to repair/replace the valve. Surgical options include a mechanical aortic valve in older children big enough to receive an adult-size valve or a Ross procedure in infants and children; the latter consists of translocating the patient's pulmonary valve to the aortic position and placing an RV-to-pulmonary artery conduit.

Discrete subvalvular aortic stenosis is surgically removed, often at lower gradients than valvular stenosis to prevent progressive damage to the aortic valve by turbulent flow which may produce aortic insufficiency. Unfortunately, simple resection is followed by recurrence in up to 20%; additional muscle resection lowers this risk but is associated with potential heart block or iatrogenic VSD creation.

Supravalvar aortic stenosis requiring repair is usually addressed with surgical patch augmentation of the affected area. Recurrent stenosis is common, as is new stenosis development beyond repair sites.

Course & Prognosis

All forms of LV outflow tract obstruction tend to be progressive. Despite this, with the exception of those with critical aortic stenosis in infancy, patients are usually asymptomatic. Symptoms such as angina, syncope, or HF are rare but imply serious disease. Children often have normal oxygen consumption and exercise capacity with less-than-moderate stenosis. Children with mild stenosis and normal exercise stress tests may safely participate in vigorous physical activity, including non-isometric competitive sports. Those with moderate stenosis may have restrictions based on symptoms and exercise testing. Children with severe aortic stenosis are predisposed to ventricular dysrhythmias and should refrain from vigorous activity and all isometric exercise.

Feltes TF et al: Indications for cardiac catheterization and intervention in pediatric cardiac disease: a scientific statement from the American Heart Association. Circulation 2011 Jun 7;123(22):2607–2652. doi: 10.1161/CIR.0b013e31821b1f10 [PMID: 21536996].

Nishimura RA et al: 2014 AHA/ACC guideline for the management of patients with valvular heart disease: a report of the American College of Cardiology/American Heart Association Task Force on Practice Guidelines. J Am Coll Cardiol 2014 Jun 10;63(22):e57–185. doi: 10.1016/j.jacc.2014.02.536 [PMID: 24603191].

Soulatges C et al: Long-term results of balloon valvuloplasty as primary treatment for congenital aortic valve stenosis: a 20-year review. Pediatr Cardiol 2015 Aug;36(6):1145–1152. doi: 10.1007/s00246-015-1134-4 [PMID: 25788411].

3. Mitral Valve Prolapse

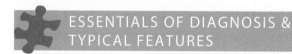

ESSENTIALS OF DIAGNOSIS & TYPICAL FEATURES

► Midsystolic click.

► Late systolic "whooping" or "honking" murmur.

► Typical symptoms include chest pain, palpitations, and dizziness.

► Often overdiagnosed on routine cardiac ultrasound.

General Considerations

In this condition as the mitral valve closes during systole, it moves posteriorly or superiorly (prolapses) into the left atrium. Mitral valve prolapse (MVP) occurs in about 2% of thin female adolescents, a minority of whom have concomitant mitral insufficiency. Although MVP is usually an isolated lesion, it can occur in association with connective tissue disorders such as Marfan, Loeys-Dietz, and Ehlers-Danlos syndromes.

Clinical Findings

A. Symptoms and Signs

Most patients with MVP are asymptomatic. Chest pain, palpitations, and dizziness may be reported, but it is unclear whether these symptoms are more common in affected patients than in the normal population. Chest pain on exertion is rare and should be assessed with cardiopulmonary stress testing. Significant dysrhythmias have been reported, including increased ventricular ectopy and nonsustained ventricular tachycardia. If significant mitral regurgitation (MR) is present, atrial arrhythmias may also occur. Standard auscultation technique must be modified to diagnose MVP. A midsystolic click (with or without a systolic murmur) is elicited best in the standing position and is the hallmark of this entity. Conversely, maneuvers that increase LV volume, such as squatting or handgrip exercise, will cause delay or obliteration of the click-murmur complex. The systolic click usually is heard at the apex but may be audible at the left sternal border. A late, short systolic murmur after the click implies mitral insufficiency and is much less common than isolated prolapse. The murmur is not holosystolic, in contrast to rheumatic mitral insufficiency.

B. Imaging

Most chest radiographs are normal and are not usually indicated in this condition. In the rare case of significant mitral valve insufficiency, the left atrium may be enlarged.

C. Electrocardiography

The ECG is usually normal. Diffuse flattening or inversion of T waves may occur in the precordial leads. U waves are sometimes prominent.

D. Echocardiography

Echocardiography assesses the degree of myxomatous change of the mitral valve and the degree of mitral insufficiency. Significant posterior systolic movement of the mitral valve leaflets to the atrial side of the mitral annulus is diagnostic.

E. Other Testing

Invasive procedures are rarely indicated. Holter monitoring or event recorders may be useful in establishing the presence of ventricular dysrhythmias in patients with palpitations.

Treatment & Prognosis

Propranolol may be effective in treatment of coexisting arrhythmias. Prophylaxis for infectious endocarditis is no longer indicated, based on 2007 AHA guidelines. The natural course of this condition is not well defined. Twenty years of observation indicate that isolated MVP in childhood is usually a benign entity. Surgery for mitral insufficiency is rarely needed.

Delling FN, Vasan RS: Epidemiology and pathophysiology of mitral valve prolapse: new insights into disease progression, genetics, and molecular basis. Circulation 2014 May 27; 129(21):2158–2170 [PMID: 24867995].

4. Other Congenital Left Heart Valvular Lesions

A. Congenital Mitral Stenosis

Congenital mitral stenosis is a rare disorder in which the valve leaflets are thickened and/or fused, producing a diaphragm- or funnel-like structure with a central opening. In many cases, the subvalve apparatus (papillary muscles and chordae) is also abnormal. When mitral stenosis occurs with other left-sided obstructive lesions, such as subaortic stenosis and coarctation of the aorta, the complex is called Shone syndrome. Most patients develop symptoms early in life with tachypnea, dyspnea, and failure to thrive. Physical examination reveals an accentuated S_1 and a loud pulmonary closure sound. No opening snap is heard. In most cases, a presystolic crescendo murmur is heard at the apex. Occasionally, only a mid-diastolic murmur can be heard. ECG shows right-axis deviation, biatrial enlargement, and RVH. Chest radiograph reveals left atrial enlargement and frequent pulmonary venous congestion. Echocardiography shows abnormal mitral valve structures with reduced leaflet excursion and left atrial enlargement. Cardiac catheterization reveals an elevated pulmonary capillary wedge pressure and PH, owing to the elevated left atrial pressure.

Mitral valve repair or mitral valve replacement with a prosthetic mitral valve may be performed, even in young infants, but it is a technically difficult procedure. Mitral valve repair is the preferred surgical option, as valve replacement can have a poor outcome in infants.

B. Cor Triatriatum

Cor triatriatum is a rare abnormality in which the pulmonary veins join in a confluence that is not completely incorporated into the left atrium. The pulmonary vein confluence communicates with the left atrium through an opening of variable size and may be obstructed. Patients may present in a similar way as those with mitral stenosis. Clinical findings depend on the degree of obstruction of pulmonary venous flow into the left atrium. If the communication between the confluence and the left atrium is small and restrictive to flow, symptoms develop early in life. Echocardiography reveals a linear density in the left atrium with a pressure gradient present between the pulmonary venous chamber and the true left atrium. Cardiac catheterization may be needed if the diagnosis is in doubt. High pulmonary wedge pressure and low left atrial pressure (with the catheter passed through the foramen ovale into the true left atrium) support the diagnosis. Angiocardiography identifies the pulmonary vein confluence and the anatomic left atria. Surgical repair is always required in the presence of an obstructive membrane, and long-term results are good. Coexisting mitral valve abnormalities may be noted, including a supravalvular mitral ring or a dysplastic mitral valve.

Brown JW, Fiore AC, Ruzmetov M, Eltayeb O, Rodefeld MD, Turrentine MW: Evolution of mitral valve replacement in children: a 40-year experience. Ann Thorac Surg 2012 Feb; 93(2):626–633 [PMID: 22153051].

DISEASES OF THE AORTA

Patients at risk for progressive aortic dilation and dissection include those with isolated bicuspid aortic valve, Marfan syndrome, Loeys-Dietz syndrome, Turner syndrome, and type IV Ehlers-Danlos syndrome.

1. Bicuspid Aortic Valve

Patients with bicuspid aortic valves have an increased incidence of aortic dilation and dissection, regardless of the presence of aortic stenosis. Histologic examination demonstrates cystic medial degeneration of the aortic wall, similar to that seen in patients with Marfan syndrome. Patients with an isolated bicuspid aortic valve require regular follow-up even in the absence of aortic insufficiency or aortic stenosis. Significant aortic root dilation requiring surgical intervention typically does not occur until adulthood.

2. Marfan & Loeys-Dietz Syndromes

Marfan syndrome is an autosomal dominant disorder of connective tissue caused by a mutation in the fibrillin-1 gene. Spontaneous mutations account for 25%–30% of cases, and thus family history is not always helpful. Patients are diagnosed by the Ghent criteria and must have at a minimum, major involvement of two body systems plus involvement of a third body system or a positive family history. Body systems involved include cardiovascular, ocular, musculoskeletal, pulmonary, and integumentary. Cardiac manifestations include aortic root dilation and MVP, which may be present at birth. Patients are at risk for aortic dilation and dissection and are restricted from competitive athletics, contact sports, and isometric activities. β-Blockers (eg, atenolol), ACE inhibitors, or angiotensin receptor blockers (eg, losartan) are used to lower blood pressure and slow the rate of aortic dilation. A recent study of atenolol versus losartan in children and young adults with Marfan syndrome showed no difference in the rate of aortic dilation between the two medications. Elective surgical intervention is performed in patients of adult size when the aortic root dimension reaches 50 mm or if there is an increase of greater than 1 cm in root dimension in 1 year. The ratio of actual to expected aortic root dimension is used to determine the need for surgery in the young child. Surgical options include replacement of the dilated aortic root with a composite valve graft (Bentall technique) or a David procedure in which the patient's own aortic valve is spared and a Dacron tube graft is used to replace the dilated ascending aorta. Young age at diagnosis was previously thought to confer a poor prognosis; however, early diagnosis with close follow-up and early medical therapy has more recently been associated with more favorable outcome. Ventricular dysrhythmias may contribute to the mortality in Marfan syndrome.

Loeys-Dietz syndrome is a connective tissue disorder first described in 2005. Many patients with Loeys-Dietz were thought to have Marfan syndrome in the past. Loeys-Dietz is a result of a mutation in the transforming growth factor β (TGFβ) receptor and is associated with musculoskeletal, skin, and cardiovascular abnormalities. Cardiovascular involvement includes mitral and tricuspid valve prolapse, aneurysms of the PDA, and aortic and pulmonary artery dilation. Dissection and aneurysm formation of arteries throughout the body can occur including in the head and neck vessels.

3. Turner Syndrome

Cardiovascular abnormalities are common in Turner syndrome. Patients are at risk for aortic dissection, typically during adulthood. Risk factors include hypertension regardless of cause, aortic dilation, bicuspid aortic valve, and coarctation of the aorta. There are rare reports of aortic dissection in adult Turner syndrome patients in the absence of any risk factors suggesting that there is a vasculopathic component to this syndrome. Patients with Turner syndrome require routine follow-up from adolescence onward to monitor for this potentially lethal complication.

Lacro RV et al: Atenolol versus losartan in children and young adults with Marfan's syndrome. N Engl J Med 2014 Nov 27; 371(22):2061–2071 [PMID: 25405392].

Nishimura RA et al: 2014 AHA/ACC guideline for the management of patients with valvular heart disease: executive summary: a report of the American College of Cardiology/American Heart Association Task Force on Practice Guidelines. J Am Coll Cardiol 2014 Jun 10;63(22):2438–2488 [PMID: 24603192].

CORONARY ARTERY ABNORMALITIES

Several anomalies involve the origin, course, and distribution of the coronary arteries. Abnormal origin or course of the coronary arteries are often asymptomatic and can go undetected. However, in some instances these children are at risk for sudden death. The most common congenital coronary artery abnormality in infants is anomalous origin of the left coronary artery from the pulmonary artery (ALCAPA) and is discussed in more detail here.

Anomalous Origin of the Left Coronary Artery From the Pulmonary Artery

In this condition, the left coronary artery arises from the pulmonary artery rather than the aorta. In neonates, whose PAP is high, perfusion of the left coronary artery may be adequate and the infant may be asymptomatic. By age 2 months the pulmonary arterial pressure falls, causing a progressive decrease in myocardial perfusion provided by the anomalous left coronary artery. Ischemia and infarction of the LV is the result. Immediate surgery is indicated to reimplant the left coronary artery and restore myocardial perfusion.

▶ Clinical Findings

A. Symptoms and Signs

Neonates appear healthy and growth and development are relatively normal until PAP decreases. Detailed questioning may disclose a history of intermittent abdominal pain (fussiness or irritability), pallor, wheezing, and sweating, especially during or after feeding. Presentation may be subtle, with nonspecific complaints of "fussiness" or intermittent "colic." The colic and fussiness are probably attacks of true angina. Presentation may be fulminant at age 2–4 months with sudden, severe HF due to LV dysfunction and mitral insufficiency. On physical examination, the infants are usually well developed and well nourished. The pulses are typically weak but equal. A prominent left precordial bulge is present. A gallop and/or holosystolic murmur of MR is sometimes present, though frequently auscultation alone reveals no obvious abnormalities.

B. Imaging

Chest radiographs show cardiac enlargement, left atrial enlargement, and may show pulmonary venous congestion if LV function has been compromised.

C. Electrocardiography

On the ECG, there is T-wave inversion in leads I and aVL. The precordial leads also show T-wave inversion from V_4–V_7. Deep and wide Q waves are present in leads I, aVL, and sometimes in V_4–V_6. These findings of myocardial infarction are similar to those in adults.

D. Echocardiography

The diagnosis can be made with two-dimensional echo techniques by visualizing a single large right coronary artery arising from the aorta and visualization of the anomalous left coronary artery arising from the main pulmonary artery. Flow reversal in the left coronary (heading *toward* the pulmonary artery, rather than away from the aorta) confirms the diagnosis. LV dysfunction, echo-bright (ischemic) papillary muscles, and MR are commonly seen.

E. Cardiac Catheterization and Angiocardiography

Angiogram of the aorta fails to show the origin of the left coronary artery. A large right coronary artery fills directly from the aorta, and contrast flows from the right coronary system via collaterals into the left coronary artery and finally into the pulmonary artery. Angiogram of the RV or main pulmonary artery may show the origin of the anomalous vessel. Rarely, a left-to-right shunt may be detected as oxygenated blood passes through the collateral system without delivering oxygen to the myocardium, and passes into the pulmonary artery.

▶ Treatment & Prognosis

The prognosis of ALCAPA depends in part on the clinical appearance of the patient at presentation. Medical management with diuretics and afterload reduction can help stabilize a critically ill patient, but surgical intervention should not be delayed. Surgery involves reimplantation of the anomalous coronary button onto the aorta. The mitral valve may have to be replaced, depending on the degree of injury to the papillary muscles and associated mitral insufficiency. Although a life-threatening problem, cardiac function nearly always recovers if the infant survives the surgery and postoperative period.

Imamura M et al: Reoperation and mechanical circulatory support after repair of anomalous origin of the left coronary artery from the pulmonary artery: a twenty-year experience. Ann Thorac Surg 2011;92(1):167–172; discussion 172–173 [PMID: 21592461].

Neumann A et al: Long-term results after repair of anomalous origin of left coronary artery from the pulmonary artery: Takeuchi repair versus coronary transfer. Eur J Cardiothorac Surg 2017 Feb 1;51(2):308–315. doi: 10.1093/ejcts/ezw268 [PMID: 28186291].

▼ CYANOTIC CONGENITAL HEART DISEASE

TETRALOGY OF FALLOT

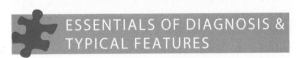

ESSENTIALS OF DIAGNOSIS & TYPICAL FEATURES

▶ Hypoxemic spells during infancy.

▶ Right-sided aortic arch in 25% of patients.

▶ Systolic ejection murmur at the upper left sternal border.

▶ General Considerations

In tetralogy of Fallot (ToF), anterior deviation of the infundibular (pulmonary outflow) septum causes narrowing of the RV outflow tract. This deviation also results in a VSD and the aorta then overrides the crest of the ventricular septum. The RV hypertrophies, not because of pulmonary stenosis, but because it is pumping against systemic resistance across a (usually) large VSD. ToF is the most common cyanotic cardiac lesion and accounts for 10% of all congenital heart disease. A right-sided aortic arch is present in 25% of cases, and ASD occurs in 15%.

Obstruction to RV outflow with a large VSD causes a right-to-left shunt at the ventricular level with arterial desaturation. The greater the obstruction and the lower the systemic vascular resistance, the greater is the right-to-left shunt. ToF is associated with deletions in the long arm of chromosome 22 (22q11, DiGeorge syndrome) in as many as 15% of affected children. This is especially common in those with an associated right aortic arch.

▶ Clinical Findings

A. Symptoms and Signs

Clinical findings vary with the degree of RV outflow obstruction. Patients with mild obstruction are minimally cyanotic or acyanotic. Those with severe obstruction are deeply cyanotic from birth. Few children are asymptomatic. In those with significant RV outflow obstruction, many have cyanosis at birth, and nearly all have cyanosis by age 4 months. The cyanosis usually is progressive, as subvalvular obstruction increases. Growth and development are not typically delayed, but easy fatigability and dyspnea on exertion are common. The fingers and toes show variable clubbing depending on age and severity of cyanosis. Historically, older children with ToF would frequently squat to increase systemic vascular resistance. This decreased the amount of right-to-left shunt, forcing blood through the pulmonary circuit, and would help ward off cyanotic spells. Squatting is rarely seen as the diagnosis is now made in infancy.

Hypoxemic spells, also called cyanotic or "Tet spells," are one of the hallmarks of severe ToF. These spells can occur spontaneously and at any time but in infants occur most commonly with crying or feeding, while in older children they can occur with exercise. They are characterized by (1) sudden onset of cyanosis or deepening of cyanosis; (2) dyspnea; (3) alterations in consciousness, from irritability to syncope; and (4) decrease in or disappearance of the systolic murmur (as RV the outflow tract becomes completely obstructed). These episodes most commonly start at age 4–6 months. Cyanotic spells are treated acutely by administration of oxygen and placing the patient in the knee-chest position (to increase systemic vascular resistance). Intravenous morphine should be administered cautiously but is helpful for its sedative effect. Propranolol produces β-blockade and may reduce the obstruction across the RV outflow tract through its negative inotropic action. Acidosis, if present, should be corrected with intravenous sodium bicarbonate. Chronic oral prophylaxis of cyanotic spells with propranolol may be useful to delay surgery, but the onset of Tet spells usually prompts surgical intervention. In fact, in the current era, elective surgical repair generally occurs around the age of 3 months so as to avoid the development of Tet spells.

On examination, an RV lift is palpable. S_2 is predominantly aortic and single. A grade II–IV/VI, rough, systolic ejection murmur is present at the left sternal border in the third intercostal space and radiates well to the back.

B. Laboratory Findings

Hemoglobin, hematocrit, and red blood cell count are usually elevated in older infants or children secondary to chronic arterial desaturation.

C. Imaging

Chest radiographs show a normal-size heart. The RV is hypertrophied, often shown by an upturning of the apex (boot-shaped heart). The main pulmonary artery segment is usually concave, and if there is a right aortic arch, the aortic knob is to the right of the trachea. The pulmonary vascular markings are usually decreased.

D. Electrocardiography

The QRS axis is rightward, ranging from +90 to +180 degrees. The P waves are usually normal. RVH is always present, but RV strain patterns are rare.

E. Echocardiography

Two-dimensional imaging is diagnostic, revealing thickening of the RV wall, overriding of the aorta, and a large subaortic VSD. Obstruction at the level of the infundibulum and pulmonary valve can be identified, and the size of the proximal pulmonary arteries measured. The anatomy of the coronary arteries should be visualized, as abnormal branches crossing the RV outflow tract are at risk for transection during surgical enlargement of the area.

F. Cardiac Catheterization and Angiocardiography

Cardiac catheterization is generally done mainly in those patients with hypoplastic pulmonary arteries. If a catheterization is done, it reveals a right-to-left shunt at the ventricular level in most cases. Arterial desaturation of varying degrees is present. The RV pressure is at systemic levels and the pressure tracing in the RV is identical to that in the LV if the VSD is large. The PAP is invariably low. Pressure gradients may be noted at the pulmonary valvular level, the infundibular level, or both. RV angiography reveals RV outflow obstruction and a right-to-left shunt at the ventricular level. The major indications for cardiac catheterization are to establish coronary artery and distal pulmonary artery anatomy if not able to be clearly defined by echocardiography.

▶ Treatment

A. Palliative Treatment

Most centers currently advocate complete repair of ToF during the neonatal or infant period regardless of patient size. However, some centers prefer palliative treatment for small neonates in whom complete correction is deemed risky. Surgical palliation consists of the insertion of a GoreTex shunt from the subclavian artery to the ipsilateral pulmonary artery [modified Blalock-Taussig (BT) shunt] to replace the ductus arteriosus (which is ligated and divided) or stenting of the ductus. This secures a source of pulmonary blood flow regardless of the level of infundibular or valvular obstruction and, as some believe, allows for growth of the patient's pulmonary arteries (which are usually small) prior to complete surgical correction.

B. Total Correction

Open-heart surgery for repair of ToF is performed at ages ranging from birth to 2 years, depending on the patient's anatomy and the experience of the surgical center. The current surgical trend is toward earlier repair for symptomatic infants. The major limiting anatomic feature of total correction is the size of the pulmonary arteries. During surgery, the VSD is closed and the obstruction to RV outflow removed. Although a valve sparing procedure is preferred, in many cases a transannular patch is placed across the RV outflow tract as the pulmonary valve is contributing to the obstruction. When a transannular patch repair is done, the patient has PI that is usually well tolerated for years. However, pulmonary valve replacement is eventually necessary once symptoms (usually exercise intolerance) and RV dilation occur. Surgical mortality is low.

▶ Course & Prognosis

Infants with severe ToF are usually deeply cyanotic at birth. These children require early surgery. Complete repair before age 2 years usually produces a good result, and patients are currently living well into adulthood. Depending on the extent of the repair required, patients frequently require additional surgery 10–15 years after their initial repair for replacement of the pulmonary valve. Transcatheter pulmonary valves are now performed in some adolescents and young adults with a history of ToF, avoiding the need for open heart surgery. Patients with ToF are at risk for sudden death due to ventricular dysrhythmias. A competent pulmonary valve without a dilated RV appears to diminish arrhythmias and enhance exercise performance.

Valente AM et al: Multimodality imaging guidelines for patients with repaired tetralogy of Fallot: a report from the American Society of Echocardiography: developed in collaboration with the Society for Cardiovascular Magnetic Resonance and the Society for Pediatric Radiology. J Am Soc Echocardiogr 2014 Feb; 27(2):111–141 [PMID: 24468055].

PULMONARY ATRESIA WITH VENTRICULAR SEPTAL DEFECT

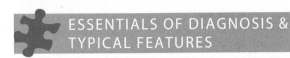

ESSENTIALS OF DIAGNOSIS & TYPICAL FEATURES

▶ Symptoms depend on degree of pulmonary blood flow.

▶ Pulmonary blood flow via PDA and/or aortopulmonary collaterals.

Complete atresia of the pulmonary valve in association with a VSD is essentially an extreme form of ToF. Because there is no antegrade flow from the RV to the pulmonary artery, pulmonary blood flow must be derived from a PDA or from multiple aortopulmonary collateral arteries (MAPCAs). Symptoms depend on the amount of pulmonary blood flow. If flow is adequate, patients may be stable. If pulmonary flow is inadequate, severe hypoxemia occurs and immediate palliation is required. Newborns are stabilized with intravenous prostaglandin E_1 (PGE$_1$) to maintain the PDA while being prepared for surgery. Rarely, if the ductus does not contribute significantly to pulmonary blood flow (eg, the MAPCAs alone are sufficient), PGE$_1$ may be discontinued. Once stabilized, a BT shunt, stenting of the ductus or complete repair is undertaken. The decision to perform palliation or complete repair in a newborn is dependent on surgical expertise and preference in combination with pulmonary artery anatomy. In many centers, a palliative shunt is performed in newborns with severely hypoplastic pulmonary arteries or in those with only MAPCAs as a source of pulmonary blood flow. The goal of the shunt is to augment pulmonary blood flow and encourage vascular growth, and open-heart surgical correction is planned several months later. In children with MAPCAs, relocation of the MAPCAs is performed so that they are connected to the pulmonary artery (unifocalization) to complete the repair.

Echocardiography is usually diagnostic. Cardiac catheterization and angiocardiography or cardiac MRI can confirm the source(s) of pulmonary blood flow and document size of the distal pulmonary arteries.

Pulmonary vascular disease is common in PA with VSD, due both to intrinsic abnormalities of the pulmonary vasculature and to abnormal amounts of pulmonary blood flow. Even patients who have undergone surgical correction as infants are at risk. Pulmonary vascular disease is a common cause of death as early as the third decade of life.

Mainwaring RD: Hemodynamic assessment after complete repair of pulmonary atresia with major aortopulmonary collaterals. Ann Thorac Surg 2013 Apr;95(4):1397–1402 [PMID: 23453744].

Ten Cate FA: Stenting the arterial duct in neonates and infants with congenital heart disease and duct-dependent pulmonary blood flow: a multicenter experience of an evolving therapy over 18 years. Catheter Cardiovasc Interv 2013 Sep 1;82(3): E233–E243 [PMID: 23420699].

PULMONARY ATRESIA WITH INTACT VENTRICULAR SEPTUM

ESSENTIALS OF DIAGNOSIS & TYPICAL FEATURES

▶ Completely different lesion from pulmonary atresia with VSD.

▶ Cyanosis at birth.

▶ Pulmonary blood flow is always ductal dependent with rare aortopulmonary collateral arteries being present.

▶ RV-dependent coronary arteries sometimes are present.

▶ **General Considerations**

Although pulmonary atresia with intact ventricular septum (PA/IVS) sounds as if it might be related to PA with VSD, it is a distinct cardiac condition. As the name suggests, the pulmonary valve is atretic. The pulmonic annulus usually has a small diaphragm consisting of the fused valve cusps. The ventricular septum is intact. The main pulmonary artery segment is usually present and closely approximated to the atretic valve but is somewhat hypoplastic. Although the RV is always reduced in size, the degree of reduction is variable. The size of the RV is critical to the success of surgical repair. In some children with PA/IVS, the RV is adequate for an ultimate two-ventricular repair. A normal RV has three component parts (inlet, trabecular or body, and outlet). The absence of any one of the components makes adequate RV function unlikely and a single ventricle palliative approach is necessary. Even with all three components, some RVs are inadequate.

After birth, the pulmonary flow is provided by the ductus arteriosus. MAPCAs are usually not present in this disease, in contrast to PA with VSD. A continuous infusion of PGE$_1$ must be started as soon as possible after birth to maintain ductal patency.

▶ **Clinical Findings**

A. Symptoms and Signs

Neonates are usually cyanotic and become more so as the ductus arteriosus closes. A blowing systolic murmur resulting from the associated PDA may be heard at the pulmonary area. A holosystolic murmur is often heard at the lower left sternal border, as many children develop tricuspid insufficiency if the RV is of good size and egress from that ventricle is only through the tricuspid valve. A PFO or ASD is essential for decompression of the right side of the heart.

B. Imaging

The heart size varies depending on the degree of tricuspid insufficiency. With severe tricuspid insufficiency, right atrial enlargement may be massive and the cardiac silhouette may fill the chest on radiograph. In patients with an associated hypoplastic tricuspid valve and or RV, most of the systemic venous return travels right-to-left across the ASD, and so the heart size can be normal.

C. Electrocardiography

ECG reveals a left axis for age (45–90 degrees) in the frontal plane. LV forces dominate the ECG, and there is a paucity of RV forces, particularly with a hypoplastic RV. Findings of right atrial enlargement are usually striking.

D. Echocardiography

Echocardiography shows atresia of the pulmonary valve with varying degrees of RV cavity and tricuspid annulus hypoplasia. Patency of an intra-atrial communication and ductus are verified by echocardiography.

E. Cardiac Catheterization and Angiocardiography

RV pressure is often suprasystemic. Angiogram of the RV reveals no filling of the pulmonary artery. Unrestricted flow through the ASD is a necessity, since egress of blood from the right heart can only occur across the atrial defect and into the left atrium. A Rashkind balloon atrial septostomy may be required to open any inadequate existing communication across the atrial septum. Some children with PA and IVS have sinusoids between the RV and the coronary arteries. In some patients, the coronary circulation may depend on high RV pressure. Any attempt to decompress the RV in patients with RV-dependent coronary circulation causes myocardial infarction and death because of the precipitous decrease in coronary perfusion, so precise coronary angiography is required to evaluate the anatomy. If the RV is tripartite, coronary circulation is not RV-dependent and an eventual two-chamber repair is planned. The pulmonary valve plate may be perforated and dilated during cardiac catheterization in the newborn to allow antegrade flow from the RV to the pulmonary artery and thus encourage RV cavity growth.

Treatment & Prognosis

As in all ductal-dependent lesions, PGE$_1$ is used to stabilize the patient and maintain patency of the ductus until surgery can be performed. Surgery is usually undertaken in the first week of life. If the RV is hypoplastic, significant sinusoids are present, there is RV-dependent coronary circulation (lack of antegrade filling of the coronaries from the aorta), or the pulmonic valve cannot be opened successfully during cardiac catheterization, a BT shunt or ductal stenting is performed to establish pulmonary blood flow. Later in infancy, a communication between the RV and pulmonary artery can be created to stimulate RV cavity growth. If either RV dimension or function is inadequate for two-ventricular repair, an approach similar to that taken for a single ventricle pathway best serves these children (see section Hypoplastic Left Heart Syndrome). Children with significant sinusoids or coronary artery abnormalities are considered for cardiac transplantation because they are at risk for coronary insufficiency and sudden death.

The prognosis in this condition is guarded.

Lowenthal A et al: Prenatal tricuspid valve size as a predictor of postnatal outcome in patients with severe pulmonary stenosis or pulmonary atresia with intact ventricular septum. Fetal Diagn Ther 2014;35(2):101–107 [PMID: 24457468].

Mallula K, Vaughn G, El-Said H, Lamberti JJ, Moore JW: Comparison of ductal stenting versus surgical shunts for palliation of patients with pulmonary atresia and intact ventricular septum. Catheter Cardiovasc Interv 2015 Jun;85(7):1196–1202. doi: 10.1002/ccd.25870 [PMID: 25639613].

Schneider AW et al: More than 25 years of experience in managing pulmonary atresia with intact ventricular septum. Ann Thorac Surg 2014 Nov;98(5):1680–1686 [PMID: 25149048].

TRICUSPID ATRESIA

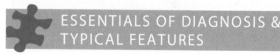

ESSENTIALS OF DIAGNOSIS & TYPICAL FEATURES

► Marked cyanosis present from birth.
► ECG with left-axis deviation, right atrial enlargement, and LVH.

General Considerations

In tricuspid atresia, there is complete atresia of the tricuspid valve with no direct communication between the right atrium and the RV. There are two types of tricuspid atresia based on the relationship of the great arteries (normally related or transposed great arteries). The entire systemic venous return must flow through the atrial septum (either ASD or PFO) to reach the left atrium. The left atrium thus receives both the systemic venous return and the pulmonary venous return. Complete mixing occurs in the left atrium, resulting in variable degrees of arterial desaturation.

Because there is no flow to the RV, development of the RV depends on the presence of a ventricular left-to-right shunt. Severe hypoplasia of the RV occurs when there is no VSD or when the VSD is small.

► Clinical Findings

A. Symptoms and Signs

Symptoms usually develop in early infancy with cyanosis present at birth in most infants. Growth and development are poor, and the infant usually exhibits exhaustion during feedings, tachypnea, and dyspnea. Patients with increased pulmonary blood flow may develop HF with less prominent cyanosis. The degree of pulmonary blood flow is most dependent on PVR. Those patients with low PVR will have increased pulmonary blood flow. A murmur from the VSD is usually present and heard best at the lower left sternal border. Digital clubbing is present in older children with long-standing cyanosis.

B. Imaging

The heart is slightly to markedly enlarged. The main pulmonary artery segment is usually small or absent. The size of the right atrium is moderately to massively enlarged, depending on the size of the communication at the atrial level. The pulmonary vascular markings are usually decreased. Pulmonary vascular markings may be increased if pulmonary blood flow is not restricted by the VSD or pulmonary stenosis.

C. Electrocardiography

The ECG shows marked left-axis deviation. The P waves are tall and peaked, indicative of right atrial hypertrophy. LVH or LV dominance is found in almost all cases. RV forces on the ECG are usually low or absent.

D. Echocardiography

Two-dimensional echocardiography is diagnostic and show absence of the tricuspid valve, the relationship between the great arteries, the anatomy of the VSD, presence of an ASD or PFO, and the size of the pulmonary arteries. Color-flow Doppler imaging can help identify atrial level shunting and levels of restriction of pulmonary blood flow, either at the VSD or in the RV outflow tract.

E. Cardiac Catheterization and Angiocardiography

Catheterization reveals a right-to-left shunt at the atrial level. Because of mixing in the left atrium, oxygen saturations in the LV, RV, pulmonary artery, and aorta are identical to those in the left atrium. Right atrial pressure is increased if the ASD is restrictive. LV and systemic pressures are normal. The catheter cannot be passed through the tricuspid valve

from the right atrium to the RV. A balloon atrial septostomy is performed if a restrictive PFO or ASD is present.

► Treatment & Prognosis

In infants with unrestricted pulmonary blood flow, conventional anticongestive therapy with diuretics and afterload reduction should be given until the infant begins to outgrow the VSD. Sometimes, a pulmonary artery band is needed to protect the pulmonary bed from excessive flow and development of pulmonary vascular disease.

Staged palliation of tricuspid atresia is the usual surgical approach. In infants with diminished pulmonary blood flow, PGE$_1$ is given until an aortopulmonary shunt (BT shunt or ductal stent) can be performed. A Glenn procedure (SVC to pulmonary artery anastomosis) is done with takedown of the aortopulmonary/BT shunt at 4–6 months when saturations begin to fall, and completion of the Fontan procedure (redirection of IVC and SVC to pulmonary artery) is performed when the child reaches around 15 kg.

The long-term prognosis for children treated by the Fontan procedure is unknown, although patients now are living into their late 20s and early 30s. In the short term, the best results for the Fontan procedure occur in children with low PAPs prior to open-heart surgery.

Wald RM et al: Outcome after prenatal diagnosis of tricuspid atresia: a multicenter experience. Am Heart J 2007;153:772–778 [PMID:17452152].

HYPOPLASTIC LEFT HEART SYNDROME

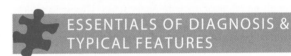

ESSENTIALS OF DIAGNOSIS & TYPICAL FEATURES

► Mild cyanosis at birth.
► Minimal auscultatory findings.
► Rapid onset of shock with ductal closure.

► General Considerations

Hypoplastic left heart syndrome (HLHS) includes several conditions in which obstructive lesions of the left heart are associated with hypoplasia of the LV. The syndrome occurs in 1.4%–3.8% of infants with congenital heart disease.

Stenosis or atresia of the mitral and aortic valves is the rule. In the neonate, survival depends on a PDA because antegrade flow into the systemic circulation is inadequate or nonexistent. The PDA provides the only flow to the aorta and coronary arteries. Children with HLHS are usually stable at birth, but they deteriorate rapidly as the ductus closes in the first week of life. Untreated, the average age at death is the first week of life. Rarely, the ductus remains patent and infants may survive for weeks to months without PGE$_1$ therapy.

The diagnosis is often made prenatally by fetal echocardiography. Prenatal diagnosis aids in counseling for the expectant parents and planning for the delivery of the infant at or near a center with experience in treating HLHS.

▶ Clinical Findings

A. Symptoms and Signs

Neonates with HLHS appear stable at birth because the ductus is patent. They deteriorate rapidly as the ductus closes, with shock and acidosis secondary to inadequate systemic perfusion. Oxygen saturation may actually increase for a period of time as the ductus closes due to increased blood flowing to the lungs.

B. Imaging

Chest radiograph in the first day of life may be relatively unremarkable, with the exception of a small cardiac silhouette. Later, chest radiographs demonstrate cardiac enlargement with severe pulmonary venous congestion if the PDA has begun closing or if the baby has been placed on supplemental oxygen increasing pulmonary blood flow.

C. Electrocardiography

The ECG shows right-axis deviation, right atrial enlargement, and RVH with a relative paucity of LV forces. The small Q wave in lead V$_6$ may be absent, and a qR pattern is often seen in lead V$_1$.

D. Echocardiography

Echocardiography is diagnostic. A hypoplastic aorta and LV with atretic or severely stenotic mitral and aortic valves are diagnostic. The systemic circulation is dependent on the PDA. Color-flow Doppler imaging shows retrograde flow in the ascending aorta, as the coronary arteries are supplied by the ductus via the small native aorta.

▶ Treatment & Prognosis

Initiation of PGE$_1$ is essential and lifesaving, as systemic circulation depends on a PDA. Later management depends on balancing pulmonary and systemic blood flow both of which depend on the RV. At a few days of age the pulmonary resistance falls, favoring pulmonary overcirculation and systemic underperfusion. Therapy is then directed at encouraging systemic blood flow. Despite hypoxia and cyanosis, supplemental oxygen is avoided as this will decrease pulmonary resistance and lead to further increases in pulmonary blood flow. In some centers, nitrogen is used to decrease inspired oxygen to as low as 17%. This therapy must be carefully monitored but results in increased pulmonary arterial resistance,

which encourages systemic blood flow and improves systemic perfusion. Systemic afterload reduction will also increase systemic perfusion. Adequate perfusion can usually be obtained by keeping systemic O$_2$ saturation between 65% and 80%, or more accurately a Po$_2$ of 40 mm Hg.

Staged surgical palliation is the most common management approach. In the Norwood procedure, the relatively normal main pulmonary artery is transected and connected to the small ascending aorta. The entire aortic arch must be reconstructed due to its small size. Then, either a BT shunt (from the subclavian artery to the pulmonary artery) or a Sano shunt (from the RV to the pulmonary artery) must be created to restore pulmonary blood flow. Children who have a Norwood procedure will later require a Glenn anastomosis (SVC to pulmonary artery with takedown of the systemic-pulmonary shunt) and then a Fontan (IVC to pulmonary artery, completing the systemic venous bypass of the heart) at ages 6 months and 2–3 years, respectively. Despite advances in surgical technique and postoperative care, HLHS remains one of the most challenging lesions in pediatric cardiology, with 1-year survival as low as 70%.

Orthotopic heart transplantation is also a treatment option for newborns with HLHS but in the current era is typically performed only in infants who are considered poor Norwood candidates. Heart transplantation is more commonly utilized in the event of a failed surgical palliation or if the systemic RV fails (often in adolescence or young adulthood).

Recently, some centers offer a "hybrid" approach to HLHS as a result of collaboration between surgeons and interventional cardiologists. In the hybrid procedure, the chest is opened surgically and the branch pulmonary arteries are banded, to limit pulmonary blood flow. Then, also through the open chest, a PDA stent is placed by the interventionalist to maintain systemic output. The second stage is considered a "comprehensive Glenn," in which the pulmonary artery bands and ductal stent are taken down, the aortic arch is reconstructed and the SVC is surgically connected to the pulmonary arteries. Short-term (30 day) survival after the first-stage "hybrid" is greater than 90% at the most experienced centers, but second-stage risks and complications mitigate some of that initial survival advantage. Long-term follow-up data are not yet available.

Alsoufi B et al: Results of heart transplantation following failed staged palliation of hypoplastic left heart syndrome and related single ventricle anomalies. Eur J Cardiothorac Surg 2015 Nov;48(5):792–798; discussion 798. doi: 10.1093/ejcts/ezu547 [PMID: 25602055].

Oster ME et al: Association of interstage home monitoring with mortality, readmissions, and weight gain: a multicenter study from the National Pediatric Cardiology Quality Improvement Collaborative. Circulation 2015 Aug 11;132(6):502–508. doi: 10.1161/CIRCULATIONAHA.114.014107 [PMID: 26260497].

Sharma V et al: In search of the ideal pulmonary blood source for the Norwood procedure: a meta-analysis and systematic review. Ann Thorac Surg 2014 Jul;98(1):142–150 [PMID: 24793687].

TRANSPOSITION OF THE GREAT ARTERIES

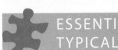

ESSENTIALS OF DIAGNOSIS & TYPICAL FEATURES

▶ Cyanotic newborn without respiratory distress.

▶ More common in males.

General Considerations

Transposition of the great arteries (TGA) is the second most common cyanotic congenital heart disease, accounting for 5% of all cases of congenital heart disease. The male-to-female ratio is 3:1. It is caused by an embryologic abnormality in the spiral division of the truncus arteriosus in which the aorta arises from the RV and the pulmonary artery from the LV. This is referred to as "ventriculoarterial discordance." Patients may have a VSD, or the ventricular septum may be intact. Left unrepaired, transposition is associated with a high incidence of early pulmonary vascular obstructive disease. Because pulmonary and systemic circulations are in parallel, survival is impossible without mixing between the two circuits. Specifically an interatrial communication (PFO or ASD) is critically important. The majority of mixing occurs at the atrial level (some mixing can occur at the level of the ductus as well), so even in the presence of a VSD an adequate interatrial communication is needed. If the atrial communication is inadequate at birth, the patient is severely cyanotic.

Clinical Findings

A. Symptoms and Signs

Many neonates are large (up to 4 kg) and profoundly cyanotic without respiratory distress or a significant murmur. Infants with a large VSD may be less cyanotic, and they usually have a prominent murmur. The findings on cardiovascular examination depend on the intracardiac defects. Obstruction to outflow from either ventricle is possible, and coarctation must be ruled out.

B. Imaging

The chest radiograph in transposition is usually nondiagnostic. Sometimes there is an "egg on a string" appearance because the aorta is directly anterior to the main pulmonary artery, giving the image of a narrow mediastinum.

C. Electrocardiography

Because the newborn ECG normally has RV predominance, the ECG in transposition is of little help, as it will frequently look normal.

D. Echocardiography

Two-dimensional imaging and Doppler evaluation demonstrate the anatomy and physiology well. The aorta arises from the RV, and the pulmonary artery arises from the LV. Associated defects, such as a VSD, RV, or LV outflow tract obstruction, or coarctation, must be evaluated. The atrial septum should be closely examined, as any restriction could prove detrimental as the child awaits repair. The coronary anatomy is variable and must be defined prior to surgery.

E. Cardiac Catheterization and Angiocardiography

A Rashkind balloon atrial septostomy is frequently performed in complete transposition if the interatrial communication is restrictive. This procedure can be done at the bedside with echocardiographic guidance in most cases. The coronary anatomy can be delineated by ascending aortography if not well seen by echocardiography.

Treatment

Early corrective surgery is recommended. The arterial switch operation (ASO) has replaced the previously performed atrial switch procedures (Mustard and Senning operations). The ASO is performed at age 4–7 days. The arteries are transected above the level of the valves and switched, while the coronaries are separately reimplanted. Small associated VSDs may be left to close on their own, but large VSDs are repaired. The ASD is also closed. Early surgical repair (< 14 days of age) is vital for patients with TGA and an IVS to avoid potential deconditioning of the LV as it pumps to the low-resistance pulmonary circulation. If a large, unrestrictive VSD is present, LV pressure is maintained at systemic levels, the LV does not become deconditioned, and corrective surgery can be delayed for a few months. Surgery should be performed by age 3–4 months in those with TGA and a VSD because of the high risk of early pulmonary vascular disease associated with this defect.

Operative survival after the ASO is greater than 95% in major centers. The main advantage of the *arterial* switch procedure in comparison to the *atrial* switch procedures (Mustard and Senning operations) is that the systemic ventricle is the LV. Patients who have undergone an *atrial* switch undergo surgical patch placement to baffle the venous return through the atria to the opposite ventricle. They then have an RV as their systemic ventricle, leaving them with significant late risk of RV failure, and need for heart transplantation and are at risk for atrial baffle obstruction.

Cohen MS: Multimodality imaging guidelines of patients with transposition of the great arteries: a report from the American Society of Echocardiography Developed in Collaboration with the Society for Cardiovascular Magnetic Resonance and the Society of Cardiovascular Computed Tomography. J Am Soc Echocardiogr 2016 Jul;29(7):571–621. doi: 10.1016/j.echo.2016.04.002 [PMID: 27372954].

Villafañe J et al: D-transposition of the great arteries: the current era of the arterial switch operation. J Am Coll Cardiol 2014 Aug; 64(5):498–511 [PMID: 25082585].

1. Congenitally Corrected Transposition of the Great Arteries

Congenitally corrected transposition of the great arteries (ccTGA) is a relatively uncommon congenital heart disease. Patients may present with cyanosis, HF, or be asymptomatic, depending on the associated lesions. In ccTGA, both atrioventricular and ventriculoarterial discordance occurs so that the right atrium connects to a morphologic LV, which supports the pulmonary artery. Conversely, the left atrium empties via a tricuspid valve into a morphologic RV, which supports the aorta. Common associated lesions are VSD and pulmonary stenosis. A dysplastic left-sided tricuspid valve is almost always present. In the absence of associated lesions, patients with ccTGA are often undiagnosed until adulthood when they present with left-sided AV valve insufficiency or arrhythmias.

Previously, surgical repair was directed at VSD closure and relief of pulmonary outflow tract obstruction—a technique that maintained the RV as the systemic ventricle with outflow to the aorta. It is now recognized that these patients have a reduced life span due to systemic RV failure; thus other surgical techniques have been advocated. The double-switch procedure is one such technique. An atrial level switch (Mustard or Senning technique) is performed, in which pulmonary and systemic venous blood are baffled such that they drain into the contralateral ventricle (systemic venous return drains into the RV and pulmonary venous return drains into the LV). An ASO then restores the morphologic LV to its position as systemic ventricle.

Patients with ccTGA have an increased incidence of complete heart block with an estimated risk of 1% per year and an overall frequency of 50%.

Malhotra SP et al: The hemi-Mustard/bidirectional Glenn atrial switch procedure in the double-switch operation for congenitally corrected transposition of the great arteries: rationale and midterm results. J Thorac Cardiovasc Surg 2011;141(1):162–170 [PMID: 21055773].

2. Double-Outlet Right Ventricle

In this uncommon malformation, both great arteries arise from the RV. There is always a VSD that allows blood to exit the LV. Presenting symptoms depend on the relationship of the VSD to the semilunar valves. The VSD can be in variable positions, and the great arteries could be normally related or malposed. In the absence of outflow obstruction, a large left-to-right shunt exists and the clinical picture resembles that of a large VSD. Pulmonary stenosis may be present, particularly if the VSD is remote from the pulmonary

artery. This physiology is similar to ToF. Alternatively, if the VSD is nearer the pulmonary artery, aortic outflow may be obstructed (called the Taussig-Bing malformation). Early primary correction is the goal. LV flow is directed to the aorta across the VSD (closing the VSD), and an RV to pulmonary artery conduit is placed to maintain unobstructed flow through the pulmonary circulation. If the aorta is far from the VSD, an arterial switch may be necessary. Echocardiography is usually sufficient to make the diagnosis and determine the orientation of the great vessels and their relationship to the VSD.

Mahle WT et al: Anatomy, echocardiography, and surgical approach to double outlet right ventricle. Cardiol Young 2008; 18(Suppl 3):39–51 [PMID: 19094378].

Pushparajah K et al: A systematic three-dimensional echocardiographic approach to assist surgical planning in double outlet right ventricle. Echocardiography 2013 Feb;30(2):234–238. doi: 10.1111/echo.12037 [PMID: 23167820].

TOTAL ANOMALOUS PULMONARY VENOUS RETURN

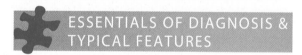

ESSENTIALS OF DIAGNOSIS & TYPICAL FEATURES

▶ Abnormal pulmonary venous connection leading to cyanosis.

▶ Occurs with or without a murmur and may have accentuated P_2.

▶ Right atrial enlargement and RVH.

▶ General Considerations

This malformation accounts for 2% of all congenital heart lesions. Instead of the pulmonary veins draining into the left atrium, the veins empty into a confluence that usually is located behind the left atrium. However, the confluence is not connected to the left atrium and instead the pulmonary venous blood drains into the systemic venous system. Therefore, there is complete mixing of the systemic and pulmonary venous blood at the level of the right atrium. The presentation of a patient with total anomalous pulmonary venous return (TAPVR) depends on the route of drainage into the systemic circulation and whether or not this drainage route is obstructed.

The malformation is classified as either intra-, supra-, or infracardiac. Intracardiac TAPVR occurs when the pulmonary venous confluence drains directly into the heart, usually via the coronary sinus into the right atrium (rarely direct drainage into the right atrium). Supracardiac (or supradiaphragmatic) return is defined as a confluence that drains into the right SVC, innominate vein, or persistent left SVC. In infracardiac (or infradiaphragmatic) return, the confluence drains below the diaphragm usually into the portal venous system, which empties into the IVC. Infracardiac pulmonary venous return is very frequently obstructed. This obstruction to pulmonary venous drainage makes this lesion a potential surgical emergency. Supracardiac veins may also be obstructed, though less commonly. Rarely, the pulmonary venous confluence drains to more than one location, called mixed TAPVR.

Because the entire venous drainage from the body returns to the right atrium, a right-to-left shunt must be present at the atrial level, either as an ASD or a PFO. Occasionally, the atrial septum is restrictive and balloon septostomy is needed at birth to allow filling of the left heart.

▶ Clinical Findings

A. Unobstructed Pulmonary Venous Return

Patients with unobstructed TAPVR and a large atrial communication tend to have high pulmonary blood flow and typically present with cardiomegaly and HF rather than cyanosis. Oxygen saturations in the high 80s or low 90s are common. Most patients in this group have mild to moderate elevation of PAP owing to elevated pulmonary blood flow. In most instances, PAP does not reach systemic levels.

1. Symptoms and signs—Patients may have mild cyanosis and tachypnea in the neonatal period and early infancy. Examination discloses dusky nail beds and mucous membranes, but overt cyanosis and digital clubbing are usually absent. An RV heave is palpable, and P_2 is increased. A systolic and diastolic murmur may be heard as a result of increased flow across the pulmonary and tricuspid valves, respectively.

2. Imaging—Chest radiography reveals cardiomegaly involving the right heart and pulmonary artery. Pulmonary vascular markings are increased.

3. Electrocardiography—ECG shows right-axis deviation and varying degrees of right atrial enlargement and RVH. A qR pattern is often seen over the right precordial leads.

4. Echocardiography—Demonstration by echocardiography of a discrete chamber posterior to the left atrium and an obligatory right-to-left atrial level shunt is strongly suggestive of the diagnosis. The availability of two-dimensional echocardiography plus color-flow Doppler has increased diagnostic accuracy such that diagnostic cardiac catheterization is rarely required.

B. With Obstructed Pulmonary Venous Return

This group includes many patients with infracardiac TAPVR and a few of the patients in whom venous drainage is into a systemic vein above the diaphragm. The pulmonary venous return is usually obstructed at the level of the ascending or descending vein that connects the confluence to the systemic veins to which it is draining. Obstruction can be caused from extravascular structures (such as the diaphragm), or by inherent stenosis within the ascending or descending vein.

1. Symptoms and signs—Infants usually present shortly after birth with severe cyanosis and respiratory distress and require early corrective surgery. Cardiac examination discloses a striking RV impulse. S_2 is markedly accentuated and single. Although there is often no murmur, sometimes, a systolic murmur is heard over the pulmonary area with radiation over the lung fields. Diastolic murmurs are uncommon.

2. Imaging—The heart is usually small and pulmonary venous congestion severe with associated air bronchograms. The chest radiographic appearance may lead to an erroneous diagnosis of severe lung disease. In less severe cases, the heart size may be normal or slightly enlarged with mild pulmonary venous congestion.

3. Electrocardiography—The ECG shows right-axis deviation, right atrial enlargement, and RVH.

4. Echocardiography—Echocardiography shows a small left atrium and LV, a dilated right heart with high RV pressure. For infracardiac TAPVR, appearance of a vessel lying parallel and anterior to the descending aorta and to the left of the IVC may represent the vein draining the confluence caudally toward the diaphragm. Color-flow Doppler echocardiography will demonstrate a right-to-left atrial level shunt and may reveal flow disturbance, commonly near the confluence or in the liver, where flow is obstructed.

5. Cardiac catheterization and angiocardiography—If echocardiography does not confirm the anatomy, cardiac catheterization and angiography demonstrate the site of entry of the anomalous veins, determine the degree of PH, and calculate PVR.

▶ Treatment

Surgery is always required for TAPVR. If pulmonary venous return is obstructed, surgery must be performed immediately (obstructed TAPVR represents one of the few surgical emergencies in congenital heart disease). If early surgery is not required and the atrial septum is restrictive, a balloon atrial septostomy can be performed in newborns, to be followed shortly by less emergent surgical repair.

▶ Course & Prognosis

Most children with TAPVR do well after surgery. However, some surgical survivors develop late stenosis of the pulmonary veins. Pulmonary vein stenosis is an intractable condition that is difficult to treat either with interventional catheterization or surgery and has a poor prognosis.

A heart-lung transplant may be the only remaining option available to those with severe pulmonary vein stenosis. By avoiding direct suturing at the pulmonary venous ostia, the chance of recurrent stenosis at the anastomotic site is lessened. Unfortunately, any manipulation of the pulmonary veins increases the risk of stenosis.

Marino BS et al: Neurodevelopmental outcomes in children with congenital heart disease: evaluation and management: a scientific statement from the American Heart Association. Circulation 2012 Aug 28;126(9):1143–1172. doi: 10.1161/CIR.0b013e318265ee8a [PMID: 22851541].

Seale AN et al: Total anomalous pulmonary venous connection: outcome of postoperative pulmonary venous obstruction. J Thorac Cardiovasc Surg 2013 May;145(5):1255–1262 [PMID: 22892140].

TRUNCUS ARTERIOSUS

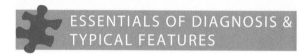

ESSENTIALS OF DIAGNOSIS & TYPICAL FEATURES

► Early HF with or without cyanosis.
► Systolic ejection click.

General Considerations

Truncus arteriosus accounts for less than 1% of congenital heart malformations. A single great artery arises from the heart, giving rise to the systemic, pulmonary, and coronary circulations. Truncus develops embryologically as a result of failure of the division of the common truncus arteriosus into the aorta and the pulmonary artery. A VSD is almost always present. The number of truncal valve leaflets varies from one to six, and the valve may be insufficient or stenotic.

Truncus arteriosus is divided into subtypes by the anatomy of the pulmonary circulation. A single main pulmonary artery may arise from the base of the trunk and gives rise to branch pulmonary arteries (type 1). Alternatively, the pulmonary arteries may arise separately from the common trunk, either in close association with one another (type 2) or widely separated (type 3). This lesion can occur in association with an interrupted aortic arch.

In patients with truncus, blood from both ventricles leaves the heart through a single exit. Thus, oxygen saturation in the pulmonary artery is equal to that in the systemic arteries. The degree of systemic arterial oxygen saturation depends on the ratio of pulmonary to systemic blood flow. If PVR is normal, the pulmonary blood flow is greater than the systemic blood flow and the saturation is relatively high. If PVR is elevated because of pulmonary vascular obstructive disease or small pulmonary arteries, pulmonary blood flow is

reduced and oxygen saturation is low. The systolic pressures are systemic in both ventricles.

► Clinical Findings

A. Symptoms and Signs

High pulmonary blood flow characterizes most patients with truncus arteriosus. These patients are usually minimally cyanotic and present in HF. Examination of the heart reveals a hyperactive precordium. A systolic thrill is common at the lower left sternal border. A loud early systolic ejection click is commonly heard. S_2 is single and accentuated. A loud holosystolic murmur is audible at the left lower sternal border. A diastolic flow murmur can often be heard at the apex due to increased pulmonary venous return crossing the mitral valve. An additional diastolic murmur of truncal insufficiency may be present.

Patients with decreased pulmonary blood flow are more profoundly cyanotic early. The most common manifestations are growth retardation, easy fatigability, and HF. The heart is not hyperactive. S_1 and S_2 are single and loud. A systolic murmur is heard at the lower left sternal border. No mitral flow murmur is heard, as pulmonary venous return is decreased. A loud systolic ejection click is commonly heard. In the current era, this lesion is often diagnosed by prenatal screening echocardiography.

B. Imaging

The common radiographic findings are cardiomegaly, absence of the main pulmonary artery segment, and a large aorta that has a right arch 30% of the time. The pulmonary vascular markings vary with the degree of pulmonary blood flow.

C. Electrocardiography

The axis is usually normal. RVH or combined ventricular hypertrophy is commonly present.

D. Echocardiography

Images generally show override of a single great artery (similar to ToF, but no second great artery arises directly from the heart). The origin of the pulmonary arteries and the degree of truncal valve abnormality can be defined. Color-flow Doppler can aid in the description of pulmonary flow and the function of the truncal valve, both of which are critical to management. Echocardiography is critical in identifying associated lesions, which will impact surgical planning, such as the presence of an interrupted aortic arch.

E. Angiocardiography

Cardiac catheterization is not routinely performed but may be of value in older infants in whom pulmonary vascular disease must be ruled out. The single most important angiogram would be from the truncal root, as both the origin of the pulmonary arteries and the amount of truncal insufficiency would be seen from one injection.

▶ Treatment

Anticongestive measures are needed for patients with high pulmonary blood flow and congestive failure. Surgery is always required in this condition. Because of HF and the risk of development of pulmonary vascular disease, surgery is usually performed in the neonatal period or early infancy. The VSD is closed to allow LV egress to the truncal valve. The pulmonary artery (type 1) or arteries (types 2–3) are separated from the truncus as a block, and a valved conduit is fashioned from the RV to the pulmonary circulation.

▶ Course & Prognosis

Children with a good surgical result generally do well. Outcome is also dependent to some degree on anatomy and integrity of the truncal valve, which becomes the "neoaortic" valve. Patients with a dysplastic valve may eventually require surgical repair or replacement of this valve. In addition, similar to patients with ToF, they eventually outgrow the RV-to-pulmonary artery conduit placed in infancy and require revision of the conduit in later childhood. The risk of early pulmonary vascular obstructive disease is high in the unrepaired patient and a decision to delay open-heart surgery beyond age 4–6 months is not wise even in stable patients.

O'Byrne ML et al: Morbidity in children and adolescents after surgical correction of truncus arteriosus communis. Am Heart J 2013 Sep;166(3):512–518. doi: 10.1016/j.ahj.2013.05.023 [PMID: 24016501].

▼ QUALITY IMPROVEMENT IN CONGENITAL HEART DISEASE

The National Pediatric Cardiology Quality Improvement Collaborative (NPC-QIC) was formed in response to the Joint Council on Congenital Heart Disease (JCCHD) initiative to improve outcomes of children with heart disease. The mission of the NPC-QIC is to build a collaborative network of pediatric cardiologists and an associated database to serve as the foundation for improvement projects such as improving survival and quality of life in infants with HLHS. As outcomes improve and children with complex congenital heart disease are surviving into adulthood, subspecialty clinics addressing the needs of adults with repaired or palliated congenital heart disease are required to assess and advise patients regarding adult issues such as impact of pregnancy, risks of anticoagulation during pregnancy, and appropriate adult career choices. The Adult Congenital Pediatric Cardiology (ACPC) section of the American College of Cardiology

has implemented quality metrics for various aspects of congenital heart disease, including ambulatory metrics for evaluation of chest pain, infection prevention, KD, ToF with genetic testing, evaluation of coarctation, TGA, preventative cardiology, and noninvasive imaging (https://cvquality.acc.org/initiatives/ACPC-Quality-Network).

Baker-Smith CM et al: Predictors of prolonged length of intensive care unit stay after stage I palliation: a report from the National Pediatric Cardiology Quality Improvement Collaborative. Pediatr Cardiol 2014 Mar;35(3):431–440 [PMID: 24104215].

▼ ACQUIRED HEART DISEASE

RHEUMATIC FEVER

ESSENTIALS OF DIAGNOSIS & TYPICAL FEATURES

▶ Preceding group A streptococcal infection.

▶ Diagnosis: initial acute rheumatic fever: two major manifestations or one major plus two minor manifestations.

▶ Diagnosis: recurrent acute rheumatic fever: two major or one major and two minor or three minor manifestations.

▶ Major criteria:
- Carditis
- Arthritis
- Chorea
- Erythema marginatum
- Subcutaneous nodules

▶ Minor criteria:
- Polyarthralgia or monoarthralgia
- Fever (≥ 38.5°C)
- Elevated inflammatory markers
- Prolonged PR interval on ECG

Rheumatic fever remains a major cause of morbidity and mortality in developing countries that suffer from poverty, overcrowding, and poor access to health care. Even in developed countries, rheumatic fever has not been entirely eradicated. The overall incidence in the United States is less than 1 per 100,000. Group A β-hemolytic streptococcal infection of the upper respiratory tract is the essential trigger in predisposed individuals. Only certain serotypes of group A streptococcus cause rheumatic fever. The latest attempts to define host susceptibility implicate immune response genes that are present in approximately 15% of the population. The immune response triggered by infection of the pharynx with group A streptococci consists of (1) sensitization of B lymphocytes by streptococcal antigens, (2) formation of anti-streptococcal antibody, (3) formation of immune complexes that cross-react with cardiac sarcolemma antigens, and (4) myocardial and valvular inflammatory response.

The peak age of risk in the United States is 5–15 years. The disease is slightly more common in girls and in African Americans. The annual death rate from rheumatic heart disease in school-aged children (whites and non-whites) recorded in the 1980s was less than 1 per 100,000.

▶ Clinical Findings

Two major or one major and two minor manifestations (plus supporting evidence of streptococcal infection) based on the modified Jones criteria are needed for the diagnosis of acute rheumatic fever (Table 20–13). Except in cases of rheumatic fever manifesting solely as Sydenham chorea or long-standing carditis, there should be clear evidence of a streptococcal infection such as scarlet fever, a positive throat culture for group A β-hemolytic streptococcus, and increased antistreptolysin O or other streptococcal antibody titers. The antistreptolysin O titer is significantly higher in rheumatic fever than in uncomplicated streptococcal infections.

A. Carditis

Carditis is the most serious consequence of rheumatic fever and varies from minimal to life-threatening HF. The term *carditis* implies pancardiac inflammation, but it may be limited to valves, myocardium, or pericardium. Valvulitis is frequently seen, with the mitral valve most commonly affected. Mitral insufficiency is the most common valvular

---

Table 20–13. Jones criteria (modified) for diagnosis of rheumatic fever.

Major manifestations
Carditis
Polyarthritis
Sydenham chorea
Erythema marginatum
Subcutaneous nodules
Minor manifestations
Clinical
Previous rheumatic fever or rheumatic heart disease
Polyarthralgia
Fever
Laboratory
Acute phase reaction: elevated erythrocyte sedimentation rate, C-reactive protein, leukocytosis
Prolonged PR interval
Plus
Supporting evidence of preceding streptococcal infection, ie, increased titers of antistreptolysin O or other streptococcal antibodies, positive throat culture for group A streptococcus

---

residua of acute rheumatic carditis. Mitral stenosis after acute rheumatic fever is rarely encountered until 5–10 years after the first episode. Thus, mitral stenosis is much more commonly seen in adults than in children.

An early decrescendo diastolic murmur consistent with aortic insufficiency is occasionally encountered as the sole valvular manifestation of rheumatic carditis. The aortic valve is the second most common valve affected in polyvalvular as well as in single-valve disease. The aortic valve is involved more often in males and in African Americans. Dominant aortic stenosis of rheumatic origin does not occur in pediatric patients. In one large study, the shortest length of time observed for a patient to develop dominant aortic stenosis secondary to rheumatic heart disease was 20 years.

B. Polyarthritis

The large joints (knees, hips, wrists, elbows, and shoulders) are most commonly involved, and the arthritis is typically migratory. Joint swelling and associated limitation of movement should be present. This is one of the more common major criteria, occurring in 80% of patients. Arthralgia alone is not a major criterion.

C. Sydenham Chorea

Sydenham chorea is characterized by involuntary and purposeless movements and is often associated with emotional lability. These symptoms become progressively worse and may be accompanied by ataxia and slurring of speech. Muscular weakness becomes apparent following the onset of the involuntary movements. Chorea is self-limiting, although it may last up to 3 months. Chorea may not be apparent for months to years after the acute episode of rheumatic fever.

D. Erythema Marginatum

A macular, serpiginous, erythematous rash with a sharply demarcated border appears primarily on the trunk and the extremities. The face is usually spared.

E. Subcutaneous Nodules

These usually occur only in severe cases, and then most commonly over the joints, scalp, and spinal column. The nodules vary from a few millimeters to 2 cm in diameter and are nontender and freely movable under the skin.

▶ Treatment & Prophylaxis

A. Treatment of the Acute Episode

1. Anti-infective therapy—Eradication of the streptococcal infection is essential. Long-acting benzathine penicillin is the drug of choice. Depending on the age and weight of the patient, a single intramuscular injection of 0.6–1.2 million units is effective; alternatively, give penicillin V, 250–500 mg orally two to three times a day for 10 days, or amoxicillin, 50 mg/kg (maximum 1 g) once daily for 10 days. Narrow-spectrum cephalosporins, clindamycin, azithromycin, or clarithromycin are used in those allergic to penicillin.

2. Anti-inflammatory agents

A. ASPIRIN—Aspirin, 30–60 mg/kg/day, is given in four divided doses. This dose is usually sufficient to affect dramatic relief of arthritis and fever. Higher dosages carry a greater risk of side effects, and there are no proven short- or long-term benefits of high doses that produce salicylate blood levels of 20–30 mg/dL. The duration of therapy is tailored to meet the needs of the patient, but 2–6 weeks of therapy with reduction in dose toward the end of the course is usually sufficient. Other nonsteroidal anti-inflammatory agents used because of concerns about Reye syndrome are less effective than aspirin.

B. CORTICOSTEROIDS—There is no clear evidence to support the use of corticosteroids, but they are occasionally used for those with severe carditis.

3. Therapy in heart failure—
Treatment for HF is based on symptoms and severity of valve involvement and cardiac dysfunction (see section Heart Failure).

4. Bed rest and ambulation—
Bed rest is not required in most cases. Activity level should be commensurate with symptoms and children should be allowed to self-limit their activity level while affected. Most acute episodes of rheumatic fever are managed on an outpatient basis.

B. Treatment After the Acute Episode

1. Prevention—
Prevention is critical, as patients who have had rheumatic fever are at greater risk of recurrence if future group A β-hemolytic streptococcal infections are inadequately treated. Follow-up visits are essential to reinforce the necessity for prophylaxis, with regular intramuscular long-acting benzathine penicillin injections preferred to oral medication due to better adherence. Long-term (possibly lifelong) prophylaxis is recommended for patients with residual rheumatic heart disease. More commonly, with no or transient cardiac involvement, 5–10 years of therapy or discontinuance in early adulthood (age 21) (whichever is longer) is an effective approach.

The following preventive regimens are in current use:

A. PENICILLIN G BENZATHINE—600,000 units for less than 27 kg, 1.2 million units for more than 27 kg intramuscularly every 4 weeks is the drug of choice.

B. PENICILLIN V—250 mg orally twice daily is much less effective than intramuscular penicillin benzathine G (5.5 vs 0.4 streptococcal infections per 100 patient-years).

C. SULFADIAZINE—500 mg for less than 27 kg and 1 g for more than 27 kg, once daily. Blood dyscrasias and lesser

effectiveness in reducing streptococcal infections make this drug less satisfactory than penicillin benzathine G. This is the recommended regimen for penicillin-allergic patients.

D. ERYTHROMYCIN—250 mg orally twice a day may be given to patients who are allergic to both penicillin and sulfonamides. Azithromycin or clarithromycin may also be used.

2. Residual valvular damage—
As described above, the mitral and aortic valves are most commonly affected by rheumatic fever and the severity of carditis is quite variable. In the most severe cases, cardiac failure or the need for a valve replacement can occur in the acute setting. In less severe cases, valve abnormalities can persist, requiring lifelong medical management and eventual valve replacement. Other patients fully recover without residual cardiac sequelae.

Although antibiotic prophylaxis to protect against endocarditis used to be recommended for those with residual valvular abnormalities, the criteria for prevention of IE were revised in 2007 and routine prophylaxis is recommended only if a prosthetic valve is in place.

Cilliers A et al: Anti-inflammatory treatment for carditis in acute rheumatic fever. Cochrane Database Syst Rev 2012 Jun 13; 6:CD003176 [PMID: 22696333].

Gewitz MH et al: Revision of the Jones Criteria for the diagnosis of acute rheumatic fever in the era of Doppler echocardiography: a scientific statement from the American Heart Association. Circulation 2015 May 19;131(20):1806–1818. doi: 10.1161/CIR.0000000000000205 [PMID: 25908771].

KAWASAKI DISEASE

ESSENTIALS OF DIAGNOSIS & TYPICAL FEATURES

▶ At least 5 days of fever + 4/5 of following:
  - Conjunctival injection without exudate
  - Mucous membrane changes (lips/tongue/pharynx)
  - Peripheral extremity changes (hand/foot erythema and/or swelling)
  - Polymorphous generalized rash
  - Unilateral enlarged cervical lymph node (> 1.5 cm)
▶ Exclusion of other causes of these findings
▶ Dilated coronary arteries from echocardiograms can help with diagnosis in incomplete Kawasaki disease (KD)

KD was first described in Japan in 1967 and was initially called mucocutaneous lymph node syndrome. The cause is unclear, and there is no specific diagnostic test. KD is the leading cause of acquired heart disease in children in the United States. Eighty percent of patients are younger than

5 years (median age at diagnosis is 2 years), and the male-to-female ratio is 1.5:1. Diagnostic criteria are fever for more than 5 days and at least four of the following features: (1) bilateral, painless, nonexudative conjunctivitis; (2) lip or oral cavity changes (eg, lip cracking and fissuring, strawberry tongue, and inflammation of the oral mucosa); (3) cervical lymphadenopathy greater than or equal to 1.5 cm in diameter and usually unilateral; (4) polymorphous exanthema; and (5) extremity changes (redness and swelling of the hands and feet with subsequent desquamation). In the presence of more than four principal clinical criteria, the diagnosis can be made with only 4 days of fever. Clinical features not part of the diagnostic criteria, but frequently associated with KD, are shown in Table 20–14.

The potential for cardiovascular complications is the most serious aspect of KD. Complications during the acute illness include myocarditis, pericarditis, valvular heart disease (usually mitral or aortic regurgitation), and coronary arteritis. Patients with fever for at least 5 days but fewer than four of the diagnostic features can be diagnosed with incomplete KD, especially if they have coronary artery abnormalities detected by echocardiography. Comprehensive recommendations regarding the evaluation for children with suspected incomplete KD were outlined in a 2017 Statement by the American Heart Association (see references at the end of this section).

Coronary artery lesions range from mild transient dilation of a coronary artery to large aneurysms. Aneurysms rarely form before day 10 of illness. Untreated patients have a 15%–25% risk of developing coronary aneurysms. Those at greatest risk for aneurysm formation are males, young infants (< 6 months), and those not treated with intravenous immunoglobulin (IVIG). Most coronary artery aneurysms resolve within 5 years of diagnosis; however, as aneurysms resolve,

associated obstruction or stenosis (19% of all aneurysms) may develop, which may result in coronary ischemia. Giant aneurysms (> 8 mm) are less likely to resolve, and nearly 50% eventually become stenotic. Of additional concern, acute thrombosis of an aneurysm can occur, resulting in myocardial infarction that is fatal in approximately 20% of cases.

▶ Treatment

Immediate management of KD includes IVIG and high-dose aspirin. This therapy is effective in decreasing the incidence of coronary artery dilation and aneurysm formation. The currently recommended regimen is 2 g/kg of IVIG administered over 10–12 hours and 80–100 mg/kg/day (some centers use 30–50 mg/kg/day) of aspirin in four divided doses. The duration of high-dose aspirin is institution-dependent: many centers reduce the dose once the patient is afebrile for 48–72 hours; others continue through 5 afebrile days or day 14 of the illness. Once high-dose aspirin is discontinued, low-dose aspirin (3–5 mg/kg/day) is given through the subacute phase of the illness (6–8 weeks) or until coronary artery abnormalities resolve. If fever recurs within 48–72 hours of the initial treatment course and no other source of the fever is detected, a second dose of IVIG is often recommended; however, the effectiveness of this approach has not been clearly demonstrated. Corticosteroids or other anti-inflammatory therapy (eg, infliximab) should be considered for patients with persistent fever despite one or two infusions of IVIG. Follow-up of patients with treated KD depends on the degree of coronary involvement (Table 20–15).

McCrindle BW et al: Diagnosis, treatment, and long-term management of Kawasaki disease: a scientific statement for health professionals from the American Heart Association [review]. Circulation 2017 Apr 25;135 (17):e927–e999. doi: 10 1161/CIR 0000000000000484. Epub 2017 Mar 29 [PMID: 28356445].

Newburger JW, Takahashi M, Burns JC: Kawasaki disease. J Am Coll Cardiol 2016 Apr 12;67(14):1738–1749. doi: 10.1016/j.jacc.2015.12.073 [PMID: 27056781].

INFECTIVE ENDOCARDITIS

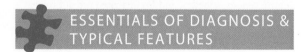

ESSENTIALS OF DIAGNOSIS & TYPICAL FEATURES

▶ Positive blood culture.

▶ Intracardiac oscillating mass, abscess, or new valve regurgitation on echocardiogram.

▶ Fever.

▶ Elevated erythrocyte sedimentation rate or C-reactive protein.

Table 20–14. Noncardiac manifestations of Kawasaki disease.

System	Associated Signs and Symptoms
Gastrointestinal	Vomiting, diarrhea, gallbladder hydrops, elevated transaminases
Blood	Elevated ESR or CRP, leukocytosis, hypoalbuminemia, mild anemia in acute phase and thrombocytosis in subacute phase (usually second to third week of illness)
Renal	Sterile pyuria, proteinuria
Respiratory	Cough, hoarseness, infiltrate on chest radiograph
Joint	Arthralgia and arthritis
Neurologic	Mononuclear pleocytosis of cerebrospinal fluid, irritability, facial palsy

CRP, C-reactive protein; ESR, erythrocyte sedimentation rate.

Table 20–15. Long-term management in Kawasaki disease.

Risk Level	Definition	Management Guidelines
I	No coronary artery changes at any stage of the illness	No ASA is needed beyond the subacute phase (6–8 wk). No follow-up beyond the first year.
II	Coronary dilation only (Z-score[a] 2–2.5)	Same as above or clinical follow-up every 2–5 y if persistent coronary dilation.
III	Small coronary aneurysms (Z-score > 2.5 to < 5)	ASA until abnormality resolves. Assess at 6 mo and every 2–3 y thereafter with ECG and echo if < 7 y and every other-year stress testing if > 7 y.
IV	Medium aneurysms (Z-score > 5 to < 10 and absolute dimension < 8 mm)	Long-term ASA ± clopidogrel. Annual follow-up with ECG, echo, and stress testing.
V	Large and giant aneurysms (Z-score > 10 or absolute dimension > 8 mm) or coronary artery obstruction	Long-term ASA ± clopidogrel ± warfarin ± calcium channel blocker to reduce myocardial oxygen consumption. Echo and ECG every 6 mo. Stress testing and Holter examination annually.

ASA, acetyl salicylic acid; ECG, electrocardiogram; echo, echocardiogram.
[a]Coronary artery size assessments are based on standard deviation (Z-score) compared to the normal population.

General Considerations

Bacterial or fungal infection of the endocardium of the heart is rare and usually occurs in the setting of a preexisting abnormality of the heart or great arteries. It may occur in a normal heart during septicemia or as a consequence of infected indwelling central catheters.

The frequency of infective endocarditis (IE) appears to be increasing for several reasons: (1) increased survival in children with congenital heart disease, (2) greater use of central venous catheters, and (3) increased use of prosthetic material and valves. Pediatric patients without preexisting heart disease are also at increased risk for IE because of (1) increased survival rates for children with immune deficiencies, (2) long-term use of indwelling lines in ill newborns and patients with chronic diseases, and (3) increased intravenous drug abuse.

Patients at greatest risk are children with unrepaired or palliated cyanotic heart disease (especially in the presence of an aorta to pulmonary shunt), those with implanted prosthetic material, and patients who have had a prior episode of IE. Common organisms causing IE are viridans streptococci (30%–40% of cases), *Staphylococcus aureus* (25%–30%), and fungal agents (about 5%).

▶ Clinical Findings

A. History

The majority of patients with IE have a history of heart disease. There may or may not be an antecedent infection or surgical procedure (cardiac surgery, tooth extraction, tonsillectomy). Transient bacteremia occurs frequently during normal daily activities such as flossing or brushing teeth, using a toothpick and even when chewing food. Although dental and nonsterile surgical procedures also can result in transient bacteremias, these episodes are much less frequent for a given individual. This may be why a clear inciting event is often not identified in association with IE and also underlies the recent changes in guidelines for antibiotic prophylaxis to prevent IE (for details, see Wilson et al reference).

B. Symptoms, Signs, and Laboratory Findings

Although IE can present in a fulminant fashion with cardiovascular collapse, often it presents in an indolent manner with fever, malaise, and weight loss. Joint pain and vomiting are less common. On physical examination, there may be a new or changing murmur, splenomegaly, and hepatomegaly. Classic findings of Osler nodes (tender nodules, usually on the pulp of the fingers), Janeway lesions (nontender hemorrhagic macules on palms and soles), splinter hemorrhages, and Roth spots (retinal hemorrhage) are uncommonly noted in children. Laboratory findings include multiple positive blood cultures, elevated erythrocyte sedimentation rate or C-reactive protein, and hematuria. Transthoracic echocardiography can identify large vegetations in some patients, but transesophageal imaging has better sensitivity and may be necessary if the diagnosis remains in question.

▶ Prevention

In 2007, the AHA revised criteria for patients requiring prophylaxis for IE (Table 20–16). Only the high-risk patients listed require antibiotics before dental work (tooth extraction or cleaning) and procedures involving the respiratory

Table 20–16. Conditions requiring antibiotic prophylaxis for the prevention of infective endocarditis (IE).

Prosthetic cardiac valves
Prior episode of IE
Congenital heart disease (CHD)
   Palliated cyanotic CHD
   For 6 months postprocedure if CHD repair involves implanted
      prosthetic material
   Repair of CHD with residual defect bordered by prosthetic material
Cardiac transplant with valvulopathy

tract or infected skin or musculoskeletal structures. IE prophylaxis is not recommended for gastrointestinal or genitourinary procedures, body piercing, or tattooing. The impact of changes in the guideline in children is still uncertain.

Recommended prophylaxis is 50 mg/kg of oral amoxicillin for patients less than 40 kg and 2000 mg for those more than 40 kg. This dose is to be given 1 hour prior to procedure. If the patient is allergic to amoxicillin, alternative prophylactic antibiotics are recommended in the AHA guidelines.

▶ Treatment

In general, appropriate antibiotic therapy should be initiated as soon as IE is suspected and several large volume blood cultures have been obtained via separate venipunctures. Therapy can be tailored once the pathogen and sensitivities are defined. Vancomycin or a β-lactam antibiotic, with or without gentamicin, for a 6-week course is the most common regimen. If HF occurs and progresses in the face of adequate antibiotic therapy, surgical excision of the infected area and prosthetic valve replacement must be considered.

▶ Course & Prognosis

Factors associated with a poor outcome are delayed diagnosis, presence of prosthetic material, perioperative associated IE, and *S aureus* infection. Mortality for bacterial endocarditis in children ranges from 10% to 25%, with fungal infections having a much greater mortality (50% or more).

Baltimore RS et al: Infective endocarditis in childhood: 2015 update: a scientific statement from the American Heart Association. Circulation 2015 Oct 13;132(15):1487–1515. doi: 10.1161/CIR.0000000000000298 [PMID: 26373317].

Dixon G et al: Infective endocarditis in children: an update. Curr Opin Infect Dis 2017 Jun;30 (3):257–267 [PMID: 28319472].

PERICARDITIS

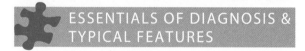

ESSENTIALS OF DIAGNOSIS & TYPICAL FEATURES

▶ Chest pain made worse by deep inspiration and decreased by leaning forward.

▶ Fever and tachycardia.

▶ Shortness of breath.

▶ Pericardial friction rub.

▶ ECG with elevated ST segments.

▶ General Considerations

Pericarditis is an inflammation of the pericardium and is commonly related to an infectious process. The most common cause of pericarditis in children is viral infection (eg, coxsackievirus, mumps, Epstein-Barr, adenovirus, influenza, and human immunodeficiency virus [HIV]). Purulent pericarditis results from bacterial infection (eg, pneumococci, streptococci, staphylococci, and *Haemophilus influenzae*) and is less common but potentially life threatening.

In some cases, pericardial disease occurs in association with a generalized process. Associations include rheumatic fever, rheumatoid arthritis, uremia, systemic lupus erythematosus, malignancy, and tuberculosis. Pericarditis after cardiac surgery (postpericardiotomy syndrome) is most commonly seen after surgical closure of an ASD. Postpericardiotomy syndrome appears to be autoimmune in nature with high titers of antiheart antibody and evidence of acute or reactivated viral illness. The syndrome is often self-limited and responds well to short courses of aspirin or corticosteroids.

▶ Clinical Findings

A. Symptoms and Signs

Childhood pericarditis usually presents with sharp stabbing mid chest, shoulder, and neck pain made worse by deep inspiration or coughing, and decreased by sitting up and leaning forward. Shortness of breath and grunting respirations are common. Physical findings depend on the presence of fluid accumulation in the pericardial space (effusion). In the absence of significant accumulation, a characteristic scratchy, high-pitched friction rub may be heard. If the effusion is large, heart sounds are distant and muffled and a friction rub may not be present. In the absence of cardiac tamponade, the peripheral, venous, and arterial pulses are normal.

Cardiac tamponade occurs in association with a large effusion, or one that has rapidly accumulated. Tamponade is characterized by jugular venous distention, tachycardia, hepatomegaly, peripheral edema, and pulsus paradoxus, in which systolic blood pressure drops more than 10 mm Hg during inspiration. Decreased cardiac filling and subsequent decrease in cardiac output result in signs of right HF and the potential for cardiovascular collapse.

B. Imaging

In pericarditis with a significant pericardial effusion, the cardiac silhouette is enlarged. The cardiac silhouette can appear normal if the effusion has developed over an extremely short period of time.

C. Electrocardiography

The ST segments are commonly elevated in acute pericarditis and PR segment depression may be present. Low voltages or electrical alternans (alteration in QRS amplitude between beats) can be seen with large pericardial effusions.

D. Echocardiography

Serial echocardiography allows a direct, noninvasive estimate of the volume of pericardial fluid and its change over time. Cardiac tamponade is associated with compression of the atria or respiratory alteration of ventricular inflow demonstrated by Doppler imaging.

▶ Treatment

Treatment depends on the cause of pericarditis and the size of the associated effusion. Viral pericarditis is usually self-limited, and symptoms can be improved with nonsteroidal anti-inflammatory therapy. Purulent pericarditis requires immediate evacuation of the fluid and appropriate antibiotic therapy. Cardiac tamponade from any cause must be treated by immediate removal of the fluid, usually via pericardiocentesis. Pericardiocentesis should also be considered if the underlying cause is unclear or identification of the pathogen is necessary for targeted therapy. In the setting of recurrent or persistent effusions, a surgical pericardiectomy or pericardial window may be necessary. Diuretics should be avoided in the patient with cardiac tamponade because they reduce ventricular preload and can exacerbate the degree of cardiac decompensation.

▶ Prognosis

Prognosis depends to a great extent on the cause of pericardial disease. Constrictive pericarditis can develop following infectious pericarditis (especially if bacterial or tuberculous) and can be a difficult problem to manage. Cardiac tamponade will result in death unless the fluid is evacuated.

Adler Y et al: 2015 ESC guidelines for the diagnosis and management of pericardial diseases: the Task Force for the Diagnosis and Management of Pericardial Diseases of the European Society of Cardiology (ESC) endorsed by: The European Association for Cardio-Thoracic Surgery (EACTS). Eur Heart J 2015 Nov 7;36(42): 2921–2964. doi: 10.1093/eurheartj/ehv318 [PMID: 26320112].

Ratnapalan S, Brown K, Benson L: Children presenting with acute pericarditis to the emergency department. Pediatr Emerg Care 2011 Jul;27(7):581–585 [PMID: 21712753].

CARDIOMYOPATHY

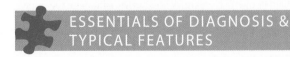

ESSENTIALS OF DIAGNOSIS & TYPICAL FEATURES

▶ Failure to thrive.

▶ Poor appetite, abdominal pain, and/or vomiting.

▶ Exercise intolerance.

▶ Tachypnea, cough, orthopnea, and/or shortness of breath.

▶ Diaphoresis.

▶ Edema.

▶ Tachycardia.

▶ Fainting or aborted sudden death event.

▶ Diagnosis based on echocardiographic findings.

There are five classified forms of cardiomyopathy in children: (1) dilated, (2) hypertrophic, (3) restrictive, (4) arrhythmogenic right ventricular dysplasia (ARVD), and (5) LV noncompaction. Discussion will be limited to the first three forms, which are the most common.

1. Dilated Cardiomyopathy

This most frequent of the childhood cardiomyopathies occurs with an annual incidence of 4–8 cases per 100,000 population in the United States and Europe. Although usually idiopathic, identifiable causes of dilated cardiomyopathy (DCM) include viral myocarditis, untreated tachyarrhythmias, left heart obstructive lesions, congenital abnormalities of the coronary arteries, medication toxicity (eg, anthracycline), and genetic (eg, dystrophin gene defects, sarcomeric mutations) and metabolic diseases (inborn errors of fatty acid oxidation and mitochondrial oxidative phosphorylation defects). Genetic causes are being discovered at an increasing rate with commercial testing now available for some of the more common genes.

▶ Clinical Findings

A. Signs and Symptoms

As myocardial function fails and the heart dilates, cardiac output falls, and affected children develop decreased exercise tolerance, failure to thrive, diaphoresis, and tachypnea. As the heart continues to deteriorate, congestive signs such as hepatomegaly and rales develop, and a prominent gallop can be appreciated on examination. The initial diagnosis in a previously healthy child can be difficult, as presenting symptoms can resemble a viral respiratory infection, pneumonia, or asthma.

B. Imaging

Chest radiograph shows generalized cardiomegaly with or without pulmonary venous congestion.

C. Electrocardiography

Sinus tachycardia with ST-T segment changes is commonly seen on ECG. The criteria for RVH and LVH may also be met, and the QT interval may be prolonged. Evaluation for the presence of supraventricular arrhythmias on ECG is critical, as this is one of the few treatable and reversible causes of DCM in children.

D. Echocardiography

The echocardiogram shows LV and left atrial enlargement with decreased LV-shortening fraction and ejection fraction. The calculated end-diastolic and end-systolic dimensions are increased, and mitral insufficiency is commonly seen. A careful evaluation for evidence of structural abnormalities (especially coronary artery anomalies or left heart obstructive lesions) must be performed, especially in infant patients.

E. Other Testing

Cardiac catheterization is useful to evaluate hemodynamic status and coronary artery anatomy. Endomyocardial biopsies can aid in diagnosis. Biopsy specimens may show inflammation consistent with acute myocarditis, abnormal myocyte architecture, and myocardial fibrosis. Electron micrographs may reveal evidence of mitochondrial or other metabolic disorders. Polymerase chain reaction (PCR) testing may be performed on biopsied specimens to detect viral genome products in infectious myocarditis. Cardiopulmonary stress testing is useful for measuring response to medical therapy and as an objective assessment of the cardiac limitations on exercise.

▶ Treatment & Prognosis

Outpatient management of pediatric DCM usually entails combinations of afterload-reducing agents and diuretics (see section Heart Failure). In 2007, Shaddy et al published the results of a multicenter, placebo-controlled, double-blind trial of carvedilol in children with HF. Children did not receive the same beneficial effects of β-blocker therapy as adults with HF, possibly due to the heterogenous nature of HF in children and increasing evidence that there are inherent differences in pediatric and adult HF. Aspirin or warfarin may be used to prevent thrombus formation in the dilated and poorly contractile cardiac chambers. Arrhythmias are more common in dilated hearts and antiarrhythmic therapy is sometimes necessary. Despite widespread use of internal defibrillators in the adult population, the technical difficulty of implanting internal defibrillators, the risk of adverse events (eg, high frequency of inappropriate discharge, vascular obstruction), and the low incidence of sudden cardiac death (SCD) in children limit their use.

Therapy of the underlying cause of cardiomyopathy is always indicated if possible. Unfortunately despite complete evaluation, a diagnosis is discovered in less than 30% of patients with DCM. If medical management is unsuccessful, cardiac transplantation is considered.

2. Hypertrophic Cardiomyopathy

The most common cause of hypertrophic cardiomyopathy (HCM) is familial HCM, which is found in 1 in 500 individuals. HCM is the leading cause of SCD in young persons. The most common presentation is in an older child, adolescent, or adult, although it may occur in neonates. Causes of non-familial HCM in neonates and young children include glycogen storage disease, Noonan syndrome (including related syndromes such as LEOPARD and Costello syndrome), Friedreich ataxia, maternal gestational diabetes, mitochondrial disorders, and other metabolic disorders.

A. Familial Hypertrophic Cardiomyopathy

In the familial form, HCM is most commonly caused by a mutation in one of the several genes that encode proteins of the cardiac sarcomere (β-myosin heavy chain, cardiac troponin T or I, α-tropomyosin, and myosin-binding protein C).

1. Clinical findings—Patients may be asymptomatic despite having significant hypertrophy, or may present with symptoms of inadequate coronary perfusion or HF such as angina, syncope, palpitations, or exercise intolerance. Patients may experience SCD as their initial presentation, often precipitated by sporting activities. Although the cardiac examination may be normal on presentation, some patients develop a left precordial bulge with a diffuse point of maximal impulse. An LV heave or an S_4 gallop may be present. If outflow tract obstruction exists, a systolic ejection murmur will be audible. A murmur may not be audible at rest but may be provoked by exercise or positional maneuvers that decrease LV volume (standing), thereby increasing the outflow tract obstruction.

A. ECHOCARDIOGRAPHY—The diagnosis of HCM is usually made by echocardiography and in most familial cases demonstrates asymmetrical septal hypertrophy. Young patients with metabolic or other nonfamilial causes are more likely to have concentric hypertrophy. Systolic anterior motion of the mitral valve leaflet may occur and contribute to LV outflow tract obstruction. The mitral valve leaflet may become distorted and result in mitral insufficiency. LV outflow tract obstruction may be present at rest or provoked with monitored exercise. Systolic function is most often hypercontractile in young children but may deteriorate over time, resulting in poor contractility and LV dilation. Diastolic function is almost always abnormal.

B. ELECTROCARDIOGRAPHY—The ECG may be normal but more typically demonstrates deep Q waves in the inferolateral leads (II, III, aVF, V_5, and V_6) secondary to the increased mass of the hypertrophied septum. ST-segment abnormalities may be seen in the same leads. Age-dependent criteria for LVH are often present as criteria for left atrial enlargement.

C. OTHER TESTING—Cardiopulmonary stress testing is valuable to evaluate for provocable LV outflow tract obstruction, ischemia, and arrhythmias, and to determine prognosis. Extreme LVH and a blunted blood pressure response to exercise have both been associated with increased mortality in children. Cardiac MRI is useful for defining areas of myocardial fibrosis or scarring. Patients are at risk for myocardial ischemia, possibly as a result of systolic compression of the intramyocardial septal perforators, myocardial bridging of epicardial coronary arteries, or an imbalance of coronary artery supply and demand due to the presence of massive myocardial hypertrophy.

D. CARDIAC CATHETERIZATION—Cardiac catheterization may be performed in patients with HCM who have angina, syncope, resuscitated sudden death, or a worrisome stress test. Hemodynamic findings include elevated left atrial pressure secondary to impaired diastolic filling. If midcavitary LV outflow tract obstruction is present, an associated pressure gradient will be evident. Provocation of LV outflow tract obstruction with either rapid atrial pacing or isoproterenol may be sought, but this is not commonly done in children. Angiography demonstrates a "ballerina slipper" configuration of the LV secondary to the midcavitary LV obliteration during systole. Although uncommonly done in the current era, myocardial biopsy demonstrates myofiber disarray.

2. Treatment and prognosis—Treatment varies depending on symptoms and phenotype. Affected patients are restricted from competitive athletics and isometric exercise due to associated risk of SCD. Patients with resting or latent LV outflow tract obstruction may be treated with β-blockers, verapamil, or disopyramide with variable success in alleviating obstruction. Patients with severe symptoms despite medical therapy and an LV outflow tract gradient may require additional intervention. Surgical myectomy with resection of part of the hypertrophied septum has been used in symptomatic patients with good results. At the time of myectomy, the mitral valve may require repair or replacement in patients with a long history of systolic anterior motion of the mitral valve. Ethanol ablation is used in adults with HCM and LV outflow tract obstruction. This procedure involves selective infiltration of ethanol in a coronary septal artery branch to induce a small targeted myocardial infarction. This leads to a reduction in septal size and improvement of obstruction. The long-term effects of this procedure are unknown, and it is not commonly employed in children. Dual-chamber pacing to relieve obstruction has been used in children, but data to support its use are lacking. Risk stratification with respect to sudden death is important in HCM. Consideration for placement of internal defibrillators in adult patients are based on the known risk factors for SCD: severe hypertrophy (> 3 cm septal thickness in adults), documented ventricular arrhythmias, syncope, abnormal blood pressure response to exercise, resuscitated sudden death, or a strong family history of HCM with associated sudden death. The criteria for defibrillator placement in children are not as well defined.

B. Glycogen Storage Disease of the Heart

There are at least 10 types of glycogen storage disease. The type that primarily involves the heart is Pompe disease (GSD IIa) in which acid maltase, necessary for hydrolysis of the outer branches of glycogen, is absent. There is marked deposition of glycogen within the myocardium. Affected infants are well at birth, but symptoms of growth and developmental delay, feeding problems, and cardiac failure occur by the sixth month of life. Physical examination reveals generalized muscular weakness, a large tongue, and cardiomegaly without significant heart murmurs. Chest radiographs reveal cardiomegaly with or without pulmonary venous congestion. The ECG shows a short PR interval and LVH with ST depression and T-wave inversion over the left precordial leads. Echocardiography shows severe concentric LVH. Although historically children with Pompe disease usually died before age 1 year, recent enzyme replacement clinical trials have shown some promise in reversing hypertrophy and preserving cardiac function. Death may be sudden or result from progressive HF.

3. Restrictive Cardiomyopathy

Restrictive cardiomyopathy is a rare entity in the pediatric population, accounting for less than 5% of all cases of cardiomyopathy. The cause is usually idiopathic but can be familial or secondary to an infiltrative process (eg, amyloidosis).

▶ Clinical Findings

Patients present with signs of congestive HF as a consequence of diastolic dysfunction in the setting of preserved systolic function. The LV is more severely affected than the RV in restrictive cardiomyopathy, but the RV is also affected in most cases resulting in signs and symptoms consistent with biventricular congestion. Patients often present with exercise intolerance, fatigue, chest pain, and orthopnea. Physical examination is remarkable for a prominent S_4 and jugular venous distention.

A. Electrocardiography

ECG demonstrates marked right and left atrial enlargement with normal ventricular voltages. ST-T–wave abnormalities including a prolonged QTc interval may be present.

B. Echocardiography

The diagnosis is confirmed echocardiographically by the presence of normal-sized ventricles with normal systolic function and massively dilated atria. Cardiac MRI is useful in ruling out pericardial abnormalities (restrictive or constrictive pericarditis) and infiltrative disorders.

▶ Treatment & Prognosis

Anticongestive therapy is used for symptomatic relief. The risk of sudden death in restrictive cardiomyopathy and the propensity for rapid progression of irreversible PH warrant close follow-up with early consideration of cardiac transplantation.

Chen LR et al: Reversal of cardiac dysfunction after enzyme replacement in patients with infantile-onset Pompe disease. J Pediatr 2009 Aug;155(2):271–275, e272 [PMID: 19486996].

Decker JA et al: Risk factors and mode of death in isolated hypertrophic cardiomyopathy in children. J Am Coll Cardiol 2009 Jul 14;54(3):250–254 [PMID: 19589438].

Shaddy RE et al: Carvedilol for children and adolescents with heart failure: a randomized controlled trial. JAMA 2007 Sep 12;298(10):1171–1179 [PMID: 17848651].

Towbin JA et al: Incidence, causes, and outcomes of dilated cardiomyopathy in children. JAMA 2006 Oct 18;296(15):1867–1876 [PMID: 17047217].

MYOCARDITIS

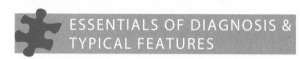

ESSENTIALS OF DIAGNOSIS & TYPICAL FEATURES

▶ Often occurs in association with a viral infection.

▶ Signs and symptoms of cardiomyopathy as outlined earlier.

▶ Echocardiogram will demonstrate a poorly functioning ventricle with varying degrees of ventricular dilation.

▶ May see diffusely low voltages on ECG.

▶ Elevated inflammatory markers may be present (eg, ESR, CRP).

▶ Cardiac MRI is an evolving diagnostic tool.

▶ Endomyocardial biopsy will demonstrate lymphocytic infiltrate and viral PCR positivity.

The most common causes of viral myocarditis are adenoviruses, coxsackie A and B viruses, echoviruses, parvovirus, cytomegalovirus, and influenza A virus. HIV can also cause myocarditis. The ability to identify the pathogen has been enhanced by PCR technology, which replicates identifiable segments of the viral genome from the myocardium of affected children.

▶ Clinical Findings

A. Symptoms and Signs

There are two major clinical patterns. In the first, sudden-onset HF occurs in an infant or child who was relatively healthy in the hours to days previously. This malignant form of the disease is usually secondary to overwhelming viremia with tissue invasion in multiple organ systems including the heart. In the second pattern, the onset of cardiac symptoms is gradual, and there may be a history of upper respiratory tract infection or gastroenteritis in the previous month. This more insidious form may have a late postinfectious or autoimmune component. Acute and chronic presentations occur at any age and with all types of myocarditis.

The signs of HF are variable, but in a decompensated patient with fulminant myocarditis, they include pale gray skin; rapid, weak, and thready pulses; and breathlessness. In those with a more subacute presentation signs include increased work of breathing such as orthopnea, difficulty with feeding in infants, exercise intolerance and edema of the face and extremities. The patient is usually tachycardic and heart sounds may be muffled and distant; an S_3 or S_4 gallop (or both) are common. Murmurs are usually absent, although a murmur of tricuspid or mitral insufficiency may be heard. Moist rales are usually present at both lung bases. The liver is enlarged and frequently tender.

B. Imaging

Generalized cardiomegaly is seen on radiographs along with moderate to marked pulmonary venous congestion.

C. Electrocardiography

The ECG is variable. Classically, there is low-voltage QRS in all frontal and precordial leads with ST-segment depression and inversion of T waves in leads I, III, and aVF (and in the left precordial leads during the acute stage). Dysrhythmias are common, and AV and intraventricular conduction disturbances may be present.

D. Echocardiography

Echocardiography demonstrates four-chamber dilation with poor ventricular function and AV valve regurgitation. A pericardial effusion may be present. Patients with a more acute presentation may have less ventricular dilation than those with a longer history of HF-related symptoms.

E. Myocardial Biopsy

An endomyocardial biopsy may be helpful in the diagnosis of viral myocarditis. An inflammatory infiltrate with myocyte damage can be seen by hematoxylin and eosin staining. Viral PCR testing of the biopsy specimen may yield a positive result in 30%–40% of patients suspected to have myocarditis. However, myocarditis is thought to be a "patchy" process, so it is possible that biopsy results are falsely negative if the area of active myocarditis was missed.

F. Cardiac MRI

Cardiac MRI is increasing in use as a potential diagnostic modality for myocarditis. Abnormalities in T2-weighted imaging (consistent with myocardial edema, inflammation) and global relative enhancement (evidence of capillary leak) are evident in patients with acute myocarditis. This imaging method requires general anesthesia in infants and young children, which is associated with significant risk in those with HF and must be a consideration when ordering this test.

Treatment

The inpatient cardiac support measures outlined previously in section Heart Failure are used in the treatment of these patients. The use of digitalis in a rapidly deteriorating child with myocarditis is dangerous and should be undertaken with great caution, as it may cause ventricular dysrhythmias.

Administration of immunomodulating medications such as corticosteroids for myocarditis is controversial. Subsequent to the successful use of IVIG in children with KD, there have been several trials of IVIG in presumed viral myocarditis. The therapeutic value of IVIG remains unconfirmed. Initiation of mechanical circulatory support in those with fulminant or severe myocarditis is another therapeutic option as a bridge to transplantation or recovery.

Prognosis

The prognosis of myocarditis is determined by the age at onset and the response to therapy. Children presenting with fulminant myocarditis and severe hemodynamic compromise have a 75% early mortality. Those at highest risk for a poor outcome are those presenting in the first year of life. Complete recovery is possible, although some patients recover clinically but have persistent LV dysfunction and require ongoing medical therapy for HF. It is possible that subclinical myocarditis in childhood is the pathophysiologic basis for some of the "idiopathic" DCMs later in life. Children with myocarditis whose ventricular function fails to return to normal may be candidates for cardiac transplantation if they remain symptomatic or suffer growth failure despite maximal medical management.

Pettit MA et al: Myocarditis. Pediatr Emerg Care 2014 Nov; 30(11):832–835 [PMID: 25373572].

▼ PREVENTIVE CARDIOLOGY

HYPERTENSION

Blood pressure should be determined at every pediatric visit beginning at 3 years. Because blood pressure is being more carefully monitored, systemic hypertension has become more widely recognized as a pediatric problem. Pediatric standards for blood pressure have been published. Blood pressures in children must be obtained when the child is relaxed and an appropriate-size cuff must always be used. The widest cuff that fits between the axilla, and the antecubital fossa should be used (covers 60%–75% of the upper arm). Most children aged 10–11 years need a standard adult cuff (bladder width of 12 cm), and many high school students need a large adult cuff (width of 16 cm) or leg cuff (width of 18 cm). The pressure coinciding with the onset (K_1) and the loss (K_5) of the Korotkoff sounds determines the systolic and diastolic blood pressure, respectively. If a properly measured blood pressure exceeds the 95th percentile, the measurement should be repeated several times over a 2- to 4-week interval. If it is elevated persistently, a search for the cause should be undertaken. Although most hypertension in children is essential, the incidence of treatable causes is higher in children than in adults; these include conditions such as coarctation of the aorta, renal artery stenosis, chronic renal disease, and pheochromocytoma, as well as medication side effects (eg, steroids). If no cause is identified, and hypertension is deemed essential, antihypertensive therapy should be initiated and nutritional and exercise counseling given. β-Blockers or ACE inhibitors are the usual first-line medical therapies for essential hypertension in children.

Flynn JT et al: Update: ambulatory blood pressure monitoring in children and adolescents: a scientific statement from the American Heart Association. Hypertension 2014 May;63(5): 1116–1135 [PMID: 24591341].

ATHEROSCLEROSIS & DYSLIPIDEMIAS

Awareness of coronary artery risk factors in general, and atherosclerosis in particular, has risen dramatically in the general population since the mid-1970s. Although coronary artery disease is still the leading cause of death in the United States, the age-adjusted incidence of death from ischemic heart disease has been decreasing as a result of improved diet, decreased smoking, awareness and treatment of hypertension, and an increase in physical activity. The level of serum lipids in childhood usually remains constant through adolescence. Biochemical abnormalities in the lipid profile appearing early in childhood correlate with higher risk for coronary artery disease in adulthood. Low-density lipoprotein (LDL) is atherogenic, while its counterpart, high-density lipoprotein (HDL) has been identified as an anti-atherogenic factor.

Routine lipid screening of children at age 3 years remains controversial. The National Cholesterol Education Program recommends selective screening in children with high-risk family members, defined as a parent with total cholesterol greater than 240 mg/dL or a parent or grandparent with early-onset cardiovascular disease. When children have LDL levels greater than 130 mg/dL on two successive tests, dietary lifestyle counseling is appropriate. Dietary modification may decrease cholesterol levels by 5%–20%. If the patient is unresponsive to diet change and at extreme risk (eg, LDL > 160 mg/dL, HDL < 35 mg/dL, and a history of cardiovascular disease in a first-degree relative at an age < 40 years), drug therapy may be indicated. Cholestyramine, a bile acid–binding resin, is rarely used today due to poor adherence. The 3-hydroxy-3-methylglutaryl coenzyme A (HMG-CoA) reductase inhibitors (statins) are more commonly used in the pediatric population. Niacin is useful for treatment of hypertriglyceridemia.

Daniels SR et al: Expert panel on integrated guidelines for cardiovascular health and risk reduction in children and adolescents: summary report. Pediatrics 2011 Dec;128 Suppl 5:S21356 [PMID: 22084329].

▼ CHEST PAIN

ESSENTIALS OF DIAGNOSIS & TYPICAL FEATURES

▶ Location, severity, intensity, and modulating factors will help with diagnosis.

▶ Often musculoskeletal or reflux in origin.

▶ Chest pain on exertion likely cardiac in origin.

Overview

Chest pain is a common pediatric complaint, accounting for 3–6 in 1000 visits to urban emergency departments and urgent care clinics, with median age of 12–13 years and a male predominance (1–1.6:1). Although children with chest pain are commonly referred for cardiac evaluation, chest pain in children is uncommonly cardiac in origin, with a cardiac etiology found in only 2–5% of emergency department visits and 3–7% of cardiology clinic visits. Detailed history and physical examination should guide the pediatrician to the appropriate workup of chest pain. The location, duration, intensity, frequency, and radiation of the pain should be documented, as well as associated symptoms and any possible worsening or alleviating factors. The presence of triggering events preceding the pain should be explored. Chest pain during or immediately following exertion should lead to a more elaborate evaluation for a cardiac disorder. Associated symptoms should be evaluated, including syncope, palpitations, nausea/vomiting, shortness of breath, cough, or wheezing. Relation of pain to meals should be investigated. Detailed social history may reveal psychosocial stressors or exposures such as smoking or drug abuse. On physical examination, attention must be placed on the following: vital signs; general appearance of the child; the chest wall morphology and musculature; cardiac, pulmonary, and abdominal examination findings; and quality of peripheral pulses. If the pain can be reproduced through direct palpation of the chest wall, it is almost always musculoskeletal in origin.

Etiology

Chest pain is typically noncardiac and may be due to a multitude of conditions. Most commonly, no identifiable cause is found (idiopathic chest pain), despite sometimes extensive evaluations. Musculoskeletal etiologies are the most common identifiable cause of chest pain and include costochondritis, muscular strain, skeletal abnormality, and trauma, among others. Costochondritis (or Tietze syndrome) accounts for 26–41% of chest pain cases, is caused by inflammation of the costochondral joints, and is reproducible on examination. Respiratory causes include reactive airway disease, pneumonia, pleuritis, and pneumothorax. Gastrointestinal causes of chest pain include reflux, esophagitis, gastritis, foreign-body ingestion, hiatal hernia, cholecystitis, and referred abdominal pain. Hematology-oncology conditions include pulmonary embolism, sickle cell anemia, and tumors. Psychological conditions are more common in adolescents than younger children and include stress, anxiety, panic attacks, somatoform disorder, and depression.

Cardiac disease is itself an infrequent cause of chest pain; however, if misdiagnosed, it may be life threatening. Although myocardial infarction very rarely occurs in children, it is possible. Often, it is related to substance abuse and/or coronary vasospasm. Abnormal origins of the coronary arteries can be associated with chest pain and SCD. Coronary arteries may arise from the wrong sinus of Valsalva in the aortic root, with a slit-like orifice and narrowed, intramural course within the wall of the aorta. They may also arise from another coronary artery with a course that traverses between the aorta and pulmonary artery, which can limit flow during exercise. Even in the setting of normal coronary artery origins, particular medical conditions can put one at increased risk for myocardial infarction. A history of KD with coronary artery involvement puts one at risk for future myocardial infarction secondary to thrombosis of coronary aneurysms. Arrhythmias can also elicit chest pain, and young children may simply describe the palpitations associated with an arrhythmia as chest pain. Arrhythmias that can be associated with chest pain include the following: supraventricular tachycardia (SVT), including atrioventricular reentrant tachycardia (AVRT), atrioventricular nodal reentrant tachycardia (AVNRT), atrial flutter, and ectopic atrial tachycardia; ventricular tachycardia; complete heart block; or simple ectopy, including PACs or PVCs. Structural lesions that can cause chest pain include LV outflow tract obstruction, including aortic stenosis, and pulmonary stenosis. Other cardiac conditions that can cause chest pain include DCM, myocarditis, pericarditis, rheumatic carditis, and aortic dissection.

Evaluation

In most cases, sophisticated testing is not required. However, if a cardiac origin is suspected, a pediatric cardiologist should be consulted. Evaluation in these instances may include an ECG, chest radiograph, echocardiogram, Holter or transient arrhythmia monitor, or serum troponin levels if there are known risk factors for ischemia. In a 10-year study of

3700 patients evaluated in a pediatric cardiology clinic, only 1% of patients were found to have a cardiac etiology to their chest pain; the vast majority of these patients had suggestive symptoms (eg, exertional chest pain), concerning family/medical history, abnormal examination, or abnormal ECG. Forty percent of patients underwent echocardiography; incidental cardiac findings (unrelated to chest pain) were found in 4% of all patients and a positive finding potentially related to the complaint of chest pain was found in only 0.3% of patients. Rhythm monitors were positive in only 0.4% of patients, most of whom had complaints of palpitations. Exercise stress test was not additive to making a diagnosis. There were no SCDs in any of the 3700 patients who presented with chest pain; children were more likely to die from suicide, confirming that depression and anxiety are potential serious causes of chest pain.

Friedman KG et al: Management of pediatric chest pain using a standardized assessment and management plan. Pediatrics 2011 Aug;128(2):239–245. doi: 10.1542/peds.2011-0141 [PMID: 21746719].

Mahle WT, Campbell RM, Favaloro-Sabatier J: Myocardial infarction in adolescents. J Pediatr 2007 Aug;151(2):150–154. doi: 10.1016/j.jpeds.2007.02.045 [PMID: 17643766].

Saleeb SF, Li WY, Warren SZ, Lock JE: Effectiveness of screening for life-threatening chest pain in children. Pediatrics 2011 Nov;128(5):e1062–e1068. doi: 10.1542/peds.2011-0408. [PMID: 21987702].

Thull-Freedman J: Evaluation of chest pain in the pediatric patient. Med Clin North Am 2010 Mar;94(2):327–347. doi: 10.1016/j.mcna.2010.01.004 [PMID: 20380959].

▼ CARDIAC TRANSPLANTATION

Cardiac transplantation is an effective therapeutic modality for infants and children with end-stage cardiac disease. Indications for transplantation include (1) progressive HF despite maximal medical therapy, (2) complex congenital heart diseases that are not amenable to surgical repair or palliation, or in instances in which the surgical palliative approach has an equal or higher risk of mortality compared with transplantation, and (3) malignant arrhythmias unresponsive to medical therapy, catheter ablation, or automatic implantable cardiodefibrillator. Approximately 300–400 pediatric cardiac transplant procedures are performed annually in the United States. Infant (< 1 year of age) transplants account for 30% of pediatric cardiac transplants. The current estimated graft half-life for children undergoing cardiac transplantation in infancy is over 19 years, while overall pediatric heart transplant graft half-life is approximately 14 years.

Careful evaluation of the recipient and the donor is performed prior to cardiac transplantation. Assessment of the recipient's PVR is critical, as irreversible and severe PH is a risk factor for posttransplant right HF and early death. End-organ function of the recipient may also influence posttransplant outcome and should be evaluated. Donor-related factors that can have an impact on outcome include cardiac function, amount of inotropic support needed, active infection (HIV and hepatitis B and C are contraindications to donation), donor size, and ischemic time to transplantation.

Immunosuppression

The ideal posttransplant immunosuppressive regimen allows the immune system to continue to recognize and respond to foreign antigens in a productive manner while avoiding graft rejection. Although there are many different regimens, calcineurin inhibitors (eg, cyclosporine and tacrolimus) remain the mainstay of maintenance immunosuppression in pediatric heart transplantation. Calcineurin inhibitors may be used in isolation in children considered to be at low risk for graft rejection. Double-drug therapy includes the addition of antimetabolite or antiproliferative medications such as azathioprine, mycophenolate mofetil, or sirolimus. Because of the significant adverse side effects of corticosteroids in children, chronic steroid use is avoided if possible. Growth retardation, susceptibility to infection, impaired wound healing, hypertension, diabetes, osteoporosis, and a cushingoid appearance are some of the consequences of long-term steroid use.

Graft Rejection

Despite advances in immunosuppression, graft rejection remains the leading cause of death in the first 3 years after transplantation. Because graft rejection can present in the absence of clinical symptomatology, monitoring for and diagnosing rejection in a timely fashion can be difficult. Screening regimens include serial physical examinations, ECG, echocardiography, and cardiac catheterization with endomyocardial biopsy.

▶ Rejection Surveillance

A. Symptoms and Signs

Acute graft rejection may not cause symptoms in the early stages. With progression, patients may develop tachycardia, tachypnea, rales, a gallop rhythm, or hepatosplenomegaly. Infants and young children may present with irritability, poor feeding, vomiting, or lethargy. There is 50% mortality within 1 year for those suffering an episode of rejection associated with hemodynamic compromise, so early detection is critical.

B. Imaging

In an actively rejecting patient, chest radiographs may show cardiomegaly, pulmonary edema, or pleural effusions.

C. Electrocardiography

Abnormalities in conduction, reduced QRS voltages, and atrial and ventricular arrhythmias can occur in rejection.

D. Echocardiography

Echocardiography is a useful noninvasive rejection surveillance tool. Changes in ventricular compliance and function may initially be subtle but are progressive with increasing duration of the rejection episode. A new pericardial effusion or worsening valvular insufficiency may also indicate rejection.

E. Cardiac Catheterization and Endomyocardial Biopsy

Hemodynamic assessment including ventricular filling pressures, cardiac output, and oxygen consumption can be obtained via cardiac catheterization. The endomyocardial biopsy is useful in diagnosing acute graft rejection but not all episodes of symptomatic rejection result in a positive biopsy result. The appearance of infiltrating lymphocytes with myocellular damage on the biopsy is the hallmark of cell-mediated graft rejection and is helpful if present.

▶ Treatment of Graft Rejection

The goal of graft rejection treatment is to reverse the immunologic inflammatory cascade. High-dose corticosteroids are the first line of treatment. Frequently additional therapy with antithymocyte biologic preparations such as antithymocyte globulin (a rabbit-based polyclonal antibody) is needed to reverse rejection. Most rejection episodes can be treated effectively if diagnosed promptly. Usually graft function returns to its baseline state, although severe rejection episodes can result in chronic graft failure, graft loss, and patient death even with optimal therapy. Antibody-mediated rejection is another form of acute rejection that is treated in a similar fashion as T-cell–mediated rejection, but the addition of plasmapheresis and IVIG to the treatment regimen may improve outcomes. The diagnosis of antibody-mediated rejection is complicated but is based on a combination of clinical symptoms, evidence of complement deposition on endomyocardial biopsy, and new or increasing antibody production (typically anti-human lymphocyte antigen [HLA] antibodies) in the circulation.

▶ Course & Prognosis

The quality of life of pediatric heart transplant recipients is usually quite good. The risk of infection is low after the immediate posttransplant period in spite of chronic immunosuppression. Cytomegalovirus is the most common pathogen responsible for infection-related morbidity and mortality in heart transplant recipients. Most children tolerate environmental pathogens well. Nonadherence with lifetime immunosuppression is of great concern especially in adolescent patients. Several recent studies have identified nonadherence as the leading cause of late death. Posttransplant lymphoproliferative disorder, a syndrome related to Epstein-Barr virus infection, can result in a Burkitt-like lymphoma that usually responds to a reduction in immunosuppression but occasionally must be treated with chemotherapy and can be fatal. The overwhelming majority of children are not physically limited and do not require restrictions related to the cardiovascular system.

The most common cause of late graft loss is cardiac allograft vasculopathy (transplant coronary artery disease). Cardiac allograft vasculopathy results from intimal proliferation within the lumen of the coronary arteries that can ultimately result in complete luminal occlusion. These lesions are diffuse and often involve distal vessels, and thus are usually not amenable to bypass grafting, angioplasty, or stent placement. The etiology of these lesions has an immune basis, but the specifics are not known making targeted therapy challenging. Newer, more specific, and more effective immunosuppressive agents are currently being tried in clinical studies or are being evaluated in preclinical studies, making the future promising for children after cardiac transplantation.

▼ QUALITY IMPROVEMENT FOR PEDIATRIC HEART TRANSPLANTATION

The Pediatric Heart Transplant Study (PHTS) group is a consortium of over 40 pediatric heart transplant centers in North America and Europe that maintains an event-driven database that is used to support research aimed at improving treatment options and outcomes for children in need of a heart transplant or who have had a transplant. Each participating center receives an annual report that details center-specific outcomes compared to the collaborative group as a whole. This report is utilized for internal quality assurance purposes and as a performance benchmark.

Canter CE et al: Indications for heart transplantation in pediatric heart disease: a scientific statement from the American Heart Association Council on Cardiovascular Disease in the Young; the Councils on Clinical Cardiology, Cardiovascular Nursing, and Cardiovascular Surgery and Anesthesia; and the Quality of Care and Outcomes Research Interdisciplinary Working Group. Circulation 2007 Feb 6;115(5):658–676 [PMID: 17261651].

International Society for Heart and Lung Transplant Registry Slides: http://www.ishlt.org/registries/slides.asp?slides=heartLungRegistryPHTSwebsite:http://www.uab.edu/phts/.

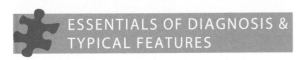

PULMONARY HYPERTENSION

ESSENTIALS OF DIAGNOSIS & TYPICAL FEATURES

► Often subtle with symptoms of dyspnea, fatigue, chest pain, and syncope.

► Loud pulmonary component of S_2; ECG with RVH.

► Rare, progressive, and often fatal disease without treatment.

▶ General Considerations

Pulmonary hypertension (PH) is defined as an increase in mean PAP 25 mm Hg or greater. The etiology of PH in children is very different from adults, with a predominance of idiopathic pulmonary arterial hypertension (IPAH) and pulmonary arterial hypertension (PAH) associated with congenital heart disease. PAH, a subset of PH, affects the pulmonary arterial tree and is defined as a sustained mean PAP 25 mm Hg or greater with a mean pulmonary capillary wedge pressure 15 mm Hg or less and PVR more than 3 Wood units. A diagnostic classification has been developed and modified at the World Symposium on Pulmonary Hypertension (WSPH). This clinical classification system identifies five categories of disorders that cause PH, with each group sharing similar hemodynamic, pathologic, and management features: PAH (group 1); PH due to left heart disease (group 2); PH due to chronic lung disease and/or hypoxia (group 3); chronic thromboembolic PH (group 4); and PH due to multifactorial mechanisms (group 5). The incidence of IPAH and PAH associated with congenital heart disease is 1–2 persons per million. PH is difficult to diagnose in the early stages because of its subtle manifestations. Although the outcome for pediatric PH is improving due to the advent of new therapies, prognosis remains guarded, with only 74% survival at 5 years. Familial PH occurs in 6%–12% of affected individuals. When a clear familial association is known, the disease shows evidence of genetic anticipation, presenting at younger ages in subsequent generations.

▶ Clinical Findings

A. Symptoms and Signs

The clinical picture varies with the severity of PH, and usually early symptoms are subtle, delaying the diagnosis. Initial symptoms may be dyspnea, palpitations, or chest pain, often brought on by strenuous exercise or competitive sports. Syncope may be the first symptom, which usually implies severe disease. As the disease progresses, patients have signs of low cardiac output and right HF. Right HF may be manifested by hepatomegaly, peripheral edema, and an S_3 gallop on examination. Murmurs of pulmonary regurgitation and tricuspid regurgitation may be present, and the pulmonary component of S_2 is usually pronounced.

B. Imaging

The chest radiograph most often reveals a prominent main pulmonary artery, and the RV may be enlarged. The peripheral pulmonary vascular markings may be normal or diminished. However, in 6% of patients with confirmed PH, the chest radiograph is normal.

C. Electrocardiography

The ECG usually shows RVH with an upright T wave in V_1 (when it should be negative in young children) or a qR complex in lead V_1 or V_{3R}. Also present may be evidence of right-axis deviation and right atrial enlargement.

D. Echocardiography

The echocardiogram is an essential tool for excluding congenital heart disease as a cause of PH. It frequently shows RVH and dilation. In the absence of other structural disease, tricuspid and PI velocity can be used to estimate pulmonary artery systolic and diastolic pressures, respectively. Other echocardiographic measures such as tissue Doppler imaging, myocardial performance index, systolic-to-diastolic ratio from tricuspid regurgitation velocity, RV-to-LV ratio in end systole, and tricuspid annular plane systolic excursion are used in the evaluation of PH.

E. Cardiac Catheterization and Angiocardiography

Cardiac catheterization is the best method for determining the severity of disease. The procedure is performed to rule out cardiac (eg, restrictive cardiomyopathy) or vascular (eg, pulmonary vein stenosis) causes of PH, determine the severity of disease, and define treatment strategies. The reactivity of the pulmonary vascular bed to short-acting vasodilator agents (oxygen, nitric oxide, or prostacyclin) can be assessed and used to determine treatment options. Angiography may show a decrease in the number of small pulmonary arteries with tortuous vessels.

F. Other Evaluation Modalities

Cardiac MRI is used in some patients to evaluate RV function, pulmonary artery anatomy, and hemodynamics, as well as thromboembolic phenomena. Cardiopulmonary exercise testing using cycle ergometry correlates with disease severity. More simply, a 6-minute walk test, in which distance walked and perceived level of exertion are measured, has a strong independent association with mortality in late disease.

Treatment

The goal of therapy is to reduce PAP, increase cardiac output, and improve quality of life. Cardiac catheterization data are used to determine the proper treatment. Patients responsive to pulmonary vasodilators are given calcium channel blockers such as nifedipine or diltiazem. Patients unresponsive to vasodilators initially receive one of three classes of drugs: prostanoids (such as epoprostenol), endothelin receptor antagonists (such as bosentan), or phosphodiesterase-5 inhibitors (such as tadalafil). All of these agents have distinct mechanisms of action that can reduce PVR. Warfarin is commonly used for anticoagulation to prevent thromboembolic events, usually with a goal to maintain the INR between 1.5 and 2.0.

Atrial septostomy is indicated in some patients with refractory PH and symptoms. Cardiac output falls as PVR rises, so an interatrial shunt can preserve left heart output, albeit with deoxygenated blood. Lung transplantation should be considered in patients with intractable PH and in those with associated anatomic lesions that contribute to high pulmonary arterial pressure, like pulmonary vein stenosis. Heart-lung transplant procedures appear to have survival benefits over isolated lung transplantation in patients with PH. Recurrence of PH is rare after heart-lung transplant.

Abman SH et al: Pediatric pulmonary hypertension: guidelines from the American Heart Association and American Thoracic Society. Circulation 2015 Nov 24;132(21):2037–2099. 10.1161/CIR.0000000000000329 [PMID: 26534956].

Ivy DD et al: Pediatric pulmonary hypertension. J Am Coll Cardiol 2013 Dec 24;62(25 Suppl):D11276 [PMID: 24355636].

Pulmonary Hypertension Association: www.phassociation.org/.

▼ DISORDERS OF RATE & RHYTHM

Cardiac rhythm abnormalities can occur in two different patient populations: (1) healthy children with structurally normal hearts who have an intrinsic abnormality of the electrical conduction system; and (2) children with congenital heart disease who are at risk for a cardiac rhythm abnormalities based on the underlying heart defect itself. In the latter population, changes in cardiac muscle cells associated with a chronic state of altered cardiac hemodynamics and any operative procedures with surgical suture lines/scars place the patients at higher risk for certain types of arrhythmias.

The evaluation and treatment of cardiac rhythm disorders have advanced significantly over the last several decades. Arguably, the most significant advancements in the last few years have continued in the area of the genetic basis of rhythm disorders such as long QT syndrome (LQTS) that is discussed at the end of this chapter. Treatment for cardiac rhythm abnormalities includes clinical monitoring with no intervention, antiarrhythmic medications, invasive electrophysiology study and ablation procedures, pacemakers, and internal cardioverter/defibrillators.

Deal BJ et al: Arrhythmic complications associated with the treatment of patients with congenital cardiac disease: consensus definitions from the Multi-Societal Database Committee for Pediatric and Congenital Heart Disease. Cardiol Young 2008 Dec; 18(Suppl 2):202–205.

DISORDERS OF THE SINUS NODE

Sinus Arrhythmia

Phasic variation in the heart rate (sinus arrhythmia) is normal. Typically, the sinus rate varies with the respiratory cycle (heart rate increases with inspiration and decreases with expiration), whereas P-QRS-T intervals remain stable. Sinus arrhythmia may occur in association with respiratory distress or increased intracranial pressure, or it may be present in normal children. In isolation, it never requires treatment; however, it may be associated with sinus node dysfunction or autonomic nervous system dysfunction.

Sinus Bradycardia

Sinus bradycardia is defined as a heart rate below the normal limit for age (neonates to 6 years, 60 beats/min; 7–11 years, 45 beats/min; > 12 years, 40 beats/min). Sinus bradycardia is often seen in athletic children. Causes of sinus bradycardia include hypoxia, central nervous system damage, eating disorders, and medication side effects. Symptomatic bradycardia (syncope, low cardiac output, or exercise intolerance) requires treatment (atropine, isoproterenol, or cardiac pacing).

Sinus Tachycardia

The heart rate normally accelerates in response to stress such as exercise, anxiety, fever, hypovolemia, anemia, or HF. Although sinus tachycardia in the normal heart is well tolerated, symptomatic tachycardia with decreased cardiac output warrants evaluation for structural heart disease, cardiomyopathy or true tachyarrhythmias. The first evaluation should be made with a 12-lead ECG to determine the precise mechanism of the rapid rate. Treatment may be indicated for correction of the underlying cause of sinus tachycardia (eg, transfusion for anemia or correction of hypovolemia or fever).

Sinus Node Dysfunction

Sinus node dysfunction is a clinical syndrome of inappropriate sinus nodal function and rate. The abnormality may be a true anatomic defect of the sinus node or its surrounding tissue, or it may be an abnormality of autonomic input. It is defined as one or more of the following: severe sinus bradycardia, sinus pause or arrest, chronotropic incompetence (inability of the heart rate to increase with activity or other demands), or combined bradyarrhythmias and tachyarrhythmias. It is a common late finding after repair of congenital heart disease (most commonly the Mustard or Senning repair for complete TGA or the Fontan procedure), but it is also seen in normal hearts, in unoperated congenital heart disease, and in acquired heart diseases. Symptoms usually manifest between ages 2 and 17 years and consist of episodes of presyncope, syncope, palpitations, pallor, or exercise intolerance.

The evaluation of sinus node dysfunction may involve the following: baseline ECG, 24-hour ambulatory ECG monitoring, exercise stress test, and transient event monitoring. Treatment for sinus node dysfunction is indicated only in symptomatic patients. Bradyarrhythmias are treated with vagolytic (atropine or glycopyrrolate) or adrenergic (aminophylline) agents or permanent cardiac pacemakers.

PREMATURE BEATS

Atrial Premature Beats

Atrial premature beats are triggered by an ectopic focus in the atrium. They are one of the most common premature beats occurring in pediatric patients, particularly during the fetal and newborn periods. The premature beat may be conducted to the ventricle and therefore followed by a QRS complex, or it may be nonconducted, as the beat has occurred so early that the AV node is still refractory (Figure 20–4). A brief pause usually occurs until the next normal sinus beat occurs. As an isolated finding, atrial premature beats are benign and require no treatment.

Junctional Premature Beats

Junctional premature beats arise in the AV node or the bundle of His. They induce a normal QRS complex with no preceding P wave. Junctional premature beats are usually benign and require no specific therapy.

Ventricular Premature Beats

Ventricular premature beats or premature ventricular contractions (PVCs) are relatively common, occurring in 1%–2% of patients with normal hearts. They are characterized by an early beat with a wide QRS complex, without a preceding P wave, and with a full compensatory pause following this early beat (Figure 20–5).

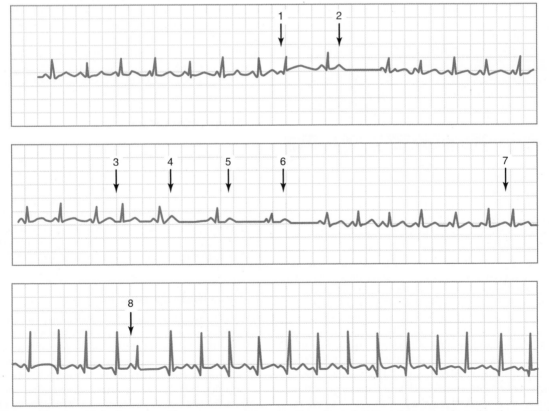

▲ **Figure 20–4.** Lead II rhythm strip with premature atrial contractions. Beats 1, 3, 7, and 8 are conducted to the ventricles, whereas beats 2, 4, 5, and 6 are not.

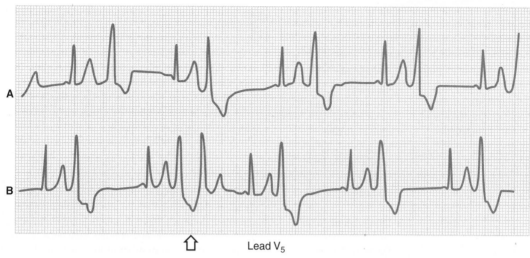

Lead V$_5$

▲ **Figure 20–5.** Lead V$_5$ rhythm strip with unifocal premature ventricular contractions in a bigeminy pattern. The arrow shows a ventricular couplet.

Ventricular premature beats originating from a single ectopic focus all have the same configuration, while those of multifocal origin show varying configurations. The consecutive occurrence of two PVCs is referred to as a ventricular couplet and of three or more as ventricular tachycardia. Most PVCs in otherwise normal patients are usually benign. However, patients with frequent PVCs are usually evaluated with tests such as a 24-hour ambulatory ECG or with exercise testing to rule out concerning arrhythmias. An echocardiogram may be performed to evaluate ventricular function. Frequent PVCs may result in decreased ventricular function, a phenomenon known as PVC-induced cardiomyopathy. The exact frequency of PVCs necessary to cause a cardiomyopathy is incompletely understood but is most commonly greater than 20% of the total daily beats. The significance of PVCs can also be evaluated by having the patient exercise. As the heart rate increases, benign PVCs usually disappear. If exercise results in an increase or coupling of contractions, underlying disease may be present. Multifocal PVCs are always abnormal and may be more dangerous. They may be associated with drug overdose (tricyclic antidepressants or digoxin toxicity), electrolyte imbalance, myocarditis, or hypoxia. Treatment is directed at correcting the underlying disorder.

SUPRAVENTRICULAR TACHYCARDIA

Supraventricular tachycardia (SVT) is a term used to describe any rapid rhythm originating from the atrium, the AV node, or an accessory pathway. These tachycardias are rapid, narrow complex tachycardias. The mode of presentation depends on the heart rate, the presence of underlying

cardiac structural or functional abnormalities, coexisting illness, and patient age. An otherwise healthy child with SVT may complain of intermittent periods of rapid heartbeat. An infant with SVT may have poor feeding and increased fatigue (manifesting as less awake time). Incessant tachycardia, even if fairly slow (120–150 beats/min), may cause myocardial dysfunction and HF if left untreated. In children with preexisting HF or an underlying systemic disease such as anemia or sepsis, SVT may result in decreased heart function and further signs of hemodynamic instability much more rapidly than in a healthy child.

The mechanisms of tachycardia are generally divided into reentrant and automatic mechanisms and can be described by the location of tachycardia origination (Table 20–17).

Reentrant tachycardias represent approximately 80% of pediatric arrhythmias. Reentrant tachycardias have the following characteristics: they initiate abruptly, they have a fixed rate, they have little variation with fever or internal catecholamines, and they terminate abruptly. They can be terminated to sinus rhythm with maneuvers such as vagal maneuvers, administration of adenosine, pacing maneuvers, or DC cardioversion.

Reentrant tachycardia mechanisms involve two connections where electrical conduction travels down one of the pathways and then backs up the other, creating a sustained repetitive circular loop. The circuit can be confined to the atrium (*atrial flutter* in a normal heart or *intra-atrial reentrant tachycardia* in a patient with congenital heart disease) (Figure 20–6). It may be confined within the AV node (*AV nodal reentrant tachycardia*), or it may encompass an accessory connection between atria and ventricle (*accessory pathway–mediated tachycardia*). If, during tachycardia, the

Table 20–17. Mechanism of supraventricular tachycardia.

Site of Origination	Automatic Mechanisms	Reentrant Mechanisms
Sinus node	Sinus tachycardia	Sinoatrial node reentry
Atrium	Ectopic atrial tachycardia Multifocal atrial tachycardia	Atrial flutter Intra-atrial reentrant tachycardia Atrial fibrillation
Atrioventricular node	Junctional ectopic tachycardia	Atrioventricular nodal reentrant tachycardia (AVNRT)
Accessory pathways		Concealed accessory pathways Wolff-Parkinson-White (WPW) syndrome Permanent form of junctional reciprocating tachycardia (PJRT) Mahaim fiber tachycardia

electrical impulse travels antegrade (from atria to ventricles) through the AV node and retrograde (from ventricle to atria) back up the accessory pathway, orthodromic reciprocating tachycardia is present. If, instead, the impulse travels antegrade through the accessory pathway and retrograde up through the AV node, antidromic reciprocating tachycardia is present. This latter tachycardia would present as a wide complex tachycardia. *Wolff-Parkinson-White* (WPW) *syndrome* is a subclass of reentrant tachycardia in which, during sinus rhythm, the impulse travels antegrade down the accessory connection, bypassing the AV node and creating ventricular preexcitation (early eccentric activation of the ventricle with a short PR interval and slurred upstroke of the QRS, a delta wave) (Figure 20–7). Most patients with WPW have otherwise structurally normal hearts. However, WPW

has been noted to occur with increased frequency in association with the following congenital cardiac lesions: tricuspid atresia, Ebstein anomaly of the tricuspid valve, HCM, and ccTGA. Different than other causes of tachycardias described above where the arrhythmia is not life threatening, there have been rare cases of sudden collapse from WPW syndrome. The mechanism of this sudden event is the development of atrial fibrillation, conducting down a rapid accessory pathway to the ventricle leading to ventricular fibrillation and sudden death. For this reason, most centers recommend that even asymptomatic patients undergo an invasive procedure to assess the conduction properties of the WPW accessory pathway (described under treatment for tachyarrhythmias).

Improved surgical survival for patients with congenital heart disease has created a new, increasingly prevalent, chronic arrhythmia that is similar to atrial flutter in a normal heart structure. These arrhythmias have been referred to by many names: intra-atrial reentrant tachycardia, incisional tachycardia, macroreentry, or postoperative atrial flutter. In this tachycardia, electrically isolated corridors of atrial myocardium (eg, the tricuspid valve–IVC isthmus, or the region between an atrial incision and the crista terminalis) act as pathways for sustained reentrant circuits of electrical activity. These tachycardias are chronic, medically refractory, and clinically incapacitating.

The *automatic tachycardias* represent approximately 20% of childhood arrhythmias. The characteristics of automatic arrhythmias include gradual onset, rate variability, variations in rate with fever or increasing internal catecholamines, and gradual offset. Maneuvers such as vagal maneuvers, adenosine, and attempt pacing can alter the rhythm temporarily, but they do not result in termination of the rhythm to sinus rhythm as would be seen in the reentrant tachycardias. Automatic tachycardias can be episodic or incessant. They are usually under autonomic influence. When they are incessant, they are usually associated with HF and a clinical picture of DCM. Automatic tachycardias are created when a focus of cardiac tissue develops an abnormally

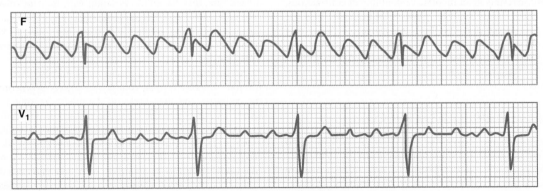

▲ **Figure 20–6.** Leads aVF (F) and V$_1$ showing atrial flutter with "sawtooth" atrial flutter waves.

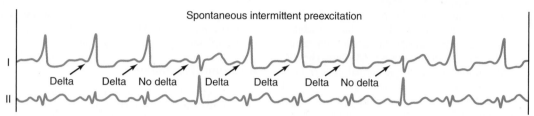

Spontaneous intermittent preexcitation

▲ **Figure 20–7.** Leads I and II with spontaneous intermittent ventricular preexcitation (Wolff-Parkinson-White syndrome).

fast spontaneous rate of depolarization. For ectopic atrial tachycardia, the ECG demonstrates a normal QRS complex preceded by an abnormal P wave (Figure 20–8). Junctional ectopic tachycardia does not have a P wave preceding the QRS waves and may be associated with AV dissociation or 1:1 retrograde conduction.

Cohen MI et al: PACES/HRS expert consensus statement on the management of the asymptomatic young patient with a Wolff-Parkinson-White (WPW, ventricular preexcitation) electro-cardiographic pattern: developed in partnership between the Pediatric and Congenital Electrophysiology Society (PACES) and the Heart Rhythm Society (HRS). Heart Rhythm 2012;9(6): 1006–1024 [PMID: 22579340].

► **Clinical Findings**

A. Symptoms and Signs

Presentation varies with age. Infants tend to turn pale and mottled with onset of tachycardia and may become irritable.

With long duration of tachycardia, symptoms of HF develop. Older children complain of dizziness, palpitations, fatigue, and chest pain. Heart rates range from 240–300 beats/min in the younger child to 150–180 beats/min in the teenager. HF is less common in children than in infants. Tachycardia may be associated with either congenital heart defects or acquired conditions such as cardiomyopathies and myocarditis.

B. Imaging

Chest radiographs are normal during the early course of tachycardia and therefore are usually not obtained. If HF is present, the heart is enlarged and pulmonary venous congestion is evident.

C. Electrocardiography

ECG is the most important tool in the diagnosis of SVT and to define the precise tachycardia mechanism. Findings include a heart rate that is rapid and out of proportion to the patient's physical status (eg, a rate of 140 beats/min with an abnormal

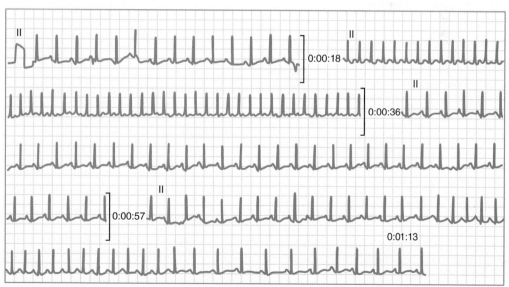

▲ **Figure 20–8.** Lead II rhythm strip of ectopic atrial tachycardia. The tracing demonstrates a variable rate with a maximum of 260 beats/min, an abnormal P wave, and a gradual termination.

P wave while quiet and asleep). For reentrant mechanisms, the rhythm would be extremely regular with little variability. For automatic mechanisms, the rhythm would be irregular with a gradual increasing and decreasing of the rate. The QRS complex is usually the same as during normal sinus rhythm. However, the QRS complex is occasionally widened (SVT with aberrant ventricular conduction), in which case the condition may be difficult to differentiate from ventricular tachycardia. The presence of P waves and their association with the QRS are important in determining tachycardia mechanism. With automatic tachycardias, there is often a 1:1 or 2:1 A:V relationship with P waves preceding the QRS. With reentrant tachycardias, such as accessory pathway–mediated tachycardias, a small retrograde P wave can often be seen just after the QRS. With AVNRT, P waves cannot be identified as they are occurring at the same time as the QRS.

▶ Treatment

A. Acute Treatment

During the initial episodes of SVT, patients require close monitoring. Correction of acidosis and electrolyte abnormalities is also indicated. The following acute treatments are effective in terminating tachycardia only for patients with reentrant SVT. Acute treatment for automatic SVT is aimed at rate control, usually with a β-blocker.

1. Vagal maneuvers—The "diving reflex" produced by placing an ice bag on the nasal bridge for 20 seconds (for infants) will increase parasympathetic tone and terminate some tachycardias. The Valsalva maneuver, which can be performed by older compliant children, may also terminate reentrant tachycardias.

2. Adenosine—Adenosine transiently blocks AV conduction and terminates tachycardias that incorporate the AV node or may aid in the diagnosis of arrhythmias confined to the atrium by causing a pause in ventricular conduction, so one can identify the presence of multiple P waves. The dose is 0.1–0.2 mg/kg by rapid intravenous bolus. It is antagonized by aminophylline and should be used with caution in patients with sinus node dysfunction or asthma. Patient's status postorthotopic heart transplant should not be administered adenosine due to an exaggerated response that results in prolonged block of AV conduction.

3. Transesophageal atrial pacing—Atrial overdrive pacing and termination can be performed from a bipolar electrode-tipped catheter positioned in the esophagus adjacent to the left atrium. Overdrive pacing at rates approximately 30% faster than the tachycardia rate will interrupt a reentrant tachycardia circuit and restore sinus rhythm.

4. Direct current cardioversion—Direct current cardioversion (0.5–2 synchronized J/kg) should be used immediately when a patient presents in cardiovascular collapse. This will convert a reentrant mechanism to sinus. Automatic tachycardia will not respond to cardioversion.

B. Chronic Treatment

Once the patient has been diagnosed with SVT and the mechanism has been evaluated, then long-term treatment options can be considered. Options include monitoring clinically for tachycardia recurrences, medical management with antiarrhythmic medications, or an invasive electrophysiology study and ablation procedure. In infancy and early childhood, antiarrhythmic medications are the mainstay of therapy. Medications such as digoxin and β-blockers are the first-line therapies. Other antiarrhythmic medications (eg, verapamil, flecainide, propafenone, sotalol, and amiodarone) have increased pharmacologic actions and are extremely effective. However, these medications also have serious side effects, including induction of arrhythmias and sudden death, and should be used only under the direction of a pediatric cardiologist.

Tachycardias, both automatic and reentrant, can be more definitively addressed with an invasive electrophysiology study and ablation procedure. This is a nonsurgical transvascular catheter technique that desiccates an arrhythmia focus or accessory pathway and permanently cures an arrhythmia. The ablation catheters can utilize either a heat source (radiofrequency) or a cool source (cryoablation). The latter has been reported to be safer around the normal conduction pathway and thus decreases the risk of inadvertent AV block. The success rate from an ablation procedure in a patient with a normal heart structure is more than 90%, with a recurrence risk of less than 10%. The procedure can be performed in infants or adults. In patients less than 15 kg, the risks of procedural complications or failed ablation are potentially higher, and the procedure should be reserved for those whose arrhythmias are refractory to medical management. The high success rate, low complication and low recurrence rates, in addition to the elimination of the need for chronic antiarrhythmic medications have made ablation procedures the primary treatment option in most pediatric cardiovascular centers. In patients with congenital heart disease, electrophysiology study and ablation procedures are also utilized to address arrhythmia substrates. The success rate of these procedures is lower than in patients with a normal heart structure, often reported in the 75%–80% range.

▶ Prognosis

SVT in infants and children generally carries an excellent prognosis. It can be treated with medical management or with the potentially curative ablation procedures. There are, however, rare cases of incessant SVT leading to HF, and there is reported sudden collapse from atrial fibrillation in the presence of WPW. All patients with complaints of rapid heartbeats or other symptoms where there is a concern for tachyarrhythmia should be referred for evaluation.

Pflaumer A: Perspectives in ablation of arrhythmias in children and patients with congenital heart disease. Intern Med J 2012;42(Suppl 5):70–76 [PMID: 23035686].

VENTRICULAR TACHYCARDIA

Ventricular tachycardia is uncommon in childhood (Figure 20–9). It is usually associated with underlying abnormalities of the myocardium (myocarditis, cardiomyopathy, myocardial tumors, or postoperative congenital heart disease) or toxicity (hypoxia, electrolyte imbalance, or drug toxicity). On occasion, it can be secondary to a primary electrical abnormality in an otherwise normal heart. Sustained ventricular tachycardia can be an unstable situation, and if left untreated, it could degenerate into ventricular fibrillation and sudden collapse.

Ventricular tachycardia must be differentiated from accelerated idioventricular rhythm. The latter is a sustained ventricular tachycardia occurring in neonates with normal hearts, with a ventricular tachycardia rate within 10% of the preceding sinus rate. This is a self-limiting arrhythmia that requires no treatment. Because of the consequences of sustained ventricular tachycardia, however, a symptomatic patient with a wide complex tachycardia should be considered to have ventricular tachycardia (not an accelerated idioventricular rhythm) until proven otherwise.

Acute termination of ventricular tachycardia involves restoration of the normal myocardium when possible (correction of electrolyte imbalance, drug toxicity, etc) and direct current cardioversion (1–4 J/kg), cardioversion with lidocaine (1 mg/kg), or with amiodarone (5 mg/kg load).

Chronic suppression of ventricular arrhythmias with antiarrhythmic drugs has many side effects (including proarrhythmia and death), and it must be initiated in the hospital under the direction of a pediatric cardiologist. If the etiology of the tachycardia is a primary electrical abnormality, catheter ablation procedures can be offered in select patients as a potentially curative treatment option. Ablation for ventricular tachycardia in the pediatric population is much less commonly performed compared to ablation for SVT.

Hayashi M et al: Incidence and risk factors of arrhythmic events in catecholaminergic polymorphic ventricular tachycardia. Circulation 2009 May 12;119(18):2426–2434 [PMID: 9398665].
McCammond AN, Balaji S: Management of tachyarrhythmias in children. Curr Treat Options Cardiovasc Med 2012;14(5):490–502 [PMID: 22923097].

LONG QT SYNDROME

Long QT syndrome (LQTS) is a malignant disorder of cardiac conduction in which cardiac repolarization is prolonged (QTc measurement on ECG), predisposing the patient to sudden episodes of syncope, seizures, or sudden death (5% per year if untreated). The mechanism is a pause-dependent initiation of torsades de pointes, a multifocal ventricular tachycardia. It can be congenital or acquired. Congenital LQTS is inherited in an autosomal dominant (more common) or recessive pattern or it may occur spontaneously (less likely). The recessive inheritance pattern is associated with congenital deafness and the Jervell and Lange-Nielsen syndrome (bilateral sensorineural hearing loss and long QTc > 500 milliseconds resulting in torsades de pointes). Congenital LQTS is caused by a defect in one of several genes that code for potassium or sodium channels in cardiac

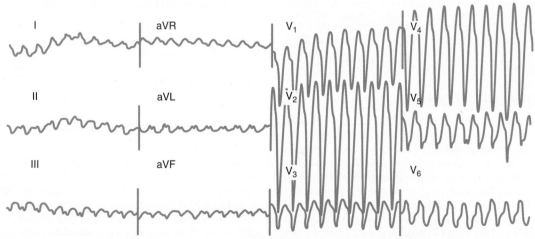

▲ **Figure 20–9.** Twelve-lead ECG from a child with imipramine toxicity and ventricular tachycardia.

myocytes. The gene mutations result in subtypes of LQTS that have differing presentations and associations. Overall risk and environmental conditions and activities associated with ventricular arrhythmias and SCD have been shown to be gene specific. The risk of SCD is greatest in those with LQT3 and occurs most commonly during exercise among patients with LQT1. Auditory and emotional stimuli are provocative in LQT2, with SCD occurring during sleep in LQT3. The genetic and phenotypic heterogeneity contributes to the difficulty in diagnosing and managing patients with congenital LQTS. The wide range of QTc values in both unaffected and affected individuals, as well as age related variation, also confounds the diagnosis. Although a QTc of greater than 460 milliseconds is a reasonable threshold, the majority of individuals in this range are not affected.

Evaluation includes an ECG that shows a long QTc measurement, 24-hour ambulatory ECG, and, possibly, an exercise test. There is a commercially available genetic test for the primary genes that cause LQTS. This test is most helpful in determining who in an affected family has LQTS. Unfortunately, this test cannot completely rule out LQTS due to a 25% false-negative rate.

The mainstay of treatment for LQTS has been exercise restriction, treatment with β-blockade, and, possibly, placement of an internal cardioverter/defibrillator. Within the next several years, more gene-specific therapies are anticipated.

LQTS resulting from altered ventricular repolarization can also be acquired secondary to myocardial toxins, ischemia, or inflammation. This condition also predisposes to ventricular arrhythmias. Numerous medications can also cause QT prolongation.

Ackerman MJ et al: HRS/EHRA expert consensus statement on the state of genetic testing for the channelopathies and cardiomyopathies this document was developed as a partnership between the Heart Rhythm Society (HRS) and the European Heart Rhythm Association (EHRA). Heart Rhythm 2011 Aug;8(8):1308–1339. doi: 10.1016/j.hrthm.2011.05.020 [PMID: 21787999].

Kirsh JA: Finding the proverbial "needle in a haystack": identifying presymptomatic individuals with long QT syndrome. Heart Rhythm 2013;10(2):239–240 [PMID: 23219703].

SUDDEN CARDIAC DEATH

Sudden cardiac death (SCD) can be defined as biologic death resulting from abrupt, unexpected cardiovascular collapse from which an individual does not recover or regain consciousness. The precise incidence of SCD in young persons is unknown, though an estimated 4000–8000 children in the United States die from SCD annually, compared to more than 300,000 older individuals. SCD in athletic, competitive young persons is rare, with the risk in a high school male athlete of less than 1 in 100,000 patient-years; the risk in female athletes is even lower. The causes of SCD vary

with age. In infants (≤ 1 year), approximately one-half of cases may have coronary anomalies, and in the other half, no structural cause is found. The latter group, described as having "sudden infant death syndrome" (SIDS), may have a genetic cardiac ion channel mutation, and up to one-third of SIDS cases are thought to be caused by congenital LQTS. Beyond infancy, in patients 21 years or younger, the most frequent causes are HCM, myocarditis, primary electrical disturbances, coronary artery abnormalities, and preexisting structural congenital heart disease.

As many of causes of SCD are genetic, it is necessary to investigate cases by conducting detailed family histories, looking for seizures, syncope, or early sudden death. Family members should be examined with an arrhythmia screen consisting of a physical examination, ECG, and echocardiography to detect arrhythmias or cardiomyopathies. Depending on the history, cardiac MRI, signal-averaged ECG, and genetic screening may be helpful.

Harmon KG et al: Incidence of sudden cardiac death in athletes: a state-of-the-art review. Heart 2014 Aug;100(16):122734 [PMID: 25049314].

Pilmer CM et al: Sudden cardiac death in children and adolescents between 1 and 19 years of age. Heart Rhythm 2014 Feb;11(2):23945 [PMID: 24239636].

DISORDERS OF ATRIOVENTRICULAR CONDUCTION

▶ General Considerations

The AV node is the electrical connection between the atrium and the ventricles. AV blocks involve a slowing or disruption of this connection and are described according to the degree of this slowing or disruption.

First-Degree Atrioventricular Block

First-degree AV block is an ECG diagnosis of prolongation of the PR interval. The block does not, in itself, cause problems. It may be associated with structural congenital heart defects, namely AV septal defects and ccTGA, and with diseases such as rheumatic carditis. The PR interval is prolonged in patients receiving digoxin therapy.

Second-Degree Atrioventricular Block

Mobitz type I (Wenckebach) AV block is recognized by progressive prolongation of the PR interval until there is no QRS following a P wave (Figure 20–10). Mobitz type I block occurs in normal hearts at rest and is usually benign. In Mobitz type II block, there is no progressive lengthening of the PR interval before the dropped beat (Figure 20–11). Mobitz type II block is frequently associated with organic heart disease, and a complete evaluation is necessary.

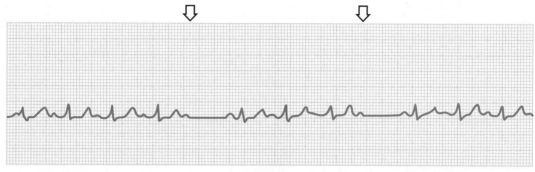

Lead I

▲ **Figure 20–10.** Lead I rhythm strip with Mobitz type I (Wenckebach) second-degree heart block. There is progressive lengthening of the PR interval prior to the nonconducted P wave (*arrows*).

Complete Atrioventricular Block

In complete AV block, the atria and ventricles beat independently. Ventricular rates can range from 40 to 80 beats/min, whereas atrial rates are faster (Figure 20–12). The most common form of complete AV block is congenital complete AV block that occurs in a fetus or infant with an otherwise normal heart. There is a very high association with maternal systemic lupus erythematosus antibodies, and therefore it is recommended to screen the mother of an affected infant even if the mother has no symptoms of collagen vascular disease. Congenital complete AV block is also associated with some forms of congenital heart disease (congenitally corrected transposition of the great vessels and AV septal defect). Acquired complete AV block may be secondary to acute myocarditis, drug toxicity, electrolyte imbalance, hypoxia, and cardiac surgery.

▶ Clinical Findings

The primary finding in infants and children with complete AV block is a significantly low heart rate for age. The diagnosis is often made prenatally when fetal bradycardia is documented. An ultrasound is then conducted as well as a fetal echocardiogram of the heart. With the fetal echocardiogram, atrial and ventricular contractions can be distinguished and the atrial rate is documented as being higher than the ventricular rate with no relationship to each other. If the heart rates are sufficiently low, there will be low cardiac output, decreased cardiac function, and the development of hydrops fetalis. Postnatal adaptation largely depends on the heart rate; infants with heart rates less than 55 beats/min are at significantly greater risk for low cardiac output, HF, and death. Wide QRS complexes and a rapid atrial rate are also poor prognostic signs. Most patients have an innocent flow murmur from increased stroke volume. In symptomatic patients, the heart can be quite enlarged, and pulmonary edema may be present.

Complete AV block can also occur in older patients. Patients may be asymptomatic or may present with presyncope, syncope, or fatigue. Complete cardiac evaluation, including ECG, echocardiography, and Holter monitoring, is necessary to assess the patient for ventricular dysfunction and to relate any symptoms to concurrent arrhythmias.

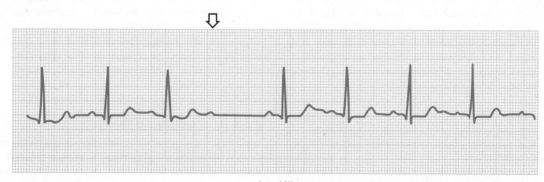

Lead III

▲ **Figure 20–11.** Lead III rhythm strip with Mobitz type II second-degree heart block. There is a consistent PR interval with occasional loss of AV conduction (*arrow*).

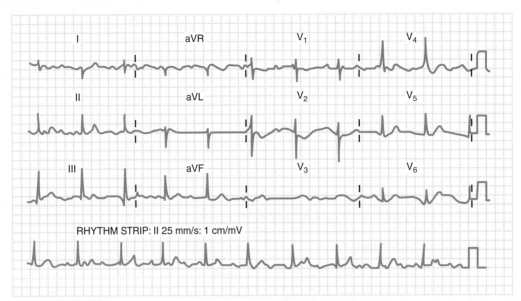

▲ **Figure 20–12.** Twelve-lead ECG and lead II rhythm strip of complete heart block. The atrial rate is 150 beats/min, and the ventricular rate is 60 beats/min.

Treatment

When diagnosis of complete AV block is made in a fetus, the treatment depends on gestational age, ventricular rate, and the presence or absence of hydrops. Some centers have advocated the administration of steroids, IVIG, and/or β-adrenergic stimulation treatment of the mother in some instances (fetuses that have associated HF). Emergent delivery is sometimes warranted. Postnatal treatment for neonates or older patients who present with significant symptoms and require immediate intervention includes temporary support by the infusions of isoproterenol, temporary transvenous pacing wires, or by temporary transcutaneous pacemakers if needed. The relationship of complete congenital AV block to auto-antibody production and cardiomyopathy is the basis for the consideration of immune modulation with steroids and IVIG in neonates in addition to their mothers. Long-term treatment involves the placement of a permanent pacemaker.

Trucco SM et al: Use of intravenous gamma globulin and corticosteroids in the treatment of maternal autoantibody-mediated cardiomyopathy. J Am Coll Cardiol 2011 Feb 8:57(6):715–723 [PMID: 21292131].

Villain E: Indications for pacing in patients with congenital heart disease. Pacing Clin Electrophysiol 2008 Feb;31(Suppl 1):S17–S20 [PMID: 18226027].

SYNCOPE (FAINTING)

INTRODUCTION

Syncope is defined as the transient loss of consciousness and postural tone resulting from an abrupt, temporary decrease in cerebral blood flow. It is one of the most common referrals to pediatric cardiology. There is an estimated 30% lifetime risk. The majority of episodes are self-limited and benign and are known as vasovagal syncope or "simple fainting." It is a disorder of heart rate and blood pressure control by the autonomic nervous system that causes hypotension or bradycardia. Rarely, syncope can be the first warning sign of a serious condition such as arrhythmia, structural heart disease, or noncardiac disease. Even vasovagal syncope, if recurrent, can cause a major impact on lifestyle, interfering with school and/or sports. Many states impose driving restrictions following syncope. Therefore, accurate diagnosis and counseling are important.

DIAGNOSTIC EVALUATION

Given the many possible causes of syncope, a carefully planned approach is preferred to avoid an involved and expensive diagnostic evaluation. The patient history, family history, physical examination, and an ECG are fundamental and direct the remainder of the evaluation. Important historical details include the age of the patient (syncope is rare before 10 years of age except for breathing holding syncope), time of day (early morning is typical), the state of hydration and nutrition at the time of the event (last fluid or food intake), the environmental conditions (ambient temperature), the patient's activity or body position immediately prior to the syncope episode, the frequency and duration of the episodes, and any aura, prodrome, or specific symptoms prior to the episode. Witnesses should provide details regarding the patient's condition prior to syncope, duration of loss of consciousness, any injuries or seizure-like movements, loss of bowel or bladder function, heart rate during episode, and duration and nature of recovery. Medication history (prescription and over the counter supplements) is critical and may point to proarrhythmic potential. Additionally, a history of severe viral illness such as infectious mononucleosis frequently precedes the development of vasovagal syncope. Pertinent positives of the past medical history include neurologic disorders, traumatic brain injury, and neurosurgical interventions.

It is not uncommon to elicit a history of multiple family members who experienced syncope during adolescence that subsequently resolved. However, if the family history is positive for recurrent syncope, it is also important to consider familial disorders and question about the presence of HCM or DCM, LQTS, Brugada syndrome, exertional syncope (to consider catecholaminergic polymorphic ventricular tachycardia), primary PH, or arrhythmogenic RV cardiomyopathy. Additionally, families should be asked about sudden unexplained death in children or young adults (drownings, single car accidents, SCD, and SIDS), seizures, and congenital deafness. A genetic counselor can frequently be helpful in organizing the family history.

On physical examination, the general condition should be noted, with particular emphasis on hydration, nutritional status (evidence of eating disorders), and manifestations of thyroid disease. Orthostatic vital signs should be obtained, but care must be taken to follow a strict protocol to avoid false positives. Orthostatic hypotension is defined as a decrease in systolic blood pressure of 20 mm Hg or a decrease in diastolic blood pressure of 10 mm Hg after 3 minutes of standing when compared with blood pressure in the supine or sitting position. Pulse strength, rate, and any differences between upper and lower extremities should be noted. The presence of heart murmurs suggesting anatomic disease should prompt an echocardiogram. Finally, a phenotype of inherited connective tissue disorders (ie, Marfan syndrome) should be considered.

An ECG should be obtained, particularly if syncope is recurrent or occurs with exercise. It should be evaluated for heart rate, corrected QT interval, T-wave abnormalities (including T-wave alternans), or any ventricular arrhythmias, as well as for ventricular preexcitation, AV conduction disturbances, or features consistent with Brugada syndrome. All patients with exertional syncope, even those with positive orthostatic vital signs, should undergo additional evaluation with an echocardiogram and exercise stress testing. Echocardiograms are necessary to examine for cardiomyopathy, myocarditis, anomalous coronary arteries, PAH, and arrhythmogenic RV cardiomyopathy. An exercise test is necessary for catecholaminergic polymorphic ventricular tachycardia. Additionally testing may include a signal averaged ECG, Holter monitor, MRI, cardiac catheterization, and invasive electrophysiologic testing. Tilt table testing is less commonly performed in pediatric patients as the diagnosis of vasovagal syncope does not require a positive tilt test and results of unclear significance (ie, prolonged asystolic pauses) are common.

VASOVAGAL/NEUROCARDIOGENIC SYNCOPE

Pathophysiology/Clinical Presentation

By far the most common etiology for syncope in pediatrics is vasovagal or neurocardiogenic syncope. While the pathophysiologic mechanisms are heterogenous and not completely understood, it is thought to be primarily a response of the cardiac-central nervous system reflex. The most common initiating event is prolonged or rapid assumption of an upright position that results in gravitationally mediated venous pooling in the lower extremities. This causes central hypovolemia leading to decreased venous return and stroke volume. Alternatively, an emotional or physical stress (pain or fright) or a reflex mechanism related to hair grooming, glutination (swallowing), or micturition can trigger this sequence by creating a sympathetic response characterized by tachycardia and vasoconstriction. This increased sympathetic output may result in a subsequent parasympathetic response characterized by bradycardia or asystole. Additionally, the abrupt withdrawal of sympathetically mediated tachycardia despite persistent peripheral vasodilation causes a decrease in systemic blood pressure and venous return/stroke volume.

As a result of loss of consciousness, the patient falls into a supine state that restores venous return and central blood volume. The loss of consciousness is short (< 1–2 minutes), with rapid return to baseline behavior. Bowel or bladder incontinence is uncommon, and although seizures rarely occur, myoclonic "jerks" are common. A prodrome consisting of nausea, epigastric pain, clammy sensation, pallor, dizziness, lightheadedness, tunnel vision, and weakness is very characteristic of vasovagal or neurocardiogenic syncope. Some patients with profound bradycardia or asystole may have little to no warning and will typically require additional evaluation to confirm the diagnosis. If the prodrome is of sufficient duration, patients may learn to recognize it and lie down to prevent complete loss of consciousness.

Therapy

Maintaining adequate intravascular volume is the mainstay of treatment of vasovagal syncope. While choosing a fluid volume goal is acceptable, having patients target clear urine at least five times per day ensures appropriate intake. Increased salt intake with salt tablets or simply increased dietary sources (a handful of salted peanuts or crackers) is also recommended. Counter regulatory maneuvers such as leg pumping, leg crossing, and squatting can ameliorate the presyncopal symptoms and frequently avoid complete loss of consciousness. Finally, regular aerobic exercise should be encouraged as it strengths the muscles of the lower extremities and improves vascular tone. Medications can be useful although these frequently rely on adequate hydration for effectiveness.

There are only limited randomized studies of medications in pediatric patients. Fludrocortisone is a mineralocorticoid that results in renal salt resorption and thus increases intravascular volume. α-Agonist agents such as midodrine work through their vasoconstrictor effects. Their utility is limited by the necessity for three times daily administration. Although β-blockers have been used for treatment of syncope by targeting the increased sympathetic output with resultant parasympathetic response, the side effects may mask the therapeutic benefits and there is a paucity of data regarding their effectiveness. Vagolytic agents (disopyramide) help control hypervagotonia, and the selective serotonin reuptake inhibitors have also been effective in alleviating symptoms in select patients.

Mosqueda-Garcia R et al: The elusive pathophysiology of neurally mediated syncope. Circulation 2000;102(23):2898–2906.

Strickberger SA et al: AHA/ACCF scientific statement on the evaluation of syncope: from the American Heart Association Councils on Clinical Cardiology, Cardiovascular Nursing, Cardiovascular Disease in the Young, and Stroke, and the Quality of Care and Outcomes Research Interdisciplinary Working Group; and the American College of Cardiology Foundation: in collaboration with the Heart Rhythm Society: endorsed by the American Autonomic Society. Circulation 2006 Jan 17;113(2):316–327. doi: 10.1161/CIRCULATIONAHA.105.170274 [PMID: 16418451].

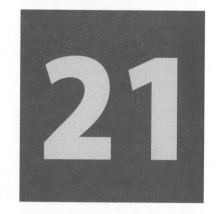

Gastrointestinal Tract

David Brumbaugh, MD

Glenn T. Furuta, MD

Edward J. Hoffenberg, MD

Gregory E. Kobak, MD

Robert E. Kramer, MD

Seth Septer, MD

Mary Shull, MD

Jason Soden, MD

Thomas Walker, MD

▼ DISORDERS OF THE ESOPHAGUS

GASTROESOPHAGEAL REFLUX & GERD

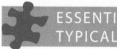

ESSENTIALS OF DIAGNOSIS & TYPICAL FEATURES

- ▶ Key definitions:
- ▶ **Gastroesophageal reflux (GER)** refers to uncomplicated recurrent spitting and vomiting in healthy infants that resolves spontaneously.
- ▶ **Gastroesophageal reflux disease (GERD)** is present when reflux causes secondary symptoms or complications.
- ▶ **Esophageal manifestations of GERD** include symptoms (heartburn, regurgitation) and mucosal complications (esophagitis, stricture, Barrett esophagus) primarily related to acid exposure in the upper gastrointestinal (GI) tract, primarily the esophagus itself.
- ▶ **Extraesophageal manifestations of GERD** include a myriad of clinical disorders that may be linked to reflux, including upper and lower airway symptoms and findings, as well as dental erosions. In most settings, objective confirmation of extraesophageal reflux complications is challenging.

▶ Clinical Findings

A. Infants With Gastroesophageal Reflux

Gastroesophageal (GE) reflux is common in young infants and is a physiological event. Frequent postprandial regurgitation, ranging from effortless to forceful, is the most common infant symptom. Infant GER is usually benign, and it is expected to resolve by 12–18 months of life.

Reflux of gastric contents into the esophagus occurs during spontaneous relaxations of the lower esophageal sphincter that are unaccompanied by swallowing. Factors promoting reflux in infants include small stomach capacity, frequent large-volume feedings, short esophageal length, supine positioning, and slow swallowing response to the flow of refluxed material up the esophagus. Infants' individual responses to the stimulus of reflux, particularly the maturity of their self-settling skills, are important factors determining the severity of reflux-related symptoms.

When infants develop symptoms such as failure to thrive, food refusal, pain behavior, GI bleeding, upper or lower airway-associated respiratory symptoms, or Sandifer syndrome, these indicate gastroesophageal reflux disease (GERD).

B. Older Children With Reflux

Older children with GERD complain of adult-type symptoms such as regurgitation into the mouth, heartburn, and dysphagia. Esophagitis can occur as a complication of GERD and requires endoscopy with biopsy for diagnostic confirmation. Children with asthma, cystic fibrosis, developmental handicaps, hiatal hernia (HH), and repaired tracheoesophageal fistula are at increased risk of GERD and esophagitis.

C. Extraesophageal Manifestations of Reflux Disease

Upper airway symptoms (hoarseness, sinusitis, laryngeal erythema, and edema), apnea or apparent life-threatening events (ALTEs), lower airway symptoms (asthma, recurrent pneumonia, recurrent cough), dental erosions, and Sandifer syndrome have all been linked to GERD, although proof of cause-and-effect relationship is challenging.

D. Diagnostic Studies

History and physical examination alone should help differentiate infants with benign, recurrent vomiting (physiologic GER) from those who have red flags for GERD or other underlying primary conditions that may present with recurrent emesis at this age. Warning signs that warrant further investigation in the infant with recurrent vomiting include bile-stained emesis, GI bleeding, onset of vomiting after 6 months, failure to thrive, diarrhea, fever, hepatosplenomegaly, abdominal tenderness or distension, or neurologic changes.

An upper GI series should be considered when anatomic etiologies of recurrent vomiting are considered, but should not be considered to be a test for GERD.

In older children with heartburn or frequent regurgitation, a limited trial of acid-suppressant therapy may be both diagnostic and therapeutic. If a child has symptoms requiring ongoing acid suppressant therapy, or if symptoms fail to improve with empiric therapy, consider referral to a pediatric gastroenterologist to assist in evaluation for complicated GERD, or nonreflux diagnoses including eosinophilic esophagitis (EoE).

Esophagoscopy and mucosal biopsies are useful to evaluate for mucosal injury secondary to GERD (Barrett esophagus, stricture, erosive esophagitis), or to evaluate for nonreflux diagnoses that present with reflux-like symptoms, including EoE. Endoscopic evaluation is not requisite for the evaluation of all infants and children with suspected GERD.

Intraluminal esophageal pH monitoring (pH probe) and combined multiple intraluminal impedance and pH monitoring (pH impedance probe) are indicated to quantify reflux, and to evaluate for objective evidence of symptom associations with regards to atypical reflux presentations. pH impedance studies may have higher diagnostic yield in evaluating for respiratory or atypical complications of reflux disease, or in evaluating for breakthrough reflux symptoms while a patient is on acid-suppressant therapy.

▶ Treatment & Prognosis

Reflux resolves spontaneously in 85% of affected infants by 12 months of age, coincident with assumption of erect posture and initiation of solid feedings. Until then, regurgitation volume may be reduced by offering small feedings at frequent intervals and by thickening feedings with rice cereal (2–3 tsp/oz of formula). In infants with unexplained crying or fussy behavior, no evidence supports empiric use of acid suppression.

Acid suppression may be used to treat suspected esophageal or extraesophageal complications of acid reflux in infants and older children. Therapeutic options include histamine-2 (H_2)–receptor antagonists or proton pump inhibitors (PPIs). PPI therapy has been shown to significantly heal both esophageal mucosal injury and symptoms from GERD within 8–12 weeks. Potential risk factors associated with long-term PPI therapy include risk for infection (pneumonia, *Clostridium difficile*–associated diarrhea), and an increased risk for osteoporosis has been demonstrated in adults. Although

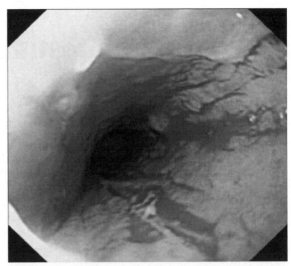

▲ **Figure 21–1.** Esophagitis associated with GERD. Mucosa is erythematous with loss of vascular pattern.

there are no standardized recommendations regarding prophylaxis or surveillance for these complications in pediatric patients on long-term PPI therapy, one should consider weaning or discontinuing treatment if it is no longer required. There is no sufficient evidence to support the routine use of prokinetic agents for treatment of pediatric GERD.

Spontaneous resolution is less likely in older children with GERD and those with underlying neurodevelopmental disorders. Episodic symptoms may be controlled with intermittent use of acid blockers and those with persistent symptoms may require chronic acid suppression. Complications of reflux esophagitis or chronic GERD include feeding dysfunction, esophageal stricture, and anemia (Figure 21–1). Barrett esophagus, a precancerous condition, is very uncommon in children, but it may occur in patients with an underlying primary diagnosis that offers high risk for GERD.

Antireflux surgery (Nissen fundoplication) may be considered in a child with GERD who (1) fails medical therapy; (2) is dependent on persistent, aggressive medical therapy; (3) is symptomatic and nonadherent to medical therapy; and (4) has persistent, severe respiratory complications of GERD or other life-threatening complications of GERD. Potential complications after antireflux surgery include dumping syndrome, gas bloat syndrome, persistent retching or gagging, or wrap failure.

Lightdale JR et al: Gastroesophageal reflux: management guidance for the pediatrician. Pediatrics 2013 May;131(5):e1684–e1695 [PMID: 23629618].

Martin K et al: Outcomes of pediatric laparoscopic fundoplication: a critical review of the literature. Can J Gastroenterol Hepatol 2014 Feb;28(2):97–102 [PMID: 24288692].

Mousa H, Hassan M: Gastroesophageal reflux disease. Pediatr Clin North Am 2017 Jun; 64(3):487–505 [PMID: 28502434].

Smits MJ et al: Association between gastroesophageal reflux and pathologic apneas in infants: a systematic review. Neurogastroenterol Motil 2014 Nov;26(11):1527–1538 [PMID: 25080836].

Vandenplas Y, Hauser B: An updated review on gastro-esophageal reflux in pediatrics. Expert Rev Gastroenterol Hepatol 2015; 9(12):1511–1521. doi: 10.1586/17474124.2015.1093932. Review [PMID: 26414355].

EOSINOPHILIC ESOPHAGITIS

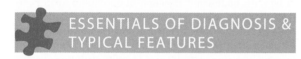

ESSENTIALS OF DIAGNOSIS & TYPICAL FEATURES

▶ Feeding dysfunction, dysphagia, esophageal food impaction, and heartburn are common symptoms.

▶ Must rule out other causes for esophageal eosinophilia before assigning diagnosis of EoE.

▶ Esophageal food impaction and esophageal stricture are two most common complications.

▶ Elimination of food allergens or swallowed topical steroids are effective treatments.

▶ Clinical Findings

A. Symptoms and Signs

This recently recognized entity occurs in all ages and more frequently affects boys. Common initial presentations in young children include feeding dysfunction and vague non-specific symptoms of GERD such as abdominal pain, vomiting, and regurgitation. If a history of careful and lengthy chewing, long mealtimes, washing food down with liquid or avoiding highly textured foods is encountered, one may suspect EoE. In adolescent's symptoms of solid food dysphagia, and acute and recurrent food impactions predominate. If a child's symptoms are unresponsive to medical and/or surgical management of GERD, EoE should be strongly considered as a diagnostic possibility. A family or personal history of atopy, asthma, dysphagia, esophageal dilation, or food impaction is often present.

B. Laboratory Findings

Peripheral eosinophilia may or may not be present. The esophageal mucosa usually appears abnormal with features of thickening, mucosal fissures, strictures, and rings. The esophagus is often sprinkled with pinpoint white exudates that superficially resemble *Candida* infection. On microscopic examination the white spots are composed of eosinophils (Figure 21–2). A lengthy stricture can be seen at the time of endoscopy but esophagrams may capture this more often. Serum IgE may be elevated, but this is not a diagnostic

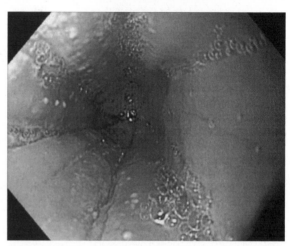

▲ **Figure 21–2.** Esophagitis associated with EoE. Mucosa contains linear folds, white exudate, and has loss of vascular pattern.

finding. Specific allergens can often be identified by skin testing, and patient can sometimes identify foods that precipitate pain and dysphagia.

▶ Differential Diagnosis

The most common differential conditions are peptic esophagitis, congenital esophageal stricture, and *Candida* esophagitis. Patients with eosinophilic gastroenteropathy can also present with gastric outlet obstruction or intestinal caused by large local infiltrates of eosinophils in the antrum, duodenum, and cecum.

▶ Diagnosis

The diagnosis of EoE is based on both clinical and histopathological features. Symptoms referable to esophageal dysfunction must be seen in association with esophageal eosinophilia and a normal gastric and duodenal mucosa. Other causes for esophageal eosinophilia, in particular, GERD, must be ruled out. A preendoscopy trial of PPIs is not required to make the diagnosis.

▶ Treatment

Dietary exclusion of offending allergens (elemental diet, removal of allergenic foods) is effective treatment, but adherence in older children can be difficult. Topical corticosteroids are an effective treatment. Steroids are puffed in the mouth and swallowed from a metered dose pulmonary inhaler; this method of administration is completely opposite of how topical steroids are administered for the treatment of asthma. Patients should not rinse their mouth or eat for 30 minutes to maximize the effectiveness. The association of EoE and esophageal malignancy has not been identified. Parent and family support is available at American Partnership for Eosinophilic Disorders APFED.org.

Furuta GT, Katzka DA: Eosinophilic esophagitis. N Engl J Med 2015 Oct 22;373(17):1640–1648 [PMID: 26488694].

Inage E, Furuta GT, Menard-Katcher C, Masterson JC: Eosinophilic esophagitis: pathophysiology and its clinical implications. Am J Physiol Gastrointest Liver Physiol 2018 Nov 1;315(5):G879–G886 [PMID: 30212252].

Menard-Katcher C et al: Significance of feeding dysfunction in eosinophilic esophagitis. World J Gastroenterol 2014 Aug 21;20(31):11019–11022 [PMID: 25152606].

Ruffner MA, Spergel JM: Pediatric eosinophilic esophagitis: updates for the primary care setting. Curr Opin Pediatr 2018 Dec;30(6):829–836 [PMID: 3023937].

ACHALASIA OF THE ESOPHAGUS

A. Symptoms and Signs

Achalasia occurs rarely in pediatrics, with an incidence of 0.11 per 100,000 and most commonly in children who are older than 5 years. Cases during infancy have been reported, but overall less than 5% of achalasia occurs in patients less than 15 years of age. Common symptoms reported were emesis (84.6%), dysphagia (69.2%), weight loss (46.0%), and chronic cough (46.1%). Patients may eat slowly and often require large amounts of fluid when ingesting solid food. Familial cases occur in Allgrove syndrome (alacrima, adrenal insufficiency, and achalasia) and familial dysautonomia.

B. Imaging and Manometry

Barium esophagram shows a dilated esophagus with a tapered "beak" at the GE junction. Fluoroscopy shows irregular tertiary contractions of the esophageal wall, indicative of disordered esophageal peristalsis. Esophageal manometry classically shows high resting pressure of the lower esophageal sphincter, failure of sphincter relaxation after swallowing, and abnormal esophageal peristalsis, though these findings may be sporadic, with partial or normal relaxations present in some swallows. Use of high-resolution manometry has become the standard in diagnosis and the Chicago classification into types I, II, and III have been used to indicate prognosis.

C. Differential Diagnosis

Congenital or peptic stricture, webs, and masses of the esophagus may mimic achalasia. EoE commonly presents with symptoms of dysphagia and food impaction, similar to achalasia. Cricopharyngeal achalasia or spasm is a rare cause of dysphagia in children, but it shares some clinical features of primary achalasia of the LES. Intestinal pseudo-obstruction, multiple endocrine neoplasia type 2b, systemic amyloidosis, and postvagotomy syndrome cause esophageal dysmotility similar to achalasia. Teenage girls may be suspected of having an eating disorder. In Chagas disease, caused by the parasite *Trypanosoma cruzi*, nNOS and ganglion cells are diminished or absent in the muscular layers of the LES causing an acquired achalasia.

▶ Treatment & Prognosis

Based on studies in adults, prognosis is typically best in patients with type II achalasia, followed by type I and worst in type III. Endoscopic injection of botulinum toxin paralyzes the lower esophageal sphincter and may temporarily relieve obstruction but in a recent small study in adults was no better than sham operation and has only been recommended as a short-term bridge to more definitive therapy in medically unstable patients. Pneumatic dilation trials in children are limited, but a single-center experience of endoscopic dilation showed a long-term success rate of up to 87% with one to three dilations. However, a large recent cohort of pediatric to young adult achalasia patients comparing surgical treatment with a Heller myotomy to endoscopic dilation found a similar complication rate but with increased need for reintervention (65% vs 16%) and propose that surgical myotomy be considered the treatment for pediatric achalasia. Postoperative GERD is common, and in the meta-analysis fundoplication was performed in 82% cases, though rates of postoperative GERD were not significantly different between those with and without fundoplication. In a large retrospective pediatric study, general response rates of pneumatic dilation compared to Heller myotomy were not significantly different, though some suggest that children older than 6 years may have better outcomes with pneumatic dilation. Per-oral endoscopic myotomy (POEM) has been increasingly utilized as a less invasive alternative to surgical treatment, with several studies now showing long-term resolution of symptoms and similar rates of adverse events, as well as improved durability of response compared to balloon dilation. Self-expanding metal stents has been reported in childhood refractory cases but have not been recommended in adults.

Hung YC, Westfal ML, Chang DC, Kelleher CM: Heller myotomy is the optimal index procedure for esophageal achalasia in adolescents and young adults. Surg Endosc 2018. [Epub ahead of print] [PMID: 30552502].

Liu ZQ, Chen WF, Wang Y, Xu XY, et al: Mast cell infiltration associated with loss of interstitial cells of Cajal and neuronal degeneration in achalasia. Neurogastroenterol Motil 2019 May;31(5):e13565 [PMID: 30868687].

Miao S, Wu J, Lu J, Wang Y, Tang Z, Zhou Y, Huang Z, Ying H, Zhou P: Peroral endoscopic myotomy in children with achalasia: a relatively long-term single-center study. J Pediatr Gastroenterol Nutr 2018;66(2):257–262 [PMID: 28691974].

Zaninotto G, Bennett C, Boeckxstaens G, Costantini M, et al: The 2018 ISDE achalasia guidelines. Dis Esophagus 2018;31(9) [PMID: 30169645].

CAUSTIC BURNS OF THE ESOPHAGUS

ESSENTIALS OF DIAGNOSIS & TYPICAL FEATURES

▶ Reported history of ingestion, with or without evidence of oropharyngeal injury.

▶ Painful swallowing, drooling, and food refusal typical of esophageal injury.

▶ Endoscopic evaluation of severity and extent of injury at 24–48 hours postingestion.

▶ Significant risk for development of esophageal strictures, especially in second- and third-degree lesions.

▶ Clinical Findings

A. Symptoms and Signs

Ingestion of caustic solids or liquids (pH < 2 or pH > 12) produces esophageal lesions ranging from superficial inflammation to deep necrosis with ulceration, perforation, mediastinitis, or peritonitis. Meta-analysis encompassing more than 11,000 ingestions indicates a slight male predominance and a mean age of ingestion of 2.78 years. Acidic substances typically have a sour taste and therefore lead to limited injury because of the small volume ingested. Their pathogenesis is due to superficial coagulative necrosis with eschar formation. Conversely, the more benign taste of alkali ingestions may allow for larger volume ingestions and subsequent liquifactive necrosis that can lead to deeper mucosal penetration. Factors that determine the severity of injury include the amount ingested, the physical state of the agent, and the duration of mucosal exposure time, making powdered or gel formulations of dishwashing detergent especially dangerous. Ingestions of liquid detergent capsules or pods have become more common, due in part to their bright coloring and benign taste. They tend to cause more respiratory than esophageal injury, though a recent study found endoscopic injury present in 24%. The lips, mouth, and airway should be examined in suspected caustic ingestion, although up to 12% of children without oral lesions can have significant esophageal injury.

B. Imaging Studies

Esophagoscopy is often performed; however, timing is important as endoscopy may not indicate the true severity of injury if it is performed too early (< 24–48 hours) and may increase the risk of perforation if it is performed too late (> 72 hours) due to formation of granulation tissue. Grading of esophageal lesions into first degree (superficial injury, erythema only), second degree (transmucosal with erythema,

ulceration, and sloughing), and third degree (transmural with circumferential sloughing and deep mucosal ulceration) can help predict prognosis. Circumferential lesions carry the highest risk of stricture formation. In a recent large single-center study, 34% of ingestions in children were grade 2 or 3, with 50% of these requiring one or more endoscopic dilations. If dilation is felt to be necessary, it should not be performed in the acute phase of injury, though a recent study showed that early initiation of dilations by 15 days decreased the duration and number of dilations ultimately needed. Among elements of the CBC, elevation of red cell distribution width (RDW) above a cutoff of 12.2 was shown to be the most sensitive indicator of esophageal injury at endoscopy with sensitivity of 84.2% and OR of 7.74. In addition, even without clinical findings, endoscopic esophageal lesions have been found in up to 35% and gastric lesions in up to 14% of patients. Plain radiographs of the chest and abdomen may be performed if there is clinical suspicion of perforation. Contrast studies of the esophagus should be performed when endoscopic evaluation is not available, though they are unlikely to detect grades 1 and 2 lesions. Recent data has shown the utility of a 99mTc sucralfate scan in predicting the presence of significant esophageal injury on endoscopy after caustic ingestion.

▶ Treatment & Prognosis

Clinical observation is always prudent, as it is often difficult to predict the severity of esophageal injury at presentation. A large study of almost 1000 pediatric ingestions treated conservatively without steroids, endoscopy, or nasogastric tube showed a stricture rate of 23%. Vomiting should not be induced and administration of buffering agents should be avoided to prevent an exothermic reaction in the stomach. Intravenous corticosteroids (eg, methylprednisolone, 1–2 mg/kg/day) are given immediately to reduce oral swelling and laryngeal edema. A study using high dose (1 g/1.73 m^2) methylprednisone for the first 3 days after ingestion, however, showed a significant decrease in the occurrence of esophageal strictures. Treatment may be stopped if there are only first-degree burns at endoscopy. Broad-spectrum antibiotic coverage with third-generation cephalosporins may be considered to decrease stricture formation by preventing bacterial colonization into necrotic tissue. Acid-blockade is often used to decrease additional injury from acid reflux.

Nonobstructive esophageal narrowings occur at the thoracic inlet, GE junction, or point of compression where the left bronchus crosses the esophagus. Strictures occur only with full-thickness esophageal necrosis and prevalence of stricture formation varies from 10% to 50%. In refractory cases, fully covered, self-expanding, removable esophageal stents, now available in pediatric sizes, may offer additional options for recurrent caustic strictures. Topical mitomycin-C has been effective in treatment of refractory caustic strictures of the esophagus and a recent randomized, prospective trial showed benefit in terms of number of dilations (3.25 vs 6.25), cost and ultimate success rate (81.6% vs 40%). Animal models utilizing 5-fluorouracil in the early management of caustic esophageal injuries have also shown promise in preventing fibrosis and stricture formation. Surgical replacement of the esophagus by colonic interposition or gastric tube may be needed for long strictures resistant to dilation, though stricture rates may be as high as 47% and leaks as high as 18%. Study of histopathology of caustic injuries in children has shown changes of chronic esophagitis in 85%, reactive atypia in 13% and squamous dysplasia in 2%. Patients with history of caustic esophageal injury are estimated to have as much as a 1000-fold increase risk for esophageal carcinoma, though no formal surveillance guidelines have been established.

Aydin E, Beser OF, Sazak S, Duras E: Ingestion. Children (Basel) 2017;5(1) [PMID: 29286326].

Eskander A et al: Histopathological changes in the oesophageal mucosa in Egyptian children with corrosive strictures: a single-centre vast experience. World J Gastroenterol 2019;25(7):870–879 [PMID: 30809086].

Ghobrial CM, Eskander AE. Prospective study of the effect of topical application of Mitomycin C in refractory pediatric caustic esophageal strictures. Surg Endosc 2018;32(12):4932–4938. Epub 2018 Jun 4 [PMID: 29869087].

Nondela BB, Cox SG, Brink A, Millar AJW, Numanoglu A: Correlation of 99mTc sucralfate scan and endoscopic grading in caustic oesophageal injury. Pediatr Surg Int 2018;34(7):781–788 [PMID: 29761251].

Singh A, Anderson M, Altaf MA: Clinical and endoscopy findings in children with accidental exposure to concentrated detergent pods. J Pediatr Gastroenterol Nutr 2019. [Epub ahead of print] [PMID: 30664563].

FOREIGN BODIES IN THE ALIMENTARY TRACT

ESSENTIALS OF DIAGNOSIS & TYPICAL FEATURES

▶ Dysphagia, odynophagia, drooling, regurgitation, and chest/abdominal pain are typical symptoms of esophageal foreign body.

▶ Esophageal foreign bodies should be removed within 24 hours of ingestion.

▶ Esophageal button batteries must be removed emergently because of their ability to cause lethal injury.

▶ Most foreign bodies in the stomach will pass spontaneously.

Accidental foreign body ingestions are a common occurrence in pediatrics. The rate of children presenting to Emergency Department with foreign body ingestion has increased in the last two decades in the United States. Fortunately, 80%–90% of foreign bodies pass spontaneously with only 10%–20% requiring endoscopic or surgical management. At presentation the most common symptoms of an ingested foreign body are dysphagia, odynophagia, drooling, regurgitation, and chest or abdominal pain, but patients may be completely asymptomatic. Respiratory symptoms, such as cough, become prominent for foreign bodies retained in the esophagus for more than 1 week. A high index of suspicion should be maintained for toddlers presenting with these symptoms, even without a witnessed ingestion. If the ingestion is witnessed, the timing of the event is important to note as it will have implications for the timing of endoscopic removal.

Coins are the most common foreign body ingested by children (Figure 21–3). Ingested foreign bodies tend to lodge in narrowed areas—valleculae, thoracic inlet, GE junction, pylorus, ligament of Treitz, and ileocecal junction, or at the site of congenital or acquired intestinal stenoses. Evaluations to detect swallowed foreign body start with plain radiography. Radio-opaque objects will be easily visualized. Non–radio-opaque objects, such as plastic toys, may not appear on standard radiograph. If there is particular concern, based on patient symptoms, for a retained esophageal foreign body that is non–radio-opaque, a contrast esophagram is a useful test. Use of contrast, however, may delay or increase the risk of anesthesia due to aspiration concerns.

Most foreign bodies can be removed from the esophagus or stomach of a child by flexible endoscopy. During removal of an esophageal foreign body, the increased risk of

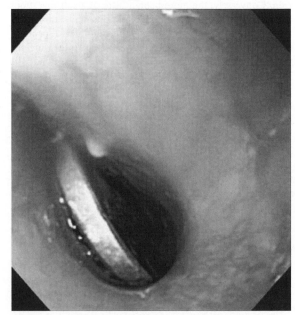

▲ **Figure 21–3.** Foreign body in esophagus. Coin is lodged in the esophageal lumen.

airway aspiration supports intubation with an endotracheal tube. Esophageal foreign bodies should be removed within 24 hours to avoid injury to the esophagus. The urgency of removal of esophageal foreign bodies is dictated by the severity of patient symptoms and the ability to swallow oral secretions.

Disk-shaped button batteries lodged in the esophagus are especially concerning and should be removed immediately. Button batteries may cause an electrical thermal injury in as little as 2 hours and can cause many severe complications including death, aortoesophageal fistula, tracheoesophageal fistula, esophageal perforation, esophageal stricture, vocal cord paralysis, and discitis. Although most button batteries in the stomach will pass uneventfully, greater attention is required for larger batteries (> 20 mm) in younger children (< 5 years of age), as there is greater risk for injury sustained to the esophagus and the battery is less likely to successfully traverse the pylorus. In these cases, endoscopic evaluation with gastric batteries may still be considered in order to evaluate the esophagus for signs of injury and to remove the gastric battery. Rates of significant injury and death due to swallowed button batteries have increased in recent years with the transition toward production of higher-voltage lithium batteries.

Esophageal food impaction should always raise the question of underlying esophagitis. In particular, EoE has been shown to be present in up to 75% of pediatric patients presenting initially with esophageal food impaction.

Smooth foreign bodies in the stomach, such as buttons or coins, may be monitored without attempting removal for up to several weeks if the child is free of symptoms. Screws and nails are examples of objects with a blunt end that is heavier than the sharp end. These asymmetrically weighted objects will generally pass without incident and so need for endoscopic removal must be considered on a case-by-case basis. In contrast, double-sided sharp objects that are weighted equally on each end, such as fishbones and wooden toothpicks, should be removed as they can migrate through the wall of the GI tract into the pericardium, liver, and inferior vena cava. Large, open safety pins should be removed from the stomach because they may not pass the pyloric sphincter and may cause perforation. Objects longer than 5 cm may be unable to pass the ligament of Treitz and should be removed. Magnets require consideration for removal only if there has been more than one ingested, or if a single magnet was ingested along with a metallic object, because of the risk of fistula or erosion of mucosal tissue trapped between two adherent foreign bodies. Rare earth metal magnets, or neodymium magnets, are very powerful small magnets that are sold in bulk and have caused multiple cases of bowel perforation necessitating surgical intervention. Ingestion of multiple magnets should lead to immediate endoscopic removal if technically feasible. If not, their migration through the GI tract should be followed radiographically until they are passed.

The use of balanced electrolyte lavage solutions containing polyethylene glycol may help the passage of small, smooth foreign bodies lodged in the intestine. Lavage is especially useful in hastening the passage of foreign bodies that may contain an absorbable toxic material such as a heavy metal.

Brumbaugh DE et al: Management of button battery-induced hemorrhage in children. J Pediatr Gastroenterol Nutr 2011;52(5): 585–589 [PMID: 215028305].

Hussain SZ et al: Management of ingested magnets in children. J Pediatr Gastroenterol Nutr 2012 Sep;55(3):239–242 [PMID: 22785419].

Kramer et al: Management of Ingested Foreign Bodies in Children: A Clinical Report of the NASPGHAN Endoscopy Committee [PMID: 25611037]

Litovitz T, Whitaker N, Clark L, White NC, Marsolec M: Emerging battery-ingestion hazard: clinical implications. Pediatrics 2010; 125(6):1168–1177 [PMID: 20498173].

Orsagh-Yentis D, McAdams RJ, Roberts KJ, McKenzie LB: Foreign-body ingestions of young children treated in US Emergency Departments: 1995-2015. Pediatrics 2019 Apr 12; 143(5): pii: e20181988 [PMID: 3079810].

▼ DISORDERS OF THE STOMACH & DUODENUM

HIATAL & PARAESOPHAGEAL HERNIA

Hiatal hernias (HHs) are classified into four types, encompassing both sliding hiatal hernias and paraesophageal hiatal hernias. Type I is a sliding hiatal hernia, in which the GE junction and a portion of the proximal stomach is displaced above the diaphragmatic hiatus. Sliding HHs are common, with a recent study showing a prevalence of nearly 21% of all EGD's performed and a correlation between HHs and clinical symptoms of heartburn and regurgitation in children > 48 months. Paraesophageal hiatal hernias encompass types II, III, and IV of HHs, in which the esophagus and GE junction are in their normal anatomic position, but the gastric cardia is herniated through the diaphragmatic hiatus. In type II, the gastric fundus herniates alongside the thoracic esophagus while the GE junction remains within the abdomen. In type III there is some sliding of the GE junction up into the chest, thus is a hybrid of type I and II. In type IV there is herniation of other abdominal contents, such as colon, omentum, or spleen into the chest as well. Most hiatal hernias are acquired, with congenital paraesophageal hernias being rare in childhood. Patients may present with recurrent pulmonary infections, vomiting, anemia, failure to thrive, or dysphagia. The most common cause of acquired paraesophageal hernia is previous fundoplication surgery, though they have also been described following blunt abdominal trauma and EA/TEF repair. Following fundoplication, the degree of circumferential surgical dissection of the esophageal hiatus is the most important risk factor, with one prospective study demonstrating a reduction in the 5 year herniation rate from 36.5% to 12.2% with limited dissection.

Radiographic studies typically reveal a cystic mass in the posterior mediastinum or a dilated esophagus. The diagnosis is typically made with an upper GI series or a CT scan of the chest and abdomen, though diagnosis via ultrasound in the prenatal period has been reported. Presence of a ring in the lower esophagus on upper GI has been found to be associated with HH in 96% of children and should increase the index of suspicion. Recently, use of pH Impedance probe testing has been proposed as an effective method to identify HH in children, where inversion of the usual acid:nonacid reflux ratio to > 1.0 had a sensitivity of 93.8% and specificity of 79.6%. Treatment in symptomatic cases is generally surgical, with laparoscopic repair being used more commonly. Controversy exists about using biosynthetic mesh for repair, as it decreases the risk of recurrent hernia but also increases esophageal erosion in children. Fundoplication is generally indicated at the time of repair, as rates of significant GERD requiring surgical intervention have been reported as high as 60%.

Garvey EM, Ostlie DJ: Hiatal and paraesophageal hernia repair in pediatric patients. Semin Pediatr Surg 2017;26(2):61–66 [PMID 28550872].

PYLORIC STENOSIS

ESSENTIALS OF DIAGNOSIS & TYPICAL FEATURES

▶ Postnatal muscular hypertrophy of the pylorus.

▶ Progressive gastric outlet obstruction, nonbilious vomiting, dehydration, and alkalosis in infants younger than 12 weeks.

▶ Upper GI contrast radiographs or abdominal ultrasound are diagnostic.

The cause of postnatal pyloric muscular hypertrophy with gastric outlet obstruction is unknown. The incidence is 1–8 per 1000 births, with a 4:1 male predominance. Recent studies suggest that erythromycin in the neonatal period is associated with a higher incidence of pyloric stenosis.

▶ Clinical Findings

A. Symptoms and Signs

Projectile postprandial vomiting usually begins between 2 and 4 weeks of age but may start as late as 12 weeks. Vomiting starts at birth in about 10% of cases and onset of symptoms may be delayed in preterm infants. Vomitus is rarely bilious but may be blood-streaked. Infants are usually hungry and nurse avidly. The upper abdomen may be distended after feeding, and prominent gastric peristaltic waves from left to right may be seen. An oval mass, 5–15 mm in longest dimension can be felt on deep palpation in the right upper abdomen, especially after vomiting. This palpable "olive," however, was only present in 13.6% of patients studied.

B. Laboratory Findings

Hypochloremic alkalosis with potassium depletion is the classic metabolic findings, though low chloride may be seen in as few as 23% and alkalosis in 14.4%. These findings may not be as common in younger infants and their absence should not dissuade from the diagnosis in the appropriate clinical setting. Dehydration causes elevated hemoglobin and hematocrit. Mild unconjugated bilirubinemia occurs in 2%–5% of cases.

C. Imaging

Ultrasonography shows a hypoechoic muscle ring greater than 4 mm thickness with a hyperdense center and a pyloric channel length greater than 15 mm. A barium upper GI series reveals retention of contrast in the stomach and a long narrow pyloric channel with a double track of barium. The hypertrophied muscle mass produces typical semilunar filling defects in the antrum. Infants presenting younger than 21 days may not fulfill these classic ultrasonographic criteria and may require clinical judgment to interpret "borderline" measures of pyloric muscle thickness.

▶ Treatment & Prognosis

Pyloromyotomy is the treatment of choice and consists of incision down to the mucosa along the pyloric length. Treatment of dehydration and electrolyte imbalance is mandatory before surgical treatment, even if it takes 24–48 hours. Patients often vomit postoperatively as a consequence of gastritis, esophagitis, or associated GE reflux. The outlook after surgery is excellent, though patients may show as much as a four times greater risk for development of chronic abdominal pain of childhood.

El-Gohary Y, Abdelhafeez A, Paton E, Gosain A, Murphy AJ: Pyloric stenosis: an enigma more than a century after the first successful treatment. Pediatr Surg Int 2018 Jan;34(1):21–27 [PMID: 29030700].

Vinycomb TI, Laslett K, Gwini SM, Teague W, Nataraja RM: Presentation and outcomes in hypertrophic pyloric stenosis: an 11-year review. J Paediatr Child Health 2019 Jan 24; [PMID: 30677197].

GASTRIC & DUODENAL ULCER

ESSENTIALS OF DIAGNOSIS & TYPICAL FEATURES

▶ Localized erosions of gastric or duodenal mucosa.

▶ Pain, vomiting, and bleeding are the most common symptoms.

▶ Underlying severe illness, Helicobacter pylori infection, and nonsteroidal anti-inflammatory drugs (NSAIDs) are the most common causes.

▶ Successful eradication of *H pylori* infection requires knowledge of regional antimicrobial resistance patterns.

▶ Diagnosis by endoscopy.

▶ General Considerations

Gastric and duodenal ulcers occur at any age. In the United States, most childhood gastric and duodenal ulcers are associated with underlying illness, toxins, or drugs such as NSAIDS that cause breakdown in mucosal defenses.

Worldwide, the most common cause of gastric and duodenal ulcer is mucosal infection with the bacterium *H pylori*. The prevalence of *H Pylori* infection varies greatly by country and increases with poor sanitation, crowded living conditions, and family exposure. Infection is thought to be acquired in childhood, but only in a small percentage of infected persons will infection lead to nodular gastritis, peptic ulcer, or in the case of long-standing infection, gastric lymphoid tumors and gastric ·adenocarcinoma. Some bacterial virulence factors have been identified, but the host and bacterial characteristics that contribute to disease progression are still largely unknown. In contrast to ulcers secondary to *H pylori*, non–*H pylori* ulcers tend to present at a younger age and are more likely to recur. In a large study of over 1000 children undergoing endoscopy, 5.4% had ulcers, with 47% of these due to *H pylori*, 16.5% related to NSAIDs, and 35.8% unrelated to either H *pylori* or NSAIDs. Recent evidence suggests that the prevalence of non–*H pylori* peptic ulcers is increasing.

Illnesses predisposing to secondary ulcers include central nervous system (CNS) disease, burns, sepsis, multiorgan system failure, chronic lung disease, Crohn disease (CrD), cirrhosis, and rheumatoid arthritis. The most common drugs causing secondary ulcers are aspirin, alcohol, and NSAIDs. NSAID use may lead to ulcers throughout the GI tract but most often in the stomach and duodenum. Severe ulcerative lesions in full-term neonates have been found to be associated with maternal antacid use in the last month of pregnancy.

▶ Clinical Findings

A. Symptoms and Signs

In children younger than 6 years, vomiting and upper GI bleeding are the most common symptoms. Older children are more likely to complain of epigastric abdominal pain. Ulcers in the pyloric channel may cause gastric outlet obstruction. Chronic blood loss may cause iron-deficiency anemia. Deep penetration of the ulcer may erode into a mucosal arteriole and cause acute hemorrhage. Penetrating duodenal ulcers (especially common during cancer chemotherapy, immunosuppression, and in the intensive care setting) may perforate the duodenal wall, resulting in peritonitis or abscess.

B. Diagnostic Studies

Upper GI endoscopy is the most accurate diagnostic examination. The typical endoscopic appearance of an ulcer is a white exudative base with erythematous margins (Figure 21–4). Histopathologic assessment of biopsies obtained at endoscopy provides the opportunity to distinguish between different causes of ulcer disease, including *H pylori* infection, eosinophilic GI disease, celiac disease (CD), and Crohn disease. Endoscopic diagnosis of active *H pylori* infection may be achieved by histologic examination of gastric biopsies or measurement of urease activity on gastric tissue specimens. Additional noninvasive methods of diagnosis of active *H pylori* infection include evaluation of breath for radiolabeled carbon dioxide after administration of radiolabeled urea by mouth and detection of *H pylori*

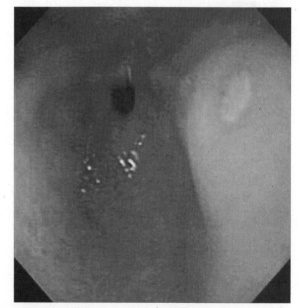

▲ **Figure 21–4.** Gastric ulcer. White exudate coats the ulcer bed of antral ulcer that is surrounded by an erythematous margin.

antigen in the stool. False-negative results for the latter two tests have been described when the patient is taking a PPI. Serum antibodies against *H pylori* have poor sensitivity and specificity, and do not prove that there is active infection or that treatment is needed. For severe or recurrent ulcerations not caused by *H pylori*, stress, or medications, a serum gastrin level may be considered to evaluate for a gastrin-secreting tumor (Zollinger-Ellison syndrome), though mild to moderate elevation in gastrin levels can be seen with use of PPI drugs. Upper GI barium radiographs may show an ulcer crater. Radiologic signs suggestive of peptic disease in adults (duodenal spasticity and thick irregular folds) are not reliable indicators in children.

▶ Treatment

Treatment of symptomatic *H pylori* infection requires eradication of the organism, a goal that remains elusive in children. The optimal medical regimen is still undetermined. Standard first-line triple therapy for eradication of *H pylori* has traditionally been a 7–10 day treatment course involving simultaneous use two oral antibiotics (most commonly, amoxicillin and clarithromycin) and PPI. However, rising rates of resistance to clarithromycin have rendered this combination ineffective in certain parts of the world. As a result, alternative combinations of antimicrobials (metronidazole and tetracycline) have been evaluated. The addition of bismuth to two antibiotics and PPI (bismuth quadruple therapy) may increase efficacy. Because resistance to antibiotics varies greatly by country, regional antibiotic resistance patterns for *H pylori* should be a guide in selecting initial therapy. Antimicrobial susceptibility testing can be performed on gastric biopsy specimens using a variety of techniques. Test of cure can be achieved by either the urease breath test or fecal *H pylori* antigen test.

Federico A et al: Eradication of *Helicobacter Pylori* infection: which regimen first? World J Gastroenterol 2014; 20(3):665–672 [PMID: 24574740].

Tam YH et al: *Helicobacter pylori*-positive versus *Helicobacter pylori*-negative idiopathic peptic ulcers in children with their long-term outcomes. J Pediatr Gastroenterol Nutr 2009;48(3):299–305 [PMID: 19274785].

CONGENITAL DIAPHRAGMATIC HERNIA

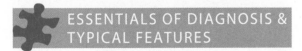

ESSENTIALS OF DIAGNOSIS & TYPICAL FEATURES

▶ Congenital diaphragmatic hernia (CDH) typically is diagnosed prenatally by screening ultrasound.

▶ Pulmonary hypoplasia and cardiovascular dysfunction are clinical challenges in the postnatal period.

▶ After surgical repair, chronic pulmonary disease and GER can be lifelong morbidities.

Herniation of abdominal contents through the diaphragm usually occurs through a posterolateral defect involving the left side of the diaphragm (foramen of Bochdalek). In about 9% of cases, the diaphragmatic defect is retrosternal (foramen of Morgagni). In eventration of the diaphragm, a subtype of CDH, a leaf of the diaphragm with hypoplastic muscular elements balloons into the chest and is asymptomatic or leads to milder symptoms. Hernias result from failure of the embryologic diaphragmatic anlagen to fuse and divide the thoracic and abdominal cavities at 8–10 weeks' gestation. The herniation of abdominal contents into the thoracic cavity can lead to pulmonary hypoplasia and significant cardiovascular dysfunction after birth, in particular severe persistent pulmonary hypertension.

Diagnosis of CDH is typically made prenatally by ultrasound. Associated congenital malformations, most commonly cardiovascular, may be detected prenatally. With the advent of improved care of the immediate complication of cardiopulmonary disease in the newborn period, including the use of inhaled nitric oxide, high-frequency oscillatory ventilation, and extracorporeal membrane oxygenation, survival has improved for infants with CDH and is as high as 70%–90% in some centers. Antenatal intervention with fetal tracheal occlusion may improve survival in CDH associated with severe pulmonary hypoplasia. Operative repair of the diaphragmatic defect is usually performed in the newborn period once cardiopulmonary stabilization is achieved, with increasing utilization of laparoscopic and thoracoscopic minimally invasive approaches. Long-term health issues in CDH survivors include chronic pulmonary disease, pulmonary hypertension, neurodevelopmental delays, hearing loss, and GER.

CONGENITAL DUODENAL OBSTRUCTION

▶ General Considerations

Obstruction is generally classified into intrinsic and extrinsic causes, although rare cases of simultaneous intrinsic and extrinsic anomalies have been reported.

Etiologies of extrinsic duodenal obstruction include congenital peritoneal bands associated with intestinal malrotation, annular pancreas, or duodenal duplication. Intrinsic duodenal obstruction is more common and is typically associated with congenital atresia, stenosis, or mucosal webs (so-called "wind sock deformity"). In about two-thirds of patients with congenital duodenal obstruction, there are other associated anomalies.

▶ Imaging Studies

Diagnosis of congenital duodenal obstructions is often made prenatally by ultrasound. Prenatal diagnosis predicts complete obstruction in 77% of cases and is associated with polyhydramnios, prematurity, and higher risk of maternal-fetal complications. Presence of a "double bubble" on ultrasound and an echogenic band in the second portion of the duodenum are 100% sensitive and specific for an annular pancreas. Postnatal abdominal plain radiographs show gaseous distention of the stomach and proximal duodenum (the "double-bubble" radiologic sign). With protracted vomiting, there is less air in the stomach and less abdominal distention. Absence of distal intestinal gas suggests atresia or severe extrinsic obstruction, whereas a pattern of intestinal air scattered over the lower abdomen may indicate partial duodenal obstruction. Barium enema may be helpful in determining the presence of malrotation or atresia in the lower GI tract, as well as evaluating for radiographic evidence of Hirschsprung disease, which may also present with abdominal distension and vomiting.

▶ Clinical Findings

A. Duodenal Atresia

Maternal polyhydramnios is common and often leads to prenatal diagnosis by ultrasonography. Vomiting (usually bile-stained) and epigastric distention begin within a few hours of birth. Meconium may be passed normally. Duodenal atresia is often associated with other congenital anomalies (30%), including esophageal atresia, intestinal atresias, and cardiac and renal anomalies. Preterm birth (25%–50%) and Down syndrome (20%–30%) are also associated with duodenal atresia.

B. Duodenal Stenosis

In this condition, duodenal obstruction is not complete. Onset of obvious obstructive symptoms may be delayed for weeks or years. Although the stenotic area is usually distal to the ampulla of Vater, the vomitus does not always contain bile. Duodenal stenosis or atresia is the most common GI tract malformation in children with Down syndrome, occurring in 3.9%.

C. Annular Pancreas

Annular pancreas is a rotational defect in which normal fusion of the dorsal and ventral pancreatic anlagen does not occur, and a ring of pancreatic tissue encircles the duodenum. The presenting symptom is duodenal obstruction. Down syndrome and congenital anomalies of the GI tract occur frequently. Polyhydramnios is common. Symptoms may develop late in childhood or even in adulthood if the obstruction is not complete in infancy. Treatment consists of duodenoduodenostomy or duodenojejunostomy without operative dissection or division of the pancreatic annulus. Pancreatic function is normal.

▶ Treatment & Prognosis

In almost all settings, surgical intervention (either laparoscopic or open) is required for congenital duodenal obstructive lesions. Typically, duodenoduodenostomy is performed to bypass the area of stenosis or atresia. For duodenal stenoses, however, there have been isolated reports of successful endoscopic treatment with balloon dilation. Thorough surgical exploration is typically done to ensure that no lower GI tract anomalies are present. More recent reports document the safety and utility of a laparoscopic approach. The mortality rate is increased in infants with preterm birth, Down syndrome, and associated congenital anomalies. Duodenal dilation and hypomotility from antenatal obstruction may cause duodenal dysmotility with obstructive symptoms even after surgical treatment. Placement of transanastomotic feeding tubes at the time of the initial repair has been found to result in more rapid progression to full enteral feeds and decreased need for parenteral nutrition (PN). The overall prognosis for these patients is good, with the majority of their mortality risk due to associated anomalies other than duodenal obstruction.

Adams SD, Stanton MP: Malrotation and intestinal atresias. Early Hum Dev 2014 Dec;90(12):921–925 [PMID: 25448782].

Brinkley MF, Tracy ET, Maxfield CM: Congenital duodenal obstruction: causes and imaging approach. Pediatr Radiol 2016 Jul;46(8):1084–1895. doi: 10.1007/s00247-016-3603-1. Review [PMID: 27324508].

Mustafawi AR, Hassan ME: Congenital duodenal obstruction in children: a decade's experience. Eur J Pediatr Surg 2008;18:93–97 [PMID: 18437652].

▼ DISORDERS OF THE SMALL INTESTINE

INTESTINAL ATRESIA & STENOSIS

Excluding anal anomalies, intestinal atresia or stenosis accounts for one-third of all cases of neonatal intestinal obstruction (see Chapter 2). Antenatal ultrasound can identify intestinal atresia in utero; polyhydramnios occurs in most affected pregnancies. Sensitivity of antenatal ultrasound is greater in more proximal atresias. Other congenital anomalies may be present in up to 54% of cases and 52% are delivered preterm. In apparently isolated atresia cases, occult congenital cardiac anomalies have been reported in as many as 30%. In one large population-based study, the prevalence was 2.9 per 10,000 births, although there is some evidence that the prevalence may be increasing. The localization and relative incidence of atresias and stenoses are listed in Table 21–1. Although jejunal and ileal atresias are often grouped together, there are data to suggest that jejunal atresias are associated with increased morbidity and mortality compared to ileal atresia. These differences may be related to increased compliance of the jejunal wall, resulting in more proximal dilation and subsequent loss in peristaltic activity.

Bile-stained vomiting and abdominal distention begin in the first 48 hours of life. Multiple sites in the intestine may be affected and the overall length of the small intestine may be

Table 21–1. Localization and relative frequency of congenital gastrointestinal atresias and stenoses.

	Area Involved	Type of Lesion	Relative Frequency (%)
Pylorus		Atresia; web or diaphragm	1
Duodenum	80% are distal to the ampulla of Vater	Atresia, stenosis; web or diaphragm	45
Jejunoileal	Proximal jejunum and distal ileum	Atresia (multiple in 6%–29%); stenosis	50
Colon	Left colon and rectum	Atresia (usually associated with atresias of the small bowel)	5–9

significantly shortened. Radiographic features include dilated loops of small bowel and absence of colonic gas. Barium enema reveals narrow-caliber microcolon because of lack of intestinal flow distal to the atresia. In over 10% of patients with intestinal atresia, the mesentery is absent and the superior mesenteric artery (SMA) cannot be identified beyond the origin of the right colic and ileocolic arteries. The ileum coils around one of these two arteries, giving rise to the so-called Christmas tree deformity on contrast radiographs. The tenuous blood supply often compromises surgical anastomoses. The differential diagnosis of intestinal atresia includes Hirschsprung disease, paralytic ileus secondary to sepsis, midgut volvulus, and meconium ileus. Surgery is mandatory. Postoperative complications include short bowel syndrome (SBS) in 15% and small bowel hypomotility secondary to antenatal obstruction. Overall mortality has been reported at 8%, with increased risk in low-birth-weight and premature infants.

Adams SD, Stanton MP: Malrotation and intestinal atresias. Early Hum Dev 2014 Dec;90(12):921-925 [PMID: 25448782].

Best KE et al: Epidemiology of small intestinal atresia in Europe: a register-based study. Arch Dis Child Fetal Neonatal Ed 2012 Sep;97(5):F353-F358 [PMID: 22933095].

INTESTINAL MALROTATION

▶ General Considerations

The midgut extends from the duodenojejunal junction to the mid-transverse colon. It is supplied by the SMA, which runs in the root of the mesentery. During gestation, the midgut elongates into the umbilical sac, returning to an intra-abdominal position during the 10th week of gestation. The root of the mesentery rotates in a counterclockwise direction during retraction causing the colon to cross the abdominal cavity ventrally. The cecum moves from the left to the right lower quadrant, and the duodenum crosses dorsally becoming partly retroperitoneal. When rotation is incomplete, the dorsal fixation of the mesentery is defective and shortened, so that the bowel from the ligament of Treitz to

the mid-transverse colon may rotate around its narrow mesenteric root and occlude the SMA (volvulus). From autopsy studies it is estimated that up to 1% of the general population may have intestinal malrotation, which is diagnosed in the first year of life in 70%–90% of patients.

▶ Clinical Findings

A. Symptoms and Signs

Malrotation with volvulus accounts for 10% of neonatal intestinal obstructions. Most infants present in the first 3 weeks of life with bile-stained vomiting or with overt small bowel obstruction. Intrauterine volvulus may cause intestinal obstruction or perforation at birth. The neonate may present with ascites or meconium peritonitis. Later presenting signs include intermittent intestinal obstruction, malabsorption, protein-losing enteropathy, or diarrhea. Associated congenital anomalies, especially cardiac, occur in over 25% of symptomatic patients. Many of these may be found in a subgroup of malrotation patients with heterotaxy syndromes, with associated asplenia or polysplenia. Older children and adults with undiagnosed malrotation typically present with chronic GI symptoms of nausea, vomiting, diarrhea, abdominal pain, dyspepsia, bloating, and early satiety.

B. Imaging

An upper GI series is considered the gold standard for diagnosis, with a reported sensitivity of 96%, and classically shows the duodenojejunal junction and the jejunum on the right side of the spine. The diagnosis of malrotation can be further confirmed by barium enema, which may demonstrate a mobile cecum located in the midline, right upper quadrant, or left abdomen. Plain films of the abdomen in the newborn period may show a "double-bubble" sign, resulting in a misdiagnosis of duodenal atresia. CT scan and ultrasound of the abdomen may be used to make the diagnosis as well and are characterized by the "whirlpool sign" denoting midgut volvulus. Reversal of the normal position of the SMA and superior mesenteric vein (SMV) may be seen in malrotation, though normal position may be found in up to 29% of patients. Identification of the third portion of the duodenum within the retroperitoneum makes malrotation very unlikely.

Treatment & Prognosis

Surgical treatment of malrotation is the Ladd procedure. In young infants the Ladd procedure should be performed even if volvulus has not occurred. The duodenum is mobilized, the short mesenteric root is extended, and the bowel is then fixed in a more normal distribution. Treatment of malrotation discovered in children older than 12 months is uncertain. Because volvulus can occur at any age, surgical repair is usually recommended, even in asymptomatic children. Laparoscopic repair of malrotation is possible but is technically difficult and is never performed in the presence of volvulus.

Midgut volvulus is a surgical emergency. Bowel necrosis results from occlusion of the SMA. When necrosis is extensive, it is recommended that a first operation include only reduction of the volvulus with lysis of mesenteric bands. Resection of necrotic bowel should be delayed if possible until a second-look operation 24–48 hours later can be undertaken in the hope that more bowel can be salvaged. The prognosis is guarded if perforation, peritonitis, or extensive intestinal necrosis is present. Mid-gut volvulus is one of the most common indications for small bowel transplant in children, responsible for 10% of cases in a recent series.

Adams SD, Stanton MP: Malrotation and intestinal atresias. Early Hum Dev 2014 Dec;90(12):921–925 [PMID: 25448782].
Langer JC: Intestinal rotation abnormalities and midgut volvulus. Surg Clin North Am 2017 Feb;97(1):147–159. doi: 10.1016/j. suc.2016.08.011. Review [PMID: 27894424].

SHORT BOWEL SYNDROME

General Considerations

Short bowel syndrome (SBS) is defined as a condition resulting from reduced intestinal absorptive surface that leads to alteration in intestinal function that compromises normal growth, fluid/electrolyte balance, or hydration status. The vast majority of pediatric patients with SBS have undergone neonatal surgical resection of intestine. The most common etiologies in children are necrotizing enterocolitis (45%); intestinal atresias (23%); gastroschisis (15%); volvulus (15%); and, less commonly, congenital short bowel, long-segment Hirschsprung disease, and ischemic bowel. In many instances, infants with SBS require PN in order to provide adequate caloric, fluid, and electrolyte delivery in the setting of insufficient intestinal absorptive function. The requirement of supplemental PN for more than 2–3 months in the setting of SBS or any other underlying disorder qualifies the diagnosis of intestinal failure (IF).

The goal in management of the patient with SBS is to promote growth and adaptation of the intestine such that adequate nutrition can be delivered and absorbed enterally. Many factors, including patient's gestational age, postsurgical anatomy (including residual small bowel length and presence of ileocecal valve and/or colon), presence of small bowel bacterial overgrowth, and underlying surgical disease, influence the process and likelihood of bowel adaptation and achievement of enteral autonomy. No specific anatomic bowel length measurements offer 100% certainty in predicting clinical outcomes in SBS.

Symptoms & Signs

Typical signs for the patient with SBS are related to their underlying malabsorptive state, including diarrhea, dehydration, electrolyte or micronutrient deficiency states, and growth failure. Patients with SBS are also at risk for small bowel obstruction, bowel dilation and dysmotility (with secondary small bowel bacterial overgrowth), hepatobiliary disorders including cholelithiasis, nephrolithiasis due to calcium oxalate stones, oral feeding challenges, and GI mucosal inflammatory problems including noninfectious colitis and anastomotic ulcerations. For patients with IF, complications related to underlying PN therapy are common and can be life threatening. PN-associated liver disease (PNALD) is a progressive cholestatic liver injury that occurs in pediatric patients on PN and may progress to end-stage liver disease in 10% of affected patients. Recurrent catheter-related bloodstream infections are relatively common in pediatric patients with SBS and IF. Other complication-related central venous catheters including occlusions may require intervention.

Treatment & Prognosis

Goal in management of SBS is to promote growth and adaptation while minimizing and/or treating complications of the underlying intestinal disorder or PN therapy. Intestinal rehabilitation for the child with SBS and IF refers to the multidisciplinary team approach to individual patient care, involving gastroenterology, nutrition, and surgery, and has been shown to improve outcomes. Enteral nutrition should be catered to favor absorption, commonly requiring continuous delivery of an elemental formula through a gastrostomy tube. Commonly prescribed pharmacologic adjuncts include acid suppressive therapy, antimotility and antidiarrheal agents, and antibiotics for the treatment of small bowel bacterial overgrowth. Recently, a glucagon-like peptide-2 analog (teduglutide) has been approved for use in pediatric patients, having been shown to reduce the volume of PN prescribed in patients with IF/SBS. This therapy offers the potential to accelerate intestinal adaptation and PN weaning.

Management for the patient with SBS and IF should include strategies to manage or prevent complications related to PN therapy, including infection and liver disease. Antimicrobial lock solutions distilled into central venous catheters using either ethanol or antibiotics may have a role in reducing infection rates. Compelling evidence over the past several years suggests that modification of parenteral lipid solution, either through reduction in dose of soy-based intralipid or replacement with a third-generation lipid solution (Omegaven or SMOF lipid), improves outcomes associated with PNALD in pediatric patients.

Autologous bowel reconstructive surgery (bowel lengthening) should be considered in a patient who is failing to advance enterally and has anatomy amendable to surgical intervention, typically with regards to adequate bowel dilation. Both the serial transverse enteroplasty (STEP) procedure and longitudinal intestinal lengthening and tailoring (Bianchi) procedure have been successful in allowing weaning from TPN in up to 50% of patients in reported series. In recent years, the STEP procedure has gained favor as being potentially less technically demanding and repeatable, if the bowel dilates sufficiently after the initial procedure.

When medical, nutritional, and surgical managements fail, intestinal transplantation may be considered for a child with refractory and life-threatening complications of IF. Current outcome data after pediatric intestinal transplantation suggest 1- and 3-year survival rates of 83% and 60%, respectively.

Carter BA, Cohran VC, Cole CR, et al: Outcomes from a 12-week, open-label, multicenter clinical trial of teduglutide in pediatric short bowel syndrome. J Pediatr 2017 Feb;181:102–111.e5. doi: 10.1016/j.jpeds.2016.10.027 [PMID: 27855998].

D'Antiga L, Goulet O: Intestinal failure in children: the European view. J Pediatr Gastroenterol Nutr 2013 Feb;56(2):118–126 [PMID: 22820123].

Duggan CP, Jaksic T: Pediatric intestinal failure. N Engl J Med 2017 Aug 17;377(7):666–675 [PMID: 28813225].

Gosselin KB, Duggan C: Enteral nutrition in the management of pediatric intestinal failure. J Pediatr 2014 Dec;165(6):1085–1090 [PMID: 25242686].

Jeppesen PB, Gabe SM, Seidner DL, Lee HM, Olivier C: Factors associated with response to teduglutide in patients with short-bowel syndrome and intestinal failure. Gastroenterology 2018 Mar;154(4):874–885 [PMID: 29174926].

Langer JC: Intestinal rotation abnormalities and midgut volvulus. Surg Clin North Am 2017 Feb;97(1):147–159. doi: 10.1016/j.suc.2016.08.011. Review [PMID: 27894424].

Martinez Rivera A, Wales PW: Intestinal transplantation in children: current status. Pediatr Surg Int 2016 Jun;32(6):529–540. doi: 10.1007/s00383-016-3885-2. Review [PMID: 27033524].

Piper HG, Wales PW: Prevention of catheter-related blood stream infections in children with intestinal failure. Curr Opin Gastroenterol 2013 Jan;29(1):16 [PMID: 22954690].

Soden JS: Clinical assessment of the child with intestinal failure. Semin Pediatr Surg 2010 Feb;19(1):10–19 [PMID: 20123269].

INTUSSUSCEPTION

ESSENTIALS OF DIAGNOSIS & TYPICAL FEATURES

▶ Intussusception is the most common cause of bowel obstruction in the first 2 years of life.

▶ The most common location for intussusception is ileo-colic and 85% of cases are idiopathic.

▶ Ultrasound is the most sensitive and specific diagnostic modality for intussusception.

▶ Air enema is the best therapeutic approach in the stable patient, with successful reduction in 75% of cases.

Intussusception is the invagination of one segment of intestine into another. Intussusception can occur anywhere along the small and large bowel and usually starts just proximal to the ileo-cecal valve and extends for varying distances into the colon. It is the most frequent cause of intestinal obstruction in the first 2 years of life and three times more common in males. Symptoms related to obstruction and ischemia are due to swelling, hemorrhage, vascular compromise, and necrosis of the intussuscepted ileum. In 85% of cases the cause is idiopathic but the likelihood of identifying a cause of intussusception increases with the age of the patient. Implicated primary causes of intussusception include small bowel polyp, Meckel diverticulum, omphalomesenteric remnant, duplication, lymphoma, lipoma, parasites, foreign bodies, and viral enteritis with hypertrophy of Peyer patches. Intussusception of the small bowel can also be seen in celiac disease, cystic fibrosis, and Henoch-Schönlein purpura. In children older than 6 years, lymphoma is the most common cause of intussusception.

▶ Clinical Findings

Classically, a previously healthy infant 3–12 months of age develops recurring paroxysms of abdominal pain with screaming and drawing up of the knees. Vomiting and diarrhea occur soon afterward (90% of cases), and bloody bowel movements with mucus appear within the next 12 hours (50%). The child is characteristically lethargic between paroxysms and may be febrile. The abdomen is tender and often distended. A sausage-shaped mass may be palpated, usually in the upper mid abdomen. In older children, sudden attacks of abdominal pain may be related to chronic recurrent intussusception with spontaneous reduction.

Diagnosis & Treatment

The constellation of abdominal pain, lethargy, vomiting, and a suspicious abdominal radiograph was found to have a sensitivity of 95% in identifying intussusceptions in children. Abdominal radiographs alone, however, are poorly sensitive for the diagnosis of intussusception. Abdominal ultrasound carries sensitivity for diagnosis of intussusception of 98%–100%. Barium enema and air enema are both diagnostic and therapeutic. Reduction of the intussusception by barium enema should not be attempted if signs of strangulated bowel, perforation, or toxicity are present. Air insufflation of the colon under fluoroscopic guidance is a safe alternative to barium enema that has excellent diagnostic sensitivity and specificity without the risk of contaminating the abdominal cavity with barium. Rates of successful reduction by air enema approach 75%. When initial enema reduction is successful, recurrence of intussusception within 24–48 hours occurs in less than 5% of patients. The rate of perforation with either liquid or air enema is approximately 1%. Care is required in patient selection for either air or barium enema because if ischemic damage to the intestine is suspected based on symptom severity (shock or sepsis), the risk of perforation increases and surgical reduction is preferred. Surgery is thus required for extremely ill patients, in patients with evidence of bowel perforation, or in those in whom hydrostatic or pneumatic reduction has been unsuccessful (25%). Surgery has the advantage of identifying a lead point such as Meckel diverticulum, lymphoma, or small bowel polyp. Surgical reduction of intussusception is associated with a lower recurrence rate than pneumatic reduction.

Prognosis

The likelihood of successful reduction by enema decreases if symptom duration is greater than 24 hours. Of those requiring surgical reduction, the risk of subsequent bowel resection increased from 17% to 39% in patients with symptoms greater than 24 hours. Overall mortality rate with treatment is 1%–2%.

Gray MP et al: Recurrence rates after intussusception enema reduction: a meta-analysis. 2014 Jul;134(1):110–119. doi: 10.1542/peds.2013-3102 [PMID 24935997].

INGUINAL HERNIA

Inguinal hernias may present at any age, are most often indirect, and occur more frequently (9:1) in boys. The incidence in preterm male infants is close to 5% and is reported in 30% of male infants weighing 1000 g or less.

Clinical Findings

In most cases, a hernia is a painless inguinal swelling. Parents may be the only one to see the mass, as it may retract when the infant is active, cold, frightened, or agitated. A history of inguinal fullness associated with coughing or long periods of standing, or presence of a firm, globular, and tender swelling, sometimes associated with vomiting and abdominal distention are clinical clues. In some instances, a herniated loop of intestine may become partially obstructed leading to severe pain. Rarely, bowel becomes trapped in the hernia sac, and complete intestinal obstruction occurs. Gangrene of the hernia contents or testis may occur. In girls, the ovary may prolapse into the hernia sac presenting as a mass below the inguinal ligament. A suggestive history often is the only criterion for diagnosis, along with the "silk glove" feel of the rubbing together of the two walls of the empty hernia sac.

Differential Diagnosis

Inguinal lymph nodes may be mistaken for a hernia. Nodes are usually multiple with more discrete borders. A hydrocele of the cord should transilluminate. An undescended testis is usually mobile in the canal and is associated with absence of the gonad in the scrotum.

Treatment

Incarceration of an inguinal hernia is more likely to occur in boys and in children younger than 10 months. Manual reduction of incarcerated inguinal hernias can be attempted after the sedated infant is placed in the Trendelenburg position with an ice bag on the affected side. Manual reduction is contraindicated if incarceration has been present for more than 12 hours or if bloody stools are noted. Surgery is indicated if a hernia has ever incarcerated. Hydroceles frequently resolve by age 2 years.

Esposito C et al: Laparoscopic versus open inguinal hernia repair in pediatric patients: a systematic review. J Laparoendosc Adv Surg Tech A 2014 Nov;24(11):811–818 [PMID: 25299121].
Gause CD et al: Laparoscopic versus open inguinal hernia repair in children ≤3: a randomized controlled trial. Pediatr Surg Int 2017 Mar;33(3):367–376. doi: 10.1007/s00383-016-4029-4 [PMID: 28025693].

UMBILICAL HERNIA

Umbilical hernias are more common in full-term, African-American infants. Small bowel may incarcerate in small-diameter umbilical hernias. Most umbilical hernias regress spontaneously if the fascial defect has a diameter of less than 1 cm. Hernias persisting after age 4 years should be treated surgically.

PATENT OMPHALOMESENTERIC DUCT

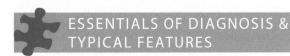

ESSENTIALS OF DIAGNOSIS & TYPICAL FEATURES

▶ Persistent umbilical discharge in an infant may represent a patent omphalomesenteric duct.

▶ Ultrasound is the preferred diagnostic method for patent omphalomesenteric duct.

▶ Surgical excision of the omphalomesenteric remnant is required.

The omphalomesenteric duct connects the fetal yolk sac to the developing gut. This duct is usually obliterated early in embryologic development, but failure of this process can lead to a variety of structures that originate from the embryonic duct remnant connecting the ileum to the undersurface of the umbilicus. If the remnant is patent, it can lead to herniation of intestinal contents into the umbilical cord or lead to fecal discharge from the umbilicus. A fibrous cord may become the focal point for volvulus and resulting intestinal obstruction. Mucoid umbilical discharge may indicate a mucocele in the omphalomesenteric remnant with an opening at the umbilicus. A closed mucocele may protrude through the umbilicus and appear as a polypoid mass that may be mistaken for an umbilical granuloma because it is firm and bright red. Surgical excision of omphalomesenteric remnants is indicated. Ultrasound examination or abdominal computed tomography (CT) can help confirm the diagnosis of an omphalomesenteric duct remnant.

Kadian YS, Verma A, Rattan KN, Kajal P: Vitellointestinal duct anomalies in infancy. *J Neonatal Surg* 2016 Jul 3;5(3):30. doi: 10.21699/jns.v5i3.351 [PMID: 27433448].

Kelly KB et al: Pediatric abdominal wall defects. *Surg Clin North Am* 2013 Oct;93(5):1255–1267 [PMID: 24035087].

MECKEL DIVERTICULUM

Meckel diverticulum is the most common form of omphalomesenteric duct remnant. It occurs in 1.5% of the population and in the majority of cases causes no symptoms. If complications occur, they are three times more common in males than in females. More than 50% of complications occur in the first 2 years of life.

▶ Clinical Findings

A. Symptoms and Signs

Forty to 60% of symptomatic patients have painless episodes of maroon or melanotic rectal bleeding. Bleeding is due to deep ileal ulcers adjacent to the diverticulum caused by acid secreted by heterotopic gastric tissue and may be voluminous enough to cause shock and anemia. Occult bleeding is less common. Intestinal obstruction occurs in 25% of symptomatic patients as a result of ileocolonic intussusception. Intestinal volvulus may occur around a fibrous remnant of the vitelline duct extending from the tip of the diverticulum to the abdominal wall. Meckel diverticula may be trapped in an inguinal hernia.

B. Imaging

Diagnosis of Meckel diverticulum is made with a Meckel scan. Technetium-99m (^{99m}Tc)-pertechnetate is taken up by the heterotopic gastric mucosa in the diverticulum and outlines the diverticulum on a nuclear scan. Giving pentagastrin or cimetidine before administering the radionuclide increases ^{99m}Tc-pertechnetate uptake and retention by the heterotopic gastric mucosa, and can increase the sensitivity of the test.

▶ Treatment & Prognosis

Treatment is surgical and the prognosis for Meckel diverticulum is good.

ACUTE APPENDICITIS

▶ General Considerations

Acute appendicitis is the most common indication for emergency abdominal surgery in childhood. The frequency increases with age and peaks between 15 and 30 years. Obstruction of the appendix by fecalith (25%) is a common predisposing factor. Parasites may rarely cause obstruction (especially ascarids). Most of the remaining cases are idiopathic. The incidence of perforation is high in childhood (40%), especially in children younger than 2 years, in whom pain is often poorly localized and symptoms nonspecific. To avoid delay in diagnosis, it is important to maintain close communication with parents and perform a thorough initial physical examination with sequential examinations at frequent intervals over several hours to correctly interpret the evolving symptoms and signs.

▶ Clinical Findings

A. Symptoms and Signs

Typical patients have fever and periumbilical abdominal pain, which then localizes to the right lower quadrant with signs of peritoneal irritation. Anorexia, vomiting, constipation, and diarrhea also occur. Contrary to the vomiting of acute gastroenteritis, which usually precedes abdominal pain, vomiting in appendicitis usually follows the onset of pain and is often bilious. The clinical picture is frequently atypical, especially in young children and infants. A rectal examination may clarify the site of tenderness or reveal a localized appendiceal mass. Serial examinations are critical in differentiating appendicitis from the many other conditions that transiently mimic its symptoms.

B. Laboratory Findings

The white blood cell count is seldom higher than 15,000/μL. Pyuria, fecal leukocytes, and guaiac-positive stool are sometimes present. The combination of elevated C-reactive protein (CRP) and leukocytosis has been reported to have positive predictive value of 92% for acute appendicitis, although having normal values for both measures does not exclude the diagnosis.

C. Imaging

A radio-opaque fecalith reportedly is present in two-thirds of cases of ruptured appendix. In experienced hands, ultrasonography of the appendix shows a noncompressible, thickened appendix in 93% of cases. Abdominal CT after rectal instillation of contrast with thin cuts in the area of the appendix may be diagnostic. An otherwise normal abdominal CT scan with a nonvisualized appendix has still been reported to have a negative predictive value of 99%. Analysis of diagnostic strategies for pediatric patients with suspected appendicitis has shown abdominal ultrasound, followed by CT scan for negative studies, to be the most cost-effective diagnostic approach compared to CT or ultrasound alone.

▶ Differential Diagnosis

Pneumonia, pleural effusion, urinary tract infection, right-sided kidney stone, cholecystitis, perihepatitis, and pelvic inflammatory disease may mimic appendicitis. Acute gastroenteritis with *Yersinia enterocolitica* may present as pseudoappendicitis in 17% of cases. Other medical and surgical conditions causing acute abdomen should also be considered (see Table 21–7).

▶ Treatment & Prognosis

Exploratory laparotomy or laparoscopy is indicated when the diagnosis of acute appendicitis cannot be ruled out after a period of close observation. Postoperative antibiotic therapy is reserved for patients with gangrenous or perforated appendix. The mortality rate is less than 1% during childhood, despite the high incidence of perforation. In uncomplicated nonruptured appendicitis, a laparoscopic approach is associated with a shortened hospital stay.

Bansal S, Banever GT, Karrer FM, Partrick DA: Appendicitis in children less than 5 years old: influence of age on presentation and outcome. Am J Surg 2012 Dec;204(6):1031–1035 [PMID: 23231939].

Linnaus ME, Ostlie DJ: Complications in common general pediatric surgery procedures. Semin Pediatr Surg 2016 Dec;25(6): 404–411. doi: 10.1053/j.10.002 [PMID: 27989365].

DUPLICATIONS OF THE GASTROINTESTINAL TRACT

Enteric duplications are congenital spherical or tubular structures found most commonly in the ileum but can also be found in the duodenum, rectum, and esophagus. Most duplications do not communicate with the intestinal lumen. Some duplications (neuroenteric cysts) are attached to the spinal cord and are associated with hemivertebrae and anterior or posterior spina bifida. Symptoms of vomiting, abdominal distention, colicky pain, rectal bleeding, partial or total intestinal obstruction, or an abdominal mass may start in infancy. Diarrhea and malabsorption may result from bacterial overgrowth in communicating duplications. Physical examination may reveal a rounded, smooth, movable mass, and barium radiograph or CT of the abdomen may show a noncalcified cystic mass displacing other organs. ^{99m}Tc-pertechnetate scan may help identify duplications containing gastric mucosa. Duplications of the ileum can give rise to an intussusception. Prompt surgical treatment is indicated.

Erginel B et al: Enteric duplication cysts in children: a single-institution series with forty patients in twenty-six years. World J Surg 2017 Feb;41(2):620–624. doi: 10.1007/s00268-016-3742-4 [PMID: 27734079].

▼ DISORDERS OF THE COLON

CONGENITAL AGANGLIONIC MEGACOLON (HIRSCHSPRUNG DISEASE)

▶ General Considerations

Hirschsprung disease results from an absence of ganglion cells in the mucosal and muscular layers of the colon. Neural crest cells fail to migrate into the gut mesodermal layers during gestation, possibly secondary to abnormal end-organ cell surface receptors or local deficiency of nitric oxide synthesis. Ganglion cell absence results in failure of the colonic muscles to relax in front of an advancing bolus. In 80% of individuals, aganglionosis is restricted to the rectosigmoid colon (short-segment disease); in 15%–20%, aganglionosis extends proximal to the sigmoid colon (long-segment disease); in about 5%, aganglionosis affects the entire large intestine (total colonic aganglionosis). Segmental aganglionosis is possible but rare.

Aganglionic segments have normal or slightly narrowed caliber with dilation of the normal colon proximal to the obstructing aganglionic segment. The mucosa of the dilated colonic segment may become thin and inflamed, causing diarrhea, bleeding, and protein loss (enterocolitis).

A familial pattern has been described, particularly in total colonic aganglionosis. The incidence of Hirschsprung disease is 1 in 5000 live births; it is four times more common in boys than girls. A chromosomal abnormality is present in approximately 12% of individuals with Hirschsprung disease.

Mutations in the ret proto-oncogene have been identified in about 15% of nonsyndromic cases. The most common chromosomal abnormality associated with Hirschsprung disease is Down syndrome; 2%–10% of all individuals with Down syndrome may have Hirschsprung disease.

▶ Clinical Findings

A. Symptoms and Signs

Failure of the newborn to pass meconium, followed by vomiting, abdominal distention, and reluctance to feed suggest the diagnosis of Hirschsprung disease. Most children with Hirschsprung disease do not pass stool in the first 24 hours of their life. Enterocolitis manifested by fever, explosive diarrhea, and prostration is reported in approximately 50% of affected newborns. Enterocolitis may lead to inflammatory and ischemic changes in the colon, with perforation and sepsis. In some patients, especially those with short segments involved, symptoms are not obvious at birth. In later infancy, alternating obstipation and diarrhea predominate. The older child is more likely to have constipation alone. Symptoms can include foul-smelling or ribbon-like stools, a distended abdomen with prominent veins and visible peristaltic waves with palpable fecal masses. Intermittent bouts of intestinal obstruction, hypoproteinemia, and failure to thrive are common. Encopresis is rare. On digital rectal examination, the anal canal and rectum are devoid of fecal material despite obvious retained stool on abdominal examination or radiographs. If the aganglionic segment is short, there may be a gush of flatus and stool as the finger is withdrawn. Infants of diabetic mothers may have similar symptoms, and in this setting small left colon syndrome should be suspected. Meglumine diatrizoate (Gastrografin) enema is both diagnostic and therapeutic in small left colon syndrome as it reveals a meconium plug in the left colon, which is often passed during the diagnostic radiograph. The left colon is narrow but usually functional.

B. Laboratory Findings

On rectal suction biopsy samples, ganglion cells are absent in both the submucosal and muscular layers of involved bowel. Special stains may show nerve trunk hypertrophy and increased acetylcholinesterase activity. Ganglionated bowel above the aganglionic segment is sometimes found to contain more than normal numbers of ganglion cells in abnormal locations (neuronal dysplasia).

C. Imaging

Plain abdominal radiographs may reveal dilated proximal colon and absence of gas in the pelvic colon. Barium enema using a catheter without a balloon and with the tip inserted barely beyond the anal sphincter usually demonstrates a narrow distal segment with a sharp transition to the proximal dilated (normal) colon. Transition zones may not be seen in neonates since the normal proximal bowel has not had time to become dilated. Retention of barium for 24–48 hours is not diagnostic of Hirschsprung disease in older children as it typically occurs in retentive constipation as well.

D. Special Examinations

Rectal manometric testing reveals failure of rectoanal inhibitory reflex (**RAIR**), relaxation of the internal anal sphincter after distention of the rectum in all patients with Hirschsprung disease, regardless of the length of the aganglionic segment. In some patients, a nonrelaxing internal anal sphincter is the only abnormality. This condition is often called "ultrashort segment Hirschsprung disease."

▶ Differential Diagnosis

Hirschsprung disease accounts for 15%–20% of cases of neonatal intestinal obstruction. It must be differentiated from the small left colon syndrome by biopsy. In childhood, Hirschsprung disease must be differentiated from retentive constipation, hypothyroidism, intestinal pseudo-obstruction, and other motility disorders. In older infants and children, it can also be confused with CD because of the striking abdominal distention and failure to thrive.

▶ Treatment & Prognosis

Treatment is surgical. Depending on the child's size and state of health, a diverting colostomy (or ileostomy) may be performed or the surgeon may undertake a primary repair. In unstable infants, resection of the aganglionic segment may be postponed. At the time of definitive surgery, the transition zone between ganglionated and nonganglionated bowel is identified. Aganglionic bowel is resected, and a pull-through of ganglionated bowel to the preanal rectal remnant is made. In children with ultrashort segment disease, an internal anal sphincter myotomy, or botulinum toxin injection of the internal anal sphincter may control symptoms.

Complications after surgery include fecal retention, fecal incontinence, anastomotic breakdown, or anastomotic stricture. Postoperative obstruction may result from inadvertent retention of a distal aganglionic colon segment or postoperative destruction of ganglion cells secondary to vascular impairment. Neuronal dysplasia of the remaining bowel may produce a pseudo-obstruction syndrome. Enterocolitis occurs postoperatively in 15% of patients. Recent studies have shown that patients even after surgical correction have an altered microbiome; the role this may play in enterocolitis or other long-term issues for children is still under investigation.

Frykman PK, Short SS: Hirschsprung-associated enterocolitis: prevention and therapy. Semin Pediatr Surg 2012 Nov;21(4):328–335 [PMID: 22985838].

Neuvonen MI et al: Intestinal microbiota in Hirschsprung disease. J Pediatr Gastroenterol Nutr 2018 Nov;67(5):594–600 [PMID: 29652728].

Rintala RJ, Pakarinen MP: Long-term outcomes of Hirschsprung's disease. Semin Pediatr Surg 2012 Nov;21(4):336–343 [PMID: 22985839].

CONSTIPATION

Chronic constipation in childhood is defined as two or more of the following characteristics for 2 months: (1) fewer than three bowel movements per week; (2) more than one episode of encopresis per week; (3) impaction of the rectum with stool; (4) passage of stool so large it obstructs the toilet; (5) retentive posturing and fecal withholding; and (6) pain with defecation. Retention of feces in the rectum can result in overflow incontinence (encopresis) in 60% of children with constipation. Most constipation in childhood is a result of voluntary or involuntary retentive behavior (chronic retentive constipation). About 2% of healthy primary school children have chronic retentive constipation. The ratio of males to females may be as high as 4:1.

▶ Clinical Findings

Infants younger than 3 months often grunt, strain, and turn red in the face while passing normal stools. Failure to appreciate this normal developmental pattern may lead to the unwise use of laxatives or rectal stimulation. Infants and children may, however, develop the ability to ignore the sensation of rectal fullness and retain stool. Many factors reinforce this behavior, which results in impaction of the rectum and overflow incontinence. Among these are painful defecation; skeletal muscle weakness; psychological issues, especially those relating to control and authority; modesty and distaste for school bathrooms; medications; and other factors listed in Table 21–2. The dilated rectum gradually becomes less sensitive to fullness, thus perpetuating the problem.

▶ Differential Diagnosis

One must distinguish between chronic retentive constipation from Hirschsprung disease as summarized in Table 21–3.

▶ Treatment

In children with poor diets increased intake of high-residue foods such as bran, whole wheat, fruits and vegetables, and water may be sufficient therapy in mild constipation. If diet change alone is ineffective, medications may be required. Polyethylene glycol solution (MiraLax™), 0.8–1 g/kg/day, lactulose 1–2 g/kg/day, and milk of magnesia for 2–5 years old: 400–1200 mg/day, 6–11 years old: 1200–2400 mg/day are safe stool softeners in infants and children. Stimulant laxatives such as Senna or Bisacodyl can be considered as an additional or second-line treatment. A recent study showed

Table 21–2. Causes of constipation.

Functional or retentive causes	Abnormalities of myenteric ganglion cells
Dietary causes	
Undernutrition, dehydration	Hirschsprung disease
Excessive milk intake	Waardenburg syndrome
Lack of bulk	Multiple endocrine neoplasia 2a
Cathartic abuse	**Hypo- and hyperganglionosis**
Drugs	von Recklinghausen disease
Narcotics	Multiple endocrine neoplasia 2b
Antihistamines	Intestinal neuronal dysplasia
Some antidepressants	Chronic intestinal
Vincristine	pseudo-obstruction
Structural defects of	**Spinal cord defects**
gastrointestinal tract	**Metabolic and endocrine**
Anus and rectum	**disorders**
Fissure, hemorrhoids, abscess	Hypothyroidism
Anterior ectopic anus	Hyperparathyroidism
Anal and rectal stenosis	Renal tubular acidosis
Presacral teratoma	Diabetes insipidus
Small bowel and colon	(dehydration)
Tumor, stricture	Vitamin D intoxication
Chronic volvulus	(hypercalcemia)
Intussusception	Idiopathic hypercalcemia
Smooth muscle diseases	**Skeletal muscle weakness or**
Scleroderma and	**incoordination**
dermatomyositis	Cerebral palsy
Systemic lupus erythematosus	Muscular dystrophy/myotonia
Chronic intestinal	
pseudo-obstruction	

Modified with permission from Silverman A, Roy CC: *Pediatric Clinical Gastroenterology*, 3rd ed. Philadelphia, PA: Mosby; 1983.

Table 21–3. Differentiation of retentive constipation and Hirschsprung disease.

	Retentive Constipation	Hirschsprung Disease
Onset	2–3 y	At birth
Abdominal distention	Rare	Present
Nutrition and growth	Normal	Poor
Soiling and retentive behavior	Intermittent or constant	Rare
Rectal examination	Ampulla full	Ampulla may be empty
Rectal biopsy	Ganglion cells present	Ganglion cells absent
Rectal manometry	Normal rectoanal reflex	Nonrelaxation of internal anal sphincter after rectal distention
Barium enema	Distended rectum	Narrow distal segment with proximal megacolon

lubiprostone was efficacious and well tolerated in children and adolescents with functional constipation. Lubiprostone is a prostone that, acting locally as a specific activator of chloride channel protein-2 in the GI epithelium, promotes intestinal secretion of chloride ions and fluid, enhancing GI motility. If encopresis is present, treatment should start with relieving fecal impaction. Disimpaction can be achieved in several ways, including medications such as saline enemas, and nonabsorbable osmotic agents such as polyethylene glycol, (1 g/kg/day) and milk of magnesia (1–2 mL/kg/day). Effective stool softeners should thereafter be given regularly in doses sufficient to induce very soft daily bowel movements. After several weeks to months of regular soft stools, stool softeners can be tapered and stopped. Mineral oil should not be given to nonambulatory infants, physically handicapped or bed-bound children, or any child with GE reflux. Aspiration of mineral oil may cause lipid pneumonia. Recurrence of encopresis is common and should be treated promptly with a short course of stimulant laxatives or an enema. Psychiatric consultation may be indicated for patients with resistant symptoms or severe emotional disturbances.

Pärtty A, Rautava S, Kalliomäki M: Probiotics on pediatric functional gastrointestinal disorders. Nutrients 2018 Nov 29;10(12) [PMID: 30501103].

Shin A, Preidis GA, Shulman R, Kashyap PC: The gut microbiome in adult and pediatric functional gastrointestinal disorders. Clin Gastroenterol Hepatol 2019 Jan;17(2):256–274 [PMID: 30153517].

Tabbers, MM et al: Evaluation and treatment of functional constipation in infants and children: evidence-based recommendations from ESPGHAN and NASPGHAN. J Pediatr Gastroenterol Nutr 58(2):258–274, February 2014 [PMID: 24345831].

ANAL FISSURE

Anal fissure is a slit-like tear in the squamous epithelium of the anus, which usually occurs secondary to the passage of large, hard fecal masses, typically at the superior and inferior aspects of the anus. Anal stenosis, anal crypt abscess, and trauma can be contributory factors. Sexual abuse must be considered in children with large, irregular, or multiple anal fissures. Anal fissures may be the presenting sign of Crohn disease in older children.

The infant or child with anal fissure typically cries with defecation and will try to hold back stools. Sparse, bright red bleeding is seen on the outside of the stool or on the toilet tissue following defecation. The fissure can often be seen if the patient is examined in a knee-chest position with the buttocks spread apart. When a fissure cannot be identified, it is essential to rule out other causes of rectal bleeding such as juvenile polyp, perianal inflammation due to group A β-hemolytic streptococcus, or inflammatory bowel disease (IBD). Anal fissures should be treated promptly to break the constipation, fissure, pain, retention, and constipation cycle.

A stool softener should be given. Warm sitz baths after defecation may be helpful. Rarely, silver nitrate cauterization or surgery is indicated. Anal surgery should be avoided in patients with Crohn disease because of the high risk of recurrence and progression after surgery.

CONGENITAL ANORECTAL ANOMALIES

1. Anterior Displacement of the Anus

Anterior displacement of the anus is a common anomaly of infant girls. Its usual presentation in infants is constipation and straining with stool with the introduction of solids. On physical examination, the anus looks normal but is ventrally displaced, located close to the vaginal fourchette (in females) or to the base of the scrotum (in males). The diagnosis is made in girls if the distance from the vaginal fourchette to the center of the anal opening is less than 34% of the total distance from fourchette to coccyx. In boys, the diagnosis is made if the distance from the base of the scrotum to the anal aperture is less than 46% of the total distance from scrotum to coccyx. Often on internal digital examination a posterior "rectal shelf" will be appreciated. In severe anterior displacement, when the anal opening is located less than 10% of the distance from the vaginal fourchette to the coccyx, the anal sphincter muscle may not completely encircle the anal opening and severe obstipation similar to that seen in imperforate anus may occur. Indeed, extreme anterior displacement of the anus may be a form of imperforate anus. Surgery is not needed in most cases. Stool softeners or occasional glycerin suppositories usually relieve straining. This problem improves significantly by age 3–4 years as normal toddler lordosis disappears.

2. Anal Stenosis

Anal stenosis usually presents in the newborn period. The anal aperture may be very small and filled with a dot of meconium. Defecation is difficult, with ribbon-like stools, blood and mucus per rectum, fecal impaction, and abdominal distention. Anal stenosis occurs in about 3 of 10,000 live births, with slightly more males affected. Anal stenosis may not be apparent at birth because the anus looks normal. Rectal bleeding in a straining infant often leads to a rectal examination, which reveals a tight ring in the anal canal. Dilation of the anal ring is usually curative but may have to be repeated daily for several weeks.

3. Imperforate Anus

Imperforate anus typically develops during the fifth to seventh week of pregnancy and occurs in 1 of 5000 live births, slightly more common males. Almost 50% of babies with imperforate anus have additional defects, often in association with a particular syndrome.

Defects are generally classified as low (rectoperineal malformation) where the rectum may not connect to the anus, a membrane may be present over the anal opening, or the anal opening may be narrow or misplaced. A high lesion is classified where the rectum may connect to part of the urinary tract or the reproductive system through a fistula. Infants with low imperforate anus fail to pass meconium. There may be a greenish bulging membrane obstructing the anal aperture. Perforation of the anal membrane is a relatively simple surgical procedure. A skin tag shaped like a "bucket handle" is seen on the perineum of some males below which a stenotic aperture can be seen. The aperture is sometimes surrounded by normal anal musculature, but in many cases the aperture is a rectoperineal fistula and the anal musculature is displaced posteriorly or is absent. Eighty to 90% of patients with low imperforate anus are continent after surgery.

In high imperforate anus, physical examination usually shows no anal musculature. There may be a rectoperineal, rectovesicular, rectourethral, or rectovaginal fistula; hypoplastic buttocks; cloacal anomalies; and sometimes evidence of distal neurologic deficit. It is critical in these cases to fully evaluate the complex anatomy and neurologic function before attempting corrective surgery. A diverting colostomy is usually performed to protect the urinary tract and relieve obstruction. After reparative surgery, only 30% of patients with high imperforate anus achieve fecal continence.

Levitt MA, Pena A: Outcomes from the correction of anorectal malformations. Curr Opin Pediatr 2005;17:394 [PMID: 15891433].
Reisner SH, Sivan Y, Nitzan M, Merlob P: Determination of anterior displacement of the anus in newborn infants and children. Pediatrics 1984;73:216–217 [PMID: 6694879].

CLOSTRIDIUM DIFFICILE INFECTION IN CHILDREN

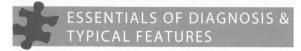

ESSENTIALS OF DIAGNOSIS & TYPICAL FEATURES

▶ *C difficile* in children leads to a spectrum of clinical disease, from asymptomatic colonization to severe pseudomembranous colitis with fever, severe abdominal pain, and bloody diarrhea.

▶ Risk factors for *C difficile* disease include previous antibiotic use and a variety of chronic diseases, including immunodeficiency, cystic fibrosis, Hirschsprung disease, IBD, oncology patients, and solid-organ transplant recipients.

▶ Community-acquired *C difficile* disease in healthy hosts is increasing in incidence.

▶ Pathogenesis

C difficile is a spore-forming gram-positive bacillus that causes human disease via the secretion of enterotoxins that cause necrotizing inflammation of the colon. Interestingly, asymptomatic *C difficile* colonization of the human GI tract occurs commonly in infants and can occur in older children and adults as well. To some extent, *C difficile* may reside in balance with the constituent intestinal microbiome in a health host. Disruption of normal commensal intestinal bacteria or interruption of host immune defense, via intestinal injury or host immune suppression, then appears to give *C difficile* a potential foothold in the human gut where it can lead to disease. Hospitalization is a critical risk factor for *C difficile* disease. Additional risk factors in children include previous antibiotic use and a variety of chronic diseases including IBD, cystic fibrosis, Hirschsprung disease, solid-organ transplant recipients, oncology patients, and immunodeficient hosts. For reasons that are incompletely understood, community-acquired symptomatic *C difficile* infection in healthy children is increasing in incidence.

In recent years there has been an alarming increase in the incidence, morbidity, and mortality of *C difficile* reported in Europe, Canada, and the United States. At least a portion of this increase seems to be due to the expansion of a new strain of *C difficile*, identified as the North American Pulsed Field type 1 (NAP1) *C difficile*, which has been found to have increased toxin production, sporulation, and antibiotic resistance. Surveillance from children's hospitals seems to mirror the increase in incidence of *C difficile* in adults but not necessarily the increase in morbidity and mortality. Pediatric hospitalizations in the United States due to *C difficile* have almost doubled between 1997 and 2006. The NAP1 strain was identified in 19% of *C difficile* isolates in a recent pediatric study.

▶ Clinical Findings

C difficile disease in children represents a spectrum of clinical symptoms, ranging from asymptomatic colonization to persistent, watery diarrhea to pseudomembranous colitis. Recognizing that antibiotic exposure remains a critical risk factor, the onset of colitis ranges from 1 to 14 days after initiation of antibiotic therapy to as many as 30 days after antibiotics have been discontinued. Clindamycin was one of the first antibiotics associated with pseudomembranous colitis, but all antibiotics are now recognized to be potential causes, although erythromycin seems less likely than most. In pediatric patients, amoxicillin and cephalosporins are commonly associated with pseudomembranous enterocolitis, probably because of their widespread use.

The patient with pseudomembranous colitis characteristically has fever, abdominal distention, tenesmus, diarrhea, and generalized abdominal tenderness. Chronic presentations with low-grade fever, diarrhea, and abdominal pain have been described. Diarrheal stools contain sheets of

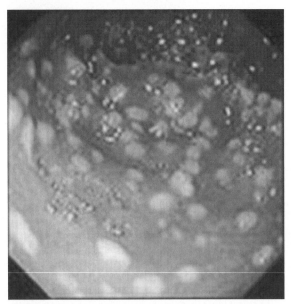

▲ **Figure 21–5.** *C difficile*–associated pseudomembranes. Colonic mucosa is covered with plaques coated with white exudates.

neutrophils and sometimes gross blood. Plain abdominal radiographs show a thickened colon wall and ileus. Endoscopically, the colon appears to be covered by small, raised white plaques (pseudomembranes) with areas of apparently normal bowel in between (Figure 21–5). Biopsy specimens show "exploding crypts or volcano lesion"—an eruption of white cells that appears to be shooting out of affected crypts. Stool cultures often show overgrowth of *Staphylococcus aureus*, which is probably an opportunistic organism growing in the necrotic tissue. *C difficile* can be cultured in specialized laboratories. Identification of stool toxins is the usual method of diagnosis. Use of real-time polymerase chain reaction (PCR) for toxin identification has been replacing more traditional enzyme immunoassay (EIA) methods of stool toxin detection, because of improved sensitivity. Interpretation of *C difficile* diagnostic testing in infants remains controversial because asymptomatic colonization is well recognized in the first year of life.

▶ Treatment

Standard treatment of pseudomembranous colitis consists of stopping antibiotics and instituting therapy with oral metronidazole (30 mg/kg/day) or vancomycin (30–50 mg/kg/day). Vancomycin is many times more expensive than metronidazole and no more efficacious. Metronidazole can be given intravenously in patients with vomiting or ileus. With increasing virulence and antibiotic resistance being reported,

alternative therapies, such as rifaximin and nitazoxanide, are being used and show similar response rates as oral vancomycin. Relapse occurs after treatment in 10%–50% of patients because of exsporulation of residual spores in the colon. Spores are very hardy and may remain viable on inanimate surfaces for up to 12 months. Retreatment with the same antibiotic regimen is usually effective, but multiple relapses are possible and may be a significant management problem. Adjunctive strategies, such as *Saccharomyces boulardii* probiotic therapy, cholestyramine as a toxin-binder, and pulsed courses of antibiotics, have been used for refractory disease. Fecal bacteriotherapy, known popularly as *fecal microbiota transplantation*, is now a widely accepted and effective treatment for the treatment of recurrent *C difficile* infection in adults, and is increasingly being utilized in the pediatric population. As clinical experience increases with this novel therapy, a more accurate understanding of appropriate indications, contraindications, and potential risks may be further realized.

Borali E, De Giacomo C: *Clostridium difficile* infection in children: a review. J Pediatr Gastroenterol Nutr 2016 Dec;63(6):e130–e140 [PMID: 27182626].

Cammarota G, Ianiro G, Tilg H, Rajilić-Stojanović M, et al; European FMT Working Group: European consensus conference on faecal microbiota transplantation in clinical practice. Gut 2017 Apr;66(4):569–580. doi: 10.1136/gutjnl-2016-313017 [PMID: 28087657].

Khalaf N, Crews JD, DuPont HL, Koo HL: *Clostridium difficile*: an emerging pathogen in children. Discov Med 2012 Aug; 14(75):105–113 [PMID: 22935207].

Kim J et al: Epidemiological features of *Clostridium difficile*-associated disease among inpatients at children's hospitals in the United States, 2001–2006. Pediatrics 2008;122(6):1266–1270 [PMID: 19047244].

Toltzis P et al: Presence of the epidemic North American Pulsed Field type 1 *Clostridium difficile* strain in hospitalized children. J Pediatr 2009;154(4):607–608 [PMID: 19324222].

▼ DISORDERS OF THE PERITONEAL CAVITY

PERITONITIS

Primary bacterial peritonitis accounts for less than 2% of childhood peritonitis. The most common causative organisms are *Escherichia coli*, other enteric organisms, hemolytic streptococci, and pneumococci. Primary peritonitis occurs in patients with splenectomy, splenic dysfunction, or ascites (nephrotic syndrome, advanced liver disease, kwashiorkor). It can also occur in infants with pyelonephritis or pneumonia.

Secondary peritonitis is much more common. It is associated with peritoneal dialysis, abdominal trauma, or ruptured viscus. The organisms associated with secondary peritonitis vary with the cause. Organisms such as *Staphylococcus epidermidis* and *Candida* may cause secondary peritonitis in patients receiving peritoneal dialysis. Multiple enteric organisms may be isolated after abdominal injury, bowel perforation, or ruptured appendicitis. Intra-abdominal abscesses may form in pelvic, subhepatic, or subphrenic areas.

Symptoms of peritonitis include abdominal pain, fever, nausea, vomiting, acidosis, and shock. The abdomen is tender, rigid, and distended, with involuntary guarding. Bowel sounds may be absent. Most peritonitis is an acute medical emergency. In patients receiving peritoneal dialysis, peritonitis can be a chronic infection causing milder symptoms.

Leukocyte count is high initially (> 20,000/μL) and later it may fall to neutropenic levels, especially in primary peritonitis. Abdominal imaging can confirm the presence of ascites. Bacterial peritonitis should be suspected if paracentesis fluid contains more than 500 leukocytes/μL or more than 32 mg/dL of lactate; if it has a pH less than 7.34; or if the pH is over 0.1 pH unit less than arterial blood pH. Diagnosis is made by Gram stain and culture, preferably of 5–10 mL of fluid for optimal yield.

Antibiotic treatment and supportive therapy for dehydration, shock, and acidosis are indicated. Surgical treatment of the underlying cause of secondary peritonitis is critical. Removal of infected peritoneal dialysis catheters in patients with secondary peritonitis is sometimes necessary and almost always required if *Candida* infection is present.

European Association for the Study of the Liver: EASL clinical practice guidelines on the management of ascites, spontaneous bacterial peritonitis and hepatorenal syndrome in cirrhosis. J Hepatol 2010 Sep;53(3):397–417 [PMID: 20633946].

CHYLOUS ASCITES

Neonatal chylous ascites may be due to congenital infection or developmental abnormality of the lymphatic system (intestinal lymphangiectasia). If the thoracic duct is involved, chylothorax may be present. Later in life, chylous ascites may result from congenital lymphangiectasia, retroperitoneal or lymphatic tumors, peritoneal bands, abdominal trauma, intestinal malrotation or infection, or it may occur after cardiac or abdominal surgery.

Both congenital and acquired lymphatic obstructions cause chylous ascites, diarrhea, and failure to thrive. The abdomen is distended, with a fluid wave and shifting dullness. Unilateral or generalized peripheral edema may be present. Laboratory findings include hypoalbuminemia, hypogammaglobulinemia, and lymphopenia. Ascitic fluid contains lymphocytes and has the biochemical composition of chyle if the patient has just been fed; otherwise, it is indistinguishable from ascites secondary to cirrhosis. Chylous ascites must be differentiated from ascites due to liver disease

and in the older child, from constrictive pericarditis, chronically elevated right heart pressure, malignancy, infection, or inflammatory diseases causing lymphatic obstruction. In the newborn, urinary ascites from anatomic abnormalities of the kidney or collecting system must be considered. A simple test to diagnose urinary ascites is a urea nitrogen or creatinine concentration of abdominal fluid. Neither of these is present in chylous or hepatic ascites.

Chylous ascites is associated with fat malabsorption and protein loss with resultant edema. Little can be done to correct congenital abnormalities due to hypoplasia, aplasia, or ectasia of the lymphatics unless they are surgically resectable. More recently, somatostatin and fibrin glue have been tried with varying success. Treatment is supportive, consisting mainly of a high-protein diet and careful attention to infections. Shunting of peritoneal fluid into the venous system is sometimes effective. A fat-free diet supplemented with medium-chain triglycerides decreases the formation of chylous ascites. Total parenteral nutrition (TPN) may rarely be necessary. Infusions of albumin generally provide only temporary relief and are rarely used for chronic management. In the neonate, congenital chylous ascites may spontaneously disappear following one or more paracenteses and a medium-chain triglyceride diet.

Densupsoontorn N et al: Congenital chylous ascites: the roles of fibrin glue and CD31. Acta Paediatr 2009 Nov;98(11):1847–1849 [PMID: 19627262].

Moreira D de A et al: Congenital chylous ascites: a report of a case treated with hemostatic cellulose and fibrin glue. J Pediatr Surg 2013 Feb;48(2):e17–e19 [PMID: 23414895].

Olivieri C, Nanni L, Masini L, Pintus C: Successful management of congenital chylous ascites with early octreotide and total parenteral nutrition in a newborn. BMJ Case Rep 2012 Sep 25 [PMID: 23010459].

▼ GASTROINTESTINAL TUMORS & MALIGNANCIES

JUVENILE POLYPS

Juvenile polyps belong to the hamartomatous category of polyps and are usually pedunculated and solitary (Figure 21–6). The head of the polyp is composed of hyperplastic glandular and vascular elements, often with cystic transformation. Juvenile polyps are benign, and 80% occur in the rectosigmoid. Juvenile polyps are the most common type of intestinal polyps in children and occur most commonly between ages 3 and 5 years of age and rarely before 1 year. The painless passage of small amounts of bright red blood with mucus on a normal or constipated stool is the most frequent manifestation. Abdominal pain is rare, but low-lying polyps may prolapse during defecation. Colonoscopy is diagnostic and therapeutic when polyps are suspected.

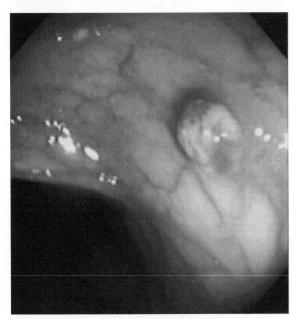

▲ **Figure 21–6.** Juvenile polyp. Solitary, smooth polyp coated with exudate and erythematous pattern that lies on the surface of a normal colonic mucosa.

After removal of a single juvenile polyp by electrocautery, nothing further should be done if histologic findings confirm the diagnosis. Risk of developing further juvenile polyps is low. Other polyposis syndromes are summarized in Table 21–4.

Rarely, many juvenile polyps may be present in the colon, causing anemia, diarrhea with mucus, and protein loss. An individual may be diagnosed with juvenile polyposis syndrome (JPS) if there are more than five juvenile polyps in the colon, multiple juvenile polyps elsewhere in the GI tract, or any number of juvenile polyps with a family history of juvenile polyposis syndrome. JPS does confer an increased risk of colorectal cancer and surveillance with endoscopy is required. Other hamartomatous polyp syndromes include Peutz-Jeghers syndrome and the PTEN hamartoma tumor syndrome. Peutz-Jeghers syndrome is associated with polyps commonly in the small intestine and colon but can also been seen in the stomach and in other organs. A distinctive mucocutaneous pigmentation (freckling) may appear along the vermillion border of the lips, buccal mucosa, and hands and feet but can disappear by age 5. Due to the higher risk of both GI and non-GI malignancies, routine cancer surveillance is necessary. In addition, 50% will develop intussusception at some point in their lifetime and prompt investigation for intussusception is needed in the case of symptoms suggesting intestinal obstruction. Phosphatase and tensin homolog (PTEN) hamartoma syndrome involves a spectrum of hamartomatous conditions that are associated with mutations in the PTEN gene such as Cowden syndrome, Bannayan-Riley-Ruvalcaba syndrome, and Proteus syndrome. Besides hamartomas and other benign tumors throughout the body, an increased risk of intestinal and extraintestinal cancers in those with PTEN mutations exists.

Barnard J: Screening and surveillance recommendations for pediatric gastrointestinal polyposis syndrome. J Pediatr Gastroenterol Nutr 2009 Apr;48(Suppl 2):575–578 [PMID: 19300132].

Thakkar K, Fishman DS, Gilger MA: Colorectal polyps in childhood. Curr Opin Pediatr 2012 Oct;24(5):632–637. doi: 10.1097/MOP.0b013e328357419f [PMID: 22890064].

Zbuk KM, Eng C: Hamartomatous polyposis syndromes: Nat Clin Pract Gastroenterol Hepatol 2007 Sep;4(9):492–502 [PMID: 17768394].

CANCERS OF THE ESOPHAGUS, SMALL BOWEL, & COLON

Esophageal cancer is rare in childhood. Cysts, leiomyomas, and hamartomas predominate. Caustic injury of the esophagus increases the very long-term risk of squamous cell carcinoma. Chronic peptic esophagitis is associated with Barrett esophagus, a precancerous lesion. Simple GE reflux in infancy without esophagitis is not a risk for esophageal cancer. The most common gastric or small bowel cancer in children is lymphoma or lymphosarcoma. Intermittent abdominal pain, abdominal mass, intussusception, or a celiac-like presentation may be present. Carcinoid tumors are usually benign and most often an incidental finding in the appendix. The carcinoid syndrome (flushing, sweating, hypertension, diarrhea, and vomiting), associated with serotonin secretion, only occurs with rare metastatic carcinoid tumors. Colonic adenocarcinoma is rare in childhood. The low 5-year survival rate relates to the nonspecificity of presenting complaints and the large percentage of undifferentiated types. Children with a family history of colon cancer, chronic ulcerative colitis (UC), or familial polyposis syndromes including familial adenomatous polyposis or JPS are at greater risk.

MESENTERIC CYSTS

Mesenteric and omental cysts are rare intra-abdominal masses in children. These cysts may be small or large, single or multiloculated. They are thin-walled and contain serous, chylous, or hemorrhagic fluid. They are commonly located in the small bowel mesentery but are also found in the mesocolon. Most mesenteric cysts cause no symptoms and are found incidentally. Traction on the mesentery may lead to colicky abdominal pain, which can be mild and recurrent but may appear acutely with vomiting. Volvulus may occur around a cyst, and hemorrhage into a cyst may be mild or hemodynamically significant. A rounded mass can occasionally be palpated or seen on radiograph displacing adjacent intestine. Abdominal ultrasonography is usually diagnostic.

Table 21–4. Gastrointestinal polyposis syndromes.

	Location	Number	Histology	Extraintestinal Findings	Malignant Potential	Recommended Therapy
Juvenile polyps	Colon	Single (70%) Several (30%)	Hyperplastic, hamartomatous	None	None	Remove polyp for continuous bleeding or prolapse.
Juvenile polyposis syndrome[a]	Colon, stomach, small bowel	≥ 5	Hyperplastic, hamartomatous, can have focal adenomatous change	None	Up to 50%	Remove all polyps. Consider colectomy if very numerous or adenomatous.
PTEN hamartoma tumor syndrome[a]	Colon, stomach, small bowel	Multiple	Hyperplastic, hamartomatous	Skin, eyes, GU, CNS. Cancers especially for breast, thyroid, and endometrium	16% colorectal cancer risk	Surveillance colonoscopies
Peutz-Jeghers syndrome[a]	Small bowel, stomach, colon	Multiple	Hamartomatous	Pigmented cutaneous and oral macules; ovarian cysts and tumors; bony exostoses	2%–3%	Remove accessible polyps or those causing obstruction or bleeding.
Cronkhite-Canada syndrome	Stomach, colon; less commonly, esophagus and small bowel	Multiple	Hamartomatous	Alopecia; onychodystrophy; hyperpigmentation	Rare	None.
Familial adenomatous polyposis[a]	Colon; less commonly, stomach and small bowel	Multiple	Adenomatous	None	95%–100%	Colectomy by age 18 years.

[a]Autosomal dominant.

Surgical removal is indicated. Malignant transformation of mesenteric cysts has been reported in adults, and therefore surgical removal is indicated even in asymptomatic cases.

Tan JJ, Tan KK, Chew SP: Mesenteric cysts: an institution experience over 14 years and review of the literature. World J Surg 2009 Sep;33(9):1961–1965 [PMID: 19609826].

INTESTINAL HEMANGIOMAS & VASCULAR MALFORMATIONS

GI hemangiomas and vascular malformations are uncommon causes of bleeding. Like their skin counterparts, intestinal hemangiomas are typically not present at birth. They tend to appear in the first 2 months of life, cause bleeding in the first year as they undergo a rapidly proliferating growth phase, and then can involute. Vascular malformations include capillary, arterial, venous, and mixed lesions, and are present from birth with risk of bleeding throughout life. The physically largest subtype of vascular lesion is the cavernous malformation, which may protrude into the lumen as a polypoid lesion or may invade the intestine from mucosa to serosa.

▶ Clinical Presentation

Intestinal vascular lesions are most often found in the small bowel. These lesions may cause acute or occult blood loss or may present as intussusception, intestinal narrowing, or intramural hematoma. Thrombocytopenia and consumptive coagulopathy are complications of rapidly growing hemangiomas. Intestinal vascular lesions are usually found in isolation, but associated syndromes include the Blue rubber bleb nevus syndrome, the Osler-Rendu-Weber syndrome, and the Klippel-Trenaunay-Weber syndrome. The diagnosis of GI bleeding can be challenging, particularly when bleeding is occult or intermittent. Physical examinations are typically not helpful unless there are other skin hemangiomas present in the young child that may point to an intestinal hemangioma. Vascular protocols with CT or magnetic resonance imaging (MRI) may identify larger vascular lesions.

Endoscopic techniques remain crucial to the diagnosis of intestinal vascular lesions. Video capsule endoscopy and small bowel enteroscopy techniques have allowed for diagnosis and potential therapy of small bowel vascular lesions that were previously inaccessible using conventional endoscopy.

▶ Treatment

Vascular malformations of the skin and liver have been treated medically with corticosteroids, propranolol, sirolimus, angiotensin converting enzyme inhibitors, interferon, and vincristine. There is relatively little experience with using these medical techniques for intestinal hemangiomas. Endoscopic techniques for treatment of vascular lesions include banding, submucosal injections of sclerosants, and electrocautery methods. Vascular embolization is a consideration for rapid blood loss in the setting of gastrointestinal vascular malformations. Finally, surgical resection of the vascular lesion and surrounding bowel may be required for lesions in the mid-small bowel that are not accessible by endoscopy or for large lesions that are not amenable to endoscopic therapies.

Yoo S: GI-associated hemangiomas and vascular malformations. Clin Colon Rectal Surg 2011 Sep;24(3):193–200 [PMID: 22942801].

▼ MAJOR GASTROINTESTINAL SYMPTOMS & SIGNS

ACUTE DIARRHEA

Viruses are the most common cause of acute gastroenteritis in developing and developed countries. Bacterial and parasitic enteric infections are discussed in Chapters 42 and 43. Of the viral agents causing enteric infection, Rotavirus and Caliciviridae (Norovirus and Sapovirus) are the most common, followed by enteric adenovirus, and Astrovirus. As with most viral pathogens, rotavirus affects the small intestine, causing voluminous watery diarrhea without leukocytes or blood. In the United States, rotavirus primarily affects infants between 3 and 15 months of age. The peak incidence in the United States is in the winter with sporadic cases occurring at other times. The virus is transmitted via the fecal-oral route and survives for hours on hands and for days on environmental surfaces. Rotavirus had been the most common viral source accounting for between 1/3 and 2/3 of hospitalizations prior to vaccine introduction.

1. Rotavirus Infection

The incubation period for rotavirus is 1–3 days. Symptoms caused by rotavirus are similar to other viral pathogens. Vomiting is the first symptom in 80%–90% of patients, followed within 24 hours by low-grade fever and watery diarrhea. Diarrhea is often preceded by vomiting and usually lasts 4–8 days but may last longer in young infants or

immunocompromised patients. Fever is present in up to a third of patients. Rotavirus and adenoviruses can be detected in feces using EIA or latex agglutination. The specific identification of rotavirus is not required in every case, however, as treatment is nonspecific. Additional laboratory testing is also generally unnecessary but, when obtained, it will usually show a normal white blood cell count. Hyper- or hyponatremia may occur with dehydration. Metabolic acidosis can occur from bicarbonate loss in the stool, ketosis from poor intake, and in severe cases lactic acidemia occurs from hypotension and hypoperfusion. Stools do not contain blood or white blood cells.

As is with most other viral causes of acute diarrhea, treatment is nonspecific and supportive. Replacement of fluid and electrolyte deficits, along with ongoing losses, especially in small infants is necessary. (Oral and intravenous therapies are discussed in Chapter 23.) The use of oral rehydration solutions is appropriate in most cases. The use of clear liquids or hypocaloric (dilute formula) diets for more than 48 hours is not advisable. Early initiation of refeeding is recommended. Intestinal lactase levels may be reduced during rotavirus infection. Therefore, the brief use of a lactose-free diet may be associated with a shorter period of diarrhea but is not critical to successful recovery in healthy infants. Reduced fat intake during recovery may decrease nausea and vomiting.

Antidiarrheal medications are ineffective (kaolin-pectin combinations) and in some circumstances can be dangerous (loperamide, tincture of opium, diphenoxylate with atropine). Bismuth subsalicylate preparations may reduce stool volume but are not critical to recovery and are generally not recommended especially in young children due to the salicylate component and potential risk of Reye syndrome. Oral immunoglobulin or specific antiviral agents have occasionally been useful in limiting duration of disease in immunocompromised patients.

Most children are infected with rotavirus more than once, with the first infection being the most severe. Some protective immunity is imparted by the first infection. Prevention of infection occurs primarily by good hygiene and prevention of fecal-oral contamination. As treatment for rotavirus is nonspecific, prevention of illness is critical. The American Academy of Pediatrics issued guidelines in January 2007 recommending the routine use of bovine-based pentavalent rotavirus vaccine to be given orally to infants at 2, 4, and possibly 6 months of age, depending on which vaccine is used. Prevention is the key, and two rotavirus vaccines are commercially available, which are administered in multiple doses typically from 2 to 6 months of age.

2. Other Viral Infections Causing Acute Diarrhea

Other viral pathogens causing diarrhea in children can be identified in stool by electron microscopy, viral culture, or enzyme-linked immunoassay. Depending on the geographic norovirus and enteric adenoviruses are the next most common viral pathogens in infants. The symptoms of enteric adenovirus infection are similar to those of rotavirus, but infection is not seasonal and the incubation period more prolonged (8–10 days) with more prolonged duration of illness of typically 8–10 days, but up to 2 weeks.

Norovirus is now thought to be the leading source of community acquired diarrhea, and is highly contagious. Recent estimates suggest it is responsible for up to 800 deaths, 71,000 hospitalizations, 400,000 emergency department visits, 1.9 million outpatient visits, and 21 million morbidities annually. Norovirus is a small RNA virus that mainly causes vomiting but can also cause diarrhea in older children and adults, usually in common source outbreaks. The duration of symptoms is short, usually 24–48 hours. Other potentially pathogenic viruses include astroviruses, corona-like viruses, and other small round viruses. There is no FDA-approved assay for norovirus.

Cytomegalovirus rarely causes diarrhea in immunocompetent children but may cause erosive enteritis or colitis in immunocompromised hosts. Cytomegalovirus enteritis is particularly common after solid-organ and bone marrow transplant and in the late stages of human immunodeficiency virus (HIV) infection, but can be seen in patients taking immunosuppressive medication.

Probiotics may be effective in treating acute viral gastroenteritis in healthy children with potential reduction in duration and frequency of the illness. A diversity of opinions exist that range from the Center for Disease Control that states "not recommended" to that from the European Society for Pediatric Gastroenterology, Hepatology, and Nutrition that "strongly" recommends use. Probiotics should be used with caution, however, in immunocompromised or seriously ill children, in particular those with a central venous catheter.

Bernstein DT: Rotavirus overview. Pediatric Infect Dis J 2009 Mar;28(Suppl 3):S50–S53 [PMID: 19252423].

Chiejina M, Samant H: Viral diarrhea. [Updated 2019 Apr 10]. In: StatPearls. Treasure Island (FL): StatPearls Publishing; 2019 Jan: https://www.ncbi.nlm.nih.gov/books/NBK470525/.

O'Ryan M et al: An update on management of severe acute infectious gastroenteritis in children. Expert Rev Anti Infect Ther 2010 Jun;8(6):671–682 [PMID: 20521895].

Shane AL, Mody RK et al: 2017 Infectious Diseases Society of America clinical practice guidelines for the diagnosis and management of infectious diarrhea. Clin Infect Dis 2017 Nov 29;65(12):e45–e80 [PMID: 29194529].

Suez J, Zmaro N et al: The pros, cons, and many unknowns of probiotics. Nat Med 2019;25(5): 716–729 [PMID: 31061539].

CHRONIC DIARRHEA

Bowel habits are variable, making the specific diagnosis of chronic diarrhea difficult. Some healthy infants may have five to eight stools daily. A gradual or sudden increase in the number and volume of stools to more than 15 g/kg/day combined with an increase in fluidity should raise a suspicion that an organic cause of chronic diarrhea is present. Diarrhea may result from (1) interruption of normal cell transport processes for water, electrolytes, or nutrients; (2) decrease in surface area available for absorption secondary to shortened bowel or mucosal disease; (3) increase in intestinal motility; (4) increase in unabsorbable, osmotically active molecules in the intestinal lumen; (5) increase in intestinal permeability, leading to increased loss of water and electrolytes; and (6) stimulation of enterocyte secretion by toxins or cytokines. The most common entities causing chronic diarrhea are listed as follows. Malabsorption syndromes, which also cause chronic or recurrent diarrhea, are considered separately.

1. Causes of Chronic Diarrhea

A. Antibiotic Therapy

Acute and chronic diarrhea is reported in up to 60% of children receiving antibiotics. Only a small fraction of these patients have *C difficile*–related pseudomembranous enterocolitis. Eradication of normal gut flora and overgrowth of other organisms may cause antibiotic-associated diarrhea. Most antibiotic-associated diarrhea is watery, is not associated with systemic symptoms, and decreases when antibiotic therapy is stopped. Data are mixed regarding the use of probiotics, though some suggest their use may decrease the incidence and severity of this diarrhea by helping to restore intestinal microbial balance.

B. Extraintestinal Infections

Infections of the urinary tract and upper respiratory tract (especially otitis media) are at times associated with diarrhea, though the mechanism is incompletely understood. Antibiotic treatment of the primary infection, toxins released by infecting organisms, and local irritation of the rectum (in patients with bladder infection) may play a role.

C. Malnutrition

Malnutrition is associated with an increased frequency of enteral infections. Decreased bile acid synthesis, decreased pancreatic enzyme output, decreased disaccharidase activity, altered motility, and changes in the intestinal flora all may contribute to diarrhea. In addition, severely malnourished children are at higher risk of enteric infections because of depressed cellular and humoral immune functions. Protein-calorie malnutrition can result in villous atrophy, and represent an important cause of malabsorption.

D. Diet and Medications

Relative deficiency of pancreatic amylase in young infants causes osmotic diarrhea after starchy foods. Fruit juices, especially those high in fructose or sorbitol, produce diarrhea because these osmotically active sugars are poorly absorbed. Intestinal irritants (spices and foods high in fiber) and histamine-containing or histamine-releasing foods (eg, citrus fruits, tomatoes, fermented cheeses, red wines, and scombroid fish) may also cause diarrhea.

FODMAPs (Fermentable, Oligo-, Di-, Mono-saccharides And Polyols) are a group of poorly absorbed short-chain carbohydrates that are not uncommonly malabsorbed. Lactose and fructose are classic examples of FODMAPs. Malabsorption of foods higher in FODMAPs can cause symptoms of chronic intermittent diarrhea. It has been implicated as a cause of diarrhea and other symptoms (bloating, gassiness, abdominal pain) in certain individuals with a prior diagnosis of irritable bowel syndrome. Removal of certain FODMAPS from the diet may improve symptoms.

Laxative abuse in association with eating disorders or Munchausen syndrome by proxy can cause unpredictable diarrhea. A high concentration of magnesium in the stool may indicate overuse of milk of magnesia or other magnesium-containing laxatives. Detection of other laxative preparations in the stool or circulation requires sophisticated analysis not available in most laboratories. A high index of suspicion and careful observation may be required to make this diagnosis.

E. Allergic Diarrhea

Diarrhea resulting from allergy to dietary proteins is a frequently entertained but rarely proven diagnosis. GI symptoms from cow's milk protein allergy are more common in infants younger than 12 months.

In contrast to the self-limited cow's milk protein hypersensitivity of infancy, infants and older children may develop more severe diarrhea caused by a systemic allergic reaction. For instance, food protein–induced enterocolitis syndrome (FPIES) is a life-threatening condition occurring during infancy manifested by large-volume diarrhea, acidosis, and shock as a result of an allergic reaction to common food proteins such as milk and soy. Patients require hospitalization for volume resuscitation and strict avoidance of allergens. Reintroduction of allergens should be performed in a controlled setting by an experienced allergist.

Infants and children may develop an enteropathy secondary to milk protein, resulting in flattening of small bowel villi, steatorrhea, hypoproteinemia, occult blood loss, and chronic diarrhea. Skin testing is not reliable since it detects circulating antibodies, not the T-cell–mediated responses that are likely responsible for food sensitivity reactions. Double-blind oral challenge with the suspected food under careful observation is often necessary to confirm this intestinal protein allergy. Small bowel biopsy findings are nonspecific. The diagnosis is often confirmed by either double-blind oral challenge with the suspected food or dietary elimination of the food followed by disappearance of occult blood in the stool and improvement in other symptoms. Consultation with an allergist is recommended for long-term management of patients with this disease.

Anaphylactic, immunoglobulin E (IgE)–mediated reactions to foods can occur in both young and older children. After ingestion, the patient quickly develops vomiting, then diarrhea, pallor, and hypotension. In these cases, radioallergosorbent test (RAST) and skin testing are positive. Food challenges should be undertaken in a setting in which resuscitation can be performed as there is often a progressively more severe reaction with subsequent ingestions. The close association between ingestion and symptoms usually leaves little doubt about the diagnosis.

F. Chronic Nonspecific Diarrhea

Chronic nonspecific diarrhea, also called *toddler's diarrhea*, is the most common cause of loose stools in otherwise thriving children. The typical patient is a healthy, thriving child aged 6–20 months who has three to six loose stools per day during the waking hours. They do not have blood in their stools. They grow normally and may have a family history of functional bowel disease. No organic etiology is found for their diarrhea, with stool tests for blood, white blood cells, fat, parasites, and bacterial pathogens being negative. Diarrhea may worsen with a low-residue, low-fat, or high-carbohydrate diet and during periods of stress and infection. Excessive fruit juice ingestion seems to worsen symptoms. This syndrome resolves spontaneously usually by age 3½ years or after potty training. Possible causes of this diarrhea include abnormalities of bile acid absorption in the terminal ileum, excess intake of osmotically active carbohydrates, and abnormal motor function. A change in dietary fiber (either increasing fiber if deficient or decreasing fiber if excessive), a slight increase in dietary fat, and restriction of osmotically active carbohydrates like fruit juices will often help control symptoms. If these measures fail, loperamide (0.1–0.2 mg/kg/day in two or three divided doses) can be used as needed for symptomatic relief. Cholestyramine has also been used in some cases.

G. Immunologic Causes of Chronic Diarrhea

Chronic diarrhea is common in immune deficiency states, especially immunoglobulin A (IgA) deficiency and T-cell abnormalities. It can be due to an autoimmune enteropathy associated with the immune deficient state or could be due to chronic infection. The infectious causes of the diarrhea include common bacterial, viral, fungal, or parasitic organisms usually considered nonpathogenic (rotavirus, *Blastocystis hominis*, *Candida*), or unusual organisms (cytomegalovirus, *Cryptosporidium*, *Isospora belli*, *Mycobacterium* spp., microsporidia).

Between 50% and 60% of patients with common variable immune deficiency have enteropathy characterized by intestinal villous atrophy. Lymphonodular hyperplasia of the small intestine is also prominent. Patients with congenital or Bruton-type agammaglobulinemia usually have diarrhea and abnormal intestinal morphology. Patients with isolated IgA deficiency can have chronic diarrhea, a celiac disease–like picture, lymphoid nodular hyperplasia, and are prone to giardiasis. Patients with isolated defects of cellular immunity, combined cellular and humoral immune incompetence, and HIV infection may have severe chronic diarrhea leading to malnutrition but often the cause cannot be identified. Chronic granulomatous disease may be associated with intestinal symptoms suggestive of chronic IBD. Specific treatments are available for many of the unusual pathogens causing diarrhea in the immunocompromised host. Thus, a vigorous diagnostic search for specific pathogens is warranted in these individuals. In addition, treatment must be directed toward correcting the immunologic defect.

H. Other Causes of Chronic Diarrhea

Most infections of the GI tract are acute and resolve spontaneously or with specific antibiotic therapy. Organisms most prone to cause chronic or recurrent diarrhea in immunocompetent children are *Giardia lamblia*, *Entamoeba histolytica*, *Salmonella* species, and *Yersinia*. Infection with these organisms requires a small inoculum. Some patients may develop a postinfectious diarrhea, with persistent diarrhea present despite the eradication of the offending organism, either viral or bacterial. Bacterial overgrowth of the small bowel in patients with SBS, those undergoing chemotherapy, or with anatomic abnormalities may experience chronic diarrhea.

Pancreatic insufficiency due to cystic fibrosis or Shwachman-Diamond syndrome may result in chronic diarrhea, typically in conjunction with failure to thrive. Certain tumors of childhood (neuroblastoma, ganglioneuroma, metastatic carcinoid, pancreatic VIPoma, or gastrinoma) may secrete substances such as gastrin and vasoactive intestinal polypeptide (VIP) that promote small intestinal secretion of water and electrolytes. Conditions that result in increased or disordered intestinal motility such as hyperthyroidism or irritable bowel syndrome may also present with diarrhea. Children may present with large-volume, chronic, and intermittent watery diarrhea that does not cease when they discontinue oral feedings.

Dennehy PH: Acute diarrheal disease in children: epidemiology, prevention, and treatment. Infect Dis Clin North Am 2005 Sep;19(3):585–602 [PMID: 16102650].

Grimwood K et al: Acute and persistent diarrhea. Pediatr Clin North Am 2009 Dec;56(6):1343–1361 [PMID: 19962025].

GASTROINTESTINAL BLEEDING

At the first evaluation of a child with GI bleeding history, physical examination, and initial examination are key to identifying the bleeding source. In large-volume, acute GI

Table 21–5. Identification of sites of gastrointestinal bleeding.

Symptom or Sign	Location of Bleeding Lesion
Effortless bright red blood from the mouth	Nasopharyngeal or oral lesions; tonsillitis; esophageal varices; lacerations of esophageal or gastric mucosa (Mallory-Weiss syndrome)
Vomiting of bright red blood or of "coffee grounds"	Lesion proximal to ligament of Treitz
Melanotic stool	Lesion proximal to ligament of Treitz, upper small bowel. Blood loss in excess of 50–100 mL/24 h
Bright red or dark red blood in stools	Lesion in the ileum or colon (Massive upper gastrointestinal bleeding may also be associated with bright red blood in stool.)
Streak of blood on outside of a stool	Lesion in the rectal ampulla or anal canal

bleeding the primary focus, however, should center on stabilizing the patient to ensure adequate hemodynamic support.

▶ History

A number of substances simulate hematochezia or melena (Table 21–5). The presence of blood should be confirmed chemically with guaiac testing. Coughing, tonsillitis, lost teeth, menarche, or epistaxis may cause what appears to be occult or overt GI bleeding. A careful history of the specifics surrounding the bleeding is critical, including the site, volume and color of blood, history of NSAID use, and use of other medications should be ascertained. Inquiry about associated dysphagia, epigastric pain, or retrosternal pain should be made and, if present, suggest GER or a peptic cause of bleeding.

Other important aspects of the history include foreign-body/caustic ingestion, history of chronic illnesses (especially liver/biliary disease), personal or family history of food allergy/atopy, associated symptoms (pain, vomiting, diarrhea, fever, weight loss), and family history of GI disorders (IBD, CD, liver disease, bleeding/coagulation disorder). In the presence of massive upper GI bleeding in the toddler, a high index of suspicion for button battery injury must be maintained despite the lack of any known history of ingestion. Other, more obscure causes of GI bleeding in children include Dieulafoy syndrome and heterotopic pancreas. Table 21–6 lists more common causes of GI bleeding by age and presentation.

▶ Physical Examination

The first objective of the examination is to determine if the child is acutely or chronically ill and initiate supportive

Table 21–6. Differential diagnosis of gastrointestinal bleeding in children by symptoms and age at presentation.

	Infant	Child (2–12 y)	Adolescent (> 12 y)
Hematemesis	Swallowed maternal blood	Epistaxis	Esophageal ulcer
	Peptic esophagitis	Peptic esophagitis	Peptic esophagitis
	Mallory-Weiss tear	Caustic ingestion	Mallory-Weiss tear
	Gastritis	Mallory-Weiss tear	Esophageal varices
	Gastric ulcer	Esophageal varices	Gastric ulcer
	Duodenal ulcer	Gastritis	Gastritis
		Gastric ulcer	Duodenal ulcer
		Duodenal ulcer	Hereditary hemorrhagic telangiectasia
		Hereditary hemorrhagic telangiectasia	Hemobilia
		Hemobilia	Henoch-Schönlein purpura
		Henoch-Schönlein purpura	
Painless melena	Duodenal ulcer	Duodenal ulcer	Duodenal ulcer
	Duodenal duplication	Duodenal duplication	Leiomyoma (sarcoma)
	Ileal duplication	Ileal duplication	
	Meckel diverticulum	Meckel diverticulum	
	Gastric heterotopia[a]	Gastric heterotopia[a]	
Melena with pain, obstruction, peritonitis, perforation	Necrotizing enterocolitis	Duodenal ulcer	Duodenal ulcer
	Intussusception[b]	Hemobilia[c]	Hemobilia[c]
	Volvulus	Intussusception[b]	Crohn disease (ileal ulcer)
		Volvulus	
		Ileal ulcer (isolated)	
Hematochezia with diarrhea, crampy abdominal pain	Infectious colitis	Infectious colitis	Infectious colitis
	Pseudomembranous colitis	Pseudomembranous colitis	Pseudomembranous colitis
	Eosinophilic colitis	Granulomatous (Crohn) colitis	Granulomatous (Crohn) colitis
	Hirzschsprung enterocolitis	Hemolytic-uremic syndrome	Hemolytic-uremic syndrome
		Henoch-Schönlein purpura	Henoch-Schönlein purpura
		Lymphonodular hyperplasia	
Hematochezia without diarrhea or abdominal pain	Anal fissure	Anal fissure	Anal fissure
	Eosinophilic colitis	Solitary rectal ulcer	Hemorrhoid
	Rectal gastric mucosa heterotopia	Juvenile polyp	Solitary rectal ulcer
	Colonic hemangiomas	Lymphonodular hyperplasia	Colonic arteriovenous malformation

[a]Ectopic gastric tissue in jejunum or ileum without Meckel diverticulum.
[b]Classically, "currant jelly" stool.
[c]Often accompanied by vomiting and right upper quadrant pain.
Reproduced with permission from Treem WR: Gastrointestinal bleeding in children. Gastrointest Endosc Clin N Am 1994 Jan;4(1):75–97.

measures as needed. Physical signs of portal hypertension, intestinal obstruction, or coagulopathy are particularly important. The nasal passages should be inspected for signs of recent epistaxis, the vagina for menstrual blood, and the anus for fissures and hemorrhoids. Skin examination should assess for hemangiomas, eczema, petechiae, or purpura. Clinical assessment of vital signs and perfusion should be assessed to establish need for transfusion.

▶ Laboratory Findings

Initial laboratory tests should include a complete blood cell count (CBC), prothrombin time (PT), and partial thromboplastin time (PTT), at minimum. In specific cases, it may be prudent to add a liver profile (with suspected variceal bleeding), erythrocyte sedimentation rate (ESR)/CRP (with possible IBD), BUN/creatinine (for possible hemolytic uremic syndrome). A BUN to creatinine ratio of more than 30 has been shown to indicate a 10-fold increase in the risk of upper versus lower GI bleeding. In patients with Henoch-Schonlein Purpura, a neutrophil-to-lymphocyte ratio of > 2.86 was found to be a predictor of subsequent GI bleeding, with sensitivity of 73% and specificity of 68%. Low MCV in association with anemia suggests chronic GI losses and may warrant addition of iron studies. Serial determination of hematocrit is essential to assess ongoing bleeding. Detection of blood in the gastric aspirate confirms a bleeding site proximal to the ligament of Treitz. However, its absence does not rule out the duodenum as the source. Testing the stool for occult blood will help monitor ongoing losses. In a large study of over 600 cases of pediatric upper GI bleeding, only 4% who were found to have significant drop in hemoglobin levels required transfusion or emergent endoscopic or surgical intervention. In this series, having one or more risk factors, including melena, hematochezia, unwell appearance, and/or large amount of fresh blood in the emesis, had a sensitivity of 100% in identifying the significant bleeds. Elevation of fecal calprotectin levels have been associated with bleeding from both IBD and juvenile polyposis.

▶ Imaging Studies

In infants with acute onset of bloody stools, multiple-view plain x-rays of the abdomen are helpful in assessing for pneumatosis intestinalis or signs of obstruction. Children younger than 2 years with a history and examination suggestive of intussusception should undergo air or water-soluble contrast enema. Painless, large-volume bleeding may prompt performance of a ^{99}Tc-pertectnetate nuclear scan to assess for a Meckel diverticulum. Pretreatment with an H_2-receptor antagonist may be helpful in increasing the sensitivity of this study; however, a negative scan does not preclude the diagnosis. CT scan of the abdomen with oral and IV contrast may be indicated to look for structural and inflammatory causes of bleeding. More recently, CT enterography has been proposed as a useful tool in cases of lower GI bleeding in children. Persistent bleeding without a clear source may prompt consideration of a radioisotope-tagged red blood cell (RBC) scan with ^{99m}Tc-sulfur colloid, though the bleeding must be active at the time of the study, with a rate of at least 0.1 mL/min. Angiography is generally less sensitive, requiring 1–2 mL/min.

▶ Treatment

In severe bleeding, the ABCs of resuscitation should be performed. Adequate IV access is critical in these cases. If a hemorrhagic diathesis is detected, vitamin K and additional blood products should be administered to correct any underlying coagulopathy. In severe bleeding, the need for volume replacement is monitored by measurement of central venous pressure. In less severe cases, vital signs, serial hematocrits, and gastric aspirates are sufficient.

In suspected upper GI bleeding, gastric lavage with saline should be performed, but there is no value of lavage in controlling bleeding. After stabilization, EGD may be considered to identify the bleeding site, and performance of endoscopy has been associated with lower readmission rates after an initial GI bleeding event. A large retrospective study of endoscopy performed for upper GI bleeding in children found that a definitive source for bleeding was identified in 57%, with a suspected source in another 30%. Risk factors for a nondiagnostic endoscopy in this series were a history of bleeding of less than 1 month and a delay of greater than 48 hours between presentation and endoscopy. Acid suppression with intravenous H_2-antagonists or, preferably PPIs, may be helpful in suspected peptic causes of bleeding. A recent randomized trial of pediatric patients with endoscopically treated bleeding compared continuous esomeprazole therapy for 72 hours to second-look endoscopy and bolus esomeprazole and showed them to have no significant difference in rebleeding rates (4.6% vs 6.3%). Colonoscopy may identify the source of bright red rectal bleeding, but it should be performed emergently only if the bleeding is severe and if abdominal radiographs show no signs of obstruction. Colonoscopy on an unprepped colon is often inadequate for making a diagnosis. Capsule endoscopy may help identify the site of bleeding if colonoscopy and upper endoscopy findings are negative. Push or balloon enteroscopy may be helpful to perform therapeutic interventions, obtain biopsies, or mark small bowel lesions (prior to laparotomy/laparoscopy) identified on capsule endoscopy. Use of balloon enteroscopy in conjunction with capsule endoscopy in children with occult GI bleeding has been found to have a diagnostic yield of 95%.

Persistent vascular bleeding (varices [Figure 21–7], vascular anomalies) may be relieved temporarily using intravenous octreotide (1–4 mcg/kg/h) and may be used for up to 48 hours with careful monitoring of glucose homeostasis. Bleeding from esophageal varices may be stopped by compression with a Sengstaken-Blakemore tube. Endoscopic sclerosis or banding of bleeding varices are both effective, with equivalent success rates (87%–89%) and complication rates (10%–19%) between methods. Use of cyanoacrylate for gastric varices in children has been shown to be safe and effective in small, single-center studies.

If conservative measures are ineffective in stopping ulcer bleeding, endoscopic therapy with argon plasma coagulation, local injection of epinephrine, electrocautery, or application of hemostatic clips may be employed. Newer, over-the-scope clips have recently been shown to be safe and effective in pediatric patients as young as 4 years of age and as small as 17.4 kg. Though there are no studies yet published in children, use of hemostatic powder shows promise as effective and less technically challenging then other forms of endoscopic hemostasis. As in adults, use of only one modality in

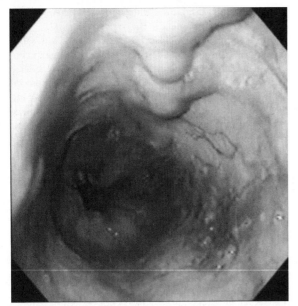

▲ **Figure 21–7.** Esophageal varices. Serpiginous esophageal varix extending to the esophageal lower esophageal sphincter.

nonvariceal bleeding has been shown to increase the risk of rebleeding. If bleeding remains refractory to therapy, emergency surgery may be necessary. Alternatively, endovascular therapy with selective coiling of involved vessels by interventional radiology has been shown to be effective in children with refractory bleeding. A single dose of cyclophosphamide has been shown to be effective in steroid-resistant GIB in Henoch-Schönlein purpura. In some cases, angiography and selective embolization have been used successfully in unidentified and refractory bleeding.

Belei O, Olariu L, Puiu M, et al: Continuous esomeprazole infusion versus bolus administration and second look endoscopy for the prevention of rebleeding in children with a peptic ulcer. Rev Esp Enferm Dig 2018;110(6):352–357 [PMID: 29465250].

Henderson L, Nour S, Dagash H: Heterotopic pancreas: a rare cause of gastrointestinal bleeding in children. Dig Dis Sci 2018;63(5):1363–1365 [PMID: 29468375].

Hong SH, Kim CJ, Yang EM: Neutrophil-to-lymphocyte ratio to predict gastrointestinal bleeding in Henoch: Schönlein purpura. Pediatr Int 2018;60(9):791–795 [PMID: 29947449].

Komissarov IA, Borisova NA, Komissarov MI, Aleshin IJ: Successful endovascular treatment of a 13-month-old child with gastrointestinal bleeding due to Dieulafoy syndrome of duodenum. Radiol Case Rep 2018;13(3):685–688 [PMID: 29682140].

Ramírez-Polo AI, Casal-Sánchez J, Hernández-Guerrero A, et al: Treatment of gastrointestinal bleeding with hemostatic powder (TC-325): a multicenter study. Surg Endosc. 2019 [Epub ahead of print] [PMID: 30820658].

Rao KA, Al-Hakim R, Scagnelli T, et al: Gastroduodenal artery coiling to curb upper gastrointestinal bleeding. J Pediatr Surg 2017;52(10):1699–1701 [PMID: 28756909].

Tran P, Carroll J, Barth BA, Channabasappa N, Troendle DM: Over the scope clips for treatment of acute nonvariceal gastrointestinal bleeding in children are safe and effective. J Pediatr Gastroenterol Nutr 2018;67(4):458–463 [PMID: 29927862].

VOMITING

Vomiting is an extremely complex activity that is triggered by stimulation of chemoreceptors and mechanoreceptors in the wall of the GI tract, activated by contraction and distension. The vomiting center, paraventricular nuclei, in the brain controls the emetic response. These nuclei receive afferent input from abdominal splanchnic nerves, the vagus nerve, vestibulolabyrinthine receptors, the cerebral cortex, and chemoreceptor trigger zone (CTZ). Vagal afferents from the gut to brain are stimulated by ingested drugs and toxins, mechanical stretch, inflammation, and local neurotransmitters. Once the vomiting response is triggered, a pattern of somatic muscle action occurs with abdominal, thoracic, and diaphragm muscles contracting against a closed glottis. The resulting increased intra-abdominal pressure reverses the negative pressure of the esophagus and forces gastric contents upward. The vomiting response also alters intestinal motility by generating a retroperistaltic contractile complex that moves intestinal contents toward the esophagus.

Vomiting is the presenting sign of many pediatric conditions. The most common cause of vomiting in childhood is acute viral gastroenteritis. However, obstruction and acute or chronic inflammation of the GI tract are also major causes. CNS inflammation, increased intracranial pressure, or mass effect may cause vomiting. Metabolic derangements associated with inborn errors of metabolism, sepsis, and drug intoxication can stimulate either the CTZ or the brain directly to promote vomiting.

Control of vomiting with medication is rarely necessary in acute gastroenteritis, but it may relieve nausea and vomiting and decrease the need for intravenous fluids and/or hospitalization. Antihistamines and anticholinergics are appropriate for motion sickness because of their labyrinthine effects. 5-HT$_3$–receptor antagonists (ondansetron, granisetron) are useful for vomiting associated with surgery and chemotherapy. Benzodiazepines, corticosteroids, and substituted benzamides are also used in chemotherapy-induced vomiting. Butyrophenones (droperidol, haloperidol) are powerful drugs that block the D$_2$ receptor in the CTZ and are used for intractable vomiting in acute gastritis, chemotherapy, and after surgery. Phenothiazines are helpful in chemotherapy, cyclic vomiting, and acute GI infection but are not recommended for outpatient use because of extrapyramidal side effects.

DeCamp LR et al: Use of anti-emetic agents in acute gastroenteritis: a systematic review and meta-analysis. Arch Pediatr Adolesc Med 2008 Sep;162(9):858–865 [PMID: 18762604].

Levine DA: Anti-emetics for acute gastroenteritis in children. Curr Opin Pediatr 2009 Jun;21(3):294–298 [PMID: 19381093].

1. Cyclic Vomiting Syndrome

▶ Clinical Findings

Cyclic vomiting syndrome (CVS) is defined as three or more recurrent episodes of stereotypical vomiting in children usually older than 1 year. The emesis is forceful and frequent, occurring up to six times per hour for up to 72 hours or more. Episode frequency ranges from two to three per month to less than one per year. Nausea, retching, and small-volume bilious emesis continue even after the stomach is emptied. Hematemesis secondary to forceful vomiting and a Mallory-Weiss tear (tear or laceration of the mucous membrane at the gastroesophageal junction) may occur. Patients experience abdominal pain, anorexia, and, occasionally, diarrhea. Autonomic symptoms, such as pallor, sweating, temperature instability, and lethargy, are common and give the patient a very ill appearance. The episodes end suddenly, often after a period of sleep. In some children, dehydration, electrolyte imbalance, and shock may occur. Between episodes, the child is completely healthy.

The cause of CVS is unknown; however, a relationship to migraine headaches has long been recognized. Family history is positive for migraine in 50%–70% of cases, and many patients develop migraine headaches as adults. Research suggests that abnormalities of neurotransmitters and hormones provoke CVS. About one-quarter of patients have typical migraine symptoms during episodes: premonitory sensation, headache, photophobia, and phonophobia. Identifiable triggers are similar to migraines and include infection, positive or negative emotional stress, diet (chocolate, cheese, monosodium glutamate), menses, sleep deprivation, or motion sickness.

▶ Differential Diagnosis

Conditions that mimic CVS include drug toxicity, increased intracranial pressure, seizures, brain tumor, Chiari malformation, recurrent sinusitis, choledochal cyst, gallstones, recurrent small-bowel obstruction, IBD, familial pancreatitis, obstructive uropathy, recurrent urinary infection, diabetes, mitochondrial diseases, disorders of fatty and organic acid metabolism, adrenal insufficiency, and Munchausen syndrome by proxy. Chronic marijuana use has been associated with chronic vomiting (cannabinoid hyperemesis syndrome) and can mimic CVS. Although tests for reflux are often positive in these patients, it is unlikely that reflux and CVS are related.

▶ Treatment

Avoidance of triggers prevents episodes in some patients. Sleep can also end an episode although some children awaken and resume vomiting. Diphenhydramine or lorazepam is used at the onset of spells in some children to reduce nausea and induce sleep. Early use of antimigraine medications (sumatriptan), antiemetics (ondansetron), or antihistamines can abort spells in some patients. Once a spell is well established, intravenous fluids may be required to end it. With careful supervision, some children with predictable spells can receive intravenous fluids at home. Several approaches usually are tried before an effective therapy is found. Preventing spells with prophylactic propranolol, amitriptyline, antihistamines, or anticonvulsants are effective in some patients with frequent or disabling spells. Some patients require the additions of the mitochondrial-targeted cofactors coenzyme Q10 and L-carnitine to help manage their vomiting episodes.

Blohm E, Sell P, Neavyn M: Cannabinoid toxicity in pediatrics. Curr Opin Pediatr 2019 Apr;31(2):256–261 [PMID: 30694824].

Boles RG: High degree of efficacy in the treatment of cyclic vomiting syndrome with combined co-enzyme Q10, L-carnitine and amitriptyline, a case series. BMC Neurol 2011 Aug 16;11:102 [PMID: 21846334].

Kovacic K, Sood M, Venkatesan T: Cyclic vomiting syndrome in children and adults: what is new in 2018? Curr Gastroenterol Rep 2018 Aug 29;20(10):46 [PMID: 30159612].

Sorensen CJ, DeSanto K, Borgelt L, Phillips KT, Monte AA: Cannabinoid hyperemesis syndrome: diagnosis, pathophysiology, and treatment—a systematic review. J Med Toxicol 2017 Mar;13(1):71–87 [PMID: 28000146].

ABDOMINAL PAIN

Approximately 2%–4% of all pediatric office visits occur because of unexplained, recurrent abdominal pain. Functional GI disorders have been reported in roughly 10%–30% of children/adolescents and 30%–40% of infants and toddlers. Criteria were published in 2016 in order to incorporate new findings in the literature including new information on gut-brain interactions and microenvironments. The descriptive term "recurrent abdominal pain" has been discarded for the more meaningful terms. Those with pain as a significant component have been termed functional abdominal pain disorder (FAPD) that encompasses several entities: functional dyspepsia (with subtypes of epigastric pain vs postprandial distress), irritable bowel syndrome (characterized by altered form and frequency of stools and improvement with defecation), abdominal migraines, and functional abdominal pain.

▶ Clinical Findings

A. Symptoms and Signs

Children with functional abdominal pain experience recurrent attacks of abdominal pain or discomfort at least once per week for at least 2 months. Functional abdominal pain used to be lumped into a broad category of abdominal pain without a source and without any red flag signs. Classifications of the abdominal pain depend on the characteristics of the pain such as location of pain, association with bowel habits, and associated symptoms. The pain is usually localized to the periumbilical area but may also be more generalized. The pain occurs primarily during the day but may prevent children from falling asleep at night. It may be associated with pallor, nausea, or vomiting, and also with dramatic reactions such as frantic crying, clutching the abdomen, and doubling over. Parents may become alarmed and take their children into the emergency departments, where the evaluation is negative for an acute abdomen. School attendance may suffer, and enjoyable family events may be disrupted.

Alarm symptoms that would suggest a more severe organic etiology are absent. These include dysphagia, persistent vomiting, GI blood loss, associated rashes, or joint complaints, weight loss, stunting, or fevers.

Functional abdominal pain usually bears little relationship to bowel habits and physical activity. However, some patients have a symptom constellation suggestive of irritable bowel syndrome, including bloating, postprandial pain, lower abdominal discomfort, and erratic stool habits with a sensation of obstipation or incomplete evacuation of stool. A precipitating or stressful situation in the child's life at the time the pains began can sometimes be elicited. School phobia may be a precipitant.

A careful and thorough physical examination that includes a rectal examination is essential and usually normal. Complaints of abdominal tenderness elicited during palpation may be inconsistent, out of proportion to visible signs of distress, and distractable.

B. Laboratory Findings

Complete blood count, sedimentation rate, and stool test for occult blood are usually a sufficient evaluation. Extraintestinal sources such as kidney, spleen, and genitourinary tract may require assessment. In the adolescent female patient, ultrasound of the abdomen and pelvis may be helpful to detect gallbladder or ovarian pathology. If the pain is atypical, further testing suggested by symptoms and family history should be done. This may include additional imaging studies or endoscopic analysis. Any concern for lower tract inflammation, and IBD in particular may prompt consideration for the use fecal inflammatory markers such as lactoferrin and calprotectin.

▶ Differential Diagnosis

Abdominal pain secondary to disorders causing acute abdomen are listed in Table 21–7. Pinworms, mesenteric lymphadenitis, and chronic appendicitis are improbable causes of recurrent abdominal pain. *H pylori* infection does not cause

Table 21–7. Differential diagnosis of acute abdomen.

Gastrointestinal causes	Hepatobiliary causes
Appendicitis	Cholecystitis
Bowel obstruction	Cholangitis
Perforated ulcer	Hepatic abscess
Ischemic colitis	Splenic rupture
Volvulus	Splenic infarction
Intussusception	**Urologic/gynecologic causes**
Pancreatitis	Acute cystitis
Incarcerated hernia	Nephrolithiasis
Toxic megacolon	Ruptured ectopic pregnancy
Abdominal vasculitis	Ovarian torsion
Intra-abdominal abscess	Testicular torsion
Other causes	Acute salpingitis
Diabetic ketoacidosis	Pelvic inflammatory disease
Lead poisoning	
Porphyria	
Abdominal sickle cell crisis	

recurrent abdominal pain. Lactose intolerance usually causes abdominal distention, gas, and diarrhea with milk ingestion. At times, however, abdominal discomfort may be the only symptom. The incidence of peptic gastritis, esophagitis, duodenitis, and ulcer disease is probably underappreciated. Though esophageal eosinophilia typically presents with dysphagia and primarily esophageal symptoms in adolescents and adults, it can present with abdominal pain in younger children. Abdominal migraine and cyclic vomiting are conditions with an episodic character often associated with headaches or vomiting.

▶ Treatment & Prognosis

Treatment of FAPD consists of reassurance based on a thorough history and physical examination and a sympathetic, age-appropriate explanation of the nature of functional pain. It is important to acknowledge that the child is experiencing pain. The concept of "visceral hyperalgesia" or increased pain signaling from physiologic stimuli such as gas, acid secretion, or stool is one that parents can understand and helps them respond appropriately to the child's complaints. Another analogy might be to compare a child's abdominal pain to usual headaches that another person may experience, in that the workup can be normal even though there is pain. Reassurance without education is rarely helpful. Regular activity should be resumed, especially school attendance. Therapy for psychosocial stressors, including biofeedback therapy, may be necessary. In specific patients, targeted therapy based on symptoms may be helpful. For abdominal migraines, treatments for migraine headaches may also be of benefit.

Numerous dietary modifications have been proposed as treatment for functional disorders, but data is a lacking as to their effectiveness. For instance, restriction of lactose and fructose and low fermentable oligo-di-mono-saccharides and polyols (FODMAP) diets may benefit some patients, whereas a positive impact of fiber, prebiotics, and probiotics on symptoms has not been shown. Biopsychosocial therapy, cognitive behavioral therapy, and hypnosis may offer benefit.

Likewise, pharmacologic studies of pediatric patients with FAPD have been underpowered and yielded inconsistent results. For instance, peppermint oil has shown benefit in reducing frequency and severity of pain, a finding that may be attributed to inhibition of calcium channels and reduction in colonic spasm. In contrast, although studies examining the impact of antispasmotic medications in adults have shown promise, these have yet to be replicated in children. One prospective study and other retrospective studies suggest efficacy for some patients with the use of cyproheptadine. Studies examining the impact of tricyclic antidepressants, calcium channel blockers, serotonin antagonists, melatonin, and antibiotics have been studied in the treatment of FAPDs have shown no significant improvement on symptoms. Interestingly, pooled data from a recent systematic review examining the placebo effect shows improvement in pain scales in 41% and resolution of pain in 17%.

Beinvogl B et al: Multidisciplinary treatment reduces pain and increases function in children with functional gastrointestinal disorders. Clin Gastroenterol Hepatol 2019 Apr;17(5):994–996 [PMID: 30055266].

Benninga MA et al: Childhood functional gastrointestinal disorders: neonate/toddler. Gastroenterology 2016 Feb 15; [PMID: 27144631].

Chiou E et al: Management of functional abdominal pain and irritable bowel syndrome in children and adolescents. Expert Rev Gastroenterol Hepatol 2010 Jun;4(3):293–304 [PMID: 20528117].

Grover M: Functional abdominal pain. Curr Gastroenterol Rep 2010 Oct;12(5):391–398 [PMID: 20694840].

Robin SG et al: Prevalence of pediatric functional gastrointestinal disorders utilizing the Rome IV criteria. J Pediatr 2018 Apr;195:134–139. doi: 10.1016/j.jpeds.2017.12.012 [PMID: 29398057].

ACUTE ABDOMEN

An acute abdomen is a constellation of findings indicating an intra-abdominal process that may require surgery. When this develops, a high degree of urgency exists to identify an underlying cause. The localized or generalized pain of an acute abdomen intensifies over time and is rarely relieved without definitive treatment. The abdomen may be distended and tense, and bowel sounds are often reduced or absent. Patients appear ill and are reluctant to be examined or moved. The acute abdomen is usually a result of infection of intra-abdominal or pelvic organs, but can also occur with intestinal obstruction, appendicitis intestinal perforation, inflammatory conditions, trauma, and some metabolic disorders. Some of the conditions causing acute abdomen are listed in Table 21–7. Reaching a timely and accurate diagnosis is critical and requires skill in physical diagnosis, recognition of the symptoms of a large number of conditions, and a

judicious selection of laboratory and radiologic tests. (Acute appendicitis is discussed earlier in the section Disorders of the Small Intestine.)

MALABSORPTION SYNDROMES

Malabsorption of ingested food has many causes (Table 21–8). Shortened length (usually via surgical resection) and mucosal damage (CD) both reduce surface area. Impaired motility interferes with normal propulsive movements and with mixing of food with pancreatic and biliary secretions and permits anaerobic bacterial overgrowth. Bacterial overgrowth may lead to increased carbohydrate fermentation and acidic diarrhea. Bacterial overgrowth may also increase bacterial bile acid deconjugation leading to fat malabsorption as seen in intestinal pseudo-obstruction or postoperative blind loop syndrome. Impaired intestinal lymphatic (congenital lymphangiectasia) or venous drainage also causes malabsorption. Diseases reducing pancreatic exocrine function (cystic fibrosis, Shwachman syndrome) or the production and flow of biliary secretions (biliary atresia) cause nutrient malabsorption. Malabsorption of specific nutrients may also be genetically determined (acrodermatitis enteropathica, disaccharidase deficiency, glucose-galactose malabsorption, and abetalipoproteinemia).

▶ Clinical Findings

Diarrhea, vomiting, anorexia, abdominal pain, failure to thrive, and abdominal distention are common. With fat malabsorption, stools are typically bulky, foul, greasy, and pale;

Table 21–8. Malabsorption syndromes.

Intraluminal abnormalities	Graft-vs-host disease
Acid hypersecretion (eg,	Mucosal injury
Zollinger-Ellison syndrome)	Celiac disease
Exocrine pancreatic insufficiency	Allergic enteropathy
Cystic fibrosis	IBD
Shwachman syndrome	Radiation enteritis
Malnutrition	Enzyme deficiency
Enzyme deficiency	Lactase deficiency
Enterokinase deficiency	Sucrase-isomaltase
Trypsinogen deficiency	deficiency
Co-lipase deficiency	Short bowel syndrome
Decreased intraluminal bile	**Vascular abnormalities**
acids	Ischemic bowel
Chronic parenchymal liver	Vasculitis: lupus, mixed
disease	connective tissue
Biliary obstruction	disorder
Bile acid loss (short gut, ileal	Congestive heart failure
disease)	Intestinal lymphangiectasia
Bile acid deconjugation by	**Metabolic genetic disease**
bacterial overgrowth	Abetalipoproteinemia
Mucosal abnormalities	Congenital secretory diarrhea
Infection (eg, *Giardia*,	Lysinuric protein intolerance
Cryptosporidium)	Cystinosis

in contrast, osmotic diarrhea stools are loose, watery, and acidic. Stool microscopic examination for neutral fat (pancreatic insufficiency as in cystic fibrosis) and fatty acids (as in mucosal injury, liver disease) may be useful.

Fat-soluble vitamin deficiency occurs with long-standing fat malabsorption and is manifested by prolonged PT (vitamin K) and low levels of serum carotene (vitamin A), vitamin E, and 25-hydroxy vitamin D. Loss of serum proteins is suggested by elevated fecal α1-antitrypsin levels. Disaccharide or monosaccharide malabsorption manifests by acidic stool with pH less than 5.5 due to lactic acid and reducing substances. Specific enzyme deficiencies may be evaluated by breath hydrogen test, or specific disaccharidase activity measurement from small intestinal biopsy. Other screening tests suggesting a specific diagnosis include sweat chloride concentration (cystic fibrosis), intestinal mucosal biopsy (celiac disease, lymphangiectasia, IBD), liver and gallbladder function tests, and fecal elastase. Common disorders associated with malabsorption in pediatric patients are detailed below.

1. Protein-Losing Enteropathy

Loss of plasma proteins into the GI tract occurs in association with intestinal inflammation, intestinal graft-versus-host disease, acute and chronic intestinal infections, venous and lymphatic obstruction or malformations, and intestinal malignancy (Table 21–9). Chronic elevation of venous

Table 21–9. Disorders associated with protein-losing enteropathy.

Cardiac disease
Congestive heart failure
Constrictive pericarditis
Cardiomyopathy
Post-Fontan procedure with elevated right atrial pressure
Lymphatic disease
Primary congenital lymphangiectasia
Secondary lymphangiectasia
Malrotation
Malignancy: lymphoma, retroperitoneal tumor
Other: sarcoid, arsenic poisoning
Inflammation
Giant hypertrophic gastritis (Ménétrier disease), often secondary to cytomegalovirus infection or *Helicobacter pylori*
Infection: TB, *Clostridium difficile*, parasite (eg, *Giardia*), bacteria (eg, *Salmonella*)
Allergic enteropathy
Celiac disease
Radiation enteritis
Graft-vs-host disease
Inflammatory bowel disease
Hirschsprung disease
Necrotizing enterocolitis
Vascular disorders
Systemic lupus erythematosus and mixed connective tissue disorder

pressure in children with the Fontan procedure and elevated right-sided heart pressures may produce protein-losing enteropathy.

▶ **Clinical Findings**

Signs and symptoms are mainly caused by hypoproteinemia or fat malabsorption: edema, ascites, poor weight gain, anemia, lymphopenia, and fat-soluble vitamins (A, D, E, K) and mineral deficiencies. Serum albumin and globulins may be decreased. Fecal α_1-antitrypsin is elevated (> 3 mg/g dry weight stool; slightly higher in breast-fed infants). In the presence of intestinal bleeding, fecal α_1-antitrypsin measurements are falsely high.

▶ **Differential Diagnosis**

Hypoalbuminemia may be due to increased catabolism, poor protein intake, impaired hepatic protein synthesis, or congenital malformations of lymphatics outside the GI tract, and protein losses in the urine from nephritis and nephrotic syndrome.

▶ **Treatment**

Albumin infusion, diuretics, and a high-protein, low-fat diet may control symptoms. Nutritional deficiencies should be corrected, and the underlying cause treated.

2. Celiac Disease (Gluten Enteropathy)

Celiac disease (CD) is an immune-mediated enteropathy triggered by gluten, a protein in wheat, rye, and barley. CD presents any time after gluten is introduced in the diet. Disease frequency approaches 1 in 100. Risk factors include type 1 diabetes (4%–10%), Down syndrome (5%–12%), Turner syndrome (4%–8%), IgA deficiency (2%–8%), autoimmune thyroiditis (8%), and family history of CD (5%–10%). Almost all CD patients express HLA-DQ2 or DQ8 tissue antigens.

▶ **Clinical Findings**

A. Symptoms and Signs

1. Gastrointestinal manifestations—In the classic form of CD, GI symptoms begin soon after gluten-containing foods are introduced in the diet, between 6 and 24 months of age. Chronic diarrhea, abdominal distention, irritability, anorexia, vomiting, and poor weight gain are typical. Celiac crisis, with dehydration, hypotension, hypokalemia, and explosive diarrhea, is rare. Older children may have oral ulcers, chronic abdominal pain, vomiting, diarrhea or constipation, and bloating.

2. Nongastrointestinal manifestations—Adolescents with CD may present with delayed puberty or short stature, and females with delayed menarche. CD should be considered in children with unexplained iron-deficiency anemia, decreased bone mineral density, elevated liver function enzymes, arthritis, epilepsy with cerebral calcifications, or intensely pruritic rash typically on the elbows, forearms, and knees suggestive of dermatitis herpetiformis. The benefit of early screening and treatment in asymptomatic individuals is unclear.

B. Laboratory Findings

1. Serologic and genetic testing—Patients over 2 years old who are suspected of celiac disease should be screened with serum IgA and tissue transglutaminase (TTG) IgA, which is highly sensitive and specific. In children under 2 years old, the deamidated gliadin peptide IgG should also be sent. In IgA deficiency, the deamidated gliadin peptide IgG or the IgG-based versions of the TTG or antiendomysial antibodies should also be sent. Testing for HLA-DQ2 and DQ8 has a high negative predictive value, and family members who test negative are unlikely to ever develop CD.

2. Stools—May have partially digested fat or be acidic.

3. Hypoalbuminemia—Can be severe enough to lead to edema.

4. Anemia—Low MCV and evidence of iron deficiency is common.

5. Insufficient Hepatitis B surface Ab after immunization—Up to 30%–70% of patients with CD are estimated to be non-responsive to hepatitis B vaccination before treatment with gluten-free diet.

C. Biopsy Findings

Characteristic duodenal biopsy findings on light microscopy are oftentimes patchy villous atrophy with increased numbers of intraepithelial lymphocytes.

▶ Differential Diagnosis

The differential diagnosis includes food allergy, non-celiac gluten sensitivity, Crohn disease, postinfectious diarrhea, primary lactose intolerance, functional abdominal pain, irritable bowel syndrome, immunodeficiencies, and graft-versus-host disease.

▶ Treatment

A. Diet

Treatment is strict dietary gluten restriction for life. All sources of wheat, rye, and barley are eliminated. Most, but not all, patients tolerate oats as long as the manufacturer takes precautions to avoid cross-contamination in processing. The intestinal mucosa improves after 6–12 months of treatment while secondary lactose intolerance resolves within a few weeks. Supplemental calories, vitamins, and minerals are indicated only in the acute phase. CD-related antibody titers decrease on a gluten-free diet, but may take 12 months or longer to normalize.

▶ Prognosis

Adherence to gluten-free diet is difficult and difficult to assess, but is associated with regrowth of villi, resolution of symptoms, and normal life. Individuals with poor adherence to gluten-free diet may be at increased risk for fractures, iron deficiency anemia, infertility, and enteropathy-associated T-cell lymphoma.

Celiac Disease Foundation: www.celiac.org. Beyond Celiac: www.beyondceliac.org.

Hill ID et al: NASPGHAN clinical report on the diagnosis and treatment of gluten-related disorders. J Pediatr Gastroenterol Nutr 2016;63:156–165 [PMID: 27035374].

Snyder J et al: Evidence-informed expert recommendations for the management of celiac disease in children. Pediatrics 2016;138(3):e20153147 [PMID: 27565547].

3. Carbohydrate Malabsorption

Carbohydrate malabsorption is typically a nonimmune-mediated intolerance to dietary carbohydrates due to a deficiency in an enzyme or transporter, or due to excess consumption overloading a functional transporter. These systems are located on the small bowel epithelial brush border. The non-absorbed molecules cause osmotic diarrhea and are fermented in the gut producing gas. As a result, clinical symptoms include abdominal distention, bloating, flatulence, abdominal discomfort, nausea, and watery diarrhea. Stools will test positive for reducing substances, except for sucrose, which is not a reducing sugar.

Berni Canani R et al: Diagnosing and treating intolerance to carbohydrates in children. Nutrients 2016;8:157 [PMID: 26978392].

A. Disaccharidase Deficiency

Starches and the disaccharides sucrose and lactose are the most important dietary carbohydrates. Dietary disaccharides and the oligosaccharide products of pancreatic amylase action on starch require hydrolysis by intestinal brush border disaccharidases for absorption. Disaccharidase levels are highest in the jejunum and proximal ileum. Characteristics of primary disaccharidase deficiency include permanent disaccharide intolerance, absence of intestinal injury, and frequent positive family history.

B. Lactase Deficiency

All human ethnic groups are lactase-sufficient at birth making congenital lactase deficiency extremely rare. Genetic or familial lactase deficiency appears after 5 years of age. Genetic lactase deficiency develops in virtually all Asians, Alaskan natives, Native Americans, 80% of Africans, 70% of African Americans, and 30%–60% of Caucasian Americans. Transient or secondary lactase deficiency caused by mucosal injury such as an acute viral gastroenteritis is common and resolves within a few weeks. Lactose ingestion in lactase deficient individuals causes variable degrees of diarrhea, abdominal distention, flatus, and abdominal pain. Stools are liquid or frothy and acidic, and may test positive for reducing substances. Diagnostic tests include genetic testing and lactose breath test. Symptoms resolve with dietary avoidance of lactose or with lactase supplementation.

C. Sucrase-Isomaltase Deficiency

This condition is inherited in a rare autosomal recessive fashion and found most commonly in Greenland, Iceland, and among Alaskan natives. Infants may present with abdominal distention, failure to thrive, and watery, acidic diarrhea. Diagnosis is made by oral sucrose breath hydrogen testing (1 g/kg), or by testing a snap frozen intestinal biopsy for enzyme activity. Treatment is avoidance of sucrose and starches rich in amylopectin, or the use of sacrosidase enzyme supplement.

CSID parent support group: www.csidinfo.com.
QOL Medical, LLC: www.sucraid.net.
Treem WR: Clinical aspects and treatment of congenital sucrose-isomaltase deficiency. J Pediatr Gastroenterol Nutr 2012;55(Suppl 2):S7–S13 [PMID: 23103658].

4. Monosaccharide Malabsorption

The most important monosaccharides are fructose, glucose, and galactose.

A. Glucose-Galactose Malabsorption

Glucose-galactose malabsorption is a rare disorder in which the sodium-glucose transport protein is defective. Transport of glucose in the intestinal epithelium and renal tubule is impaired. Diarrhea begins with the first feedings, accompanied by reducing sugar in the stool and acidosis. Glycosuria and aminoaciduria may occur and the glucose tolerance test is abnormal. Small bowel histology appears normal. Diarrhea subsides promptly on withdrawal of glucose and galactose from the diet and is mandatory treatment for the congenital disease. The acquired, transient form of glucose-galactose malabsorption occurs mainly in infants younger than 6 months, usually following acute viral or bacterial enteritis, and may require PN until healing. A carbohydrate-free base formula is used with added fructose. Prognosis is good if diagnosed early. Tolerance for glucose and galactose improves with age.

B. Dietary Fructose Intolerance

Fructose malabsorption occurs when fructose is in excess of glucose, often with consumption of high-fructose corn syrup. Malabsorbed fructose leads to symptoms such as abdominal pain, bloating, flatulence, and diarrhea. Diagnosis is made with a fructose breath hydrogen test.

C. Intestinal Lymphangiectasia

This form of protein-losing enteropathy results from obstruction of intestinal lymphatics and leakage of lymph into the bowel lumen. Congenital lymphangiectasia is associated with abnormalities of the lymphatics in the extremities. Malrotation with volvulus can also cause intestinal lymphangiectasia.

▶ Clinical Findings

Peripheral edema, diarrhea, abdominal distention, chylous effusions, and repeated infections are common. Laboratory findings include low calcium, magnesium, albumin, immunoglobulin levels, lymphocytopenia, and anemia and elevated fecal α_1-antitrypsin. Imaging may show bowel wall edema, and biopsy may reveal dilated lacteals in the villi and lamina propria. If only the lymphatics of the deeper layers of bowel or intestinal mesenteries are involved, laparotomy may be necessary to establish the diagnosis. Capsule endoscopy shows diagnostic brightness secondary to the fat-filled lacteals.

▶ Differential Diagnosis

Causes of protein losing enteropathy should be considered.

▶ Treatment & Prognosis

A high-protein diet (6–7 g/kg/day may be needed) enriched with medium-chain triglycerides as a fat source usually allows for adequate nutrition and growth. Vitamin and calcium supplements should be given. Parenteral nutritional supplementation may be needed temporarily. Surgery may be curative if the lesion is localized to a small area of the bowel or in cases of constrictive pericarditis or obstructing tumors. IV albumin and immune globulin may be needed but usually not chronically. The serum albumin may not normalize. The prognosis is not favorable, although remission may occur with age. Malignant degeneration of the abnormal lymphatics may occur, and intestinal B-cell lymphoma may develop.

5. Cow's Milk Protein Intolerance

Milk protein intolerance refers to nonallergic food sensitivity and is more common in males than females and in young infants with a family history of atopy. The estimated prevalence is 0.5%–1.0%. Symptoms may occur while an infant is still exclusively breast-fed. The most commonly heard history reports a healthy, well appearing infant, who when fed formula or breast milk with cow's milk protein, develops flecks of blood in the stool or loose mucoid, blood streaked stools. A family history of atopy is common but skin testing is not reliable or indicated since this is not thought to be an IgE-mediated disease. Removal of cow's milk protein is the treatment. Maternal avoidance of milk protein will usually suffice if breast-fed. If formula-fed, substituting a protein hydrolysate formula for cow's milk–based formula is indicated. Allergic colitis in young infants is self-limited, usually disappearing by 8–12 months of age. Since no long-term consequences of this problem have been identified, when symptoms are mild and the infant is thriving, no treatment may be needed. Histology, not required for diagnosis, shows mild lymphonodular hyperplasia, mucosal edema, and eosinophilia on rectal biopsy.

In older children, milk protein sensitivity may induce eosinophilic gastroenteritis with protein-losing enteropathy, iron deficiency, hypoalbuminemia, and hypogammaglobulinemia. A celiac-like syndrome with villous atrophy, malabsorption, hypoalbuminemia, occult blood in the stool, and anemia can occur.

Sacnhez-Garcia S et al: Food allergy in childhood. Pediatric Allergy Immunol 2015;26(8):711–720 [PMID: 26595763].

6. Pancreatic Insufficiency

The most common cause of pancreatic exocrine insufficiency in childhood is cystic fibrosis. Decreased secretion of pancreatic digestive enzymes is caused by obstruction of the exocrine ducts by thick secretions, which destroys pancreatic acinar cells. Other conditions associated with exocrine pancreatic insufficiency are discussed in Chapter 22.

7. Other Genetic Disorders Causing Malabsorption

A. Abetalipoproteinemia

Abetalipoproteinemia is a rare autosomal recessive condition in which the secretion of triglyceride-rich lipoproteins from the small intestine (chylomicrons) and liver (very low-density lipoproteins) is limited or absent. Profound steatosis of intestinal enterocytes (and hepatocytes) and severe fat malabsorption occur. Deficiencies of fat-soluble vitamins develop with neurologic complications of vitamin E deficiency and atypical retinitis pigmentosa. Serum cholesterol level is very low, and red cell membrane lipids are abnormal, causing acanthosis of red blood cells, two findings that may be the key to diagnosis.

B. Acrodermatitis Enteropathica

Acrodermatitis enteropathica is an autosomal recessive condition in which the intestine has a selective inability to absorb zinc. The condition usually becomes obvious at the time of weaning from breast-feeding and is characterized by rash on the extremities, rashes around the body orifices, eczema, profound failure to thrive, steatorrhea, diarrhea, and immune deficiency. Zinc supplementation by mouth results in rapid improvement.

INFLAMMATORY BOWEL DISEASE

▶ General Considerations

IBD, a chronic relapsing inflammatory disease, is most commonly differentiated into Crohn disease (CrD) and ulcerative colitis (UC). The etiology is multifactorial, involving a complex interaction of environmental and genetic factors leading to maladaptive immune responses to flora in the GI tract. With 5%–30% of patients identifying a family member with IBD, and a 10–20 relative risk of a sibling developing IBD, a genetic association is certain in most. Very early onset IBD, before age 2, is more likely to be monogenic and severe.

▶ Clinical Findings

A. Symptoms and Signs

Inflammation causes abdominal pain, diarrhea, bloody stools, fever, anorexia, fatigue, and weight loss. CrD may also present as a stricturing process with abdominal pain and intestinal obstruction, or as a penetrating/fistulizing form with abscess, perianal disease, or symptoms similar to acute appendicitis. UC usually presents with abdominal pain and bloody diarrhea.

CrD can affect any part of the GI tract from lips to anus. Childhood CrD most often affects the terminal ileum and colon. UC is limited to the colon, and in children it usually involves the entire colon (pancolitis). The younger the age at onset, the more severe the course is likely to be.

Extraintestinal manifestations are common in both forms of IBD and may precede the intestinal complaints. These include uveitis, recurrent oral aphthous ulcers, arthritis, growth and pubertal delay, liver involvement (typically primary sclerosing cholangitis), rash (erythema nodosa and pyoderma gangrenosum), and iron deficiency anemia.

B. Diagnostic Testing

Diagnosis is based on symptoms, relapsing course, radiographic, endoscopic, and histologic findings, and exclusion of other disorders. No single test is diagnostic. Patients often have low hemoglobin, iron, and serum albumin levels, and elevated ESR and CRP and fecal calprotectin. IBD-related serum antibodies are frequently present; antibodies to *Saccharomyces cerevisiae* (ASCA) in 60% of CrD, and perinuclear antineutrophil cytoplasmic antibodies (pANCAs) in 70% of UC. These, and other IBD-related antibodies, may be helpful in differentiating CrD from UC, but they are neither sensitive nor specific enough to be diagnostic. Abdominal imaging with CT, magnetic resonance enterography, US, and video capsule may reveal small bowel disease and exclude other etiologies. Findings include thickening of the bowel wall, stricturing, mucosal ulceration, enteric fistulas, and mucosal and mural edema.

Upper endoscopy and ileocolonoscopy are the most useful diagnostic modalities, revealing severity and extent of upper intestinal, ileal, and colonic involvement. Granulomas are found in 25%–50% of CrD cases. Deep linear ulcers, white exudate (Figure 21–8), aphthous lesions (Figure 21–9), patchy involvement, and perianal disease suggest CrD. Superficial and continuous involvement of the colon sparing the upper GI tract are most consistent with UC. Both forms of IBD may have mild gastritis.

▶ Differential Diagnosis

When extraintestinal symptoms predominate, CrD can be mistaken for rheumatoid arthritis, systemic lupus erythematosus or other vasculitides, CD, or hypopituitarism. The acute onset of ileocolitis may be mistaken for intestinal obstruction,

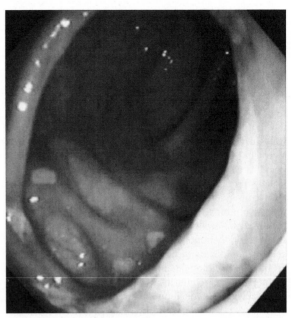

▲ **Figure 21–9.** Crohn colitis. Discrete aphthous lesions are scattered across a thickened mucosa with some areas with normal vascular pattern.

appendicitis, lymphoma, infectious diarrhea. Malabsorption symptoms suggest CD, peptic ulcer, *Giardia*, food protein allergy, anorexia nervosa, or growth failure from endocrine causes. Perianal disease may suggest child abuse. Crampy diarrhea and blood in the stool can also occur with infection such as *Shigella*, *Salmonella*, *Yersinia*, *Campylobacter*, *E histolytica*, enteroinvasive *E coli* (*E coli* O157), *Aeromonas hydrophila*, *C difficile*, and, if immunocompromised, CMV. Mild IBD mimics irritable bowel syndrome, or lactose intolerance. Consider Behçet disease if there are deep intestinal ulcers, oral aphthous ulcerations along with at least two of the following: genital ulcers, synovitis, posterior uveitis, meningoencephalitis, and pustular vasculitis. Chronic granulomatous disease and sarcoidosis also cause granulomas.

▶ Complications

A. Crohn Disease

Nutritional complications include failure to thrive, short stature, decreased bone mineralization, and specific nutrient deficiencies, including iron, calcium, zinc, vitamin B_{12}, and vitamin D. Prolonged corticosteroid therapy may impact growth and bone mineral density. Intestinal obstruction, fistulae, abdominal abscess, perianal disease, pyoderma gangrenosum, arthritis, and amyloidosis occur. Crohn colitis increases risk for colon adenocarcinoma.

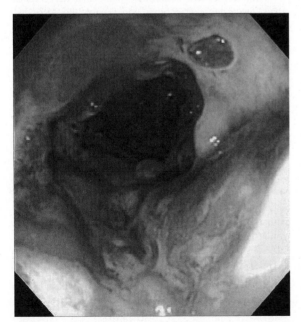

▲ **Figure 21–8.** Ulcerative colitis. White exudate is present overlying an abnormal colonic mucosa that has lost its typical vascular pattern.

B. Ulcerative Colitis

Even with the typical presentation of UC, up to 35% will develop CrD. Arthritis, uveitis, pyoderma gangrenosum, and malnutrition can occur. Growth failure and delayed puberty are less common than in CrD, while liver disease (chronic active hepatitis, sclerosing cholangitis) is more common. Adenocarcinoma of the colon occurs with an incidence of 1%–2% per year after the first 7–8 years of disease in patients with pancolitis and is significantly higher in patients with UC and sclerosing cholangitis.

▶ Treatment

A. Medical Treatment

Therapy for pediatric IBD involves induction of remission, maintenance of remission, and addressing nutritional deficiencies to promote normal growth and development. Treatment includes diet, anti-inflammatory, immunomodulatory, antidiarrheal, antibiotic, and biological options. No medical therapy is uniformly effective in all patients. In severe CrD, growth hormone may be needed to attain full height potential.

1. Diet—Enteral nutrition with liquid formula providing more than 85% of caloric needs is an effective therapy for induction and maintenance for CrD and promotes linear growth. Diet therapies are less effective in UC. Ensuring adequate nutrition for replenishing deficits and promoting normal growth (including pubertal growth) can be challenging. In addition to total calories, micronutrient, calcium, and vitamin deficiencies should be replenished. Restrictive or bland diets are counterproductive because they usually result in poor intake. A high-protein, high-carbohydrate diet with decreased fiber may reduce symptoms during active colitis or partial intestinal obstruction; however, once the colitis is controlled, increased fiber may benefit mucosal health via bacterial production of fatty acids. Low-lactose diet or lactase replacement may be needed temporarily for small bowel CrD. Ileal disease may require antibiotics to treat bacterial overgrowth and extra fat-soluble vitamins due to increased losses. In severe CrD, supplemental calories from formulas taken orally or by NG tube promote catch-up growth.

2. Aminosalicylates (ASA)—Multiple preparations of 5-ASA derivatives are available and used to induce and maintain remission in mild CrD and UC. Common preparations including 5-ASA products such as sulfasalazine (50 mg/kg/day), or balsalazide (0.75–2.5 g PO tid) or mesalamine products (adult dose range 2.4–4.8 g/day), are available in tablets, granules, and delayed release formulations targeting specific locations in the GI tract. Side effects include skin rash; nausea; headache and abdominal pain; hair loss; diarrhea; and rarely nephritis, pericarditis, serum sickness, hemolytic anemia, aplastic anemia, and pancreatitis. Sulfasalazine, in which sulfa delivers the 5-ASA, may cause sulfa-related side effects including photosensitivity and rash.

3. Corticosteroids—Patients with moderate to severe CrD and UC generally respond quickly to corticosteroids. Methylprednisolone (1 mg/kg/day) may be given intravenously when disease is severe. For moderate disease, prednisone (1 mg/kg/day, orally in one to two divided doses), or budesonide in preparations targeting the ileocecal area or colon may quickly improve symptoms but should be tapered over 4–8 weeks. Budesonide, due to "single pass" liver clearance, may have less side effects than prednisone. Steroid dependence is an indication for escalating therapy. Corticosteroid enemas and foams are useful topical agents for distal proctitis or left-sided colitis. While on systemic corticosteroids, consideration should be given to calcium and vitamin D supplementation as well as acid suppression to prevent gastritis.

4. Immunomodulators: azathioprine (AZA), 6-mercaptopurine (6MP), and methotrexate (MTX)—If patients experience moderate to severe or are steroid-dependent, immunomodulators may be used as effective agents to maintain remission and reduce corticosteroids use. AZA (2–3 mg/kg/day PO) or 6MP (1–2 mg/kg/day PO) provides effective maintenance therapy for moderate to severe CrD. The optimal dose of AZA or 6MP depends on the enzyme thiopurine methylene transferase (TPMT), which should be measured before starting therapy. For individuals deficient in TPMT, MTX should be used; for intermediate enzyme activity, dose is reduced by 50%. In cases when adherence may be an issue, or when dose adjustments may be necessary, AZA or 6MP metabolites may be measured. Maximum therapeutic efficacy may not be seen for 2–3 months after beginning treatment. Side effects include pancreatitis, hepatotoxicity, and bone marrow suppression.

MTX is effective in CrD but not UC, and with onset of action within 2–3 weeks. Weekly oral or intramuscular dosage ranges from 15 mg/m² up to 25 mg. The most common side effect is nausea, managed with folate 1 mg a day, while serious adverse events include bone marrow, liver, lung, and kidney toxicities. MTX is well known to cause fetal death and deformities.

5. Antibiotics—Metronidazole (15–30 mg/kg/day in three divided doses) and ciprofloxacin treat perianal CrD and bacterial overgrowth. Peripheral neuropathy may occur with prolonged use of metronidazole.

6. Biologicals—Antibody against tumor necrosis factor-α (TNFα) is used for moderate to severe CrD and UC, and for fistulizing or penetrating disease. Formulations are available for IV (infliximab) or intramuscular (adalimumab) administration. Disease recurrence is usually within 12 months of stopping therapy. New biologicals include vedolizumab, an alpha4/beta7 anti-integrin, and ustekinumab, an anti IL12/23 agent. Use of biologics is associated with risk for infusion reactions, injection site reactions, and increased risk for opportunistic infections and for malignancy. Rarely, hepatosplenic T-cell lymphoma is associated with anti-TNF agents and concomitant AZA/6MP.

7. Other agents—Cyclosporine or tacrolimus may be used as a "bridge" to more definitive therapy (such as colectomy for UC). Probiotics and prebiotics are frequently used but with very limited data on efficacy. Tofactinib, an oral JAK inhibitor, has recently received approval for adults with UC.

8. Surveillance—After 7–8 years of colitis, cancer screening with routine colonoscopy and multiple biopsies is recommended. Persistent metaplasia, aneuploidy, or dysplasia indicates need for colectomy.

B. Surgical Treatment

1. Crohn disease—Ileocecal resection is the most common surgery but recurrence is expected. Indications for surgery in CrD include stricture, obstruction, uncontrollable bleeding, perforation, abscess, fistula, and failure of medical management. Up to 50% of patients with CrD eventually require a surgical procedure.

2. Ulcerative colitis—Total colectomy is curative and is recommended for patients with steroid dependence or steroid resistance, uncontrolled hemorrhage, toxic megacolon, high-grade dysplasia, or malignant tumors; elective colectomy may be chosen for prevention of colorectal cancer after 7–8 years of disease. A J-pouch provides better continence, but pouchitis develops in up to 25% of patients, manifested by diarrhea and cramping, and is treated with metronidazole or ciprofloxacin. Liver disease associated with IBD is not improved by colectomy.

Amil-Dias J et al: Surgical management of Crohn disease in children: guidelines from the Paediatric IBD Porto Group of ESPGHAN. J Pediatr Gastroenterol Nutr 2017;64(5):818. [PMID: 28267075].

Levine A et al: ESPGHAN revised porto criteria for the diagnosis of inflammatory bowel disease in children and adolescents. J Pediatr Gastroenterol Nutr 2014;58(6):795 [PMID: 24231644].

Ruemmele FM et al: Consensus guidelines of ECCO/ESPGHAN on the medical management of pediatric Crohn's disease. J Crohns Colitis 2014;8(10):1179 [PMID: 24909831].

Turner D et al: Management of paediatric ulcerative colitis, part 1: ambulatory care—an evidence-based guideline from European Crohn's and Colitis Organization and European Society of Paediatric Gastroenterology, Hepatology and Nutrition. J Pediatr Gastroenterol Nutr 2018;67(2):257. [PMID: 30044357].

Turner, D et al: Management of paediatric ulcerative colitis, part 2: acute severe colitis—an evidence-based consensus guideline from the European Crohn's and Colitis Organization and the European Society of Paediatric Gastroenterology, Hepatology and Nutrition. J Pediatr Gastroenterol Nutr 2018;67(2):292 [PMID: 30044358].

Web Resources

http://www.crohnscolitisfoundation.org/.

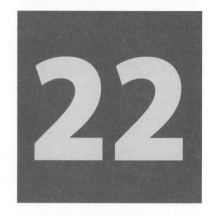

Liver & Pancreas

Ronald J. Sokol, MD

Michael R. Narkewicz, MD

Jacob A. Mark, MD

Cara L. Mack, MD

Amy G. Feldman, MD, MSCS

Shikha S. Sundaram, MD, MSCI

▼ LIVER DISORDERS

NEONATAL CHOLESTATIC JAUNDICE

Key clinical features of disorders causing prolonged neonatal cholestasis are (1) jaundice with elevated serum conjugated (or direct) bilirubin fraction (> 1.0 mg/dL and > 20% of total bilirubin), (2) variably acholic stools, (3) dark urine, and (4) hepatomegaly.

Neonatal cholestasis (conditions with decreased bile flow) is caused by both intrahepatic and extrahepatic diseases. Specific clinical clues (Table 22–1) distinguish these two major categories of jaundice in 85% of cases. Patients with intrahepatic cholestasis frequently appear ill and are failing to thrive, whereas infants with extrahepatic cholestasis typically do not appear ill, have stools that are usually completely acholic, and have an enlarged, firm liver. Histologic examination of percutaneous liver biopsy specimens increases the accuracy of differentiation to 85%–95% (Table 22–2).

INTRAHEPATIC CHOLESTASIS

ESSENTIALS OF DIAGNOSIS & TYPICAL FEATURES

▶ Elevated total and conjugated bilirubin.

▶ Hepatomegaly and dark urine.

▶ Patency of extrahepatic biliary tree.

▶ General Considerations

Intrahepatic cholestasis is characterized by impaired hepatocyte secretion of bile and patency of the extrahepatic biliary system. A specific cause can be identified in about 60%–80% of cases, the remainder being labeled as idiopathic neonatal hepatitis or transient neonatal cholestasis. Patency of the extrahepatic biliary tract is suggested by pigmented stools and lack of bile duct proliferation and portal tract bile plugs on liver biopsy. Bile duct patency can be confirmed least invasively by hepatobiliary scintigraphy using technetium-99m (^{99m}Tc)-dimethyliminodiacetic acid (diethyl-IDA [DIDA]). Radioactivity in the bowel within 4–24 hours is evidence of bile duct patency, as is finding bilirubin in duodenal aspirates. However, these tests are rarely needed in the clinical setting. Patency can also be determined, when clinically indicated, by cholangiography carried out either intraoperatively, percutaneously by transhepatic cholecystography, or by endoscopic retrograde cholangiopancreatography (ERCP) using a pediatric-size side-viewing endoscope. Magnetic resonance cholangiopancreatography in infants is of limited use and highly dependent on the operator and equipment.

1. Perinatal or Neonatal Hepatitis Resulting From Infection

This diagnosis is considered in infants with jaundice, hepatomegaly, vomiting, lethargy, fever, and petechiae. It is important to identify perinatally acquired viral, bacterial, or protozoal infections (Table 22–3) as they may be treatable. Infection may occur transplacentally, by ascent through the cervix into amniotic fluid, from swallowed contaminated fluids (maternal blood, urine, vaginal secretions) during delivery, from blood transfusions administered in the early neonatal period, or from breast milk or environmental exposure. Infectious agents include herpes simplex virus, varicella virus, picornaviruses (enteroviruses and human parechoviruses), cytomegalovirus (CMV), rubella virus, adenovirus, parvovirus, human herpesvirus type 6 (HHV-6), hepatitis B virus (HBV), human immunodeficiency virus (HIV), *Treponema pallidum*, and *Toxoplasma gondii*. Although hepatitis C may be transmitted vertically, it rarely causes

Table 22–1. Characteristic clinical features of intrahepatic and extrahepatic neonatal cholestasis.

Intrahepatic	Extrahepatic
Preterm infant, small for gestational age, appears ill	Full-term infant, seems well
Hepatosplenomegaly, other organ or system involvement	Hepatomegaly (firm to hard)
Stools with some pigment	Acholic stools
Associated cause identified (infections, metabolic, familial, etc)	Polysplenia or asplenia syndromes, midline liver

neonatal cholestasis. The degree of liver cell injury caused by these agents is variable, ranging from massive hepatic necrosis (herpes simplex, picornavirus) to focal necrosis and mild inflammation (CMV, HBV). Serum bilirubin, alanine aminotransferase (ALT), aspartate aminotransferase (AST), alkaline phosphatase, and bile acids are typically elevated. The infant is jaundiced, may have petechiae or rash, and generally appears ill.

▶ Clinical Findings

A. Symptoms and Signs

Clinical symptoms typically present in the first 2 weeks of life, but may appear as late as age 2–3 months. Poor oral intake, poor sucking reflex, lethargy, hypotonia, and vomiting are frequent. Stools may be normal to pale in color, but are seldom acholic. Dark urine stains the diaper. Firm hepatomegaly may be present and splenomegaly is variably present. Macular, papular, vesicular, or petechial rashes may occur. Unusual presentations include neonatal liver failure,

Table 22–2. Characteristic histologic features of intrahepatic and extrahepatic neonatal cholestasis.

	Intrahepatic	Extrahepatic
Giant cells	+++	+
Lobules	Disarray	Normal
Portal reaction	Inflammation, minimal fibrosis	Fibrosis, lymphocytic infiltrate
Neoductular proliferation	Rare	Marked
Other	Steatosis, extramedullary hematopoiesis, iron deposition	Portal bile duct plugging, bile lakes

hypoproteinemia, anasarca (nonhemolytic hydrops), and hemorrhagic disease of the newborn.

B. Diagnostic Studies

Neutropenia, thrombocytopenia, and mild hemolysis are common. Mixed hyperbilirubinemia, elevated aminotransferases with near-normal alkaline phosphatase and gamma-glutamyl transpeptidase (GGT), prolongation of clotting studies, mild acidosis, and elevated cord serum IgM suggest congenital infection. Nasopharyngeal washings, urine, stool, serum, and cerebrospinal fluid (CSF) should be cultured for virus and/or tested for pathogen-specific nucleic acid. Specific IgM antibody may be useful, as are long-bone radiographs to determine the presence of "celery stalking" in the metaphyseal regions of the humeri, femurs, and tibias. When indicated, computed tomography (CT) scans can identify intracranial calcifications (especially with CMV and toxoplasmosis). Hepatobiliary scintigraphy shows decreased hepatic clearance of the circulating isotope with intact excretion into the gut. Gallbladder is present on ultrasonography. Careful ophthalmologic examination may be useful for diagnosis of herpes simplex virus, CMV, toxoplasmosis, and rubella.

A percutaneous liver biopsy may be useful in distinguishing infectious cholestasis, but may not identify a specific infectious agent (see Table 22–2). Exceptions are the typical inclusions of CMV in hepatocytes or bile duct epithelial cells, the presence of multinucleated giant cells and intranuclear acidophilic inclusions of herpes simplex or varicella-zoster virus, the presence of adenovirus basophilic intranuclear inclusions, or positive immunohistochemical stains for several viruses. Variable degrees of lobular disarray characterized by focal necrosis, multinucleated giant-cell transformation, and ballooned pale hepatocytes with loss of cord-like arrangement of liver cells are usual. Intrahepatocytic and canalicular cholestasis may be prominent. Portal changes are not striking, but modest neoductular proliferation and mild fibrosis may occur. Viral cultures, immunohistochemical stains, or polymerase chain reaction (PCR) testing of biopsy material may be helpful.

▶ Differential Diagnosis

Great care must be taken to distinguish infectious causes of intrahepatic cholestasis from genetic or metabolic disorders because the clinical presentations are similar and may overlap. Galactosemia, hereditary fructose intolerance, and tyrosinemia must be investigated promptly, because specific therapy is available. These infants may also have concomitant gram-negative bacteremia. α_1-Antitrypsin deficiency, cystic fibrosis, bile acid synthesis defects, progressive familial intrahepatic cholestasis (PFIC), mitochondrial respiratory chain disorders, and neonatal iron storage disease must also be considered. Specific physical features may suggest Alagille syndrome, arthrogryposis/renal dysfunction/

Table 22–3. Infectious causes of neonatal hepatitis.

Infectious Agent	Diagnostic Tests	Specimens	Treatment
Cytomegalovirus	Culture and PCR, liver histology, IgM/[a]IgG	Urine, blood, liver, saliva	Ganciclovir (Foscarnet)[b]
Herpes simplex	PCR and culture, liver histology, Ag (skin)	Liver, blood, eye, throat, rectal, CSF, skin	Acyclovir
Rubella	Culture, IgM/[a]IgG	Liver, blood, urine	Supportive
Varicella	Culture, PCR, Ag (skin)	Skin, blood, CSF, liver	Acyclovir (Foscarnet)[b]
Parvovirus	Serum IgM/[a]IgG, PCR	Blood	Supportive, IVIG
Enteroviruses	Culture and PCR	Blood, urine, CSF, throat, rectal, liver	IVIG may have value; experimental drugs being tested
Adenovirus	Culture and PCR	Nasal/throat, rectal, blood, liver, urine	No established therapy, Cidofovir or IVIG may have value
Hepatitis B virus (HBV)	HBsAg, HBcAg IgM, HBV DNA	Serum	Supportive for acute infection
Hepatitis C virus (HCV)	HCV PCR, HCV IgG	Serum	Supportive for acute infection
Treponema pallidum	Serology	Serum, CSF	Penicillin
Toxoplasma gondii	IgM/[a]IgG, PCR, culture	Serum, CSF, liver	See Chapter 43, Parasites
Mycobacterium tuberculosis	Chest radiograph, liver tissue histologic stains, culture or PCR, gastric aspirate stain, culture or PCR	Serum, liver, gastric aspirate	INH, pyrazinamide, rifampin, ethambutol (if multiple drug-resistant TB is present, consult a specialist)
Bacterial infection	Cultures or PCR and other rapid methods	Blood, urine, other tissues or surfaces	Appropriate antibiotics

Ag, viral antigen testing; CSF, cerebrospinal fluid; HBcAg, hepatitis B core antigen; HBsAg, hepatitis B surface antigen; INH, isoniazid; IVIG, intravenous immune globulin; PCR, polymerase chain reaction test for viral DNA or RNA; PPD, purified protein derivative.
[a]IgG = positive indicates maternal infection and transfer of antibody transplacentally; negative indicates unlikelihood of infection in mother and infant.
[b]Use foscarnet for resistant viruses, which should be rare in the neonate. Treat only if symptomatic.

cholestasis (ARC) syndrome, or Zellweger syndrome. Idiopathic neonatal hepatitis (transient neonatal cholestasis) can be indistinguishable from infectious causes.

▶ **Treatment**

Infections with herpes simplex virus, varicella, CMV, parvovirus, and toxoplasmosis have specific treatments (see Table 22–3). Penicillin for suspected syphilis, specific antiviral therapy, or antibiotics for bacterial hepatitis or urinary tract infections need to be administered promptly. Intravenous dextrose is needed if feedings are not well tolerated. The consequences of cholestasis are treated as indicated (Table 22–4). Vitamin K orally or by injection and vitamins D and E orally should be provided. Choleretics (ursodeoxycholic acid [UDCA]) are used if cholestasis persists. Corticosteroids are contraindicated.

▶ **Prognosis**

Multiple organ involvement portends a poor outcome. Hepatic or cardiac failure, intractable acidosis, or intracranial hemorrhage is associated with fatal outcome in herpesvirus, adenovirus, or enterovirus infections, and occurs occasionally in CMV or rubella infection. HBV rarely causes fulminant neonatal hepatitis; most infected infants are immunotolerant to hepatitis B. The neonatal liver usually recovers without fibrosis after acute infections. Chronic cholestasis, although rare following infections, may lead to dental enamel hypoplasia, failure to thrive, biliary rickets, severe pruritus, and xanthoma.

Bilavsky E, Schwarz M, Bar-Sever Z, Pardo J, Amir J: Hepatic involvement in congenital cytomegalovirus infection—infrequent yet significant. J Viral Hepat 2014 Dec 12. doi: 10.1111/jvh.12374 [PMID: 25496231].

Feldman AG, Sokol RJ: Neonatal cholestasis: emerging molecular diagnostics and potential novel therapeutics. Nat Rev Gastroenterol Hepatol 2019 Jun;16(6):346–360 [PMID: 30903105].

Goel A, Chaudhari S, Sutar J, Bhonde G, Bhatnagar S, Patel V, Bhor V, Shah I: Detection of cytomegalovirus in liver tissue by polymerase chain reaction in infants with neonatal cholestasis. Pediatr Infect Dis J 2018 Jul;37(7):632–636 [PMID: 29389827].

Table 22–4. Treatment of complications of chronic cholestatic liver disease.

Indication	Treatment	Dose	Toxicity
Intrahepatic cholestasis	Phenobarbital	3–10 mg/kg/day	Drowsiness, irritability, interference with vitamin D metabolism
	Cholestyramine or colestipol hydrochloride	250–500 mg/kg/day	Constipation, acidosis, binding of drugs, increased steatorrhea
	Ursodeoxycholic acid	15–20 mg/kg/day	Transient increase in pruritus
Pruritus	Phenobarbital	3–10 mg/kg/day	Drowsiness, irritability, interference with vitamin D metabolism
	Cholestyramine or colestipol	250–500 mg/kg/day	Constipation, acidosis, binding of drugs, increased steatorrhea
	Diphenhydramine hydrochloride	5–10 mg/kg/day	Drowsiness
	Hydroxyzine	2–5 mg/kg/day	Drowsiness
	Ultraviolet light B	Exposure as needed	Skin burn
	Rifampicin	10 mg/kg/day	Hepatotoxicity, bone marrow suppression
	Ursodeoxycholic acid	15–20 mg/kg/day	Transient increase in pruritus
	Naltrexone	1 mg/kg/day	Irritability, vomiting
	Plasmapheresis	Each 2–4 wk	Central venous access, expensive
Steatorrhea	Formula containing medium-chain triglycerides (eg, Pregestimil or Alimentum)	120–150 kcal/kg/day for infants	Expensive
	Oil supplement containing medium-chain triglycerides	1–2 mL/kg/day	Diarrhea, aspiration
Malabsorption of fat-soluble vitamins	Vitamin A	10,000–25,000 U/day	Hepatitis, pseudotumor cerebri, bone lesions
	Vitamin D_2 or D_3	800–8000 U/day (up to 1000 U/kg/day for infants)	Hypercalcemia, hypercalciuria
	25-Hydroxy-cholecalciferol (25-OH vitamin D)	3–5 mcg/kg/day	Hypercalcemia, hypercalciuria
	1,25-Dihydroxy-cholecalciferol (1,25 OH_2 vitamin D)	0.05–0.2 mcg/kg/day	Hypercalcemia, hypercalciuria
	Vitamin E (oral)	25–200 IU/kg/day	Potentiation of vitamin K deficiency
	Vitamin E (oral, TPGS[a])	15–25 IU/kg/day	Potentiation of vitamin K deficiency
	Vitamin E (intramuscular)	1–2 mg/kg/day	Muscle calcifications
	Vitamin K (oral)	2.5 mg twice per wk to 5 mg/day	
	Vitamin K (intramuscular)	2–5 mg each 4 wk	
Malabsorption of other nutrients	Multiple vitamin	One to two times the standard dose	
	Calcium	25–100 mg/kg/day	Hypercalcemia, hypercalciuria
	Phosphorus	25–50 mg/kg/day	Gastrointestinal intolerance
	Zinc	1 mg/kg/day	Interference with copper and iron absorption

[a]D-α-Tocopheryl polyethylene glycol-1000 succinate.

2. Specific Infectious Agents

A. Neonatal Hepatitis B Virus Disease

Vertical transmission of HBV may occur at any time during perinatal life. Most cases are acquired from mothers who are asymptomatic carriers of HBV. Although HBV has been found in most body fluids, including breast milk, neonatal transmission occurs primarily from exposure to maternal blood at delivery and only occasionally transplacentally (< 5%–10% of cases). In chronic HB surface antigen (HBsAg)–carrier mothers, neonatal acquisition risk is greatest if the mother: (1) is also HB "e" antigen (HBeAg)–positive and HB "e" antibody (HBeAb)–negative, (2) has high serum levels of hepatitis B core antibody (HBcAb), or (3) has high blood levels of HBV DNA (> 10^7 copies/mL). The infant has a 70%–90% chance of acquiring HBV at birth from an HBsAg/HBeAg-positive mother if the infant does not receive prophylaxis. Most infected infants develop a prolonged asymptomatic immune-tolerant phase of HBV infection. Fulminant hepatic necrosis and liver failure rarely occur in infants. Other patients develop immune active chronic hepatitis with focal hepatocyte necrosis and a mild portal inflammatory response. Chronic hepatitis may persist for years, with serologic evidence of persisting HBeAg and mildly elevated or normal serum aminotransferases. Most infected infants have only mild biochemical evidence, if any, of liver injury and do not appear ill. Most infants remain asymptomatic in an immune-tolerant state of HBV infection; 3%–5% per year develop acute or chronic hepatitis (see section on Hepatitis B).

To prevent perinatal transmission, all infants of mothers who are HBsAg-positive (regardless of HBeAg status) should receive hepatitis B immunoglobulin (HBIG) and hepatitis B vaccine within the first 24 hours after birth and vaccine again at ages 1 and 6 months (see Chapter 10). This prevents HBV infection in 85%–95% of infants. If not given at birth, HBIG can be administered as late as 7 days postpartum as long as the infant has received the vaccine. Universal HBV immunization during infancy is recommended for all infants regardless of maternal HBV status. Universal screening of pregnant women for HBsAg is conducted to determine which infants will also need HBIG. Pregnant women with greater than 200,000 IU/mL of HBV DNA should be considered for third trimester anti-viral therapy to lower HBV levels and reduce risk for vertical transmission.

B. Neonatal Bacterial Hepatitis

Most bacterial liver infections in newborns are acquired by transplacental invasion from amnionitis with ascending spread from maternal vaginal or cervical infection. Onset is abrupt, usually within 48–72 hours after delivery, with signs of sepsis and often shock. Jaundice appears early with direct hyperbilirubinemia. The most common organisms involved are *Escherichia coli*, *Listeria monocytogenes*, and group B streptococci. Neonatal liver abscesses caused by *E coli* or *Staphylococcus aureus* may result from omphalitis or umbilical vein catheterization. These infections require specific antibiotics in optimal doses and combinations and, rarely, surgical or interventional radiologic drainage. Deaths are common, but survivors show no long-term consequences of liver disease.

C. Neonatal Jaundice With Urinary Tract Infection

Urinary tract infections typically present with cholestasis between the second and fourth weeks of life. Lethargy, fever, poor appetite, jaundice, and hepatomegaly may be present.

Except for mixed hyperbilirubinemia, other liver function tests (LFTs) are only mildly abnormal. Leukocytosis is frequently present, and infection is confirmed by urine culture. The liver impairment is caused by the action of endotoxin and cytokines on bile secretion.

Treatment of the infection leads to resolution of the cholestasis without hepatic sequelae. Metabolic liver diseases, such as galactosemia and tyrosinemia, may present with gram-negative bacterial urinary tract infection and must be excluded.

Cheung KW, Seto MTY, Lao TT: Prevention of perinatal hepatitis B virus transmission. Arch Gynecol Obstet 2019 Aug;300(2): 251–259 [PMID: 31098821].

Gentile I et al: Prevention of mother-to-child transmission of hepatitis B virus and hepatitis C virus. Expert Rev Anti Infect Ther 2014 Jul;12(7):775–782 [PMID: 24840817].

Pinninti SG, Kimberlin DW: Management of neonatal herpes simplex virus infection and exposure. Arch Dis Child Fetal Neonatal Ed 2014 May;99(3):F240–F244 [PMID: 24589428].

Terrault NA, Lok ASF, McMahon BJ, Chang KM, Hwang JP, Jonas MM, Brown RS Jr, Bzowej NH, Wong JB: Update on prevention, diagnosis, and treatment of chronic hepatitis B: AASLD 2018 hepatitis B guidance. Hepatology 2018 Apr;67(4): 1560–1599 [PMID: 29405329].

3. Intrahepatic Cholestasis Resulting From Inborn Errors of Metabolism, Familial, & "Toxic" Causes

Cholestasis caused by specific enzyme deficiencies, other genetic disorders, or certain toxins share findings of intrahepatic cholestasis (jaundice, hepatomegaly, and normal to completely acholic stools). Specific clinical conditions have characteristic clinical signs.

A. Inborn Errors of Metabolism

Establishing the specific diagnosis as early as possible is important because dietary or pharmacologic treatment may be available (Table 22–5), and Parents of the affected infant should be offered genetic counseling. For some disorders, prenatal genetic diagnosis is available.

Cholestasis caused by metabolic diseases (eg, galactosemia, hereditary fructose intolerance, and tyrosinemia) is frequently accompanied by vomiting, lethargy, poor feeding, hypoglycemia, or irritability. The infants often appear septic; gram-negative bacteria can be cultured from blood in 25%–50% of symptomatic cases, especially in galactosemia with cholestasis. Neonatal screening programs for galactosemia and tyrosinemia usually detect the disorder before cholestasis develops. Other metabolic and genetic causes of neonatal intrahepatic cholestasis are outlined in Table 22–5. Treatment of these disorders is discussed in Chapter 36.

Table 22–5. Metabolic and genetic causes of neonatal cholestasis.

Disease	Inborn Error	Hepatic Pathology	Diagnostic Studies
Galactosemia	Galactose-1-phosphate uridyltransferase	Cholestasis, steatosis, necrosis, pseudoacini, fibrosis	Galactose-1-phosphate uridyltransferase assay of red blood cells or genotyping[a]
Fructose intolerance	Fructose-1-phosphate aldolase	Steatosis, necrosis, pseudoacini, fibrosis	Liver fructose-1-phosphate aldolase assay or genotyping[a]
Tyrosinemia	Fumarylacetoacetase	Necrosis, steatosis, pseudoacini, portal fibrosis	Urinary succinylacetone, fumarylacetoacetase assay of red blood cells
Cystic fibrosis	Cystic fibrosis transmembrane conductance regulator gene	Cholestasis, neoductular proliferation, excess bile duct mucus, portal fibrosis	Sweat test and genotyping[a]
Hypopituitarism	Deficient production of pituitary hormones	Cholestasis, giant cells	Thyroxin, TSH, cortisol levels
α$_1$-Antitrypsin deficiency	Abnormal α$_1$-antitrypsin molecule (PiZZ or PiSZ phenotype)	Giant cells, cholestasis, steatosis, neoductular proliferation, fibrosis, PAS-positive diastase–resistant cytoplasmic globules	Serum α$_1$-antitrypsin phenotype or genotype
Gaucher disease	β-Glucosidase	Cholestasis, cytoplasmic inclusions in Kupffer cells (foam cells)	β-Glucosidase assay in leukocytes or genotyping[a]
Niemann-Pick type C disease	Lysosomal sphingomyelinase	Cholestasis, cytoplasmic inclusions in Kupffer cells	Sphingomyelinase assay of leukocytes or liver or fibroblasts (type C); genotyping[a]
Glycogen storage disease type IV	Branching enzyme	Fibrosis, cirrhosis, PAS-diastase–resistant cytoplasmic inclusions	Branching enzyme analysis of leukocytes or liver, genotyping[a]
Neonatal hemochromatosis	Transplacental alloimmunization	Giant cells, portal fibrosis, hemosiderosis, cirrhosis	Histology, iron stains, lip biopsy, chest and abdominal MRI
Peroxisomal disorders (eg, Zellweger syndrome)	Deficient peroxisomal enzymes or assembly	Cholestasis, necrosis, fibrosis, cirrhosis, hemosiderosis	Plasma very-long-chain fatty acids, qualitative bile acids, plasmalogen, pipecolic acid, liver electron microscopy, genotyping[a]
Bile acid synthesis and metabolism disorders	Nine enzyme deficiencies defined	Cholestasis, necrosis, giant cells	Urine, serum, duodenal fluid analyzed for bile acids by fast atom bombardment–mass spectroscopy, genotyping[a]
Byler disease and syndrome (PFIC types I and II)	FIC-1 (ATP8B1) and BSEP (ABCB11) genes	Cholestasis, necrosis, giant cells, fibrosis	Histology, family history, normal cholesterol, low or normal γ-glutamyl transpeptidase, genotyping[a]
Arthrogryposis/ renal dysfunction/ cholestasis syndrome	VPS33B and VIPAR genes	Cholestasis, fibrosis	Genotyping[a]
MDR3 deficiency (PFIC type III)	MDR3 (ABCB4) gene	Cholestasis, bile duct proliferation, portal fibrosis	Bile phospholipid level, genotyping[a]
TJP2 deficiency (PFIC type IV)	TJP2 gene	Cholestasis, necrosis, giant cells, fibrosis	Genotyping[a]
FXR deficiency (PFIC type V)	NRIH4 gene	Cholestasis, necrosis, giant cells, fibrosis	Genotyping[a]
MYO5B deficiency (PFIC type VI)	MYO5B gene	Cholestasis, necrosis, giant cells, fibrosis	Genotyping[a]

(Continued)

Table 22–5. Metabolic and genetic causes of neonatal cholestasis. (*Continued*)

Disease	Inborn Error	Hepatic Pathology	Diagnostic Studies
Alagille syndrome (syndromic paucity of interlobular bile ducts)	*JAGGED1* gene and *NOTCH2* mutations	Cholestasis, paucity of interlobular bile ducts, increased copper levels	Three or more clinical features, liver histology, genotyping[a]
Mitochondrial hepatopathies (respiratory chain diseases and mtDNA depletion syndrome)	*POLG, BCS1I, SCO1, DGUOK,* Twinkle and *MPV17* and other gene mutations	Cholestasis, steatosis, portal fibrosis, abnormal mitochondria on electron microscopy	mtDNA depletion studies, respiratory chain studies on liver or muscle, genotyping[a]

IV, intravenous; MDR3, multiple drug resistance protein type 3; MRI, magnetic resonance imaging; mtDNA, mitochondrial DNA; PAS, periodic acid–Schiff; PFIC, progressive familial intrahepatic cholestasis; TSH, thyroid-stimulating hormone.
[a]Performed on leukocyte DNA.

B. "Toxic" Causes of Neonatal Cholestasis

1. Neonatal ischemic-hypoxic conditions—Perinatal events that result in hypoperfusion or hypoxia of the gastrointestinal system are sometimes followed within 1–2 weeks by cholestasis. This occurs in infants with birth asphyxia, acute cardiac dysfunction, severe hypoxia, hypoglycemia, shock, and acidosis. When these perinatal conditions develop in association with gastrointestinal lesions, such as ruptured omphalocele, gastroschisis, or necrotizing enterocolitis, a subsequent cholestatic picture is common (25%–50% of cases). Mixed hyperbilirubinemia, elevated alkaline phosphatase and γ-glutamyl transpeptidase (GGT) values, and variable elevation of the aminotransferases are common. Stools are seldom persistently acholic.

The mainstays of treatment are choleretics (UDCA), introduction of enteral feedings using special formulas as soon as possible, and nutrient supplementation until the cholestasis resolves (see Table 22–4). As long as no severe intestinal problem or ongoing sepsis is present (eg, short gut syndrome or intestinal failure), resolution of the hepatic abnormalities is the rule, although this may take many weeks.

2. Parenteral nutrition-associated cholestasis (PNAC)—Cholestasis may develop after 1–2 weeks in premature newborns receiving parenteral nutrition, especially those with necrotizing enterocolitis. Even full-term infants with significant intestinal atresia, resections, congenital absorptive deficiencies, or dysmotility (intestinal failure) may develop PNAC, also called Intestinal Failure Associated Cholestasis when it occurs in term infants. Contributing factors include toxicity of intravenous soy lipid emulsions (eg, plant sterols), diminished stimulation of bile flow from prolonged absence of feedings, frequent episodes of bacterial or fungal infection, small intestinal bacterial overgrowth with translocation of intestinal bacteria and their cell wall products, missing nutrients or antioxidants, photooxidation of amino acids, and the "physiologic cholestatic" propensity of the infant. Activation of innate immune pathways in the liver by endotoxin and plant sterols appears to be involved. Histology of the liver may be identical to that of biliary atresia. Early introduction of feedings, surgical/medical therapies to induce intestinal adaptation, and modifications of intravenous lipid emulsions have reduced the frequency/severity of this disorder. The prognosis is generally good; however, in infants with intestinal failure cases may progress to cirrhosis, liver failure, or hepatoma. These infants may require liver and intestinal, or multivisceral transplantation. Oral erythromycin as a pro-motility agent may reduce the incidence of cholestasis in very-low-birth-weight infants. Substituting intravenous fish oil-based lipid emulsions or multiple constituent lipid emulsions, or reducing the amount of soy-oil-based lipid emulsions may reverse PNAC and prevent need for liver transplantation and delay the need for intestinal transplantation.

3. Inspissated bile syndrome—This syndrome is the result of accumulation of bile in canaliculi and in the small- and medium-sized bile ducts in hemolytic disease of the newborn (Rh, ABO) and in some infants receiving parenteral nutrition. The same mechanisms may cause intrinsic obstruction of the common bile duct. An ischemia-reperfusion injury may also contribute to cholestasis in Rh incompatibility. Stools may become acholic and levels of bilirubin, primarily conjugated, may reach 40 mg/dL. If inspissation of bile occurs within the extrahepatic biliary tree, differentiation from biliary atresia may be difficult. Although most cases improve slowly over 2–6 months, persistence of complete cholestasis (acholic stools) for more than 1–2 weeks requires further studies (ultrasonography, liver biopsy) with possible cholangiography. Irrigation of the common bile duct is sometimes necessary to dislodge the obstructing inspissated biliary material.

Courtney CM, Warner BW: Pediatric intestinal failure-associated liver disease. Curr Opin Pediatr 2017;29:363–370 [PMID: 28333693].

El Kasmi KC et al: Phytosterols promote liver injury and Kupffer cell activation in parenteral nutrition-associated liver disease. Sci Transl Med 2013 Oct 9;5(206):206ra137 [PMID: 24107776].

Mitra A, Ahn J: Liver disease in patients on total parenteral nutrition. Clin Liver Dis 2017 Nov;21(4):687–695. doi: 10.1016/j.cld.2017.06.008. Epub 2017 Aug 19. Review. [PMID: 28987256].

4. Idiopathic Neonatal Hepatitis (Transient Neonatal Cholestasis)

This idiopathic type of cholestatic jaundice, which has a typical liver biopsy appearance, accounts for up to 20%–30% of cases of neonatal intrahepatic cholestasis, but is decreasing in frequency as new genetic causes of cholestasis are discovered. The degree of cholestasis is variable, and the disorder may be indistinguishable from extrahepatic causes in 10% of cases. Viral infections, α_1-antitrypsin deficiency, Alagille syndrome, Niemann-Pick type C disease (NPC), PFIC disorders, citrin deficiency, neonatal hemochromatosis, mitochondrial disorders, and bile acid synthesis defects may present with similar clinical and histologic features and should be excluded. In idiopathic neonatal hepatitis, PFIC types I and II and ARC syndrome, and disease due to bile acid synthesis defects, the GGT levels are normal or low. Electron microscopy of the liver biopsy and genotyping will help distinguish NPC and PFIC. It is likely that a heterozygous state or mild missense mutations for known or yet to be discovered causative genes are responsible for the vast majority of idiopathic cases.

Intrauterine growth retardation, prematurity, poor feeding, emesis, poor growth, and partially or intermittently acholic stools are characteristic. Serious hemorrhage from vitamin K deficiency may also be present. Patients with neonatal lupus erythematosus may present with giant-cell hepatitis; however, thrombocytopenia, rash, or congenital heart block is usually also present.

In cases of suspected idiopathic neonatal hepatitis (diagnosed in the absence of infectious, known genetic, metabolic, and toxic causes), patency of the biliary tree may need to be verified to exclude extrahepatic disorders. HIDA scanning and ultrasonography may be helpful in this regard if stools are acholic. Liver biopsy findings are usually diagnostic after age 6–8 weeks (see Table 22–2), but may be misleading before age 6 weeks as there is overlap with biliary atresia histology. Failure to detect patency of the biliary tree, nondiagnostic liver biopsy findings, or persisting complete cholestasis (acholic stools) are indications for intraoperative cholangiography performed by an experienced surgeon, ERCP, or percutaneous cholecystography. Occasionally, a small but patent (hypoplastic) extrahepatic biliary tree is demonstrated (as in Alagille syndrome). It is probably the result, rather than the cause, of diminished bile flow, so

surgical reconstruction of hypoplastic biliary trees in Alagille syndrome should not be attempted.

Therapy should include choleretics, a special formula with medium-chain triglycerides (eg, Pregestimil, Alimentum) or breast milk (if growth is adequate), and supplemental fat-soluble vitamins in water-soluble form (see Table 22–4). This therapy is continued as long as significant cholestasis remains (conjugated bilirubin > 1 mg/dL). Fat-soluble vitamin serum levels and INR should be monitored at regular intervals while supplements are given and repeated at least once after their discontinuation.

Around 80% of patients recover without significant hepatic fibrosis. However, failure to resolve the cholestatic picture by age 6–12 months is associated with progressive liver disease and evolving cirrhosis, most likely caused by known or yet to be defined underlying genetic/metabolic disorder. Liver transplantation has been successful when signs of hepatic decompensation are noted (rising bilirubin, coagulopathy, intractable ascites).

Liu LY et al: Association of variants of ABCB11 with transient neonatal cholestasis. Pediatri Int 2013;55:138–344 [PMID: 23279303].

Torbenson M et al: Neonatal giant cell hepatitis: histological and etiological findings. Am J Surg Pathol 2010 Oct;34(10):1498–1503 [PMID: 20871223].

5. Paucity of Interlobular Bile Ducts

Forms of intrahepatic cholestasis caused by decreased numbers of interlobular bile ducts (< 0.5 bile ducts per portal tract) may be classified according to whether they are associated with other malformations. Alagille syndrome (syndromic paucity or arteriohepatic dysplasia) is caused by mutations in the gene JAGGED1, located on chromosome 20p, which codes for a ligand of the notch receptor, or more rarely in the gene NOTCH2. Alagille syndrome is recognized by the characteristic facies, which becomes more obvious with age. The forehead is prominent with deep-set eyes and sometimes hypertelorism. The chin is small and slightly pointed and ears are prominent. The stool color varies with the severity of cholestasis. Pruritus begins by age 6 months. Firm, smooth hepatomegaly may be present or the liver may be of normal size. Cardiac murmurs are present in 90% of patients, and butterfly vertebrae (incomplete fusion of the vertebral body or anterior arch) are present in 50%. Xanthomas develop as hypercholesterolemia becomes a problem.

Conjugated hyperbilirubinemia may be mild to severe (2–15 mg/dL). Serum alkaline phosphatase, GGT, and cholesterol may be markedly elevated, especially early in life. Serum bile acids are always elevated, aminotransferases are mildly increased, but clotting factors and other liver proteins are usually normal.

Cardiac involvement includes peripheral pulmonary artery, branch pulmonary artery, or pulmonary valvular stenoses, atrial septal defect, coarctation of the aorta, and tetralogy of Fallot. Up to 10%–15% of patients have intracranial vascular or cystic abnormalities or may develop intracranial hemorrhage or stroke early in childhood.

Eye findings (posterior embryotoxon or a prominent Schwalbe line in 90%) are common and renal abnormalities (dysplastic kidneys, renal tubular ectasia, single kidney, renal tubular acidosis, hematuria) may occur in 40% of patients. Growth retardation with normal to increased levels of growth hormone (growth hormone resistance) is common. Although variable, the intelligence quotient is frequently low. Hypogonadism with micropenis may be present. A weak, high-pitched voice may develop. Neurologic disorders resulting from vitamin E deficiency (areflexia, ataxia, ophthalmoplegia), which eventually develop in many unsupplemented children, may be profound.

In the nonsyndromic form, paucity of interlobular bile ducts occurs associated with α1-antitrypsin deficiency, Zellweger syndrome, in association with lymphedema (Aagenaes syndrome), PFIC, cystic fibrosis, CMV or rubella infection, and inborn errors of bile acid metabolism.

High doses (250 mg/kg/day) of cholestyramine may control pruritus, lower cholesterol, and clear xanthomas. UDCA (15–20 mg/kg/day) appears to be more effective and causes fewer side effects than cholestyramine. Rifampicin may also reduce pruritus. Naltrexone (1 mg/kg/day) is occasionally required. Partial external or internal biliary diversion or ileal exclusion surgery may reduce pruritus in about half of severe cases as long as significant hepatic fibrosis is absent. Nutritional therapy to prevent wasting and deficiencies of fat-soluble vitamins is of particular importance because of the severity of cholestasis (see Table 22–4).

Prognosis is more favorable in the syndromic than in the nonsyndromic varieties. In the former, only 40%–50% of patients have significant complications of disease, whereas over 70% of patients with nonsyndromic varieties progress to cirrhosis. Many of this latter group likely have forms of PFIC that are yet to be categorized genetically. In Alagille syndrome, cholestasis may improve by age 2–4 years, with minimal residual hepatic fibrosis. Survival into adulthood despite raised serum bile acids, aminotransferases, and alkaline phosphatase occurs in about 50% of cases, however progressive portal hypertension may ensue. Several patients have developed hepatocellular carcinoma. Hypogonadism has been noted; however, fertility is not often affected. Cardiovascular anomalies and intracranial vascular lesions may shorten life expectancy. Some patients have persistent, severe cholestasis, rendering their quality of life poor. Recurrent bone fractures may result from metabolic bone disease. Liver transplantation has been successfully performed under these circumstances. Intracranial hemorrhage, moyamoya disease, or stroke may occur in up to 10%–12% of affected children. Blockers of the ileal bile acid transporter have shown promise as agents to reduce pruritus.

Mouzaki M et al: Early life predictive markers of liver disease outcome in an International, Multicentre Cohort of children with Alagille syndrome. Liver Int 2016;36:755–760 [PMID: 26201540].

Saleh M, Kamath BM, Chitayat D: Alagille syndrome: clinical perspectives. Appl Clin Genet 2016 Jun 30;9:75–82 [PMID: 27418850].

Shneider BL et al: Placebo-controlled randomized trial of an intestinal bile salt transport inhibitor for pruritus in Alagille syndrome. Hepatol Commun 2018 Sep 24;2(10):1184–1198 [PMID: 30288474]

6. Progressive Familial Intrahepatic Cholestasis (Byler Disease & Byler Syndrome)

PFIC is a group of disorders presenting as pruritus, diarrhea, jaundice, fat-soluble vitamin deficiencies, and failure to thrive in the first 6–12 months of life. PFIC type I (Byler disease), caused by biallelic mutations in *ATP8B1* coding FIC1, an aminophospholipid transporting ATPase is associated with low to normal serum levels of GGT and cholesterol and elevated levels of bilirubin, aminotransferases, and bile acids. Pancreatitis and hearing loss may develop. Liver biopsy demonstrates cellular cholestasis, sometimes with a paucity of interlobular bile ducts and centrilobular fibrosis that progresses to cirrhosis. Giant cells are absent. Electron microscopy shows characteristic granular "Byler bile" in canaliculi. Treatment includes administration of UDCA, partial biliary diversion or ileal exclusion if the condition is unresponsive to UDCA, and liver transplantation if unresponsive to these therapies. Ileal bile acid transporter blockers show promise as therapy in a subset of patients. With partial biliary diversion or ileal exclusion surgery, many patients show improved growth and liver histology, reduction in symptoms, and, thus, avoid liver transplantation. Following liver transplantation, chronic diarrhea and fatty liver may complicate recovery.

PFIC type II is caused by biallelic mutations in *ABCB11* coding the bile salt export pump (BSEP), the adenosine triphosphate–dependent canalicular bile salt transport protein. These patients are clinically and biochemically similar to PFIC type I patients, but liver histology includes numerous multinucleated "giant cells" and they have higher elevations of AST and ALT. There is an increased incidence of hepatocellular carcinoma in patients with severe *ABCB11* mutations. Treatment is similar to PFIC type I although close monitoring for hepatocellular carcinoma is essential. Ileal bile acid transporter blockers show promise as therapy in a subset of patients. Following liver transplantation, recurrent disease has been described in patients who developed autoantibody-mediated BSEP dysfunction.

PFIC type III is caused by mutations in *ABCB4* coding the multiple drug resistance protein type 3 (MDR3), a canalicular protein that pumps phospholipid into bile. Serum GGT and bile acid levels are both elevated, bile duct proliferation and portal tract fibrosis are seen in liver biopsies (resembling biliary atresia), and bile phospholipid levels are low. Treatment is similar to that for other forms of PFIC except that partial biliary diversion is not recommended and liver transplantation is inevitable.

PFIC type 4 is a low GGT form of neonatal cholestasis caused by mutations in tight junction protein 2 (*TJP2*) with rapid progression to cirrhosis and need for liver transplantation in early childhood. PFIC type 5 (FXR deficiency) and type 6 (*MYO5B* deficiency) have recently been described and resemble clinically the other PFICs. About one-third of PFIC patients have negative genotyping for the above genes and likely have yet-to-be discovered genetic etiologies.

Bile acid synthesis defects are clinically similar to PFIC types I and II, with low serum levels of GGT and cholesterol; however, the serum level of total bile acids is inappropriately normal or low, pruritus is generally absent, and urine bile acid analysis may identify a synthesis defect. Milder defects cause fat-soluble vitamin deficiency without severe liver disease. Treatment of most bile acid synthesis defects is with oral cholic acid and for conjugation defects with oral glycocholic acid.

Feldman AG, Sokol RJ: Neonatal cholestasis: emerging molecular diagnostics and potential novel therapeutics. Nat Rev Gastroenterol Hepatol 2019 Jun;16(6):346–360 [PMID: 30903105].

Henkel SA, Squires JH, Ayers M, Ganoza A, Mckiernan P, Squires JE: Expanding etiology of progressive familial intrahepatic cholestasis. World J Hepatol 2019 May 27;11(5):450–463 [PMID: 31183005].

Sambrotta M et al: Mutations in TJP2 cause progressive cholestatic liver disease. Nat Genet 2014 Apr;46(4):326–328 [PMID: 24614073].

Wang K et al: Analysis of surgical interruption of the enterohepatic circulation as a treatment for pediatric cholestasis. Hepatology 2017;65:1645–1654 [PMID: 28027587].

EXTRAHEPATIC NEONATAL CHOLESTASIS

Extrahepatic neonatal cholestasis is characterized by complete and persistent cholestasis (acholic stools) in the first 3 months of life; lack of patency of the extrahepatic biliary tree demonstrated by intraoperative, percutaneous, or endoscopic cholangiography; firm to hard hepatomegaly; and typical features on histologic examination of liver biopsy tissue (see Table 22–2). Causes include biliary atresia, choledochal cyst, spontaneous perforation of the extrahepatic ducts, neonatal sclerosing cholangitis, and intrinsic or extrinsic obstruction of the common duct.

1. Biliary Atresia

▶ General Considerations

Biliary atresia (BA) is a progressive fibroinflammatory obliteration of the lumen of all, or part of, the extrahepatic biliary tree presenting within the first 3 months of life. BA occurs in 1:6,600 (Taiwan)–1:18,000 (Europe) births, and in the United States the incidence is approximately 1:12,000. The incidence is highest in Asians, African Americans, and preterm infants,

and there is a slight female predominance. There are four types of BA: isolated BA (84% of cases), BA with at least one malformation but without laterality defects (6%; CV, GI, or GU defects), BA splenic malformation (BASM) syndrome associated with laterality defects and polysplenia or asplenia (4%–10%), and cystic BA which includes a hilar choledochal cyst. The etiology of BA is likely multifactorial, encompassing an initial viral, toxin or environmental injury to the bile duct epithelium, leading to inflammatory and autoimmune responses targeting the bile ducts in the genetically predisposed individual, and culminating in aggressive fibrosis of the biliary system.

▶ Clinical Findings

A. Symptoms and Signs

All infants with BA will have jaundice that may be noted in the newborn period or by age 2–3 weeks. Therefore, all jaundiced infants ≥ 2 weeks of age should have conjugated bilirubin measured to identify cholestasis. Stools are pale yellow, gray, or acholic. Firm hepatomegaly is common at diagnosis and infants are at risk for failure to thrive due to fat malabsorption. Symptoms of portal hypertension (splenomegaly, ascites, variceal bleeding) may develop in the first year of life. Pruritus, digital clubbing, bone fractures, and variceal bleeding complications may occur later in childhood.

B. Laboratory Findings and Imaging

No single laboratory test will consistently differentiate BA from other causes of complete obstructive jaundice. Although BA is suggested by persistent elevation of serum GGT in addition to conjugated/direct bilirubin, these findings have also been reported in severe neonatal hepatitis, α_1-antitrypsin deficiency, cystic fibrosis, MDR3 deficiency, neonatal sclerosing cholangitis, and bile duct paucity. Furthermore, these tests will not differentiate the location of the obstruction within the extrahepatic system. Generally, the aminotransferases are only moderately elevated in BA and serum albumin and blood clotting factors are normal early in the disease. Ultrasonography of the biliary system should be performed to exclude the presence of choledochal cyst and identify intra-abdominal anomalies associated with BA. In the majority of cases of BA, the gallbladder is not visualized or is small; however, the presence of a normal gallbladder on ultrasound does not exclude BA.

▶ Differential Diagnosis

The major diagnostic dilemma is distinguishing between this entity and bile duct paucity, genetic and metabolic liver diseases (particularly α_1-antitrypsin deficiency and PFIC), choledochal cyst, neonatal sclerosing cholangitis, or intrinsic bile duct obstruction (inspissated bile syndrome). Although spontaneous perforation of extrahepatic bile ducts leads to jaundice and acholic stools, the infants in such cases are usually quite ill with chemical peritonitis from biliary ascites.

The diagnosis of BA is suggested based on histologic findings of obstruction (bile duct plugs, bile duct proliferation, portal fibrosis). Once the diagnosis of α-1 antitrypsin deficiency and Alagille syndrome are excluded, a cholangiogram (intraoperative [IOC], endoscopic or transcholycystographic) to confirm the diagnosis of BA should be performed as soon as possible. Radiographic visualization of cholangiographic contrast in the duodenum excludes obstruction to the distal extrahepatic ducts. In the majority of cases of BA, the entire extrahepatic biliary system including the gall bladder is obstructed and no cholangiographic contrast will be visible within the biliary tree.

▶ Treatment

In the absence of surgical correction or transplantation, biliary cirrhosis, hepatic failure, and death occur uniformly by age 18–24 months. The standard procedure at the time of IOC diagnosis of BA is the hepatoportoenterostomy (Kasai procedure) to achieve drainage of bile from liver to intestine. The Kasai procedure is best done in specialized centers where experienced surgical, pediatric, and nursing personnel are available. For best results, surgery should be performed as early as possible (ideally before 30–45 days of life); the Kasai procedure should generally not be undertaken in infants older than age 4 months because the likelihood of bile drainage at this age is very low. Orthotopic liver transplantation is indicated for patients who do not undergo the Kasai procedure, who fail to drain bile after the Kasai procedure, or who progress to end-stage biliary cirrhosis despite surgical treatment. Timing of liver transplant evaluation and care prior to transplant has recently been reviewed.

Supportive medical treatment consists of vitamin and caloric support (vitamins A, D, E, and K supplements and formulas containing high amounts of medium-chain triglycerides [Pregestimil or Alimentum]) (see Table 22–4). Nasogastric tube feedings or parenteral nutrition may be required in patients failing oral caloric supplementation. Monitoring of serum fat-soluble vitamin levels is essential to ensure adequate supplementation. UDCA as a choloretic agent is routinely given post-Kasai and continued up to 3 years of age. UDCA should not be used in the setting of a "failed Kasai" whereby bile flow is not established, as UDCA in this setting is potentially hepatotoxic. Suspected ascending cholangitis (based on fever, jaundice, acholic stools, abdominal pain, leukocytosis, elevated bilirubin and liver enzymes) should be treated promptly with antibiotics that treat gram-negative bacterial infections. Antibiotic prophylaxis may reduce the recurrence rate of cholangitis. Ascites can be managed initially with spironolactone; furosemide is added in severe or unresponsive cases. There is no therapy that prevents the progression of biliary disease and portal fibrosis that occurs

in the majority of patients post-Kasai, including the use of corticosteroids.

▶ Prognosis

In general, outcomes of post-Kasai include failure to reestablish bile flow in one-third and improvement in bile flow in up to two-thirds of patients. Approximately 50% of BA patients will require liver transplantation in the first 2 years of life, some despite achieving good bile drainage. The best predictor of the need for liver transplant in the first 2 years is the total serum bilirubin value at 3 months post-Kasai: if the total bilirubin is less than 2 mg/dL, then it is unlikely that child will need transplant in the first 2 years; if the bilirubin is greater than 6 mg/dL, then a liver transplant will likely be necessary in the first 2 years. Even in the setting of reestablished bile flow following Kasai surgery, the majority of patients will progress to biliary cirrhosis and need a liver transplantation at some point in childhood (~ 80% of all BA patients). Death is usually caused by liver failure, sepsis, intractable variceal bleeding, or respiratory failure secondary to intractable ascites. Esophageal variceal hemorrhage develops in 40% of patients, yet terminal hemorrhage is unusual. Occasional long-term survivors develop hepatopulmonary syndrome (intrapulmonary right to left shunting of blood resulting in hypoxia) or portopulmonary hypertension (pulmonary arterial hypertension in patients with portal hypertension). Liver transplantation is indicated for all of the above-noted complications and long-term survival post-transplant is ~ 80%–90%.

Bezerra JA et al: Biliary atresia: clinical and research challenges for the 21st century. Hepatology 2018. [Epub ahead of print] [PMID: 29604222].

Feldman AG, Sokol RJ: Neonatal cholestasis: emerging molecular diagnostics and potential novel therapeutics. Nat Rev Gastroenterol Hepatol 2019 Jun;16(6):346–360 [PMID: 30903105].

Sundaram SS et al: Biliary atresia: indications and timing of liver transplantation and optimization of pretransplant care. Liver Transpl 2017;23(1):96–109 [PMID: 27650268].

2. Choledochal Cyst

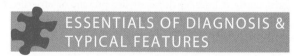

ESSENTIALS OF DIAGNOSIS & TYPICAL FEATURES

▶ Abnormal abdominal ultrasound with cyst of the biliary tree.

▶ Clinical Features

A. Symptoms and Signs

Choledochal cysts (CDC) are cystic lesions of all or part of the extrahepatic biliary system, which in rare cases can include the intrahepatic bile duct branches. Abdominal ultrasound imaging will detect all cases of CDC. In most cases presenting in infancy, the clinical manifestations and basic laboratory findings are indistinguishable from those associated with biliary atresia. Furthermore, a rare form of biliary atresia, termed "cystic biliary atresia" can mimic a CDC in the neonatal period. Clues to the diagnosis of CDC (versus cystic biliary atresia) include the presence of intrahepatic biliary dilation and a normal or distended gallbladder. In older children, CDC presents as recurrent episodes of right upper quadrant abdominal pain, fevers, vomiting, obstructive jaundice, pancreatitis, or as a right abdominal mass. Infants and children with CDC are at increased risk for developing bacterial cholangitis. CDC represent only 2%–5% of cases of extrahepatic neonatal cholestasis; the incidence is higher in girls and patients of Asian descent.

B. Diagnosis and Treatment

▶ Diagnosis

Ultrasonography is used to screen for CDC and an MRCP will confirm the diagnosis and the extent of the cystic lesion.

▶ Treatment

Timely surgery is indicated once abnormalities in clotting factors have been corrected and bacterial cholangitis, if present, has been treated with intravenous antibiotics. Excision of the cyst and its mucosa and choledocho–Roux-en-Y jejunal anastomosis are recommended. Anastomosis of cyst to jejunum or duodenum is not recommended due to the continued risks of cholangitis and bile duct carcinoma (cholangiocarcinoma).

▶ Prognosis

If an isolated extrahepatic cyst is encountered, the outcome is generally excellent, with resolution of the jaundice and return to normal liver architecture after cyst excision. However, bouts of ascending cholangitis may occur, particularly if intrahepatic cysts are present or stricture of the anastomotic site develops. The risk of cholangiocarcinoma developing within the cyst is about 5%–15% in adulthood.

Aspelund G et al; American Academy of Pediatrics Section on Surgery's Delivery of Surgical Care Committee: Transitional care for patients with surgical pediatric hepatobiliary disease: choledochal cysts and biliary atresia. J Gastroenterol Hepatol 2019 Jun;34(6):966–974 [PMID: 30552863].

Soares KC et al: Pediatric choledochal cysts: diagnosis and current management. Ped Surg Int 2017;33(6):637–650 [PMID: 28364277].

3. Spontaneous Perforation of the Extrahepatic Bile Ducts

The sudden appearance of obstructive jaundice, acholic stools, and abdominal enlargement with ascites in a sick newborn is suggestive of this condition. The liver is usually normal in size, and a yellow-green discoloration can often be discerned under the umbilicus or in the scrotum. In 24% of cases, stones or sludge obstructs the common bile duct. HIDA scan or ERCP shows leakage from the biliary tree, and ultrasonography confirms ascites or fluid around the bile duct.

Treatment is surgical. Simple drainage, without attempts at oversewing the perforation, is sufficient in primary perforations. A diversion anastomosis is constructed in cases associated with choledochal cyst or stenosis. The prognosis is generally good.

Jeanty C et al: Spontaneous biliary perforation in infancy: management strategies and outcomes. J Pediatr Surg 2015; 50(7):1137–1141 [PMID: 25783338].

OTHER NEONATAL HYPERBILIRUBINEMIC CONDITIONS (NONCHOLESTATIC NONHEMOLYTIC)

Two other groups of disorders are associated with hyperbilirubinemia: (1) unconjugated hyperbilirubinemia is characteristic of breast-feeding and breast milk jaundice, congenital hypothyroidism, red blood cell hemolysis, upper intestinal obstruction, Gilbert disease, Crigler-Najjar syndrome, and drug-induced hyperbilirubinemia; and (2) conjugated noncholestatic hyperbilirubinemia is characteristic of the Dubin-Johnson syndrome and Rotor syndrome.

1. Unconjugated Hyperbilirubinemia

A. Breast Milk Jaundice

Jaundice at 2 weeks of age is relatively common affecting up to 15% of newborns. Enhanced β-glucuronidase activity in breast milk is one factor that increases absorption of unconjugated bilirubin. Substances (eg, L-aspartic acid) in casein hydrolysate formulas inhibit this enzyme. The increased enterohepatic shunting of unconjugated bilirubin exceeds the normal conjugating capacity in the liver of these infants. The mutation for Gilbert syndrome (UDP-glucuronyltransferase 1A1 [UGT1A1]) predisposes to breast milk jaundice and to more prolonged jaundice. Neonates who carry the 211 and 388 variants in the UGT1A1 and OATP 2 genes, respectively, or the UGT1A1*6 allele and feed with breast milk, are at high risk to develop severe hyperbilirubinemia. Low volumes of ingested breast milk may also contribute to jaundice in the first week of life. Finally, breast milk may suppress UGT1A1 expression in the infant's intestines which may also lead to unconjugated hyperbilirubinemia.

Hyperbilirubinemia does not usually exceed 20 mg/dL, with most cases in the range of 10–15 mg/dL. Jaundice is noticeable by the fifth to seventh day of breast-feeding. It may accentuate the underlying physiologic jaundice—especially early, when total fluid intake may be less than optimal. Except for jaundice, the physical examination is normal; urine does not stain the diaper, and the stools are golden yellow.

The jaundice peaks before the third week of life and clears before age 3 months in almost all infants, even when breast-feeding is continued. All infants who remain jaundiced past age 2–3 weeks should have measurement of conjugated bilirubin to exclude cholestasis and hepatobiliary disease.

Kernicterus has rarely been reported in association with this condition. In special situations, breast-feeding may be discontinued temporarily and replaced by formula feedings for 2–3 days until serum bilirubin decreases by 2–8 mg/dL. Cow's milk formulas inhibit the intestinal reabsorption of unconjugated bilirubin. When breast-feeding is reinstituted, the serum bilirubin may increase slightly, but not to the previous level. Phototherapy is not indicated in the healthy full-term infant with this condition unless bilirubin levels meet high-risk levels as defined by the American Academy of Pediatrics.

Bratton S, Stern M: Breast milk jaundice. *StatPearls [Internet]*. Treasure Island, FL: StatPearls Publishing; 2019 Jan–2019 Nov [PMID: 30726019].

Fujiwara R et al: Reduced expression of UGT1A1 in intestines of humanized UGT1 mice via inactivation of NF-κB leads to hyperbilirubinemia. Gastroenterology 2012;142:109 [PMID: 21983082].

Maruo Y et al: Bilirubin uridine diphosphate-glucuronosyltransferase variation is a genetic basis of breast milk jaundice. J Pediatr 2014 Jul;165(1):36–41 [PMID: 24650397].

Preer GL, Philipp BL: Understanding and managing breast milk jaundice. Arch Dis Child Fetal Neonatal Ed 2011;96:F461 [PMID: 20688866].

B. Congenital Hypothyroidism

Although the differential diagnosis of indirect hyperbilirubinemia should always include congenital hypothyroidism, the diagnosis is usually identified by the newborn screening results or by clinical and physical clues. The jaundice clears quickly with replacement thyroid hormone therapy, although the mechanism is unclear. Hypopituitarism can also present with neonatal cholestasis and can be associated with septo-optic dysplasia, a congenital malformation syndrome featuring underdevelopment of the optic nerve, pituitary gland dysfunction, and absence of the septum pellucidum.

Tiker F: Congenital hypothyroidism and early severe hyperbilirubinemia. Clin Pediatr (Phila) 2003;42:365 [PMID: 12800733].

C. Upper Intestinal Obstruction

The association of indirect hyperbilirubinemia with high intestinal obstruction (eg, duodenal atresia, annular pancreas, pyloric stenosis) in the newborn has been observed repeatedly; the mechanism is unknown. Diminished levels of hepatic glucuronyl transferase are found on liver biopsy in pyloric stenosis, and genetic studies suggest that this indirect hyperbilirubinemia may be an early sign of Gilbert syndrome. Treatment is that of the underlying obstructive condition (usually surgical). Jaundice disappears once adequate nutrition is achieved.

Hua L et al: The role of UGT1A1*28 mutation in jaundiced infants with hypertrophic pyloric stenosis. Pediatr Res 2005;58:881 [PMID: 16257926].

D. Gilbert Syndrome

Gilbert syndrome is a common form of familial hyperbilirubinemia present in 3%–7% of the population. It is associated with a partial reduction of hepatic bilirubin uridine diphosphate-glucuronyl transferase activity. Affected infants may have more rapid increase in jaundice in the newborn period, accentuated breast milk jaundice, and jaundice with intestinal obstruction. During puberty and beyond, mild fluctuating jaundice, especially with illness and vague constitutional symptoms, is common. Shortened red blood cell survival in some patients is thought to be caused by reduced activity of enzymes involved in heme biosynthesis (protoporphyrinogen oxidase). Reduction of hyperbilirubinemia has been achieved in patients by administration of phenobarbital (5–8 mg/kg/day), although this therapy is not needed.

The disease is inherited as an abnormality of the promoter region of uridine diphosphate-glucuronyl transferase-1 (*UDGT1*) coded by *UGT1A1*; however, another factor appears to be necessary for disease expression. The homozygous (16%) and heterozygous states (40%) are common. Males are affected more often than females (4:1) for reasons that are not clear. Serum unconjugated bilirubin is generally less than 3–6 mg/dL, although unusual cases may exceed 8 mg/dL. The findings on liver biopsy and most LFTs are normal. An increase of 1.4 mg/dL or more in the level of unconjugated bilirubin after a 2-day fast (300 kcal/day) is consistent with the diagnosis of Gilbert syndrome. Gilbert syndrome, conferred by the donor liver, can occur following liver transplantation. Genetic testing is available but rarely needed. No treatment is necessary.

Erlinger S et al: Inherited disorders of bilirubin transport and conjugation: new insights into molecular mechanisms and consequences. Gastroenterology 2014 Jun;146(7):1625–1638 [PMID: 24704527].

Kathemann S et al: Gilbert syndrome—a frequent cause of unconjugated hyperbilirubinemia in children after orthotopic liver transplantation. Pediatr Transplant 2012;16:20 [PMID: 22360405].

Travan L et al: Severe neonatal hyperbilirubinemia and UGT1A1 promoter polymorphism. J Pediatr 2014 Jul;165(1):42–45 [PMID: 24726540].

E. Crigler-Najjar Syndrome

Infants with type 1 Crigler-Najjar syndrome usually develop rapid severe unconjugated hyperbilirubinemia (> 30–40 mg/dL) with neurologic consequences (kernicterus). The deficiency in UGT1A1 is inherited in an autosomal recessive pattern. Consanguinity is often present. Genetic testing of *UGT1A1* is definitive. Prompt recognition of this entity and treatment with exchange transfusions are required, followed by phototherapy. Phenobarbital administration does not significantly alter these findings, nor does it lower serum bilirubin levels. A combination of aggressive phototherapy and cholestyramine may keep bilirubin levels below 25 mg/dL. Orlistat therapy may decrease bilirubin in a subset of patients. Liver transplantation is curative and may prevent kernicterus if performed early. Auxiliary orthotopic transplantation also relieves the jaundice while the patient retains native liver. Hepatocyte transplantation through the portal vein has been tried in the past but is hampered by the requirement of multiple infusions of cells over time. Clinical trials using an adeno-associated virus vector to mediate gene therapy or using mesenchymal stem cells are underway.

A milder form (type 2) with both autosomal dominant and recessive inheritance is rarely associated with neurologic complications. Hyperbilirubinemia is less severe, and the bile is pigmented and contains small amounts of bilirubin monoglucuronide and diglucuronide. Patients with this form respond to phenobarbital (4 mg/kg/day in infants) with lowering of serum bilirubin levels. An increased proportion of monoconjugated and diconjugated bilirubin in the bile follows phenobarbital treatment. Liver biopsy findings and LFTs are consistently normal in both types.

Bartlett MG, Gourley GR: Assessment of UGT polymorphisms and neonatal jaundice. Semin Perinatol 2011;35:127 [PMID: 21641485].

Collaud et al: Preclinical development of an AAV8-hUGT1A1 vector for the treatment of Crigler-Najjar syndrome. Mol Ther Methods Clin Dev 2018;12:157–174 [PMID: 30705921].

Erlinger S et al: Inherited disorders of bilirubin transport and conjugation: new insights into molecular mechanisms and consequences. Gastroenterology 2014 Jun;146(7):1625–1638 [PMID: 24704527].

Smets F et al: Phase I/II trial of liver derived mesenchymal stem cells in pediatric liver based metabolic disorders: a prospective, open label, multicenter, partially randomized, safety study of one cycle of heterologous human adult liver-derived progenitor cells (HepaStem) in urea cycle disorders and Crigler-Najjar syndrome patients. Transplantation 2019;103(9):1903–1915 [PMID: 30801523].

F. Drug-Induced Hyperbilirubinemia

Vitamin K_3 (menadiol) may elevate indirect bilirubin levels by causing hemolysis. Vitamin K_1 (phytonadione) can be used safely in neonates. Carbamazepine can cause conjugated hyperbilirubinemia in infancy. Rifampin and antiretroviral protease inhibitors (atazanavir) may cause unconjugated hyperbilirubinemia. Pancuronium bromide and chloral hydrate have been implicated in causing neonatal jaundice. Other drugs (eg, ceftriaxone, sulfonamides) may displace bilirubin from albumin, potentially increasing the risk of kernicterus—especially in the sick premature infant.

2. Conjugated Noncholestatic Hyperbilirubinemia (Dubin-Johnson Syndrome & Rotor Syndrome)

These diagnoses are suspected when persistent or recurrent conjugated hyperbilirubinemia and jaundice occur and LFTs are normal. The basic defect in Dubin-Johnson syndrome is in the multiple organic anion transport protein 2 (*MRP2*) of the bile canaliculus, causing impaired hepatocyte excretion of conjugated bilirubin into bile. A variable degree of impairment in uptake and conjugation complicates the clinical picture. Transmission is autosomal recessive, so a positive family history is occasionally obtained. In Rotor syndrome, the defect lies in hepatic uptake and storage of bilirubin. OATP1B1 (coded by *SLCO1B1*) and OATP1B3 (*SLCO1B3*) are the two transporters that are deficient. Bile acids are metabolized normally, so that cholestasis does not occur. Bilirubin values range from 2 to 5 mg/dL, and other LFTs are normal.

In Rotor syndrome, the liver is normal; in Dubin-Johnson syndrome, it is darkly pigmented on gross inspection and may be enlarged. Microscopic examination reveals numerous dark-brown pigment granules consisting of polymers of epinephrine metabolites, especially in the centrilobular regions. However, the amount of pigment varies within families, and some jaundiced family members may have no demonstrable pigmentation in the liver. Otherwise, the liver is histologically normal. Oral cholecystography fails to visualize the gallbladder in Dubin-Johnson syndrome, but is normal in Rotor syndrome. Differences in the excretion patterns of bromosulfophthalein, in results of HIDA cholescintigraphy, in urinary coproporphyrin I and III levels, and in the serum pattern of monoglucuronide and diglucuronide conjugates of bilirubin can help distinguish between these two conditions. Clinical genotyping of *MRP2*, *SLCO1B1*, and *SLCO1B3* is available. No treatment is needed for either condition. Choleretic agents (eg, UDCA) may help reduce the cholestasis in infants with Dubin-Johnson syndrome.

Jirsa M et al: Rotor syndrome. In: Pagon RA et al. (eds): *GeneReviews™* [Internet]. 2012 Dec 13 [PMID: 23236639].

Keppler D: The roles of MRP2, MRP3, OATP1B1, and OATP1B3 in conjugated hyperbilirubinemia. Drug Metab Dispos 2014 Apr;42(4):561–565 [PMID: 24459177].

HEPATITIS VIRUS ABBREVIATIONS

HAV	Hepatitis A virus
HBV	Hepatitis B virus
HBcAg	HBV core antigen
Anti-HBs	Antibody to HBsAg
Anti-HBc IgM	IgM antibody to HBcAg
HCV	Hepatitis C virus
HDV	Hepatitis D (delta) virus
HEV	Hepatitis E virus
Anti-HAV IgM	IgM antibody to HAV
HBsAg	HBV surface antigen
HBeAg	HBV e antigen
Anti-HBc	Antibody to HBcAg
Anti-HBe	Antibody to HBeAg
Anti-HCV	Antibody to HCV
Anti-HDV	Antibody to HDV
Anti-HEV	Antibody to HEV

HEPATITIS A

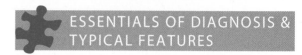

ESSENTIALS OF DIAGNOSIS & TYPICAL FEATURES

▶ Gastrointestinal upset (anorexia, vomiting, diarrhea).

▶ Jaundice.

▶ Liver tenderness and enlargement.

▶ Abnormal LFTs.

▶ Local epidemic of hepatitis A infection.

▶ Positive anti–hepatitis A virus (HAV) IgM antibody.

▶ Pathogenesis

Hepatitis A virus (HAV) infection occurs in both epidemic and sporadic fashion and is transmitted by the fecal-oral route (Table 22–6). HAV viral particles are found in stool during the acute phase of hepatitis A infection. Epidemic outbreaks are caused by contaminated food or water supplies, including by food handlers, while sporadic cases usually result from contact with an infected individual. Transmission through

Table 22–6. Hepatitis viruses.

	HAV	HBV	HCV	HDV	HEV
Type of virus	Enterovirus (RNA)	Hepadnavirus (DNA)	Flavivirus (RNA)	Deltavirus (RNA)	Hepevirus (RNA)
Transmission routes	Fecal-oral	Parenteral, sexual, vertical	Parenteral, sexual, vertical	Parenteral, sexual	Fecal-oral
Incubation period (days)	15–40	45–160	30–150	20–90	14–65
Diagnostic test	Anti-HAV IgM	HBsAg, anti-HBc IgM, DNA PCR	Anti-HCV, RNA PCR	Anti-HDV antibody	Anti-HEV IgM, HEV PCR
Mortality rate (acute)	0.1%–0.2%	0.5%–2%	1%–2%	2%–20%	1%–2% (10%–20% in pregnant women)
Carrier state	No	Yes	Yes	Yes	Rare (in immunocompromised)
Vaccine available	Yes	Yes	No	Yes (HBV)	Yes (experimental)
Treatment	None	Interferon-α (pegylated interferon in adults), nucleoside analogues (lamivudine or entecavir > 2 y old, tenofovir or, adefovir > 12; telbivudine > 16)	Pegylated interferon plus ribavirin[a]	Treatment for HBV	None

HAV, hepatitis A virus; HBc, hepatitis B core; HBsAg, hepatitis B surface antigen; HBV, hepatitis B virus; HDV, hepatitis D (delta) virus; HEV, hepatitis E virus; PCR, polymerase chain reaction.
[a]Ongoing pediatric clinical trials of direct-acting antiviral agents.

blood products obtained during the viremic phase is a rare event, although it has occurred in a newborn nursery.

Prevention

Isolation of an infected patient during initial phases of illness is indicated, although most patients with hepatitis A are noninfectious by the time the disease becomes overt. Stool, diapers, and other fecally stained clothing should be handled with care for 1 week after the appearance of jaundice.

Passive-active immunization of exposed susceptible persons younger than 12 months or older than 40 years: anyone who is immunocompromised or who has chronic liver disease is recommended with immune globulin, 0.02 mL/kg intramuscularly. Illness is prevented in more than 85% of individuals if immune globulin is given within 2 weeks of exposure. For individuals 12 months to 40 years old, HAV vaccine is recommended following exposure. Infants younger than 12 months traveling to endemic disease areas should receive HAV vaccine or 0.02 or 0.06 mL/kg (for trip > 3 months) of immune globulin as prophylaxis. Older individuals should receive the HAV vaccine. All children older than 12 months with chronic liver disease should receive two doses of HAV vaccine 6 months apart. It is also currently recommended that all children 12–18 months of age receive two doses of HAV vaccine in the United States. If an emigrant child from an endemic area is adopted, the immediate family members should be immunized. Lifelong immunity to HAV follows infection.

Antibody to HAV appears within 1–4 weeks of clinical symptoms. Although the great majority of children with infectious hepatitis are asymptomatic or have mild disease and recover completely, some will develop fulminant hepatitis leading to death or requiring liver transplantation.

Clinical Findings

A. History

Historical risk factors may include direct exposure to a previously jaundiced individual or recently arrived individual from a high-prevalence country, consumption of seafood, contaminated water or imported fruits or vegetables, attendance in a day care center, or recent travel to an area of endemic infection. Following an incubation period of 15–40 days, nonspecific symptoms usually precede the development of jaundice by 5–10 days. In developing countries, hepatitis A is common and most children are exposed to HAV by age 10 years, while only 20% are exposed by age 20 years in developed countries.

B. Symptoms and Signs

The overt form of the disease is easily recognized by the clinical manifestations. However, two-thirds of children are asymptomatic, and two-thirds of symptomatic children are anicteric. Therefore, the presenting symptoms in children with HAV often resemble gastroenteritis. Fever, anorexia, vomiting, headache, and abdominal pain are typical and dark urine precedes jaundice, which peaks in 1–2 weeks and then begins to subside. The stools may become light- or clay-colored. Clinical improvement can occur as jaundice develops. Tender hepatomegaly and jaundice are typically present in symptomatic children; splenomegaly is variable.

C. Laboratory Findings

Serum aminotransferases and conjugated and unconjugated bilirubin levels are elevated. Although unusual, hypoalbuminemia, hypoglycemia, and marked prolongation of PT (international normalized ratio [INR] > 2.0) are serious prognostic findings. Diagnosis is made by a positive anti-HAV IgM, whereas anti-HAV IgG persists after recovery.

Percutaneous liver biopsy is rarely indicated. "Balloon cells" and acidophilic bodies are characteristic histologic findings. Liver cell necrosis may be diffuse or focal, with accompanying infiltration of inflammatory cells containing polymorphonuclear leukocytes, lymphocytes, macrophages, and plasma cells, particularly in portal areas. Some bile duct proliferation may be seen in the perilobular portal areas alongside areas of bile stasis. Regenerative liver cells and proliferation of reticuloendothelial cells are present. Occasionally, massive hepatocyte necrosis portends a poor prognosis.

Differential Diagnosis

Before jaundice appears, the symptoms are those of nonspecific viral enteritis. Other diseases with somewhat similar onset include pancreatitis, infectious mononucleosis, leptospirosis, drug-induced hepatitis, Wilson disease, autoimmune hepatitis (AIH), and infection with other hepatitis viruses. Acquired CMV disease may also mimic HAV, although lymphadenopathy is usually present in the former.

Treatment

No specific treatment measures are required although bed rest is reasonable for the child who appears ill. Sedatives and corticosteroids should be avoided. During the icteric phase, lower-fat foods may diminish gastrointestinal symptoms but do not affect overall outcome. Drugs and elective surgery should be avoided. Hospitalization is recommended for children with coagulopathy, encephalopathy, or severe vomiting. Hospitalization rates for hepatitis A have decreased over the last decade, with those who require hospitalization being older adults or those with concurrent other liver disease and/or comorbid conditions.

Prognosis

Around 99% of children recover without sequelae. Persons with underlying chronic liver disease have an increased risk of death. In rare cases of acute liver failure (ALF) due to

HAV hepatitis, the patient may die within days to weeks or require evaluation for liver transplantation. The prognosis is poor if hepatic coma or ascites develop; liver transplantation is indicated under these circumstances and is life-saving. Incomplete resolution can cause a prolonged hepatitis, but resolution invariably occurs without long-term hepatic sequelae. Rare cases of aplastic anemia following acute infectious hepatitis have been reported. A benign relapse of symptoms may occur in 10%–15% of cases after 6–10 weeks of apparent resolution.

Collier MG et al: Hepatitis A hospitalizations in the United States, 2002–2011. Hepatology 2015;61:481 [PMID: 25266085].

Dorell CG et al: Hepatitis A vaccination coverage among adolescents in the United States. Pediatrics 2012;129:213 [PMID: 22271690].

Hepatitis A in Red Book: 2012 report of the committee on infectious diseases. 29th ed. Elk Grove Village, IL. American Academy of Pediatrics; 2012.

Lee HW et al: Clinical factors and viral load influencing severity of acute hepatitis A. PLoS One 2015 Jun 19;10(6) [PMID: 26090677].

Murphy TV et al: Progress toward eliminating hepatitis A disease in the United States. MMWR Supple 2016 Feb 12;65(1): 29–41 [PMID: 26916458].

HEPATITIS B

ESSENTIALS OF DIAGNOSIS & TYPICAL FEATURES

▶ The vast majority of patients with vertically acquired HBV infection will be asymptomatic and have a normal physical exam.

▶ Acute HBV infection may be associated with anorexia, vomiting, diarrhea, jaundice, tender hepatomegaly, and abnormal LFTs.

▶ Serologic evidence of hepatitis B disease: positive HBsAg, HBeAg, anti-HBc IgM.

▶ History of parenteral, sexual, or household exposure or maternal HBsAg carriage.

General Considerations

Hepatitis B virus (HBV) is a DNA virus whose infection has an incubation period of 45–160 days (see Table 22–6). HBV is either acquired perinatally from a carrier mother, or later in life from exposure to contaminated blood through shared needles, needle sticks, skin piercing, tattoos, or sexual transmission.

Pathophysiology

The HBV particle is composed of a core that is found in the nucleus of infected liver cells and a double outer shell (surface antigen or HBsAg). The nomenclature for the viral antigens and antibodies is found in the table of Hepatitis Virus Abbreviations provided above. HBeAg, a truncated soluble form of HBcAg, correlates with active virus replication. Persistence of HBeAg is a marker of infectivity, whereas the appearance of anti-HBe generally implies a lower level of viral replication. However, HBV mutant viruses (precore mutant) may replicate with negative HBeAg tests and positive tests for anti-HBe antibody (HBeAg-negative chronic hepatitis). Such cases are associated with a more virulent form of hepatitis. Circulating HBV DNA (measured by PCR) also indicates viral replication.

Prevention

HBV vaccination is the preferred method for prevention. Universal immunization of all infants is recommended. Other control methods include screening of blood donors and pregnant women, use of properly sterilized needles and surgical equipment, avoidance of sexual contact with carriers, general adoption of safe sex practices, and vaccination of household contacts, sexual partners, medical personnel, and those at high risk. For postexposure prophylaxis, HBV vaccine is given alone (see Chapter 10) or together with administration of hepatitis B immune globulin (HBIG) (0.06 mL/kg intramuscularly, given as soon as possible after exposure, up to 7 days). The risk of vertical transmission is dramatically reduced with the combination of newborn vaccination and HBIG administration. For infected pregnant women with high viral loads, use of oral antivirals in the last half of pregnancy combined with postdelivery prophylaxis can further reduce perinatal prophylaxis failures from 5% to 1.5%.

Clinical Findings

A. Symptoms and Signs

Most infants and young children are asymptomatic, especially if the infection is acquired vertically. Symptoms of acute HBV infection may include a slight fever, malaise, and mild gastrointestinal upset. Visible jaundice is usually the first significant finding and hepatomegaly is frequently present. Rare presentations include immune complex-mediated rash, arthritis, glomerulonephritis, or nephrotic syndrome.

B. Laboratory Findings

The diagnosis of acute HBV infection is confirmed by the presence of HBsAg and anti-HBc IgM. Recovery from acute infection is accompanied by HBsAg clearance and appearance of anti-HBs and anti-HBc IgG. Individuals who are immune by vaccination are positive for anti-HBs, but negative for anti-HBc IgG. Chronic infection is defined as the presence of HBsAg for at least 6 months. Vertical transmission to newborns is documented by positive HBsAg. The various phases of chronic HBV infection are shown in Table 22–7.

Table 22–7. Phases of chronic hepatitis B infection.

Phase	HBeAg/Anti-HBeAb	HBsAg/Anti-HBsAb	ALT	HBV DNA
Immune tolerant	Positive/negative	Positive/negative	Normal	> 20,000 IU/mL
Immune active	Positive/negative	Positive/negative	Elevated	High
Chronic HBsAg carrier	Negative/positive	Positive/negative	Normal	< 2000 IU/mL
HBeAg negative hepatitis/ reactivation	Negative/positive	Positive/negative	Elevated	> 2000 IU/mL
HBsAg clearance	Negative/positive	Negative/positive	Normal	Undetectable

Differential Diagnosis

The differentiation between HAV and HBV disease is aided by a history of parenteral exposure, a HBsAg-positive parent, or an unusually long period of incubation. HBV and hepatitis C virus (HCV) infection or Epstein-Barr virus (EBV) infection are differentiated serologically. Other diseases to consider in the differential diagnosis include autoimmune hepatitis, Wilson disease, hemochromatosis, nonalcoholic fatty liver disease (NAFLD), or α₁-antitrypsin deficiency.

Treatment

There is no therapy that is highly curative for Hepatitis B. For children with vertically acquired HBV infection and normal LFTs and physical exam (immunotolerant phase), treatment is not recommended. For acute infection complicated by ALF, or for chronic infection with elevated LFTs for more than 6 months (immunoactive phase), nucleos(t)ide therapy may be helpful. Orally administered nucleoside analog therapy includes entecavir or tenofovir. A significant decrease in viral load with these nucleos(t)ide therapies can be seen in up to 75% of treated children, with minimal side effects, but may require long-term treatment. Resistant virus mutants rarely emerge. Liver transplantation is successful in ALF due to hepatitis B; however, reinfection is common following liver transplantation for chronic hepatitis B unless long-term HBIG or antivirals are used.

Prognosis

The prognosis for acute HBV infection is good in older children, although ALF (< 0.1%) or chronic hepatitis and cirrhosis (up to 10%) may supervene. The course of the acute disease is variable, but jaundice seldom persists for more than 2 weeks. HBsAg disappears in 95% of cases at the time of clinical recovery. Individuals who have cleared HBV (HBsAg negative, anti-HBcIgG positive) are at risk for reactivation of HBV infection with significant immunosuppression (eg, chemotherapy). Chronic infection is particularly common in children with vertical transmission, Down syndrome, or leukemia, and in those undergoing chronic hemodialysis.

Persistence of neonatally acquired HBsAg occurs in 70%–90% of infants without immunoprophylaxis or vaccination. The presence of HBeAg in the HBsAg carrier indicates ongoing viral replication. However, 1%–2% of children infected at birth will show spontaneous seroconversion of HBeAg each year. If HBV infection is acquired later in childhood, HBV is cleared and recovery occurs in 90%–95% of patients. Chronic HBV disease predisposes the patient to development of hepatocellular carcinoma. Once chronic HBV infection is established, surveillance for development of hepatocellular carcinoma with serum α-fetoprotein is performed biannually and ultrasonography every 1–3 years. Routine HBV vaccination of newborns in endemic countries has reduced the incidence of ALF, chronic hepatitis, and hepatocellular carcinoma in children.

Defresne F, Sokol E: Chronic hepatitis B in children: therapeutic challenges and perspectives. J Gastroenterol Hepatol 2017:368–71 [PMID: 27262164].
Jonas M et al: Antiviral therapy in management of chronic hepatitis B viral infection in children: a systematic review and meta-analysis. Hepatology 2016;63:307 [PMID: 26566163].

HEPATITIS C

General Considerations

Hepatitis C virus (HCV) is the most common cause of non-B chronic hepatitis (see Table 22–6). HCV is a single-stranded RNA flavivirus with at least seven genotypes. Risk factors in adults and adolescents include illicit use of intravenous drugs, occupational or sexual exposure, and a history of transfusion of blood products prior to 1992. Most cases in children are associated with transmission from an infected mother (vertical transmission) or rarely from other household contacts, and in adolescents from IV drug use or sexual contact. Vertical transmission from HCV-infected mothers occurs more commonly with mothers who are HIV-positive (15%–20%) compared with those who are HIV-negative (5%–6%). Approximately, 0.2% of children, 0.4% of adolescents, and 1.5% of adults in the United States have serologic evidence of infection.

Prevention

At present, the only effective means of prevention is avoidance of exposure through elimination of risk-taking behaviors such as illicit use of intravenous drugs. There is no effective prevention for vertical transmission, but avoidance of fetal scalp monitoring in infant of mothers with HCV has been suggested. Elective Caesarean section is not recommended for HCV-monoinfected women, as it confers no reduction in the rate of mother-to-infant HCV transmission. Breast-feeding does not promote HCV transmission from mother to infant. It is advised to avoid breast-feeding if the nipples are bleeding, if mastitis is present or if the mother is experiencing a flare of hepatitis with jaundice postpartum. There is no vaccine, and no benefit from using immune globulin in infants born to infected mothers.

Clinical Findings

A. Symptoms and Signs

The majority of childhood cases, especially those acquired vertically, are asymptomatic despite development of chronic hepatitis. The incubation period is 1–5 months, with insidious onset of symptoms. Flu-like prodromal symptoms and jaundice occur in less than 25% of cases. Hepatosplenomegaly may or may not be evident. Ascites, clubbing, palmar erythema, or spider angiomas are rare and indicate progression to cirrhosis. In adults, chronic HCV infection has been associated with mixed cryoglobulinemia, polyarteritis nodosa, a sicca-like syndrome, and membranoproliferative glomerulonephritis, as well as hepatocellular carcinoma.

B. Laboratory Findings

Since anti-HCV IgG crosses the placenta, testing anti-HCV IgG is not informative until the infant is 18 months old, at which time antibody testing should be performed. Patients older than 18 months with positive anti-HCV IgG should have subsequent testing for serum HCV RNA in order to determine active infection. Serum HCV RNA can be tested prior to 18 months of age, but should not be tested before 2 months old. If serum HCV RNA is positive in infancy, it should be rechecked when the infant is 12 months of age in order to determine presence of chronic infection. Fluctuating mild to moderate elevations of aminotransferases over long periods are characteristic of chronic HCV infection; however, normal aminotransferases are common in children. Cirrhosis in adults generally requires 20–30 years of chronic HCV infection, but it has occasionally developed sooner in children.

Differential Diagnosis

HCV disease should be distinguished from HAV and HBV disease by serologic testing. Other causes of chronic hepatitis in children should be considered, including Wilson disease, α_1-antitrypsin deficiency, AIH, primary sclerosing cholangitis, drug-induced hepatitis, or steatohepatitis.

Treatment

The treatment for chronic HCV has rapidly changed in the past decade, with the advent of direct-acting antiviral therapies (DAA), which when used for 12–24 weeks have resulted in HCV eradication rates of more than 90%. The use of subcutaneous injections of pegylated interferon-α and oral ribavirin is no longer recommended. In April of 2017, the FDA approved the combination of Sofosbuvir (400 mg) plus Ledipasvir (90 mg) (Harvoni) once daily for 12 weeks for the treatment of genotype 1, 4, 5, or 6 in children greater than 12 years of age, or 35 Kg in weight. For genotypes 2 and 3, 12 weeks of Sofosbuvir (400 mg daily, Sovaldi) plus Ribavirin (15 mg/kg in two divided doses), was approved for the treatment of children greater than 12 years of age, or 35 Kg in weight. Current clinical trials of Sofosbuvir plus Ledipasvir and Sofosbuvir plus Ribavirin are underway in children as young as 3 years of age. Most recently, in April of 2019, the FDA approved the DAA combination of Glecaprevir (GLE) and Pibrentasvir (PIB) to treat all six genotypes of HCV in children ages 12–17 (DORA Study, Part 1, ClinicalTrials.gov Identifier: NCT03067129). End-stage liver disease secondary to HCV responds well to liver transplantation, although reinfection of the transplanted liver is very common; the new DAA therapies appear to be effective at eradicating HCV post-liver transplant as well. A website provides up-to-date guidance for suggested therapies in this era of rapidly evolving approval of new drugs for HCV (http://www.hcvguidelines.org).

Prognosis

Following an acute infection with HCV, 70%–80% of adults and older children develop a chronic infection. Around 20% of adults with chronic HCV develop cirrhosis by 30 years. Infants infected by vertical transmission have a high rate of spontaneous resolution, approaching 25%–40%. Most have spontaneous resolution by 24 months of age, but some may have spontaneous resolution as late as 7 years after vertical infection. The majority of children with chronic HCV have mild inflammation and fibrosis on liver biopsy, although cirrhosis may develop rapidly in rare cases. Limited 30-year follow-up of infants exposed to HCV by transfusion suggests a lower rate of progression to cirrhosis compared to adults. The prognosis for infants infected at birth with concomitant HIV infection is unknown, but the course appears benign for the first 10 years of life.

AASLD/IDSA: Recommendations for testing, managing and treating hepatitis C. http://www.hcvguidelines.org. Accessed June 1, 2019.

Modin L et al: Epidemiology and natural history of hepatitis C virus infection among children and young people. J Hepatol 2019 Mar;70(3) [PMID: 30496763].

Squires JE et al: Hepatitis C virus infection in children and adolescents. Hepatol Commun 2017 Mar;23(1) [PMID: 29404447].

HEPATITIS D (DELTA AGENT)

The hepatitis D virus (HDV) is a 36-nm virus that requires the presence of HBsAg to be infectious (see Table 22–6). Thus, HDV infection can occur only in the presence of HBV infection. Transmission is by parenteral exposure or intimate contact. HDV is rare in North America, but common in Africa, South America, Turkey, Mongolia, southern Italy, and Russia. HDV can infect simultaneously with HBV, causing acute hepatitis, or can superinfect a patient with chronic HBV infection, predisposing the individual to chronic hepatitis or fulminant hepatitis. In children, the association between chronic HDV coinfection with HBV and chronic hepatitis and cirrhosis is strong. Vertical HDV transmission is rare. HDV can be detected by anti-HDV IgG, which indicates active or previous infection; active infection is confirmed by detecting HDV RNA by PCR or by detecting HDV IgM antibody. Treatment is limited to interferon therapy but new treatments are being explored.

Wranke A, Wedemeyer H: Antiviral therapy of hepatitis delta virus infection—progress and challenges towards cure. Curr Opin Virol 2016;20:112 [PMID: 27792905].

HEPATITIS E

Hepatitis E virus (HEV) infection causes acute hepatitis (see Table 22–6). The World Health Organization estimates that one-third of the world's population has been exposed to HEV. Epidemics have occurred mainly in developing regions secondary to contamination of drinking water; however, recently HEV has increasingly been recognized as endemic in some developed regions where infections occur through zoonotic transmission or contaminated blood products. The routes of HEV transmission include fecal-oral (consumption of contaminated water and food), vertical, person-to-person, and, rarely, parenteral transmission. The majority of cases are asymptomatic; if symptomatic, the clinical manifestations resemble those of HAV infection. HEV infection in pregnancy is associated with a high mortality (10%–20%), particularly when acquired in the third trimester. HEV infection in individuals with chronic liver disease can cause acute deterioration. Immunocompromised individuals infected with HEV are at increased risk for the development of chronic infection, with higher rates of ALF and rapid onset of cirrhosis. Diagnosis is established by detecting anti-HEV IgM antibody or by HEV PCR. HEV is usually self-limited. Treatment is supportive care for healthy individuals and

lowering of immunosuppressive medications and ribavirin in immunosuppressed individuals.

Hartl J et al: Acute hepatitis E: two sides of the same coin. Viruses 2016;8:E299 [PMID: 27827877].

Kamar N et al: Hepatitis E virus infection. Nat Rev Dis Primers 2017 Nov l6;3:17086 [PMID: 29154369].

OTHER HEPATITIS VIRUSES

Other viruses including enterovirus, adenovirus, parvovirus, varicella, influenza, cytomegalovirus, herpes simplex virus, HHV-6, HIV, brucella, Q-fever, and leptospirosis may cause severe acute hepatitis or acute liver failure (ALF) in children, in some cases in association with aplastic anemia. Aplastic anemia occurs in a small proportion of patients recovering from hepatitis and in 10%–20% of those undergoing liver transplantation for ALF of unknown etiology. Infectious mononucleosis (EBV) is commonly associated with acute hepatitis and rare cases of EBV-associated ALF have been reported. Primary EBV infection in an immunocompromised solid organ transplant recipient may result in a lymphoproliferative disorder.

Jha HC et al: Epstein-Barr virus: diseases linked to infection and transformation. Front Microbiol 2016;7:1602 [PMID: 27826287].

ACUTE LIVER FAILURE

ESSENTIALS OF DIAGNOSIS & TYPICAL FEATURES

► Acute hepatitis with deepening jaundice.
► Extreme elevation of AST and ALT.
► Prolonged PT and INR.
► Encephalopathy and cerebral edema.
► Asterixis.

► General Considerations

Acute liver failure (ALF) is defined as acute liver dysfunction associated with significant hepatic synthetic dysfunction evidenced by vitamin K–resistant coagulopathy (INR > 2.0) within 8 weeks of onset of liver injury. This is often associated with encephalopathy, but in young children, encephalopathy may be difficult to detect. Without liver transplantation, mortality approaches 40% in children. In many cases, an identifiable cause is not found but is postulated to be an unusually virulent infectious agent or aggressive host immune response. Common identifiable causes of ALF are shown in Table 22–8.

Table 22–8. Common identifiable causes a of acute liver failure by age.

Neonates	Infections: herpesviruses and enteroviruses. Metabolic: neonatal iron storage disease, galactosemia, fructosemia, tyrosinemia, FAO, mitochondrial disorders. Ischemia: congenital heart disease.
Infants 1–24 mo	Infections: HAV, HBV. Metabolic: FAO, mitochondrial disorders, tyrosinemia, fructosemia, bile acid synthesis defects. Drug: acetaminophen, valproate. Immune: AIH, HLH.
Children	Infections: EBV, HAV. Metabolic: FAO, Wilson disease. Drug: acetaminophen, valproate, others. Immune: AIH.
Adolescents	Infections: EBV, HAV. Metabolic: FAO, Wilson disease, acute fatty liver of pregnancy. Drug: acetaminophen, valproate, herbs, "ecstasy," others. Immune: AIH.

AIH, autoimmune hepatitis; EBV, Epstein-Barr virus; FAO, fatty acid oxidation defects; HAV, hepatitis A; HBV, hepatitis B; HLH, hemophagocytic lymphohistiocytosis.
[a]Unknown cause of ALF remains the most common etiology.

▶ Clinical Findings

A. History

In some patients, ALF presents with the rapid development of deepening jaundice, bleeding, confusion, and progressive encephalopathy, while others are asymptomatic at the onset and then suddenly become severely ill during the second week of the disease. Jaundice, fever, anorexia, vomiting, and abdominal pain are the most common symptoms. A careful history of drug and toxin exposure may identify a drug-induced cause.

B. Symptoms and Signs

Children may present with flu-like symptoms, including malaise, myalgias, jaundice, nausea, and vomiting. Tender hepatomegaly is common, which may be followed by progressive shrinking of the liver, often with worsening hepatic function. Other physical findings (splenomegaly, spider hemangiomata) should suggest an underlying chronic liver disease. Hyper-reflexia and positive extensor plantar responses are seen in the early stages of hepatic encephalopathy.

C. Laboratory Findings

Characteristic findings include elevated serum bilirubin levels (usually > 10 mg/dL), sustained elevations of AST and ALT (often > 3000 U/L), low serum albumin, hypoglycemia,

and prolonged PT and INR. Blood ammonia levels may become elevated. Prolonged PT from disseminated intravascular coagulation (DIC) can be differentiated by determination of factor V (low in ALF and DIC) and VIII (normal to high in ALF and low in DIC). Rapid decreases in AST and ALT, together with shrinking hepatomegaly, due to massive necrosis and collapse, combined with worsening coagulopathy portend a poor prognosis.

▶ Differential Diagnosis

Severe hepatitis, with or without coagulopathy, due to infections, metabolic disease, AIH or drug toxicity can initially mimic ALF. Acute leukemia, cardiomyopathy, and Budd-Chiari syndrome can mimic severe hepatitis. Patients with Reye syndrome or urea cycle defects are typically anicteric.

▶ Complications

The development of renal failure and depth of hepatic coma are major prognostic factors. Patients in stage 4 coma (unresponsiveness to verbal stimuli, decorticate or decerebrate posturing) rarely survive without liver transplantation and may have residual central nervous system deficits even after transplant. Cerebral edema, which usually accompanies coma, is frequently the cause of death. Extreme prolongation of PT or INR greater than 3.5 predicts poor recovery, except with acetaminophen overdose. Sepsis, hemorrhage, renal failure, and cardiorespiratory arrest are common terminal events.

▶ Treatment

Excellent critical care is paramount, including careful management of hypoglycemia, bleeding and coagulopathy, hyperammonemia, cerebral edema, and fluid balance, while systematically investigating for potentially treatable causes. Several therapies have failed to affect outcome, including exchange transfusion, plasmapheresis with plasma exchange, total body washout, charcoal hemoperfusion, and hemodialysis using a special high-permeability membrane. While spontaneous survival may occur in up to 50% of patients, liver transplant may be lifesaving in patients without signs of spontaneous recovery. Therefore, early transfer of patients in ALF to centers where liver transplantation can be performed is recommended. Criteria for deciding when to perform transplantation are not firmly established; however, serum bilirubin over 20 mg/dL, INR greater than 4, and factor V levels less than 20% indicate a poor prognosis. Prognosis is better for acetaminophen ingestion, particularly when *N*-acetylcysteine treatment is given. *N*-acetylcysteine is not recommended in non–acetaminophen-induced liver failure, as it does not improve survival and may, in fact, negatively impact survival in those younger than 2 years.

Corticosteroids may be harmful, except in AIH for which steroids may reverse ALF. Acyclovir is essential in herpes simplex or varicella-zoster virus infection. For hyperammonemia, oral antibiotics such as neomycin or rifaximin, and lactulose (1–2 mL/kg three or four times daily) are used to reduce blood ammonia levels and trap ammonia in the colon.

Close monitoring of fluid and electrolytes is mandatory and requires a central venous line. Adequate dextrose should be infused (6–8 mg/kg/min) to maintain normal blood glucose and cellular metabolism. Diuretics, sedatives, and tranquilizers should be used sparingly. Comatose patients should be intubated, given mechanical ventilatory support, and monitored for signs of infection. Coagulopathy accompanied by bleeding and is treated with fresh-frozen plasma, recombinant factor VIIa, other clotting factor concentrates, platelet infusions. Hemodialysis may help stabilize a patient while awaiting liver transplantation. Monitoring for increased intracranial pressure (hepatic coma stages 3 and 4) in patients awaiting liver transplantation is advocated by some. Continuous venous-venous dialysis may be helpful to maintain fluid balance.

▶ Prognosis

Prognosis is primarily dependent on the etiology of ALF and depth of coma. Only 20%–30% of children with stage 3 or 4 hepatic encephalopathy will have a spontaneous recovery. Children with acute acetaminophen toxicity have a high rate of spontaneous survival, while 40% of children with indeterminate ALF (of unknown etiology) will have a spontaneous recovery. A recent large study suggests that the spontaneous recovery rate is about 40%–50% when all causes of ALF are combined; 30% of patients will receive a liver transplant; and 20% will die without a transplant. Exchange transfusions or other modes of heroic therapy do not improve survival figures. Indeterminate ALF, non-acetaminophen drug-induced ALF, and ALF in infants are associated with a poorer prognosis. Acetaminophen and autoimmune hepatitis etiologies of ALF and rising levels of factors V and VII, coupled with rising levels of serum α-fetoprotein, may signify a more favorable prognosis. The 1-year survival rate in patients who undergo liver transplantation for ALF is 60%–85%.

Alonso EM et al: Pediatric acute liver failure of undetermined cause: a research workshop. Hepatology, 2017 Mar;65(3) [PMID: 17862115].

Feldman AG et al: Lactate and lactate:pyruvate ratio in the diagnosis and outcomes of pediatric acute liver failure. J Pediatr 2017 Mar;182 [PMID: 28088395].

Squires JE et al: Liver transplant listing in pediatric acute liver failure: practices and participant characteristics. Heaptology 2108 Dec;68(6):2338–2347 [PMID: 30070372].

Sundaram SS et al: Characterization and outcomes of young infants with acute liver failure. J Pediatr 2011;159:813 [PMID: 21621221].

AUTOIMMUNE HEPATITIS

ESSENTIALS OF DIAGNOSIS & TYPICAL FEATURES

▶ Acute or chronic hepatitis.

▶ Hypergammaglobulinemia.

▶ Positive antinuclear antibodies (ANA), anti–smooth muscle (or actin) antibodies (ASMA), or anti–liver-kidney microsomal (LKM) antibodies.

▶ Clinical Findings

A. History

Autoimmune hepatitis (AIH) is a progressive inflammatory disorder. It is characterized histologically by portal tract inflammation that extends into the parenchyma; serologically by the presence of nonorgan-specific autoantibodies; biochemically by elevated aminotransferases and serum IgG; and clinically by response to immunosuppressive treatment in the absence of other known causes of liver disease. A family history of autoimmune diseases is present in approximately 40% of cases.

B. Symptoms and Signs

Pediatric patients are often asymptomatic early in the disease process and come to medical attention based on an incidental finding of elevated liver tests. Lethargy as well as malaise are common symptoms, and patients may also complain of jaundice, recurrent fevers, abdominal pain, or distension. Other complaints at the time of presentation may include a recurrent rash, arthritis, chronic diarrhea, or amenorrhea. Hepatomegaly and/or splenomegaly may be found on examination. In more advanced cases, jaundice and ascites may develop. Cutaneous signs of chronic liver disease may be noted (eg, spider angiomas, palmar erythema, and digital clubbing). In ~ 10% of cases, AIH patients present with ALF.

C. Laboratory Findings

Liver tests reveal moderate elevations of serum AST, ALT, and variable elevations of alkaline phosphatase, bilirubin, and total IgG. Two subtypes of disease have been described based on the autoantibodies present: type 1 AIH—ANA and/or ASMA (anti-actin); type 2 AIH—anti-LKM (anti–liver-kidney microsomal). Type 1 AIH is the most common form of AIH in the United States. Type 2 AIH is more common in Europe, presents at a younger age, and is more likely to present with ALF compared to type 1. A genetic susceptibility to AIH is suggested by the increased incidence of the histocompatibility alleles HLA DR*0301 (type 1 AIH) or HLA DR*0701 (type 2 AIH). Liver biopsy remains the gold standard in diagnosis, revealing the typical histological picture of interface hepatitis: a dense infiltration of the portal tracts consisting mainly of lymphocytes and plasma cells that extends into the liver lobules with destruction of the hepatocytes at the periphery of the lobule and erosion of the limiting plate. There may be bridging fibrosis or cirrhosis evident as well.

▶ Differential Diagnosis

Laboratory and histologic findings differentiate other types of chronic hepatitis (eg, HBV, HCV; steatohepatitis; Wilson disease; α_1-antitrypsin deficiency; primary sclerosing cholangitis [PSC]). PSC occasionally presents in a manner similar to AIH, including the presence of autoantibodies. Up to 30% of pediatric patients have an "overlap syndrome" of AIH and PSC. Drug-induced chronic hepatitis (minocycline, isoniazid, methyldopa, pemoline) should be ruled out. In addition, minocycline has been reported as a potential "trigger" of type 1 AIH.

▶ Complications

Untreated disease that continues for months to years eventually results in cirrhosis, with complications of portal hypertension and liver synthetic dysfunction. Untreated AIH can also lead to ALF. Bleeding from esophageal varices and development of ascites usually signal impending hepatic failure.

▶ Treatment

Corticosteroids (prednisone, 2 mg/kg/day; maximum 60 mg) as induction therapy decreases the mortality rate during the early active phase of the disease. Recent data suggests that oral budesonide may be as efficacious as prednisone at inducing remission with less steroid side effects. Budesonide, however, is not as potent an anti-inflammatory as prednisone and studies suggest that budesonide should be reserved for mild cases at presentation (ie, mild elevation of liver transaminases and minimal/no fibrosis on liver histology). Maintenance therapy with azathioprine or 6-mercaptopurine (6-MP), 1–2 mg/kg/day, is recommended in order to facilitate weaning off of steroids. Thiopurine methyltransferase activity in red blood cells or genotype should be assessed prior to starting azathioprine or 6-MP to prevent extremely high blood levels and severe bone marrow toxicity. Steroids are reduced over a 3- to 6-month period and azathioprine is continued for at least 2 years. At that point, if AST and ALT have been consistently normal, then one can consider a future wean off of therapy. A liver biopsy must be performed before stopping azathioprine or 6-MP therapy; if any inflammation persists, then azathioprine or 6-MP is continued. The majority of pediatric patients will require chronic azathioprine or 6-MP therapy, but up to 30% can be taken off of azathioprine or 6-MP eventually. Mycophenolate mofetil can be substituted for azathioprine or 6-MP if there is a contraindication or side effect

from these medications. The calcineurin inhibitors, cyclosporine or tacrolimus, are highly effective in cases refractory to standard therapies. Liver transplantation is indicated when disease progresses to decompensated cirrhosis or in cases presenting in ALF that do not respond to steroid therapy.

▶ Prognosis

The overall prognosis for AIH has improved significantly with early therapy; approximately 90% of patients with type 1 AIH will enter remission. Some studies report permanent remission (normal histologic findings) in up to 30% of patients. Relapses (seen clinically and histologically) occur in 40%–50% of patients after cessation of therapy; remissions follow repeat treatment. Complications of portal hypertension (bleeding varices, ascites, spontaneous bacterial peritonitis, and hepatopulmonary syndrome) require specific therapy or liver transplant. Disease recurs after transplantation in ~ 20% of cases and is treated by adding azathioprine or mycophenolate mofetil to the post-transplant immunosuppressant regimen.

Mieli-Vergani G et al: Autoimmune hepatitis. Nat Rev Dis Primers 2018;12;4:18017. [PMID: 29644994].

NONALCOHOLIC FATTY LIVER DISEASE

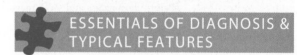

ESSENTIALS OF DIAGNOSIS & TYPICAL FEATURES

- ▶ Hepatomegaly in patient with BMI more than 95th percentile.
- ▶ Elevated ALT > AST.
- ▶ Histologic evidence of fat in the liver.

Nonalcoholic fatty liver disease (NAFLD), a clinicopathologic condition of abnormal hepatic fat deposition in the absence of alcohol, is the most common cause of abnormal LFTs in the United States. NAFLD ranges from bland steatosis, to fat and inflammation, with or without scarring (also referred to as nonalcoholic steatohepatitis, NASH) to cirrhosis. Trends in NAFLD parallel trends in obesity, with up to 10% of all children, and 38% of obese children affected in the United States. Many children with NAFLD are also affected by type 2 diabetes mellitus, hypertension, hyperlipidemia, obstructive sleep apnea, and the metabolic syndrome. Most children are 11–13 years of age at diagnosis, with males (ratio of 2:1) and Hispanics at highest risk.

▶ Prevention

The most effective therapy is prevention of the overweight or obese state.

Clinical Findings

A. History

Most patients with NAFLD are asymptomatic and discovered upon routine screening. Some may complain of fatigue or right-upper quadrant pain. Obesity and insulin resistance are known risk factors. Moderate sleep apnea is also common in children with NAFLD. NAFLD screening (using ALT) should be considered in children beginning at age 9–11 years if they are obese or overweight with additional risk factors.

B. Symptoms and Signs

Patients with NAFLD may present with asymptomatic soft hepatomegaly, though abdominal adiposity may make this difficult to assess. Physical findings of insulin resistance (acanthosis nigricans and a buffalo hump) are frequently present.

C. Laboratory Findings

Serum aminotransferases will not identify bland steatosis, so NAFLD patients may have completely normal AST and ALT. If elevated, the AST and ALT are typically elevated less than 1.5 times the upper limit of normal, with an ALT:AST ratio of greater than 1. Alkaline phosphatase and GGT may be mildly elevated, but bilirubin is normal. Hyperglycemia and hyperlipidemia are also common. If performed, the liver biopsy may show micro- or macrovesicular steatosis, hepatocyte ballooning, Mallory bodies, and lobular or portal inflammation. In addition, varying degrees of fibrosis from portal focused to cirrhosis may be present. Obstructive sleep apnea and hypoxia appear to contribute to NAFLD disease severity. There are no established reliable biochemical predictors of the degree of hepatic fibrosis. Currently, surrogate markers and scores developed to predict NAFLD are not accurate enough nor sufficiently validated to be used in the clinical setting.

D. Imaging

Ultrasonography, CT scan, or MRI can be used to confirm fatty infiltration of the liver. Ultrasound, however, is of lower cost and lacks radiation exposure, although it may be insensitive with severe central adiposity or if less than 30% steatosis is present. Currently, radiologic imaging cannot distinguish bland steatosis from the more severe NASH, nor reliably identify fibrosis. Transient elastography and MR elastography are increasingly available as clinical tools that show promise in accurately estimating both hepatic fat and fibrosis.

Differential Diagnosis

Steatohepatitis is also associated with Wilson disease, hereditary fructose intolerance, tyrosinemia, HCV hepatitis, cystic fibrosis, fatty acid oxidation defects, kwashiorkor, Reye syndrome, respiratory chain defects, total parenteral nutrition associated liver disease, and toxic hepatopathy (ethanol and others).

Complications

Untreated, NAFLD with hepatic inflammation can progress to cirrhosis with complications that include portal hypertension. Dyslipidemia, hypertension, insulin resistance, and obstructive sleep apnea are more common in children and adolescents with NAFLD.

Treatment

Multiple potential therapies, including metformin, UDCA, and lipid-lowering agents, have been tested without therapeutic success. Therefore, treatment is focused on lifestyle modifications, through both dietary changes and exercise, to induce slow weight loss. A 10% decrease in body weight can significantly improve NAFLD. Vitamin E, an antioxidant, has shown promise in clinical trials in improving histologically confirmed NASH.

Prognosis

Although untreated NAFLD can progress to cirrhosis and liver failure; there is a very high response rate to weight reduction. However, success in achieving long-term weight reduction is low in children and adults.

Chalasani A et al: The diagnosis and management of nonalcoholic fatty liver disease: practice guidance from the American Association for the Study of Liver Diseases. Hepatology 2018 Jan;67(1):328–357 [PMID: 28714183].

Mann J et al: Non-alcoholic fatty liver disease in children. Semin Liver Dis 2018 Feb;38(1) [PMID: 29471561].

Sundaram SS: Obstructive Sleep apnea and hypoxemia are associated with advanced liver histology in pediatric nonalcoholic fatty liver disease. J Pediatr 2014;164:699 [PMID: 24321532].

Vos MB et al: NASPGHAN clinical practice guideline for the diagnosis and treatment of nonalcoholic fatty liver disease in children: recommendations from the expert committee on NAFLD (ECON) and the North American Society of Pediatric Gastroenterology, Hepatology and Nutrition (NASPGHAN). J Pediatr Gastroenterol Nutr 2017 Feb;64(2) [PMID: 28107283].

α₁-ANTITRYPSIN DEFICIENCY LIVER DISEASE

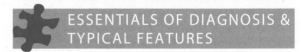

ESSENTIALS OF DIAGNOSIS & TYPICAL FEATURES

► Serum α₁-antitrypsin level < 50–80 mg/dL.

► Identification of a specific protease inhibitor (PI) phenotype (PIZZ, PISZ) or genotype.

▶ Detection of PAS positive, diastase-resistant glycoprotein deposits in periportal hepatocytes.

▶ Family history of early-onset pulmonary disease or liver disease.

General Considerations

The disease is caused by a deficiency in α_1-antitrypsin, a protease inhibitor (Pi), predisposing patients to chronic liver disease, and an early onset of pulmonary emphysema. Liver disease is associated only with the Pi phenotypes ZZ and SZ. The accumulation of misfolded aggregates of α_1-antitrypsin protein in the liver causes liver injury by unclear mechanisms. α_1-Antitrypsin is a common genetic disorder affecting up to 1 in 1600 to 1 in 2000 live births, especially among those of Northern European heritage.

Clinical Findings

A. Symptoms and Signs

α_1-Antitrypsin deficiency should be considered in all infants with neonatal cholestasis. About 10%–20% of affected individuals present with neonatal cholestasis. Serum GGT is usually elevated. Jaundice, acholic stools, and malabsorption may also be present. Infants are often small for gestational age, and may have pruritus, hepatosplenomegaly, ascites and/or easy bleeding and bruising. The family history may be positive for emphysema or cirrhosis.

Toddlers and older children may present with signs of chronic liver disease, including failure to thrive, hepatosplenomegaly, gastrointestinal bleeding, or ascites. Very few children have significant pulmonary involvement. Most affected children are completely asymptomatic, with no laboratory or clinical evidence of liver or lung disease.

B. Laboratory Findings

Serum α_1-antitrypsin level is low (< 50–80 mg/dL) in homozygotes (PiZZ). Specific Pi phenotyping or genotyping should be done to confirm the diagnosis. LFTs often reflect underlying hepatic pathologic changes. Hyperbilirubinemia (mixed) and elevated aminotransferases, alkaline phosphatase, and GGT are present early. Hyperbilirubinemia generally resolves, while aminotransferase and GGT elevation may persist. Signs of cirrhosis and hypersplenism may develop even when LFTs are normal.

Liver biopsy findings after age 6 months show diastase resistant, periodic acid–Schiff staining intracellular globules, particularly in periportal zones. These may be absent prior to age 6 months, but when present are characteristic of α_1-antitrypsin deficiency.

Differential Diagnosis

In newborns, other specific causes of neonatal cholestasis need to be considered, including biliary atresia. In older children, other causes of insidious cirrhosis (eg, HBV or HCV infection, AIH, Wilson disease, cystic fibrosis, and glycogen storage disease) should be considered.

Complications

Of all infants with PiZZ α_1-antitrypsin deficiency, only 15%–20% develop liver disease in childhood, and many have clinical recovery. Thus, other genetic or environmental modifiers must be involved. An associated abnormality in the microsomal disposal of accumulated aggregates may contribute to the liver disease phenotype. The complications of portal hypertension, cirrhosis, and chronic cholestasis predominate in affected children. An increased susceptibility to hepatocellular carcinoma has been noted in cirrhosis associated with α_1-antitrypsin deficiency. α_1-Antitrypsin deficiency is the most common genetic cause of pediatric liver disease and the most frequent inherited indication for liver transplantation in the pediatric population.

Early-onset pulmonary emphysema occurs in young adults (age 30–40 years), particularly in smokers.

Treatment

There is no specific treatment for the liver disease of this disorder. The neonatal cholestatic condition is treated with choleretics, medium-chain triglyceride–containing formula, and water-soluble preparations of fat-soluble vitamins (see Table 22–4). UDCA may reduce AST, ALT, and GGT, but its effect on outcome is unknown. Portal hypertension, esophageal bleeding, ascites, and other complications are treated as described elsewhere. Hepatitis A and B vaccines should be given to children with α_1-antitrypsin deficiency. Genetic counseling is indicated when the diagnosis is made. Diagnosis by prenatal screening is possible. Liver transplantation, performed for end-stage liver disease cures the deficiency with excellent long-term survival and prevents the development of pulmonary disease. Pediatric patients should be referred to a pulmononologist by 18 years of age for education and to establish baseline pulmonary function tests (PFTs). Passive and active cigarette smoke exposure should be eliminated to help prevent pulmonary manifestations, and obesity should be avoided. Replacement of the protein by infusion therapy is used to prevent or treat pulmonary disease in affected adults. In the future, novel treatments including chemical chaperones, authophagy inducers, hepatocyte transplantation, and gene transfer therapy may be available.

Prognosis

Of those patients presenting with neonatal cholestasis, approximately 10%–25% will need liver transplantation in the first 5 years of life, 15%–25% during childhood or adolescence, and 50%–75% will survive into adulthood with variable degrees of liver fibrosis. A correlation between histologic patterns and clinical course has been documented in the infantile form of the disease. Liver failure can be expected 5–15 years after development of cirrhosis. Recurrence or persistence of hyperbilirubinemia along with worsening coagulation studies indicates the need for evaluation for liver transplantation. Decompensated cirrhosis caused by this disease is an indication for liver transplantation. Pulmonary involvement is prevented by liver transplantation. Heterozygotes may have a slightly higher incidence of liver disease. The exact relationship between low levels of serum α_1-antitrypsin and the development of liver disease is unclear. Emphysema develops because of a lack of inhibition of neutrophil elastase, which destroys pulmonary connective tissue.

Feldman AG, Sokol RJ: Alpha-1-antitrypsin deficiency: an important cause of pediatric liver disease. Lung Health Prof Mag 2013;4(2):8–11 [PMID: 27019872].

Lomas DA, Hurst JR, Gooptu B: Update on alpha-1 antitrypsin deficiency: new therapies. J Hepatol 2016;65:413 [PMID: 27034252].

WILSON DISEASE (HEPATOLENTICULAR DEGENERATION)

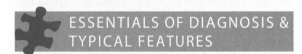

ESSENTIALS OF DIAGNOSIS & TYPICAL FEATURES

► Acute or chronic liver disease.

► Deteriorating neurologic status.

► Kayser-Fleischer rings.

► Elevated liver copper.

► Abnormalities in levels of ceruloplasmin and serum and urine copper.

► General Considerations

Wilson disease is caused by mutations in the gene *ATP7B* on chromosome 13 coding for a specific P-type adenosine triphosphatase involved in copper transport. This results in impaired bile excretion of copper and incorporation of copper into ceruloplasmin by the liver. The accumulated hepatic copper causes oxidative (free-radical) damage to the liver. Subsequently, copper accumulates in the basal ganglia and other tissues. The disease should be considered in all children older than age 1–2 years with evidence of liver disease (especially with hemolysis) or with suggestive neurologic signs. A family history is often present, and 25% of patients are identified by screening asymptomatic homozygous family members. The disease is autosomal recessive and occurs in 1:30,000 live births in all populations.

► Clinical Findings

A. Symptoms and Signs

Hepatic involvement may present as ALF, acute hepatitis, chronic liver disease, cholelithiasis, fatty liver disease, or as cirrhosis with portal hypertension. Findings may include jaundice, hepatomegaly early in childhood, splenomegaly, and Kayser-Fleischer rings. The disease is generally considered after 3 years of age. However, liver involvement occurs early in life and may be present by age 1–2 years. The later onset of neurologic or psychiatric manifestations after age 10 years may include tremor, dysarthria, and drooling. Deterioration in school performance can be the earliest neurologic expression of disease. The Kayser-Fleischer ring is a brown band at the junction of the iris and cornea, generally requiring slit-lamp examination for detection. Absence of Kayser-Fleischer rings does not exclude this diagnosis.

B. Laboratory Findings

The laboratory diagnosis can be challenging. Plasma ceruloplasmin levels are usually less than 20 mg/dL. (Normal values are 23–43 mg/dL.) Low values, however, occur normally in infants younger than 3 months, and in at least 10%–20% of homozygotes the levels may be within the lower end of the normal range (20–30 mg/dL), particularly since immunoassays are commonly used to measure ceruloplasmin. Rare patients with higher ceruloplasmin levels have been reported. Serum copper levels are low, but the overlap with normal is too great for satisfactory discrimination. In acute fulminant Wilson disease, serum copper levels are elevated markedly, owing to hepatic necrosis and release of copper. The presence of anemia, hemolysis, very high serum bilirubin levels (> 20–30 mg/dL), low alkaline phosphatase, and low uric acid are characteristic of acute Wilson disease. Urine copper excretion in children older than 3 years is normally less than 30 mcg/day; in Wilson disease, it is generally greater than 100 mcg/day although it can be as low as > 40 mcg/day. Finally, the tissue content of copper from a liver biopsy, normally less than 40–50 mcg/g dry tissue, is greater than 250 mcg/g in most Wilson disease patients, but may be as low as > 75 mcg/g.

Glycosuria and aminoaciduria have been reported. Hemolysis and gallstones may be present; bone lesions simulating those of osteochondritis dissecans have also been found.

The coarse nodular cirrhosis, macrovesicular steatosis, and glycogenated nuclei in hepatocytes seen on liver biopsy may distinguish Wilson disease from other types of cirrhosis. Early in the disease, vacuolation of liver cells, steatosis, and lipofuscin granules can be seen, as well as Mallory bodies. The presence of Mallory bodies in a child is strongly suggestive of Wilson disease. Stains for copper may sometimes be negative despite high copper content in the liver. Therefore, quantitative liver copper levels must be determined biochemically on biopsy specimens. Electron microscopy findings of abnormal mitochondria may be helpful.

▶ Differential Diagnosis

During the icteric phase, acute or chronic viral hepatitis, α_1-antitrypsin deficiency, AIH, and drug-induced hepatitis are the usual diagnostic possibilities. Nonalcoholic steatohepatitis may have similar histology and be confused with Wilson disease in overweight patients. Later, other causes of cirrhosis and portal hypertension require consideration. Laboratory testing for plasma ceruloplasmin, 24-hour urine copper excretion, liver quantitative copper concentration, and a slit-lamp examination of the cornea will help differentiate Wilson disease from the others. Urinary copper excretion during penicillamine challenge (500 mg twice a day in the older child or adult) may also be helpful. Genetic testing of *ATP7B* is available and is helpful if two disease-causing mutations are present. Other copper storage diseases that occur in early childhood include Indian childhood cirrhosis, Tyrolean childhood cirrhosis, and idiopathic copper toxicosis. However, ceruloplasmin concentrations are normal to elevated in these conditions.

▶ Complications

Cirrhosis, hepatic coma, progressive neurologic degeneration, and death are the rule in the untreated patient. The complications of portal hypertension (variceal hemorrhage, ascites) may be present at diagnosis. Progressive central nervous system disease and terminal aspiration pneumonia were common in untreated older people. Acute hemolytic disease may result in acute renal failure and profound jaundice and coma as part of the presentation of fulminant hepatitis.

▶ Treatment

Copper chelation with D-penicillamine or trientine hydrochloride, 750–1500 mg/day orally, is the treatment of choice, whether or not the patient is symptomatic. The target dose for children is 20 mg/kg/day; begin with 250 mg/day and increase the dose weekly by 250 mg increments. Strict dietary restriction of copper intake is not practical; however, selected high copper foods should be minimized. Supplementation with zinc acetate (25–50 mg orally, three times daily) may reduce copper absorption but must not be given at same time as copper chelators. Copper chelation or zinc therapy is continued for life, although doses of chelators may be reduced transiently at the time of surgery or early in pregnancy. Vitamin B_6 (25 mg) is given daily during therapy with penicillamine to prevent optic neuritis. In some countries, after a clinical response to penicillamine or trientine, zinc therapy is substituted and continued for life. Derivatives of tetrathiomolybdate are being tested as an alternative therapy.

Noncompliance with any of the drug regimens (including zinc therapy) can lead to sudden fulminant liver failure and death.

Liver transplantation is indicated for all cases of acute fulminant disease (with hemolysis and renal failure), for progressive hepatic decompensation despite several months of therapy, and severe progressive hepatic insufficiency in patients who inadvisedly discontinue penicillamine, triene, or zinc therapy.

▶ Prognosis

The prognosis of untreated Wilson disease is poor. The fulminant presentation is fatal without liver transplantation in almost all cases. Copper chelation reduces hepatic copper content, reverses many of the liver lesions, and can stabilize the clinical course of established cirrhosis. Neurologic symptoms generally respond to therapy and following liver transplantation. All siblings should be immediately screened and homozygotes given treatment with copper chelation or zinc acetate therapy, even if asymptomatic. Recent data suggest that zinc monotherapy may not be as effective for hepatic Wilson disease as copper chelation. Genetic testing (*ATP7B* genotyping) is available clinically if there is any doubt about the diagnosis and is particularly useful for screening family members.

European Association for Study of Liver: EASL clinical practice guidelines: Wilson's disease. J Hepatol 2012 Mar;56(3):671–685 [PMID: 22340672].

Roberts EA: Update on the diagnosis and management of Wilson disease. Curr Gastroenterol Rep 2018 Nov 5;20(12):56 [PMID: 30397835].

Roberts EA, Schilsky ML; American Association for Study of Liver Diseases (AASLD): Diagnosis and treatment of Wilson disease: an update. Hepatology 2008;47:2089–2111 [PMID: 18506894].

Socha P et al: Wilson's disease in children: a position paper by the Hepatology Committee of the European Society for Paediatric Gastroenterology, Hepatology and Nutrition. J Pediatr Gastroenterol Nutr 2018 Feb;66(2):334–344 [PMID: 29341979].

DRUG-INDUCED LIVER DISEASES

▶ General Considerations

Drug-induced liver injury (DILI) may be predictable or unpredictable. Predictable hepatotoxins cause liver injury in a dose-dependent manner. Unpredictable hepatotoxins cause liver injury in an idiosyncratic manner, which may be influenced by the genetic and environmental characteristics of particular individuals. DILI has been described with a wide variety of medications, including antihypertensives, acetaminophen, anabolic steroids, antibiotics, anticonvulsants, antidepressants, antituberculosis medications, antipsychotics, antivirals, herbals, dietary supplements, and weight loss agents.

Symptoms

Many people with DILI are asymptomatic and only detected because aminotransferases are performed for other reasons. If symptomatic, indicating more severe DILI, patients may have malaise, anorexia, pruritus, nausea and vomiting, right-upper quadrant pain, jaundice, acholic stools, and dark urine. If the DILI is a hypersensitivity reaction, fever and rash may also occur.

When submassive hepatic necrosis and fulminant failure occur, mortality can exceed 50%.

Diagnosis

No specific testing for DILI is available, with diagnosis requiring a causality assessment. This assessment should determine if the patient was exposed to the drug during a logical time period; if the drug has previously been reported to cause DILI; and if the symptom complex is consistent with DILI. In addition, other explanations for liver injury should be sought, including viral hepatitis, AIH, and alcohol use.

Treatment

Primary therapy is supportive care, discontinuation of the offending drug, and avoiding reexposure. This typically results in rapid and complete resolution of symptoms. However, DILI severe enough to cause ALF has a poor prognosis without urgent liver transplant. Specific therapies for some DILI etiologies include *N*-acetylcysteine for acetaminophen poisoning and L-carnitine for valproic acid hepatotoxicity. The use of ursodeoxycholic acid may speed resolution of jaundice. The use of corticosteroids for DILI remains controversial but may have a role in immune-mediated disease. An NIH-sponsored website provides up-to-date information about each drug and herbal substance associated with DILI (LiverTox).

Amin MD et al: Drug induced liver injury in children. Curr Opin Pediatr 2015 Oct;27(5) [PMID: 26208237].

LiverTox: Clinical and research information on drug-induced liver injury. http://www.livertox.nih.gov/. Accessed August 1, 2017.

CIRRHOSIS

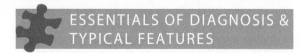

ESSENTIALS OF DIAGNOSIS & TYPICAL FEATURES

▶ Underlying liver disease.

▶ Nodular hard liver and splenomegaly.

▶ Nodular liver on abdominal imaging.

▶ Liver biopsy demonstrating cirrhosis.

General Considerations

Cirrhosis is defined by the World Health Organization as a diffuse process whereby the architecture of the liver has been replaced by structurally abnormal nodules due to fibrosis. It may be micronodular or macronodular in appearance. It is the vasculature distortion that leads to increased resistance to blood flow, producing portal hypertension, and its consequences.

Many liver diseases may progress to cirrhosis in children, including metabolic and genetic disorders, infectious diseases, autoimmune and inflammatory diseases, cholestatic diseases and biliary malformations, vascular lesions, and drugs/toxins. In the first year of life, biliary atresia and genetic-metabolic diseases are the most common cause of cirrhosis. In older children, cirrhosis is most commonly caused by chronic viral hepatitis, Wilson's disease, primary sclerosing cholangitis, AIH, and α_1-antitrypsin deficiency. Regardless of etiology, cirrhosis can lead to liver failure and death.

Clinical Findings

A. History

Many children with cirrhosis may be asymptomatic early in the course. Malaise, loss of appetite, failure to thrive, and nausea are frequent complaints, especially in anicteric varieties. Easy bruising may be reported. Jaundice may or may not be present.

B. Symptoms and Signs

The first indication of underlying liver disease may be splenomegaly, ascites, gastrointestinal hemorrhage, or hepatic encephalopathy. Variable hepatomegaly, spider angiomas, warm skin, palmar erythema, or digital clubbing may be present. A small, shrunken liver may be present. Most often, the liver is enlarged slightly, especially in the subxiphoid region, where it has a firm to hard quality and an irregular edge. Splenomegaly generally precedes other complications of portal hypertension. Ascites, gynecomastia in males, digital clubbing, pretibial edema, and irregularities of menstruation in females may be present. In biliary cirrhosis, patients often also have jaundice, dark urine, pruritus, hepatomegaly, and sometimes xanthomas. Malnutrition and failure to thrive due to steatorrhea may be more apparent in biliary cirrhosis.

C. Laboratory Findings

Mild abnormalities of AST and ALT are often present, with a decreased level of albumin. PT is prolonged and may be unresponsive to vitamin K administration. Burr and target red cells may be noted on the peripheral blood smear. Anemia, thrombocytopenia, and leukopenia are present if hypersplenism exists. However, blood tests may be normal in patients with cirrhosis. In biliary cirrhosis, increased levels of conjugated bilirubin, bile acids, GGT, alkaline phosphatase, and cholesterol are common.

D. Imaging

Hepatic ultrasound, CT, or MRI examination may demonstrate abnormal hepatic texture and nodules. In biliary cirrhosis, abnormalities of the biliary tree may be apparent. Elastography and fibroscan will demonstrate increased liver stiffness.

E. Pathologic Findings

Liver biopsy findings of regenerating nodules and surrounding fibrosis are hallmarks of cirrhosis. Pathologic features of biliary cirrhosis also include canalicular and hepatocyte cholestasis, as well as plugging of bile ducts. The interlobular bile ducts may be increased or decreased, depending on the cause and the stage of the disease process.

▶ Differential Diagnosis

In the pediatric population, multiple diseases can result in cirrhosis, including biliary obstruction (biliary atresia, choledochal cyst, bile duct stenosis), inborn errors of metabolism and genetic conditions (PFIC, α_1-antitrypsin deficiency, galactosemia, fructosemia, GSD type III and IV, cystic fibrosis, mitochondrial hepatopathies, Wilson's disease), viral and parasitic infections (HBV, HCV, *Opisthorchis sinensis*, *Fasciola*, Schistosoma, and *Ascaris*), chronic drug and toxin exposure, AIH, primary sclerosising cholangitis, vascular alertations, and NAFLD. Most cases of biliary cirrhosis result from congenital abnormalities of the bile ducts (biliary atresia, choledochal cyst), tumors of the bile duct, Caroli disease, progressive familial intrahepatic cholangitis, primary sclerosing cholangitis, paucity of the intrahepatic bile ducts, and cystic fibrosis. The evolution to cirrhosis may be insidious, with no recognized icteric phase. At the time of diagnosis of cirrhosis, the underlying liver disease may be active, with abnormal LFTs; or it may be quiescent, with normal LFTs.

▶ Complications

Major complications of cirrhosis in childhood include progressive nutritional disturbances, hormonal disturbances, infections, and the evolution of portal hypertension and its complications (GI bleeding, ascites, and encephalopathy). Hepatocellular carcinoma occurs with increased frequency in the cirrhotic liver, especially in patients with the chronic form of hereditary tyrosinemia or after long-standing HBV or HCV disease. Some children with cirrhosis may develop hepatopulmonary syndrome characterized by intrapulmonary vasodilation and hypoxia, portal-pulmonary hypertension, or hepatorenal syndrome characterized by progressive deterioration of renal function.

▶ Treatment

At present, there is no proven medical treatment for cirrhosis, but whenever a treatable condition is identified (eg, Wilson disease, galactosemia, AIH) or an offending agent eliminated (HBV, HCV, drugs, toxins), disease progression can be altered; occasionally regression of fibrosis has been noted. Recent evidence suggests that cirrhosis from HCV and HBV may be reversed by successful antiviral therapy. Children with cirrhosis should receive the hepatitis A and B vaccines and be monitored for the development of hepatocellular carcinoma with serial serum α-fetoprotein determinations annually and abdominal ultrasound for hepatic nodules annually. Liver transplantation may be appropriate in patients with cirrhosis caused by a progressive disease; evidence of worsening hepatic synthetic function; or complications of cirrhosis that are no longer manageable.

▶ Prognosis

Cirrhosis has an unpredictable course. Without transplantation, affected patients may die from liver failure within 10–15 years. Patients with a rising bilirubin, a vitamin K–resistant coagulopathy, or diuretic refractory ascites usually survive less than 1–2 years. The terminal event in some patients may be generalized hemorrhage, sepsis, or cardiorespiratory arrest. For patients with biliary cirrhosis, the prognosis is similar, except for those with surgically corrected lesions that result in regression or stabilization of the underlying liver condition. With liver transplantation, the long-term survival rate is 70%–90%.

Hsu EK, Murray KF: Cirrhosis and chronic liver failure. In: Suchy FJ, Sokol RJ, Balistreri WF (eds): *Liver Disease in Children*. 4th ed. Cambridge University Press; 2014:51–67.

Pinto RB, Schneider AC, da Silveira TR: Cirrhosis in children and adolescents: an overview. World J Hepatol 2015 Mar 27;7(3):392–405. doi: 10.4254/wjh.v7.i3.392 [PMID: 25848466].

PORTAL HYPERTENSION

ESSENTIALS OF DIAGNOSIS & TYPICAL FEATURES

- ▶ Splenomegaly.
- ▶ Recurrent ascites.
- ▶ Variceal hemorrhage.
- ▶ Hypersplenism.

▶ General Considerations

Portal hypertension is defined as an increase in the portal venous pressure to more than 5 mm Hg greater than the inferior vena caval pressure. Portal hypertension is most commonly a result of cirrhosis. Portal hypertension may be divided into prehepatic, suprahepatic, and intrahepatic causes. Although the specific lesions vary somewhat in their clinical signs and symptoms, the consequences of portal hypertension are common to all.

A. Prehepatic Portal Hypertension

Prehepatic portal hypertension from acquired abnormalities of the portal and splenic veins accounts for 30%–50% of cases of variceal hemorrhage in children. A history of neonatal omphalitis, sepsis, dehydration, or umbilical vein catheterization may be present. Causes in older children include local trauma, peritonitis (pylephlebitis), hypercoagulable states, and pancreatitis. Symptoms may occur before age 1 year, but in most cases the diagnosis is not made until age 3–5 years. Patients with a positive neonatal history tend to be symptomatic earlier.

A variety of portal or splenic vein malformations, some of which may be congenital, have been described, including defects in valves and atretic segments. Cavernous transformation is the result of attempted collateralization around the thrombosed portal vein rather than a congenital malformation. The site of the venous obstruction may be anywhere from the hilum of the liver to the hilum of the spleen.

B. Suprahepatic Vein Occlusion or Thrombosis (Budd-Chiari Syndrome)

No cause can be demonstrated in most instances in children, while tumor, medications, and hypercoagulable states are common causes in adults. The occasional association of hepatic vein thrombosis in inflammatory bowel disease favors the presence of endogenous toxins traversing the liver. Vasculitis leading to endophlebitis of the hepatic veins has been described. In addition, hepatic vein obstruction may be secondary to tumor, abdominal trauma, hyperthermia, or sepsis, or it may occur following the repair of an omphalocele or gastroschisis. Congenital vena caval bands, webs, a membrane, or stricture above the hepatic veins are sometimes causative. Hepatic vein thrombosis may be a complication of oral contraceptive medications. Underlying thrombotic conditions (deficiency of antithrombin III, protein C or S, or factor V Leiden; antiphospholipid antibodies; or mutations of the prothrombin gene) are common in adults.

C. Intrahepatic Portal Hypertension

1. Cirrhosis—See previous section.

2. Veno-occlusive disease (acute stage)—This entity occurs most frequently in bone marrow or stem cell transplant recipients. Additional causes include high-dose thiopurines, ingestion of pyrrolizidine alkaloids ("bush tea") or other herbal teas, and a familial form of the disease occurring in congenital immunodeficiency states. The acute form of the disease generally occurs in the first month after bone marrow transplantation and is heralded by the triad of weight gain (ascites), tender hepatomegaly, and jaundice.

3. Congenital hepatic fibrosis—This is a rare autosomal recessive cause of intrahepatic presinusoidal portal hypertension (see Table 22–10). Liver biopsy is generally diagnostic, demonstrating Von Meyenburg complexes (abnormal clusters of ectatic bile ducts). On angiography, the intrahepatic branches of the portal vein may be duplicated. Autosomal recessive polycystic kidney disease is frequently associated with this disorder.

4. Other rare causes—Hepatoportal sclerosis (idiopathic portal hypertension, noncirrhotic portal fibrosis), focal nodular regeneration of the liver, and schistosomal hepatic fibrosis are also rare causes of intrahepatic presinusoidal portal hypertension.

▶ Clinical Findings

A. Symptoms and Signs

For prehepatic portal hypertension, splenomegaly in an otherwise well child is the most common physical sign. Ascites may be noted. The usual presenting symptoms are hematemesis and melena.

The presence of prehepatic portal hypertension is suggested by (1) an episode of severe infection in the newborn period or early infancy—especially omphalitis, sepsis, gastroenteritis, severe dehydration, or prolonged or difficult umbilical vein catheterizations; (2) no previous evidence of liver disease; (3) a history of well-being prior to onset or recognition of symptoms; and (4) normal liver size and liver tests with splenomegaly.

Most patients with suprahepatic portal hypertension present with abdominal pain, tender hepatomegaly of acute onset, and ascites. Jaundice is present in only 25% of patients. Vomiting, hematemesis, and diarrhea are less common. Cutaneous signs of chronic liver disease are often absent, as the obstruction is usually acute. Distended superficial veins on the back and the anterior abdomen, along with dependent edema, are seen when inferior vena cava obstruction affects hepatic vein outflow. Absence of hepatojugular reflux (jugular distention when pressure is applied to the liver) is a helpful clinical sign.

The symptoms and signs of intrahepatic portal hypertension are generally those of cirrhosis (see earlier section on Cirrhosis).

B. Laboratory Findings and Imaging

Most other common causes of splenomegaly or hepatosplenomegaly may be excluded by appropriate laboratory tests.

Cultures, EBV and hepatitis serologies, blood smear examination, bone marrow studies, and LFTs may be necessary. In prehepatic portal hypertension, LFTs are generally normal. In Budd-Chiari syndrome and veno-occlusive disease, mild to moderate hyperbilirubinemia with modest elevations of AST, ALT, and PT/INR are often present. Significant early increases in fibrinolytic parameters (especially plasminogen activator inhibitor 1) have been reported in veno-occlusive disease. Hypersplenism with mild leukopenia and thrombocytopenia is often present. Upper endoscopy may reveal varices in symptomatic patients.

Doppler-assisted ultrasound scanning of the liver, portal vein, splenic vein, inferior vena cava, and hepatic veins may assist in defining the vascular anatomy. In prehepatic portal hypertension, abnormalities of the portal or splenic vein may be apparent, whereas the hepatic veins are normal. When noncirrhotic portal hypertension is suspected, angiography often is diagnostic. Selective arteriography of the superior mesenteric artery or MRI is recommended prior to surgical shunting to determine the patency of the superior mesenteric vein.

For suprahepatic portal hypertension, an inferior vena cavogram using catheters from above or below the suspected obstruction may reveal an intrinsic filling defect, an infiltrating tumor, or extrinsic compression of the inferior vena cava by an adjacent lesion. A large caudate lobe of the liver suggests Budd-Chiari syndrome. Care must be taken in interpreting extrinsic pressure defects of the subdiaphragmatic inferior vena cava if ascites is significant.

Simultaneous wedged hepatic vein pressure and hepatic venography are useful to demonstrate obstruction to major hepatic vein ostia and smaller vessels. In the absence of obstruction, reflux across the sinusoids into the portal vein branches can be accomplished. Pressures should also be taken from the right heart and supradiaphragmatic portion of the inferior vena cava to eliminate constrictive pericarditis and pulmonary hypertension from the differential diagnosis.

▶ Differential Diagnosis

All causes of splenomegaly must be included in the differential diagnosis. The most common ones are infections, immune thrombocytopenic purpura, blood dyscrasias, lipidosis, reticuloendotheliosis, cirrhosis of the liver, and cysts or hemangiomas of the spleen. When hematemesis or melena occurs, other causes of gastrointestinal bleeding are possible, such as gastric or duodenal ulcers, tumors, duplications, and inflammatory bowel disease.

Because ascites is almost always present in suprahepatic portal hypertension, cirrhosis resulting from any cause must be excluded. Other suprahepatic (cardiac, pulmonary) causes of portal hypertension must also be ruled out. Although ascites may occur in prehepatic portal hypertension, it is uncommon.

▶ Complications

The major manifestation and complication of portal hypertension is bleeding from esophageal varices. Fatal exsanguination is uncommon, but hypovolemic shock or resulting anemia may require prompt treatment. Hypersplenism with leukopenia and thrombocytopenia occurs, but seldom causes major symptoms.

Without treatment, complete and persistent hepatic vein obstruction in suprahepatic portal hypertension leads to liver failure, coma, and death. A nonportal type of cirrhosis may develop in the chronic form of hepatic veno-occlusive disease in which small- and medium-sized hepatic veins are affected. Death from renal failure may occur in rare cases of congenital hepatic fibrosis.

▶ Treatment

Definitive treatment of noncirrhotic portal hypertension is generally lacking. Aggressive medical treatment of the complications of prehepatic portal hypertension is generally quite effective. Excellent results are also seen with either portosystemic shunt or the mesorex (mesenterico–left portal bypass) shunt. When possible (there must be an open left portal vein and no underlying liver disease on biopsy), the mesorex shunt is the preferred technique. Veno-occlusive disease may be prevented somewhat by the prophylactic use of UDCA or defibrotide prior to conditioning for bone marrow transplantation. Treatment with defibrotide and withdrawal of the suspected offending agent, if possible, may increase the chance of recovery. Transjugular intrahepatic portosystemic shunts have been successful in bridging to recovery in veno-occlusive disease. For suprahepatic portal hypertension, efforts should be directed at correcting the underlying cause, if possible. Either surgical or angiographic relief of obstruction should be attempted if a defined obstruction of the vessels is apparent. Liver transplantation, if not contraindicated, should be considered early if direct correction is not possible. In most cases, management of portal hypertension is directed at management of the complications (Table 22–9).

▶ Prognosis

For prehepatic portal hypertension, the prognosis depends on the site of the block, the effectiveness of variceal eradication, the availability of suitable vessels for shunting procedures, and the experience of the surgeon. In patients treated by medical means, bleeding episodes seem to diminish with adolescence. Portacaval encephalopathy is unusual after shunting except when protein intake is excessive, but neurologic outcome may be better in patients who receive a mesorex shunt when compared with medical management alone.

The mortality rate of hepatic vein obstruction is very high (95%). In veno-occlusive disease, the prognosis is better,

Table 22–9. Treatment of complications of portal hypertension.

Complication	Diagnosis	Treatment
Bleeding esophageal varices	Endoscopic verification of variceal bleeding.	Endosclerosis or variceal band ligation. Octreotide, 30 mcg/m² BSA/h intravenous. Pediatric Sengstaken-Blakemore tube. Surgical portosystemic shunt, TIPS, surgical variceal ligation, selective venous embolization, OLT. Propranolol (nonselective β-blockers) may be useful to prevent recurrent bleeding.
Ascites	Clinical examination (fluid wave, shifting dullness), abdominal ultrasonography.	Sodium restriction (1–2 mEq/kg/day), spironolactone (3–5 mg/kg/day), furosemide (1–2 mg/kg/day), intravenous albumin (0.5–1 g/kg per dose), paracentesis, peritoneovenous (LeVeen) shunt, TIPS, surgical portosystemic shunt, OLT.[a]
Hepatic encephalopathy	Abnormal neurologic examination, elevated plasma ammonia.	Protein restriction (0.5–1 g/kg/day), intravenous glucose (6–8 mg/kg/min), neomycin (2–4 g/m²BSA PO in four doses), rifaximin (200 mg three times a day in children > 12 y), lactulose (1 mL/kg per dose [up to 30 mL] every 4–6 h PO), plasmapheresis, hemodialysis, OLT.[a]
Hypersplenism	Low WBC count, platelets, and/ or hemoglobin. Splenomegaly.	No intervention, partial splenic embolization, surgical portosystemic shunt, TIPS, OLT. Splenectomy may worsen variceal bleeding.

BSA, body surface area; OLT, orthotopic liver transplantation; PO, by mouth; TIPS, transjugular intrahepatic portosystemic shunt; WBC, white blood cell.
[a]In order of sequential management.

with complete recovery possible in 50% of acute forms and 5%–10% of subacute forms.

Chapin C, Bass LM: Cirrhosis and portal hypertension in the pediatric population. Clin Liver Dis 2018; 22(4):735–752 [PMID: 30266160].

Giouleme O, Theocharidou E: Management of portal hypertension in children with portal vein thrombosis. J Pediatr Gastroenterol Nutr 2013;57:419–425 [PMID: 23820400].

McKiernan P, Abdel-Hady M: Advances in the management of childhood portal hypertension. Expert Rev Gastroenterol Hepatol 2015 May;9(5):575–583. doi: 10.1586/17474124.2015. 993610 [PMID: 25539572].

BILIARY TRACT DISEASE

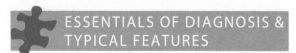

ESSENTIALS OF DIAGNOSIS & TYPICAL FEATURES

► Episodic right-upper quadrant abdominal pain.
► Elevated bilirubin, alkaline phosphatase, and GGT.
► Stones or sludge seen on abdominal ultrasound.

1. Cholelithiasis

General Considerations

Gallstones may develop at all ages in the pediatric population and in utero. Gallstones may be divided into cholesterol

stones (> 50% cholesterol) and pigment (black [sterile bile] and brown [infected bile]) stones. Pigment stones predominate in the first decade of life, while cholesterol stones account for up to 90% of gallstones in adolescence. The process is reversible in some patients.

► Clinical Findings

A. History

Most symptomatic gallstones are associated with acute or recurrent episodes of moderate to severe, sharp right upper quadrant, or epigastric pain. The pain may radiate substernally or to the right shoulder. On rare occasions, the presentation may include a history of jaundice, back pain, or generalized abdominal discomfort, when it is associated with pancreatitis, suggesting stone impaction in the common duct or major ampulla. Nausea and vomiting may occur during attacks. Pain episodes often occur postprandially, especially after ingestion of fatty foods. The groups at risk for gallstones include patients with known or suspected hemolytic disease; females; teenagers with prior pregnancy; obese individuals; individuals with rapid weight loss; children with portal vein thrombosis; certain racial or ethnic groups, particularly Native Americans (Pima Indians) and Hispanics; infants and children with ileal disease (Crohn disease) or prior ileal resection; patients with cystic fibrosis or Wilson disease; infants on prolonged parenteral nutrition and those with bile acid transporter defects. Other, less certain risk factors include a positive family history, use of birth control pills, and diabetes mellitus.

B. Symptoms and Signs

During acute episodes of pain, tenderness is present in the right-upper quadrant or epigastrium, with a positive inspiratory arrest (Murphy sign), usually without peritoneal signs. While rarely present, scleral icterus is helpful. Evidence of underlying hemolytic disease in addition to icterus may include pallor (anemia), splenomegaly, tachycardia, and high-output cardiac murmur. Fever is unusual in uncomplicated cases and should raise concern for cholangitis or cholecystitis.

C. Laboratory Findings

Laboratory tests are usually normal unless calculi have lodged in the extrahepatic biliary system, in which case the serum bilirubin and GGT (or alkaline phosphatase) may be elevated. Amylase and lipase levels may be increased if stone obstruction occurs at the major papilla and causes gallstone pancreatitis.

D. Imaging

Ultrasound evaluation is the best imaging technique, showing abnormal intraluminal contents (stones, sludge) as well as anatomic alterations of the gallbladder or dilation of the biliary ductal system. The presence of an anechoic acoustic shadow differentiates calculi from intraluminal sludge or sludge balls. In selected cases, ERCP, MRCP, or endoscopic ultrasound may be helpful in defining subtle abnormalities of the bile ducts and locating intraductal stones.

▶ Differential Diagnosis

Other abnormal conditions of the biliary system with similar presentation are summarized in Table 22–10. Liver disease (hepatitis, abscess, or tumor) can cause similar symptoms or signs. Peptic disease, reflux esophagitis, paraesophageal hiatal hernia, cardiac disease, and pneumomediastinum must be considered when the pain is epigastric or substernal in location. Renal or pancreatic disease is a possible explanation if the pain is localized to the right flank or mid back. Subcapsular or supracapsular lesions of the liver (abscess, tumor, or hematoma) or right-lower lobe infiltrate may also be a cause of nontraumatic right shoulder pain.

▶ Complications

Major problems are related to stone impaction in either the cystic or common duct, which may lead to stricture formation or perforation and subsequent bile leak. Stones impacted at the level of the major ampulla often cause gallstone pancreatitis.

▶ Treatment

Symptomatic cholelithiasis is treated by laparoscopic cholecystectomy or open cholecystectomy in selected cases. Intraoperative cholangiography via the cystic duct or preoperative endoscopic ultrasound can be considered in select patients so that the physician can be certain the biliary system is free of retained stones. Calculi in the extrahepatic bile ducts may be removed via ERCP.

Gallstones developing in premature infants on parenteral nutrition can be followed by ultrasound examination. Most of the infants are asymptomatic, and the stones will resolve in 3–36 months. Gallstone dissolution using cholelitholytics (UDCA) or mechanical means (lithotripsy) has not been approved for children. Asymptomatic gallstones do not usually require treatment, as less than 20% will eventually cause problems.

▶ Prognosis

The prognosis is excellent in uncomplicated cases that come to standard or laparoscopic cholecystectomy.

Fradin K et al: Obesity and symptomatic cholelithiasis in childhood: epidemiologic and case-control evidence for a strong relation. J Pediatr Gastroenterol Nutr 2014;58:102–106 [PMID: 23969538].

Langballe KO, Bardram L: Cholecystectomy in Danish children—a nationwide study. J Pediatr Surg 2014;49:626–630 [PMID: 24726126].

Svensson J et al: Gallstone disease in children. Semin Pediatr Surg 2012;21:255 [PMID: 22800978].

2. Primary Sclerosing Cholangitis

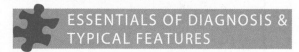

ESSENTIALS OF DIAGNOSIS & TYPICAL FEATURES

- ▶ Pruritus and jaundice.
- ▶ Elevated GGT.
- ▶ Associated with inflammatory bowel disease.
- ▶ Abnormal ERCP or MRCP.

▶ General Considerations

Primary sclerosing cholangitis (PSC) is a progressive liver disease characterized by chronic inflammation and fibrosis of the intrahepatic and/or extrahepatic bile ducts, leading to fibrotic strictures and saccular dilations of all or parts of the biliary tree. The etiology of PSC is likely multifactorial, including genetic predispositions, with alterations in innate and autoimmunity. PSC is more common in males, and has a strong relationship to inflammatory bowel disease,

Table 22–10. Biliary tract diseases of childhood.

	Acute Hydrops/Transient Dilation of Gallbladder[a,b]	Choledochal Cyst[c] (see Figure 22–1)	Acalculous Cholecystitis[d]	Caroli Disease[e] (Idiopathic Intrahepatic Bile Duct Dilation)	Congenital Hepatic Fibrosis[f]	Biliary Dyskinesia[g] and Functional Dyspepsia
Predisposing or associated conditions	Premature infants with prolonged fasting or systemic illness. Hepatitis. Abnormalities of cystic duct. Kawasaki disease. Bacterial sepsis, EBV.	Congenital lesion. Female sex. Asians. Rarely with Caroli disease or congenital hepatic fibrosis.	Systemic illness, sepsis (*Streptococcus, Salmonella, Klebsiella,* etc.), EBV or HIV infection. Gallbladder stasis, obstruction of cystic duct (stones, nodes, tumor).	Congenital lesion. Also found in congenital hepatic fibrosis or with choledochal cyst. Female sex. Autosomal recessive polycystic kidney disease.	Familial (autosomal recessive), 25% with autosomal recessive polycystic kidney disease (PKHD1 mutation). Choledochal cyst. Caroli disease. Meckel-Gruber, Ivemark, or Jeune syndrome.	School ages and adolescents.
Symptoms	Absent in premature infants. Vomiting, abdominal pain in older children.	Abdominal pain, vomiting, jaundice.	Acute severe abdominal pain, vomiting, fever.	Recurrent abdominal pain, vomiting. Fever, jaundice when cholangitis occurs.	Hematemesis, melena from bleeding esophageal varices.	Intermittent epigastric or RUQ pain.
Signs	RUQ abdominal mass. Tenderness in some.	Icterus, acholic stools, dark urine in neonatal period. RUQ abdominal mass or tenderness in older children.	Tenderness in mid and right upper abdomen. Occasional palpable mass in RUQ.	Icterus, hepatomegaly.	Hepatosplenomegaly.	Usually normal examination.
Laboratory abnormalities	Most are normal. Increased WBC count during sepsis (may be decreased in premature infants). Abnormal LFTs in hepatitis.	Conjugated hyperbilirubinemia, elevated GGT, slightly increased AST. Elevated pancreatic serum amylase common.	Elevated WBC count, normal or slight abnormality of LFTs.	Abnormal LFTs. Increased WBC count with cholangitis. Urine abnormalities if associated with congenital hepatic fibrosis.	Low platelet and WBC count (hypersplenism), slight elevation of AST, GGT. Inability to concentrate urine.	Usually normal.
Diagnostic studies most useful	Gallbladder US.	Gallbladder US, MRCP, endoscopic ultrasound.	Scintigraphy to confirm nonfunction of gallbladder. US or abdominal CT scan to rule out other neighboring disease.	Transhepatic cholangiography, MRCP, ERCP, scintigraphy, US	Liver biopsy. US of liver and kidneys. Upper endoscopy.	Normal US, HIDA scans have not predicted improvement after cholecystectomy in pediatrics

Treatment	Treatment of associated condition. Needle or tube cystostomy rarely required. Cholecystectomy seldom indicated.	ERCP if acute obstruction. Definitive treatment is surgical resection and choledochojejunostomy.	Broad-spectrum antibiotic coverage, then cholecystectomy.	Antibiotics and surgical or endoscopic drainage for cholangitis. Liver transplantation for some. Lobectomy for localized disease.	Treatment of portal hypertension. Liver and kidney transplantation for some.	Symptomatic therapy. Cholecystectomy may be considered in well-selected cases.
Complications	Perforation with bile peritonitis rare.	Progressive biliary cirrhosis. Increased incidence of cholangiocarcinoma. Cholangitis in some.	Perforation and bile peritonitis, sepsis, abscess or fistula formation. Pancreatitis.	Sepsis with episodes of cholangitis, biliary cirrhosis, portal hypertension. Intraductal stones. Cholangiocarcinoma.	Bleeding from varices. Splenic rupture, severe thrombocytopenia. Progressive renal failure.	Continued pain after surgery. Complications from surgery.
Prognosis	Excellent with resolution of underlying condition. Consider cystic duct obstruction if disorder fails to resolve.	Depends on anatomic type of cyst, associated condition, and success of surgery. Liver transplantation required in some.	Good with early diagnosis and treatment.	Poor, with gradual deterioration of liver function. Multiple surgical drainage procedures expected. Liver transplantation should improve long-term prognosis.	Good in absence of serious renal involvement and with control of portal hypertension. Slightly increased risk of cholangiocarcinoma.	Similar to other functional gastrointestinal disorders. Unclear if surgery is beneficial for biliary dyskinesia.

AST, aspartate aminotransferase; CCK, cholecystokinin; CT, computed tomography; EBV, Epstein-Barr virus; ERCP, endoscopic retrograde cholangiopancreatography; GGTx, γ-glutamyl transpeptidase; HIDA, hepatobiliary iminodiacetic acid; HIV, human immunodeficiency virus; LFT, liver function test; MRCP, magnetic resonance cholangiopancreatography; RUQ, right upper quadrant; US, ultrasound; WBC, white blood cell.

aCrankson S et al: Acute hydrops of the gallbladder in childhood. Eur J Pediatr 1992;151:318 [PMID: 9788647].

bMathai SS et al: Gall bladder hydrops—a rare initial presentation of Kawasaki disease. Indian J Pediatr 2013;80:616–617 [PMID: 23180399].

cRonnekleiv-Kelly SM, Soares KC, Ejaz A, Pawlik TM. Management of choledochal cysts. Curr Opin Gastroenterol 2016 May;32(3):225–231 [PMID: 26885950].

dImamoglu M et al: Acute acalculous cholecystitis in children: diagnosis and treatment. J Pediatr Surg 2002;37:36 [PMID: 11781983].

eLiang JJ, Kamath PS: Caroli syndrome. Mayo Clin Proc 2013;88(6):e59 [PMID: 23726409].

fHoyer PF: Clinical manifestations of autosomal recessive polycystic kidney disease. Curr Opin Pediatr 2015 Apr;27(2):186–192 [PMID: 25689455].

gSantucci NR, Hyman PE, Harmon CM, Schiavo JH, Hussain SZ: Biliary dyskinesia in children: a systematic review. J Pediatr Gastroenterol Nutr 2017 Feb;64(2):186–193 [PMID: 27472474].

particularly ulcerative colitis. A PSC-like condition can also be seen with histiocytosis X, AIH, IgG4 autoimmune pancreatitis, sicca syndromes, congenital and acquired immunodeficiency syndromes, and cystic fibrosis. Sclerosing cholangitis due to Cryptosporidia may occur in immunodeficiency syndromes.

Clinical Findings

A. Symptoms and Signs

PSC often has an insidious onset and may be asymptomatic. Clinical symptoms may include abdominal pain, fatigue, pruritus, jaundice, and weight loss. Acholic stools, steatorrhea, hepatomegaly, and splenomegaly can occur.

B. Laboratory Findings

The earliest finding may be asymptomatic elevation of the GGT. Subsequent laboratory abnormalities include elevated levels of alkaline phosphatase and bile acids. Later, cholestatic jaundice and elevated AST and ALT may occur. Markers of autoimmune liver disease (ANA and ASMA) are often found, but are not specific for PSC and may actually be due to concurrent overlap with AIH (overlap syndrome or autoimmune cholangitis).

C. Diagnosis

Ultrasound is often normal in PSC, but may detect dilated bile ducts related to dominant biliary strictures. MRCP is the diagnostic study of choice for medium/large duct PSC, demonstrating irregularities of the biliary tree, including saccular dilation of normal intrahepatic bile ducts with segmental strictures ("beads on a string"), dominant strictures of large ducts, or "pruning" of the smaller bile duct branches. ERCP may be more sensitive for the diagnosis of irregularities of the intrahepatic biliary tree and allow for therapeutic interventions. In ~ 15% of cases, the MRCP will be normal and the disease manifests only in the small bile ducts ("small duct PSC"). Small duct PSC is diagnosed based on the liver histology finding of concentric fibrosis surrounding the bile ducts ("onion skinning").

Differential Diagnosis

The differential diagnosis includes infectious hepatitis, secondary sclerosing cholangitis, AIH, progressive familial intrahepatic cholestasis type 3, cystic fibrosis, choledochal cyst, or other anomalies of the biliary tree, including Caroli disease (see Table 22–10).

Complications

Complications include refractory pruritus, bacterial cholangitis, biliary fibrosis, cirrhosis, and complications of portal hypertension. Slow progression to end-stage liver disease is likely, and patients are at increased risk of cholangiocarcinoma.

Treatment

Treatment of PSC focuses on supportive care. UDCA is often used in pediatrics, though high doses may worsen disease in adults. Pruritus may improve with UDCA, rifampin, or naltrexone. Patients with autoimmune sclerosing cholangitis or IgG4 cholangitis should benefit from treatment with corticosteroids and azathioprine. Antibiotic treatment of cholangitis and dilation and stenting of dominant bile duct strictures can reduce symptoms. Liver transplantation is effective for patients with end-stage complications, but the disease may recur in up to 20% after transplant.

Prognosis

The majority of patients will eventually require liver transplantation in adulthood. PSC is the fifth leading indication for liver transplantation in adults in the United States.

Mieli-Vergani G, Vergani D: Sclerosing cholangitis in children and adolescents. Clin Liver Dis 2016;20(1):99–111 [PMID: 26593293].

3. Other Biliary Tract Disorders

For a schematic representation of the various types of choledochal cysts, see Figure 22–1. For summary information

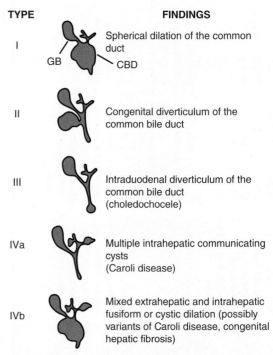

▲ **Figure 22–1.** Classification of cystic dilation of the bile ducts. Types I, II, and III are extrahepatic choledochal cysts. Type IVa is solely intrahepatic, and type IVb is both intrahepatic and extrahepatic.

on acute hydrops, choledochal cyst, acalculous cholecystitis, Caroli disease, biliary dyskinesia, and congenital hepatic fibrosis, see Table 22–10.

PYOGENIC & AMEBIC LIVER ABSCESS

ESSENTIALS OF DIAGNOSIS & TYPICAL FEATURES

▶ Fever and painful enlarged liver.

▶ Ultrasound of liver demonstrating an abscess.

▶ Positive serum ameba antibody or positive bacterial culture of abscess fluid.

▶ General Considerations

Pyogenic liver abscesses are rare in developed countries, but remain a significant issue in developing countries. The most common cause is *S aureus*, with enteric bacteria less common; fungal abscesses also occur. The resulting lesion tends to be solitary and located in the right hepatic lobe. Unusual causes include omphalitis, subacute infectious endocarditis, pyelonephritis, Crohn disease, and perinephric abscess. In immunocompromised patients, *S aureus*, gram-negative organisms, and fungi may seed the liver from the arterial system. Multiple pyogenic liver abscesses are associated with severe sepsis. Children receiving anti-inflammatory and immunosuppressive agents and children with defects in white blood cell function (chronic granulomatous disease) are prone to pyogenic hepatic abscesses, especially those caused by *S aureus*.

Amebic liver abscess can occur when *Entamoeba histolytica* invasion occurs via the large bowel, although a history of diarrhea (colitis-like picture) is not always obtained.

▶ Clinical Findings

A. History

With any liver abscess, nonspecific complaints of fever, chills, malaise, and abdominal pain are frequent. Amebic liver abscess is rare in children. An increased risk is associated with travel in areas of endemic infection within 5 months of presentation.

B. Symptoms and Signs

Weight loss is very common, especially when diagnosis is delayed. A few patients have shaking chills and jaundice. The dominant complaint is a constant dull pain over an enlarged liver that is tender to palpation. An elevated hemidiaphragm with reduced or absent respiratory excursion may be demonstrated on physical examination and confirmed by fluoroscopy.

Fever and abdominal pain are the two most common symptoms of amebic liver abscess. Abdominal tenderness and hepatomegaly are present in over 50%. An occasional prodrome may include cough, dyspnea, and shoulder pain when rupture of the abscess into the right chest occurs.

C. Laboratory Findings

Laboratory studies show leukocytosis and, at times, anemia. LFTs may be normal or reveal mild elevation of transaminases and alkaline phosphatase. Blood cultures may be positive. The distinction between pyogenic and amebic abscesses in developed countries is best made by indirect hemagglutination test for specific antibody (which is positive in more than 95% of patients with amebic liver disease) and the prompt clinical response of the latter to anti-amebic therapy (metronidazole). Examination of material obtained by needle aspiration of the abscess using ultrasound guidance is often diagnostic.

D. Imaging

Ultrasound is the most useful diagnostic aid in evaluating pyogenic and amebic abscesses, detecting lesions as small as 1–2 cm. MRI, CT, or nuclear scanning may be useful in differentiating tumor or hydatid cyst. Consolidation of the right lower lobe of the lung is common (10%–30% of patients) in amebic abscess.

▶ Differential Diagnosis

Hepatitis, hepatoma, hydatid cyst, gallbladder disease, or biliary tract infections can mimic liver abscess. Subphrenic abscesses, empyema, and pneumonia may give a similar picture. Inflammatory disease of the intestines or of the biliary system may be complicated by liver abscess.

▶ Complications

Spontaneous rupture of the abscess may occur with extension of infection into the subphrenic space, thorax, peritoneal cavity, and, occasionally, the pericardium. Bronchopleural fistula with large sputum production and hemoptysis can develop in severe cases. Simultaneously, the amebic liver abscess may be secondarily infected with bacteria (in 10%–20% of patients). Metastatic hematogenous spread to the lungs and the brain has been reported.

▶ Treatment

Small bacterial liver abscesses (< 5 cm) or those with a solid appearance can be treated medically. Ultrasound- or CT-guided percutaneous needle aspiration for aerobic and anaerobic culture with simultaneous placement of a catheter for drainage, combined with appropriate antibiotic therapy, is the treatment of choice for solitary larger or liquid pyogenic liver abscess. Multiple liver abscesses may also be treated successfully by this method. Surgical intervention may be indicated if rupture occurs outside the capsule of the liver or if enterohepatic fistulae are suspected.

Amebic abscesses in uncomplicated cases should be treated with oral metronidazole, 35–50 mg/kg/day, in three divided doses for 10 days. Intravenous metronidazole can be used for patients unable to take oral medication. Needle aspiration or surgical drainage is indicated for failure of medical management or cysts greater than 10 cm. Once oral feedings can be tolerated, a luminal amebicide such as iodoquinol should be initiated. Resolution of the abscess cavity occurs over 3–6 months.

▶ Prognosis

With drainage and antibiotics, the cure rate is about 90%. Mortality rates have improved, but remain at 4% for pyogenic liver abscess, especially with extrahepatic complications, and less than 1% for amebic abscess.

Jain M, Jain J, Gupta S: Amebic liver abscess in children-experience from Central India. Indian J Gastroenterol 2016 May;35(3):248–249 [PMID: 27260285].

Roy Choudhury S, Khan NA, Saxena R, Yadav PS, Patel JN, Chadha R: Protocol-based management of 154 cases of pediatric liver abscess. Pediatr Surg Int 2017 Feb;33(2):165–172 [PMID: 27826650].

LIVER TUMORS

ESSENTIALS OF DIAGNOSIS & TYPICAL FEATURES

▶ Abdominal enlargement and pain, weight loss, anemia.

▶ Hepatomegaly with or without a definable mass.

▶ Mass lesion on imaging studies.

▶ Laparotomy and tissue biopsy.

▶ General Considerations

Primary neoplasms of the liver represent 0.3%–5% of all solid tumors in children. Of these, two-thirds are malignant, with hepatoblastoma being most common (79% of all pediatric liver cancers). Hepatoblastoma typically occurs in children ages 6 months to 3 years, with a male predominance. Most children present with an asymptomatic abdominal mass, though with more advanced disease, weight loss, anorexia, abdominal pain, and emesis may occur. Children with Beckwith-Wiedemann syndrome and familial adenomatosis polyposis coli are at increased risk of hepatoblastoma,

and should undergo routine screening with α-fetoprotein determinations and abdominal ultrasound until the age of 5 years. In addition, low-birth-weight infants (< 1000 g) have a 15 times increased risk of hepatoblastoma, as compared to infants weighing more than 2500 g. Differentiation from hepatocellular carcinoma, the other major malignant tumor of the liver, may be difficult.

Hepatocellular carcinoma most commonly occurs between the ages of 10 and 12 years and is more common in males. Children are more likely to have advanced disease at presentation, and therefore be symptomatic, with abdominal distension, pain, anorexia, and weight loss. Patients with chronic HBV or HCV infection, cirrhosis, glycogen storage disease type I, tyrosinemia, and α_1-antitrypsin deficiency are at increased risk for developing hepatocellular carcinoma. The late development of hepatocellular carcinoma in patients receiving androgens for treatment of Fanconi syndrome and aplastic anemia must be kept in mind. The use of anabolic steroids by body-conscious adolescents poses a risk of hepatic neoplasia. In addition, Wilms tumors, neuroblastoma, and lymphoma may metastasize to the liver.

▶ Clinical Findings

A. History

Noticeable abdominal distension, with or without pain, is the most constant feature. A parent may note a bulge in the upper abdomen or report feeling a hard mass. Constitutional symptoms (eg, anorexia, weight loss, fatigue, fever, and chills) may be present. Jaundice or pruritus may occur with obstruction of the biliary tree. Virilization has been reported as a consequence of gonadotropic activity of tumors. Feminization with bilateral gynecomastia may occur in association with high estradiol levels in the blood, the latter a consequence of increased aromatization of circulating androgens by the liver. Leydig cell hyperplasia without spermatogenesis has also been reported.

B. Symptoms and Signs

Weight loss, pallor, and abdominal pain in association with a large abdomen are common. Physical examination reveals hepatomegaly with or without a definite tumor mass, usually to the right of the midline. In the absence of cirrhosis, signs of chronic liver disease are usually absent.

C. Laboratory Findings

Normal LFTs are the rule. Anemia frequently occurs, especially in cases of hepatoblastoma. α-Fetoprotein levels are typically elevated, especially in hepatoblastoma. Estradiol levels are sometimes elevated. Tissue diagnosis is best obtained at laparotomy, although ultrasound- or CT-guided needle biopsy of the liver mass can be used.

D. Imaging

Ultrasonography, CT, and MRI are useful for diagnosis, staging, and following tumor response to therapy. A chest CT is generally part of the preoperative workup to evaluate metastatic disease.

▶ Differential Diagnosis

In the absence of a palpable mass, the differential diagnosis is that of hepatomegaly with or without anemia or jaundice. Hematologic and nutritional conditions should be ruled out, as well as HBV and HCV infection, α_1-antitrypsin deficiency disease, lipid storage diseases, histiocytosis X, glycogen storage disease, tyrosinemia, congenital hepatic fibrosis, cysts, adenoma, focal nodular hyperplasia, and hemangiomas. If fever is present, hepatic abscess (pyogenic or amebic) must be considered. Veno-occlusive disease and hepatic vein thrombosis are rare possibilities. Tumors in the left lobe may be mistaken for pancreatic pseudocysts.

▶ Complications

With progressive enlargement of the tumor, abdominal discomfort, ascites, respiratory difficulty, and widespread metastases (especially to the lungs and the abdominal lymph nodes) may occur. Rupture of the neoplastic liver and intraperitoneal hemorrhage have been reported.

▶ Treatment

For tumors that are resectable, an aggressive surgical approach with complete resection of the lesion offers the only chance for cure. Individual lung metastases should also be surgically resected. Radiotherapy and chemotherapy have been disappointing in the treatment of hepatocellular carcinoma, although hepatoblastomas are generally more responsive. Chemotherapy may be used for initial cytoreduction of tumors (especially hepatoblastoma) found to be unresectable at the time of primary surgery (see Chapter 31 for additional discussion). Liver transplantation can be an option in hepatoblastoma with unresectable disease limited to the liver, with an 85% 10-year survival. For hepatocellular carcinoma, the survival rate is poor due to the typically advanced stage at diagnosis. The survival rate may be better for those patients in whom the tumor is incidental to another disorder (tyrosinemia, biliary atresia, cirrhosis) or is less than a total of 7 cm diameter without vascular invasion. In HBV-endemic areas, childhood HBV vaccination has reduced the incidence of hepatocellular carcinoma.

▶ Prognosis

If the tumor is completely removed, the survival rate is 90% for hepatoblastoma and 33% for hepatocellular carcinoma. If metastases that cannot be surgically resected are present,

survival is reduced to 40% for hepatoblastoma. In well-selected candidates with unresectable hepatoblastoma, survival after liver transplantation approaches 65%.

Aronson DC, Meyers RL: Malignant tumors of the liver in children. Semin Pediatr Surg 2016 Oct;25(5) [PMID: 27955729].

Khanna R et al: Pediatric hepatocellular carcinoma. World J Gastroenterol 2018 Sept;24(35) [PMID: 30254403].

Meyers RL: Hepatoblastoma state of the art: pre-treatment extent of disease, surgical resection guidelines and the role of liver transplantation. Curr Opin Pediatr 2014 Feb;26:29 [PMID: 24362406].

LIVER TRANSPLANTATION

Orthotopic liver transplantation is indicated in children with end-stage liver disease, acute fulminant hepatic failure, non-resectable liver tumors, or complications from metabolic liver disorders. Approximately 600 pediatric liver transplants are performed annually, with excellent 1-year (83%–91%) and 5-year (82%–84%) survival rates. The multitude of immunosuppression options, ability to individualize immunosuppression, improved candidate selection, refinements in surgical techniques, anticipatory monitoring for complications (eg, CMV and EBV infections, hypertension, renal dysfunction, and dyslipidemias), and experience in postoperative management have all contributed to improved outcomes over time. The major indications for childhood transplantation are shown in Table 22–11.

Table 22–11. Indications for pediatric liver transplantation.

Indication	Percentage of Pediatric Transplants
Biliary atresia (failed Kasai or decompensated cirrhosis)	39.6
Metabolic diseases (α_1-antitrypsin deficiency, urea cycle enzyme defects, Wilson disease, tyrosinemia)	14.6
Non-biliary atresia cholestatic disorders (eg, Alagille syndrome, PFIC)	13.6
Acute liver failure	13.2
Cirrhosis (autoimmune hepatitis, hepatitis B and C)	8.0
Hepatic malignancies (unresectable hepatoblastoma, HCC, others)	5.8
Other	5.2

HCC, hepatocellular carcinoma; PFIC, progressive familial intrahepatic cholestasis.

Children who are potential candidates for liver transplantation should be referred to a pediatric transplant center early for evaluation. In addition to full-sized cadaveric organs, children may also receive reduced segment or split cadaveric livers and live donor transplants, all of which have expanded the potential donor pool. Lifetime immunosuppression therapy, using combinations of tacrolimus, prednisone, azathioprine, mycophenolate mofetil, or sirolimus, with its incumbent risks, is generally necessary to prevent rejection. Small studies have examined the potential for complete immunosuppression withdrawal, with a more definitive multicenter study currently underway. Currently, the minimal amount of immunosuppression that will prevent allograft rejection should be chosen. The overall quality of life for children with a transplanted liver appears to be excellent. There is an increased risk (up to 25%) of renal dysfunction and low intelligence scores. The lifelong risk of EBV-induced lymphoproliferative disease, which is approximately 5%, is related to age and EBV exposure status at time of transplantation, and intensity of immunosuppression.

Rawal et al: Pediatric liver transplantation. Pediatr Clin North Am 2017;64(3) [PMID: 28502445].

Squires RH et al: Evaluation of the pediatric patient for liver transplantation: 2014 practice guideline by the American Association for the Study of Liver Diseases, American Society of Transplantation and the North American Society for Pediatric Gastroenterology, Hepatology and Nutrition. Hepatology 2014;60:362–398 [PMID: 25185661].

▼ PANCREATIC DISORDERS

ACUTE PANCREATITIS

ESSENTIALS OF DIAGNOSIS & TYPICAL FEATURES

Two out of three of the following:

▶ Abdominal pain, nausea, vomiting, or upper back pain.

▶ Elevated serum lipase and/or amylase ≥ 3 times the upper limit of normal.

▶ Evidence of pancreatic inflammation by imaging (usually CT or ultrasound).

▶ General Considerations

The incidence of acute pancreatitis in children is now about 1 per 10,000. Acute pancreatitis is defined as at least two of the following three: abdominal pain consistent with acute pancreatitis; amylase and/or lipase greater than three times the upper limit of normal; and US, CT, or MRI imaging consistent with acute pancreatitis. Most cases of acute pancreatitis are the result of drugs, viral infections, systemic diseases, abdominal trauma, or obstruction of pancreatic flow. More than 20% are idiopathic. Causes of pancreatic obstruction include stones, choledochal cyst, tumors of the duodenum, pancreas divisum, and ascariasis. Acute pancreatitis has been seen following treatment with many different medications, including sulfasalazine, thiazides, valproic acid, azathioprine, mercaptopurine, asparaginase, antiretroviral drugs, high-dose corticosteroids, and other drugs. It may also occur in cystic fibrosis, systemic lupus erythematosus, diabetes mellitus, Crohn disease, glycogen storage disease type I, hyperlipidemia, hyperparathyroidism, Henoch-Schönlein purpura, Reye syndrome, organic acidopathies, Kawasaki disease, or chronic renal failure; during rapid refeeding in cases of malnutrition; following spinal fusion surgery; and certain genetic mutations. Alcohol-induced pancreatitis should be considered in adolescents.

▶ Clinical Findings

A. History

An acute onset of persistent (hours to days), moderate to severe upper abdominal and midabdominal pain occasionally referred to the back, frequently associated with vomiting, or nausea is the common presenting picture.

B. Symptoms and Signs

The abdomen is tender, but not rigid. Abdominal distention is common in infants and younger children, and classic symptoms of abdominal pain, tenderness, and nausea are less common in this age group. Jaundice is unusual. Ascites may be noted, and a left-sided pleural effusion is present in some patients. Periumbilical and flank bruising are rare and indicate hemorrhagic pancreatitis.

C. Laboratory Findings

An elevated serum amylase or lipase (more than three times normal) is the key laboratory finding. The elevated serum lipase persists longer than serum amylase. Infants younger than 6 months may not have an elevated amylase or lipase. In this setting, an elevated immunoreactive trypsinogen may be more sensitive. Pancreatic lipase can help differentiate nonpancreatic causes (eg, salivary, intestinal, or tuboovarian) of serum lipase elevation. Leukocytosis, hyperglycemia (serum glucose > 300 mg/dL), hypocalcemia, falling hematocrit, rising blood urea nitrogen, hypoxemia, and acidosis may occur in severe cases and imply a worse prognosis.

D. Imaging

Ultrasonography is the initial imaging of choice and is primarily used to assess for biliary tract disease leading to pancreatitis, but can show decreased echodensity of the pancreas in comparison with the left lobe of the liver. The pancreas (especially the body and tail) is often difficult to image with ultrasound due to overlying gas. CT scan images the pancreas more consistently and is better for detecting pancreatic phlegmon, pseudocyst, or necrosis. ERCP or MRCP may be useful in confirming patency of the main pancreatic duct in cases of abdominal trauma; in recurrent acute pancreatitis; or in revealing stones, ductal strictures, and pancreas divisum.

Differential Diagnosis

There are many other causes of acute upper abdominal pain include gastritis, peptic ulcer disease, duodenal ulcer, hepatitis, liver abscess, cholelithiasis, cholecystitis, choledocholithiasis, acute gastroenteritis, functional gastrointestinal disorders such as functional dyspepsia, atypical appendicitis, pneumonia, volvulus, intussusception, and nonaccidental trauma.

Complications

Early complications include shock, fluid and electrolyte disturbances, ileus, acute respiratory distress syndrome, and hypocalcemia. Hypervolemia due to renal insufficiency related to renal tubular necrosis may occur. Early predictors of a more aggressive course include renal dysfunction, significant fluid requirements, and multisystem organ dysfunction. Around 5%–20% of patients can develop pancreatic fluid collections (pseudocysts are completely fluid filled and walled off necrosis cavities contain fluid and solid necrotic debris) that may be asymptomatic or present with recurrence of abdominal pain, vomiting, or nausea. Up to 60%–70% of pseudocysts resolve spontaneously. Infection, hemorrhage, rupture, or fistulization may occur. Phlegmon formation is rare in children, but when present may extend from the gland into the retroperitoneum or into the lesser sac. Infection may occur in this inflammatory mass. Mature symptomatic fluid collections (pseudocyst or pancreatic walled-off necrosis) may be treated with endoscopic ultrasound-guided cystgastrostomy. Chronic pancreatitis and exocrine or endocrine pancreatic insufficiency are rare sequelae of acute pancreatitis.

Treatment

Medical management includes careful attention to fluid, electrolytes, and respiratory status. Data in adults suggest lactated ringers may be preferred for initial volume expansion in acute pancreatitis. Pain should be aggressively treated with opioid and non-opioid medications. Historically patients were kept NPO, but more recent studies have shown that early enteral nutrition by mouth decreases hospital length of stay in mild-moderate pediatric pancreatitis. Early supplemental enteral nutrition via nasogastric or nasojejunal

tube has better outcomes than parenteral nutrition in severe pancreatitis. Broad-spectrum antibiotic coverage is only beneficial in necrotizing pancreatitis. Drugs known to produce acute pancreatitis should be discontinued. Surgical treatment is reserved for traumatic disruption of the gland, other anatomic obstructive lesions, and unresolved or infected pseudocysts or abscesses not amenable to endoscopic or radiographically-guided drainage. Early endoscopic decompression of the biliary system reduces the morbidity associated with pancreatitis caused by obstruction of the common bile duct.

Prognosis

In the pediatric age group, the prognosis is good with conservative management with mortality less than 0.4%. Up to 42% of children hospitalized with their initial episode of acute pancreatitis will have one or more subsequent admissions for pancreatitis.

Abu-El-Haija et al: Management of acute pancreatitis in the pediatric population: a clinical report from the North American Society for Pediatric Gastroenterology, Hepatology and Nutrition Pancreas Committee. J Pediatr Gastroenterol Nutr 2018 Jan;66(1):159–176. doi: 10.1097/MPG.0000000000001715 [PMID: 29280782].

Gariepy CE et al: Causal evaluation of acute recurrent and chronic pancreatitis in children: consensus from the INSPPIRE Group. J Pediatr Gastroenterol Nutr 2017 Jan;64(1):95–103. doi: 10.1097/MPG.0000000000001446 [PMID: 27782962].

Morinville VD: Definitions of pediatric pancreatitis and survey of present clinical practices. J Pediatr Gastroenterol Nutr 2012 Sep;55(3):261–265. doi: 10.1097/MPG.0b013e31824f1516 [PMID: 22357117].

Pant C, Sferra TJ, Lee BR, Cocjin JT, Olyaee M: Acute recurrent pancreatitis in children: a study from the pediatric health information system. J Pediatr Gastroenterol Nutr 2016 Mar;62(3):450–452. doi: 10.1097/MPG.0000000000001058 [PMID: 26704865].

CHRONIC PANCREATITIS

Chronic pancreatitis does not imply long-standing pancreatitis, but denotes that the pancreas has permanent parenchymal or ductal changes from inflammation.

The causes are similar to acute pancreatitis, but children with chronic pancreatitis are more likely to have underlying genetic or anatomic risk factors for pancreatitis.

Clinical Findings

A. History

The diagnosis often is delayed by the nonspecificity of symptoms and the lack of persistent laboratory abnormalities. There is usually a prolonged history of recurrent upper abdominal pain and/or nausea of variable severity. Radiation of the pain into the back is a frequent complaint.

B. Symptoms and Signs

Fever and vomiting are rare. Diarrhea, due to steatorrhea, and symptoms of diabetes may develop later in the course. Malnutrition due to acquired exocrine pancreatic insufficiency may also occur.

C. Laboratory Findings

Serum amylase and lipase levels are usually elevated during early acute attacks, but are often normal in the chronic phase. Pancreatic insufficiency may be diagnosed by demonstration of a low fecal pancreatic elastase 1. Increasingly, multiplex genetic testing panels are used to screen for the expanding number of identified genetic causes for chronic pancreatitis. Some identified genes include those for cationic trypsinogen (PRSS1), the pancreatic secretory trypsin inhibitor, the cystic fibrosis transmembrane conductance regulator (CFTR), carboxypeptidase A1, and chymotrypsin C. Screening for pancreatogenic (type 3c) diabetes should be considered. Sweat chloride should be checked for cystic fibrosis and serum calcium for hyperparathyroidism.

D. Imaging

Ultrasound or CT examination may demonstrate an abnormal gland (enlargement, atrophy or calcifications), ductal dilation, and/or calculi in up to 80% in advanced disease. MRCP or ERCP can show ductal dilation, stones, strictures, or stenotic segments. Endoscopic ultrasound may show early changes of chronic pancreatitis.

▶ Differential Diagnosis

Other causes of recurrent abdominal pain must be considered. Specific causes of pancreatitis such as autoimmune pancreatitis, hyperparathyroidism, systemic lupus erythematosus, infectious disease, traumatic pancreatitis, and ductal obstruction by tumors, stones, or helminths must be excluded by appropriate tests.

▶ Complications

Disabling abdominal pain, steatorrhea, malnutrition, pancreatic pseudocysts, and diabetes are the most frequent long-term complications. Pancreatic carcinoma occurs more frequently in patients with chronic pancreatitis, and in up to 40% of patients with hereditary pancreatitis (PRSS1 mutations) by age 70.

▶ Treatment

Medical management of acute attacks is indicated (see section on Acute Pancreatitis). If ductal obstruction is strongly suspected, endoscopic therapy (balloon dilation, stenting, stone removal, or sphincterotomy) should be pursued. Relapses occur in most patients. There are no proven therapies which modify disease course of chronic pancreatitis. Pancreatic enzyme therapy should be used in patients with exocrine insufficiency. Mature fluid collections may be drained with endoscopic ultrasound-guided cystgastrostomy, or if this is unavailable, interventional radiology, or surgical approaches if they fail to regress spontaneously.

Surgical treatment includes pancreatic ductal decompression procedures as well as total pancreatectomy and islet cell autotransplantation (TPIAT). TPIAT is performed in specialized centers and is curative for the pancreatic inflammation, resolves risk of pancreatic cancer, and may significantly improve or resolve pain. However, it carries risks of surgical morbidity, causes lifelong exocrine insufficiency, and many patients progress to need lifelong insulin. Previous pancreatic surgery decreases the amount of islet cells which can be isolated from the pancreas and increases risk of diabetes after TPIAT.

▶ Prognosis

In the absence of a correctable lesion, the prognosis is not good. Disabling episodes of pain, pancreatic insufficiency, diabetes, and pancreatic cancer may ensue. Narcotic addiction and suicide are risks in teenagers with disabling disease. TPIAT may significantly improve quality of life in pediatric patients with severe chronic pancreatitis pain. Given the complexity of chronic pancreatitis, a multidisciplinary approach is often beneficial, and referral to centers with expertise with management of pancreatic disorders should be considered.

Awano H et al: Childhood-onset hereditary pancreatitis with mutations in the CT gene and SPINK1 gene. Pediatr Int 2013;55: 646–649 [PMID: 24134754].

Ceppa EP et al: Hereditary pancreatitis: endoscopic and surgical management. J Gastrointest Surg 2013;17:847–856 [PMID: 23435738].

Masamune A: Genetics of pancreatitis: the 2014 update. Tohoku J Exp Med 2014;232:69–77 [PMID: 24522117].

GASTROINTESTINAL & HEPATOBILIARY MANIFESTATIONS OF CYSTIC FIBROSIS

Pulmonary and pancreatic involvement dominate the clinical picture for most patients with cystic fibrosis (see Chapter 19), however, various other organs can be involved. Table 22–12 lists the important gastrointestinal, pancreatic, and hepatobiliary conditions that may affect patients with cystic fibrosis along with their clinical

Table 22–12. Gastrointestinal and hepatobiliary manifestations of cystic fibrosis.

Organ	Condition	Symptoms	Age at Presentation	Prevalence (%)	Diagnostic Evaluation	Management
Esophagus	Gastroesophageal reflux, esophagitis	Pyrosis, dysphagia, epigastric pain, hematemesis.	All ages.	10–20	Endoscopy and biopsy, overnight pH study.	H_2 blockers, PPIs, surgical antireflux procedure.
	Varices in those with cirrhosis	Hematemesis, melena.	Childhood and adolescents.	3–5	Endoscopy.	Endosclerosis, band ligation, drugs (see text), TIPS, surgical shunt, liver transplantation (see Table 22–9).
Stomach	Gastritis	Upper abdominal pain, vomiting, hematemesis.	School age and older.	10–25	Endoscopy and biopsy.	H_2 blockers, PPIs.
	Hiatal hernia	Reflux symptoms (see above), epigastric pain.	School age and older.	3–5	UGI; endoscopy.	As above. Surgery in some.
Intestine	Meconium ileus	Abdominal distention, bilious emesis.	Neonate.	10–15	Radiologic studies, plain abdominal films; contrast enema shows microcolon.	Dislodgement of obstruction with Gastrografin enema. Surgery if unsuccessful or if case complicated by atresia, perforation, or volvulus.
	Distal intestinal obstruction syndrome	Abdominal pain, acute and recurrent; distention; occasional vomiting.	Any age, usually school age through adolescence.	5–10	Palpable mass in right lower quadrant, radiologic studies.	Gastrografin enema, intestinal lavage solution, diet, bulk laxatives, adjustment of pancreatic enzyme intake.
	Intussusception	Acute, intermittent abdominal pain; distention; emesis.	Infants through adolescence.	1–3	Radiographic studies, barium enema.	Reduction by barium or air enema or surgery if needed. Diet. Bulk laxatives. Adjustment of pancreatic enzyme intake.
	Rectal prolapse	Anal discomfort, rectal bleeding.	Infants and children to age 4–5 y.	15–25	Visual mass protruding from anus.	Manual reduction, adjustment of pancreatic enzyme dosage, reassurance as problem resolves by age 3–5 y.
	Carbohydrate intolerance	Abdominal pain, flatulence, continued diarrhea with adequate enzyme replacement therapy.	Any age.	10–25	Intestinal mucosal biopsy and disaccharidase analysis. Lactose breathe hydrogen test.	Reduce lactose intake; lactase; reduction of gastric hyperacidity if mucosa shows partial villous atrophy. Beware concurrent celiac disease or *Giardia* infection.
	Small bowel bacterial overgrowth	Abdominal pain, flatulence, continued diarrhea with adequate enzyme replacement therapy.	Any age: Higher risk with previous intestinal surgery.	Unknown	Culture of duodenal fluid, glucose breath hydrogen test.	Probiotic therapy, oral antibiotics (metronidazole, trimethoprim-sulfamethoxazole).
Pancreas	Total exocrine insufficiency	Diarrhea, steatorrhea, malnutrition, failure to thrive. Fat-soluble vitamin deficiency.	Neonate through infancy.	85–90	72-h fecal fat evaluation, fecal pancreatic elastase, direct pancreatic function tests.	Pancreatic enzyme replacement, may need elemental formula, fat-soluble vitamin supplements.

(Continued)

Table 22–12. Gastrointestinal and hepatobiliary manifestations of cystic fibrosis. (*Continued*)

Organ	Condition	Symptoms	Age at Presentation	Prevalence (%)	Diagnostic Evaluation	Management
	Pancreatic sufficiency (partial exocrine insufficiency)	Occasional diarrhea, mild growth delay.	Any age.	10–15	72-h fecal fat evaluation, direct pancreatic function tests, fecal pancreatic elastase.	Pancreatic enzyme replacement in selected patients. Fat-soluble vitamin supplements as indicated by biochemical evaluation.
	Pancreatitis	Recurrent abdominal pain, vomiting.	Older children through adolescence. Primarily in patients with partial pancreatic sufficiency.	0.1	Increased serum lipase and amylase, CT, MRCP, ERCP.	Endoscopic removal of sludge or stones if present, endoscopic papillotomy.
	Diabetes	Weight loss, polyuria, polydipsia.	Older children through adolescence.	Increases with age up to 35%	Glucose tolerance test and insulin levels.	Diet, insulin.
Liver	Steatosis	Hepatomegaly, often in setting of malnutrition, elevated ALT.	Neonates and infants, but can be seen at all ages.	20–60	US showing homogeneous increased echogenicity. Liver biopsy.	Improved nutrition, replacement of pancreatic enzymes, vitamins, and essential fatty acids.
	Hepatic fibrosis	Hepatomegaly, firm liver. May have abnormal AST, ALT.	Infants and older patients.	10–70	US showing heterogeneous echogenicity. Liver biopsy.	As above. UDCA
	Cirrhosis	Hepatosplenomegaly, hematemesis from esophageal varices; hypersplenism, jaundice, ascites late in course.	Infants through adolescence.	5–10	US showing nodular liver, signs of portal hypertension. Liver biopsy, endoscopy.	Improved nutrition, UDCA endosclerosis or band ligation of varices, or partial splenic embolization, liver transplantation.
	Neonatal jaundice	Cholestatic jaundice hepatomegaly; often seen with meconium ileus.	Neonates.	0.1–1	Sweat chloride test, liver biopsy	Nutritional support, special formula with medium-chain triglyceride–containing oil, pancreatic enzyme replacement, vitamin supplements.
Gallbladder	Microgallbladder	None.	Congenital—present at any age.	30	US or hepatobiliary scintigraphy.	None needed.
	Cholelithiasis	Recurrent right upper quadrant abdominal pain, rarely jaundice.	School age through adolescence.	1–10	US.	Surgery if symptomatic and low-risk, trial of cholelitholytics in others.
Extrahepatic bile ducts	Intraluminal obstruction (sludge, stones, tumor)	Jaundice, hepatomegaly, abdominal pain.	Neonates, then older children through adolescence.	Rare in neonates (< 0.1)	US and hepatobiliary scintigraphy, MRCP.	Surgery in neonates; ERCP in older patients or surgery.
	Extraluminal obstruction (intrapancreatic compression, tumor)	As above.	Older children to adults.	Rare (< 1)	As above.	Surgical biliary drainage procedure or ERCP.

ALT, alanine aminotransferase; AST, aspartate aminotransferase; CT, computed tomography; ERCP, endoscopic retrograde cholangiopancreatography; MRCP, magnetic resonance cholangiopancreatography; PPI, proton pump inhibitor; TIPS, transjugular intrahepatic portosystemic shunt; UDCA, ursodeoxycholic acid; UGI, upper gastrointestinal; US, abdominal ultrasound.

findings, incidence, most useful diagnostic studies, and preferred treatment. In addition to the listed conditions, children with cystic fibrosis can develop functional gastrointestinal disorders like any other children.

Debray D et al: Best practice guidance for the diagnosis and management of cystic fibrosis-associated liver disease. J Cyst Fibros 2011;10:S29 [PMID: 21658639].

Flass T, Narkewicz MR: Cirrhosis and other liver disease in cystic fibrosis. J Cyst Fibros 2013;12:116 [PMID: 23266093].

Ooi CY, Durie PR: Cystic fibrosis from the gastroenterologist's perspective. Nat Rev Gastroenterol Hepatol 2016 Mar;13(3): 175–185. doi: 10.1038/nrgastro.2015.226 [PMID: 26790364].

Somaraju UR, Solis-Moya A: Pancreatic enzyme replacement therapy for people with cystic fibrosis. Cochrane Database Syst Rev 2014;10:CD008227 [PMID: 25310479].

SYNDROMES WITH PANCREATIC EXOCRINE INSUFFICIENCY

Several syndromes are associated with exocrine pancreatic insufficiency. Patients present with failure to thrive, diarrhea, fatty stools, and an absence of respiratory symptoms. Laboratory findings include low fecal pancreatic elastase 1; high fecal fat content with 72 hour fecal fat analysis using a standardized high-fat diet; and low to absent pancreatic lipase, amylase, and trypsin levels on endoscopic duodenal fluid aspiration. Each disorder has several associated clinical features that aid in the differential diagnosis. In Shwachman-Diamond syndrome, pancreatic exocrine hypoplasia with widespread fatty replacement of the glandular acinar tissue is associated with neutropenia because of maturational arrest of the granulocyte series. Metaphyseal dysostosis and an elevated fetal hemoglobin level are common; immunoglobulin deficiency and hepatic dysfunction are also reported. CT examination of the pancreas demonstrates the widespread fatty replacement. Genotyping of the *SBDS* gene is available. Serum immunoreactive trypsinogen levels are extremely low.

Other associations of exocrine pancreatic insufficiency include (1) aplastic alae, aplasia cutis, deafness (Johanson-Blizzard syndrome); (2) sideroblastic anemia, developmental delay, seizures, and liver dysfunction (Pearson bone marrow pancreas syndrome); (3) duodenal atresia or stenosis; (4) malnutrition; and (5) pancreatic hypoplasia or agenesis.

The complications and sequelae of exocrine pancreatic insufficiency are malnutrition, diarrhea, and growth failure. The degree of steatorrhea may vary by age and degree of pancreatic function. Intragastric lipolysis by lingual lipase may compensate in patients with low or absent pancreatic function. In Shwachman-Diamond syndrome, pancreatic exocrine insufficiency usually improves with age. Increased infections may result from chronic neutropenia and reduced neutrophil mobility. An increased incidence of leukemia has been noted in these patients; thus patients with myelodysplasia syndrome should be considered for hematopoietic stem cell transplantation.

Pancreatic enzyme and fat-soluble vitamin replacement are required therapy in most patients.

Almashraki N, Abdulnabee MZ, Sukalo M, Alrajoudi A, Sharafadeen I, Zenker M: Johanson-Blizzard syndrome. World J Gastroenterol 2011;17:42–47 [PMID: 22072859].

Chen R et al: Neonatal and late-onset diabetes mellitus caused by failure of pancreatic development: report of 4 more cases and a review of the literature. Pediatrics 2008;121:1541 [PMID: 18519458].

Dror Y et al: Draft consensus guidelines for diagnosis and treatment of Shwachman-Diamond syndrome. Ann N Y Acad Sci 2011;1242:40 [PMID: 22191555].

Myers KC et al: Clinical and molecular pathophysiology of Shwachman-Diamond syndrome: an update. Hematol Oncol Clin North Am 2013;27:117 [PMID: 23351992].

ISOLATED EXOCRINE PANCREATIC ENZYME DEFECT

Premature infants and most newborns produce little, if any, pancreatic amylase following meals or exogenous hormonal stimulation. This temporary physiologic insufficiency may persist for the first 3–6 months of life and be responsible for diarrhea when complex carbohydrates (cereals) are introduced early in the diet.

Congenital pancreatic lipase deficiency and congenital colipase deficiency are extremely rare disorders, causing diarrhea and variable malnutrition with malabsorption of dietary fat and fat-soluble vitamins. In these cases, the sweat chloride level is normal and neutropenia is absent. Treatment is oral replacement of pancreatic enzymes and a low-fat diet or formula containing medium-chain triglycerides.

Exocrine pancreatic insufficiency of proteolytic enzymes (eg, trypsinogen, trypsin, chymotrypsin) is caused by enterokinase deficiency, a duodenal mucosal enzyme required for activation of the pancreatic proenzymes. These patients present with malnutrition associated with hypoproteinemia and edema. Similar to lipase and colipase deficiencies, the sweat test and neutrophil counts are normal. Patients with enterokinase deficiency respond to pancreatic enzyme replacement therapy and feeding formulas that contain a casein hydrolysate (eg, Nutramigen, Pregestimil). Some patients may have transient exocrine pancreatic insufficiency which resolves with time.

Stormon MO, Durie PR: Pathophysiologic basis of exocrine pancreatic dysfunction in childhood. J Pediatr Gastroenterol Nutr 2002;35:8 [PMID: 12142803].

PANCREATIC TUMORS

Pancreatic tumors, whether benign or malignant, are rare. The majority of patients with malignant tumors present with abdominal pain or are found incidentally. The most common pediatric pancreatic tumors are solid pseudopapillary tumors (found predominantly in adolescent females), and neuroendocrine tumors (NET) (insulinoma, gastrinoma, glucagonoma, VIPoma, and nonfunctioning NET). NET present in the pancreas in pediatric patients should prompt evaluation for MEN1 syndrome. NET can produce diverse symptoms if they are producing biologically active polypeptides or be asymptomatic. The clinical features of these tumors are summarized in Table 22–13.

Table 22–13. Pancreatic tumors.

	Age	Major Findings	Diagnosis	Treatment	Associated Conditions
Solid Pseudopapillary Tumor	Adolescents, usually female	Single solid mass in pancreas found incidentally or in evaluation of abdominal pain	CT scan, MRI, EUS	Surgery	
Adenocarcinoma	Older adolescents	Epigastric pain, mass, weight loss, anemia, biliary obstruction	CT scan, MRI, EUS	Chemotherapy, surgery	Chronic pancreatitis
Lymphoma	Any age	Solid round tumors, enlarged lymph nodes	CT scan, MRI, EUS	Chemotherapy	
Pancreaticoblastoma	2–20, mean 7 y	Heterogeneous, may appear pancreatic or liver origin on imaging, metastases	CT scan, MRI, EUS	Chemotherapy, surgery	
Pancreatic Neuroendocrine Tumors					
Nonfunctioning	Any age	Incidental finding, abdominal pain	CT scan, EUS, MRI	Observation or surgery depending size	MEN1
Insulinoma	Any age	Hypoglycemia, seizures; high serum insulin; weight gain; abdominal pain and mass infrequent	CT scan, MRI, PET, EUS, SRS	Surgery, diazoxide, SSTA	MEN1
Gastrinoma	> 5–8 y	Male sex, gastric hypersecretion, peptic symptoms, multiple ulcers, gastrointestinal bleeding, anemia, diarrhea	Elevated fasting gastrin and post secretin suppression test (> 300 pg/mL), CT scan, MRI, EUS, SRS, laparotomy	PPI, surgical resection, total gastrectomy, SSTA	Zollinger-Ellison syndrome, MEN1, neurofibromatosis
VIPoma	Any age (more common 2–4 y old)	Secretory diarrhea, hypokalemia, hypochlorhydria, weight loss, flushing	Elevated VIP levels (> 75 pg/mL); sometimes, elevated serum gastrin and pancreatic polypeptide; CT, EUS, SRS	Surgery, SSTA, IV fluids	
Glucagonoma	Older patients	Diabetes, necrolytic migratory erythema, diarrhea, anemia, thrombotic events, depression	Elevated glucagon, hyperglycemia, gastrin, VIP, CT, MRI, EUS, SRS	Surgery, SSTA	

CT, computed tomography; EUS, endoscopic ultrasound; IV, intravenous; MEN1, multiple endocrine neoplasia syndrome type I; MRI, magnetic resonance imaging; NET, neuroendocrine tumor; PET, Positron emission tomography; PPI, proton pump inhibitor; SRS, somatostatin-receptor scintigraphy; SSTA, somatostatin analogue; VIP, vasoactive intestinal polypeptide.

The differential diagnosis of pancreatic tumors includes Wilms tumor, neuroblastoma, pancreaticoblastoma, and lymphoma. Endoscopic ultrasonography with fine needle biopsy can aid in making definitive diagnoses and guiding surgical planning.

Klimstra DS, Adsay V: Acinar neoplasms of the pancreas—a summary of 25 years of research. Semin Diagn Pathol 2016;33(5):307–318 [PMID: 27320062].

Rojas Y et al: Primary malignant pancreatic neoplasms in children and adolescents: a 20 year experience. J Pediatr Surg 2012;47:2199 [PMID: 23217876].

REFERENCES

Kleinman R et al (eds): *Walker's Pediatric Gastrointestinal Disease: Physiology, Diagnosis, Management.* 6th ed. BC Decker Inc; 2014.

Suchy FJ, Sokol RJ, Balistreri WF (eds): *Liver Disease in Children.* 4th ed. Cambridge University Press; 2014.

Wyllie R, Hyams JS (eds): *Pediatric Gastrointestinal and Liver Disease.* 4th ed. Elsevier; 2011.

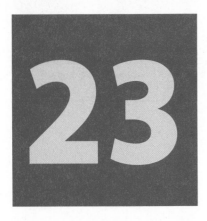

23

Fluid, Electrolyte, & Acid–Base Disorders & Therapy

Melisha G. Hanna, MD, MS

Margret E. Bock, MD, MS

▼ REGULATION OF BODY FLUIDS, ELECTROLYTES, & TONICITY

Total body water (TBW) constitutes 50%–75% of the total body mass, depending on age, sex, and fat content. After an initial brisk postnatal diuresis, the TBW slowly decreases to the adult range near puberty. TBW is divided into the intracellular and extracellular spaces. Intracellular fluid (ICF) accounts for two-thirds of the TBW and extracellular fluid (ECF) for one-third. The ECF is further compartmentalized into plasma (intravascular) volume and interstitial fluid (ISF).

The principal constituents of plasma are sodium, chloride, bicarbonate, and protein (primarily albumin). The ISF is similar to plasma but lacks significant amounts of protein. Conversely, the ICF is rich in potassium, magnesium, phosphates, sulfates, and protein.

An understanding of osmotic shifts between the ECF and ICF is fundamental to understanding disorders of fluid balance. Iso-osmolality is generally maintained between fluid compartments. Because the cell membrane is water-permeable, abnormal fluid shifts occur if the concentration of solutes that cannot permeate the cell membrane in the ECF does not equal the concentration of such solutes in the ICF. Thus, NaCl, mannitol, and glucose (in the setting of hyperglycemia) remain restricted to the ECF space and contribute effective osmoles by obligating water to remain in or be drawn into the ECF compartment. In contrast, a freely permeable solute such as urea does not contribute effective osmoles because it is not restricted to the ECF and readily crosses cell membranes. Tonicity, or effective osmolality, differs from measured osmolality in that it accounts only for osmotically active impermeable solutes rather than all osmotically active solutes, including those that are permeable to cell membranes. Osmolality may be estimated by the following formula:

$$mOsm/kg = 2[Na^+(mEq/L)] + \frac{Glucose\,(mg/dl)}{18} + \frac{BUN\,(mg/dL)}{2.8}$$

Although osmolality and osmolarity differ, the former being an expression of osmotic activity per weight (kg) and the latter per volume (L) of solution, for clinical purposes they are similar and occasionally used interchangeably. Oncotic pressure, or colloid osmotic pressure, represents the osmotic activity of macromolecular constituents such as albumin in the plasma and body fluids. The importance of albumin in maintaining intravascular volume status is reflected in the setting of the nephrotic syndrome, protein losing enteropathy, and other low serum albumin states wherein fluids accumulate in the interstitial compartment leading to edema.

The principal mechanisms that regulate ECF volume and tonicity are thirst, vasopressin or antidiuretic hormone (ADH), aldosterone, and atrial natriuretic peptide (ANP), the latter three exerting their influence by their effects on renal water and sodium handling.

Thirst

Water intake is commonly determined by cultural and behavioral factors. Thirst is not physiologically stimulated until plasma osmolality reaches 290 mOsm/kg, a level at which ADH release induces maximal antidiuresis. Thirst provides control over a wide range of fluid states and allows maintenance of appropriate intravascular volume, even in polyuric states (such as central or nephrogenic DI, or obstructive uropathy). An adequate thirst mechanism is central to maintaining adequate fluid balance.

Antidiuretic Hormone

In the kidney, ADH increases water reabsorption in the cortical and medullary collecting ducts, leading to formation of concentrated urine. In the absence of ADH, dilute urine is produced. Typically, ADH secretion is regulated by the tonicity of body fluids rather than intravascular fluid volume; it becomes detectable at a plasma osmolality of 280 mOsm/kg or greater. Tonicity may, however, be sacrificed to preserve ECF volume (ie, with hyponatremic dehydration), wherein ADH secretion and renal water retention are maximal, despite comparatively lower plasma osmolality.

Aldosterone

Aldosterone is released from the adrenal cortex in response to (1) decreased effective circulating volume and resultant stimulation of the renin-angiotensin-aldosterone axis or (2) in response to increasing plasma K^+. Aldosterone enhances renal tubular reabsorption of Na^+ in exchange for K^+, and to a lesser degree H^+. At a constant osmolality, retention of Na^+ leads to expansion of ECF volume and suppression of aldosterone release.

Atrial Natriuretic Peptide

ANP, a polypeptide hormone secreted principally by the cardiac atria in response to atrial dilation, contributes to regulation of blood volume and blood pressure. ANP inhibits renin secretion and aldosterone synthesis and causes an increase in glomerular filtration rate and renal sodium excretion. ANP also guards against excessive plasma volume expansion in the face of increased ECF volume by shifting fluid from the vascular to the interstitial compartment. ANP inhibits angiotensin II and norepinephrine-induced vasoconstriction and acts in the brain to decrease the desire for salt and inhibit the release of ADH. Thus, the net effect of ANP is a decrease in blood volume and blood pressure associated with natriuresis and diuresis.

Danziger J, Zeidel ML: Osmotic homeostasis. Clin J Am Soc Nephrol 2015 May 7;10(5):852–862 (Epub ahead of print) [PMID: 25078421].
Finberg L et al: *Water and Electrolytes in Pediatrics: Physiology, Pathophysiology and Treatment.* 2nd ed. WB Saunders; 1993.
Friedman A: Fluid and electrolyte therapy: a primer. Pediatr Nephrol 2010;25:842–846 [PMID: 19444484].

▼ ACID–BASE BALANCE

The pH of arterial blood is maintained between 7.38 and 7.42 to ensure that pH-sensitive enzyme systems function normally. Acid-base balance is maintained by interaction of the lungs, kidneys, and systemic buffering systems. Over 50% of the blood's buffering capacity is provided by the carbonic acid–bicarbonate system, roughly 30% by hemoglobin, and the remainder by phosphates and ammonium. The carbonic acid–bicarbonate system, depicted chemically as

$$CO_2 + H_2O \leftrightarrow H_2CO_3 \leftrightarrow H^+ + HCO_3^-$$

interacts via the lungs and kidneys, and in conjunction with the nonbicarbonate systems, to stabilize systemic pH. The concentration of dissolved CO_2 in blood is established by the respiratory system and that of HCO_3^- by the kidneys. Disturbances in acid–base balance are initially stabilized by chemical buffering, compensated for by pulmonary or renal regulation of CO_2, and ultimately corrected when the primary cause of the acid–base disturbance is eliminated.

Renal regulation of acid–base balance is accomplished by the reabsorption of filtered HCO_3^-, primarily in the proximal tubule, and the excretion of H^+ or HCO_3^- in the distal nephron to match the net input of acid or base. When urine is alkalinized, HCO_3^- enters the kidney and is ultimately lost in the urine. However, urinary alkalinization will not occur if there is a deficiency of urine Na^+ or K^+, as electroneutrality must be maintained. In contrast, the urine may be acidified if an absolute or relative decrease occurs in systemic HCO_3^-. In this setting, proximal tubular HCO_3^- reabsorption and distal tubular H^+ excretion are maximal. A "paradoxical aciduria" with low urinary pH may be seen in the setting of hypokalemic metabolic alkalosis and systemic K^+ depletion wherein H^+ is exchanged and excreted in preference to K^+ in response to mineralocorticoid. Some of the processes involved in acid–base regulation are shown in Figure 23–1.

Fall PJ: A stepwise approach to acid-base disorders. Practical patient evaluation for metabolic acidosis and other conditions. Postgrad Med 2000;107:249 [PMID: 10728149].
Seifter JL: Integration of acid-base and electrolyte disorders. N Engl J Med 2014;371:1821–1831 [PMID: 25372090].

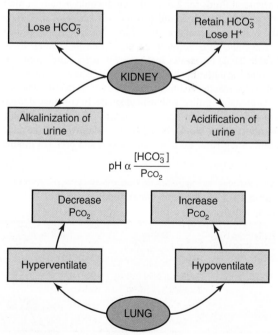

▲ **Figure 23–1.** Maintaining metabolic stability via compensatory mechanisms.

▼ FLUID & ELECTROLYTE MANAGEMENT

Therapy of fluid and electrolyte disorders should be phased to (1) expand the ECF volume and restore tissue perfusion, (2) replenish fluid and electrolyte deficits while correcting attendant acid–base abnormalities, (3) meet the patient's nutritional needs, and (4) replace ongoing losses.

The cornerstone of therapy involves a detailed understanding of "maintenance" fluid and electrolyte requirements. "Maintenance" requirements call for provision of enough water, glucose, and electrolytes to prevent deterioration of body stores for a euvolemic patient under normal conditions. During short-term parenteral therapy, sufficient glucose is provided to prevent ketosis and limit protein catabolism, although this usually provides little more than 20% of the patient's true caloric needs. Prior to the administration of "maintenance" fluids, it is important to consider the patient's volume status and to determine whether intravenous fluids are truly needed.

Various models have been devised to facilitate calculation of "maintenance" requirements based on body surface area, weight, and caloric expenditure. A system based on caloric expenditure is most helpful, because 1 mL of water is needed for each kilocalorie expended. The system presented in Table 23–1 is based on caloric needs and is applicable to children weighing more than 3 kg.

As depicted in Table 23–1, a child weighing 30 kg would need 1700 kcal or 1700 mL of water daily. If the child received parenteral fluids for 2 days, the fluid would usually contain 5% glucose, which would provide 340 kcal/day, or 20% of the maintenance caloric needs. Maintenance fluid requirements take into account normal insensible water losses (Table 23–2) and water lost in sweat, urine, and stool, and assume the patient to be afebrile, at their true dry weight, and relatively inactive. Thus, if excessive losses occur, standard "maintenance fluids" will be inadequate. In contrast, if losses are reduced for any reason, standard "maintenance fluid" administration would be excessive. Maintenance requirements are greater for low-birth-weight and preterm infants.

Table 23–1. Caloric and water needs per unit of body weight.

Body Weight (kg)	kcal/kg	mL of Water/kg
3–10	100	100
11–20	1000 kcal + 50 kcal/kg for each kg > 10 kg	1000 mL + 50 mL/kg for each kg > 10 kg
> 20	1500 kcal + 20 kcal/kg for each kg > 20 kg	1500 mL + 20 mL/kg for each kg > 20 kg

Data from Holliday MA, Segar WE: The maintenance need for water in parenteral fluid therapy. Pediatrics 1957 May;19(5):823–832.

Table 23–2. Insensible losses.

Preterm infant	40 mL/kg/day
Infant	20–30 mL/kg/day
Children, adults, and adolescents	400 mL/m²/day

Table 23–3 lists other factors that commonly alter fluid and caloric needs.

Electrolyte losses occur primarily through the urinary tract and to a lesser degree via the skin and stool. Maintenance sodium and potassium electrolyte needs have historically been approximated to be in the 3 mEq Na/100 kcal and 2 mEq K/100 kcal range, leading to the common use of hypotonic intravenous fluids with 77 mEq/L of sodium (½ normal saline) and 20 mEq/L of potassium. Over the past 10 years many authors have drawn attention to the serious problem of hospital-acquired hyponatremia in children with the use of hypotonic IV solutions; notably, hyponatremia is the most common electrolyte abnormality in children and affects approximately 25% of hospitalized pediatric patients. Furthermore, the astute clinician will bear in mind the dynamic nature of clinical context in treating patients and that the choice of IV solution (Table 23–4) and rate of infusion must be made on an individual basis and must be reassessed often. A child with profound water loss stools and hypernatremia

Table 23–3. Alterations of fluid requirements.

Increased Requirements	
Factor	Altered Requirement
Fever	12% per degree >38°C
Hyperventilation	10–60 mL/100 kcal
Sweating	10–25 mL/100 kcal
Hyperthyroidism	Variable: 25%–50%
Hyperosmolar states (eg, diabetic ketoacidosis)	Variable, assess volume status (see Chapter 35)
Gastrointestinal loss (vomiting, diarrhea, NG output)	Monitor and analyze output. Adjust therapy accordingly.
Decreased Requirements	
Factor	Altered Requirement
Hypothermia	Variable
Increased environmental humidity	Variable
Hypometabolic states	Variable
Renal failure	Restrict to insensible losses plus urine output

Table 23–4. Composition of common intravenous fluid solutions.

Fluid	Dextrose (g/L)	Na⁺ (mEq/L)	Cl⁻ (mEq/L)	K⁺ (mEq/L)	Lactate (mEq/L)
Lactated ringers (LR)	0	130	109	4	28
D5W	50	0	0	0	0
D5 0.2 NS	50	38	38	0	0
D5 0.45 NS	50	77	77	0	0
D5 0.9 NS	50	154	154	0	0
Normal saline (NS)	0	154	154	0	0
Hypertonic saline (3% NaCl)	0	513	513	0	0

who is placed on hypotonic IV fluids and whose diarrhea ceases, but is continued on hypotonic solution without close monitoring of serum electrolytes is at risk for the devastating clinical consequences related to sequelae of rapid changes in sodium balance. In recent years, there also has been a trend for total parenteral nutrition solution sodium and other electrolytes to be calculated and ordered on a milli-equivalents-per-kilogram basis rather than the more classic milliequivalents-per-liter basis (eg, 0.2 or 0.45 normal). If the administered fluid volume is decreased in this setting, as the child is weaned from supplemental IV fluids to enteral intake, the sodium and other electrolytes will need to be reduced accordingly to avoid changes in IV fluid tonicity that can result in hypernatremia or other electrolyte derangements.

Patient weight, total output, urinary output, and total fluid input should be monitored daily. Electronic medical records may calculate the net total volume in a 24 hour period but this should be interpreted cautiously as it does not account for the patient's insensible losses; obtaining daily weights is a corner-stone of appropriate monitoring of fluid and electrolyte balance. If fluid or electrolyte balance is abnormal, serial determination of serum electrolyte concentrations, blood urea nitrogen, and creatinine are necessary; for example, in patients with significant burns, anuria, oliguria, or persistent abnormal stool or urine losses. Serial labs should also be monitored in patients receiving IV fluids or parental nutrition.

DEHYDRATION

Depletion of body fluids is one of the most commonly encountered problems in clinical pediatrics. The clinical evaluation of a child with dehydration, or volume contraction, should focus on the composition and volume of fluid intake and losses (vomiting, diarrhea, urine, "insensible losses"). An updated weight is central to calculating the magnitude of volume depletion. Important clinical features in estimating the degree of dehydration include the capillary refill time, postural blood pressure, and heart rate changes; dryness of the lips and mucous membranes; lack of tears; lack of external jugular venous filling when supine; a sunken fontanelle in an infant; oliguria; and altered mental status (Table 23–5). Children generally respond to a decrease in circulating volume with a compensatory increase in pulse rate and may maintain their blood pressure in the face of severe dehydration. A low or falling blood pressure is, therefore, a late sign of shock in children, and when present should prompt emergent treatment. Salient laboratory parameters include a high urine-specific gravity (in the absence of an underlying renal concentrating defect as seen in diabetes insipidus or chronic obstructive or reflux nephropathy), a relatively greater elevation in blood urea nitrogen than in serum creatinine, a low urinary [Na⁺] excretion (< 20 mEq/L) or fractional excretion of sodium less than 0.1%, and an elevated hematocrit or serum albumin level secondary to hemoconcentration.

Emergent intravenous therapy is indicated when there is evidence of compromised perfusion (inadequate capillary refill, tachycardia, poor color, oliguria, or hypotension). The initial goal is to rapidly expand the plasma volume and to prevent circulatory collapse. A 20-mL/kg bolus of isotonic fluid should be given intravenously as rapidly as possible. Either colloid (5% albumin) or crystalloid (normal saline or Ringer lactate) may be used. Colloid is particularly useful in hypernatremic patients in shock, in malnourished infants, and in neonates. If no intravenous site is available, fluid may be administered intra-osseously through the marrow space. If there is no response to the first fluid bolus, a second bolus may be given. When adequate tissue perfusion is demonstrated by improved capillary refill, decreased pulse rate and improved mental status, deficit replacement may be instituted. If adequate perfusion is not restored after 40 mL/kg of isotonic fluids, other pathologic processes must be considered such as sepsis, occult hemorrhage, or cardiogenic shock. Isotonic dehydration may be treated by providing half of the remaining fluid deficit over 8 hours and the second half over the ensuing 16 hours in the form of 5% dextrose with 0.45% saline containing 20 mEq/L of KCl. In the presence of metabolic acidosis, the addition of sodium or potassium acetate may be considered. Serum potassium and calcium concentrations should be closely monitored, as these can decrease significantly with resolution of acidosis. Maintenance fluids and replacement of ongoing losses should also be provided. Typical electrolyte compositions of various body fluids are depicted in Table 23–6, although it may be necessary to measure the specific constituents of a patient's fluid losses to guide therapy. If the patient is unable to eat for a prolonged period, nutritional needs must be met through hyperalimentation or enteral tube feedings.

Table 23–5. Clinical manifestations of dehydration.

Clinical Signs	Degree of Dehydration		
	Mild	Moderate	Severe
Decrease in body weight	3%–5%	6%–10%	11%–15%
Skin			
Turgor	Normal ±	Decreased	Markedly decreased
Color	Normal	Pale	Markedly decreased
Mucous membranes	Dry	———————————————→	Mottled or gray; parched
Hemodynamic signs			
Pulse	Normal	Slight increase	Tachycardia
Capillary refill	2–3 s	3–4 s	> 4 s
Blood pressure	Normal	———————————————→	Low
Perfusion	Normal	———————————————→	Circulatory collapse
Fluid loss			
Urinary output	Mild oliguria	Oliguria	Anuria
Tears	Decreased		Absent
Urinary indices			
Specific gravity	> 1.020	———————————————→	Anuria
Urine [Na⁺]	< 20 mEq/L	———————————————→	Anuria

Oral rehydration may be provided to children with mild to moderate dehydration and commercially available solutions provide 45–75 mEq/L of Na⁺, 20–25 mEq/L of K⁺, 30–34 mEq/L of citrate or bicarbonate, and 2%–2.5% of glucose (Table 23–7). Clear liquid beverages found in the home, such as broth, soda, juice, and tea are inappropriate for the treatment of dehydration. Frequent small aliquots (5–15 mL) should be given to provide approximately 50 mL/kg over 4 hours for mild dehydration and up to 100 mL/kg over 6 hours for moderate dehydration. Oral rehydration is contraindicated in children with altered levels of consciousness or respiratory distress who cannot drink freely; in children suspected of having an acute surgical abdomen; in infants with greater than 10% volume depletion; in children with hemodynamic instability; and in the setting of severe hyponatremia ([Na⁺] < 120 mEq/L) or hypernatremia ([Na⁺] > 160 mEq/L). Failure of oral rehydration due to persistent vomiting or inability to keep up with losses mandates intravenous therapy. Successful oral rehydration requires explicit instructions to caregivers and close clinical follow-up of the child.

The type of dehydration is often characterized by the serum [Na⁺]. If relatively more solute is lost than water, the [Na⁺] falls, and hyponatremic dehydration ([Na⁺] < 130 mEq/L) ensues. This is important clinically because hypotonicity of the plasma contributes to further volume loss from the ECF into the intracellular space. Thus, tissue perfusion is more significantly impaired for a given degree of hyponatremic dehydration than for a comparable degree of isotonic or hypertonic dehydration. It is important to note, however, that significant solute losses also occur in hypernatremic dehydration. Furthermore, because plasma volume is somewhat protected in hypernatremic dehydration, it poses the

Table 23–6. Typical electrolyte compositions of various body fluids.

	Na⁺ (mEq/L)	K⁺ (mEq/L)	HCO₃⁻ (mEq/L)
Diarrhea	10–90	10–80	40
Gastric	20–80	5–20	0
Small intestine	100–140	5–15	40
Ileostomy	45–135	3–15	40

Data from Winters RW: *Principles of Pediatric Fluid Therapy.* Philadelphia, PA: Lippincott Williams & Wilkins; 1973.

Table 23–7. Composition of oral rehydration solutions.

Fluid	Carbohydrate (g/L)	Na⁺ (mEq/L)	HCO₃⁻ (mEq/L)	K⁺ (mEq/L)
Pedialyte	25	45	30	20
Enfalyte	30	50	30	25
WHO (2002)	13.5	75	30	20

Table 23–8. Estimated water and electrolyte deficits in dehydration (moderate to severe).

Type of Dehydration	H$_2$O (mL/kg)	Na$^+$ (mEq/kg)	K$^+$ (mEq/kg)	Cl$^-$ (mEq/kg)
Isotonic	100–150	8–10	8–10	16–20
Hypotonic	50–100	10–14	10–14	20–28
Hypertonic	120–180	2–5	2–5	4–10

Adapted with permission from Winters RW: *Principles of Pediatric Fluid Therapy*, 2nd ed. Philadelphia, PA: Lippincott Williams & Wilkins; 1973.

risk of the clinician underestimating the severity of dehydration. Typical fluid and electrolyte losses associated with each form of dehydration are shown in Table 23–8.

HYPONATREMIA

Hyponatremia may be factitious in the presence of high plasma lipids or proteins, which decrease the percentage of plasma volume that is water. Hyponatremia in the absence of hypotonicity also occurs when an osmotically active solute, such as glucose or mannitol, is added to the ECF. Water drawn from the ICF dilutes the serum [Na$^+$] despite isotonicity or hypertonicity.

Patients with hyponatremic dehydration generally demonstrate typical signs and symptoms of dehydration (see Table 23–5), as the vascular space is compromised as water leaves the ECF to maintain osmotic neutrality. The treatment of hyponatremic dehydration is fairly straightforward. The magnitude of the sodium deficit may be calculated by the following formula:

$$Na^+ \text{ deficit} = (Na^+ \text{ desired} - Na^+ \text{ observed}) \times \text{Bodyweight (kg)} \times 0.6$$

Half of the deficit is replenished in the first 8 hours of therapy, and the remainder is given over the following 16 hours. Maintenance and replacement fluids should also be provided. The deficit plus maintenance calculations often approximate 5% dextrose with 0.45% or higher saline. The rise in serum [Na$^+$] should not exceed 0.5 mEq/L/h or 6–8 mEq/L/24 h unless the patient demonstrates central nervous system (CNS) symptoms that warrant more rapid initial correction. The dangers of too rapid correction of hyponatremia include cerebral dehydration and injury due to fluid shifts from the ICF compartment, a condition known as osmotic demyelination syndrome.

Hypovolemic hyponatremia also occurs in cerebral salt-wasting (CSW) associated with CNS insults, a condition characterized by high urine output and elevated urinary [Na$^+$] (> 40 mEq/L) due to an increase in ANP. CWS is a diagnosis of exclusion represented by an inappropriate natriuresis in a patient with a contracted effective circulatory blood volume in the absence of other causes for Na$^+$ excretion. This must be distinguished from the syndrome of inappropriate secretion of ADH (SIADH), which may also manifest in CNS conditions and pulmonary disorders (Table 23–9). In contrast to CSW, SIADH is characterized by euvolemia or mild volume expansion and relatively low urine output due to ADH-induced water retention. Urinary [Na$^+$] is high in both conditions, though generally not as high as in SIADH. It is important to distinguish between these two conditions, because the treatment of cerebral salt wasting involves replacement of urinary salt and water losses, whereas the treatment of SIADH involves water restriction. It is also important to remember that in SIADH patients are not necessarily oliguric, and that their urine does not need to be maximally concentrated but merely inappropriately concentrated for their degree of serum tonicity.

In cases of severe hyponatremia (serum [Na$^+$] < 120 mEq/L) with CNS symptoms, intravenous 3% NaCl may be given to raise the [Na$^+$] by 5 mEq/L to alleviate CNS manifestations and sequelae. In general, 1 mL/kg of 3% NaCl will raise the serum [Na$^+$] by about 1 mEq/L. If 3% NaCl is administered, estimated Na$^+$ and fluid deficits should be adjusted accordingly. Further correction should proceed slowly, as outlined earlier.

Table 23–9. SIADH and cerebral salt wasting.

	Serum Na$^+$	Serum Osmolality	Urine Na$^+$	Urine Output	Urine Osmolality	Volume Status	Treatment
SIADH	< 135 mEq/L	< 280 mOsm/kg	> 40 mEq/L	Low	> 100 mOsm/kg[a]	Euvolemia or mild volume expansion	Water restriction
Cerebral salt-wasting	< 135 mEq/L	< 280 mOsm/kg	> 40 mEq/L	High	Variable[b]	Hypovolemia	Sodium and water replacement

[a]Urine is inappropriately concentrated when it should be maximally dilute with a urine osmolality of <100 mOsm/kg.
[b]May be normal or maximally dilute with a urine osmolality of <100 mOsm/kg.

Hypervolemic hyponatremia may occur in edematous disorders such as nephrotic syndrome, congestive heart failure, and cirrhosis, wherein water is retained in excess of salt. Treatment involves restriction of Na^+ and water and correction of the underlying disorder. Hypervolemic hyponatremia due to water intoxication is characterized by a maximally dilute urine (specific gravity < 1.003) and is also treated with water restriction.

HYPERNATREMIA

Although diarrhea is commonly associated with hyponatremic or isonatremic dehydration, hypernatremia may develop in the presence of persistent fever or decreased fluid intake or in response to improperly mixed rehydration solutions. Extreme care is required to treat hypernatremic dehydration appropriately. If the serum $[Na^+]$ falls precipitously, the osmolality of the ECF drops more rapidly than that of the CNS and water shifts from the ECF compartment into the CNS to maintain osmotic neutrality. If hypertonicity is corrected too rapidly (a drop in $[Na^+]$ of > 0.5 mEq/L/h), cerebral edema, seizures, and CNS injury may occur. Thus, following the initial restoration of adequate tissue perfusion using isotonic fluids, a gradual decrease in serum $[Na^+]$ is desired (6–8 mEq/L/day). This is commonly achieved using 5% dextrose with 0.2% saline to replace the calculated fluid deficit over 48 hours or longer depending on the severity and chronicity of the fluid losses. Maintenance and replacement fluids should also be provided. If the serum $[Na^+]$ is not correcting appropriately, the free water deficit may be estimated as 4 mL/kg of free water for each milliequivalent of serum $[Na^+]$ above 145 mEq/L and provided as 5% dextrose. If metabolic acidosis is also present, it must be corrected slowly to avoid CNS irritability. Potassium is provided as indicated. Electrolyte concentrations should be assessed every 2 hours in order to control the decline in serum $[Na^+]$. Elevations of blood glucose and blood urea nitrogen may worsen the hyperosmolar state in hypernatremic dehydration and should also be monitored closely. Hyperglycemia is often associated with hypernatremic dehydration and may necessitate lower intravenous glucose concentrations (eg, 2.5%).

Patients with diabetes insipidus, whether nephrogenic or central in origin, are prone to develop profound hypernatremic dehydration as a result of unremitting urinary-free water losses (urine-specific gravity < 1.010), particularly during superimposed gastrointestinal illnesses associated with vomiting or diarrhea. Treatment involves restoration of fluid and electrolyte deficits as described earlier as well as replacement of excessive water losses. Formal water deprivation testing to distinguish responsiveness to ADH should only be done during daylight hours after restoration of normal fluid volume status. The evaluation and treatment of nephrogenic and central diabetes insipidus are discussed in detail in Chapters 24 and 34, respectively.

Hypervolemic hypernatremia (salt poisoning), associated with excess total body salt and water, may occur as a consequence of providing improperly mixed formula, excessive NaCl or $NaHCO_3$ administration, or as a feature of primary hyperaldosteronism. Treatment includes the use of diuretics, and potentially, concomitant water replacement or even dialysis.

POTASSIUM DISORDERS

The predominantly intracellular distribution of potassium is maintained by the actions of Na^+-K^+-ATPase in the cell membranes. Potassium is shifted into the ECF and plasma by acidemia and into the ICF in the setting of alkalosis, hypochloremia, or in conjunction with insulin-induced cellular glucose uptake. The ratio of intracellular to extracellular K^+ is the major determinant of the cellular resting membrane potential and contributes to the action potential in neural and muscular tissue. Abnormalities of K^+ balance are potentially life threatening. In the kidney, K^+ is filtered at the glomerulus, reabsorbed in the proximal tubule, and excreted in the distal tubule. Distal tubular K^+ excretion is regulated primarily by the mineralocorticoid aldosterone. Renal K^+ excretion is primarily dependent on the urinary flow rate, and continues for significant periods even after the intake of K^+ is decreased. Thus, by the time urinary $[K^+]$ decreases, the systemic K^+ pool has been depleted significantly. In general, the greater the urine flow the greater the urinary K^+ excretion.

The causes of hypokalemia are primarily renal in origin. Gastrointestinal losses through nasogastric suction or vomiting reduce total body K^+ to some degree. However, the resultant volume depletion results in an increase in plasma aldosterone, promoting renal excretion of K^+ in exchange for Na^+ reclamation to preserve circulatory volume. Diuretics (especially thiazides and loop diuretics), mineralocorticoids, and intrinsic renal tubular diseases (eg, Bartter syndrome) enhance the renal excretion of K^+. Systemic K^+ depletion in hypokalemic metabolic acidosis may lead to "paradoxic aciduria" and low urine pH wherein H^+ is preferentially exchanged for Na^+ in response to aldosterone. Clinically, hypokalemia is associated with neuromuscular excitability, decreased peristalsis or ileus, hyporeflexia, paralysis, rhabdomyolysis, and arrhythmias. Electrocardiographic changes include flattened T waves, a shortened PR interval, and the appearance of U waves. Arrhythmias associated with hypokalemia include premature ventricular contractions; atrial, nodal, or ventricular tachycardia; and ventricular fibrillation. Hypokalemia increases responsiveness to digitalis and may precipitate overt digitalis toxicity. In the presence of arrhythmias, extreme muscle weakness, or respiratory compromise, intravenous K^+ should be given. If the patient is hypophosphatemic ($[PO_4^{3-}]$ < 2 mg/dL), a phosphate salt may be used. The first priority in the treatment of hypokalemia is the restoration of an adequate serum [K^+]. Providing maintenance amounts of K^+ is usually sufficient; however, when the serum [K^+] is dangerously low and K^+ must be administered intravenously, it is imperative that the patient have a cardiac monitor. Intravenous K^+ should generally not be given faster than at a rate of 0.3 mEq/kg/h. Oral K^+ supplements may be needed for weeks to replenish depleted body stores.

Hyperkalemia—due to decreased renal K^+ excretion, mineralocorticoid deficiency or unresponsiveness, or K^+ release from the ICF compartment—is characterized by muscle weakness, paresthesias, and tetany; ascending paralysis; and arrhythmias. Electrocardiographic changes associated with hyperkalemia include peaked T waves, widening of the QRS complex, and arrhythmias such as sinus bradycardia or sinus arrest, atrioventricular block, nodal or idioventricular rhythms, and ventricular tachycardia or fibrillation. An EKG should be obtained when significant hyperkalemia is suspected. If the serum [K^+] is less than 6 mEq/L, discontinuing K^+ supplementation may be sufficient if there is no ongoing K^+ source, such as cell lysis, and if urine output continues. If the serum [K^+] is greater than 6 mEq/L or if potentiating factors such as renal failure are present, more aggressive therapy is needed (Table 23–10). If electrocardiographic changes

or arrhythmias are present, treatment must be initiated promptly. Initial treatment consists of cardiac membrane stabilization and rapid intracellular shifting of K^+ intracellularly. Intravenous calcium gluconate will rapidly ameliorate depolarization and may be repeated after 5 minutes if electrocardiographic changes persist. Calcium should be given only with a cardiac monitor in place and should be discontinued if bradycardia develops. Administering Na^+ and increasing systemic pH with bicarbonate therapy will shift K^+ from the ECF to the ICF compartment, as will therapy with a β-agonist such as albuterol. In nondiabetic patients, 0.5 g/kg of glucose over 1–2 hours will enhance endogenous insulin secretion, lowering serum [K^+] 1–2 mEq/L. Administration of intravenous glucose and insulin may be needed as a simultaneous drip given over 2 hours with monitoring of the serum glucose level every 15 minutes.

The therapies outlined above provide transient benefits and K^+ will remain elevated unless other interventions are used to decrease total body potassium. Therapy must be given to reduce K^+ to normal levels by reestablishing adequate renal excretion using diuretics or optimizing urinary flow, using ion exchange resins such as sodium polystyrene sulfonate that act in the GI tract, or by dialysis.

Table 23–10. Drugs for the treatment of hyperkalemia in children.

Drug	Dose	Actions	Notes
Calcium gluconate (10% solution)	0.2–0.5 mL/kg IV given over 2–10 min (maximum dose 20 mL).	Cardiac membrane stabilization. Does not alter the serum K^+ level.	Cardiac monitoring needed. May repeat dose if EKG changes persist. Discontinue if bradycardia develops.
Sodium polystyrene sulfonate	1 g/kg oral every 6 h or rectal every 2–6 h.	Ion exchange resin that exchanges K^+ for Na^+. Will decrease total body K^+.	Do not use in neonates and patients with bowel hypomotility or bowel obstruction due to risk of intestinal necrosis. May cause hypernatremia, hypocalcemia, and hypomagnesemia.
Sodium bicarbonate	1 mEq/kg (maximum dose 50 mEq).	Transient shift of K^+ from the ECF to the ICF compartment.	Avoid use if alkalosis or hypocalcemia is present. May cause hypernatremia, hypocalcemia.
Furosemide	1–2 mg/kg IV.	Diuretic that increases renal K^+ excretion. Will decrease total body K^+.	May need higher doses in patients with chronic kidney disease to achieve desired effect.
Albuterol (nebulized)	Infants and children < 5 years of age: 2.5 mg in 2 mL of saline. Children > 5 years of age: 5 mg in 2 mL of saline. Adolescents: 10 mg in 2 mL of saline.	Transient shift of K^+ from the ECF to the ICF compartment.	May repeat for 1 additional dose. Tachycardia may limit repeat dosing.
Insulin (regular)	Glucose 0.5–1 g/kg with 0.3 units of insulin per gram of glucose given over 2 h.	Transient shift of K^+ from the ECF to the ICF compartment.	Must be given with a glucose infusion to prevent severe hypoglycemia. Diabetic patients may not require glucose infusion. Requires close monitoring of serum glucose.

Feld LG et al: Clinical practice guideline: maintenance intravenous fluids in children. Pediatrics 2018;142(6):e20183083 [PMID: 30478247].

Hoorn EJ, Zietse R: Diagnosis and treatment of hyponatremia: compilation of guidelines. J Am Soc Nephrol 2017;28(5):1340–1349 [PMID: 28174217].

Montford JR, Linas S: How dangerous is hyperkalemia? J Am Soc Nephrol 2017;28(11):3155–3165 [PMID: 28778861].

Palmer BF: Regulation of potassium homeostasis. Clin J Am Soc Nephrol 2015;10(6):1050–1060 [PMID: 24721891].

Sterns RH: Disorders of plasma sodium—causes, consequences, and correction. N Engl J Med 2015;372:55–65 [PMID: 25551526].

Sterns RH: Treatment of severe hyponatremia. Clin J Am Soc Nephrol 2018;13(4):641–649 [PMID: 29295830].

▼ ACID–BASE DISTURBANCES

When evaluating a disturbance in acid–base balance, the systemic pH, partial carbon dioxide pressure (Pco_2), serum HCO_3^-, and anion gap must be considered. The anion gap, $[Na^+ - (Cl^- + HCO_3^-)]$, is an expression of the unmeasured anions in the plasma and is normally 12 ± 4 mEq/L. An increase above normal suggests the presence of an unmeasured anion, such as occurs in diabetic ketoacidosis, lactic acidosis, and salicylate intoxication. Although the base excess (or deficit) is also used clinically, it is important to recall that this expression of acid–base balance is influenced by the renal response to respiratory disorders and cannot be interpreted independently (as in a compensated respiratory acidosis, wherein the base excess may be quite large).

METABOLIC ACIDOSIS

Metabolic acidosis is characterized by a primary decrease in serum $[HCO_3^-]$ and systemic pH due to the loss of HCO_3^- from the kidneys or gastrointestinal tract, the addition of an acid (from external sources or via altered metabolic processes), or the rapid dilution of the ECF with nonbicarbonate–containing solution (usually normal saline). When HCO_3^- is lost through the kidneys or gastrointestinal tract, Cl^- must be reabsorbed with Na^+ disproportionately, resulting in a hyperchloremic acidosis with a normal anion gap. Thus, a normal anion gap acidosis in the absence of diarrhea or other bicarbonate-rich gastrointestinal losses suggests the possibility of renal tubular acidosis and should be evaluated appropriately (see Chapter 24). In contrast, acidosis that results from the addition of an unmeasured acid is associated with a widened anion gap. Examples are diabetic ketoacidosis, lactic acidosis, starvation, uremia, toxin ingestion (salicylates, ethylene glycol, or methanol), and certain inborn errors of organic or amino acid metabolism. Dehydration may also result in a widened anion gap acidosis as a result of inadequate tissue perfusion, decreased O_2 delivery, and subsequent lactic and keto acid production. Respiratory compensation is accomplished through an increase in minute ventilation and a decrease in Pco_2. The patient's history, physical findings, and laboratory features should lead to the appropriate diagnosis.

The ingestion of unknown toxins or the possibility of an inborn error of metabolism (see Chapter 36) must be considered in children without an obvious cause for a widened anion gap acidosis. Unfortunately, some hospital laboratories fail to include ethylene glycol or methanol in their standard toxicology screens, so assay of these toxins must be requested specifically. This is of critical importance when therapy with fomepizole (4-methylpyrazole) must be considered for either ingestion—and instituted promptly to obviate profound toxicity. Ethylene glycol (eg, antifreeze) is particularly worrisome because of its sweet taste and accounts for a significant number of toxin ingestions. Salicylate intoxication has a stimulatory effect on the respiratory center of the CNS; thus, patients may initially present with respiratory alkalosis or mixed respiratory alkalosis and widened anion gap acidosis.

Most types of metabolic acidosis will resolve with correction of the underlying disorder, improved renal perfusion, and acid excretion. Intravenous $NaHCO_3$ administration may be considered in the setting of metabolic acidosis when the pH is less than 7.2 or the $[HCO_3^-]$ is less than 6 mEq/L, but only if adequate ventilation is ensured. The dose (in milliequivalents) of $NaHCO_3$ may be calculated as

$$\text{Weight (kg)} \times \text{Base deficit} \times 0.3$$

and given as a continuous infusion over 1 hour. The effect of $NaHCO_3$ in lowering serum potassium and ionized calcium concentrations must also be considered and monitored.

METABOLIC ALKALOSIS

Metabolic alkalosis is characterized by a primary increase in $[HCO_3^-]$ and pH resulting from a loss of strong acid or gain of buffer base. The most common cause for a metabolic alkalosis is the loss of gastric juice via nasogastric suction or vomiting. This results in a Cl^--responsive alkalosis, characterized by a low urinary $[Cl^-]$ (< 20 mEq/L) indicative of a volume-contracted state that will be responsive to the provision of adequate Cl^- salt (usually in the form of normal saline). Cystic fibrosis may also be associated with a Cl^--responsive alkalosis due to the high losses of NaCl through the sweat, whereas congenital Cl^--losing diarrhea is a rare cause of Cl^--responsive metabolic alkalosis. Chloride-resistant alkaloses are characterized by a urinary $[Cl^-]$ greater than 20 mEq/L and include Bartter syndrome, Cushing syndrome, and primary hyperaldosteronism, conditions associated with primary increases in urinary $[Cl^-]$, or volume-expanded states lacking stimuli for renal Cl^- reabsorption. Thus, the urinary $[Cl^-]$ is helpful in distinguishing the nature of a metabolic alkalosis, but must be specifically requested in many laboratories because it is not routinely included in urine electrolyte panels. The serum $[K^+]$ is also low in these settings (hypokalemic metabolic alkalosis) owing to a combination of increased mineralocorticoid activity associated with volume contraction, the shift of K^+ to the ICF compartment, and preferential reabsorption of Na^+ rather than K^+ to preserve intravascular volume. A hypokalemic alkalosis seen in the setting of primary mineralocorticoid excess would be expected to be associated with systemic hypertension clinically, as observed in an adrenal adenoma and some forms of monogenic hypertension, including Liddle syndrome and apparent mineralocorticoid excess.

RESPIRATORY ACIDOSIS

Respiratory acidosis develops when alveolar ventilation is decreased, increasing Pco_2, and lowering systemic pH. The kidneys compensate for respiratory acidosis by increasing HCO_3^- reabsorption, a process that takes several days to fully manifest. Patients with acute respiratory acidosis frequently demonstrate air hunger with retractions and the use of accessory respiratory muscles. Respiratory acidosis occurs in upper or lower airway obstruction, ventilation-perfusion disturbances, CNS depression, and neuromuscular defects. Hypercapnia is not as detrimental as the hypoxia that usually accompanies these disorders. The goal of therapy is to correct or compensate for the underlying pathologic process to improve alveolar ventilation. Bicarbonate therapy is not indicated in a pure respiratory acidosis, because it will worsen the acidosis by shifting the equilibrium of the carbonic acid–bicarbonate buffer system to increase Pco_2.

RESPIRATORY ALKALOSIS

Respiratory alkalosis occurs when hyperventilation results in a decrease in Pco_2 and an increase in systemic pH. Depending on the acuity of the respiratory alkalosis, there may be an associated compensatory loss of bicarbonate by the kidneys manifested as a low serum bicarbonate level and a normal anion gap that may be misinterpreted as a normal anion gap acidosis if all acid–base parameters are not considered. Patients may experience tingling, paresthesias, dizziness, palpitations, syncope, or even tetany and seizures due to the associated decrease in ionized calcium. Causes of respiratory alkalosis include psychobehavioral disturbances, CNS irritation from meningitis or encephalitis, salicylate intoxication, and iatrogenic over ventilation in patients who are mechanically ventilated. Therapy is directed toward the causal process. Rebreathing into a paper bag will decrease the severity of symptoms in acute hyperventilation.

Al-Jaghbeer M, Kellum JA: Acid-base disturbances in intensive care patients: etiology, pathophysiology and treatment. Nephrol Dial Transplant 2015 Jul;30(7):1104–1011 [PMID: 25213433].

Berend K, de Vries AP, Gans RO: Physiological approach to acid-base disturbances. N Engl J Med 2014;371:1434–1445 [PMID: 25295502].

Carmody JB, Norwood VF: A clinical approach to paediatric acid-base disorders. Postgrad Med J 2012;88:143–151 [PMID: 22267531].

Seifter JL: Integration of acid-base and electrolyte disorders. N Engl J Med 2014;371:1821–1831 [PMID: 25372090].

White ML, Liebelt EL: Update on antidotes for pediatric poisoning. Pediatr Emerg Care 2006;22:740 [PMID: 17110870].

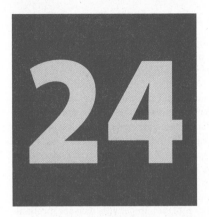

Kidney & Urinary Tract

Margret E. Bock, MD, MS

Melisha G. Hanna, MD, MS

EVALUATION OF THE KIDNEY & URINARY TRACT

HISTORY

When renal disease is suspected, the history should include the following:

1. Preceding acute or chronic illnesses (eg, urinary tract infection [UTI], pharyngitis, impetigo, endocarditis, shunt infection)

2. Rashes or joint pain/swelling

3. Growth delay or failure to thrive

4. Polyuria, polydipsia, enuresis, urinary frequency, or dysuria

5. Documentation of hematuria, proteinuria, or discolored urine

6. Pain (abdominal, costovertebral angle, or flank) or trauma

7. Sudden weight gain or loss or edema

8. Drug or toxin exposure

9. Birth history including prenatal ultrasonographic studies, oligo- or polyhydramnios, birth asphyxia, dysmorphic features and other congenital anomalies, abdominal masses, voiding patterns, and umbilical artery catheterization

10. Family history of cystic renal disease, hypertension including early-onset, hereditary nephritis, deafness, dialysis, or renal transplantation

PHYSICAL EXAMINATION

Important aspects of the physical examination include the height, weight, growth percentiles, skin lesions (café au lait, ash leaf spots, or rash), pallor, edema, or skeletal deformities. Anomalies of the ears, eyes, or external genitalia may be associated with renal anomalies or disease. The blood pressure should be measured in a quiet setting with a manual cuff of the appropriate size in the right upper extremity, ideally with the child seated with feet flat on the ground. The cuff should cover two-thirds of the child's upper arm, and peripheral pulses should be assessed. The abdomen should be palpated and auscultated, with attention to nephromegaly, abdominal masses, musculature, ascites, or bruits.

LABORATORY EVALUATION OF RENAL FUNCTION

Serum Analysis

The standard indicators of renal function are serum levels of urea nitrogen and creatinine; their ratio is normally about 10:1. This ratio may increase when renal perfusion or urine flow is decreased, as in urinary tract obstruction or dehydration. Because serum urea nitrogen levels are more affected by these and other factors (eg, nitrogen intake, catabolism, use of corticosteroids) than are creatinine levels, the most reliable single indicator of glomerular function is the serum level of creatinine. For example, an increase in serum creatinine from 0.5 to 1.0 mg/dL represents a 50% decrease in GFR (glomerular filtration rate). Norms for serum creatinine relate to muscle mass. Therefore, only larger adolescents should have levels exceeding 1 mg/dL. Serum cystatin C is an additional indicator of glomerular function, independent of muscle mass. Cystatin C is a cysteine protease inhibitor that is produced by all nucleated cells and released in the blood. It is reabsorbed and catabolized by renal tubular cells. Currently, Cystatin C is less widely available, and is less reliable in certain clinical settings, such as with corticosteroid administration or thyroid disease. Less precise but nonetheless important indicators of possible renal disease are abnormalities of serum electrolytes, pH, calcium, phosphorus, magnesium, albumin, or complement.

Glomerular Filtration Rate

The endogenous creatinine clearance (C_{Cr}) in milliliters per minute estimates the GFR. A 24-hour urine collection is the "classic" approach for determining C_{Cr}; however, it is often difficult to accurately obtain in the pediatric population, particularly in children who are not continent. The procedure for collecting a timed urine specimen should be explained carefully so that the parent or patient understands fully the rationale of (1) first emptying the bladder (discarding that urine) and noting the time and (2) putting all urine subsequently voided into the collection receptacle, including the last void, 24 hours later. Reliability of the 24-hour collection can be assessed in individuals with normal muscle mass by measuring the total 24-hour creatinine excretion in the specimen. Total daily creatinine excretion (creatinine index) should be 15–25 mg/kg, with normal values higher in males that in females, reflective of differences in muscle mass. Creatinine indices on either side of this range suggest collections that were either inadequate or excessive. Calculation by the following formula requires measurements of plasma or serum creatinine (P_{Cr}) in mg/dL, urine creatinine (U_{Cr}) in mg/dL, and urine volume (V) expressed as mL/min:

$$C_{Cr} = \frac{U_{Cr}V}{P_{Cr}}$$

Because accepted ranges of normal C_{Cr} are based on adult parameters, correction for size is needed in children. Clearance is corrected to a standard body surface area of $1.73\ m^2$ in the formula:

$$\text{"Corrected" } C_{Cr} = \frac{\text{Patient's } C_{Cr} \times 1.73\,m^2}{\text{Patient's body surface area}}$$

As 80–125 mL/min/1.73 m^2 is the normal range for C_{Cr} (for children older than 1 year), estimates at the lower end of this range may indicate problems.

A quick approximation of estimated GFR in children, the "bedside Schwartz" equation, based on plasma or serum creatinine level and length in centimeters, can be obtained as follows:

$$\text{eGFR(mL/min/1.73 } m^2) = 0.413 \times \text{height (cm)}/P_{Cr}\text{(mg/dL)}$$

This formula was developed in children with chronic kidney disease (CKD) and has more recently been validated in children with normal renal function. When cystatin C (cysC) has been assessed, the creatinine-Cystatin C-based CKiD equation may be utilized to include this variable and blood urea nitrogen (BUN):

$$\text{eGFR(mL/min/1.73 } m^2) = 39.8 \times [\text{height (m)}/P_{Cr}\text{(mg/dL)}]^{0.456}$$
$$\times [1.8/\text{cysC(mg/L)}]^{0.418} \times [30/\text{BUN}]^{0.079}$$
$$\times [1.076 \text{ (male)}] \text{ OR } [1.00 \text{ (female)}] \times [\text{ht(m)}/1]$$

This more extensive calculation may be useful as a confirmatory test in specific circumstances when eGFR based on serum creatinine is less accurate (eg, low muscle mass) or when the clinical scenario warrants a secondary test. Online tools can be utilized to facilitate this calculation.

Urine Concentrating Ability

Inability to concentrate urine causes polyuria, polydipsia, or enuresis and is often the first sign of chronic renal failure, and, in some cases, raises the possibility of diabetes insipidus. The first morning void should be concentrated (specific gravity $\geq$ 1.020), presuming cessation of fluid intake overnight. Thus, determination of the specific gravity of a first morning void is an easy and helpful test of the kidney's concentrating ability.

Urinalysis

Commercially available dipsticks can be used to screen the urine for blood, leukocytes, nitrites, protein, and specific gravity and to approximate the urine pH. Positive results for blood should always be confirmed by microscopy, which is also the only way to determine if there is significant crystalluria or casts. Hematuria is present with > 5 RBC/high-powered field (hpf). Significant proteinuria ($\geq$ 30 mg/dL) detected by dipstick should be confirmed by quantitation, either with a 24-hour urine collection or by the protein/creatinine ratio of a random specimen.

In children with asymptomatic hematuria or proteinuria, the search for renal origins will yield the most results, although urologic etiologies require consideration. Urinary red blood cell (RBC) casts suggest glomerulonephritis (GN), but the absence of casts does not exclude this disease. Urine RBC morphology may be helpful, with dysmorphic RBC arising from the kidneys. Anatomic abnormalities such as cystic disease with cyst rupture may also cause hematuria. Benign hematuria, including benign familial hematuria/thin glomerular basement membrane disease, is diagnosed by exclusion. Hematuria can also be observed in the setting of hypercalciuria or urolithiasis. Note that hypercalciuria is not associated with proteinuria. Figure 24–1 suggests an approach to the renal workup of hematuria. GN is discussed in more detail later in this chapter.

Combined proteinuria and hematuria is characteristic of more significant glomerular disease. Quantification of proteinuria is customarily accomplished by a timed collection (eg, over a 24-hour period). However, given the frequency of errors in collection in the pediatric population and the potential difficulties in timed collection in children who are not toilet trained, the degree of proteinuria may be estimated by the ratio of protein (mg/dL)/creatinine (mg/dL) in a random urine sample. A urine protein/creatinine ratio above 0.2 is abnormal. In the evaluation of asymptomatic proteinuria,

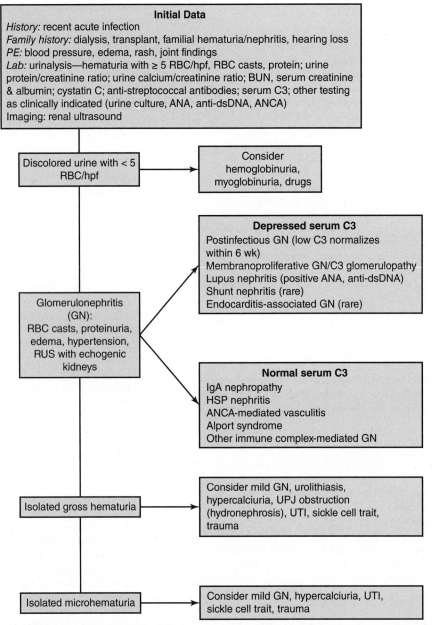

▲ **Figure 24–1.** Approach to the evaluation of hematuria. ANA, antinuclear antibody; ANCA, antineutrophil cytoplasmic antibody; BUN, blood urea nitrogen; C3, complement; dsDNA, double-stranded DNA; hpf, high-power field; HSP, Henoch-Schönlein purpura; IgA, immunoglobulin A; RBC, red blood cell; RUS, renal ultrasound; UPJ, ureteropelvic junction; UTI, urinary tract infection.

orthostatic or postural proteinuria should be excluded. This can be accomplished simply by comparing the protein/creatinine ratio of urine formed in the supine position (the first morning void accumulated in the bladder while sleeping) to a sample obtained during daily ambulation. If the "supine" sample is normal and proteinuria is occurring only during upright posture, this demonstrates postural proteinuria. Such patients typically show resolution of orthostatic proteinuria over time, but rarely an orthostatic pattern

can be seen initially in GN, so ongoing follow-up is warranted. If both samples are abnormal, proteinuria would be considered "persistent."

An approach to the workup of isolated proteinuria, including nephrotic syndrome, is shown in Figure 24–2. The presence of significant hematuria (> 20 RBC/hpf) or RBC casts should raise concern for GN (see Figure 24–1). Other renal lesions with proteinuric manifestations are discussed later in this chapter.

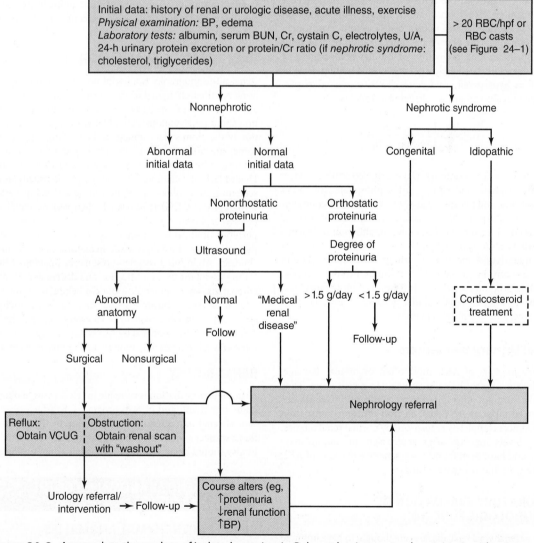

▲ **Figure 24–2.** Approach to the workup of isolated proteinuria. Rule out benign postural proteinuria with urine protein/creatine ratio of first morning void (recumbent urine) versus day void (upright). BP, blood pressure; Cr, creatinine; hpf, high-power field; RBC, red blood cell; U/A, urinalysis; VCUG, voiding cystourethrogram.

Special Tests of Renal Function

Measurements of urinary sodium, creatinine, and osmolality are useful in differentiating prerenal from renal causes of acute kidney injury (AKI). The physiologic response to decreased renal perfusion is decreased urinary output, increased urine osmolality, increased urinary solute concentration (eg, creatinine), and decreased urinary sodium (usually < 20 mEq/L).

The presence of certain substances in urine may suggest tubular dysfunction. For example, urine glucose should be less than 5 mg/dL in the setting of normal serum glucose concentration. Hyperphosphaturia occurs with significant proximal tubular abnormalities (eg, Fanconi syndrome). Measurement of the phosphate concentration of a 24-hour urine specimen and evaluation of tubular reabsorption of phosphorus (TRP) will help document renal tubular diseases as well as hyperparathyroid states. TRP (expressed as percentage of reabsorption) is calculated as follows:

$$TRP = 100 \left[1 - \frac{S_{Cr} \times U_{PO_4}}{S_{PO_4} \times U_{Cr}} \right]$$

where S_{Cr} = serum creatinine, U_{Cr} = urine creatinine, S_{PO_4} = serum phosphate, and U_{PO_4} = urine phosphate. All values for creatinine and phosphate are expressed in milligrams per deciliter for purposes of calculation. A TRP value of 85% or more is considered normal in children, although it depends somewhat on the value of S_{PO_4}.

A quantitative increase in urinary excretion of amino acids is seen in generalized proximal tubular disease. Defective proximal tubular reabsorption of bicarbonate can be seen in isolated renal tubular acidosis (RTA), Fanconi syndrome, and chronic renal failure.

Novel Urinary Biomarkers

Urinary markers of AKI, most often of tubular damage, have become more clinically available in recent years. They include, among others, Urinary Neutrophil Gelatinase-associated Lipocalin (NGAL), an iron transporting protein that is almost completely reabsorbed by normal renal tubules. NGAL levels increase after acute ischemic/nephrotoxic insults and have been found to be sensitive markers of AKI, especially in intensive care settings.

LABORATORY EVALUATION OF IMMUNOLOGIC FUNCTION

Many parenchymal renal diseases are thought to have immune causation, although the mechanisms are largely unknown. Examples include (1) deposition of circulating antigen-antibody complexes that are directly injurious or incite injurious responses and (2) formation of antibody directed against the glomerular basement membrane (rare in children).

Serum C3 and C4 complement concentrations should be measured when immune-mediated renal injury or chronic GN is suspected. Where clinically indicated, antinuclear antibodies (ANA), antineutrophil cytoplasmic antibodies (ANCA), hepatitis B surface antigen, and hepatitis C antibody should be obtained. In rare cases, cryoglobulins (very rare in childhood), C3 nephritic factor and other assessment of complement function, or antiglomerular basement membrane (anti-GBM) antibody measurements may help confirm a specific diagnosis. At some point in the workup, the diagnosis should, if possible, be confirmed by histologic examination of renal tissue.

RADIOGRAPHIC EVALUATION

Renal ultrasonography is a useful noninvasive tool for evaluating renal parenchymal disease, urinary tract abnormalities, and renal blood flow. Radioisotope studies provide information about renal anatomy, blood flow, and integrity and function of the glomerular, tubular, and collecting systems. Renal stones are often visualized by ultrasonography but are best delineated by computed tomography (CT) without contrast. Due to lack of radiation, ultrasonography is usually used for screening and follow-up of urolithiasis. Voiding cystourethrography (VCUG) is indicated when vesicoureteral reflux (VUR) or bladder outlet obstruction (eg, to visualize the posterior urethra) is suspected. Cystoscopy is rarely useful in the evaluation of asymptomatic hematuria or proteinuria in children. Abdominal magnetic resonance imaging (MRI) or CT are useful for the identification and delineation of renal or adrenal masses. Doppler ultrasound is helpful to exclude renal arterial or venous thrombosis but of variable sensitivity and specificity in the diagnosis of renal artery stenosis; the latter condition is better assessed by MR or CT angiography. Intrarenal arterial stenosis may require direct renal arteriography.

RENAL BIOPSY

Histologic information is valuable in select cases to diagnose, guide treatment, and inform prognosis. Satisfactory evaluation of renal tissue requires examination by light, immunofluorescence, and electron microscopy. The need for a renal biopsy should be determined by a pediatric nephrologist.

CONGENITAL ANOMALIES OF THE URINARY TRACT

RENAL PARENCHYMAL ANOMALIES

About 10% of children have congenital anomalies of the genitourinary tract, which range in severity from asymptomatic to lethal. Recent findings suggest that congenital anomalies of the kidney and urinary tract (CAKUT) may arise from mutations in a multitude of different single gene causes. Some asymptomatic abnormalities may have significant implications. For example, patients with "horseshoe" kidney (kidneys fused in their lower poles), although very rarely associated with reduction in kidney function, have a higher incidence of renal calculi. Unilateral agenesis or multicystic dysplasia is usually accompanied by compensatory hypertrophy of the contralateral kidney and thus is typically associated with normal renal function. Supernumerary and ectopic kidneys are often of no significance. Abnormal genitourinary tract development can be associated with varying degrees of renal dysplasia and dysfunction ranging from mild to severe; an example of the latter is in utero bilateral renal agenesis, which, without prenatal intervention to support lung development, is associated with oligoanhydramnios, abnormal facies and limb anomalies (eg, talipes equinovarus) from fetal compression, and perinatal death from pulmonary hypoplasia (Potter syndrome).

Renal Dysplasia

Renal dysplasia constitutes a spectrum of anomalies. In simple hypoplasia, which may be unilateral or bilateral, the affected kidneys are smaller than normal. In some forms of dysplasia, immature undifferentiated renal tissue persists. In some situations, the number of functional nephrons is insufficient to sustain normal renal function once the child reaches a critical body size. The lack of adequate renal tissue is not always readily discernible in the newborn period in the presence of normal or often increased urine production.

Other forms of renal dysplasia include oligomeganephronia (characterized by the presence of only a few large glomeruli) and the cystic dysplasias (characterized by the presence of renal cysts). Simple renal cysts are rare in children and are typically observed in children with a history of significant chronic medical illness. The presence of multiple "simple" cysts should raise concern for possible underlying polycystic kidney disease.

Polycystic Kidney Disease

Both forms of polycystic kidney disease (autosomal dominant [ADPKD] or recessive [ARPKD]) are increasingly diagnosed by prenatal ultrasound. In its most severe form, ARPKD kidneys are dysfunctional in utero, and therefore newborns may demonstrate Potter sequence. In less severe cases, kidney enlargement by cysts may initially be recognized when nephromegaly is noted on physical examination. Hypertension is an early problem in ARPKD. The rate of progression of renal insufficiency varies in ARPKD, but many children with a neonatal renal presentation reach end-stage renal disease (ESRD) by school age. Recent studies suggest wide variation in phenotype, even within families. Some patients present in early adulthood with liver dysfunction from congenital hepatic fibrosis with moderate nephromegaly and mild-to-moderate chronic kidney disease.

With advances in radiographic imaging, ADPKD is being diagnosed earlier in life, including prenatally. Children with ADPKD can manifest many of the same findings as adults with ADPKD, such as enlarged kidneys, pain, hematuria, proteinuria, hypertension, kidney stones, and extrarenal cysts (pancreas, spleen, liver), although renal insufficiency and intracranial aneurysms are rare in childhood. Routine monitoring for hypertension is indicated in children with or known to be at-risk for ADPKD. Because cysts grow over time, a normal renal ultrasound does not exclude ADPKD in an at-risk child (ie, parent known to have ADPKD). Approximately half of patients with ADPKD reach ESRD by 60 years of age. Rarely ADPKD can present with Potter sequence or severe neonatal manifestations.

Medullary Cystic Disease/Nephronophthisis

Medullary cystic disease and nephronophthisis are inherited conditions with similar renal morphology characterized by bilateral small corticomedullary cysts in normal to small kidneys with tubulointerstitial scarring leading to ESRD. Numerous causative genes have been identified in nephronophthisis, all of which encode for proteins expressed in the primary cilia of renal epithelial cells, leading to classification as "ciliopathies." Children with nephronophthisis manifest impaired urinary concentration leading to polyuria and polydipsia with progressive renal insufficiency in childhood or adolescence. Extrarenal involvement including retinitis pigmentosa, hepatic fibrosis, skeletal defects, cerebellar vermis aplasia, or other abnormalities can help target specific gene analysis. Several forms of autosomal-dominant medullary cystic disease exist, usually presenting with adult-onset renal failure and no extrarenal involvement. However, uromodulin-associated kidney disease with hyperuricemia and renal failure can be seen in adolescents.

Flynn JT et al; Subcommittee on Screening and Management of High Blood Pressure in Children: Clinical practice guideline for screening and management of high blood pressure in children and adolescents. *Pediatrics* 2017;140(3):e20171904 [PMID: 28827377].

Guay-Woodford LM et al: Consensus expert recommendations for the diagnosis and management of autosomal recessive polycystic kidney disease: report of an international conference. J Pediatr 2014;165(3):611–617 [PMID: 25015577].

Hildebrandt F, Benzing T, Katsanis N: Ciliopathies. N Engl J Med 2011;364(16):1533–1543 [PMID: 21506742].

Malhotra R, Siew ED: Biomarkers for the acute detection and acute prognosis of acute kidney injury. Clin J Am Soc Nephrol 2017;12(1):149–173 [PMID: 27827308].

National Kidney Foundation GFR calculators: https://www.kidney.org/professionals/KDOQI/gfr.

Vivante A, Hildebrandt F: Exploring the genetic basis of early-onset chronic kidney disease. Nat Rev Nephrol 2016;12(3):133–146 [PMID: 26750453].

Vivante A, Kohl S, Hwang DY, Dworschak GC, Hildebrandt F: Single-gene causes of congenital anomalies of the kidney and urinary tract (CAKUT) in humans. Pediatr Nephrol 2014;29(4):695–704 [PMID: 24398540].

DISTAL URINARY TRACT ANOMALIES

Obstructive Uropathy

Obstruction at the ureteropelvic junction may be the result of intrinsic muscle abnormalities, aberrant vessels, or fibrous bands. The lesion can cause hydronephrosis and usually presents as prenatal hydronephrosis, an abdominal mass in the newborn, or recurrent abdominal pain with vomiting in an older child (Dietl's crisis). Obstruction can occur in other parts of the ureter, especially at the ureterovesical junction, causing proximal hydroureter and hydronephrosis. Renal radionuclide scan with furosemide "wash-out" will reveal or rule out ureteral obstruction as the cause of the hydronephrosis. Whether intrinsic or extrinsic, urinary tract obstruction should be relieved as soon as possible to minimize damage to the kidneys and warrants referral to a pediatric urologist.

Severe bladder malformations such as exstrophy are clinically obvious and a surgical challenge. More subtle—but urgent in terms of diagnosis—is obstruction of urine flow from vestigial posterior urethral valves (PUV). This anomaly, which occurs almost exclusively in males, may be detected prenatally with an enlarged muscular bladder and hydroureteronephrosis. Neonates may demonstrate a poor voiding stream or eventual UTI. The kidneys and bladder may be easily palpable. Leakage (ureteric perforation, although rare) proximal to the obstruction may produce urinary ascites. Decompression of the bladder, most often accomplished via urethral catheterization, is critical in children with PUV to prevent irreversible kidney damage.

Eagle-Barrett (Prune Belly) syndrome is an association of urinary tract anomalies with cryptorchidism and absent abdominal musculature. Renal dysplasia and/or functional urinary tract obstruction may lead to ESRD. Timely urinary diversion is essential to sustain renal function.

Other complex malformations and external genital anomalies are beyond the scope of this text. The challenge presented by urologic abnormalities resulting in severe compromise and destruction of renal tissue is to preserve all remaining renal function, prevent UTI and potential related renal scarring, and treat the complications of progressive chronic renal failure. Collaboration between the pediatric urologist and nephrologist, ideally in a multidisciplinary clinic, in early management is essential.

Reflux Nephropathy

The retrograde flow of urine from the bladder into the ureter (vesicoureteral reflux, VUR), when high grade, may cause renal scarring and subsequent renal insufficiency or hypertension, or both, especially in the setting of UTIs. Hydronephrosis on renal ultrasound suggests the possibility of VUR or obstruction. Absence of hydronephrosis on ultrasonography does not, however, rule out the possibility of VUR. VUR is most often diagnosed with a voiding cystourethrogram. Low-grade VUR typically resolves spontaneously over time. Prophylactic antibiotics may be administered depending on the child's age, degree of VUR, and frequency of UTI while awaiting spontaneous resolution. Surgery may be required for chronic severe reflux. Appropriate management of reflux nephropathy includes prevention and prompt treatment of UTI, monitoring and management of hypertension and complications of chronic renal insufficiency, and consideration of angiotensin-converting enzyme (ACE) inhibition to prevent glomerular hyperfiltration.

Peters CA et al: Summary of the AUA guideline on management of primary vesicoureteral reflux in children. J Urol 2010;184(3):1134–1144 [PMID: 20650499].

Tekgul S et al: EAU guidelines on vesicoureteral reflux in children. Eur Urol 2012;62(3):534–542 [PMID: 22698573].

▼ HEMATURIA & GLOMERULAR DISEASE

MICROHEMATURIA

Children with painful hematuria should be investigated for UTI or direct injury to the urinary tract. Dysuria is common in cystitis or urethritis; associated back pain and/or fever suggests the possibility of pyelonephritis; and colicky flank pain may indicate the passage of a stone. Bright red blood or clots in the urine can also be associated with bleeding disorders, trauma, and arteriovenous malformations. Abdominal masses suggest the presence of urinary tract obstruction, cystic disease, or tumors of the renal or perirenal structures.

Asymptomatic hematuria is a challenge because clinical and diagnostic data are required to decide whether nephrology evaluation is needed. The diagnosis of hematuria should not rely solely on a urine "dipstick" evaluation, but it must be verified by a microscopic RBC count (normal < 5 RBC/hpf). Ruling out hypercalciuria as a cause of hematuria with a random urine calcium/creatinine ratio (both values in mg/dL) is one of the initial steps in the evaluation of hematuria. A value above 0.2 requires verification with a 24-hour urine collection when possible, and should prompt referral to pediatric nephrology. Hypercalciuria is present with excretion of calcium in excess of 4 mg/kg/day. Figure 24–1 delineates the outpatient approach to renal hematuria. The primary concern in the differential diagnosis of hematuria is the possible presence of glomerular disease.

GLOMERULONEPHRITIS

ESSENTIALS OF DIAGNOSIS & TYPICAL FEATURES

Classic features of glomerulonephritis:

▶ Hematuria

▶ Edema

▶ Hypertension

▶ RBC casts in the urine

The various types of glomerulonephritis (GN) have similar clinical manifestations. The defining features of GN include hematuria, urinary RBC casts, hypertension, and edema. Hematuria may be microscopic or gross (often coffee- or tea-colored) in nature. While RBC casts are often present, their absence does not exclude the diagnosis of GN. Urine protein excretion may range from normal (Pr/Cr ratio < 0.2) to nephrotic range (Pr/Cr ratio > 2). Edema (periorbital, facial, extremities, ascites) occurs due to salt and water retention with impaired glomerular function and contributes to systemic hypertension, which is further exacerbated by the glomerular inflammation and associated renin production. Therefore, diuretics followed by blockade of the renin-angiotensin-aldosterone system are the pillars of hypertension management. Affected children require evaluation of blood pressure, renal function, serum albumin, and urine protein excretion. Serum C3 concentration is helpful to distinguish certain types of GN (depressed in postinfectious and membranoproliferative (MPGN)/C3 glomerulopathy (C3GN), GN due to SLE, and GN related to ventriculoatrial shunt infection or endocarditis [the latter two conditions are rarely seen in childhood but are typically evident by history and examination]). Renal biopsy may be indicated when the etiology of GN is not otherwise clear from history and preliminary testing.

Severe glomerular histopathologic and clinical entities such as anti-GBM antibody disease (Goodpasture syndrome), granulomatosis with polyangiitis, microscopic polyangiitis, and crescentic IgA nephropathy may be considered in the differential diagnosis of acute GN; it should be recognized that these disorders are unusual in children. Many of these diagnoses may be rapidly progressive in nature,

Acute Postinfectious Glomerulonephritis

The diagnosis of acute poststreptococcal GN is supported by a recent history (typically within the preceding 7–14 days, with range of 1 day to 6 weeks) of group A β-hemolytic streptococcal infection, usually as pharyngitis or, less commonly, impetigo. If a positive culture is not available, recent infection may be supported by an elevated titer of antistreptococcal antibodies. However, documentation of elevated antistreptococcal antibodies alone does not confirm that GN is poststreptococcal in nature. Other infections can cause similar glomerular injury; thus "postinfectious" GN may be a preferred term for this type of acute glomerulonephritis (AGN). Postinfectious GN is associated with depressed serum C3 complement. The manifestations range from asymptomatic microhematuria to gross hematuria with nephrotic range proteinuria and marked renal insufficiency. However, in most cases, full recovery occurs and is usually complete within weeks.

Typical postinfectious GN has no specific treatment. Antibiotic therapy is indicated if an active infection is documented. Disturbances in renal function and resulting hypertension may require close monitoring, reduction in salt intake, diuretics, or other antihypertensive drugs such as ACE inhibitors. In cases of severe renal failure, hemodialysis or peritoneal dialysis may be necessary. Corticosteroids may also be considered in an attempt to influence the course of severe GN. Serum C3 may normalize as early as 24 hours or as late as 8 weeks after onset. In postinfectious GN, microscopic hematuria may persist for as long as a year; 85% of children recover completely. Persistent deterioration in renal function, chronic proteinuria, and presentation complicated by nephrotic syndrome are concerning signs for long-term prognosis.

IgA Nephropathy

When asymptomatic gross hematuria with or without proteinuria occurs concurrently with a minor acute illness or other stressful occurrence, the diagnosis of IgA nephropathy may be entertained. IgA nephropathy is the most common cause of GN. Serum complement is normal in this condition. IgA nephropathy may be accompanied by flank pain or dysuria. Gross hematuria typically resolves within days, and there are no serious sequelae in 85% of children. Treatment is not generally indicated, and the prognosis is good in most cases. Prognosis is guarded, however, if severe proteinuria, hypertension, or renal insufficiency is present or develops. In such instances, although no treatment is universally accepted, corticosteroids and other immunosuppressive drugs are used after confirmatory kidney biopsy solidifies the diagnosis. Omega-3 fatty acids from fish oils are also thought to be helpful by inhibiting macrophage infiltration of the glomerular mesangium.

Henoch-Schönlein Purpura

The diagnosis of Henoch-Schönlein purpura (HSP) rests on the presence of a typical maculopapular and purpuric rash found primarily, but not exclusively, on the dependent surfaces of the lower extremities and buttocks. Many children have abdominal pain, and bloody diarrhea may be present. Joint pain and swelling are common. Hypertension may be present. Kidney biopsy is rarely required due to the constellation of clinical findings, but lupus and ANCA-mediated vasculitis should be considered in the appropriate setting, particularly in adolescents. The renal histologic lesion of HSP is identical to that of IgA nephropathy. The condition is usually self-limited. Joint and abdominal pain responds to treatment with short courses of corticosteroids. Renal involvement ranges from none to mild GN with microhematuria to severe GN with associated nephrosis and renal insufficiency. More severe renal involvement is associated with worse long-term prognosis, including potential for progression to ESRD. There is no universally accepted treatment, but corticosteroids and other immunosuppressive agents are often administered (see Chapter 30).

Membranoproliferative Glomerulonephritis/C3 Glomerulopathy

The most common "chronic" form of GN in childhood is membranoproliferative GN (MPGN). The diagnosis is established from the histologic appearance of the glomeruli on biopsy. Recent studies have led to reclassification of these conditions, recognizing that abnormalities of complement regulation may be the primary etiology. There is a wide phenotypic spectrum of these conditions. These conditions typically are associated with depressed serum C3. Immunosuppressive treatment, including targeted blockade of components of the complement system, is recommended but response may vary depending on the underlying etiology.

Lupus Glomerulonephritis

The diagnosis of systemic lupus erythematosus (SLE) is based on its numerous clinical features and abnormal laboratory findings that include a positive antinuclear antibody test, depressed serum complement, and increased serum antibodies to double-stranded DNA. Renal involvement is indicated by varying degrees of hematuria and proteinuria and should be assessed via renal biopsy. More severe cases are accompanied by renal insufficiency and hypertension. Significant renal involvement requires treatment with various combinations of immunosuppressive drugs, including prednisone, azathioprine, cyclophosphamide, mycophenolate, tacrolimus, and rituximab, a monoclonal antibody against the B-cell surface antigen CD20. ESRD develops in 10%–15% of patients with childhood SLE.

Hereditary Glomerulonephritis

The most commonly encountered hereditary GN is Alport syndrome. This condition is due to mutations in type IV collagen found in basement membranes of the glomeruli, cochlea, and lens, and is characterized by progressive GN, high-frequency sensorineural hearing loss, and lens abnormalities. Although the condition can be inherited in autosomal dominant or recessive manners, the vast majority of cases are X-linked in transmission. Thus, males are typically more severely affected. Such boys present very early in life, even in infant and toddler years, with persistent microhematuria and recurrent gross hematuria associated with intercurrent illness, followed by chronic proteinuria and then deterioration in renal function. A family history may be present, but there is a spontaneous mutation rate of about 20%. In males with X-linked or children with autosomal recessive disease, ESRD usually occurs in the second to third decade of life. Females with X-linked Alport syndrome show a wide spectrum of disease manifestation from asymptomatic hematuria to ESRD. Although currently there is no treatment for this disorder, careful management of associated hypertension may slow the process.

Bertsias GK et al: Joint European League Against Rheumatism and European Renal Association-European Dialysis and Transplant Association (EULAR/ERA-EDTA) recommendations for the management of adult and pediatric lupus nephritis. Ann Rheum Dis 2012 November;71(11):1771–1782 [PMID: 22851469].

Davin JC, Coppo R: Henoch-Schönlein purpura nephritis in children. Nat Rev Nephrol 2014;10(10):563–573 [PMID: 25072122].

Eison TM, Ault BH, Jones DP, Chesney RW, Wyatt RJ: Poststreptococcal acute glomerulonephritis in children: clinical features and pathogenesis. Pediatr Nephrol 2011;26(2):165–180. doi: 10.1007/s00467-010-1554-6 [PMID: 20652330].

Vogt B: Nephrology update: glomerular disease in children. FP Essent 2016 May;444:30–40; quiz 41 [PMID: 27163763].

▼ TUBULOINTERSTITIAL DISEASE

ACUTE INTERSTITIAL NEPHRITIS

Acute interstitial nephritis is characterized by diffuse or focal inflammation and edema of the renal interstitium and secondary involvement of the tubules. The condition is most commonly drug related (eg, β-lactam–containing antibiotics or nonsteroidal anti-inflammatory drugs [NSAIDs]), but infectious etiologies, including Epstein-Barr virus, also occur.

Fever, rash, and eosinophilia may occur in drug-associated cases. Urinalysis usually reveals leukocyturia and, potentially, mild hematuria and proteinuria. Hansel staining of the urinary sediment may demonstrate eosinophils. The inflammation can cause significant deterioration of renal function and systemic hypertension. The association between tubulointerstitial nephritis and uveitis (TINU) is occasionally seen in childhood. If the diagnosis is unclear because of the absence of a history of drug or toxin exposure or acute infection, or the absence of eosinophils in the urine, a renal biopsy may be performed to demonstrate the characteristic tubular and interstitial inflammation. Immediate identification and removal of the causative agent whenever possible is imperative and may be all that is necessary. Treatment with corticosteroids or other immunomodulatory agents may be helpful in patients with progressive renal insufficiency or associated nephrotic syndrome. Dialysis support is occasionally required.

González E et al: Early steroid treatment improves the recovery of renal function in patients with drug-induced acute interstitial nephritis. Kidney Int 2008;73(8):940–946 [PMID: 18185501].

▼ PROTEINURIA & RENAL DISEASE

Urine is rarely completely protein free, but the average excretion is well below 150 mg/24 h. As noted previously, small increases in urinary protein can accompany febrile illnesses or exertion and in some cases occur while in the upright posture (orthostatic proteinuria).

An algorithm for investigation of isolated proteinuria is presented in Figure 24–2. In idiopathic nephrotic syndrome without associated features of GN, treatment with corticosteroids may be initiated after a comprehensive evaluation is completed in consultation with a pediatric nephrologist.

CONGENITAL NEPHROSIS (FINNISH TYPE)

Congenital nephrosis of the Finnish type is a rare autosomal recessive disorder characterized by microcystic dilations of the proximal tubules and glomerular abnormalities including proliferation, crescent formation, and thickening of capillary walls. The condition is associated with genetic mutations in *NPHS1*, which codes for nephrin, a transmembrane protein and structural component of the glomerular basement membrane.

Infants with congenital nephrosis commonly have markedly elevated maternal serum α-fetoprotein concentration, a large placenta, wide cranial sutures, and delayed ossification. Progressive edema may be seen after the first few weeks of life. Massive urine protein losses lead to other risks, including recurrent infection due to hypogammaglobulinemia (urinary loss of immunoglobulin G), thrombosis (urinary loss of antithrombin III, Protein C and S), and eventual clinical hypothyroidism (urinary loss of thyroid-binding globulin). Such children usually require nightly high-dose albumin infusions and once to twice weekly intravenous immunoglobulin (IVIG) infusions. Nephrectomies may be required to prevent complications of the high-grade protein losses. Progressive renal failure requiring dialysis and transplantation are anticipated, although historically affected infants often succumbed to serious bacterial infection in the first year of life.

IDIOPATHIC NEPHROTIC SYNDROME OF CHILDHOOD

ESSENTIALS OF DIAGNOSIS & TYPICAL FEATURES

Classic features of nephrotic syndrome:

▶ Proteinuria

▶ Hypoalbuminemia

▶ Edema

▶ Hyperlipidemia

▶ Clinical Findings

Affected patients are generally younger than 10 years at onset. Typically, periorbital swelling and oliguria are noted, often following intercurrent illness. Within a few days, increasing edema—even anasarca—becomes evident. Most children have few complaints other than vague malaise or abdominal pain. With significant hypoalbuminemia, some children experience symptoms of intestinal malabsorption. With marked edema, dyspnea due to pleural effusions or massive ascites may also occur.

Despite heavy proteinuria, the urine sediment is usually normal, although microscopic hematuria may be present. Gross hematuria is occasionally seen but more often with FSGS than minimal change disease (MCD). Plasma albumin concentration is low and lipid levels increased. When azotemia occurs, it is usually secondary to intravascular volume depletion from "third space" leak and low oncotic pressure.

▶ Complications

Infections (eg, peritonitis, sepsis) sometimes occur, and encapsulated bacteria such as *Streptococcus pneumoniae* are frequently the cause. Hypercoagulability may be present, and thromboembolic phenomena such as deep venous thrombosis, renal vein thrombosis, or sagittal sinus thrombosis are reported. Hypertension can occur, and renal insufficiency can result from decreased renal perfusion. Hyperlipidemia resolves when affected children enter remission but is of concern in treatment-resistant nephrotic syndrome.

▶ Treatment & Prognosis

When the diagnosis of idiopathic nephrotic syndrome is made, corticosteroid treatment should be started as the vast majority of children will enter remission in response to such treatment, thus avoiding the need for kidney biopsy that neither predicts response to treatment nor long-term renal function. Prednisone, 60 mg/m² or 2 mg/kg/day (maximum,

60 mg/day), is given for 6 weeks as a single daily dose. A dose of $40 mg/m^2$ or 1.5 mg/kg/day is then administered on an alternate-day schedule for 6 weeks. Thereafter, the corticosteroids are discontinued or the dose tapered gradually and discontinued over the ensuing few months depending on local practice. The goal of this regimen is the disappearance of proteinuria. If remission is not achieved during the initial 4 weeks of corticosteroid treatment, steroid-sparing therapy and kidney biopsy should be considered. If remission is achieved, only to be followed by relapse, the treatment course may be repeated. A renal biopsy is often considered when there is little or no response to treatment. One should take into account, however, that the histologic findings may not necessarily alter the treatment plan, which is designed to eliminate the nephrotic syndrome regardless of underlying renal histology.

Careful clinical assessment of intravascular volume status is indicated to guide diuretic therapy in children with idiopathic nephrotic syndrome. While those with obvious evidence of volume overload will benefit from diuretics, some children, particularly those with MCD, will show evidence of intravascular volume depletion due to third space fluid leak. The latter group of children will experience hypotension and prerenal azotemia with aggressive diuresis; thus, careful restoration of compromised circulating volume with intravenous 25% albumin infusion with consideration of a diuretic such as furosemide is most helpful in mobilizing edema. Infections such as peritonitis should be treated promptly to reduce morbidity. Immunization with pneumococcal conjugate and polysaccharide vaccines is advised due to the increased risk of invasive pneumococcal disease with active relapse.

Resolution of proteinuria with corticosteroid treatment suggests a good prognosis. Early relapse usually heralds a prolonged series of relapses; frequent relapses increase corticosteroid exposure and should lead to consideration of alternate immunosuppressive therapy to maintain remission. Historically, chlorambucil or cyclophosphamide was added to corticosteroid treatment in steroid-responsive but-dependent children to achieve corticosteroid discontinuance while maintaining remission. Because of potential significant side effects associated with these drugs, calcineurin inhibitors (most commonly tacrolimus) or mycophenylate mofetil are now added instead in steroid-dependent cases. Children who fail to respond to corticosteroids have a more guarded long-term prognosis for renal function yet may still attain remission with alternative immunosuppressive agents. Increasing reports and experience suggest that cases in which nephrotic syndrome is poorly responsive to or "dependent" upon corticosteroids, even with an added agent such as tacrolimus, may respond to rituximab, although no controlled trials have been conducted and the long-term effects of repeated courses of rituximab in this setting are not known.

FOCAL SEGMENTAL GLOMERULOSCLEROSIS

Focal segmental glomerulosclerosis (FSGS) is a cause of idiopathic nephrotic syndrome in children but can also cause chronic asymptomatic proteinuria. The condition is concerning as up to 15%–20% of cases can progress to end-stage renal failure. The response to corticosteroid treatment is variable. Treatment in the setting of active nephrotic syndrome is reviewed above, but the benefits of chronic immunosuppressive therapy are less clear in the asymptomatic child.

Recurrence of FSGS is common following renal transplantation. Fortunately, most children respond well to treatment with plasmapheresis and/or rituximab after kidney transplantation; the latter agent is also showing encouraging utility in treating the nephrotic syndrome of membranous or mesangial nephropathy as well as refractory nephrotic syndrome associated with other forms of glomerular disease or vasculitis.

MEMBRANOUS NEPHROPATHY (MEMBRANOUS GLOMERULONEPHRITIS)

Although largely idiopathic in nature, membranous nephropathy can be found in association with infections, including hepatitis B, hepatitis C, and congenital syphilis; with immunologic disorders such as autoimmune thyroiditis and SLE (in contrast to other forms of lupus nephritis, serum C3 is often normal with membranous lupus); and with administration of drugs such as penicillamine. Recent studies suggest a high frequency of antibodies to podocyte antigens in affected patients.

The onset of membranous nephropathy may be insidious or may resemble that of idiopathic nephrotic syndrome of childhood (see earlier section). It occurs more often in older children and adults. The proteinuria of membranous nephropathy may respond poorly to corticosteroid therapy and secondary immunomodulatory agents are often prescribed. Historically, alkylating agents such as cyclophosphamide were used in conjunction with corticosteroid therapy, while more recently calcineurin inhibitors, mycophenylate mofetil and rituximab have been explored with some success. The diagnosis is made by renal biopsy.

Lombel RM, Gipson DS, Hodson EM: Treatment of steroid-sensitive nephrotic syndrome: new guidelines from KDIGO. Pediatr Nephrol 2013;28(3):415–426 [PMID: 23052651].

Pasini A et al: Best practice guidelines for idiopathic nephrotic syndrome: recommendations versus reality. Pediatr Nephrol 2015 January;30(1):91–101 [PMID: 25127916].

Trautmann A et al: Spectrum of steroid-resistant and congenital nephrotic syndrome in children: the PodoNet registry cohort. Clin J Am Soc Nephrol 2015 April 7;10(4):592–600 [PMID: 25635037].

Waldman M, Austin H: Treatment of idiopathic membranous nephropathy. J Am Soc Nephrol 2012;23(10):1617–1630 [PMID: 22859855].

▼ DISEASES OF THE RENAL VESSELS

RENAL VEIN THROMBOSIS

In newborns, renal vein thrombosis may complicate sepsis or dehydration. It may be observed in infants of diabetic mothers, may be associated with umbilical vein catheterization, or may result from any condition that produces a hypercoagulable state (eg, clotting factor deficiency, or thrombocytosis). Renal vein thrombosis is less common in older children and adolescents. It may develop following trauma, with a procoagulant state (such as antiphospholipid antibody positivity in SLE or treatment-resistant nephrotic syndrome), or without any apparent predisposing factors. Spontaneous renal vein thrombosis has been associated with membranous nephropathy.

▶ Clinical Findings

Renal vein thrombosis in newborns is generally characterized by the sudden development of an abdominal mass. If the thrombosis is bilateral, oliguria may be present. In older children, flank pain, sometimes with a palpable mass, is a common presentation.

No single laboratory test is diagnostic of renal vein thrombosis. Hematuria usually is present and may occasionally be gross in nature; proteinuria is less constant. In the newborn, thrombocytopenia may be found, but it is rare in older children. The diagnosis is made by ultrasonography and Doppler flow studies.

▶ Treatment

Anticoagulation with heparin is the treatment of choice in newborns and older children. In the newborn, a course of heparin combined with treatment of the underlying problem is usually all that is required; the risks of systemic anticoagulation in the newborn, particularly if preterm, must be considered. Evaluation for thrombophilia may be needed. In children with a known tendency for recurrence, more long-term anticoagulation may be required.

▶ Course & Prognosis

The mortality rate in newborns from renal vein thrombosis depends on the underlying cause. With unilateral renal venous thrombosis at any age, the prognosis for adequate renal function is good. Bilateral disease is of course more concerning, and long-term renal follow-up focusing on renal function and growth is warranted in such children. Renal vein thrombosis may rarely recur in the same kidney or in the other kidney years after the original episode of thrombus formation. Extension into the vena cava with pulmonary emboli is possible.

RENAL ARTERIAL DISEASE

Arterial disease (eg, fibromuscular dysplasia, congenital renal artery or midaortic stenosis, Takayasu arteritis) is a rare cause of hypertension in children. Although few clinical clues are specific to underlying arterial lesions, they should be suspected in children with severe hypertension, with onset at or before age 10 years, or in children who demonstrate increasingly difficult to control hypertension. The diagnosis is established by MR or CT angiography and confirmed by renal arteriography or direct intraoperative visualization. When vasculitis is present, immunosuppressive treatment is the first approach. Other lesions may be approached by transluminal angioplasty or surgery (see section Hypertension), but repair may be technically impossible in small children. In such cases, medical management of hypertension pending somatic growth is indicated. Although thrombosis of renal arteries is rare, it should be considered in a patient with acute onset of hypertension and hematuria in an appropriate setting (eg, in association with hyperviscosity or umbilical artery catheterization). Early diagnosis and treatment provides the best chance of reestablishing renal blood flow.

HEMOLYTIC-UREMIC SYNDROME

ESSENTIALS OF DIAGNOSIS & TYPICAL FEATURES

Classic features of hemolytic-uremic syndrome:

▶ Microangiopathic hemolytic anemia

▶ Thrombocytopenia

▶ Renal dysfunction

Hemolytic-uremic syndrome (HUS) is the most common glomerulovascular cause of acute renal failure in childhood. The diarrhea-associated form is usually the result of infection with Shiga toxin–producing strains of *Shigella* or *Escherichia coli*. Ingestion of under-cooked ground beef or unpasteurized foods is a common source. There are many serotypes, but the most common pathogen in the United States is *E coli* O157:H7. Bloody diarrhea is the usual presenting complaint, followed by hemolysis, thrombocytopenia, and renal failure. Circulating toxin causes endothelial damage, which leads to platelet deposition/consumption and microvascular occlusion with subsequent hemolysis. Similar microvascular endothelial activation may also be triggered by drugs (eg, calcineurin inhibitors or mammalian target of rapamycin inhibitors); by viruses (human immunodeficiency virus [HIV]); and by pneumococcal infections, in which bacterial neuraminidase exposes the Thomsen-Friedenreich antigen on RBCs, platelets, and endothelial cells, with associated cell lysis. Rare cases are caused by genetic factors causing complement dysregulation (eg, factor H deficiency).

▶ Clinical Findings

HUS due to *Shigella* or *E coli* begins with a prodrome of abdominal pain, diarrhea, and vomiting. Oliguria, pallor, and bleeding manifestations, principally gastrointestinal, occur next. Children with pneumococcal-associated HUS typically have documented pneumococcal pneumonia, sepsis, or meningitis. Children with atypical HUS associated with complement dysregulation often develop an episode of HUS following intercurrent illness and present with malaise and pallor. Hypertension and seizures develop in some children—especially those who develop severe renal failure and fluid overload. There may also be significant endothelial involvement in the central nervous system (CNS), heart, and pancreas. Anemia may be profound, and RBC fragments are seen on blood smears. A high reticulocyte count confirms the hemolytic nature of the anemia but may not be noted in the presence of renal failure. Thrombocytopenia is often severe, but other coagulation abnormalities are less consistent. Serum fibrin split products are often present, but fulminant disseminated intravascular coagulation is rare. Hematuria and proteinuria are often present. Hemoglobinuria is occasionally observed due to marked RBC hemolysis.

▶ Complications

Complications of AKI occur. Neurologic problems, particularly seizures, may result from hyponatremia, hypertension, or CNS vascular disease. Despite thrombocytopenia, many children are prone to thrombosis due to the underlying endothelial damage.

▶ Treatment

Meticulous attention to fluid and electrolyte status is crucial. The use of antimotility agents and antibiotics for HUS caused by gastrointestinal infection is believed to worsen the disease. Antibiotics may upregulate and increase the release of large amounts of bacterial Shiga toxin. Timely dialysis improves the prognosis. RBC transfusions are often necessary. Platelet transfusions should be avoided unless there is active bleeding. Erythropoietin (epoetin alfa) treatment may reduce RBC transfusion needs and is indicated in the setting of renal failure. Atypical HUS due to complement dysregulation may benefit from plasmapheresis or plasma infusion (by replacing missing factors or removing factor H autoantibodies), but these therapies have been more recently replaced by the anti-C5a monoclonal antibody, eculizumab. Whether eculizumab may be of benefit in other forms of HUS remains to be determined. Plasma therapy should be avoided in pneumococcal HUS as it provides the patient with anti–Thomsen-Friedenreich antibody and thereby drives the HUS process. Although no therapy is universally accepted, strict control of hypertension and fluid balance, adequate nutrition support, and the timely use of dialysis reduce morbidity and mortality. If renal failure is nonoliguric and if urine output is sufficient to ensure against fluid overload and electrolyte abnormalities, management of renal failure without dialysis is possible.

▶ Course & Prognosis

Most commonly, children recover from the acute episode within 2–3 weeks. Some residual renal disease (including hypertension, proteinuria, or chronic renal insufficiency) occurs in about 30%, and end-stage renal failure occurs in about 15%. The risk of ESRD is higher in children with atypical or pneumococcal-induced HUS. Follow-up of children recovering from HUS should include serial determinations of renal function with frequency dictated by the etiology, course, and subsequent findings and routine monitoring of blood pressure. Overall mortality (about 3%–5%) is most likely in the early phase, primarily resulting from CNS or cardiac complications. As with most renal conditions, chronic proteinuria, hypertension, or abnormal renal function are associated with worse long-term renal prognosis and require follow-up.

Loirat C, Fakhouri F, Ariceta G: An international consensus approach to the management of atypical hemolytic uremic syndrome in children. Pediatr Nephrol 2016 Jan;31(1):15–39 [PMID: 25859752].

Nayer A, Asif A: Atypical hemolytic-uremic syndrome: a clinical review. Am J Ther 2016;23(1):e151–e158 [PMID: 24681522].

▼ RENAL FAILURE

ACUTE KIDNEY INJURY

The term "acute kidney injury (AKI)" denotes the sudden inability to excrete urine of sufficient quantity or composition to maintain body fluid homeostasis. Explanations include quickly reversible problems such as dehydration or urinary tract obstruction, as well as new-onset renal disease (eg, AGN), drug-related toxic nephropathies, or renal ischemia; the latter is primarily suspected in settings of significant hemodynamic instability or other circumstances resulting in decreased renal perfusion. Table 24–1 lists prerenal, renal, and postrenal causes of AKI.

▶ Clinical Findings

The hallmark of early AKI is oliguria with subsequent variable rise in serum creatinine and BUN; these observations are more likely to be the initial concern in a hospitalized patient.

Table 24–1. Classification of AKI.

Prerenal
  Intravascular volume depletion (gastrointestinal, skin, or renal losses; significantly diminished intake; hemorrhage)
  Diminished effective circulating volume (low-output cardiac failure, nephrotic syndrome, capillary leak, cirrhosis)
  Aortic or renal vessel injury
  Renal arterial thrombosis
Renal
  Hemolytic-uremic syndrome
  Renal vascular thrombosis
  Glomerulonephritis
  Nephrotoxins
  Acute tubular necrosis
  Renal (cortical) necrosis
  Tubular crystalluria (sulfonamide uric acid, tumor lysis)
  Pigment nephropathy (ATN)
  Contrast nephropathy
  Interstitial nephritis
  Trauma
Postrenal
  Obstruction due to tumor, hematoma, posterior urethral valves, ureteropelvic junction stricture, ureterovesical junction stricture, ureterocele, other bladder outlet, narcotic-induced urinary retention, stones, obstructed bladder catheter

Note: Any of the prerenal etiologies of renal failure can evolve into acute tubular nephropathy when prolonged.

Table 24–2. Urine studies.

	Prerenal Failure	Acute Tubular Necrosis
Urine osmolality	> 500	< 350
Urine-specific gravity	> 1.020	~ 1.010
Urine sodium	< 20 mEq/L	> 40 mEq/L
Fractional excretion of sodium	< 1%	> 3%
Ratio of urine creatinine to plasma creatinine	> 40:1	< 20:1
Ratio of blood urea nitrogen (BUN) to plasma creatinine	> 20:1	< 10–15

Note: Urine osmolality and sodium concentration should be interpreted in light of the child's age-related capacity for these parameters (eg, newborns have limited urinary concentrating capacity and excrete more sodium than older children).

Although an exact etiologic diagnosis may be unclear at the onset, classifying AKI as outlined in Table 24–1 is helpful in determining if an immediately reversible cause is present.

Entities that can be quickly addressed and corrected, for example, intravascular volume depletion or urinary tract obstruction, should be considered first. Once normal renal perfusion and lack of urinary tract obstruction is ensured, if there is no clinical evidence for de novo renal disease, a diagnosis of acute tubular necrosis may be entertained.

A. Prerenal Causes

The most common cause of acute decreased renal function in children is compromised renal perfusion. It is usually secondary to true intravascular volume depletion or a decrease in effective circulating volume, as may be seen in cardiac failure, cirrhosis, or nephrotic syndrome. Table 24–2 lists the urinary indices helpful in distinguishing these "prerenal" conditions from true renal parenchymal insult, such as acute tubular necrosis.

B. Renal Causes

Causes of AKI intrinsic to the kidneys include acute glomerulonephritides, HUS, acute interstitial nephritis, and nephrotoxic injury. The diagnosis of acute tubular necrosis, which is reserved for those cases in which renal ischemic insult is believed to be the likely cause, should be considered when correction of prerenal or postrenal problems does not improve renal function and there is no evidence of de novo renal disease.

C. Postrenal Causes

Postrenal failure, usually found in newborns with urologic anatomic abnormalities, is accompanied by varying degrees of renal insufficiency. One should always keep in mind the possibility of acute urinary tract obstruction in AKI, especially in the setting of anuria of acute onset. Whatever the cause, ensuring urine drainage is the first step toward reversibility of oliguria.

▶ Complications

The severity of the complications of AKI depends on the degree of renal functional impairment and oliguria. Common complications include: (1) fluid overload (hypertension, congestive heart failure, and pulmonary edema), (2) electrolyte disturbances (hyperkalemia), (3) metabolic acidosis, (4) hyperphosphatemia, and (5) uremia.

▶ Treatment

Prerenal and/or postrenal factors should be excluded and rectified. Normal circulating volume should be maintained and normal blood pressure and cardiac performance established with appropriate fluid or pressor support. Strict measurement of input and output must be maintained, with input adjusted as reduction in output dictates. Placement of a Foley bladder catheter can aid in timely measurement of the output. However, in cases where oligo/anuric renal failure is well established (ie, insignificant urine volume), the foreign body should be removed to minimize bladder infection risk. Measurement of central venous pressure may be indicated. Routine assessment of weight is helpful to assess fluid balance in children in whom this is possible. Increasing urine output with diuretics, such as furosemide (1–2 mg/kg per dose, intravenously, maximum of 200 mg every 6 hours), can be attempted. The effective dose will depend on the amount of functional compromise. If a response does not occur within 1 hour and the urine output remains low (< 0.5 mL/kg/h), the furosemide dose should be maximized and a continuous infusion may be considered. In some cases, the addition of a long-acting thiazide diuretic, such as metolazone, may improve the response. If no diuresis occurs with maximum dosing, further administration of diuretics should cease and fluid intake should be restricted accordingly. The child should be monitored closely for indications for acute dialysis.

All medication dosages should be adjusted as appropriate for the degree of renal clearance.

A. Acute Dialysis: Indications

Immediate indications for dialysis are: (1) hyperkalemia refractory to medical management; (2) unrelenting metabolic acidosis (usually in a situation where fluid overload or hypernatremia prevent repeated sodium bicarbonate administration); (3) fluid overload (which may be manifest as significant hypertension, congestive heart failure, pulmonary edema, or simply inability to provide appropriate medication and nutritional support due to fluid restriction); (4) symptoms of uremia, usually manifested in children by CNS depression (rare); and (5) ingestions of drugs/substances removed by hemodialysis. In cases in which one is concerned about the so-called "uremic" bleeding, it is important to keep in mind that despite the use of the clinical term uremia, it is not the BUN which contributes to platelet dysfunction in renal failure. Accumulation of metabolic end products that contribute to bleeding correlates better with the degree of renal function as reflected by the serum creatinine. This is especially true in cases in which the BUN, which is potentially affected by many things in an ill patient, appears to be disproportionately elevated with respect to the serum creatinine.

B. Methods of Dialysis

Peritoneal dialysis is often preferred in children because of ease of performance and patient tolerance. Although peritoneal dialysis is technically less efficient than hemodialysis, hemodynamic stability and metabolic control can be better sustained because this technique can be applied on a relatively continuous basis. Hemodialysis should be considered (1) if rapid removal of toxins is desired, (2) if the hemodynamic status will tolerate the intermittent solute and fluid removal, or (3) if impediments to efficient peritoneal dialysis are present (eg, postoperative abdomen, adhesions). If vascular access and potential usage of anticoagulation are not impediments, a slow, continuous hemodialytic process, continuous renal replacement therapy (CRRT), may be applied in hemodynamically unstable, critically ill patients, including those on extracorporeal membrane oxygenation. Typically, either systemic or regional anticoagulation is provided to maintain the extracorporeal circuit. Nutritional support and medication doses should be reviewed and adjusted accordingly for patients receiving dialytic therapies.

C. Dialysis Management and Complications

Intravascular volume depletion can be observed in any dialytic therapy; thus, close attention to the patient's hemodynamic status with adjustment in dialytic fluid removal is indicated. Significant intravascular volume depletion can contribute to acute tubular nephropathy and limit the timely recovery of intrinsic renal function. Complications specific to peritoneal dialysis include peritonitis and technical complications such as dialysate leakage or respiratory compromise from intra-abdominal dialysate fluid. Peritonitis risk can be diminished by strict aseptic technique. Peritoneal fluid cultures should be obtained as clinically indicated. Leakage is reduced by good catheter placement technique and appropriate intra-abdominal dialysate volumes. Adjustment of the electrolyte concentration of dialysate is important to maintain electrolyte balance. Potassium and phosphate, absent from standard dialysate solutions, can be added to the dialysate as clinically required. Several antibiotics can be added to the dialysate for intraperitoneal administration with associated systemic absorption. This scenario is usually reserved for treatment of peritonitis or with limited vascular access for drug administration. Correction of fluid overload is accomplished with high osmolar dialysis fluids. Higher dextrose concentrations (maximum 4.25%) can correct fluid overload rapidly at the risk of causing hyperglycemia. Fluid removal may also be increased with more frequent exchanges of the dialysate, but rapid osmotic transfer of water may result in hypernatremia. Because fluid removal is dependent on many factors (osmolar load of dialysate, individual peritoneal membrane transport characteristics, peritoneal membrane perfusion, etc), it is not possible to exactly control the hourly rate of fluid removal during peritoneal dialysis.

Even in small infants, hemodialysis can rapidly correct major metabolic and electrolyte disturbances as well as volume overload. The process is highly efficient. Systemic anticoagulation, usually with heparin, is typically required. Careful monitoring of the appropriate biochemical parameters is important. Note that during or immediately following the procedure, blood sampling will produce misleading results because equilibration between extravascular compartments and the blood will not yet have been achieved. Appropriate vascular access must be maintained.

Hemodialysis is generally intermittent, daily to three times per week. If need be, CRRT may be used to maintain more minute-to-minute, continuous metabolic and fluid control especially in the hemodynamically unstable or septic patient. The choice of anticoagulation is typically based upon institutional preference and the clinical situation. Appropriately trained staffs are needed to administer any dialytic therapy to children.

Course & Prognosis

The course and prognosis of AKI vary with the etiology. If severe oliguria occurs in acute tubular necrosis, it usually lasts about 10 days. Anuria or oliguria lasting longer than 6 weeks is concerning for progression to cortical necrosis and associated limited renal recovery. The diuretic phase of recovery from AKI begins with an increase in urinary output to large volumes of isosthenuric urine containing sodium levels of 80–150 mEq/L. The associated polyuria may persist for several days or weeks, and the care provider must ensure appropriate hydration to prevent prerenal azotemia or acute tubular necrosis. Urinary abnormalities usually disappear completely within a few months. If renal recovery does not ensue within about 6 weeks of oligoanuria, arrangements should be made for chronic dialysis and possible eventual renal transplantation. Some children requiring prolonged (> 1 month) dialysis support will demonstrate recovery to varying degrees of CKD but are obviously at high risk for eventual progression to ESRD. Children who have experienced significant AKI require long-term follow-up with a nephrologist.

Mammen C et al: Long-term risk of CKD in children surviving episodes of acute kidney injury in the intensive care unit: a prospective cohort study. Am J Kidney Dis 2012 Apr;59(4):523–530 [PMID: 22206744].

Rewa O, Bagshaw SM: Acute kidney injury—epidemiology, outcomes and economics. Nat Rev Nephrol 2014;10(4):193–207 [PMID: 24445744].

Ricci Z, Goldstein SL: Pediatric continuous renal replacement therapy. Contrib Nephrol 2016;187:121–130 [PMID: 26881430].

Sutherland SM, Alexander SR: Continuous renal replacement therapy in children. Pediatr Nephrol 2012;27(11):2007–2016 [PMID: 22366896].

CHRONIC RENAL FAILURE

Chronic renal failure in children most commonly results from congenital abnormalities of the kidneys or urinary tract (CAKUT). Renal hypoplasia/dysplasia, obstructive uropathy, or severe VUR without (or despite) surgical intervention is often associated with progressive renal insufficiency in children. In older children, the chronic glomerulonephritides and nephroses, irreversible nephrotoxic injury, or HUS may also cause chronic renal failure. Early evaluation and close follow-up by a pediatric nephrology team in these situations is advised.

Complications

ESSENTIALS OF DIAGNOSIS & TYPICAL FEATURES

Complications of chronic renal failure:

▶ Anemia of chronic renal failure

▶ Hyperphosphatemia/secondary hyperparathyroidism

▶ Metabolic acidosis

▶ Growth failure

▶ Hypertension

▶ Uremia

Any remaining unaffected renal tissue can compensate for gradual loss of functioning nephrons in progressive chronic renal failure, but complications of renal insufficiency appear when this compensatory ability is overwhelmed. In children who have structural kidney lesions associated with impaired urinary concentration, polyuria and dehydration are more likely to be problems than fluid overload until very late in the course of renal insufficiency. Some such children can continue to produce generous volumes of poor quality urine even though they require dialysis. A salt-wasting state can also occur. In contrast, children who develop chronic renal failure due to glomerular disease or renal injury will characteristically retain sodium and water with associated hypertension and eventual loss of urine output.

Metabolic acidosis and growth retardation occur early in chronic renal failure. Disturbances in calcium, phosphorus, and vitamin D metabolism leading to renal osteodystrophy and rickets require prompt attention. Increases in parathyroid hormone occur in response to decreased serum calcium from lack of renally activated vitamin D and/or rising serum phosphorus. The increase in parathyroid hormone, which improves renal tubular excretion of phosphorous, can maintain normal serum calcium and phosphate levels early in the course, but at the expense of the skeleton. Anemia due to decreased erythropoietin production can occur relatively early on as well.

Symptoms such as anorexia, nausea, and malaise occur late in chronic renal failure (generally < 30% renal function). These symptoms can be minimized if chronic renal failure has been detected early and associated complications treated, but refractory symptoms remain indications for renal replacement therapy. CNS abnormalities such as confusion and lethargy are very late symptoms, followed even later by stupor and coma. Such findings are unusual as children usually seek medical attention before deteriorating to this point, and the rise in BUN is typically gradual. Other late complications of untreated renal failure are platelet dysfunction and bleeding tendencies, pericarditis, and chronic fluid overload leading to congestive heart failure, pulmonary edema, and worsening hypertension.

► Treatment

A. Management of Complications

Treatment of chronic renal failure is primarily aimed at controlling the associated complications. Acidosis may be treated with sodium citrate or bicarbonate solutions, as long as the added sodium does not aggravate hypertension. Sodium restriction is advisable when hypertension is present. Hyperphosphatemia is controlled by dietary restriction and dietary phosphate binders (eg, calcium carbonate, sevelamer). Supplementation with vitamin D (cholecalciferol or ergocalciferol) and calcitriol is typically required. These measures target the prevention of renal osteodystrophy or rickets. Dietary potassium restriction will be necessary as the GFR falls. Diet must be maintained to provide the child's daily requirements for optimal growth. Routine input from a renal dietitian is helpful in this regard. Protein restriction in children is not recommended; rather, appropriate quantities of protein required for age and growth are targeted as part of dietary plans.

Renal function must be monitored regularly (creatinine and BUN), and serum electrolytes, calcium, phosphorus, intact PTH, 25-OH-vitamin D, iron and ferritin, and hemoglobin and hematocrit levels monitored to guide changes in fluid and dietary management as well as dosages of phosphate binder, citrate buffer, vitamin D supplements, blood pressure medications, iron supplements, and epoetin alfa. Linear growth failure may be treated with daily subcutaneous human recombinant growth hormone; an adult height in the low-normal range is targeted. Care must be taken to avoid medications that aggravate hypertension; increase the body burden of sodium, potassium, or phosphate; or increase production of BUN. Successful management relies greatly on education of the patient and family. Attention must also be directed toward the psychosocial needs of the patient and family as they adjust to chronic illness and the eventual need for dialysis and kidney transplantation. The multidisciplinary nephrology team works with each child/family to determine appropriate timing for chronic dialysis and/or kidney transplantation.

B. Dialysis and Transplantation

Chronic peritoneal dialysis (home-based) and hemodialysis provide lifesaving treatment for children prior to kidney transplantation. The best measure of the success of chronic dialysis in children is the level of physical and psychosocial rehabilitation achieved, such as continued participation in day-to-day activities and school attendance. The goal for all children with chronic or end-stage kidney disease is to achieve kidney transplantation, using dialysis as a life-saving bridge, when necessary. Pre-emptive kidney transplantation in a child with known progressing CKD should be considered if possible, given improved long-term graft and patient survival, as compared to peers transplanted after receiving dialysis.

At present, the graft survival rate for living donor kidney transplants is 96.4% at 1 year, 93.4% at 3 years, and 86.4% at 5 years. With deceased donor transplantation, graft survivals are 95%, 90%, and 79%, respectively. Five-year patient survival remains well above 95% at 5 years after transplant. Adequate growth and well-being are directly related to acceptance of the graft, the degree of normal function, and the side effects of medications.

Shellmer D, Brosig C, Wray J: The start of the transplant journey: referral for pediatric solid organ transplantation. Pediatr Transplant 2014;18(2):125–133 [PMID: 24438194].

Smith JM, Martz K, Blydt-Hansen TD: Pediatric kidney transplant practice patterns and outcome benchmarks, 1987-2010: a report of the North American Pediatric Renal Trials and Collaborative Studies. Pediatr Transplant 2013;17(2):149–157 [PMID: 23281637].

Warady BA, Neu AM, Schaefer F: Optimal care of the infant, child, and adolescent on dialysis: 2014 update. Am J Kidney Dis 2014;64(1):128–142 [PMID: 24717681].

▼ HYPERTENSION

Hypertension in children is commonly of renal origin, although the prevalence of obesity-related hypertension is rapidly rising in the pediatric population. Systemic hypertension is anticipated as a complication of known renal parenchymal disease, but it may be found on routine physical examination in an otherwise healthy-appearing child. Increased understanding of the roles of water and salt retention and overactivity of the renin-angiotensin system has done much to guide therapy; nevertheless, not all forms of hypertension can be explained by these two mechanisms.

The causes of renal hypertension in the newborn period include: (1) congenital anomalies of the kidneys or renal vasculature, (2) obstruction of the urinary tract, (3) thrombosis of renal vasculature or kidneys, and (4) volume overload. Some instances of apparent paradoxical elevations of blood pressure have been reported in clinical situations in which chronic diuretic therapy is used, such as bronchopulmonary dysplasia. Chronic hypoxia may have a role in vascular alterations, similar to what is seen with hypertension in older children with obstructive sleep apnea. Umbilical artery catheterization continues to be an important contributor to hypertension in infants and young children.

Infants and children with hypertension require careful evaluation to exclude a secondary cause of hypertension. These can include renal parenchymal or renovascular disease (renal arterial or venous thrombosis, congenital vascular stenosis), other vascular diseases (vasculitis, aortic coarctation), endocrine disorders (thyroid disease, cortisol excess, pheochromocytoma, congenital adrenal hyperplasia), monogenic hypertension (glucocorticoid remediable aldosteronism, Liddle syndrome, etc), and primary hyperaldosteronism. The family history of hypertension and cardiovascular disease should be reviewed with particular attention to early-onset hypertension. Primary or essential hypertension is becoming increasingly common with a Western diet and limited routine exercise.

▶ Clinical Findings

A child is normotensive if the average recorded systolic and diastolic blood pressures are lower than the 90th percentile for age, sex, and height. The 90th percentile in the newborn period is approximately 85–90/55–65 mm Hg for both sexes. In the first year of life, the acceptable levels are 90–100/60–67 mm Hg. Incremental increases with growth occur, gradually approaching young adult ranges of 100–120/65–80 mm Hg in the late teens. A blood pressure between the 90–95th percentile or exceeding 120/80 in adolescents is consistent with elevated blood pressure. Careful measurement of blood pressure requires correct cuff size and reliable equipment. The cuff should be wide enough to cover two-thirds of the upper arm and should encircle the arm completely without an overlap in the inflatable bladder. Ideally the child should be sitting quietly for 5 minutes with feet flat on the floor before blood pressure is measured in the right arm, upon which norms are based. Although an anxious child may have an elevation in blood pressure, abnormal readings must not be too hastily attributed to this cause. Repeat measurement is helpful, especially after the child has been consoled. Manual blood pressure measurement should be pursued when automated readings are concerning. In cases where more detailed assessment is needed, 24-hour ambulatory blood pressure monitoring can be very valuable, for example, in aiding with the diagnosis of white coat hypertension or loss of normal 24-hour variation in blood pressures.

Routine laboratory studies include serum BUN, creatinine, and electrolytes and urinalysis. Abnormal BUN and creatinine would support underlying renal disease as the cause, and serum electrolytes demonstrating hypokalemic alkalosis suggest excess mineralocorticoid effect. Depending on the age of the child, routine assessment of serum lipids, glucose, A_{1C} hemoglobin, thyroid function tests, renin, and aldosterone is indicated. Screening of plasma/urine catecholamines and metanephrines and/or serum cortisol should be obtained as clinically indicated. Pheochromocytoma is unusual in the setting of increasing obesity. Echocardiogram has been recommended for routine assessment of hypertension in children. Careful assessment of distal pulses is necessary to exclude aortic coarctation clinically, and echocardiogram may be of value in select patients to exclude left ventricular hypertrophy. Renal ultrasonography with Doppler flow is helpful in determining the possible presence of renal scarring, urinary tract obstruction, or renovascular flow disturbances as a cause of hypertension. However, the sensitivity and specificity of Doppler ultrasound for renal artery stenosis vary widely between institutions. Renal MRA or CTA is indicated when there is high suspicion for renal artery stenosis. A renal biopsy (which rarely reveals the cause of hypertension unless clinical evidence of renal disease is present) should be undertaken with special care in the hypertensive patient and preferably after pressures have been controlled by therapy. Figure 24–3 presents a suggested approach to the outpatient workup of hypertension.

▶ Treatment

A. Acute Hypertensive Emergencies

A hypertensive emergency exists when CNS signs of hypertension appear, such as papilledema, encephalopathy, or seizures. Retinal hemorrhages or exudates also indicate a need for prompt and effective control. Such children require appropriate management in the intensive care setting with consideration of continuous arterial BP monitoring and intravenous antihypertensive therapy. Whatever method is used to control emergent hypertension, medications for sustained control should also be initiated so that normal blood pressure will be maintained when the emergent measures are discontinued. The primary classes of useful antihypertensive drugs are: (1) ACE inhibitors and angiotensin receptor blockers (the latter used less frequently in children based on less clinical experience and limitations in accurate dosing for smaller children), (2) calcium channel blockers, (3) α- and β-adrenergic blockers, (4) diuretics, and (5) vasodilators. Acute elevations of blood pressure not exceeding the 99th percentile in the asymptomatic patient may be treated with oral antihypertensives, aiming for progressive improvement and control within 48 hours.

Sublingual nifedipine is a rapid-acting calcium channel blocker that can be administered to acutely decrease severe hypertension. However, its use has fallen out of favor for acute management of hypertension in adults in whom an abrupt decline in blood pressure can significantly diminish perfusion of the coronary and cerebral arteries in the setting of underlying atherosclerosis. Alternatively, nicardipine is a very effective and generally well-tolerated antihypertensive that is administered via continuous intravenous infusion for control of systemic hypertension in children. Sodium nitroprusside is a very effective infusion to gain control of malignant hypertension, but long-term usage is limited by concern for rare thiocyanate toxicity, of particular concern when renal failure is present. Hydralazine is a vasodilator that can be administered intermittently by the intravenous route. Any vasodilator can induce reflex tachycardia and sodium retention, so concomitant administration of a β-blocker or diuretic may be indicated. Intravenous forms of β-blockers

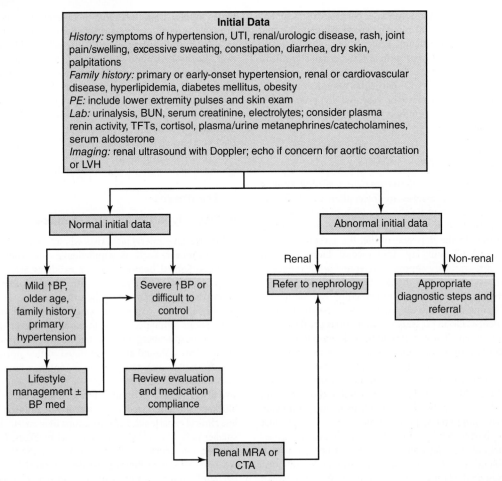

▲ Figure 24–3. Approach to the outpatient workup of hypertension. BP, blood pressure; BUN, blood urea nitrogen; CTA, computed tomography angiography; LVH, left ventricular hypertrophy; MRA, magnetic resonance angiography; TFT, thyroid function test; UTI, urinary tract infection.

such as esmolol or labetalol (both available as continuous infusions) are useful when there are no cardiac or respiratory contraindications to their use.

Diuretics such as furosemide can be useful in the acute setting when there is evidence of intravascular volume overload.

B. Sustained Hypertension

For children with sustained hypertension, rate of correction of blood pressure needs to be taken into account. Too rapid reduction in blood pressure in children with chronic hypertension places them at risk for loss of adequate cerebral and renal perfusion pressure. Therefore, reductions in blood pressure to goal measurements based on age, gender, and height by no more than 25% for each 24–48-hour period

are recommended. Several choices are available for treatment (Table 24–3). A single drug such as an ACE inhibitor or a β-blocker (unless contraindicated, eg, with underlying asthma) may be adequate to treat mild hypertension. ACE inhibitors are often the preferred choice of pediatric nephrologists given the frequent renal etiology of hypertension. Diuretics are useful to treat renal insufficiency that is often associated with sodium and fluid retention, but the disadvantages of possible electrolyte imbalance must be considered. Calcium channel blockers are increasingly useful and appear well tolerated in children. Direct vasodilators such as hydralazine and minoxidil often require diuretics and/or β-blockers to combat associated sodium and fluid retention and reflex tachycardia. Although minoxidil is extremely effective in control of hypertension of a variety of etiologies, hirsutism is a significant side effect. The advice of a pediatric

Table 24–3. Antihypertensive drugs for ambulatory treatment in children ages 1–17 years.

Class	Drug	Oral Dose	Major Side Effects[a]
Angiotensin- converting enzyme inhibitor	Captopril	1–6 mg/kg/day ÷ tid	Rash, hyperkalemia, cough, decreased GFR
	Lisinopril	0.1–0.6 mg/kg/day ÷ qd-bid	
Calcium channel blocker	Amlodipine	0.1–0.6 mg/kg/day ÷ qd-bid	Higher doses relative to body weight may be required in younger children; headache, facial flushing, pretibial edema
	Nifedipine, extended-release	0.5–3 mg/kg/day ÷ tid	Flushing, tachycardia
Diuretic	Furosemide	2–20 mg/kg/day ÷ qd-qid (maximum 5 mg/kg/dose up to 200 mg)	Potassium and volume depletion
	Hydrochlorothiazide	1–3 mg/kg/day ÷ qd-bid	Potassium and volume depletion, hyperuricemia
Sympathetic nervous system blockade	Propranolol	0.6–4 mg/kg/day ÷ bid-tid (maximum 640 mg/day)	Syncope, bradycardia; use with caution in asthma or overt heart failure
	Metoprolol	1–6 mg/kg/day ÷ qd-bid (maximum 200 mg/day)	Syncope, bradycardia; use with caution in asthma or overt heart failure
Vasodilator	Hydralazine	0.75–7.5 mg/kg/day ÷ tid-qid (maximum 200 mg/day)	Lupus-like syndrome in slow acetylators; tachycardia, fluid retention, headache
	Minoxidil	0.3–1 mg/kg/day ÷ qd-bid	Tachycardia, fluid retention, hirsutism

bid, twice a day; GFR, glomerular filtration rate; qd, daily; qid, four times a day; tid, three times a day.
[a]Not all side effects are listed.

nephrologist should be sought in the management of acute and chronic hypertension in children.

Ferguson MA, Flynn JT: Rational use of antihypertensive medications in children. Pediatr Nephrol 2014;29(6):979–988 [PMID: 23715784].

Flynn JT: Assessment of blood pressure in children: it's all in the details. J Clin Hypertens (Greenwich) 2013;15(11):772–773 [PMID: 24283595].

Flynn JT et al: Clinical practice guideline for screening and management of high blood pressure in children and adolescents. Pediatrics 2017;140(3) [PMID: 28827377].

▼ INHERITED OR DEVELOPMENTAL DEFECTS OF THE KIDNEYS

There are many developmental, hereditary, or metabolic defects of the kidneys and collecting system. The clinical consequences include metabolic abnormalities, failure to thrive, nephrolithiasis, renal glomerular or tubular dysfunction, and chronic renal failure. Table 24–4 lists some of the major entities.

DISORDERS OF THE RENAL TUBULES

Three subtypes of renal tubular acidosis (RTA) are recognized: (1) the classic form, called type I or distal RTA; (2) the bicarbonate-wasting form, called type II or proximal RTA; and (3) type IV, or hyperkalemic RTA, which is associated with hyporeninemic hypoaldosteronism or inherited in an autosomal manner. Types I and II and their variants are encountered most frequently in children. Type III is described historically as a combination of types I and II. Other primary tubular disorders in childhood, such as glycinuria, hyperuricosuria, or renal glycosuria, may result from a defect in a single tubular transport pathway (see Table 24–4).

Distal Renal Tubular Acidosis (Type I)

The most common form of distal RTA in childhood is the hereditary form. The clinical presentation is one of failure to thrive, anorexia, vomiting, and dehydration. Hyperchloremic metabolic acidosis, hypokalemia, and a urinary pH exceeding 6.5 are found. Concomitant hypercalciuria may lead to nephrocalcinosis, nephrolithiasis, and renal failure. Other situations that may be responsible for distal RTA are found in some of the entities listed in Table 24–4.

Distal RTA results from a defect in the distal nephron in the tubular transport of hydrogen ion or in the maintenance of a steep enough gradient for proper excretion of hydrogen ion. Historically the diagnosis could be established with an acid loading test, but this is rarely pursued currently. Instead, the findings of RTA with persistent elevation in urine pH despite acidosis, hypercalciuria or nephrocalcinosis, and relatively low requirement of alkali to normalize serum pH

Table 24–4. Inherited or developmental defects of the urinary tract.

Cystic diseases of genetic origin
  Polycystic disease
    Autosomal recessive
    Autosomal dominant
    Other syndromes that include either form
  Nephronophthisis
  Medullary cystic kidney disease
  Glomerulocystic kidney disease
  Renal cysts and diabetes (HNF1-β)
 	
Dysplastic renal diseases
  Renal agenesis
  Renal hypoplasia
  Renal dysplasia
  Cystic renal dysplasia
  Multicystic dysplastic kidney
  Oligomeganephronia
 	
Hereditary diseases associated with nephritis
  Hereditary nephritis with deafness and ocular defects
    (Alport syndrome)
  Nail-patella syndrome
  Familial hyperprolinemia
  Hereditary osteolysis with nephropathy
 	
Hereditary diseases associated with intrarenal deposition of metabolites
  Fabry disease
  Zellweger syndrome
  Various storage diseases (eg, G_{M1} monosialogangliosidosis, Hurler syndrome, Niemann-Pick disease, familial metachromatic leukodystrophy, glycogenosis type I [von Gierke disease], glycogenosis type II [Pompe disease])
	Hereditary amyloidosis (familial Mediterranean fever, heredofamilial urticaria with deafness and neuropathy, primary familial amyloidosis with polyneuropathy)
	
	Hereditary renal diseases associated with tubular transport defects
	  Hartnup disease
	  Oculocerebrorenal syndrome of Lowe
	  Cystinosis (infantile, adolescent, adult types)
	  Wilson disease
	  Galactosemia
	  Hereditary fructose intolerance
	  Renal tubular acidosis
	  Hereditary tyrosinemia
	  Renal glycosuria
	  Vitamin D–resistant rickets
	  Pseudohypoparathyroidism
	  Nephrogenic diabetes insipidus
	  Bartter syndrome
	  Gitelman syndrome
	  Liddle syndrome
	  Hypouricemia
	
	Hereditary diseases associated with lithiasis
	  Hyperoxaluria
	  L-Glyceric aciduria
	  Xanthinuria
	  Lesch-Nyhan syndrome and variants, gout
	  Nephropathy due to familial hyperparathyroidism
	  Cystinuria (types I, II, III)
	  Glycinuria
	  Dent disease

and bicarbonate concentration (1–3 mEq/kg/day) support a distal defect. Some forms of genetic distal RTA are associated with hearing loss. Correction of acidosis with citrate or less commonly bicarbonate reduces complications and improves growth. Distal RTA is often permanent. However, if renal damage from calcinosis is prevented, the prognosis with treatment is good.

Proximal Renal Tubular Acidosis (Type II)

Proximal RTA, the most common form of RTA in childhood, is characterized by failure to reabsorb bicarbonate appropriately in the proximal tubule with associated reduced serum bicarbonate concentration and normal anion gap hyperchloremic metabolic acidosis. Once a steady state is reached, the intact distal nephron appropriately excretes hydrogen ion, leading to a low urine pH.

Proximal RTA is often an isolated defect, and in the newborn can be considered an aspect of renal immaturity which improves with increasing gestational age. Proximal RTA in infants is accompanied by failure to thrive and sometimes hypokalemia. Secondary forms result from reflux

or obstructive uropathy or occur in association with other tubular disorders (see Table 24–4). Due to bicarbonate wasting, children with proximal RTA typically require 5–20 mEq/kg/day citrate/bicarbonate to achieve normal serum pH and bicarbonate concentration.

Evaluation & Treatment

The diagnosis of RTA is made with the finding of normal anion gap, hyperchloremic metabolic acidosis in the absence of diarrhea, or intravascular volume depletion. A concomitant urine pH is helpful in many cases, as it is elevated in distal RTA despite the metabolic acidosis. The finding of hypophosphatemia or glycosuria should lead to further investigation of proximal tubular function (eg, Fanconi syndrome). A renal ultrasound should be obtained to exclude urinary tract obstruction (which can be seen with either proximal or distal RTA) and nephrocalcinosis (seen in distal RTA). A urine calcium to creatinine ratio may be helpful in the latter condition. In either proximal or distal RTA, citrate or bicarbonate supplementation is provided to target a serum bicarbonate level of 20–24 mEq/L, as an index of normal serum pH. Citrate solutions are more effective and often better tolerated than sodium bicarbonate. Sodium citrate contains 1 mEq/mL of Na^+ and citrate. Potassium citrate contains 2 mEq/mL of citrate and 1 mEq/mL each of Na^+ and K^+. The medication is administered two to three times per day, targeting a trough serum bicarbonate at goal. Potassium supplementation may be required (and can often be accomplished simply with a change from sodium citrate to potassium citrate) because the added sodium load presented to the distal tubule may exaggerate potassium losses.

The prognosis is excellent in cases of isolated proximal RTA, especially when the problem is related to renal immaturity. Alkali therapy can usually be discontinued after several months to a few years. Growth should be normal, and the gradual increase in the serum bicarbonate level to greater than 24 mEq/L heralds the normalization of the threshold for proximal tubular bicarbonate reabsorption. If the defect is part of Fanconi syndrome or distal RTA, the prognosis depends on the underlying disorder or syndrome.

CYSTINOSIS

Cystinosis, most often transmitted via autosomal recessive inheritance, is the most common cause of Fanconi syndrome in children and results from mutations in the *CTNS* gene, which encodes the cystine transporter. There are three types of cystinosis: adult, adolescent, and infantile. The adult form is characterized by ocular cystinosis without renal involvement. In the adolescent and infantile types, cystine accumulation in lysosomes causes cell death in numerous organs, including the kidneys. Treatment with oral cysteamine aids in the metabolic conversion of cystine (unable to exit cells) to cysteine (able to exit cells) and delays intracellular accumulation and associated complications, which include Fanconi syndrome with salt-wasting and functional nephrogenic diabetes insipidus (NDI), proximal RTA, hypophosphatemic rickets, eventual progression to ESRD, hypothyroidism, ocular cystinosis with eventual blindness, and neurologic deterioration. The infantile type is most common and the most severe. Characteristically, children present in the first or early second year of life with Fanconi syndrome, polyuria and polydipsia, and failure to thrive. If left untreated, ESRD is reached by 7–10 years of age in the infantile form. Whenever the diagnosis of cystinosis is suspected, slit-lamp examination of the corneas should be performed. Cystine crystal deposition causes an almost pathognomonic ground-glass "dazzle" appearance. Increased white blood cell cystine levels are diagnostic. The condition does not recur in transplanted kidneys, but ongoing cysteamine therapy is required to prevent complications in other organs.

Emma F et al: Nephropathic cystinosis: an international consensus document. Nephrol Dial Transplant 2014;29 Suppl 4:iv87–iv94 [PMID: 25165189].

OCULOCEREBRORENAL SYNDROME (LOWE SYNDROME)

Lowe syndrome results from various mutations in the *OCRL1* gene, which codes for a Golgi apparatus phosphatase. Affected males have anomalies involving the eyes, brain, and kidneys. The physical stigmata and degree of mental retardation vary with the location of the mutation. In addition to congenital cataracts and buphthalmos, the typical facies includes prominent epicanthal folds, frontal prominence, and a tendency to scaphocephaly. Muscle hypotonia is a prominent finding. The renal abnormalities are tubular and include hypophosphatemic rickets with low serum phosphorus levels, low to normal serum calcium levels, elevated serum alkaline phosphatase levels, proximal RTA, and aminoaciduria. Renal treatment includes alkali therapy, phosphate replacement, and vitamin D support. Progressive glomerulosclerosis likely results from progressive renal tubular injury and may lead to chronic renal failure and end-stage renal disease between the second and fourth decades of life.

HYPOKALEMIC ALKALOSIS (BARTTER SYNDROME, GITELMAN SYNDROME, & LIDDLE SYNDROME)

There are a number of genetic tubular disorders which result in hypokalemic metabolic alkalosis. Bartter syndrome is characterized by severe hypokalemic, hypochloremic metabolic alkalosis, extremely high levels of circulating renin and aldosterone, and a paradoxical absence of hypertension. On renal biopsy (rarely pursued in the current era), a striking juxtaglomerular hyperplasia is seen. A neonatal form of Bartter syndrome is thought to result from mutations in two genes (*NKCC2, ROMK*) affecting nephron Na^+-K^+ or K^+ transport. These patients typically have a history of polyhydramnios and following birth have recurrent life-threatening episodes of fever and dehydration with the aforementioned electrolyte and acid–base disturbances, hypercalciuria, and early-onset nephrocalcinosis. Classic Bartter syndrome presenting in infancy with polyuria and growth retardation (but not nephrocalcinosis) is thought to result from mutations in a chloride channel gene. Gitelman syndrome occurs in older children and features episodes of muscle weakness and tetany associated with severe hypokalemia, and hypomagnesemia. These children have hypocalciuria. Treatment with prostaglandin inhibitors and potassium-conserving diuretics (eg, amiloride) and potassium and magnesium supplements where indicated is beneficial in Bartter or Gitelman syndrome. These are lifelong conditions which require ongoing electrolyte supplementation.

Liddle syndrome is associated with constitutive activation of the epithelial sodium channel with associated salt and water retention. Thus, the initial presenting abnormality is often hypertension associated with hypokalemia and metabolic alkalosis. Serum renin and aldosterone are suppressed due to the sodium and fluid retention. Treatment in Liddle syndrome is with a low-sodium diet and blockade of the epithelial sodium channel with amiloride or triamterene. Spironolactone is ineffective in this condition as aldosterone is typically suppressed.

NEPHROGENIC DIABETES INSIPIDUS

Hereditary nephrogenic (vasopressin-resistant) diabetes insipidus is most often caused by X-linked mutations in the *AVPR2* gene that encodes the vasopressin V_2 receptor. Autosomal (recessive and dominant) forms of NDI occur less commonly due to mutations of the *AQP2* gene that codes for the collecting tubule water channel protein, aquaporin-2. Affected children often have a profound impairment in maximal urinary concentrating capacity, which rarely exceeds 100 mOsm/kg H_2O. Genetic counseling and mutation testing are available.

Acquired NDI is observed in numerous conditions including sickle cell anemia, chronic pyelonephritis, hypokalemia, hypercalcemia, Fanconi syndrome, obstructive uropathy, chronic renal insufficiency, and lithium treatment.

The symptoms of NDI include polyuria and polydipsia. In severe cases, water intake is preferred to formula, leading to failure to thrive. In some children, particularly if the solute intake is unrestricted, adjustment to an elevated serum osmolality may develop. Children with genetic NDI are particularly susceptible to episodes of dehydration, fever, vomiting, and hypernatremia when access to free water is limited.

The diagnosis can be suspected on the basis of a history of polydipsia and polyuria. The family history may be informative in hereditary cases while a review of the patient's medical history, medications, and serum chemistries can help identify a source of acquired NDI. The diagnosis is confirmed by performing a water deprivation test, during which time serum and urine osmolality are assessed and either arginine vasopressin or desmopressin administered to assess tubular response. When hereditary NDI is suspected, it is imperative that a water deprivation test be performed in the hospital in a controlled setting. Due to the severe concentrating defect, restricting water intake overnight at home in such children can lead to severe intravascular volume depletion and hyperosmolality. In addition to hyperglycemia, the differential diagnosis of polydipsia and polyuria includes primary polydipsia, which occurs in children as young as infancy.

In infants with NDI, it is usually best to allow water as demanded and to restrict salt intake. Caregivers must be aware of the risks of dehydration and hypernatremia if fluid intake is restricted either due to lack of provision by the caregiver or inability to keep fluids down (eg, vomiting). A low-salt diet limits the amount of urine that must be produced for daily solute excretion. Due to the need for high-volume free-water intake, caloric intake may be limited and affected children often benefit from routine follow-up with a renal

dietitian. Treatment with hydrochlorothiazide decreases urine volume by limiting the amount of free water delivered to the distal nephron for excretion. Prostaglandin inhibitors such as indomethacin are efficacious by decreasing renal blood flow, thereby diminishing GFR, and by preventing reclamation of the AQP2 water channel from the apical membrane of the collecting duct cell. Prostaglandin inhibitors, however, are associated with risk of gastritis/ulceration.

Bockenhauer D, Bichet DG: Urinary concentration: different ways to open and close the tap. Pediatr Nephrol 2014;29(8): 1297–1303 [PMID: 23736674].

Wong LM, Man SS: Water deprivation test in children with polyuria. J Pediatr Endocrinol Metab 2012;25(9–10):869–874 [PMID: 23426815].

NEPHROLITHIASIS

Renal calculi in children may result from products of hereditary errors of metabolism, such as cystine in cystinuria, glycine in hyperglycinuria, urates in Lesch-Nyhan syndrome, and oxalates in primary hyperoxaluria. Stones in children are most often calcium oxalate and calcium phosphate in composition, resulting most commonly from hypercalciuria or hypocitraturia. These diagnoses are best established via 24-hour urine collection to assess for common biochemical risk factors for stone formation. Large stones are quite often seen in children with spina bifida who have paralyzed lower limbs or in any situation where immobilization promotes calcium mobilization from the bones or there is recurrent UTI with urease-producing organisms (struvite calculi). Treatment is focused on the primary condition, if possible. Most cases are initially addressed with attention toward maintaining optimal hydration and targeting the inciting cause of stone formation with appropriate medical therapy. Surgical removal of stones or lithotripsy should be considered for obstruction, intractable severe pain, and chronic infection.

Tasian GE, Copelovitch L: Evaluation and medical management of kidney stones in children. J Urol 2014;192(5):1329–1336 [PMID: 24960469].

Cystinuria

Cystinuria is primarily an abnormality of amino acid transport across both the enteric and proximal renal tubular epithelium. There are at least three biochemical types. In the first type, the bowel transport of basic amino acids and cystine is impaired, but transport of cysteine is not impaired. In the renal tubule, basic amino acids are again rejected by the tubule, but cystine absorption appears to be normal. The reason for cystinuria remains obscure. Heterozygous individuals have no aminoaciduria. The second type is similar to the first except that heterozygous individuals excrete excess cystine and lysine in the urine, and cystine transport in the bowel is normal. In the third type, only the nephron is involved. The only clinical manifestations are related to stone formation: ureteral colic, dysuria, hematuria, proteinuria, and secondary UTI. Urinary excretion of cystine, lysine, arginine, and ornithine is increased.

The most reliable way to prevent stone formation is to maintain a constantly high free-water clearance. This involves generous fluid intake. Alkalinization of the urine is helpful. If these measures do not prevent significant renal lithiasis, the use of tiopronin is recommended.

Sumorok N, Goldfarb DS: Update on cystinuria. Curr Opin Nephrol Hypertens 2013;22(4):427–431 [PMID: 23666417].

Primary Hyperoxaluria

Oxalate in humans is derived from the oxidative deamination of glycine to glyoxylate, the serine-glycolate pathway, and from ascorbic acid. At least two enzymatic blocks have been described. Type I is a deficiency of liver-specific peroxisomal alanine–glyoxylate aminotransferase. Type II is glyoxylate reductase deficiency. Recently a type III primary hyperoxaluria has been described in association with increased mitochondrial 4-hydroxy-2-oxoglutarate aldolase activity; this type appears to be milder than types I or II.

Excess oxalate combines with calcium to form insoluble deposits in the kidneys, lungs, and other tissues, beginning during childhood. The joints are occasionally involved, but the main effect is on the kidneys, where progressive oxalate deposition leads to fibrosis and eventual renal failure.

A low-oxalate diet with normal calcium intake and high fluid intake is recommended. High-dose pyridoxine can be administered in type I primary hyperoxaluria as it is a cofactor for the defective pathway, but the overall prognosis is poor, with half of patients developing ESRD by 15 years of age. Renal transplantation is not very successful because of destruction of the transplant kidney with continued oxalate overproduction. However, encouraging results have been obtained with concomitant liver transplantation that corrects the metabolic defect. Types II and III primary hyperoxaluria appear to have better long-term renal outcomes.

Secondary hyperoxaluria with associated urolithiasis can be a consequence of severe ileal disease or ileal resection due to excessive absorption of dietary oxalate.

URINARY TRACT INFECTIONS

It is estimated that 8% of girls and 2% of boys will acquire urinary tract infections (UTIs) in childhood. Girls older than 6 months have UTIs far more commonly than boys, whereas uncircumcised boys younger than 3 months have more UTIs than girls. Circumcision reduces the risk of UTI in boys. The density of distal urethral and periurethral bacterial colonization with uropathogenic bacteria correlates with the risk of UTI in children. Most UTIs are ascending infections. Specific adhesins present on the fimbria of uropathogenic bacteria allow colonization of the uroepithelium in the urethra and bladder and increase the likelihood of UTI. The organisms most commonly responsible for UTI are fecal flora, most frequently *E coli* (> 85%), *Klebsiella*, *Proteus*, other gram-negative bacteria, and, less frequently, *Enterococcus* or coagulase-negative staphylococci.

▶ Pathogenesis

Dysfunctional voiding, which is uncoordinated relaxation of the urethral sphincter during voiding, leads to incomplete emptying of the bladder, increasing the risk of bacterial colonization. Similarly, any condition that interferes with complete emptying of the bladder, such as constipation, VUR, urinary tract obstruction, or neurogenic bladder, increases the risk of UTI. Poor perineal hygiene, structural abnormalities of the urinary tract, catheterization, instrumentation of the urinary tract, and sexual activity increase the risk as well.

The inflammatory response to pyelonephritis may produce renal parenchymal scars. Such scars in infancy and childhood may contribute to hypertension, renal disease, and renal failure later in life.

▶ Clinical Findings

A. Symptoms and Signs

Newborns and infants with UTI have nonspecific signs, including fever, hypothermia, jaundice, poor feeding, irritability, vomiting, failure to thrive, and sepsis. Strong, foul-smelling or cloudy urine may be noted. Preschool children may have abdominal or flank pain, vomiting, fever, urinary frequency, dysuria, urgency, or enuresis. School-aged children commonly have classic signs of cystitis (frequency, dysuria, and urgency) or pyelonephritis (fever, vomiting, and flank pain). Costovertebral tenderness is unusual in young children, but may be demonstrated by school-aged children. Physical examination should include attention to blood pressure determination, abdominal examination, and a genitourinary examination. Urethritis, poor perineal hygiene, herpes simplex virus infection, or other genitourinary infections may be apparent on examination.

B. Laboratory Findings

Screening urinalysis indicates pyuria (> 5 WBCs/hpf) in most children with UTI, but some children can have sterile pyuria without UTI. White cells from the urethra or vagina may be present in urine or white cells may be in the urine because of a renal inflammatory process. The leukocyte esterase test correlates well with pyuria, but has a similar false-positive rate. The detection of urinary nitrite by dipstick is highly correlated with enteric organisms being cultured from urine.

Most young children (70%) with UTI have negative nitrite tests, however. They empty their bladders frequently, and it requires several hours for bacteria to convert ingested nitrates to nitrite in the bladder.

The gold standard for diagnosis remains the culture of a properly collected urine specimen. Collection of urine for urinalysis and culture is difficult in children due to frequent contamination of the sample. In toilet-trained, cooperative, older children, a midstream, clean-catch method is usually satisfactory. Although cleaning of the perineum does not improve specimen quality, straddling of the toilet to separate the labia in girls, retraction of the foreskin in boys, and collecting midstream urine significantly reduce contamination. In infants and younger children, bladder catheterization or suprapubic collection is necessary in most cases to avoid contaminated samples. Bagged urine specimens are helpful only if negative. Specimens that are not immediately cultured should be refrigerated and kept cold during transport. Any growth is considered significant from a suprapubic culture. Quantitative recovery of 10^5 cfu/mL or greater is considered significant from clean-catch specimens, and 10^4–10^5 is considered significant from catheterized specimens. Usually, the recovery of multiple organisms indicates contamination.

Asymptomatic bacteriuria is detected in 0.5%–1.0% of children who are screened with urine culture. Asymptomatic bacteriuria, as seen commonly in children requiring chronic bladder catheterization, is believed to represent colonization of the urinary tract with nonuropathogenic bacteria. Treatment in such cases may increase the risk of symptomatic UTI by eliminating nonpathogenic colonization. Screening urine cultures in asymptomatic children are, therefore, generally discouraged.

C. Imaging

Because congenital urologic abnormalities increase the risk of UTI, a renal ultrasound, which is a noninvasive study, is recommended for children with UTI. The finding of significant hydronephrosis or other concerning urinary tract abnormalities on screening ultrasound warrants further imaging. A voiding cystourethrogram is no longer routinely recommended following first UTI in childhood, although the sensitivity of the renal ultrasound for detection of significant VUR varies widely in medical literature. VUR, a congenital abnormality present in about 1% of the population beyond infancy, is graded using the international scale (I—reflux into ureter; II—reflux to the kidneys; III—reflux to kidneys with dilation of ureter only; IV—reflux with dilation of ureter and mild blunting of renal calyces; V—reflux with dilation of ureter and blunting of renal calyces). Reflux is detected in 30%–50% of children presenting with a UTI at 1 year of age and younger. The natural history of reflux is to improve, and 80% of reflux of grades I, II, or III will resolve or significantly improve within 3 years following detection.

Significant debate exists in the literature regarding appropriate radiographic imaging for UTI and best management of VUR, including indications for and value of surgical intervention and/or prophylactic antibiotics.

▶ Treatment

A. Antibiotic Therapy

Management of UTI is influenced by clinical assessment. Very young children (age < 3 months) and children with dehydration, toxicity, or sepsis continue to be admitted to the hospital and treated with parenteral antimicrobials. Older infants and children who are not seriously ill can be treated as outpatients. Initial antimicrobial therapy is based on prior history of infection and antimicrobial use, as well as presumed location of the infection in the urinary tract.

Most uncomplicated cystitis can be treated with amoxicillin, trimethoprim-sulfamethoxazole, or a first-generation cephalosporin. These antimicrobials are concentrated in the lower urinary tract, and high cure rates are common. There is significant variation in rates of antimicrobial resistance, so knowledge of the rates in the local community is important. More seriously ill children are initially treated parenterally with a third-generation cephalosporin or less commonly aminoglycoside. The initial antimicrobial choice is adjusted after culture and susceptibility results are known. The recommended duration of antimicrobial therapy for uncomplicated cystitis is 7–10 days. For sexually mature teenagers with cystitis, fluoroquinolones such as ciprofloxacin and levofloxacin for 3 days are effective and cost-effective. Short-course therapy of cystitis is not recommended in children, because differentiating upper and lower tract disease may be difficult and higher failure rates are reported in most studies of short-course therapy.

Acute pyelonephritis is usually treated for 10 days. In nontoxic children older than 3 months of age who are not vomiting, oral treatment with an appropriate agent can be used. In sicker children, parenteral therapy may be required initially. Most of these children can complete therapy orally once symptomatic improvement has occurred. A repeat urine culture 24–48 hours after beginning therapy is not needed if the child is improving and doing well.

B. Prophylactic Antimicrobials

Selected children with frequently recurring UTI may benefit from prophylactic antimicrobials. In children with high-grade VUR, prophylactic antimicrobials may be beneficial in reducing UTI, as an alternative to surgical correction, or in the interval prior to surgical therapy. Some experts recommend surgical correction of higher-grade reflux, particularly grade V. Trimethoprim—sulfamethoxazole and nitrofurantoin are approved for prophylaxis. The use of broader-spectrum antimicrobials leads to colonization and infection with resistant strains.

Children with dysfunctional voiding may benefit from prophylactic antimicrobials; however, addressing the underlying dysfunctional voiding is most important.

Awais M, Rehman A, Baloch NU, Khan F, Khan N: Evaluation and management of recurrent urinary tract infections in children: state of the art. Expert Rev Anti Infect Ther 2015;13(2):209–231 [PMID: 25488064].

Subcommittee on Urinary Tract Infection, Steering Committee on Quality Improvement and Management, Roberts KB: Urinary tract infection: clinical practice guidelines for the diagnosis and management of the initial UTI in febrile infants and children 2 to 24 months. Pediatrics 2011;128(3):595–610 [PMID: 21873693].

▼ QA/QI IN PEDIATRIC NEPHROLOGY

The *North American Pediatric Renal Trials & Collaborative Study* (NAPRTCS) (www.naprtcs.org) has collected clinical information on children undergoing kidney transplant since 1987 and expanded the registry in 1994 to include patients with CKD and dialysis. Since the first data analysis in 1989, NAPRTCS reports have documented marked improvements in outcomes after kidney transplantation in addition to identifying factors associated with both favorable and poor outcomes. Since 2009, NAPRTCS data have been used as a source of benchmarking for pediatric nephrology centers, providing center-specific outcomes for CKD, dialysis, and transplant patients for comparison with national statistics.

The *Standardized Care to Improve Outcomes in Pediatric ESRD* (SCOPE) *Collaborative* helps pediatric dialysis centers minimize dialysis-related infections in peritoneal dialysis and hemodialysis patients through encouragement of multi-center adherence to recommended best practices. As of 2018, SCOPE has demonstrated a 41% reduction in peritonitis rates and 47.5% reduction in hemodialysis-associated bloodstream infections.

Since 1997, the National Kidney Foundation (NKF) (https://www.kidney.org) has published clinical practice guidelines in nephrology known as KDOQI—Kidney Disease Outcomes Quality Initiative. There are numerous guidelines addressing the best practice care of patients with CKD.

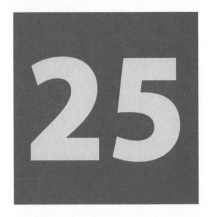

Neurologic & Muscular Disorders

Ricka Messer, MD, PhD

Teri L. Schreiner, MD, MPH

Diana Walleigh, MD

Michele L. Yang, MD

Jan A. Martin, MD

Scott Demarest, MD

NEUROLOGIC ASSESSMENT & NEURODIAGNOSTICS

HISTORY & EXAMINATION

History

Even in this era of increasingly sophisticated neurodiagnostic testing, the assessment and diagnosis of a child with a possible neurologic disorder still hinges on a detailed history and examination. The standard pediatric history and physical examination are presented in Chapter 9. In particular, the temporal progression of the neurologic signs and symptoms (acute vs chronic, progressive vs static, episodic vs continuous) can direct the evaluation. Episodic events, such as headaches or seizures, warrant emphasis on the symptoms preceding, during, and succeeding the event. Spells can also be videotaped, allowing the examiner to observe important details. Both acute and chronic neurologic symptoms may be associated with other organ system involvement, such as joint pain, changes in appetite or bowel/bladder habits, or a preceding viral illness. Birth history should include assessment of fetal movement and whether the infant was breech or vertex. A thorough past medical history and family history can illuminate risk factors for certain neurologic disorders. Social history should include school performance, preferred activities, and travel history.

Neurologic Examination

A general physical examination is essential in any neurologic assessment. Growth parameters and head circumference should be charted (see Chapter 3). A developmental assessment, often with an appropriate screening tool, is fundamental for every neurologic evaluation of an infant or young child (see Chapter 3 for details of developmental landmarks and example screening tools). The specifics of the neurologic examination are determined by the age of the child and the ability to cooperate with the examination. Expected infant reflexes and other age-related examination findings are included in Chapter 2. The hallmark of neurologic diagnosis is *localization*—determining where within the nervous system the "lesion" is located. While not all childhood neurologic disorders are easily localized, the part of the nervous system involved—for example, central versus neuromuscular—can often guide further evaluation and diagnosis.

Table 25–1 outlines components of the neurologic examination—mental status, cranial nerves, motor (including tone, muscle bulk, and strength), reflexes, sensation, coordination, and gait. Much of the examination of the frightened or active child is, by necessity, observational, and the examiner must capitalize on moments of opportunity while maintaining a systematic approach to avoid overlooking a key component. Playing games engages a toddler or preschooler; activities such as throwing a ball, stacking blocks, jumping, running, counting, and drawing (circles, lines) can reduce anxiety and allow assessment of motor coordination, balance, and handedness. In the older child, "casual" conversation can reveal both language and cognitive competence.

DIAGNOSTIC TESTING

Electroencephalography

Electroencephalography (EEG) is a noninvasive method for recording neuronal electrical activity. EEG background patterns vary by both age (infant, toddler, or adolescent) and clinical state (awake, drowsy, or asleep). The EEG has its greatest clinical applicability in the evaluation of seizure disorders. An EEG may demonstrate "epileptiform activity," interictal patterns that can indicate a general risk for seizures, or in some cases, can be diagnostic for a particular type of epilepsy, such as the hypsarrhythmia pattern seen in infantile spasms (West syndrome) or generalized 3-Hz spike-wave activity seen in childhood absence epilepsy. EEG also can be

Table 25–1. Neurologic examination: toddler age and up.

Category	Operation	Assesses
Mental status	Level of consciousness; level of awareness; orientation, language, development/cognition; affect	Cortical and subcortical pathways, executive functioning
Cranial nerves	CN I: Smell (usually omitted) CN II: Pupillary light reflex (sensory), visual acuity, visual fields, fundi CN III, IV, VI: Pupillary light reflex (motor), eye opening, extraocular movements, convergence CN V: Facial sensation (upper, middle, lower; V_1, V_2, V_3); muscles of mastication (clench jaw) CN VII: Upper—eye closure, brow raise; Lower—smile, grimace, show teeth CN VIII: Finger rub at each ear; Rinne and Weber tests when appropriate CN IX, X: Palate elevation (gag—often omitted); strength of vocalizations CN XI: Head turn (sternocleidomastoid) and shoulder shrug (trapezius) CN XII: Tongue protrusion and bulk	Cortical pathways, brainstem (midbrain, pons, medulla), and peripheral cranial nerves
Motor	Tone: head control and body posture, passive range of motion of the limbs Muscle bulk: palpate for atrophy, pseudohypertrophy, or fibrosis Strength: proximal (shoulder abduction/hip flexion) to distal (finger movement, ankle movement). Grading: 0 = no movement, 1 = trace movement, 2 = movement in lateral plane but not against gravity, 3 = against gravity, 4 (4−/4/4+) = some resistance with mild weakness, 5 = normal strength	Upper motor neurons: motor cortex, corticospinal tracts → Lesions cause spastic tone Lower motor neurons: anterior horn cells in the spinal cord, spinal nerve roots, peripheral nerves → Lesions cause flaccid tone
Reflexes	Tendon stretch reflexes: biceps, triceps, brachioradialis, patella, Achilles. Grading: 0 = reflex absent; 1 = reflex present only with augmentation maneuver; 2 = reflex present without spread to adjacent muscle groups (if movement is large amplitude, can describe as "brisk"); 3 = reflex spreads to adjacent muscle groups; 4 = clonus Cutaneous sensory reflexes: abdominal, cremasteric	Corticospinal tracts → Lesions cause hyperreflexia Spinal cord and peripheral nerves → Lesions cause hyporeflexia
Gait	Assess casual stance for excessive wide base. Walking, running, walking on heels/toes, tandem gait (forward, backward)	Cerebellum (vermis), spinocerebellar tracts, sensory pathways, others
Coordination (truncal, limb)	Smooth eye pursuit; reaching for objects; finger-to-nose and heel-to-shin movements; rapid alternating movements. Other abnormal movements should be noted.	Cerebellum (hemisphere or vermis), sensory pathways, others
Sensory	Light touch, vibration (with tuning fork), proprioception. temperature, pinprick Romberg test: truncal balance and recovery Cortical: two-point discrimination, object identification	Peripheral nerves Posterior columns Spinothalamic tracts Thalamus Parietal lobe

very useful in the evaluation of altered mental status and in some encephalopathies.

EEG is rarely diagnostic in isolation, but rather is only one part of the child's clinical picture. Routine EEG, obtained in the outpatient setting, is brief (<30 minutes). Therefore, events of interest are usually not recorded. EEG may be difficult to obtain or interpret if the child is unable to cooperate, but sedating medications, such as barbiturates and benzodiazepines, may alter the EEG, confuse interpretation, and decrease the likelihood of recording abnormalities. In addition, children without epilepsy may also have an abnormal EEG. EEG findings such as those occasionally seen in migraine, learning disabilities, or behavior disorders are often nonspecific and do not reflect structural brain damage or dysfunction. When questions arise regarding the clinical significance of EEG findings, consultation with a pediatric neurologist is appropriate.

Prolonged ambulatory EEG (obtained over 24–72 hours) can be useful in capturing and assessing events to ascertain if they are due to epileptic seizures. Likewise, recording a full montage EEG during nocturnal polysomnograms can help differentiate nonepileptic sleep-related events from nocturnal epileptic seizures.

Prolonged or continuous inpatient EEG recordings are useful in the assessment of patients with altered mental status, suspected nonconvulsive status epilepticus, and drug-induced coma, as well as patients with hypoxic ischemic brain injury or traumatic brain injury.

A continuous video-EEG recording, obtained in conjunction with inpatient admission to an epilepsy monitoring unit (EMU), allows assessment of the patient with medically intractable epilepsy. Localization of the seizure focus by EEG recording during seizures can determine candidacy for surgical resection or other surgical procedures. Correlating video with EEG has also proven useful in characterizing spells that may or may not be seizures, such as staring.

Evoked Potentials

Visual-, auditory-, or somatosensory-evoked potentials (evoked responses) can be obtained by repetitive stimulation of the retina by light flashes, the cochlea by sounds, or a nerve by galvanic stimuli. These stimuli result in cortical responses recorded from the scalp surface. The presence or absence of evoked potential waves and their latencies from the time of the stimuli can be useful in some specific situations, such as the use of visual-evoked potentials (VEP) in patients with optic neuritis, multiple sclerosis (MS), or other demyelinating diseases, as well as somatosensory-evoked potentials (SSEP) in the monitoring of patients during spinal surgery for rapid identification of potentially reversible spinal cord injury. However, evoked potentials are not routinely obtained for evaluation of neurologic disorders. One important exception is the use of brainstem auditory-evoked responses (BAER), which are now considered standard for screening hearing in neonates.

Lumbar Puncture

Cerebrospinal fluid (CSF) can be obtained by inserting a small-gauge needle through the L3–L4 intervertebral space into the thecal sac, while the patient is lying in a lateral recumbent position. Radiographic guidance and sedation may be necessary in some patients. After an opening pressure is measured, fluid is removed to examine for evidence of infection, inflammation, or metabolic disorders (Table 25–2). Special staining techniques can be used for mycobacterial and fungal infections, and further testing can be performed for specific viral agents, antibody titer determinations, cytopathologic studies, lactate and pyruvate concentrations, amino acid levels, and neurotransmitter analysis. Lumbar puncture is imperative when bacterial meningitis is suspected. However, papilledema or focal neurologic deficits are relative contraindications to lumbar puncture prior to imaging, due to the risk of precipitating tentorial or tonsillar herniation.

Genetic/Metabolic Testing

The diagnostic yield of genetic and metabolic evaluation of children with global developmental delay or intellectual disability (GDD/ID) depends on the specific testing done. Chromosomal microarray testing is diagnostic in almost 8%

of children with GDD/ID and in other appropriate clinical situations; tests for metabolic disorders have a yield of up to 5%. Thus, focused assessments for genetic disorders should be part of the evaluation of the child with GDD/ID.

Electromyography & Nerve Conduction Velocity Testing

Electromyography (EMG) and nerve conduction study (NCS) testing can assess for disorders of the motor neuron, nerve, neuromuscular junction, and muscle.

NCS is performed by applying small current to peripheral nerves and calculating the response amplitude and conduction velocity. EMG requires placement of recording electrodes into selected muscles to record spontaneous and volitional electrical activity of skeletal muscle tissue. For more details, refer to section within this chapter entitled Disorders of Childhood Affecting Muscles.

PEDIATRIC NEURORADIOLOGIC PROCEDURES

Computed Tomography

Computed Tomography (CT) scanning allows visualization of intracranial contents by obtaining a series of cross-sectional X-ray images. Current scanning techniques allow rapid acquisition of data, often without sedation. CT scanning has high sensitivity (88%–96% of lesions larger than 1–2 cm can be seen), but low specificity (tumor, infection, or infarct may look the same). CT is particularly useful for assessment of head trauma, allowing excellent visualization of intracranial blood, skull fractures, and the ventricular system, as well as evaluating for intracranial calcifications, such as those associated with intrauterine infections or tubers in patients with tuberous sclerosis complex. Intravenous injection of iodized contrast media may be helpful to visualize the arteries (CTA) or veins (CTV) but is typically not helpful for assessment of the brain parenchyma. When ordering a CT scan of the head, as well as repeated CT scans, consider radiation exposure. A single CT scan of the head is approximately 2 millisieverts (mSv; typical chest X-ray PA view = 0.02 mSv), which equates to ~8 months of exposure to the naturally occurring radiation in the environment. The risk of malignancy is thought to be 1 brain tumor per 10,000 patients in the 10 years following CT exposure, and the lifetime risk of brain tumor after head CT is likely higher, particularly in younger children.

Magnetic Resonance Imaging

Magnetic resonance imaging (MRI) provides high-resolution images of soft tissues by detecting the response (resonance) of hydrogen protons to electromagnetic radiation. The strength of MRI signals varies with the relationship of water to protein and lipid in tissue. MRI can provide information about the histological, physiological, and biochemical status

Table 25–2. Characteristics of cerebrospinal fluid in the normal child and in central nervous system infections and inflammatory conditions.

Condition	Initial Pressure (mm H$_2$0)	Appearance	Cells/μL	Protein (mg/dL)	Glucose (mg/dL)	Other Tests	Comments
Normal	<160	Clear	0–5 lymphocytes; first 3 mo, 1–3 PMNs; neonates, up to 30 lymphocytes, rare RBCs	15–35 (lumbar), 5–15 (ventricular); up to 150 (lumbar) for short time after birth; to 6 mo up to 65	50–80 (two-thirds of blood glucose); may be increased after seizure	CSF-IgG index[a] < 0.7[a], LDH 2–27 U/L	CSF protein in first month may be up to 170 mg/dL in small-for-date or premature infants; no increase in WBCs due to seizure
Bloody tap	Normal or low	Bloody (sometimes with clot)	One additional WBC/700 RBCs[b]; RBCs not created	One additional milligram per 800 RBCs[b]	Normal	RBC number should fall between 1st and 3rd tubes	Spin down fluid, supernatant will be clear and colorless[c]
Bacterial meningitis, acute	200–750+	Opalescent to purulent	Up to thousands, mostly PMNs; early, few cells	Up to hundreds	Decreased; may be none	Smear and culture mandatory; LDH > 24 U/L	Very early, glucose may be normal; PCR meningococci and pneumococci in plasma, CSF may aid diagnosis Elevated CSF lactate, IL-8, and TNF may correlate with prognosis
Bacterial meningitis, partially treated	Usually increased	Clear or opalescent	Usually increased; PMNs usually predominate	Elevated	Normal or decreased	LDH usually > 24 U/L; PCR may still be positive	Smear and culture may be negative if antibiotics have been in use
Tuberculous meningitis	150–750+	Opalescent; fibrin web or pellicle	250–500, mostly lymphocytes; early, more PMNs	45–500; parallels cell count; increases over time	Decreased; may be none	Smear for acid-fast organism; CSF culture and inoculation; PCR	Consider AIDS, a common comorbidity of tuberculosis
Fungal meningitis	Increased	Variable; often clear	10–500; early, more PMNs; then mostly lymphocytes	Elevated and increasing	Decreased	India ink preparations, cryptococcal antigen, PCR, culture, inoculations, immunofluorescence tests	Often superimposed in patients who are debilitated or on immunosuppressive therapy

(Continued)

Table 25–2. Characteristics of cerebrospinal fluid in the normal child and in central nervous system infections and inflammatory conditions. (*Continued*)

Condition	Initial Pressure (mm H₂O)	Appearance	Cells/µL	Protein (mg/dL)	Glucose (mg/dL)	Other Tests	Comments
Aseptic meningoencephalitis (viral meningitis, or parameningeal disease); encephalitis is similar	Normal or slightly increased	Clear unless cell count > 300/µL	None to a few hundred, mostly lymphocytes; PMNs predominate early	20–125	Normal; may be low in mumps, herpes, or other viral infections	CSF, stool, blood, throat washings for viral cultures; LDH < 28 U/L; PCR for HSV, CMV, EBV, enterovirus, etc	Acute and convalescent antibody titers for some viruses; in mumps, up to 1000 lymphocytes; serum amylase often elevated; up to 1000 cells present in enteroviral infection
Parainfectious encephalomyelitis (ADEM)	80–450, usually increased	Usually clear	0–50+, mostly lymphocytes; lower numbers, even 0, in MS	15–75	Normal	CSF-IgG index, oligoclonal bands variable; in MS, moderate increase	No organisms; fulminant cases resemble bacterial meningitis
Polyneuritis	Normal and occasionally increased	Early: normal; late: xanthochromic if protein high	Normal; occasionally slight increase	Early: normal; late: 45–1500	Normal	CSF-IgG index may be increased; oligoclonal bands variable	Try to find cause (viral infections, toxins, lupus, diabetes, etc)
Meningeal carcinomatosis	Often elevated	Clear to opalescent	Cytologic identification of tumor cells	Often mildly to moderately elevated	Often depressed	Cytology	Seen with leukemia, medulloblastoma, meningeal melanosis, histiocytosis X
Brain abscess	Normal or increased	Usually clear	5–500 in 80%; mostly PMNs	Usually slightly increased	Normal; occasionally decreased	Imaging study of brain (MRI)	Cell count related to proximity to meninges; findings as in purulent meningitis if abscess ruptures

ADEM, acute disseminated encephalomyelitis; AIDS, acquired immunodeficiency syndrome; CMV, cytomegalovirus; CSF, cerebrospinal fluid; EBV, Epstein-Barr virus; HSV, herpes simplex virus; IL-8, interleukin 8; LDH, lactate dehydrogenase; MRI, magnetic resonance imaging; MS, multiple sclerosis; PCR, polymerase chain reaction; PMN, polymorphonuclear neutrophil; RBC, red blood cell; TNF, tumor necrosis factor; WBC, white blood cell.

[a]CSF-IgG index = (CSF IgG/serum IgG)/(CSF albumin/serum albumin).

[b]Many studies document pitfalls in using these ratios due to WBC lysis. Clinical judgment and repeat lumbar punctures may be necessary to rule out meningitis in this situation.

[c]CSF WBC (predicted) = CSF RBC × (blood WBC/blood RBC). O:P ratio = (observed CSF WBC)/(predicted CSF WBC). Also, do WBC:RBC ratio. If O:P ratio ≤ 0.01, and WBC:RBC ratio ≤ 1:100, meningitis is absent.

of tissues, as well as gross anatomic features. Sedation is usually necessary for MRI in children who are unable to lie still for 45 minutes to avoid movement artifact. Abbreviated MRI protocols are being increasingly used to rule out hemorrhage and hydrocephalus, sparing the patient from unnecessary ionizing radiation exposure from a CT.

MRI is used to assess a wide variety of neurologic disorders such as tumors, edema, ischemic and hemorrhagic lesions, vascular disorders, inflammation, demyelination, CNS infection, metabolic disorders, and degenerative processes. Because bone does not produce artifact in the images, the posterior fossa contents can be studied far better with MRI than with CT scans, allowing imaging of the brainstem, blood vessels, and cranial nerves.

Magnetic resonance angiography (MRA) or venography (MRV) is used to visualize large extra- and intracranial blood vessels, though they are not as sensitive as conventional angiography. Perfusion-weighted imaging and diffusion-weighted imaging (DWI) (measuring random motion of water molecules) are used to evaluate brain ischemic penumbra and cytotoxic edema in acute stroke, as well as toxic and metabolic brain disorders.

MR spectroscopy (MRS) assesses biochemical changes in CNS tissue, measuring signals of increased cellular activity and oxidative metabolism such as occur, for example, in brain tumors.

Newer functional MRI (fMRI) can localize various brain functions, such as language and motor activity, by assessing blood oxygenation changes in an area of interest during language or motor tasks. The axonal tracts of neurologic pathways, such as the optic radiations or motor system, can be identified using diffusion tensor imaging (DTI). These techniques generally require a team involving a neuropsychologist and radiologist to derive specific paradigms for testing and evaluation of imaging, as well as a cooperative patient.

Positron Emission Tomography

Positron emission tomography (PET) uses radiolabeled substrates such as intravenously administered fluorodeoxyglucose to measure the metabolic rate at given sites within the brain, producing three-dimensional reconstructions for localization of CNS function. PET is most often performed in the interictal state (during a seizure). The information is aligned with traditional CT scan, MRI, or SPECT (single-photon emission computerized tomography) to allow precise localization of the epileptogenic zone ("focus") of a patient's seizures, for example, in preoperative evaluation for epilepsy surgery.

Single-Photon Emission Computerized Tomography (SPECT Scans)

SPECT scans image cerebral blood flow using a radioactive tracer (typically technetium-99m), similar to CT. This allows virtual three-dimensional visualization of vascular blood flow. It is useful in assessment of patients for epilepsy surgery, aiding in identification of increased blood flow in a seizure focus during a seizure. In children with brain tumors, SPECT can help differentiate tumor recurrence from post-treatment changes, assessing the response to treatment, directing biopsy, and planning therapy. Regional cerebral blood flow can be assessed in children with strokes due to vascular stenosis and moyamoya syndrome.

Ultrasonography

Ultrasonography (US) allows assessment of brain structures quickly with easily portable equipment, without ionizing radiation, and at about one-fourth the cost of CT scanning. Sedation is usually not necessary, and the procedure can be repeated as often as needed without risk to the patient. The thin skull and the open anterior fontanel in neonates facilitate imaging of the brain to screen for intracranial hemorrhage, hydrocephalus, periventricular ischemic lesions, major brain and spine malformations, and calcifications. Once the fontanels start to close, this modality is no longer useful due to inability of ultrasound waves to penetrate bone.

Conventional Cerebral Angiography

Arteriography remains useful in the diagnosis of cerebrovascular disorders, particularly ischemic and hemorrhagic stroke, as well as potentially operable vascular malformations and brain tumors. Since cerebral angiography uses traditional X-ray to produce images, there is significant exposure to ionizing radiation, and the process also requires catheterization, typically via the femoral vessels.

Cakir B et al: Inborn errors of metabolisms presenting in childhood. J Neuroimaging 2011;21(2)e117–e133 [PMID: 21435076].

Dahmoush HM, Vossough A, Roberts TP: Pediatric high-field magnetic resonance imaging. Neuroimaging Clin N Am 2012;22:297–313 [PMID: 22548934].

Haslam, RHA: Clinical neurological examination of infants and children. Handbook of Clinical Neurology, Vol III (3rd series) Pediatric Neurology Part 1; 2013 [PMID: 23622147].

Michelson DJ, Shevell MI, Sherr EH, Moeschler JB, Gropman AL, Ashwal S: Evidence report: genetic and metabolic testing on children with global developmental delay: report of the Quality Standards Subcommittee of the American Academy of Neurology and the Practice Committee of the Child Neurology Society. Neurology 2011 Oct 25;77(17):1629–1635 [PMID: 21956720].

Pitt MC: Nerve conduction studies and needle EMG in very small children. Eur J Paediatr Neurol 2012;16:285–291 [PMID: 21840229].

Sables-Baus S, Robinson MV: Pediatric neurologic exam. Int Emerg Nurs 2011 Oct;19(4):199–205 [PMID: 21968413].

Yock-Corrales A, Barnett P: The role of imaging studies for evaluation of stroke in children. Pediatr Emerg Care 2011;27:966–974 [PMID: 21975501].

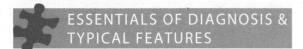

DISORDERS AFFECTING THE NERVOUS SYSTEM IN INFANTS & CHILDREN

ALTERED STATES OF CONSCIOUSNESS (COMA)

ESSENTIALS OF DIAGNOSIS & TYPICAL FEATURES

▶ Reduction or alteration in cognitive and affective mental functioning and in arousability or attentiveness.

▶ Acute onset.

Consciousness encompasses both the patient's level of wakefulness and the patient's ability to interact with the environment. The neurologic substrate for consciousness is the ascending reticular activating system (RAS), comprised of the reticular formation in the brainstem, thalamic intralaminar nuclei, and portions of the hypothalamus. Dysfunction of the cerebral cortex, especially bilateral lesions, can also cause coma.

▶ Clinical Findings

A. Symptoms and Signs

Many terms, including obtundation, lethargy, somnolence, stupor, and coma, are used to describe the continuum from fully alert and aware to complete unresponsiveness. Providers can use a scale, such as the Glasgow Coma Scale (Table 12–4), but they should also provide qualitative descriptions such as, "opens eyes with painful stimulus, but does not respond to voice." These descriptions help subsequent observers evaluate the severity of the disorder of consciousness (Table 25–3).

- *Coma* is defined by the complete absence of wakefulness and interaction with the environment for at least 1 hour. When coma persists, evaluation for the presence of sleep-wake cycles or absence of all brain function can further delineate the severity.

- *Persistent or permanent vegetative state* (PVS) denotes a chronic condition (persistent if > 4 weeks; permanent if > 3–12 months, depending on etiology) in which sleep-wake cycles are preserved, but the patient has no awareness of self or the environment. PVS is sometimes referred to as "wakefulness without awareness."

- *Minimally conscious state* (MCS) denotes patients who demonstrate sleep-wake cycles and some residual degree of interaction with the environment. For instance, these patients occasionally may have purposeful movements. Thus, MCS involves "partial preservation of consciousness."

- *Brain death* (death by neurologic criteria) refers to patients in coma who have cessation of all brain function, including cortical activity, brainstem reflexes, and spontaneous respirations.

B. Laboratory and Imaging Diagnostics

Medical causes account for 90% of cases of coma in children; structural causes comprise the remaining 10% (Table 25–4). If the cause of the coma is not obvious, emergency laboratory tests must be obtained, such as blood glucose, complete blood count, urine studies, pH and electrolytes (including bicarbonate), serum urea nitrogen, liver function tests, and ammonia. Urine, blood, and even gastric contents can be sent for toxin screens if the underlying cause is not obvious. Infection is a common cause (30%), and blood cultures and lumbar puncture are often necessary. In obscure cases of coma, additional testing might include oxygen and carbon dioxide partial pressures, serum and urine osmolality, porphyrins, lead, amino acids, and urine organic acids.

If severe head trauma, intracranial hemorrhage, or increased intracranial pressure is suspected, an emergency CT scan or MRI is necessary. CT is typically faster and superior to MRI for detecting small hemorrhages, but MRI is more sensitive in detecting stroke and anoxic brain injury. Bone windows on CT or skull radiographs may demonstrate skull fractures better. The absence of skull fracture does not rule out coma caused by closed head trauma, such as from abusive head trauma. Treatment of head injury associated with coma is discussed in detail in Chapter 12.

Table 25–3. The spectrum of consciousness/unconsciousness.

	Conscious	MCS	PVS	Coma	Brain Death
Awake?	Yes	Yes	Yes	No	No
Aware?	Yes	Partially	No	No	No
Motor responses?	Present	Present	Present	Absent	Absent
Brainstem reflexes?	Present	Present	Present	Present	Absent

MCS, minimally conscious state; PVS, persistent or permanent vegetative state.

Table 25–4. Some causes of coma in childhood.

Mechanism of Coma	Likely Cause	
	Newborn Infant	**Older Child**
Anoxia Asphyxia Respiratory obstruction Severe anemia	Birth asphyxia, HIE, meconium aspiration, infection (especially respiratory syncytial virus) Hydrops fetalis	CO poisoning Croup, tracheitis, epiglottitis Hemolysis, blood loss
Ischemia Cardiac Shock	Shunting lesions, hypoplastic left heart Asphyxia, sepsis	Shunting lesions, aortic stenosis, myocarditis, blood loss, infection
Head trauma (structural cause)	Birth contusion, hemorrhage, AHT	Falls, auto accidents, athletic injuries
Infection (**most common cause in childhood**)	Gram-negative meningitis, enterovirus, herpes encephalitis, sepsis	Bacterial meningitis, viral encephalitis, postinfectious encephalitis, sepsis, typhoid, malaria
Vascular (stroke, often of unknown cause)	Intraventricular hemorrhage, cerebral venous sinus thrombosis, perinatal arterial ischemic stroke	Vascular occlusion with congenital heart disease, head or neck trauma, childhood arterial ischemic stroke
Neoplasm (structural cause)	Rare this age. Choroid plexus papilloma with severe hydrocephalus	Brainstem glioma, increased pressure with posterior fossa tumors
Drugs (toxidrome)	Maternal sedatives; injected pudendal and paracervical analgesics	Overdose, salicylates, lithium, sedatives, psychotropic agents
Toxins (toxidrome)	Maternal sedatives or injections	Arsenic, CO, pesticides, mushrooms, lead
Epilepsy	Constant focal motor seizures, electrographic seizures without motor manifestations, medication side effect	Nonconvulsive or absence status epilepticus, postictal state, medication side effect
Hypoglycemia	Birth injury, diabetic progeny, toxemic progeny	Diabetes, "prediabetes," hypoglycemic agents
Increased intracranial pressure (metabolic or structural cause)	Anoxic brain injury, hydrocephalus, metabolic disorders (urea cycle; amino or organic acidurias)	Toxic encephalopathy, Reye syndrome, head trauma, tumor of posterior fossa
Hepatic causes	Hepatic failure, inborn metabolic errors in bilirubin conjugation	Hepatic failure, inborn errors of metabolism
Renal causes, hypertensive encephalopathy	Hypoplastic kidneys	Nephritis, acute (AGN) and chronic; uremia, uremic syndrome
Hypothermia, hyperthermia	Iatrogenic (therapeutic hypothermia)	Cold weather exposure, drowning; heat stroke
Hypercapnia	Congenital lung anomalies, bronchopulmonary dysplasia	Cystic fibrosis (hypercapnia, anoxia)
Electrolyte changes Hyper- or hyponatremia Hyper- or hypocalcemia Severe acidosis, lactic acidosis	Iatrogenic ($NaHCO_3$ use), salt poisoning (formula errors) SIADH, adrenogenital syndrome, dialysis (iatrogenic) Septicemia, metabolic errors	Diarrhea, dehydration Lactic acidosis Infection, diabetic coma, poisoning (eg, aspirin), hyperglycemic nonketotic coma

AGN, acute glomerulonephritis; AHT, abusive head trauma; CO, carbon monoxide; HIE, hypoxic-ischemic encephalopathy; SIADH, syndrome of inappropriate antidiuretic hormone secretion.
Modified with permission from Conn H, Conn R: *Current Diagnosis*, 5th ed. Philadelphia, PA: WB Saunders; 1977.

EEG can sometimes aid in diagnosing the cause of coma, such as with nonconvulsive status epilepticus, a specific abnormality (such as periodic lateralized epileptiform discharges seen with herpes encephalitis), or focal slowing (such as with stroke or cerebritis). EEG may correlate with the stage of coma and add prognostic information.

Differential Diagnosis

Conditions mistaken for coma:

- *Locked-in syndrome* describes patients who are conscious (awake and aware) but cannot demonstrate interactiveness with their environment due to a massive loss of motor function, typically from a lesion in the pons. Vertical eye movements may be preserved.

- *Akinetic-mutism* denotes a patient who is awake and aware, but does not speak, initiate movements, or follow commands, typically due to lesions of the frontal lobes.

- *Catatonia* refers to patients with abnormal alertness and awareness (though typically not completely absent) secondary to psychiatric illness. Patients often retain the ability to maintain trunk and limb postures.

Treatment

As with any emergency, the clinician must first stabilize the comatose child using the ABCs of resuscitation. Signs of intracranial pressure and impending brain herniation are another priority of the initial assessment. Bradycardia, high blood pressure, and irregular breathing (Cushing's Triad) or third nerve palsy (with the eye deviated down and out), or a "blown" pupil (large, fixed/unreactive pupil) indicate prompt neurosurgical consultation and head CT. Initial treatment of impending herniation includes elevating the head of the bed to 15–30 degrees and providing moderate hyperventilation. The use of mannitol, hypertonic saline, pharmacologic coma, hypothermia, and drainage of cerebrospinal fluid (CSF) are covered in detail in Chapter 14.

Prognosis

About 50% of children with nontraumatic causes of coma have a good outcome. Outcome can be successfully predicted at an early stage in approximately two-thirds of patients by assessing coma severity, extraocular movements, pupillary reactions, motor patterns, blood pressure, temperature, and seizure type. In patients with severe head trauma, a Glasgow Coma Scale ≤ 5, hypothermia, hyperglycemia, and coagulation disorders are factors associated with an increased risk of mortality. Other characteristics such as the need for assisted respiration, the presence of increased intracranial pressure, and the duration of coma are not significantly predictive.

Hirschberg R, Giacino JT: The vegetative and minimally conscious states: diagnosis, prognosis and treatment. Neurol Clin 2011;20:773–786 [PMID: 22032660].

Kirkham FJ, Ashwal S: Coma and brain death. Handb Clin Neurol 2013;111:43–61 [PMID: 23622150].

MacNeill EC, Vashist S: Approach to syncope and altered mental status. Pediatr Clin North Am 2013;60(5):1083–1106 [PMID: 24093897].

Nakagawa TA et al: Clinical Report-Guidelines for the determination of brain death in infants and children: an update of the 1987 taskforce recommendations. Pediatrics 2011;128(3):e720–e740 [PMID: 21873704].

SEIZURES & EPILEPSY

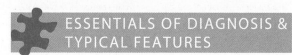

ESSENTIALS OF DIAGNOSIS & TYPICAL FEATURES

▶ Recurrent unprovoked seizures or a single seizure with an EEG and/or risk factors suggesting high risk for recurrent events.

▶ Often, interictal EEG changes.

A seizure is a sudden, transient disturbance of brain function, manifested by involuntary motor, sensory, autonomic, or psychic phenomena, alone or in any combination, often accompanied by alteration or loss of consciousness. Seizures can be caused by any factor that disturbs brain function. They may occur after a metabolic, traumatic, anoxic, or infectious insult to the brain (classified as symptomatic seizures), or spontaneously without prior known CNS insult. Genetic mutations are increasingly identified in many patients without prior known cause of seizures.

Epilepsy is defined as two seizures that are separated by at least 24 hours or a single seizure associated with a greater than 60% risk of recurrence or the diagnosis of an epilepsy syndrome. During childhood, the incidence is highest in the newborn period. Prevalence flattens out after age 10–15 years. The chance of having a second seizure after an initial unprovoked episode in a child is about 50%. The risk of recurrence after a second unprovoked seizure is 85%. Up to 70% of children with epilepsy will achieve seizure remission with their first appropriate medication.

Classification

The International League Against Epilepsy (ILAE) has established classifications of seizures and epilepsy syndromes. Seizures are classified as either focal, previously called partial (with suspected seizure onset that can be localized to one part of the brain), generalized (likely involving the whole brain or a network of the brain), or "unknown" if it is not clear if they are focal or generalized.

There are several types of generalized seizures that are recognized with the new classification: tonic-clonic, absence (typical, atypical, and with special features), myoclonic, myoclonic atonic, tonic, clonic, and atonic seizures. New nomenclature is suggested for focal seizures that is based on the presentation of the seizure. The description of the seizure is most beneficial with suggested terms such as "with or without alteration of awareness," "motor" vs "non motor (autonomic, emotional, or sensory)" seizure. Such descriptions allow better classification of seizures.

Epilepsy syndromes are defined by the nature of the seizures, age of onset, EEG findings, and other clinical factors. New terminology has been developed for epilepsy syndromes to reflect our growing understanding of underlying etiology. The newest classification allows for a hierarchical classification approach identical to the seizure guidelines. In parallel, patients may have an etiologic diagnosis (structural, genetic, infectious, etc) and may have comorbid diagnoses (ADHD, depression, anxiety, etc). Tools to aid in the classification of seizures and epilepsy syndromes can be found at the International League Against Epilepsy website https://www.ilae.org/.

1. Seizures & Epilepsy in Childhood

Characterizing the seizure and subsequent epilepsy syndrome is necessary for accurate diagnosis, which will determine the nature of further evaluation and treatment. This also assists with prognostication (Table 25–5) and research of specific syndromes.

▶ Clinical Findings

A. Symptoms and Signs

Seizures are stereotyped paroxysmal clinical events; the key to diagnosis is usually in the history. Not all paroxysmal events are epileptic. A detailed description of seizure onset is important in determining if an event is a seizure and if there is a localized onset (focal seizure). Events prior to, during, and after the seizure need to be ascertained. Although observers often initially recall little except generalized convulsive activity because of its dramatic appearance, careful detailed questions can lead to a better description of the event and situation in which it occurred. An aura may precede the clinically apparent seizure. The patient may describe a feeling of fear, numbness or tingling in the fingers, or bright lights in one visual field. The specific symptoms may help define the location of seizure onset (eg, déjà vu suggests temporal lobe onset). Often, the child does not recall or cannot define the aura, though the family may note alterations in behavior at the onset. Video of events have been extremely useful.

Postictal states can be helpful in diagnosis. After many focal seizures and most generalized convulsive seizures, postictal sleep typically occurs. However, postictal changes are not seen after generalized absence, myoclonic, or atonic seizures.

It also helps to determine if there was a loss of speech after the seizure (suggesting a left hemisphere involvement) or if the patient was able to respond and speak in short order. The parent may report lateralized motor activity (eg, the child's eyes may deviate to one side or the child may experience dystonic posturing of a limb). Motor activity without impaired awareness supports the diagnosis of focal seizures, as does impaired awareness and automatisms previously defined as a "complex partial seizure."

In contrast, generalized convulsive seizures usually manifest with acute loss of consciousness, with generalized motor activity. Tonic posturing, tonic-clonic activity, or myoclonus may occur. In children with generalized absence seizures, behavioral arrest may be associated with automatisms such as blinking, chewing, or hand movements, making it difficult to differentiate between absence seizures and focal seizures.

Frequently, the child presenting with a presumed unprovoked first seizure has experienced unrecognized seizures before the event that brings the child to medical attention. Focal, atonic, myoclonic, and absence seizures may not be recognized except in retrospect. Thus, careful questioning regarding prior events is important. Events that are perceived as seizures but are not epileptic, such as syncopal events, can also be determined by careful questioning.

B. Diagnostic Evaluation

Many factors determine the extent and urgency of the diagnostic evaluation, such as the child's age, the severity and type of seizure, whether the child is ill or injured, and the clinician's suspicion about the underlying cause. Seizures in early infancy often have an underlying cause that is structural, genetic, or metabolic and will guide prognosis and management. Therefore, the younger the child, the more extensive must be the diagnostic assessment.

Any child younger than 3 years with new onset of *unprovoked* seizures should be evaluated with an EEG and MRI, although the need is not emergent. EEG is very unlikely to yield clinically useful information in the child with a febrile seizure. Other diagnostic studies should be used selectively.

Metabolic abnormalities are seldom found in the well child with seizures. Unless there is a high clinical suspicion of serious medical conditions (eg, uremia, hyponatremia, hypocalcemia, and hypoglycemia), "routine" laboratory tests are typically not necessary. Special studies may be necessary in circumstances that suggest an acute systemic etiology for a seizure, for example, in the presence of apparent renal failure, sepsis, or substance abuse. Emergent imaging of the brain is usually not needed in the absence evidence of trauma or acute abnormalities on examination.

C. Electroencephalography

The limitations of EEG are considerable. A 20–30 minute routine EEG is useful primarily for defining interictal activity

Table 25–5. Seizures by age at onset, pattern, and preferred treatment.

Seizure Type Epilepsy Syndrome	Age at Onset	Clinical Manifestations	Causative Factors	EEG Pattern	Other Diagnostic Studies	Treatment and Comments
Neonatal seizures	Birth–2 wk	Can be any seizure type, can be very subtle.	Neurologic insults (hypoxia/ischemia; intracranial hemorrhage) present more in first 3 days or after 8th day; metabolic disturbances alone between 3rd and 8th days; hypoglycemia, hypocalcemia, hyper- and hyponatremia. Drug withdrawal. Pyridoxine dependency. Other metabolic disorders, CNS infections. Structural abnormalities. Genetic causes increasing recognized.	May correlate poorly with clinical seizures. Focal spikes or slow rhythms; multifocal discharges. Electroclinical dissociation may occur: electrical seizure without clinical manifestations.	Lumbar puncture; CSF PCR for herpes, enterovirus; serum Ca^{2+}, PO_4^{3-}, serum and CSF glucose, Mg^{2+}; BUN, amino acid screen, blood ammonia, organic acid screen, TORCHS, other metabolic testing if suspected. Ultrasound or CT/MRI for suspected intracranial hemorrhage and structural abnormalities.	Benzodiazepines, phenobarbital, IV or IM; if seizures not controlled, add phenytoin IV. Recent experience with levetiracetam and topiramate. Treat underlying disorder. Seizures due to brain damage often resistant to anticonvulsants. When cause in doubt, stop protein feedings until enzyme deficiencies of urea cycle or amino acid metabolism ruled out.
Epileptic spasms (aka infantile spasms or West syndrome)	3–18 mo, usually about 6 mo	Abrupt, usually but not always symmetric; adduction or flexion of limbs with flexion of head and trunk; or abduction and extensor movements (similar to Moro reflex). Occur in clusters typically upon awakening. Associated irritability and regression in development.	Etiology identified in approximately two-thirds, structural/metabolic or genetic. Tuberous sclerosis in 5%–10%. TORCHS, homeobox gene mutations, *ARX*, and other genetic mutations.	Hypsarrhythmia (chaotic high-voltage slow waves or random spikes) [90%]; other abnormalities in 10%. Rarely normal at onset. EEG improvement is required for treatment efficacy.	Funduscopic and skin examination, amino and organic acid screen. Chromosomal analysis, TORCHS screen, brain MRI scan. Trial of pyridoxine. Consider gene panels.	ACTH, prednisolone, vigabatrin (especially if tuberous sclerosis). B_6 (pyridoxine) trial. In resistant cases, topiramate, zonisamide, valproic acid, lamotrigine, ketogenic diet. Early treatment leads to improved outcome. Occasionally, surgical resection of cortical malformation.
Febrile convulsions	3 mo–6 y (peak 6–18 mo); most common childhood seizure (incidence 2%)	Usually generalized seizures, rarely focal in onset; < 15 min. May lead to status epilepticus. Recurrence risk of second febrile seizure 30% (50% if < 1 y of age); recurrence risk is same after status epilepticus.	Nonneurologic febrile illness (temperature rises to 39°C or higher). Risk factors: positive family history, day care, developmental delay, prolonged neonatal hospitalization.	Normal interictal EEG, especially when obtained 8–10 days after seizure. Therefore, not useful unless complicating features.	Lumbar puncture in infants or whenever suspicion of meningitis exists.	Treat underlying illness, fever. Diastat rectally for prolonged (> 5 min) seizure. Prophylaxis with oral diazepam, phenobarbital, or valproic acid is rarely needed.

	Age of onset	Seizure types/clinical features	Etiology/genetics	EEG findings	Diagnosis/workup	Treatment
Lennox-Gastaut syndrome)	Any time in childhood (usually 2–7 y)	Multiple seizure types including tonic, myoclonic (shock-like contractions of muscle groups); rare atonic ("drop attacks"), and atypical absence with episodes of absence status epilepticus.	Multiple causes, usually resulting in diffuse neuronal damage. History of infantile spasms; prenatal or perinatal brain damage; viral meningoencephalitis; CNS degenerative disorders; structural cerebral abnormalities (eg, migrational abnormalities).	Atypical slow (1–2.5 Hz) spike-wave complexes and bursts of high-voltage generalized spikes, often with diffusely slow background frequencies. Electrodecrement and fast spikes during sleep.	Dictated by index of suspicion: genetic testing; inherited metabolic disorders, neuronal ceroid lipofuscinosis, others. MRI scan, WBC lysosomal enzymes. Skin or conjunctival biopsy for electron microscopy; nerve conduction studies if degenerative disease suspected.	Difficult to treat, consider topiramate, ethosuximide, felbamate, levetiracetam, zonisamide, valproate, clonazepam, rufinamide, clobazam (approval pending) ketogenic diet; VNS. Avoid phenytoin, carbamazepine, oxcarbazepine, gabapentin.
Doose syndrome	Any time in childhood (usually 2–7 y)	Multiple seizure types including atonic, myoclonic atonic, atypical absence, tonic and generalized tonic-clonic	Rarely is etiology found, likely genetic, < 5% with SCN1A mutation large percentage with family history of febrile seizures.	Generalized spike wave discharges, central theta slowing	Genetic testing	Can be difficult to treat, consider topiramate, felbamate, levetiracetam, zonisamide, valproate, rufinamide, ketogenic diet, VNS. Avoid phenytoin, carbamazepine, oxcarbazepine, and gabapentin.
Dravet syndrome	First to second year of life	Initially prolonged febrile seizure that may be hemiconvulsions; after 1 y of age with multiple seizure types; typically sensitive to change in temperature	85% with SCN1a, mutation others with SCN1B, GABA receptor mutations.	Multifocal epileptiform discharges, generalized epileptiform discharges, mild slowing	Abnormal genetic testing also associated with abnormal gait in adolescent, requiring supportive therapy	Can be difficult to treat, consider topiramate, zonisamide, valproic acid, levetiracetam, ketogenic diet, clobazam, stiripentol. Avoid Na channel blockers such as phenytoin, carbamazepine, oxcarbazepine as maintenance.

(Continued)

Table 25–5. Seizures by age at onset, pattern, and preferred treatment. (*Continued*)

Seizure Type Epilepsy Syndrome	Age at Onset	Clinical Manifestations	Causative Factors	EEG Pattern	Other Diagnostic Studies	Treatment and Comments
Childhood absence epilepsy	3–12 y	Lapses of consciousness or vacant stares, lasting 3–10 s, often in clusters. Automatisms of face and hands; clonic activity in 30%–45%. Often mimics focal seizures but no aura or postictal confusion.	Unknown. Genetic component. Abnormal thalamocortical circuitry.	3-Hz spike and wave discharges, bilateral, synchronous, symmetric, high-voltage, provoked by hyperventilation. EEG always abnormal. EEG normalization correlates with seizure control.	Hyperventilation often provokes attacks. Imaging studies rarely of value.	Ethosuximide most effective and best tolerated; valproic acid. Lamotrigine, in resistant cases, zonisamide, topiramate, levetiracetam, acetazolamide, ketogenic diet. Some risk for developing GTCs.
Juvenile absence epilepsy	10–15 y	Absence seizures less frequent than in childhood absence epilepsy. May have greater risk of convulsive seizures.	Unknown (idiopathic), possibly genetic.	3-Hz spike wave and atypical generalized discharges.	Not always triggered by hyperventilation.	Same as childhood absence epilepsy but may be more difficult to treat successfully.
Focal seizures (previously called partial seizures)	Any age	Seizure may involve any part of body; may spread in fixed pattern.	Often unknown; brain tumor, birth trauma, vascular pathology, meningitis, cortical malformations (dysplasia), etc.	EEG may be normal; focal spikes or slow waves in appropriate cortical region; Possibly genetic.	MRI, repeat if seizures poorly controlled or progressive. Consider Rasmussen encephalitis if patient develops focal status epilepticus.	Oxcarbazepine, carbamazepine; lamotrigine, gabapentin, topiramate, levetiracetam, zonisamide, lacosamide, and phenytoin. Valproic acid useful adjunct. If medications fail, surgery may be an option.
Self-limited/BECTS, previously called benign rolandic epilepsy)	5–16 y	Focal seizures of face, tongue, hand +/– secondary generalization. Usually nocturnal. Similar seizure patterns may be observed in patients with focal cortical lesions. Almost always remits by puberty.	Seizure history or abnormal EEG findings in relatives of 40% of affected probands and 18%–20% of parents and siblings, suggesting a single autosomal dominant gene, possibly with age-dependent penetrance.	Centrotemporal spikes or sharp waves ("rolandic discharges") appearing paroxysmally against a normal EEG background.	Seldom need CT or MRI.	Often no medication is necessary, especially if seizure is exclusively nocturnal and infrequent. Oxcarbazepine, carbamazepine, or others. (See focal seizures.)

	Age	Clinical Features	Etiology	EEG	Imaging/Evaluation	Treatment
Juvenile myoclonic epilepsy (of Janz)	Late childhood and adolescence, peaking at 13 y	Mild myoclonic jerks of neck and shoulder flexor muscles after awakening. GTCs; sometimes absence seizures. Intelligence usually normal. Rarely resolves but usually remits on medications.	40% of relatives have myoclonias, especially in females; 15% have the abnormal EEG pattern with clinical attacks.	Interictal EEG shows variety of spike-and-wave sequences or 4–6-Hz multispike-and-wave complexes ("fast spikes").	Imaging may not be necessary. If course is unfavorable, consider progressive myoclonic syndromes	Lamotrigine, valproic acid, topiramate, levetiracetam, zonisamide.
GTCs (previously called grand mal)	Any age	Loss of consciousness; tonic-clonic movements, often preceded by vague aura or cry. Incontinence in 15%. Postictal confusion and somnolence. Often mixed with or masking other seizure patterns.	Often unknown. Genetic component. May be seen with metabolic disturbances, trauma, infection, intoxication, degenerative disorders, brain tumors.	Bilateral synchronous, symmetric multiple high-voltage spikes, spikes waves (eg, 3 Hz). EEG often normal in those < 4 y. Focal spikes may become "secondarily generalized."	Imaging; metabolic and infectious evaluation may be appropriate.	Levetiracetam; topiramate, lamotrigine, zonisamide, valproic acid, felbamate. Combinations may be necessary. Carbamazepine, oxcarbazepine or valproic acid; phenytoin may also be effective.

ACTH, adrenocorticotropic hormone; BECTS, benign epilepsy of childhood with centrotemporal spikes; BUN, blood urea nitrogen; CNS, central nervous system; CSF, cerebrospinal fluid; CT, computed tomography; EEG, electroencephalogram; GTC, generalized tonic-clonic seizures; IM, intramuscularly; IV, intravenously; MRI, magnetic resonance imaging; PCR, polymerase chain reaction; PET, positron emission tomography; SPECT, single-photon emission tomography; TORCHS, toxoplasmosis, other infections, rubella, cytomegalovirus, herpes simplex, and syphilis; VNS, vagus nerve stimulation; WBC, white blood cell.

(except for the fortuitous recording of a clinical seizure or in situations when seizures are easily provoked such as childhood absence epilepsy). A seizure is a clinical phenomenon; an EEG showing epileptiform activity may confirm and clarify the clinical diagnosis (for instance, defining an epilepsy syndrome), but it is only occasionally diagnostic (see Electroencephalography under Diagnostic Testing section).

▶ Differential Diagnosis

The diagnosis of epilepsy will carry profound implications for the patient; thus, sufficient proof and accuracy are imperative. To the layperson, epilepsy often has connotations of brain damage and limitation of activity. A person so diagnosed may be excluded from certain occupations in later life.

Various nonepileptic paroxysmal events are outlined in Table 25–6. Psychogenic nonepileptic spells are much less common in children than in adults but must be considered, even in the young or cognitively impaired child. More common seizure "mimics" include inattention in school-aged children, stereotypies, sleep-related movements, habit movements such as head-banging and so-called infantile masturbation (sometimes referred to as self-gratification movements), and gastroesophageal reflux in very young (often impaired) infants.

▶ Complications & Sequelae

A. Psychosocial Impact

Emotional disturbances, especially depression but also anxiety, anger, and feelings of guilt and inadequacy, often occur in the patient, as well as the parents of a child with epilepsy. Actual or perceived stigmas as well as issues regarding "disclosure" are common. School-aged children and adults with epilepsy have an increased risk of suicide, secondary to comorbid depression. The discussion of comorbid mental health concerns should start at the time of diagnosis. Schools often limit activities of children with epilepsy inappropriately, perpetuating the stigma.

Epilepsy with onset in childhood has an impact on adult function. Adults with early onset of epilepsy, even when well controlled, are less likely to complete high school, have less adequate employment, and are less likely to marry. Persistent epilepsy results in significant dependence; even when epilepsy is successfully treated, patients with long-standing epilepsy often do not become independent due to driving restrictions and safety concerns.

B. Cognitive Impairment

Children living with epilepsy, particularly with untreated or poorly controlled seizures, can develop reduced cognition and memory. Clearly, epileptic encephalopathy (ie, epileptic activity or frequent seizures are contributing to worse

neurocognitive function) does occur, particularly in young children with epilepsies such as infantile spasms (West syndrome), Dravet syndrome, and Lennox-Gastaut syndrome. The impact of persistent focal seizures on development is less clear, although persistent temporal lobe seizures in adults are associated with cognitive dysfunction. Increased epileptiform burden has been demonstrated to cause mild cognitive problems in some disorders previously thought to be benign, such as childhood epilepsy with centrotemporal spikes, formally BECTS. In general, interictal epileptiform activity is not felt to contribute to cognitive impairment. Continuous epileptiform activity in sleep is associated with Landau-Kleffner syndrome (acquired epileptic aphasia) and the syndrome of electroencephalographic status epilepticus in sleep (ESES), both of which are associated with cognitive decline and developmental/behavioral regression.

Depression is a common cause of impaired cognitive function in children with epilepsy. Most antiseizure medications (ASMs) do not have cognitive side effects at usual therapeutic doses, but phenobarbital, topiramate, and zonisamide may produce reversible cognitive impairment. Psychosis also can occur after seizures or as a side effect of certain seizure medications.

C. Injury and Death

Children with epilepsy are at far greater risk of injuries than the general pediatric population. Physical injuries are particularly frequent in atonic seizures (so-called drop attacks), at times necessitating protective headgear. Injuries as a direct result of other seizure types are not as common, although drowning, injuries related to working in kitchens, and falls from heights remain potential risks for all children with epilepsy—highlighting the need for "seizure precautions," especially water safety. Showers are recommended over bathing. Ultimately, patients with epilepsy should not participate in activities that could result in serious injury in the case of sudden loss of consciousness, without taking precautions to address that possibility. However, for most activities, simple accommodations allow individuals with epilepsy to lead very normal lives.

The greatest fear of a parent of a child with new-onset of epilepsy is the possibility of death or brain injury. Children with epilepsy do have an increased risk of premature death, but most deaths are related to the underlying neurologic disorder, not the seizures. Sudden unexpected death with epilepsy (SUDEP) is a rare event in children, occurring in only 1–2:10,000 patient-years. The greatest risk for SUDEP is in children with medically uncontrolled epilepsy. The etiology of SUDEP is not yet known, and the only proven strategy to prevent SUDEP is seizure control. Identifying life-threatening disorders (eg, identifying patients with cardiac arrhythmias, especially prolonged QT syndrome) as the cause of misdiagnosed epilepsy is clearly of utmost importance. While SUDEP is rare, increased mortality in children with epilepsy should be mentioned when counseling families.

Table 25–6. Nonepileptic paroxysmal events.

Breath-holding attacks (cyanotic and pallid) (see below)

Cyanotic: Age 6 mo–3 y. Always precipitated by trauma and fright. Cyanosis; sometimes stiffening, tonic (or jerking-clonic) convulsion (anoxic seizure). Patient may sleep following attack. Family history positive in 30%. Electroencephalogram (EEG) is not useful. No medication treatment is useful but if the patient is found to be iron-deficient supplementation may reduce events. However, in general reassurance is most important.

Pallid: Usually, there is no apparent precipitant although fright may precipitate. Pallor may be followed by seizure (anoxic-ischemic). Vagally mediated (heart-slowing), like adult syncope. EEG is not useful.

Tics (Tourette syndrome)

Simple or complex stereotyped jerks or movements, coughs, grunts, sniffs. Worse at repose or with stress. May be suppressed during physician visit. Family history often positive for tics or for obsessive compulsive disorder. Diagnosis is clinical. Magnetic resonance imaging (MRI) and EEG are negative. Medications may benefit.

Parasomnias (night terrors, sleep talking, walking, "sit-ups")

Ages 3–10 y. Usually occur in first sleep cycle (30–90 min after going to sleep), with crying, screaming, and autonomic discharge (pupils dilated, perspiring, etc). May last only a few minutes or be more prolonged. Child goes back to sleep and has no recall of event next day. Sleep studies (polysomnogram and EEG) are normal. Sleep talking and walking and short "sit-ups" in bed are fragmentary arousals. If a spell is recorded, EEG shows arousal from deep sleep, but behavior seems wakeful. Child needs to be protected from injury and gradually settled down and taken back to bed. Medications may be considered in rare instances.

Nightmares

Nightmares or vivid dreams occur in subsequent cycles of sleep, often in early morning hours, and generally are partially recalled the next day. The bizarre and frightening behavior may sometimes be confused with complex partial seizures but occurs during REM (rapid eye movement) sleep, whereas epilepsy usually does not. In extreme or difficult cases, an all-night sleep EEG may help differentiate seizures from nightmares. Frontal lobe epilepsy with sleep related "hypermotor" seizures should be considered.

Migraine

On occasion, migraine can be associated with an acute confusional state. Usual migraine prodrome of spots before the eyes, dizziness, visual field defects, followed by headache and then agitated confusion is present. History of other, more typical migraine with severe headache and vomiting but without confusion may aid in diagnosis. Severe headache with vomiting as child comes out of spell may aid in distinguishing the attack from epilepsy. However, partial seizures, while brief, may be associated with more prolonged postictal agitation and confusion. Other seizure manifestations are practically never seen (eg, tonic-clonic movements, falling, complete loss of consciousness). EEG in migraine is usually normal and seldom has epileptiform abnormalities often seen in patients with epilepsy. Migraine and epilepsy are sometimes linked: Benign occipital epilepsy may present with migraine-like visual aura and headache. There may be migraine-caused cortical ischemia which leads to later epilepsy. Postictal headache can be confused with migraine.

Benign nocturnal myoclonus

Common in infants and may last even up to school age. Focal or generalized jerks (the latter also called hypnic or sleep jerks) may persist from onset of sleep on and off all night. A video record for physician review can aid in diagnosis. EEG taken during jerks is normal, proving that these jerks are not epilepsy. Treatment is reassurance.

Shuddering

Shuddering or shivering attacks can occur in infancy and may be a forerunner of essential tremor in later life. Often, family history is positive for tremor. Shivering may be very frequent. EEG is normal. There is no clouding or loss of consciousness.

Gastroesophageal reflux (Sandifer syndrome)

Seen more commonly in children with cerebral palsy or brain damage; reflux of acid gastric contents may cause pain that cannot be described by child. Unusual posturing (dystonic or other) of head and neck or trunk may occur, an apparent attempt to stretch the esophagus or close the opening. There is no loss of consciousness, but eye rolling, apnea, and occasional vomiting may simulate a seizure. An upper gastrointestinal series, cine of swallowing, sometimes even an EEG (normal during episode) may be necessary to distinguish from seizures.

Infantile masturbation/gratification movements

Rarely in infants, repetitive rocking or rubbing motions may simulate seizures. Infant may look out of contact, be poorly responsive to environment, and have autonomic expressions (eg, perspiration, dilated pupils) that may be confused with seizures. Observation by a skilled individual, sometimes even in a hospital setting, may be necessary to distinguish from seizures. EEG is normal between and during attacks. Interpretation and reassurance are the only necessary treatment.

Conversion reaction/psychogenic nonepileptic seizures

Up to 50% of patients with nonepileptic seizures also have epilepsy. Episodes may involve writhing, pelvic thrusting, tonic movements, bizarre jerking and thrashing, or even apparently sudden unresponsiveness. Children may be developmentally delayed. Spells must often be seen or recorded with a videorecorder to distinguish from epilepsy but are sometimes so bizarre they are easily differentiated. A normal EEG during a spell is a key diagnostic feature. Combativeness is common; self-injury and incontinence, rare. Within the pediatric population, most patients with psychogenic nonepileptic seizures have a good prognosis without deep seated psychological trauma.

Temper tantrums and rage attacks

Child often reports amnesia for events during spell. Attacks are usually precipitated by frustration or anger, often directed either verbally or physically, and subside with behavior modification and isolation. EEGs are generally normal but seldom obtained during an attack. It should be noted that directed violence is very uncommon following partial seizures but severe agitation can occur.

Staring spells

Teachers often make referral for absence or "petit mal" seizures in children who stare or seem preoccupied at school. Helpful in the history is the lack of these spells at home (eg, before breakfast, a common time for absence seizures). Lack of other epilepsy in child or family history often is helpful. These children often have difficulties with school and cognitive or learning disabilities. Child can generally be brought out of spell by a firm command or touch and if event is interruptible they are unlikely to be seizures. EEG is sometimes necessary to confirm that absence seizures are not occurring.

▶ Treatment

The ideal treatment of acute seizures is the correction of specific causes. However, even when a biochemical disorder, tumor, meningitis, or another specific cause is being treated, ASMs are often still required.

A. First Aid

Caregivers should be instructed to protect the patient against self-injury. Turning the child to the side is useful for preventing aspiration. Placing any objects in the mouth of a convulsing patient or trying to restrain tonic-clonic movements may cause worse injuries than a bitten tongue or bruised limb and could potentially become a choking hazard. Parents are often concerned that cyanosis will occur during generalized convulsive seizures, clinically significant hypoxia is rare. Mouth-to-mouth resuscitation is rarely necessary and is unlikely to be effective.

For prolonged seizures (those lasting over 5 minutes), acute home treatment with benzodiazepines such as rectal diazepam gel (Diastat) or intranasal midazolam may be administered to prevent the development of status epilepticus and has proven to be safe even when administered by nonmedical professionals.

B. Antiseizure Medication Therapy

1. Drug selection—Several issues should be considered when choosing an antiseizure medication (ASM), no longer called antiepileptic drugs (AEDs) in recognition that no ASM actually prevents or cures epilepsy. Some ASMs are effective for focal seizures but can make generalized seizures worse (eg, oxcarbazepine and carbamazepine), while other medications are effective for most seizure types and are relatively safe (levetiracetam). It is worth noting that most of this "knowledge" is based on experience and expert opinion rather than comparative effectiveness or randomized control trials. In some cases, side effects can help guide treatment; for example, topiramate tends to suppress appetite; whereas, valproic acid often precipitates weight gain. When balancing risks, side effects, and potential effectiveness, one must consider the impact on the patient and their family's life.

2. Treatment strategy—The goal of antiseizure treatment is "no seizures and no side effects." The child with a single seizure has a 50% chance of seizure recurrence. Thus, ASMs are not necessary until the diagnosis of epilepsy is established, that is, until there is a second seizure or evidence of a high probability of additional seizures. The seizure type and epilepsy syndrome, as well as potential side effects, will determine which drug to initiate as discussed earlier. If monotherapy fails, a second, and when necessary, a third medication may be required to help reduce seizure frequency. Care must be taken when using multiple ASMs, which increases the chance of side effects and often does not substantially improve seizure control. There is some evidence that ASMs with different mechanisms of action may improve their combined tolerability and effectiveness.

3. Long-term management and discontinuation of treatment—Therapy should be continued until the patient is free of seizures for at least 1–2 years. In about 75% of patients, seizures will not recur following discontinuation of medication after 2 years of remission. Variables such as younger age at onset, normal EEG, undetermined etiology, and ease of controlling seizures carry a favorable prognosis, whereas identified etiology, later onset, continued epileptiform EEG, difficulty in establishing initial control of the seizures, polytherapy, generalized tonic-clonic or myoclonic seizures, and an abnormal neurologic examination are associated with a higher risk of recurrence. Most ASMs (with the exception of barbiturates and benzodiazepines) can be withdrawn over 6–8 weeks. There does not appear to be an advantage to slower withdrawal.

Recurrent seizures affect up to 25% of children who attempt withdrawal from medications. Recurrence of seizures is most likely within 6–12 months of discontinuing medications. Therefore, seizure safety precautions will need to be reinstituted, including driving restriction. If seizures recur during or after withdrawal, ASM therapy should be reinstituted and maintained for at least another 1–2 years. The majority of children will again achieve remission of their seizures.

C. Alternative Treatments

1. Adrenocorticotropic hormone (ACTH) and corticosteroids—Treatment with ACTH or oral corticosteroids is the standard of care for infantile spasms. Duration of therapy is guided by cessation of clinical seizures and normalization of the EEG. Vigabatrin is an alternative treatment that is also considered standard of care for infantile spasms and has been shown to be superior for infantile spasms resulting from tuberous sclerosis. All other treatments for infantile spasms have a lower likelihood of being effective.

Precautions: It is important to guard against infections, provide GI prophylaxis, and follow for possible hypertension, and discuss the cushingoid appearance and its disappearance. Oral corticosteroids should not be withdrawn suddenly. Side effects in some series occur in up to 9% of patients. In some regions of the country, prophylaxis against *Pneumocystis* infection may be required. Careful and frequent follow-up is necessary. Visiting nurse services and partnering with a medical home can be very helpful in surveillance, such as monitoring blood pressure, weight, and potential adverse effects.

2. Ketogenic diet—Fasting has been described to stop seizures for centuries and a diet high in fat and low in protein and carbohydrates will result in ketosis and simulate a fasting state. Such a diet has been observed to decrease and even control seizures in some children. This diet should be monitored very carefully (by a clinical team familiar with the ketogenic diet) to ensure sufficient nutrients, including vitamins and minerals, to maintain overall health. Recent reports suggest potential efficacy with a modified Atkins diet or a low-glycemic index diet in older and higher functioning children who will not accept the ketogenic diet.

The mechanism for the anticonvulsant action of the ketogenic diet is not understood. The ketogenic diet requires close adherence and full cooperation of all family members. However, when seizure control is achieved by this method, acceptance of the diet is usually excellent. Families must be cautioned that abrupt withdrawal (accidental or purposeful) of the diet can precipitate seizures and even status epilepticus. Increased use of the ketogenic diet and family support groups have increased the number of palatable recipes for patients and families on the ketogenic diet.

As with all therapies, potential adverse effects can occur with the ketogenic diet. These include acidosis and hypoglycemia, particularly on initiation of the diet. The child should be admitted to a center well versed in managing ketogenic diet to start this treatment. Close follow-up will help prevent risk for renal stones, pancreatitis, and acidosis. In addition, vitamin and minerals need to be followed carefully to avoid deficiencies, especially carnitine, iron, and vitamin D.

3. Vagus nerve stimulator (VNS)—The VNS is a pacemaker-like device that is implanted below the clavicle and attached to the left vagus nerve. A cycle of electrical stimulation of the nerve is established, which has an anticonvulsant effect, reducing seizures by at least 50% in over half the children treated. In addition, an emergency mode that is activated by swiping a magnet (of abrupt tachycardia on newer models) may interrupt a seizure. With current technology, the battery in the stimulator may last 7 or more years in many patients.

D. Epilepsy Surgery

An evaluation for epilepsy surgery is indicated for all children with medically intractable focal epilepsy (generally defined as failure of two antiseizure medications at effective doses). The evaluation and surgery should be performed at a center with expertise in epilepsy surgery and which has a dedicated neurosurgeon, epileptologists and neuropsychologists with experience in epilepsy surgery.

The first surgery for treatment of epilepsy took place over 100 years ago, and surgery is now established as an appropriate treatment option for adults and children with epilepsy refractory to medical treatment. Evaluation for possible surgical treatment should begin as soon as it is apparent that a child with focal onset seizures is not responding to standard therapy. Medication resistant ("refractory") epilepsy is usually defined as failure of two or three anti-epileptic

drugs alone or as combination therapy to control seizures. Advances in technology allow for definition and removal of the epileptogenic focus even in young infants. Many centers now have access to variety of resources for identifying the region of seizure onset. Ultimately, the chance of seizure freedom can range from 50% to 95% depending on the clinical circumstance. Some children with more generalized seizures may qualify for other types of surgery, such as corpus callosotomy, that aim to reduce seizure burden, but are not expected to make the patient seizure free.

E. General Management of the Child With Epilepsy

1. Education—The initial diagnosis of epilepsy is often devastating for families. The patient and parents must be helped to understand the nature of epilepsy and its management, including etiology, prognosis, safety issues, and treatment options.

Excellent educational materials are available for families of a child with epilepsy, both in print and online. An excellent website is http://www.epilepsy.com. Materials on epilepsy—including pamphlets, monographs, films, and videotapes suitable for children and teenagers, parents, teachers, and medical professionals—may be purchased through the Epilepsy Foundation: 8301 Professional Place, Landover, MD 20785; (800) 332–1000. The foundation's local chapter and other community organizations are able to provide guidance and other services. Support groups exist in many regions for older children and adolescents and for their parents and others concerned.

2. Privileges and precautions in daily life— *"No seizures and no side effects"* is a motto established by the Epilepsy Foundation. The child should be encouraged to live as normal a life as possible. Children should engage in physical activities appropriate to their age and social group. There are no absolute contraindications to any other sports, although some physicians recommend against contact sports. There is some literature that suggests that exercise decreases overall seizure burden and may also be helpful to maintain good bone health.

Depression, anxiety, and attentional difficulties are common comorbidities of epilepsy, particularly in adolescents, and need to be treated as they can be as (or more) debilitating as the seizures. Sleep deprivation and alcohol should be avoided as they can be triggers for seizures for patients with epilepsy. Prompt attention should be given to intercurrent illnesses that can also trigger seizures.

Although every effort should be made to control seizures, treatment must not interfere with a child's ability to function normally. A child may do better having an occasional mild seizure than being so heavily sedated that function at home, in school, or at play is impaired. Therapy and medication adjustment often require much art and fortitude on the physician's part.

3. Driving—Driving becomes important to most young people at age 15 or 16 years. Restrictions for persons with epilepsy and other disturbances of consciousness vary from state to state. In most states, a learner's permit or driver's license will be issued to an individual with epilepsy if he or she has been under a physician's care and free of seizures for at least 6–12 months provided that the treatment or basic neurologic problems do not interfere with the ability to drive. A guide to this and other legal matters pertaining to persons with epilepsy is published by the Epilepsy Foundation, and its legal department may be able to provide additional information.

4. Pregnancy—Contraception (especially interaction of oral contraceptive with some ASMs), childbearing, potential teratogenicity of ASMs, and the management of pregnancy should be discussed as soon as appropriate with the adolescent young woman with epilepsy. Daily use of vitamin preparations and high-dose folic acid can be protective against neural tube defects. For the pregnant teenager with epilepsy, management by an obstetrician conversant with the use of ASMs in pregnancy is appropriate. The patient should be cautioned against discontinuing her medications during pregnancy. The possibility of teratogenic effects of ASMs, such as facial clefts (two to three times increased risk), must be weighed against the risks from seizures. All ASMs appear to have some risk for teratogenicity, although valproate carries a particularly high risk for spinal dysraphism as well as being associated with cognitive issues in children exposed to valproate in utero. Dosing may need to be adjusted frequently during pregnancy as blood volume expands. Frequent ASM blood levels may be helpful in making these adjustments.

5. School intervention and seizure response plans—Schools are required by federal law to work with parents to establish a seizure action plan for their child with epilepsy. A template for such a plan is available on the Epilepsy Foundation website at https://www.epilepsy.com/living-epilepsy/toolbox/seizure-forms. These plans usually require the approval of the child's physician. Schools are sometimes hesitant to administer rescue medications. Often, information from the physician, especially that obtained from the Epilepsy Foundation website, will relieve anxieties. School authorities should be encouraged to avoid needless restrictions and to address the emotional and educational needs of all children with disabilities, including epilepsy. The local affiliates of the Epilepsy Foundation can often provide support and education for both families and schools.

2. Status Epilepticus

Status epilepticus is usually defined as a clinical or electrical seizure lasting at least 15 minutes, or a series of seizures without complete recovery over a 30-minute period. Importantly, this time cut-off keeps getting shorter as more evidence accrues that even relatively short seizures may be harmful to the brain. After 30 minutes of seizure activity, hypoxia and acidosis occur, with depletion of energy stores, cerebral edema, and structural damage. Eventually, high fever, hypotension, respiratory depression, and even death may occur. Status epilepticus is a medical emergency. Aggressive treatment of prolonged seizures may prevent development of status epilepticus. Treatment with benzodiazepines, including rectal valium, intranasal midazolam, sublingual lorazepam, and intramuscular diazepam, at home for prolonged seizures should be initiated 5 minutes after onset of a seizure.

Status epilepticus is classified as (1) convulsive (the common generalized tonic-clonic type) or (2) nonconvulsive (characterized by altered mental status or behavior with subtle or absent motor components). Absence status, or spike-wave stupor, and focal status epilepticus are examples of the nonconvulsive type. An EEG may be necessary to aid in diagnosing nonconvulsive status because patients sometimes appear merely stuporous and lack typical convulsive movements. Status epilepticus that has not responded to two medications is considered refractory status epilepticus and often requires care in an intensive care unit.

▶ **Treatment**

For treatment options, see Table 25–7.

3. Febrile Seizures

▶ **Clinical Findings**

A. Symptoms and Signs

Criteria for febrile seizures are: (1) age 3 months to 6 years (most occur between ages 6 and 18 months), (2) fever of greater than 38.8°C, and (3) non-CNS infection. More than 90% of febrile seizures are generalized, last less than 5 minutes, and occur early in the illness causing the fever. Often the fever is not noted until after the seizure occurs. Febrile seizures occur in 2%–3% of children. Acute respiratory illnesses are most commonly associated with febrile seizures. Gastroenteritis, especially when caused by *Shigella* or *Campylobacter*, and urinary tract infections are less common causes. Roseola infantum is a rare but classic cause. One study implicated viral causes in 86% of cases. HHV-6 and HHV-7 are common causes for febrile status epilepticus, both accounting for one-third of cases. Febrile seizures rarely (1%–3%) evolve to recurrent unprovoked seizures (epilepsy) in later childhood and adult life (risk is increased two- to fivefold compared with children who do not have febrile seizures). The chance of later epilepsy is higher if the febrile seizures have complex features, such as duration longer than 15 minutes, more than one seizure in the same day, or focal features. Other predictive factors are an abnormal neurologic status preceding the seizures (eg, cerebral palsy or mental retardation), early onset of febrile seizure (before

Table 25–7. Status epilepticus treatment.

1. ABCs
   a. Airway: maintain oral airway; intubation may be necessary.
   b. Breathing: oxygen.
   c. Circulation: assess pulse, blood pressure; support with IV fluids, drugs. Monitor vital signs.
2. Start glucose-containing IV (unless patient is on ketogenic diet); evaluate serum glucose, electrolytes, HCO_3^-, CBC, BUN, anticonvulsant levels.
3. Consider arterial blood gases, pH.
4. Give 50% glucose if serum glucose low (1–2 mL/kg).
5. Begin IV drug therapy; goal is to control status epilepticus in 20–60 min.
   a. Diazepam, 0.3–0.5 mg/kg over 1–5 min (20 mg max); may repeat in 5–20 min; or lorazepam, 0.05–0.2 mg/kg (less effective with repeated doses, longer-acting than diazepam); or midazolam: IV, 0.1–0.2 mg/kg; intranasally, 0.2 mg/kg.
   b. Phenytoin, 10–20 mg/kg IV (not IM) over 5–20 min; (1000 mg maximum); monitor with blood pressure and ECG. Fosphenytoin may be given more rapidly in the same dosage and can be given IM; order 10–20 mg/kg of "phenytoin equivalent" (PE).
   c. Phenobarbital, 5–20 mg/kg (sometimes higher in newborns or refractory status in intubated patients).
6. Correct metabolic perturbations (eg, low-sodium, acidosis). Administer fluids judiciously.
7. Other drug approaches in refractory status:
   a. Repeat phenytoin, phenobarbital (10 mg/kg). Monitor blood levels. Support respiration, blood pressure as necessary.
   b. Other medications: valproate sodium, available as 100 mg/mL for IV use; give 15–30 mg/kg over 5–20 min.
   c. Levetiracetam may be helpful (20–40 mg/kg/dose IV).
   d. For patients who fail initial intervention consider: midazolam drip: 1–5 mcg/kg/min (even to 20 kg/min); pentobarbital coma; propofol and general anesthetic.
8. Consider underlying causes:
   a. Structural disorders or trauma: MRI or CT scan.
   b. Infection: lumbar puncture, blood culture, antibiotics.
   c. Metabolic disorders: consider lactic acidosis, toxins, and uremia if child is being treated with chronic AEDs, obtain medication levels. Toxin screen.
9. Initiate maintenance drug treatment with IV medications: phenytoin (10 mg/kg); phenobarbital (5 mg/kg); valproate IV 30 mg/kg; levetiracetam 20–30 mg/kg. Transition to oral medication when patient can safely take them.

BUN, blood urea nitrogen; CBC, complete blood count; CT, computed tomography; ECG, electrocardiogram; IM, intramuscularly; IV, intravenously; MRI, magnetic resonance imaging.

age 1 year), and a family history of epilepsy. Even with adverse factors, the risk of epilepsy after febrile seizures is still only in the range of 15%–20%, although it is increased if more than one risk factor is present. Recurrent febrile seizures occur in 30%–50% of cases. Therefore, families should be prepared to expect more seizures. In general, recurrence of febrile seizures does not worsen the long-term outlook.

B. Diagnostic Evaluation

The child with a febrile seizure must be evaluated for the source of the fever, in particular to exclude CNS infection. Routine studies such as serum electrolytes, glucose, calcium, skull radiographs, or brain imaging are seldom helpful unless warranted based on clinical history or suspicion of abuse. History and the examination should guide the workup and any treatment amenable underlying infection should be addressed. Meningitis and encephalitis must be considered. Signs of meningitis (eg, bulging fontanelle, stiff neck, stupor, and irritability) may be absent, especially in a child younger than 18 months.

C. Lumbar Puncture

After controlling the fever and stopping an ongoing seizure, the physician must decide whether to do a lumbar puncture. The fact that the child has had a previous febrile seizure does not rule out meningitis as the cause of the current episode. It is very important, especially in younger children, to exclude CNS infection as a source; these children are not classified as having a febrile seizure. A recent study demonstrated that 96% of children with febrile status epilepticus who received an LP had less than three WBCs in the CSF. Therefore, seizure should not be an acceptable explanation for elevated cells in the CSF. Although the yield is low, a lumbar puncture should probably be considered if the child is younger than 18 months, and has been pretreated with antibiotics or is underimmunized. Certainly, any child with meningeal signs, fever and seizure should have a CSF examination. Occasionally, observation in the emergency department for several hours obviates the need for a lumbar puncture, but in general, one should have a low threshold for performing this potentially life-saving test.

D. EEG

EEG may be considered if the febrile seizure is complicated, focal, or otherwise unusual, but has little predictive value. In simple febrile seizures, the EEG is usually normal. If performed, the EEG should be done at least a week after the illness to avoid transient changes due to fever or the seizure itself.

▶ Treatment

Prophylactic ASMs are not recommended after a febrile seizure. Only phenobarbital and valproic acid have demonstrated efficacy in preventing febrile seizures, but with significant side effects; phenytoin and carbamazepine have been shown to be ineffective. Newer ASMs have not been studied. Diazepam started at the first onset of fever for the duration of the febrile illness (0.5 mg/kg two or three times per day orally or rectally) may be effective but will sedate a child and possibly complicate the evaluation for a source of the fever.

Measures to control fever such as sponging, tepid baths, or antipyretics including ibuprofen and acetaminophen have been shown to be ineffective at preventing recurrent febrile seizures and, thus, should not be recommended solely for this purpose.

▶ Prognosis

Simple febrile seizures do not have any long-term adverse consequences. As noted earlier, there is only a small increase in the risk of developing epilepsy. Cognitive function is not significantly different from that of siblings without febrile seizures.

Abend NS, Gutierrez-Colina AM, Dlugos DJ: Medical treatment of pediatric status epilepticus. Semin Pediatr Neurol 2010; 17:169–175 [PMID: 20727486].

Chu-Shore CJ, Thiele EA: New drugs for pediatric epilepsy. Semin Pediatr Neurol 2010;17:214–223 [PMID: 21183127].

Duffner P et al: Clinical Practice Guideline—febrile seizures: guideline for the neurodiagnostic evaluation of the child with a simple febrile seizure. Pediatrics 2015;127(2):389–394 [PMID: 21285335].

Frank LM et al: Cerebrospinal fluid findings in children with fever-associated status epilepticus: results of the consequences of prolonged febrile seizures (FEBSTAT) study. J Pediatr 2012;161:1169–1171 [PMID: 22985722].

Freeman JM, Kossoff EH: Ketosis and the ketogenic diet, 2010: advances in treating epilepsy and other disorders. Adv Pediatr 2010;57:315–329 [PMID: 21056745].

Go CY et al: Evidence based guideline update: medical treatment of infantile spasms. Report of the guideline development subcommittee of the American Academy of Neurology and the practice committee of the Child Neurology Society. Neurology 2012 Jun 12;78(24):1974–1980 [PMID: 22689735].

Holthausen H, Pieper T, Kudernatsch M: Towards early diagnosis and treatment to save children from catastrophic epilepsy—focus on epilepsy surgery. Brain Dev 2013;35(3)730–741 [PMID: 23791480].

Ostrowsky K: Outcome and prognosis of status epilepticus in children. Semin Pediatr Neurol 2010;17:195 [PMID: 20727490].

Ramos-Lizana J et al: Recurrence risk after withdrawal of antiepileptic drugs in children with epilepsy: a prospective study. Eur J Paediatr Neurol 2009; [Epub ahead of print] [PMID: 19541516].

Rennie J, Boylan G: Treatment of neonatal seizures. Arch Dis Child Fetal Neonatal Ed 2007;92:F148 [PMID: 17337664].

Riviello JJ et al: Practice parameter: diagnostic assessment of the child with status epilepticus (an evidence-based review): report of the Quality Standards Subcommittee of the American Academy of Neurology and the Practice Committee of the Child Neurology Society. Neurology 2006;67:1542 [PMID: 17101884].

Scheffer IE et al: ILAE classification of the epilepsies: Position paper of the ILAE Commission for Classification and Terminology. Epilepsia 2017;58(4):512–521. doi:10.1111/epi.13709 [PMID: 28276062].

Shinnar S et al: Phenomenology of prolonged febrile seizures: results of the FEBSTAT study. Neurology 2008;71:170–176 [PMID: 18525033].

Sillanpää M, Shinnar S: SUDEP and other causes of mortality in childhood-onset epilepsy. Epilepsy Behav 2013;28(2):249–255 [PMID: 23746924].

Wheless JW: Managing severe epilepsy syndromes of early childhood. J Child Neurol 2009;24:24S [PMID: 19666880].

SLEEP DISORDERS

Sleep disorders can originate from abnormalities within the respiratory system, the neurologic system and the coordination (or lack thereof) between these two systems. In order to understand abnormal sleep, one must understand normal sleep, which changes as the child develops. Sleep and its development are reviewed in Chapter 3. Chapter 3 also discusses behavioral considerations in the treatment of sleep disorders. Respiratory abnormalities that are associated with sleep such as obstructive sleep apnea are described in Chapter 19. This discussion focuses on neurologic features of several sleep disorders affecting children.

1. Narcolepsy

Narcolepsy, a primary disorder of sleep, is characterized by chronic, inappropriate daytime sleep that occurs regardless of activity or surroundings and is not relieved by increased sleep at night. One half of individuals affected by narcolepsy experience their initial symptoms in childhood. Of children with narcolepsy, 4% are under age 5, 18% are younger than age 10, and 60% are between puberty and their late teens.

The *International Classification of Sleep Disorders*, 3rd Edition (ICSD-3) describes two forms of narcolepsy:

Type 1 (narcolepsy with cataplexy): In addition to narcolepsy, patients develop cataplexy at onset or very soon thereafter. Cataplexy is a transient partial or total loss of muscle tone, often triggered by laughter, or other heightened emotional states. Consciousness is preserved during these spells, which can last several minutes in duration. The pathophysiology of Type 1 is deficiency of hypocretin-1 (orexin), a peptide essential for maintaining alertness.

Type 2 (narcolepsy without cataplexy): In addition to narcolepsy, patients may experience hypnagogic hallucinations and sleep paralysis, but they do not have cataplexy. Hypocretin-1 levels are normal. Hypnagogic hallucinations are intense visual or auditory hallucinations noted while falling asleep, whereas hypnopompic hallucinations occur while waking from sleep. Sleep paralysis is a brief loss of voluntary muscle control typically occurring at sleep-wake transitions and lasting for minutes.

Abnormally short latency between sleep onset and transition into rapid eye movement (REM) sleep occurs in subjects with narcolepsy. The first cycle of REM sleep usually occurs after 80–100 minutes in normal children. Nocturnal polysomnography and Multiple Sleep Latency Testing (MSLT) can demonstrate abnormal REM latency and are used to diagnose narcolepsy. Human leukocyte antigen (HLA) subtypes DQB1*0602 and DRB1*1501 are associated with narcolepsy, as well as absence of a hypothalamic neuropeptide, hypocretin, which can be measured in CSF. Sleep hygiene and behavior modification are used to treat patients with narcolepsy. Medications used for the treatment of narcolepsy in children are off label. CNS stimulants such as amphetamine mixtures are typically used to treat excessive daytime sleepiness. Modafinil, armodafinil, atomoxetine, and sodium oxybate are an effective treatment in adults; controlled studies in children are lacking. Cataplexy is treated with sodium oxybate, tricyclic antidepressants, selective serotonin reuptake inhibitors, and serotonin norepinephrine reuptake inhibitors.

2. Benign Neonatal Sleep Myoclonus

Benign neonatal sleep myoclonus is characterized by myoclonic jerks, usually bilateral and synchronous, which occur only during sleep and stop abruptly when the infant is aroused. It is a benign condition that is frequently confused with epileptic seizures. Onset is typically in the first 2 weeks of life and resolves spontaneously in the first months of life, although these may occur as late as 10 months. Clusters of jerks may last from a few seconds up to 20 minutes.

3. Nocturnal Frontal Lobe Epilepsy

Nocturnal frontal lobe epilepsy (NFLE) is characterized by paroxysmal arousals from NREM sleep with hypermotor seizures characterized by bizarre stereotyped hyperkinetic of dystonic motor movements lasting up to 5 minutes. NFLE is a heterogeneous disorder which includes both sporadic and familial forms. Lack of definitive epileptiform abnormalities on EEG recordings may lead to misdiagnoses of a parasomnia, such as night terrors or somnambulism.

4. Parasomnias

Parasomnias are complex movements and behaviors that occur in association with various sleep stages or the transition between sleeping and waking. The parasomnias of childhood are divided into those occurring in non-REM sleep (NREM) and REM sleep. The NREM parasomnias consist of partial arousals, disorientation, and motor disturbances and include sleep-walking (somnambulism), sleep talking, confusional arousals, and night terrors, among others. These are discussed in more detail in Chapter 3. The REM sleep parasomnias include nightmares, hypnagogic and hypnopompic hallucinations (as can occur in narcolepsy), and REM sleep behavior disorder, which is characterized by physical and sometimes violent movements during the dream state, and is primarily seen in adulthood. These typically occur during the second half of sleep, when REM comprises a larger part of the sleep cycle.

5. Restless Legs Syndrome

Restless legs syndrome refers to a feeling of needing to move the legs (dysesthesia) that often starts when resting at night. Movement of the legs temporarily relieves the symptoms, though this can interfere with the ability to fall asleep. This disorder can be familial; therefore, a detailed family history may be helpful. Occasionally, anemia (low ferritin) has been noted in adults and children with the disorder; in these cases, improvement has occurred with ferrous sulfate treatment. These are discussed in more detail in Chapter 3.

Ahmed I, Thorpy M: Clinical features, diagnosis, and treatment of narcolepsy. Clin Chest Med 2010;31:371–381 [PMID: 20488294].

American Academy of Sleep Medicine: *International Classification of Sleep Disorders.* 3rd ed. Darien, IL: American Academy of Sleep Medicine; 2014.

Aran A, Einen M, Lin L, Plazzi G, Nishino S, Mignot E: Clinical and therapeutic aspects of childhood narcolepsy-cataplexy: a retrospective study of 51 children. Sleep 2010;33:1457–1464 [PMID: 21102987].

Aurora RN et al: Practice parameters for the non-respiratory indications for polysomnography and multiple sleep latency testing for children. Sleep 2012;35:1467–1473 [PMID: 23115395].

Caraballo RH et al: The spectrum of benign myoclonus of early infancy: clinical and neurophysiologic features in 102 patients. Epilepsia 2009;50:1176–1183 [PMID: 19175386].

Hoban T: Sleep disorders in children. Ann N Y Acad Sci 2010;1184(1):1–14 [PMID: 20146688].

Kotagal S et al: Non-respiratory indications for polysomnography and related procedures in children: an evidence-based review. Sleep 2012;35:1451–1466 [PMID: 23115394].

HEADACHES

ESSENTIALS OF DIAGNOSIS & TYPICAL FEATURES

▶ The two most common causes of primary headaches in children are migraine and tension-type headache. Headaches are a common feature of viral illnesses.

▶ Diagnosis is based upon a thorough history and physical, excluding secondary causes such as mass or idiopathic intracranial hypertension (IIH).

▶ Warning signs that may require further investigation include headache in a young child, new onset and worsening headache, unexplained fever, awakening with headache or vomiting, headache worse with straining or position change, posterior headaches, neurologic deficit, or neurocutaneous stigmata.

Headaches are common in children and adolescents. Healthcare providers need to recognize and differentiate

Table 25–8. Red flags for children with headaches.

Headache in child aged < 5 years
New ("explosive onset") and worsening headache in a previously healthy child
Worst headache of life
Unexplained fever
Headache occurring in the middle of the night or early morning with or without vomiting
Headache worse with straining or Valsalva
Posterior headaches
Neurological deficit
Postural/positional headache
Worse when lying
Worse when standing
Neurocutaneous stigmata (café au lait spots, hypopigmented macules)

Table 25–9. Classification of tension type headache and migraine.

	Migraine Without Aura	Tension-Type Headache
Duration	2–72 h[a]	30 min to 7 days
Quality	Throbbing/pounding	Pressure, tight band
Severity	Moderate to severe	Mild to moderate
Location	Unilateral/bilateral[a]	Bilateral
Physical activity	Worsens headache	No effect
Associated factors		
a. Nausea +/− vomiting	a or b	Can be present (rare)
b. Photo and phonophobia		Photo or phonophobia but not both

[a]Modified for children based on the IHCD-III Beta classification criteria.

the common from the more serious causes of headaches in order to ensure the correct treatment. Approximately 45% of children experience at least one debilitating headache, and up to 28% of adolescents have migraines. First, the clinician must determine if the headache is primary or secondary. Red flags (Table 25–8) may prompt further workup and evaluation.

▶ Clinical Findings

A. Symptoms and Signs

Based on the 2013 International Classification of Headache Disorders, 3rd Edition (ICHD-III), primary headaches are divided into three major categories: migraine, tension-type, and trigeminal autonomic cephalalgias. Clinical features of migraine without aura and tension-type headache are compared in Table 25–9. Individuals with greater than 15 headaches (migraine or tension-type) per month are considered chronic, and medication overuse must be excluded. Triggers of head pain can include stress, sleep deprivation, dehydration, skipped meals, caffeine, and possibly specific foods (eg, monosodium glutamate or nitrites). Trigeminal autonomic cephalalgias (or sub-category, cluster headache) are rare in children. They present as recurrent, unilateral severe headaches with autonomic dysfunction (watery eye, congestion, facial sweating, miosis, ptosis).

According to the ICHD-III, migraines include childhood periodic syndromes such as cyclic vomiting, abdominal migraine, and benign paroxysmal vertigo of childhood. History of these periodic syndromes may be discovered in children and adolescents with migraines.

B. Laboratory Findings

Routine laboratory testing has not been found to be helpful, though the evidence is limited. History and examination

may prompt screening for general medical conditions as indicated.

C. Imaging Studies

Routine neuroimaging is not indicated for children presenting with recurrent headaches and a normal neurologic examination. Red flags as noted in Table 25–8 should prompt consideration of imaging. The type of imaging (CT vs MRI) depends on the urgency of evaluation (ie, acute onset severe headache vs worsening headache over 1–2 weeks).

▶ Differential Diagnosis

Secondary causes of headache include broad categories such as head trauma, infection, vascular, intracranial pressure changes, structural, metabolic, toxic, medication, illicit drug related, and hematologic (Table 25–10). Headaches associated with head trauma are those that start within 2 weeks of closed head injury. They can have features of migraines or tension-type headaches. Neck pain and headache after head trauma warrant evaluation for a dissection, especially if examination is suggestive for a connective tissue disorder such as Marfan syndrome. Headaches that worsen with lying down or vomiting without nausea are concerning for increased intracranial hypertension such as IIH, sinus venous clot producing increased CSF pressure, hydrocephalus, or mass. It is worth noting that, in studies evaluating the utility of imaging in pediatric headache, up to 98% of patients with intracranial process requiring surgical intervention had an

Table 25–10. Differential diagnosis of headaches.

Primary Headaches	Secondary Headaches	
• Migraine without aura • Migraine with aura • Childhood periodic syndromes • Tension-type headache • Trigeminal autonomic cephalgias including Cluster headaches	• Trauma • Hypertension • Arterial dissection • Medication overuse headache • Idiopathic intracranial hypertension (IIH) • Intracranial hypotension • Chiari malformation (rare) • Seizure • Mass/neoplasm • Sleep apnea	• Substance use or withdrawal • Infection • Sinusitis • Hypoxia • Hypercapnia • Mitochondrial disorders • Thyroid dysfunction • Anemia • Asthenopia (eye strain) • Tempomandibular joint dysfunction

abnormal neurologic examination. Headaches that worsen with standing and improve with lying down are suggestive of low-pressure headaches caused by a tear in the dura from a preceding LP or spontaneous leak.

Medication and illicit drug ingestion and withdrawal are both culprits to secondary headaches. Steroids, vitamin A toxicity, oral contraceptives, and tetracycline are all associated with IIH. Medications that are commonly associated with medication overuse headache include aspirin, acetaminophen, NSAIDs, triptans, and combination analgesics such as acetaminophen, butalbital, and caffeine. Other toxins such as lead, carbon monoxide, or organic solvent poisoning cannot be overlooked.

CNS or systemic infections are associated with new onset headaches. Additionally, common systemic or other focal infections may cause headaches such as viral upper respiratory infections, strep pharyngitis (especially in younger children), rhinosinusitis (sinus headache), influenza, and Lyme disease. Migraines are frequently misdiagnosed as sinus headaches and physicians should carefully obtain history of pain in the face, ears, or teeth and evaluate for signs of rhinosinusitis on either physical examination or imaging.

Any cause of hypoxia (eg, cardiac, respiratory, altitude, anemia) may cause a bifrontal throbbing headache that may be worsened with exertion, straining, or laying down. Hypercapnia causes a nonspecific headache and may be secondary to sleep apnea or other underlying metabolic or respiratory disorder.

Although eye strain and temporal mandibular joint dysfunction are rare causes of recurrent headaches, they can be simply treated; therefore, when suspected, evaluation by ophthalmology or dentistry, respectively, is indicated. Examination in temporomandibular joint dysfunction can include local pain, deviation of the mandible, jaw clicking, and limitations of chewing motion.

A thorough history and physical examination helps diagnose most of these conditions.

▶ **Complications**

Migraines and tension-type headaches are episodic headache disorders but may transform into chronic headaches when a child has more than 15 headache days per month for three or more months. Risk factors for chronicity include psychological comorbidity, obesity, and excessive medication.

Depression and anxiety are both comorbid with headaches and are associated with increased headache burden and disability, such as school absenteeism and poor school performance. Children with psychiatric disorders also have increased rates of primary headaches. Maintaining school attendance in children with headaches is a key factor in limiting chronicity and further disability from headaches.

▶ **Treatment**

Treatment is divided into two categories: acute/abortive and preventative. Management of headaches should emphasize the necessity for early and adequate treatment during a headache, in addition to self-management skills to reduce frequency and disability such as life-style modification and headache diaries. Pharmacologic preventative treatment can be considered if frequency or disability is significant.

A. Acute/Abortive Treatment

Acute treatment for pediatric migraine includes use of simple analgesics and migraine-specific medications. Any medication used to abort a headache (abortive medication) should be given as early as possible after the onset of headache. Simple analgesics include acetaminophen (15 mg/kg; max dose 650 mg) and ibuprofen (10 mg/kg; max dose 800 mg), often used as first-line therapy. The United States FDA has approved almotriptan (ages 12–17) and rizatriptan (ages 6–17). Studies have shown significant benefit for pediatric migraine using rizatriptan oral (5 mg for 20–39 kg, 10 mg for > 40 kg), almotriptan oral (6.25 or 12.5 mg), zolmitriptan nasal (5 mg > 12 y), and sumatriptan nasal (10 mg for < 40 kg, 20 mg for > 40 kg).

Sumatriptan may be used independently or combined with naproxen. Occasionally home treatment fails and patients may need IV medications either in an emergency department or infusion center. When a patient fails emergency room treatments, IV dihydroergotamine can be effective. Nausea as the most common side effect. All medications used for abortive treatment should be used cautiously to avoid medication overuse headache. Simple analgesics should be limited to two to three times per week and migraine-specific medications to less than one to two times per week. During a headache biobehavioral techniques include rest, relaxation, and cold/hot packs. Providing the child with a cool dark room in which to rest may provide added benefit.

B. Prevention

Any child with headaches should have biobehavioral management as a center point to treatment. This includes sleep hygiene (such as bedtime routine, adequate duration, and good quality of sleep), improved fluid intake, elimination of caffeine, regular nutritional meals, regular exercise and stretching, and stress management. Preventative treatment can be considered in individuals with headache frequency of one or more per week. Treatments should be chosen by optimizing wanted side-effects and minimizing unwanted side effects (eg, using topiramate in an obese child given its side-effect of weight loss).

Treatments are categorized into ASMs (eg, topiramate, valproic acid, levetiracetam), antihypertensive (eg, β-blockers, calcium channel blockers), antidepressants (eg, amitriptyline), antihistamine/antiserotonergic (eg, cyproheptadine), and nutraceuticals. Only small randomized double-blinded or open-label studies have tested these agents.

Topiramate, amitriptyline, and cyproheptadine are the most commonly prescribed medications for pediatric headache. If topiramate is started slowly and at low doses, cognitive side effects can be avoided. Peripheral tingling is uncommon and when present usually can be tolerated by most children. Decreased appetite and weight loss should be monitored at routine appointments. Amitriptyline is usually dosed at nighttime given its side effect of sedation, in addition to other common side effects including constipation, dry mouth, and prolonged QT (typically at higher doses). Cyproheptadine is a good medication to use in younger children given its small side-effect profile of primary increased appetite and sedation. The 24-week CHAMP study of migraine prevention in children 8–17 years old showed that topiramate was better than amitriptyline or placebo for headache prevention. Divalproex sodium has not shown efficacy and side effects including weight gain, tremor, hair loss, and teratogenicity warrant caution in adolescent female patients.

Cognitive behavioral therapy is efficacious in significantly decreasing migraine frequency and disability in youth. Coenzyme q10 and magnesium oxide have shown some efficacy in childhood migraine. They may be a useful option for children with low-frequency headache, low disability, or individuals who favor nonpharmaceutical options.

▶ Prognosis

From the few studies regarding long-term prognosis in adolescents presenting with migraines, approximately 25%–40% of adolescents will have remission of migraine symptoms, 40%–50% have persistence, and 20%–25% convert to tension-type headache. Of those with TTH, 20% convert to migraine. Headache severity at diagnosis is thought to be predictive of headache outcome in the long term.

El-Chammas K et al: Pharmacologic treatment of pediatric headaches: a meta-analysis. JAMA Pediatr 2013 Mar 1;167(3):111 [PMID: 23358935].

Evers S: The efficacy of triptans in childhood and adolescence migraine. Cur Pain Headache Rep 2013 Jul;17(7):342 [PMID: 23709234].

Gelfand A: Episodic syndromes that may be associated with migraine: A.K.A. The "Childhood Periodic Syndromes". Headache 2015;55:1358–1364 [PMID: 26234380].

Headache Classification Committee of the International Headache Society: The International Classification of Headache Disorders, 3rd edition (beta version). Cephalalgia 2013 Jul;33(9):629–808 [PMID: 23771276].

Hershey AD: Current approaches to the diagnosis and management of paediatric migraine. Lancet Neurol 2010;9:190 [PMID: 20129168].

Lewis DW et al: Headache evaluation in children and adolescents: when to worry? When to scan? Pediatr Ann 2010;39:399 [PMID: 20666345].

Orr SL, Venkateswaren S: Nutraceuticals in the prophylaxis of pediatric migraine: evidence-based review and recommendations. Cephalalgia 2014;34:568–583 [PMID: 24443395].

Powers SW, Coffey CS, et al: Trial of amitriptyline, topiramate and placebo for pediatric migraine. N Engl J Med 2017;376(2) [PMID: 27788026].

Richer L et al: Drugs for the acute treatment of migraine in children and adolescents. Cochrane Database of Syst Rev 2016;4:CD005220. doi: 10.1002/14651858.CD005220.pub2 [PMID: 27091010].

PSEUDOTUMOR CEREBRI (IDIOPATHIC INTRACRANIAL HYPERTENSION)

ESSENTIALS OF DIAGNOSIS & TYPICAL FEATURES

▶ Signs and symptoms of increased intracranial pressure: chronic or progressive positional headache, vomiting, tinnitus, papilledema, double vision, blurry vision.

▶ Normal MRI/MRV of the head.

▶ Elevated opening pressure on lumbar puncture performed in the lateral decubitus position.

Pathogenesis

Pseudotumor cerebri, or more appropriately named idiopathic intracranial hypertension (IIH), is characterized by increased intracranial pressure, as documented in the absence of an identifiable intracranial mass, infection, metabolic derangement, or hydrocephalus. The pathogenesis of IIH is poorly understood. Multiple risk factors have been identified, but obesity is the most common. Interestingly, multiple medications have also been associated with IIH, including tetracycline, steroids, and retinol (Table 25–11).

Clinical Findings

Presenting features include new or chronic positional headache (worse when supine), vomiting, pulsatile tinnitus, papilledema, blurry vision, and diplopia (typically secondary to cranial nerve VI palsy limiting lateral movement of one or both eyes). Later findings may include visual loss and optic atrophy. Transient visual obscurations (TVOs), which are brief (< 1 minute) and reversible alterations of vision, can also occur. In contrast, visual field deficits can be permanent.

Differential Diagnosis

All patients with signs/symptoms of increased intracranial pressure should receive imaging, typically with MRI and MRV to fully evaluate for hydrocephalus, tumor/mass lesion, and cerebral venous sinus thrombosis. Once a mass lesion is ruled out, lumbar puncture should be performed in the lateral decubitus position to confirm the presence of increased pressure (above 180–250 mm H_2O depending on technique and anesthetic used) and also to assess the CSF white blood cell count, glucose, and protein (looking for an infectious mimicker, such as chronic meningitis). A variety of medications, metabolic disorders, and infectious disorders are associated with or mimic IIH (see Table 25–11), but typically, no specific cause is found.

Complications

Poorly treated IIH and chronic papilledema may lead to permanent optic nerve damage and vision loss, which usually occurs in the blind spot and/or nasal aspects of the visual field, prior to affecting central vision. Headache, TVOs, cranial nerve VI palsy, and malaise are usually reversible.

Treatment

Treatment of IIH is aimed at correcting the identifiable predisposing condition and preventing vision loss. Sequential ophthalmologic evaluation is important. Many patients benefit from the use of acetazolamide or topiramate to decrease CSF production. Obese patients will benefit significantly from weight loss. If a program of medical management and ophthalmologic surveillance fail, neurosurgical intervention such as shunt placement or optic nerve fenestration may be necessary. Dural venous stenting is rarely warranted.

Prognosis

With appropriate workup and treatment, most patients recover from IIH without long-term sequela including visual outcome. Reoccurrence risk is greatest within 18 months.

Table 25–11. Conditions associated with idiopathic intracranial hypertension and idiopathic intracranial hypertension mimickers.

Medications and metabolic-toxic disorders
Hypervitaminosis A, including use of retinoids
Obesity
Steroid therapy
Hormonal therapy
Steroid withdrawal
Tetracycline, minocycline toxicity
Nalidixic acid toxicity
Iron deficiency
Clotting disorders
Hypocalcemia
Hyperparathyroidism or hyperthyroidism
Adrenal insufficiency
Systemic lupus erythematosus
Chronic CO_2 retention
Infectious and parainfectious disorders
Chronic otitis media (lateral sinus thrombosis)
Guillain-Barré syndrome
Lyme disease
Cerebral venous sinus thrombosis (CVST)
Minor head injury

Avery RA et al: CSF opening pressure in children with optic nerve head edema. Neurology 2011;76(19):1658 [PMID: 21555733].

Kosmorsky GS: Idiopathic intracranial hypertension: pseudotumor cerebri. Headache 2014 Feb;54(2):389–393 [PMID: 24512582].

Rogers DL: A review of pediatric idiopathic intracranial hypertension. Pediatr Clin North Am 2014 Jun;61(3):579–590 [PMID: 24852154].

Soiberman U et al: IIH in children: visual outcome and risk of recurrence. Childs Nerv Syst 2011 Nov;27(11):1913–1918 [PMID: 21538129].

CEREBROVASCULAR DISEASE

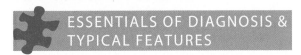

ESSENTIALS OF DIAGNOSIS & TYPICAL FEATURES

▶ Perinatal arterial ischemic stroke (perinatal AIS) occurs in neonates younger than 28 days old.

▶ Childhood AIS occurs in children between 28 days and 18 years old.

▶ Neuroimaging is required to make the diagnosis of stroke.

▶ Revascularization therapies, such as thrombolytic agents and mechanical thrombectomy, could be successfully used in childhood AIS with close guidance from urgent pediatric neurology consultation, as treatment approaches are rapidly evolving and multidisciplinary care is critical.

Pediatric AIS is subdivided into two categories: perinatal AIS (28 weeks' gestation to 28 days of life) and childhood AIS (28 days to 18 years of age).

1. Childhood Arterial Ischemic Stroke

Childhood AIS affects 1.6 per 100,000 children per year, with numerous adverse outcomes, including death (10%), neurologic deficits or seizures (70%–75%), and recurrent ischemic stroke (20%). Childhood AIS represents a neurologic emergency—prompt diagnosis can affect treatment considerations and long-term outcomes. Recanalization with thrombolytic agents or mechanical thrombectomy is increasingly used in eligible children, even 6–24 hours after symptom onset. When possible, urgent consultation with a neurologist should be obtained within 24 hours for any child who presents with concern for acute ischemic stroke, and the patient should ultimately be transferred to a tertiary care center that specializes in pediatric stroke management. Unfortunately, most pediatric AIS is not recognized until more than 24 hours after onset.

▶ Clinical Findings

A. Symptoms and Signs

Manifestations of arterial ischemic stroke in childhood vary according to the cerebral vascular territory that is involved. Children may present with acute hemiplegia, aphasia, or acute vertigo, similarly to ischemic stroke in adults. Unilateral weakness, sensory disturbance, dysarthria, and/or dysphagia may develop over a period of minutes, but at times, progressive worsening of symptoms may evolve over several hours. New onset focal seizure accompanied by focal neurologic deficits is a common presentation of childhood AIS.

Providers should carefully determine the time of the patient's "last known normal (LKN)." Importantly, the LKN is often different than the time that the symptoms were first noticed. All clinical trials have utilized LKN to determine appropriate "treatment windows." The evaluation should also include a thorough history of prior illnesses, preceding viral infection, minor head or neck trauma, and familial clotting tendencies, as well as any cardiac, vascular, hematologic, or intracranial disorders (Table 25–12).

Physical examination of the patient initially focuses on identifying the specific deficits related to impaired cerebral blood flow. The National Institutes of Health Stroke Scale (NIHSS) is a rapid neurologic exam designed to identify acute arterial stroke. In addition, the patient should be evaluated for evidence of any predisposing cardiac, vascular, hematologic, infectious, or intracranial disorders (see Table 25–12). Retinal hemorrhages, splinter hemorrhages in the nail beds, cardiac murmurs, rash, fever, neurocutaneous stigmata, and signs of trauma are especially important findings. Congenital heart disease is the most common predisposing condition, followed by hematologic and neoplastic disorders, though most patients are not found to have a specific disorder.

B. Laboratory Findings and Ancillary Testing

In the acute phase, complete blood count, complete metabolic panel, PT/PTT, and a pregnancy test, as well as brain imaging, should be carried out emergently. Additional testing to consider urgently includes disseminated intravascular coagulation (DIC) panel, fibrin split products, erythrocyte sedimentation rate, C-reactive protein, prothrombin time/partial thromboplastin time, anti-factor Xa activity, chest radiography, ECG, and urine toxicology. Subsequent studies can be carried out systemically, with particular attention to disorders involving the heart, blood vessels, platelets, red cells, hemoglobin, and coagulation proteins. Twenty to fifty percent of pediatric ischemic stroke patients have a prothrombotic state. Additional laboratory tests for systemic disorders such as vasculitis, mitochondrial disorders, and metabolic disorders are sometimes indicated.

Examination of CSF is indicated in patients with suspected infection, rheumatologic disease, or subarachnoid hemorrhage, but is otherwise rarely helpful in the acute setting. Patients with seemingly idiopathic AIS may benefit from serum and CSF testing for HSV and VZV, both of which can cause stroke secondary to focal vasculopathies/arteriopathies, even years after the initial infection.

EEG may help in patients with severely depressed consciousness. ECG and echocardiography are useful both in evaluating stroke etiology as well as for ongoing monitoring and management, particularly when hypotension or cardiac arrhythmias complicate the clinical course or when the stroke is thought to be embolic in nature.

Table 25–12. Etiologic risk factors for ischemic and/or hemorrhagic ischemic stroke.

Cardiac disorders
  Structural heart disease
  Valvular disease
  Endocarditis
  Cardiomyopathy
  Arrhythmias
Vascular occlusive disorders
  Cervical/cerebral arterial dissection
  Homocystinuria/homocystinemia
  Vasculitis
    Meningitis
    Polyarteritis nodosa
    Systemic lupus erythematosus
    Drug abuse (amphetamines)
  Varicella
  Mycoplasma
  Human immunodeficiency virus
  Fibromuscular dysplasia
  Moyamoya disease
  Diabetes
  Nephrotic syndrome
  Systemic hypertension
  Dural sinus and cerebral venous thrombosis
  Cortical venous thrombosis
Hematologic disorders
  Iron deficiency anemia
  Polycythemia
  Thrombotic thrombocytopenia
  Thrombocytopenic purpura
  Leukemia
  Hemoglobinopathies
    Sickle cell disease
  Coagulation defects
    Hemophilia
    Vitamin K deficiency
  Hypercoagulable states
    Prothrombin gene mutation
    Methylenetetrahydrofolate reductase mutation
    Lipoprotein (a) derangements
    Factor V Leiden deficiency
    Antiphospholipid antibodies
    Hypercholesterolemia
    Hypertriglyceridemia
    Factor VIII elevation
    Pregnancy
    Systemic lupus erythematosus
    Use of oral contraceptives
    Antithrombin III deficiency
    Protein C and S deficiencies
Intracranial vascular anomalies
  Moyamoya
  Arteriovenous malformation
  Arterial aneurysm
  Carotid-cavernous fistula
  Focal cerebral arteriopathy
  Connective tissue diseases

C. Imaging

Urgent CT and MRI scans of the brain are necessary to determine the extent of cerebral involvement with ischemia or hemorrhage. Importantly, CT scans may be normal within the first 24 hours of an ischemic stroke and are performed to exclude intracranial hemorrhage, which may influence the patient's eligibility for anticoagulation, thrombolytic agents, or mechanical thrombectomy. Given the high incidence of ischemic stroke mimickers in the pediatric population (migraine with aura, Todd's paralysis, encephalitis, etc), urgent MRI with DWI is increasingly employed to quickly determine whether an arterial ischemic stroke has occurred.

In addition, vascular imaging of the head and neck is an important part of pediatric ischemic stroke diagnosis and may include CTA, MRA, or conventional angiography. Evidence of large-vessel occlusion (ie, carotid artery or proximal middle cerebral artery) is a key criterion for mechanical thrombectomy, in select cases. Up to 80% of pediatric patients with idiopathic childhood-onset arterial ischemic stroke have a demonstrated vascular abnormality on imaging, and these patients have a much greater recurrence risk than patients with normal vessels. Vascular imaging can detect transient cerebral arteriopathy, focal vasculopathy, arteriopathy associated with sickle cell disease, moyamoya disease, arterial dissection, aneurysm, fibromuscular dysplasia, and vasculitis. When vessel imaging is performed, all major vessels should be examined, starting at the aortic arch.

▶ Differential Diagnosis

Patients with acute onset of neurologic deficits must also be evaluated for other disorders that can cause focal neurologic deficits. Hypoglycemia, prolonged focal seizures, a prolonged postictal paresis (Todd's paralysis), acute disseminated encephalomyelitis (ADEM), meningitis, hemorrhagic stroke, encephalitis, hemiplegic migraine, ingestion, and brain abscess should all be considered. In particular, migraine with focal neurologic deficits may be difficult to differentiate initially from ischemic stroke—urgent imaging is typically warranted. The possibility of drug abuse and other toxic exposures must be investigated diligently in any patient with acute mental status changes.

▶ Treatment

The initial management of ischemic stroke in a child focuses on quickly determining whether the patient is candidate for urgent intervention. Approaches to the pediatric use of thrombolytic agents (such as intravenous tissue plasminogen activator, tPA) and mechanical thrombectomy with interventional radiologic techniques are rapidly changing, and an increasing number of pediatric patients are benefiting from these treatments. Therefore, neurology consultation should be obtained emergently, including discussion of the patient's LKN and NIHSS, as well as other pertinent history and exam findings. Bedside providers should simultaneously support pulmonary, cardiovascular, and renal function. Patients should be administered oxygen if necessary. Typically, isotonic maintenance fluids are indicated to augment vascular volume. Pyrexia should be treated aggressively. Meningitis and other infections should be treated. Sickle cell patients require hematologists to perform urgent exchange transfusion.

Specific treatment of ischemic stroke, including blood pressure management, fluid management, and antiplatelet/anticoagulation measures, depends partly on the underlying pathogenesis and timeline. Guidelines for the role of anticoagulation or aspirin therapy are also rapidly evolving. In general, the Royal College of Physicians Pediatric Ischemic Stroke Working Group recommends aspirin, 5 mg/kg daily, as soon as the diagnosis is made. Aspirin use in pediatric patients appears safe, but the American Heart Association (AHA) does recommend yearly flu shots and close monitoring for Reye syndrome in pediatric patients taking aspirin for long periods. In some situations, such as arterial dissection or cardioembolic events, anticoagulation with heparin should be considered, particularly if evidence of persistent thrombus is present (eg, on ECHO or CTA). Some disorders require additional special considerations. For example, patients with vasculitis are often given anti-inflammatory therapy, such as steroids. Patients with moyamoya are at high risk for hemorrhage and may require surgical revascularization after the acute period has ended.

Long-term management requires intensive rehabilitation efforts and therapy aimed at improving the child's language, motor, educational, and psychological performance. Constraint therapy may be particularly helpful in cases of hemiparesis. Length of treatment with anticoagulation or antiplatelet agents, such as low-molecular-weight heparin and aspirin, is often determined on a case-by-case basis.

▶ **Prognosis**

The outcome of ischemic stroke in infants and children is variable, depending on the presence of underlying predisposing conditions and the vascular territory involved. Roughly one-third may have minimal or no deficits, one-third are moderately affected, and one-third are severely affected. When the ischemic stroke involves extremely large portions of one hemisphere or large portions of both hemispheres, and cerebral edema develops, the patient's level of consciousness may deteriorate rapidly, and death may occur within the first few days. In contrast, some patients may achieve complete recovery of neurologic function within a few days if the cerebral territory is small. Seizures, either focal or generalized, may occur in 30%–50% of patients at some point in their course. Stroke recurrence is 14%–20%, and is more prominent in some conditions, such as protein C

deficiency, lipoprotein (a) abnormalities, and arteriopathies. Chronic problems with learning, behavior, and activity are common. Long-term follow-up with a pediatric neurologist is indicated and, if possible, a multidisciplinary ischemic stroke team.

2. Perinatal Arterial Ischemic Stroke

Perinatal arterial ischemic stroke is more common than childhood ischemic stroke, affecting 1:3500 children. Perinatal ischemic stroke has two distinct presentations: acute and delayed. Most patients with an acute presentation develop neonatal seizures during the first week of life, particularly focal motor seizures of the contralateral arm and/or leg. The presentation is stereotypical because of the predilection of perinatal ischemic stroke to occur in the middle cerebral artery. The presence of diffusion-weighted abnormalities on an MRI scan confirms an acute perinatal ischemic stroke during the first week of life. Other patients present with delayed symptoms, typically with hemiparesis that became notable at 4–8 months. These patients are termed "presumed perinatal arterial ischemic stroke."

Acute treatment of a perinatal ischemic stroke is usually limited to supportive care, including normalizing glucose levels, monitoring blood pressure, optimizing oxygenation, and managing seizures. Treatable causes such as infection, cardiac embolus, metabolic derangement, and inherited thrombophilia must be ruled out, in some cases with echocardiography, thrombophilia evaluation, or lumbar puncture. Unless an embolic source is identified, aspirin and anticoagulation are almost never prescribed.

Long-term management of perinatal ischemic stroke usually starts with identifying risk factors, which might include coagulation disorders, cardiac disease, drugs, and dehydration. Prothrombotic abnormalities with the best evidence of association are factor V Leiden, protein C deficiency, and high lipoprotein (a), though many practitioners perform an extensive hematologic workup, particularly once the patient has reached at least 6 months of age. Maternal risk factors such as infertility, antiphospholipid antibodies, placental infection, premature rupture of membranes, and cocaine exposure are independently associated with perinatal ischemic stroke.

The prognosis for children who sustain perinatal ischemic strokes has been considered better than for children or adults with ischemic strokes, presumably because of the plasticity of the neonatal brain. The range of cognitive and motor outcomes after perinatal stroke is broad. Twenty to forty percent of patients have no neurologic deficits. Motor impairment affects about 40%–60% of patients and is predominantly hemiplegic cerebral palsy. In acute presentations, MRI can be predictive of motor impairment, as descending corticospinal tract diffusion-weighted MRI signal is associated with a higher incidence of hemiplegia.

Language delays, behavioral abnormalities, and cognitive deficits are seen in up to 55% of infants who experience perinatal ischemic strokes. Patients are also at an increased lifelong risk for seizures. Ischemic stroke recurs in 3% of neonates and is usually associated with a prothrombotic abnormality or an underlying illness, such as cardiac malformation or infection. Given the low incidence of recurrence, long-term management is largely rehabilitative, including constraint therapies.

Barry M et al: What is the role of mechanical thrombectomy in childhood stroke? Pediatr Neurol 2019;95:19–25 [PMID: 30795888].

Giglia T et al: Prevention and treatment of thrombosis in pediatric and congenital heart disease: a scientific statement from the American Heart Association. Circulation 2013;128:2622–2703 [PMID: 2426806].

Kirton A et al: Symptomatic neonatal arterial ischemic stroke: the international Pediatric Stroke Study. Pediatrics 2011; 128:1402–1410 [PMID: 22123886].

Kirton A, deVeber G: Paediatric stroke: pressing issues and promising directions. Lancet 2015 Jan;14(1):92–102 [PMID: 25496900].

Mallick AA et al: childhood arterial ischaemic stroke incidence, presenting features, and risk factors: a prospective population-based study. Lancet Neurol 2014;13:35–43 [PMID: 2430498].

Monagle P et al: Antithrombotic therapy in neonates and children: antithrombotic therapy and prevention of thrombosis 9th ed: American College of Chest Physicians evidence-based clinical guidelines. Chest 2012;141:e737S–801S [PMID: 22315277].

Powers WJ et al: 2015 American Heart Association/American Stroke Association focused update of the 2013 Guidelines for the early management of patients with acute ischemic stroke regarding endovascular treatment: a guideline for healthcare professionals. Stroke 2015;46:3020–3035 [PMID: 26123479].

CONGENITAL MALFORMATIONS OF THE NERVOUS SYSTEM

Malformations of the nervous system occur in 3% of living neonates and are present in 40% of infants who die in the first year of life. Structural malformation of the CNS may result from a variety of causes, including infectious, toxic, genetic, metabolic, and vascular insults. The specific type of malformation that results from such insults depends on the gestational period during which the insult. The period of induction, days 0–28 of gestation, is the period during which the neural plate appears and the neural tube forms and closes. Insults during this phase can result in a major absence of neural structures, such as anencephaly, or in a defect of neural tube closure, such as spina bifida, meningomyelocele, or encephalocele. Cellular proliferation and migration characterize neural development that occurs from 12 to 20 weeks' gestation. During this period, lissencephaly, pachygyria, agyria, and agenesis of the corpus callosum (ACC) may arise depending on the type of developmental disruption.

1. Abnormalities of Neural Tube Closure

Defects of neural tube closure constitute some of the most common congenital malformations affecting the nervous system, occurring in 1:1000 live births prior to the introduction of folate supplementation (which decreased incidence by 50%–75%). Up to 6% of fetuses with isolated spinal cord defects have an associated chromosomal abnormality (typically Trisomy 13 or 18), which should be screened for upon identification of the defect. Spina bifida with associated myelomeningocele or meningocele is commonly found in the lumbar region. Depending on the extent and severity of the involvement of the spinal cord and peripheral nerves, lower extremity weakness, bowel and bladder dysfunction, and hip dislocation may be present. Delivery via cesarean section followed by early surgical closure of meningoceles and meningomyeloceles is usually indicated. Additional treatment is necessary to manage chronic abnormalities of the urinary tract, orthopedic abnormalities such as kyphosis and scoliosis, and paresis of the lower extremities. Hydrocephalus is very common and usually requires ventriculoperitoneal shunting. For selected patients, pre-natal repair has been shown to reduce the need for VP shunt at 1 year and result in improved motor function at 30 months of age, though pregnancy and delivery-related complications were higher. This is a promising option for patients who meet the surgical criteria.

▶ Diagnosis & Prevention

In general, the diagnosis of neural tube defects is obvious at the time of birth. The diagnosis may be strongly suspected prenatally on the basis of ultrasonographic findings and the presence of elevated α-fetoprotein and acetylcholinesterase in the amniotic fluid. All women of childbearing age should take prophylactic folate, which can prevent these defects and decrease the risk of recurrence by 70%.

2. Disorders of Cortical Development

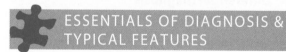

ESSENTIALS OF DIAGNOSIS & TYPICAL FEATURES

► Malformations of cortical development (MCD) can be diffuse, unilateral, or focal, which is dependent on the timing and type of the disruption of brain development.

► Clinical presentation is variable and can be divided into two large groups: diffuse MCD with poor neurodevelopmental outcomes and focal or multifocal MCD with variable, but generally less severe, outcomes.

Malformations of cortical development are known causes of a wide spectrum of developmental and cognitive disabilities as well as epilepsy. They are a diverse group of disorders characterized by disruption of the cortex primarily identified on MRI. Although MCD was historically classified based on stages of brain development disrupted, the field of neurogenetics has revealed over a hundred genetic mutations leading to a wide variety of overlapping structural phenotypes.

▶ Pathogenesis

MCD can occur when one of the three primary stages of cortical development are disrupted: (1) neuronal proliferation, (2) neuronal migration, or (3) postmigrational development. The genes associated with MCD include cell-cycle regulation, angiogenesis, protein synthesis, apoptosis, cell-fate specification, cytoskeletal structure and function, neuronal migration and basement-membrane function, and inborn errors of metabolism.

▶ Clinical Findings

Clinical presentation is variable and can be divided into those children who present early with severe neurodevelopmental deficits and diffuse MCD, and those children who present later in childhood with focal seizures or milder developmental and intellectual disabilities and are found to have focal or multifocal MCD.

Diffuse MCD is typically associated with a variety of signs including seizures, GDD, feeding, hearing, and vision impairments, poor sleep, abnormal head size, hydrocephalus, behavior problems, autonomic dysregulation, and movement disorders. Typically, there is a higher risk for shortened lifespan in these children.

Focal MCD can be associated with normal development or mild developmental delays. Focal seizures are a common presentation. Neurodevelopmental disabilities may include mild learning disabilities and behavioral concerns (including ADHD). Sometimes, focal MCD is found incidentally when neuroimaging is done for other reasons.

▶ Differential Diagnosis

A. Megalencephaly

Megalencephaly is an example of neuronal proliferation dysfunction and results in a brain size that is greater than three standard deviations above the mean. On MRI megalencephaly can be associated with normal cortical development, polymicrogyria, and hemimegalencephaly. Associated neurologic outcomes can include normal development, developmental delay, intellectual disability, and seizures. There are several genes and syndromes associated including Neurofibromatosis 1.

B. Lissencephaly and Subcortical Band Heterotopia

Lissencephaly is an example of abnormal migration and increased apoptosis. This severe malformation of the brain is characterized by a smooth cortical surface with minimal sulcal and gyral development. Lissencephalic brains have a primitive cortex with less than the normal six-layered cortical mantle. The pattern of pachygyria (thick gyri) and agyria (absence of gyri) may vary in an anterior to posterior gradient and help guide genetic diagnosis. Patients with lissencephaly usually have severe neurodevelopmental delay, microcephaly, and seizures (including infantile spasms), although there is significant phenotypic heterogeneity. These disorders are autosomal recessive and X-linked. *LIS1* mutations on chromosome 17 are sometimes associated with dysmorphic features (Miller-Dieker syndrome). Mutations in the *RELN* gene, results in a lissencephaly with severe hippocampal and cerebellar hypoplasia. X-linked syndromes involving mutations in *DCX* and *ARX* (associated with ambiguous genitalia) affect males with lissencephaly and females with band heterotopias or ACC.

Lissencephaly with hydrocephalus, cerebellar malformations, or muscular dystrophy may occur in Walker-Warburg syndrome (*POMT1* mutations and others), Fukuyama muscular dystrophy (*FKTN* mutation), and muscle-eye-brain disease (*POMGnT1* mutation). It is particularly important to identify these syndromes not only because clinical tests are available, but also because of their genetic implications. Lissencephaly may be a component of Zellweger syndrome, a peroxisomal disorder with elevated concentrations of very-long-chain fatty acids in the serum. No specific treatment for lissencephaly is available.

C. Polymicrogyria With or Without Schizencephaly

Polymicrogyria is a postmigrational disorder characterized by an overfolded and malformed cortex that can be associated with schizencephaly, diffuse, or focal, such as bilateral perisylvian polymicrogyria (the classic form). Patients with bilateral perisylvian polymicrogyria may have bulbar dysfunction, variable cognitive deficits, developmental delay, and epilepsy. Etiologies of polymicrogyria vary including genetic mutations, infectious, and vascular causes.

▶ Treatment

Treatment of MCD center on early child development intervention and focused symptomatic treatment (eg, attention deficit, hearing impairment, physical therapy for gait abnormalities).

3. Disorders of Cerebellum Development

A. Arnold-Chiari Malformations

Arnold-Chiari malformation type I consists of elongation and displacement of the caudal end of the brainstem into the spinal canal with protrusion of the cerebellar tonsils through the foramen magnum. In association with this hindbrain malformation, minor to moderate abnormalities of the base of the skull can occur, including basilar impression (platy-basia) and small foramen magnum. Arnold-Chiari malformation type I typically remains asymptomatic for years, but in older children and young adults it may cause progressive cerebellar signs (vertigo, ataxia), paresis of the lower cranial nerves or neck/posterior head pain exacerbated by straining; rarely may it present with apnea or disordered breathing. Posterior cervical laminectomy may be necessary to provide relief from symptoms.

Arnold-Chiari malformation type II consists of the malformations found in Arnold-Chiari type I plus an associated myelomeningocele. Hydrocephalus develops in approximately 90% of children with Arnold-Chiari malformation type II. These patients may also have hydromyelia, syringomyelia, and cortical dysplasias. The clinical manifestations of Arnold-Chiari malformation type II are most commonly caused by the associated hydrocephalus and meningomyelocele. In addition, dysfunction of the lower cranial nerves may be present. Up to 25% of patients may have epilepsy, likely secondary to the cortical dysplasias. Higher lesions of the thoracic or upper lumbar cord are associated with mild intellectual disability in about half of patients, while over 85% of patients with lower level lesions have normal intelligence quotients (IQs).

Arnold-Chiari malformation type III is characterized by herniation of the cerebellum through the foramen magnum with associated cervical spinal cord defect. Hydrocephalus is extremely common with this malformation.

B. Dandy-Walker Malformation

Despite being described over a century ago, the exact definition of the Dandy-Walker malformation is still debated. Classically, it is characterized by aplasia of the vermis, cystic enlargement of the fourth ventricle, and rostral displacement of the tentorium. Although hydrocephalus is usually not present congenitally, it develops within the first few months of life. Ninety percent of patients who develop hydrocephalus do so by age 1 year.

On physical examination, a rounded protuberance or exaggeration of the cranial occiput often exists. In the absence of hydrocephalus and increased intracranial pressure, few physical findings may be present to suggest neurologic dysfunction. An ataxic syndrome occurs in fewer than 20% of patients and is usually late in appearing. Many long-term neurologic deficits result directly from hydrocephalus. CT or MRI scanning of the head confirms diagnosis of Dandy-Walker syndrome. Treatment is directed at the management of hydrocephalus.

4. Agenesis of the Corpus Callosum

Agenesis of the corpus callosum (ACC), once thought to be a rare cerebral malformation, is more frequently diagnosed with modern neuroimaging techniques, occurring in 1:4000 to 1:5000 live births. There does not appear to be a single cause of this malformation. Rather, multiple single and mutigene mutations have been associated. An underlying genetic cause can be found in up to 45% of cases. It has been found in X-linked conditions, such as ARX mutations (lissencephaly and ambiguous genitalia), recessive conditions such as Andermann syndrome (neuropathy and dementia), and polygenic conditions such as Aicardi syndrome (chorioretinal lacunae, infantile spasms, skeletal abnormalities). No specific clinical picture is typical of ACC, although many patients have seizures, developmental delay, microcephaly, or neurobehavioral problems (autism, difficulties with social interactions). Interestingly, the malformation may be found coincidentally by neuroimaging studies in otherwise normal patients.

5. Hydrocephalus

Hydrocephalus is an increased volume of CSF with progressive ventricular dilation. Hydrocephalus may be communicating or non-communicating. In communicating hydrocephalus, CSF circulates through the ventricular system and into the subarachnoid space without obstruction. In noncommunicating hydrocephalus, an obstruction blocks the flow of CSF within the ventricular system or blocks the egress of CSF from the ventricular system into the subarachnoid space. A wide variety of disorders, such as hemorrhage, infection, tumors, and congenital malformations, may play a causal role in the development of hydrocephalus. Clinical features of hydrocephalus include macrocephaly, an excessive or rapid head growth, irritability, bulging or full fontanelle, vomiting, loss of appetite, impaired upgaze (known as "sun setting" phenomenon), impaired extraocular movements, hypertonia of the lower extremities, and generalized hyperreflexia. Without treatment, optic atrophy may occur. In infants, papilledema may not be present, whereas older children with closed cranial sutures can eventually develop swelling of the optic disk. Hydrocephalus can be diagnosed on the basis of the clinical course, findings on physical examination, and CT or MRI scan.

Treatment of hydrocephalus is directed at providing an alternative outlet for CSF from the intracranial compartment. The most common method is ventriculoperitoneal shunting. Other treatment should be directed, if possible, at the underlying cause of the hydrocephalus.

Barkovich AJ, Guerrini R, Kuzniecky RI, Jackson GD, Dobyns WB: A developmental and genetic classification for malformations of cortical development: update 2012. Brain 2012;135 (Pt 5):1348–1369 [PMID: 22427329].

Guerrini R, Dobyns W: Malformations of cortical development: clinical features and genetic causes. Lancet Neurol 2014;13: 710–726 [PMID: 24932993].

Liu JS: Molecular genetics of neuronal migration disorders. Curr Neurol Neurosci Rep 2011;11:171 [PMID: 21222180].

ABNORMAL HEAD SIZE

The skull bone plates have almost no intrinsic capacity to enlarge or grow; they depend on extrinsic forces to stimulate new bone formation at the suture lines. The single most important stimulus for head growth during infancy and childhood is brain growth. Therefore, accurate assessment of head growth is one of the most important aspects of the neurologic examination of young children. A head circumference that is two standard deviations above or below the mean for age requires investigation and explanation.

1. Craniosynostosis

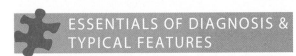

ESSENTIALS OF DIAGNOSIS & TYPICAL FEATURES

▶ Abnormal head shape.
▶ When craniosynostosis occurs with other dysmorphologies, it is considered syndromic craniosynostosis.

Craniosynostosis, or premature closure of cranial sutures, occurs in 1 in 2000 live births. Both idiopathic etiologies are much more common than genetic etiologies.

▶ Clinical Findings

Children with syndromic craniosynostosis, that is, those with other physical anomalies, are more likely to have a genetic etiology, such as Apert syndrome and Crouzon disease, which are also associated with abnormalities of the digits, extremities, and heart. Craniosynostosis may be associated with an underlying metabolic disturbance, such as hyperthyroidism and hypophosphatasia.

▶ Differential Diagnosis

The most common form of craniosynostosis involves the sagittal suture and results in scaphocephaly, an elongation of the head in the anterior to posterior direction. Premature closure of the coronal sutures causes brachycephaly, an increase in cranial growth from left to right. Importantly, closure of only one or a few sutures will not cause impaired brain growth or neurologic dysfunction.

A common complaint is abnormal head shape secondary to positional plagiocephaly due to supine sleep position. A skull film or neurosurgical consultation is typically not necessary, since plagiocephaly from occipital lambdoid suture craniosynostosis is quite rare. Repositioning the head during naps (eg, alternating which direction the child faces) and "tummy time" when awake are remedies, and most children do not require a helmet for reshaping. Most positional non-synostotic plagiocephaly resolves by age 2 years.

▶ Treatment

Management of craniosynostosis is directed at preserving normal skull shape and consists of excising the fused suture and applying material to the edge of the craniectomy to prevent reossification of the bone edges. The best cosmetic effect on the skull is achieved when surgery is performed during the first 6 months of life. An ongoing interdisciplinary approach is commonly required to assess for developmental delays, oral health, visual abnormalities, hearing and middle ear abnormalities, and speech delays.

2. Microcephaly

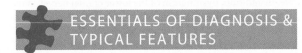

ESSENTIALS OF DIAGNOSIS & TYPICAL FEATURES

▶ Head circumference more than two standard deviations below the mean for age and sex.
▶ Often associated with developmental delay and learning difficulties.

Microcephaly is defined as a head circumference more than two standard deviations below the mean for age and sex. More important than a single head circumference measurement is the rate or pattern of head growth over time. Head circumference measurements that progressively drop to lower percentiles with increasing age are indicative of a process or condition that has impaired the brain's capacity to grow. Primary microcephaly is present at birth and secondary microcephaly develops postnatally. The causes of microcephaly are numerous. Some examples are listed in Table 25–13.

▶ Clinical Findings

A. Symptoms and Signs

Head circumference should be monitored at every well-child check. However, microcephaly may be discovered when the child is examined because of delayed developmental milestones or neurologic problems, such as seizures or spasticity. There may be a marked backward slope of the forehead (as in familial microcephaly) with narrowing of the bitemporal diameter. The fontanelle may close earlier than expected, and sutures may be prominent. Parents' heads may need measurement to rule out a rare dominantly inherited familial microcephaly. Eye, cardiac, and bone abnormalities may also be clues to congenital infection.

Table 25–13. Causes of microcephaly.

Causes	Examples
Chromosomal	Trisomies 13, 18, 21
Malformation	Lissencephaly, schizencephaly
Syndromes	Rubenstein-Taybi, Cornelia de Lange, Angelman
Toxins	Alcohol, anticonvulsants (?), maternal phenylketonuria (PKU)
Infections (intrauterine)	TORCHS[a]
Radiation	Maternal pelvis, first and second trimester
Placental insufficiency	Toxemia, infection, small for gestational age
Familial	Autosomal dominant, autosomal recessive
Perinatal hypoxia, trauma	Birth asphyxia, injury
Infections (perinatal)	Bacterial meningitis (especially group B streptococci), viral encephalitis (enterovirus, herpes simplex)
Metabolic	Glut-1 deficiency, PKU, maple syrup urine disease
Degenerative disease	Tay-Sachs, Krabbe

[a]TORCHS is a mnemonic for toxoplasmosis, other infections, rubella, cytomegalovirus, herpes simplex, and syphilis.

B. Laboratory Findings

Laboratory findings vary with the cause. In the newborn, IgM antibody titers for toxoplasmosis, rubella, CMV, herpes simplex virus, and syphilis and urine culture for CMV may be assessed for sign of congenital infection. Genetic testing can be targeted based on history and physical examination and should typically involve consultation with a genetics/metabolics expert. Most metabolic disorders present either as congenital syndromic microcephaly (ie, dysmorphisms present on examination) or with postnatal microcephaly and GDD, though nonsyndromic microcephaly presenting at birth can also be associated with fetal or maternal metabolic disorders.

C. Imaging Studies

CT or MRI scans may aid in diagnosis and prognosis. These studies may demonstrate calcifications, malformations, or atrophic patterns that suggest specific congenital infections or genetic syndromes. Plain skull radiographs are of limited value. MRI is most helpful in definitive diagnosis, prognosis, and genetic counseling.

► Differential Diagnosis

Common forms of craniosynostosis involving sagittal, coronal, and lambdoidal sutures are associated with abnormally shaped heads but do not typically cause microcephaly. Recognizing treatable causes of undergrowth of the brain, such as hypopituitarism, hypothyroidism, and severe protein-calorie undernutrition, is critical so that therapy can be initiated early. Refer to Table 25–13 for examples of causes of microcephaly.

► Treatment & Prognosis

Genetic counseling should be offered to the family of any infant with significant microcephaly. Many children with microcephaly are developmentally delayed. The notable exceptions are found in cases of hypopituitarism (rare) or familial autosomal dominant microcephaly. Individuals may need screening for vision and hearing abnormalities, as well as supportive therapies for developmental delay.

3. Macrocephaly

A head circumference more than two standard deviations above the mean for age and sex denotes macrocephaly. Rapid head growth rate suggests increased intracranial pressure, most likely caused by hydrocephalus, extra-axial fluid collections, or neoplasms. Macrocephaly with normal head growth rate suggests familial macrocephaly or true megalencephaly (enlarged brain), as might occur in neurofibromatosis. Other causes and examples of macrocephaly are listed in Table 25–14.

► Differential Diagnosis

A. Catch-up Growth

This can be seen when a neurologically intact preterm infant has rapid head enlargement in the first weeks of life. As the expected normal size is reached, head growth slows and then resumes a normal growth pattern.

B. Familial Macrocephaly

This condition may exist when another family member has an unusually large head with no signs or symptoms referable to such disorders as neurocutaneous dysplasias (especially neurofibromatosis) or cerebral gigantism (Sotos syndrome), or when there are no significant neurologic abnormalities in the child.

C. Hydrocephalus

See section on Congenital Malformations of the Nervous System.

Other causes of macrocephaly are dependent on the etiology such as metabolic or genetic causes.

Table 25–14. Causes of macrocephaly.

Causes	Examples
Pseudomacrocephaly, pseudohydrocephalus, catch-up growth crossing percentiles	Growing premature infant; recovery from malnutrition, congenital heart disease, postsurgical correction
Increased intracranial pressure With dilated ventricles With other mass	Progressive hydrocephalus, subdural effusion Arachnoid cyst, porencephalic cyst, brain tumor
Benign familial macrocephaly (idiopathic external hydrocephalus)	External hydrocephalus, benign enlargement of the subarachnoid spaces (synonyms)
Megalencephaly (large brain) With neurocutaneous disorder With gigantism With dwarfism Metabolic Lysosomal Other leukodystrophy	Neurofibromatosis, tuberous sclerosis, etc Sotos syndrome Achondroplasia Mucopolysaccharidoses Metachromatic leukodystrophy (late) Canavan spongy degeneration
Thickened skull	Fibrous dysplasia (bone), hemolytic anemia (marrow), sicklemia, thalassemia

► Clinical Findings

Clinical and laboratory findings vary with the underlying process. In neonates and young infants, ultrasound can be used to evaluate for subdural effusions, hydrocephalus, hydranencephaly, and cystic defects. A surgically or medically treatable condition must be ruled out.

A. Imaging Studies

An imaging study is necessary if signs or symptoms of increased intracranial pressure are present. If the fontanelle is open, cranial ultrasonography can assess ventricular size and diagnose or exclude hydrocephalus. CT or MRI scans are used to define any structural cause of macrocephaly and to identify an operable disorder. Even when the condition is untreatable (or does not require treatment), the information gained may permit more accurate diagnosis and prognosis, guide management and genetic counseling, and serve as a basis for comparison should future abnormal cranial growth or neurologic changes necessitate a repeat study.

Ashwal S, Michelson D, Plawner L, Dobyns W: Practice parameter: evaluation of the child with microcephaly (an evidence-based review): report of the Quality Standards Subcommittee of the American Academy of Neurology and the Practice Committee of the Child Neurology Society. Neurology 2009;73(11):887–897 [PMID: 19752457].

McCarthy JG et al: Parameters of care for craniosynostosis. Cleft Palate Craniofac J 2012;49:1S–24S [PMID: 21848431].

Olney AH: Macrocephaly syndromes. Semin Pediatric Neurol 2007;14(3):128–135 [PMID: 17980309].

Puruggganan OH: Abnormalities in head size. Pediatr Rev 2006;27:473 [PMID: 17142470].

Rogers GF: Deformational plagiocephaly, brachycephaly, and scaphocephaly. Part I: terminology, diagnosis, and etiopathogenesis. J Craniofac Surg 2011;22:9 [PMID: 21187783].

Von der Hagen et al: Diagnostic approach to microcephaly in childhood: a two-center study and review of the literature. Dev Med Child Neurol 2014;56:732 [PMID: 24617602].

NEUROCUTANEOUS DYSPLASIAS

Neurocutaneous dysplasias are diseases of the neuroectoderm and sometimes involve endoderm and mesoderm. Tissues that share a common embryologic origin may be impacted by the disorder; thus, characteristic birthmarks can be a clue to brain, spinal cord, and eye disease, and other organ systems may be involved as well. Benign and even malignant tumors may also develop in these conditions.

1. Neurofibromatosis Type 1

 ESSENTIALS OF DIAGNOSIS & TYPICAL FEATURES

► Six or more café au lait spots ≥ 5 mm in prepubertal individuals and ≥ 15 mm in postpubertal individuals.

► Peripheral nerve sheath tumors: Two or more neurofibromas of any type or one plexiform neurofibroma.

► Freckling in the axillary or inguinal regions.

► Optic pathway glioma.

► Two or more Lisch nodules (iris hamartomas).

► Distinctive bony lesions, such as sphenoid dysplasia or thinning of long bone, with or without pseudarthroses.

► First-degree relative with neurofibromatosis type 1.

Neurofibromatosis Type 1 (NF-1) is a multisystem disorder with a prevalence of 1:3000. Fifty percent of cases are due to new mutations in the *NF1* gene, which is located on chromosome 17q11.2 encoding neurofibromin. Forty percent of patients develop medical complications over their lifetime. Two or more positive criteria are diagnostic; others may appear over time. Children with six or more café au lait spots and no other positive criteria should be followed; most will develop NF-1 by 8 years of age.

Clinical Findings

A. Symptoms and Signs

The most common presenting symptoms are cognitive or psychomotor problems. Café au lait spots are seen in most affected children by age 1 year. The typical skin lesion is 10–30 mm, ovoid, and smooth-bordered. Discrete well-demarcated neurofibromas or lipomas can occur at any age. Plexiform neurofibromas are congenital but are frequently detected during periods of rapid growth.

Clinicians should evaluate head circumference, blood pressure, vision, hearing, spine for scoliosis, and limbs for pseudarthroses. The eye examination should include checking for strabismus, amblyopia, proptosis, iris Lisch nodules, optic atrophy, or papilledema. Short stature and precocious puberty are occasional findings.

Parents should be examined in detail. Family history is important in identifying dominant gene manifestations.

B. Laboratory Findings

Genetic testing can be helpful in cases of uncertainty. Selected patients require brain MRI with special attention to the optic nerves to rule out optic glioma. MRI may show "unidentified bright objects" ("UBOs")—hyperintense, non-mass lesions which often disappear with time. Hypertension necessitates evaluation of renal arteries for dysplasia and stenosis. Cognitive and school achievement testing may be indicated. Scoliosis or limb abnormalities should be studied by appropriate imaging.

Differential Diagnosis

Patients with McCune-Albright syndrome often have larger café au lait spots with precocious puberty, polyostotic fibrous dysplasia, and hyperfunctioning endocrinopathies. Legius syndrome has overlapping features of café au lait spots and inguinal/axillary freckling, but is not associated with neurofibromas. One or two café au lait spots are often seen in normal children. A large solitary café au lait spot is usually innocent.

Complications

Neurodevelopmental sequela are common—40% have learning disabilities, and 8% have intellectual disability. Seizures, hearing impairment, short stature, early puberty, and hypertension occur in less than 25% of patients with NF-1. Optic gliomas occur in about 15%; these rarely cause functional problems and are usually nonprogressive. Patients have a 5% lifetime risk for developing various malignancies, which can be a cause of early death. Even benign tumors may cause significant morbidity and mortality. For example, plexiform neurofibromas can be disfiguring or impair spinal cord, renal, or pelvic/leg function. Strokes from NF-1 cerebral arteriopathy are rare but need to be noted; arteriopathy of renal arteries can cause reversible hypertension in childhood.

Treatment

Genetic counseling is important, and 50% of cases are familial. Prenatal diagnosis is likely on the horizon. The disease may be progressive, but with serious complications only occasionally seen. Annual or semiannual visits are important in the early detection of school problems, as well as screening for bone, vision, hearing, puberty, cardiac (including hypertension), or neurologic abnormalities. Health care surveillance guidelines are regularly updated, and clinical trials are ongoing. Multidisciplinary clinics at medical centers around the United States can be excellent resources, and information is available from the National Neurofibromatosis Foundation (http://www.nf.org).

2. Neurofibromatosis Type 2

Neurofibromatosis Type-2 (NF-2) is a dominantly inherited neoplasial syndrome manifested as bilateral vestibular schwannomas (VIII nerve tumors), which may present in childhood with loss of hearing. Other tumors of the brain and spinal cord are common: meningiomas, other cranial nerve schwannomas, and ependymomas. Posterior lens cataracts are a third risk. Café au lait spots are not part of NF-2. In 50% of the patients, the mutation occurs de novo.

3. Tuberous Sclerosis

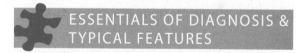

ESSENTIALS OF DIAGNOSIS & TYPICAL FEATURES

▶ At least three hypomelanotic macules, each at least 5 mm in diameter.

▶ Angiofibromas, ungual fibromas, intraoral fibromas.

▶ Shagreen patch.

▶ CNS manifestations: subependymal nodules, cortical dysplasias, subependymal giant cell astrocytoma.

▶ Cardiac rhabdomyomas and angiomyolipomas.

▶ Hamartomas.

Tuberous sclerosis complex (TSC) is a dominantly inherited disease. Almost all individuals have deletions on chromosome 9 (*TSC1* gene) or 16 (*TSC2* gene). The gene products hamartin and tuberin have tumor-suppressing effects; therefore, patients with TSC are more susceptible to hamartomas in many organs and brain tubers and tumors.

Clinical Findings

TSC has a wide phenotypic expression, from asymptomatic carriers to patients with refractory epilepsy and significant intellectual disability. Seizures in early infancy, such as infantile spasms, correlate with developmental delay. The triad of seizures, intellectual disability, and adenoma sebaceum occurs in only 33% of patients.

A. Symptoms and Signs (Table 25–15)

1. Dermatologic features—Skin findings bring most patients to the physician's attention (Table 25–16). Ninety-six percent of patients have one or more hypomelanotic macules, facial angiofibromas, ungual fibromas, or shagreen (leathery orange peel) patches. Adenoma sebaceum (facial skin hamartomas) may first appear in early childhood, often on the cheek, chin, and dry sites of the skin where acne is not usually seen. Ash-leaf spots are off-white hypomelanotic macules, are often oval or "ash leaf" in shape, and follow the dermatomes. A Wood lamp (ultraviolet light) shows the macules more clearly. The equivalent to an ash leaf spot in the scalp is poliosis (whitened hair patch). Subungual and periungual fibromas are more common in the toes. Fibrous

Table 25–15. Major and minor criteria for tuberous sclerosis.

Major Features	Minor Features
Facial angiofibromas or forehead plaque	Multiple, randomly distributed pits in dental enamel
Nontraumatic ungula or periungual fibroma	Hamartomatous rectal polyps
Hypomelanotic macules (three or more)	Bone cysts
Shagreen patch (connective tissue nevus)	Cerebral white matter radial migration lines
Multiple retinal nodular hamartomas	Gingival fibromas
Glioneuronal hamartoma (cortical tuber)	Nonrenal hamartoma
Subependymal nodule	Retinal achromic patch
Subependymal giant cell astrocytoma	"Confetti" skin lesions
Cardiac rhabdomyoma, single or multiple	Multiple renal cysts
Lymphangiomyomatosis	
Renal angiomyolipoma	

Definite tuberous sclerosis complex: either two major features or one major feature plus two minor features

Probable tuberous sclerosis complex: one major plus one minor feature

Possible tuberous sclerosis complex: either one major feature or two or more minor features

or raised plaques may resemble coalescent angiofibromas. Café au lait spots are occasionally seen.

2. Neurologic features—Seizures are the most common neurologic sequela. Virtually any kind of symptomatic seizure (eg, atypical absence, partial complex, and generalized tonic-clonic seizures) may occur. Up to 20% of patients with infantile spasms have TSC. Thus, any patient presenting with infantile spasms should be evaluated for TSC. Intellectual disability occurs in up to 50% of patients referred to tertiary care centers; the incidence is probably much lower in randomly selected patients.

3. Renal lesions—Renal cysts or angiomyolipomas may be asymptomatic, though hematuria or obstruction of urine flow sometimes occurs. Ultrasonography of the kidneys should be done in any patient suspected of TSC, both to aid in diagnosis if lesions are found and to rule out renal obstructive disease.

4. Cardiopulmonary involvement—Rarely, cystic lung disease may occur. Cardiac rhabdomyomas may be asymptomatic but can lead to outflow obstruction, conduction difficulties, and death. Cardiac rhabdomyoma may be detected on prenatal ultrasound examination or postnatal chest radiographs or echocardiograms. Rhabdomyomas typically regress with age; thus, symptomatic presentations are typically in the perinatal period.

5. Eye involvement—Retinal hamartomas are often near the disk and are usually asymptomatic.

6. Skeletal involvement—Cystic rarefactions can be found in the bones of the fingers or toes.

B. Imaging Studies and Special Tests

Plain radiographs may detect areas of thickening within the skull, spine, and pelvis, and cystic lesions in the hands and feet. Chest radiographs may show lung honeycombing. Head CT scan may show the virtually pathognomonic calcified subependymal nodules; brain MRI may show hypomyelinating white matter lesions, brain tumors, widened gyri, or cortical tubers. EEG should be considered in any TSC patient with new-onset spells concerning for seizures.

Treatment

Therapy is as indicated by underlying disease (eg, seizures and tumors of the brain, kidney, and heart). Treatment of refractory epilepsy may lead to surgical extirpation of epileptiform tuber sites. Skin lesions on the face may need dermabrasion or laser treatment. Genetic counseling emphasizes identification of the carrier. The risk of appearance in offspring if either parent is a carrier is 50%. The patient should be seen annually for counseling and reexamination in childhood. Identification of the chromosomes (9,16; TSC1 and TSC2 genes) may in the future make intrauterine diagnosis possible.

Table 25–16. Common central nervous system degenerative disorders of infancy.

Disease	Genetic Defect and Enzyme	Clinical Presentation	Laboratory Tests	Prognosis/Treatment
Early Infantile (0–1 y)				
Globoid cell leukodystrophy (Krabbe)	Autosomal recessive galactocerebroside β-galactosidase deficiency. GALC gene on chromosome 14q31	Infantile form first 6 mo Late-onset form 2–6 y Feeding difficulty Irritability with shrill cry Seizures Axial hypotonia	Elevated CSF protein, prolonged sural nerve conduction, enzyme deficiency in leukocytes, cultured skin fibroblasts. Demyelination and gliosis on MRI	Poor. Death usually by 1.5–2 y Late-onset cases may live 5–10 y Hematopoietic stem cell transplantation (HSCT) can halt progression Enzyme replacement therapy are experimental
Canavan disease/ Aspartoacylase deficiency.	Autosomal recessive. ASPA gene: 17pter-p13	Prevalent in Ashkenazi Jewish Lethargy Weak cry Feeding difficulty Macrocephaly	NAA elevated in blood Pathology: spongiform degeneration	Poor. Progressive. Supportive treatment. Intraparenchymal gene therapy and a recombinant adeno-associated virus serotype 2 shows promise in trials
Vanishing white matter/ Childhood ataxia with CNS hypomyelination	Autosomal recessive Mutation to any of five genes encoding eIF2B	Stepwise deterioration with infection or trauma Ataxia Spasticity Optic atrophy Seizures	Normal CSF Genetic testing and characteristic MRI features are diagnostic	Poor. Prevention of infection and trauma.
Megalencephalic leukodystrophy with cysts	MLC1 and HEPACAM genes	Macrocephaly in the first year Developmental Delay Ataxia Spasticity	MRI shows fronto-parietal white matter abnormalities with cysts.	Poor Antiepileptic drugs to control seizures Physical therapy
Pelizaeus Merzbacher	X-linked recessive; PLP1 gene mutation	Nystagmus, hypotonia, poor vision, ataxia, seizures	MRI with symmetric, confluent white matter signal abnormalities	Poor Supportive treatment
Aicardi-Goutieres Syndrome	Autosomal recessive; one subtype is autosomal dominant; TREX1, RNASEH2A/B/C, SAMHD1, ADAR1, IFIH1 gene mutations	Microcephaly, spasticity, developmental delay/regression, autoimmune complications	Calcification, MRI with white matter signal abnormalities, elevated levels of CSF interferon-α	Poor Supportive treatment

(Continued)

Table 25–16. Common central nervous system degenerative disorders of infancy. *(Continued)*

Disease	Genetic Defect and Enzyme	Clinical Presentation	Laboratory Tests	Prognosis/Treatment
Late Infantile (1–5 y)				
Metachromatic leukodystrophy	Recessive Arylsulfatase A (ASA) deficiency 22q13 Variant: Saposin B deficiency	Infantile form at 18–24 mo; Juvenile and adult forms Incoordination Regression Optic nerve atrophy Demyelinating neuropathy	CSF protein elevated. Urine sulfatide increased. Enzyme deficiency in leukocytes and fibroblasts. Imaging: diffuse white matter	Poor Slowly progressive Infantile form death by 3–8 y Juvenile form death by 10–15 y. Hematopoietic stem cell transplantation is an experimental treatment
Alexander disease	Autosomal dominant; Often de novo Mutations in *GFAP* gene.	Megalencephaly Psychomotor retardation Spasticity Ataxia	Contrast enhancement of gray and white matter Genetic testing	Neonatal form: death by 2 y Later-onset may have slower course
Leukoencephalopathy with brainstem and spinal cord involvement and elevated lactate (LBSL)	Autosomal recessive *DARS2*	Progressive cerebellar ataxia Spasticity Sensory deficits (vibration)	Characteristic MRI findings Genetic testing	Wheelchair dependent in adolescence, early adulthood Supportive therapy.
Late infantile neuronal ceroid lipofuscinosis, type 2	Autosomal recessive TPP1 deficiency	Seizures, ataxia, myoclonus, vision loss, developmental regression	Genetic testing	Cerliponase alfa is FDA approved for pediatric patients ≥ 3 y; administered via intraventricular injection every 2 weeks
Juvenile				
X-linked adrenoleukodystrophy	X-linked recessive; ABCD1 mutation	Behavioral changes, chronic progressive spastic paraparesis; hyperpigmentation and adrenocortical insufficiency	ACTH elevated Very-long-chain fatty acids in plasma	Variable progression; HSCT halts progression when done early in demyelination
Neuroaxonal leukoencephalopathy with axonal spheroids	Most cases sporadic. Familial cases reported	Prominent psychiatric features; seizures, dementia, ataxia.	Brain biopsy: cerebral white matter degeneration including loss of myelin and axons, gliosis, macrophages, and axonal spheroids	Poor. Supportive treatment

ACTH, adrenocorticotropic hormone; AR, autosomal recessive; CNS, central nervous system; CSF, cerebrospinal fluid; CT, computed tomography; EEG, electroencephalogram; ERG, electroretinogram; HSCT, hematopoietic stem cell therapy; MRI, magnetic resonance imaging; WBC, white blood cell.

Dysfunction of tuberin or hamartin has been proposed to disinhibit the "mammalian target of rapamycin" (mTOR), allowing abnormal cell proliferation. Ongoing studies are investigating whether mTOR inhibitors (such as rapamycin and everolimus) can shrink dysplasias/tubers, tumors, and adenoma sebacea. In April 2018, the FDA approved everolimus, an mTOR inhibitor, for the adjunctive treatment of epilepsy in patients with TSC.

4. Encephalofacial Angiomatosis (Sturge-Weber Syndrome)

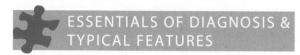

ESSENTIALS OF DIAGNOSIS & TYPICAL FEATURES

► Port-wine birthmark.
► Capillary-venous malformation in the eye (choroidal angioma) and brain (leptomeningeal angioma).

Sturge-Weber syndrome (SWS) is a sporadic neurovascular disease which consists of a facial port wine nevus involving the upper part of the face (in the first division of cranial nerve V), a venous angioma of the meninges in the occipito-parietal regions, and choroidal angioma. Rarely, the syndrome has been described without the facial nevus (type III, exclusive leptomeningeal angioma). Recently, SWS was determined to be caused by somatic mutation of the GNAQ gene.

▶ Clinical Findings

A. Symptoms and Signs

In infancy, the eye may show congenital glaucoma, or buphthalmos, with a cloudy, enlarged cornea. Initially, the facial nevus may be the only indication. Facial nevi can involve the lower face, mouth, lip, neck, and even torso. Over time, the patient may develop radiographic and clinical evidence of brain involvement. Seizures are common, particularly in infancy. Hemiparesis and/or hemiatrophy on the side contralateral to the cerebral lesion may occur. Cognitive impairment, headache and migraines, stroke, and stroke-like episodes are other neurologic manifestations.

B. Imaging and Special Tests

Radiologic studies may show calcification of the cortex; CT scanning may show this much earlier than plain radiographic studies. MRI eventually shows underlying brain involvement—cortical atrophy, calcifications, and meningeal angiomatosis. EEG often shows voltage attenuation over the involved area in early stages; later, epileptiform abnormalities may be present focally.

▶ Differential Diagnosis

The differential diagnosis includes (rare) PHACES syndrome: **P**osterior fossa malformation, segmental (facial) **H**emangioma, **A**rterial abnormalities, **C**ardiac defects, **E**ye abnormalities, and **S**ternal (or ventral) defects; often, only portions of that list are present.

▶ Management, Treatment, & Prognosis

Bilateral brain involvement is associated with poorer cognitive outcomes; whereas, larger nevus size is strongly correlated with subsequent epilepsy, which can also impact neurodevelopment, indicating a need for prompt treatment. Careful ophthalmologic assessment to detect early glaucoma is indicated. Rarely, surgical removal of the involved meninges and the involved portion of the brain, even hemispherectomy, may be indicated. Glaucoma, stroke, and stroke-like episodes can occur.

5. Von Hippel-Lindau Disease (Retrocerebellar Angiomatosis)

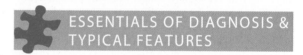

ESSENTIALS OF DIAGNOSIS & TYPICAL FEATURES

► Retinal, central nervous, renal hemangioblastomas.
► Visceral cysts.
► Less frequently adrenal and extra-adrenal pheochromocytomas, pancreatic endocrine cancers, and endolymphatic sac tumors.

Von Hippel-Lindau disease is a rare, dominantly inherited neurocutaneous disorder. The diagnostic criteria for the disease are a retinal or cerebellar hemangioblastoma with or without a positive family history, intra-abdominal cyst (kidneys, pancreas), or renal cancer. The patient may present with ataxia, slurred speech, and nystagmus due to a hemangioblastoma of the cerebellum or with a medullary spinal cord cystic hemangioblastoma. Retinal detachment may occur from hemorrhage or exudate in the retinal vascular malformation. Rarely, a pancreatic cyst or renal tumor may be the presenting symptom.

Asthagiri AR et al: Neurofibromatosis type 2. Lancet 2009;373:1974 [Epub May 22].

Cotter JA: An update on the central nervous system manifestations of tuberous sclerosis complex. Acta Neuropathol 2019 April 11; [PMID: 30976976].

Day AM et al: Physical and family history variables associated with neurological and cognitive development in Sturge-Weber Syndrome. Pediatr Neurol 2019;96:30–36 [PMID: 30853154].

Gutmann DH et al: Neurofibromatosis type 1. Nat Rev Dis Primers 2017:23:3 [PMID: 28230061].

Krueger DA, Northrup H; International Tuberous Sclerosis Complex Consensus Group: Tuberous sclerosis complex surveillance and management: recommendations of the 2012 International Tuberous Sclerosis Complex Consensus Conference. Pediatr Neurol 2013;49(4):255–265 [PMID: 24053983].

Maher ER, Neumann HP, Richard S: von Hippel-Lindau disease: a clinical and scientific review. Eur J Hum Genet 2011;19(6):617 [PMID: 21386872].

CENTRAL NERVOUS SYSTEM DEGENERATIVE DISORDERS OF INFANCY & CHILDHOOD

The CNS degenerative disorders of infancy and childhood are characterized by developmental arrest and loss, usually progressive but at variable rates, of cognitive, motor, and visual functioning (see Table 25–16). Seizures are common, especially in those with gray matter involvement. Symptoms and signs vary with age at onset and primary sites of involvement.

These disorders are fortunately rare. Referral for sophisticated biochemical testing is usually necessary before a definitive diagnosis can be made. Patients with metachromatic leukodystrophy, Krabbe disease, and adrenoleukodystrophy are candidates for bone marrow transplantation. Treatment of some lysosomal storage diseases, such as Gaucher disease, with enzyme replacement therapy (ERT) has shown promising results.

Costello DJ et al: Leukodystrophies: classification, diagnosis, and treatment. Neurologist 2009;15:319 [PMID: 19901710].

Koehler W: Leukodystrophies with late disease onset: an update. Curr Opin Neurol 2010;23:234 [PMID: 20216214].

Kohlschutter A, Eichler F: Childhood leukodystrophies: a clinical perspective. Expert Rev Neurother 2011;11(10):1485–1469 [PMID: 21955203].

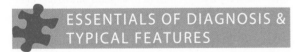

ATAXIAS OF CHILDHOOD

ESSENTIALS OF DIAGNOSIS & TYPICAL FEATURES

► Ataxia is defined as difficulty coordinating voluntary movements of the limbs and/or trunk.

► Ataxia is most commonly due to cerebellar dysfunction but can be caused by abnormalities at almost any component of the nervous system.

► Acute, episodic, and subacute/chronic ataxias have different etiologies, which can guide the evaluation, management, and outcome.

► A detailed history and evaluation of truncal versus limb ataxia, mental status, and eye movements can provide the most useful diagnostic points in the formulation of the differential diagnosis.

Ataxia can be divided into categories based on the chronicity of symptoms. Acute ataxia is a common reason for emergent neurologic consultation. Typically, the patient was previously healthy, without developmental delay or neurologic deficits, and then developed symptoms within 72 hours of presentation. The evaluation should include a detailed history of the antecedent events and current symptoms, as well as a comprehensive neurologic examination. In contrast, a patient with a subacute, episodic, or chronic ataxia often has developmental delay, other neurologic deficits, or other organ system involvement. In this section, a brief overview of the most common causes of ataxia, and the evaluation and the management of each, is provided.

ACUTE ATAXIAS OF CHILDHOOD

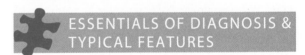

ESSENTIALS OF DIAGNOSIS & TYPICAL FEATURES

► Symptoms may include sudden development of a wide-based, "drunken" gait or possibly refusal to walk.

► Families may not notice unsteady arm movements, truncal swaying, or dysarthria, but these symptoms are often present and are essential to localization.

► Serious causes such as ingestion, CNS infection, stroke, or intracranial mass lesion, must be excluded, either by clinical history/examination or with lumbar puncture and brain MRI.

▶ Pathogenesis

Causes of acute ataxia that require emergent evaluation include toxic ingestion, CNS infection, mass lesion, trauma, or stroke. Therefore, a detailed history should assess for exposures, fever, altered mental status, irritability, headaches, developmental regression, blurry or double vision, nausea/vomiting, and other neurologic deficits.

▶ Clinical Findings

A thorough examination should be performed, with attention to signs suggesting a serious central nervous system disorder, such as altered mental status, papilledema, or cranial nerve palsies. The evaluation of an acutely ataxic patient can be difficult as the patient may refuse to participate due to the discomfort of being ataxic or associated mental status changes. Therefore, distinguishing between weakness, sensory loss, and ataxia can be difficult, but is nonetheless essential. For example, asymmetry in the examination would be unusual for acute cerebellar ataxia. Ataxia from a sensory lesion worsens with the eyes closed; whereas, ataxia from a cerebellar lesion does not. Cerebellar lesions are often associated with additional findings such as nystagmus, dysarthria, truncal titubations (oscillatory swaying and corrective postural movements), dysmetria, tremor, hypotonia, or a tendency to fall toward the side of the lesion.

▶ Laboratory & Imaging Findings

Red flags in the history or examination should prompt timely and targeted testing. These include trauma, abrupt onset of signs/symptoms (over minutes), progressive or prolonged time course, headache, altered mental status, seizures or myoclonic jerks, and opsoclonus. A recent study found that for children older than 3 years who presented with more than 3 days of symptoms, brain imaging demonstrated clinically urgent intracranial pathology (such as brain tumor or ADEM) in 10%–20%. Younger children and children with no more than 3 days of symptoms warrant close observation but may not need urgent brain imaging. Lumbar puncture should be performed if an inflammatory, demyelinating, or infectious etiology is possible.

▶ Differential Diagnosis

A. Acute Cerebellar Ataxia

Acute (postinfectious) cerebellar ataxia (ACA) causes approximately 40% of cases of acute ataxia and typically affects children aged 2–4 years. Clinical signs occur abruptly (over hours), evolve rapidly, and typically include unsteady gait, truncal swaying, dysmetria, tremor, or abnormal eye movements. Mental status is essentially normal, though some patients are mildly irritable. Sensation, strength, and reflex testing are normal. In 70% of patients, a prodromal illness, such as influenza, occurs within 3 weeks of onset. Diagnostic testing should include lumbar puncture and brain imaging. CSF opening pressure, protein, and glucose levels are typically normal, though a mild pleocytosis with lymphocytic predominance can be seen. Significant elevation in WBC or protein level suggests an alternative diagnosis, such as CNS infection or Guillain-Barre syndrome (GBS). Brain MRI is typically normal, but can show T2 hyperintensities in the cerebellum. Treatment for ACA is typically supportive. Intravenous immunoglobulin (IVIg) has been used in severe cases. Steroids are not effective. Physical therapy can

be helpful. Most patients recover without sequelae within 8 months, though some may have neurologic sequelae.

B. Toxic Cerebellar Syndrome

Toxic ingestion accounts for one-third of cases of acute ataxia in children. Common substances include ASMs, benzodiazepines, alcohol, marijuana, and cough syrup (dextromethorphan). Environmental agents, such as heavy metals (bismuth, mercury, and lead), can also cause ataxia. Mental status changes, nystagmus, pupillary changes, tremor, or other toxidromal symptoms may also occur. Urine toxicology screen may not detect specific medications or illicit substances. Imaging is typically normal. Therefore, a detailed history is required to guide testing for specific substances or make an empiric diagnosis. Treatment is guided by the ingested agent and requires toxicology consultation.

C. Intracranial Mass Lesions

Posterior fossa tumors (arising from the cerebellum or brainstem) comprise up to 60% of childhood brain tumors. Most patients experience gradual onset of progressive ataxia and clinical signs and symptoms of increased intracranial pressure, such as lethargy, headache, vomiting, or eye movement abnormalities. However, some children can present with a more rapid evolution of signs and symptoms, and even children with a large tumor and obstructive hydrocephalus may present with minor deficits. Therefore, any patient with a history of nocturnal headaches, nocturnal emesis, focal neurologic deficits, visual changes, or other signs concerning for mass lesion should have neuroimaging performed immediately.

D. Posterior Circulation Stroke (Ischemic or Hemorrhagic)

Though rare, stroke should be considered in the differential for acute ataxia, particularly if a history of neck trauma or family history of vascular or hematologic abnormalities is present. Due to the brainstem/cerebellar involvement of a posterior circulation stroke, the patient may also have significant vertigo, nausea/vomiting, nystagmus, cranial nerve palsies, hearing changes, hiccups, sensory loss, hemiparesis, or even quadriparesis. Cerebral venous sinus thrombosis should also be considered.

E. CNS Infections—Cerebellitis, Brainstem Encephalitis, and Meningitis

Some infectious agents, such as Listeria, varicella, and enterovirus 71, have a predilection for the brainstem and cerebellum, either via leptomeningeal involvement or direct invasion of the parenchyma. In some cases, postinfectious inflammation can be quite severe. Patients are typically quite ill and encephalopathic. Brain MRI may demonstrate cerebellar edema, which in some cases has required decompressive craniectomy.

F. Acute Demyelinating Encephalomyelitis

Ataxia can be a presenting symptom of acute demyelinating encephalomyelitis (ADEM), an immune-mediated, transient demyelinating disorder. ADEM often occurs after a viral infection or vaccination, most commonly in children aged 2–10 years. Unlike ACA, ADEM is typically associated with additional deficits, such as a dramatic change in mental status (encephalopathy), seizures, cranial nerve palsies, or extremity weakness. Refer to section Noninfectious Inflammatory Disorders of the Central Nervous System for more detail.

G. Sensory Ataxia

Pathology within the spinal cord, spinal nerve roots, or peripheral nerves can disrupt sensory input to the cerebellum, resulting in a sensory ataxia. Etiologies may include poliomyelitis-like infections, spinal cord demyelinating process (such as ADEM, transverse myelitis, MS, or neuromyelitis optica spectrum disorder), vitamin B_{12} deficiency, GBS (also called acute inflammatory demyelinating polyneuropathy, AIDP) or its variant, Miller-Fisher syndrome, or toxins. In addition to ataxia, patients typically have hypotonia or hypertonia, weakness, abnormal tendon reflexes, abnormal Romberg sign, loss of proprioception and vibratory sensation, or a high "steppage" gait (see the section Syndromes Presenting as Acute Flaccid Weakness for additional discussion). Autonomic instability or bowel/bladder dysfunction can also be notable. Diffuse or difficult to localize pain can be a predominate feature. Testing for suspected GBS should include a lumbar puncture to evaluate for elevated CSF protein with normal CSF white blood cell count, known as albuminocytologic dissociation, but early in the course, CSF can be normal in up to 50% of children. Antibodies against GQ1b may be positive in Miller-Fisher syndrome. Screening for toxins and vitamin deficiencies may be appropriate if the history is suggestive. Spine MRI may show enhancement of the nerve roots in GBS or infectious radiculoneuritis (such as Lyme disease). Posterior column lesions suggest demyelination, myelitis, or neurodegenerative changes. Nerve conduction studies and EMG may be helpful, though these are often normal during the acute period. GBS can be treated with either IVIg (2 g/kg divided over 3–5 days) or plasmapheresis, which have similar efficacies. Steroids have no benefit in GBS. Most patients with GBS will make a full recovery within 6–12 months. Treatment and outcome for myelopathy/myelitis will depend on etiology.

H. Paraneoplastic Syndromes

Acute ataxia can occasionally be seen in opsoclonus-myoclonus-ataxia syndrome (OMS), a rare paraneoplastic/autoimmune disorder that primarily affects young children. Proposed diagnostic criteria for OMS include opsoclonus (rapid, multidirectional conjugate abnormal eye movements), myoclonus (nonepileptic jerks of the face, head, or extremities) or ataxia, behavioral changes or sleep disruption, and/or neuroblastoma. Cognitive dysfunction can also be seen. Many patients do not immediately meet diagnostic criteria, and a high index of suspicion is needed to ultimately make the diagnosis. Aggressive treatment with immune modulation may be needed to prevent recurrence and developmental impact.

I. Migraine With Brainstem Aura (Formerly Called "Basilar Migraine")

Migraine with brainstem aura can be associated with ataxia. Most patients will have other neurologic signs and symptoms, such as vertigo, nausea, vomiting, cranial nerve dysfunction, and/or headache. Positive visual phenomenon (such as flashing lights or "zig-zag" lines) or a "marching" progression of symptoms (reflecting cortical spreading depression) can provide clues to the diagnosis of migraine. However, migraine with aura is a diagnosis of exclusion, and the initial presentation warrants a prompt workup for possible stroke.

J. Vestibular Pathology

Disturbances in the vestibular system can cause ataxia, often accompanied by dramatic vertigo, nausea/vomiting, eye movement abnormalities (such as skew deviation or nystagmus), or hearing changes. Causes can include labyrinthitis/vestibular neuritis or benign paroxysmal vertigo, as well as posterior circulation stroke or migraine with brainstem aura.

K. Functional Ataxia (Also Called Pseudoataxia or Conversion Disorder)

In functional ataxia, the patient appears to lurch and stagger when walking, the gait is not wide-based, and falls are rare. The findings on the neurologic examination are often inconsistent and incompatible with neuroanatomic localization, meeting DSM-V criteria for functional symptoms.

Caffarelli M, Kimia AA, Torres AR: Acute ataxia in children: a review of the differential diagnosis and evaluation in the emergency department. Pediatr Neurol 2016;65:12–30 [PMID: 27789117].

Desai J, Mitchell WG: Acute cerebellar ataxia, acute cerebellitis, and opsoclonus-myoclonus syndrome. J Child Neurol 2012;11:1482–1488 [PMID: 22805251].

Gray MP, Gorelick MH: Acute disseminated encephalomyelitis. Pediatr Emerg Care 2016;6:395–400 [PMID: 27253358].

Rudloe T et al: The yield of neuroimaging in children presenting to the emergency department with acute ataxia in the post-varicella vaccine era. J Child Neurol 2015;10:1333–1339 [PMID: 25535060].

Thakkar K, Maricich SM, Alper G: Acute ataxia in childhood: 11-year experience at a major pediatric neurology referral center. J Child Neurol 2016;9:1156–1560 [PMID: 27071467].

CHRONIC & EPISODIC ATAXIAS

▶ Differential Diagnosis

1. Inborn Errors of Metabolism

Inborn errors of metabolism should be strongly considered for both intermittent and chronic ataxia. Metabolic disorders known to cause episodic or progressive ataxia include amino-acidopathies, urea cycle defects, primary lactic acidoses, leukodystrophies, lysosomal disorders, peroxisomal disorders, and disorders of glycosylation. Since some of these disorders are treatable, consider sending screening labs such as complete blood count with peripheral smear, compete metabolic panel, thyroid panel, serum organic acids, urine organic acids, lactate, and pyruvate. Depending on these results, additional testing may involve immunoglobulin panel, alpha-fetoprotein, ammonia, vitamin B_{12}, MMA, homocysteine, biotinidase, phytanic acid, homocysteine, vitamin E, copper, ceruloplasmin, lipid panel, acylcarnitine profile, carnitine, or very long-chain fatty acids. Ideally, testing is sent when the patient is symptomatic. Brain MRI may also demonstrate characteristic features in some metabolic disorders. For more details, refer to Chapter 36 on Inborn Errors of Metabolism.

2. Autosomal Dominant Hereditary Ataxias (Chronic and Episodic)

Most forms of spinocerebellar ataxia (SCA) and episodic ataxia are dominantly inherited, and many are due to channelopathies. Channelopathies are a broad category of disorders that result from altered function of ion channels and membrane excitability in neurons and other cells. Examples include episodic ataxia type 1 (EA1), which is due to a mutation in *KCNA1*, a potassium channel, and episodic ataxia type 2 (EA2) which is caused by a mutation in *CACNA1A*, a calcium channel. Interestingly, *CACNA1A* mutations can also cause spinocerebellar ataxia type 6 (SCA6), as well as hemiplegic migraine and epilepsy. Over 40 dominantly inherited spinocerebellar ataxias have been described.

3. Autosomal Recessive Hereditary Ataxias

The two most common autosomal recessive hereditary ataxias affecting children are Friedreich ataxia followed by ataxia-telangiectasia (discussed below). Other rare, but treatable, autosomal recessive ataxias include ataxia with vitamin E deficiency, cerebrotendinous xanthomatosis, mitochondrial disorders, Refsum disease, and abetalipoproteinemia.

A. Friedreich Ataxia

The classic presentation of Friedreich Ataxia is a school-aged/adolescent with clumsiness, sensory loss, absent tendon reflexes, positive Babinski sign (upgoing toes), and progressive weakness that ultimately leads to loss of ambulation by young adulthood. Patients can develop orthopedic deformities, including scoliosis, as well as dysarthria, hearing and visual impairment, hypertrophic cardiomyopathy, and diabetes mellitus. Friedrich ataxia is caused by a triplet GAA expansion in the frataxin gene (*FXN*).

B. Ataxia-Telangiectasia

Ataxia-telangiectasia is a multisystem disorder arising from a defect in DNA repair typically due to mutations in the ATM gene. Patients present between 1 and 4 years of age with ataxia, oculomotor apraxia, recurrent infections (due to immunoglobulin deficiencies), and conjunctival telangiectasias. Choreoathetosis and sensorimotor neuropathy are also quite common. Serum alpha-fetoprotein is typically elevated but can be normal early in the course. Patients are at increased risk of malignancy.

Ashizawa T, Xia G: Ataxia. Continuum (Minneap Minn) 2016;22(4):1208–1226 [PMID: 27495205].

Jayadev S, Bird TD: Hereditary ataxias. Genet Med 2013; 15(9):673–683 [PMID: 23538602].

Kullmann DM: Neurologic channelopathies. Annu Rev Neurosci 2010;33:151–172 [PMID: 20331364].

Marmolino D: Friedrich's ataxia. Brain Res Rev 2011;67(1–2): 311–330 [PMID: 21550666].

Storey E: Genetic cerebellar ataxias. Semin Neurol 2014; 34(3):280–292 [PMID: 25192506].

MOVEMENT DISORDERS

Movement disorders (also called extrapyramidal disorders) are characterized by the presence in the waking state of excessive, unwanted movements: dyskinesias, athetosis, chorea, ballismus, tremors, rigidity, tics, and dystonias. The precise pathologic and anatomic localizations of these disorders are not understood. Motor pathways in the striatum (putamen and caudate nucleus), globus pallidus, red nucleus, substantia nigra, and the subthalamic nucleus are involved. This system is modulated by pathways originating in the cortex, thalamus, cerebellum, and reticular formation.

1. Chorea & Athetosis

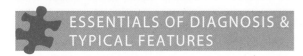

ESSENTIALS OF DIAGNOSIS & TYPICAL FEATURES

▶ Chorea is characterized by brief, random involuntary uncoordinated movements of the limbs and face which can flow from one muscle group to the next, resulting in a "dance-like" motion.

▶ Athetosis involves slow, involuntary writhing or twisting movements.

▶ Sydenham chorea, a major Jones criteria for rheumatic fever, is a common cause of acute choreoathetoid movements in children, but other etiologies should also be considered.

▶ Clinical Findings

Sydenham chorea is a common cause of acute onset of choreoathetoid movements and is major Jones criteria for rheumatic fever (see Chapter 20 for additional information about rheumatic fever). Hemichorea (involving only one side of the body) occurs in up to 35% of patients. Other symptoms and signs include behavior changes, sleep disturbances, hypotonia, and motor impersistence, such as inability to sustain grip ("milkmaid's sign") or tongue protrusion ("tongue darting"). Diagnostic testing should include CBC, ESR, CRP, antistreptolysin O titers, and anti-DNase titer. Strep throat culture should be obtained but is often negative due to the delay between infection and development of chorea. ECG and echocardiography are critical to evaluate for cardiac involvement, which is seen in up to 80% of patients.

▶ Differential Diagnosis

Brain MRI should be obtained in all children with chorea to rule out basal ganglia pathology. Though pediatric autoimmune neuropsychiatric disorder associated with Streptococcal infections (PANDAS) is a controversial diagnosis, other paraneoplastic and other autoimmune disorders can certainly cause acquired movement disorders. Additional laboratory testing should be considered to exclude other causes, such as antineuronal antibodies (to evaluate for lupus), antiphospholipid antibodies (to screen for other autoimmune causes), thyroid screening tests, serum calcium for hypocalcemia, HIV, parvovirus B19, and Epstein-Barr virus infection. Benign hereditary chorea (BHC) is an autosomal dominant genetic disorder that can be associated with intellectual disability, hypotonia, congenital hypothyroidism, and chronic lung disease. Tics can mimic chorea. Rare causes, such as drug-induced extrapyramidal syndromes, dyskinetic cerebral

palsy, Huntington chorea, hepatolenticular degeneration (Wilson disease), typically cause subacute-chronic symptoms.

▶ Treatment & Prognosis

Patients with Sydenham chorea require appropriate antibiotic prophylaxis for rheumatic fever, but no other specific treatment for Syndenham chorea has been developed. Prednisone and, in severe cases, IVIg have been successful. ASMs, such as sodium valproate or levetiracetam, can reduce chorea symptoms. Emotional lability and depression sometimes require psychologic and pharmacologic treatment. Sydenham chorea is a self-limited disease that may last from a few weeks up to 18 months. In follow-up studies, valvular heart disease occurred in about one-third of patients, particularly if other rheumatic manifestations had been present as part of the childhood illness. Neuropsychologic disturbances were also present in many patients.

2. Tics/Tourette Syndrome

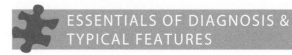

ESSENTIALS OF DIAGNOSIS & TYPICAL FEATURES

▶ Tics are paroxysmal, repetitive, rapid, involuntary movements, or vocalizations. Tics "wax and wane" and are variable over time.

▶ Tourette syndrome is characterized by multiple motor tics and at least one vocal tic with onset before age 21 years and occurring for at least 1 year.

▶ Clinical Findings

Tics are quick, repetitive but irregular, involuntary movements, which are often stereotyped and briefly suppressible. Tics affect up to 20% of school-aged children. Transient tic disorder lasts from 1 month to 1 year. Chronic tic disorder requires more than 1 year of motor or vocal tics. Tourette syndrome is characterized by both motor and vocal tics with no obvious cause, lasting more than 1 year. A premonitory urge ("I have to do it"), transient but effortful suppressibility, and sense of relief after completing the tic are characteristic for tic disorders. Tics generally wax and wane in frequency, and the type of movement evolves over time. Like many movement disorders, tics can be exacerbated by stress or excitement and generally resolve during sleep. Important common comorbidities are attention deficit hyperactivity disorder (ADHD), obsessive-compulsive disorder, academic difficulties, migraine, sleep difficulties, anxiety, and depression.

Motor tics can occur anywhere on the body, but most commonly affect the head, neck, and upper body. Facial tics can include grimaces, twitches, and eye blinking. Complex motor tics are coordinated, sequenced movements that can mimic voluntary motor acts, such as ear/nose scratching or jumping. Vocal tics can manifest as sniffing, grunting, throat clearing, barking, and, in complex forms, involve the use of words. Coprolalia and echolalia are relatively infrequent. Vocal tics are less common and are highly suggestive of Tourette syndrome. Self-injurious behavior can also occur in Tourette syndrome.

Most patients presenting with tics do not require further diagnostic workup. However, a careful history should screen for secondary causes as well as comorbidities and investigate further as indicated.

▶ Differential Diagnosis

Tics may be a symptom of other neurologic diseases such as brain injury, autism, Rett syndrome, and numerous genetic neurodevelopmental disorders. Acute brain lesion such as tumor, stroke, or infection will typically be associated with other symptoms. Postinfectious causes such as PANDAS or pediatric acute-onset neuropsychiatric symptoms (PANS) have been long debated, but can be considered if history suggests.

▶ Treatment & Prognosis

The cornerstone of treatment is reassurance and education for the patient, family, and school about the nature of tic disorders. Importantly, if the tics are not bothersome to the child and are not causing physical or social impairment, *no pharmacologic treatment is necessary*. However, screening for and treating common comorbidities, such as ADHD, obsessive-compulsive symptoms, and anxiety, can significantly improve quality of life and sometimes lesson tic severity. Stimulant medications do not need to be avoided due to concern that tics might be exacerbated—recent studies have shown that medications such as methylphenidate improved ADHD symptoms without worsening tics. Habit reversal therapy and Comprehensive Behavioral Intervention for Tics (CBIT) can be effective approaches for tics and various comorbidities. Most pediatric patients will have significant improvement or resolution of tics later in life. Tourette syndrome is considered a life-long disorder and may wax and wane, and in some severe cases may be disabling.

If pharmacologic treatment is warranted, the choice of therapy can be tailored to the child's needs and comorbidities. Clonidine and guanfacine are considered first-line, especially in a child with comorbid ADHD. Topiramate has a mild side effect profile and may be indicated if the patient has headaches or epilepsy. If tics are refractory to first-line agents, pimozide and fluphenazine are recommended next options, followed by antipsychotics, such as risperidone and aripiprazole. Haloperidol is FDA-approved for Tourette syndrome; however, due to the risk of tardive dyskinesia, it is typically reserved for refractory cases.

3. Primary Dystonia & Paroxysmal Dyskinesias

Dystonia is sustained or intermittent involuntary muscle contractions, frequently resulting in twisting movements or abnormal postures. Not all dystonias are due to co-contraction of opposing muscle groups. Secondary causes include cerebral palsy, stroke, tumor, and medication effect. However, primary dystonia can be mistakenly diagnosed as cerebral palsy. Any child with dystonia of unknown cause should have a trial of low-dose L-DOPA; a prompt improvement suggests dopa-responsive dystonia (DYT5, also called Segawa disease). Oppenheim's dystonia (DYT1) is another genetic cause of dystonia that can manifest in childhood.

Paroxysmal dyskinesias (Table 25–17) are sudden-onset, short-duration choreoathetosis or dystonia episodes. Most often, these episodes are familial or genetic in origin. Episodes may occur spontaneously or may be triggered by actions ("kinesigenic," or movement-induced) such as standing up suddenly.

4. Tremor

Tremor is a rhythmic, involuntary oscillatory movement across a joint axis and is often due to alternating contraction of opposing muscle groups. Resting tremors are most prominent when the involved muscles are completely at rest. In contrast, action tremors become more prominent when the affected muscles are engaged, for example to maintain a posture (postural tremor) or to move to a target (intention tremor). The most common causes of tremor in the pediatric population are enhanced physiologic tremor, essential

Table 25–17. Paroxysmal movement disorders (genetics).

Name	PKD[a]	PNKD[b]	PED[c]
Duration	Few minutes	2–10 min	5–40 min
Occurrence	Frequent	Occasional	Hyperventilation, exercise
Precipitants	Stress	Alcohol, caffeine, stress	Stress
Treatment	Anticonvulsants	Meds problematic, clonazepam?	Acetazolamide

[a]Paroxysmal kinesigenic dyskinesia.
[b]Paroxysmal non-kinesigenic dyskinesia.
[c]Paroxysmal exercise-induced dyskinesia.

tremor, and psychogenic tremor. Numerous medications can exacerbate physiologic tremor, such as asthma medications, antidepressants, stimulants, antipsychotics, and ASMs. Patients with essential tremor often have a family history of tremor, note worsening with caffeine, and have transient improvement with alcohol. Differential diagnosis includes birth asphyxia, Wilson disease, hyperthyroidism, and hypocalcemia; history and laboratory tests rule out these rare possibilities.

Cardoso F: Movement disorders in childhood. Parkinsonism Relat Disord 2014;20:S13–S16 [PMID: 24262164].

Kurlan R: Clinical practice: Tourette syndrome. N Engl J Med 2010;363:23–32 [PMID: 21142535].

Panzar J, Dalmau J: Movement disorders in paraneoplastic and autoimmune disease. Curr Opin Neurol 2011;24:346 [PMID: 21577108].

Sanger TD et al: Definition and classification of hyperkinetic movements in childhood. Mov Disord 2010;25:15–38 [PMID: 20589866].

Singer HS: Treatment of tics and Tourette syndrome. Curr Treat Options Neurol 2010;12(6):539–61 [PMID: 20848326].

Singer HS, Gilbert DL, Wolf DS: Moving from PANDAS to CANS. J Pediatr 2012;160:725 [PMID: 22197466].

Williams KA, Swedo SE: Post-infectious autoimmune disorders: Sydenham's chorea, pandas and beyond. Brain Res 2014;S00068993(14):144–154 [PMID: 25301689].

CEREBRAL PALSY

The term *cerebral palsy* is a nonspecific term used to describe a chronic, static impairment of muscle tone, strength, coordination, or movements. Cerebral palsy is nonprogressive, originating from some type of cerebral insult or injury in the perinatal period, with a wide spectrum of manifestations. Importantly, while cerebral palsy is, by definition, a static disorder, the full degree of impairment may not be apparent until the child has at least reached the ages of 3–4 years, when more is expected of the child developmentally. Some form of cerebral palsy occurs in about 0.2% of live births.

▶ Clinical Findings

A. Symptoms and Signs

Spastic cerebral palsy is most common form of cerebral palsy (75% of cases). Various terms denote the limbs affected: monoplegia (one limb); hemiplegia (arm and leg on same side of body); paraplegia/diplegia (both legs affected with arms unaffected); quadriplegia (all four limbs affected). In patients with hemiplegia, the affected arm and leg may be smaller and shorter than the unaffected limbs. Ataxic cerebral palsy is the second most common form, accounting for about 15% of cases. The ataxia frequently affects the upper extremities but may also involve lower extremities and trunk. Athetoid or dyskinetic cerebral palsy (with choreoathetosis or dystonia)

accounts for 5% of cases, and persistent hypotonia without spasticity for 1%.

Depending on the type and severity of the motor deficits, associated neurologic deficits or disorders may occur: epilepsy in 25%, intellectual disability in 50% (severe in 25%), and disorders of language, speech, vision, hearing, and sensory perception are found in varying degrees and combinations. Cataracts, retinopathy, and congenital heart defects may be indicative of congenital infections such as CMV and rubella.

B. Laboratory and Imaging Tests

Appropriate studies depend on the history and physical findings. MRI is helpful in understanding the full extent of cerebral injury in about 90% of cases and sometimes suggests specific etiologies (eg, periventricular calcifications in congenital CMV, perinatal strokes, or brain malformations). Genetic and metabolic testing should be targeted based on history or MRI findings.

▶ Differential Diagnosis

The diagnosis of cerebral palsy is a descriptor and implies that some underlying etiology has led to the constellation of symptoms. If identifiable, etiology can guide prognosis, but no definite etiologic diagnosis is found in 25% of cases. The incidence is high among infants small for gestational age or those born extremely preterm. Intrauterine hypoxia is a frequent cause. Other known causes are intrauterine bleeding, infections, toxins, congenital brain malformations, obstetric complications (including birth hypoxia), neonatal infections, kernicterus, extremely severe and prolonged neonatal hypoglycemia, metabolic disorders, and a small number of genetic syndromes.

▶ Treatment & Management

Treatment and management are directed at assisting the child to attain maximal neurologic functioning with appropriate physical, occupational, and speech therapy. Orthopedic monitoring and intervention and special educational assistance may all contribute to an improved outcome. Treatment of spasticity (with medications for tone or botulinum toxin) and seizures are needed in many children. Constraint-induced movement therapy can help with the affected extremity. Also important is the general support of the parents and family with counseling, educational programs, and support groups.

▶ Prognosis

The prognosis for patients with cerebral palsy depends greatly on the child's IQ, severity of the motor deficits, etiology of CP, and degree of disability. In severely affected children, aspiration, pneumonia, or other intercurrent infections are the most common causes of death.

In contrast, patients with mild cerebral palsy may improve with age. Some patients experience resolution of their motor deficits by age 7 years. Ambulatory status at 12 years of age is most predictive of adult functional ability. Many children may have normal intellect, normal life spans, and are able to lead productive, satisfying lives.

Delgado MR et al: Practice parameter: pharmacologic treatment of spasticity in children and adolescents with cerebral palsy (an evidence-based review). Neurology 2010;74:336 [PMID: 20101040].

Deon LL, Gaebler-Spira D: Assessment and treatment of movement disorders in children with cerebral palsy. Orthop Clin North Am 2010;41:507 [PMID: 20868881].

Dong VA et al: Studies comparing the efficacy of constraint-induced movement therapy and bimanual training in children with unilateral cerebral palsy: a systematic review. Dev Neurorehabil 2013;16(2):133–143 [PMID: 22946588].

Novak I et al: Clinical prognostic messages from a systematic review on cerebral palsy. Pediatrics 2012 Nov;130:e1285–e1312. doi: 10.1542/peds. 2012-0924 [PMID: 23045562].

Rethlefsen SA: Classification systems in cerebral palsy. Orthop Clin North Am 2010;41:457 [PMID: 20868878].

INFECTIONS & INFLAMMATORY DISORDERS OF THE CENTRAL NERVOUS SYSTEM

Infections and inflammation of the CNS are among the most treatable neurologic conditions. However, they also have a very high potential for causing catastrophic destruction of the nervous system. It is imperative for the clinician to recognize infections and inflammatory disorders of the CNS early to treat and prevent massive tissue destruction.

▶ Clinical Findings

A. Symptoms and Signs

Patients with CNS infections, whether caused by bacteria, viruses, or other microorganisms, present with similar manifestations. These include systemic signs of infection, such as fever, malaise, chills, and organ dysfunction, and specific features suggesting CNS infection, including headache, stiff neck, fever or hypothermia, changes in mental status (ranging from hyperirritability to lethargy and coma), seizures, and focal sensory and motor deficits. Meningeal irritation is indicated by the presence of Kernig and Brudzinski signs. In very young infants, signs of meningeal irritation may be absent, and temperature instability and hypothermia are more common than fever. In young infants, a bulging fontanelle and an increased head circumference are common. Papilledema may eventually develop, particularly in older children and adolescents. Cranial nerve palsies may develop acutely or gradually during neurologic infections. No specific clinical sign or symptom is reliable in distinguishing bacterial infections from infections caused by other microbes.

During the initial clinical assessment, conditions that predispose the patient to infection of the CNS should be sought. Infections involving the sinuses or other structures in the head and neck region can result in direct extension of infection into the intracranial compartment. Open head injuries, recent neurosurgical procedures, immunodeficiency, and the presence of a mechanical shunt may predispose to intracranial infection.

B. Laboratory Findings

When CNS infections are suspected, blood should be obtained for a complete blood count, chemistry panel, and culture. Most important, however, is obtaining CSF. In the absence of focal neurologic deficits or signs of brainstem herniation, CSF should be obtained immediately from any patient in whom serious CNS infection is suspected. Antimicrobial treatment must be started even if lumbar puncture is delayed. Spinal fluid should be examined for the presence of red and white blood cells, protein concentration, glucose concentration, bacteria, and other microorganisms; a sample should be cultured. In addition, serologic, immunologic, and nucleic acid detection (PCR) tests may be performed on the spinal fluid. Many labs have multiplex PCR panels that allow for rapid testing of many pathogens. See Infectious Disease Chapter 42. Identification of a pathogen may allow for customized treatment. Spinal fluid that contains a high proportion of polymorphonuclear leukocytes, a high protein concentration, and a low glucose concentration strongly suggests bacterial infection (see Chapter 42). CSF containing predominantly lymphocytes, a high protein concentration, and a low glucose concentration suggests infection with mycobacteria, fungi, uncommon bacteria, and some viruses such as lymphocytic choriomeningitis virus, herpes simplex virus, mumps virus, and arboviruses (see Chapters 40 and 43). CSF that contains a high proportion of lymphocytes, normal or only slightly elevated protein concentration, and a normal glucose concentration is suggestive of viral infections and CNS inflammatory disorders, although partially treated bacterial meningitis and parameningeal infections may also result in this CSF profile. Typical CSF findings in a variety of infectious and inflammatory disorders are shown in Table 25–2.

Herpes simplex virus infections can be confirmed using PCR to detect for herpes DNA in spinal fluid. This test has 95% sensitivity and 99% specificity. If clinical suspicion is high with a negative result, continue to treat and repeat PCR in 2–3 days. Rarely, brain biopsy may be needed to detect the rare PCR-negative case of herpes simplex, various parasitic infections, or in a suspected parainfectious or postinfectious cause with ambiguous spinal fluid findings (eg, vasculitis).

C. Imaging

Neuroimaging with CT and MRI scans may be helpful in demonstrating the presence of brain abscess, meningeal inflammation, or secondary problems such as venous and arterial infarctions, hemorrhages, and subdural effusions when these are suspected. In addition, these procedures may identify sinus or other focal infections in the head or neck region that are related to the CNS infection.

Although often nonspecific, EEGs may be helpful in the assessment of patients who have had seizures at the time of presentation. In some instances, such as herpes simplex virus or focal enterovirus infection, periodic lateralized epileptiform discharges (PLEDs) may be seen early in the course and may be one of the earliest study abnormalities to suggest the diagnosis. EEGs may also show focal slowing over regions of infarcts or (rare) abscesses.

BACTERIAL MENINGITIS

Bacterial infections of the CNS may present acutely (symptoms evolving rapidly over 1–24 hours), subacutely (symptoms evolving over 1–7 days), or chronically (symptoms evolving over > 1 week). Diffuse bacterial infections involve the leptomeninges, superficial cortical structures, and blood vessels. Although the term *meningitis* is used to describe these infections, it should not be forgotten that the brain parenchyma is also inflamed and that blood vessel walls may be infiltrated by inflammatory cells that result in endothelial cell injury, vessel stenosis, and secondary ischemia and infarction. Overall clinical characteristics of bacterial meningitis (and viral meningoencephalitis) are outlined in Table 25–18.

Acutely, this inflammatory process may result in cerebral edema or impaired CSF flow through and out of the ventricular system, resulting in hydrocephalus.

▶ Treatment

A. Specific Measures

(See also Chapters 39, 40, and the section Bacterial Infections in Chapter 42.)

While awaiting the results of diagnostic tests, the physician should start broad-spectrum antibiotic coverage. The appropriate antimicrobial varies with age to match the likely pathogens encountered at a given age. After specific organisms are identified, antibiotic therapy can be tailored based on antibiotic sensitivity patterns. See Chapter 39, Antimicorbial Therapy, for details of selecting antimicrobial coverage.

Meningitis in a child with a ventriculoperitoneal shunt is most commonly caused by coagulase-negative staphylococci, many of which are methicillin-resistant. In many of these patients who are not seriously ill, therapy should be postponed while awaiting the appropriate shunt fluid for Gram stain and culture. Seriously ill patients should initially be given vancomycin and a third-generation cephalosporin, because Staph aureus and gram-negative rods are also common causes of serious infection.

Table 25–18. Encephalitis.

Definition: Inflammation of brain parenchyma
  Clinically characterized by: fever, headache, impaired
    consciousness, seizures, focal neurologic deficit. Fatality rate > 5%
  Laboratory features include: CSF pleocytosis, elevated CSF protein.
    Evaluation should include: CSF culture; viral PCR; serology.
    Etiology identified in < 50% of cases.
  Radiographic features: focal or diffuse edema, abnormal T2
    signal on MRI, diffusion weighted abnormalities consistent
    with ischemia
  Pathologic features: perivascular cells, possible neuronophagia;
    edema, demyelination, gliosis
Infectious causes: enteroviruses, *Mycoplasma*, herpes, EBV, bacteria,
    fungi, protozoa
  Some causes are mosquito- or tick-borne; seasonal
Para/Postinfectious (ADEM)/Autoimmune: California Encephalitis
  Project identified anti-NMDAR encephalitis as the leading cause
  of encephalitis among young adults and children.
Treatment: Acutely, this inflammatory process may result in cerebral
  edema or impaired CSF flow through and out of the ventricular
  system, resulting in hydrocephalus. In addition to supportive
  measures, other treatments include:
  Herpes: acyclovir
  ADEM: high-dose steroids, IVIG or plasma exchange
  Broad-spectrum antibiotics until cultures are negative

ADEM, acute disseminated encephalomyelitis; CSF, cerebrospinal fluid; EBV, Epstein-Barr virus; IVIG, intravenous immune globulin; PCR, polymerase chain reaction.
Data from Bloch KC, Glaser CA: Encephalitis surveillance through the Emerging Infections Program, 1997–2010. Emerg Infect Dis 2015 Sep;21(9):1562–1567.

B. General and Supportive Measures

Children with bacterial meningitis are often systemically ill. The following complications should be looked for and treated aggressively: hypovolemia, hypoglycemia, hyponatremia, acidosis, septic shock, increased intracranial pressure, seizures, DIC, and metastatic infection (eg, pericarditis, arthritis, or pneumonia). Children should initially be monitored closely (cardiorespiratory monitor, strict fluid balance and frequent urine specific gravity assessment, daily weights, and neurologic assessment every few hours), not fed until neurologically stable, isolated until the organism is known, rehydrated with isotonic solutions, and then given intravenous fluids containing dextrose and sodium at no more than maintenance rate (assuming no unusual losses occur).

▶ Complications

Abnormalities of water and electrolyte balance result from either excessive or insufficient production of antidiuretic hormone and require careful monitoring and appropriate adjustments in fluid administration. Monitoring serum sodium every 8–12 hours during the first 1–2 days, and urine sodium if the inappropriate secretion of antidiuretic hormone is suspected, will usually uncover significant problems.

Seizures occur in 20%–30% of children with bacterial meningitis. Most seizures occur early during infection. Seizures tend to be most common in neonates and less common in older children. Persistent focal seizures or focal seizures associated with focal neurologic deficits strongly suggest subdural effusion, abscess, or vascular lesions such as arterial infarct, cortical venous infarcts, or dural sinus thrombosis. Because generalized seizures in a metabolically compromised child may have severe sequelae, early recognition and therapy are critical.

Subdural effusions occur in up to a third of young children with *Streptococcus pneumoniae* meningitis. Subdural effusions are often seen on CT scans of the head during the course of meningitis. They do not require treatment unless they are producing increased intracranial pressure or progressive mass effect. Although subdural effusions may be detected in children who have persistent fever, such effusions do not usually have to be sampled or drained if the infecting organism is *H influenzae*, meningococcus, or pneumococcus. These are usually sterilized with the standard treatment, and slowly waning fever during an otherwise uncomplicated recovery may be followed clinically. Under any other circumstance, however, aspiration of the fluid for documentation of sterilization or for relief of pressure should be considered. Prognosis is not worsened by subdural effusions.

Cerebral edema results in increased intracranial pressure, requiring treatment with dexamethasone, osmotic agents, diuretics, or hyperventilation; intracranial pressure monitoring may be needed.

Long-term sequelae of meningitis result from direct inflammatory destruction of brain cells, vascular injuries, or secondary gliosis. Focal motor and sensory deficits, visual impairment, hearing loss, seizures, hydrocephalus, and a variety of cranial nerve deficits can result. Sensorineural hearing loss in *H influenzae* meningitis occurs in approximately 5%–10% of patients during long-term follow-up. Early addition of dexamethasone to the antibiotic regimen may modestly decrease the risk of hearing loss in some children with *bacterial* meningitis (see Chapter 42).

In addition to the disorders mentioned, some patients with meningitis develop mild to severe cognitive impairment and severe behavioral disorders that limit their function at school and later performance in life.

BRAIN ABSCESS

▶ Clinical Findings

Patients with brain abscess often appear to have systemic illness similar to patients with bacterial meningitis, but in addition they may show signs of focal neurologic deficits, papilledema, and other evidence of increased intracranial pressure or a mass lesion. Symptoms may be present for a week

or more; children with bacterial meningitis usually present within a few days. Conditions predisposing to development of brain abscess include penetrating head trauma; chronic infection of the middle ear, mastoid, or sinuses (especially the frontal sinus); chronic dental or pulmonary infection; cardiovascular lesions allowing right-to-left shunting of blood (including arteriovenous malformations); and endocarditis.

When brain abscess is strongly suspected, either CT or MRI scan with contrast enhancement should be done prior to lumbar puncture. If a brain abscess is identified, lumbar puncture may be dangerous and rarely alters the choice of antibiotic or clinical management since the CSF abnormalities usually reflect only parameningeal inflammation or are normal. With spread from contiguous septic foci, streptococci and anaerobic bacteria are most common. Staphylococci most often enter from trauma or spread from distant infections. Enteric organisms may form an abscess from chronic otitis. Cultures from many brain abscesses are negative, but Gram stain may be informative.

The diagnosis of brain abscess is based primarily on a strong clinical suspicion and confirmed by a neuroimaging procedure. Strongly positive inflammatory markers (erythrocyte sedimentation rate, C-reactive protein) may be supportive as normal results would be unlikely in patients with brain abscess. EEG changes are nonspecific but frequently demonstrate focal slowing in the region of brain abscess.

▶ Differential Diagnosis

Differential diagnosis of brain abscess includes any condition that produces focal neurologic deficits and increased intracranial pressure, such as neoplasms, subdural effusions, cerebral infarctions, and other CNS infections.

▶ Treatment

When a primary source or contiguous focus is suspected Ceftriaxone plus metronidazole is recommended. Penicillin G is an alternative to a cephalosporin and is effective against most mouth flora. In posttraumatic and postsurgical cases, nafcillin or oxacillin plus a third-generation cephalosporin (cefotaxime or ceftriaxone) is recommended. Vancomycin should be considered as a substitute for nafcillin or oxacillin when methicillin-resistant *Staphylococcus aureus* is suspected. See Chapter 39, Antimicrobial Therapy, for further discussion. Treatment may include neurologic consultation and anticonvulsant therapy when necessary. In their early stages, brain abscesses are areas of focal cerebritis and can be treated with antibiotic therapies alone. Encapsulated abscesses require surgical drainage.

▶ Prognosis

The surgical mortality rate in the treatment of brain abscess is lower than 5%. Untreated cerebral abscesses lead to irreversible tissue destruction and may rupture into the ventricle, producing catastrophic deterioration in neurologic function and death. Because brain abscesses are often associated with systemic illness, the death rate is frequently high in these patients. Other poor prognostic indicators include rapid progression of disease and alteration of consciousness at the time of presentation.

VIRAL INFECTIONS

Viral infections of the CNS can involve meninges (meningitis) (see Chapter 40) or parenchyma (encephalitis). All patients, however, have some degree of involvement of both the meninges and cerebral parenchyma (meningoencephalitis). Many viral infections are generalized and diffuse, but some viruses, notably herpes simplex and some enteroviruses, characteristically cause prominent focal disease. Focal cerebral involvement is clear on neuroimaging procedures. Some viruses have an affinity for specific CNS cell populations. Poliovirus and other enteroviruses (A71 and D68) can selectively infect anterior horn cells and some intracranial motor neurons.

Although most viral infections of the nervous system have an acute or subacute course in childhood, chronic infections can occur. Subacute sclerosing panencephalitis, for example, represents a chronic indolent infection caused by altered measles virus and is characterized clinically by progressive neurodegeneration and seizures. SSEP commonly presents 7–10 years after infection. Risk is highest among those patients infected with the virus prior to the age of 2 years.

Treatment of CNS viral infections is usually limited to symptomatic and supportive measures, except for herpes simplex virus, and some cases of varicella-zoster virus infections where acyclovir is used (see HSV section in Chapter 40). West Nile virus is an arthropod-borne flavivirus. It is found in mosquitoes, thus the highest incidence of West Nile virus infections occurs from July to October. The infection is now endemic in United States. This disease is often asymptomatic or mild in pediatric patients; paralysis and death occur mostly in the elderly.

ENCEPHALOPATHY OF HUMAN IMMUNODEFICIENCY VIRUS INFECTION

Neurologic syndromes associated directly with HIV infection include subacute encephalitis, meningitis, myelopathy, polyneuropathy, and myositis. In addition, opportunistic infections of the CNS occur in patients with HIV-induced immunosuppression. *Pneumocystis*, *Toxoplasma*, and CMV infections are particularly common. Progressive multifocal leukoencephalopathy caused by a secondary papillomavirus infection, and herpes simplex and varicella-zoster infections also occur frequently in patients with untreated HIV infection. Various fungal (especially cryptococcal), mycobacterial, and bacterial infections occur.

Neurologic abnormalities in these patients can also be the result of noninfectious neoplastic disorders. Primary CNS lymphoma and metastatic lymphoma to the nervous system are the most frequent neoplasms of the nervous system in these patients. See Chapters 33, 39, and 41 for diagnosis and management of HIV infection.

OTHER INFECTIONS

A wide variety of other microorganisms, including *Toxoplasma*, mycobacteria, spirochetes, rickettsiae, amoebae, and mycoplasma, can cause CNS infections. CNS involvement in these infections is usually secondary to systemic infection or other predisposing factors. Appropriate cultures and serologic testing are required to diagnose these infections. Parenteral antimicrobial treatment for these infections is discussed in Chapter 39.

NONINFECTIOUS INFLAMMATORY DISORDERS OF THE CENTRAL NERVOUS SYSTEM

The differential diagnosis of bacterial, viral, and other microbial infections of the CNS includes disorders that cause inflammation but for which no specific causal organism has been identified. Sarcoidosis, Behçet disease, systemic lupus erythematosus, and other collagen-vascular disorders are examples. In these disorders, CNS inflammation usually occurs in association with characteristic systemic manifestations that facilitate diagnosis. Some CNS inflammatory disorders lead to demyelination syndromes described in Table 25–19. Management of CNS involvement

Table 25–19. Prominent features of CNS inflammatory demyelination syndromes.

ADEM	Encephalopathy and fever; may also have headache, meningismus, and seizures
CIS	Mono or multifocal lesions without encephalopathy, not meeting diagnostic criteria for multiple sclerosis
NMOSD	Characterized by longitudinally extensive transverse myelitis, optic neuritis, may also present with area postrema syndrome, acute brainstem syndrome, symptomatic narcolepsy or acute diencephalic clinical syndrome, or symptomatic cerebral syndrome, may be NMO-IgG+, MOG-IgG+ or antibody negative
Multiphasic ADEM	Rare; second event > 3 mo from onset of initial event; consider other etiologies, including anti-MOG antibody syndrome
Pediatric MS	Relapsing and remitting, may be diagnosed after one attack if MRI criteria for separation in time and space are met

ADEM, acute disseminated encephalomyelitis; anti-MOG, anti-myelin oligodendrocyte; CIS, clinically isolated syndrome; MS, multiple sclerosis; NMOSD, neuromyelitis optica spectrum disorder.

in these disorders is the same as the treatment of the systemic illness.

A. Acute Demyelinating Encephalomyelitis

Inflammatory reactions within the nervous system may occur during the convalescent stage of systemic viral infections. Parainfectious or postinfectious inflammation of the CNS results in several well-recognized disorders: acute disseminated encephalomyelitis (ADEM; 25% of encephalitis), transverse myelitis, optic neuritis, polyneuritis, and GBS.

▶ Clinical Findings

A. Imaging

MRI findings in ADEM are distinctive: demyelinating lesions, seen on T_2 and FLAIR images, are key to the diagnosis. White matter lesions can mimic findings in MS, but more likely are large and ill-defined. White matter lesions may also involve gray matter such as cortex, basal ganglia, and thalamus. Radiologic changes are usually florid when the patient presents but occasionally emerge days later. In cases of uncertain diagnosis, serial or repeat scans may be necessary. Unlike the demyelinating lesions of MS, ADEM lesions usually resolve within months of presentation.

B. Laboratory Findings

Anti-myelin oligodendrocyte (anti-MOG) antibodies should be tested in serum as persistence of antibodies indicates a risk of recurrence. Lumbar puncture findings may be normal or mildly abnormal, with mild pleocytosis and elevation of the CSF protein in 25%–50% of cases. Oligoclonal bands are not typically seen in ADEM, but rather are commonly found in chronic, relapsing conditions like MS. Oligoclonal bands may also be seen in chronic infections and viral syndromes.

▶ Treatment

Corticosteroids are the primary treatment for ADEM. Current practice is to administer high dose, followed by oral prednisone taper over 4–6 weeks. Most pediatric groups initially use intravenous methylprednisolone (10–30 mg/kg/days up to a maximum dose of 1 g/day). In refractory patients, IVIg or plasmapheresis may be effective.

▶ Prognosis

Rarely, ADEM relapses within 3 months of onset. Recurrence more than 3 months after treatment should raise suspicion of anti-MOG antibody syndrome, MS, neuromyelitis optica spectrum disorder (especially in cases of optic nerve or spinal cord involvement), or alternative cause. Congenital viral infections can also affect the CNS. CMV, herpes simplex virus, varicella, and (rare now, because of immunization)

rubella virus are the most notable causes of viral brain injury in utero.

B. Paraneoplastic Syndromes

Paraneoplastic syndromes are increasingly recognized. These immune-mediated disorders are clinically heterogeneous with neurologic effects that can be both central and peripheral. The disorders are identified by autoantibodies to either intraneuronal or cell surface antigens. While the pathogenesis of these disorders is poorly understood, they are thought to result from misdirected immune response to shared epitopes between neuronal antigens and tumor antigens. Anti-NMDA receptor encephalitis is one example of a paraneoplastic syndrome that may precede detection of neoplasm or result from postviral immune dysregulation. Recent case reports have identified HSV-1 as a trigger for anti-NMDAR encephalitis. Behavioral changes, autonomic instability, insomnia, aphasia, seizures, and movement disorders are prominent. Detection of the antibody is diagnostic. Immunotherapy, including glucocorticoids, IVIg, and/or plasma exchange are shown to be beneficial. Second-line therapies include rituximab and/or cyclophosphamide for refractory cases.

C. Multiple Sclerosis

Five to ten percent of patients with MS are diagnosed before the age of 18 years. Many patients diagnosed in adulthood report having symptoms attributable to MS prior to age of 18 years. The epidemiology, pathophysiology, diagnosis, and treatment of pediatric MS are areas of study. Several exciting discoveries have highlighted the importance of genetic and environmental risk factors for pediatric MS. Notable examples include HLA subtypes, viral exposures, smoking exposure, childhood obesity, vitamin D deficiency, and others. Importantly, diagnostic criteria, including clinical, MRI, and laboratory studies are different among prepubertal patients when compared to postpubertal patients.

▶ Clinical Findings

The diagnosis of MS in a child remains challenging as the presenting clinical signs and symptoms may be similar or identical to acute disseminated encephalomyelitis, despite the same pathophysiology. An earlier age at disease presentation may be associated with specific features such as encephalopathy, seizures, and brainstem and cerebellar symptoms.

A diagnosis of MS requires demyelination separated in time and space. However, a diagnosis of pediatric MS may be made after one episode of demyelination if the MRI scan meets criteria for dissemination in time and space as described in the McDonald 2017 diagnostic criteria Dissemination in time may also be established by the presence of oligoclonal bands in the CSF. If these criteria are not met, the child is diagnosed with clinically isolated syndrome, for example, optic neuritis; transverse myelitis; or brainstem, cerebellar, or hemispheric dysfunction. If the patient develops subsequent clinical or radiographic changes that meet criteria for MS, he/she may be diagnosed at that time. Atypical clinical features of pediatric MS include fever and involvement of the peripheral nervous system or other organ systems, elevated erythrocyte sedimentation rate or marked CSF pleocytosis. Encephalopathy is more commonly associated with ADEM. However, in young children, MS exacerbations may present with encephalopathy, making differentiation of the two disorders difficult.

The initial brain MRI scan of younger patients shows more frequent involvement of the posterior fossa and higher numbers of ovoid, ill-defined T2-bright foci that often partially resolve on the follow-up scan. At present, there are several sophisticated MRI criteria to separate pediatric MS diagnosis from alternative diagnoses (eg, ADEM).

Finally, the spinal fluid in younger patients may fail to reveal oligoclonal bands or elevated IgG index at disease onset.

▶ Differential Diagnosis

Differential diagnosis of pediatric MS includes ADEM, anti-MOG antibody syndrome, idiopathic transverse myelitis, optic neuritis, rheumatologic disorders such as systemic lupus erythematosis, Behcet and Sjogren syndrome, and neuromyelitis optica. Many other infections, metabolic disorders, and degenerative diseases can mimic MS. Anti-MOG antibody syndrome may account for cases previously thought to be atypical pediatric MS, and may be responsible for up to 40% of cases previously identified as ADEM.

▶ Treatment

Acute treatment of relapses includes high-dose intravenous methylprednisolone and occasionally plasmapheresis. Immunomodulatory treatment to prevent relapses in children includes injections, oral medications, and infusions. Injectable medications include interferon beta-1a, interferon beta-1b, and glatiramer acetate. Daclizumab has recently been taken off the market due to safety concerns. Oral medications include fingolimod, teriflunomide, dimethyl fumarate, and cladribine. Intravenous infused drugs include natalizumab, rituximab, ocrelizumab, and alemtuzumab. Cyclophosphamide may be used in refractory patients. Fingolimod is only one FDA-approved disease modifying therapy for children with MS. Pediatric clinical trials are underway for teriflunomide, dimethyl fumarate. Additional trials are planned for ocrelizumab and cladribine.

Chitnis T et al: Pediatric multiple sclerosis. Neurol Clin 2011;29:481 [PMID: 21439455].

Collongues N et al: Long-term follow-up of neuromyelitis optica with a pediatric onset. Neurology 2010;75:1084 [PMID: 20855851].

Cortese I et al: Evidence-based guideline update: plasmapheresis in neurologic disorders: report of the Therapeutics and Technology Assessment Subcommittee of the American Academy of Neurology. Neurology 2011 Jan 18;76(3):294–300 [PMID: 21242498].

Florance NR et al: Anti-N-methyl-D-aspartate receptor (NMDAR) encephalitis in children and adolescents. Ann Neurol 2009;66:11 [PMID: 19670433].

Frohman EM, Wingerchuk DM: Clinical practice. Transverse myelitis. N Engl J Med 2010;363:564–572 [PMID: 20818891].

Graus F, Saiz A, Dalmau J: Antibodies and neuronal autoimmune disorders of the CNS. J Neurol 2010;257(4):509–517 [PMID: 20035430].

Krupp LB et al: International Pediatric Multiple Sclerosis Study Group. International Pediatric Multiple Sclerosis Study Group criteria for pediatric multiple sclerosis and immune-mediated central nervous system demyelinating disorders: revisions to the 2007 definitions. Mult Scler 2013;19(10):1261–1267.

Sonneville R, Klein IF, Wolff M: Update on investigation and management of postinfectious encephalitis. Curr Opin Neurol 2010;23:300 [PMID: 20442573].

Thompson AJ et al. Diagnosis of multiple sclerosis. 2017 revisions of the McDonald Criteria. Lancet Neurol 2018 Feb;17(2) [PMID: 29275977].

Van de Beek D et al: Corticosteroids for acute bacterial meningitis. Cochrane Database Syst Rev 2007;1:CD004405 [PMID: 17253505].

Wingerchuk DM et al: International consensus diagnostic criteria for neuromyelitis optica spectrum disorders. Neurology 2015 Jul 14;85(2):177–189 [PMID: 26092914].

Yeh EA et al: Multiple sclerosis therapies in pediatric patients with refractory multiple sclerosis. Arch Neurol 2011;68:437 [PMID: 21149803].

▼ SYNDROMES PRESENTING AS ACUTE FLACCID WEAKNESS

▶ Pathogenesis

Flaccid paralysis in a child can occur because of a lesion anywhere along the neuroaxis. The key to diagnosis is localizing the lesion. Associated changes in reflexes, sensory changes, abnormal reflexes such as a positive Babinski's sign, and bowel and bladder changes can help in localizing the lesion (see the section Sensory Ataxia for additional discussion). Mass lesions, infectious or postinfectious causes, toxins (eg, from a tick or due to botulism), and metabolic causes are only a few of the etiologies that can cause acute weakness. A review of some of the more common causes of acute flaccid weakness and their associated findings are listed in Table 25–20.

▶ Clinical Findings

A. Symptoms and Signs

Features assisting diagnosis are age, a history of preceding illness, rapidity of progression, cranial nerve findings, bowel and bladder changes, and sensory findings (see Table 25–20). The finding of increased reflexes and upgoing toes suggests

Table 25–20. Acute flaccid paralysis in children.

	Acute Flaccid Myelitis	Guillain-Barré Syndrome (AIDP)	Botulism	Tick-Bite Paralysis	Transverse Myelitis
Etiology	Poliovirus types I, II, and III; other enteroviruses, eg, EV-71; EV-68, vaccine strain poliovirus (rare); West Nile virus.	Likely delayed hypersensitivity—with T-cell–mediated antiganglioside antibodies. Mycoplasma and viral infections (EBV, CMV), Campylobacter jejuni, hepatitis B; surgery, pregnancy can be precipitants	Clostridium botulinum toxin. Block at neuromuscular junction. Under age 1, toxin synthesized in bowel by organisms in ingested spores or honey. At older ages toxin ingested in food. Rarely from wound infection.	Neurotoxin in tick saliva.	Idiopathic transverse myelitis often postinfectious. May occur as constellation of findings with multiple sclerosis, neuromyelitis optica spectrum disorder and anti-MOG antibody syndrome.
History	None, or inadequate polio immunization. May have preceding upper respiratory or GI symptoms. Often in summer and early fall epidemics.	Nonspecific respiratory or GI symptoms in preceding 5–14 days common. Any season, though slightly lower incidence in summer.	Infants: dusty environment (eg, construction area), honey. Older: food poisoning, with symptoms hours to days after ingesting contaminated food.	Exposure to ticks (dog tick in eastern United States; wood ticks). Irritability 12–24 h before onset of a rapidly progressive ascending paralysis.	Progression from onset to paresis often rapid.
Presenting complaints	May be febrile at time of paralysis. Meningeal signs, muscle tenderness, and spasm. Asymmetrical weakness widespread or segmental (cervical, thoracic, lumbar). Bulbar symptoms may precede extremity weakness.	Symmetric weakness of legs, with rapid ascension to arms, trunk, and face. Verbal child may complain of paresthesias. Fever uncommon. Facial weakness early. Diplopia possible.	Infancy: constipation, poor suck and weak cry due to bulbar weakness. "Floppy." Respiratory weakness or failure Older: blurred vision, diplopia, ptosis, choking, and weakness.	Rapid onset and progression of ascending flaccid paralysis; often accompanied by pain and paresthesias. Paralysis of upper extremities 2nd day after onset. Sometimes acute ataxia presentation.	Back pain in about 30%–50% of cases. Sensory loss below level of lesion accompanying rapidly developing paralysis. Sphincter difficulties common. Fever (58%).
Findings	Flaccid weakness, usually asymmetric. Cranial nerve dysfunction; Encephalopathy possible, but not common; MRI with T2 signal change in anterior gray matter.	Flaccid, usually symmetric weakness of the extremities, with variable respiratory and bulbar weakness in severe cases. Miller-Fisher variant: ophthalmoplegia, ataxia. Bulbar involvement may occur.	In both infants and older children usually appear alert, but with flaccid weakness, decreased/absent reflexes, ophthalmoparesis, and weak/absent gag. Respiratory failure can occur. Pupils typically dilated and nonreactive to light.	Flaccid, symmetric paralysis. Cranial nerve and bulbar (respiratory) paralysis, ataxia, sphincter dysfunction, and sensory deficits may occur. Occasional fever. Diagnosis rests on finding tick, which is especially likely to be on occipital scalp.	Paraplegia with areflexia below level of lesion early; later, may have hyperreflexia and spasticity. Sensory loss below and hyperesthesia or normal sensation above level of lesion. Paralysis of bladder and rectum. MRI with T2 signal change in spinal cord, often with edema.

(Continued)

Table 25–20. Acute flaccid paralysis in children. (Continued)

	Acute Flaccid Myelitis	Guillain–Barré Syndrome (AIDP)	Botulism	Tick-Bite Paralysis	Transverse Myelitis
CSF	Pleocytosis (20–500 + cells) with PMN predominance in 1st few days, later monocytic preponderance. Protein frequently elevated (50–150 mg/dL). Virus may be identified with encephalitis panel.	Cytoalbuminologic dissociation; 10 or fewer mononuclear cells with high protein after 1st week. Normal glucose. IgG may be elevated.	Normal.	Normal.	Usually normal opening pressure; CSF may show increased protein, pleocytosis with predominantly mononuclear cells, increased IgG.
EMG/NCS	EMG shows denervation after 10–21 days. No sensory NCS abnormalities	NCSs may be normal early (within 1st week). Earliest changes: slowed to absent F or H reflexes. Demyelinating changes are typically seen 7–10 days after onset of symptoms.	EMG distinctive: BSAP (brief small abundant potentials). High-frequency stimulation may increase in CMAP amplitude but is painful to perform in awake infant.	Nerve conduction velocity slowed; returns rapidly to normal after removal of tick.	Normal early. Can have denervation at level of lesion after 10–21 days.
Other studies	Polio virus in stool and throat. Enterovirus D68 in nasal secretions. Serial serologic titers IgG, IgM in West Nile. Hyponatremia 30% in West Nile.	Search for specific cause such as infection, intoxication, autoimmune disease. Anti GM₁ antibodies seen in AMANᵃ. Anti-GQ1b antibodies seen in Miller-Fisher syndrome.	Infancy: stool culture, toxin. Rare serum toxin positive. Older: serum (or wound) toxin.	Leukocytosis, often with moderate eosinophilia.	MRI to rule out cord-compressive lesions.
Course and prognosis	Paralysis usually maximal 3–5 days after onset. Transient bladder symptoms may occur. Outlook varies with extent and severity of involvement.	Course progressive over a few days to about 2 wk.	Infancy: supportive.	Total removal of tick is followed by rapid improvement and recovery. Otherwise, mortality rate due to respiratory paralysis is very high.	Large degree of functional recovery possible. Corticosteroids, plasmapheresis and IVIg have been used to shorten the course
	Note: Mortality greatest from respiratory failure and superinfection.	**Note:** Morbidity greatest from respiratory failure (10%), autonomic crises (eg, widely variable blood pressure, arrhythmia), and superinfection. Majority recover completely. Plasmapheresis and IVIg can shorten the hospitalization. Relapses occasionally occur.	Botulism immune globulin intravenous (BIGIV). Respiratory support, gavage feeding. Avoid aminoglycosides. Prognosis: excellent. Fatality 3%.		

AIDP, acute inflammatory demyelinating neuropathy; CMAP, compound muscle action potentials; CMV, cytomegalovirus; CSF, cerebrospinal fluid; EBV, Epstein-Barr virus; EMG, electromyogram; EV-71, enterovirus 71; GI, gastrointestinal; IVIg, intravenous immunoglobulin; MRI, magnetic resonance imaging; NCS, nerve conduction studies; PMN, polymorphonuclear neutrophil; SIDS, sudden infant death syndrome.

ᵃAMAN is acute motor axonal neuropathy (uncommon variant in the United States).

a CNS lesion. Fatigability when drinking from a bottle and constipation may be seen in infants with botulism. In GBS, patients may initially present with an ascending paresthesia and loss of reflexes before they develop overt weakness. Patients with the Miller Fisher variant of GBS may present with a classic constellation of symptoms including ophthalmoplegia, ataxia, and loss of reflexes. Back pain is suggestive of a spinal cord lesion, such as in transverse myelitis or a spinal cord mass.

B. Laboratory Findings

When a spinal cord or brain lesion is suspected, MRI imaging may be helpful, and in fact is essential if a mass lesion is suspected. Once a mass lesion is excluded by imaging, CSF studies, including opening pressure, can be obtained. Viral cultures (CSF, throat, and stool) and titers aid in diagnosing poliomyelitis. A high sedimentation rate may suggest tumor, abscess, or autoimmune disorder.

EMG and nerve conduction studies (NCSs) can be helpful in diagnosing GBS. NCSs are particularly helpful after the first week when delayed or absent H or F reflexes are the first changes. Later, motor NCSs show prolonged distal latency, conduction block or temporal dispersion, with these changes seen in 50% of patients by 2 weeks and 85% by 3 weeks. EMG findings of fibrillation potentials and increased compound muscle action potential amplitudes with high-frequency stimulation are suggestive of botulism. Rarely, elevation of muscle enzymes or even myoglobinuria may aid in diagnosis of acute myopathic weakness.

▶ Differential Diagnosis

Atypical presentations of viral infections such as with influenza A, West Nile virus, and enterovirus should be considered when a patient presents with symptoms of poliomyelitis. Ascending paresthesias and absent reflexes are often early signs of GBS. The weakness of the extremities, respiratory muscles and bulbar muscles can be followed rapidly thereafter. In previously healthy infants who present with acute weakness, botulism should be considered, particularly in endemic areas or with a history of ingesting honey or canned foods. Tick paralysis can be rapidly corrected with removal of the tick but requires an index of suspicion and a careful search for the offending insect. Patients with transverse myelitis may present with acute weakness and absent reflexes, but in the ensuing weeks will develop hyperreflexia and increased tone in the regions below the area of the lesion.

▶ Complications

A. Respiratory Weakness and Failure

Early careful attention to ventilation is essential, especially in those patients with bulbar weakness and early signs of respiratory failure. Administration of oxygen, intubation,

mechanical respiratory assistance, and careful suctioning of secretions may be required. Increasing anxiety and a rise in diastolic and systolic blood pressures are early signs of hypoxia. Cyanosis is a late sign. Deterioration of spirometry testing: forced expiratory volume in 1 second and total vital capacity, may indicate the need for controlled intubation and respiratory support. At the bedside, measurement of negative inspiratory force (NIF) is recommended at frequent intervals in the acute course as this may be more sensitive to early respiratory failure than blood gases.

B. Infections

Pneumonia is common, especially in patients with respiratory weakness. Antibiotic therapy is best guided by results of cultures. Bladder infections occur when an indwelling catheter is required because of bladder paralysis. Recovery from myelitis may be delayed by urinary tract infection.

C. Autonomic Crisis

This may be a cause of death in GBS. Strict attention to vital signs to detect and treat hypotension or hypertension and cardiac arrhythmias in an intensive care setting is advisable, at least early in the course and in severely ill patients.

▶ Treatment

Ticks causing paralysis must be removed. Botulism immune globulin administration shortens the hospitalization course in infant botulism, as can treatment with IVIg or plasmapheresis in GBS. Steroids, IVIg, and/or plasmapheresis have been used in transverse myelitis. Comorbid associated disorders (eg, endocrine, neoplastic, or toxic) should be treated by appropriate means. Supportive treatment is of the essence for all of the diagnoses, including pulmonary toilet, adequate fluids and nutrition, bladder and bowel care, prevention of decubitus ulcers, and in many cases, psychiatric support.

Ayscue P et al: Acute flaccid paralysis with anterior myelitis-California, June 2012-June 2014. MMWR Morb Mortal Wkly Rep 2014;63(40):903–906 [PMID: 25299608].

Cortese I et al: Evidence-based guideline update: plasmapheresis in neurologic disorders: report of the Therapeutics and Technology Assessment Subcommittee of the American Academy of Neurology. Neurology 2011;76:294 [PMID: 21242498].

Devia K et al: Acute idiopathic transverse myelitis in children: early predictors of relapse and disability. Neurology 2014; [PMID: 25540303].

Hughes RA et al: Intravenous immunoglobulin for Guillain-Barré syndrome. Cochrane Database Syst Rev 2010 Jun 16;CD002063 [PMID: 20556755].

Messacar K et al: A cluster of acute flaccid paralysis and cranial nerve dysfunction temporally associated with an outbreak of enterovirus D68 in children in Colorado, USA. Lancet 2015 Apr 25;385(9978):1662–1671 [PMID: 25638662].

Mori M, Kuwabara S: Fisher syndrome. Curr Treat Options Neurol 2011;13:71 [PMID: 21104459].

Pastula DM et al: Acute neurologic illness of unknown etiology in children-Colorado, August-September 2014. MMWR Morb Mortal Wkly Rep 2014 10;63(40):901–902 [PMID: 25299607].

Pifko E, Price A, Sterner S: Infant Botulism and indications for administration of botulism immune globulin. Pediatr Emerg Care 2014;30(2):120 [PMID: 24488164].

Roodbol J et al: Recognizing Guillain-Barre syndrome in preschool children. Neurology 2011;76:807 [PMID: 21357832].

Walgaard C et al: Early recognition of poor prognosis in Guillain-Barre syndrome. Neurology 2011;968–975 [PMID: 21403108].

DISORDERS OF CHILDHOOD AFFECTING MUSCLES

 ESSENTIALS OF DIAGNOSIS & TYPICAL FEATURES

▶ Usually symmetric proximal more than distal muscle weakness (positive Gowers sign, excessive lordosis with walking, waddling gait).

▶ Deep tendon reflexes are typically preserved until late in the disease course, and typically lost in proportion of the degree of weakness

▶ Normal to elevated serum creatine kinase (CK) levels.

▶ Generally normal NCSs; myopathic findings on EMG.

▶ Clinical Findings

A. Laboratory Findings and Special Tests

1. Serum enzymes—Serum creatine kinase (CK) levels reflect muscle damage or "leaks" from muscle into plasma. Generally, CK levels are normal to mildly elevated in myopathies, and markedly elevated in muscular dystrophies up to 50–100 times, as in Duchenne muscular dystrophy (DMD). Medications and activity level may affect CK levels, for instance after an EMG or muscle biopsy procedure. Corticosteroids may decrease levels despite very active muscle disease, for example, as in polymyositis.

2. Electrophysiologic studies—Nerve conduction study (NCS) and needle electromyography (EMG) are often helpful in differentiating myopathic from neurogenic processes. Generally, NCSs are normal in muscle disorders. In demyelinating polyneuropathies, NCSs may show slowing of conduction velocities or conduction block. EMG involves inserting a needle electrode into muscle to record muscle electrical potentials. The examination includes assessment of abnormal spontaneous activity (eg, fibrillation and fasciculation potentials and myotonic discharges) and motor unit action potentials (MUAPs). In the myopathies, MUAPs during contraction characteristically are of short duration, polyphasic, and increased in number for the strength of the contraction (increased interference pattern). In neuropathic processes, MUAPs are polyphasic, are of large amplitude, and show decreased recruitment.

3. Muscle biopsy—A muscle biopsy can be helpful in the diagnosis of a muscle disorder, if properly executed. It is important to consider the timing of the biopsy, and the biopsied muscle should be chosen based upon the degree of weakness (ie, weaker muscles will show more pathology than strong muscles). Imaging with MRI or ultrasound may guide the choice of an appropriate site. Biopsies performed in the newborn period may be of limited utility as pathologic changes may not be evident in immature muscle. Care should be taken to avoid sites of prior needle EMG examinations or injections as this may cause spurious areas of focal inflammation pathologically. Findings common to the muscular dystrophies include variation in the size and shape of muscle fibers, increase in connective tissue, interstitial infiltration of fatty tissue, areas of degeneration and regeneration, and focal areas of inflammatory changes. Myopathies typically do not have the vigorous cycles of degeneration/regeneration and inflammation is seen in dystrophies. Immunostaining for proteins of the sarcolemmal membrane, surrounding collagen matrix, and intracellular components of the myofiber is a valuable tool.

4. Genetic testing and carrier detection—Mutation analysis for Duchenne muscular dystrophy and Becker muscular dystrophy (BMD) is considered the initial step in diagnosis, though it should be noted that readily available commercial testing is not exhaustive, and an initial negative result does not exclude the diagnosis. Full characterization of the mutation is recommended, as treatments targeting specific mutations are emerging. Carrier testing should be offered to all mothers, not only for genetic counseling purposes but also because carriers are at increased risk for developing cardiomyopathy.

Genetic testing for other myopathies and muscular dystrophies should be guided by the clinical findings, serum CK levels, and muscle biopsy results. Commercially available genetic panels are available for many of these disorders (Table 25–21).

▶ Complications

Though skeletal muscle weakness may be profound in muscle disorders, the greatest morbidity and mortality arises from cardiorespiratory complications. Advances in supportive care, especially in critical care management of these patients, have had a tremendous impact in the care of these patients. Noninvasive ventilation, better management of secretions, and generation of effective cough are a few examples. Other complications include delayed gastrointestinal motility which can lead to debilitating constipation or pseudo-obstruction. Contractures

Table 25–21. Muscular dystrophies, myopathies, myotonias, and anterior horn diseases of childhood.

Disease	Genetic Pattern	Age at Onset	Early Manifestation	Involved Muscles	Reflexes	Muscle Biopsy Findings	Other Diagnostic Tests	Treatment	Prognosis
Muscular dystrophies									
Duchenne muscular dystrophy	X-linked recessive; Xp21; 30%–50% have no family history and are spontaneous mutations.	2–6 y; rarely in infancy.	Clumsiness, and delayed motor milestones are early signs. Difficulty climbing stairs Walking on toes; waddling gait with excessive lumbar lordosis. Positive Gowers maneuver.	Proximal (pelvic > shoulder girdle) muscles; pseudohypertrophy typically of gastrocnemius. Second decade, progressive scoliosis, cardiomyopathy and respiratory weakness develop.	Knee jerks +/– or 0; ankle jerks + to ++	Areas of degeneration and regeneration, variation in fiber size, inflammatory changes, proliferation of connective tissue. Immunostaining for dystrophin absent.	Myopathic EMG. CK levels can be up to 50–100× normal, but decrease with increasing disease severity, reflecting replacement of muscle with fat/connective tissue. Genetic testing will show deletion 60% of time, while 5%–15% are duplications, and 20%–30% are point mutations, intronic deletions, or repeats.	Corticosteroids may prolong extend independent ambulation by 2.5 y if started between age 4 and 8 y; management is largely supportive. Close pulmonary and cardiac follow-up should be maintained due to risk of cardio-respiratory failure in 2nd–3rd decade of life. Osteoporosis should be treated with calcium and vitamin D.	Patients are wheelchair bound by 12 y old. Death from cardiorespiratory causes usually occurs by the 20s.
Becker muscular dystrophy (late onset)	X-linked recessive; Xp21.	Variable: childhood to adulthood.	Similar to Duchenne.	Similar to Duchenne.	Similar to Duchenne	Same as above except dystrophin immunostaining is reduced, not absent.	As above.	As above.	Variable. Patients may remain ambulant 15–20 y after 1st symptoms. Near-normal life expectancies.
Limb-girdle muscular dystrophy	Autosomal dominant, autosomal recessive, and X-linked forms.	Variable; early childhood to adulthood.	Weakness, with distribution according to type. Waddling gait, difficulty climbing stairs. Excessive lumbar lordosis.	Slowly progressive, symmetric proximal muscle involvement; characteristically involves shoulder and pelvic muscles.	Usually present	Necrosis and fiber splitting, increased endomysial connective tissue and inflammation, absent immunostaining for various DGC proteins by subtype.	Myopathic EMG. CK often > 5000 IU/L. MRI of the legs may show selective involvement (eg, peroneal muscles in Miyoshi myopathy).	Physical therapy. Echocardiogram to screen for cardiomyopathy. PFTs to screen to respiratory weakness. No curative treatment available.	Variable by subtype.

(Continued)

Table 25–21. Muscular dystrophies, myopathies, myotonias, and anterior horn diseases of childhood. (Continued)

Disease	Genetic Pattern	Age at Onset	Early Manifestation	Involved Muscles	Reflexes	Muscle Biopsy Findings	Other Diagnostic Tests	Treatment	Prognosis
Facioscapulo-humeral muscular dystrophy	Most are autosomal dominant inherited deletions of D4Z4 on 4q35	Usually late in 1st–5th decade depending on size of deletion.	Diminished facial movements with inability to close eyes, smile, or whistle. Difficulty in raising arms over head.	Face, shoulder girdle muscles (biceps, triceps), asymmetric. Deltoid and forearm spared. 75% sensorineural hearing loss; 60% Coats disease	Present	Nonspecific myopathic changes: variation in fiber size, moderate increased endomysial connective tissue, mild inflammatory changes.	Nonspecific chronic myopathic changes. CK mild to moderately elevated (< 1500 IU/L).	No curative treatments available. Management of pain important. Identify and treat hearing loss, retinal telangiectasias, respiratory insufficiency (1% cases).	Variable and inversely related to age at symptom onset. Life-threatening bulbar, respiratory and cardiac problems rare, so life expectancy normal.
Congenital myopathies									
Myotubular myopathy	X-linked recessive, due to MTM1 mutation	Neonatal period.	Floppy infant; severe hypotonia and respiratory insufficiency.	Ptosis, ophthalmoplegia; severe symmetric distal and proximal weakness.	+ to –	Small rounded myotube-like myofibers. Patchy central clearing with radial spokes.	Normal to mildly elevated CK. Myopathic EMG with fibrillations and complex repetitive discharges.	No curative treatment. Respiratory, nutritional support. Liver and peritoneal hemorrhage reported in cases.	Generally death before 5 mo of age.
Metabolic myopathies									
Pompe disease	Autosomal recessive; 17q23.	Classic infantile presentation: present by 6 mo of age. Juvenile: 2–18 y.	Severe hypotonia, hepatomegaly, cardiomyopathy, hypoventilation. Proximal muscle weakness.	Proximal more than distal muscles, bulbar and respiratory muscles. Recurrent respiratory infections; nocturnal hypoventilation.	0	Cytoplasmic lysosomal vacuoles stain positive with acid phosphatase.	High CK in infants (< 10 × normal). Mildly high CK in teens.	Enzyme replacement therapy with alglucosidase alfa (Myozyme). Respiratory and nutritional support. Monitor cardiomyopathy. As above.	Significant but variable with treatment, with improved survival, cardiorespiratory status and motor skills. Variable, some become nonambulatory and most require ventilatory support.

	Genetics	Onset	Clinical features	Distribution		Pathology	Labs/Tests	Treatment	Prognosis
Ion channel disorders									
Hyperkalemic periodic paralysis	Autosomal dominant 17q35.	Childhood, usually by 1st decade.	Episodic flaccid weakness, precipitated by rest after exercise, stress, fasting or cold.	Proximal and symmetric muscles, distal muscles may be involved if exercised.	Normal, may be 0 with episode	Hyperkalemic periodic paralysis.	CK normal to 300 IU/L; attacks associated with high serum K⁺; NCS show increased CMAP amplitude after 5 min exercise.	Many attacks are brief and do not need treatment; treat acute attack with carbohydrates; if needed, chronic treatment with acetazolamide.	Attacks may be more frequent with increasing age.
Congenital muscular dystrophies (CMD)									
CMD without CNS involvement: includes laminin a/c mutations, collagen VI myopathies	Autosomal recessive, autosomal dominant.	Birth to 1st mo.	Hypotonia, generalized weakness. Contractures proximally and lax hypermobility distally.	Generalized and respiratory muscle weakness.	0 to +	Laminin $\alpha2$ deficiency: absent/reduced laminin $\alpha2$ staining. Collagen VI myopathies: reduced/absent COLVI.	CK normal to 10 × normal. Laminin α_2 deficiency: mild neuropathy. Skin changes in collagen VI myopathies: follicular hyperkeratosis.	Most never walk or lose ability to walk early. Respiratory support required early.	Variable: death by 1st–2nd decade secondary to respiratory failure in more severely affected patients.
CMD with CNS involvement: dystroglycanopathies including Fukayama (FCMD), Walker-Warburg (WW), Muscle-eye-brain (MEB)	Recessive; 14 genes identified associated with abnormalities of glycosylation of α-dystroglycan.	Birth to 9 mo.	Severe weakness; profound motor delay; severe intellectual disability. MEB with severe congenital myopia, retinal hypoplasia.	Severe generalized weakness.	Variable	Variability in fiber size, internalized nuclei, decreased immunostaining of α-dystroglycan.	CK 400–4000 IU/L, myopathic EMG, small evoked response on electroretinogram, MRI shows white matter changes, migrational abnormalities, lissencephaly, cerebellar hypoplasia.	No curative treatment. Respiratory and nutritional support. Treatment of seizures.	Variable, but generally poor with death by 2nd decade secondary to respiratory failure.

(Continued)

Table 25–21. Muscular dystrophies, myopathies, myotonias, and anterior horn diseases of childhood. *(Continued)*

Disease	Genetic Pattern	Age at Onset	Early Manifestation	Involved Muscles	Reflexes	Muscle Biopsy Findings	Other Diagnostic Tests	Treatment	Prognosis
Myotonic disorders									
Myotonic dystrophy type 1 (DM1)	Autosomal dominant, expanded CTG triple repeat on chromosome 19q13.	Congenital presentation.	Decreased fetal movement, respiratory insufficiency, difficulties in feeding, sucking, and swallowing.	Generalized weakness; facial and pharyngeal involvement prominent; mental retardation.	Decreased to 0	Mild myopathic changes, centralized nuclei, variation in fiber size, ring fibers.	Usually normal CK. Electrical myotonia on EMG. Cataracts on slit lamp exam. Reduced testosterone levels. ECG shows conduction defects, like ventricular arrhythmias. Insulin resistance. Sleep study shows hypercapnia and hypoventilation.	No curative treatment. Patients should avoid medications that predispose to arrhythmia such as quinine, amitriptyline, and digoxin. Should be closely followed by pulmonologist for risk of apnea, by cardiologist for risk of arrhythmia, by endocrinologist for insulin resistance, and by ophthalmologist for cataracts. May have GI hypomotility with constipation and pseudoobstruction.	Reduced survival to age 65; mean survival to 60 y. 50% patients are wheelchair bound before death.
Myotonia congenita (Thomsen)	Autosomal dominant or autosomal recessive on chromosome 7q35 on CLCN1 gene.	Early infancy to adulthood.	Muscle hypertrophy. Difficulty in relaxing muscles after contracting them, especially with cold or stress.	Mild fixed proximal muscle weakness or mild functional difficulties (like climbing stairs).	Normal	Usually normal though there may be absence of 2B fibers.	Myotonia and mild myopathic changes on EMG; CK may be slightly elevated 3-4x normal	Symptom treatment with quinine, mecliletine, Dilantin, carbamazepine. May improve with exercise. Worsened with β₂ agonists, monocarboxylic amino acids, depolarizating muscle relaxants.	Normal life expectancy; muscle stiffness may interfere with activity but improves with exercise.

Spinal muscular atrophy

	Inheritance	Age	Presentation	Weakness	Reflexes	Muscle biopsy	EMG/CK	Treatment	Prognosis
SMA type 1	Autosomal recessive, 5q.	1st 6 mo of life.	Hypotonia, "floppy" infant, with alert look, fasciculations may be noted of tongue.	Severe progressive, symmetric proximal muscle weakness; face spared.	0	Large areas of grouped muscle fiber atrophy, most larger fibers are type I.	EMG shows fibrillation and fasciculation potentials, large amplitude motor unit potentials. Normal to mildly elevated CK.	Respiratory and nutritional support. Improved gross motor control and respiratory function with nusinersin (Spinraza). One time gene therapy with onasemnogene abeparvovec-xioi (Zolgensma)	Without treatment, no independent sitting or standing. Life expectancy < 2 y without respiratory or nutritional support. Likely improved with introduction of nusinersin in 2017.
SMA type 2		1st 18 mo.	Motor delays.	Progressive symmetric proximal muscles, mild to moderate respiratory weakness, limited cough and secretion control.	0 to +	As above.	EMG also shows fibrillation potentials and large amplitude motor unit potentials, but fasciculations not as common as in SMA type 1; tremor of fingers.	Improved gross motor control and respiratory function with nusinersin (Spinraza). One time gene therapy with onasemnogene abeparvovec-xioi (Zolgensma)	If untreated, will achieve independent sitting but not standing. 75% alive at 25 y old if untreated.
SMA type 3		Recognized after 18 mo of age.	Motor delays, difficulty with climbing stairs, may achieve independent walking but may lose this.	Progressive symmetric proximal muscle weakness, +/– tremor of hands.	0 to +	As above.	EMG similar to SMA type 2.	Improved gross motor control and respiratory function with nusinersin (Spinraza). One time gene therapy with onasemnogene abeparvovec-xioi (Zolgensma)	Independent ambulation may be achieved If untreated. Normal life expectancy.
SMA type 4		Adulthood.	Clumsy gait.	Mild progressive proximal muscle weakness.	0 to ++	As above.	EMG similar to SMA type 2; tremor of hands often noted.	Improved gross motor control and respiratory function with nusinersin (Spinraza). One time gene therapy with onasemnogene abeparvovec-xioi (Zolgensma)	Slow progression of muscle weakness if untreated. Normal life expectancy.

ASA, acetylsalicylic acid; CK, creatine kinase; CPT, carnitine palmityl transferase; CSF, cerebrospinal fluid; CT, computed tomography; ECG, electrocardiogram; EMG, electromyogram; MRI, magnetic resonance imaging; PCR, polymerase chain reaction; SIDS, sudden infant death syndrome.

are a particularly frustrating complication which can limit mobility of these patients, cause pain, and affect quality of life. Some DMD patients may have a nonprogressive intellectual disability with IQ scores one standard deviation below normal means.

▶ Treatment

Treatment for patients with muscle disorders is predominantly supportive, and medications altering disease progression are, at this time, limited. A few examples of treatable conditions include DMD/BMD and Pompe's disease.

Patients with Duchenne muscular dystrophy (DMD)/BMD should be offered treatment with corticosteroids (prednisone/prednisolone 0.75mg/kg/day or deflazacort 0.9mg/kg/day) which have been shown to extend the period of independent ambulation by approximately 2.5 years and to preserve respiratory strength and cardiac function into the second decade. Instituting steroid treatment between 4 and 8 years, when motor function plateaus or is in decline, appears to have the greatest impact on muscle strength and cardiorespiratory function, according to practice parameter guidelines. Additional treatments targeting specific mutations have been developed over the last decade, including commercial treatments with exon-skipping (eteplirsen) and read-through strategies (ataluren) that target specific mutations.

In the past, the prognosis for infantile Pompe disease was uniformly grim, with death by age 1 year, but ERT with recombinant alglucosidase alfa has changed the outlook for many of these patients. Treatment with ERT in these patients show overall benefit and increased survival, though in the long-term patients may have residual or progressive weakness.

Until curative treatments for muscle diseases are available, the emphasis on management ought to be on slowing the progressive deterioration in muscle strength and cardiorespiratory function, and to improve quality of life.

Aartsma-Rus A et al: Evidence-based consensus and systematic review on reducing time to diagnosis of Duchenne muscular dystrophy. J Pediatr 2019;204:305–313 [PMID: 30579468].

Birnkrant DJ et al: Diagnosis and management of Duchenne muscular dystrophy part 3: primary care, emergency management, psychosocial care and transition of care across the lifespan. Lancet Neurol 2018;17(5):445–455 [PMID: 29398641].

Bushby K et al: Diagnosis and management of Duchenne muscular dystrophy part 1. Lancet Neurol 2010;9(2):77–93 [PMID: 19945913].

Bushby K et al. Diagnosis and management of Duchenne muscular dystrophy part 2. Lancet Neurol 2010;9(2):177–189 [PMID: 19945914].

Kishnani PS, Hwu WL: Introduction to the new born screening, diagnosis, and treatment of Pompe disease guidance supplement. Pediatrics 2017;140(Suppl 1):S1–S3 [PMID: 29162672].

Nortiz G et al: Primary care and emergency department management of the patient with Duchenne. Pediatrics 2018;142(Suppl 2): 890–898 [PMID: 30275253].

Wang CH et al: Consensus statement on standard of care for congenital muscular dystrophies. J Child Neurol 2010;25(12): 1559–1581 [PMID: 21078917].

Wang CH et al: Consensus statement on standard of care for congenital myopathies. J Child Neurol 2012;27(3):363–382 [PMID: 22431881].

BENIGN ACUTE CHILDHOOD MYOSITIS

Benign acute childhood myositis (myalgia cruris epidemica) is characterized by transient severe muscle pain and weakness affecting mainly the calves and occurring 1–2 days following an upper respiratory tract infection. Although symptoms involve mainly the gastrocnemius muscles, all skeletal muscles appear to be invaded directly by virus. Children are typically between the ages of 6 and 8 years. The course is usually self-limited, but management of rhabdomyolysis and myoglobinuria is occasionally warranted, with supportive treatment with IV fluids and pain management. Follow-up of serum CK levels is recommended to ensure that they return to normal. Patients with persistently elevated CKs or recurrent episodes of rhabdomyolysis require further workup for underlying disorders such as metabolic myopathies or muscular dystrophies.

Rosenberg T et al: Outcome of benign acute childhood myositis. Pediatr Emerg Care 2018;34(6):400–402 [PMID: 27548740].

DISORDERS OF NEUROMUSCULAR TRANSMISSION

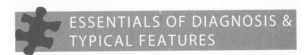

ESSENTIALS OF DIAGNOSIS & TYPICAL FEATURES

▶ Asymmetric, fluctuating weakness, usually coming on or increasing with use (fatigue).

▶ Involves extraocular, bulbar, and respiratory muscles, in addition to appendicular muscles.

▶ Positive response to neostigmine and edrophonium.

▶ General Considerations

Myasthenic syndromes are characterized by easy fatigability of muscles, particularly the extraocular, bulbar, and respiratory muscles. In the neonatal period or in early infancy, the weakness may be so constant and general that an affected infant may present nonspecifically as a "floppy infant." Three general categories of myasthenic syndromes are recognized: transient neonatal myasthenia, autoimmune myasthenia gravis, and congenital myasthenia.

▶ Clinical Findings

A. Symptoms and Signs

1. Neonatal (transient) myasthenia—This disorder occurs in 12%–19% of infants born to myasthenic mothers as a result of passive transfer of maternal acetylcholine receptor antibody across the placenta. Neonates present before the third day of life with bulbar weakness, difficulty feeding, weak cry, and hypotonia.

2. Juvenile myasthenia gravis—Like the adult form of myasthenia gravis, autoimmune juvenile myasthenia gravis is characterized by fatigable and asymmetric weakness. However, more than half of patients present with ocular symptoms (ptosis or ophthalmoplegia), unlike adult patients who typically present with limb weakness. Weakness may remain limited to the extraocular muscles in 10%–15% of patients, but approximately half of children develop systemic or bulbar symptoms within 2 years and 75% within 4 years. Symptoms of weakness tend to recur and remit, and can be precipitated by illness or medications such as aminoglycoside antibiotics. Typical signs include difficulty chewing foods like meat, dysphagia, nasal voice, ptosis, ophthalmoplegia, and proximal limb weakness. Other autoimmune disorders such as rheumatoid arthritis and thyroid disease may be associated findings.

3. Congenital myasthenic syndromes—These syndromes are a heterogenous group of hereditary, nonimmune disorders of presynaptic, synaptic, or postsynaptic neuromuscular transmission. Patients present with symptoms similar to that of myasthenia gravis, but onset is earlier, before the age of 2 years, and can vary from mild motor delay to dramatic episodic apnea. Serum acetylcholine receptor antibody testing is negative. Response to anticholinesterases is variable, depending on the type of congenital myasthenic syndrome, and some forms may paradoxically worsen. The distinction between this group of disorders and myasthenia gravis is important, as these patients will not benefit from a thymectomy, steroids, or immunosuppressants, but it may be clinically difficult to distinguish between the two. Additionally, certain subtypes of congenital myasthenic syndrome may show a paradoxical response to cholinesterase inhibitors, with worsening of the weakness. Therefore, cholinesterase inhibitors must be used with caution in patients with suspected congenital myasthenic syndromes.

B. Laboratory Findings

1. Anticholinesterase inhibitor testing

A. NEOSTIGMINE TEST—In newborns and very young infants, the neostigmine test may be preferable to the edrophonium (Tensilon) test because the longer duration of its response permits better observation, especially of sucking and swallowing movements. There is a delay of about 10 minutes before the effect may be manifest. The physician should be prepared to suction secretions, and administer atropine if necessary.

B. EDROPHONIUM TEST—Testing with edrophonium is used in older children who are capable of cooperating in certain tasks and who exhibit easily observable clinical signs, such as ptosis, ophthalmoplegia, or dysarthria. Maximum improvement occurs within 2 minutes. Both cholinesterase inhibitor tests can be limited by patient cooperation and lack of an easily observable clinical sign.

2. Antibody testing—Serum acetylcholine receptor binding, blocking, and modulating antibodies typically, though not always, are found in autoimmune juvenile myasthenia gravis. Though not specifically studied in the pediatric population, in the general myasthenia gravis population at large, about 40% of the seronegative patients have muscle-specific receptor tyrosine kinase (MuSK) antibodies. Serum acetylcholine receptor antibodies or MuSK antibodies are often found in the neonatal and juvenile forms. In juveniles, thyroid studies are appropriate.

3. Genetic testing—Commercial genetic testing is available for patients with congenital myasthenic syndromes.

C. Electrophysiologic Studies

Electrophysiologic studies may be helpful when myasthenic syndromes are considered. Repetitive stimulation of a motor nerve at slow rates of 2–3 Hz with recording over an appropriately chosen muscle reveals a progressive fall in compound muscle action potentials by the fourth to fifth repetition in myasthenic patients. At higher rates of stimulation of 50 Hz, there may be a transient repair of this defect before the progressive decline is seen. Both studies may be technically difficult to perform in infants and younger children as repetitive stimulation can be painful and requires cooperation. If this study is negative, single-fiber EMG in older cooperative children may be helpful diagnostically, but it is technically challenging and time intensive, and requires concentration on the part of the child. Stimulated single-fiber EMG may be performed by trained electromyographers.

D. Imaging

Chest radiograph and CT scanning in older children may show thymic hyperplasia. Thymomas are rare in children.

▶ Treatment

A. General and Supportive Measures

In the newborn or in a child in myasthenic or cholinergic crisis (see the following section Complications), supportive care is essential and the child should be monitored in a critical care setting. A careful search for signs of respiratory failure is crucial: simple bedside tests include evaluation of cough and counting to 20 in a single breath. An inability to do either signals respiratory failure. Neck flexion weakness, nasal speech, and drooling are other important signs of respiratory problems. Management of secretions and respiratory assistance should be monitored by trained critical care staff.

B. Symptomatic Treatment: Anticholinesterase Inhibitors

1. Pyridostigmine bromide—Pyridostigmine is the first-line symptomatic treatment in patients with juvenile myasthenia gravis and mild weakness. Anticholinesterase inhibitors do not modify disease progression but transiently improve muscle strength. For younger children, the starting dose is 0.5–1 mg/kg every 4–6 hours. In older children, the initial dose is 30–60 mg every 4–6 hours. The maximal daily dose is 7 mg/kg/days with an absolute maximum dose of 300 mg/day. The dosage must be adjusted for each patient based on clinical symptoms and side effects. Care must be taken in using this medication in patients suspected of having congenital myasthenic syndrome, as its use could potentially precipitate weakness.

2. Neostigmine—Fifteen milligrams of neostigmine are roughly equivalent to 60 mg of pyridostigmine bromide. Neostigmine often causes gastric hypermotility with diarrhea, but it is the drug of choice in newborns, in whom prompt treatment may be lifesaving. It may be given parenterally.

C. Immunomodulatory Treatment

Patients with autoimmune myasthenia gravis and more severe weakness not responding to cholinesterase inhibitors alone require long-term treatment with immunomodulation. There are four therapeutic options in this category: (1) plasmapheresis, (2) IVIg, (3) steroids, and (4) immunosuppressants. The mainstay of treatment is steroids, but some patients who either cannot tolerate or do not respond to steroids require treatment with other immunosuppressants such as azathioprine, cyclosporine, or mycophenolate mofetil. Both plasmapheresis and IVIg may be given on a long-term basis, depending on the severity of symptoms, as well as in the acute setting, with myasthenic crises. Special note must be made to the use of steroids, which can transiently worsen symptoms before any benefit is noted, particularly with large starting doses.

D. Surgical Treatment

There are few data for efficacy of thymectomy in the pediatric population. Some studies suggest that thymectomy within 2 years of diagnosis results in a higher rate of remission in Caucasian children. Experienced surgical and postsurgical care are prerequisites.

▶ Complications

A. Myasthenic Crisis

Respiratory failure can develop swiftly due to critical weakness of respiratory muscle, bulbar muscles or both, resulting in a myasthenic crisis. Crises are generally not fatal as long as patients receive timely respiratory support and appropriate immunotherapy. Vigilance, however, needs to be maintained as crises can occur in the setting of medical illnesses or surgical procedures. Patients and their caregivers should also be alerted that certain medications can exacerbate myasthenia gravis, including aminoglycoside antibiotics, muscle relaxants, and anesthetics.

B. Cholinergic Crisis

Cholinergic crisis may result from overmedication with anticholinesterase drugs. The resulting weakness may be similar to that of myasthenic crises, and the muscarinic side effects (diarrhea, sweating, lacrimation, miosis, bradycardia, and hypotension) are often absent or difficult to evaluate. If suspected, cholinesterase inhibitors should be discontinued immediately, and improvement afterward suggests cholinergic crisis. As in myasthenic crisis, supportive respiratory care and appropriate immunotherapy should be given.

▶ Prognosis

Prognosis for neonatal (transient) myasthenia is generally good, with complete resolution of symptoms in 2–3 weeks. However, immediate treatment with appropriate respiratory support in the acute presentation period is crucial, primarily because of the risk of secretion aspiration. No further treatment is required thereafter. The prognosis for congenital myasthenic syndromes is variable by subtype. Some subtypes show improvement in weakness with age. Others demonstrate life-threatening episodic apnea, including those with rapsyn mutations, fast-channel mutations, and choline acetyltransferase mutations. Patients with childhood and juvenile myasthenia gravis generally do well, with greater spontaneous remission rates than adult patients. Improvements in respiratory and critical care support have improved prognosis for these patients.

Cortese I et al: Evidence-based guideline update: plasmapheresis in neurologic disorders: report of the Therapeutics and Technology Assessment Subcommittee of the American Academy of Neurology. Neurology 2011;76(3):294–300 [PMID: 21242498].

Hantai D et al: Congenital myasthenic syndromes. Curr Opin Neurol 2013;26(5):561–568 [PMID: 23995276].

Hennessey IA et al: Thymectomy for inducing remission in juvenile myasthenia gravis. Pediatr Surg Int 2011;27(6):591–594 [PMID: 21243366].

Liew WK et al: Comparison of plasmapheresis and intravenous immunoglobulin as maintenance therapies for juvenile myasthenia gravis. JAMA Neurol 2014;71(5):575–580 [PMID: 24590389].

Liew WK, Kang PB: Update on juvenile myasthenia gravis. Curr Opin Pediatr 2013;25(6):694–700 [PMID: 24141560].

Mehndiratta MM, Pandey S, Kuntzer T: Acetylcholinesterase inhibitor treatment for myasthenia gravis. Cochrane Database Syst Rev 2011;16(2):CD006986 [PMID: 21328290].

LESIONS OF THE PERIPHERAL NERVE

Facial Weakness

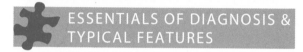

ESSENTIALS OF DIAGNOSIS & TYPICAL FEATURES

▶ Central versus peripheral facial nerve lesions need to be distinguished to determine workup, treatment, and prognosis. The inability to raise the eyebrows indicates peripheral involvement of the facial nerve.

Pathogenesis

The most common cranial mononeuropathy is facial nerve palsy. Cranial nerve VII is a complex nerve that carries several different nerve fibers, including motor fibers to all muscles of facial expression, parasympathetic motor fibers supplying the mucosa of the soft palate and the salivary and lacrimal glands, taste fibers to the anterior two-thirds of the tongue, parasympathetic sensory fibers for visceral sensation from the salivary glands and the nasal and pharyngeal mucosa, and somatic sensory fibers supplying a small part of the external auditory meatus and the skin of the ear. Facial weakness can occur as the result of a lesion anywhere along the path of the nerve. A central lesion such that of a stroke, proximal to the facial nerve nuclei, causes contralateral weakness of the lower face, sparing the forehead and orbicularis oculi muscles which are bilaterally innervated. Peripheral lesions such that of Bell's Palsy, at or distal to the facial nerve nuclei, cause ipsilateral facial weakness that affects both the upper and lower facial muscles, resulting in an inability to wrinkle the forehead, close the eye or smile. In addition, there may be dysfunction in the ability of tearing and saliva production, hyperacusis, and absent taste sensation over the anterior two-thirds of the tongue.

Clinical Findings

The inability to wrinkle the forehead may be demonstrated in infants and young children by getting them to follow a light moved vertically above the forehead. Loss of taste of the anterior two-thirds of the tongue on the involved side may be demonstrated in cooperative children by age 4 or 5 years. Playing with a younger child and the judicious use of a tongue blade may enable the physician to note whether the child's face puckers up when something sour (eg, lemon juice) is applied with a swab to the anterior tongue.

Differential Diagnosis

Injuries to the facial nerve at birth occur in 0.25%–6.5% of consecutive live births. Forceps delivery is the cause in some cases; in others, the side of the face affected may have abutted in utero against the sacral prominence. Often, no cause can be established.

Acquired peripheral facial weakness (Bell palsy) is common in children. Some cases are postinfectious, although an increasing body of evidence suggests that Bell palsy is a viral-induced cranial neuritis. It may be a presenting sign of Lyme disease, infectious mononucleosis, herpes simplex, or GBS and is usually diagnosable by the history, physical examination, and appropriate laboratory tests. Chronic cranial nerve VII palsy may be a sign of brainstem tumor.

Bilateral facial weakness in early life may be due to agenesis of the facial nerve nuclei or muscles (part of Möbius syndrome) or may even be familial. Myasthenia gravis, Miller-Fisher syndrome, fascioscapulohumeral muscular dystrophy, and myotonic dystrophy must be considered.

Asymmetrical crying facies, in which one side of the lower lip depresses with crying (ie, the normal side) and the other does not, is usually an autosomal dominantly inherited congenital malformation. The defect in the parent (the asymmetry often improves with age) may be almost inapparent. EMG suggests congenital absence of the depressor angularis muscle of the lower lip. Forceps pressure is often erroneously incriminated as a cause of this innocent congenital anomaly. Occasionally, other major (eg, cardiac septal defects) congenital defects accompany the palsy. Congenital unilateral lower lip paralysis with asymmetric crying facies, most often attributed to congenital absence of the depressor anguli oris, is associated with major malformations, most commonly heart defects, in 10% of cases.

Treatment & Prognosis

In the vast majority of cases of isolated peripheral facial palsy—both those due to birth trauma and those acquired later—improvement begins within 1–2 weeks, and near or total recovery of function is observed within 2 months. In severe palsy with inefficient blinking, methylcellulose drops, 1%, should be instilled into the eyes to protect the cornea during the day; at night the lid should be taped down with cellophane tape. Upward massage of the face for 5–10 minutes three or four times a day may help maintain muscle tone. Prednisone therapy (2–4 mg/kg orally for 5–7 days) likely does not aid recovery. In the older child, acyclovir or valacyclovir (herpes antiviral agent) therapy or antibiotics (Lyme disease) may have a role in Bell palsy.

In the few children with permanent and cosmetically disfiguring facial weakness, plastic surgical intervention at age 6 years or older may be of benefit. New procedures, such as attachment of facial muscles to the temporal muscle and transplantation of cranial nerve XI, are being developed.

Gronseth GS, Paduga R; American Academy of Neurology: Evidence-based guideline update: steroids and antivirals for Bell palsy: report of the Guideline Development Subcommittee of the American Academy of Neurology. Neurology 2012;79(22):2209–2213 [PMID: 23136264].

Kennedy PG: Herpes simplex virus type 1 and Bell's palsy-a current assessment of the controversy. J Neurovirol 2010;16(1):1–5 [PMID: 20113184].

Pavlou E et al: Facial nerve palsy in childhood. Brain Dev 2011;33(8):644–650 [PMID: 21144684].

Rioja-Mazza et al: Asymmetric crying facies. J Matern Fetal Neonatal Med 2005;18(4):275–277 [PMID: 16318980].

PERIPHERAL NEUROPATHY

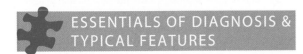

ESSENTIALS OF DIAGNOSIS & TYPICAL FEATURES

► Weakness in neuropathies typically occurs in the distal limbs

► Reflexes are typically lost early in the disease course, out of proportion to the degree of weakness.

► Sensory changes usually accompany a neuropathy.

▶ General Considerations

Lesions of the peripheral nerve typically progress in a distal to proximal fashion, with weakness and muscle atrophy occurring in the distal extremities first. Children can present with disturbances of gait, such as tripping over their toes, and easy fatigability in walking or running, and slightly less often, weakness or clumsiness of the hands. Pain, tenderness, or paresthesia is mentioned less frequently, but positive symptoms suggest an acquired neuropathy. On neurologic examination, patients often have more weakness in the lower legs than thighs and in the hands more than the arms. Reflexes typically are depressed in a distal to proximal fashion. Sensory deficits occur in a stocking-and-glove distribution. Trophic changes such as glassy or parchment skin and absent sweating may occur if the course has been chronic. Rarely, thickening of the ulnar and peroneal nerves may be felt. In small fiber sensory neuropathy, the patient may not feel minor trauma or burns, leading to traumatic injuries.

The history is crucial in determining whether the cause of a chronic polyneuropathy is genetic or acquired, as this determines management and treatment. In the hereditary sensorimotor polyneuropathies (eg, Charcot-Marie-Tooth disease), there may be a family history of gait or orthopedics

abnormalities but no systemic involvement. Other genetic causes of polyneuropathies associated with systemic involvement include storage disorders or leukodystrophies. A careful history may reveal an exposure to toxins known to cause neuropathies such as lead or arsenic, or use of medications such as vincristine. Neuropathies can be the late manifestations of systemic disorders like diabetes and autoimmune disorders. Treatment of these underlying disorders can improve or slow the progression of the neuropathy. AIDP has been discussed in another section, but a similar disorder, chronic inflammatory demyelinating polyneuropathy (CIDP) is an immune-mediated disorder with a more slowly progressive course. Recognition of this diagnosis by electrophysiologic testing, CSF studies, and occasionally nerve biopsy, is important as it is responsive to treatment with immunomodulating and immunosuppressant treatments, as with AIDP.

▶ Clinical Findings

Hereditary neuropathy is the most common documented cause of chronic neuropathy in childhood. A careful genetic history (pedigree) and examination and electrophysiologic testing (motor and sensory nerve conduction and EMG) of patient and relatives are keys to diagnosis. Genetic tests are available for many of the variants. Nerve biopsy is rarely necessary.

Other hereditary neuropathies may have ataxia as a prominent finding, often overshadowing the neuropathy. Examples are Friedreich ataxia, adrenoleukodystrophy, and Krabbe disease. Finally, some hereditary neuropathies are associated with identifiable and occasionally treatable metabolic errors (see Tables 25–21 and 25–22). These disorders are described in more detail in Chapter 36.

Laboratory diagnosis of chronic polyneuropathies is made by electrophysiologic testing with EMG/NCS. CSF protein levels can be elevated, sometimes with an increased IgG index. Nerve biopsy, with teasing of the fibers and staining for metachromasia, may demonstrate loss of myelin, and to a lesser degree, loss of axons and increased connective tissue or concentric lamellas (so-called onion bulb appearance) around the nerve fiber. Muscle biopsy may show the pattern associated with denervation. Other laboratory studies directed toward specific causes mentioned above include screening for heavy metals and for metabolic, renal, or vascular disorders.

▶ Treatment & Prognosis

Therapy is directed at specific disorders whenever possible. In patients with CIDP, treatment includes corticosteroid treatment, which may be prescribed alone or in combination with immunosuppressant agents and immunomodulatory treatments. Identification of secondary causes of CIDP is important as autoimmune disorders, thyroid disease, and infectious etiologies can be associated with CIDP and should be treated independently. For chronic neuropathies, physical therapy and management of pain and discomfort are the mainstays of management.

The long-term prognosis varies with the cause and the ability to offer specific therapy. There are few studies evaluating the long-term prognosis in pediatric patients with CIDP, but children with DIDP typically have a more favorable outcome than adult patients. Genetic counseling of patients with inherited polyneuropathies is important for not only the patients, but their families as well. Generally, the course of patients with inherited polyneuropathies is one of slow progression of distal weakness, but the phenotypic and genotypic variability of the inherited polyneuropathies is broad.

Eftimov F et al: Intravenous immunoglobulin for chronic inflammatory demyelinating polyradiculoneuropathy. Cochrane Database Syst Rev 2013;12 [PMID: 24379104].

Harada Y et al: Pediatric CIDP: Clinical features and response to treatment. J Clin Neuromuscul Dis 2017;19(2):57–65 [PMID: 29189550].

Mahdi-Rogers M et al: Immunomodulatory treatment other than corticosteroids, immunoglobulin and plasma exchange for chronic inflammatory demyelinating polyraducloneuropathy. Cochrane Database Syst Rev 2013;6 [PMID: 23771584].

McMillan HJ et al: Childhood chronic inflammatory demyelinating polyradiculoneuropathy. Neuromuscul Disord 2013;23(2):103–111 [PMID: 23140945].

Shy M, Gutmann L: Update on Charcot-Marie-Tooth disease. Curr Opin Neurol 2015;28(5):462–467 [PMID: 26263471].

MOTOR NEURON DISORDERS

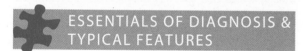

ESSENTIALS OF DIAGNOSIS & TYPICAL FEATURES

▶ Spinal muscular atrophy (SMA) is the most common cause of lower motor neuron disease.

▶ Commercially available treatments are available for SMA and therefore early diagnosis is crucial for treatment.

▶ Weakness, hypotonia, absent reflexes, and fasciculations in an alert and bright eyed child should suggest SMA.

Pathogenesis

SMA occurs in about 1 in 11,000 live births and is cause by autosomal recessive mutations in *SMN1*. The lack of survival motor neuron (SMN) protein results in progressive degeneration of the lower motor neurons in the spinal cord and brainstem. Infants and children develop progressive weakness of the limbs, bulbar muscles, and respiratory muscles.

Clinical Findings

A. Signs and Symptoms

There is a broad range of phenotypes in patients with SMA, classified as type 0–4 by their best functional ability. In patient SMA0, patients have severe weakness with neonatal onset of symptoms. These patients often have joint contractures due to the severe weakness, and often die in utero or shortly after birth. SMA type 1 is the most common type and is characterized by onset prior to 6 months of age. These patients develop progressive hypotonia and weakness, and never achieve the ability to sit. They develop progressive difficulty with feeding and respiratory weakness. Patients with SMA type 2 typically have delayed motor milestones, and while they may achieve the ability to sit independently, may lose the ability to do so. Patients with SMA type 3 achieve the ability to walk but typically lose that skill. Finally, patients with SMA type 4 present in adulthood with weakness. In general, the phenotype of patients with SMA is modified by the number of copies of the *SMN2*. *SMN2* encodes the same protein but contains an exonic splice enhancer variant that results in skipping of exon 7, leading to an unstable, truncated protein product that provides about 10%–20% of total SMN function. The higher the copy number of *SMN2*, the milder the clinical phenotype. While this is not an absolute correlation, this can be a predictor of clinical course. For instance, generally SMA type 1 patients typically have no more than 2 copies of SMN2, while type 3 and 4 patients have 4 or more copies.

B. Laboratory Findings

A. Commercially available genetic testing for *SMN1* deletions and duplications and sequence variants has allowed rapid diagnosis of SMA. Several states already include SMA in their newborn screening, and more are in progress. Electrophysiologic testing and muscle biopsy are therefore no longer used in the diagnosis of this disorder. Serum CK, if obtained, can be normal to mildly increased to the 500IU/L range.

Differential Diagnosis

The diagnostic considerations for a hypotonia infant with absent reflexes includes other primary neuromuscular disorders such as congenital myopathies, congenital muscular dystrophies, and congenital myasthenia syndromes. Patients with central nervous system disorders typically are encephalopathic, in contrast to patients with SMA who appear bright-eyed and alert.

Treatment

Historically, only supportive care was offered to patients with SMA. With rapid advancements in neuromuscular research, the treatment landscape has changed markedly for these patients. Nusinersen (Spinraza) is a commercially available treatment that is an antisense oligonucleotide designed to target the *SMN2* gene product to include exon 7 and produce a full-length SMN protein. It is administered intrathecally, and must be administered lifelong. It has been shown to improve motor and respiratory function in patients. Gene therapy with onasemnogene abeparvovec-xioi (Zolgensma) replaces full-length *SMN1* as a single intrathecal treatment. For both treatments, early treatment produces better outcomes. This underscores the importance of early recognition and diagnosis. While these treatments are available, supportive care is still the mainstay in the management of these patients. Monitoring and management of respiratory insufficiency, nutrition, and orthopedic issues are crucial to the care of these patients.

Finkel RS et al: Nusinersen versus sham control in infantile-onset spinal muscular atrophy. N Negl J Med 2017;377(18):1723–1732 [PMID: 29091570].

Finkel RS et al: Diagnosis and management of spinal muscular atrophy: part 1. Neuromuscul Disord 2018;28(3):197–207 [PMID: 29290580].

Mendell JR et al: Single-dose gene-replacement therapy for spinal muscular atrophy. N Engl J Med 2017;377(18):1713–1722 [PMID: 209091557].

Mercuri E et al: Diagnosis and management of spinal muscular atrophy: part 2. Neuromuscul Disord 2018;28(2):103–115 [PMID: 29305137].

Wang CH et al: Consensus statement for standard of care in spinal muscular atrophy. J Child Neurol 2007;22:1027–1049 [PMID: 17761659].

▼ MISCELLANEOUS NEUROMUSCULAR DISORDERS

FLOPPY INFANT SYNDROME

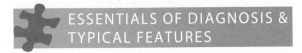

ESSENTIALS OF DIAGNOSIS & TYPICAL FEATURES

► Classic maneuvers to evaluate a floppy infant include checking vertical suspension, horizontal suspension, and traction response.

► Correct interpretation of neurologic findings in a hypotonic infant is dependent on a thorough knowledge of normal childhood development.

▶ Pathogenesis

An infant may present with hypotonia due to dysfunction at any place along the neuroaxis, from the brain, spinal cord, nerve, neuromuscular junction, and muscle. Additionally, systemic disorders, metabolic disease, and genetic disorders may cause an infant to appear "floppy." The evaluation of the hypotonic infant is therefore one of the most challenging diagnostic problems that a pediatrician is often faced with. The diagnostic workup requires a thorough knowledge of normal developmental milestones at each stage of a developing infant and child, and careful assessment of the pre- and perinatal history, family history, developmental history, and presence of other systemic involvement (Table 25–22).

▶ Clinical Findings

A. Signs and Symptoms

In the young infant, horizontal suspension (ie, supporting the infant with a hand under the chest) normally results in the infant's holding its head slightly up (45 degrees or less), the back straight or nearly so, the arms flexed at the elbows and slightly abducted, and the knees partly flexed. The "floppy" infant droops over the hand like an inverted U. The normal newborn attempts to keep the head in the same plane as the body when pulled up from supine to sitting by the hands (traction response). Marked head lag is characteristic of the floppy infant. In vertical suspension, the hypotonic infant will slip through the examiner's hands when held under the armpits. Hyperextensibility of the joints is not a dependable criterion.

B. Laboratory Findings

A general rule for laboratory testing is to localize the etiology of the hypotonia. For instance, if a lower motor neuron etiology is suspected, a serum CK, EMG/NCS, and/or muscle biopsy may be appropriate as first-tier testing. Many neuromuscular disorders may be diagnosed by clinical findings alone, as is often the case with SMA and congenital myotonic dystrophy, and in those cases, genetic testing is often the first testing warranted. If the hypotonic is accompanied by language or cognitive delay, a CNS or genetic disorder is most likely, and MR imaging of the brain may be the most useful diagnostic test.

▶ Differential Diagnosis

The most common etiology of hypotonia in the neonate is hypoxic-ischemic encephalopathy (HIE). Dysmorphic features may suggest a genetic etiology such as Down syndrome and Prader-Willi syndrome. Abnormalities of the hair or skin, which form from the neuroectoderm in development with the brain, may prompt an evaluation for brain malformations. Often seizures or language or cognitive delay may be accompanying features. Regression in development is often a clue for mitochondrial or metabolic disorders. Neuromuscular disorders, including congenital myotonic dystrophy and

Table 25–22. Floppy infant.

Lower Motor Neuron Causes		
Disease	Causes	Manifestations
SMA	Autosomal recessive; diagnose by deletion exons 7 and 8 in the SMN gene (98% of cases).	In-utero movements decreased in one-third. Gradual weakness, delay in gross motor milestones. Weak cry. Abdominal breathing. Few spontaneous movements except of the distal extremities. No deep tendon reflexes. Fasciculations of tongue. Normal personal-social behavior.
Infantile botulism	Acquired, younger than age 1 y (mostly before age 6 mo); botulism spore in stool makes toxin.	Poor feeding. Constipation. Weak cry. Failure to thrive. Lethargy. Facial weakness, ptosis, ocular muscle palsy. Inability to suck, swallow. Apnea. Source: soil dust, honey. EMG may be helpful.

Myasthenia gravis
  Neonatal transient
  Congenital
	12% of infants born from a myasthenic mother.
	Mother normal. Rare inherited disorder.
		Floppiness. Poor sucking and feeding; choking. Respiratory distress. Weak cry. Autoimmune antibodies from mother.
		As above; may improve and later exacerbate.

Myotonic dystrophy type 1	Autosomal dominant: In 99% mother transmits gene. DNA testing 98% accurate.	Polyhydramnios; failure of suck, respirations. Facial diplegia. Ptosis. Arthrogryposis. Thin ribs. Later, developmental delay. Examine mother for myotonia, physiognomy. EMG variable in infant.
Congenital myopathy and muscular dystrophy myopathy	Multiple genetic causes.	Clinical features often include respiratory failure, facial or bulbar weakness, joint contractures. Severe mental retardation. Seizures. Brain structural abnormalities; MRI helpful to distinguish muscle disorders with CNS involvement. Muscle biopsy for definitive diagnosis.
Infantile neuropathy Hypomyelinating/dysmelinating	Multiple genetic causes.	Demyelinating or axonal; a rare cause. Can appear similar to SMA EMG/NCS is helpful as is MRI brain to evaluate for central demyelination/dysmeylination
Central Causes		
	Causes	Manifestations
Structural CNS causes		
Hypoxic-ischemic encephalopathy	Multiple causes, detailed prenatal and perinatal history crucial	Limpness, stupor; poor suck, cry, Moro reflex, and grasp; later, irritability, increased tone and reflexes.
Brain malformations	Multiple causes, including genetic, exposures, infections	Seizures may be seen. Cognitive and language delay when older.
Syndromes with hypotonia (CNS origin)		
Trisomy 21	Genetic	All have hypotonia early.
Prader-Willi syndrome	Genetic deletion 15q11.	Hypotonia, hypomentia, hypogonadism, obesity
Marfan syndrome	Autosomal dominant.	Arachnodactyly.
Dysautonomia	Autosomal recessive.	Respiratory infections, corneal anesthesia.
Turner syndrome	45X, or mosaic.	Somatic stigmata (see Chapter 36).
Degenerative disorders		
Tay-Sachs disease	Autosomal recessive.	Cherry-red spot on macula.
Metachromatic leukodystrophy	Autosomal recessive.	Deep tendon reflexes increased early, polyneuropathy late; mental retardation.

(Continued)

Table 25–22. Floppy infant. (*Continued*)

	Central Causes	
	Causes	**Manifestations**
Systemic diseases[a]		
Malnutrition	Deprivation, cystic fibrosis.	
Chronic illness	Congenital heart disease; chronic pulmonary disease (eg, bronchopulmonary dysplasia); uremia, renal acidosis.	
Metabolic disease	Mitochondrial; Lowe, Pompe, Leigh disease; hypercalcemia.	
Endocrinopathy	Hypothyroidism	

AD, autosomal dominant; AR, autosomal recessive; EMG, electromyogram; HSMN, hereditary sensory motor neuropathy; MRI, magnetic resonance imaging; NCV, nerve conduction velocity; SMA, Spinal muscular atrophy; SMN, survival motor neuron.
[a]See elsewhere in text for manifestations.

SMA, can present as hypotonia in the infant. While the list of differential diagnosis in Table 25–22 is not complete, it describes the clinical features of some of the more common causes of hypotonia in infants and children.

► Treatment

Treatment for many of these disorders is supportive. Physical and occupational therapy can facilitate some progress to a varying degree. Accompanying seizures and other systemic manifestations should be controlled to optimize development.

Birdi K et al: The floppy infant: retrospective analysis of clinical experience (1990–2000) in a tertiary care facility. J Child Neurol 2005;20:803 [PMID: 16417874].

Paro-Panjan D, Neubauer D: Congenital hypotonia: is there an algorithm? J Child Neurol 2005;19:439 [PMID: 15446393].

Richer LP et al: Diagnostic profile of neonatal hypotonia: an 11-year study. Pediatr Neurol 2001;25:32 [PMID: 11483393].

Vasta I et al: Can clinical signs identify newborns with neuromuscular disorders? J Pediatr 2005;146:73 [PMID: 1564482].

Web Resources

American Academy of Neurology: http://www.aan.com.
Provides both adult and child neurology practice parameters.
American Epilepsy Society: http://www.aesnet.org.
Includes general information about epilepsy, and a comprehensive section about antiepileptic drugs.
Child Neurology Foundation: http://www.childneurologyfoundation.org/index.html.
Describes resources and tests related to child neurology and provides a comprehensive list of child neurology–related website links.
Child Neurology Society: http://www.childneurologysociety.org.
Provides research updates and organizational information and has child neurology–specific practice parameters.
Cure CMD: http://curecmd.org/.
Epilepsy Foundation of America: http://www.epilepsyfoundation.org.
Includes tutorials about epilepsy and living with epilepsy.
Families of SMA: http://www.fsma.org/.
Gene tests: http://www.genetests.org.
Provides detailed information about available genetic testing, research, literature/disorder reviews, and resources for most genetically determined neurologic disorders.
Muscular Dystrophy Association: http://www.mda.org.
Contains research updates, organizational information, and detailed information regarding neuromuscular disorders.
National Institute of Neurologic Disorders and Stroke: http://www.ninds.nih.gov.
Provides brief descriptions of neurologic disorders, related research, research opportunities, and relevant organizations.
National Ataxia Foundation http://www.ataxia.org/.
Resource for providers and patients with ataxia including research and support groups.
National MS Society http://nmss.org.
Provides resources for providers, schools, patients, and families on pediatric onset multiple sclerosis.
Neurofibromatosis Foundation: http://www.nf.org.
Provides detailed information for parents and providers about neurofibromatosis.
Washington University, St. Louis, Neuromuscular Disease Center: http://neuromuscular.wustl.edu.
Includes detailed descriptions of neuromuscular disorders and differential diagnoses.
Tuberous Sclerosis Association: http://www.tsalliance.org.
Contains detailed information for parents and providers about Tuberous Sclerosis.
We Move: worldwide education and awareness for movement disorders: http://wemove.org.
Descriptions of movement disorders, related research, and research opportunities.

Orthopedics

Jason T. Rhodes, MD, MS

Alex Tagawa, BS

Cameron Niswander, BA

Wade Coomer, BS

Mark A. Erickson, MD, MMM

Sayan De, MD

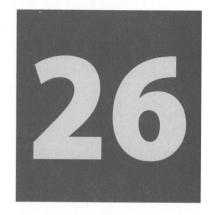

INTRODUCTION

Orthopedics is the medical discipline that deals with disorders of the musculoskeletal system. Patients with orthopedic problems generally present with one or more of the following complaints: pain, swelling, loss of function, or deformity. While the history reveals the patient's expectation, physical examination and radiographic imaging are vitally important features of orthopedic diagnosis.

DISTURBANCES OF PRENATAL ORIGIN

ESSENTIALS OF DIAGNOSIS & TREATMENT

▶ Conditions are present at birth (congenital).

▶ Multiple organ systems may be involved.

▶ Treatment is aimed at maximizing function.

CONGENITAL AMPUTATIONS & LIMB DEFICIENCIES

▶ Clinical Findings

A. Symptoms and Signs

The specific etiology of many congenital amputations is not clear, but a genetic association has been suggested. Some congenital amputations may be due to teratogens (eg, drugs or viruses), amniotic bands, or metabolic diseases (eg, maternal diabetes). Limb deficiencies are rare with an overall prevalence for all types of limb deficiencies of 0.79 per 1000. The most common cause of limb deficiencies is vascular disruption defects (prevalence of 0.22 per 1000). As a group, upper limb deficiencies occur more frequently than lower limb deficiencies, but the single most frequent form of limb deficiency is congenital longitudinal deficiency of the fibula. Children with congenital limb deficiencies generally also have a high incidence of other congenital anomalies, including genitourinary, cardiac, and palatal defects. Deficiencies have a wide spectrum, ranging from mild limb length discrepancy to significant deformity. They usually consist of a partial absence of structures in the extremity along one side. For example, in radial club hand, the entire radius is absent, but the thumb may be either hypoplastic or completely absent. The effect on structures distal to the deficiency varies. Complex tissue defects are virtually always associated with longitudinal bone deficiency since associated nerves and muscles are not completely represented when a bone is absent.

▶ Treatment

The overall goal of treatment is to achieve a functional extremity. If the deficiency is in a weight-bearing limb, the goal is to ensure equal loading after treatment. Limb lengthening and/or contralateral limb shortening or guided growth (epiphysiodesis, which tethers or slows the growth of one limb while the other limb continues to grow to equalize leg length discrepancy) can be used to treat less severe deficiencies. More severe deficiencies are treated with a prosthesis or orthosis to compensate for the length discrepancy. For certain severe anomalies, operative treatment to remove a portion of the malformed extremity (eg, foot) is indicated to allow for early prosthetic fitting. In these instances, early prosthetic fitting allows for maximization of function.

Typically, a lower extremity prosthesis would be fit as the child begins to stand, allowing the child to begin ambulation at an appropriate developmental age. The prosthesis is well accepted since it becomes necessary for balancing and walking. In unilateral upper extremity amputation, the child may benefit from the use of a passive mitten-type prosthesis starting earlier than 6 months of age. Typically, adaptive prostheses, which are designed specifically for a particular activity such as skiing, biking, or running sports, are used to participate in physical activity. Although myoelectric prostheses have a technologic appeal, the majority of patients find the simplest construct to be the most functional. Children quickly learn how to function with their prostheses and can lead active lives.

Curran B, Hambrey R: The prosthetic treatment of upper limb deficiency. Prosthet Orthot Int 1991;15:82–87 [PMID: 1923727].

Gold NB, Westgate MN, Holmes LB: Anatomic and etiological classification of congenital limb deficiencies. Am J Med Genet Part A 2011;155:1225–1235 [PMID: 21557466].

Hamdy RC, Makhdom AM, Saran N, Birch J: Congenital fibular deficiency. J Am Acad Orthop Surg 2014;22:246–255 [PMID: 24668354].

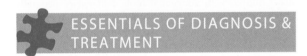

▼ DEFORMITIES OF THE EXTREMITIES

ESSENTIALS OF DIAGNOSIS & TREATMENT

▶ Many represent normal physiologic growth patterns.

▶ Key to diagnosis is recognition of abnormal patterns that deviate from normal development.

▶ Treatment is varied depending on condition.

COMMON FOOT PROBLEMS

Metatarsus Adductus

▶ **Clinical Findings**

A. Symptoms and Signs

Metatarsus adductus, a common congenital foot deformity, is characterized by inward deviation of the forefoot. It is the most common foot abnormality, observed in newborns at a rate of 1–2 per 1000 live births. When the deformity is more rigid, it is characterized by a vertical crease in the medial aspect of the arch. Angulation occurs at the base of the fifth metatarsal causing prominence of this bone. Most flexible deformities are secondary to intrauterine positioning and usually resolve spontaneously. Several investigators have noticed that 10%–15% of children with metatarsus adductus have hip dysplasia; therefore, a careful hip examination is necessary. The etiology of rigid deformities is unknown.

▶ **Treatment**

Fully flexible deformity requires no treatment. If the deformity is rigid and cannot be manipulated past the midline, it is worthwhile to perform serial casting, with cast changes in 1- to 2-week intervals, to correct the deformity. Orthoses and corrective shoes do not improve symptoms; however, they can be used to maintain the correction obtained by casting.

Gonzales AS, Mendez MD: Intoeing (Pigeon Toes, Femoral Anteversion, Tibial Torsion, Metatarsus Adductus); *National Center for Biotechnology Information*, U.S. National Library of Medicine, 27 Oct. 2018 [PMID: 29763169].

Williams CM, James AM, Tran T: Metatarsus adductus: development of a non-surgical treatment pathway. J Paediatr Child Health 2014;49(9):428–433 [PMID: 23647850].

Clubfoot (Talipes Equinovarus)

▶ **Clinical Findings**

A. Symptoms and Signs

Classic talipes equinovarus, or clubfoot, requires three features for diagnosis: (1) plantar flexion of the foot at the ankle joint (equinus), (2) inversion deformity of the heel (varus), and (3) medial deviation of the forefoot (adductus) (Figure 26–1). Clubfoot occurs in approximately 1 to 2 per 1000 live births. The three major categories of clubfoot are idiopathic, neurogenic, and those associated with syndromes such as arthrogryposis and Larsen syndrome. Infants with a clubfoot should be examined carefully for associated anomalies, especially of the spine. Idiopathic club feet may be hereditary.

▶ **Treatment**

Manipulation of the foot to stretch the contracted tissues on the medial and posterior aspects, followed by casting to hold the correction is the preferred treatment. Serial castings are typically performed on a weekly basis for 6–8 weeks. When instituted shortly after birth, correction is rapid. If treatment is delayed, the foot tends to become more rigid within

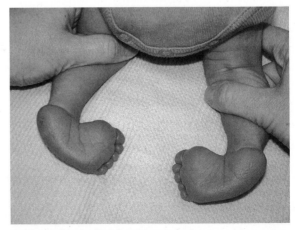

▲ **Figure 26–1.** Clubfoot in an infant.

a matter of days. Casting treatment requires patience and experience, but fewer patients require surgery when attention is paid to details of the Ponseti technique. If there is remaining equinus, surgery may be required in the form of a percutaneous Achilles tenotomy in order to achieve full correction. After full correction is obtained, a night brace is necessary for long-term maintenance of correction. Recent studies indicate that there is poor compliance with brace use following intervention with the Ponseti technique; however, many patients undergoing this treatment are able to independently ambulate only 2 months later than infants with no deformity. The French method is another nonsurgical method of treatment, which is commonly performed by physical therapists. The feet are stretched and manipulated several times per week and a combination of taping and a plastic splint are used to hold the correction after each session. If the foot is rigid and resistant to correction through the Ponseti or French techniques, extensive surgical release and correction are occasionally needed to improve the functional position of the foot. Approximately 15%–50% of patients require a surgical release.

Chen C, Kaushal N, Scher DM, Doyle SM, Blanco JS, Dodwell ER: Clubfoot etiology: a meta-analysis and systematic review of observational and randomized trials. J Pediatr Orthop 2018;38(8):e462–e469 [PMID: 29917009].

Graf A, Wu KW, Smith PA, Kuo KN, Krzak J, Harris G: Comprehensive review of the functional outcome evaluation of clubfoot treatment: a preferred methodology. J Pediatr Orthop 2012;27(1):93–104 [PMID: 19963172].

Miller NH et al: Does strict adherence to the Ponseti method improve isolated clubfoot treatment outcomes? A two-institution review. Clin Orthop Relat Res 2015:1–7. doi: 10.1007/s11999-015-4559-4 [PMID: 26394639].

Flatfoot

Clinical Findings

A. Symptoms and Signs

Flatfoot is normal in infants. If the heel cord is of normal length, full dorsiflexion is possible when the heel is in the neutral position. If the heel cord is of normal length and a longitudinal arch is noted when the child is sitting in a non–weight-bearing position, a normal arch will generally develop.

Younger children who are male, obese, and have excessive joint laxity are more likely to be flatfooted. Around 15% of flatfeet do not resolve spontaneously. There is usually a familial incidence of relaxed flatfeet in children who have no apparent arch. In any child with a shortened heel cord or stiffness of the foot, other causes of flatfoot such as tarsal coalition (congenital fusion of the tarsal bones) should be ruled out by a complete orthopedic examination, radiographs and advanced imaging.

Treatment

For an ordinary correctable flatfoot, no active treatment is indicated unless calf or leg pain is present. In children who have leg pains attributable to flatfoot, a supportive shoe, such as a good-quality sports shoe, is useful. An orthotic that holds the heel in neutral position and supports the arch may relieve discomfort if more support is needed. An arch insert should not be prescribed unless passive correction of the arch is easily accomplished; otherwise, the skin over the medial side of the foot will be irritated. Surgical correction can be done; however, surgery has been found to only improve symptoms associated with shoe or brace wear such as pain, calluses, or skin breakdown, with limited improvement of the planovalgus deformity.

Bouchard M, Mosca VS: Flatfoot deformity in children and adolescents: surgical indications and management. J Am Acad Orthop Surg 2014;10:623–632 [PMID: 25281257].

Ford SE, Scannell BP: Pediatric flatfoot: pearls and pitfalls. Foot Ankle Clin 2017 Sep; 22(3):643–656 [PMID: 28779814].

Talipes Calcaneovalgus

Clinical Findings

A. Symptoms and Signs

Talipes calcaneovalgus is characterized by excessive dorsiflexion at the ankle and eversion of the foot (Figure 26–2). This disorder can be associated with posteromedial bowing of the tibia and is due to intrauterine position and is often present at birth. The deformity occurs in 0.4–1.0 per 1000 live births.

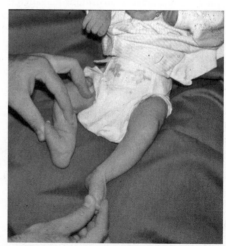

▲ **Figure 26–2.** Excessive dorsiflexion and eversion of the foot in talipes calcaneovalgus.

Treatment

Treatment consists of passive exercises, such as stretching the foot into plantar flexion. With or without treatment, the deformity usually resolves by age 3–6 months. In rare instances, it may be necessary to use plaster casts to help with manipulation and positioning. Complete correction is the rule.

"Calcaneovalgus Foot." Orthobullets, Lineage Medical Inc, 2 May 2018, www.orthobullets.com/pediatrics/4067/calcaneovalgus-foot.
Sankar WN, Weiss J, Skaggs DL: Orthopedic conditions in the newborn. J Am Acad Orthop Surg 2009;17(2):112–122 [PMID: 19202124].

Cavus Foot

Clinical Findings

A. Symptoms and Signs

Cavus foot consists of an unusually high longitudinal arch of the foot. It may be hereditary or associated with neurologic conditions such as poliomyelitis, hereditary sensory motor neuropathies, tethered spinal cord, cerebral palsy, and diastematomyelia (congenital splitting of the spinal cord). Typically, there is an associated contracture of the toe extensors, producing a claw toe deformity in which the metatarsal phalangeal joints are hyperextended and the interphalangeal joints acutely flexed. Cavus foot presents with diffuse and localized pain in the lower legs and is commonly associated with an inflexible foot deformity. Any child presenting with progressive cavus feet should receive a careful neurologic examination as well as radiographs and magnetic resonance imaging (MRI) of the spine and possible electromyography workup for neuromuscular disorder.

Treatment

Conservative therapy, such as an orthotic to realign the foot, can be effective in milder cases. In symptomatic cases, surgery may be necessary to lengthen the contracted extensor and flexor tendons and to release the plantar fascia and other tight plantar structures, but tethered cord or other spinal anomalies should be addressed first. Associated varus heel deformities cause more problems than the high arch.

Eleswarapu AS, Yamini B, Bielski RJ: Evaluating the Cavus Foot. Pediatr Ann 2016 Jun 1;45(6):e218-22. doi: 10.3928/00904481-20160426-01 [PMID: 27294497].
Grice J, Willmontt J, Taylor H: Assessment and Management of Cavus Foot Deformity. Orthop Trauma 2016;30(1):68–74. doi: 10.1016/j.mporth.2016.02.001.

Bunions (Hallux Valgus)

Clinical Findings

A. Symptoms and Signs

With a prevalence of 23%–35%, hallux valgus (bunion) is the most common forefoot deformity. The etiology is unknown.

Adolescents may present with lateral deviation of the great toe associated with a prominence over the head of the first metatarsal. Around 60% of patients have a family history of this condition. The deformity is painful with shoe wear and almost always relieved by fitting shoes that are wide enough in the toe area. Since further growth tends to cause recurrence of the deformity, surgery should be avoided in the adolescent.

Treatment

Therapeutic treatments are aimed at correcting the muscular and weight-bearing forces that act on the joint. While conservative treatment provides symptomatic relief, it does not reverse the natural history, as these deformities will typically continue to progress until corrected surgically. A high percentage of these patients ultimately have surgery in adulthood due to a continued progression of the deformity through childhood and adolescence. Surgical treatment should be delayed until the patient is mature, due do the risk of recurrence of deformity. Surgery leads to satisfactory outcomes in 95% of patients.

Greene JD, Nicholson AD, Sanders JO, Cooperman DR, Liu RW: Analysis of serial radiographs of the foot to determine normative values for the growth of the first metatarsal to guide hemiepiphysiodesis for immature hallux valgus. J Pediatr Orthop 2017;37(5):338–343 [PMID: 26509315].
Sabah Y et al: Lateral hemiepiphysiodesis of the first metatarsal for juvenile hallux valgus. J Orthop Surg (Hong Kong) 2018; 26(3):2309499018801135 [PMID: 30270740].
Wulker N, Mittag F: The treatment of hallux valgus. Dtsch Arztebl Int 2012;109(49):857–867; quiz 868 [PMID: 23267411].

GENU VARUM & GENU VALGUM

Clinical Findings

A. Symptoms and Signs

Genu varum (bowleg) is normal from infancy through 3 years of age. The alignment then changes to genu valgum (knock-knee, Figure 26–3) until about age 8 years, at which time adult alignment of 5–9 degrees of anatomic valgus is attained. If bowing persists beyond age 2, increases rather than decreases, occurs in only one leg, or if a patient is knock-kneed in association with short stature, the patient should be referred to an orthopedist. Genu varum is usually secondary to tibial rotation (Blount disease, Figure 26–4), while genu valgum may be caused by skeletal dysplasia or rickets.

Treatment

Individuals with genu varum may be at a greater risk for future osteoarthritis due to possible changes in gait kinematics. Bracing may be appropriate. An osteotomy may be necessary for severe problems, such as occurs in Blount disease (proximal tibial epiphysial dysplasia).

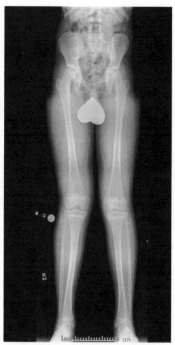

▲ **Figure 26–3.** Idiopathic genu valgum.

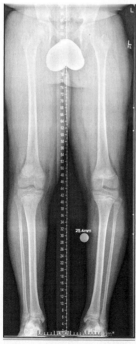

▲ **Figure 26–4.** Blount's disease with genu varum.

American Academy of Orthopaedic Surgeons: "Bowed Legs (Blount's Disease)–OrthoInfo AAOS." *OrthoInfo*, Feb. 2015, orthoinfo. aaos.org/en/diseases–conditions/bowed-legs-blounts-disease/.

TIBIAL TORSION & FEMORAL ANTEVERSION

▶ Clinical Findings

A. Symptoms and Signs

"Toeing in" in small children is a common parental concern. Tibial torsion refers to rotation of the leg between the knee and the ankle. Internal rotation amounts to about 20 degrees at birth but decreases to neutral rotation by age 16 months. The deformity may be accentuated by laxity of the knee ligaments, which allows excessive internal rotation of the leg in small children. This condition is largely self-limiting and usually resolves spontaneously with further growth and development. Toeing in beyond age 2 or 3 years is usually secondary to femoral anteversion, characterized by more internal rotation of the hip than external rotation. This femoral alignment decreases toward neutral during growth.

▶ Treatment

Treatment for tibial torsion is focused on educating the families to the benign nature and expected resolution with observation. In older children suspected to have femoral anteversion, there is no long-term improvement with treatment with shoes or braces. Osteotomy for rotational correction is occasionally required when symptoms such as knee and hip pain are present. However, the vast majority go on to resolve spontaneously.

Davids JR, Davis RB, Jameson LC, Westberry DE, Hardin JW: Surgical management of persistent intoeing gait due to increased internal tibial torsion in children. J Pediatr Orthop 2014;34(4):467–473 [PMID: 24531409].

Lincoln TL, Suen PW: Common rotational variations in children. J Am Acad Orthop Surg 2003;11:312 [PMID: 14565753].

Nourai MH, Fadaei B, Rizi AM: In-toeing and out-toeing gait conservative treatment; hip anteversion and retroversion: 10-year follow-up. J Res Med Sci 2015;20(11):1084–1087 [PMID: 26941813].

DEVELOPMENTAL DYSPLASIA OF THE HIP JOINT

▶ Clinical Findings

Developmental dysplasia of the hip (DDH) encompasses a spectrum of conditions where an abnormal relationship exists between the proximal femur and the acetabulum. In the most severe condition, the femoral head is not in contact with the acetabulum and is classified as a *dislocated hip*. In a *dislocatable hip*, the femoral head is within the acetabulum

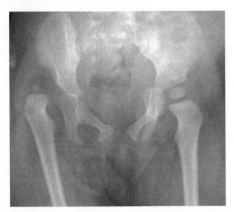

▲ **Figure 26–5.** Radiographic evidence of underdeveloped acetabulum and femur in developmental dysplasia of the hip.

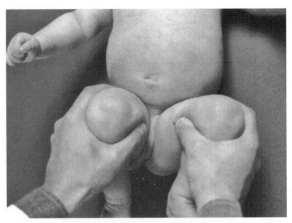

▲ **Figure 26–6.** Ortolani/Barlow examination technique.

but can be dislocated with a provocative maneuver. A *subluxatable hip* is one in which the femoral head comes partially out of the joint with a provocative maneuver. *Acetabular dysplasia* is used to denote insufficient acetabular development and is a radiographic diagnosis. Congenital dislocation of the hip more commonly affects the left hip, occurring in approximately 1%–3% of newborns. At birth, both the acetabulum and femur are underdeveloped (Figure 26–5). The four major risk factors for DDH are first-born child, female gender, breech presentation, and family history of DDH.

A. Symptoms and Signs

Clinical diagnosis of dislocations in newborns is dependent on demonstrating the instability of the joint by placing the infant on his or her back and obtaining complete relaxation. As these clinical signs can be subtle, they can be easily missed with a crying or upset infant. The examiner's long finger is placed over the greater trochanter and the thumb over the inner side of the thigh. Both hips are flexed 90 degrees and then slowly abducted from the midline, one hip at a time. With gentle pressure, an attempt is made to lift the greater trochanter forward. A feeling of slipping as the head *relocates* is a sign of instability (Ortolani sign). When the joint is more stable, the deformity must be provoked by applying slight pressure with the thumb on the medial side of the thigh as the thigh is adducted, thus slipping the hip posteriorly and eliciting a palpable clunk as the hip *dislocates* (Barlow sign, Figure 26–6). Limited hip abduction of less than 60 degrees while the knee is in 90 degrees of flexion is believed to be the most sensitive sign for detecting a dysplastic hip. Asymmetrical skin folds are present in about 25% of normal newborns and therefore are not particularly helpful to diagnosing hip dislocation.

The signs of instability become less evident after the first month of life. If the knees are at unequal heights when the hips and knees are flexed, the dislocated hip will be on the side with the lower knee. This is called a Galeazzi sign. If dysplasia of the hip has not been diagnosed before the child begins to walk, there will be a painless limp and/or a lurch to the affected side. When the child stands on the affected leg, a dip of the pelvis will be evident on the opposite side, due to weakness of the gluteus medius muscle. This is called the Trendelenburg sign and accounts for the unusual swaying gait. As a child with bilateral dislocation of the hips begins to walk, the gait is waddling.

B. Imaging Studies

Clinical signs of instability are more reliable than radiographs for diagnosing developmental dislocation of the hip in the newborn. Ultrasonography is most useful in newborns, and can be helpful for screening high-risk infants, such as those with breech presentation or positive family history. Radiological examination becomes more valuable after the first 6 weeks of life, with lateral displacement of the femoral head being the most reliable sign. In children with incomplete abduction during the first few months of life, a radiograph of the pelvis is indicated.

▶ Treatment

Dysplasia is progressive with growth unless the instability is corrected. If the dislocation is corrected in the first few weeks of life, the dysplasia can be completely reversible and a normal hip will more likely develop. If the dislocation or subluxation persists with age, the deformity will worsen until it is not completely reversible, especially after the walking age. For this reason, it is important to diagnose the deformity and institute treatment early.

A Pavlik harness, which maintains reduction by placing the hip in a flexed and abducted position, can be easily used to treat dislocation or dysplasia diagnosed in the first few weeks

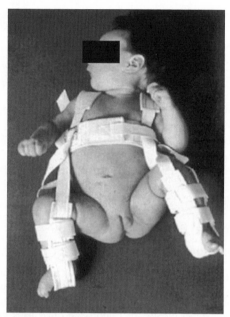

▲ **Figure 26–7.** A Pavlik harness used to treat developmental dysplasia of the hip.

Murphy RF, Kim YJ: Surgical management of pediatric developmental dysplasia of the hip. J Am Acad Orthop Surg 2016 Sep; 24(9):615–624 [PMID: 27509038].

Novais EN, Sanders J, Kestel LA, Carry PM, Meyers ML: Graf Type-IV hips have a higher risk of residual acetabular dysplasia at 1 year of age following successful Pavlik harness treatment for developmental hip dysplasia. J Pediatr Orthop 2016;38(10):498–502 [PMID: 27662383].

Omeroglu H: Use of ultrasonography in developmental dysplasia of the hip. J Child Orthop 2014;8(2):105–113 [PMID: 24510434].

Wang TM, Wu KW, Shih SF, Huang SC, Kuo KN: Outcomes of open reduction for developmental dysplasia of the hip: does bilateral dysplasia have a poorer outcome? J Bone Joint Surg Am 2013;95(12):1081–1086 [PMID: 23783204].

SLIPPED CAPITAL FEMORAL EPIPHYSIS

▶ **Clinical Findings**

A. Symptoms and Signs

Slipped capital femoral epiphysis (SCFE) is caused by displacement of the proximal femoral epiphysis due to disruption of the growth plate (Figure 26–8). The head of the femur is usually displaced medially and posteriorly relative to the femoral neck. This condition is most commonly seen in adolescent, obese males. It occurs when stress increases across the proximal femoral physis (growth plate) or resistance to shear is reduced. Factors that can lead to this increase in stress or decrease in resistance include endocrine or renal disorders, obesity, coxa profunda (a deep acetabular socket), and femoral or acetabular retroversion. Retroversion of the femur occurs when the proximal femoral segment is angled posteriorly relative to the shaft of the femur. Acetabular retroversion refers to when the alignment of the opening of the acetabulum does not face the normal anterolateral direction, but inclines more posterolaterally.

Clinically, SCFE is classified as stable or unstable. SCFE is considered stable if the child is able to bear weight on the

or months of life (Figure 26–7). In order to be safely treated in a Pavlik harness, hips must be manually reducible with only gentle manipulation. Treatment with a Pavlik harness in the face of a dislocated hip that does not reduce easily on clinical exam and with mild manipulation leads to Pavlik disease, which causes damage to the femoral head and acetabulum and can make relocation and reconstruction much more difficult. Forced abduction, or reduction requiring extremes of motion for stability, can lead to avascular necrosis of the femoral head and is contraindicated. The use of double or triple diapers is ineffective. An orthopedic surgeon with experience managing the problem is best to supervise treatment.

If a hip cannot be reduced and have a stable reduction with Pavlik treatment, then a closed reduction with arthrogram is appropriate treatment. A hip spica cast is used after reduction. If the hip is not stable within a reasonable range of motion after closed reduction, open reduction is indicated.

Closed treatment is possible in the first year of life, but results are superior with early treatment (within the first 6 months of life). In patients older than 18 months, more aggressive surgeries to correct the deformities of the acetabulum and femur, as well as open reduction, are often necessary to create a more normal orientation and shape of the hip joint. Children of walking age, as well as children who are bilaterally affected, are more likely to experience complications from more extensive procedures.

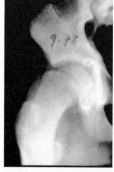
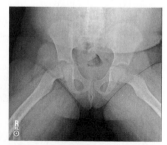

▲ **Figure 26–8.** Radiographic evidence of slipped capital femoral epiphysis.

affected extremity. In unstable SCFE, the child is unable to bear weight. An increased rate of avascular necrosis is correlated with the inability to bear weight.

Temporally, SCFE can be classified as acute or chronic. Acute SCFE occasionally occurs following a fall or direct trauma to the hip, with symptoms present for less than 3 weeks. More commonly, in a chronic SCFE, vague symptoms occur over a protracted period in an otherwise healthy child who presents with pain and limp. The pain can be referred into the thigh or the medial side of the knee, making examination of the hip joint important in any obese child complaining of knee pain. Physical examination consistently reveals a limitation of internal rotation of the hip. Appropriate diagnostic workup should include an AP and lateral pelvis radiograph.

► Treatment

Initial management consists of making the patient non–weight bearing on crutches and immediate referral to an orthopedic surgeon. Treatment is based on the same principles that govern treatment of any fracture of the femoral neck: the head of the femur is internally fixated in situ to the neck of the femur and the physeal injury allowed to heal. In situ fixation without closed reduction is considered the standard of care for SCFE treatment due to the high risk of AVN of the femoral head associated with attempted closed reduction. For a SCFE that is significant in terms of displacement, specialized centers are beginning to perform open reduction through a surgical dislocation of the hip, but due to the risk of avascular necrosis of the femoral head, this should only be employed by an orthopedic surgeon with experience in this procedure.

► Prognosis

The long-term prognosis is guarded because most of these patients continue to be overweight and overstress their hip joints. Follow-up studies have shown a high incidence of premature degenerative arthritis, even in those who do not develop avascular necrosis. The development of avascular necrosis almost guarantees a poor prognosis, because new bone does not readily replace the dead bone at this late stage of skeletal development. About 30% of patients have bilateral involvement, which may occur as late as 1 or 2 years after the primary episode.

Kohno Y et al: Is the timing of surgery associated with avascular necrosis after unstable slipped capital femoral epiphysis? A multicenter study. J Orthop Sci 2017;22(1):112–115 [PMID: 27629912].

Novais EN, Millis MB: Slipped capital femoral epiphysis: prevalence, pathogenesis, and natural history. Clin Orthop Relat Res 2012;470(12):3432–3438 [PMID: 23054509].

▼ COMMON SPINE CONDITIONS

ESSENTIALS OF DIAGNOSIS & TREATMENT

► Conditions most often present with a neck or back deformity.

► Treatment varies and is based on risk factors for progression.

BACK PAIN

► Clinical Findings

A. Symptoms and Signs

Back pain in a child may be the result of an acute traumatic event, but could also be the only symptom of significant disease and warrants clinical investigation. Inflammation, infection, renal disease, or tumors can cause back pain in children, and sprain should not be accepted as a routine diagnosis. A thorough history and physical examination is warranted to elucidate the etiology of the back pain.

Gurd DP: Back pain in the young athlete. Sports Med Arthrosc Rev 2011;19:7–16 [PMID: 21293233].

TORTICOLLIS

► Clinical Findings

A. Symptoms and Signs

Injury to the sternocleidomastoid muscle during delivery or disease affecting the cervical spine in infancy, such as congenital vertebral anomalies, may cause torticollis. When contracture of the sternocleidomastoid muscle causes torticollis, the chin is rotated to the side opposite of the affected muscle, causing the head to tilt toward the side of the contracture (Figure 26–9). A mass felt in the midportion of the sternocleidomastoid muscle in a newborn is likely a hematoma or developmental fibroma, rather than a true tumor.

Acute torticollis may follow upper respiratory infection or mild trauma in children. Upper respiratory infections may lead to swelling in the upper cervical spine, particularly at the C1-C2 region. This swelling renders the C1-C2 articulation susceptible to rotatory subluxation, which commonly presents as a clinical picture of torticollis. Rotatory subluxation of the upper cervical spine requires computed tomography for accurate assessment. Other causes of torticollis include spinal cord and cerebellar tumors, syringomyelia, and rheumatoid arthritis.

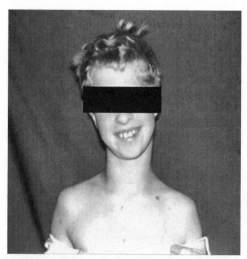

▲ **Figure 26–9.** Torticollis in a young male.

Treatment

If torticollis in early infancy is left untreated, a striking facial asymmetry can persist. Passive stretching is an effective treatment in up to 97% of all cases. If the deformity does not correct with passive stretching during the first year of life, surgical release of the muscle origin and insertion can be an effective treatment option. Excising the "tumor" of the sternocleidomastoid muscle is unnecessary and creates an unsightly scar.

For acquired torticollis in childhood, traction or a cervical collar usually results in resolution of the symptoms within 1 or 2 days.

Prognosis

Torticollis is occasionally associated with congenital deformities of the cervical spine. Radiographs of the spine are indicated in most cases where such anomalies are suspected. In addition, there is a 15%–20% incidence of associated hip dysplasia.

Lee K, Chung E, Lee BH: A study on asymmetry in infants with congenital muscular torticollis according to head rotation. J Phys Ther Sci 2017;29(1):48–52 [PMID: 28210037].
Tomczak KK, Rosman NP: Torticollis. J Child Neurol 2013; 28(3):365–378 [PMID: 23271760].

SCOLIOSIS

Scoliosis is characterized by lateral curvature of the spine associated with rotation of the involved vertebrae and classified by its anatomic location, in either the thoracic or lumbar spine. There are four main categories of scoliosis: idiopathic, congenital, neuromuscular (associated with a neurological or muscular disease), and syndromic (associated with a known syndrome). Idiopathic scoliosis accounts for around 80% of cases. It is more common in girls and typically develops around 10–12 years of age, but can occur earlier. There is a genetic component, but the etiology is multifactorial. Congenital scoliosis accounts for 5%–7% of cases and is a result of vertebral abnormalities due to a failure of formation or segmentation of the affected vertebrae. Cervical spine involvement is rare, and is manifested most commonly as Klippel-Feil syndrome. Failure of segmentation of some or all of the cervical vertebrae in this syndrome may be accompanied by multiple other congenital spinal anomalies. The neck is short and stiff, the hairline is low, and the ears are low set. Cervical rib, spina bifida, torticollis, web neck, high scapula, renal anomalies, and deafness are commonly associated defects. Renal ultrasound as well as a hearing test is indicated if there is evidence of abnormal renal function.

▶ Clinical Findings

A. Symptoms and Signs

Scoliosis in adolescents does not typically cause significant pain. If a patient has significant pain, she/he should be evaluated to rule out the possibility of some other disorder such as infection or tumor. Deformity of the rib cage and asymmetry of the waistline are clinically evident for curvatures of 30 degrees or more. Lesser curves may be detected through a forward bending test, which is designed to detect early abnormalities of rotation that may not be apparent when the patient is standing erect. Rotation of the spine may be measured with a scoliometer. Rotation is associated with a marked rib hump as the lateral curvature increases in severity.

B. Imaging

Radiographs taken of the entire spine in the standing position in both the posterior anterior (PA) and lateral planes are the most valuable for diagnosis (Figure 26–10). Usually, a primary curve is evident with compensatory curvature to balance the body.

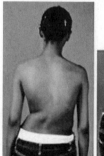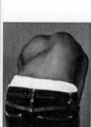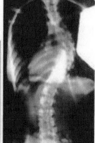

▲ **Figure 26–10.** Clinical and radiographic representation of scoliosis.

Treatment

Treatment of scoliosis depends on the curve magnitude, skeletal maturity, and risk of progression. Specific management is dependent on the Cobb angle, measured on a standing PA x-ray of the spine. Curvatures of less than 20 degrees typically do not require treatment unless they show progression. Bracing is indicated for curvatures of 20–40 degrees in a skeletally immature child. Curvatures greater than 40 degrees are resistant to treatment by bracing. Thoracic curvatures greater than 70 degrees have been correlated with poor pulmonary function in adult life, leading treatment algorithms toward preventing progression to this extreme. Curvatures reaching a magnitude of 40–60 degrees are indicated for surgical correction as they are highly likely to continue to progress. Surgical intervention consists of spinal instrumentation and fusion. Spinal instrumentation (rods, screws, hooks, etc) are applied to the region of the spine to be corrected and bone graft is added. Definitive spinal fusions should be delayed as long as possible in young children through the use of casting, bracing, and growth modulating surgeries such as growing rods, vertical expandable prosthetic titanium ribs (VEPTR), or magnetic expansion (MAGEC) rods to reduce anesthetic events and incisional complications.

Prognosis

Compensated small curves that do not progress may cause minor deformities but are well tolerated throughout life. Patients should be counseled about the genetic transmission of scoliosis and cautioned that their children's backs should be examined as part of routine physicals. Early detection allows for simple brace treatment. Severe scoliosis may require correction by spinal fusion.

Erickson MA, Baulesh DM: Pathways that distinguish simple form complex scoliosis repair and their outcomes. Curr Opin Pediatr 2011;23(3):339–345 [PMID: 21508841]

Kim HJ: Cervical spine anomalies in children and adolescents. Curr Opin Pediatr 2013;25(1):72–77 [PMID: 23263023].

Xue X et al: Klippel-Feil syndrome in congenital scoliosis. Spine (Phila Pa 1976) 2014;39(23):E1353–E1358 [PMID: 25202932].

KYPHOSIS

Clinical Findings

A. Symptoms and Signs

When looking at the sagittal view of a spine, there are two normal curves to be noticed. In the lumbar region, the normal curve with an anterior convexity is known as lumbar lordosis. In the thoracic region, a normal curve with a posterior convexity is called kyphosis. Excessive kyphosis is pathologic and known as hyperkyphosis. Clinically, a visible deformity may

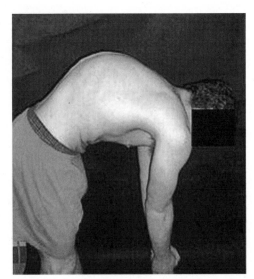

▲ **Figure 26–11.** Kyphosis in an adolescent.

be visible on the back, exacerbated by the forward bend test (Figure 26–11). Kyphosis can often accompany scoliosis, in which case the two conditions may share a common etiology. Additionally, excessive kyphosis can be caused by trauma and degenerative and inflammatory conditions. Congenital and developmental abnormalities, including Scheuermann disease, are the most common cause of severe kyphosis. In congenital kyphosis, abnormal vertebrae arise from either a failure of segmentation or formation and commonly result in wedge-shaped vertebrae that cause severe kyphosis.

B. Imaging

Standing radiographs taken in the lateral plane are necessary to measure the angle of the curve of the spine and quantify the severity of the curve. The curve is typically measured across the thoracic region from T1 to T12. Normal values for this measurement fall in the 20–45 degree range. Anything in excess of 45 degrees is considered pathologic (Figure 26–12).

Treatment

Treatment for kyphosis is similar to that of scoliosis. Mild forms of the deformity may undergo treatment with bracing. Depending on etiology, however, the effectiveness and indications for doing so are fraught with mixed results. Surgical intervention with spinal instrumentation and fusion may be indicated for more severe deformities. In patients who have congenital, wedge-shaped abnormal vertebrae, vertebral column resection may be indicated.

Yaman O, Dalbayrak S: Kyphosis and review of the literature. Turk Neurosurg 2014;24(4):455–465 [PMID: 25050667].

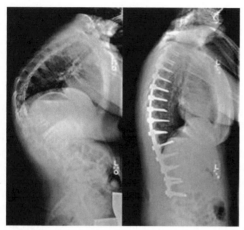

▲ **Figure 26–12.** Lateral radiograph showing severe kyphosis.

▼ INFLAMMATORY CONDITIONS

ESSENTIALS OF DIAGNOSIS & TREATMENT

▶ Chronic conditions generally related to overuse.

▶ Rule out more serious conditions first.

▶ Activity restriction is the treatment.

▼ SYNDROMES WITH MUSCULOSKELETAL INVOLVEMENT

ESSENTIALS OF DIAGNOSIS & TREATMENT

▶ Many genetic syndromes include a musculoskeletal component or association.

▶ Resulting deformity can result in a lack of function.

ARTHROGRYPOSIS MULTIPLEX CONGENITA (AMYOPLASIA CONGENITA)

▶ Clinical Findings

A. Symptoms and Signs

Arthrogryposis multiplex congenita (AMC) consists of incomplete fibrous ankylosis (usually bilateral) of many or all joints of the body. AMC affects both genders equally

and occurs in approximately 1 in 2–3000 live births. Upper extremity contractures usually consist of adduction of the shoulders; extension of the elbows; flexion of the wrists; and stiff, straight fingers with poor muscle control of the thumbs. Common deformities of the lower extremities include dislocation of the hips, extension contractures of the knees, and severe club feet. The joints are fusiform and the joint capsules decreased in volume due to lack of movement during fetal development. Muscle development is poor and may be represented only by fibrous bands. Various investigations have attributed the basic defect to an abnormality of muscle or lower motor neurons.

▶ Treatment

Passive mobilization of joints is the early treatment. Prolonged casting results in further stiffness and is not indicated. Removable splints combined with vigorous therapy are the most effective conservative treatment; however, surgical release of the affected joints is often necessary. Clubfoot associated with arthrogryposis is very stiff and nearly always requires surgical correction. Knee surgery, including capsulotomy, osteotomy, and tendon lengthening, is used to correct deformities. In young children, a dislocated hip may be reduced operatively by a medial approach. Multiple operative hip procedures are contraindicated, as they may further stiffen the hip dislocation with consequent impairment of motion. Osteotomies are successful in treating some deformities by improving mechanical alignment to improve the function of a lower extremity. Affected children are often able to walk despite dislocations and contractures, but functional gait improves with treatment. The long-term prognosis for physical and vocational independence is guarded. These patients have normal intelligence, but they have such severe physical restrictions that gainful employment is hard to find.

Kalampokas E, Kalampokas T, Sofoudis C, Deligeoroglou E, Botsis D: Diagnosing arthrogyrposis multiplex congenital: a review. ISRN Obstet Gynecol 2012;2012:264918 [PMID: 23050160].

Ma L, Yu X: Arthrogryposis multiplex congenital: classification, diagnosis, perioperative care, and anesthesia. Front Med 2017; 11(1):48–52 [PMID: 28213879].

Marfan Syndrome

▶ Clinical Findings

A. Symptoms and Signs

Marfan syndrome is a connective tissue disorder characterized by unusually long fingers and toes (arachnodactyly); hypermobility of the joints; subluxation of the ocular lenses; other eye abnormalities, including cataract, coloboma, megalocornea, strabismus, and nystagmus; a high-arched palate; a strong tendency to scoliosis; pectus carinatum (an outward protrusion of the sternum); and thoracic aortic aneurysms due to weakness of the media of the vessels (see Chapter 37). Fibrillin-1 gene mutations are commonly associated with Marfan syndrome. Serum mucoproteins may be decreased, and urinary excretion of hydroxyproline increased. The condition is easily confused with homocystinuria, because the phenotypic presentation is nearly identical. The two diseases are differentiated by detecting homocystine in the urine of patients with homocystinuria.

Treatment

Treatment is usually supportive and includes management of blood pressure and restriction of physical activity. Scoliosis may require more vigorous treatment by bracing or spine fusion. The long-term prognosis has improved for patients since the development of better treatment of their aortic aneurysms.

Dietz HC: Marfan syndrome. GeneReviews 2017; Internet: [PMID: 20301510].

Lebreiro A et al: Marfan syndrome clinical manifestations, pathophysiology and, new outlook on drug therapy. Rev Port Cardiol 2010;29(6):1021–1036 [PMID: 20964113].

Sprengel Deformity

Clinical Findings

A. Symptoms and Signs

Sprengel deformity is a congenital condition where one or both scapulas are elevated and hypoplastic. The deformity prevents the arm from raising completely on the affected side, and torticollis may be an associated finding. The deformity occurs alone or in association with Klippel-Feil syndrome or scoliosis and rib abnormalities. If the deformity is functionally limiting, the scapula may be surgically relocated closer to the normal anatomic position. Surgical intervention improves cosmetic appearance and function.

Dhir R, Chin K, Lambert S: The congenital undescended scapula syndrome: sprengel and the cleithrum: a case series and hypothesis. J Shoulder Elbow Surg 2018;27(2):252–259 [PMID: 28964675].

Harvey EJ, Bernstein M, Desy NM, Saran N, Ouellet JA: Sprengel deformity: pathogenesis and management. J Am Acad Orthop Surg 2012;20(3):177–186 [PMID: 22382290].

Osteogenesis Imperfecta

Clinical Findings

A. Symptoms and Signs

Osteogenesis imperfecta is a rare genetic connective tissue disease characterized by multiple and recurrent fractures. The estimated incidence is 1 in 12,000–15,000. Clinical features of the disease lead to diagnosis in the majority of cases. There are several forms of osteogenesis imperfecta, designated type I to type XII. Types I–V are the result of autosomal dominant mutations, whereas types VI–XII are autosomal recessive. Each type is associated with a mutation of a different gene, varying levels of severity, and a range of characteristic features. The severe fetal type (osteogenesis imperfecta congenita) is distinguished by multiple intrauterine or perinatal fractures. Moderately affected children have numerous fractures and exhibit dwarfism as a result of their acquired bone deformities and growth retardation. Fractures begin to occur at different times and in variable patterns after the perinatal period, resulting in fewer fractures and deformities relative to severe cases. Cortical thickness is reduced in the shafts of the long bones, and accessory skull bones that are completely surrounded by cranial sutures (wormian bones) are present in the skull. Blue sclerae, thin skin, hyperextensibility of ligaments, otosclerosis with significant hearing loss, and hypoplastic and deformed teeth are characteristic of osteogenesis imperfecta. Cardiovascular and respiratory problems are the most common causes of morbidity and mortality in adulthood. Intelligence is not affected.

Affected patients are sometimes suspected of having suffered abuse. Osteogenesis imperfecta should be ruled out in any case of potential nonaccidental trauma. Of note, an olecranon fracture in a child is rare and can be indicative of osteogenesis imperfecta.

Treatment

Surgical treatment involves deformity correction of the long bones. Multiple intramedullary rods have been used to decrease the incidence of fractures and prevent deformity from fracture malunion. Patients are often confined to wheelchairs during adulthood. Bisphosphonates have been shown to decrease the incidence of fractures.

Biggin A, Munns CF: Osteogenesis imperfecta: diagnosis and treatment. Curr Osteoporos Rep 2014;12(3):279–288 [PMID: 24964776].

Harrington J, Sochett E, Howard A: Update on the evaluation and treatment of osteogenesis imperfecta. Pediatr Clin North Am 2014;61(6):1243–1257 [PMID: 25439022].

Achondroplasia (Classic Chondrodystrophy)

Clinical Findings

A. Symptoms and Signs

Achondroplasia is the most common form of short-limbed dwarfism. The upper arms and thighs are proportionately shorter than the forearms and legs. Skeletal dysplasia is suspected based on abnormal stature, disproportion, dysmorphism, or deformity. Measurement of height is an excellent clinical screening tool. Findings frequently include bowing of the extremities, a waddling gait, limitation of motion of major joints, relaxation of the ligaments, short stubby fingers of almost equal length, frontal bossing, midface hypoplasia, otolaryngeal system dysfunction, moderate hydrocephalus, depressed nasal bridge, and lumbar lordosis. Intelligence and sexual function are normal. While this disorder has an autosomal dominant transmission pattern, 80% of cases result from a random mutation in the fibroblast growth factor receptor-3 (*FGFR3*) gene.

B. Imaging

Radiographs demonstrate short, thick tubular bones and irregular epiphysial plates. The ends of the bones are thick, with broadening and cupping. Epiphysial ossification may be delayed. Due to diminished growth in the spinal pedicles, the spinal canal is narrowed (congenital stenosis), and a herniated disk in adulthood may lead to acute paraplegia.

► Treatment

Growth hormone is given to some children with bone dysplasia. Limb lengthening is possible to achieve a more normal proportion of extremities but is controversial.

Ornitz DM, Legeai-Mallet L: Achondroplasia: development, pathogenesis and therapy. Dev Dyn 2017;246(4):291–309 [PMID: 27987249].

Shirley ED, Ain MC: Achondroplasia: manifestations and treatment. J Am Acad Orthop Surg 2009;(17):231–241 [PMID: 19307672].

▼ NEUROLOGIC DISORDERS INVOLVING THE MUSCULOSKELETAL SYSTEM

ESSENTIALS OF DIAGNOSIS & TREATMENT

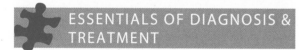

► Take a detailed birth history.

► Assess functional status of patient.

► Management geared to maximize function.

Orthopedic Aspects of Cerebral Palsy

► Clinical Findings & Treatment

Cerebral palsy is defined as a nonprogressive brain injury causing muscle control issues that occurs while a child's brain is developing. Early physical therapy encouraging completion of normal developmental patterns may benefit patients with cerebral palsy.

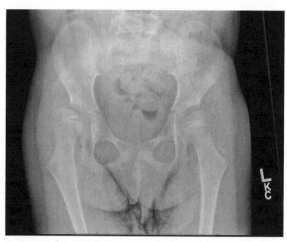

▲ **Figure 26–13.** Neuromuscular hip subluxation in a patient with spastic quadriplegic cerebral palsy.

Bracing and splinting are of questionable benefit, although ankle and foot orthoses (AFOs) or night splints may be useful in preventing equinus deformity of the ankle, the most common deformity found in this population, or adduction contractures of the hips. Orthopedic surgery is useful for treating joint contractures that interfere with function. Muscle transfers are effective in carefully selected patients with cerebral palsy, and most orthopedic procedures are directed at tendon lengthening or bony stabilization by osteotomy or arthrodesis.

Flexion and adduction of the hip due to hyperactivity of the adductors and flexors may produce a progressive neuromuscular dislocation of the hip (Figure 26–13). This can lead to pain and dysfunction, with treatment being difficult and unsatisfactory. Treatment can include abduction bracing, supplemented by release of the adductors and hip flexors but this has been shown to only delay the need for osteotomy. Osteotomy of the femur and/or pelvis may be necessary to correct bony deformities of femoral anteversion, coxa valga, and acetabular dysplasia that are invariably present.

Surgeons must examine patients on several occasions before any operative procedure as it is difficult to predict the surgical outcome in individuals diagnosed with cerebral palsy. Follow-up care with a physical therapist can maximize the anticipated long-term gains and should be arranged before surgery.

Wynter M et al: Australian Hip Surveillance Guidelines for Children with Cerebral Palsy 2014. AusACPDM 2014. https://www.ausacpdm.org.au/wp-content/uploads/2017/05/2014-Aus-Hip-Surv-Guidelines_booklet_WEB.pdf.

Orthopedic Aspects of Myelodysplasia (Spina Bifida)

▶ Clinical Findings & Treatment

Patients with myelodysplasia (spina bifida) should be examined early by an orthopedic surgeon. The level of neurologic involvement determines the muscle imbalance that will be present to produce deformity with growth. The involvement is often asymmetrical and tends to change during the first 12–18 months of life. Associated musculoskeletal problems may include clubfoot, congenital dislocation of the hip, arthrogryposis-type changes of the lower extremities, and congenital scoliosis and kyphosis. Spina bifida lesions are most common at the L3–L4 level and tend to affect the hip joint, with progressive dislocation occurring during growth due to unopposed hip flexion and adduction forces. Foot deformities are complicated by the fact that sensation is generally absent; these deformities may be in any direction depending on the muscle imbalance present. Spinal deformities develop in a high percentage of these children, with scoliosis present in approximately 40%.

Ambulation may require long leg braces. In children who have a reasonable likelihood of walking, operative treatment consists of reduction of the hip, alignment of the feet in the weight-bearing position, as well as stabilization of the scoliosis. In children who lack active quadriceps function and extensor power of the knee, the likelihood of ambulation is greatly decreased. In such patients, aggressive surgery to the foot and hip region is usually not indicated as it may result in stiffening of the joints and prevent sitting. The overall treatment of the child with spina bifida should be coordinated in a multidisciplinary clinic where various medical specialists work with therapists, social workers, and teachers to provide the best possible care.

▼ TRAUMA

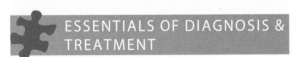

ESSENTIALS OF DIAGNOSIS & TREATMENT

- ▶ Fall on outstretched hand (FOOSH) is the most common mechanism.
- ▶ Directed physical examination (eg, swelling, tenderness, deformity, instability) and radiographic examination.
- ▶ Rule out physeal fracture.
- ▶ Early protected motion for sprains and strains.
- ▶ Reduction and immobilization for fractures.

Soft Tissue Trauma

A sprain is the stretching of a ligament and a strain is a stretch of a muscle or tendon. Contusions are generally due to tissue compression, with damage to blood vessels within the tissue and the formation of a hematoma.

In a severe sprain, the ligament is completely disrupted resulting in instability of the joint. Incomplete tearing of the ligament, with local pain and swelling but no joint instability, is considered a mild or moderate sprain.

The initial treatment of any sprain consists of rest, ice, compression, and elevation. Brief splinting followed by early range of motion exercises of the affected joint protect against further injury and relieves swelling and pain. Nonsteroidal anti-inflammatory drugs (NSAIDs) are useful for pain. If more severe trauma occurs, resulting in complete tearing of a ligament, instability of the joint may be demonstrated by gross examination or by stress testing with radiographic documentation. Such deformity of the joint may cause persistent instability resulting in other injuries. If instability is evident, surgical repair of the torn ligament may be indicated. If a muscle is torn at its tendinous insertion, it can be repaired surgically.

Knee Sprains
▶ Clinical Findings
A. Symptoms and Signs

Sprains of the collateral and cruciate ligaments are uncommon in children. These ligaments are so strong that it is more common to have bony injury. In adolescence, rupture of the anterior cruciate ligament can result from a rotational injury.

▶ Treatment

Effusion of the knee after trauma deserves referral to an orthopedic specialist. The differential diagnosis includes torn ligament, torn meniscus, and osteochondral fracture. If an injury produces avulsion of the tibial spine, associated injuries can include meniscal and chondral injuries, and anatomic reduction and fixation are often required. Nontraumatic effusion should be evaluated for inflammatory conditions (eg, juvenile rheumatoid arthritis) or patellar malalignment or instability.

Internal Derangements of the Knee
▶ Clinical Findings
A. Symptoms and Signs

Meniscal injuries are uncommon in children younger than 12 years. Clicking or locking of the knee may occur in young children as a result of a discoid lateral meniscus, which is a rare congenital anomaly that has a higher risk of meniscal tear.

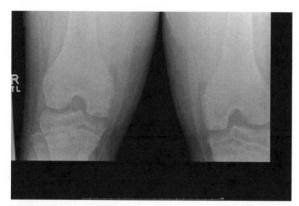

▲ **Figure 26–14.** Bilateral medial femoral condyle osteo-chondritis dissecans.

As the child approaches adolescence, internal damage to the knee from a torsion weight-bearing injury may result in locking of the knee if tearing and displacement of a meniscus occurs. Osteochondritis dissecans, avascular necrosis of subchondral bone that can lead to cartilage cracking, instability and degeneration, also presents as swelling, pain, and mechanical symptoms of the knee in adolescence (Figure 26–14). This can be seen in all synovial joints, but the most common presentation is in the medial femoral condyle of the knee. Posttraumatic synovitis may mimic a meniscal lesion. Epiphysial injury should be suspected in any severe injury to the knee or when there is tenderness on both sides of the femoral metaphysis after injury. Stress films will sometimes demonstrate separation of the distal femoral epiphysis.

Contusions

▶ Clinical Findings

A. Symptoms and Signs

Muscle contusions with hematoma formation produce the familiar "charley horse" injury.

▶ Treatment

Treatment includes application of ice, compression, and rest. Exercise should be avoided for 5–7 days. Local heat may hasten healing once the acute phase of tenderness and swelling has passed.

Myositis Ossificans

▶ Clinical Findings

A. Symptoms and Signs

Myositis ossificans, ossification within muscle, occurs when sufficient trauma causes a hematoma that later heals in the manner of a fracture. Contusions of the quadriceps of the thigh or the triceps of the arm are the most common injuries. Disability is great, with local swelling, heat and extreme pain with the slightest provocation of the adjacent joint.

▶ Treatment

The limb should be rested until the local reaction has subsided (5–7 days). When local heat and tenderness have decreased, gentle active exercises may be initiated. Passive stretching exercises are not indicated as they may stimulate the ossification reaction. If an extremity experiences a severe injury with a hematoma, it should be splinted and further activity should be avoided until the acute reaction has subsided. If additional trauma causes recurrent injury, ossification may reach spectacular proportions and resemble an osteosarcoma. Surgery to excise the ossification may restart the process and lead to an even more severe reaction and should not be attempted before 9 months to 1 year after injury.

Sferopoulos NK, Kotakidou R, Petropoulos AS: Myositis ossificans in children: a review. Eur J Orthop Surg Traumatol 2017;27(4):491–502. doi: 10.1007/s00590-017-1932-x [PMID: 28275867].

TRAUMATIC SUBLUXATIONS & DISLOCATIONS

▶ Clinical Findings

Dislocation or Separation of the Shoulder

A. Symptoms, Signs, and Treatment

Shoulder dislocations usually following traumatic injury. Patients almost always present with shoulder pain, but can be with or without weakness or lack of function. The vast majority (~ 90%) of shoulder dislocations occur anteriorly and can have obvious deformity of the shoulder with anterior displacement of the humoral head. Posterior dislocation is rare. It is important to examine and evaluate both shoulders for any asymmetry between the two. Range of motion testing should be limited if a dislocation is suspected to limit further ligament and joint damage. Appropriate radiographic evaluation, including anteroposterio, Grashey, and axillary views, is important for confirming a dislocation or separation diagnosis.

Acromioclavicular separation—Acromioclavicular (AC) separations involve partial or complete tearing of the ligament complex of the AC joint. They are among the most common shoulder injuries, but vary significantly in severity (grade I–VI, with the latter the most severe) and treatment. Grade I–III acromioclavicular separations are most common and generally treated nonsurgically (which includes early physical therapy), while grades IV–VI are usually the result of high energy impacts and are treated surgically. The amount of displacement distinguishes grade III from higher grades. There is controversy about whether grade III AC separations should be treated surgically or nonsurgically.

Allemann F, Halvachizadeh S, Waldburger M, Schaefer F, Pothmann C, Pape HC, Rauer T: Different treatment strategies for acromioclavicular dislocation injuries: a nationwide survey on open/minimally invasive and arthroscopic concepts. Eur J Med Res 2019;24(1):18 [PMID: 30904018].

Kraus N, Hann C, Gerhardt C, Scheibel M: Dynamic instability of the acromioclavicular joint: a new classification for acute AC joint separation. Obere Extremitat 2018;13(4):279–285 [PMID: 30546493].

Subluxation of the Radial Head (Nursemaid's Elbow)

A. Symptoms, Signs, and Treatment

Infants may sustain subluxation of the radial head as a result of being lifted or pulled by the hand. The child appears with the elbow fully pronated and painful. The usual complaint is that the child's elbow will not bend. Radiographic findings are normal, but there is point tenderness over the radial head. A **subluxated** radial head (nursemaid's elbow) can be reduced by placing the elbow in full supination and slowly moving the arm from full extension to full flexion or by holding the elbow at a 90-degree angle of flexion, then slowly hyperpronating the wrist to complete reduction; a click may be palpated at the level of the radial head. Relief of pain is remarkable, as the child usually stops crying immediately. The elbow may be immobilized in a sling for comfort for a day. Occasionally, symptoms last for several days, requiring more prolonged immobilization. A pulled elbow may be a clue to battering. This should be considered during examination, especially if the problem is recurrent.

Bexkens R, Washburn FJ, Eygendaal D, Van Den Bekerom MP, Oh LS: Effectiveness of reduction maneuvers in the treatment of nursemaid's elbow: a systematic review and meta-analysis. Am J Emerg Med 2017;35(1):159–163 [PMID: 27836316].

Dislocation of the Patella

A. Symptoms and Signs

Complete patellar dislocations nearly always dislocate laterally. Pain is severe, and the patient will present with the knee slightly flexed and an obvious bony mass lateral to the knee joint associated with a flat area over the anterior knee. Radiologic examination, including sunrise views, confirms the diagnosis. When subluxation of the patella occurs, symptoms may be more subtle, and the patient will complain that the knee "gives out" or "jumps out of place."

Recurrent dislocations more commonly occur in individuals with hyperlaxity, especially adolescent girls. Factors that affect risk for recurrence include length of patellar tendon, the depth of trochlear groove, and position of the patella in relation to the trochlear groove that is affected by axial and coronal boney alignment.

▶ Treatment of Dislocations

In contrast to fracture reduction, which may be safely postponed, most dislocations must be reduced immediately in order to minimize further joint damage. Dislocations can usually be reduced by gentle sustained traction. Often, no anesthetic is needed for several hours after the injury due to the protective anesthesia produced by the injury. A thorough neurovascular examination should be performed and documented pre- and postreduction. Radiographs should be obtained postreduction to document congruency and assess for the presence of associated osteochondral fractures. Following reduction, the joint should be splinted for transportation of the patient. NSAIDs may be used along with ice for pain control and to reduce inflammation. The dislocated joint should be treated by immobilization, followed by graduated active exercises through a full range of motion. Vigorous passive manipulation of the joint by a therapist may be harmful, but muscle strengthening is the key in long-term treatment.

A dislocated patella can be reduced by extending the knee and placing slight pressure on the patella while gentle traction is exerted on the leg. For first-time dislocation, initial treatment after reduction should be nonoperative, consisting of physical therapy to strengthen the quadriceps, hips, and core stabilizers. Surgery is reserved for individuals with reparable osteochondral injuries, loose bodies, and recurrent dislocation following appropriate nonoperative therapy. Around one-third of patients report a repeated dislocation after rehabilitation.

Longo UG, Ciuffreda M, Locher J, Berton A, Salvatore G, Denaro V: Treatment of primary acute patellar dislocation: systematic review and quantitative synthesis of the literature. Clin J Sport Med 2017;27(6):511–523 [PMID: 28107220].

Nwachukwu BU, So C, Schairer WW, Green DW, Dodwell ER: Surgical versus conservative management of acute patellar dislocation in children and adolescents: a systematic review. Knee Surg Sports Traumotol Arthrsc 2016;24(3):760–767 [PMID: 26704809].

▼ FRACTURES

Epiphyseal Separations

▶ Clinical Findings

A. Symptoms and Signs

Epiphyseal separations (also referred to as epiphyseal fractures) are more common than ligamentous injuries in children since the ligaments of the joints are generally stronger than their associated growth plates. Radiographs should be taken whenever a dislocation is suspected in order to rule out epiphyseal fracture. Radiographs of the opposite extremity, especially for injuries around the elbow, are valuable for comparison. Fractures across the growth plate may produce bony bridges that will cause premature cessation of growth or angular deformities of the extremity. These bridges are due to trauma to the growth plate and can occur even with adequate reductions. Epiphyseal separations in a nonambulatory child should be concerning for non-accidental trauma.

Treatment

Reduction of a fractured epiphysis should be done under anesthesia to align the growth plate with the least amount of force. Epiphyseal fractures around the shoulder, wrist, and fingers can usually be treated by closed reduction, but fractures of the epiphyses around the elbow often require open reduction. In the lower extremity, accurate reduction of the epiphyseal plate is necessary to prevent joint deformity when a joint surface is involved. If angular deformities result, corrective osteotomy may be necessary. Multiple attempts at closed reduction are not recommended due to higher risk of physeal damage.

Dwek JR: The radiographic approach to child abuse. Clin Orthop Relat Res 2011;469:776–789 [PMID: 20544318].

Torus Fractures
Clinical Findings & Treatment

Torus fractures consist of "buckling" of the cortex due to compression of the bone. They are most common in the distal radius or ulna. Alignment is usually satisfactory, and simple immobilization for 3 weeks is sufficient. Soft bandage therapy and cast therapy are effective in preventing further angulation. It is important that the fracture is not misdiagnosed as a greenstick fracture (see next) at initial presentation. Children with a torus fracture who are misdiagnosed with a greenstick fracture report having more pain after application of a soft bandage or cast.

Jiang N, Cao ZH, Ma YF, Lin Z, Yu B: Management of pediatric forearm torus fractures: a systematic review and meta-analysis. Pediatr Emerg Care 2016;32(11):773–778 [PMID: 26555307].

Greenstick Fractures
Clinical Findings & Treatment

Greenstick fractures involve frank disruption of the cortex on one side of the bone but no discernible cleavage plane on the opposite side. The term "greenstick" implies similarity to what happens when one tries to break a twig/stick from a live tree; commonly bark will break on one side of the stick, while remaining intact on the opposite side. Bone ends are not separated, making these fractures angulated but not displaced. Reduction is achieved by straightening the arm into normal alignment and maintaining alignment with a snugly fitting cast. It is necessary to obtain radiographs of greenstick fractures again in 7–10 days to make certain that the reduction has been maintained in the cast. A slight angular deformity can be corrected by remodeling of the bone. The farther the fracture is from the growing end of the bone, the longer the time required for remodeling. The fracture can be considered healed when no tenderness is present and a bony callus is seen on a radiograph.

Fracture of the Clavicle
Clinical Findings & Treatment

Clavicular fractures are very common injuries in infants and children. The patient can be immobilized in a sling for comfort. The healing callus will be apparent when the fracture has consolidated, but this unsightly lump will generally resolve over a period of months to a year via bone remodeling. Operative fixation of clavicle fractures in children and adolescents is rarely indicated.

Shetty SK, Chandran R, Ballal A, Mathias LJ, Hedge A, Shetty A: To operate or not to operate the mid-shaft fractures of the clavicle: a comparative study of functional outcomes of the two methods of management. J Clin Diag Res 2017;11(1):RC01–RC03 [PMID: 28274008].
Stepanyan H, Gendelberg D, Hennrikus W: Management of simple clavicle fractures by primary care physicians. Clin Pediatr (Phila) 2017;56(5):467–471 [PMID: 27496001]

Supracondylar Fractures of the Humerus
Clinical Findings

A. Symptoms and Signs

The condyles of the distal humerus form the proximal half of the elbow joint. There is a concavity in the posterior distal humerus that is present anatomically to accommodate the olecranon when the elbow reaches full extension. This anatomic accommodation, located in what is referred to as the supracondylar region of the humerus, also creates a thinner area of cortical bone that is more susceptible to injury/fracture (Figure 26–15). Supracondylar fractures tend to occur in children age 3–6 years and are the most common elbow fracture in children. The proximity to the brachial artery in the distal arm creates a potential danger when dealing with these types of fractures. Absence of a distal pulse is a strong indicator of a secondary arterial injury. Swelling may be severe as these injuries are usually associated with a significant amount of trauma.

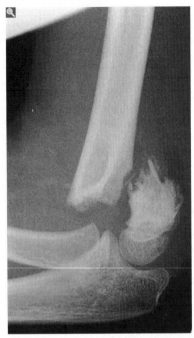

▲ **Figure 26–15.** Supracondylar fracture of the humerus.

▶ Treatment

Most often, these fractures are treated by closed reduction and percutaneous pinning performed under general anesthesia. Complications associated with supracondylar fractures include Volkmann ischemic contracture of the forearm due to vascular compromise and cubitus varus (decreased carrying angle, "gunstock deformity") secondary to poor reduction. The "gunstock deformity" of the elbow may be somewhat unsightly but does not usually interfere with joint function.

Kumar V, Singh A: Fracture supracondylar humerus: A review. J Clin Diag Res 2016;10(12):RE01–RE06 [PMID: 28208961].

General Comments on Other Fractures in Children

Reduction of fractures in children can usually be accomplished by simple traction and manipulation; open reduction is indicated if a satisfactory alignment is not obtained. Remodeling of the fracture callus generally produces an almost normal appearance of the bone over a matter of months. The younger the child, the more remodeling is possible. Angular deformities in the plane of joint motion remodel reliably while rotational malalignment does not remodel well.

There should be suspicion of child abuse whenever the age of a fracture does not match the history given or when the severity of the injury is more than the alleged accident would have produced. In suspected cases of battering in which no fracture is present on the initial radiograph, a repeat radiograph 10 days later is in order. Bleeding beneath the periosteum will be calcified by 7–10 days, and the radiographic appearance can be diagnostic of severe closed trauma characteristic of a battered child.

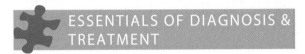

▼ INFECTIONS OF THE BONES & JOINTS

ESSENTIALS OF DIAGNOSIS & TREATMENT

▶ Movement of the extremity causes pain, resulting in pseudoparalysis.

▶ Soft tissue swelling.

▶ Elevated erythrocyte sedimentation rate (ESR) and C-reactive protein (CRP).

▶ Surgical drainage of abscess plus antibiotics.

▶ Antibiotic therapy for early osteomyelitis without abscess.

Osteomyelitis

Osteomyelitis is an infectious process that usually starts in the spongy or medullary bone and extends into compact or cortical bone. Commonly preceded by trauma, the lower extremities are more likely to be affected. Osteomyelitis is most commonly caused by hematogenous spread of bacteria from other infected or colonized areas (eg, pyoderma or upper respiratory tract) but it may occur as a result of direct invasion from the outside (exogenous), through a penetrating wound (nail) or open fracture. *Staphylococcus aureus* is the most common infecting organism and has a tendency to infect the metaphyses of growing bones. Anatomically, the arterial supply to the metaphysis in the long bones includes end arteries just below the growth plate which turn sharply and end in venous sinusoids, causing relative stasis that predisposes to bacterial localization. In the infant (< 1 year), there is direct vascular communication with the epiphysis across the growth plate. Bacterial spread occurs from the metaphysis to the epiphysis and into the joint. In the older child, the growth plate provides an effective barrier and the epiphysis is usually not infected. Infection spreads retrograde from the metaphysis into the diaphysis, and by rupture through the cortical bone, down along the diaphysis beneath the periosteum.

In hematogenous osteomyelitis, 85% of cases are due to *S aureus*. Streptococci (group B *Streptococcus* in neonates and young infants, *Streptococcus pyogenes* in older children) are a less common cause of osteomyelitis. *Pseudomonas aeruginosa* is common in cases of nail puncture wounds. Children with sickle cell anemia are especially prone to osteomyelitis caused by *Salmonella* species.

▶ Clinical Findings

A. Symptoms and Signs

Osteomyelitis may be subtle in infants, presenting as irritability, diarrhea, or failure to feed properly; temperature may be normal or slightly low; and white blood cell count may be normal or only slightly elevated. There may be pseudoparalysis of the involved limb. Manifestations are more striking in older children, with severe local tenderness and pain and, often, but not invariably, high fever, rapid pulse, and elevated white blood cell count, ESR, and CRP. Osteomyelitis of a lower extremity often occurs around the knee joint in children age 7–10 years. Tenderness is most marked over the metaphysis of the bone where the process has its origin. For a child who refuses to bear weight, osteomyelitis is high in the differential diagnosis.

B. Laboratory Findings

Blood cultures are often positive early. The most important test is the aspiration of pus or biopsy of involved bone. It is useful to insert a needle into the bone in the area of suspected infection and aspirate any fluid present. Fluid should be stained for organisms and cultured. Even edema fluid can be useful for determining the causative organism. Elevation of the ESR above 50 mm/h is typical for osteomyelitis. CRP is elevated earlier than the ESR.

C. Imaging

Osteomyelitis should be diagnosed clinically before significant plain radiographic findings are present. Plain film findings progress from nonspecific local swelling, to elevation of the periosteum, with formation of new bone from the cambium layer of the periosteum occurring after 3–6 days. As infection becomes chronic, areas of cortical bone are isolated by pus spreading down the medullary canal, causing rarefaction and demineralization of the bone. Isolated pieces of cortex become ischemic and form sequestra (dead bone fragments). These radiographic findings are specific, but late. Bone scan is sensitive (before plain radiographic findings are apparent) but nonspecific and should be interpreted in the clinical context. MRI can demonstrate early edema and subperiosteal abscess and is helpful to confirm and localize disease prior to plain film changes.

▶ Treatment

A. Specific Measures

Intravenous antibiotics should be started as soon as the diagnosis of osteomyelitis is made and diagnostic specimens have been obtained. Transition to oral antibiotics occurs when tenderness, fever, white cell count, and CRP are all resolved/decreasing and is facilitated by a positive culture. Agents that cover *S aureus* and *S pyogenes* (eg, oxacillin, nafcillin, cefazolin, and clindamycin) are appropriate for most cases of hematogenous osteomyelitis. Alternative antistaphylococcal therapy (eg, vancomycin) may be needed if methicillin-resistant and clindamycin-resistant *S aureus* is suspected or isolated. Methicillin-resistant *S aureus* infection should be suspected in patients with severe cases of hematogenous osteomyelitis. Coverage for other pathogens is also appropriate in specific circumstances (eg, group B *Streptococcus* in neonates and young infants, *P aeruginosa* for nail puncture-associated osteomyelitis, *Salmonella* species in children with sickle cell anemia). Surgical debridement and broader antibiotic coverage (guided by cultures of infected bone) are often indicated for osteomyelitis resulting from penetrating injury. Consultation with an infectious disease specialist is very helpful and standard in many facilities. For specific recommendations, see Chapter 42.

Acute osteomyelitis is usually treated for a minimum of 4–6 weeks and until normalization of the physical examination and inflammatory markers. Chronic infections are treated for months. Following surgical debridement, *Pseudomonas* foot infections usually respond to 1–2 weeks of antibiotic treatment.

B. General Measures

Splinting minimizes pain and decreases spread of the infection through lymphatic channels in the soft tissue. The splint should be removed periodically to allow active use of adjacent joints and prevent stiffening and muscle atrophy. In chronic osteomyelitis, splinting may be necessary to guard against fracture of the weakened bone.

C. Surgical Measures

Aspiration of the metaphysis for culture and Gram stain is the most useful diagnostic measure in any case of suspected osteomyelitis. If frank pus is aspirated from the bone, surgical drainage is indicated. If the infection has not shown a significant response within 24 hours, surgical drainage is also indicated. It is important that all devitalized soft tissue be removed and adequate exposure of the bone be obtained to permit free drainage. Excessive amounts of bone should not be removed when draining acute osteomyelitis as it will not be completely replaced by the normal healing process. Bone damage is limited by surgical drainage, whereas failure to evacuate pus in acute cases may lead to widespread damage.

▶ Prognosis

When osteomyelitis is diagnosed in the early clinical stages and prompt antibiotic therapy is begun, the prognosis is excellent. If the process has been unattended for a week to 10 days, there is almost always some permanent loss of bone structure, as well as the possibility of future growth abnormality due to physeal injury.

Bouchoucha S et al: Epidemiology of acute hematogenous osteomyelitis in children: a prospective study over a 32 months period. Tunis Med 2012;90(6):473–480 [PMID: 22693089].

Pyogenic (Septic) Arthritis

The source of pyogenic arthritis (septic arthritis) varies according to the child's age. Infantile pyogenic arthritis often develops from adjacent osteomyelitis. In older children, it presents as an isolated infection, usually without bony involvement. In teenagers with pyogenic arthritis, an underlying systemic disease or an organism that has an affinity for joints (eg, *Neisseria gonorrhoeae*) may be present.

The most frequent infecting organisms similarly vary with age: group B *Streptococcus* and *S aureus* in those younger than 4 months; *Haemophilus influenzae B* (if unimmunized) and *S aureus* in those aged 4 months to 4 years; and *S aureus* and *S pyogenes* in older children and adolescents. *Streptococcus pneumoniae* and *Neisseria meningitidis* are occasionally implicated, and *N gonorrhoeae* is a cause in adolescents. *H influenzae B* is now uncommon in the United States because of effective immunization. *Kingella kingae* is a gram-negative bacterium that is increasingly recognized as a cause of pyarthrosis (and, occasionally, osteomyelitis) in children younger than 5 years.

The initial effusion of the joint rapidly becomes purulent in pyogenic arthritis. A joint effusion may accompany osteomyelitis in the adjacent bone, but a white cell count exceeding 50,000/μL in the joint fluid indicates a purulent infection involving the joint. Generally, spread of infection is from bone into a joint, but unattended pyogenic arthritis may also affect adjacent bone. The ESR is often above 50 mm/h.

► Clinical Findings

A. Symptoms and Signs

In older children, signs may be striking, with fever, malaise, vomiting, and restriction of motion, in addition to joint swelling, warmth, erythema, and/or tenderness. In infants, paralysis of the limb due to inflammatory pseudoparalysis may be evident. Infection of the hip joint in infants should be suspected if decreased abduction of the hip is present in an infant who is irritable or feeding poorly. A history of umbilical catheter treatment in the newborn nursery should alert the physician to the possibility of pyogenic arthritis of the hip.

B. Imaging

Early distention of the joint capsule is nonspecific and difficult to measure by plain radiograph. In infants with unrecognized pyogenic arthritis, dislocation of the joint may follow within a few days as a result of distention of the capsule by purulent effusion. Destruction of the joint space, resorption of epiphysial cartilage, and erosion of the adjacent bone of the metaphysis occur later. Bone scan shows increased flow and increased uptake about the joint. MRI and ultrasound imaging are useful adjuncts for detecting joint effusions, which can be helpful in assessing potential joint sepsis. MRI is recommended if the clinical presentation does not fit the expected picture of septic synovitis and also is beneficial to evaluate for associated bone or soft tissue infection.

► Treatment

Aspiration of the joint is the key to diagnosis. The need for aspiration is evaluated through the Kocher criteria that include fever, inability to bear weight, elevated WBC, ESR, and CRP. Surgical drainage followed by the appropriate antibiotic therapy provides the best treatment for pyogenic arthritis. Antibiotics can be selected based on the child's age and results of the Gram stain and culture of aspirated pus. Reasonable empiric therapy in infants and young children is nafcillin or oxacillin plus a third-generation cephalosporin. An antistaphylococcal agent alone is usually adequate for children older than 5 years, unless gonococcal or meningococcal infection is suspected. Alternative antistaphylococcal therapy (eg, clindamycin or vancomycin) may be needed if methicillin-resistant *S aureus* is suspected or isolated. Consultation with an infectious disease specialist can be helpful in managing antibiotic treatment.

► Prognosis

The prognosis for the patient with pyogenic arthritis is excellent if the joint is drained before damage to the articular cartilage has occurred. If infection is present for more than 24 hours, dissolution of the proteoglycans in the articular cartilage takes place, with subsequent arthrosis and fibrosis of the joint. Damage to the growth plate may occur, especially within the hip joint, where the epiphyseal plate is intracapsular.

Kocher MS, Zurakowski D, Kasser JR: Differentiating between septic arthritis and transient synovitis of the hip in children: an evidence-based clinical prediction algorithm. J Bone Joint Surg Am 1999;81(21):1662–1670 [PMID: 10608376].

Montgomery NI, Epps HR: Pediatric septic arthritis. Orthop Clin North Am 2017;48(2):209–216 [PMID: 28336043].

Diskitis

Diskitis is pyogenic infectious spondylitis in children. Although many infections are culture-negative, *S aureus* is considered to be the most frequent etiologic pathogen. The typical clinical presentation includes avoidance of activity, back pain, and malaise over a several weeks to months duration. Younger children, less than 5 years, may not be able to localize their complaints and commonly present with "abdominal" pain. Supportive treatment and appropriate antibiotics are likely to lead to rapid relief of symptoms and signs without recurrence.

Early SD, Kay RM, Tolo VT: Childhood diskitis. J Am Acad Orthop Surg 2003;11:413–420 [PMID: 14686826].
Gouliouris T, Aliyu SH, Brown NM: Spondylodiscitis: update on diagnosis and management. J Antimicrob Chemother 2010; 65:11–24 [PMID: 20876624].

Transient (Toxic) Synovitis (Versus Septic Arthritis of the Hip)

▶ Clinical Findings

A. Symptoms and Signs

The most common cause of limping and hip pain in children in the United States is transient synovitis. This acute inflammatory reaction often follows an upper respiratory or gastrointestinal infection and is generally self-limited. Classically affecting children aged 3–10 years, it is more common in boys than girls. The hip joint experiences limitation of motion, particularly internal rotation, and radiographic changes are nonspecific, with some swelling apparent in the soft tissues around the joint.

It is important for the provider to differentiate between transient synovitis and septic arthritis upon initial presentation. Early in the disease both conditions have similar symptoms but each requires a different treatment plan. Generally, toxic synovitis of the hip is not associated with elevation of the ESR, white blood cell count, or temperature above 38.3°C. In questionable cases, aspiration of the hip yields only yellowish fluid in transient synovitis rather than purulent fluid in pyogenic arthritis. Transient synovitis can be distinguished from septic arthritis with a dynamic contrast enhanced MRI (DCE-MRI).

▶ Treatment

Rest and nonsteroidal anti-inflammatory medications are the preferred treatments for transient synovitis, whereas patients afflicted with septic arthritis of the hip are treated with operative drainage followed by antibiotic treatment. NSAIDs shorten the course of the transient synovitis, although even with no treatment, the disease usually runs its course in days. Radiographic follow-up is essential as toxic synovitis may be the precursor of avascular necrosis of the femoral head (described in the next section) in a small percentage of patients. Radiographs can be obtained at 6 weeks, or earlier if either a persistent limp or pain is present.

Ryan DD: Differentiating transient synovitis of the hip from more urgent conditions. Pediatr Ann 2016;45(6): e209–e2013 [PMID: 27294495].
Whitelaw CC, Varacallo M: Transient Synovitis. StatPearls. 2019: Treasure Island (FL) [PMID: 29083677].

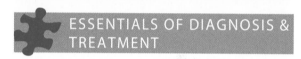

▼ VASCULAR LESIONS & AVASCULAR NECROSIS (OSTEOCHONDROSES)

ESSENTIALS OF DIAGNOSIS & TREATMENT

▶ Diagnosis made by characteristic radiographic findings.

▶ Radiographic resolution lags behind symptomatic resolution.

▶ Treatment for most cases is supportive.

Osteochondrosis (degeneration of an ossification center) due to vascular lesions may affect various growth centers. Table 26–1 indicates the common sites and the typical ages at presentation.

In contrast to other body tissues that undergo infarction, bone removes necrotic tissue and replaces it with living bone through creeping substitution (a process where necrotic bone is replaced by viable bone). This replacement of necrotic bone may be so complete that a normal bone results.

Table 26–1. The osteochondroses.

Ossification Center	Eponym	Typical Age (y)
Capital femoral	Legg-Calvé-Perthes disease	4–8
Tarsal navicular	Köhler bone disease	6
Second metatarsal head	Freiberg disease	12–14
Vertebral ring	Scheuermann disease	13–16
Capitellum	Panner disease	9–11
Tibial tubercle	Osgood-Schlatter disease	11–13
Calcaneus	Sever disease	8–9

Adequacy of replacement depends on the patient's age, the presence or absence of associated infection, the congruity of the involved joint, and other physiologic and mechanical factors.

Rapid growth of the secondary ossification centers in the epiphyses in relation to their blood supply subject them to avascular necrosis. Despite the number of different names referring to avascular necrosis of the epiphyses (see Table 26–1), the process is identical: necrosis of bone followed by replacement.

Even though the pathologic and radiographic features of avascular necrosis of the epiphyses are well known, the cause is not generally agreed upon. Necrosis may follow known causes such as trauma or infection, but idiopathic lesions usually develop during periods of rapid growth of the epiphyses.

Brewer P, Fernandes JA: Osteochondroses. Orthop Trauma 2016; 30(6):553–561.

Avascular Necrosis of the Proximal Femur (Legg-Calvé-Perthes Disease)

▶ Clinical Findings

A. Symptoms and Signs

The highest incidence of Legg-Calvé-Perthes disease occurs between 4 and 8 years of age and occurs when the vascular supply to the proximal femur is interrupted. Persistent pain is the most common symptom, and the patient may present with limp or limitation of motion.

B. Imaging

Radiographic findings correlate with progression of the disease and the extent of necrosis. Effusion of the joint associated with slight widening of the joint space and periarticular swelling are the early findings. Decreased bone density in and around the joint is apparent after a few weeks. The necrotic ossification center appears denser than the surrounding viable structures, and the femoral head is collapsed or narrowed. As replacement of the necrotic ossification center occurs, rarefaction of the bone begins in a patchwork fashion, producing alternating areas of rarefaction and relative density, referred to as "fragmentation" of the epiphysis. Widening of the femoral head may be associated with flattening, or coxa plana. If infarction has extended across the growth plate, a radiolucent lesion will be evident within the metaphysis. If the growth center of the femoral head has been damaged and normal growth arrested, shortening of the femoral neck results. Eventually, complete replacement of the epiphysis develops as living bone replaces necrotic bone by creeping substitution. The final shape of the head depends on the extent of the necrosis and collapse of weakened bone. Serial radiographs help to distinguish this disease from transient synovitis of the hip.

▶ Treatment

Protection of the joint by minimizing impact is the principal treatment. Nonoperative (casting) and surgical approaches are geared to promoting containment of the femoral head within the acetabulum and abduction of the hip.

▶ Prognosis

The prognosis for complete replacement of the necrotic femoral head in a child is excellent, but the functional result depends on the amount of deformity that has developed. Better outcomes are observed for patients with an onset of symptoms before the age of 6. Generally, a poorer prognosis is expected for patients who develop the disease late in childhood, those with more completed involvement of the epiphysial center, those with metaphysial defects and those who have more complete involvement of the femoral head.

Chaudhry S, Phillips D, Feldman D: Legg-Calve-Perthes disease: an overview with recent literature. Bull Hosp Jt Dis 2014; 72(1):18–27 [PMID: 25150324].

Kim HW, Herring JA: Pathophysiology, classifications, and natural history of Perthes disease. Orthop Clin N Am 2011;42:285–295 [PMID: 21742140].

Osteochondritis Dissecans

▶ Clinical Findings

A. Symptoms and Signs

In osteochondritis dissecans, a wedge-shaped necrotic area of subchondral bone can lead to significant chondral damage. The fragment of bone may break off from the host bone and displace into the joint as a loose body. If it remains attached, the necrotic fragment may be completely replaced through creeping substitution. The pathologic process is the same as that for avascular necrosing lesions of ossification centers. Joint damage may occur because of the proximity of these lesions to adjacent articular cartilage.

The knee (medial femoral condyle, see Figure 26–14), the elbow joint (capitellum), and the talus (superior lateral dome) are the most common sites for these lesions. Joint pain is the usual presenting complaint; however, local swelling or locking may be present, particularly if a fragment is free in the joint. Laboratory studies are normal.

▶ Treatment

Treatment consists of protection of the involved area from mechanical damage. Stable/attached lesions are generally treated with activity modification and immobilization for

3–6 months. Unstable/dislodged lesions are treated surgically with arthroscopic drilling, in order to bring new blood flow to the area, and fixation to stabilize the lesion. For some marginal lesions, it may be worthwhile to drill the necrotic fragment to encourage more rapid vascular in-growth and replacement. If a fragment is free within the joint as a loose body, it must be removed. If large areas of a weight-bearing joint are involved, secondary degenerative arthritis may result. Adolescents have less favorable outcomes with nonoperative therapy.

Pascual-Garrido C, Southworth TM, Slabaugh MA, Naveen NB, Friel NA, Nwachukwu BU, Cole BJ: Osteochondritis Dissecans. 2019.

Wall EJ et al: Research on Osteochondritis dissecans of the knee (ROCK) study group. Am J Sports Med 2015;43(2):303–309 [PMID: 25583756].

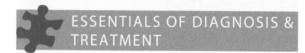

NEOPLASIA OF THE MUSCULO-SKELETAL SYSTEM

ESSENTIALS OF DIAGNOSIS & TREATMENT

▶ Most typically present with unresolving pain.

▶ Reassess *any* child with unresolved pain previously thought benign in origin.

▶ Obtain radiographs.

▶ Refer any suspicious lesions for specialty evaluation.

The poor prognosis of malignant tumors arising in the bone or other tissues derived from the mesoderm makes neoplastic diseases of the musculoskeletal system a serious problem. Fortunately, few benign lesions undergo malignant transformation. Accurate diagnosis depends on correlation of the clinical, radiographic, and microscopic findings. Complaints about the knee should be investigated for tumor, although the usual causes of knee pain are traumatic, infectious, or developmental in origin.

Hashefi M: Ultrasound in the diagnosis of noninflammatory musculoskeletal conditions. Semin Ultrasound CT MR 2011; 32(2):74–90 [PMID: 21414544].

Osteochondroma

Clinical Findings

A. Symptoms and Signs

Osteochondroma is the most common benign bone tumor in children. It usually presents as a pain-free mass. When present, pain is caused by bursitis or tendinitis due to irritation by the tumor. Lesions may be single or multiple. Pathologically, the lesion is a bone mass capped with cartilage. These masses result from a developmental defect of the growth plate and tend to grow during childhood and adolescence in proportion to the child's growth. Males are more affected than females. Generally, the tumors are present on radiographs in the metaphyseal region of long bones and may be pedunculated or sessile. The cortex of the underlying bone "flows" into the base of the tumor.

Treatment

An osteochondroma should be excised if it interferes with function, is frequently traumatized, or is large enough to be deforming. The prognosis is excellent. Malignant transformation is very rare.

Osteoid Osteoma

Clinical Findings

A. Symptoms and Signs

Osteoid osteoma is a benign bone-forming lesion of unclear etiology.

It classically produces night pain that can be relieved by NSAIDs. On physical examination, there usually is tenderness over the lesion. An osteoid osteoma in the upper femur may cause referred pain to the knee.

The radiographic lesion consists of a radiolucent nidus surrounded by dense osteosclerosis that may obscure the nidus. Bone scan shows intense uptake in the lesion. CT scans are confirmatory and delineate the nidus well.

Treatment

Surgical excision or radiofrequency ablation of the nidus is curative and may be done using computed tomography imaging and a minimally invasive technique. The prognosis is excellent, with no known cases of malignant transformation, although the lesion has a tendency to recur if incompletely excised.

Noordin S, Allana S, Hilal K, Nadeem N, Lakdawala R, Sadruddin A, Uddin N: Osteoid osteoma: contemporary management. Orthop Rev (Pavia) 2018;10(3):7496 [PMID: 30370032].

Enchondroma

Clinical Findings & Treatment

Enchondroma (nest of benign cartilage within long bones) is usually a silent lesion unless it produces a pathologic fracture. On radiograph it is radiolucent, usually in a long bone. Speckled calcification may be present. The classic lesion looks as though someone dragged his or her fingernails through clay, making streaks in the bones. Enchondroma is treated by surgical curettage and bone grafting. The prognosis is excellent. Malignant transformation may occur but is very rare in childhood.

Chondroblastoma

▶ Clinical Findings & Treatment

The presenting complaint in chondroblastoma (benign chondral origin lesions typically in the epiphyses [joint ends] of long bones) is pain around a joint. This neoplasm may produce a pathologic fracture. On radiograph, the lesion is radiolucent and usually located in the epiphysis. With little to no reactive bone, calcification is unusual. The lesion is treated by surgical curettage and bone grafting. The prognosis is excellent if complete curettage is performed. There is no known malignant transformation.

Chen W, DiFrancesco LM: Chondroblastoma: an update. Arch Pathol Lab Med 2017; 141(6):867–871 [PMID: 28557595].

Nonossifying Fibroma

▶ Clinical Findings & Treatment

Nonossifying fibroma, or benign cortical defect, is nearly always an incidental finding on radiograph. Nonossifying fibroma is a radiolucent lesion eccentrically located in the metaphyseal region of the bone. Usually a thin sclerotic border is evident. Multiple lesions may be present. The most frequent sites are the distal femur and proximal tibia. In general, no treatment is needed because these lesions heal as they ossify with maturation and growth. Rarely, pathologic fractures result from large lesions.

Osteosarcoma

▶ Clinical Findings

A. Symptoms and Signs

Osteosarcoma is an aggressive form of cancer characterized by chromosomal instability. It is suspected that micro RNAs (noncoding, single-stranded molecules of RNA that regulate gene expression) play an important role in cancer development. The presenting complaint is usually pain in a long bone; however, the patient may present with, loss of function, mass, or limp. Pathological fracture is uncommon. The malignant osseous tumor produces a destructive, expanding, and invasive lesion. A triangle may be adjacent to the tumor, produced by elevated periosteum and subsequent tumor ossification. The lesion may contain calcification and violates the cortex of the bone. Femur, tibia, humerus, and other long bones are the sites usually affected.

▶ Treatment

Surgical excision (limb salvage) or amputation is indicated based on the extent of the tumor. Adjuvant chemotherapy is routinely used prior to and after surgical excision. The prognosis is improving, with greater than 65%long-term survival rates reported in modern series. Death usually occurs as a result of lung metastasis. Patients with osteosarcoma complicated by pathological fracture have lower long-term survival rates than patients with osteosarcoma and no pathological fracture.

Heare T, Hensley MA, Dell'Orfano S: Bone tumors: osteosarcoma and Ewing's sarcoma. Curr Opin Pediatr 2009;21(3):365–672 [PMID: 19421061].

Misaghi A Goldin A, Awad M, Kulidjian AA: Osteosarcoma: a comprehensive review. SICOT J 2018;4:12 [PMID: 29629690].

Ewing Sarcoma

▶ Clinical Findings

A. Symptoms and Signs

In Ewing sarcoma, the presenting complaint is usually pain and tenderness, but fever and leukocytosis may be present. Osteomyelitis is the main differential diagnosis. The lesion may be multicentric. Ewing sarcoma is radiolucent and destroys the cortex, frequently in the diaphyseal region. Reactive bone formation may occur about the lesion, seen as successive layers of the so-called onion skin layering.

▶ Treatment

Treatment is with multiagent chemotherapy, radiation, and surgical resection. Large tumor size, pelvic lesions, and inadequate response to chemotherapy portend a poor prognosis.

Parida L et al: Clinical management of Ewing sarcoma of the bones of the hands and feet: a retrospective single-institution review. J Pediatr Surg 2012;47(10):1806–1810 [PMID: 23084188].

▼ MISCELLANEOUS DISEASES OF BONE & JOINT

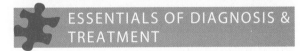

ESSENTIALS OF DIAGNOSIS & TREATMENT

- ▶ Rule out malignant process.
- ▶ Obtain radiographs when indicated.
- ▶ Treatment based on symptoms and location.

FIBROUS DYSPLASIA

Dysplastic fibrous tissue replacement of the medullary canal is accompanied by the formation of metaplastic bone in areas with fibrous dysplasia. Three forms of the disease are recognized: monostotic, polyostotic, and polyostotic with endocrine disturbances (precocious puberty in females, hyperthyroidism, and hyperadrenalism [Albright syndrome]).

▶ Clinical Findings

A. Symptoms and Signs

The lesion or lesions may be asymptomatic. If present, pain is probably due to pathologic fractures (Figure 26–16). In females, endocrine disturbances may be present in the polyostotic variety and are associated with café au lait spots.

B. Imaging

The lesion begins centrally within the medullary canal, usually of a long bone, and expands slowly. Pathologic fracture may occur. If metaplastic bone predominates, the contents of the lesion have the density of bone. The disease is often asymmetrical, and limb length disturbances may occur as a result of stimulation of epiphysial cartilage growth. Marked deformity of the bone may result, and a shepherd's crook deformity of the upper femur is a classic feature of the disease.

▶ Treatment

If the lesion is small and asymptomatic, no treatment is needed. If the lesion is large and produces or threatens pathologic fracture, curettage and bone grafting are indicated. The prognosis is good, as malignant transformation is rare.

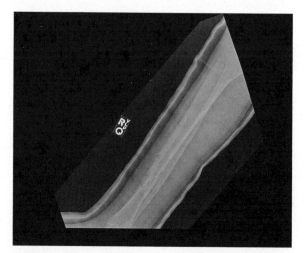

▲ **Figure 26–16.** Tibia fracture with fibrous dysplasia.

Boyce AM, Florenzano P, Castro L, Collins MT: Fibrous Dysplasia/McCune-Albright Syndrome. In: GeneReviews (R), Adam MP, et al (eds); 1993: Seattle (WA) Updated 2018, [PMID: 25719192]

BONE CYSTS, BAKER CYST, & GANGLIONS

▶ Clinical Findings

A. Symptoms and Signs

Unicameral Bone Cyst

Unicameral bone cysts occur in the metaphysis of a long bone, usually in the femur or humerus. A cyst begins in the medullary canal adjacent to the epiphysial cartilage. It probably results from some fault in enchondral ossification (the process where bone is formed from cartilaginous precursors). The cyst is considered active as long as it abuts onto the metaphysial side of the epiphysial cartilage, and there is a risk of growth arrest with or without treatment. When a border of normal bone exists between the cyst and the epiphysial cartilage, the cyst is inactive. The lesion is usually identified when a pathologic fracture occurs, producing pain. Laboratory findings are normal. On radiograph, the cyst is identified centrally within the medullary canal, producing expansion of the cortex and thinning over the widest portion of the cyst.

Aneurysmal Bone Cyst

Aneurysmal bone cyst is similar to unicameral bone cyst, except it contains blood rather than clear fluid. It usually occurs in a slightly eccentric position in a long bone, expanding the cortex of the bone but not breaking the cortex. Involvement of the flat bones of the pelvis is less common. On radiographs, the lesion appears somewhat larger than the width of the epiphysial cartilage, distinguishing it from a unicameral bone cyst.

Chromosomal abnormalities have been associated with aneurysmal bone cysts. The lesion may appear aggressive histologically, and it is important to differentiate it from osteosarcoma or hemangioma.

Baker Cyst

A Baker cyst is a herniation of the synovium in the knee joint into the popliteal region. In children, the diagnosis may be made by aspiration of mucinous fluid, but the cyst nearly always disappears with time.

Ganglion

A ganglion is a smooth, small cystic mass connected by a pedicle to the joint capsule, usually on the dorsum of the wrist.

It may also occur in the tendon sheath over the flexor or extensor surfaces of the fingers. Ganglia may interfere with function or cause persistent pain.

▶ Treatment

Treatment of bone cysts and ganglion can be by curettage and bone grafting. Baker cysts usually require no surgical treatment. Ganglia can be excised if they cause symptoms.

Mascard E, Gomez-Brouchet A, Lambot K: Bone cysts: unicameral and aneurysmal bone cyst. Orthop Traumatol Surg Res 2015; 101(1 Suppl): 119–127 [PMID: 25579825].

QUALITY ASSURANCE/IMPROVEMENT INITIATIVES IN ORTHOPEDICS

The Pediatric Orthopedic Society of North America (POSNA) has an ongoing, well-developed quality, safety, and value initiative (QSVI). QSVI research is included during the POSNA annual scientific meeting.

Pediatric Orthopaedic Society of North America (POSNA). QSVI: Quality, safety and value initiative. Retrieved March 27, 2017 from https://posna.org/Resources/QSVI.

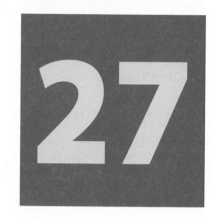

Sports Medicine

Katherine S. Dahab, MD, FAAP, CAQSM

Stephanie W. Mayer, MD

Kyle B. Nagle, MD, MPH, FAAP, CAQSM

Armando Vidal, MD

Sports medicine as a separate discipline has grown since the 1980s in response to an expanding body of knowledge in the areas of exercise physiology, biomechanics, and musculoskeletal medicine. As more children participate in recreational and competitive activities, pediatric health care providers are encountering more young athletes in their practice. Familiarity with the common medical and orthopedic issues faced by athletically active children and knowledge of which injuries necessitate referral to a sports medicine specialist are essential.

▼ BASIC PRINCIPLES

Pediatric Injury Patterns

Although young athletes have injuries and issues similar to those of adults, there are many injuries that are unique to the pediatric and adolescent athlete. An understanding of the differences between adult and pediatric injury patterns is important to foster an appropriate index of suspicion for situations unique to pediatrics.

Components of a long bone include the diaphysis, metaphysis, and epiphysis. In the pediatric bone architecture, the presence of cartilaginous growth plates and apophyses predispose children to unique injury patterns that are different from their adult counterparts. Open growth plates or physes and their various stages of development are important factors to consider when treating young athletes. The physes are located at the ends of the long bones and are the primary ossification centers where length is added to the immature skeleton. The physis is a weak link in the musculoskeletal complex and has a high risk of fracture during periods of rapid growth. The surrounding soft tissues, including ligaments and tendons, are relatively stronger than the physis. The epiphyses are secondary centers of ossification that also contribute to long bone formation and, like the adjacent articular cartilages, are vulnerable to trauma. Injuries that involve the epiphysis can lead to joint deformity. The apophyses are secondary centers of ossification that add contour but not length to the bone. The apophysis is the attachment site of the muscle-tendon unit and is vulnerable to both acute and chronic overuse traction injury during times of rapid growth. Unlike injuries to the physis and epiphysis, however, apophyseal injuries do not result in long-term growth disturbance. Recognizing injuries to growth centers is important because of the risk for partial or complete physeal arrest. Complications of growth plate injury can lead to limb length discrepancy or angular deformity.

FITNESS & CONDITIONING

Compared to children who are sedentary, physically active youth tend to develop greater agility and skills and maintain better fitness throughout their lifetime. Young children and adolescents should participate in physical activity for 60 minutes or more each day. To improve overall fitness and reduce the risk of injury, children and adolescents should focus on three different components of exercise:

1. Integrative training (curriculum of diverse skills, increasing fitness, and appropriate rest periods). Examples include developing fundamental skills and technique, learning proper movement mechanics, and aerobic and anaerobic conditioning.

2. Neuromuscular conditioning (mixture of basic fundamental and specialized motor control exercises aimed at improving general health and sports performance). Examples include core strength exercises, agility, and plyometrics.

3. Resistance (strength) training (progressive resistive loads in a variety of modalities).

Periodization is a training concept that emphasizes variations in the volume and intensity of training throughout the year in a conditioning program. Continuously varying the specific type and goals of training provides adequate recovery from each strenuous exercise session and avoids overtraining, burnout, and overuse injuries.

Strength Training

Strength is defined as the peak force that can be generated during a single maximal contraction. Strength training uses progressive resistance to improve an athlete's ability to resist or exert force. This can be achieved by a variety of techniques, including body weight, free weight, or machine resistance. The benefits of strength training include improved performance, endurance, and muscular strength. Strength training can be safely started in prepubescent athletes as early as 7 and 8 years old if designed appropriately with a focus on lighter resistance, increased repetitions, proper technique and mechanics, coordination, and building self-confidence. During preadolescence, it is thought that strength training leads to increased strength largely through improved neuromuscular adaptation as opposed to muscular hypertrophy. As such, attempts to gain fat-free mass through maximal weight lifting and high weight, low repetition resistance training regimens may not have that desired effect. Children mature at varying paces, and strength training programs should be individualized to accommodate for these unique differences. All strength training regimens should be modified as needed to remain age-appropriate and pain-free. Tanner staging (see Chapter 34) helps define readiness for progression to more strenuous programs. Power lifting and maximal weight lifting should be restricted to athletes who have reached or passed Tanner stage V. To prevent injuries, care should be taken to instruct children on the proper use of weight-training equipment at home. Children and adults with disabilities can benefit from weight-training programs modified to meet their specific needs.

Faigenbaum AD et al: Youth resistance training: updated position statement paper from the national strength and conditioning association. J Strength Cond Res 2009;23(Suppl):S60–S79 [PMID: 19620931].

Myer GD et al: When to initiate integrative neuromuscular training to reduce sports-related injuries and enhance health in youth? Curr Sports Med Rep 2011;10(3):155–166 [PMID: 21623307].

SPORTS NUTRITION

Proper nutrition in young athletes focuses on maintaining an appropriate energy balance; creating healthy eating and hydration habits; and avoiding harmful food, drink, and supplement choices. Keeping an adequate nutritional intake will increase lean muscle mass, maximizing strength, endurance, immunity, and training benefit. Athletes should be encouraged to balance caloric intake with energy expenditure, eat whole grains, avoid processed foods, focus on healthy fats and proteins, and maintain proper hydration. Carbohydrates should compose 50%–60% of a young athlete's diet, with fat and protein making up 25%–30% and 15%–25%, respectively. Hydration can come mainly from water if the exercise lasts less than 1 hour, after which time a carbohydrate-containing sports drink is appropriate. Water or sports drinks should be consumed every 15–20 minutes during prolonged exercise greater than 1 hour or in hot playing conditions. For bouts of exercise lasting greater than 1 hour, some carbohydrates should be ingested as well. These carbohydrates can be in the liquid form as sports drinks or solids combined with water. A light snack and hydration are recommended prior to and immediately after an extended workout. To avoid excessive caloric and sugar intake, sports drinks are not recommended at meals or times other than prolonged exercise. The average athlete eats a well-balanced diet not necessitating nutritional supplementation. However, if food allergies or improper dietary intake is confirmed, an athlete may benefit from a daily multivitamin. In general, nutritional sports supplements are not recommended and extreme caution is suggested when considering their use. The supplement industry is not well regulated and contamination with toxic and banned substances has been noted in the past. Similarly, energy drinks are not recommended for use in any youth younger than 18 years due to high levels of caffeine and other stimulants contained in such beverages.

Committee on Nutrition and Council on Sports Medicine and Fitness: Sports drinks and energy drinks for children and adolescents: are they appropriate? Pediatrics 2011;127(6):1182–1189 [PMID: 21624882].

Kleinman R (ed): *Pediatric Nutrition Handbook*. 6th ed. AAP; 2009.

Rodriguez NR, Di Marco NM, Langley S: American College of Sports Medicine position stand. Nutrition and athletic performance. Med Sci Sports Exerc 2009;41(3):709–731 [PMID: 19225360].

PREPARTICIPATION PHYSICAL EVALUATION

The ultimate goal of the preparticipation physical evaluation (PPE) is to promote the health and safety of athletes. Its primary objectives are to screen for conditions that may be life threatening or disabling and for conditions that may predispose to injury or illness. Secondary objectives of the PPE include establishing a medical home, determining the general health of the individual, assessing fitness for specific sports, and counseling on injury prevention and health-related issues. The ideal timing of the examination is at least 6–8 weeks before training starts. This allows time to further evaluate, treat, or rehabilitate any identified problems.

Preparticipation History

The medical history is the most important part of the encounter, identifying 65%–77% of medical and musculoskeletal conditions. Therefore, obtaining a thorough and accurate history is essential in identifying conditions that may affect a child's ability to safely participate in sports. Many key elements should be explored with the athlete. A standardized PPE form, endorsed by six medical societies, including the American Academy of Pediatrics (AAP), is available in the fourth edition of the PPE monograph (Bernhardt and Roberts 2010) or on the Internet (https://www.aap.org/en-us/about-the-aap/Committees-Councils-Sections/Council-on-sports-medicine-and-fitness/Pages/PPE.aspx). This monograph, formulated based on current literature, policies, consensus statements, expert opinion, and extensive peer review, is currently the recommended standard for the preparticipation physical examination in the United States. The history includes the following areas:

A. Cardiovascular History

The routine use of electrocardiogram (ECG) and echocardiography in the preparticipation cardiovascular screening in athletes remains a highly debated topic in sports medicine and sports cardiology. Despite ongoing controversy, the American Heart Association (AHA) currently recommends against its routine usage in asymptomatic athletes because of its low sensitivity, high false-positive rate, limited resources, lack of trained physicians to interpret the ECG, and poor cost-effectiveness due to the low prevalence of disease. In 2014, the AHA updated its consensus statement on cardiovascular screening stating its position to this effect. According to the AHA, the goal of the PPE is to reduce cardiovascular risk associated with physical activity. The 2007 AHA recommendations for cardiovascular screening are incorporated in the fourth edition PPE monograph and include the following 12-point screen:

Personal Medical History:

1. Chest pain or discomfort with exercise

2. Syncope or near syncope associated with exercise

3. Excessive shortness or breath or fatigue associated with exertion

4. History of heart murmur

5. History of elevated blood pressure

Family Medical History:

6. Premature death before age 50 years due to heart disease

7. Disability from heart disease in a close relative younger than 50 years

8. Knowledge of specific cardiac conditions: hypertrophic or dilated cardiomyopathy, long QT syndrome, other ion channelopathies, Marfan syndrome, or arrhythmias

Physical Examination:

9. Auscultation of heart murmur in supine and standing position

10. Palpation of radial and femoral pulses

11. Physical stigmata of Marfan syndrome

12. Brachial blood pressure taken in seated position

Sudden cardiac arrest is the leading medical cause of sudden death in young athletes. Addressing these areas may help identify potentially life-threatening cardiac lesions. However, clinicians should keep in mind that there are currently no outcome-based studies that demonstrate the effectiveness of the PPE in preventing sudden cardiac death in athletes. In the United States, the most common causes of sudden cardiac death on the playing field are hypertrophic cardiomyopathy (HCM) and congenital coronary artery anomalies, with HCM accounting for one-third of sudden cardiac deaths in young athletes. Any athletes with cardiovascular symptoms require further evaluation before allowing them to participate in sports. Any activity restrictions or sports disqualification for an athlete should be made in consultation with a cardiologist.

B. History of Hypertension

Any history of hypertension requires investigation for secondary causes of hypertension and target organ disease. An athlete with hypertension who exercises may cause their blood pressure to rise even higher, placing them at increased risk for complications. Athletes should also be asked about the use of stimulants (ie, caffeine, nicotine, attention deficit disorder medications) and a family history of hypertension. The diagnosis of hypertension in children younger than 18 years is based on gender, age, and height, and the blood pressure must be measured on three separate occasions. Blood pressure measurements with values from 90% to 95% of gender, age, and height-based norms are considered prehypertension; values from 95% to 5 mm Hg above the 99% of norms are defined as stage 1 hypertension; and values greater than 5 mm Hg above the 99% of norms are defined as stage 2 hypertension.

Athletes with prehypertension are eligible to participate in sports. Counseling regarding lifestyle modifications should be made, including healthy dietary changes, weight management, and daily physical activity. Those with stage 1 hypertension, in the absence of end-organ damage, may also participate in competitive sports but with appropriate subspecialist referral if the individual is symptomatic, have associated heart disease or structural abnormality, or have persistent elevated blood pressure on two additional occasions despite lifestyle modifications. Athletes who have stage 2 hypertension or end-organ damage should not be cleared to participate in competitive sports until their blood pressure is evaluated, treated, and is under control.

C. Central Nervous System

A history of frequent or exertional headaches, seizure disorders, concussions or head injuries, recurrent stingers or burners, or cervical cord neurapraxia may affect an athlete's ability to participate in sports. These conditions require further evaluation, rehabilitation, or informed decision making prior to clearance for sports participation. The fourth edition PPE monograph provides an updated review and recommendations on concussions in sports. (See also section Concussion.)

D. History of Chronic Diseases

Diseases such as reactive airway disease, exercise-induced asthma, diabetes, renal disease, liver disease, chronic infections, or hematologic diseases should be noted.

E. Surgical History

Surgical history may influence participation in certain sports. Full recovery with no long-term impact on athletic performance is required prior to clearance.

F. Infectious Mononucleosis

Ask about infectious mononucleosis in the last 4 weeks. The risk for splenic rupture is highest within the first 3 weeks of illness and can occur in the absence of trauma. Therefore, physical activity should be avoided during the first 3–4 weeks after the infection starts. The athlete may return to play once clinical symptoms are resolved and risk for splenic rupture is assessed as minimal. The use of serial abdominal ultrasound to assess spleen size to aid in return to play decisions is likely not useful or recommended. Parameters for spleen size based on ethnicity, sex, height, and weight have not yet been established, so determining when spleen size has normalized based on imaging becomes difficult.

G. Musculoskeletal Limitations and Prior Injuries

The physician should inquire about joints with limited range of motion, muscle weakness, and prior injuries that may affect future performance. Chronic pain or soreness long after activity may reflect overuse syndromes that should be evaluated.

H. Menstrual History in Females

The physician should pay particular attention to the so-called female athlete triad: amenorrhea, disordered eating, and osteoporosis.

I. Nutritional Issues

The physician should record methods the athlete uses to maintain, gain, or lose weight. Eating disorders or inadequate nutritional intake could lead to persistent or recurrent injury, including stress fractures. Vitamin D deficiency has become increasingly common in athletes due to inadequate dietary intake or decreased sunlight exposure.

J. Medication History

Inquire about the use of prescription medications, over-the-counter medications, and supplements. Not only will medications reveal problems omitted in the medical history, but the information will also provide data on current medications whose side effects may suggest activity modifications. Documenting drug use may provide the opportunity to explore with the patient the drawbacks of performance-enhancing compounds such as anabolic steroids, creatine, stimulants, and narcotics.

Physical Examination

The physical examination should be focused on the needs of the athlete. It may be the only time an athlete has contact with medical personnel and can be used to promote wellness along with screening for physical activity. An example of a preparticipation physical examination form is endorsed in the fourth edition of the PPE monograph (Bernhardt and Roberts 2010) and is available at https://www.aap.org/en-us/about-the-aap/Committees-Councils-Sections/Council-on-sports-medicine-and-fitness/Pages/PPE.aspx. The examination should include routine vital signs, including blood pressure measurements obtained in the upper extremity. The cardiovascular examination should include palpation of pulses, auscultation for murmurs while sitting and standing, evaluation for physical stigmata of Marfan syndrome, and assessment of any cardiovascular symptoms as previously described. The musculoskeletal examination is used to determine strength, range of motion, flexibility, and previous injuries. Included is a quick guide that can be used to screen for musculoskeletal abnormalities (Table 27–1). The remainder of the examination should emphasize the following areas:

A. Skin

Are there any contagious lesions such as herpes or impetigo?

B. Vision

Are there any visual problems? Is there any evidence of retinal problems? Are both eyes intact?

C. Abdomen

Is there any evidence of hepatosplenomegaly?

D. Genitourinary System

Are any testicular abnormalities or hernias present?

Table 27–1. The screening sports examination.[a]

General evaluation	Have patient stand in front of examiner; evaluate both front and back along with posture. Look at general body habitus. Look for asymmetry in muscle bulk, scars, or unusual postures. Watch how patient moves when instructed.
Neck evaluation	Evaluate ROM by having patient bend head forward (chin to chest), rotate from side to side, and laterally bend (ear to shoulder). Observe for asymmetry, lack of motion, or pain with movement.

Shoulder and upper extremity evaluation	Observe clavicles, shoulder position, scapular position, elbow position, and fingers.
	ROM screening:
	    Fully abduct arms with palms in jumping jack position.
	    Internally and externally rotate shoulder.
	    Flex and extend wrist, pronate and supinate wrist, flex and extend fingers.
	Do the following manual muscle testing:
	    Have patient shrug shoulders (testing trapezius).
	    Abduct to 90 degrees (testing deltoid).
	    Flex elbow (testing biceps).
	    Extend elbow over head (testing triceps).
	    Test wrist flexion and extension.
	    Have patient grasp fingers.

Back evaluation	General inspection to look for scoliosis or kyphosis.
	ROM screening:
	    Bend forward touching toes with knees straight (spine flexion and hamstring range).
	    Rotation, side bending, and spine extension.

Gait and lower extremity evaluation	General observation while walking. Have patient walk short distance normally (look at symmetry, heel-toe gait pattern, look at all joints involved in gait and leg lengths, any evidence of joint effusions or pain). Have patient toe-walk and heel-walk for short distance and check tandem walking (balance beam walking).

ROM, range of motion.

[a]If any abnormalities are found, a more focused evaluation is required.

E. Neurologic System

Are there any problems with coordination, gait, or mental processing?

F. Sexual Maturity

What is the individual's Tanner stage?

Recommendations for Participation

After completing the medical evaluation, the physician can make recommendations about sports clearance. The options include the following:

- Cleared for all sports without restrictions
- Cleared for all sports without restrictions with recommendations for further evaluation or treatment
- Not cleared: pending further evaluation, for any sports, or for certain sports

Table 27–2 is a composite of recommendations for sports participation organized by body system. Recommendations for sports participation with specific medical conditions can be found on the AAP website.

Bernhardt DT, Roberts WO: *Preparticipation Physical Evaluation.* 4th ed. American Academy of Pediatrics; 2010.

Harmon KG et al: Incidence of sudden cardiac death in National Collegiate Athletic Association athletes. Circulation 2011;123:1594–1600 [PMID: 21464047].

Harris G et al: Diabetes in the competitive athlete. Curr Sports Med Rep 2012 Nov/Dec;11(6):309–315 [PMID: 23147019].

Hull J et al: Managing respiratory problems in athletes. Clin Med 2012;12(4):351–356 [PMID: 22930882].

Jaworski C et al: Infectious disease. Clin Sports Med 2011;30:575–590 [PMID: 21658549].

Maron BJ et al: Assessment of the 12-lead electrocardiogram as a screening test for detection of cardiovascular disease in healthy general populations of young people (12–25 years of age). J Am Coll Cardiol 2014;64:1479–1514.

Maron BJ et al: Sudden deaths in young competitive athletes: analysis of 1866 deaths in the United States, 1980–2006. Circulation 2009;119:1085–1092 [PMID: 19221222].

Table 27–2. Recommendations and considerations for participation in sports.

Disorders	Considerations and Recommendations	References
Cardiac		
Anticoagulation treatment	Need to avoid all contact sports.	
Aortic stenosis	Individualize treatment based on extent of disease and systolic gradient: Mild: < 20 mm Hg, all sports if asymptomatic. Moderate: limited sports. Severe: no competitive sports.	
Arrhythmias	Long-QT syndrome, malignant ventricular arrhythmias, symptomatic WPW syndrome, advanced heart block, family history of sudden death or previous sudden cardiac event, and implantation of a cardioverter-defibrillator. May participate: qualified yes. Consult with cardiologist.	Rice 2008
Arrhythmogenic right ventricular cardiomyopathy	May participate: qualified no. Consult with cardiologist.	Rice 2008
Carditis	May participate: qualified no. May result in sudden death with exertion.	Rice 2008
Congenital heart disease	May participate: qualified yes. Consult with cardiologist. Mild, moderate, and severe diseases for cardiac lesions are defined by the 36th Bethesda Conference. Those with mild lesions may fully participate in most cases. Those with moderate or severe lesions or who have undergone surgery need further evaluation.	Maron et al 2005
Coronary artery anomalies	May participate: qualified no. Consult with cardiologist.	Rice 2008
Ehlers-Danlos syndrome, vascular form	May participate: qualified no. Consult with cardiologist.	Rice 2008
Heart failure	Screen patient with LVEF < 30% for ischemia. Use AHA risk stratification criteria to define exercise capacity.	Braith 2002
Heart implants	No jumping, swimming, or contact sports.	
Hypertrophic cardiomyopathy	May participate: qualified no. Athletes should not participate in sports except possibly low-intensity forms (eg, golf, bowling). Consult with cardiologist.	Maron 2002a, b
Hypertension	May participate: qualified yes. Those with hypertension > 5 mm Hg above 99th percentile for age, gender, and height should avoid heavy weightlifting and power lifting, bodybuilding, and high-static component sports.	Rice 2008
Marfan syndrome	Aortic root dilation is associated with mitral valve prolapse and regurgitation. May participate: qualified yes. Participate in sports with minimal physical demands.	Salim and Alpert 2001
Mitral valve prolapse	May participate: qualified yes. No restrictions unless there is a history of syncope, positive family history of sudden death, arrhythmias with exercise, or moderate regurgitation.	
Syncope	Unexplained syncopal episodes during exercise must be evaluated by ECG, echocardiograph, Holter and tilt test prior to resumption of any activities.	Firoozi et al 2003
Vasculitis/vascular disease	Kawasaki disease, pulmonary hypertension. May participate: qualified yes. Consult with cardiologist.	Rice 2008

(Continued)

Table 27–2. Recommendations and considerations for participation in sports. (*Continued*)

Disorders	Considerations and Recommendations	References
Endocrine		
Diabetes mellitus type 1	No restrictions to activity. However, athletes are at risk for hypoglycemia and ketoacidosis, so ensure proper hydration and caloric intake. As exercise enhances insulin sensitivity, the quantity and duration of aerobic and anaerobic exercise and intensity of practices and games need to be assessed. In general: Short-term exercise = no insulin changes. Vigorous exercise may require 25% reduction in insulin with 15–30 g of carbohydrates before and every 30 min during exercise. Strenuous exercise = may require up to an 80% reduction in insulin with extra carbohydrates. Generally, monitor blood glucose frequently during exercise. Diabetic athletes typically perform best with glucose levels between 70 and 150 mg/dL.	Draznin 2000, Harris et al 2012
Eye		
Detached retina	May participate in sport, but athlete may have increased risk of injury because of weakened eye tissue. Therefore, participation should be determined on an individual basis.	Rice 2008
Functionally one eyed	Defined as having best corrected visual acuity worse than 20/40 in the poorest seeing eye. Consider avoiding contact sports, although if patient participates, use of eye protection is mandatory.	Rice 2008
Genitourinary		
One testicle	Need to wear protective cups in collision and contact sports.	
Solitary kidney	May participate: qualified yes. Protective equipment may reduce risk of injury to remaining kidney sufficiently to allow participation in most sports.	Rice 2008
Hematologic		
Hemophilia	Avoid contact and collision sports.	
Sickle cell disease	May participate: qualified yes. If illness status permits, all sports may be played. However, any sport or activity that entails overexertion, overheating, dehydration, or chilling should be avoided. Participation at high altitude poses risk for sickle cell crisis.	Rice 2008
Sickle cell trait	Currently, no recommendations for universal screening in athletes. However, the NCAA now requires screening for athletes if their sickle cell status is unknown. May participate: yes. Under normal environmental conditions, no increased risk of sudden death or other medical problems. Ensure acclimatization to extreme environment conditions (eg, altitude, heat, humidity) and adequate hydration during participation to reduce risk of heat illness and/or rhabdomyolysis.	Seto 2011 Rice 2008
Infectious disease		
Fever	May participate: no. Cardiopulmonary effort is increased while maximum exercise capacity is decreased during febrile illnesses. Risk of heat illness is also increased.	Rice 2008
Infectious mononucleosis	Splenic rupture is most important consideration. Risk of spleen rupture highest during first 3 wk of illness. No athletic participation during the first 3–4 wk after the infection starts. Too early a return to sports increases risk of splenic rupture or could cause EBV reactivation and relapse. If symptoms resolve by third week, light activities can be started during the fourth week with graded increases in intensity. Full contact activity participation may resume at week 5.	Putukian et al 2008

(Continued)

Table 27–2. Recommendations and considerations for participation in sports. (*Continued*)

Disorders	Considerations and Recommendations	References
Skin infections	Herpes simplex, molluscum contagiosum, warts, staphylococcal and streptococcal infections, impetigo, scabies, and tinea. May participate: qualified yes. During contagious periods, participation in gymnastics or cheerleading with mats, martial arts, wrestling, or other collision, contact or limited contact sports is not allowed.	Rice 2008
Upper respiratory infections (including common cold)	May participate in sports if tolerated. Exceptions include those with fever, severe bacterial infections (sinusitis, pharyngitis), or those with symptoms below the neck. "Neck check" guide allows athletes to return to sports if symptoms are "above the neck" (eg, rhinorrhea, congestion, or sore throat). If symptoms "below the neck" (eg, fever or malaise) are present, the athlete should not participate.	Jaworski et al 2011
Neurologic		
Epilepsy	Majority of sports are safe for those with good seizure control; contact sports are allowed with proper protection. Definitely wear a helmet. Fitness may reduce number of seizures. Swimming and water sports should be supervised. Sports such as free climbing, hang gliding, and scuba are not recommended.	Howard et al 2004
Herniated disk (with cord compression)	Avoid contact and collision sports.	
Muscle disease or myopathy	Exercise within physical limits. Low- to moderate-intensity activity is appropriate for patients with slow progressive disorders. Patients with disorders that are rapidly progressing should avoid high-resistance and eccentric muscle activity. With eccentric exercise, muscles elongate during contraction and oppose the force of gravity (eg, lowering of weights), resulting in high levels of tension in the muscle. Modification of exercise with intercurrent illness is also necessary.	Tarnopolsky 2002, Ansved 2003
Spinal stenosis	Avoid contact and collision sports.	
Orthopedic		
Scoliosis	No restrictions unless severe.	
Spondylolisthesis	Grade 2 and above should avoid contact sports or sports with lumbar hyperextension.	
Spondylolysis	No restrictions if pain-free.	
Respiratory		
Asthma	No activity restrictions. Using an inhaled short-acting β_2-agonist 15 min before exercise is recommended to help prevent exercise-induced bronchoconstriction. For athletes with asthma symptoms unassociated with exercise or who have frequent use of β_2-agonists (> 3 times per week), a regular inhaled corticosteroid should be considered. Antidoping regulations need to be considered for athletes using β_2-agonists.	Hull et al 2012
Pneumothorax	Can occur spontaneously in sports, especially in young, tall males. Athlete may present with atypical symptoms such as chest pain. Therefore, have a low threshold for obtaining chest x-ray. Management is per standard guideline recommendations. Athlete may return to sports when there is evidence of radiographic resolution. Increased risk for recurrence; should consider not participating in strenuous and contact sports.	Hull et al 2012
Tuberculosis	Active infection: not allowed to participate because of exposure to other athletes.	

(*Continued*)

Table 27-2. Recommendations and considerations for participation in sports. (*Continued*)

Disorders	Considerations and Recommendations	References
Other		
Cerebral palsy	Full participation with modifications.	
Developmental disabilities	Athletes with developmental disabilities often have associated medical problems including diabetes, obesity, and hypokinesis.	Platt 2001
Down syndrome	10%–40% have atlantoaxial instability. Head or neck trauma in these patients may cause catastrophic spinal cord injury.	Sanyer 2006
	Correlation of radiographic findings of atlantoaxial instability with neurologic abnormalities has not been well established. At present, there are no evidence-based guidelines for screening and activity restrictions. However, the Special Olympics requires radiographic screening in all athletes with Down syndrome and the American Academy of Pediatrics, while acknowledging the lack of evidence to support routine screening, also recommends plain films of the cervical spine to assess for atlantoaxial instability. If x-rays are abnormal, participation in contact sports or sports that entail high risk of head or neck trauma should not be allowed.	
	40%–50% of persons with Down syndrome have cardiac anomalies. Evaluation of underlying congenital heart disorders should be considered in this population.	
Remote spinal cord injury or spina bifida	Full participation.	
	Consider modification of equipment to accommodate activity or modification of activity to accommodate disability.	
	Consider how modification affects performance.	
	Be aware of thermoregulatory dysfunction, medications, and pressure areas.	

AHA, American Heart Association; EBV, Epstein-Barr virus; ECG, electrocardiogram; LVEF, left ventricular ejection fraction; NCAA, National Collegiate Athletic Association; WPW, Wolff-Parkinson-White syndrome.

McCambridge TM et al: Council on Sports Medicine and Fitness: policy statement—athletic participation by children and adolescents who have systemic hypertension. American Academy of Pediatrics. Pediatrics 2010 Jun;125(6):1287–1294 [PMID: 20513738].

Roberts WO et al: Advancing the preparticipation physical examination: an ACSM and FIMS Joint Consensus Statement. Clin J Sport Med 2014;24;442–447.

Seto C: The preparticipation physical examination: an update. Clin Sports Med 2011;30:491–501 [PMID: 21658544].

REHABILITATION OF SPORTS INJURIES

Participation in sports benefits children not only by promoting physical activity but also by the acquisition of motor and social skills. All sports participation, however, carries an inherent risk of injury. Injuries are classified as either acute or chronic. Chronic injuries occur over time as a result of overuse, repetitive microtrauma, and inadequate repair of injured tissue. When the demands of exercise exceed the body's ability to recover, overuse injury may occur. Overuse injury accounts for up to 50% of all injuries in pediatric sports medicine. Risk factors for overuse may include year round participation, participation in more than one team at a time, early specialization in one sport, poor mechanics, and training errors such as increasing exercise volume, load, frequency, or intensity too quickly. To avoid overuse injury, athletes should train with a regular variety of resistances, power, speed, agility, skills, and distance. Adequate periods of rest and recovery should be incorporated into every training regimen in order to ensure proper healing of stressed tissues. Treatment measures such as corticosteroid or platelet-rich plasma injections are more commonly used in skeletally mature athletes.

Present trends in injury rehabilitation and prevention focus on core stability training and dynamic warm-up and stretching. Core exercises emphasize isometric holds that activate the core and pelvis. They utilize light single limb movements to challenge endurance over protracted time periods. Programs should be age appropriate and modified as needed to exercise in a pain-free range. The development of back pain during a core program signifies poor technique, overly complicated curriculum, or a prior back injury. Exercise programs can be obtained from the website resource: http://www.webexercises.com.

Dynamic warm-up and stretching programs concentrate on light movement prior to exercise. Dynamic programs use controlled, full active range of motion of each joint for an overall excitatory and stretching effect prior to exercise. The aim is to initiate light perspiration and increase heart rate, peripheral circulation, and connective tissue suppleness through simple excitatory activity. In contrast to traditional static stretching regimens in which athletes hold a stretching position for a distinct period of time, an appropriate dynamic curriculum will incorporate aerobic activity and moving stretches into sport-specific movement preparation. Areas of focus include joint range of motion, proprioception, coordination, balance, flexibility, muscular contraction, and stimulation of the central nervous system and energy resources. For example, athletes may work through a series of exercises such as side shuffle, high knee stepping, bear crawls, and double-leg hopping over cones three times. Static stretching is appropriate after exercise is complete. A useful website to design a dynamic stretching program can be found at: http://www.webexercises.com.

Acute injuries or macrotrauma are one-time events that can cause alterations in biomechanics and physiology. Response to an acute injury occurs in predictable phases. The first week is characterized by an acute inflammatory response. During this time, initial vasoconstriction is followed by vasodilation. Chemical mediators of inflammation are released, resulting in the classical physical findings of local swelling, warmth, pain, and loss of function. This phase is essential in healing of the injury. The proliferative phase occurs over the next 2–4 weeks and involves repair and clean-up. Fibroblasts infiltrate and lay down new collagen. Last, the maturation phase allows for repair and regeneration of the damaged tissues.

The management of acute sports injuries focuses on optimizing healing and restoring function. The goals of immediate care are to minimize the effects of the injury by reducing pain and swelling, educate the athlete about the nature of the injury and how to treat it, and maintain the health and fitness of the rest of the body. The treatment for an acute injury is captured in the acronym PRICE:

- **P**rotect the injury from further damage (taping, splints, braces)
- **R**est the area
- **I**ce
- **C**ompression of the injury
- **E**levation immediately

Nonsteroidal anti-inflammatory drugs (NSAIDs) may reduce the inflammatory response and reduce discomfort. These medications may be used immediately after the injury. When safely and appropriately managed, therapeutic use of physical modalities, including early cold and later heat, hydrotherapy, massage, electrical stimulation, iontophoresis, and ultrasound, can enhance recovery in the acute phase.

The recovery phase can be lengthy and requires athlete participation. Physical therapy prescription is a common treatment modality. Initial treatment is focused on joint range of motion and flexibility. Range-of-motion exercises should follow a logical progression of starting with passive motion, then active assistive and finally active movement. Active range of motion is initiated once normal joint range has been reestablished. Flexibility exercises, particularly dynamic stretches, are sport-specific and aimed at reducing tightness of musculature. Strength training can begin early in this phase of rehabilitation. Initially only isometric exercises (static muscle contraction against stable resistance without movement of a joint or change in length of a muscle) are encouraged. As recovery progresses and flexibility increases, isotonic (change in length of a muscle without varying resistance) and isokinetic (change in length of a muscle against variable resistance without varying speed) exercises can be added to the program. These should be done at least three times per week.

As the athlete approaches near-normal strength and is pain-free, the final maintenance phase can be introduced. During this phase, the athlete continues to build strength and work on endurance. The biomechanics of sport-specific activity need to be analyzed and retraining incorporated into the exercise program. Generalized cardiovascular conditioning should continue during the entire rehabilitation treatment. Typically, return-to-play guidelines after an injury include the attainment of full joint range of motion, nearly full and symmetric strength, full speed, and nearly full sport-specific agility and skill.

Brooks GP et al: Musculoskeletal injury in children and skeletally immature adolescents: overview of rehabilitation for nonoperative injuries. UpToDate 2013. http://www.uptodate.com.hsl-ezproxy.ucdenver.edu/contents/musculoskeletal-injury-in-children-and-skeletally-immature-adolescents-overview-of-rehabilitation-for-nonoperative-injuries. Accessed February 11, 2016.

DiFiori JP et al: Overuse injuries and burnout in youth sports: a position statement from the American Medical Society for Sports Medicine. Clin J Sport Med 2014;24(1):3–20 [PMID: 24366013].

Faccioni A: Dynamic warm-up routines for sports. www.ptonthenet.com. 2001. http://www.ptonthenet.com/content/articleprint.aspx?p=1&ArticleID=MTAzNyA3ZHVRU20yM2MzVmRLRmVxeXRzY3NBPT0=. Accessed February 11, 2016.

Jayanthi N et al: Sports specialization in young athletes: evidence based recommendations. Sports Health 2013;5(3):251–257 [PMID: 24427392].

▼ COMMON SPORTS MEDICINE ISSUES & INJURIES

INFECTIOUS DISEASES

Infectious diseases are common in both recreational and competitive athletes. These illnesses have an effect on basic physiologic function and athletic performance. Physicians, parents, and coaches can adopt the guidelines listed in Table 27–3.

Active skin infections are common reasons to exclude athletes from sports participation. Herpes simplex, staphylococcal, molluscum, and tinea skin infections are commonly

Table 27–3. Sports participation guidelines: infectious diseases.

Bacterial dermatoses (including impetigo, furuncles, cellulitis, folliculitis, and abscesses)
> Athlete may participate when no new lesions for 48 h, no moist or draining lesions, and has completed oral antibiotics for at least 72 h

Diarrhea, infectious
> May participate: No.
> May increase risk of dehydration and heat illness. No participation is permitted unless symptoms are mild and athlete is fully hydrated.

Fever
> May participate: No.
> Cardiopulmonary effort increases with fever and maximum exercise capacity is reduced. Heat illness also more likely to occur.

Hepatitis, infectious
> May participate: Qualified yes.
> Minimal risk to others. May participate in all sports if health allows. Use universal precautions when handling blood or bodily fluids. Athlete should have skin lesions covered properly.

Herpes gladiatorum
> Transmission occurs by skin-to-skin contact. Athlete may participate when free of systemic symptoms, has no new lesions for 72 h, and has been on oral antiviral treatment for 120 h. Any open wounds must be properly covered.

Human immunodeficiency virus infection
> May participate: Yes.
> Minimal risk to others. May participate in all sports if health allows. Use universal precautions when handling blood or bodily fluids. Athletes should have skin lesions covered properly with an occlusive dressing. They should also be instructed to report bleeding wounds.

Infectious mononucleosis
> Splenomegaly is present in almost all cases and risk of splenic rupture is highest in the first 3 wk of illness. Once clinical symptoms resolve, gradual return to activity 3 wk after symptom onset is reasonable. Contact sports should be avoided until 4 weeks post illness onset.

Methicillin-resistant *Staphylococcus aureus* (MRSA) skin infections
> Athletes with suspected MRSA should be cultured and treated accordingly with antibiotics. Abscesses should be treated with incision and drainage. Athlete may return to sport when no new lesions for 48 h, no moist or draining lesions, and has been on oral antibiotics for at least 72 h.

Molluscum contagiosum
> Require appropriate covering for participation.

Streptococcal pharyngitis
> Athletes can resume activity once treatment has been provided for 24 h, and they are afebrile.

Upper respiratory infections
> May participate in sports if tolerated. Exceptions include those with fever, severe bacterial infections (sinusitis, pharyngitis), or those with symptoms below the neck. "Neck check" guide allows athletes to return to sports if symptoms are "above the neck" (eg, rhinorrhea, congestion, or sore throat). If symptoms "below the neck" (eg, fever or malaise) are present, the athlete should not participate.

Warts
> Require appropriate covering for participation.

seen and most easily transmitted in sports with skin-to-skin contact and shared equipment usage. In particular, athletes are at high risk for infection with community-associated methicillin-resistant *Staphylococcus aureus* (CA-MRSA). Recent reports of outbreaks in sports teams have prompted many sports organizations to adopt specific protocols to deal with the problem. Transmission is primarily by skin-to-skin contact and clinical manifestations are most commonly skin infections and soft tissue abscesses. Early treatment of CA-MRSA soft tissue infections by incision and drainage followed by appropriate antibiotic treatment is important to prevent significant morbidity and possible mortality.

Rice SG; Council on Sports Medicine and Fitness, American Academy of Pediatrics: Medical conditions affecting sports participation. Pediatrics 2008;121(4):841–848 [PMID: 18381550].

Selected Issues for the Adolescent Athlete and the Team Physician: A consensus statement. Med Sci Sports Exerc 2008 Nov;40(11):1997–2012 [PMID: 19430330].

HEAD & NECK INJURIES

Head and neck injuries occur most commonly in contact and individual sports. The sports with the highest incidence of brain injury are football, bicycling, baseball, and horseback riding. Concussions most commonly occur in football, ice hockey, rugby, boxing, basketball, lacrosse, soccer, bicycling, judo, and baseball/softball. The optimal treatment of these injuries has not been established and multiple guidelines have been developed. As a general rule, treatment of head and neck injuries in young children should be more conservative because of their developing central nervous systems.

1. Concussion

ESSENTIALS OF DIAGNOSIS & TYPICAL FEATURES

► Symptoms appear after a traumatic blow causing sudden movement to the head.

► Headache, dizziness, light or noise sensitivity, balance issues, fatigue, fogginess, and concentration difficulties are commonly present.

► Focal neurologic symptoms should raise concern for acute intracranial process or bleed and prompt more immediate workup.

► Efforts should be made to normalize activities of daily life as soon as possible by following the return to learn steps.

► Return to contact sports should take place only after the patient is back to normal with no symptoms and has successfully completed the return to play protocol.

Concussion is a complex process that occurs when a direct blow to the body or head translates forces into the brain, causing a transient alteration of neurologic function. Even in the presence of neurologic symptoms, concussions are usually not associated with structural changes in brain tissue detectable by standard imaging studies. Instead, they may cause metabolic and vascular changes in cerebral tissues. Consequently, there are complex alterations in physiologic function, such as catecholamine surges and failure of cerebral blood flow autoregulation, leading to the common symptoms we ascribe to this type of injury. Symptoms may appear and evolve over the first few hours after injury. Confusion, headache, visual disturbance, posttraumatic amnesia, and balance problems are common symptoms. It is important to note that concussion does not have to involve loss of consciousness. Concussion should be suspected in any athlete with somatic, cognitive, or behavioral complaints as listed in Table 27–4. Observers may notice physical signs, behavioral changes, or cognitive impairment in the injured athlete. Diagnosis may be aided by the use of the Sport Concussion Assessment Tool v.3 (SCAT5) and the Child-SCAT5 (ages 5–12 years), which also provide standardized patient handouts (available at: https://bjsm.bmj.com/content/51/11/851 and https://bjsm.bmj.com/content/bjsports/early/2017/04/26/bjsports-2017-097492childscat5.full.pdf). Regardless of level of participation or elite status, any athlete suspected of sustaining a concussion in a practice or competition should be immediately removed from play. The athlete should not be left alone in the initial hours after the injury in order to monitor for deterioration. An athlete diagnosed with a concussion should not be permitted to return to sport on the day of injury. In the acute setting, computed tomography (CT) is rarely indicated beyond the first 24 hours after injury. CT should be considered during initial evaluation if the patient displays deteriorating or altered mental status, prolonged loss of consciousness, repeated vomiting, severe headache, signs of skull fracture, or focal neurologic deficit or if he/she experienced a severe mechanism of injury.

Symptoms associated with concussions usually follow a predictable pattern and most resolve in 7–10 days. Children and adolescents tend to have a longer recovery interval. Acute management of concussion includes an early period of physical and cognitive rest (1–2 days), the exact duration of which is currently unknown. Return to school and light noncontact physical activity may be reasonable early during the recovery period if symptoms are not exacerbated. In young athletes, interventions may include modified school attendance, decreased school work, reduction in technological stimulation (television, Internet, computer games, cellular phone use), proper nutrition and hydration, and adequate rest and sleep. Before athletes are allowed to return to sports participation, symptoms should be resolved both at rest and during exercise without the aid of medication and a graduated return-to-play protocol should be completed. Return to play is a six-step progression with each step lasting 24 hours: (1) when asymptomatic at rest for 24 hours, progress to (2) light aerobic exercise, followed by (3) sport-specific exercise, then begin (4) noncontact drills, followed by (5) contact practice drills, and finally (6) release to game play. If any symptoms recur during any of the steps, the athlete should not move to the next stage and should rest for 24 hours, thereafter restarting at the previous step where the athlete was asymptomatic. Commonly, it is recommended that an athlete follow-up with a medical provider for clearance for return to contact or collision sports, and many states have passed legislation requiring medical assessment of concussed youth and medical clearance for return to play. Current expectations are that children should return to school prior to return to sport. In general, conservative return to play guidelines should be used in children.

Among commonly used assessment tools are the SCAT5, Standardized Assessment of Concussion (SAC), Balance Error Scoring System (BESS), computerized testing, and symptoms checklist (see Table 27–4). Neuropsychological testing may be helpful in assessing the cognitive function of concussed athletes, but it should not be used as the only source of clinical decision making. It may assist in management decisions for athletes with complex cases or severe or prolonged symptoms and is best performed and interpreted by a qualified neuropsychologist. Preseason testing may provide a comparison to help practitioners assess acute concussive status, but there is no solid evidence currently to support the use of baseline neuropsychological testing.

The long-term effects of concussions or contact/collision sports have yet to be established; specifically, a cause-and-effect relationship has not been proven between

Table 27–4. Concussion: symptom checklist.

Headache
Confusion
Amnesia: classically anterograde
Dizziness
Balance problems
Nausea
Vomiting
Visual disturbances
Light sensitivity
Noise sensitivity
Ringing in the ears
Fatigue or excessive sleepiness
Sleep abnormalities
Memory problems
Concentration difficulties
Irritability
Behavioral changes

concussions and chronic traumatic encephalopathy (CTE). Second impact syndrome is a controversial diagnosis primarily based on anecdotal reports. There is no universal agreement on the existence of this reported phenomenon. Advocates endorse a rare but potentially deadly complication of repeated head injury, causing loss of vascular autoregulation, catecholamine surge, increased cerebral blood pressure, and subsequent malignant cerebral edema without intracranial hematoma. Consequences include massive brain swelling and herniation leading to seizure, coma, and, possibly, death. Opponents suggest the phenomenon is actually the well-established condition of diffuse cerebral swelling, a known complication of head injury, particularly in younger individuals. The decision to retire an athlete from high risk or contact/collision sport is a sensitive and challenging one. There is currently little evidence to support a standardized approach to retirement decisions. However, considerations should include total number of concussions; increasing frequency; occurrence with serially less force; and prolonged, more severe, or permanent symptoms/signs.

Davis GA et al: The Child Sport Concussion Assessment Tool 5th Edition (Child SCAT5): background and rationale. Br J Sports Med 2017;51:859–861 [PMID: 28446452].

Davis GA et al: SCAT5. Br J Sports Med 2017. https://bjsm.bmj.com/content/bjsports/early/2017/04/26/bjsports-2017-097506SCAT5.full.pdf.

McCrory P, Davis G, Makdissi M: Second impact syndrome or cerebral swelling after sporting head injury. Curr Sports Med Rep 2012;11:21–23 [PMID: 22236821].

McCrory P et al: Consensus statement on concussion in sport: the 4th international conference on concussion in sport held in Zurich, November 2012. Br J Sports Med 2013;47:250–258 [PMID: 23479479].

Randolph C: Baseline neuropsychological testing in managing sport-related concussion: does it modify risk? Curr Sports Med Rep 2011;10(1):21–26 [PMID: 21228656].

Schatz P, Moser RS: Current issues in pediatric sports concussion. Clin Neuropsychol 2011:1–16 [PMID: 21391151].

2. Atlantoaxial Instability

Atlantoaxial instability is common in children with Down syndrome because of hypotonia and ligamentous laxity, especially including the annular ligament of C1. Consequently, this condition causes increased mobility at C1 and C2. Most cases are asymptomatic. Lateral cervical neck films in flexion, extension, and neutral position evaluate the atlantodens interval (ADI). ADI is normally less than 2.5 mm, but up to 4.5 mm is acceptable in this population. Children with an ADI greater than 4.5 mm or who have neurologic symptoms with neck flexion or extension should be restricted from contact and collision activities, as well as any sport requiring excessive neck flexion or extension until evaluation by an orthopedic specialist.

Dimberg EL: Management of common neurologic conditions in sports. Clin Sports Med 2005;24:637 [PMID: 16004923].

Klenck C, Gebke K: Practical management: common medical problems in disabled athletes. Clin J Sport Med 2007;17(1):55–60 [PMID: 17304008].

Winell J: Sports participation of children with Down syndrome. Orthop Clin North Am 2003;34:439 [PMID: 12974493].

3. Burners or Stingers

ESSENTIALS OF DIAGNOSIS & TYPICAL FEATURES

▶ Symptoms appear on the same side as an injury to the neck and shoulder.

▶ Burning pain or numbness in the shoulder and arm.

▶ Weakness may be present.

Burners or stingers are common injuries in contact sports, especially football. The two terms are used interchangeably to describe transient unilateral pain and paresthesias in the upper extremity. These cervical radiculopathies or brachial plexopathies typically occur when the head is laterally bent and the shoulder depressed, causing exacerbation of a degenerative cervical disk or stenosis, a compressive injury to a cervical nerve root on the symptomatic upper extremity, or a traction injury to the brachial plexus of the ipsilateral shoulder. Symptoms include immediate burning pain and paresthesias down one arm generally lasting only minutes. Unilateral weakness in the muscles of the upper trunk—supraspinatus, deltoid, and biceps—also tends to resolve quickly, but can persist for weeks. The most important part of the workup is a thorough neurologic assessment to differentiate this injury from a more serious brain or cervical spine injury. The key distinguishing feature of the stinger is its unilateral nature. If symptoms persist or include bilateral complaints, headache, change in mental status, or severe neck pain, a diagnostic evaluation should include a careful neurologic examination and possibly cervical spine radiographs, including flexion/extension views, magnetic resonance imaging (MRI) scans, and electromyography (EMG).

Treatment consists of removal from play and observation. The athlete can return to play once symptoms have resolved, neck and shoulder range of motion is pain-free, reflexes and strength are normal, and the Spurling test is negative. The Spurling test is performed by having the neck extended, rotated, and flexed to the ipsilateral shoulder while applying an axial load. Restriction of same day return to play should be considered in athletes with a history of multiple stingers, particularly if sustained in the same season.

Preventive strategies include always wearing well-fitting protective gear, proper blocking and tackling techniques, and maintaining neck and shoulder strength. Long-term complications are possible, including permanent neurologic injury or repeated occurrence of stingers, which would necessitate further workup and possible lifetime exclusion from contact or collision sports.

Ahearn BM, Starr HM, Seiler JG: Traumatic brachial plexopathy in athletes: current concepts for diagnosis and management of stingers. J Am Acad Orthop Surg 2019;27(18):677–684 [PMID: 30741724].

Cantu RC, Li YM, Abdulhamid M, Chin LS: Return to play after cervical spine injury in sports. Curr Sports Med Rep 2013;12:14–17 [PMID: 23314078].

Standaert CJ, Herring SA: Expert opinion and controversies in musculoskeletal and sports medicine: stingers. Arch Phys Med Rehabil 2009;90:402–406 [PMID: 19254603].

SPINE INJURIES

As children have become more competitive in sports, spine injuries have become more common. Sports with a fairly high incidence of spine injuries include golf, gymnastics, football, dance, wrestling, and weightlifting. Back pain lasting more than 2 weeks indicates a possible structural problem that should be investigated.

Acute injury to the spine often results from an axial load injury. Patients present with focal tenderness of the thoracic or thoracolumbar spine. Evaluation includes plain radiography that may demonstrate anterior wedging of the thoracic vertebra, representing a compression fracture. When significant spinal tenderness or any neurologic abnormalities are present, radiographs are often followed by CT or MRI. Treatment of minor compression fractures includes pain control, bracing, rest from high-risk sports, and physical therapy. With appropriate rehabilitation, athletes can usually return to contact activity within 8 weeks.

1. Spondylolysis

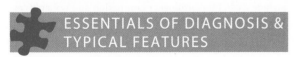

ESSENTIALS OF DIAGNOSIS & TYPICAL FEATURES

► Injury to the pars interarticularis.
► Usually presents as lower back pain with extension.

Spondylolysis is an injury to the pars interarticularis of the vertebral complex, resulting in a stress reaction or an acquired stress fracture. The pars interarticularis is the bony connection between the inferior and superior articulating facets.

Injuries to the pars interarticularis, or pars defects for short, are present in 4%–6% of the population. In adolescent athletes, however, the incidence of spondylolysis in those presenting with lower back pain is close to 50%. As such, it should be high on the differential when evaluating lower back pain in this population. The incidence of pars defects in athletes such as gymnasts, dancers, divers, and wrestlers is significantly increased because of the repetitive flexion/extension motions combined with rotation. Repetitive overload results in stress fractures. Spondylolysis occurs at L5 in 85% of cases. The athlete presents with midline low back pain that is aggravated by extension, such as arching the back in gymnastics. There may be palpable tenderness over the lower lumbar vertebrae, with pain on the single leg hyperextension test (Stork test). Tight hamstrings are another common physical finding. Evaluation includes anteroposterior (AP) and lateral radiographs of the lumbar spine. Although oblique radiographic views of the lumbar spine are helpful to look for the so-called Scottie dog sign, they are falling out of favor because they do not significantly improve diagnostic accuracy and increase radiation exposure. Single-photon emission computed tomography (SPECT) scan, CT scan, and MRI can be useful to determine the presence of an active spondylotic lesion. Bone/SPECT scan shows stress reaction or pars injury before other radiographic changes. CT provides excellent definition of bony anatomy and can document healing. MRI is an alternative to detect pars interarticularis problems. With the use of high magnetic field strength and fat saturation techniques, high-resolution MRI scans can now show subtle bone marrow edema of early stress injuries and are becoming popular, particularly for pediatric patients because of the lack of radiation exposure. There is currently no gold standard for the treatment of spondylolysis. The goal is to alleviate painful symptoms and allow the athlete a safe return to play. Management includes refraining from hyperextension and high-impact sporting activities, stretching of the hamstrings, and core and back stabilization exercises. Athletes can cross-train with low-impact activity and neutral or flexion-based physical therapy. Bracing is controversial. Outcome studies show similar results regarding return to sports and bony healing whether or not braces are worn. It is important to note also that clinical outcome does not necessarily correlate with healed pars fracture versus bony nonunions (when the fractured bone fails to heal). Satisfactory outcomes (asymptomatic patients and return to sports) can be achieved regardless of bony healing status. Typically, return to play is often delayed 8–12 weeks or longer based on clinical signs of healing. Most symptomatic spondylolysis improves with rest and activity modifications (with or without radiologic evidence of healing). Once asymptomatic, an athlete can usually return to sports without restrictions. Surgery is reserved for refractory cases that fail conservative measures.

2. Spondylolisthesis

ESSENTIALS OF DIAGNOSIS & TYPICAL FEATURES

▶ Bilateral pars interarticularis injury resulting in forward slippage of one vertebra over the one below it.

▶ Usually presents as back pain with extension.

▶ Hyperlordosis or possible step-off of lumbar spine.

When a bilateral pars stress fracture (spondylolysis) occurs, slippage of one vertebra over another causes a spondylolisthesis. Patients present with hyperlordosis, kyphosis, pain with hyperextension, and, in severe cases, a palpable step-off. A standing lateral radiograph is used to make the diagnosis and to monitor for any progression of slippage. These injuries are graded from 1 to 4 based on the percentage of slippage: grade 1 (0%–24%), grade 2 (25%–49%), grade 3 (50%–74%), and grade 4 (75%–100%).

Treatment is often symptom based. Asymptomatic athletes with less than 25% slippage often have no restrictions and are followed on a routine basis for radiograph assessment. Management of symptomatic spondylolisthesis requires a period of activity modifications, particularly protection from spine extension and impact activities, coupled with a regimen of stretching of the hamstrings and core and back stabilization exercises. Bracing may also be considered. Surgical intervention is considered for slippage greater than 50%, progressive spondylolisthesis, or intractable pain despite nonoperative treatment. If surgery is required, the athlete must understand that he or she cannot return to activities for at least 1 year and may not be able return to previous sporting activities.

3. Disk Herniation

ESSENTIALS OF DIAGNOSIS & TYPICAL FEATURES

▶ Back pain worse with flexion and sitting.

▶ Radiculopathy can be present.

▶ Positive straight leg raise.

Discogenic back pain accounts for a small percentage of back injuries in children. These injuries are almost unheard of in preadolescence. Back pain can originate from disk bulging, disk herniation, or disk degeneration. Most injuries occur at L4–L5 and L5–S1 vertebrae. Not all disk bulges found on MRI are symptomatic. In adolescents, most disk herniations are central rather than posterolateral. Risk factors include heavy lifting,

excessive or repetitive axial loading of the spine, rapid increases in training, or trauma. Symptoms include back pain, which may be increased with activities such as bending, sitting, and coughing. Although not as common as in adults, radicular symptoms of pain down the leg can also occur and are often associated with large disk herniations. Evaluation includes physical and neurologic examinations, including straight leg testing, sensory testing, and checking reflexes. If symptoms persist, evaluation usually begins with radiographs and an MRI, which is the imaging test of choice for diagnosing disk herniation. EMG may also be considered in the presence of radiculopathy.

Treatment usually is conservative as most disk herniations, even if large, improve spontaneously. The athlete can rest the back for a short period, with avoidance of prolonged sitting, jumping, or hyperextension and hyperflexion of the spine, as these activities may increase pressure on the disk, leading to aggravation of symptoms. After a short period of rest, a structured physical therapy program should begin, focusing on core and pelvic stabilization, peripelvic flexibility and sports or activity specific conditioning. If symptoms persist, a short course of oral steroids or epidural steroid injection may be indicated. Surgery is recommended for patients who fail conservative therapy, have significant or progressive radiculopathy, or who have progressive neurologic deficit.

Kim H, Green D: Spondylolysis in the adolescent athlete. Curr Opinion Ped 2011;23:68–72 [PMID: 21150440].

Lavelle W et al: Pediatric disk herniation. J Am Acad Orthop Surg 2011;19:649–656 [PMID: 22052641].

Selected issues for the adolescent athlete and the team physician: a consensus statement. Med Sci Sports Exerc Nov 2008;40(11):1997–2012 [PMID: 19430330].

SHOULDER INJURIES

Shoulder injury is usually a result of acute trauma or chronic overuse. Acute injuries around the shoulder include contusions, fractures, sprains (or separations), and dislocations. The age of the patient affects the injury pattern, as younger patients are more likely to sustain fractures instead of sprains. Sprains (ligaments) and strains (muscle and tendon) are generally defined as low-grade soft tissue injuries that do not result in functional compromise of a structure.

1. Fracture of the Clavicle

ESSENTIALS OF DIAGNOSIS & TYPICAL FEATURES

▶ Injury by fall on to the shoulder or outstretched hand.

▶ Severe pain in the shoulder.

▶ Tenderness, swelling, and/or deformity over the clavicle.

Clavicular fractures occur from a fall or direct trauma to the shoulder. Focal swelling, deformity, and tenderness are present over the clavicle. The diagnosis is made by radiographs of the clavicle; the fractures are most common in the middle third of the bone.

Initial treatment is focused on pain control and protection with a sling and swathe. Early range of motion is permitted based on pain level. Progressive rehabilitation is important. Athletes cannot return to contact sports for 8–12 weeks. Absolute surgical indications for acute clavicular fractures include open fractures or neurovascular compromise. Fracture nonunion is unusual in young patients. However, there is recent evidence in the adult population recommending surgical stabilization for fractures that are very displaced or shortened. The role of acute surgical stabilization in the pediatric and adolescent population in regards to shortening is still being defined. Patients with recurrent fractures or nonunion typically will also require surgical fixation.

2. Acromioclavicular Separation

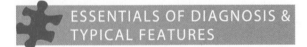

▶ Injury with fall on the shoulder.

▶ Severe pain in the shoulder.

▶ Tenderness, swelling, and/or deformity over the acromioclavicular joint.

A fall on the point of the shoulder is the most common cause of acromioclavicular (AC) separation. Tearing of the acromioclavicular joint capsule and possibly the coracoclavicular ligaments occurs. The injury is classified by the extent of the injuries to these ligaments. Athletes present with focal soft tissue swelling and tenderness over the acromioclavicular joint. More severe injuries are associated with deformity. Patients have a positive cross-arm test, in which pain is localized to the acromioclavicular joint. Radiographs are necessary in this setting to assess the degree of injury and to evaluate for a coexisting fracture or growth plate injury.

Treatment of low-grade AC injuries is supportive, with rest and immobilization in a sling followed by progressive rehabilitation. Return to activity can be accomplished in 1–6 weeks depending on the severity of the injury and the persistence of symptoms. Full range of motion and full strength must be achieved prior to being cleared to return to sports. More severe injuries may require surgical intervention.

3. Fracture of the Humerus

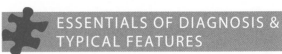

▶ Injury with significant fall on outstretched arm.

▶ Severe pain in the proximal humerus.

▶ Tenderness, swelling, and/or deformity over the proximal humerus.

Fractures of the humerus occur from a severe blow or fall on the shoulder. Pain and swelling are localized to the proximal humeral region. The fractures can include the physes or may be extraphyseal. A significant amount of displacement and angulation can be tolerated in this location because of the young athlete's potential for remodeling and because of the intrinsic range of motion of the shoulder. Careful assessment of the brachial plexus and radial nerves are needed to rule out associated nerve damage.

Treatment consists of a sling and often a hanging arm cast to allow for gravity to reduce the fracture for 4–6 weeks followed by progressive rehabilitation with return to play at 8–12 weeks when bony healing, full range of motion, and strength have been achieved.

4. Acute Traumatic Anterior Shoulder Instability (Anterior Shoulder Dislocation/Subluxation)

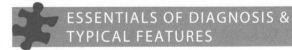

▶ Injury with an abducted and externally rotated arm.

▶ Severe pain in the shoulder.

▶ Squared-off shoulder on examination.

▶ Reduced range of motion of the shoulder.

Acute traumatic anterior shoulder instability occurs when significant force is applied to the abducted and externally rotated shoulder. Most often, the humeral head is dislocated in an anterior and inferior direction. The patient has severe pain and a mechanical block to motion. Some patients will spontaneously reduce within seconds or minutes of their injury. Most patients, however, require immediate closed reduction on the field or in the emergency room. Radiographs are helpful to confirm the position of the humeral head as well as to evaluate for coexisting fracture. MRI may be required for accurate visualization of fractures and cartilaginous injury.

Optimal follow-up treatment for glenohumeral dislocation in young athletes has not been established. Initially, the shoulder is immobilized for comfort. Range-of-motion exercises and progressive rehabilitation are initiated. Prolonged immobilization does not decrease the risk of recurrence and is discouraged. Return to play in-season can be considered with appropriate counseling and when rehabilitation has achieved full range of motion and strength. A brace is often used when an athlete returns to sport in season. Because of the high risk of recurrence in the adolescent population, options for treatment should be individualized, with consideration given to both nonoperative and surgical management.

5. Rotator Cuff Injury

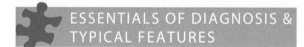

ESSENTIALS OF DIAGNOSIS & TYPICAL FEATURES

▶ Injury can be acute or chronic.
▶ Pain is described as diffuse or anterior and lateral.
▶ Overhead activities exacerbate the pain.

Shoulder injuries are often a consequence of repetitive overuse and tissue failure. Rotator cuff tendonitis and bursitis are the most commonly observed rotator cuff injuries in youth sports. Rotator cuff tears, including traumatic tears, in children and adolescents are exceedingly rare. Most commonly, rotator cuff injuries are overuse injuries and typically occur in sports requiring repetitive overhead motions. Muscle imbalances and injury can cause the position of the humeral head to be abnormal, which may cause entrapment of the supraspinatus tendon under the acromial arch. Patients with nontraumatic shoulder instability due to ligamentous and capsular laxity (also known as multidirectional instability) are prone to overuse rotator cuff injury. These athletes present with chronic pain in the anterior and lateral shoulder, which is increased with overhead activities. Diagnostic workup includes plain radiographs and an outlet view to look for anatomic variability. The rehabilitation of this injury is geared toward reduction of inflammation, improved flexibility, and core stabilization and strengthening of the scapular stabilizers and rotator cuff muscles. A biomechanics evaluation can assist athletes in the recovery process by building

sport-specific skills and eliminating substitution patterns. Surgery is rarely indicated.

6. Little League Shoulder

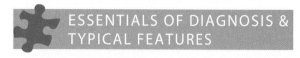

ESSENTIALS OF DIAGNOSIS & TYPICAL FEATURES

▶ Participation in a throwing sport.
▶ Pain with throwing.
▶ Pain in the lateral aspect of the humerus.
▶ Swelling around the shoulder.
▶ Widening of the proximal humeral physis on radiographs.

Proximal humeral epiphysitis, or "Little League shoulder," is an overuse injury that occurs in children aged 11–14 years who play overhead sports such as baseball. The patient presents with activity-related pain in the lateral aspect of the proximal humerus. Examination often shows tenderness over the proximal humerus. Absence of findings on office examination does not preclude this diagnosis. The hallmark feature is pain with throwing. Radiographs show widening, sclerosis, and irregularity of the proximal humeral physis. Comparison views are often helpful when considering this diagnosis.

Treatment consists of rest from throwing or other aggravating activity. Physical therapy is initiated during the rest period. Return to play can only be considered after a period of rest has significantly decreased the pain and the athlete has proceeded through a progressive throwing program. Healing can take several months. Signs of radiographic healing may lag behind the athlete's clinical progress and normal radiographs are not necessarily required to return an athlete to play. Permanent sequelae such as fracture, growth arrest, or deformity is extremely rare but can occur in chronic cases that are not treated appropriately.

Brophy RH, Marx RG: The treatment of traumatic anterior instability of the shoulder: nonoperative and surgical treatment. Arthroscopy 2009;25:298–304 [PMID: 19245994].
Mariscalco MW, Saluan P: Upper extremity injuries in the adolescent athlete. Sports Med Arthrosc Rev 2011;19:17–26 [PMID: 21293234].

ELBOW INJURIES

Injuries in the elbow are quite common and have both chronic and acute etiologies. They often occur in athletes involved in throwing or overhead sports. Although acute injuries to the elbow are common, chronic overuse injuries are becoming more and more prevalent in young athletes. Risk factors leading to overuse elbow injury include single sport specialization, year-round participation, longer competitive seasons, insufficient rest, and poor biomechanics. The term *Little League elbow* is used loosely to encompass a variety of causes of elbow pain in young throwing athletes. These injuries include medial epicondylitis, apophysitis, medial epicondyle avulsion fracture, Panner disease, and osteochondritis dissecans (OCD) of the capitellum. It is intended, however, to refer to medial epicondyle apophysitis, an overuse elbow injury resulting from repetitive valgus stress from overhead throwing.

When the elbow is evaluated, it is helpful to divide the examination into specific anatomic areas, discussed as follows.

1. Medial Epicondyle Apophysitis (Little League Elbow)

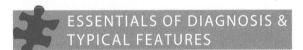

ESSENTIALS OF DIAGNOSIS & TYPICAL FEATURES

▶ Participation in a throwing sport.
▶ Pain over the medial epicondyle, especially with pitching.
▶ Tenderness and swelling of the medial elbow.

Little League elbow is a traction injury to the medial epicondylar physis, which develops in young overhead throwing athletes, particularly baseball pitchers, between the ages of 9 and 12 years. The biomechanical forces generated around the elbow during throwing, namely repetitive valgus stress, can result in shearing, inflammation, traction, and abnormal bone development. The symptoms are primarily swelling, medial elbow pain, performance difficulties, and weakness. The pain localizes to the medial epicondyle, which may be tender to palpation, and worsens with valgus stress. Wrist flexion and forearm pronation may increase symptoms. The physician should inquire about the exposure to throwing, including pitch counts, the number of practices and games, and the duration of the season. Workup includes elbow radiographs, with comparison films of the unaffected side, to look for widening of the apophysis. Rarely, MRI is used to confirm the diagnosis.

Treatment of the injury includes complete rest from throwing activities. It is not uncommon for a player to be restricted from throwing for up to 6 weeks. Competition can be resumed once the player is asymptomatic and has progressed through a graduated, age-appropriate throwing program. The key approach for this injury is prevention. Children should be properly conditioned and coached in

Table 27–5. Guidelines for pitching limits in youth baseball.

Age (y)	Pitches per Day
7–8	50
9–10	75
11–12	85
13–16	95
17–18	105

correct throwing biomechanics. Guidelines for Little League pitching limits in youth baseball have been developed and are outlined in Table 27–5.

2. Panner Disease

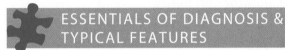

ESSENTIALS OF DIAGNOSIS & TYPICAL FEATURES

▶ Participation in a throwing sport.
▶ Pain over the lateral elbow.
▶ Swelling and flexion contracture.

Panner disease refers to developmental osteochondrosis of the capitellum that results from overuse injury. The lesion involves disordered ossification of the capitellum, which is the lower end of the humerus that articulates with the radius. This condition occurs in children aged 5–12 years who play sports that involve overhead throwing and in gymnasts. The repetitive lateral compressive forces from loading the elbow in these sports compromises the blood supply to the growing epiphysis, leading to degeneration of the ossification center, or osteochondrosis. The child may have dull aching in the lateral elbow that worsens with throwing. Swelling and reduced elbow extension usually are present. Radiocapitellar compression test will also elicit pain—with elbow fully extended, arm is actively pronated and supinated. Radiographs show an abnormal, flattened capitellum, with fragmentation and areas of sclerosis. This should be distinguished from OCD of the capitellum, which typically occur in older children (see as follows). Treatment is conservative, using rest, ice, and splinting. Avoid activities that load the elbow for 3–6 months. The child can return to play once symptoms resolve, and there is evidence of healing on follow-up radiographs. The natural history of this condition is one of complete resolution of symptoms and, ultimately, normal ossification of the capitellum.

3. Ulnar Collateral Ligament Tear

ESSENTIALS OF DIAGNOSIS & TYPICAL FEATURES

▶ Sudden forceful tensile stress on ligament from a fall or from valgus stress to elbow during overhead throw.

▶ Feeling a pop or sensation of elbow giving out.

▶ Medial elbow pain.

▶ Tenderness distal to medial epicondyle.

Once the medial epicondylar physis closes in a skeletally mature athlete, valgus forces are then transmitted to the ulnar collateral ligament, resulting in a sprain or tear. Patients present with medial elbow pain and are often unable to fully extend the elbow. Examination reveals tenderness just distal to the medial epicondyle, and there may be instability with valgus stressing. Treatment is conservative, including rest, ice, and physical therapy directed at range of motion and strengthening. Surgery may be suggested for those with persistent pain or instability and who desire to continue participating in overhead sports.

4. Osteochondritis Dissecans

ESSENTIALS OF DIAGNOSIS & TYPICAL FEATURES

▶ Participation in a throwing sport.

▶ Pain over the lateral elbow, especially with pitching.

▶ Tenderness over the radiocapitellar joint.

▶ Elbow flexion contracture.

Lateral elbow pain in a slightly older throwing athlete, usually aged 13–15 years, can be secondary to osteochondritis dissecans (OCD), which is a more worrisome diagnosis than Panner disease. Unlike Panner disease, which is self-limiting, OCD lesions can lead to permanent destruction of the bone. It is an injury to the subchondral bone and its overlying articular cartilage can then become involved. Although it can involve different sites of the elbow, including the olecranon, radial head, or trochlea, it most commonly affects the capitellum. Repetitive valgus compressive forces can lead to avascular necrosis of the capitellum, which can ultimately result in the formation of loose bodies in the joint. The athlete presents with lateral pain, swelling, lack of full extension, and

occasionally locking. Radiographs show lucency of the capitellum with surrounding sclerotic bone. MRI can more fully delineate the lesion. The prognosis for high-grade lesions is guarded.

A child with OCD should be seen by either a sports medicine specialist or an orthopedic surgeon with expertise in upper extremity injuries. Treatment is based on stability of the lesion and can be either conservative or surgical. For early or stable OCD lesions, particularly in skeletally immature individuals, management includes throwing activity restrictions and range of motion exercises. More advanced lesions or those with persistent symptoms despite conservative treatment may require surgical intervention.

5. Lateral Epicondylitis

Lateral epicondylitis (also known as *tennis elbow*) is common in skeletally mature athletes participating in racquet sports. It is a tendinopathy of the extensor muscles in the forearm, which inserts onto the lateral epicondyle causing lateral elbow pain. The pain is increased by wrist extension. Initial treatment is aimed at inflammation control. Stretching and strengthening of forearm muscles are the primary interventions during the subsequent phases. Stroke mechanics may need to be altered and a forearm brace used to decrease the forces in the extensor muscles.

6. Posterior Elbow Pain

Posterior elbow pain is uncommon. Etiologies include dislocations, impingement, fractures, triceps avulsions and tendinitis, olecranon apophysitis, and olecranon bursitis.

Gerbino PG: Elbow disorders in throwing athletes. Orthop Clin North Am 2003;34:417 [PMID: 12974491].

Kobayashi K et al: Lateral compression injuries in the pediatric elbow: Panner's disease and osteochondritis dissecans of the capitellum. J Am Acad Orthop Surg 2004;12:246–254 [PMID: 15473676].

Little League: http://www.littleleague.org. Accessed January 31, 2018.

HAND & WRIST INJURIES

The hand and wrist are the most common area of injury in children and account for a large proportion of emergency room visits. All hand and wrist injuries have the potential for serious long-term disability and deserve thorough evaluation. A thorough neurovascular examination as well as evaluation of rotational or angular deformity or malalignment is critical. Examples of complications include loss of range of motion, dysfunction, deformity, limb length discrepancy, and arthritis.

1. Distal Phalanx Injury

Tuft injury requires splinting for 3–6 weeks or until the patient is pain free. If there is significant displacement, a surgical K-wire can be used for reduction. Nail-bed injury often requires nail-bed suturing, splinting, and drainage of subungual hematomas. Nail avulsions should be replaced into the nail fold, and if not possible, a substitute material should be interposed into the nail bed as a stent. Patients with nail-bed injuries should be advised that nail regrowth may appear irregular or may not occur at all.

2. Distal Interphalangeal Injury

Mallet finger or extensor tendon avulsion occurs more commonly in ball-handling sports. The mechanism of injury is an axial load or forced flexion against an actively extending finger, causing avulsion fracture or rupture of the extensor digitorum tendon. Athletes present with a flexion contracture at the distal interphalangeal (DIP) joint and inability to actively extend the distal phalanx. Referral to an orthopedic surgeon is necessary. Conservative treatment consists of splinting in extension for 4 weeks for fractures and 6–8 weeks for tendon rupture. Surgery may be required if the initial fracture involves greater than 30% of the joint space or poor healing with loss of function occurs.

Jersey finger, or flexor tendon avulsion, occurs in contact sports, particularly American football. The mechanism of injury is forced extension against an actively flexed finger. The fourth ("ring") finger is the most commonly injured digit. Athletes present with tenderness, swelling, and inability to flex at the DIP. The examiner can test the function of the flexor tendon by holding the proximal interphalangeal joint in extension while having the injured athlete attempt flexion at the DIP joint. The injured finger should be splinted in a comfortable position and immediately referred to an orthopedic surgeon, as definitive treatment is often surgical.

3. Thumb Injury

Gamekeeper's or skier's thumb is an injury to the ulnar collateral ligament from forced abduction of the thumb metacarpophalangeal (MCP) joint. It is a common skiing injury to those who fall while holding on to their ski poles. Patients will complain of pain over the medial aspect of the MCP joint and pain with apposition or pinching. If a radiograph shows an avulsed fragment that is displaced less than 2 mm, a thumb spica cast can be used. If there is no fragment, less than 35 degrees of lateral joint space opening, or less than 15 degrees difference in joint space opening compared to the uninjured thumb, a spica cast for 4–6 weeks is indicated. Surgery is required for more serious injuries.

4. Hand Fractures

All finger fractures should be assessed for growth plate involvement, rotation, angulation, and displacement. If stable and not displaced, these fractures can be splinted for 3–4 weeks and buddy-taped for immediate return to sports. However, spiral or oblique fractures of the middle phalanx, intra-articular fractures, and severely angulated physeal fractures are considered unstable and should be referred to an orthopedic surgeon.

Boxer's fracture is a neck fracture of the fourth or fifth metacarpal, typically caused by poor punching technique or punching into a hard surface. Less than 40 degrees of volar/dorsal angulation in the fourth or fifth metacarpals is acceptable. Assessment of displacement and rotational deformity by looking at the cascade of the fingers while the patient holds a loose fist is critical, as displaced or rotated fractures require reduction and fixation. Prior to definitive treatment with hand-based casting for 4 weeks, boxer's fractures may be temporarily immobilized with an ulnar gutter splint with the MCP joints flexed to 70 degrees.

5. Wrist Injury

Most swollen wrists without evidence of gross deformity or instability can be splinted temporarily for several days. Distal radial and ulnar fractures, which are fairly common in children, must be ruled out. Particular attention should be paid to the growth plates and the scaphoid bone. Typically, distal radius and ulna fractures require casting for 3–6 weeks in either a short or long arm cast, depending on the involvement of one or both bones and the severity of displacement or angulation. Torus, or buckle, fractures may be placed in a rigid wrist brace or short arm cast for 3–4 weeks. Scaphoid fractures are caused by a force applied to a hyperextended wrist, most commonly a fall onto an outstretched hand. Despite normal radiographs, if evidence of snuffbox tenderness and swelling is present, there is tenderness along the volar aspect of the scaphoid, or there is pain with radial wrist deviation or active wrist range of motion; the wrist must be further evaluated, either by MRI acutely or immobilized for 10 days and then reassessed both clinically and with follow-up radiographs. A nondisplaced scaphoid fracture requires at least 6 weeks of immobilization in a thumb spica cast. Nonunion can occur, particularly in fractures of the proximal pole of the scaphoid, related to the poor blood supply of this area of the bone. Displacement requires operative management. Gymnast's wrist is chronic wrist pain due to repetitive overloading of the distal radial physis. Athletes complain of dorsal wrist pain, worsened with weight bearing on the affected upper extremity or active extension of the wrist. This overuse stress injury may cause long-term growth abnormalities or degenerative wrist joint changes, which may ultimately require surgical intervention. Athletes should be placed in a rigid wrist brace or short arm cast for 4 weeks and undergo a period of relative rest and activity modification.

Anz AW et al: Pediatric scaphoid fractures. J Am Acad Orthop Surg 2009;17:77–87 [PMID: 19202121].

Cornwall R, Ricchetti ET: Pediatric phalanx fractures: unique challenges and pitfalls. Clin Orthop Relat Res 2006 Apr;445:146–156 [PMID: 16505727].

Mariscalco MW, Saluan P: Upper extremity injuries in the adolescent athlete. Sports Med Arthrosc Rev 2011;19(1):17–26 [PMID: 21293234].

Williams AA, Lochner HV: Pediatric hand and wrist injuries. Current Rev Musculoskeletal Med 2013;6:18–25 [PMID: 23264097].

HIP INJURIES

Because the pelvis and hip articulate with both the lower extremities and the spine, this area is rich in ligaments, muscle attachments, and nerves. Injuries in young children are rare, but sprains, strains, and avulsion fractures can occur. Additionally, athletes can be susceptible to overuse injury involving the hip.

1. Hip Avulsion Fractures

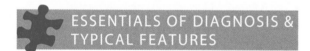

ESSENTIALS OF DIAGNOSIS & TYPICAL FEATURES

▶ Fractures at apophyseal areas.

▶ Pain with weight bearing.

▶ Focal pain over the site of injury.

Avulsion fractures around the hip in adolescents occur at apophyseal regions such as the ischial tuberosity, anterior superior iliac spine, anterior inferior iliac spine, and iliac crest. The mechanism of injury is a forceful, unbalanced muscle contraction that causes avulsion of the muscle tendon insertion. The athlete presents with a history of an acute traumatic incident; often a "pop" is felt and the athlete is immediately unable to bear weight. Range of motion of the hip is limited secondary to pain, and focal tenderness is present over the apophysis.

Treatment is usually conservative. Surgical management is reserved for significantly displaced fractures. The athlete is typically placed on crutches for the first couple of weeks for pain control and to normalize gait. After the acute phase, an athlete can progress to weight bearing as tolerated. The rehabilitation phase focuses on regaining motion, flexibility

training and pelvic, and core strengthening. Progressive return to activity can often be accomplished in 4–6 weeks, if full range of motion, full strength, and sport-specific skills have been achieved.

2. Slipped Capital Femoral Epiphysis

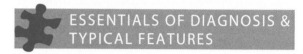

ESSENTIALS OF DIAGNOSIS & TYPICAL FEATURES

▶ Pain in the hip or knee, or both.

▶ Loss of internal rotation of the hip.

▶ Radiographs in the frog-leg position show widening of the physis and epiphyseal slippage.

Slipped capital femoral epiphysis occurs in children aged 11–16 years and is associated with obesity and some endocrinopathies such as hypothyroidism. The physis is weakened during times of rapid growing and is susceptible to shearing failure either acutely secondary to a traumatic injury or insidiously from chronic overload. Patients complain of groin, thigh, or knee pain and often have a limp or, in unstable cases, they may not be able to bear weight. Examination shows painful range of motion of the hip, limited internal rotation, and obligatory external rotation when the hip is flexed. Radiographs include AP and frog-leg lateral films, which demonstrate widening of the physis and epiphyseal slippage or displacement of the femoral head relative to the femoral neck.

Treatment consists of immediate non–weight-bearing and urgent referral to an orthopedic specialist for surgical stabilization. Failure to identify this injury can increase the chance of avascular necrosis resulting in early arthritis. Rehabilitation is a component of the postsurgical treatment. Return to activity is progressive over months. (See also Chapter 26.)

3. Acetabular Labral Tears

Acetabular labral tears are an increasingly recognized cause of anterior hip and groin pain in athletes. The majority of hip labral tears occur as a result of an underlying anatomical abnormality such as femoroacetabular impingement (FAI) or hip dysplasia. Because of the stress and range of motion requirements for most athletics, these injuries tend to present and be more symptomatic in the athletic population. Athletes with this injury typically do not report an acute traumatic event that precipitated their symptoms. Symptoms often develop insidiously rather than acutely.

Athletes often present with deep anterior hip or groin pain that worsens with activity and is resistant to treatment. Radiographic imaging generally shows no acute findings but will outline the structural aberrances that may have caused the labral tear over time. An MRI is used to demonstrate the tear. Treatment typically starts conservatively and requires rest and physical therapy. Ultimately, treatment is tailored to the athlete's particular needs and symptoms. Arthroscopy to repair the tear and address any underlying structural issue that caused the tear is often required.

4. Adductor Strain

An adductor strain or a groin pull is generally caused by forced abduction during running, falling, twisting, or tackling. Sports that require quick directional changes place athletes at risk for these types of injuries. The associated pain is in the adductor muscle. There is often pain with hip adduction or flexion and tenderness over the adductor tubercle. Treatment includes rest, ice, and protection—often with crutches, and strengthening of the muscle when it heals.

5. Hamstring Strain

ESSENTIALS OF DIAGNOSIS & TYPICAL FEATURES

▶ Mechanism is forced knee extension.
▶ Pain with tearing or popping sensation in the posterior leg.
▶ Pain with resisted knee extension.

Hamstring strain is a common injury in athletes. The majority of these injuries occur in the muscle belly and can be treated successfully with nonoperative management. The mechanism of injury is forced extension of the knee or directional changes. Typically, the athlete with a hamstring strain suddenly stops playing and grabs the back of the thigh. There are three grades of injury. Examination reveals pain on palpation of the muscle and occasionally a defect. Pain also occurs with knee flexion against resistance.

Initial treatment is focused on minimizing swelling, bruising, and pain. The thigh should be iced and compression applied. In moderate and severe injuries, crutches may be needed for a short duration. The athlete can walk as soon as he or she can tolerate the activity. It is particularly important to stretch the hamstring because, as a two-joint muscle, it is more susceptible to injury than other types of muscle. Eccentric strengthening is an important component of rehabilitation.

6. Quadriceps Contusion

Quadriceps contusion is caused by a direct injury to the muscle that causes bruising, swelling, and pain. The amount of damage is directly related to the amount of force. The anterior and lateral thigh regions are most commonly injured, often in contact sports such as football and lacrosse.

Treatment is rest, ice, and protection for the first 24 hours. The knee should be kept in a fully flexed position to tamponade any further hematoma formation. Two to 3 days after the injury, range-of-motion exercises may begin in both flexion and extension. Once 120 degrees of motion has been established and movement does not cause pain, the athlete may return to competitive activity. If the muscle remains firm on examination after 2 weeks, radiographs of the thigh should be obtained to rule out myositis ossificans, an abnormal deposition of calcium in the muscle that may be induced by aggressive stretching of the muscle too early in the clinical course.

7. Hip Dislocation

ESSENTIALS OF DIAGNOSIS & TYPICAL FEATURES

▶ Usually produces posterior dislocation.
▶ Leg is flexed, adducted, and internally rotated.
▶ Hip pain is severe.
▶ This is an on-site emergency and must be treated quickly.

The hip is a very constrained joint and is inherently very stable. Therefore, hip dislocations are rare and typically occur only in high energy or forceful injuries. Most hip dislocations occur in the posterior direction. Athletes with this injury typically have severe pain and any motion of the hip or leg is poorly tolerated. Classically, these athletes present with an acutely painful hip with inability to move or weight bear on the limb following a major impact, and the hip is locked in flexion, adduction, and internal rotation. Hip dislocations in skeletally mature athletes are often associated with acetabular and femoral neck fractures. The preadolescent, skeletally immature competitor may have an isolated dislocation without fracture. Hip radiographs and advanced imaging such as a CT or MRI scan are needed to completely evaluate the injury.

This injury is an emergency. The athlete should be transported immediately to the nearest facility that has an orthopedic surgeon available. Severe bleeding, avascular necrosis, and nerve damage can result with delay in relocation. Most athletes can be relocated in a closed fashion. Once reduction has been established in an uncomplicated case, protected weight bearing on crutches for 6 weeks is recommended followed by another 6 weeks of range-of-motion and strengthening exercises. An athlete may return gradually to competition after 3 months, when strength and motion are normal.

Surgery can be necessary if there is an associated fracture, labral tear, loose body, or if a concentric reduction cannot be achieved in a closed fashion.

8. Pelvic Apophysitis

Pelvic apophysitis occurs in competitive adolescent athletes who typically are participating consistently, often year round, in their sport. Common locations are the ischial tuberosity and iliac crest. The athlete presents with pain over the apophysis and pain with resisted hip motion specific to the muscle insertion. Radiographs can show irregularity over the apophysis, or be normal. Treatment consists of relative rest, progressive rehabilitation focusing on flexibility, and pelvis and core stabilization.

9. Iliotibial Band Syndrome

ESSENTIALS OF DIAGNOSIS & TYPICAL FEATURES

▶ Overuse running injury.

▶ Pain over lateral knee or hip.

▶ Positive Ober test.

Iliotibial (IT) band syndrome and associated trochanteric bursitis result when the bursa and IT band become inflamed because of repetitive friction from the underlying greater trochanter and lateral femoral condyle. This condition can cause pain when the hip or knee is flexed as a result of reduced flexibility of the IT band and gluteus medius tendons. The bursa is a structure that normally allows for improved motion by reducing friction but becomes pathologic in this condition. Movement is painful and may be limited. Pain is reproduced when the hip or knee is actively flexed from a fully extended position. Patients may also have a positive Ober test. The Ober test is used to measure flexibility of the IT band. The patient lies on his or her side with the affected leg on top. The examiner stabilizes the pelvis with one hand while the other hand moves the tested leg into knee flexion, hip abduction and extension and then lowers the leg into adduction until it stops via soft tissue stretch, posterior rotation of the pelvis, or both. The test is positive if the tested leg fails to adduct parallel to the table in a neutral position.

Initial treatment is to alter the offending activity and then start a stretching program geared at the IT band and hip abductors. Core and pelvic stabilization are also important. Ultrasound can be beneficial and corticosteroid injections may be used after conservative treatment has failed.

10. Femoral Neck Stress Fractures

Femoral neck stress fractures are generally the result of repetitive microtrauma. They commonly occur in running athletes who have rapidly increased their mileage. Athletes with this type of injury present with persistent pain in the groin and pain with internal and external rotation. Symptoms often are present with sports, but as the fracture progresses, symptoms often develop during activities of daily living. Athletes with a history of previous stress fracture, disordered eating, or any disorder of calcium metabolism and groin pain should alert the provider to the possibility of this diagnosis. Special attention to the risk of stress fracture should be given to the female athlete with the triad of energy imbalance and possible disordered eating, amenorrhea or oligomenorrhea, and low bone density.

On physical examination, range of motion may be limited in hip flexion and internal rotation. A limp may be present. Pain with hopping on the affected leg is universally present. If plain radiographs are negative, an MRI is indicated.

Treatment is based on the type of fracture. A tension-sided fracture (on the superior aspect of the femoral neck) generally requires internal fixation to prevent completion of the fracture or displacement and reduce the risk of avascular necrosis. A compression-sided fracture (on the inferior aspect of the femoral neck) is less likely to become displaced; treatment is conservative and involves a period of 6 weeks on crutches.

Jacoby L, Yi-Meng Y, Kocher MS: Hip problems and arthroscopy: adolescent hip as it relates to sports. Clin Sports Med 2011;30:435–451 [PMID: 21419965].
Kovacevic D, Mariscalco M, Goodwin RC: Injuries about the hip in the adolescent athlete. Sports Med Arthrosc Rev 2011;19:64–74 [PMID: 21293240].

KNEE INJURIES

Knee injuries are some of the most common sports-related problems. The knee is stabilized through a variety of ligaments, tendons, and menisci. Knee injuries can be divided into two groups: those resulting from acute or chronic causes. Acute injuries occur during a well-defined traumatic incident. The mechanism of injury is an important historical feature, although many young patients have difficulty describing the details of the inciting event. The onset of rapid swelling after a traumatic event indicates the presence of a hemarthrosis and likely internal derangements such as fracture, rupture of the anterior cruciate ligament (ACL), meniscal tear, or patellar dislocation.

1. Anterior Knee Pain

The most common knee complaint is anterior knee pain. This complaint can have multiple etiologies but should always include hip pathology as a possible source. Patellofemoral dysfunction (defined as follows) is a common cause of anterior knee pain. The differential diagnosis of anterior knee pain is extensive and requires a thorough examination. The following are the most common knee diagnoses responsible for anterior knee pain.

A. Patellofemoral Overuse Syndrome

Patellofemoral overuse syndrome occurs during running and sports that involve repetitive stress in the lower extremity. The athlete presents with activity-related pain in the anterior knee. In young athletes, it is occasionally associated with swelling and crepitus of the knee joint.

Evaluation of these injuries is comprehensive and requires a "top-down" evaluation of the athlete's leg from the hip to the foot. Most athletes with this condition, regardless of level or physical condition, typically have hip/core weakness that results in altered knee biomechanics. A comprehensive evaluation of hip alignment and rotation, muscle development, tightness in the hamstrings and IT band, and foot mechanics is necessary to fully understand and treat the cause of this disorder. Most athletes with this complaint often have a multifactorial cause for their symptoms.

Treatment should be geared toward identifying the cause. Often, athletes are overtraining and need to modify current activities. Cross-training may help. Addressing hip and pelvic stability is now a mainstay of treatment for this disorder. Stretching and strengthening of the hamstrings and quadriceps are recommended. The use of braces providing proprioceptive feedback during competition is controversial.

B. Patellar Tendonitis ("Jumper's Knee")

Patellar tendonitis is an overuse injury is caused by repetitive loading of the quadriceps during running or jumping. This diagnosis is common in jumping sports such as basketball and volleyball. Tenderness is located directly over the patellar tendon at its insertion site at the inferior pole of the patella. Physical therapy, icing, and activity modification can help facilitate healing.

C. Osgood-Schlatter Disease (Tibial Tubercle Apophysitis)

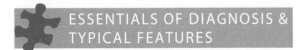

ESSENTIALS OF DIAGNOSIS & TYPICAL FEATURES

► Insidious onset of activity-related anterior knee pain in adolescents.

► Swelling and pain over the tibial tubercle.

► Progressive fragmentation of tibial tubercle apophysis.

Osgood-Schlatter disease is caused by the recurrent traction on the tibial tubercle apophysis (growth plate) that occurs in jumping and running sports. Fragmentation and microfractures of the tibial tubercle occur during its time of rapid growth. The condition occurs in the pre-teen and adolescent years and is most common in boys aged 12–15 years and girls aged 11–13 years. Pain is localized to the tibial tubercle and is aggravated by activities using eccentric quadriceps muscle movement. The pain can become so severe that routine activity must be curtailed. Radiographs typically demonstrate fragmentation or irregular ossification of the tibial tubercle.

Typically, the condition resolves spontaneously as the athlete reaches skeletal maturity. In the interim, pain control using NSAIDs is indicated. Physical therapy and stretching the hamstrings and application of ice after workouts are helpful.

D. Sinding-Larsen-Johansson Disease (Apophysitis of the Inferior Pole of the Patella)

Sinding-Larsen-Johansson disease involves a process similar to that in Osgood-Schlatter disease but occurs in younger athletes between ages 9 and 12 years. Traction from the patellar tendon on the inferior pole of the patella results in fragmentation of the inferior patella that is often obvious on a lateral knee radiograph. Treatment and prognosis is similar to Osgood-Schlatter disease.

► Treatment

The treatment of the above knee disorders is similar. As with many injuries, control of pain and inflammation is essential. This begins with relative rest from offending activity and application of ice. Alignment problems and mechanics across the anterior knee can be improved with an effective rehabilitation program that includes flexibility and strengthening. Quadriceps, pelvic, and core strengthening are all important components of this program. Orthotics, in theory, can have an impact on mechanics across the knee joint if they correct excessive pronation or supination. Knee bracing is controversial, and the major benefits are proprioceptive feedback and patellar tracking. Return to activity is often based on symptoms.

2. Posterior Knee Pain

Posterior knee pain often results from an injury to the gastrocnemius-soleus complex caused by overuse. Other causes include a Baker cyst (benign synovial fluid filled cyst in the posterior aspect of the knee), tibial stress fracture, or tendonitis of the hamstring. Treatment is rest, ice, and strengthening exercises after symptoms have improved. Intra-articular injuries such as meniscal tears and cartilage injuries can also cause posterior knee pain and should be considered if symptoms do not improve.

3. Meniscal Injuries

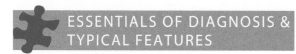

ESSENTIALS OF DIAGNOSIS & TYPICAL FEATURES

▶ Medial or lateral knee pain.

▶ Effusion and joint line tenderness.

▶ Feeling of locking or of the knee giving way.

▶ Positive McMurray, Apley, and Thessaly tests.

The meniscus of the knee cushions forces in the knee joint, increases nutrient supply to the cartilage, and stabilizes the knee. Most injuries are related to directional changes on a weight-bearing extremity. Medial meniscus injuries have a history of tibial rotation in a weight-bearing position. This injury happens frequently in ball-handling sports. Lateral meniscus injuries occur with tibial rotation with a flexed knee, as in exercises such as squatting or certain wrestling maneuvers. These injuries are uncommon in children younger than 10 years.

▶ Clinical Findings

The athlete with such an injury has a history of knee pain, swelling, snapping, or locking and may report a feeling of the knee giving way. Physical examination often reveals effusion; joint line tenderness; and a positive McMurray hyperflexion-rotation test, Apley test, and/or positive Thessaly test. The McMurray test is performed by having the examiner place his/her fingers across the joint lines while flexing the knee maximally. The knee is then rotated while it is brought out into extension. A positive test is evoked when the patient reports pain and the examiner feels an associated click or catch along the joint line. The Apley test is performed by having the patient lie prone with the knee flexed to 90 degrees. The examiner applies an axial load on the knee and rotates the tibia at the same time. A positive test is evoked when the patient reports pain. The Thessaly test is performed by having the patient stand on the injured leg. The examiner supports the patient by holding his or her outstretched arms. The patient is instructed to flex the knee to 5 degrees and then rotate his or her body and knee internally and externally three times. This is repeated with the knee at 20 degrees of flexion. A test is positive if the patient has joint line pain or a sense of locking or catching in the knee. The diagnostic test of choice is MRI of the knee, although standard knee radiographs should be obtained initially. It is important to note that the increased vascularity of the meniscus in the pediatric population often causes increased signal changes on MRI that can be confused with a tear. Therefore,

an MRI diagnosis of a meniscal tear in a young athlete needs to be correlated with the patient's clinical symptoms and examination.

▶ Treatment

Treatment of these injuries is typically surgical because of the limited ability of the meniscus to heal without surgical intervention. Nonoperative management can be considered if the tear is minor and symptoms are minimal. Surgery can entail repairing the tear or removing the torn portion of the meniscus. Typically, every attempt is made to preserve the meniscal tissue in young athletes because of their favorable healing rates and the long-term concern over the development of arthritis in meniscal deficient patients. Meniscectomy (removal of torn tissue) patients can often return to sports 3–6 weeks after surgery. Meniscal repair patients require a period of crutch protection followed by physical therapy. Return to sport after a repair is typically 4–6 months.

4. Medial & Lateral Collateral Ligament Injuries

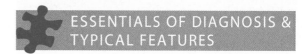

ESSENTIALS OF DIAGNOSIS & TYPICAL FEATURES

▶ Pain on the medial or lateral portion of the knee.

▶ Tenderness along the ligament.

▶ Positive valgus or varus stress test at 0 and 30 degrees.

The medial collateral ligament (MCL) and lateral collateral ligament (LCL) are positioned along either side of the knee and act to stabilize the knee during varus and valgus stress. Medial injuries occur either with a blow to the lateral aspect of the knee, as seen in a football tackle, or with a noncontact rotational stress.

▶ Clinical Findings

The athlete may feel a pop or pain sensation along the medial or lateral aspect of the knee. The examination reveals a mild effusion and tenderness medially or laterally along the course of the ligament. A valgus stress test performed in 20–30 degrees of flexion reproduces pain and possibly instability in MCL injuries. A varus stress test performed in 20–30 degrees of flexion reproduces pain and possible instability in LCL injuries.

MCL and LCL injuries are graded on a scale of 1–3. Grade 1 injury represents a stretching injury. Grade 2 injury involves partial disruption of the ligament. Grade 3 injury is a complete disruption of the ligament. Radiographs are useful, especially in the skeletally immature athlete, to look for distal femoral or proximal tibial bone injury. MRI scans are used if grade 2–3 injury or concomitant intra-articular derangement is suspected.

▶ Treatment

Treatment is generally conservative. Initial injuries should be iced and elevated. A protective brace is worn and full knee motion in the brace can be permitted within a few days. Weight bearing is allowed and a strengthening program can be started. The athlete should use the brace until pain and range of motion have improved. The use of a functional brace is often required when a player returns to competition. Bracing is temporary until the ligament heals completely and the athlete has no subjective feelings of instability. Return to sports is variable and is dependent on the severity of the tear and other associated injuries. Most isolated, low-grade MCL injuries can return to play in 3–5 weeks.

5. Anterior Cruciate Ligament Injuries

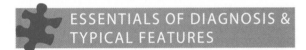

ESSENTIALS OF DIAGNOSIS & TYPICAL FEATURES

► Pain and effusion of the knee.
► Pain along the lateral joint line.
► Positive Lachman test.

The anterior cruciate ligament (ACL) consists of two bundles that prevent anterior subluxation and rotation of the tibia. Most ACL injuries are noncontact and occur with deceleration, twisting, and cutting motions. ACL injuries can also occur with knee hyperextension or from a direct blow to the knee—typically on the lateral side—which causes an extreme valgus stress with both ACL and MCL disruption.

▶ Clinical Findings

The athlete often reports hearing or feeling a "pop" followed by swelling that occurs within hours of the injury. Evaluation of the knee begins with examination of the uninjured knee. The Lachman test provides the most accurate information about knee stability in relation to the ACL. The Lachman test is performed by holding the knee in 30 degrees of flexion while supporting the tibia and femur. The proximal tibia is pulled anteriorly, and the degree of excursion and the firmness of the endpoint are assessed and compared to the contralateral side. All other structures of the knee should be examined to rule out concomitant injuries. Imaging of the knee includes plain radiographs and an MRI scan. In skeletally immature athletes, a tibial spine avulsion is frequently seen on radiographs rather than a midsubstance ACL tear.

▶ Treatment

Initial treatment focuses on controlling swelling and pain. Structured physical therapy can be instituted early to assist in regaining range of motion and strength. Conservative treatment includes bracing, strengthening, and restricting physical activity. Knee braces enhance proprioception and control terminal extension. Conservative management can be complicated by continued instability and damage to meniscal and articular cartilage.

Surgical reconstruction is typically indicated for young athletes in cutting sports and is also required for persistent instability. Surgery can be performed 2–6 weeks following the injury if the swelling and motion of the knee have improved. Recent advances in surgical treatment of the skeletally immature athlete have been helpful in dealing with the complicated management of young athletes with ACL tears. Rehabilitation of the knee starts immediately after surgery. A structured ACL physical therapy protocol is initiated with the goals of building strength, muscle reeducation, endurance, agility, and coordination. Return to cutting and pivoting sports can be achieved by 6–9 months after surgery if certain criteria are met, although many young athletes will need 12 months or more before they are ready to return to sports.

6. Posterior Cruciate Ligament Injuries

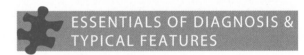

ESSENTIALS OF DIAGNOSIS & TYPICAL FEATURES

► Pain and swelling of the knee.
► Increased pain with knee flexion.
► Positive posterior Drawer test.

The posterior cruciate ligament (PCL) runs from the medial femoral condyle to the posterior tibial plateau and has two bundles. Its main function is to prevent posterior tibial subluxation. Injury to the PCL is uncommon; it occurs when the individual falls on a flexed knee with the ankle in plantarflexion or with forced hyperflexion of the knee. The most common sports in which PCL injuries are sustained are football and hockey.

▶ Clinical Findings

The athlete presents with swelling and pain in the posterior and lateral knee. The examination begins with the uninjured knee and proceeds to the injured side. Confirmatory testing includes the posterior drawer test, performed with the patient supine, the knee flexed to 90 degrees, and the foot stabilized. Grading is based on the amount of translation. Grade 1 (mild) is up to 5 mm, grade 2 (moderate) is 5–10 mm, and grade 3 (severe) is more than 10 mm. Grade 3 injuries are typically indicative that another ligament is injured in addition to the PCL and should alert the provider to an associated injury. Diagnostic imaging includes plain radiographs and MRI scan.

Treatment

Isolated PCL injuries are almost universally treated nonoperatively. The exception is bony avulsions of the PCL off the femur or tibia. Generally, surgical fixation is recommended for these injuries. Ligamentous PCL injuries in isolation are remarkably well tolerated in athletes and can be treated with bracing and a progressive rehabilitation program. PCL injuries with injury to other structures are complex and often require surgical stabilization. Surgical stabilization of these injuries is complicated, and return to sports at the previous level is uncertain after combined injuries that involve the PCL.

Francavilla ML, Restrepo R, Zamora KW, Sarode V, Swirsky SM, Mintz D: Meniscal pathology in children: differences and similarities with the adult meniscus. Pediatr Radiol 2014;44:910–925 [PMID: 25060615].

Frank JS, Gambacorta PL: Anterior cruciate ligament injuries in the skeletally immature athlete: diagnosis and management. J Amer Acad Orthop Surg 2013;21:78–87.

Kocher MS, Shore B, Nasreddine AY, Heyworth BE: Treatment of posterior cruciate ligament injuries in pediatric and adolescent patients. J Pediatr Orthop 2012;32:553–560 [PMID: 22892615].

Schub D, Saluan P: Anterior cruciate ligament injuries in the young athlete: evaluation and treatment. Sports Med Arthrosc Rev 2011;19:34–43 [PMID: 21293236].

FOOT & ANKLE INJURIES

Injuries to the lower leg, ankle, and foot are common in pediatric athletes. The types of injuries sustained typically depend on the age group. Young children tend to have diaphyseal injuries, in contrast to older children in rapid growth, who tend to have epiphyseal and apophyseal injuries. Skeletally mature adolescents are prone to adult-pattern ligamentous injury. Although fractures of the ankle are possible with inversion and eversion mechanisms, the most common acute injury involving the ankle is the lateral ankle sprain.

1. Ankle Sprain

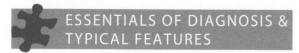

ESSENTIALS OF DIAGNOSIS & TYPICAL FEATURES

▶ Mechanism is usually inversion and plantarflexion.

▶ Swelling and pain in the ankle over the ligament.

▶ Bruising over the ankle.

When a ligament is overloaded, tearing occurs. These injuries are graded on a scale of 1–3. Grade 1 injury is a stretch without instability; grade 2 is a partial tear with some instability; and grade 3 is a total disruption of the ligament with instability of the joint. The ankle has three lateral ligaments (anterior talofibular, calcaneofibular, and posterior talofibular) and a medial deltoid ligament. Inversion of the foot generally damages the anterior talofibular ligament, whereas eversion injures the deltoid ligament. Lateral ankle sprains are far more common than medial ankle sprains because the deltoid ligament is stronger mechanically than the lateral ligaments. However, medial ankle sprains may have more severe complications, including syndesmotic tearing and instability of the ankle joint requiring surgical stabilization. High ankle sprains involve injury to the tibiofibular syndesmosis, a movable connection in which the adjacent tibia and fibula bones are bound together by ligamentous structures. The syndesmosis supports the integrity of the ankle mortise joint. The ankle mortise is defined as the bony arc formed by the tibial plafond, the medial and lateral malleoli, and the roof of the talus. The mortise provides the wide range of flexibility and motion of the ankle, but its injury causes instability and pain. Syndesmotic injuries do not typically require surgery but do involve longer healing times than low-grade medial or lateral ankle sprains.

Clinical Findings

Physical examination often reveals swelling, bruising, and pain. Diagnostic testing should be done when a bony injury is suspected. Obtaining radiographs is especially important when evaluating skeletally immature athletes who are more prone to growth plate injury. Medial ankle swelling, tenderness, and bruising warrant ankle three-view radiographs (AP, lateral, mortise) to evaluate asymmetry and instability of the ankle mortise.

The adult Ottawa Ankle Rules are used to determine whether obtaining x-rays are necessary and appear to be reliable in patients older than 5 years. Tenderness over the malleoli, tenderness beyond ligament attachments, and excessive swelling are additional reasons to obtain radiographs in young athletes.

Differential Diagnosis

Other injuries to consider include injuries to the fifth metatarsal, which can occur with an inversion mechanism. In this injury, the athlete presents with localized swelling and tenderness over the base of the fifth metatarsal. Fractures at the base of the fifth metatarsal can be divided into avulsion, Jones, and diaphyseal fractures. High-ankle sprains (a.k.a. syndesmotic injuries) occur most commonly with dorsiflexion and external rotation. Radiographs are required, and the syndesmotic squeeze test and Kleiger test (external rotation of the foot in dorsiflexion) are positive. Fractures of the tibial epiphysis, malleoli, fibula, talar dome, or calcaneus may also mimic an ankle sprain.

▶ **Treatment**

Appropriate treatment of ligamentous ankle injuries is imperative to ensure full recovery and should begin immediately after the injury. Fractures and instability of the ankle mortise require immediate orthopedic surgical referral. Nonoperative management is typical of the vast majority of ankle sprains. Phase 1 care involves immediate compressive wrapping and icing to control swelling and inflammation. Protected weight bearing is encouraged as tolerated in the early phase of rehabilitation. Severe ankle sprains may benefit from a short period of treatment in a lower leg walking boot or cast. Phase 2 begins when the athlete can ambulate without pain. Supervised physical therapy prescription may be beneficial. During this time, ankle range of motion is emphasized, along with isometric contractions of the ankle dorsiflexors. Once 90% of strength has returned, active isotonic (eccentric and concentric exercises) and isokinetic exercises can be added. Phase 3 is designed to increase strength, improve proprioception, and add ballistic activity (more complex movement patterns), as well as sport-specific agility and function. The "foot alphabet" and "balance board" are excellent methods to improve ankle range of motion and proprioception. To restore range of motion, the patient is asked to actively move the ankle by drawing letters of the alphabet with the toes. To restore proprioception, the ability to maintain proper balance and control, balance exercises are performed on a balance board (or wobble board). This could also be done by having the patient stand on one leg while playing catch with a ball. This program can be effective in returning athletes to activity within a few weeks, although up to 6 weeks may be required for return to full activity. The athlete should wear a protective brace for 3–4 months, continue phase 3 home exercises, and ice after exercising.

2. Sever Disease

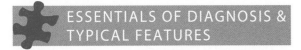

ESSENTIALS OF DIAGNOSIS & TYPICAL FEATURES

▶ Activity-related heel pain in preadolescents.
▶ Pain localized to the calcaneal apophysis and Achilles insertion.
▶ Positive calcaneal squeeze test.

Sever disease, or calcaneal apophysitis, occurs in athletes aged 8–12 years who are typically involved in high-impact activities, such as gymnastics and soccer. Causes include overuse, improper footwear, and tightness in the calf musculature

and Achilles tendon. Pain occurs about the heel and at the point of muscle tendon insertion onto the growth center of the calcaneus. The athlete presents with activity-related heel pain and examination reveals focal tenderness over the calcaneal apophysis. Tenderness created by pressing forcefully on the lateral and medial heel constitutes a positive "calcaneal squeeze test."

Treatment is symptomatic and consists of reassurance and education, relative rest, heel cord stretching, eccentric calf strengthening, ice massage, heel cups, NSAIDs for pain control, and progression to activity as tolerated based on pain level. Activity restriction is not required. Heel cups are rubber or gel infused shoe inserts that provide heel lift and cushion to decrease both tension and impact on the calcaneal apophysis. Refractory cases may benefit from brief immobilization and partial or non–weight-bearing in a walking boot or cast followed by supervised physical therapy.

3. Plantar Fasciitis

Plantar fasciitis is a common problem that manifests as heel pain in the adolescent or older athlete. It typically occurs in runners who log more than 30 miles per week and in athletes who have tight Achilles tendons or wear poorly fitting shoes. It is also common in people with cavus feet and in those who are overweight. The pain is worse upon first standing up in the morning and taking a few steps. Differential diagnosis includes navicular or calcaneal stress fracture. A bone spur is often found on examination. Treatment involves local massage, stretching of the gastrocnemius-soleus-Achilles complex, NSAIDs, arch supports, and local steroid injections. Runners may need to cut back on their weekly mileage until these measures eliminate pain.

Bahr R: Prevention of ankle sprains in adolescent athletes. Clin J Sports Med 2007;17:4 [PMID: 17620800].

Dowling S et al: Accuracy of Ottawa Ankle Rules to exclude fractures of the ankle and midfoot in children: a meta-analysis. Acad Emerg Med 2009;16(4):277–287 [PMID: 19187397].

Pontell D, Hallivis R, Dollard MD: Sports injuries in the pediatric and adolescent foot and ankle: common overuse and acute presentations. Clin Podiatr Med Surg 2006;23:209–231 [PMID: 16598916].

Seah R, Mani-Babu S: Managing ankle sprains in primary care: what is best practice? A systematic review of the last 10 years of evidence. Br Med Bull 2011;97:105–135 [PMID: 20710025].

▼ **PREVENTION**

As in all activities, many sports-related injuries can be prevented by education, reducing dangerous behaviors, use of protective equipment, and proper training. Early recognition of injuries, proper treatment, and appropriate rehabilitation are also crucial to ensure safe sports participation. Protective equipment should be properly fitted and maintained by an individual with training and instruction. Helmets should be used in football, baseball, hockey, bicycling, skiing, in-line skating, skateboarding, or any sport with risk of head injury. Eye protection should be used in sports that have a high incidence of eye injuries. Proper protective padding should be identified and used, including chest pads for catchers; shin guards in soccer; shoulder, arm, chest, and leg padding in hockey; and wrist and elbow protectors in skating. Other primary prevention strategies should also be addressed by coaches, parents, and physicians in order to ensure the safety of children participating in sports. These include inspecting playing fields for potential hazards, adapting rules to the developmental level of the participants, and matching opponents equally in skill level and size.

The use of the preparticipation history and physical examination can identify potential problems and allow for prevention and early intervention. Proper training techniques reduce injuries by encouraging flexibility, promoting endurance, and teaching correct biomechanics. Sports education reinforces the concepts of fitness and a healthy lifestyle along with sport-specific training. Early identification of an injury allows the athlete to modify techniques and avoid micro- and macrotrauma. Once an injury has occurred, it needs to be identified properly and appropriate measures used to minimize morbidity. Rehabilitation of the injury starts as soon as it has been identified. Early and appropriate care offers the athlete an optimal chance for full recovery and return to full participation.

Emery CA: Injury prevention and future research. Med Sport Sci 2005;49:170–191 [PMID: 16247266].

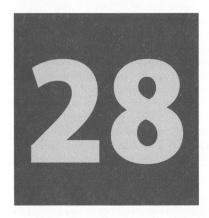

Rehabilitation Medicine

Pamela E. Wilson, MD

Gerald H. Clayton, PhD

Rehabilitation medicine is the multispecialty discipline involved in diagnosis and therapy of individuals with congenital and acquired disabilities. The goals of rehabilitation medicine are to maximize functional capabilities and improve quality of life. Disabilities are described using the World Health Organization's International Classification of Function, Health, and Disability. Three aspects are evaluated in every patient: (1) the impact of the disability on body structure and function, (2) the impact of the disability on activity and participation in society, and (3) the environmental factors with an impact on the individual's function. These three areas are the common framework for discussion of a disabling condition and its therapy.

PEDIATRIC BRAIN INJURY

ESSENTIALS OF DIAGNOSIS & TYPICAL FEATURES

▶ Severe head injury: Glasgow coma scale (GCS) of < 9.

▶ Moderate head injury: GCS of 9–13.

▶ Mild head injury: GCS of 13–15.

Various estimates indicate that there are up to 500,000 pediatric traumatic brain injuries in the United States every year, resulting in 37,000–50,000 hospitalizations. Mortality rates vary significantly by region (relative risk 1.19–4.2 nationally), but, overall, pediatric brain injuries result in 2000–3000 deaths annually. The cost of these injuries is significant, particularly when also considering that survivors of pediatric brain injury may have long-term deficits with lifetime needs.

▶ Pathogenesis

Brain injury is classically divided into two categories based on the timing of the pathologic findings: primary and secondary injury.

Primary injury occurs at the time of trauma, causing focal and diffuse mechanical damage to both the neurons and glia as well as the vasculature and is typically irreversible. *Focal damage* includes skull fracture, parenchymal bruising or contusion, extraparenchymal or intraparenchymal hemorrhage, blood clots, tearing of blood vessels, or penetrating injury. *Diffuse damage* includes diffuse axonal injury and edema. Consequences of primary injury, either focal or diffuse, include cellular disruption with release of excitatory amino acids, opiate peptides, and inflammatory cytokines.

Secondary injury is the loss of cellular function accompanying primary injury that results in loss of cerebrovascular regulation, altered cellular homeostasis, or cell death and functional dysregulation. Mitochondrial dysfunction due to dysregulation of Ca++ and other cations and anions leads to depletion of ATP to drive homeostatic cellular pumps. This leads to oxidation of cellular DNA, protein and lipids causing among other things cell death. These multiple mechanisms can also lead to increased extracellular glutamate resulting in excess depolarization further stressing compromised cells. A primary injury can initiate the processes of secondary programmed cell death (apoptosis), which further exacerbates the primary injury. Secondary injury may develop hours or days after the initial insult. It appears to be precipitated by elevated intracranial pressure, cerebral edema, and release of neurochemical mediators. Current treatment paradigms are focused on treating and preventing secondary injury.

▶ Clinical Findings

Classification & Assessment of Injury Severity

Traumatic brain injury is usually categorized as open or closed. *Open injuries* are the result of penetration of the skull by missile or sharp object or deformation of the skull with exposure of the underlying intracranial tissues. *Closed injuries* are the result of blunt trauma to the head, which causes movement (intracranial acceleration or deceleration and rotational forces) and compression of brain tissue. Brain contusions are referred to as *coup* (occurring at the site of injury) or *contra-coup* (occurring on the side of the brain opposite the injury). Rating the severity of injury and eventual outcomes is important in medical management. Included below are the two most commonly used scales relevant to clinical care of these injuries in rehabilitation medicine.

A. Glasgow Coma Scale (GCS)

The GCS is the most commonly used system to assess the depth and duration of impaired consciousness in the acute setting. The score is derived from three areas of evaluation: motor responsiveness (maximum score 6), verbal performance (maximum score 5), and eye opening to stimuli (maximum score 6). The scale has been modified for use in infants and children younger than 5 years, allowing for their lack of verbal responsiveness and understanding. Cumulative scores define injury as mild (13–15), moderate (9–12), and severe (≤ 8). The concept of posttraumatic amnesia is used to gauge severity of injury and is an adjunct to the GCS. Posttraumatic amnesia is the period after an injury during which new memory cannot be incorporated and the person appears confused or disoriented. Amnesia can be retrograde, anterograde, or both.

B. Rancho Los Amigos Levels of Cognitive Function

The Rancho Los Amigos Levels of Cognitive Function (LCFS or "Rancho") is used to gauge the overall severity of cognitive deficit and can be used serially during recovery as a rough gauge of improvement. The scale has 10 levels of functioning ranging from "no response" to "purposeful, appropriate."

Common Sequelae of Brain Injury

Depending on the severity of brain injury, there may be deficits in cognition and behavior, as well as physical impairments. Injuries can also produce changes in sensory and motor function, emotional stability, social behavior, speed of mental processing, memory, speech, and language. The consequences of mild brain injuries may be difficult to discern. Small intraparenchymal injuries, easily identified by computed tomographic (CT) or magnetic resonance imaging (MRI) scans, may not cause obvious signs or symptoms. The following are common problems associated with brain injury.

A. Seizures

Seizures occurring in the first 24 hours after injury are referred to as *immediate seizures*. Those occurring during the first week are *early seizures*, and those starting more than 1 week after injury are referred to as *late seizures*. Seizure prophylaxis with medications is recommended in the first week

after brain injury in children at high risk for seizures and in very young children. Seizure prophylaxis is also recommended for 1 week after any penetrating brain trauma. Seizure prophylaxis is probably not effective for prevention of late-onset seizures; these may require long-term treatment.

B. Neuromotor Deficits/Movement Disorders

Neuromotor deficits after brain injury include movement disorders, spasticity, paralysis, and weakness. The type of disorder will be influenced by the areas damaged. The most common movement disorders are tremors and dystonias. These deficits can result in impaired ambulation, coordination, impaired ability to use upper extremities, and speech problems. Physical therapy is the primary means of treating these problems.

C. Communication Disorders

Language and communication disorders are common. Aphasia, difficulty in understanding and producing written and spoken language, is categorized as fluent, nonfluent, or global. Individuals with fluent aphasia or Wernicke-type disorder can produce speech but have little content associated. The nonfluent aphasias or Broca's type have a paucity of speech and may have word finding difficulties. Global aphasias have extensive injuries and the most severe language disorders.

D. Paroxysmal Sympathetic Hyperactivity

Severe brain injuries may be associated with excessive sympathetic outflow and results in a constellation of symptoms known as paroxysmal sympathetic hyperactivity (PSH). Symptoms of PSH are tachycardia, tachypnea, sweating, hyperthermia, hypertension, agitation, and posturing. Common medications used to treat PSH include dopamine agonists (eg, bromocriptine), β-blockers (eg, propranolol), and α-agonists (eg, clonidine).

E. Cognitive and Behavioral Deficits

After brain injury, cognitive and behavioral deficits are a frequent occurrence. Cognitive disorders depend on the location and severity of the injury. Damage to the frontal lobes can disrupt executive function along with initiation delays. Neuropsychiatric sequelae are common, and depression, anxiety disorders, and posttraumatic stress disorders (PTSD) are present in one-third of those injured. Testing by a neuropsychologist may help to identify problem areas, allowing for development of accommodations in school and use of behavioral strategies.

F. Hypothalamic-Pituitary-Adrenal Axis Dysfunction

Dysfunction of the hypothalamic-pituitary-adrenal axis is common after head injury. The syndrome of inappropriate secretion of antidiuretic hormone (SIADH) and diabetes insipidus (DI) from a posterior pituitary injury can result in significant electrolyte and osmolality imbalance. Amenorrhea that typically resolves spontaneously is common in females. Injury near the onset of puberty can complicate normal development, and endocrine status should be monitored closely.

G. Cranial Nerve Injuries

The sensory and motor components of the cranial nerves are often damaged, resulting in a wide variety of deficits not centrally mediated. The most commonly injured nerves are I, IV, VII, and VIII. Hyposmia or anosmia (cranial nerve I) can occur if the shearing forces at the cribriform plate disrupt the afferent olfactory nerves. Injury to cranial nerves IV (trochlear) is common as it has the longest intracranial length. Superior oblique injuries typically cause a head tilt and vertical diplopia. Facial nerve injuries (cranial nerve VII) are common especially with temporal bone fractures. This impacts the ability to use the facial muscles, causes dryness in the eye and salivary glands along with decreasing taste in the anterior part of the tongue. The cochlear nerve (VIII) is also frequently damaged in temporal bone fractures and can result in vertigo and dizziness.

Developmental Considerations

Much of what we know of traumatic brain injury is based on adult experience. The confounding effects of age and the etiologies unique to the pediatric population (eg, child abuse) make care of the pediatric head-injured patient very complex.

The assumption that younger children will fare better than older children or adults after a brain injury is a myth. The fact that in a child a significant amount of development and synaptic reorganization has yet to occur does not guarantee an improved chance for functional recovery. Indeed, disruption of developmental processes, especially in very young infants or neonates, may be catastrophic. These processes often cannot be recapitulated.

The mechanism of injury plays an important role in determining the severity of brain injury in very young children. Mechanisms associated with nonaccidental injury such as shaking often result in global diffuse damage. The weak neck musculature, large head-body mass ratio, immature blood-brain barrier, and high intracranial fluid-brain mass ratio all contribute to widespread damage.

During puberty, major hormonal changes have an impact on the outcome of brain injury. Behavioral problems may be pronounced in brain-injured adolescents. Precocious puberty and precocious development of sexual activity may occur in preadolescents and should be carefully monitored.

Careful consideration should be given to the developmental progress of the brain-injured child and adolescent. Delays can be anticipated after moderate and severe brain injuries related to abnormalities of cognition and behavior.

Educational programs should include an individualized educational program (IEP) to support the child with significant remediation and assistance during their school years. Programs should also include a 504 plan (Section 504 of the Rehabilitation Act and the Americans with Disabilities Act). The 504 plan identifies the accommodations necessary in regular school settings for students with lesser disabilities so that they may be educated in a setting with their peers.

▶ Treatment

The primary goal of rehabilitation after childhood brain injury is to maximize functional independence. Rehabilitative care can be divided into three phases: acute, subacute, and long term. The acute and subacute phases typically occur in the inpatient setting while the long-term phase is an outpatient endeavor.

A. Acute Care

Therapy in the acute phase consists mainly of medical, surgical, and pharmacologic measures to decrease brain edema, treat increased intracranial pressure, and normalize laboratory values. Nutrition is essential for the healing process, and either parenteral nutrition or supplemental enteral feedings are employed. Current research suggests that transitioning to enteral nutrition (eg, nasogastric tube feeding) as soon as possible after brain injury is associated with improved outcomes. Placement of a gastrostomy tube for supplemental enteral feeding is often performed in patients with severe brain injuries when recovery will be protracted, and swallowing function is inadequate for safe oral feeding.

B. Subacute Care

Therapy in the subacute phase is characterized by early, intensive participation in rehabilitative therapies promoting functional recovery. Treatment should be planned after consultation with physical therapy, occupational therapy, speech-language specialists, and neuropsychologists. Nursing staff members are a primary interface with the patient and often serve as educators for family-directed care. Pharmacologic approaches may be used to enhance arousal and focus in patients with traumatic brain injury to enable them to more fully participate in therapies or to deal with other subacute sequelae such as agitation. Most children and adolescents with brain injuries can be discharged home to continue with treatment on an outpatient basis.

C. Long-Term Care

Long-term follow-up starts immediately after discharge. Annual multidisciplinary evaluation, including neuropsychological testing is important as the child approaches school age so strategies to deal with noted deficits can be implemented to improve outcomes within the educational environment.

Medication is often required for cognitive and behavioral issues. Attention deficit and fatigue may be amenable to treatment with stimulants such as methylphenidate and modafinil. Dopaminergic agents such as amantadine, levodopa, and bromocriptine can be useful in improving cognition, processing speed, and agitation. Antidepressants such as selective serotonin reuptake inhibitors can be helpful in treating depression and mood lability. Anticonvulsants can be used as mood stabilizers and in treating agitation and aggression. Tegretol and valproic acid are typical agents for this purpose.

Attention and arousal can also be successfully addressed by utilizing behavioral techniques to reinforce desired behaviors and by identifying environmental situations to facilitate success. Gains made in the behavioral realm often have a positive impact on therapies designed to address physical issues.

▶ Prognosis & Outcomes

Directly after brain injury, poor pupillary reactivity, low blood pH, absence of deep tendon reflexes, and low GCS all correlate with poor outcome. Coalescing lesions noted on imaging and increased depth and duration of coma suggest more severe injury and poor functional recovery. Children younger than 1 year tend to have worse outcomes.

Functional outcome assessment is important for judging the efficacy of rehabilitation therapy. Global multidomain measures (eg, FIM/WeeFIM) are used to provide a functional "snapshot in time" of select functions—motor function and mobility, self-care, cognition, socialization, and communication. Simpler, single-domain, functional assessment tools such as the Glasgow Outcome Scale (GOS) and its pediatric cousin, the Kings Outcome Scale for Childhood Head Injury (KOSCHI), may also be of use. The National Institute of Neurological Disorders & Stroke (NINDS) is coordinating an effort to validate and promote the use of "common data elements" for evaluating outcomes of brain injury (www.commondataelements.ninds.nih.gov). The goal of this effort is to promote the use of common measures that will facilitate comparison of results across studies and generalizable conclusions.

Outcome associated with mild brain injury is often quite favorable. Most patients recover normal function within a short time. A small percentage develop persistent problems such as chronic headache, poor focusing ability, altered memory, and vestibular abnormalities which may last for many weeks or months. Differentiating between musculoskeletal and central nervous system (CNS) etiologies of persistent symptoms such as headache is important and can influence prognosis and care planning.

In children, recovery may not be fully achieved for many months or years after the initial injury. The impact of the injury on developmental processes and its future consequences are difficult to predict. Long-term follow-up is required, particularly as the child approaches school age.

Baquley IJ et al: Paroxysmal sympathetic hyperactivity after acquired brain injury: consensus on conceptual definition, nomenclature and diagnostic criteria. J Neurotrauma 2014;31(17):1515 [PMID: 24731076].

Boake C et al: Brain injury rehabilitation. In: Braddom RL (ed). *Physical Medicine & Rehabilitation*. Philadelphia, PA: Saunders; 1996:1073–1116.

Kochanek PM et al: Guidelines for the management of pediatric severe traumatic brain injury, third edition: update of the brain trauma foundation guidelines, executive summary. Pediatr Crit Care Med 2019;20(3):280–289 [PMID: 30830016].

Prins M et al: The pathophysiology of traumatic brain injury at a glance. Dis Model Mech 2013;6(6):1307 [PMID: 3820255].

Walker KR, Tesco G: Molecular mechanisms of cognitive dysfunction following traumatic brain injury. Front Aging Neurosci 2013;5:29 [PMID: 23847533].

Wat R et al: The effectiveness of antiepileptic medications as prophylaxis of early seizure in patients with traumatic brain injury compared with placebo or no treatment: a systematic review and meta-analysis. World Neurosurger 2019;122:433–440 [PMID: 30465951].

SPINAL CORD INJURY

ESSENTIALS OF DIAGNOSIS & TYPICAL FEATURES

▶ Spinal cord injury (SCI) is an alteration in normal motor, sensory, or autonomic function secondary to spinal insult.

▶ Characterized as either complete (total loss of function) or incomplete (some preservation of function below the level of lesion).

Epidemiologic studies of SCI suggest that there will be about 10,000 new injuries per year and that 20% will be in those younger than 20 years. Motor vehicle accidents are the leading cause of SCI in all ages. Falls are common causes in young children. The phenomenon of SCI without obvious radiologic abnormality (SCIWORA) can be present in 20%–40% of young children. Children from birth to 2 years tend to have high-level injuries to the cervical spine because of anatomical features of their spine. The facets tend to be shallower and oriented horizontally, and the boney spine is more flexible than the spinal cord. In addition, the head is disproportionately large and the neck muscles are weak.

▶ Clinical Findings

A. Classification and Assessment of Injury Severity

SCI is classified using the International Standards for Neurological Classification of Spinal Cord Injury (ISNCSCI), formerly known as the American Spinal Injury Association (ASIA) classification system.

This classification evaluates motor and sensory function, defines the neurologic level of the injury, and assesses the completeness (level of motor or sensory sparing) of the deficit. The 72-hour examination is used in predicting recovery. A complete lesion identified on examination at 72 hours predicts a poor recovery potential. The ISNCSCI classification is as follows:

1. Class A is a complete SCI, with no motor or sensory function in the lowest sacral segments.

2. Class B is an incomplete injury, with preserved sensory function but no motor function in the sacral segments.

3. Class C is an incomplete lesion in which the strength of more than 50% of key muscles below the injury level is graded less than 3/5 on manual muscle testing.

4. Class D is an incomplete lesion in which the strength of more than 50% of key muscles below the injury level is graded greater than 3/5 on manual muscle testing.

5. Class E is an injury in which full motor and sensory function is preserved.

B. Clinical Patterns of Spinal Cord Injury

1. Brown-Séquard injury—The cord is hemisected causing motor paralysis, loss of proprioception and vibration on the ipsilateral side, and loss of pain and temperature on the contralateral side.

2. Central cord syndrome—Injury is to the central part of the cord and results in greater weakness in the arms than the legs.

3. Anterior cord syndrome—Disruption of the anterior spinal artery causes motor deficits and loss of pain and temperature sensation. Proprioception and fine touch are spared.

4. Conus medullaris syndrome—Injury or tumor of the conus, the lower conical shaped end of the spinal cord, can cause minimal motor impairment but significant sensory, bowel, and bladder abnormalities.

5. Cauda equina syndrome—Injury to the nerve roots produces flaccid bilateral weakness in the legs, sensory abnormalities in the perineum, and lower motor neuron bowel and bladder dysfunction.

C. Imaging

The diagnosis and anatomic description of SCI is made mainly through imaging techniques. Initial studies should include radiographs of the entire spine (including cervical spine) and special studies for boney structures. MRI is required to evaluate soft tissues. CT scans, including three-dimensional reconstructions, may be used to further define the injured elements.

▶ Treatment

A. Initial Management

The two primary precepts of SCI treatment are early identification and immediate stabilization of the spine. The approach used to stabilize the spine is determined by the type of injury, location of injury, and underlying condition of the spinal cord. Stabilizing the spine may prevent further damage to the spinal cord. External traction devices such as halo traction and orthotics are often used. Some injuries require internal stabilization. The benefit of methylprednisolone administration in acute SCI has recently come into question. Based on the ongoing controversy regarding efficacy and outcomes, steroids remain an option, but their administration is not considered standard of care.

B. Functional Expectations After Spinal Cord Injury

The lesions associated with SCI have a predictable impact on motor and sensory function. It is helpful to understand these concepts when discussing functional expectations with patients and parents (Table 28–1).

C. Special Clinical Problems Associated With Spinal Cord Injury

1. Autonomic hyperreflexia or dysreflexia—This condition occurs in spinal injuries above the T6 level. Noxious stimuli in the injured patient cause sympathetic vasoconstriction below the level of injury. Vasoconstriction produces hypertension and then a compensatory, vagal-mediated bradycardia. Symptoms include hypertension, bradycardia, headaches, and diaphoresis. This response may be severe enough to be life threatening. Treatment requires identification and relief of the underlying noxious stimulus. Bowel, bladder, and skin problems are the most common stimuli. The patient should be placed in an upright position and antihypertensive medication used if conservative measures fail.

2. Hypercalcemia—Hypercalcemia, in response to immobilization, often occurs in male adolescents within the first 2 months of becoming paraplegic or tetraplegic. Patients complain of abdominal pain and malaise. Behavioral problems may occur. Initial treatment is focused on hydration and forced diuresis using fluids and furosemide to increase urinary excretion of calcium. In severe cases, especially in older children, calcitonin and etidronate may be required.

3. Thermoregulation problems—These problems are common in higher-level injuries and usually result in a poikilothermic state where body temperature changes with that of the environment. The ability to vasoconstrict and vasodilate below the injury level is impaired. The person with an SCI above T6 is particularly susceptible to environmental temperature and is at risk for hypothermia and hyperthermia.

Table 28–1. Functional expectations related to spinal cord injury.

Level of Injury and Key Muscle Function	Functional Skills
C1–C4 (no upper extremity function)	Dependent for all skills, can use voice-activated computer, mouth stick; can drive power wheelchair with technology devices such as sip and puff, chin drive, or head array
C5 (biceps function)	Can assist with ADLs, power wheelchair with joy stick, push manual wheelchair short distances, use modified push rims
C6 (wrist extension)	More ADL skills; can push manual wheelchair indoors, perform level transfers; hand function augmented with adapted equipment
C7 (elbow extension)	ADLs independent; hand function augmented with adapted equipment; can push manual wheelchair indoor and outdoor
C8 (finger flexors)	ADLs independent; independent manual wheelchair skills; increased transfer skills
T1 (little finger abduction)	
T2–T12 (chest, abdominal, and spinal extensors)	ADLs independent; independent manual wheelchair skills; improved transfer; standing with braces
L1 and L2 (hip flexors)	Standing and walking with long leg braces, KAFO, and RGO; swing-through gait; manual wheelchair main form of mobility
L3 (knee extension)	Home and limited community ambulation; long leg or short leg braces
L4 (ankle dorsiflexion)	Community ambulation with short leg braces, AFO
L5 (long toe extensors)	Community ambulation; may be slower than peers and have some endurance issues
S1 (ankle plantar flexors)	

ADLs, activities of daily living; AFO, ankle-foot orthosis; KAFO, knee-ankle-foot orthosis; RGO, reciprocal gait orthosis.

4. Deep vein thrombosis—Thrombosis is a common complication of SCI, especially in postpubescent children. Deep vein thrombosis should be suspected in children with any unilateral extremity swelling, palpable cords in the calf muscles, fevers, erythema, or leg pain. Diagnosis is confirmed by Doppler ultrasound, and full evaluation may require spiral CT scan or ventilation-perfusion scan if pulmonary embolus is suspected. Preventative measures include elastic stockings and compression devices. Anticoagulation prophylaxis may be required using medications such as low-molecular-weight heparins (eg, enoxaparin).

5. Heterotopic ossification—This complication occurs in both spinal cord and traumatic brain injuries. Ectopic calcium deposits usually appear around joints in the first 6 months after injury. They may cause swelling, decreased range of motion, pain with motion, palpable firm masses, fever, elevated sedimentation rate, and abnormal triple phase bone scan. Nonsteroidal anti-inflammatory drugs or bisphosphonates such as Etidronate should be started at the time of diagnosis. Surgical removal of ectopic deposits is controversial and usually performed only in cases of extreme loss of motion, pressure sores, or severe pain.

Evaniew N et al: Methylprednisolone for the treatment of patients with acute spinal cord injuries: a systematic review and meta-analysis. J Neurotrauma 2016;33(5):468–481 [PMID: 26529320].

Grant RA et al: Management of acute traumatic spinal cord injury. Curr Treat Options Neurol 2015;17(2):334 [PMID: 25630995].

Powell A, Davidson L: Pediatric spinal cord injury: a review by organ system. Phys Med Rehabil Clin N Am 2015;26(1):109 [PMID: 25479784].

Rozelle CJ et al: Spina Cord injury without radiographic abnormality (SCIWORA). Neurosurgery 2013;71(Suppl 2):227 [PMID: 23417193].

BRACHIAL PLEXUS LESIONS & TYPICAL FEATURES

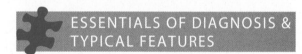

ESSENTIALS OF DIAGNOSIS & TYPICAL FEATURES

► Upper trunk (C5 and C6) is the most common area injured and results in the classic Erb palsy.

► Injury to the lower trunk (C7–T1) produces Klumpke palsy.

► Pan plexus lesion involves all roots.

Pathogenesis

Brachial plexus lesions associated with delivery are related to traction applied to the nerves and is often associated with shoulder dystocia. The nerve injury can range from simple neuropraxia (stretch) to complete avulsion. Acquired brachial plexus injuries from sports, surgery, and accidents also have a mechanism that stretches or injures the plexus.

Prevention

Identification of factors associated with shoulder dystocia, such as macrosomia, or proper positioning during surgical procedures to decrease traction on the brachial plexus may reduce the incidence of these lesions.

Clinical Findings

Erb palsy has been described as the "waiter's tip posture" and is characterized by shoulder weakness with internal rotation and adduction of the upper arm. The elbow is extended and the wrist flexed. There is good preservation of hand function. Klumpke palsy is characterized by good shoulder function but decreased or absent hand function. Brachial plexus injuries may also cause a Horner syndrome (unilateral miosis, ptosis, and facial anhidrosis) due to disruption of cervical sympathetic nerves. The physical examination should include inspection of the humerus and clavicle for fractures. There may be injuries to the phrenic and facial nerves. The diagnosis of a brachial plexus lesion should be based on the history and clinical examination. Diagnostic testing helps confirm, localize, and classify the lesion. Electromyography is helpful 3–4 weeks after the injury. This test not only is used diagnostically, but it also can track recovery. MRI, myelography, and CT scan can help to locate the lesion and determine its extent.

Complications

The development of complications reflects the degree of nerve recovery. Severe injuries are at risk for shoulder contractures, muscle atrophy, osseous deformities, functional deficits, pain, and maladapted postures.

Treatment & Prognosis

The treatment for brachial plexus lesions will depend on the severity of the lesion. Many will heal on their own and no interventions are needed. For persistent injuries, physical/occupational therapy is the major treatment and includes stretching, bracing, strengthening, electrical stimulation, and functional training. Primary surgery to the nerves of the plexus is indicated for children who have no spontaneous recovery of biceps function by 6–9 months. Secondary procedures to maximize function include muscle transfers and orthopedic interventions.

Many factors are used to predict recovery. The anatomic location of the lesion impacts recovery, as upper trunk lesions do better than lower trunk lesions. If a Horner syndrome is present, these injuries always have a poor recovery. Children in whom antigravity function returns within 2 months of injury will usually have a good recovery of function. If antigravity function is delayed until 6 months, recovery will probably be limited. If antigravity function is absent at 6–9 months, there will be no recovery of function and surgery should be considered.

Chang KW et al: A systematic review of evaluation methods for neonatal brachial plexus palsy: a review. J Neurosurg Pediatr 2013;12(4):395 [PMID: 23930602].

Hale HB et al: Current concepts in the management of brachial plexus birth palsy. J Hand Surg Am 2010 Feb;35(2):322 [PMID: 20141905].

COMMON REHABILITATION PROBLEMS

ESSENTIALS OF DIAGNOSIS & TYPICAL FEATURES

▶ Neurogenic bladder may be caused by trauma or disease affecting central or peripheral connections and can be classified depending on the type of dysfunction.

▶ Neurogenic bowel may be caused by upper or lower motor neuron damage with loss of sensation and sphincter control, with or without reflexive bowel activity depending on injury.

▶ Spasticity, a velocity dependent increase in tone and loss of isolated muscle function, is commonly graded using the Ashworth scale.

1. Neurogenic Bladder

During the first year of life, the bladder is a reflex-driven system that empties spontaneously. After the first year, control begins to develop and most children achieve continence by age 5 years. Children with damage to the central or peripheral nervous system may develop a neurogenic bladder. The diagnosis of neurogenic bladder requires a complete history and physical examination and is usually classified as follows:

1. *Uninhibited* neurogenic bladder occurs after upper motor neuron injuries at the level of the brain or spinal cord that result in failure to inhibit detrusor contractions. This results in a hyperreflexive voiding pattern.

2. *Reflex* neurogenic bladder results from damage to the sensory and motor nerves above the S3 and S4 level. The bladder empties reflexively, but coordination may not be present and dyssynergia (contraction of the bladder musculature against a closed sphincter) can occur. Increased intravesicular pressure and vesicourethral reflux may be consequences of dyssynergia.

3. *Autonomous* neurogenic bladder is a flaccid bladder and is associated with lower motor neuron damage. Bladder volumes are usually increased and overflow incontinence can occur.

4. *Motor paralytic* neurogenic bladder results from injury to the motor nerves of the S2–S4 roots. Sensation is intact, but there is motor dysfunction. The child has the sensation to void but has difficulty with the voluntary contractions.

5. *Sensory paralytic* neurogenic bladder results when sensory roots are disrupted. Affected patients do not have sensation of the full bladder but are able to initiate voiding.

The type of neurologic damage should be identified as this will help to predict anticipated voiding issues. The upper tracts should be assessed using ultrasound, intravenous pyelogram, or renogram (isotope) studies. Lower tract testing includes urinalysis, postvoid residuals, urodynamics, cystography, and cystoscopy.

▶ Treatment

Treatment is geared to the type of bladder dysfunction. The simplest methods, such as timed voiding, can be effective for children with uninhibited bladders. In this technique, children are reminded verbally or use a cueing device (watch with a timer) to void every 2–3 hours before bladder capacity is reached. The Credé and Valsalva maneuvers are used in patients with an autonomous bladder to assist in draining a flaccid bladder. There is a risk of provoking vesicoureteral reflux by increasing intravesicular pressure during these maneuvers that should never be used in a patient with a reflex neurogenic bladder.

Medications are often employed to treat neurogenic bladder. Anticholinergics are commonly used to reduce detrusor contractions, decrease the sense of urgency, and increase bladder capacity. Medications include oxybutynin, tolterodine, and hyoscyamine. The side effects of these medications include sleepiness, nausea, and constipation. Absorbent pads and diapers, external catheters, indwelling catheters, and intermittent catheterization are also effective. A young child with a high-pressure bladder is at particular risk for reflux and may need medication, intermittent catheterization, or vesicostomy to prevent hydrostatic renal damage and infection. An older child may require reconstructive bladder surgery (bladder augmentation) to increase the capacity of the bladder or an intestinal conduit from bladder to skin surface (Mitrofanoff procedure) to relieve bladder distention. If an incompetent urethral sphincter causes urinary leakage, injections, slings, or implants may be used to increase the urethral barrier. Recently, electrical stimulation of sacral roots has been used to initiate voiding. Biofeedback training is also used to improve voiding.

2. Neurogenic Bowel

Control of bowel function depends on an intact autonomic (sympathetic and parasympathetic) and somatic nervous system. Goals of treatment for patients with neurogenic bowel are to establish a predictable and reliable bowel habit and prevent incontinence and complications. There are two types of neurogenic bowel dysfunction: upper motor and lower motor dysfunction. The upper neuron bowel results from damage above the conus. Affected patients usually have reflex bowel contractions of high amplitude, absence of sensation, and no voluntary sphincter control. Patients with the lower motor neuron bowel have no voluntary sphincter control and no reflex contraction of the external anal sphincter (anocutaneous reflex). It has been described as a flaccid

bowel. In general, establishing a bowel program is easier in patients with upper motor neuron lesions.

▶ Treatment

Fiber intake and fluids are critical elements for maintaining a soft stool consistency, although some patients try to keep themselves constipated to prevent accidents. A predictable and scheduled bowel program is essential. Bowel movements should be scheduled to occur with meals, as the gastrocolic reflex can trigger defecation.

Laxative and stool softening medications are usually included in a comprehensive bowel program. Stool softeners such as docusate retain stool water. Mineral oil is an acceptable stool softener in patients not at risk for pulmonary aspiration. Bulking agents such as Metamucil increase fiber and water content of stool and reduce transit time. Stimulants such as senna fruit extract or bisacodyl increase peristalsis. Osmotic agents such as polyethylene glycol keep stools soft by retaining stool water. Suppositories and enemas are often used when other methods have not been successful. Upper motor neuron bowel management programs may include digital rectal stimulation. When conservative methods are ineffective, options may include surgical implantation of sacral nerve stimulators or techniques to facilitate antegrade flushing of the colon. For example, the ACE (antegrade continence enema) or Malone procedure approximates the appendix to the surface of the abdomen providing a conduit for flushing. Also, a capped cecostomy tube can be placed into the cecum through which fluids can be administered in an antegrade fashion to remove fecal matter from the colon.

3. Spasticity

Spasticity is a velocity-dependent increase in muscle tone and a loss of isolated muscle function. Whereas tone is the resistance felt in a muscle as it is moved in space, spasticity occurs when there is damage to the CNS from trauma or injury. It is included in the upper motor neuron syndrome (hyperactive and exaggerated reflexes, increased tone, clonus, positive Babinski sign). Spasticity is evaluated using the Ashworth scale, with 0 indicating no increase in muscle tone and 4 indicating complete rigidity of the extremity.

▶ Treatment

Treatment is goal directed and influenced by the functional status of the client. Options for therapy range from conservative to aggressive. Children should be positioned properly and have appropriate equipment to prevent nociceptive input and facilitate physical therapy. Physical therapy can reduce the long-term effects of spasticity by use of stretching and range-of-motion exercises. Heat and cold are useful in improving tone, but their effects are not long lived. Casting of both upper and lower extremities can decrease tone and increase range of motion. Constraint therapy can be used to try to improve upper extremity function.

Pharmacologic support with medications, such as baclofen, diazepam, dantrolene, and tizanidine, can be effective. Baclofen (a direct γ-aminobutyric acid type B [GABA$_B$] agonist) is a first-line medication, which produces effects at the spinal cord level. Side effects are primarily sleepiness and weakness. Seizure threshold may be reduced by baclofen. Baclofen, delivered directly to the CNS through an intrathecal pump, has been used successfully in children with brain injury, cerebral palsy, and SCI. Diazepam, an allosteric modulator of postsynaptic GABA$_A$ receptors in both the brain and the spinal cord, can be effective, but its central CNS effects can cause drowsiness and dependence. Dantrolene inhibits excitation contraction coupling but use can result in weakness or, rarely, hepatotoxicity. Tizanidine is a newer agent and works at the α$_2$-adrenergic receptors presynaptically. It can cause dry mouth and sedation, and liver function tests can be elevated.

Relief of focal spasticity can be achieved by using chemodenervation techniques. Botulinum toxin A and B can be injected in selected muscles to block acetylcholine release at the neuromuscular junction and thereby improve range of motion. Enhanced function, improved hygiene, reduced pain, and deformity are the result. Botulinum toxins have also been used to treat drooling, hyperhidrosis, and chronic pain. The effects are temporary, lasting only 3–6 months, and repeat injections are often needed. Technically more challenging phenol injection denatures proteins in both myelinated and unmyelinated fibers and produces neurolysis or myolysis, depending on the site of injection. The effects may last longer than botulinum toxins but carry a risk of sensory dysesthesia if mixed nerves are injected.

Surgical options include orthopedic procedures geared toward improving function and ambulation and alleviating deformities produced over time by spasticity. Contractures are common in the Achilles tendon, hamstrings, and adductors. Upper extremity contractures occur in the elbow, wrist, and finger flexors. Scoliosis is common and bracing or surgery may be needed. Gait analysis may be helpful in evaluating the child with functional spasticity as a guide for the use of orthotics, therapy, and surgery. Neurosurgical techniques such as selective dorsal rhizotomy, sectioning afferent sensory nerve fibers, are used in a very select group of children to permanently alter spasticity patterns and improve ambulation.

Vadivelu S et al: Pediatric tone management. Phys Med Rehabil Clin N Am 2015;26(1):69 [PMID: 25479780].

Wheeler TL et al: Translating promising strategies for bowel and bladder management in spinal cord injury. Exp Neurol 2018;306:169–176 [PMID: 29753647].

QUALITY ASSURANCE/IMPROVEMENT INITIATIVES IN REHABILITATION MEDICINE

Working with the Accreditation Council for Graduate Medical Education (ACGME), the American Academy of Physical Medicine and Rehabilitation (AAPM&R) fosters acquisition of knowledge regarding the use of quality assurance/improvement techniques in its training programs. This is now one of six competencies required for board certification. The AAPM&R feels that these skills endow the practitioner with the capacity to maintain and improve the quality of care provided to the public.

Rheumatic Diseases

Jennifer B. Soep, MD

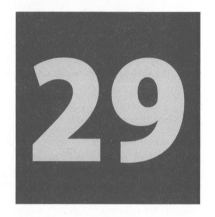

29

JUVENILE IDIOPATHIC ARTHRITIS

ESSENTIALS OF DIAGNOSIS & TYPICAL FEATURES

▶ Arthritis, involving pain, swelling, warmth, tenderness, morning stiffness, and/or decreased range of motion of one or more joints, lasting at least 6 weeks.

▶ May have associated systemic manifestations, including fever, rash, uveitis, serositis, anemia, and fatigue.

Juvenile idiopathic arthritis (JIA) is characterized by chronic arthritis in one or more joints for at least 6 weeks. There are four main subtypes of JIA: (1) oligoarticular, (2) polyarticular, (3) systemic, and (4) enthesitis associated. The exact cause of JIA is not known, but there is substantial evidence that it is an autoimmune process with genetic susceptibility factors.

▶ Clinical Findings

A. Symptoms and Signs

The most common type of JIA is the oligoarticular form, which constitutes approximately 40%–60% of patients and is characterized by arthritis of four or fewer joints. This type often affects medium to large joints. Because the arthritis is often asymmetrical, children may develop a leg-length discrepancy in which the involved leg may grow longer due to increased blood flow and growth factors. Systemic features are uncommon except for inflammation in the eye. Approximately 20% of children with oligoarticular arthritis develop insidious, asymptomatic uveitis, which may cause blindness if untreated. The activity of the eye disease does not correlate with that of the arthritis. Therefore, routine ophthalmologic screening with slit-lamp examination must be performed at 3-month intervals when the antinuclear antibody (ANA) test is positive, and at 6-month intervals if the ANA test is negative, for at least 4 years after the onset of arthritis, as this is the period of highest risk.

Polyarticular disease, which is defined as arthritis involving five or more joints, accounts for 20%–35% of JIA. Both large and small joints are involved, typically in a symmetrical pattern. Systemic features are not prominent, although low-grade fever, fatigue, rheumatoid nodules, and anemia may be present. This group is further divided into rheumatoid factor (RF)–positive and RF-negative disease. The former resembles adult rheumatoid arthritis with more chronic, destructive arthritis.

The systemic form comprises 10%–15% of patients with JIA. The arthritis can involve any number of joints and affects both large and small joints but may be absent at disease onset. One of the classic features is a high fever, often as high as 39°C–40°C, typically occurring one to two times per day. In between fever spikes, the temperature usually returns to normal or subnormal. Around 80%–90% patients have a characteristic evanescent, salmon-pink macular rash that is most prominent on pressure areas and when fever is present. Other systemic features that may be present include hepatosplenomegaly, lymphadenopathy, leukocytosis, and serositis.

Enthesitis-associated arthritis is most common in males, older than 10 years of age, and is typically associated with lower extremity, large joint arthritis. The hallmark of this form is inflammation of tendinous insertions (enthesitis), such as the tibial tubercle or the heel. Low back pain and sacroiliitis are also commonly seen. This form of arthritis comprises approximately 5%–10% of patients with JIA.

There are two additional subtypes of JIA. Children with psoriatic arthritis may have typical psoriasis but may also present prior to the onset of the classic thick scaly plaques and have more subtle changes such as nail pitting. Patients with psoriatic arthritis may also present with dactylitis or "sausage digit," which is painful swelling of an entire finger or toe. Undifferentiated JIA, comprising 10% of patients, includes children with chronic arthritis who do not meet criteria for any of the other subgroups or meet more than one criterion and therefore could be classified into multiple subgroups.

B. Laboratory Findings

There is no diagnostic test for JIA. A normal erythrocyte sedimentation rate (ESR) does not exclude the diagnosis of JIA. However, patients with systemic JIA typically have significantly elevated markers of inflammation, including ESR, C-reactive protein (CRP), white blood cell count, and platelets. RF is positive in about 5% of patients, usually when the onset of polyarticular disease occurs after age 8 years. The anti-cyclic citrullinated peptide (anti-CCP) antibody has a very high specificity for rheumatoid arthritis and may be detectable prior to the RF. ANAs are associated with an increased risk of uveitis in patients with oligoarticular disease and are also fairly common in patients with the late-onset RF-positive form of the disease. Carriage of HLAB27 antigen is associated with an increased risk of developing enthesitis-associated arthritis.

Table 29–1 lists the general characteristics of joint fluid in various conditions. The main indication for joint aspiration and synovial fluid analysis is to rule out infection. A positive Gram stain or culture is the only definitive test for infection. A leukocyte count over 2000/μL suggests inflammation; this may be due to infection, rheumatologic diseases, leukemia, or reactive arthritis. A very low glucose concentration (< 40 mg/dL) or very high polymorphonuclear leukocyte count (> 60,000/μL) is highly suggestive of bacterial arthritis.

C. Imaging Studies

In the early stages of the disease, only soft tissue swelling and possibly periarticular osteoporosis may be seen. Magnetic resonance imaging (MRI) of involved joints may show early joint damage and, if obtained with gadolinium, can confirm the presence of synovitis. Ultrasound is now used to detect synovitis, tenosynovitis, and bony erosions without radiation and without requiring sedation. Later in the course of the disease, particularly in patients with RF-positive disease, plain films may demonstrate joint space narrowing due to cartilage thinning and erosive changes of the bone related to chronic inflammation.

▶ Differential Diagnosis

Table 29–2 lists the most common causes of limb pain in childhood. JIA is a diagnosis of exclusion; therefore, it is important to rule out other causes of the clinical signs and symptoms

Table 29–2. Differential diagnosis of limb pain in children.

Orthopedic
Stress fracture
Chondromalacia patellae
Osgood-Schlatter disease
Slipped capital femoral epiphysis
Legg-Calvé-Perthes disease
Hypermobility syndrome
Reactive arthritis
Henoch-Schönlein purpura
Transient synovitis
Rheumatic fever
Poststreptococcal arthritis
Infections
Bacterial
Lyme arthritis
Osteomyelitis
Septic arthritis
Discitis
Viral (including parvovirus, Epstein-Barr virus, hepatitis B, dengue, chikungunya)
Rheumatologic
Juvenile idiopathic arthritis
Systemic lupus erythematosus
Dermatomyositis
Chronic recurrent multifocal osteomyelitis
Neoplastic
Leukemia
Lymphoma
Neuroblastoma
Osteoid osteoma
Bone tumors (benign or malignant)
Pain syndromes
Growing pains
Fibromyalgia
Complex regional pain syndrome

Table 29–1. Joint fluid analysis.

Disorder	Cells/μL	Glucose[a]
Trauma	More red cells than white cells; usually < 2000 white cells	Normal
Reactive arthritis	3000–10,000 white cells, mostly mononuclear cells	Normal
Juvenile idiopathic arthritis and other inflammatory arthritides	5000–60,000 white cells, mostly neutrophils	Usually normal or slightly low
Septic arthritis	> 60,000 white cells, > 90% neutrophils	Low to normal

[a]Normal value is ≥ 75% of the serum glucose value.

prior to settling on this diagnosis. The differential diagnosis is often quite broad, including orthopedic conditions, infectious diseases, and malignancies. A few key features can help distinguish these different entities, including the timing of the pain and associated signs and symptoms. In inflammatory conditions, patients frequently have increased symptoms in the morning with associated stiffness, whereas patients with an orthopedic abnormality typically have increased symptoms later in the day and with activity. Growing pains, a common cause of leg pain in childhood, are characterized by poorly localized pain at night, which frequently wakes the child from sleep; no objective signs of inflammation; and no daytime symptoms. Patients with growing pains often ask to be massaged, which is not typical of those with arthritis.

It is particularly important to establish the diagnosis in the case of monoarticular arthritis. Bacterial arthritis is usually acute and monoarticular except for arthritis associated with gonorrhea, which may be associated with a migratory pattern and hemorrhagic pustules, usually on the distal extremities. Fever, leukocytosis, and increased ESR with an acute process in a single joint demand synovial fluid examination and culture to rule out an infection. Pain in the hip or lower extremity is a frequent symptom of childhood cancer, especially leukemia, neuroblastoma, and rhabdomyosarcoma. Radiographs of the affected site and examination of the blood smear for unusual cells and thrombocytopenia are necessary. An elevated lactate dehydrogenase value should also raise concern about an underlying neoplastic process. In doubtful cases, bone marrow examination or biopsies are indicated.

Reactive arthritis is joint pain and swelling triggered by an infection. The infection is nonarticular and can be either viral or bacterial. A preceding illness is identified in approximately half of cases. Patients often have acute onset of arthritis, and there may be a migratory pattern. The duration of symptoms is a very important distinction between reactive arthritides and JIA. Symptoms associated with reactive arthritis typically resolve within 4–6 weeks. In contrast, to meet criteria for chronic arthritis, symptoms must be present for at least 6 weeks.

The arthritis of rheumatic fever is migratory, transient, and often more painful than that of JIA. (see Chapter 20). In suspected cases, evidence of rheumatic carditis should be sought based on examination and electrocardiographic findings. Evidence of recent streptococcal infection is essential to the diagnosis. The fever pattern in rheumatic fever is low grade and persistent compared with the spiking fever that characterizes the systemic form of JIA. Lyme arthritis resembles oligoarticular JIA, but the former usually occurs as discrete, recurrent episodes of arthritis lasting 2–6 weeks and children should have a history of being in an endemic area. The typical bull's-eye rash, erythema chronicum migrans, is reported for approximately 70%–80% of patients, although it is resolved by the time the arthritis appears. For children suspected of having Lyme disease, testing for antibodies against

Borrelia burgdorferi should be performed, with confirmatory testing by Western blot.

▶ Treatment

The objectives of therapy are to restore function, relieve pain, maintain joint motion, and prevent damage to cartilage and bone.

A. Nonsteroidal Anti-Inflammatory Medications

Nonsteroidal anti-inflammatory drugs (NSAIDs) are frequently used for symptomatic relief. A wide range of agents is available, but only a few are approved for use in children, including naproxen (10 mg/kg per dose twice daily), ibuprofen (10 mg/kg per dose three to four times daily), and meloxicam (0.125–0.25 mg/kg once daily). NSAIDs are generally well tolerated in children, as long as they are taken with food and adequate hydration. The average time to symptomatic improvement is 1 month, but in some patients, a response is not seen for 8–12 weeks.

B. Disease-Modifying and Biologic Agents

Most patients with JIA require treatment with a disease-modifying medication, most commonly weekly methotrexate. Symptomatic response usually begins within 3–4 weeks. The low dosages used (5–10 mg/m²/wk or up to 1 mg/kg/wk as a single dose) are generally well tolerated. Potential side effects include nausea, vomiting, hair thinning, stomatitis, leukopenia, immunosuppression, and hepatotoxicity. A complete blood count and liver function tests should be obtained every 2–3 months. Several additional disease-modifying agents are available for use in patients with persistently active disease or those intolerant to methotrexate. Leflunomide is an antipyrimidine medication that is administered orally. Side effects may include diarrhea and alopecia. Biological-modifying medications that inhibit tumor necrosis factor, a cytokine known to play an important role in the pathogenesis of JIA, include etanercept, infliximab, and adalimumab. These drugs are generally quite effective in controlling disease and preventing cartilage and bone damage and have been associated with healing based on radiologic changes. However, their potential long-term effects are less well understood, they are very expensive, and require parenteral administration. Anakinra and tocilizumab, which block interleukin 1 and 6, respectively, are particularly effective for systemic JIA. Other biologic agents, including rituximab and abatacept, have demonstrated some efficacy in patients who have not responded to other treatments.

C. Corticosteroids

Local steroid joint injections may be helpful in patients who have arthritis in one or a few joints. Triamcinolone acetonide is a long-acting steroid that can be used for injections and is often associated with at least several months of disease control. Oral or parenteral steroids are reserved for children with severe involvement, primarily patients with systemic disease.

D. Uveitis

Inflammation of the uveal tract (uveitis or iridocyclitis) should be closely monitored by an ophthalmologist. Typically, treatment is initiated with corticosteroid eye drops and dilating agents to prevent scarring between the iris and the lens. In patients who fail topical treatments, methotrexate, cyclosporine, mycophenolate mofetil, and/or a tumor-necrosis factor inhibitor such as infliximab or adalimumab may be used.

E. Rehabilitation

Physical and occupational therapies are important to focus on range of motion, stretching, and strengthening. These exercises, as well as other modalities such as heat and water therapy, can help control pain, maintain and restore function, and prevent deformity and disability. Young children with oligoarticular disease affecting asymmetrical lower extremity joints can develop a leg-length discrepancy, which may require treatment with a shoe lift on the shorter side.

▶ Prognosis

The course and prognosis for JIA is variable, depending on the subtype of disease. Children with persistent oligoarticular JIA have the highest rate of clinical remission, while patients with RF-positive disease are the least likely to achieve this status and are at highest risk for chronic, erosive arthritis that may continue into adulthood. The systemic features associated with systemic arthritis tend to remit within months to years. The prognosis in systemic disease is worse in patients with persistent systemic disease after 6 months, thrombocytosis, and more extensive arthritis.

Giancane G et al: Recent therapeutic advances in juvenile idiopathic arthritis. Best Pract Res Clin Rheumatol 2017;31(4):476–487 [PMID: 29773268].
Palman J et al: Update on the epidemiology, risk factors and disease outcomes of juvenile idiopathic arthritis. Best Pract Res Clin Rheumatol 2018;32(2):206–222 [PMID: 30527427].
www.arthritis.org. Accessed June 17, 2019.

SYSTEMIC LUPUS ERYTHEMATOSUS

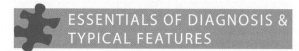

ESSENTIALS OF DIAGNOSIS & TYPICAL FEATURES

▶ Multisystem inflammatory disease of the joints, serosal linings, skin, kidneys, blood, and central nervous system.

▶ Pathogenesis

Systemic lupus erythematosus (SLE) is the prototype of immune complex diseases; its pathogenesis is related to the formation of antibody–antigen complexes that exist in the circulation and deposit in the involved tissues. The spectrum of symptoms is due to tissue-specific autoantibodies as well as the damage to tissues by lymphocytes, neutrophils, and complement evoked by the deposition of immune complexes.

▶ Clinical Findings

A. Symptoms and Signs

The onset of pediatric SLE is most common in girls between the ages of 9 and 15 years. Signs and symptoms depend on the organs affected by immune complex deposition. The American College of Rheumatology has established classification criteria for SLE; 4 of the following 11 criteria are necessary to be classified as SLE:

1. Malar rash—photosensitive, "butterfly rash" on the cheeks and nasal bridge
2. Discoid rash—annular, scaly rash on the scalp, face, and extremities that can lead to scarring
3. Photosensitivity—increased rash or other disease symptoms in response to sunlight exposure
4. Mucous membrane ulcers—painless ulcers on the hard palate and/or nasal septum
5. Arthritis—nonerosive arthritis of large and small joints, typically in a symmetrical distribution
6. Serositis—pericarditis and/or pleuritis, often associated with chest pain and difficulty breathing
7. Renal abnormalities—proteinuria (> 0.5 g/day) and/or cellular casts
8. Neurologic abnormalities—seizures and/or psychosis
9. Blood count abnormalities—low white blood cell count (< 4000/mm³), Coombs test–positive hemolytic anemia, and/or thrombocytopenia (< 100,000/mm³)
10. Positive ANA—seen in almost 100% of patients with SLE
11. Autoantibodies—positive double-stranded DNA antibody, anti-Smith antibody, anticardiolipin antibodies, lupus anticoagulant, and/or false-positive blood test for syphilis

More recent classification criteria, established by the SLE International Collaborating Clinics Group (SLICC) in 2012, are now being used for pediatric rheumatology research studies (Table 29–3). These are similar to the above, but more inclusive, including low complements and a positive Coombs test in the absence of hemolytic anemia.

Table 29–3. SLICC classification criteria for systemic lupus erythematosus

Clinical Criteria	Laboratory/Immunologic Criteria
1. Acute cutaneous lupus	1. ANA
2. Chronic cutaneous lupus	2. Anti-dsDNA
3. Oral or nasal ulcers	3. Anti-Sm
4. Nonscarring alopecia	4. Antiphospholipid antibodies
5. Arthritis	5. Low complement (C3, C4, CH50)
6. Serositis	6. Direct Coombs' test in the absence of hemolytic anemia
7. Renal	
8. Neurologic	
9. Hemolytic anemia	
10. Leukopenia	
11. Thrombocytopenia (< 100,000)	

SLICC, SLE International Collaborating Clinics Group.
Requirements: Four or more criteria (at least one clinical and one laboratory criteria).
OR biopsy-proven lupus nephritis with positive ANA or anti-dsDNA.

Other common signs and symptoms include fever, fatigue, weight loss, anorexia, Raynaud phenomenon, myositis, and vasculitis.

B. Laboratory Findings

Blood count abnormalities are common, including leukopenia, anemia, and thrombocytopenia. Approximately 15% of patients are Coombs test positive, but many patients develop anemia due to other causes, including chronic disease and blood loss. Patients with significant renal involvement may have electrolyte disturbances, elevated kidney function tests, and hypoalbuminemia. The ESR is frequently elevated during active disease. In contrast, many patients with active SLE have a normal CRP. When the CRP is elevated, it is important to investigate possible infectious causes, particularly bacterial infections. It is critical to monitor the urinalysis in patients with SLE for proteinuria and hematuria, as the renal disease may be otherwise clinically silent. In immune complex diseases, complement is consumed; therefore, levels of C3 and C4 are depressed with active disease.

The ANA test is positive in almost 100% of patients, usually at titers of 1:320 or above. In patients with suspected SLE, it is important to obtain a full ANA profile—including antibodies directed against double-stranded DNA, Smith, ribonucleic protein, and Sjögren-specific antibody A and B to better characterize their serologic markers of disease. Because approximately 50%–60% of pediatric SLE patients have antiphospholipid antibodies and are therefore at increased risk of thrombosis, it is important to screen all patients with SLE for anticardiolipin antibodies and lupus anticoagulant.

Differential Diagnosis

Because there is such a wide spectrum of disease with SLE, the differential diagnosis is quite broad, including systemic JIA, mixed connective tissue disease (MCTD), rheumatic fever, vasculitis, malignancies, and bacterial and viral infections. A negative ANA test essentially excludes the diagnosis of SLE. Anti–double-stranded DNA and Smith antibodies are very specific for SLE. The preceding classification criteria, which can be very helpful in establishing the diagnosis of SLE, have a specificity and sensitivity of 96%.

MCTD, an overlap syndrome with features of several rheumatologic diseases, shares many signs and symptoms with SLE. The symptom complex is diverse and often includes arthritis, fever, skin tightening, Raynaud phenomenon, muscle weakness, and rash. The ANA test is typically positive in very high titers. The ANA profile is negative except for antibodies directed against ribonucleic protein.

Treatment

The treatment of SLE should be tailored to the organ system involved so that toxicities may be minimized. Prednisone is the mainstay of treatment and has significantly lowered the mortality rate in SLE. Patients with severe, life-threatening, or organ-threatening disease are typically treated with intravenous pulse methylprednisolone, 30 mg/kg per dose (maximum of 1000 mg) daily for 3 days, and then switched to 2 mg/kg/day of prednisone. The dosage should be adjusted using clinical and laboratory parameters of disease activity, and the minimum amount of corticosteroid to control the disease should be used. Skin manifestations, arthritis, and fatigue may be treated with antimalarials such as hydroxychloroquine, 5 to 7 mg/kg/day orally. Pleuritic pain or arthritis can often be managed with NSAIDs.

Most patients are also started on a steroid-sparing agent, such as mycophenolate mofetil, azathioprine, cyclophosphamide or rituximab. Patients who have evidence of antiphospholipid antibodies are often treated with a baby aspirin every day to help prevent thrombosis. Thrombotic events due to these antibodies require long-term anticoagulation.

The toxicities of the regimens must be carefully considered. Growth failure, osteoporosis, Cushing syndrome, adrenal suppression, infections, and aseptic bone necrosis are serious side effects of chronic use of prednisone. Cyclophosphamide can cause bone marrow suppression, bladder epithelial dysplasia, hemorrhagic cystitis, and sterility. Azathioprine has been associated with liver damage and bone marrow suppression. Rituximab can be associated with infusion reactions and can lead to long-term hypogammaglobulinemia. Retinal damage from hydroxychloroquine is generally not observed with recommended dosages, but patients should have routine visual field testing to screen for retinal toxicity.

Prognosis

The disease has a natural waxing and waning cycle; it may flare at any time and spontaneous remission may rarely occur. The 5-year survival rate has improved from 51% in 1954 to 90% today. Factors that have contributed to improved prognosis include earlier diagnosis, more aggressive treatments with cytotoxic/immunosuppressive agents, pulse high-dose steroids, and advances in the treatment of hypertension, infections, and renal failure.

Couture J, Silverman ED: Update on the pathogenesis and treatment of childhood-onset systemic lupus erythematosus. Curr Opin Rheumatol 2016;28(5):488–496 [PMID: 27341622].

Hedrick C et al: Juvenile-onset systemic lupus erythematosus (jSLE)—pathophysiological concepts and treatment options. Best Pract Res Clin Rheumatol 2017;31(4):488–504 [PMID: 29773269].

Thakral A, Klein-Gitelman MS: An update on treatment and management of pediatric systemic lupus erythematosus. Rheumatol Ther 2016;3(2):209–219 [PMID: 27747587].

www.lupus.org. Accessed June 18, 2019.

DERMATOMYOSITIS

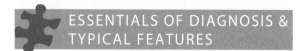

ESSENTIALS OF DIAGNOSIS & TYPICAL FEATURES

▶ Pathognomonic skin rashes.

▶ Weakness of proximal muscles and occasionally of pharyngeal and laryngeal groups.

▶ Pathogenesis related to vasculopathy.

Clinical Findings

A. Symptoms and Signs

The predominant symptom is proximal muscle weakness, particularly affecting pelvic and shoulder girdle muscles. Tenderness, stiffness, and swelling may be found. Pharyngeal involvement, manifested as voice changes and difficulty swallowing, is associated with an increased risk of aspiration. Intestinal vasculitis can be associated with ulceration and perforation of involved areas. Flexion contractures and muscle atrophy may produce significant residual deformities. Calcinosis may follow the inflammation in muscle and skin.

Several characteristic rashes are seen in dermatomyositis. Patients often have a heliotrope rash with a reddish-purple hue on the upper eyelids, along with a malar rash that may be accompanied by edema of the eyelids and face. Gottron papules are shiny, erythematous, scaly plaques on the extensor surfaces of the knuckles, elbows, and knees. Dilated nail-bed vessels are commonly seen with active disease. Thrombosis and dropout of periungual capillaries may identify patients with a more severe, chronic disease course.

B. Laboratory Findings/Imaging Studies/Special Tests

Determination of muscle enzyme levels, including aspartate aminotransferase, alanine aminotransferase, lactate dehydrogenase, creatine phosphokinase, and aldolase, is helpful in confirming the diagnosis, assessing disease activity, and monitoring the response to treatment. Even in the face of extensive muscle inflammation, the ESR and CRP may be normal. An MRI scan of the quadriceps muscle can be used in equivocal cases to confirm the presence of inflammatory myositis. Electromyography is useful to distinguish myopathic from neuropathic causes of muscle weakness. Muscle biopsy is indicated in cases of myositis without the pathognomonic rash.

Treatment

Treatment is aimed at suppression of the inflammatory response and prevention of the loss of muscle function and joint range of motion. Acutely, it is very important to assess the adequacy of the ventilatory effort and swallowing and to rule out intestinal vasculitis. Corticosteroids are the initial therapy of choice. Treatment is usually initiated with prednisone, 2 mg/kg/day, and continued until signs and symptoms of active disease are controlled; the dosage is then gradually tapered. In severe cases, intravenous pulse methylprednisolone for 3 days is indicated. Therapy is guided by the physical examination findings and muscle enzyme values. Methotrexate is often used concomitantly to achieve better control of the disease and minimize the steroid side effects. If patients continue to have active disease, additional steroid-sparing agents, such as mycophenolate mofetil, cyclosporine, intravenous immunoglobulin, and, in severe cases, rituximab or cyclophosphamide may be considered.

Hydroxychloroquine and intravenous immunoglobulin may be particularly helpful in managing the skin manifestations. As the rashes are photosensitive, sun protection is very important. Physical and occupational therapy should be initiated early in the course of disease. Initially, passive range-of-motion exercises are performed to prevent loss of motion. Later, once the muscle enzymes have normalized, a graduated program of stretching and strengthening exercises is introduced to restore normal strength and function.

Prognosis

Patients may have a monocyclic course, chronic or recurrent course. Factors that influence the outcome include the rapidity of symptom onset, extent of weakness, presence of cutaneous or gastrointestinal vasculitis, timeliness of diagnosis, initiation of therapy, and response to treatment. Dermatomyositis in children is not associated with cancer as it is in adults.

Enders FB et al: Consensus-based recommendations for the management of juvenile dermatomyositis. Ann Rheum Dis 2017;76(2):329–340 [PMID: 27515057].

Huber A: Juvenile idiopathic inflammatory myopathies. Pediatr Clin North Am 2018;65(4):739–756 [PMID: 30031496].

Wu Q et al: Juvenile dermatomyositis: latest advances. Best Pract Res Clin Rheumatol 2017;31(4):535–557 [PMID: 29773272]. www.curejm.org. Accessed June 18, 2019.

VASCULITIS

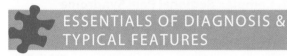

ESSENTIALS OF DIAGNOSIS & TYPICAL FEATURES

▶ Cutaneous involvement with nonblanching, tender skin lesions.

▶ Frequent presence of systemic inflammation, particularly in the lungs and kidneys.

▶ Gold standard for diagnosis is demonstration of vasculitis on biopsy.

The vasculitides are a group of conditions that involve inflammation of blood vessels. They are classified by the size of the blood vessels affected (Table 29–4). The two most common forms of vasculitis in childhood—Henoch-Schönlein purpura (HSP) and Kawasaki disease—are acute, self-limited forms of vasculitis. In contrast, there are idiopathic, chronic forms of vasculitis, such as granulomatosis with polyangiitis (GPA) and microscopic polyangiitis (MPA), which are rare in childhood.

Table 29–4. Classification of vasculitides by vessel size involved.

Large vessel
Takayasu arteritis
Giant cell arteritis
Medium vessel
Kawasaki disease
Granulomatosis with polyangiitis (previously called Wegener granulomatosis)
Polyarteritis nodosa
Eosinophilic granulomatosis with polyangiitis (previously called Churg-Strauss syndrome)
Small vessel
Henoch-Schönlein purpura
Microscopic polyarteritis

▶ **Clinical Findings**

A. Symptoms and Signs

Signs and symptoms vary by disease, but most children with chronic vasculitis have persistent fever, fatigue, weight loss, and signs of pulmonary, renal, musculoskeletal, gastrointestinal, and/or skin inflammation.

Granulomatosis with polyangiitis (previously called Wegener granulomatosis) often causes nephritis and involves the lungs, manifesting as chronic cough, hemorrhage, and/or cavitating lesions. This form of vasculitis also frequently affects the upper respiratory tract, causing chronic otitis media, sinusitis, and/or inflammation of the trachea; saddle nose deformity may occur.

Children with polyarteritis nodosa (PAN) often present with skin lesions such as purpura, nodules or ulcers, and evidence of organ involvement with abdominal pain, testicular pain, hypertension, hematuria, and/or neurologic symptoms. MPA typically presents with pulmonary-renal syndrome with features of pulmonary hemorrhage and rapidly progressive kidney inflammation.

B. Laboratory Findings/Imaging Studies/Special Tests

Patients with vasculitis often have elevated inflammatory markers. If they have significant renal involvement, they may have elevated renal function tests and abnormal urinary sediment. Anemia is common, due to chronic disease and/or renal insufficiency. Low hemoglobin may also be an indicator of pulmonary hemorrhage in a patient with cough, hemoptysis, respiratory distress, and/or infiltrates on chest x-ray.

Antineutrophil cytoplasmic antibodies (ANCA) may be present in patients with small vessel vasculitis. Cytoplasmic ANCA (c-ANCA), which is usually directed against proteinase 3 and is quite sensitive and specific for GPA, is positive in 80%–95% of patients. Perinuclear ANCA (p-ANCA) is typically directed against myeloperoxidase; is associated with MPA; and can also be seen in HSP, eosinophilic granulomatosis with polyangiitis (previously known as Churg-Strauss syndrome), and inflammatory bowel disease.

The diagnosis is made based on a typical clinical presentation and laboratory findings. If the diagnosis remains uncertain, attempting to establish the diagnosis with a biopsy of involved tissue is warranted. A biopsy in patients with GPA typically demonstrates necrotizing granulomatous vasculitis. Biopsies of involved areas will confirm the presence of vasculitis in small vessels in patients with MPA and small and medium arteries in PAN. If a biopsy is not feasible, additional imaging studies such as an angiogram, which can demonstrate characteristic patterns of inflammation in affected blood vessels, should be considered.

Treatment

The treatment of the various forms of chronic vasculitis is based on the severity of illness and the organs involved. Typically, corticosteroids are the initial therapy. Patients with severe disease are usually treated with intravenous pulse methylprednisolone, 30 mg/kg per dose (maximum of 1000 mg) daily for 3 days, and then switched to 2 mg/kg/day of prednisone. The dosage is then gradually tapered as tolerated based on clinical and laboratory markers of disease activity. Patients are usually treated with other immunosuppressant medications to gain and maintain control of the disease and minimize the steroid side effects. Standard treatment has included cyclophosphamide for induction, followed by maintenance with methotrexate, azathioprine, or mycophenolate. More recent studies in patients with ANCA-positive vasculitis suggest that rituximab can be used for induction therapy with potentially fewer side effects and risks than cyclophosphamide.

Prognosis

Immunosuppressive medications have improved survival and remission rates for patients with chronic vasculitis. Conditions such as GPA had almost always been fatal. Since introducing the regimen of high-dose steroids and cyclophosphamide (or other cytotoxic agents), patients with vasculitides have greatly improved outcomes, with 5-year survival ranging from 50% to 100%. Because relapses are common when therapy is weaned or stopped, maintenance immunosuppression is commonly required.

Calatroni M et al: ANCA-associated vasculitis in childhood: recent advances. Ital J Pediatr 2017;43(1):46 [PMID: 28476172].

Sag E et al: Childhood systemic vasculitis. Best Pract Res Clin Rheumatol 2017;31(4):558–575 [PMID: 29773273].

RAYNAUD PHENOMENON

Raynaud phenomenon is an intermittent vasospastic disorder of the extremities. As much as 5%–10% of the adult population has this disorder, and onset in childhood is not uncommon. The classic triphasic presentation is cold-induced pallor, then cyanosis, followed by hyperemia, but incomplete forms are frequent. In adults older than 35 years who are ANA-positive, Raynaud phenomenon may be a harbinger of rheumatic disease. This progression is rarely seen in childhood. Evaluation should include a detailed history with review of systems relevant to rheumatic disease. Examination of the cuticle edge, using an otoscope or a special microscope called a capillaroscope, is important to screen for dilated and/or tortuous capillaries that may suggest an underlying rheumatic disease such as lupus or scleroderma. In the absence of positive findings, Raynaud phenomenon is likely to be idiopathic.

Treatment involves education about keeping the extremities and core body warm and the role of stress, which may be a precipitant. In very symptomatic patients, treatment with vasodilators, such as calcium channel blockers, can be effective.

Pain CE et al: Raynaud's syndrome in children: systematic review and development of recommendations for assessment and monitoring. Clin Exp Rheumatol 2016;34:200–206 [PMID: 27494080].

Rigante D et al: Handy hints about Raynaud's phenomenon in children: a critical review. Pediatr Dermatol 2017;34(3):235–239 [PMID: 28523890].

NONINFLAMMATORY PAIN SYNDROMES

1. Complex Regional Pain Syndrome

Complex regional pain syndrome, previously known as reflex sympathetic dystrophy, is a painful condition that is frequently confused with arthritis. Prevalence and recognition of the condition is increasing. Severe extremity pain leading to nearly complete loss of function is the hallmark of the condition. Evidence of autonomic dysfunction is demonstrated by pallor or cyanosis, temperature differences (with the affected extremity cooler than surrounding areas), and generalized swelling. On examination, allodynia, which is marked cutaneous hyperesthesia to even the slightest touch, is often evident. Results of laboratory tests are normal, without evidence of systemic inflammation. Radiographic findings are normal except for late development of osteoporosis. Bone scans may be helpful and may demonstrate either increased or decreased blood flow to the painful extremity.

The cause of this condition remains elusive. Treatment includes physical therapy to focus on restoration of function, maintenance of range of motion, and pain relief. NSAIDs can be helpful for pain control; in patients with more chronic disease, gabapentin or pregabalin are frequently effective. Persistent disease may respond to local nerve blocks. Counseling is helpful to identify potential psychosocial stressors and to assist with pain management. Long-term prognosis is good if recovery is rapid; recurrent episodes imply a less favorable prognosis.

http://stopchildhoodpain.org/. Accessed June 18, 2019.

Rabin J et al: Update in the treatment of chronic pain within pediatric patients. Curr Probl Pediatr Adolesc Health Care 2017;47(7):167–172 [PMID: 28716513].

Weissmann R, Uziel Y: Pediatric complex regional pain syndrome: a review. Pediatr Rheumatol Online J 2016;14:29 [PMID: 27130211].

2. Fibromyalgia

Fibromyalgia is a chronic pain syndrome characterized by diffuse musculoskeletal pain, fatigue, sleep disturbance, and chronic headaches. Weather changes, lack of sleep, and stress exacerbate symptoms. Patients have a normal examination except for characteristic trigger points at the insertion of muscles, especially along the neck, spine, and pelvis.

Treatment centers on physical therapy, nonnarcotic pain medications, improving sleep, and counseling. Low-dose amitriptyline or trazodone can help with sleep and may produce remarkable reduction in pain. Physical therapy should emphasize a graded rehabilitative approach to stretching and exercise and promote regular aerobic exercise. Pregabalin recently became the first medication to be approved by the Food and Drug Administration for the treatment of fibromyalgia. Use of the drug is associated with decreased pain in adults with fibromyalgia, and studies are planned to test safety and efficacy in children with the condition. The prognosis for children with fibromyalgia is not clear, and long-term strategies may be necessary to enable them to cope with the condition.

Namerow LB, Kutner EC, Wakefield EC, Rzepski BR, Sahl RA: Pain amplification syndrome: a biopsychosocial approach. Semin Pediatr Neurol 2016;23(3):224–230 [PMID: 27989330].

Weiss JE, Stinson JN: Pediatric pain syndromes and noninflammatory musculoskeletal pain. Pediatr Clin North Am 2018;65(4):801–826 [PMID: 30031499].

www.myalgia.com. Accessed June 18, 2019.

Zemel L, Blier PR: Juvenile fibromyalgia: a primary pain, or pain processing, disorder. Semin Pediatr Neurol 2016;23(3):231–241 [PMID: 27989331].

3. Hypermobility Syndrome

Ligamentous laxity is a common cause of joint pain. Patients with hypermobility present with episodic joint pain and occasionally with swelling that lasts a few days after increased physical activity. Depending on the activity, almost any joint may be affected. Five criteria have been established: (1) passive opposition of the thumb to the flexor surface of the forearm, (2) passive hyperextension of the fingers so that they are parallel to the extensor surface of the forearm, (3) hyperextension of the elbow, (4) hyperextension of the knee, and (5) palms on floor with knees extended. Results of laboratory tests are normal. The pain associated with the syndrome is produced by improper joint alignment caused by the laxity during exercise. Treatment consists of a graded conditioning program designed to provide muscular support of the joints to compensate for the loose ligaments and to train patients to protect their joints from hyperextension.

Armon K: Musculoskeletal pain and hypermobility in children and young people: is it benign joint hypermobility syndrome? Arch Dis Child 2015;100(1):2–3 [PMID: 25336435].

Cattalini M, Khubchandani R, Cimaz R: When flexibility is not necessarily a virtue: a review of hypermobility syndromes and chronic or recurrent musculoskeletal pain in children. Pediatr Rheumatol Online J 2015;13(1):40 [PMID: 26444669].

Revivo G et al: Interdisciplinary pain management improves pain and function in pediatric patients with chronic pain associated with joint hypermobility syndrome. PM R 2019;11(2):150–157 [PMID: 30010052].

Hematologic Disorders

Michael Wang, MD

Christopher McKinney, MD

Rachelle Nuss, MD

Daniel R. Ambruso, MD

▼ NORMAL HEMATOLOGIC VALUES

The normal ranges for peripheral blood counts vary significantly with age. Normal neonates have a hematocrit of 45%–65%. The reticulocyte count at birth is relatively high at 2%–8%. Within the first few days of life, erythrocyte production decreases, and the values for hemoglobin and hematocrit fall to a nadir at about 6–8 weeks. During this period, known as physiologic anemia of infancy, normal infants have hemoglobin values as low as 10 g/dL and hematocrits as low as 30%. Thereafter, the normal values for hemoglobin and hematocrit gradually increase until adult values are reached after puberty. Premature infants can reach a nadir hemoglobin level of 7–8 g/dL at 8–10 weeks. Anemia is defined as a hemoglobin concentration two standard deviations below the mean for a normal population of the same gender and age.

Newborns have larger red cells than children and adults, with a mean corpuscular volume (MCV) at birth of more than 94 fL. The MCV subsequently falls to a nadir of 70–84 fL at about age 6 months. Thereafter, the normal MCV increases gradually until it reaches adult values after puberty.

The normal number of white blood cells (WBCs) is higher in infancy and early childhood than later in life. Neutrophils predominate in the differential white count at birth and in the older child. Lymphocytes predominate (up to 80%) between about ages 1 month and 6 years.

Normal values for the platelet count are 150,000–400,000/μL and vary little with age.

▼ BONE MARROW FAILURE

Failure of the marrow to produce adequate numbers of circulating blood cells may be congenital or acquired and may cause pancytopenia or involve only one cell line (single cytopenia). Constitutional and acquired aplastic anemias are discussed in this section and the more common single cytopenias in later sections. Bone marrow failure caused by malignancy or other infiltrative disease is discussed in this chapter. It is important to remember that many drugs and toxins may affect the marrow and cause single or multiple cytopenias.

Suspicion of bone marrow failure is warranted in children with pancytopenia and in children with single cytopenias who lack evidence of peripheral red cell, white cell, or platelet destruction. Macrocytosis often accompanies bone marrow failure. Many of the constitutional bone marrow disorders are associated with a variety of congenital anomalies. Not all are discussed.

▼ CONSTITUTIONAL APLASTIC ANEMIA (FANCONI ANEMIA)

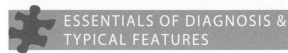

ESSENTIALS OF DIAGNOSIS & TYPICAL FEATURES

▶ Progressive pancytopenia.

▶ Macrocytosis.

▶ Multiple congenital anomalies in two-thirds.

▶ Increased chromosome breakage in peripheral blood lymphocytes.

▶ General Considerations

Fanconi anemia, which is the most common inherited bone marrow failure syndrome, is caused by germline mutations in the repair genes of the *FA/BRCA* pathway Inheritance is generally autosomal recessive, and the disease occurs in all ethnic groups; 75%–90% of affected individuals develop bone marrow failure in the first 10 years of life.

Clinical Findings

A. Symptoms and Signs

Symptoms are determined principally by the degree of hematologic abnormality. Thrombocytopenia may cause purpura, petechiae, and bleeding; neutropenia may cause severe or recurrent infections; and anemia may cause weakness, fatigue, and pallor. Congenital anomalies are present in at least two-thirds of patients. The most common anomalies include abnormal pigmentation of the skin (generalized hyperpigmentation, café au lait or hypopigmented spots), short stature with delicate features, and skeletal malformations (hypoplasia, anomalies, or absence of the thumb and radius). More subtle anomalies are hypoplasia of the thenar eminence or a weak or absent radial pulse. Associated renal anomalies include aplasia, horseshoe kidney, and duplication of the collecting system. Other anomalies are microcephaly, microphthalmia, strabismus, ear anomalies, and hypogenitalism.

B. Laboratory Findings

Thrombocytopenia or leukopenia typically occurs first, followed over the course of months to years by anemia and progression to severe aplastic anemia. Macrocytosis, which is virtually always present, is usually associated with anisocytosis and an elevation in fetal hemoglobin levels, and is an important diagnostic clue. The bone marrow reveals hypoplasia or aplasia. The diagnosis is confirmed by demonstration of an increased number of chromosome breaks and rearrangements in peripheral blood lymphocytes. The use of diepoxybutane to stimulate the breaks and rearrangements provides a sensitive assay that is virtually always positive in children with Fanconi anemia, even before the onset of hematologic abnormalities.

Specific Fanconi genes (FANC A, B, C, and others) have been identified and transmission is generally autosomal recessive, although FANCB is X-linked.

Differential Diagnosis

Because patients with Fanconi anemia frequently present with thrombocytopenia, the disorder must be differentiated from idiopathic thrombocytopenic purpura (ITP) and other more common causes of thrombocytopenia. In contrast to patients with ITP, those with Fanconi anemia usually exhibit a gradual fall in the platelet count. Counts less than 20,000/μL are often accompanied by neutropenia or anemia. Fanconi anemia may also be manifested initially by pancytopenia, and must be differentiated from acquired aplastic anemia and other disorders, such as acute leukemia. Examination of the bone marrow and chromosome studies of peripheral blood lymphocytes (chromosomal breakage) will usually distinguish between these disorders. Alternative constitutional causes of consideration include dyskeratosis congenital, Schwachman Diamond, and congenital amegakaryocytic thrombocytopenia.

Complications

Complications are those related to thrombocytopenia and neutropenia. Endocrine dysfunction may include growth hormone deficiency, hypothyroidism, or impaired glucose metabolism. Persons with Fanconi anemia have a significantly increased risk of developing malignancies, especially acute nonlymphocytic leukemia (800-fold), head and neck cancers, genital cancers, and myelodysplastic syndromes related to defective DNA repair.

Treatment

Attentive supportive care is critical. Patients with neutropenia who develop fever require prompt evaluation and parenteral broad-spectrum antibiotics. Transfusions are important, but should be used judiciously, especially in the management of thrombocytopenia, which frequently becomes refractory to platelet transfusions as a consequence of alloimmunization. Transfusions from family members should be discouraged because of the deleterious effect on the outcome of bone marrow transplantation. At least 50% of patients with Fanconi anemia respond, albeit incompletely, to oxymetholone, and many recommend institution of androgen therapy before transfusions are needed. However, oxymetholone is associated with hepatotoxicity, hepatic adenomas, and masculinization, and is particularly troublesome for female patients.

The definitive treatment is a reduced intensity hematopoietic stem cell transplant, ideally from a human leukocyte antigen (HLA)–identical sibling donor, although matched unrelated transplant may be considered. Before transplant, a prospective sibling donor must be screened for Fanconi anemia.

Prognosis

Many patients succumb to bleeding, infection, or malignancy in adolescence or early adulthood. Hematopoietic stem cell transplantation does not reduce the increased susceptibility for malignancy; 40% develop malignancy by 20 years posttransplant.

Dufour C: How I manage patients with Fanconi anaemia. Br J Haematol 2017;178:32–47 [PMID: 28474441].

Ebens CL: Comparable outcomes after HLA-matched sibling and alternative donor hematopoietic cell transplantation for children with Fanconi anemia and severe aplastic anemia. Biol Blood Marrow Transplant 2018;24:765–771 [PMID: 2920342].

Wegman-Ostrosky T, Savage SA: The genomics of inherited bone marrow failure: from mechanism to the clinic. Br J Haematol 2017;177: 526–542 [PMID: 28211564].

ACQUIRED APLASTIC ANEMIA

ESSENTIALS OF DIAGNOSIS & TYPICAL FEATURES

▶ Weakness and pallor.

▶ Petechiae, purpura, and bleeding.

▶ Frequent or severe infections.

▶ Pancytopenia with hypocellular bone marrow.

General Considerations

Acquired aplastic anemia is characterized by peripheral pancytopenia without an abnormal infiltrate or increased reticulin and a hypocellular bone marrow. Approximately 70% of cases in childhood are idiopathic. Other cases are secondary to idiosyncratic reactions to drugs such as nifedipine, sulfonamides, nonsteroidal anti-inflammatory drugs (NSAIDs), cytotoxic drugs and anticonvulsants. Toxic causes include exposure to benzene, insecticides, and heavy metals. Infectious causes include viral hepatitis, infectious mononucleosis (Epstein-Barr virus [EBV]), and human immunodeficiency virus (HIV). In children with immune disorders, aplastic anemia has been associated with human parvovirus B19 infection. Immune dysregulation can be associated with anemia.

Clinical Findings

A. Symptoms and Signs

Weakness, fatigue, and pallor result from anemia; petechiae, purpura, and bleeding occur due to thrombocytopenia; and fevers due to generalized or localized infections are associated with neutropenia. Hepatosplenomegaly and significant lymphadenopathy are unusual.

B. Laboratory Findings

Anemia is usually normocytic, with a low reticulocyte count. The WBC count is low, with a marked neutropenia. The platelet count is typically below 50,000/μL and is frequently below 20,000/μL. Bone marrow biopsy shows a marked decrease in cellularity, typically less than 20% of normal in severe aplastic anemia and less than 50% in moderate aplastic anemia. To diagnose severe aplastic anemia at least two of the following must be present: absolute neutrophil count less than 500/μL, platelet count less than 20,000, or reticulocyte count less than 60,000.

Differential Diagnosis

Examination of the bone marrow usually excludes pancytopenia caused by peripheral destruction of blood cells or by infiltrative processes such as acute leukemia, storage diseases, and myelofibrosis. Many of these other conditions are associated with hepatosplenomegaly. Preleukemic conditions also may present with pancytopenia and hypocellular bone marrows. Cytogenetic analysis of the marrow is helpful because a clonal abnormality may predict the subsequent development of leukemia. Alternative etiologies to be considered include paroxysmal nocturnal hemoglobinuria, myelodysplasia, hemophagocytic lymphocytic histiocytosis, or infection with HIV.

Complications

Acquired aplastic anemia is characteristically complicated by infection and hemorrhage, which are the leading causes of death. Other complications are those associated with therapy.

Treatment

Comprehensive supportive care is essential. Febrile illnesses require prompt evaluation and usually parenteral antibiotics. Irradiated leukocyte-depleted red blood cell (RBC) transfusions alleviate symptoms of anemia. Irradiated leukocyte depleted platelet transfusions may be lifesaving, but they should be used sparingly because many patients eventually develop platelet alloantibodies and become refractory to platelet transfusions.

Immunomodulation, usually with antithymocyte globulin and cyclosporine, is associated with a high response rate and improved overall survival. The addition of eltrombopag, a thrombopoietin mimic, is advantageous. However, incomplete response, relapse, and progression to myelodysplasia/leukemia likely occur. Hematopoietic stem cell transplant is the treatment of choice for severe aplastic anemia when an HLA-identical sibling donor is available. Because the likelihood of success with transplant is influenced adversely by receipt of transfusions, HLA typing of family members should be undertaken at the time of diagnosis. Increasingly, patients who lack HLA-identical siblings are able to find matched donors through cord blood banks or the National Marrow Donor Program.

Prognosis

Sustained, complete remissions may be seen in 65%–80% of patients receiving immunosuppressive therapy. Children receiving early bone marrow transplant from an HLA-identical sibling have a long-term survival rate of greater than 90%. Matched unrelated donor and haploidentical transplant can be considered. Survivors are at an increased risk of myelodysplastic syndrome, acute leukemia, and other malignancies.

Bacigalupo A: Alternative donor transplants for severe aplastic anemia. Hematology Am Soc Hematol Educ Program 2018 Nov 30;2018(1):467–473 [PMID: 30504347].

Townsley DM et al: Eltrombopag added to immune suppression for aplastic anemia. N Engl J Med 2017;20;1540–1550 [PMID: 23292240].

▼ ANEMIAS

APPROACH TO THE CHILD WITH ANEMIA

Anemia is a relatively common finding, and identifying the cause is important. Even though anemia in childhood has many causes, the correct diagnosis can usually be established with relatively little laboratory cost. Frequently the cause is identified with a careful history. Nutritional causes should be sought by inquiry about dietary intake; growth and development; and symptoms of chronic disease, malabsorption, or blood loss. Hemolytic disease may be associated with a history of jaundice (including neonatal jaundice) or by a family history of anemia, jaundice, gallbladder disease, splenomegaly, or splenectomy. The child's ethnicity may suggest the possibility of certain hemoglobinopathies or deficiencies of red cell enzymes, such as glucose-6-phosphate dehydrogenase (G6PD). The review of systems may reveal clues to a previously unsuspected systemic disease associated with anemia. The patient's age is important because some causes of anemia are age related. For example, patients with iron deficiency anemia (IDA) and β-globin disorders present more commonly at ages 6–36 months than at other times in life.

The physical examination may also reveal clues to the cause of anemia. Poor growth may suggest chronic disease or hypothyroidism. Congenital anomalies may be associated with constitutional aplastic anemia (Fanconi anemia) or with congenital hypoplastic anemia (Diamond-Blackfan anemia). Other disorders may be suggested by the findings of petechiae or purpura (leukemia, aplastic anemia, hemolytic uremic syndrome), jaundice (hemolysis or liver disease), generalized lymphadenopathy (leukemia, juvenile rheumatoid arthritis, HIV infection), splenomegaly (leukemia, sickle hemoglobinopathy syndromes, hereditary spherocytosis, liver disease, hypersplenism), or evidence of chronic or recurrent infections.

The initial laboratory evaluation of the anemic child consists of a complete blood count (CBC) with differential and platelet count, review of the peripheral blood smear, and a reticulocyte count. The algorithm in Figure 30–1 uses limited laboratory information, together with the history and physical examination, to reach a specific diagnosis or to focus additional laboratory investigations on a limited diagnostic category (eg, microcytic anemia, bone marrow failure, pure red cell aplasia, or hemolytic disease). This diagnostic scheme depends principally on the MCV to determine whether the

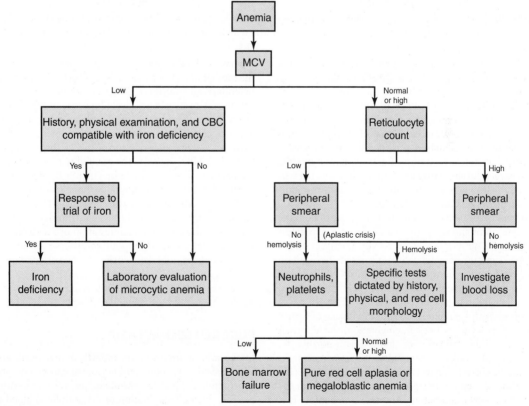

▲ Figure 30–1. Investigation of anemia.

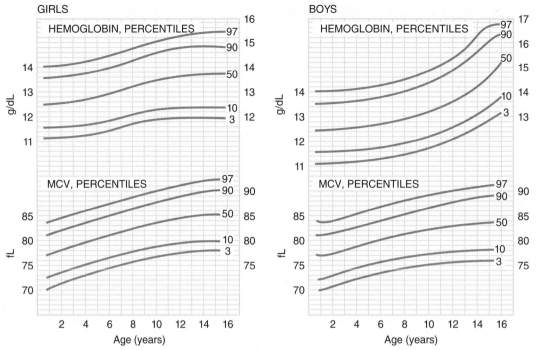

▲ **Figure 30–2.** Hemoglobin and red cell volume in infancy and childhood. (Reproduced with permission from Dallman PR, Siimes MA: Percentile curves for hemoglobin and red cell volume in infancy and childhood. J Pediatr 1979 Jan;94(1):26–31.)

anemia is microcytic, normocytic, or macrocytic, according to the percentile curves of Dallman and Siimes (Figure 30–2).

Although the incidence of IDA in the United States has decreased significantly with improvements in infant nutrition, it remains an important cause of microcytic anemia, especially at ages 6–24 months. A trial of therapeutic iron is appropriate in such children, provided the dietary history is compatible with ID and the physical examination or CBC does not suggest an alternative cause for the anemia. If a trial of therapeutic iron fails to correct the anemia and/or microcytosis, further evaluation is warranted.

Another key element of Figure 30–1 is the use of both the reticulocyte count and the peripheral blood smear to determine whether a normocytic or macrocytic anemia is due to hemolysis. Typically hemolytic disease is associated with an elevated reticulocyte count, but some children with chronic hemolysis initially present during a period of a virus-induced aplasia when the reticulocyte count is not elevated. Thus, review of the peripheral blood smear for evidence of hemolysis (eg, spherocytes, red cell fragmentation, sickle forms) is important in the evaluation of children with normocytic anemias and low reticulocyte counts. When hemolysis is suggested, the correct diagnosis may be suspected by specific abnormalities of red cell morphology or by clues from the history or physical examination. Autoimmune hemolysis is usually excluded by a negative direct antiglobulin test (DAT).

Review of blood counts and the peripheral blood smears of the mother and father may suggest genetic disorders such as hereditary spherocytosis. Children with normocytic or macrocytic anemias, with relatively low reticulocyte counts and no evidence of hemolysis on the blood smear, usually have anemias caused by inadequate erythropoiesis in the bone marrow. The presence of neutropenia or thrombocytopenia in such children suggests the possibility of aplastic anemia, malignancy, or severe folate or vitamin B_{12} deficiency, and usually dictates examination of the bone marrow.

Pure red cell aplasia may be congenital (Diamond-Blackfan anemia), acquired, and transient (transient erythroblastopenia of childhood); a manifestation of a systemic disease such as renal disease or hypothyroidism; or associated with malnutrition or mild deficiencies of folate or vitamin B_{12}.

Wood SK: Pediatric screening: development, anemia and lead. Prim Care 2019;46:69–84 [PMID: 30704661].

PURE RED CELL APLASIA

Infants and children with normocytic or macrocytic anemia, a low reticulocyte count, and normal or elevated numbers of neutrophils and platelets should be suspected of having pure red cell aplasia. Examination of the peripheral blood smear in such cases is important because signs of hemolytic disease suggest chronic hemolysis complicated by an aplastic crisis due to parvovirus infection. Appreciation of this phenomenon is important because chronic hemolytic disease may not be diagnosed until the anemia is exacerbated by an episode of red cell aplasia and subsequent rapidly falling hemoglobin level. In such cases, cardiovascular compromise and congestive heart failure may develop quickly.

1. Congenital Hypoplastic Anemia (Diamond-Blackfan Anemia)

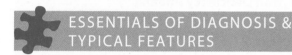

ESSENTIALS OF DIAGNOSIS & TYPICAL FEATURES

▶ Age: birth to 1 year.
▶ Macrocytic anemia with reticulocytopenia.
▶ Bone marrow with erythroid hypoplasia.
▶ Often short stature or congenital anomalies.

▶ General Considerations

Diamond-Blackfan anemia is a relatively rare cause of anemia that usually presents at 2–3 months of age but generally before 1 year of age. To date, mutations of genes encoding ribosomal proteins occur in 70%–80% tested. Early diagnosis is important because treatment with corticosteroids results in increased erythropoiesis in 80% of patients, thus avoiding the difficulties and complications of long-term chronic transfusion therapy.

▶ Clinical Findings

A. Symptoms and Signs

Signs and symptoms are generally those of chronic anemia, such as pallor and congestive heart failure. Jaundice, splenomegaly, or other evidence of hemolysis are usually absent. Short stature or other congenital anomalies are present in 50% of patients. A wide variety of anomalies have been described; craniofacial and triphalangeal thumbs are the most common.

B. Laboratory Findings

Diamond-Blackfan anemia is characterized by severe macrocytic anemia and marked reticulocytopenia. The neutrophil count is usually normal or slightly decreased, and the platelet count is normal, elevated, or decreased. The bone marrow usually shows a marked decrease in erythroid precursors but is otherwise normal. In older children, fetal hemoglobin levels are usually increased and there is evidence of persistent fetal erythropoiesis, such as the presence of the i antigen on erythrocytes.

▶ Differential Diagnosis

The principal differential diagnosis is transient erythroblastopenia of childhood. Children with Diamond-Blackfan anemia generally present at an earlier age, often have macrocytosis, and have evidence of fetal erythropoiesis and an elevated level of red cell adenosine deaminase. In addition, short stature and congenital anomalies are not associated with transient erythroblastopenia, and transient erythroblastopenia of childhood usually resolves within 6–8 weeks of diagnosis, whereas Diamond-Blackfan anemia is a lifelong affliction. Other disorders associated with decreased red cell production such as renal failure, hypothyroidism, and the anemia of chronic disease need to be considered.

▶ Treatment

Oral corticosteroids should be initiated at the time of diagnosis. Eighty percent of patients respond to prednisone, 2 mg/kg/day, and many who respond subsequently tolerate significant tapering of the dose. Patients who are unresponsive to prednisone require chronic transfusion therapy. Bone marrow transplant is an alternative definitive therapy that should be considered for transfusion-dependent patients who have HLA-identical siblings. Unpredictable spontaneous remissions occur in up to 20% of patients.

▶ Prognosis

The prognosis for patients responsive to corticosteroids is generally good, particularly if remission is maintained with low doses of alternate-day prednisone. Patients dependent on transfusion are at risk for the complications of hemosiderosis. There is an increased risk for the development of myelodysplastic syndrome, acute myeloid leukemia (AML), and solid tumors.

Da Costa L, Narla A, Mohandas N: An update on the pathogenesis and diagnosis of Diamond-Blackfan anemia. F1000Res 2018;7:F1000 Faculty Rev-1350. https://doi.org/10.12688/f1000research.15542 [PMID: 30228860].

2. Transient Erythroblastopenia of Childhood

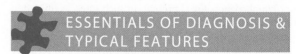

ESSENTIALS OF DIAGNOSIS & TYPICAL FEATURES

▶ Age: 6 months to 4 years.
▶ Normocytic anemia with reticulocytopenia.
▶ Absence of hepatosplenomegaly or lymphadenopathy.
▶ Erythroid precursors initially absent from bone marrow.

General Considerations

Transient erythroblastopenia of childhood is a relatively common cause of acquired anemia in early childhood. The disorder is suspected when a normocytic anemia is discovered during evaluation of pallor or when a CBC is obtained for another reason. Because the anemia is due to decreased red cell production, and thus develops slowly, the cardiovascular system has time to compensate. Therefore, children with hemoglobin levels as low as 4–5 g/dL may look remarkably well. The disorder is thought to be autoimmune in most cases, because IgG from some patients has been shown to suppress erythropoiesis in vitro.

Clinical Findings

Pallor is the most common sign, and hepatosplenomegaly and lymphadenopathy are absent. The anemia is normocytic, and the peripheral blood smear shows no evidence of hemolysis. The platelet count is normal or elevated, and the neutrophil count is normal or, in some cases, decreased. Early in the course, no reticulocytes are identified. The Coombs test is negative, and there is no evidence of chronic renal disease, hypothyroidism, or other systemic disorder. Bone marrow examination shows severe erythroid hypoplasia initially; subsequently, erythroid hyperplasia develops along with reticulocytosis, and the anemia resolves.

Differential Diagnosis

Transient erythroblastopenia of childhood must be differentiated from Diamond-Blackfan anemia, particularly in infants younger than 1 year. In contrast to Diamond-Blackfan anemia, transient erythroblastopenia is not associated with macrocytosis, short stature, or congenital anomalies, or with evidence of fetal erythropoiesis prior to the phase of recovery. Also in contrast to Diamond-Blackfan anemia, transient erythroblastopenia is associated with normal levels of red cell adenosine deaminase. Transient erythroblastopenia of childhood must also be differentiated from chronic disorders associated with decreased red cell production, such as renal failure, hypothyroidism, and other chronic states of infection or inflammation. As with other single cytopenias, the possibility of malignancy (ie, leukemia) should always be considered, particularly if fever, bone pain, hepatosplenomegaly, or lymphadenopathy is present. In such cases, examination of the bone marrow is generally diagnostic. Confusion may sometimes arise when the anemia of transient erythroblastopenia is first identified during the early phase of recovery when the reticulocyte count is high. In such cases, the disorder may be confused with the anemia of acute blood loss or with hemolytic disease. In contrast to hemolytic disorders, transient erythroblastopenia of childhood is not associated with jaundice or peripheral destruction of red cells.

Treatment & Prognosis

By definition, this is a transient disorder. Some children require red cell transfusions if cardiovascular compromise is present. Resolution of the anemia is heralded by an increase in the reticulocyte count, which generally occurs within 4–8 weeks of diagnosis. Transient erythroblastopenia of childhood is not treated with corticosteroids because of its short course.

NUTRITIONAL ANEMIAS

1. Iron Deficiency Anemia

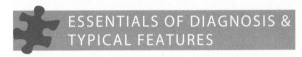

ESSENTIALS OF DIAGNOSIS & TYPICAL FEATURES

► Pallor and fatigue.
► Poor dietary intake of iron (ages 6–24 months).
► Chronic blood loss (age > 2 years).
► Microcytic hypochromic anemia.

General Considerations

Iron deficiency (ID) and iron deficiency anemia (IDA) are a worldwide concern. ID is defined as a state in which there is insufficient iron to maintain normal physiologic functions such that iron stores (serum ferritin or bone marrow iron content) are reduced. IDA is defined as a hemoglobin more than two standard deviations below normal for age and gender, which has developed as a consequence of ID.

Normal-term infants are born with sufficient iron stores to prevent ID for the first 4 months of life, whereas premature infants have reduced iron stores since iron is predominantly acquired in the last trimester. Thus premature infants, as well as those with low birth weight, neonatal anemia, perinatal blood loss, or subsequent hemorrhage may have reduced iron stores. Breast milk is low in iron relative to cow's milk and fortified formulas, and without iron supplementation, ID may develop in exclusively breast-fed children.

Clinical Findings

A. Symptoms and Signs

Symptoms and signs vary with the severity of the deficiency. ID is usually asymptomatic. IDA may be associated with, pallor, fatigue, and irritability. A history of pica is common. It is controversial whether or not ID/IDA adversely affects long-term neurodevelopment and behavior. IDA is associated with increased lead absorption and subsequent neurotoxicity.

B. Laboratory Findings

According to the American Academy of Pediatrics (AAP) guidelines, screening for anemia should be performed at about 12 months of age with determination of hemoglobin concentration and an assessment of risk factors for ID/IDA. Risks include low socioeconomic status, prematurity or low birth weight, lead exposure, exclusive breast-feeding beyond 4 months of age without iron supplementation, weaning to whole milk or complementary foods that do not include iron, feeding problems, poor growth, and inadequate nutrition. If the hemoglobin is less than 11 mg/dL or there is a high risk for ID, an iron evaluation should be performed. There is no single measurement that will document the iron status; tests to be considered include iron saturation, ferritin, C-reactive protein, and reticulocyte hemoglobin concentration.

▶ Differential Diagnosis

The differential diagnosis is that of microcytic, hypochromic anemia. The possibility of thalassemia (α-thalassemia, β-thalassemia, and hemoglobin E disorders) should be considered, especially in infants of African, Mediterranean, or Asian ethnic background. In contrast to infants with ID, those with thalassemia generally have an elevated red cell number and are less likely, in mild cases, to have an elevated RBC distribution width (the Mentzer index of the MCV divided by the red cell number is usually < 13 in thalassemia). Thalassemias are associated with normal or increased levels of serum iron and ferritin and with normal iron-binding capacity. The hemoglobin electrophoresis in β-thalassemia minor typically shows an elevation of hemoglobin A_2 levels, but coexistent ID may theoretically lower the percentage of hemoglobin A_2 into the normal range. Hemoglobin electrophoresis will also identify children with hemoglobin E, a cause of microcytosis common in Southeast Asians. In contrast, the hemoglobin electrophoresis in α-thalassemia trait is normal. Lead poisoning has also been associated with microcytic anemia, but anemia with lead levels less than 40 mg/dL is often due to coexistent ID.

The anemia of chronic inflammation or infection is normocytic but in late stages may be microcytic. This anemia is usually suspected because of the presence of a chronic systemic disorder and an elevated CRP. Relatively mild infections, particularly during infancy, may cause transient anemia. Thus, screening tests for anemia should not be obtained within 3–4 weeks of such infections.

▶ Treatment

The AAP has published guidelines for routine iron intake for children. If a child has hemoglobin of 10–11 mg/dL at the 12-month screening visit, the child can be closely monitored or empirically treated with iron supplementation with a recheck of hemoglobin in 1 month.

If a child is found to have ID/IDA, the recommended oral dose of elemental iron is 3 mg/kg/day. The dose for an adolescent is 65 mg a day. Iron therapy results in an increased reticulocyte count within 3–5 days, which is maximal between 5 and 7 days. The rate of hemoglobin rise is inversely related to the hemoglobin level at diagnosis. A rise in hemoglobin of 1 or more g/dL after 1 month of iron therapy indicates a good response. Treatment is continued for another 2 months to replenish iron stores. If unresponsive, consider underlying cow's milk protein–induced colitis, inflammatory bowel disease, menorrhagia, or poor compliance. Parenteral iron is used as first-line treatment for children receiving dialysis and erythrocyte stimulants and may be indicated for those with celiac or inflammatory bowel disease. It can be considered for children not adherent or responding to oral iron.

Powers JM: Disorders of iron metabolism. Hematol Oncol Clin North Am 2019;33:393–408. https://doi.org/10.1016/j.hoc.2019.01.006 [PMID: 31030809].

2. Megaloblastic Anemias

ESSENTIALS OF DIAGNOSIS & TYPICAL FEATURES

- ▶ Pallor and fatigue.
- ▶ Nutritional deficiency or intestinal malabsorption.
- ▶ Macrocytic anemia.
- ▶ Megaloblastic bone marrow changes.

▶ General Considerations

Megaloblastic anemia is manifest as large red cells with nuclear maturation arrest. The macrocytic anemia is caused by deficiency of cobalamin (vitamin B_{12}), folic acid, or both. Cobalamin deficiency due to dietary insufficiency may occur in infants who are breast-fed by mothers who are vegans or who have pernicious anemia. Intestinal malabsorption is the usual cause of cobalamin deficiency in children and occurs with Crohn disease, chronic pancreatitis, bacterial overgrowth of the small bowel, infection with the fish tapeworm (*Diphyllobothrium latum*), or after surgical resection of the terminal ileum. Deficiencies due to inborn errors of metabolism (transcobalamin II deficiency and methylmalonic aciduria) also have been described. Malabsorption of cobalamin due to deficiency of intrinsic factor (pernicious anemia) is rare in childhood.

Folic acid deficiency may be caused by inadequate dietary intake, malabsorption, increased folate requirements, or some combination of the three. Folate deficiency due to dietary deficiency alone is rare but occurs in severely malnourished infants and has been reported in infants fed with goat's milk not fortified with folic acid. Folic acid is absorbed in the jejunum, and deficiencies are encountered in malabsorptive syndromes such as celiac disease. Anticonvulsion medications (eg, phenytoin and phenobarbital) and cytotoxic drugs (eg, methotrexate) also have been associated with folate deficiency, caused by interference with folate absorption or metabolism. Finally, folic acid deficiency is more likely to develop in infants and children with increased requirements. This occurs during infancy because of rapid growth and also in children with chronic hemolytic anemia. Premature infants are particularly susceptible to the development of the deficiency because of low body stores of folate.

Clinical Findings

A. Symptoms and Signs

Infants with megaloblastic anemia may show pallor and mild jaundice as a result of ineffective erythropoiesis. Classically, the tongue is smooth and beefy red. Infants with cobalamin deficiency may be irritable and poor feeders. Older children with cobalamin deficiency may complain of paresthesias, weakness, or an unsteady gait, and may show decreased vibratory sensation and proprioception on neurologic examination.

B. Laboratory Findings

The laboratory findings of megaloblastic anemia include an elevated MCV and mean corpuscular hemoglobin (MCH). The peripheral blood smear shows numerous macro-ovalocytes with anisocytosis and poikilocytosis. Neutrophils are large and have hypersegmented nuclei. The white cell and platelet counts are normal with mild deficiencies but may be decreased in more severe cases. Examination of the bone marrow is not indicated, but it typically shows erythroid hyperplasia with large erythroid and myeloid precursors. Nuclear maturation is delayed compared with cytoplasmic maturation, and erythropoiesis is ineffective. The serum indirect bilirubin concentration may be slightly elevated.

Children with cobalamin deficiency often have a low serum vitamin B_{12} level, but not always. Decreased levels of serum vitamin B_{12} may also be found in about 30% of patients with folic acid deficiency. Negative results should not negate treatment if clinically compatible symptoms are present. The level of red cell folate is a better reflection of folate stores than is the serum folic acid level. Elevated serum levels of metabolic intermediates (methylmalonic acid and homocysteine) may help establish the correct diagnosis. Elevated methylmalonic acid levels are consistent with cobalamin deficiency and generally decrease with treatment, whereas elevated levels of homocysteine occur with both cobalamin and folate deficiency as well as hypothyroidism.

Differential Diagnosis

Most macrocytic anemias in pediatrics are not megaloblastic. Other causes of an increased MCV include drug therapy (eg, anticonvulsants, anti-HIV nucleoside analogues), Down syndrome, an elevated reticulocyte count (hemolytic anemias), bone marrow failure syndromes (Fanconi anemia, Diamond-Blackfan anemia), liver disease, and hypothyroidism.

Treatment

Treatment of cobalamin deficiency due to inadequate dietary intake is readily accomplished with high-dose oral supplementation that is as effective as parenteral treatment if absorption is normal. Folic acid deficiency is treated effectively with oral folic acid in most cases. Children at risk for the development of folic acid deficiencies, such as premature infants and those with chronic hemolysis, are often given folic acid prophylactically.

Green R: Vitamin B12 deficiency from the perspective of a practicing hematologist. Blood 2017;129:2603–2611 [PMID: 28360040].

ANEMIA OF CHRONIC DISORDERS

Anemia is a common manifestation of many chronic illnesses in children. In some instances, causes may be mixed. For example, children with chronic disorders involving intestinal malabsorption or blood loss may have anemia of chronic inflammation in combination with nutritional deficiencies of iron, folate, or cobalamin. In other settings, the anemia is due to dysfunction of a single organ (eg, renal failure, hypothyroidism), and correction of the underlying abnormality resolves the anemia.

1. Anemia of Chronic Inflammation

Anemia is frequently associated with chronic infections or inflammatory diseases. The anemia is usually mild to moderate in severity, with a hemoglobin level of 8–12 g/dL. In general, the severity of the anemia corresponds to the severity of the underlying disorder, and there may be microcytosis, but not hypochromia. The reticulocyte count is low. The anemia is thought to be due to inflammatory cytokines that inhibit erythropoiesis, and shunting of iron into, and impaired iron release from, reticuloendothelial cells. High levels of hepcidin, a peptide produced in the liver during infection or inflammation, reduce iron absorption by the duodenum and release from macrophages. Levels of erythropoietin are relatively low for the severity of the anemia. The serum iron concentration is low, but in contrast to ID, anemia of chronic inflammation is not associated with elevated iron-binding capacity and is associated with an elevated serum ferritin level. Treatment consists of correction of the underlying disorder, which, if controlled, generally results in improvement in hemoglobin level.

2. Anemia of Chronic Renal Failure

Severe normocytic anemia occurs in most forms of renal disease that have progressed to renal insufficiency. Although white cell and platelet production remain normal, the bone marrow shows significant hypoplasia of the erythroid series and the reticulocyte count is low. The principal mechanism is deficiency of erythropoietin, a hormone produced in the kidney, but other factors may contribute to the anemia. In the presence of significant uremia, a component of hemolysis may also be present. Recombinant human erythropoietin (epoetin alfa) and iron correct the anemia, largely eliminating the need for transfusions.

3. Anemia of Hypothyroidism

Some patients with hypothyroidism develop significant anemia. Occasionally, anemia is detected before the diagnosis of the underlying disorder. A decreased growth velocity in an anemic child suggests hypothyroidism. The anemia is usually normocytic or macrocytic, but it is not megaloblastic, and hence not due to deficiencies of cobalamin or folate. Replacement therapy with thyroid hormone is usually effective in correcting the anemia.

Fraenkel PG: Anemia of inflammation: a review. Med Clin N Am 2017;101:285–296 [PMID: 28189171].

CONGENITAL HEMOLYTIC ANEMIAS: RED CELL MEMBRANE DEFECTS

The congenital hemolytic anemias are divided into three categories: defects of the red cell membrane, hemoglobinopathies, and disorders of red cell metabolism. Red cell membrane defects are inherited and secondary to mutations in genes that encode for the membrane, cytoskeleton proteins or transmembrane transporters and channels. Hereditary spherocytosis and elliptocytosis are the most common red cell membrane disorders. The diagnosis is suggested by the peripheral blood smear, which shows characteristic red cell morphology (eg, spherocytes, elliptocytes). These disorders usually have an autosomal dominant inheritance, and the diagnosis may be suggested by family history. The hemolysis is due to the deleterious effect of the membrane abnormality on red cell deformability. Decreased cell deformability leads to entrapment of the abnormally shaped red cells in the spleen.

1. Hereditary Spherocytosis

ESSENTIALS OF DIAGNOSIS & TYPICAL FEATURES

► Anemia and jaundice.
► Splenomegaly.
► Positive family history of anemia, jaundice, or gallstones in 75%
► Spherocytosis with increased reticulocytes.
► Abnormal ektacytometry
► Increased osmotic fragility.
► Negative DAT.

► General Considerations

Hereditary spherocytosis is a relatively common inherited hemolytic anemia that occurs in all ethnic groups but most common in Caucasians of northern European ancestry, in whom the incidence is about 1:2000–5000. The disorder is marked by variable degrees of anemia, jaundice, and splenomegaly. In most persons, the disorder is mild to moderate because erythroid hyperplasia fully or partially compensates for hemolysis. The hallmark of hereditary spherocytosis is the presence of microspherocytes in the peripheral blood. The disease is inherited in an autosomal dominant fashion in about 75% of cases; the remaining cases are thought to be autosomal recessive or due to de novo mutations.

Hereditary spherocytosis is secondary to alteration of genes encoding for spectrin, band 3, ankyrin, or protein 4.2 of the red cell membrane; spectrin abnormalities are more often diagnosed in childhood and band 3 in adulthood. The vertical linkages in the membrane are impaired so that spherocytes form. These are poorly deformable, resulting in a shortened lifespan because they are trapped in the microcirculation of the spleen and engulfed by splenic macrophages.

► Clinical Findings

A. Symptoms and Signs

Hemolysis causes significant neonatal hyperbilirubinemia in 50% of affected children. Splenomegaly subsequently develops in the majority and is often present by age 5 years. Jaundice is variably present and in many patients may be noted only during infection. Patients with significant chronic anemia may complain of pallor, fatigue, or malaise. Intermittent exacerbations of the anemia are caused by increased hemolysis, splenic sequestration or by aplastic crises, and may be associated with severe weakness, fatigue, fever, abdominal pain, or even heart failure.

B. Laboratory Findings

Most patients have mild chronic hemolysis with hemoglobin levels of 9–12 g/dL. In some cases, the hemolysis is fully compensated and the hemoglobin level is in the normal range. Rare cases of severe disease require frequent transfusions. The anemia is usually normocytic and hyperchromic, and many patients have an elevated MCHC and RDW. The peripheral blood smear shows numerous microspherocytes and polychromasia. The reticulocyte count is elevated, often higher than might be expected for the degree of anemia. WBC and platelet counts are usually normal. Serum bilirubin usually shows an elevation in the unconjugated fraction. The DAT is negative. The osmotic fragility is increased, particularly after incubation at 37°C for 24 hours, and confirms the diagnosis. Alternative confirmatory tests are the acidified glycerol lysis test and osmotic gradient ektacytometry. DNA panels are available.

▶ Differential Diagnosis

Spherocytes are frequently present in persons with immune hemolysis. Thus, in the newborn, hereditary spherocytosis must be distinguished from hemolytic disease caused by ABO or other blood type incompatibilities. Older patients with autoimmune hemolytic anemia (AIHA) frequently present with jaundice, splenomegaly, and spherocytes on the peripheral blood smear. The DAT is positive in most cases of immune hemolysis and negative in hereditary spherocytosis. Occasionally, the diagnosis is confused in patients with splenomegaly from other causes, especially when hypersplenism increases red cell destruction and when some spherocytes are noted on the blood smear. In such cases, the true cause of the splenomegaly may be suggested by signs or symptoms of portal hypertension or by laboratory evidence of chronic liver disease. In contrast to children with hereditary spherocytosis, those with hypersplenism typically have some degree of thrombocytopenia or neutropenia.

▶ Complications

Severe jaundice may occur in the neonatal period and, if not controlled by phototherapy, may occasionally require exchange transfusion. Gallstones occur in 60%–70% of adults who have not undergone splenectomy and may form as early as age 5–10 years. Intermittent or persistent splenomegaly occurs in 10%–25% of patients and may require removal. Splenectomy is associated with an increased risk of overwhelming bacterial infections, particularly with pneumococci.

▶ Treatment

Supportive measures include the administration of folic acid to prevent the development of red cell hypoplasia due to folate deficiency. Acute hemolytic or aplastic crises caused by infection, often with human parvovirus, may be severe enough to require red cell transfusions. Laparoscopic splenectomy, if possible, may be indicated depending on clinical severity. Splenectomy increases survival of the red cells and results in complete correction of the anemia in most cases. Except in unusually severe cases, the procedure should be postponed until the child is at least age 5 years because of the greater risk of postsplenectomy sepsis prior to this age. All patients scheduled for splenectomy should be immunized, ideally at least 2 weeks prior, with pneumococcal, *Haemophilus influenzae* type b (Hib), and meningococcal vaccines. Prophylactic antimicrobial therapy, usually penicillin, is recommended by the RED BOOK for asplenic children younger than 5 years and for at least 1 year after splenectomy at any age. High-risk patients with asplenia could continue prophylaxis throughout childhood and into adulthood.

Asplenic patients with fever should be promptly evaluated for sepsis. Splenectomy prevents the subsequent development of cholelithiasis and eliminates the need for the activity restrictions. However, these benefits must be weighed against the risks of the surgical procedure and the subsequent lifelong risk of postsplenectomy sepsis and increased risk for thrombosis.

▶ Prognosis

Splenectomy eliminates signs and symptoms in all but the most severe cases. The abnormal red cell morphology and increased osmotic fragility persist without clinical consequence. Subtotal splenectomy can be considered for some children.

2. Hereditary Elliptocytosis

Hereditary elliptocytosis is a heterogeneous disorder that ranges in severity from an asymptomatic state with almost normal red cell morphology to about 10% having moderate to severe hemolytic anemia. Most affected persons have numerous elliptocytes on the peripheral blood smear, but mild or no hemolysis. Those with hemolysis have an elevated reticulocyte count and may have jaundice and splenomegaly. This disorder is caused by weakened horizontal linkages in the red cell membrane skeleton due to either a defective spectrin dimer-dimer interaction or a defective spectrin-actin protein 4.1R junctional complex. Inheritance is autosomal dominant. Because most patients are asymptomatic, no treatment is indicated. Patients with significant degrees of hemolytic anemia may benefit from folate supplementation or splenectomy but some degree of hemolysis persists post splenectomy.

Some infants with hereditary elliptocytosis present in the neonatal period with moderate to marked hemolysis and significant hyperbilirubinemia. This disorder has been termed transient infantile pyknocytosis because such infants exhibit bizarre erythrocyte morphology with elliptocytes, microspherocytes, and red cell fragments. The MCV is low, and the anemia may be severe enough to require red cell transfusions. Typically, one parent has hereditary elliptocytosis, usually mild or asymptomatic. The infant's hemolysis gradually abates during the first year of life, and the erythrocyte morphology subsequently becomes more typical of hereditary elliptocytosis.

Haley K: Congenital hemolytic anemia. Med Clin North Am 2017;361–374 [PMID: 28189176].

Mohandas N: Inherited hemolytic anemia: a possessive beginner's guide. Hematology Am Soc Hematol Educ Program 2018 Nov 30;2018(1):377–381 [PMID: 30504335].

CONGENITAL HEMOLYTIC ANEMIAS: HEMOGLOBINOPATHIES

The hemoglobinopathies are an extremely heterogeneous group of congenital disorders that occur in all ethnic groups. The relatively high frequency of these genetic variants is related to the malaria protection afforded to heterozygous individuals. The hemoglobinopathies are generally classified into two major groups. The first, the thalassemias, are caused by quantitative or qualitative deficiencies in the production of globin chains. Defects in globin synthesis cause microcytic and hypochromic anemias. The second group of hemoglobinopathies consists of those caused by structural abnormalities of globin chains. The most important of these, hemoglobins S, C, and E, are all the result of point mutations and single amino acid substitutions in β-globin. Many, but not all, infants with hemoglobinopathies are identified by routine neonatal screening.

Figure 30–3 shows the normal developmental changes that occur in globin-chain production during gestation and the first year of life. At birth, the predominant hemoglobin is fetal (hemoglobin F), which is composed of two α-globin chains and two γ-globin chains. Subsequently, the production of γ-globin decreases and β-globin increases so that adult hemoglobin (two α- and two β-globin chains) predominates after 2–4 months of age. Because α-globin chains are present in both fetal and adult hemoglobin, disorders of α-globin synthesis (α-thalassemia) are clinically manifest in the newborn as well as later in life. In contrast, patients with β-globin disorders such as β-thalassemia and sickle cell disease are generally asymptomatic during the first 3–4 months of age.

1. α-Thalassemia

ESSENTIALS OF DIAGNOSIS & TYPICAL FEATURES

► Predominately African, Mediterranean, Middle Eastern, Chinese, or Southeast Asian ancestry.

► Microcytic, hypochromic anemia of variable severity.

► Generally Bart's hemoglobin (γ_4) detected on neonatal screening.

► General Considerations

Most of the α-thalassemia syndromes are the result of deletions of one or more of the four α-globin genes, a pair of two closely linked genes on each chromosome 16, although nondeletional α+ mutations also occur. Excess non–α-globin chains damage the red cell membrane, causing extravascular hemolysis. The variable severity of the α-thalassemia syndromes is related to the number of gene deletions (Table 30–1). The severity of the α-thalassemia syndromes varies among affected ethnic groups. In persons of African ancestry, α-thalassemia is usually caused by the deletion of only one of the two α-globin genes on each

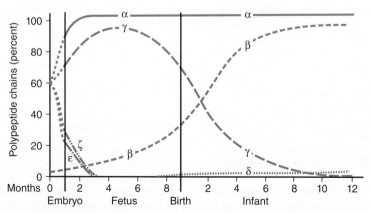

▲ **Figure 30–3.** Changes in hemoglobin polypeptide chains during human development. (Reproduced with permission from Miller DR, Baehner RL: *Blood Diseases of Infancy and Childhood*. 6th ed. Philadelphia, PA: Mosby; 1989.)

Table 30–1. The α-thalassemias.

Usual Genotypes[a]	α–Gene Deletions	Clinical Features	Hemoglobin Electrophoresis[b]	
			Birth	> 6 mo
αα/αα	0	Normal	N	N
–α/αα	1	Silent carrier	0%–3% Hb Bart's	N
–/αα or –α/–α	2	α-Thal trait/minor	2%–10% Hb Bart's[c]	N
–/–α	3	Hb H disease	15%–30% Hb Bart's	Hb; H present
–/–	4	Fetal hydrops	> 75% Hb Bart's	—

[a]α indicates presence of α-globin gene; – α indicates deletion of α-globin gene.
[b]N = normal results, Hb = hemoglobin, Hb Bart's = γ_4, Hb H = β_4.
[c]The level of Hb Bart's does not directly correlate with the number of deleted α genes.

chromosome (trans). Thus, in the African population, heterozygous individuals are silent carriers and homozygous individuals have α-thalassemia trait. In Asians, deletions of one or of both α-globin genes on the same chromosome are common (cis); heterozygous individuals are either silent carriers or have α-thalassemia trait, and homozygous individuals or compound heterozygous individuals have α-thalassemia trait, hemoglobin H disease, or hydrops fetalis. Thus, the presence of α-thalassemia in a child of Asian ancestry may have important implications for genetic counseling, whereas this is not usually the case in families of African ancestry.

▶ **Clinical Findings**

The clinical findings depend on the number of α-globin genes deleted. Table 30–1 summarizes the α-thalassemia syndromes. Persons with three α-globin genes (one-gene deletion) are asymptomatic and have no hematologic abnormalities. Hemoglobin electrophoresis in the neonatal period shows 0%–3% Bart's hemoglobin, which is a variant hemoglobin composed of four γ-globin chains. Hemoglobin electrophoresis after the first few months of life is normal. Thus, this condition is usually suspected only in the context of family studies or when a small amount of Bart's hemoglobin is detected by neonatal screening for hemoglobinopathies.

Persons with two α-globin genes (two-gene deletion) are typically asymptomatic. The MCV is usually less than 100 fL at birth. Hematologic studies in older infants and children show a normal or slightly decreased hemoglobin level with a low MCV and a slightly hypochromic blood smear with some target cells.

Persons with one α-globin gene (three-gene deletion) have hemoglobin H disease, a mild to moderately severe microcytic hemolytic anemia (hemoglobin level of 7–10 g/dL), which may be accompanied by hepatosplenomegaly, leg ulcers, hemolytic episodes, and some bony abnormalities caused by the expanded medullary space. The reticulocyte count is elevated, and the red cells show marked hypochromia and microcytosis with significant poikilocytosis and some basophilic stippling. Incubation of red cells with brilliant cresyl blue shows inclusion bodies formed by denatured hemoglobin H (β_4).

The deletion of all four α-globin genes causes severe intrauterine anemia and results in hydrops fetalis and fetal demise or neonatal death shortly after delivery. Extreme pallor and massive hepatosplenomegaly are present. With intrauterine transfusions and sophisticated prenatal support, there are a few survivors. Hemoglobin electrophoresis reveals a predominance of Bart's hemoglobin (γ_4) with a complete absence of normal fetal or adult hemoglobin. Molecular analysis can be useful in diagnosis.

▶ **Differential Diagnosis**

α-Thalassemia trait (two-gene deletion) must be differentiated from other mild microcytic anemias, including ID and β-thalassemia minor (see the next section). In contrast to children with ID, children with α-thalassemia trait have elevated red cell counts, normal or increased levels of ferritin and serum iron. In contrast to children with β-thalassemia minor, children with α-thalassemia trait have a normal hemoglobin electrophoresis after age 4–6 months. Finally, the history of a low MCV (96 fL) at birth or the presence of Bart's hemoglobin on the neonatal hemoglobinopathy screening test suggests α-thalassemia.

Children with hemoglobin H disease may have jaundice and splenomegaly, and the disorder must be differentiated from other hemolytic anemias. The key to the diagnosis is the decreased MCV and the marked hypochromia on the blood smear. With the exception of β-thalassemia, most other significant hemolytic disorders have a normal or elevated MCV and the RBCs are not hypochromic. Infants with hydrops fetalis due to severe α-thalassemia must be distinguished from those with hydrops due to other causes of anemia, such as alloimmunization or parvovirus.

▶ **Complications**

The principal complication of α-thalassemia trait is the needless administration of iron, given in the belief that a mild microcytic anemia is due to ID. Persons with hemoglobin H disease may have intermittent exacerbations of their anemia in response to oxidant stress or infection, which occasionally require blood transfusions. Splenomegaly may exacerbate the anemia. Women pregnant with hydropic α-thalassemia fetuses are subject to increased complications of pregnancy, particularly toxemia and postpartum hemorrhage.

Treatment

Persons with α-thalassemia trait require no treatment. Those with hemoglobin H disease should receive supplemental folic acid and avoid the same oxidant drugs that cause hemolysis in persons with G6PD deficiency, because exposure to these drugs may exacerbate their anemia. The anemia may also be exacerbated during periods of infection. Iron overload may occur independent of whether transfusions are given or not. Hypersplenism may develop later in childhood. Genetic counseling and prenatal diagnosis should be offered to families at risk for hydropic fetuses.

Daughety MM: Unusual anemias. Med Clin North Am 2017;101: 417–429 [PMID: 28189179].

Porter J: Beyond transfusion therapy: new therapies in thalassemia including drugs, alternate donor transplant, and gene therapy. Hematology Am Soc Hematol Educ Program 2018 Nov 30;2018(1):361–370 [PMID: 30504333].

2. β-Thalassemia

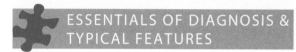

ESSENTIALS OF DIAGNOSIS & TYPICAL FEATURES

β-Thalassemia minor:

▶ Normal neonatal screening test.

▶ Predominantly African, Mediterranean, Middle Eastern, or Asian ancestry.

▶ Mild microcytic, hypochromic anemia.

▶ No response to iron therapy.

▶ Elevated level of hemoglobin A_2.

▶ β-Thalassemia intermedia:

▶ Ancestry as above.

▶ Microcytic, hypochromic anemia that usually becomes symptomatic after the first few years of life with hepatosplenomegaly.

▶ β-Thalassemia major:

▶ Neonatal screening shows hemoglobin F only.

▶ Mediterranean, Middle Eastern, or Asian ancestry.

▶ Severe microcytic, hypochromic anemia with marked hepatosplenomegaly.

General Considerations

Two β-globin genes are present, one on each chromosome 11. Excess non–β-globin chains damage the red cells, causing extravascular hemolysis. Classification of beta-thalassemia as minor, intermedia or major is complicated depending on the mutations in the hemoglobin genes and whether or not an individual produces any normal A hemoglobin or requires transfusions for survival. Individuals heterozygous for one β-thalassemia gene have β-thalassemia minor. Individuals with two non-hemoglobin A producing mutations have β-thalassemia major (Cooley anemia), a severe transfusion-dependent anemia. Thalassemia major is the most common worldwide cause of transfusion-dependent anemia in childhood. Individuals with compound mutations may have β-thalassemia major or intermedia depending on the severity of their anemia. In addition, the anemia found with thalassemia intermedia may worsen with age. Due to the complexity in diagnosis and variable course, there is a trend to classify affected individuals as either transfusion-dependent or non-transfusion dependent. β-thalassemia genes also interact with genes for structural β-globin variants, such as hemoglobin S and hemoglobin E to cause serious disease in compound heterozygous individuals. These disorders are discussed further in the sections dealing with sickle cell disease and hemoglobin E disorders.

Clinical Findings

A. Symptoms and Signs

Persons with β-thalassemia minor are usually asymptomatic with a normal physical examination. The time to presentation for those with β-thalassemia intermedia is variable. Those with β-thalassemia major are normal at birth but develop significant anemia during the first year of life. If the disorder is not identified and treated with blood transfusions, such children grow poorly and develop massive hepatosplenomegaly and enlargement of the medullary space with thinning of the bony cortex. The skeletal changes (due to ineffective erythropoiesis and marrow hyperplasia) cause characteristic facial deformities (prominent forehead and maxilla) and predispose the child to pathologic fractures.

B. Laboratory Findings

Children with β-thalassemia minor have normal neonatal screening results but subsequently develop a decreased MCV with or without mild anemia. The peripheral blood smear typically shows hypochromia, target cells, and sometimes basophilic stippling. Hemoglobin electrophoresis performed after 6–12 months of age is usually diagnostic when levels of hemoglobin A_2, hemoglobin F, or both are elevated. β-Thalassemia major is suspected when hemoglobin A is absent on neonatal screening. Such infants are hematologically normal at birth, but they develop severe anemia after the first few months of life. The peripheral blood smear typically shows a severe hypochromic, microcytic anemia with marked anisocytosis and poikilocytosis. Target cells are prominent, and nucleated RBCs often exceed the number of circulating WBCs. The hemoglobin level usually falls to 5–6 g/dL or less, and the reticulocyte count is elevated. Platelet and WBC counts may be increased, and the serum indirect bilirubin level is elevated. Hemoglobin electrophoresis shows only fetal hemoglobin and hemoglobin A_2 in children with homozygous β^0-thalassemia.

Those with β^+-thalassemia genes make a variable amount of hemoglobin A, depending on the mutation, but have a marked increase in fetal and hemoglobin A_2 levels. The diagnosis of β-thalassemia major, intermedia or minor, can be supported by DNA analysis.

▶ Differential Diagnosis

β-Thalassemia minor must be differentiated from other causes of mild microcytic, hypochromic anemias, principally ID and α-thalassemia. In contrast to patients with IDA, those with β-thalassemia minor typically have an elevated number of RBCs, and the Mentzer index of the MCV divided by the red cell count is under 13. Generally, an elevated hemoglobin A_2 level is diagnostic; occasionally, the A_2 level may be lowered by coexistent ID.

β-Thalassemia major is rarely confused with other disorders. Hemoglobin electrophoresis, DNA analysis and family studies readily distinguish it from hemoglobin E/β-thalassemia, which is the other increasingly important cause of transfusion-dependent thalassemia.

▶ Complications

The principal complication of β-thalassemia minor is the unnecessary use of iron therapy in a futile attempt to correct the microcytic anemia. Children with β-thalassemia major who are inadequately transfused experience poor growth and recurrent infections and may have hepatosplenomegaly, thinning of the cortical bone, and pathologic fractures. Without treatment, most children die within the first decade of life. The principal complications of β-thalassemia major in transfused children are hemosiderosis, splenomegaly, and hypersplenism. Transfusion-related hemosiderosis requires chelation therapy to minimize cardiac, hepatic, and endocrine dysfunction. Noncompliance with chelation in adolescents and young adults may lead to death from congestive heart failure, cardiac arrhythmias, or hepatic failure. Even with adequate transfusions, many patients develop splenomegaly and some degree of hypersplenism. Splenectomy increases the risk of thrombosis, pulmonary hypertension, and overwhelming sepsis.

▶ Treatment

β-Thalassemia minor requires no specific therapy, but the diagnosis may have important genetic implications for the family. The time to presentation for those with β-thalassemia intermedia is variable and some will become transfusion dependent over their life. For β-thalassemia major, two treatments are available: chronic transfusion with iron chelation and hematopoietic stem cell transplant. Programs of blood transfusion are generally targeted to maintain a nadir hemoglobin level of 9.5–10.5 g/dL. This approach gives increased vigor and well-being, improved growth, and fewer overall complications. However, maintenance of good health requires iron chelation. Small doses of supplemental ascorbic acid may enhance the efficacy of iron chelation.

Hematopoietic stem cell transplant is an important therapeutic option for children with β-thalassemia major. The probability of hematologic cure with an HLA-matched related donor is greater than 90% when transplant is performed prior to the development of hepatomegaly or portal fibrosis. Matched unrelated transplant is also a viable option. Gene therapy may become an alternative option.

Srivastava A: Cure for thalassemia major-from allogeneic hematopoietic stem cell transplantation to gene therapy. Haematologica 2017;102:214–223 [PMID: 27909215].

3. Sickle Cell Disease

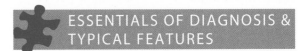

ESSENTIALS OF DIAGNOSIS & TYPICAL FEATURES

- ▶ Neonatal screening test usually with hemoglobins FS, FSC, or FSA (S > A).
- ▶ Predominantly African, Mediterranean, Middle Eastern, Indian, or Caribbean ancestry.
- ▶ Anemia, elevated reticulocyte count, usually jaundice.
- ▶ Recurrent episodes of musculoskeletal or abdominal pain.
- ▶ Often hepatomegaly and splenomegaly that resolves.
- ▶ Increased risk of bacterial sepsis.

▶ General Considerations

Sickle cell disease encompasses a family of disorders with manifestations secondary to the propensity of deoxygenated sickle hemoglobin (S) to polymerize. Sickle hemoglobin is a consequence of a change in the sixth chain of the β-globin whereby valine is substituted for glutamic acid. Polymerization of sickle hemoglobin distorts erythrocyte morphology; decreases red cell deformability; causes a marked reduction in red cell lifespan; increases blood viscosity; and predisposes to inflammation, coagulation activation, and episodes of vaso-occlusion. Sickle cell anemia, the most severe sickling disorder, is caused by homozygosity for the sickle gene and is the most common form of sickle cell disease. Other clinically important sickling disorders are compound heterozygous conditions in which the sickle gene interacts with genes for hemoglobins C, E, D_{Punjab}, O_{Arab}, C_{Harlem}, or β-thalassemia.

Overall, sickle cell disease occurs in about 1 of every 400 African-American infants. Eight percent of African Americans are heterozygous carriers of the sickle gene and thus have sickle cell trait.

▶ Clinical Findings

A. Symptoms and Signs

These are related to the hemolytic anemia, tissue ischemia, and organ dysfunction caused by vaso-occlusion. They are most severe in children with sickle cell anemia or sickle $β^0$-thalassemia. Physical findings are normal at birth, and symptoms are unusual before age 3–4 months because high levels of fetal hemoglobin inhibit sickling. A moderately severe hemolytic anemia may be present by age 1 year. This causes pallor, fatigue, and jaundice, and predisposes to the development of gallstones during childhood and adolescence. Intense congestion of the spleen with sickled cells may cause splenomegaly in early childhood and ultimately results in functional asplenia as early as age 3 months in sickle cell anemia. This places children at great risk for overwhelming infection with encapsulated bacteria, particularly pneumococci. Up to 30% of patients experience one or more episodes of acute splenic sequestration, characterized by sudden enlargement of the spleen with pooling of red cells, acute exacerbation of anemia, and, in severe cases, shock and death. Acute exacerbation of anemia also occurs with aplastic crises, usually caused by infection with human parvovirus B19 and other viruses.

Recurrent episodes of vaso-occlusion and tissue ischemia cause acute and chronic morbidity. Dactylitis, or hand-and-foot syndrome, which is the most common initial symptom of the disease, occurs in up to 50% of children with sickle cell anemia before age 3 years. Recurrent episodes of abdominal and musculoskeletal pain may occur throughout life. Historically, overt strokes occurred in about 11% of children with sickle cell anemia and without chronic transfusion tended to be recurrent; recurrence is significantly reduced with chronic red cell transfusions. The acute chest syndrome, characterized by respiratory symptoms and a new acute pulmonary infiltrate, is caused by pulmonary infection, infarction, or fat embolism from ischemic bone marrow. All tissues are susceptible to damage from vaso-occlusion, and multiple organ dysfunction is common by adulthood in those with sickle cell anemia or sickle $β^0$-thalassemia. The common manifestations of sickle cell disease are listed in Table 30–2. Manifestations are less frequent in those with SC and S $β^+$-thalassemia.

B. Laboratory Findings

Children with homozygous sickle cell anemia generally show a baseline hemoglobin level of 7–10 g/dL. This value may fall to life-threatening levels at the time of a splenic sequestration or aplastic crisis; often this occurs in association with

Table 30–2. Common clinical manifestations of sickle cell disease.

	Acute	Chronic
Children	Bacterial sepsis or meningitis Splenic sequestration Aplastic crisis Vaso-occlusive events Dactylitis Bone infarction Acute chest syndrome Stroke Priapism	Functional asplenia Delayed growth and development Avascular necrosis of the hip Hyposthenuria Cholelithiasis
Adults	Bacterial sepsis[a] Aplastic crisis Vaso-occlusive events Bone infarction Acute chest syndrome Stroke Priapism Acute multiorgan failure syndrome	Leg ulcers Proliferative retinopathy Avascular necrosis of the hip Cholecystitis Chronic organ failure Liver Lung Kidney Decreased fertility

[a]Associated with significant mortality rate.

parvovirus B19 infection. The baseline reticulocyte count is elevated. The anemia is usually normocytic or macrocytic, and the peripheral blood smear typically shows the characteristic sickle cells as well as numerous target cells. Patients with sickle β-thalassemia have a low MCV and hypochromia. Those with sickle $β^+$-thalassemia tend to have less hemolysis and anemia. Persons with sickle hemoglobin C disease have fewer sickle forms and more target cells, and the hemoglobin level may be normal or only slightly decreased because the rate of hemolysis is much less than in sickle cell anemia.

Most infants with sickle hemoglobinopathies born in the United States are identified by universal neonatal screening. Results indicative of possible sickle cell disease require prompt confirmation. Children with sickle cell anemia and with sickle $β^0$-thalassemia have only hemoglobins S, F, and A_2. Persons with sickle $β^+$-thalassemia have a preponderance of hemoglobin S with a lesser amount of hemoglobin A and elevated A_2. Persons with sickle hemoglobin C disease have about equal amounts of hemoglobins S and C although the quantity of S is greater than the C. The use of solubility tests to screen for the presence of sickle hemoglobin should be avoided because a positive result does not differentiate sickle cell trait from sickle cell disease. Solubility tests will not identify hemoglobin variants other than S. Thus, hemoglobin electrophoresis, HPLC or DNA analysis is always necessary to accurately identify sickle cell disease.

▶ Differential Diagnosis

Hemoglobin electrophoresis and sometimes hematologic studies of the parents are usually sufficient to confirm sickle cell disease, although DNA testing is available. It is critical to determine whether the child with only F and S hemoglobins on newborn screening has sickle cell anemia, sickle β⁰ thalassemia, or is a compound heterozygote for sickle hemoglobin and pancellular hereditary persistence of fetal hemoglobin. Such children, when older, typically have 30% fetal hemoglobin and 70% hemoglobin S, and are often well.

▶ Complications

Repeated tissue ischemia and infarction can cause damage to virtually every organ system. Table 30–2 lists the most important complications. Patients who require frequent red cell transfusions are at risk of developing transfusion-related hemosiderosis and infections as well as red cell antibodies. Guidelines for routine evaluation for stroke risk with transcranial Doppler screening are available followed by red cell transfusion and possibly hydroxyurea has reduced the incidence of stroke.

▶ Treatment

The cornerstone of treatment is enrollment in a sickle cell program involving patient and family education, comprehensive outpatient care, and appropriate treatment of acute complications. Important to the success of such a program are psychosocial services, blood bank services, and the ready availability of baseline patient information in the setting in which acute illnesses are evaluated and treated.

Management of sickle cell anemia and sickle β⁰-thalassemia includes daily prophylactic penicillin, which should be initiated by age 2 months and continued to age 5 years. The routine use of penicillin prophylaxis in sickle hemoglobin C disease and sickle β⁺-thalassemia is controversial. Pneumococcal conjugate and polysaccharide vaccines should be administered to all children who have sickle cell disease. Other routine immunizations, including vaccination against influenza and meningococcus, should be provided. All illnesses associated with fever greater than 38.5°C should be evaluated promptly, bacterial cultures performed, parenteral broad-spectrum antibiotics administered, and careful inpatient or outpatient observation conducted.

Treatment of painful vaso-occlusive episodes includes the maintenance of adequate hydration (with avoidance of overhydration), correction of acidosis if present, administration of adequate analgesia, maintenance of normal oxygen saturation, and the treatment of any associated infections.

Red cell transfusions play an important role in management. Transfusions are indicated to improve oxygen-carrying capacity during acute severe exacerbations of anemia, as occurs during episodes of splenic sequestration or aplastic crisis. Red cell transfusions are not indicated for the treatment of chronic steady-state anemia or for uncomplicated episodes of vaso-occlusive pain. Simple or partial exchange transfusion to reduce the percentage of circulating sickle cells is indicated for some acute events and may be lifesaving. These events include stroke, moderate to severe acute chest syndrome, and multi-organ failure. Transfusions may be administered prior to high-risk procedures such as surgery with general anesthesia and arteriograms with high ionic contrast materials. Some patients with severe complications may benefit from chronic transfusion therapy. The most common indications for transfusions are stroke or an abnormal transcranial Doppler assessment indicating an increased risk for stroke. Leukocyte depleted, red cells negative for C, E, and Kell antigens reduces the incidence of alloimmunization.

Successful hematopoietic stem cell transplant can cure sickle cell disease. Gene therapy is being evaluated as curative therapy. Daily administration of oral hydroxyurea increases levels of fetal hemoglobin, decreases hemolysis, and reduces the frequency of acute chest syndrome, hospitalization rates, and need for transfusions. The hematologic effects and short-term toxicity of hydroxyurea in children are similar to those in adults. Hydroxyurea is recommended for children and adolescents with sickle cell anemia and sickle β⁰-thalassemia beginning at 9 months of age; efficacy in SC and β⁺-thalassemia has not been formally studied. ʟ-glutamine is also Food and Drug Administration (FDA) approved to reduce the frequency of vaso-occlusive crises.

▶ Prognosis

Early identification by neonatal screening, combined with sickle cell comprehensive care that includes prescription of prophylactic penicillin, instruction on splenic palpation, and education on the need to urgently seek care when fever occurs, has markedly reduced mortality in childhood. Most patients now live well into adulthood but eventually succumb to complications with survival to 45–50 years.

Moerdler S, Manwani D: New insights into the pathophysiology and development of novel therapies for sickle cell disease. Hematology Am Soc Hematol Educ Program 2018 Nov 30;2018(1):493–506 [PMID: 30504350].

Piel FB: Sickle cell disease. New Engl J Med 2017;376:1561–1573 [PMID: 28423290].

Yawn BP: Management of sickle cell disease: summary of the 2014 evidence-based report by expert panel members. JAMA 2014;312:1033–1048 [PMID: 25203083].

4. Sickle Cell Trait

Individuals who are heterozygous for the sickle gene have sickle cell trait; neonatal screening shows hemoglobin FAS (A > S). Adults typically have about 60% hemoglobin A and 40% hemoglobin S. No anemia or hemolysis is present, and the physical examination is normal. Persons with sickle cell trait are generally healthy with normal life expectancy despite a slight increased risk for pulmonary embolism.

However, sickle trait erythrocytes are capable of sickling, with acidemia and hypoxemia. Thus, the kidney may be affected with the most common manifestation of sickle trait being hyposthenuria. Transient painless hematuria, usually microscopic, affects about 4% of those with sickle trait and does not progress to significant renal dysfunction. Sickle cell trait is a risk factor for chronic kidney disease. Fewer than 40 individuals have been reported with an exceedingly rare malignancy, renal medullary carcinoma, and the majority have had sickle trait. The incidence of bacteriuria and pyelonephritis may be increased during pregnancy, but overall rates of maternal and infant morbidity and mortality are not affected by sickle cell trait.

Exertion at moderate altitudes rarely precipitates splenic infarction. In general, exercise tolerance seems to be normal; the incidence of sickle cell trait in black professional football players is similar to that of the general African-American population. The risk for exertional rhabdomyolysis is increased 1.5 fold.

There is no reason to restrict strenuous activity for individuals with sickle cell trait. As is true for all individuals performing strenuous activity, it is important to be conditioned, dress appropriately, have access to fluids, rest periodically, and perform moderate activity in extreme heat and humidity. Sickle cell trait is most significant for its genetic implications.

5. Hemoglobin C Disorders

Hemoglobin C is detected by neonatal screening. Two percent of African-Americans are heterozygous for hemoglobin C and thus have hemoglobin C trait. They have no symptoms, anemia, or hemolysis, but the peripheral blood smear may show some target cells. Identification of persons with hemoglobin C trait is important for genetic counseling, particularly with regard to the possibility of sickle hemoglobin C disease in offspring.

Persons with homozygous hemoglobin C have a mild microcytic hemolytic anemia and may develop splenomegaly. The peripheral blood smear shows prominent target cells. As with other hemolytic anemias, potential complications of homozygous hemoglobin C include gallstones and aplastic crises.

6. Hemoglobin E Disorders

Hemoglobin E is the second most common hemoglobin variant worldwide, with a gene frequency up to 60% in northeast Thailand and Cambodia. Persons heterozygous for hemoglobin E show hemoglobin FAE by neonatal screening and are asymptomatic and usually not anemic, but they may have mild microcytosis. Individuals homozygous for hemoglobin E are also asymptomatic but may have mild anemia; the peripheral blood smear shows microcytosis and some target cells.

Compound heterozygotes for hemoglobin E and β^0-thalassemia are normal at birth and, like infants with homozygous E, show hemoglobin FE on neonatal screening. They subsequently develop mild to severe microcytic hypochromic anemia. Such children may exhibit jaundice, hepatosplenomegaly, and poor growth if the disorder is not recognized and treated appropriately. In some cases, the anemia becomes severe enough to require lifelong transfusion therapy. Even without regular transfusions, hemosiderosis may occur. In certain areas of the United States, hemoglobin E/β^0-thalassemia has become a more common cause of transfusion-dependent anemia than homozygous β-thalassemia.

7. Other Hemoglobinopathies

Hemoglobin variants are common. Heterozygous individuals, who are frequently identified during the course of neonatal screening programs, are generally asymptomatic and usually have no anemia or hemolysis. The principal significance of most hemoglobin variants is the potential for disease in compound heterozygous individuals who also inherit thalassemia or sickle hemoglobin. For example, children who are compound heterozygous for hemoglobins S and D_{Punjab} ($D_{Los\ Angeles}$) are symptomatic.

Pecker LH: The current state of sickle cell trait: implications for reproductive and genetic counseling. Hematology Am Soc Hematol Educ Program 2018 Nov 30;2018(1):474–481 [PMID: 30504348].

CONGENITAL HEMOLYTIC ANEMIAS: DISORDERS OF RED CELL METABOLISM

Erythrocytes depend on the anaerobic metabolism of glucose for the maintenance of adenosine triphosphate levels sufficient for homeostasis. Glycolysis also produces the 2,3-diphosphoglycerate (2,3-DPG) levels needed to modulate the oxygen affinity of hemoglobin. Glucose metabolism via the hexose monophosphate shunt is necessary to generate sufficient reduced nicotinamide adenine dinucleotide phosphate (NADPH) and reduced glutathione to protect red cells against oxidant damage. Congenital deficiencies of many glycolytic pathway enzymes have been associated with hemolytic anemias. In general, the morphologic abnormalities present on the peripheral blood smear are nonspecific, and the inheritance of these disorders is autosomal recessive or X-linked. Thus, the possibility of a red cell enzyme defect should be considered during the evaluation of a patient with a congenital hemolytic anemia in the following instances: when the peripheral blood smear does not show red cell morphology typical of membrane or hemoglobin defects (eg, spherocytes, sickle forms, target cells); when hemoglobin disorders are excluded by laboratory results and when family studies are inconsistent. The diagnosis is confirmed by finding a low level of the deficient enzyme. The two most common disorders of erythrocyte metabolism are G6PD deficiency and pyruvate kinase deficiency.

1. Glucose-6-Phosphate Dehydrogenase Deficiency

 ESSENTIALS OF DIAGNOSIS & TYPICAL FEATURES

▶ Predominantly African, Mediterranean, or Asian ancestry.

▶ Neonatal hyperbilirubinemia.

▶ Generally sporadic hemolysis associated with infection or with ingestion of oxidant drugs or fava beans.

▶ X-linked inheritance.

▶ General Considerations

Deficiency of glucose-6-phosphate dehydrogenase (G6PD) is the most common red cell enzyme defect that causes hemolytic anemia. The disorder has an X-linked recessive inheritance and occurs with a higher frequency among persons of African, Mediterranean, and Asian ancestry. Girls may be affected. In most instances, the deficiency is due to enzyme instability; thus, older red cells are more deficient than younger ones and are unable to generate sufficient nicotinamide adenine dinucleotide (NADH) to maintain the levels of reduced glutathione necessary to protect the red cells against oxidant stress. Thus, most persons with G6PD deficiency do not have a chronic hemolytic anemia; instead, they have episodic hemolysis at times of exposure to the oxidant stress of infection or of certain drugs or food substances. The severity of the disorder varies among ethnic groups; G6PD deficiency in persons of African ancestry usually is less severe than in other ethnic groups.

▶ Clinical Findings

A. Symptoms and Signs

Neonates with G6PD deficiency may have significant hyperbilirubinemia and require phototherapy or exchange transfusion to prevent kernicterus. The deficiency is an important cause of hyperbilirubinemia in neonates of Mediterranean or Asian ancestry, but less so in those of African ancestry. Hemolytic episodes are often triggered by infection or by the ingestion of oxidant drugs such as antimalarial compounds, rasburicase, and sulfonamide antibiotics (Table 30–3). Ingestion of fava beans may trigger hemolysis in children of Mediterranean or Asian ancestry but usually not in children of African ancestry. Episodes of hemolysis are associated with

Table 30–3. Some common drugs and chemicals that can induce hemolytic anemia in persons with G6PD deficiency.

Acetanilide	Niridazole
Doxorubicin	Nitrofurantoin
Furazolidone	Phenazopyridine
Methylene blue	Primaquine
Nalidixic acid	Sulfamethoxazole

Reproduced with permission from Beutler E: Glucose-6-phosphate dehydrogenase deficiency. N Engl J Med 1991 Jan 17;324(3):169–174.

pallor, jaundice, hemoglobinuria, and sometimes cardiovascular compromise.

B. Laboratory Findings

The hemoglobin concentration, reticulocyte count, and peripheral blood smear are usually normal in the absence of oxidant stress. Episodes of hemolysis are associated with a variable fall in hemoglobin. "Bite" cells or "blister" cells may be seen, along with a few spherocytes on blood smear. Hemoglobinuria is common, and the reticulocyte count increases within a few days. Heinz bodies may be demonstrated with appropriate stains. The diagnosis is confirmed by the finding of reduced levels of G6PD in erythrocytes. Because this enzyme is present in increased quantities in reticulocytes, the test is best performed at a time when the reticulocyte count is normal or near normal.

▶ Complications

Kernicterus is a risk for infants with significant neonatal hyperbilirubinemia. Episodes of acute hemolysis in older children may be life threatening. Rare G6PD variants are associated with chronic hemolytic anemia; the clinical course of patients with such variants may be complicated by splenomegaly and by the formation of gallstones.

▶ Treatment

The most important treatment issue is avoidance of drugs known to be associated with hemolysis (see Table 30–3). For some patients of Mediterranean, Middle Eastern, or Asian ancestry, the consumption of fava beans must also be avoided. Infections should be treated promptly and antibiotics given when appropriate. Most episodes of hemolysis are self-limiting, but red cell transfusions may be lifesaving when signs and symptoms indicate cardiovascular compromise.

2. Pyruvate Kinase Deficiency

Pyruvate kinase deficiency is an autosomal recessive disorder observed in all ethnic groups but is most common in northern Europeans. The deficiency is associated with a chronic hemolytic anemia of varying severity. Approximately one-third of those affected present in the neonatal period with jaundice and hemolysis that require phototherapy or exchange transfusion. Occasionally, the disorder causes hydrops fetalis and neonatal death. In older children, the hemolysis may require red cell transfusions or be mild enough to go unnoticed for many years. Jaundice and splenomegaly frequently occur in the more severe cases. The diagnosis of pyruvate kinase deficiency is occasionally suggested by the presence of echinocytes on the peripheral blood smear, but these findings may be absent prior to splenectomy. The diagnosis depends on the demonstration of low levels of pyruvate kinase activity in red cells.

Treatment of pyruvate kinase depends on the severity of the hemolysis. Blood transfusions may be required for significant anemia, and splenectomy may be beneficial. Although the procedure does not cure the disorder, it ameliorates the anemia and its symptoms. Characteristically, the reticulocyte count increases and echinocytes become more prevalent after splenectomy, despite the decreased hemolysis and increased hemoglobin level.

Luzzatto L: Glucose-6-phosphate dehydrogenase deficiency. Hematol Oncol Clin N Am 2016; 30:373–393 [PMID: 27040960].

ACQUIRED HEMOLYTIC ANEMIA

1. Autoimmune Hemolytic Anemia

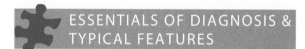
ESSENTIALS OF DIAGNOSIS & TYPICAL FEATURES

▶ Pallor, fatigue, jaundice, and dark urine.
▶ Splenomegaly.
▶ Positive DAT.
▶ Reticulocytosis and spherocytosis.

General Considerations

Acquired autoimmune hemolytic anemia (AIHA) is rare during the first 4 months of life but is one of the more common causes of acute anemia after the first year. It may arise as a primary disorder or may complicate an infection (hepatitis, upper respiratory tract infections, EBV mononucleosis, or cytomegalovirus [CMV] infection); systemic lupus erythematosus and other autoimmune syndromes; immunodeficiency states, including autoimmune lymphoproliferative syndrome (ALPS); or, very rarely, malignancies. Drugs may induce antibody-associated hemolytic anemia, and recently third-generation cephalosporins, such as ceftriaxone, have become a common cause for this adverse event of antibiotic therapy.

Clinical Findings

A. Symptoms and Signs

The disease usually has an acute onset manifested by weakness, pallor, dark urine, and fatigue. Jaundice is a prominent finding, and splenomegaly is often present. Some cases have a more chronic, insidious onset. Clinical evidence of an underlying disease may be present.

B. Laboratory Findings

The anemia is normochromic and normocytic and may vary from mild to severe (hemoglobin concentration < 5 g/dL). The reticulocyte count and index are usually increased but occasionally are normal or low. Spherocytes and nucleated red cells may be seen on the peripheral blood smear. Although leukocytosis and elevated platelet counts are common, thrombocytopenia occasionally occurs. Other laboratory data observed with hemolysis are increased indirect and total bilirubin, lactic dehydrogenase, aspartate aminotransferase, and urinary urobilinogen. Intravascular hemolysis is indicated by hemoglobinemia, hemoglobinuria, and decreased levels of haptoglobin. Examination of bone marrow shows marked erythroid hyperplasia and hemophagocytosis but is seldom required for the diagnosis.

Serologic studies are helpful in defining pathophysiology, planning therapeutic strategies, and assessing prognosis (Table 30–4). In almost all cases, the direct and indirect antiglobulin (DAT and IAT) tests are positive. Rarely patients with AIHA may have a negative DAT due to the presence of IgG bound to RBCs with low affinity or below the level of detection of the assay, affinity to an immature antigen found on reticulocytes, or IgA bound to RBCs not recognized by the Coombs reagent.

Further evaluation allows distinction into one of three syndromes. The presence of IgG and no or low level of C3 on the patient's RBCs, maximal in vitro antibody activity at 37°C, and either no antigen or an Rh-like specificity constitute warm AIHA with mostly extravascular destruction by the reticuloendothelial system. In contrast, the detection of complement alone on RBCs, optimal reactivity at 4°C, and I or i antigen specificity are diagnostic of cold AIHA with mostly intravascular and mild extravascular hemolysis. Cold agglutinins are relatively common (~ 10%) in normal individuals, but clinically significant cold (IgM) antibodies exhibit in vitro reactivity at 30°C or above.

Paroxysmal cold hemoglobinuria presents a third category of disease. The laboratory evaluation is identical to cold AIHA except for antigen specificity (P) and the exhibition of an in vitro hemolysis. Paroxysmal cold hemoglobinuria is almost always associated with significant infections, such as *Mycoplasma*, parvovirus, adenovirus, EBV, and CMV.

Table 30–4. Classification of AIHA in children.

Syndrome	Warm AIHA	Cold AIHA	Paroxysmal Cold Hemoglobinuria
Specific antiglobulin test IgG Complement	Strongly positive. Negative or mildly positive.	Negative. Strongly positive.	Negative. Strongly positive.
Temperature at maximal reactivity (in vitro)	37°C.	4°C.	4°C.
Antigen specificity	May be panagglutinin or may have an Rh-like specificity.	I or i.	P.
Other		Clinically significant if agglutination occurs ≥ 30°C.	Positive biphasic hemolysin test.
Pathophysiology	Extravascular hemolysis, destruction by the RES (eg, spleen). Rarely an intravascular component early in the course.	Intravascular hemolysis (may have extravascular component).	Intravascular hemolysis (may have extravascular component).
Prognosis	May be more chronic (> 3 mo) with significant morbidity and mortality. May be associated with a primary disorder (lupus, immunodeficiency, etc).	Generally acute (< 3 mo). Good prognosis: often associated with infection.	Acute, self-limited. Associated with infection.
Therapy	Responds to RES blockade, including steroids (prednisone, 2 mg/kg/day), IVIG (1 g/kg/day for 2 days), or with specific indication, splenectomy.	May not respond to RES blockade. Severe cases may benefit from plasmapheresis.	Usually self-limited. Symptomatic management.

AIHA, autoimmune hemolytic anemia; IgG, immunoglobulin G; IVIG, intravenous immune globulin; RES, reticuloendothelial system.

▶ Differential Diagnosis

AIHA must be differentiated from other forms of congenital or acquired hemolytic anemias. The DAT discriminates antibody-mediated hemolysis from other causes, such as hereditary spherocytosis. The presence of other cytopenias and antibodies to platelets or neutrophils suggests an autoimmune (eg, lupus) syndrome, immunodeficiency (eg, ALPS, congenital immunodeficiency), or Evans syndrome (AIHA and ITP or other cytopenias associated with autoantibodies). Over half of patients diagnosed as Evans syndrome may have ALPS or other genetic immune dysregulation disorders.

▶ Complications

The anemia may be very severe and result in cardiovascular collapse, requiring emergency management. The complications of an underlying disease, such as disseminated lupus erythematosus or an immunodeficiency state, may be present.

▶ Treatment

Medical management of the underlying disease is important in symptomatic cases. Defining the clinical syndrome provides a useful guide to treatment. Most patients (50%–80%) with warm AIHA (in which hemolysis is mostly extravascular) respond to prednisone (2 mg/kg/day). After the initial treatment, the dose of corticosteroids may be decreased slowly. Patients may respond to 1 g of intravenous immune globulin (IVIG) per kilogram per day for 2 days, but fewer patients respond to IVIG than to prednisone. In severe cases, rituximab may be a successful alternative; however, this drug should be avoided in AIHA associated with ALPS. Although remission with splenectomy may be as high as 50%–60%, in warm AIHA, this strategy should be considered only for patients older than 5 years who are refractory or resistant to first-line therapies. Short- and long-term complications are now more apparent and include infection with encapsulated organisms, increased risk for venous thromboembolism, and risk for portal and pulmonary arterial hypertension. In cases unresponsive to more conventional therapy, immunosuppressive agents such as mycophenolate, sirolimus, cyclosporine, tacrolimus, cyclophosphamide, azathioprine, or methotrexate may be tried alone or in combination with corticosteroids. The first four therapies produce less myelosuppression and risk for infection and may be helpful when hemolysis is associated with Evans syndrome or ALPS. Plasma exchange is not indicated for warm, IgG, autoantibody diseases. Transplantation, especially when hemolysis is secondary, has been used successfully in small numbers of cases.

Patients with cold AIHA and paroxysmal cold hemoglobinuria are less likely to respond to corticosteroids or IVIG. Because these syndromes are most apt to be associated with infections and have an acute, self-limited course, supportive care alone may be sufficient. Plasma exchange may be effective in severe cold autoimmune (IgM) hemolytic anemia because the offending antibody has an intravascular distribution. Rituximab or other immunosuppressive therapies may be helpful in rare cases.

Supportive therapy is crucial. Patients with cold-reacting antibodies, particularly paroxysmal cold hemoglobinuria, should be kept in a warm environment. Transfusion may be necessary because of the complications of severe anemia but should be used only when there is no alternative. In most patients, cross-match compatible blood will not be found, and the least incompatible unit among the few tested may be transfused. Transfusion must be conducted carefully, beginning with a test dose (see Transfusion Medicine section, later in this chapter). Identification of the patient's phenotype for minor red cell alloantigens may be helpful in avoiding alloimmunization or in providing appropriate transfusions if alloantibodies arise after initial transfusions. Patients with severe intravascular hemolysis may have associated disseminated intravascular coagulation (DIC), and heparin therapy should be considered in such cases.

▶ Prognosis

The outlook for AIHA in childhood usually is good unless associated diseases are present (eg, likely to have a chronic course). In general, children with warm (IgG) AIHA are at greater risk for more severe and chronic disease with higher morbidity and mortality rates. Hemolysis and positive antiglobulin tests may continue for months or years. Patients with cold AIHA or paroxysmal cold hemoglobinuria are more likely to have acute, self-limited disease (< 3 months). Paroxysmal cold hemoglobinuria is almost always associated with infection (eg, *Mycoplasma* infection, CMV, and EBV).

Bride KL et al: Sirolimus is effective in relapsed/refractory autoimmune cytopenias: results of a prospective multi-institutional trial. Blood 2016;127(1):17–28. doi: 10.1182/blood-2015-07-657981 [PMID: 26504182].

Hadjadj J et al; French Reference Center for Pediatric Autoimmune Cytopenia (CEREVANCE): Pediatric Evans syndrome is associated with a high frequency of potentially damaging variants in immune genes. Blood 2019;314(1):9–21. doi: 10.1182/blood-2018-11-887141 [PMID: 30940614].

Hill QA: Guidelines on the management of drug-induced immune and secondary autoimmune, hemolytic anaemia. Br J Haematol 2017;1772(2):208–220. doi: 10.1111/bjh.14654 [PMID: 28369704].

Ladogana S: Diagnosis and management of newly diagnosed childhood autoimmune haemolytic anaemia. Recommendations from the Red Cell Study Group of the Paediatric Haemato-Oncology Italian Association. Blood Transfus 2017;15(3):259–267. doi: 10.2450/2016.0072-16 [PMID: 28151390].

Petz LD, Garratty G: *Immune Hemolytic Anemias*. 2nd ed. Churchill Livingstone; Philadelphia, PA, 2004:341–344.

2. Nonimmune Acquired Hemolytic Anemia

Hepatic disease may alter the lipid composition of the red cell membrane. This usually results in the formation of target cells and is not associated with significant hemolysis.

Occasionally, hepatocellular damage is associated with the formation of spur cells and brisk hemolytic anemia. Renal disease may also be associated with significant hemolysis; hemolytic-uremic syndrome is one example. In this disorder, hemolysis is associated with the presence, on the peripheral blood smear, of echinocytes, helmet cells, fragmented red cells, and spherocytes.

A microangiopathic hemolytic anemia with fragmented red cells and some spherocytes may be observed in several conditions associated with intravascular coagulation and fibrin deposition within vessels. This occurs with DIC complicating severe infection, but may also occur when the intravascular coagulation is localized, as with giant cavernous hemangiomas (Kasabach-Merritt syndrome). Fragmented red cells may also be seen with mechanical damage (eg, associated with artificial heart valves and devices).

▼ POLYCYTHEMIA & METHEMOGLOBINEMIA

Polycythemia in children is defined as a hemoglobin or hematocrit greater than two standard deviations above the normal for age and is usually secondary to chronic hypoxemia. Hereditary polycythemia is rare. The most common cause of secondary polycythemia in children is cyanotic congenital heart disease, but it also occurs in chronic pulmonary disease such as cystic fibrosis. Persons living at extremely high altitudes, as well as some with methemoglobinemia, develop polycythemia. Polycythemia may occur in the neonatal period; it is particularly exaggerated in infants who are preterm or large for gestational age. It may occur in infants of diabetic mothers, in infants with trisomies 13, 18, or 21 or as a complication of congenital adrenal hyperplasia.

The disorder differs from polycythemia vera in that only RBCs are affected; the WBC and platelet counts are normal. There are usually no physical findings except for plethora and splenomegaly. Symptoms are generally limited to headache and lethargy.

ID may complicate polycythemia and aggravate the associated hyperviscosity. This complication of polycythemia should be suspected when the MCV falls below the normal range. Coagulation and bleeding abnormalities, including thrombocytopenia, mild consumption coagulopathy, and elevated fibrinolytic activity, have been described in severely polycythemic cardiac patients. Bleeding at surgery may be severe.

The ideal treatment of secondary polycythemia is correction of the underlying disorder. When this cannot be done, phlebotomy may be necessary to control symptoms. Iron sufficiency should be maintained. These measures help prevent the complications of thrombosis and hemorrhage.

METHEMOGLOBINEMIA

When heme iron is oxidized, it changes from the ferrous to the ferric state and methemoglobin is produced. Normally, methemoglobin is enzymatically reduced back to hemoglobin. Methemoglobin is unable to deliver oxygen to the tissues and causes a left shift in the oxygen dissociation curve. Cyanosis is seen with methemoglobin levels greater than 15%.

1. Hemoglobin M

This designation is given to several abnormal hemoglobins associated with methemoglobinemia due to amino acid substitutions in the globin chains. Hemoglobin M is transmitted as an autosomal dominant disorder. Hemoglobin electrophoresis at the usual pH will not always demonstrate the abnormal hemoglobin, and isoelectric focusing or DNA analysis may be needed. Affected individuals are cyanotic, but they have normal exercise tolerance and life expectancy. No treatment is indicated.

2. Congenital Methemoglobinemia Due to Enzyme Deficiencies

Congenital methemoglobinemia is caused most frequently by deficiency of the reducing enzyme cytochrome b5 reductase and is transmitted as an autosomal recessive trait. Affected individuals may have as much as 40% methemoglobin but usually have no symptoms, although a mild compensatory polycythemia may be present. Patients with diaphorase I deficiency respond to treatment with ascorbic acid and methylene blue (see the next section), but treatment is not usually indicated.

3. Acquired Methemoglobinemia

Nitrites and nitrates, chlorates, and quinines such as aniline dyes, sulfonamides, acetanilid, phenacetin, bismuth subnitrate, and potassium chlorate generate methemoglobin. Recreational use of volatile nitrites ("poppers") and cocaine may precipitate methemoglobinemia. Poisoning with a drug or chemical containing one of these substances should be suspected with sudden onset cyanosis. Methemoglobin levels in such cases may be extremely high and can produce anoxia, dyspnea, unconsciousness, circulatory failure, and death. Because of transiently deficient NADH methemoglobin reductase, newborns are more susceptible to drug- or chemical-induced methemoglobinemia especially when exposed to

lidocaine, benzocaine, or prilocaine. Infants with metabolic acidosis may also develop methemoglobinemia.

Children with acquired methemoglobinemia (other than those related to G6PD deficiency) respond dramatically to intravenous methylene blue. Ascorbic acid administered orally or intravenously also reduces methemoglobin, but the response is slower.

▼ DISORDERS OF LEUKOCYTES

NEUTROPENIA

ESSENTIALS OF DIAGNOSIS & TYPICAL FEATURES

- ► Increased frequency of infections.
- ► Ulceration of oral mucosa and gingivitis.
- ► Decreased absolute neutrophil count; normal numbers of red cells and platelets.

► General Considerations

Neutropenia is an absolute neutrophil (granulocyte) count of less than 1500/μL in childhood, or less than 1100/μL between ages 1 month and 2 years. During the first few days of life, an absolute neutrophil count of less than 3500/μL may be considered neutropenia in term infants. Neutropenia results from absent or defective myeloid stem cells; ineffective or suppressed myeloid maturation; altered production of hematopoietic cytokines or chemokines or abnormalities in their receptors; decreased marrow release; increased neutrophil apoptosis; destruction or consumption; or, in pseudoneutropenia, from an increased neutrophil marginating pool (Table 30–5). A decrease in neutrophil mass diminishes delivery of these cells to areas where the balance favors bacterial proliferation and invasion.

The severity of neutropenia may be characterized by the level of peripheral neutrophils, the number and severity of infections, and the production of mature neutrophils in the marrow. Also important is whether the neutropenia is acute (< 3 months) or chronic (> 3 months). The most severe types of chronic neutropenia include reticular dysgenesis (congenital aleukocytosis), Kostmann syndrome or severe congenital neutropenia, SCN (severe neutropenia with maturation defect in the marrow progenitor cells associated with specific gene defects), Shwachman syndrome (neutropenia with pancreatic insufficiency), neutropenia with immune deficiency states, cyclic neutropenia, and myelokathexis or dysgranulopoiesis. Genetic mutations for Chédiak-Higashi syndrome

Table 30–5. Classification of neutropenia in childhood.

Congenital neutropenia with abnormalities of stem cells or committed myeloid progenitor cells
  Reticular dysgenesis
  Chronic idiopathic neutropenia of childhood
  Severe congenital neutropenia (SCN 1-5 and X-linked)
  Cyclic neutropenia
  Shwachman-Diamond syndrome
  WHIM syndrome
  Glycogenosis Ib
  Chédiak-Higashi syndrome
  Cohen syndrome
  Barth syndrome
  Hermansky-Pudlak syndrome
  Griscelli syndrome
  Charcot-Marie-Tooth syndrome
  Cartilage-hair hypoplasia
  Dyskeratosis congenital
  Organic acidemias (eg, propionic, methylmalonic)
  Osteopetrosis
  Fanconi anemia
  Neutropenia with immunodeficiency disorders (SCID, hyper-IgM)
Acquired neutropenias affecting stem cells
  Malignancies (leukemia, lymphoma) and preleukemic disorders
  Drugs or toxic substances
  Ionizing radiation
  Aplastic anemia
Acquired neutropenias affecting committed myeloid progenitors or survival of mature neutrophils
  Ineffective myelopoiesis (vitamin B_{12}, folate, and copper deficiency)
  Infection
  Immune (neonatal alloimmune or autoimmune, autoimmune, or chronic benign neutropenia of childhood)
  Hypersplenism

(LYST (CHS1), Whim syndrome (CXCR4), SCN 1-5 (ELANE, GFl1, HAX1, G6PC3, VPS45, as well as WASP and GCSF3R), Shwachman syndrome (SBDS), and cyclic neutropenia (ELANE) have been identified. Neutropenia may also be associated with storage (GSD-Ib) and metabolic diseases, immunodeficiency states, and other disorders. At least 17 genes have been implicated in all these disorders. In many cases, neutropenia represents the sole manifestation but sometimes the disorder is also associated with multisystem involvement. The most common causes of acute neutropenia are viral infection or drugs, resulting in decreased neutrophil production in the marrow, increased peripheral turnover, or both. Severe bacterial infections may be associated with neutropenia. Although not commonly identified, neonatal alloimmune neutropenia can be severe and associated with infection. Autoimmune neutropenia occurs with chronic benign neutropenia of childhood, immunodeficiency syndromes, autoimmune disorders, or, in the newborn, as a result of passive transfer of antibody (alloimmune) from the mother to the fetus. Benign ethnic neutropenia is a common cause of neutropenia in patients of African or Middle Eastern ethnicity and has recently been attributed to single nucleotide polymorphism in the gene ACKR1/DARC. While peripheral blood neutrophil counts are moderately decreased, patients are not at increased risk for infections due to the presence of abundant neutrophils in the tissues. Malignancies, osteopetrosis, marrow failure syndromes, and hypersplenism usually are not associated with isolated neutropenia.

▶ Clinical Findings

A. Symptoms and Signs

Acute severe bacterial or fungal infection is the most significant complication of neutropenia. Although the risk is increased when the absolute neutrophil count is less than 500/μL, the actual susceptibility is variable and depends on the cause of neutropenia, marrow reserves, and other factors. The most common types of infection include septicemia, cellulitis, skin abscesses, pneumonia, and perirectal abscesses. In addition to local signs and symptoms, patients may have chills, fever, and malaise. Sinusitis, aphthous ulcers, gingivitis, and periodontal disease are also significant problems in chronic neutropenia. In most cases, the spleen and liver are not enlarged. *Staphylococcus aureus* and gram-negative bacteria are the most common pathogens.

B. Laboratory Findings

Neutrophils are absent or markedly reduced in the peripheral blood. In most forms of neutropenia or agranulocytosis, the monocytes and lymphocytes are normal and the red cells and platelets are not affected. The bone marrow usually shows a normal erythroid series, with adequate megakaryocytes, but a marked reduction in the myeloid cells or a significant delay in maturation of this series may be noted at various stages of myeloid maturation. Total cellularity may be decreased.

In the evaluation of neutropenia (eg, persistent, intermittent, cyclic), attention should be paid to the duration and pattern of neutropenia, the types of infections and their frequency, and phenotypic abnormalities on physical examination. A careful family history and blood counts from the parents may be useful. If an acquired cause, such as viral infection or drug, is not obvious as an acute cause, no other primary disease is present, and the neutropenia is chronic, WBC counts, white cell differential, and platelet and reticulocyte counts should be completed twice weekly for 6 weeks to determine the pattern of neutropenia. Bone marrow aspiration and biopsy including cytogenetic analysis are most important to characterize the morphologic features of myelopoiesis. Measuring the neutrophil counts in response to corticosteroid infusion may document the marrow reserves. Other tests that aid in the diagnosis include measurement of neutrophil antibodies, immunoglobulin levels, antinuclear antibodies, and lymphocyte phenotyping to detect immunodeficiency states. Culture of bone marrow may define myeloid progenitors or the presence of inhibitory factors. Cytokines in plasma or by mononuclear cells can be measured directly. Some neutropenia disorders have abnormal neutrophil function, but severe neutropenia may preclude collection of sufficient cells to complete assays. Analysis for gene mutations noted above may help confirm the diagnosis of a severe neutropenia syndrome. Increased apoptosis in marrow precursors or circulating neutrophils is a general characteristic described in several congenital or genetic disorders.

▶ Treatment

Underlying disorders should be identified and treated or associated agents should be eliminated. Infections should be aggressively assessed and treated. Prophylactic antimicrobial therapy is not indicated for afebrile, asymptomatic patients but may be considered in rare cases with recurrent infections. Recombinant granulocyte-colony–stimulating factor (G-CSF) will increase neutrophil counts in most patients; granulocyte-macrophage colony-stimulating factor (GM-CSF) may be considered but is less extensively used. For patients with neutrophil counts 500/μL or less G-CSF (Filgrastim) may be started at 3–5 mcg/kg/day subcutaneously or intravenously once a day, and the dose adjusted to keep the absolute neutrophil count more than 500/μL and less than 10,000/μL. The use of long-acting G-CSF (pegfilgrastim) has been used in a few patients with chronic neutropenia. In a small number of patients, G-CSF therapy has been shown to be safe for mothers throughout pregnancies and for newborns without evidence of teratogenicity. Some patients maintain adequate counts with G-CSF given every other day. Treatment will decrease infectious complications but may have little effect on periodontal disease. However, not all patients with neutropenia syndromes require G-CSF (eg, chronic benign neutropenia of childhood). Patients with cyclic neutropenia may have a milder clinical course as they grow older. Immunizations should be given if the adaptive immune system is normal. Hematopoietic stem cell transplant may be considered for patients with severe complications, especially those with severe congenital neutropenia refractory to G-CSF administration.

▶ Prognosis

The prognosis varies greatly with the cause and severity of the neutropenia. In severe cases with persistent agranulocytosis, the prognosis is poor in spite of antibiotic therapy but G-CSF has the potential to prolong life expectancy. In mild or cyclic forms of neutropenia, symptoms may be minimal and the prognosis for normal life expectancy excellent. Chronic benign neutropenia of childhood resolves spontaneously in up to 90% of children by 5 years of age. Up to 50% of patients with Shwachman syndrome may develop aplastic anemia, myelodysplasia, or leukemia during their lifetime. Patients with other SCNs also have a potential for leukemia, as do patients with neutropenia associated with some immune disorders. Hematopoietic stem cell transplant may be the only curative therapy for some disorders.

Dale D: How I manage children with neutropenia. Br J Haematol 2017;178:351–363. doi: 10.1111/bjh.14677 [PMID: 28419427].

Dale DC: An update on diagnosis and treatment of chronic idiopathic neutropenia. Curr Opin Hematol 2017;24:46 [PMID: 27841775].

Donadieu J, Beaupain B, Fenneteau O, Bellanné-Chantelot C: Congenital neutropenia in the era of genomics: classification, diagnosis, and natural history. Br J Haematol 2017;179:557–574. doi: 10.1111/bjh.14887 [PMID: 28875503].

Fioredda F: Long-term use of pegfilgrastim with severe congenital neutropenia: clinical and pharmacokinetic data. Blood 2016;128:2178 [PMID: 27621310].

Palmblad J: Ethnic benign neutropenia: a phenomenon finds an explanation. Peditar Blood Cancer 2018;65(12):e27361. doi: 10.1002/pbc.27361 [PMID: 30117263].

NEUTROPHILIA

Neutrophilia is an increase in the absolute neutrophil count in the peripheral blood to greater than 7500–8500/μL for infants, children, and adults. To support the increased peripheral count, neutrophils may be mobilized from bone marrow storage or peripheral marginating pools. Neutrophilia occurs acutely in association with bacterial or viral infections, inflammatory diseases (eg, juvenile rheumatoid arthritis, inflammatory bowel disease, Kawasaki disease), surgical or functional asplenia, liver failure, diabetic ketoacidosis, azotemia, congenital disorders of neutrophil function (eg, chronic granulomatous disease, leukocyte adherence deficiency), and hemolysis. Drugs such as corticosteroids, lithium, and epinephrine increase the blood neutrophil count. Corticosteroids cause release of neutrophils from the marrow pool, inhibit egress from capillary beds, and postpone apoptotic cell death. Epinephrine causes release of the marginating pool. Acute neutrophilia has been reported after stress, such as from electric shock, trauma, burns, surgery, and emotional upset. Tumors involving the bone marrow, such as lymphomas, neuroblastomas, and rhabdomyosarcoma, may be associated with leukocytosis and the presence of immature myeloid cells in the peripheral blood. Infants with Down syndrome have defective regulation of proliferation and maturation of the myeloid series and may develop neutrophilia. At times this process may affect other cell lines and mimic myeloproliferative disorders or acute leukemia.

The neutrophilias must be distinguished from myeloproliferative disorders such as chronic myelogenous leukemia and juvenile chronic myelogenous leukemia. In general, abnormalities involving other cell lines, the appearance of immature cells on the blood smear, and the presence of hepatosplenomegaly are important differentiating characteristics.

DISORDERS OF NEUTROPHIL FUNCTION

Neutrophils play a key role in host defenses. Circulating in the laminar flow of blood vessels, they adhere to capillary vascular endothelium adjacent to sites of infection and inflammation. Moving between endothelial cells, the neutrophil migrates toward the offending agent. Contact with a microbe that is properly opsonized with complement or antibodies triggers ingestion, a process in which cytoplasmic streaming results in the formation of pseudopods that fuse around the invader, encasing it in a phagosome. During the ingestion phase, the oxidase enzyme system assembles in the phagosomal membrane and is activated, taking oxygen from the surrounding medium and reducing it to form toxic oxygen metabolites critical to microbicidal activity. Concurrently, granules from the two main classes (azurophil and specific) fuse and release their contents into the phagolysosome. The concentration of toxic oxygen metabolites (eg, hydrogen peroxide, hypochlorous acid, hydroxyl radical) and other compounds (eg, proteases, cationic proteins, cathepsins, defensins) increases dramatically, resulting in the death and dissolution of the microbe. Complex physiologic and biochemical processes support and control these functions. Defects in any of these processes may lead to inadequate cell function and an increased risk of infection.

▶ Classification

Table 30–6 summarizes congenital neutrophil function defects. Recently reported is variant CGD with p40phox deficiency manifested by inflammatory bowel disease. Also described is a syndrome of severe neutrophil dysfunction and severe infections associated with a mutation in a GTPase signaling molecule, Rac2 (gene, RAC2). New syndromes of innate immune dysfunction include defects in interferon and interleukin (IL)-12 receptor and signaling pathways, leading to monocyte and macrophage dysfunction and defective toll-like receptor signaling pathways (IL-1 receptor–associated kinase 4 [IRAK-4] deficiency) associated with recurrent bacterial infections. Leukocyte adhesion deficiency (LAD) III is a disorder characterized by severe bleeding, impaired leukocyte adhesion, and endothelial inflammation, and is associated with mutations of *FERMT3* gene, which encodes for a protein, Kindlin-3, critical for intracellular function of β integrins and perhaps other adhesion strategies. Other congenital or acquired causes of mild to moderate neutrophil dysfunction include metabolic defects (eg, glycogen storage disease Ib, G6PC3 deficiency, other congenital neutropenia syndromes (eg, Chediak-Higashi syndrome and Shwachman-Diamond syndrome), diabetes mellitus, renal disease, and hypophosphatemia, viral infections, and certain drugs. Neutrophils from newborn infants have abnormal adherence, chemotaxis, and bactericidal activity. Cells from patients with thermal injury, trauma, and overwhelming infection have defects in cell motility and bactericidal activity similar to those seen in neonates.

▶ Clinical Findings

Recurrent bacterial or fungal infections are the hallmark of neutrophil dysfunction. Although patients will have infection-free periods, episodes of pneumonia, sinusitis, cellulitis, cutaneous and mucosal infections (including perianal or peritonsillar abscesses), and lymphadenitis are frequent. As with neutropenia, aphthous ulcers of mucous membranes, severe gingivitis, and periodontal disease are also major complications. In general, *S aureus* or gram-negative organisms are commonly isolated from infected sites; other organisms may be specifically associated with a defined neutrophil function defect. In some disorders, fungi account for an increasing number of infections. Deep or generalized infections, such as osteomyelitis, liver abscesses, pneumonitis, sepsis, meningitis, and necrotic or gangrenous soft-tissue lesions, occur in specific syndromes (eg, leukocyte adherence deficiency or chronic granulomatous disease). Patients with severe neutrophil dysfunction may die in childhood from severe infections and associated complications. Table 30–6 summarizes pertinent laboratory findings.

▶ Treatment

The mainstay of management of these disorders is anticipation of infections and aggressive attempts to identify the foci and the causative agents. Surgical procedures to achieve these goals may be both diagnostic and therapeutic. Broad-spectrum antibiotics covering the range of possible organisms should be initiated without delay, switching to specific antimicrobial agents when the microbiologic diagnosis is made. When infections are unresponsive or they recur, granulocyte transfusions may be helpful.

Chronic management may include prophylactic antibiotics. Trimethoprim-sulfamethoxazole and some other antibiotics (eg, rifampin) enhance the bactericidal activity of neutrophils from patients with chronic granulomatous disease. Some patients with Chédiak-Higashi syndrome improve clinically when given ascorbic acid. Recombinant γ-interferon decreases the number and severity of infections in patients with chronic granulomatous disease. Demonstration of this activity with one patient group raises the possibility that cytokines, growth factors, and other biologic response modifiers may be helpful in other conditions in preventing recurrent infections. Bone marrow transplant has been successfully used to cure most major congenital neutrophil dysfunction syndromes, and reconstitution with normal cells and cell function has been documented. Gene therapy techniques using autologous hematopoietic stem cells corrected by lentiviral gene insertion or gene editing techniques are promising and may provide a future strategy for curing these disorders.

Table 30–6. Classification of congenital neutrophil function deficits.

Disorder	Clinical Manifestations	Functional Defect	Biochemical Defect	Inheritance (Chromosome; Gene)
Chédiak-Higashi syndrome	Oculocutaneous albinism, photophobia, nystagmus, ataxia. Recurrent infections of skin, respiratory tract, and mucous membranes with gram-positive and gram-negative organisms. Many patients die during lymphoproliferative phase with hepatomegaly, fever, which may be a viral-associated hemophagocytic syndrome secondary to Epstein-Barr virus infection. Older patients may develop degenerative CNS disease.	Neutropenia. Neutrophils, monocytes, lymphocytes, platelets, and all granule-containing cells have giant granules. Most significant defect is in chemotaxis. Also milder defects in microbicidal activity and degranulation.	Gene (CHS1/LYST) deficit identified. Alterations in membrane fusion with formation of giant granules. Other biochemical abnormalities in cAMP and cGMP, microtubule assembly.	Autosomal recessive (1q42.1-.2; *CHS1*)
Leukocyte adherence deficiency I	Recurrent soft-tissue infections, including gingivitis, otitis, mucositis, periodontitis, skin infections. Delayed separation of the cord in newborn and problems with wound healing.	Neutrophilia. Diminished adherence to surfaces, leading to decreased chemotaxis.	Absence or partial deficiency of CD11b/CD18 cell surface adhesive glycoprotein. Defect in expression CD18 (gene, TGB2)	Autosomal recessive (12q22.3; *ITGB2*)
Leukocyte adherence deficiency II	Recurrent infections, mental retardation, craniofacial abnormalities, short stature.	Neutrophilia. Deficient "rolling" interactions with endothelial cells. Red cells have Bombay phenotype.	Deficient fucosyl transferase (gene, SLC35C1) results in deficient Sialyl-Lewis-X antigen, which interacts with P selectin. P selectin on endothelial cells is required for neutrophil rolling, a prerequisite for adherence and diapedesis.	Autosomal recessive (11p11.2; *SLC35C1*)
Leukocyte adherence deficiency III	Recurrent severe infections, life-threatening bleeding complications	Neutrophilia. Dysfunctional platelet aggregation.	Mutations in kindlin-3 impair intracellular activation of integrins	Autosomal recessive (*FERMT3*)
Chronic granulomatous disease	Recurrent purulent infections with catalase-positive bacteria and fungi. May involve skin, mucous membranes. Patients also develop deep infections (lymph nodes, lung, liver, bones) and sepsis.	Neutrophilia. Neutrophils demonstrate deficient bactericidal activity but normal chemotaxis and ingestion. Defect in the oxidase (Nox2) enzyme system, resulting in absence or diminished production of oxygen metabolites toxic to microbes.	Several molecular defects in oxidase components. Absent cytochrome b558 with decreased expression of either (1) or (2): (1) gp91-phox (gene, CYBB) (2) p22-phox (gene, CYBA) Absent p47-phox (gene, NCF1) or p67-phox (gene, NCF2) both are cytosolic components. Fourth cytosolic component defect described, p40phox deficiency (gene, NCF4)	X-linked in 60%–65% of cases (Xp21.1; *CYBB*) Autosomal recessive in < 5% of cases (16q24; *CYBA*) Autosomal recessive in 30% of cases (7q11.23; *NCF1* and 1q25; *NCF2*, respectively)

(Continued)

Table 30–6. Classification of congenital neutrophil function deficits. (*Continued*)

Disorder	Clinical Manifestations	Functional Defect	Biochemical Defect	Inheritance (Chromosome; Gene)
Myeloperoxidase deficiency	Generally healthy. Fungal infections when deficiency associated with systemic diseases (eg, diabetes in poor control).	Diminished capacity to enhance hydrogen peroxide-mediated microbicidal activity. Decreased killing of *Candida*.	Diminished or absent myeloperoxidase; posttranslational defect in processing protein.	Autosomal recessive (17q22-23)
Specific granule deficiency	Recurrent skin and deep tissue infections.	Neutropenia. Neutrophils have band-shaped or bilobed nuclei. Decreased chemotaxis and bactericidal activity.	Failure to produce specific granules or their contents during myelopoiesis. Defect in transcription factor (gene, C/EBP-epsilon).	Autosomal recessive (14q11.2; *CEBPε*)

cAMP, cyclic adenosine monophosphate; cGMP, cyclic guanosine monophosphate; CNS, central nervous system; Nox2, NADPH oxidase 2.

▶ Prognosis

For mild to moderate defects, anticipation and conservative medical management ensure a better outlook. For severe defects, excessive morbidity and significant mortality still exist. In some diseases, the development of noninfectious complications, such as the lymphoproliferative phase of Chédiak-Higashi syndrome or inflammatory syndromes in chronic granulomatous disease, may influence prognosis.

Ambruso DR: Primary immunodeficiency and other diseases with immune dysregulation. In: Wilmott RW et al, (eds): *Kendig's Disorders of the Respiratory Tract in Children*. 9th ed. Philadelphia, PA: Elsevier; 2019:909–922.

Bousfiha A et al: The 2017 IUIS phenotypic classification for primary immunodeficiencies. J Clin Immunol 2018;38(1):129–143. doi: 10.1007/s10875-017-0465-8 [PMID: 29226301].

De Ravin SS: CRISPR-Cas9 gene repair of hematopoietic stem cells from patients with X-linked chronic granulomatous disease. Sci Transl Med 2017;9(372). doi: 10.1126/scitranslmed.aah3480 [PMID: 28077679].

Jun HS: Molecular mechanisms of neutrophil dysfunction in glycogen storage disease type Ib. Blood 2014;123:2843 [PMID: 24565827].

Kuhns DB: Residual NADPH oxidase and survival in chronic granulomatous disease. N Engl J Med 2010;363:2600 [PMID: 21190454].

LYMPHOCYTOSIS

From the first week up to the fifth year of life, lymphocytes are the most numerous leukocytes in human blood. The ratio then reverses gradually to reach the adult pattern of neutrophil predominance. An absolute lymphocytosis in childhood is associated with acute or chronic viral infections, pertussis, syphilis, tuberculosis, and hyperthyroidism. Other noninfectious conditions, drugs, and hypersensitivity and serum sickness–like reactions cause lymphocytosis.

Fever, upper respiratory symptoms, gastrointestinal complaints, and rashes are clues in distinguishing infectious from noninfectious causes. The presence of enlarged liver, spleen, or lymph nodes is crucial to the differential diagnosis, which includes acute leukemia and lymphoma. Most cases of infectious mononucleosis are associated with hepatosplenomegaly or adenopathy. The absence of anemia and thrombocytopenia helps to differentiate these disorders. Evaluation of the morphology of lymphocytes on peripheral blood smear is crucial. Infectious causes, particularly infectious mononucleosis, are associated with atypical features in the lymphocytes, such as basophilic cytoplasm, vacuoles, finer and less-dense chromatin, and an indented nucleus. These features are distinct from the characteristic morphology associated with lymphoblastic leukemia. Lymphocytosis in childhood is most commonly associated with infections and resolves with recovery from the primary disease.

EOSINOPHILIA

Eosinophilia in infants and children is an absolute eosinophil count greater than 300/µL. Marrow eosinophil production is stimulated by the cytokine IL-5. Allergies, particularly those associated with asthma and eczema, are the most common primary causes of eosinophilia in children. Eosinophilia also occurs in drug reactions, with tumors (Hodgkin and non-Hodgkin lymphomas and brain tumors), and with immunodeficiency and histiocytosis syndromes. Increased eosinophil counts are a prominent feature of many invasive parasitic infections. Gastrointestinal disorders such as chronic hepatitis, ulcerative colitis, Crohn disease, and milk precipitin disease may be associated with eosinophilia. Increased blood eosinophil counts have been identified in several families without association with any specific illness. Rare causes of eosinophilia include the hypereosinophilic syndrome, characterized by counts greater than 1500/µL and organ involvement and damage (hepatosplenomegaly, cardiomyopathy, pulmonary fibrosis, and central nervous system injury).

This is a disorder of middle-aged adults and is rare in children. Eosinophilic leukemia has been described, but its existence as a distinct entity is very rare.

Eosinophils are sometimes the last type of mature myeloid cell to disappear after marrow ablative chemotherapy. Increased eosinophil counts are associated with graft-versus-host disease after bone marrow transplant, and elevations are sometimes documented during rejection episodes in patients who have solid organ grafts.

BLEEDING DISORDERS

Bleeding disorders may occur as a result of (1) quantitative or qualitative abnormalities of platelets, (2) quantitative or qualitative abnormalities in plasma procoagulant factors, (3) vascular abnormalities, or (4) accelerated fibrinolysis. The coagulation cascade and fibrinolytic system are shown in Figures 30–4 and 30–5.

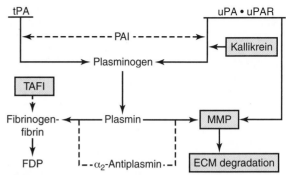

▲ **Figure 30–5.** The fibrinolytic system. Solid arrows indicate activation; dashed line arrows indicate inhibition. ECM, extracellular matrix; FDP, fibrinogen-fibrin degradation products; MMP, matrix metalloproteinases; PAI, plasminogen activator inhibitor; TAFI, thrombin activatable fibrinolysis inhibitor; tPA, tissue plasminogen activator; uPA, urokinase; uPAR, cellular urokinase receptor. (Reproduced with permission from Goodnight SH, Hathaway WE: *Disorders of Hemostasis & Thrombosis: A Clinical Guide.* 2nd ed. New York, NY: McGraw Hill; 2001.)

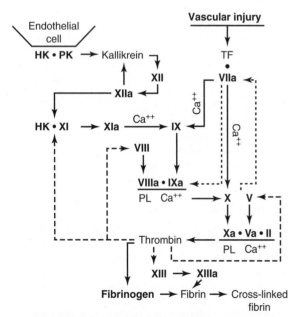

▲ **Figure 30–4.** The procoagulant system and formation of a fibrin clot. Vascular injury initiates the coagulation process by exposure of tissue factor (TF); the dashed lines indicate thrombin actions in addition to clotting of fibrinogen. The dotted lines associated with VIIa indicate the feedback activation of the VII-TF complex by Xa and IXa. Ca++, calcium; HK, high-molecular-weight kininogen; PK, prekallikrein; PL, phospholipid. (Reproduced with permission from Goodnight SH, Hathaway WE: *Disorders of Hemostasis & Thrombosis: A Clinical Guide.* 2nd ed. New York, NY: McGraw Hill; 2001.)

The most critical aspect in evaluating the bleeding patient is obtaining detailed personal and family bleeding histories, including bleeding complications associated with birth and the perinatal period, dental interventions, minor procedures, surgeries, and trauma. Excessive mucosal bleeding is suggestive of a platelet disorder, von Willebrand disease (vWD), dysfibrinogenemia, or vasculitis. Bleeding into muscles and joints may be associated with a plasma procoagulant factor abnormality. In either scenario, the abnormality may be congenital or acquired. A thorough physical examination should be performed with special attention to the skin, oro- and nasopharynx, liver, spleen, and joints. Screening and diagnostic evaluation in patients with suspected bleeding disorders may include the following laboratory testing:

1. Prothrombin time (PT) to assess clotting function of factors VII, X, V, II, and fibrinogen.

2. Activated partial thromboplastin time (aPTT) to assess clotting function of high-molecular-weight kininogen, prekallikrein, XII, XI, IX, VIII, X, V, II, and fibrinogen.

3. Platelet count and size determined as part of a CBC.

4. Platelet functional assessment by platelet function analyzer-100 (PFA-100), template bleeding time, or whole blood platelet aggregometry.

5. Fibrinogen functional level by clotting assay.

The following laboratory tests may also be useful:

1. Thrombin time to measure the generation of fibrin from fibrinogen following conversion of prothrombin to thrombin, as well as the antithrombin effects of

fibrin-split products and heparin. The thrombin time may be prolonged in the setting of a normal fibrinogen concentration if the fibrinogen is dysfunctional (ie, dysfibrinogenemia).

2. Euglobulin lysis time (ELT) to evaluate for hyperfibrinolysis if the preceding workup is nonrevealing despite documented history of bleeding. If the ELT is shortened, assess hyperfibrinolysis due to a congenital deficiency of the fibrinolytic inhibitors plasminogen activator inhibitor-1 and α_2-antiplasmin. In ill patients, measurement of fibrin degradation products may assist in the diagnosis of DIC.

Goodnight SH, Hathaway WE (eds): *Disorders of Hemostasis & Thrombosis: A Clinical Guide.* 2nd ed. McGraw-Hill, New York, NY; 2001:41–51.

ABNORMALITIES OF PLATELET NUMBER OR FUNCTION

Thrombocytopenia in the pediatric age range is often immune-mediated (eg, ITP, neonatal auto- or alloimmune thrombocytopenia) but is also caused by consumptive coagulopathy (eg, DIC, Kasabach-Merritt phenomenon), acute leukemias, or rarer disorders such as Wiskott-Aldrich syndrome and type 2b vWD, and artifactually in automated cytometers (eg, Bernard-Soulier syndrome), where giant forms may not be enumerated as platelets.

1. Idiopathic Thrombocytopenic Purpura

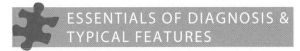

ESSENTIALS OF DIAGNOSIS & TYPICAL FEATURES

▶ Otherwise healthy child.
▶ Decreased platelet count.
▶ Petechiae, ecchymoses.

General Considerations

Acute ITP is the most common bleeding disorder of childhood. It occurs most frequently in children aged 2–5 years and often follows infection with viruses, such as rubella, varicella, measles, parvovirus, influenza, EBV, or HIV. The thrombocytopenia results from clearance of circulating IgM- or IgG-coated platelets by the reticuloendothelial system. The spleen plays a predominant role in the disease by forming the platelet cross-reactive antibodies and sequestering the antibody-bound platelets. Most patients recover spontaneously within months. Chronic ITP (> 12 months duration) occurs in 10%–20% of affected patients.

Clinical Findings

A. Symptoms and Signs

Onset of ITP is usually acute, with the appearance of multiple petechiae and ecchymoses. Epistaxis is common at presentation. No other physical findings are usually present. Rarely, concurrent infection with EBV or CMV may cause hepatosplenomegaly or lymphadenopathy, simulating acute leukemia.

B. Laboratory Findings

1. Blood—The platelet count is markedly reduced (usually < 50,000/µL and often < 10,000/µL), and large platelets are present in the peripheral blood smear, suggesting accelerated new platelet production. The WBC count and differential are normal, and the hemoglobin concentration is preserved unless hemorrhage has been significant.

2. Bone marrow—Megakaryocyte hyperplasia with normal erythroid and myeloid cellularity.

3. Other laboratory tests—Platelet-associated IgG or IgM, or both, may be demonstrated on the platelets or in the serum. PT and aPTT are normal.

Differential Diagnosis

Table 30–7 lists common causes of thrombocytopenia. ITP remains a diagnosis of exclusion. Family history or the finding of predominantly giant platelets on the peripheral blood smear is helpful in distinguishing from hereditary thrombocytopenia. Bone marrow examination should be performed if the history is atypical (ie, the child is not otherwise healthy, or there is a family history of bleeding), if abnormalities other than purpura and petechiae are present on physical examination, or if other cell lines are abnormal on the CBC. Bone marrow examination prior to treatment with corticosteroids is usually not required.

Complications

Severe hemorrhage and bleeding into vital organs are feared complications of ITP. Intracranial hemorrhage is the most serious complication, occurring in less than 1% of affected children. The most important risk factors for hemorrhage are a platelet count less than 10,000/µL and mean platelet volume less than 8 fL.

Treatment

A. General Measures

Observation is recommended for most children in the absence of bleeding regardless of platelet count. Aspirin and other medications (eg, NSAIDs such as ibuprofen, naproxen, etc) that compromise platelet function should be avoided.

Table 30–7. Common causes of thrombocytopenia.

	Increased Turnover		Decreased Production	
Antibody-Mediated	**Coagulopathy**	**Other**	**Congenital**	**Acquired**
Idiopathic thrombocy-topenic purpura	Disseminated intravascular coagulopathy	Hemolytic-uremic syndrome	Fanconi anemia Amegakaryocytic thrombocytopenia	Aplastic anemia
Infection	Sepsis	Thrombotic thrombocytopenic purpura	Wiskott-Aldrich syndrome	Leukemia and other malignancies
Immunologic diseases	Necrotizing enterocolitis Thrombosis Cavernous hemangioma	Hypersplenism Respiratory distress syndrome Wiskott-Aldrich syndrome	Thrombocytopenia with absent radii Metabolic disorders Osteopetrosis	Vitamin B_{12} and folate deficiencies Medications

Bleeding precautions (eg, restriction from physical contact activities and use of helmets) should be observed. Platelet transfusion should be avoided except in circumstances of life-threatening bleeding, in which case emergent splenectomy may be considered. In this setting, administration of corticosteroids and IVIG is also advisable.

B. Corticosteroids

Patients with clinically significant but non–life-threatening bleeding (ie, epistaxis, hematuria, and hematochezia) and those with a platelet count of less than 10,000/dL may benefit from treatment with corticosteroids. No single dose or dosing regimen has evidence to support its use above another. Prednisone 2 mg/kg/day (maximum of 60 mg/day) for 14–21 days, or alternatively, prednisone 4 mg/kg/day for 7 days, with a taper to day 14–21 are commonly used regimens. An initial higher dose (3–5 mg/kg/day) for 3–7 days may lead to faster count recovery. Long-term use of corticosteroids should be avoided because of toxicity.

C. Intravenous Immunoglobulin

Intravenous immunoglobulin (IVIG) is the treatment of choice for severe, acute bleeding, and may also be used as an alternative or adjunct to corticosteroid treatment in both acute and chronic ITP. IVIG may be effective when the patient is resistant to corticosteroids; responses are prompt and may last for several weeks. A single dose of 0.8–1 g/kg has been recommended. Platelets may be given simultaneously during life-threatening hemorrhage but are rapidly destroyed. Side effects of IVIG are common, including transient neurologic complications in one-third of patients (eg, headache, nausea, and aseptic meningitis) that mimic intracranial hemorrhage and necessitate radiologic evaluation. A transient decrease in neutrophil number may also be seen, and hemolytic anemia is rare.

D. Anti-Rh(D) Immunoglobulin

This polyclonal immunoglobulin binds to the D antigen on RBCs. The splenic clearance of anti-D–coated red cells interferes with removal of antibody-coated platelets, resulting in improvement in platelet count. This approach is effective only in Rh(+) patients with a functional spleen who are DAT negative. At doses of 50–75 mcg/kg, approximately 80% of Rh+ children with acute or chronic ITP respond; however, there is no clear difference between anti-D and IVIG in the time to reach a platelet count of 20×10^9/L. Significant hemolysis may occur in up to 5% of patients. The FDA has provided specific monitoring requirements because of reports of fatal intravascular hemolysis.

E. Splenectomy

Many children with chronic ITP have platelet counts less than 30,000/μL. Up to 70% of such children recover with a platelet count less than 100,000/μL within 1 year. For the remainder, corticosteroids, IVIG, and anti-D immunoglobulin are typically effective treatment for acute bleeding. Splenectomy produces a complete response in 70% and partial response in 20% of children with ITP, but it should be considered only after persistence of significant thrombocytopenia for more than 12 months and the failure of a preferred or alternative second-line therapy. The risk of overwhelming infection with encapsulated organisms is increased after splenectomy, particularly in the young child. Preoperative vaccination with polyvalent pneumococcal conjugate and polysaccharide vaccines, meningococcal C conjugate, and H. influenza b conjugate is recommended. If possible, the splenectomy should be postponed, until age 5 years. For patients younger than 5 years, daily penicillin prophylaxis should be started postoperatively and continued at least until 5 years of age. Postoperatively, a reactive thrombocytosis may raise the platelet count to more than 1 million/μL, but it is not associated with thrombotic complications in children. However, thrombosis is recognized as a potential post-splenectomy complication in the long term.

F. Rituximab (Anti-CD20 Monoclonal Antibody)

There have been no randomized trials for rituximab in children. The efficacy of treating childhood chronic ITP in several series and case studies has demonstrated response rates between 26% and 60%. Because of significant adverse events, this therapy may be reserved for refractory cases with significant bleeding or as an alternative to splenectomy.

G. New Agents

Thrombopoietin receptor agonists are now available for the treatment of ITP for children and are FDA-approved for children 1 year or older. A recently completed phase III clinical trial evaluating the use of eltrombopag for chronic ITP demonstrated an initial platelet response rate of 75% with significant decrease in bleeding symptoms and improvement in quality of life. In addition, as a second-line agent, they may be useful in patients for corticosteroid sparing. One pitfall of this approach is that these agents require long-term administration. While adult studies have shown adequate safety profiles with use up to 7 years, continued study in children is needed to evaluate long-term adverse effects, efficacy, and sustained response.

▶ Prognosis

Eighty percent of children with ITP will achieve a remission. Predictors of the development of chronic ITP include female gender, age greater than 10 years at presentation, insidious onset of bruising, and the presence of other autoantibodies. Treatment with combination of IVIG and corticosteroids has been associated with increased remission rates at 12 and 24 months after diagnosis as compared to single agent therapy. Older child- and adolescent-onset ITP is associated with an increased incidence of chronic autoimmune diseases or immunodeficiency states. Appropriate screening by history and laboratory studies is warranted.

Bennett CM: Predictors of remission in children with newly diagnosed immune thrombocytopenia: data from the Intercontinental Cooperative ITP Study Group Registry II participants. Pediatr Blood Cancer 2018;65(1). doi: 10.1002/pbc.26736.

Kim TO: Eltrombopag for use in children with immune thrombocytopenia. Blood Adv 2018;2(4):454–461. doi: 10.1182/bloodadvances.2017010660.

Neunert CE: Evidence-based management of immune thrombocytopenia: ASH guideline update. Hematology Am Soc Hematol Educ Program 2018;2018(1):568–575. doi: 10.1182/asheducation-2018.1.568 [PMID: 30504359].

2. Thrombocytopenia in the Newborn

Thrombocytopenia is one of the most common causes of neonatal hemorrhage and should be considered in any newborn with petechiae, purpura, or other significant bleeding. Defined by a platelet count of less than 150,000/μL, thrombocytopenia occurs in approximately 0.9% of unselected neonates; however, up to 80% of neonates in a newborn intensive care unit may experience thrombocytopenia; most of these cases are transient. Several specific entities may be responsible for more severe thrombocytopenia (see Table 30–7). Infection and DIC are the most common causes of thrombocytopenia in ill full-term newborns and in preterm newborns. In the healthy neonate, antibody-mediated thrombocytopenia (alloimmune or maternal autoimmune), viral syndromes, hyperviscosity, and major-vessel thrombosis are frequent causes of thrombocytopenia. Management is directed toward the underlying etiology. Other infants are affected by unknown mechanisms in mothers with preeclampsia. Most of these cases resolve over several days to a few weeks without treatment, but some are severe enough to warrant platelet transfusions.

A. Thrombocytopenia Associated With Platelet Alloantibodies (Fetal and Neonatal Alloimmune Thrombocytopenia [FNAIT])

FNAIT is the most common cause of thrombocytopenia in well, term infants, with a prevalence of 0.7 per 1000 pregnancies. Alloimmunization occurs when a platelet antigen of the infant from the father differs from that of the mother, and the mother is sensitized by fetal platelets that cross the placenta into the maternal circulation. In Caucasians, 80% are associated with HPA1a, and 10%–15% HPA5b. Bleeding can vary from minor skin effects to severe intracranial hemorrhage (1 in 11,000 neonates). Other platelet-specific alloantigens may be etiologic. Unlike in Rh incompatibility, 30%–40% of affected neonates are first-born. Thrombocytopenia is progressive over the course of gestation and worse with each subsequent pregnancy. The presence of antenatal maternal platelet antibodies on more than one occasion and their persistence into the third trimester is predictive of severe neonatal thrombocytopenia; a weak or undetectable antibody does not exclude thrombocytopenia. Severe intracranial hemorrhage occurs in 10%–30% of affected neonates as early as 20 weeks' gestation. Petechiae or other bleeding manifestations are usually present shortly after birth. The disease is self-limited, and the platelet count normalizes within 4 weeks.

If alloimmunization is associated with clinically significant bleeding, transfusion of irradiated platelets harvested from the mother is more effective than random donor platelets in increasing the platelet count. Transfusion with HPA-negative platelets from an unrelated donor is an option. Treatment with IVIG to acutely block macrophage uptake of sensitized platelets has also been successful in raising the platelet count and achieving hemostasis but is second line as it takes 24–48 hours to be effective. If thrombocytopenia is not severe (> 20–30,000/uL) and bleeding is absent, observation alone may be appropriate.

Intracranial hemorrhage in a previous child secondary to alloimmune thrombocytopenia is the strongest risk factor for severe fetal thrombocytopenia and hemorrhage in a subsequent pregnancy. Amniocentesis or chorionic villus sampling to obtain fetal DNA for platelet antigen typing is sometimes performed if the father is heterozygous for HPA1a. If alloimmunization has occurred with a previous pregnancy, irrespective of history of intracranial hemorrhage, screening cranial ultrasound for hemorrhage should begin at 20 weeks' gestation and be repeated regularly. In addition, if the fetal platelet count is less than 100,000/μL, the mother should be treated with weekly IVIG. Delivery near term by elective cesarean section which is recommended if the fetal platelet count is less than 50,000/μL results in less severe complications.

B. Thrombocytopenia Associated With ITP in the Mother (Neonatal Autoimmune Thrombocytopenia)

Infants born to mothers with ITP or other autoimmune diseases (eg, antiphospholipid antibody syndrome or systemic lupus erythematosus) may develop thrombocytopenia as a result of transfer of antiplatelet IgG from the mother to the infant. Unfortunately, maternal and fetal platelet counts and maternal antiplatelet antibody levels are unreliable predictors of bleeding risk. Antenatal corticosteroid administration to the mother is considered if maternal platelet count falls below 50,000/μL, with or without a concomitant course of IVIG.

Most neonates with autoimmune thrombocytopenia do not develop clinically significant bleeding, and treatment is not often required. The risk of intracranial hemorrhage is 0.2%–1.5%. If diffuse petechiae or minor bleeding are evident, a 1- to 2-week course of oral prednisone, 2 mg/kg/day, may be helpful. If the platelet count remains consistently less than 20,000/μL or if severe hemorrhage develops, IVIG should be given (1 g/kg daily for 1–2 days). Platelet transfusions are indicated only for life-threatening bleeding and may be effective only after removal of antibody by exchange transfusion. The platelet nadir is typically between the fourth and sixth day of life and improves significantly by 1 month; full recovery may take 2–4 months. Platelet recovery may be delayed in breast-fed infants because of transfer of IgG by milk.

C. Neonatal Thrombocytopenia Associated With Infections

Thrombocytopenia is commonly associated with severe generalized infections during the newborn period. Between 50% and 75% of neonates with bacterial sepsis are thrombocytopenic. Intrauterine infections such as rubella, syphilis, toxoplasmosis, HIV, CMV, herpes simplex (acquired intra- or postpartum), enteroviruses, and parvovirus are often associated with thrombocytopenia. In addition to specific treatment for the underlying disease, platelet transfusions may be indicated in severe cases.

D. Kasabach-Merritt Phenomenon

A rare but important cause of thrombocytopenia in the newborn is Kasabach-Merritt phenomenon that is associated with kaposiform hemangioendotheliomas, a benign neoplasm with histopathology distinct from that of classic infantile hemangiomas or less often, tufted angioma. Intense platelet sequestration in the lesion results in thrombocytopenia and may rarely be associated with a DIC-like picture and hemolytic anemia. The bone marrow typically shows megakaryocytic hyperplasia in response to the thrombocytopenia. Corticosteroids and vincristine or steroids and sirolimus are treatment options if significant coagulopathy is present, a vital structure is compressed, or the lesion is cosmetically unacceptable. Depending on the site, embolization may be an option. Surgery is often avoided because of the high risk of hemorrhage.

Fogerty AE: Thrombocytopenia in pregnancy: mechanism and management. Tran Med Rev 2018;32:225–229. https://www.ncbi.nlm.nih.gov/pubmed/30177431#Drolet BA.

Mahajan R, Margolin J, Iacobas I: Kasabach-Merritt phenomenon: classic presentation and management options. Clin Med Insights Blood Disord 2017;10:1–5 [PMID: 28579853].

Winkelhorst D, Oepkes D, Lopriore E: Fetal and neonatal alloimmune thrombocytopenia: evidence based antenatal and postnatal management strategies. Expert Rev Hem 2017;10:729–737 [PMID: 28644735].

3. Disorders of Platelet Function

Individuals with platelet function defects typically develop abnormal bruising and mucosal bleeding similar to that occurring in persons with thrombocytopenia. The PFA-100, which can evaluate platelet dysfunction and vWD, has replaced the template bleeding time in many institutions but is not unanimously endorsed. Although labor-intensive, platelet aggregometry remains important in selected clinical situations and is now used for in vitro assessment of platelet function, and uses agonists, such as adenosine diphosphate, collagen, arachidonic acid, and ristocetin. Unfortunately, none of these screening tests of platelet function uniformly predicts clinical bleeding severity.

Platelet dysfunction may be inherited or acquired, with the latter being more common. Acquired disorders of platelet function may occur secondary to uremia, cirrhosis, sepsis, myeloproliferative disorders, congenital heart disease, and viral infections. Many pharmacologic agents decrease platelet function. The most common offending agents in the pediatric population are aspirin and other NSAIDs, synthetic penicillins, and valproic acid. In acquired platelet dysfunction, the PFA-100 closure time is prolonged with collagen-epinephrine, while normal with collagen-ADP.

The inherited disorders are due to defects in platelet-vessel interaction, platelet-platelet interaction, platelet granule content or release (including defects of signal transduction), thromboxane and arachidonic acid pathway, and platelet-procoagulant protein interaction. Individuals with hereditary platelet dysfunction have a prolonged bleeding time with normal platelet number and morphology by light microscopy. PFA-100 closure time is typically prolonged with both collagen-ADP and collagen-epinephrine.

Congenital causes of defective platelet-vessel wall interaction include Bernard-Soulier syndrome, which is characterized by increased platelet size and decreased platelet number. The molecular defect in this autosomal recessive disorder is a deficiency or dysfunction of glycoprotein Ib-V-IX complex on the platelet surface resulting in impaired von Willebrand factor (vWF) binding, and hence impaired platelet adhesion to the vascular endothelium.

Glanzmann thrombasthenia is an example of severe platelet-platelet dysfunction. In this autosomal recessive disorder, glycoprotein IIb-IIIa is deficient or dysfunctional. Platelets do not bind fibrinogen effectively and exhibit impaired aggregation. As in Bernard-Soulier syndrome, acute bleeding is treated by platelet transfusion and with recombinant factor VIIa.

Disorders involving platelet granule content include storage pool disease and Quebec platelet disorder. In individuals with storage pool disease, platelet-dense granules lack adenosine diphosphate and adenosine triphosphate and are found to be low in number by electron microscopy. These granules are also deficient in Hermansky-Pudlak, Chédiak-Higashi, and Wiskott-Aldrich syndromes. Whereas deficiency of a second granule class, α-granules, results in the gray platelet syndrome, Quebec platelet disorder is characterized by a normal platelet α-granule number, but with abnormal proteolysis of α-granule proteins and deficiency of platelet α-granule multimerin. α-Granule abnormality in this disorder also results in increased serum levels of urokinase-type plasminogen activator. Epinephrine-induced platelet aggregation is markedly impaired.

Platelet dysfunction has also been observed in other congenital syndromes, such as Down and Noonan syndromes, without a clear understanding of the molecular defect.

▶ Treatment

Acute bleeding in many individuals with acquired or selected congenital platelet function defects responds to therapy with desmopressin acetate, likely due to an induced release of vWF from endothelial stores and/or upregulated expression of glycoprotein Ib-V-IX on the platelet surface. If this therapy is ineffective or if the patient has Bernard-Soulier syndrome or Glanzmann syndrome, the mainstay of treatment for bleeding episodes is platelet transfusion, possibly with HLA type–specific platelets. Recombinant VIIa, which has variable efficacy and may be helpful in platelet transfusion-refractory patients, is FDA-approved for patients with Glanzmann syndrome.

Matthews DC: Inherited disorders of platelet function. Pediatr Clin North Am 2013Dec;60(6):1475–1488 [PMID: 24237983].

INHERITED BLEEDING DISORDERS

Table 30–8 lists normal values for coagulation factors. The more common factor deficiencies are discussed in this section. Individuals with bleeding disorders should avoid exposure to medications that inhibit platelet function. Participation in contact sports should be considered in the context of the severity of the bleeding disorder.

1. Factor VIII Deficiency (Hemophilia A)

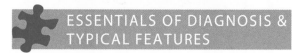

ESSENTIALS OF DIAGNOSIS & TYPICAL FEATURES

- ▶ Bruising, soft-tissue bleeding, hemarthrosis.
- ▶ Prolonged aPTT.
- ▶ Reduced factor VIII activity.

▶ General Considerations

Factor VIII activity is reported in units per milliliter, with 1 U/mL equal to 100% of the factor activity found in 1 mL of normal plasma. The normal range for factor VIII activity is 0.50–1.50 U/mL (50%–150%). Hemophilia A occurs predominantly in males as an X-linked disorder. One-third of cases are due to a spontaneous mutation. The incidence of factor VIII deficiency is 1:5000 male births.

▶ Clinical Findings

A. Symptoms and Signs

Persons with hemophilia who have less than 1% factor VIII activity have severe hemophilia A and have frequent spontaneous bleeding episodes involving skin, mucous membranes, joints, muscles, and viscera. In contrast, patients with mild hemophilia A (5%–40% factor VIII activity) mainly bleed at times of trauma or surgery. Those with moderate hemophilia A (1% to < 5% factor VIII activity) typically have intermediate bleeding manifestations but their treatment should be similar to patients with severe hemophilia. The most

Table 30–8. Physiologic alterations in measurements of the hemostatic system.

Measurement	Normal Adults	Fetus (20 wk)	Preterm (25–32 wk)	Term Infant	Infant (6 mo)	Pregnancy (term)	Exercise (acute)	Aging (70–80 y)
Platelets								
Count µL/10³	250	107–297	293	332	—	260	↑18%–40%	225
Size (fL)	9.0	8.9	8.5	9.1	—	9.6	↑	—
Aggregation ADP	N	+	→	→	—	↑	↓15%	—
Collagen	N	→	→	→	—	N	↓60%	N
Ristocetin	N	—	↑	↑	—	N	↓10%	—
BT (min)	2–9	—	3.6 ± 2	3.4 ± 1.8	—	9.0 ± 1.4	—	5.6
Procoagulant system								
PTT*	1	4.0	3	1.3	1.1	1.1	↓15%	→
PT*	1.00	2.3	1.3	1.1	1	0.95	N	—
TCT*	1	2.4	1.3	1.1	1	0.92	N	—
Fibrinogen, mg/dL	278 (0.61)	96 (50)	250 (100)	240 (150)	251 (160)	450 (100)	↓25%	↑15%
II, U/mL	1 (0.7)	0.16 (0.10)	0.32 (0.18)	0.52 (0.25)	0.88 (0.6)	1.15 (0.68–1.9)	—	N
V, U/mL	1.0 (0.6)	0.32 (0.21)	0.80 (0.43)	1.00 (0.54)	0.91 (0.55)	0.85 (0.40–1.9)	↑	N
VII, U/mL	1.0 (0.6)	0.27 (0.17)	0.37 (0.24)	0.57 (0.35)	0.87 (0.50)	1.17 (0.87–3.3)	↑200%	↑25%
VIIIc, U/mL	1.0 (0.6)	0.50 (0.23)	0.75 (0.40)	1.50 (0.55)	0.90 (0.50)	2.12 (0.8–6.0)	↑250%	1.50
vWF, U/mL	1.0 (0.6)	0.65 (0.40)	1.50 (0.90)	1.60 (0.84)	1.07 (0.60)	1.7	↑75–200%	↑
IX, U/mL	1.0 (0.5)	0.10 (0.05)	0.22 (0.17)	0.35 (0.15)	0.86 (0.36)	0.81–2.15	↑25%	1.0–1.40
X, U/mL	1.0 (0.6)	0.19 (0.15)	0.38 (0.20)	0.45 (0.3)	0.78 (0.38)	1.30	—	N
XI, U/mL	1.0 (0.6)	0.13 (0.08)	0.2 (0.12)	0.42 (0.20)	0.86 (0.38)	0.7	—	N
XII, U/mL	1.0 (0.6)	0.15 (0.08)	0.22 (0.09)	0.44 (0.16)	0.77 (0.39)	1.3 (0.82)	—	↑16%
XIII, U/mL	1.04 (0.55)	0.30	0.4	0.61 (0.36)	1.04 (0.50)	0.96	—	—
PreK, U/mL	1.12 (0.06)	0.13 (0.08)	0.26 (0.14)	0.35 (0.16)	0.86 (0.56)	1.18	—	↑27%
HK, U/mL	0.92 (0.48)	0.15 (0.10)	0.28 (0.20)	0.64 (0.50)	0.82 (0.36)	1.6	—	↑32%

Anticoagulant system								
AT, U/mL	1.0	0.23	0.35	0.56	1.04	1.02	↑14%	N
α₂-MG, U/mL	1.05 (0.79)	0.18 (0.10)	—	1.39 (0.95)	1.91 (1.49)	1.53 (0.85)	—	—
C1IN, U/mL	1.01	—	—	0.72	1.41	—	—	—
PC, U/mL	1.0	0.10	0.29	0.50	0.59	0.99	N	N
Total PS, U/mL	1.0 (0.6)	0.15 (0.11)	0.17 (0.14)	0.24 (0.1)	0.87 (0.55)	0.89	—	N
Free, PS, U/mL	1.0 (0.5)	0.22 (0.13)	0.28 (0.19)	0.49 (0.33)	—	0.25	—	—
Heparin	1.01	0.10 (0.06)	0.25 (0.10)	0.49 (0.33)	0.97 (0.59)	—	—	↓15%
Cofactor II, U/mL	(0.73)							
TFPI, ng/mL	73	21	20.6	38	—	—	—	—
Fibrinolytic system								
Plasminogen, U/mL	1.0	0.20	0.35 (0.20)	0.37 (0.18)	0.90	1.39	↓10%	N
tPA, ng/mL	4.9	—	8.48	9.6	2.8	4.9	↑300%	N
α₂-AP, U/mL	1.0	1.0	0.74 (0.5)	0.83 (0.65)	1.11 (0.83)	0.95	N	N
PAI-1, U/mL	1.0	—	1.5	1.0	1.07	4.0	↓5%	N
Overall fibrinolysis	N	↑	↑	↓	—	→	←	→

Except as otherwise indicated values are mean ±2 standard deviation (SD) or values in parentheses are lower limits (−2 SD or lower range); +, positive or present; ↓, decreased; ↑, increased; N, normal or no change;* values as ratio or subject/mean of reference range; α₂-MG, α₂-macroglobulin; α₂-AP, α₂-antiplasmin; ADP, adenosine diphosphate; AT, antithrombin; BT, bleeding time; C1IN, C1 esterase inhibitor; HK, high-molecular-weight kininogen; PAI, plasminogen activator inhibitor; PC, protein C; PreK, prekallikrein; PS, protein S; PT, prothrombin time; PTT, partial thromboplastin time; TCT, thrombin clotting time; TFPI, tissue factor pathway inhibitor; tPA, tissue plasminogen activator; vWF, von Willebrand factor. Overall fibrinolysis is measured by euglobulin lysis time.

Reproduced with permission from Goodnight SH, Hathaway WE: *Disorders of Hemostasis & Thrombosis: A Clinical Guide.* 2nd ed. New York, NY: McGraw Hill; 2001.

crippling aspect of factor VIII deficiency is the development of recurrent hemarthroses that incite joint destruction, and the sequelae of intracranial hemorrhage.

B. Laboratory Findings

Individuals with hemophilia A have a prolonged aPTT, except in some cases of mild deficiency. The PT is normal. The diagnosis is confirmed by confirming decreased factor VIII activity with normal vWF activity. In two-thirds of families of hemophilic patients, the females are carriers and may manifest symptomatic bleeding. Carriers of hemophilia can be diagnosed by DNA sequencing, and their bleeding severity by factor activity. In a male fetus or newborn with a family history of hemophilia A, cord blood sampling for factor VIII activity is accurate and important for subsequent care.

▶ Complications

Intracranial hemorrhage is the leading disease-related cause of death among persons with hemophilia. Most intracranial hemorrhages in moderate to severe deficiency are spontaneous and not associated with trauma. Hemarthroses begin early in childhood and, when recurrent, can result in joint destruction (ie, hemophilic arthropathy). Large intramuscular hematomas can lead to compartment syndrome with resultant neurologic compromise or pseudotumors. Although these complications are most common in severe hemophilia A, they may be experienced by individuals with moderate or mild disease. Acquired neutralizing antibodies to factor VIII are a potential serious complication after treatment with factor VIII concentrate. These antibodies develop in up to 30% of patients with severe hemophilia A, and especially in patients with absence or large deletions in the factor VIII gene. Inhibitors may be desensitized with regular factor VIII infusion (immune tolerance therapy). Therapy that bypasses the FVIII inhibitor with recombinant factor VIIa and/or FEIBA (factor eight inhibitor bypassing agent) is standard treatment of acute hemorrhage in patients with hemophilia A and a high-titer inhibitor. The bispecific monoclonal antibody emicizumab was recently approved for prophylaxis in all patients with hemophilia A with or without an inhibitor.

In prior decades, therapy-related complications in hemophilia A have included factor-related infection with HIV, hepatitis B virus, and hepatitis C virus. Through stringent donor selection, implementation of sensitive screening assays, use of heat or chemical methods for viral inactivation, and development of recombinant products, the risk of these infections is effectively eliminated. Inactivation methods do not eradicate viruses lacking a lipid envelope; therefore, transmission of parvovirus and hepatitis A remains a concern with the use of plasma-derived products. Immunization with hepatitis A and hepatitis B vaccines is recommended for all hemophilia patients.

▶ Treatment

The general aim of management is to raise the factor VIII activity to prevent or stop bleeding (see Table 30–8). Some patients with mild factor VIII deficiency may respond to desmopressin via release of endothelial stores of factor VIII and vWF into plasma; however, many patients still require administration of exogenous factor VIII to achieve hemostasis. The *in vivo* half-life of infused factor VIII is 6–14 hours but varies among individuals. Non–life-threatening, non–limb-threatening hemorrhage is treated with 20–30 U/kg of factor VIII, to achieve a rise in plasma factor VIII activity to 40%–60%. Joint hemarthrosis and life- or limb-threatening hemorrhage is treated with 50 U/kg of factor VIII, targeting a rise to 100% factor VIII activity. Subsequent doses are determined according to the site and extent of bleeding, and clinical response to factor VIII infusion. In circumstances of poor clinical response, recent change in bleeding frequency, or comorbid illness, monitoring the plasma factor VIII activity response is recommended. For most instances of non–life-threatening hemorrhage in experienced patients with moderate or severe hemophilia A, treatment can be administered at home, provided adequate intravenous access and management with the hemophilia treatment center.

Prophylactic factor VIII infusions prevent the development of arthropathy in severe and moderate hemophilia, and are the standard of care in pediatric hemophilia. Extended half-life factor VIII concentrates have been approved by the FDA with the hope of decreasing infusions and improving clinical outcomes. In addition, multiple nonfactor replacement strategies (eg, emicizumab, fitusiran, concizumab) are emerging that may replace factor VIII for prophylaxis and are disruptive technologies. Along with gene therapy, they look to reshape the lives and outcomes of people with hemophilia.

▶ Prognosis

The development of innovative, safe, and effective therapies for hemophilia A has resulted in improved long-term survival in recent decades. In addition, comprehensive care managed through hemophilia treatment centers has greatly improved quality of life and level of function.

2. Factor IX Deficiency (Hemophilia B, Christmas Disease)

The mode of inheritance and clinical manifestations of factor IX deficiency are the same as those of factor VIII deficiency. Hemophilia B is 15%–20% as prevalent as hemophilia A. Factor IX deficiency is associated with a prolonged aPTT but normal PT and thrombin time. However, the aPTT is slightly less sensitive to factor IX deficiency than factor VIII deficiency. Diagnosis of hemophilia B is made by assaying factor IX activity, and severity is determined similar to hemophilia A.

The mainstay of treatment in hemophilia B is exogenous factor IX. Unlike factor VIII, about 50% of the administered dose of factor IX diffuses into the extravascular space. Therefore, 1 U/kg of plasma-derived factor IX concentrate or recombinant factor IX is expected to increase plasma factor IX activity by approximately 1%. Factor IX typically has a half-life of 18–22 hours in vivo. In contrast to severe factor VIII deficiency, only 1%–3% of persons with factor IX deficiency develop a factor IX inhibitor, but patients may be at risk for anaphylaxis when receiving exogenous factor IX. The prognosis for persons with factor IX deficiency is comparable to that of patients with factor VIII deficiency. Extended half-life factor concentrates have changed treatment of severe and moderate hemophilia B. Gene therapy and nonfactor replacement technologies are in clinical trial.

Srivastava A: Guidelines for the management of hemophilia. Haemophilia 2013 Jan;19(1):e1–47 [PMID: 22776238].
Weyland AC: New therapies for hemophilia. Blood 2019 Jan 31;133(5):389–398 [PMID: 30559264].

3. Factor XI Deficiency (Hemophilia C)

Factor XI deficiency is a genetic, autosomal coagulopathy, typically of mild to moderate clinical severity. Cases of factor XI deficiency account for less than 5% of all persons living with hemophilia. Homozygous individuals generally bleed at surgery or following severe trauma, and at hyperfibrinolytic sites, but do not commonly have spontaneous hemarthroses. In contrast to factor VIII and IX deficiencies, factor XI activity is least predictive of bleeding risk. Pathologic bleeding may be seen in heterozygous individuals with factor XI activity as high as 60%. The aPTT is often considerably prolonged. In individuals with deficiency of both plasma and platelet-associated factor XI, the PFA-100 may also be prolonged. Management typically consists of perioperative prophylaxis and episodic therapy for acute hemorrhage. Treatment includes infusion of fresh frozen plasma (FFP); platelet transfusion may also be useful for acute hemorrhage in patients with deficiency of platelet-associated factor XI. Desmopressin has been used in some cases, and antifibrinolytic therapy is common.

James P: Rare bleeding disorders—bleeding assessment tools, laboratory aspects and phenotype and therapy of FXI deficiency. Haemophilia 2014 May;20 Suppl 4:71–75 [PMID: 24762279].

4. Other Inherited Bleeding Disorders

Other hereditary single clotting factor deficiencies are rare and generally autosomal. Homozygous individuals with a deficiency or structural abnormality of prothrombin, factor V, factor VII, or factor X may have excessive bleeding.

Persons with dysfibrinogenemia (ie, structurally or functionally abnormal fibrinogen) may develop recurrent venous thromboembolic episodes or bleeding. Immunologic assay of fibrinogen is normal, but clotting assay may be low and the thrombin time prolonged. The PT and aPTT may be prolonged.

Afibrinogenemia resembles hemophilia clinically but has an autosomal recessive inheritance. Affected patients experience a variety of bleeding manifestations, including mucosal bleeding, ecchymoses, hematomas, hemarthroses, and intracranial hemorrhage, especially following trauma. Fatal umbilical cord hemorrhage has been reported. The PT, aPTT, and thrombin time are all prolonged. A severely reduced fibrinogen concentration in an otherwise well child is confirmatory of the diagnosis. As in dysfibrinogenemia, fibrinogen concentrates are used for surgical prophylaxis and for acute hemorrhage.

Menegatti M: Treatment of rare factor deficiencies other than hemophilia. Blood 2019 Jan 31;133(5):415–424 [PMID: 30559262].

VON WILLEBRAND DISEASE

ESSENTIALS OF DIAGNOSIS & TYPICAL FEATURES

▶ Easy bruising and epistaxis from early childhood.

▶ Menorrhagia.

▶ Prolonged PFA-100 (or bleeding time), normal platelet count, absence of acquired platelet dysfunction.

▶ Reduced amount or abnormal activity of vWF.

▶ General Considerations

von Willebrand disease (vWD) is the most common inherited bleeding disorder among Caucasians, with a prevalence as high as 1%. vWF is a multimeric plasma protein that binds factor VIII and facilitates platelet adhesion to damaged endothelium. An estimated 70%–80% of all patients with vWD have type 1 vWD, caused by a partial quantitative deficiency of vWF. vWD type 2 involves a qualitative deficiency of (ie, dysfunctional) vWF, and vWD type 3 is characterized by a nearly complete deficiency of vWF. vWD is most often transmitted as an autosomal dominant trait, but it can be autosomal recessive. The disease can also be acquired, develop in association with hypothyroidism, Wilms tumor, cardiac disease, renal disease, or systemic lupus erythematosus, and in individuals receiving valproic acid. Acquired vWD is most often caused by the development of an antibody to vWF or increased turnover of vWF.

▶ Clinical Findings

A. Symptoms and Signs

Mucocutaneous bleeding including with increased bruising and excessive epistaxis is often present. Prolonged bleeding occurs with trauma or at surgery. Menorrhagia is often a presenting finding in females.

B. Laboratory Findings

PT is normal, and aPTT is prolonged if factor VIII is decreased. Prolongation of the PFA-100 is usually present. Platelet number may be decreased in type 2b vWD. Factor VIII and vWF antigen are decreased in types 1 and 3 but may be normal in type 2 vWD. vWF activity (eg, ristocetin cofactor, collagen binding, GB1b-binding assay) is decreased in all types. Since normal vWF antigen levels vary by blood type (type O associated with lower levels), blood type must be determined. Complete laboratory classification also requires vWF multimer assay. The diagnosis requires confirmatory laboratory testing.

▶ Treatment

Desmopressin acetate can be given intravenously or subcutaneously to prevent or halt bleeding for many patients with vWD types 1 and 2, by releasing vWF from endothelial stores. In responding patients, the increase in vWF and factor VIII in the plasma can be two- to fivefold. A high-concentration desmopressin nasal spray (150 mcg/spray), different from the preparation used for enuresis, may also be used. Because response to vWF is variable among patients, factor VIII and vWF activities are typically measured before, 30–60 minutes post, and 4 hours after desmopressin administration to document response. Desmopressin causes fluid retention which can result in hyponatremia; therefore, fluid restriction should be discussed. Because release of stored vWF is limited, tachyphylaxis often occurs after two to three administered doses of desmopressin.

If further therapy is indicated, vWF-replacement therapy (plasma derived or recombinant VWF) is recommended; such therapy is also used in patients with type 1 or 2a vWD who exhibit suboptimal laboratory response to desmopressin, and for all individuals with type 2b or 3 vWD. Antifibrinolytic agents (eg, ε-aminocaproic acid and tranexamic acid) are useful for control of mucosal bleeding. Oral or intrauterine contraceptive therapy may be helpful for menorrhagia.

▶ Prognosis

With the availability of effective treatment and prophylaxis for bleeding, life expectancy in vWD is normal.

http://practical-hemostasis.com (Excellent Practical source for Laboratory Hemostasis). Accessed June 31, 2019.

Nichols WL: von Willibrand disease (VWD): evidence-based diagnosis and management guidelines, the National Heart, Lung, and Blood Institute (NHLBI) Expert Panel report (USA). Haemophilia 2008;14(2):171–232 [PMID: 18315614].

O'Brien SH: von Willebrand disease in pediatrics: evaluation and management. Hematol Oncol Clin North Am 2019 Jun;33(3):425–438 [PMID: 31030811].

ACQUIRED BLEEDING DISORDERS

1. Disseminated Intravascular Coagulation

 ESSENTIALS OF DIAGNOSIS & TYPICAL FEATURES

▶ Presence of a disorder known to trigger DIC.

▶ Evidence for consumptive coagulopathy (prolonged aPTT, PT, or thrombin time; increase in FSPs [fibrin-fibrinogen split products]; decreased fibrinogen or platelets).

▶ General Considerations

Disseminated intravascular coagulation (DIC) is an acquired coagulopathy characterized by tissue factor–mediated coagulation activation in the host. DIC involves dysregulated, excessive thrombin generation, with consequent intravascular fibrin deposition and consumption of platelets and procoagulant factors. Microthrombi, composed of fibrin and platelets, may produce tissue ischemia and end-organ damage. The fibrinolytic system is frequently activated in DIC, leading to plasmin-mediated destruction of fibrin and fibrinogen. These fibrin-fibrinogen degradation products (FDPs) exhibit anticoagulant and platelet-inhibitory functions. While DIC commonly accompanies severe infection, other conditions known to trigger DIC include endothelial damage (eg, endotoxin, virus), tissue necrosis (eg, burns), diffuse ischemic injury (eg, shock, hypoxia acidosis), and systemic release of tissue procoagulants (eg, certain cancers, placental disorders).

▶ Clinical Findings

A. Symptoms and Signs

Signs of DIC may include (1) complications of shock, often including end-organ dysfunction, (2) diffuse bleeding tendency (eg, hematuria, melena, purpura, petechiae, persistent oozing from needle punctures or other invasive procedures), and (3) evidence of thrombosis (eg, small and large vessel thrombosis, purpura fulminans).

B. Laboratory Findings

Tests that are sensitive, easiest to perform, useful for monitoring, and reflect the hemostatic capacity of the patient are the PT, aPTT, platelet count, fibrinogen, and FDPs (including D-dimer). The PT and aPTT are typically prolonged, and the platelet count and fibrinogen concentration may be decreased. However, in children the fibrinogen level may be normal until late in the course. Levels of FSPs are increased. Elevated levels of D-dimer, a cross-linked fibrin degradation byproduct, may be helpful in monitoring the degree of activation of both coagulation and fibrinolysis. However, D-dimer is nonspecific and may be elevated in the context of a triggering event (eg, severe infection) without concomitant DIC. Often, physiologic inhibitors of coagulation, especially antithrombin III, protein C, and protein S are consumed, predisposing to thrombosis. The specific laboratory abnormalities in DIC may vary with the triggering event and the course of illness.

▶ **Differential Diagnosis**

DIC can be difficult to distinguish from the coagulopathy of liver disease (ie, hepatic synthetic dysfunction), especially when the latter is associated with thrombocytopenia secondary to portal hypertension and hypersplenism. Generally, factor VII activity is decreased markedly in liver disease due to deficient synthesis of this protein, which has the shortest half-life among the procoagulant factors, but only mildly to moderately decreased in DIC (due to consumption). Factor VIII activity is often normal or even increased in liver disease but decreased in DIC.

▶ **Treatment**

A. Therapy for Underlying Disorder

The most important aspect of therapy in DIC is the identification and treatment of the triggering event. If the pathogenic process underlying DIC is reversed, often no other therapy is needed for the coagulopathy.

B. Replacement Therapy for Consumptive Coagulopathy

Replacement of consumed procoagulant factors with FFP, cryoprecipitate, unactivated prothrombin complex concentrates (PCCs), and platelets is warranted in the setting of DIC with hemorrhagic complications, or as periprocedural bleeding prophylaxis. Infusion of 10–15 mL/kg FFP typically raises procoagulant factor activities by approximately 10%–15%. Cryoprecipitate can also be given as a rich source of fibrinogen, factor VIII, vWF, and factor XIII; one bag of cryoprecipitate per 3 kg in infants or one bag of cryoprecipitate per 6 kg in older children typically raises plasma fibrinogen concentration by 75–100 mg/dL.

C. Anticoagulant Therapy for Coagulation Activation

Continuous intravenous infusion of unfractionated heparin is sometimes given in order to attenuate coagulation activation and consequent consumptive coagulopathy. The rationale for heparin therapy is to maximize the efficacy of, and minimize the need for, replacement of procoagulants and platelets; however, clinical evidence demonstrating benefit of heparin in DIC is lacking. Prophylactic doses of unfractionated heparin or low-molecular-weight heparin (LMWH) in critically ill and nonbleeding patients with DIC may be considered for prevention of venous thromboembolism. Unfractionated heparin dosing and monitoring is listed on page 932.

D. Specific Factor Concentrates

A nonrandomized pilot study of antithrombin concentrate in children with DIC and associated acquired antithrombin deficiency demonstrated favorable outcomes, suggesting that replacement of this consumed procoagulant may be beneficial. Protein C concentrate has also shown promise in two small pilot studies of meningococci-associated DIC with purpura fulminans.

2. Liver Disease

The liver is the major synthetic site of prothrombin, fibrinogen, high-molecular-weight kininogen, and factors V, VII, IX, X, XI, XII, and XIII. Plasminogen and the physiologic anticoagulants (antithrombin III, protein C, and protein S) are synthesized in the liver, as is α_2-antiplasmin, a regulator of fibrinolysis. Deficiency of factor V and the vitamin K–dependent factors (II, VII, IX, and X) is most often a result of decreased hepatic synthesis, and is manifested by a prolonged PT and often a prolonged aPTT. Extravascular loss and increased consumption of clotting factors may also contribute to PT and aPTT prolongation. Fibrinogen production is often decreased, or an abnormal fibrinogen (dysfibrinogen) containing excess sialic acid residues may be synthesized, or both. Hypofibrinogenemia or dysfibrinogenemia is associated with prolongation of thrombin time and reptilase time. FSPs and D-dimers may be present because of increased fibrinolysis, particularly in the setting of chronic hepatitis or cirrhosis. Thrombocytopenia secondary to hypersplenism may occur. DIC and the coagulopathy of liver disease also mimic vitamin K deficiency; however, vitamin K deficiency has normal factor V activity. Treatment of acute bleeding in the setting of coagulopathy of liver disease consists of replacement with FFP or PCCs and platelets. Desmopressin may shorten the bleeding time and aPTT in patients with chronic liver disease, but its safety is not well established. Recombinant VIIa also is efficacious for life-threatening refractory hemorrhage.

3. Vitamin K Deficiency

The newborn period is characterized by physiologically depressed activity of the vitamin K–dependent factors

(II, VII, IX, and X). If vitamin K is not administered at birth, a bleeding diathesis previously called hemorrhagic disease of the newborn, now termed *vitamin K deficiency bleeding* (VKDB), may develop. Outside of the newborn period, vitamin K deficiency may occur as a consequence of inadequate intake, excess loss, inadequate formation of active metabolites, or competitive antagonism.

One of three patterns is seen in the neonatal period:

1. Early VKDB of the newborn occurs within 24 hours of birth, most often manifested by cephalohematoma, intracranial hemorrhage, or intra-abdominal bleeding. Although occasionally idiopathic, it is most often associated with maternal ingestion of drugs that interfere with vitamin K metabolism (eg, warfarin, phenytoin, isoniazid, and rifampin). Early VKDB occurs in 6%–12% of neonates born to mothers who take these medications without receiving vitamin K supplementation. The disorder is often life threatening.

2. Classic VKDB occurs at 24 hours to 7 days of age and usually is manifested as gastrointestinal, skin, or mucosal bleeding. Bleeding after circumcision may occur. Although occasionally associated with maternal drug usage, it most often occurs in well infants who do not receive vitamin K at birth and are solely breast-fed.

3. Late neonatal VKDB occurs on or after day 8. Manifestations include intracranial, gastrointestinal, or skin bleeding. This disorder is often associated with fat malabsorption (eg, in chronic diarrhea) or alterations in intestinal flora (eg, with prolonged antibiotic therapy). Like classic VKDB, late VKDB occurs almost exclusively in breast-fed infants.

The diagnosis of vitamin K deficiency is suspected based on the history, physical examination, and laboratory results. The PT is prolonged out of proportion to the aPTT (also prolonged). The thrombin time becomes prolonged late in the course. The platelet count is normal. This laboratory profile is similar to the coagulopathy of acute liver disease, but with normal fibrinogen level and absence of hepatic transaminase elevation. The diagnosis of vitamin K deficiency is confirmed by a demonstration of non-carboxylation of specific clotting factors in the absence of vitamin K in the plasma and by clinical and laboratory responses to vitamin K. Intravenous or subcutaneous treatment with vitamin K should be given immediately and not withheld while awaiting test results. In the setting of severe bleeding, additional acute treatment with FFP or PCCs may be indicated.

4. Uremia

Uremia is frequently associated with acquired platelet dysfunction. Bleeding occurs in approximately 50% of patients with chronic renal failure. The bleeding risk conferred by platelet dysfunction associated with metabolic imbalance may be compounded by decreased vWF activity and procoagulant deficiencies (eg, factor II, XII, XI, and IX) due to increased urinary losses of these proteins in some settings of renal insufficiency. In accordance with platelet dysfunction, uremic bleeding is typically characterized by purpura, epistaxis, menorrhagia, or gastrointestinal hemorrhage. Acute bleeding may be managed with infusion of desmopressin acetate, factor VIII concentrates containing vWF, or cryoprecipitate with or without coadministration of FFP. Severe anemia increases the potential for bleeding; therefore red bleed cell transfusion may be required. Recombinant VIIa may be useful in refractory bleeding.

Rajagopal R: Disseminated intravascular coagulation in paediatrics. Arch Dis Child 2017;102:187–193. [PMID: 27540263].
Shearer MJ: Vitamin K deficiency bleeding (VKDB) in early infancy. Blood Rev 2009;23:49–59 [PMID: 18804903].

VASCULAR ABNORMALITIES ASSOCIATED WITH BLEEDING

1. Immunoglobulin A vasculitis (Henoch-Schönlein Purpura)

ESSENTIALS OF DIAGNOSIS & TYPICAL FEATURES

▶ Purpuric cutaneous rash.

▶ Migratory polyarthritis or polyarthralgia.

▶ Intermittent abdominal pain.

▶ Nephritis.

▶ General Considerations

Immunoglobulin A vasculitis the most common type of small vessel vasculitis in children, primarily affects boys 2–7 years of age. Occurrence is highest in the spring and fall, and upper respiratory infection precedes the diagnosis in two-thirds of children.

Leukocytoclastic vasculitis in immunoglobulin A vasculitis principally involves the small vessels of the skin, gastrointestinal tract, and kidneys, with deposition of IgA immune complexes. The most common and earliest symptom is palpable purpura, which results from extravasation of erythrocytes into the tissue surrounding the involved venules. Antigens from group A β-hemolytic streptococci and other bacteria, viruses, drugs, foods, and insect bites have been proposed as inciting agents.

Clinical Findings

A. Symptoms and Signs

Skin involvement may be urticarial initially; progresses to a maculopapules; and coalesces to a symmetrical, palpable purpuric rash distributed on the legs, buttocks, and elbows. New lesions may continue to appear for 2–4 weeks and may extend to involve the entire body. Two-thirds of patients develop migratory polyarthralgia or polyarthritis, primarily of the ankles and knees. Intermittent, sharp abdominal pain occurs in approximately 50% of patients, and hemorrhage and edema of the small intestine can often be demonstrated. Intussusception may develop. Approximately 25%–50% develop renal involvement in the second or third week of illness with either a nephritic or, less commonly, nephrotic picture. Hypertension may accompany the renal involvement. In males, testicular torsion may also occur, and neurologic symptoms are possible due to small vessel vasculitis.

B. Laboratory Findings

The platelet count is normal or elevated, and other screening tests of hemostasis and platelet function are typically normal. Urinalysis frequently reveals hematuria, and sometimes proteinuria. Stool may be positive for occult blood. The antistreptolysin O (ASO) titer is often elevated and the throat culture positive for group A β-hemolytic streptococci. Serum IgA may be elevated.

Differential Diagnosis

The rash of septicemia (especially meningococcemia) may be similar to skin involvement in immunoglobulin A vasculitis, although the distribution tends to be more generalized. The possibility of trauma should be considered in any child presenting with purpura. Other vasculitides should also be considered. The lesions of thrombotic thrombocytopenic purpura (TTP) are not palpable.

Treatment

Generally, treatment is supportive. NSAIDs may be useful for arthritis. Corticosteroid therapy may provide symptomatic relief for severe gastrointestinal or joint manifestations but does not alter skin or renal manifestations. If culture for group A β-hemolytic streptococci is positive or if the ASO titer is elevated, a course of penicillin is warranted.

Prognosis

The prognosis for recovery is generally good, although symptoms frequently (25%–50%) recur over a period of several months. In patients who develop renal manifestations, microscopic hematuria may persist for years. Progressive renal failure occurs in fewer than 5% of patients with immunoglobulin A vasculitis, with an overall fatality rate of 3%.

Key NS: Vascular hemostasis. Haemophilia 2010 Jul;16(Suppl 5):146 [PMID: 20590874].

Ozen S: European consensus-based recommendations for diagnosis and treatment of immunoglobulin A vasculitis—the SHARE initiative. Rheumatology (Oxford). 2019 Sep 1;58(9):1607–1616 [PMID: 30879080].

2. Collagen Disorders

Mild to life-threatening bleeding occurs with some types of Ehlers-Danlos syndrome, the most common inherited collagen disorder. Ehlers-Danlos syndrome is characterized by joint hypermobility, skin extensibility, and easy bruising. Coagulation abnormalities may sometimes be present, including platelet dysfunction and deficiencies of coagulation factors VIII, IX, XI, and XIII. However, bleeding and easy bruising, in most instances, relates to fragility of capillaries and compromised vascular integrity. Ehlers-Danlos syndrome types 4 and 6 are associated with at risk for aortic dissection and spontaneous rupture of aortic aneurysms. Surgery should be avoided for patients with Ehlers-Danlos syndrome, as should medications that induce platelet dysfunction.

Malfait F: Bleeding in the heritable connective tissue disorders: mechanisms, diagnosis and treatment. Blood Rev 2009 Sep;23(5):191–197 [PMID: 19592142].

THROMBOTIC DISORDERS

General Considerations

Uncommon in children, thrombotic disorders are recognized with increasing frequency, particularly with heightened physician awareness and improved survival in pediatric intensive care settings.

Clinical Findings

Initial evaluation of the child who has thrombosis includes an assessment for potential provoking factors, as well as a family history of thrombosis and early cardiovascular or cerebrovascular disease.

A. Clinical Risk Factors

Clinical risk factors are present in more than 90% of children with acute venous thromboembolism (VTE). These conditions include the presence of an indwelling vascular catheter, cardiac disease, infection, trauma, surgery, immobilization, collagen-vascular or chronic inflammatory disease, renal disease, sickle cell anemia, and malignancy. Prospective findings employing serial radiologic evaluation as screening indicate that the risk of VTE is nearly 30% for short-term central venous catheters placed in the internal jugular veins. Retrospective data suggest that approximately 8% of children with cancer develop symptomatic VTE.

1. Inherited Thrombophilia (Hypercoagulable) States

A. PROTEIN C DEFICIENCY—Protein C is a vitamin K–dependent protein that is activated by thrombin bound to thrombomodulin, inactivating activated factors V and VIII. In addition, activated protein C promotes fibrinolysis. Two phenotypes of hereditary protein C deficiency exist. Heterozygous individuals with autosomal dominant protein C deficiency often present with VTE as young adults, but the disorder may manifest during childhood or in later adulthood. In mild protein C deficiency, anticoagulant prophylaxis is typically limited to periods of increased prothrombotic risk. Homozygous or compound heterozygous protein C deficiency is rare and phenotypically severe. Affected children generally present within the first 12 hours of life with purpura fulminans (Figure 30–6) and/or VTE. Prompt protein C replacement by infusion of protein C concentrate or FFP every 6–12 hours, along with therapeutic heparin administration, is recommended. Subsequent management requires chronic therapeutic anticoagulation, often with routine protein C concentrate infusion. Recurrent VTE is common, especially during periods of subtherapeutic anticoagulation or in the presence of conditions associated with increased prothrombotic risk.

B. PROTEIN S DEFICIENCY—Protein S is a cofactor for protein C. Neonates with homozygous protein S deficiency have a course similar to those with homozygous or compound

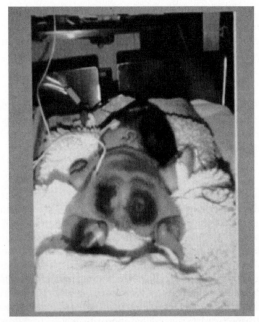

▲ **Figure 30–6.** Purpura fulminans in an infant with severe protein C deficiency.

heterozygous protein C deficiency. Lifelong anticoagulation therapy is indicated in homozygous/severe deficiency, or in heterozygous individuals who have experienced recurrent VTE. Efforts must be made to distinguish these conditions from acquired deficiency, which can be antibody-mediated or secondary to an increase in C4b-binding protein induced by inflammation.

C. ANTITHROMBIN DEFICIENCY—Antithrombin, which is the most important physiologic inhibitor of thrombin, also inhibits activated factors IX, X, XI, and XII. Antithrombin deficiency is transmitted in an autosomal dominant pattern and associated with VTE, typically with onset in adolescence or young adulthood. Therapy for acute VTE is therapeutic anticoagulation. The efficiency of heparin may be significantly diminished in the setting of severe antithrombin deficiency, and it often requires supplementation with antithrombin concentrate. Patients with homozygous/severe deficiency or recurrent VTE are maintained on lifelong anticoagulation.

D. FACTOR V LEIDEN MUTATION—An amino acid substitution in the gene coding for factor V results in factor V Leiden, a factor V polymorphism that is resistant to inactivation by activated protein C. The most common cause of activated protein C resistance in Caucasians, factor V Leiden is present in approximately 5% of the Caucasian population, 20% of Caucasian adults with deep vein thrombosis (DVT), and 40%–60% of those with a family history of VTE. VTE occurs in both heterozygous and homozygous individuals. For heterozygous individuals, thrombosis is typically triggered by a clinical risk factor (or else develops in association with additional thrombophilia traits), whereas in homozygous people, it is often spontaneous. Population studies suggest that the risk of incident VTE is increased two- to sevenfold in the setting of heterozygous factor V Leiden, 35-fold among heterozygous individuals taking the oral contraceptives, and 80-fold in those homozygous for factor V Leiden.

E. PROTHROMBIN MUTATION—The 20210 glutamine to alanine mutation in the prothrombin gene is a relatively common polymorphism in Caucasians that enhances its activation to thrombin. In heterozygous form, this mutation is associated with a two- to threefold increased risk for incident VTE. This mutation also appears to modestly increase the risk for recurrent VTE.

F. OTHER INHERITED DISORDERS—Qualitative abnormalities of fibrinogen (dysfibrinogenemias) are usually inherited in an autosomal dominant manner. Most individuals with dysfibrinogenemia are asymptomatic. Some patients experience bleeding, while others develop venous or arterial thrombosis. The diagnosis is suggested by a prolonged thrombin time with a normal fibrinogen concentration. Hyperhomocysteinemia can be an inherited or an acquired condition and is associated with an increased risk for both arterial and venous thromboses. In children, it may also serve as a risk factor for ischemic arterial stroke. Hyperhomocysteinemia is quite uncommon in the setting of dietary folate supplementation (as in the United States) and is observed almost uniquely in cases of renal insufficiency or metabolic disease (eg, homocystinuria). Methylene tetrahydrofolate reductase receptor mutations do not appear to constitute a risk factor for thrombosis in US children unless homocysteine is elevated.

Lipoprotein(a) is a lipoprotein with homology to plasminogen. In vitro studies suggest that lipoprotein(a) may both promote atherosclerosis and inhibit fibrinolysis. Some evidence suggests that elevated plasma concentrations of lipoprotein(a) are associated with an increased risk of VTEs and recurrent ischemic arterial stroke in children.

Increased factor VIII activity is a risk factor for incident VTE and is common among children with acute VTE. Most elevations in factor VIII is acquired and may persist, but it may also be inherited.

2. Acquired Disorders

A. ANTIPHOSPHOLIPID ANTIBODIES—The development of antiphospholipid antibodies is the most common form of acquired thrombophilia in children. Antiphospholipid antibodies, which include the lupus anticoagulant, anticardiolipin antibodies, and β_2-glycoprotein-1 antibodies (among others) can be present in acute childhood VTE. The lupus anticoagulant is detected in vitro by its inhibition of phospholipid-dependent coagulation assays (eg, aPTT, dilute Russell viper venom time, hexagonal phase phospholipid neutralization assay), whereas immunologic techniques (eg, enzyme-linked immunosorbent assays) are often used to detect anticardiolipin and β_2-glycoprotein-1 antibodies. More common in patients with autoimmune diseases such as systemic lupus erythematosus, antiphospholipid antibodies may also develop following certain drug exposures, infection, acute inflammation, and lymphoproliferative diseases. VTE and antiphospholipid antibodies may predate other signs of lupus. Viral illness is a common precipitant in children, and in many cases, the inciting infection may be asymptomatic.

When an antiphospholipid antibody persists for 12 weeks following the acute thrombotic event, the diagnosis of antiphospholipid syndrome (APS) is confirmed. Optimal duration of anticoagulation in this setting is unclear, such that current pediatric treatment guidelines recommend a 3-month to lifelong course.

B. DEFICIENCIES OF INTRINSIC ANTICOAGULANTS— Acquired deficiencies of proteins C and S and antithrombin may occur in the clinical context of antibodies (eg, protein S antibodies in varicella) or in excessive consumption, including sepsis, DIC, major-vessel or extensive VTE, and post–bone marrow transplant sinusoidal obstruction syndrome (formerly termed *hepatic veno-occlusive disease*). Pilot studies in children have suggested a possible therapeutic role for antithrombin or protein C concentrates in sepsis-associated DIC (eg, meningococcemia) and severe posttransplant sinusoidal obstruction syndrome.

C. ACUTE PHASE REACTANTS—As part of the acute phase response, elevations in plasma fibrinogen concentration, plasma factor VIII, and platelet count may occur, all of which may contribute to an acquired prothrombotic state. Reactive thrombocytosis is rarely associated with VTEs in children when the platelet count is less than 1 million/μL.

B. Symptoms and Signs

Presenting features of thrombosis vary with the anatomic site, extent of vascular involvement, degree of vaso-occlusion, and presence of end-organ dysfunction. The classic presentation of deep venous thrombosis of an upper or lower extremity is pain and acute or subacute extremity swelling, while that for pulmonary embolism commonly involves dyspnea and pleuritic chest pain, and in cerebral sinovenous thrombosis (CSVT) often includes severe or persistent headache, with or without neurologic deficit in otherwise well children. Arterial thrombosis of the lower extremity (eg, neonatal umbilical artery catheter–associated) as well as vasospasm without identified thrombosis, often manifests with diminished distal pulses and dusky discoloration of the limb.

C. Laboratory Findings

A comprehensive laboratory investigation for thrombophilia (ie, hypercoagulability) remains controversial with wide variation of practice. Recent trends favor thrombophilia testing in infants, children, and adolescents with unprovoked thrombosis, and in neonates/children with non–catheter-related thrombosis and stroke. There are insufficient data to recommend routine thrombophilia testing in neonates or children with catheter-related thrombosis. When indicated, thrombophilia testing can include: evaluation for intrinsic anticoagulant deficiency (proteins C and S and antithrombin), procoagulant factor excess (eg, factor VIII), proteins and genetic mutations mediating enhanced procoagulant activity or reduced sensitivity to inactivation (antiphospholipid antibodies; factor V Leiden and prothrombin 20210 polymorphisms), biochemical mediators of endothelial damage (homocysteine), and markers or regulators of fibrinolysis (eg, D-dimer, plasminogen activator inhibitor-1, and lipoprotein[a]). Interpretation of procoagulant factor and intrinsic anticoagulant levels should recognize the age-dependent normal values for these proteins. Among VTE risk factors, antiphospholipid antibodies and elevated levels of homocysteine and lipoprotein(a) have also been demonstrated as risk factors for arterial thrombotic ischemic events.

D. Imaging

Appropriate radiologic imaging is essential for objective documentation of thrombosis and to delineate the type (venous vs arterial), degree of occlusion, and extent (proximal and distal termini) of thrombosis. Depending on site, typical imaging modalities include compression ultrasound with

Doppler, computed tomographic (CT) venography, magnetic resonance venography, and conventional angiography.

Treatment

Current guidelines for the treatment of first-episode VTE in children have been largely based on adult experience and include therapeutic anticoagulation for at least 3 months. During the period of anticoagulation, bleeding precautions should be followed, as previously described (see Treatment under Idiopathic Thrombocytopenic Purpura, earlier). Initial therapy for acute VTE employs continuous intravenous unfractionated heparin or subcutaneous injections of LMWH for at least 7 days, monitored by anti-Xa activity level to maintain safe and therapeutic anticoagulant levels of 0.3–0.7 or 0.5–1.0 IU/mL, respectively. Subsequent extended anticoagulant therapy is given with LMWH or daily oral warfarin, the latter agent monitored by the PT to maintain an international normalized ratio (INR) of 2.0–3.0. During warfarin treatment, the INR optimally should be within the therapeutic range before discontinuation of heparin. Warfarin pharmacokinetics are affected by acute illness, numerous medications, and changes in diet, and can necessitate frequent monitoring. In children, warfarin dose is determined by age and weight. LMWH offers the advantage of infrequent need for monitoring but is far more expensive than warfarin. Anatomic contributions to venous stasis (eg, mastoiditis or depressed skull fracture as risk factors for cerebral sinus venous thrombosis congenital left iliac vein stenosis in DVT of proximal left lower extremity with May-Thurner anomaly) should be addressed to optimize response to anticoagulation. In cases of limb- or life-threatening VTEs, including massive proximal pulmonary embolus, and in cases of progressive VTE despite therapeutic anticoagulation, thrombolytic therapy (eg, tissue-type plasminogen activator) may be considered. Whether thrombolytic therapy may also reduce the risk of the postthrombotic syndrome (PTS) in children with veno-occlusive DVT of the proximal limbs in whom adverse prognostic biomarkers (ie, elevated factor VIII and D-dimer levels) are present at diagnosis needs prospective evaluation. In adolescent females, estrogen-containing contraceptives are relatively contraindicated in those with prior VTE if not using anticoagulation, particularly if an additional genetic cause for impairment of protein C pathway is disclosed.

Direct oral anticoagulants are now first-line therapy for adult acute VTE and for extended anticoagulation. Phase 3 clinical trials in infants and children are ongoing.

Prognosis

Registries and cohort studies have suggested that recurrent VTE occurs in approximately 10% of children within 2 years. Persistent thrombosis is evident following completion of a standard therapeutic course of anticoagulation in up to 30% of children, with unclear clinical importance. Approximately one in four children with DVT involving the extremities develop PTS, a condition of venous insufficiency of varying severity characterized by chronic skin changes, edema, and dilated collateral superficial venous formation, and often accompanied by functional limitation (pain with activities or at rest), venous stasis ulcers, and cellulitis. Complete veno-occlusion and elevated levels of factor VIII and D-dimer at VTE diagnosis have been identified as prognostic factors for PTS among children with DVT affecting the limbs. The presence of homozygous anticoagulant deficiencies, multiple thrombophilia traits, or persistent antiphospholipid antibodies following VTE diagnosis has been associated with increased risk of recurrent VTE, leading to consideration of extended anticoagulation in these instances. In cerebral sinus venous thrombosis failure to provide antithrombotic therapy has been associated with adverse neurologic outcome.

Mahajerin A: Thrombosis in children: approach to anatomic risks, thrombophilia, prevention, and treatment. Hematol Oncol Clin North Am 2019 Jun;33(3):439–453 [PMID: 31030812].

Monagle P: American Society of Hematology 2018 Guidelines for management of venous thromboembolism: treatment of pediatric venous thromboembolism. Blood Adv. 2018 Nov 27;2(22):3292–3316 [PMID: 30482766].

▼ SPLENIC ABNORMALITIES

SPLENOMEGALY & HYPERSPLENISM

The differential diagnosis of splenomegaly includes the categories of congestive splenomegaly, chronic infections, leukemia and lymphomas, hemolytic anemias, reticuloendothelioses, and storage diseases (Table 30–9).

Splenomegaly due to any cause may be associated with hypersplenism and the excessive destruction of circulating red cells, white cells, and platelets. The degree of cytopenia is variable and, when mild, requires no specific therapy. In other cases, the thrombocytopenia may cause life-threatening bleeding, particularly when the splenomegaly is secondary to portal hypertension and associated with esophageal varices or the consequence of a storage disease. In such cases, treatment with surgical splenectomy or with splenic embolization may be warranted. Although more commonly associated with acute enlargement, rupture of an enlarged spleen can be seen in more chronic conditions such as Gaucher disease.

Stirnemann J: A review of Gaucher disease pathophysiology, clinical presentation and treatments. Int J Mol Sci 2017;18(2). doi: 10.3390/ijms18020441 [PMID: 28218669].

ASPLENIA & SPLENECTOMY

Children who lack normal splenic function are at risk for sepsis, meningitis, and pneumonia due to encapsulated bacteria such as pneumococci, meningococcus, and

Table 30–9. Causes of chronic splenomegaly in children.

Cause	Associated Clinical Findings	Diagnostic Investigation
Congestive splenomegaly	History of umbilical vein catheter or neonatal omphalitis; signs of portal hypertension (varices, hemorrhoids, dilated abdominal wall veins); pancytopenia; history of hepatitis or jaundice	Complete blood count, platelet count, liver function tests, ultrasonography
Chronic infections	History of exposure to tuberculosis, histoplasmosis, coccidioidomycosis, other fungal disease; chronic sepsis (foreign body in bloodstream; subacute infective endocarditis)	Appropriate cultures and skin tests, ie, blood cultures; PPD, fungal serology and antigen tests, chest film; HIV serology
Infectious mononucleosis	Fever, fatigue, pharyngitis, rash, adenopathy, hepatomegaly	Atypical lymphocytes on blood smear, monospot, EBV antibody titers
Leukemia, lymphoma, Hodgkin disease	Evidence of systemic involvement with fever, bleeding tendencies, hepatomegaly, and lymphadenopathy; pancytopenia	Blood smear, bone marrow examination, chest film, gallium scan, LDH, uric acid
Hemolytic anemia	Anemia, jaundice; family history of anemia, jaundice, and gallbladder disease in young adults	Reticulocyte count, Coombs test, blood smear, osmotic fragility test, hemoglobin electrophoresis
Reticuloendothelioses (histiocytosis X)	Chronic otitis media, seborrheic or petechial skin rashes, anemia, infections, lymphadenopathy, hepatomegaly, bone lesions	Skeletal radiographs for bone lesions; biopsy of bone, liver, bone marrow, or lymph node
Storages diseases	Family history of similar disorders, neurologic involvement, evidence of macular degeneration, hepatomegaly	Biopsy of liver or bone marrow in search for storage cells
Splenic cyst	Evidence of other infections (postinfectious cyst) or congenital anomalies; peculiar shape of spleen	Radionuclide scan, ultrasonography
Splenic hemangioma	Other hemangiomas, consumptive coagulopathy	Radionuclide scan, arteriography, platelet count, coagulation screen

EBV, Epstein-Barr virus; HIV, human immunodeficiency virus; LDH, lactic dehydrogenase; PPD, purified protein derivative.

H influenzae. Such infections are often fulminant and fatal because of inadequate antibody production and impaired phagocytosis of circulating bacteria.

Congenital asplenia is usually suspected when an infant is born with abnormalities of abdominal viscera and complex cyanotic congenital heart disease. Howell-Jolly bodies are usually present on the peripheral blood smear, and the absence of splenic tissue is confirmed by technetium radionuclide scanning. The prognosis depends on the underlying cardiac lesions, and many children die during the first few months. Prophylactic antibiotics, usually penicillin, and pneumococcal conjugate and subsequent pneumococcal polysaccharide, Hib, and meningococcal conjugate vaccines are recommended.

The risk of overwhelming sepsis following surgical splenectomy is related to the child's age and to the underlying disorder. Because the risk is highest when the procedure is performed earlier in life, splenectomy is usually postponed until after age 5 years. The risk of postsplenectomy sepsis is also greater in children with malignancies, thalassemias, and reticuloendothelioses than in children whose splenectomy is performed for ITP, hereditary spherocytosis, or trauma.

Prior to splenectomy, children should be immunized against *Streptococcus pneumoniae*, *H influenzae*, and *Neisseria meningitidis*. Additional management should include penicillin prophylaxis and prompt evaluation for fever 38.8°C or above or signs of severe infection.

Children with sickle cell anemia develop functional asplenia during the first year of life, and overwhelming sepsis is the leading cause of early deaths in this disease. Prophylactic penicillin reduces the incidence of sepsis by 84%.

Iolascon A et al; Working Study Group on Red Cells and Iron of the EHA: Recommendations regarding splenectomy in hereditary hemolytic anemias. Haematologica 2017;102(8):1304–1313. doi: 10.3324/haematol.2016.161166 [PMID: 28550188].

Robinson CL, Bernstein H, Romero JR, Szilagyi P: Advisory Committee on Immunization Practices Recommended Immunization Schedule for Children and Adolescents Aged 18 Years or Younger—United States, 2019. MMWR Morb Mortal Wkly Rep 2019;68(5):112–114. doi: 10.15585/mmwr.mm6805a4 [PMID: 30730870].

Rubin LG: Care of the asplenic patient. New Engl J Med 2014;371:349–356 [PMID: 25054718].

▼ TRANSFUSION MEDICINE

DONOR SCREENING & BLOOD PROCESSING: RISK MANAGEMENT

Minimizing the risks of transfusion begins by screening volunteer donors with a universal donor questionnaire designed to protect the recipient from transmission of infectious agents as well as other risks of transfusions. In addition, information defining high-risk groups whose behavior increases the possible transmission of HIV, hepatitis, and other diseases is provided, with the request that persons in these groups not donate blood. This screen also decreases risk of blood donation for the donor. Positive responses may result in temporary or permanent deferral from donation.

Before blood components can be released for transfusion, donor blood is screened for hepatitis B surface antigen; antibodies to hepatitis B core antigen, hepatitis C, HIV-1 and 2, and human T-cell lymphotropic virus (HTLV) I and II; and a serologic test for syphilis (Table 30–10). Screening donor

Table 30–10. Transmission risks of infectious agents for which screening of blood products is routinely performed.

Disease Entity	Transmission	Screening and Processing Procedures	Approximate Risk of Transmission
Syphilis	Low risk: fresh blood drawn during spirochetemia can transmit infection. Organism not able to survive beyond 72 h during storage at 4°C.	Donor history. RPR or VDRL.	< 1:100,000
Hepatitis A	Units drawn during prodrome could transmit virus. Because of brief viremia during acute phase, absence of asymptomatic carrier phase, and failure to detect transmission in multiple transfused individuals, infection by this agent is unlikely.	Donor history.	1:1,000,000
Hepatitis B	Prolonged viremia during various phases of the disease and asymptomatic carrier state make HBV infection a significant risk of transfusion. Incidence has markedly decreased with screening strategies. Also, an increasing number of blood recipients have been vaccinated.	Donor history, education, and self-exclusion. HBsAg. Surrogate test for non-A, non-B hepatitis (hepatitis-B core antibody) has helped screen out population at risk for transmitting HBV.	1:500,000–1:200,000
Hepatitis C	Most cases of posttransfusion hepatitis in the past have been related to this virus.	Donor history. Surrogate tests: hepatitis B core antibody, anti-HCV. Nucleic acid testing for viral genome required.	1:2,000,000
Non-A, non-B, non-C hepatitis	Agents other than HAV, HBV, HCV, EBV, and CMV, which can cause posttransfusion hepatitis.	Donor history. Surrogate tests: anti-HBc.	Undefined
HIV (HIV-1, HIV-2) infection	Retroviruses spread by sexual contact, parenteral (including transfusion) and mother to fetus.	Donor history, education, and self-exclusion. Anti-HIV by EIA screening test. Western blot confirmatory. Nucleic acid testing for viral genome required.	1:2,000,000
HTLV-I and II infection	Retroviruses spread by sexual contact, parenteral (including transfusion) and mother to fetus.	Donor history. Anti-HTLV-I and II by enzyme immunoassay screening test. Western blot confirmatory.	1:3,000,000
Chagas disease	Transmitted by insect vector, blood transfusion (all components), organ transplant, food contaminated with parasites, and mother to fetus.	History (especially country of origin), detection of antibody in donor serum or plasma.	< 1:25,000
West Nile virus	Seasonal transmission through mosquito vector. Transmitted by blood transfusion and organ transplant.	History, nucleic acid testing for viral genome.	1:350,000
Zika virus	Transmitted by mosquito vector, sexual fluids, blood transfusion, and mother to fetus.	History, nucleic acid testing for viral genome	Undefined

CMV, cytomegalovirus; EBV, Epstein-Barr virus; EIA, enzyme-linked immunosorbent assay; HAV, HBV, HCV, hepatitis A virus, hepatitis B virus, hepatitis C virus, respectively; HIV, human immunodeficiency virus; HBsAg, hepatitis B surface antigen; HTLV, human T-cell lymphotropic virus; RPR, rapid plasma reagin; VDRL, syphilis test.

blood for viral genome (nucleic acid amplification [NAT] testing) was mandated for HIV, HCV, and West Nile virus. NAT testing for other viruses including Chagas and Zika virus can now also be performed. Positive tests are repeated.

Upon confirmation of a positive test, the unit in question is destroyed and the donor is notified and deferred from future donations. Many of the screening tests used are very sensitive and have a high rate of false-positive results. As a result, confirmatory tests have been developed to check the initial screening results and separate the false positives from the true positives, allowing for donors with repeat reactive screening tests on a specific donation to be reentered into the donor pool in the future if they meet specifications of an algorithm for further testing. Bacterial culture of apheresis or pooled platelet concentrates is included in the testing paradigm.

With these approaches, the risk of an infectious complication from blood components has been minimized (see Table 30–10). Recent addition of pathogen reduction techniques to blood components will provide an additional strategy to reduce transfusion transmitted infections and reduce the expense of additional testing for emerging infectious agents associated with blood transfusion. Autologous donation is recognized by some centers as a safe alternative to homologous blood. Issues of donor size limit the use of autologous donation difficult to apply to the pediatric population.

Primary CMV infections are significant complications of blood transfusion in transplant recipients, neonates, and immunodeficient individuals. Transmission of CMV can be avoided by using seronegative donors, apheresis platelet concentrates collected by techniques ensuring low numbers of residual white cells, or red cell or platelet products that are leukocyte-depleted by filtration (< 5 million WBCs per packed red cell unit or apheresis platelet concentrate equivalent).

STORAGE & PRESERVATION OF BLOOD & BLOOD COMPONENTS

Whole blood is routinely fractionated into packed red cells, platelets, and FFP or cryoprecipitate for most efficient use of all blood components. The storage conditions and biologic characteristics of the components are summarized in Table 30–11. The conditions provide the optimal environment to maintain appropriate recovery, survival, and function, and are different for each blood component. For example, red cells undergo dramatic metabolic changes during their 35- to 42-day storage, with a virtual disappearance of 2,3-DPG by day 14 of storage, a decrease in adenosine triphosphate, and gradual loss of intracellular potassium. After transfusion, in vivo recovery of greater than or equal to 80% transfused cells in red cells occurs even with older products.

Fortunately, these changes are reversed readily in vivo within hours to days after the red cells are transfused. However, in certain clinical conditions, these effects may define the type of components used. For example, blood less than 5–7 days old would be preferred for exchange transfusion in neonates, red cell exchanges in older patients, or replacement of red cells in persons with severe cardiopulmonary disease to ensure adequate oxygen-carrying capacity. Storage time is not usually an issue when administering transfusions to those with chronic anemia.

If extracellular potassium in older packed red cells may present a problem, one may use blood less than 10 days old, making packed cells out of an older unit of whole blood or washing blood stored as packed cells.

Platelets are stored at 22°C for a maximum of 5 days; criteria for 7-day storage are being developed. At the extremes of storage, there should be at least a 60% recovery, a survival time that approximates turnover of fresh autologous platelets, and normalization of the bleeding time or PFA-100 in proportion to the peak platelet count. Frozen components, red cells, FFP, and cryoprecipitate are outdated at 10 years, 1 year, and 1 year, respectively. Frozen red cells retain the same biochemical and functional characteristics as the day they were frozen. FFP contains 80% or more of all of the clotting factors of fresh plasma. Factors VIII and XIII, vWF, and fibrinogen are concentrated in cryoprecipitate.

PRETRANSFUSION TESTING

Donated blood and recipient samples are tested for ABO and Rh(D) antigens and screened for auto- or alloantibodies in the plasma. The cross-match is required on any component that contains red cells. In the major cross-match, washed donor red cells are incubated with the serum from the patient, and reactivity or agglutination is detected and graded after immediate centrifugation. The antiglobulin phase of the test may then be performed; Coombs reagent, which will detect the presence of IgG or complement on the surface of the red cells, is added to the mixture, and reactivity evaluated. In the presence of a negative antibody screen in the recipient, a negative immediate spin cross-match test confirms the compatibility of the blood and antiglobulin phase is not required. Further testing is required if the antibody screen or the cross-match is positive, and blood should not be given until the nature of the reactivity is delineated. An incompatible cross-match is evaluated first with a DAT or Coombs test to detect IgG or complement on the surfaces of the recipient's red cells. The indirect antiglobulin test is also used to determine the presence of antibodies that will coat red cells or activate complement, and additional studies are completed to define the antibody.

Table 30–11. Characteristics of blood and blood components.

Component	Storage Conditions	Composition and Transfusion Characteristics	Indications	Risks and Precautions	Administration
Whole blood	4°C for 35 days. RBC characteristics: *Survival:* Recovery decreases during storage but is always > 70%–80%. Cells that circulate approximate normal survival. *Function:* 2,3-DPG levels fall to undetectable after second week of storage. This defect is repaired within 12 h of transfusion. *Electrolytes:* With storage, potassium increases in plasma. This rises to high levels after 2 wk of storage.	Contains RBCs and many plasma compounds of whole blood. Leukocytes and platelets lose activity or viability after 1–3 day under these conditions. Procoagulant clotting factors (particularly VIII and V) deteriorate rapidly during storage. Each unit has about 500 mL volume and Hct 36%–40%.	Oxygen-carrying capacity (anemia). Volume replacement for massive blood loss or severe shock.	Must be ABO-identical and cross-match-compatible. Infections. Febrile or hemolytic transfusion reactions. Alloimmunization to red cell, white cell, or platelet antigens.	During acute blood loss, as rapidly as tolerated. In other settings, 2–4 h. 10 mL/kg will raise Hct by 5% and support volume.
Packed red cells	Same as for whole blood. Special preservative solutions allow storage for 42 day.	Contains RBCs; most plasma removed in preparation. Status of leukocytes, clotting factors, and platelets same as for whole blood. Hct about 70%, volume 200–250 mL. May request tighter pack to give Hct 80%–90%.	Oxygen-carrying capacity. Acute trauma or bleeding or situations requiring intensive cardiopulmonary support (Hct < 25%–30%). Chronic anemia (Hct < 21%).	Same as for whole blood.	May be given as patient will tolerate, based on cardiovascular status over 2–4 h. Dose of 3 mL packed RBC/kg will raise Hct by 3%. If cardiovascular status is stable, give 10 mL/kg over 2–4 h. If unstable, use smaller volume or do packed RBC exchange.
Washed or filtered red cells	When cells are washed, there is a 24-h outdate. Up to that time, they have the same characteristics as for packed red cells.	Same as for packed red cells.	Same as packed red cells. Depending on technique used and extent of reduction of white blood cells, leukoreduced red cells may achieve the following: Decrease in febrile reactions. Decrease in transmission of CMV. Decrease in incidence of alloimmunization to white cell antigens.	Same as whole blood. Removal of white cells diminishes the risk of febrile reactions. Filtration with high-efficiency white cell filters may decrease rate of alloimmunization to white cell antigens and transmission of CMV.	Same as for packed red cells.

Frozen red cells	Packed red cells frozen in 40% glycerol solution at < –65°C. After storage for 10 y, cells retain the same biochemical characteristics, function, and capacity for survival as on the day they were frozen; when thawed, 24-h outdate.	Same as for packed red cells.	Same as packed red cells. Useful for avoiding febrile reactions, decreasing transmission of CMV, autologous blood donation, and developing an inventory of rare red cell blood groups.	Same as for packed red cells. Risk of CMV transmission is at same level as using seronegative components.	Same as for packed red cells.
Fresh frozen plasma or 24 h frozen plasma	Plasma from whole blood stored at < –18°C for up to 1 y.	Contains > 80% of all procoagulant and anticoagulant plasma proteins. Plasma separated from stored whole blood by 24 hours has similar characteristics.	Replacement of plasma procoagulant and anticoagulant proteins. May provide "other" factors, eg, treatment of TTP. Use with deficiency of one or more clotting factors in association with bleeding, decreased liver production, or consumption (DIC) when the INR >1.5. For VIII, IX, VII, protein C, AT-III deficiency or inhibitors, use factor concentrates if available.	Need not be cross-matched; should be type-compatible. Volume overload, infectious diseases, allergic reactions. Solvent detergent-treated plasma or donor-retested plasma units have decreased risk for viral transmission.	As rapidly as tolerated by patient, but not > 4 h. Dose: 10–15 mL/kg will increase level of all clotting factors by 10%–20%.
Cryoprecipitate	Produced by freezing fresh plasma to < –65°C, then allowed to thaw 18 h at 4°C. After centrifugation, cryoprecipitable proteins are separated. May be stored at < –18°C for up to 1 y.	Contains factor VIII, vWF, fibrinogen, and fibronectin at concentrations greater than those of plasma. Also contains factor XIII, VIII > 80 IU/pack, fibrinogen 100–350 mg/pack.	Treatment of acquired or congenital deficiencies of fibrinogen, F XIII. Useful in making biologic glues that contain fibrinogen. Commercial clotting factor concentrates treatment of choice for factor VIII deficiency and vWD because sterilization procedures further reduce the risk of viral transmission.	Same as for fresh frozen plasma. ABO agglutinins may also be concentrated and can give positive direct agglutination test if not type-specific.	Cryoprecipitate can be given as a rapid infusion (30-60 min). Dose: ½ pack/kg body weight will increase factor VIII level by 80%–100% and fibrinogen by 200–250 mg/dL.

(Continued)

Table 30–11. Characteristics of blood and blood components. (*Continued*)

Component	Storage Conditions	Composition and Transfusion Characteristics	Indications	Risks and Precautions	Administration
Platelet concentrates from whole blood donation	Separated from platelet-rich plasma and stored with gentle agitation at 22–24°C for 5 days or up to 7 days with confirmation of sterility. Containers currently in use are plastic and allow for gas exchange; diffusion of CO_2 helps keep pH > 6, a major factor in keeping platelets viable and functional.	Each unit contains about 5×10^{10} platelets. *Survival:* Although there may be some loss with storage, 60%–70% recovery should be achieved, with stored platelets able to correct platelet function test in proportion to the peak counts reached.	Treatment of thrombocytopenia or platelet function defects.	No cross-match necessary. Should be ABO type–specific. Other risks as for whole blood.	Can be taken during rapid transfusion or as defined by cardiovascular status, not > 4 h. Dose: 10 mL/kg should increase platelet count by at least 50,000/μL.
Platelet concentrates by apheresis techniques	Same as random donor units.	Platelet content is equivalent to 6–10 units of concentrates from whole blood (3×10^{11} platelets); can be made relatively free of leukocytes, which is important for avoiding alloimmunization.	Same as above, particularly useful in treating patients who have insufficient production and also may have a problem with alloisoimmunization.	Same as above.	Same as above.
Granulocytes	Although they may be stored stationary at 22–24°C, transfuse as soon as possible after collection.	Contains at least 1×10^{10} granulocytes, but also platelets and red cells. When donors given 10 mcg/kg G-CSF subcutaneously and 8 mg Decadron orally 12–15 h before collection, yield increases to > 5×10^{10} granulocytes.	Severely neutropenic individuals (< 500/μL) with poor marrow reserves and suspected bacterial or fungal infections not responding to 48–72 h of parenteral antibiotics. Also in patients with neutrophil dysfunction.	Same as for platelets. Pulmonary leukostasis reactions. Severe febrile reactions.	Given in an infusion over 2–4 h. Dose: 1 unit daily for newborns and infants, 1 × 10^9 granulocytes/kg.

CMV, cytomegalovirus; DPG, diphosphoglycerate; G-CSF, granulocyte colony–stimulating factor; Hct, hematocrit; RBC, red blood cell; TTP, thrombotic thrombocytopenic purpura; vWD, von Willebrand disease; vWF, von Willebrand factor.

TRANSFUSION PRACTICE

General Rules

Several rules should be observed in administering any blood component:

1. In final preparation of the component, no solutions should be added to the bag or tubing set except for normal saline (0.9% sodium chloride for injection, USP), ABO-compatible plasma, or other specifically approved expanders. Hypotonic solutions cause hemolysis of red cells, and if these are transfused, a severe reaction will occur. Any reconstitution should be completed by the blood bank.

2. Transfusion products should be protected from contact with any calcium-containing solution (eg, lactated Ringer); recalcification and reversal of citrate effect will cause clotting of the blood component.

3. Blood components should not be warmed to a temperature greater than 37°C. If a component is incubated in a water bath, it should be enclosed in a watertight bag to prevent bacterial contamination of entry ports.

4. Whenever a blood bag is entered, the sterile integrity of the system is violated, and that unit should be discarded within 4 hours if left at room temperature or within 24 hours if the temperature is 4–6°C.

5. Transfusions of products containing red cells should not exceed 4 hours. Blood components in excess of what can be infused during this time period should be stored in the blood bank until needed.

6. Before transfusion, the blood component should be inspected visually for any unusual characteristics, such as the presence of flocculent material, hemolysis, or clumping of cells, and mixed thoroughly.

7. The unit and the recipient should be identified properly.

8. The administration set includes a standard 170- to 260-μm filter. Under certain clinical circumstances, an additional microaggregate filter may be used to eliminate small aggregates of fibrin, white cells, and platelets that will not be removed by the standard filter.

9. The patient should be observed during the entire transfusion, especially during the first 15 minutes. With the onset of any adverse symptoms or signs, the transfusion should be stopped, an evaluation initiated immediately, and the reaction reported promptly to the transfusion service. Untransfused components, blood samples from the patient, and appropriate paperwork should also be submitted to the transfusion service.

10. When cross-match–incompatible red cells or whole blood unit(s) must be given to the patient (as with AIHA), a test dose of 10% of the total volume (not to exceed 50 mL) should be administered over 15–20 minutes; the transfusion is then stopped and the patient observed. If no changes in vital signs or the patient's condition are noted, the remainder of the volume can be infused carefully.

11. Blood for exchange transfusion in the newborn period may be cross-matched with either the infant's or the mother's serum or plasma. If the exchange is for hemolysis, 1 unit of whole blood stored for less than 5–7 days will be adequate. If replacement of clotting factors is a key issue, packed red cells reconstituted with ABO type-specific FFP may be considered. Based on post-transfusion platelet counts, platelet transfusion may be considered. Other problems to be anticipated are acid–base derangements, hyponatremia, hyperkalemia, hypocalcemia, hypoglycemia, hypothermia, and hypervolemia or hypovolemia.

Choice of Blood Component

Several principles should be considered when deciding on the need for blood transfusion. Indications for blood or blood components must be well defined, and the patient's medical condition, not just the laboratory results, should be the basis for the decision. Specific deficiencies exhibited by the patient (eg, oxygen-carrying capacity, thrombocytopenia) should be treated with appropriate blood components and the use of whole blood minimized. Information about specific blood components is summarized in Table 30–11. In general, very little is known about specific indications for blood component transfusion and outcomes. In recent years the criteria have become more restrictive for transfusion of any component. A recent review evaluates what is known and presents fertile areas for investigation (see Josephson et al).

A. Whole Blood

See Table 30–11.

B. Packed Red Blood Cells

See Table 30–11.

C. Platelets

The decision to transfuse platelets depends on the patient's clinical condition, the status of plasma phase coagulation, the platelet count, the cause of the thrombocytopenia, and the functional capacity of the patient's platelets. In the face of decreased production, clinical bleeding, and platelet counts less than 10,000/μL, the risk of severe, spontaneous bleeding is increased markedly. In the presence of these factors and in the absence heparin-induced thrombocytopenia,

TTP, or antibody-mediated thrombocytopenia, transfusion may be considered. Under certain circumstances, especially with platelet dysfunction or treatment that inhibits the procoagulant system, transfusions at higher platelet counts may be necessary.

Transfused platelets are sequestered temporarily in the lungs and spleen before reaching their peak concentrations, 45–60 minutes after transfusion. A significant proportion of the transfused platelets never circulate but remain sequestered in the spleen. This phenomenon results in reduced recovery; under best conditions, only 60%–70% of the transfused platelets are accounted for when peripheral platelet count increments are used as a measure of response.

In addition to cessation of bleeding, two variables indicate the effectiveness of platelet transfusions. The first is platelet recovery, as measured by the maximum number of platelets circulating in response to transfusion. The practical measure is the platelet count at 1 hour after transfusion. In the absence of immune or drastic nonimmune factors that markedly decrease platelet recovery, one would expect a 7000/μL increment for each random donor unit and a 40,000–70,000/μL increment for each single-donor apheresis unit in a large child or adolescent. For infants and small children, 10 mL/kg of platelets will increase the platelet count by at least 50,000/μL. The second variable is the survival of transfused platelets. If the recovery is greater than 50,000/uL, transfused platelets will approach a normal half-life in the circulation. In the presence of increased platelet destruction, the lifespan may be shortened to a few days or a few hours. Frequent platelet transfusions may be required to maintain adequate hemostasis.

A particularly troublesome outcome in patients receiving long-term platelet transfusions is the development of a refractory state characterized by poor ($\leq$ 20%) recovery or no response to platelet transfusion (as measured at 1 hour). Most (70%–90%) of these refractory states result from the development of alloantibodies directed against HLA antigens on the platelet. Platelets have Class I HLA antigens, and the antibodies are primarily against HLA A or B determinants. A smaller proportion of these alloantibodies (< 10%) may be directed against platelet-specific alloantigens. The most effective approach to prevent HLA sensitization is to use leukocyte-depleted components (< 5 million leukocytes per unit of packed red cells or per apheresis or 6–10 random donor unit concentrates). For the alloimmunized, refractory patient, the best approach is to provide HLA-matched platelets for transfusion. Platelet cross-matching procedures using HLA-matched or unmatched donors may be helpful in identifying platelet concentrates most likely to provide an adequate response.

D. Fresh Frozen Plasma

See Table 30–11.

E. Cryoprecipitate

See Table 30–11.

F. Granulocytes

With better supportive care over the past 20 years, the need for granulocytes in neutropenic patients with severe bacterial infections has decreased. Indications still remain for severe bacterial or fungal infections unresponsive to vigorous medical therapy in either newborns or older children with bone marrow failure, or patients with neutrophil dysfunction. Newer mobilization schemes using G-CSF and steroids in donors result in granulocyte collections with at least 50 billion neutrophils. This may provide a better product for patients requiring granulocyte support.

G. Apheresis Products and Procedures

Apheresis equipment allows one or more blood components to be collected while the rest are returned to the donor. Apheresis platelet concentrates, which have as many platelets as 6–10 units of platelet concentrates from whole blood donations, are one example; granulocytes are another. Apheresis techniques can also be used to collect hematopoietic stem cells that have been mobilized into the blood by cytokines (eg, G-CSF) or mononuclear cells for immunotherapy. Stem cells are used for allogeneic or autologous bone marrow transplantation. Blood cell separators can be used for the collection of single-source plasma or removal of a blood component that is causing disease. Examples include red cell exchange in sickle cell disease and plasmapheresis in Goodpasture syndrome, Guillain-Barré syndrome, or other antibody-mediated disorders.

Adverse Effects

The noninfectious complications of blood transfusions are outlined in Table 30–12. Most complications present a significant risk to the recipient.

Busch MP, Bloch EM, Kleinman S: Prevention of transfusion-transmitted infections. Blood 2019;133(17):1854–1864. doi: 10.1182/blood-2018-11-833996 [PMID: 30808637].

Goodrich RP: Special considerations for the use of pathogen reduced blood components in pediatric patients: an overview. Transfusion Apher Sci 2018;57(3):374–377. doi: 10.1016/j.transci.2018.05.022 [PMID: 29773498].

Jacquot C, Mo YD, Luban NLC: New approaches and trials in pediatric transfusion medicine. Hematol Oncol Clin North Am 2019;33(3):507–520. doi: 10.1016/j.hoc.2019.01.012 [PMID: 31030816].

Schulz WL et al: Blood utilization and transfusion reactions in pediatric patients transfused with conventional or pathogen reduced platelets. J Pediatr 2019 Jun;209:220–225 doi: 10.1016/j.peds.2019.01.046 [PMID: 30885645].

Table 30–12. Adverse events following transfusions.

Event	Pathophysiology	Signs and Symptoms	Management
Acute hemolytic transfusion reaction	Preformed alloantibodies (most commonly to ABO) and infrequently autoantibodies cause rapid intravascular hemolysis of transfused cells with activation of clotting (DIC), activation of inflammatory mediators, and acute renal failure.	Fever, chills, nausea, chest pain, back pain, pain at transfusion site, hypotension, dyspnea, oliguria, hemoglobinuria.	The risk of this type of reaction overall is low (1:70,000–1:30,000), but the mortality rate is high (up to 40%). Stop the transfusion; maintain renal output with intravenous fluids and diuretics (furosemide or mannitol); treat DIC with heparin; and institute other appropriate supportive measures.
Delayed hemolytic transfusion reaction	Formation of alloantibodies after transfusion and resultant destruction of transfused red cells, usually by extravascular hemolysis.	Jaundice, anemia. A small percentage may develop chronic hemolysis.	Detection, definition, and documentation (for future transfusions). Supportive care. Risk, < 5% of transfused patients may develop alloantibody; hemolysis, 1:11,000–1:2500.
Febrile reactions	Usually caused by leukoagglutinins in recipient, cytokines, or other biologically active compounds.	Fever. May also involve chills.	Supportive. Leukocyte-reduced products decrease reactions. Risk per transfusion, 1:100 transfusions.
Allergic reactions	Most causes not identified. In IgA-deficient individuals, reaction occurs as a result of antibodies to IgA.	Itching, hives, and occasionally chills and fever. In severe reactions, may see signs of anaphylaxis: dyspnea, pulmonary edema.	Mild to moderate reactions: diphenhydramine. More severe reactions: epinephrine subcutaneously and steroids intravenously. Risk for mild to moderate allergic reactions, 1:100. Severe anaphylactic reactions, 1:50,000—1:20,000.
Transfusion-related acute lung injury	Acute lung injury occurring within 6 h after transfusion. Two sets of factors interact to produce the syndrome. Patient factors: infection, surgery, cytokine therapy. Blood component factors: lipids, antibodies, cytokines. Two groups of factors interact during transfusion to result in lung injury indistinguishable from ARDS.	Tachypnea, dyspnea, hypoxia. Diffuse interstitial markings. Cardiac evaluation normal.	May consider younger products: packed red blood cells ≤ 2 wk, platelets ≤ 3 days, washing components to prevent syndrome. Management: supportive care. Risk, 1:2000–1:3000 per transfusion. Current preventive procedures include avoiding donors at risk for alloimmunization: use of male-only FFP or white blood cell antibody-negative apheresis FFP or platelet products.
Transfusion-associated circulatory overload	Circulatory volume overload occurring within 6 hours of cessation of transfusion. Risk factors: age, history of heart failure, number of units transfused	Acute respiratory distress, elevated brain natriuretic peptide, elevated central venous pressure, left heart failure, positive fluid balance, pulmonary edema	Stop the transfusion; administer supplemental oxygen if needed; diuretics; ventilatory support.
Dilutional coagulopathy	Massive blood loss and transfusion with replacement with fluids or blood components and deficient clotting factors.	Bleeding.	Replacement of clotting factors or platelets with appropriate blood components.
Bacterial contamination	Contamination of units results in growth of bacteria or production of clinically significant levels of endotoxin.	Chills, high fever, hypotension, other symptoms of sepsis or endotoxemia.	Stop transfusion; make aggressive attempts to identify organism; provide vigorous support. Sepsis in 1:500,000–1:75,000

(Continued)

Table 30–12. Adverse events following transfusions. (*Continued*)

Event	Pathophysiology	Signs and Symptoms	Management
Graft-versus-host disease	Lymphocytes from donor transfused in an immunoincompetent host.	Syndrome can involve a variety of organs, usually skin, liver, gastrointestinal tract, and bone marrow.	Rare. Preventive management: irradiation (> 1500 cGy) of cellular blood components transfused to individuals with congenital or acquired immunodeficiency syndromes, intrauterine transfusion, very premature infants, and when donors are relatives of the recipient.
Iron overload	There is no physiologic mechanism to excrete excess iron. Target organs include liver, heart, and endocrine organs. In patients receiving red cell transfusions over long periods of time, there is an increase in iron burden.	Signs and symptoms of dysfunctional organs affected by the iron.	Significant risk with chronic transfusions. Treated with chronic administration of iron chelator such as deferoxamine given intravenously or Exjade given orally.

ARDS, adult respiratory distress syndrome; DIC, disseminated intravascular coagulation; FFP, fresh frozen plasma; IgA, immunoglobulin A.

REFERENCES

Fung MK et al: *Technical Manual.* 19th ed. AABB, Bethesda, MD; 2017.
Goodnight SH, Hathaway WE (eds): *Disorders of Hemostasis and Thrombosis: A Clinical Guide.* 2nd ed. McGraw-Hill, New York, NY; 2001.

Klein HG, Anstee DJ (eds): *Blood Transfusion in Clinical Medicine.* 12th ed. Wiley-Blackwell Hoboken, NJ; 2014.
Petz L, Garratty G: *Immune Hemolytic Anemias.* 2nd ed. Churchill Livingstone Philadelphia, PA; 2004.

Neoplastic Disease

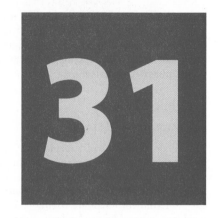

Amy K. Keating, MD

Jessica Knight-Perry, MD, MB

Kelly Maloney, MD

Jean M. Mulcahy Levy, MD

Brian S. Greffe, MD

Anna R.K. Franklin, MD

Timothy Prince Garrington, MD

Each year approximately 150 out of every 1 million children younger than 20 years are diagnosed with cancer. For children between the ages of 1 and 20 years, cancer is the fourth leading cause of death, behind unintentional injuries, homicides, and suicides. However, combined-modality therapy, including surgery, chemotherapy, and radiation therapy, has improved survival dramatically, such that the overall 5-year survival rate of pediatric malignancies is now greater than 75%. It is estimated that currently 1 in 570 adults will be a survivor of childhood cancer.

Because pediatric malignancies are rare, cooperative clinical trials have become the mainstay of treatment planning and therapeutic advances. The Children's Oncology Group (COG), representing the amalgamation of four prior pediatric cooperative groups (Children's Cancer Group, Pediatric Oncology Group, Intergroup Rhabdomyosarcoma Study Group, and the National Wilms Tumor Study Group), offers current therapeutic protocols and strives to answer important treatment questions. A child or adolescent newly diagnosed with cancer should be enrolled in a cooperative clinical trial whenever possible. Because many protocols are associated with significant toxicities, morbidity, and potential mortality, treatment of children with cancer should be supervised by a pediatric oncologist familiar with the hazards of treatment, preferably at a multidisciplinary pediatric cancer center.

Advances in molecular genetics, cell biology, and tumor immunology have contributed and are crucial to the continued understanding of pediatric malignancies and their treatment. Continued research into the biology of tumors will lead to the identification of targeted therapy for specific tumor types with, it is hoped, fewer systemic effects.

Research in supportive care areas, such as prevention and management of infection, pain, and emesis, has improved the survival and quality of life for children undergoing cancer treatment. Long-term studies of childhood cancer survivors are yielding information that provides a rationale for modifying future treatment regimens to decrease morbidity. A guide for caring for childhood cancer survivors is now available to medical providers as well as families and details suggested examinations and late effects by type of chemotherapy received.

Cure Search: Children's Oncology Group. http://www.survivor shipguidelines.org.

Seehuse DA, Baird D, Bode D: Primary care of adult survivors of childhood cancer. Am Fam Physician 2010 May 15;81(10): 1250–1255 [PMID: 20507049].

Signorelli C et al: The impact of long-term follow-up care for childhood cancer survivors: a systematic review. Crit Rev Oncol Hematol 2017 Jun;114:131–138 [PMID: 28477741].

MAJOR PEDIATRIC NEOPLASTIC DISEASES

ACUTE LYMPHOBLASTIC LEUKEMIA

▶ General Considerations

Acute lymphoblastic leukemia (ALL) is the most common malignancy of childhood, accounting for about 25% of all cancer diagnoses in patients younger than 15 years. The worldwide incidence of ALL is about 1:25,000 children per year, including 3000 children per year in the United States. The peak age at onset is 4 years; 85% of patients are diagnosed between ages 2 and 10 years. Children with Down syndrome have a 10–20 times increase in the overall rate of leukemia.

ALL results from uncontrolled proliferation of immature lymphocytes. Its cause is unknown, and genetic factors may play a role. Leukemia is defined by the presence of more than 25% malignant hematopoietic cells (blasts) in the bone marrow aspirate. Leukemic blasts from the majority of cases of childhood ALL have an antigen on the cell surface called the common ALL antigen (CALLA). These blasts derive from B-cell precursors early in their development, called B-precursor ALL. Less commonly, lymphoblasts are of T-cell origin or of mature B-cell origin. Over 70% of children receiving aggressive combination chemotherapy and early presymptomatic treatment to the central nervous system (CNS) are now cured of ALL.

▶ Clinical Findings

A. Symptoms and Signs

Presenting complaints of patients with ALL include those related to decreased bone marrow production of red blood cells (RBCs), white blood cells (WBCs), or platelets and to leukemic infiltration of extramedullary (outside bone marrow) sites. Intermittent fevers are common, as a result of either cytokines induced by the leukemia itself or infections secondary to leukopenia. Many patients present due to bruising or pallor. About 25% of patients experience bone pain, especially in the pelvis, vertebral bodies, and legs.

Physical examination at diagnosis ranges from virtually normal to highly abnormal. Signs related to bone marrow infiltration by leukemia include pallor, petechiae, and purpura. Hepatomegaly and/or splenomegaly occur in over 60% of patients. Lymphadenopathy is common, either localized or generalized to cervical, axillary, and inguinal regions. The testes may occasionally be unilaterally or bilaterally enlarged secondary to leukemic infiltration. Superior vena cava syndrome is caused by mediastinal adenopathy compressing the superior vena cava. A prominent venous pattern develops over the upper chest from collateral vein enlargement. The neck may feel full from venous engorgement. The face may appear plethoric, and the periorbital area may be edematous. A mediastinal mass can cause tachypnea, orthopnea, and respiratory distress. Leukemic infiltration of cranial nerves may cause cranial nerve palsies with mild nuchal rigidity. The optic fundi may show exudates of leukemic infiltration and hemorrhage from thrombocytopenia. Anemia can cause a flow murmur, tachycardia, and, rarely, congestive heart failure.

B. Laboratory Findings

A complete blood count (CBC) with differential is the most useful initial test because 95% of patients with ALL have a decrease in at least one cell type (single cytopenia): neutropenia, thrombocytopenia, or anemia with most patients having a decrease in at least two blood cell lines. The WBC count is low or normal (= 10,000/μL) in 50% of patients, but the differential shows neutropenia (absolute neutrophil count < 1000/μL) along with a small percentage of blasts amid normal lymphocytes. In 30% of patients, the WBC count is between 10,000/μL and 50,000/μL; in 20% of patients, it is over 50,000/μL, occasionally higher than 300,000/μL. Blasts are usually readily identifiable on peripheral blood smears from patients with elevated WBC counts. Peripheral blood smears also show abnormalities in RBCs, such as

teardrops. Most patients with ALL have decreased platelet counts (< 150,000/μL) and decreased hemoglobin (< 11 g/dL) at diagnosis. In approximately 1% of patients diagnosed with ALL, CBCs and peripheral blood smears are entirely normal, but patients have bone pain that leads to bone marrow examination. Serum chemistries, particularly uric acid and lactate dehydrogenase (LDH), are often elevated at diagnosis as a result of cell breakdown.

The diagnosis of ALL is made by bone marrow examination, which shows a homogeneous infiltration of leukemic blasts replacing normal marrow elements. The morphology of blasts on bone marrow aspirate can usually distinguish ALL from acute myeloid leukemia (AML). Lymphoblasts are typically small, with cell diameters of approximately two erythrocytes. Lymphoblasts have scant cytoplasm, usually without granules. The nucleus typically contains no nucleoli or one small, indistinct nucleolus. Immunophenotyping of ALL blasts by flow cytometry helps distinguish precursor B-cell ALL from T-cell ALL or AML. Histochemical stains specific for myeloblastic and monoblastic leukemias (myeloperoxidase and nonspecific esterase) distinguish ALL from AML. About 5% of patients present with CNS leukemia, which is defined as a cerebrospinal fluid (CSF) WBC count greater than 5/μL with blasts present on cytocentrifuged specimen.

C. Imaging

Chest radiograph may show mediastinal widening or an anterior mediastinal mass and tracheal compression secondary to lymphadenopathy or thymic infiltration, especially in T-cell ALL. Abdominal ultrasound may show kidney enlargement from leukemic infiltration or uric acid nephropathy as well as intra-abdominal adenopathy. Plain radiographs of the long bones and spine may show demineralization, periosteal elevation, growth arrest lines, or compression of vertebral bodies. Although these findings may suggest leukemia, they are not diagnostic.

▶ Differential Diagnosis

The differential diagnosis, based on the history and physical examination, includes chronic infections by Epstein-Barr virus (EBV) and cytomegalovirus (CMV), causing lymphadenopathy, hepatosplenomegaly, fevers, and anemia. Prominent petechiae and purpura suggest a diagnosis of immune thrombocytopenic purpura. Significant pallor could be caused by transient erythroblastopenia of childhood, autoimmune hemolytic anemias, or aplastic anemia. Fevers and joint pains, with or without hepatosplenomegaly and lymphadenopathy, suggest juvenile rheumatoid arthritis (JRA). The diagnosis of leukemia usually becomes straightforward once the CBC reveals multiple cytopenias and leukemic blasts. Serum LDH levels may help distinguish JRA from leukemia, as the LDH is usually normal in JRA. An elevated

WBC count with lymphocytosis is typical of pertussis; however, in pertussis lymphocytes are mature and neutropenia is rarely associated.

▶ Treatment

A. Specific Therapy

Intensity of treatment is determined by specific prognostic features present at diagnosis, the patient's response to therapy, and specific biologic features of the leukemia cells. The majority of patients with ALL are enrolled in clinical trials designed by clinical groups and approved by the National Cancer Institute; the largest group is COG. The first month of therapy consists of induction, at the end of which over 95% of patients exhibit remission on bone marrow aspirates by morphology. The drugs most commonly used in induction include oral prednisone or dexamethasone, intravenous vincristine, daunorubicin, intramuscular or intravenous asparaginase, and intrathecal methotrexate.

Consolidation is the second phase of treatment, during which intrathecal chemotherapy along with continued systemic therapy and sometimes cranial radiation therapy are given to kill lymphoblasts "hiding" in the meninges. Several months of intensive chemotherapy follows consolidation, often referred to as intensification. This intensification has led to improved survival in pediatric ALL.

Maintenance therapy can include daily oral mercaptopurine, weekly oral methotrexate, and, often, monthly pulses of intravenous vincristine and oral prednisone or dexamethasone. Intrathecal chemotherapy, either with methotrexate alone or combined with cytarabine and hydrocortisone, is usually given every 2–3 months.

Chemotherapy has significant potential side effects. Patients need to be monitored closely to prevent drug toxicities and to ensure early treatment of complications. The duration of treatment ranges between 2.2 years for girls and 3.2 years for boys in COG trials. Treatment for ALL is tailored to prognostic, or risk, groups. A child aged 1–9 years with a WBC count below 50,000/μL at diagnosis of pre B ALL and without poor biologic features [t(9;22) or an 11q23 rearrangement)] is considered to be at "standard risk" and receives less intensive therapy than a "high-risk" patient who has a WBC count at diagnosis over 50,000/μL or is 10 years of age or greater. An infant younger than 1 year at diagnosis would be considered very high risk and receive even more intensive chemotherapy. Also important is the patient's response to treatment determined by minimal residual disease (MRD) monitoring. This risk-adapted treatment approach has significantly increased the cure rate among patients with less favorable prognostic features by allowing for early intensification while minimizing treatment-related toxicities in those with favorable features. Bone marrow relapse is usually heralded by an abnormal CBC, either during treatment or following completion of therapy.

The CNS and testes are sanctuary sites for leukemia, meaning that the chemotherapy has a harder time reaching the leukemic cells in these areas. Currently, about one-third of all ALL relapses are isolated to these sanctuary sites. Systemic chemotherapy does not penetrate these tissues as well as it penetrates other organs. Thus, presymptomatic intrathecal chemotherapy is a critical part of ALL treatment, without which many more relapses would occur in the CNS, with or without bone marrow relapse. The majority of isolated CNS relapses are diagnosed in an asymptomatic child at the time of routine intrathecal injection, when CSF cell count and differential show an elevated WBC with leukemic blasts. Occasionally, symptoms of CNS relapse develop: headache, nausea and vomiting, irritability, nuchal rigidity, photophobia, changes in vision, and cranial nerve palsies. Currently, testicular relapse occurs in less than 5% of boys. The presentation of testicular relapse is usually unilateral painless testicular enlargement, without a distinct mass. Routine follow-up of boys both on and off treatment includes physical examination of the testes.

Bone marrow transplantation, now called hematopoietic stem cell transplantation (HSCT), is rarely used as initial treatment for ALL, because most patients are cured with chemotherapy alone. Patients whose blasts contain certain chromosomal abnormalities and patients with a very slow response to therapy may have a better cure rate with early HSCT from a human leukocyte antigen (HLA)-DR–matched sibling donor, or a matched unrelated donor, than with intensive chemotherapy alone. HSCT and newer cellular therapies such as Car T cells are discussed later in this chapter.

Several years ago, imatinib, a tyrosine kinase inhibitor (TKI), directed against the Philadelphia chromosome (Ph+) protein product, was combined in a backbone of intensive chemotherapy for Ph+ ALL in pediatric patients. The results of this trial showed that the patients had an increased leukemia-free survival of 78% as compared to 50% in the past without imatinib. Ongoing trials for COG in Ph+ ALL are now incorporating new TKIs. Two newer targeted agents are now used in relapsed ALL. Blinatumomab is a bispecific T-cell engager (BiTE) that brings the CD19 on a leukemia cell in direct contact with a T cell. This agent is currently being studied in relapsed childhood ALL and will be moved to upfront trials in 2020. Another targeted agent, Inotuzumab is an antibody-drug conjugate against CD22, also frequently found on the surface of the leukemia cells. This drug is also used in relapsed childhood ALL but is also moving to upfront therapy trials. As more is understood about the biology of ALL, further therapy will likely include more of these targeted agents, in order to reduce late effects potentially but maintain and improved leukemia-free survival.

B. Supportive Care

Tumor lysis syndrome, which consists of hyperkalemia, hyperuricemia, hyperphosphatemia, should be anticipated when treatment is started. Maintaining brisk urine output with intravenous fluids and treating with oral allopurinol are appropriate steps in managing tumor lysis syndrome. Rasburicase is indicated for severe tumor lysis syndrome with initial high uric acid values or high WBC at presentation. Serum levels of potassium, phosphorus, and uric acid should be monitored. If superior vena caval or superior mediastinal syndrome is present, general anesthesia is contraindicated temporarily and until there has been some decrease in the mass. If hyperleukocytosis (WBC count > 100,000/μL) is accompanied by hyperviscosity with symptoms of respiratory distress and/or mental status changes, leukapheresis may be indicated to rapidly reduce the number of circulating blasts and minimize the potential thrombotic or hemorrhagic CNS complications. Throughout the course of treatment, all transfused blood and platelet products should be irradiated to prevent graft-versus-host disease (GVHD) from the transfused lymphocytes. Whenever possible, blood products should be leuko-depleted to minimize CMV transmission, transfusion reactions, and sensitization to platelets.

Due to the immunocompromised state of the patient with ALL, bacterial, fungal, and viral infections are serious and can be life-threatening or fatal. During the course of treatment, fever (temperature = 38.3°C) and neutropenia (absolute neutrophil count < 500/μL) require prompt assessment, blood cultures from each lumen of a central line, and prompt treatment with empiric broad-spectrum antibiotics. Patients receiving ALL treatment must receive prophylaxis against *Pneumocystis jirovecii* (formerly *Pneumocystis carinii*). Trimethoprim-sulfamethoxazole given twice each day on 2 or 3 consecutive days per week is the drug of choice. Patients nonimmune to varicella are at risk for very serious—even fatal—infection. Such patients should receive varicella-zoster immune globulin (VZIG) within 72 hours after exposure and treatment with intravenous acyclovir for active infection.

▶ Prognosis

Cure rates depend on specific prognostic features present at diagnosis, biologic features of the leukemic blast, and the response to therapy. Two of the most important features are WBC count and age. Children aged 1–9 years whose diagnostic WBC count is less than 50,000/μL, standard risk ALL, have an leukemia-free survival of greater than 90% range, while children 10 years or older have about an 88% chance of being cured the first time through therapy. MRD measurements are used to determine both the rapidity of response as well as the depth of remission attained at the end of induction (first 4–6 weeks of therapy). Patients with very low levels or no MRD at the end of induction will have a superior leukemia-free survival as compared to other patients with similar initial risk factors but a higher MRD level. On the flip side, by identifying patients with an increased risk of relapse at end induction, more intensified therapy can be delivered

in order to overcome this negative prognostic feature and increase their ultimate chance at staying leukemia free.

Certain chromosomal abnormalities present in the leukemic blasts at diagnosis influence prognosis. Patients with t(9;22), the Philadelphia chromosome, had a poor chance of cure in the past, but as discussed earlier in this chapter, they now have improved outcome with the incorporation of a directed TKI. Likewise, infants younger than 6 months with *11q23* rearrangements have a poor chance of cure with conventional chemotherapy. In contrast, patients whose blasts are hyperdiploid (containing > 50 chromosomes instead of the normal 46) with trisomies of chromosomes 4, and 10, and patients whose blasts have a t(12;21) and *ETV6-AML1* rearrangement have a greater chance of cure, approaching 95%–97% event-free survival (EFS), than do children without these characteristics.

Hunger SP, Mulligan CG: Acute lymphoblastic leukemia in children. N Engl J Med 2015 Oct 15;373(16):1541–1552. doi: 10.1056/NEJMra1400972 [PMID: 26465987].

Maloney KW, Gore L. Agents in development for childhood acute lymphoblastic leukemia. Paediatr Drugs 2018 Apr;20(2): 111–120 [PMID: 29143289].

Martin A, Morgan E, Hijiya N: Relapsed or refractory pediatric acute lymphoblastic leukemia: current and emerging treatments. Paediatr Drugs 2012;14(6):377 [PMID: 22880941].

Pui CH et al: Childhood acute lymphoblastic leukemia: progress through collaboration. J Clin Oncol. 2015 Sep20;33(27): 2938–2948 [PMID: 26304874].

ACUTE MYELOID LEUKEMIA

▶ General Considerations

Approximately 500 new cases of AML occur per year in children and adolescents in the United States. Although AML accounts for only 25% of all leukemias in this age group, it is responsible for at least one-third of deaths from leukemia in children and teenagers. Congenital conditions associated with an increased risk of AML include Diamond-Blackfan anemia; neurofibromatosis (NF); Down; Wiskott-Aldrich, Kostmann, and Li-Fraumeni syndromes; as well as chromosomal instability syndromes such as Fanconi anemia. Acquired risk factors include exposure to ionizing radiation, cytotoxic chemotherapeutic agents, and benzenes. However, the vast majority of patients have no identifiable risk factors. Historically, the diagnosis of AML was based almost exclusively on morphology and immunohistochemical staining of the leukemic cells. Immunophenotypic, cytogenetic, and molecular analyses are increasingly important in confirming the diagnosis of AML and subclassifying it into biologically distinct subtypes that have therapeutic and prognostic implications. Recently the World Health Organization (WHO) classification was published to describe AML as AML with recurrent genetic abnormalities with a list of genetic abnormalities sufficient to diagnose AML and then AML not otherwise specified with morphologic descriptions of AML including similar to the FAB classification (Table 31–1). Cytogenetic clonal abnormalities occur in 80% of patients with AML and are often predictive of outcome.

WHO classification of acute myeloid leukemia (AML) and related neoplasms.

AML with recurrent genetic abnormalities	AML with t(8;21)(q22;q22), RUNX1-RUNX1T1 AML with inv(16)(p13.1q22) or t(16;16)(p13.1;p22); CBFB-MYH11 Acute promyelocytic leukemia with t(15;17)(q22;q12);PML-RARA AML with t(9;11)(p22;q23)MLLT3-MLL AML with t(6;9)(p23;q34); DEK-NUP214 AML with inv(3)(q21q26.2) or t(3.3)(q21;q26.2); RPN1-EVI1 AML (megakaryoblastic) with t(1:22)(p13;q13); RBM15-MKL1 AML with mutated NPM1 AML with mutated CEBPA
AML with myelodysplasia-related changes	
Therapy-related myeloid neoplasms	
AML, not otherwise specified	AML with minimal differentiation AML without maturation AML with maturation Acute myelomonocytic leukemia Acute monoblastic and monocytic leukemia Acute erythroid leukemia Acute megakaryoblastic leukemia Acute basophilic leukemia Acute panmyelosis with myelofibrosis
Myeloid sarcoma	
Myeloid proliferation related to Down syndrome	Transient abnormal myelopoiesis Myeloid leukemia associated with Down syndrome

Data from Vardiman JW, Thiele J, Arber DA, et al: The 2008 revision of the World Health Organization (WHO) classification of myeloid neoplasms and acute leukemia: rationale and important changes. Blood 2009 Jul 30;114(5):937–951.

Aggressive induction therapy currently results in a 75%–85% complete remission rate. However, long-term survival has improved only modestly to approximately 50%, despite the availability of several effective agents, improvements in supportive care, and increasingly intensive therapies.

► Clinical Findings

The clinical manifestations of AML commonly include anemia (44%), thrombocytopenia (33%), and neutropenia (69%). Symptoms may be few and innocuous or may be life threatening. The median hemoglobin value at diagnosis is 7 g/dL, and platelets usually number fewer than 50,000/μL. Frequently the absolute neutrophil count is under 1000/μL, although the total WBC count is over 100,000/μL in 25% of patients at diagnosis.

Hyperleukocytosis may be associated with life-threatening complications. Venous stasis and sludging of blasts in small vessels cause hypoxia, hemorrhage, and infarction, most notably in the lung and CNS. This clinical picture is a medical emergency requiring rapid intervention, such as leukapheresis, to decrease the leukocyte count. CNS leukemia is present in 5%–15% of patients at diagnosis, a higher rate of initial involvement than in ALL. Certain subtypes, such as myelomonocytic and monocytic/monoblastic leukemia, have a higher likelihood of meningeal infiltration than do other subtypes. Additionally, clinically significant coagulopathy may be present at diagnosis in patients with these two subtypes as well as acute promyelocytic leukemia. This problem manifests as bleeding or an abnormal disseminated intravascular coagulation screen and should be at least partially corrected prior to initiation of treatment, which may transiently exacerbate the coagulopathy.

► Treatment

A. Specific Therapy

AML is less responsive to treatment than ALL and requires more intensive chemotherapy. Toxicities from therapy are common and likely to be life threatening; therefore, treatment should be undertaken only at a tertiary pediatric oncology center.

Current AML protocols rely on intensive administration of anthracyclines, cytarabine, and etoposide for induction of remission. After remission is obtained, patients who have a matched sibling donor undergo allogeneic bone marrow transplant while those without an appropriate related donor are treated with additional cycles of aggressive chemotherapy for a total of four to five cycles. Inv16 and t(8;21) herald a more responsive subtype of AML. In patients with a rapid response to induction chemotherapy, intensive chemotherapy alone may be curative in patients whose blasts harbor these cytogenetic abnormalities. Additional recognized genetic risk factors that carry a poor outcome for children with AML include monosomy 7 and FLT3 internal tandem duplications (ITDs). HSCT is recommended for all these patients, using either a related or unrelated donor. Trials with risk grouping are ongoing as more is understood about the varying biologic factors.

The biologic heterogeneity of AML is becoming increasingly important therapeutically. The M3 subtype, associated with t(15;17) demonstrated either cytogenetically or molecularly, is currently treated with all *trans*-retinoic acid in addition to chemotherapy with high-dose cytarabine and daunorubicin. All *trans*-retinoic acid leads to differentiation of promyelocytic leukemia cells and can induce remission,

Table 31–1. FAB subtypes of acute myeloid leukemia.

FAB Classification	Common Name	Distribution in Childhood (Age)		Cytogenetic Associations	Clinical Features
		< 2 y (%)	> 2 y (%)		
M0	Acute myeloid leukemia, minimally differentiated	1		inv (3q26), t(3;3)	
M1	Acute myeloblastic leukemia without maturation	17	23		
M2	Acute myeloblastic leukemia with maturation	26		t(8;21), t(6;9); rare	Myeloblastomas or chloromas
M3	Acute promyelocytic leukemia	4		t(15;17); rarely, t(11;17) or (5;17)	Disseminated intravascular coagulation
M4	Acute myelomonoblastic leukemia	30	24	11q23, inv 3, t(3;3), t(6;9)	Hyperleukocytosis, CNS involvement, skin and gum infiltration
M4Eo	Acute myelomonoblastic leukemia with abnormal eosinophils			inv16, t(16;16)	
M5	Acute monoblastic leukemia	46	15	11q23, t(9;11), t(8;16)	Hyperleukocytosis, CNS involvement, skin and gum infiltration
M6	Erythroleukemia	2			
M7	Acute megakaryoblastic leukemia	7	5	t(1;22)	Down syndrome frequent (< age 2 y)

CNS, central nervous system; FAB, French-American-British classification.

but cure requires conventional chemotherapy as well. The use of arsenic trioxide has also been investigated in the treatment of this subtype of AML with favorable results. This subtype has an increased EFS over other AML subtypes.

Another biologically distinct subtype of AML occurs in children with Down syndrome, almost exclusively megakaryocytic AML. Using less intensive treatment, remission induction rate and overall survival of these children are dramatically superior to non–Down syndrome children with AML. It is important that children with Down syndrome receive appropriate treatment specifically designed to be less intensive due to their increased rate of toxicity with chemotherapeutic agents.

As with ALL, newer biologic agents with more specific targeting are available and undergoing clinical trials. One such agent, sorafenib, appears to be active against AML with Flt3 ITDs. Combining sorafenib with AML therapy has been useful in relapsed disease and is now being studied in to upfront trials.

B. Supportive Care

Tumor lysis syndrome rarely occurs during induction treatment of AML. Nevertheless, when the diagnostic WBC cell count is greater than 100,000/μL or significant adenopathy or organomegaly is present, one should maintain brisk urine output, and follow potassium, uric acid, and phosphorous laboratory values closely. Hyperleukocytosis (WBC > 100,000/μL) is a medical emergency and, in a symptomatic patient, requires rapid intervention such as leukapheresis to rapidly decrease the number of circulating blasts and thereby decrease hyperviscosity. Delaying transfusion of packed RBCs until the WBC can be decreased to below 100,000/μL avoids exacerbating hyperviscosity. It is also important to correct the coagulopathy commonly associated with M3, M4, or M5 subtypes prior to beginning induction chemotherapy. As with the treatment of ALL, all blood products should be irradiated and leukodepleted; *Pneumocystis* prophylaxis must be administered during treatment and for several weeks afterward; patients not immune to varicella must receive VZIG within 72 hours of exposure and prompt treatment with intravenous acyclovir for active infection.

Onset of fever (temperature ≥ 38.3°C) or chills associated with neutropenia requires prompt assessment, blood cultures from each lumen of a central venous line, other cultures such as throat or urine as appropriate and prompt initiation of broad-spectrum intravenous antibiotics. Infections in this population of patients can rapidly become life-threatening. Because of the high incidence of invasive fungal infections, there should be a low threshold for initiating antifungal therapy. Filgrastim (granulocyte colony-stimulating factor) may be used to stimulate granulocyte recovery during the treatment of AML and results in shorter periods of neutropenia and hospitalization. It must be stressed that the supportive care for this group of patients is as important as the leukemia-directed therapy and that this treatment should be carried out only at a tertiary pediatric cancer center.

Prognosis

Published results from various centers show a 50%–60% survival rate at 5 years following first remission for patients who do not have matched sibling hematopoietic stem cell donors. Patients with matched sibling donors fare slightly better, with 5-year survival rates of 60%–70% after allogeneic HSCT.

As treatment becomes more sophisticated, outcome is increasingly related to the subtype of AML. Currently, AML in patients with t(8;21), t(15;17), inv 16, or Down syndrome has the most favorable prognosis, with 65%–75% long-term survival using modern treatments, including chemotherapy alone. The least favorable outcome occurs in AML patients with monosomy 7 or 5, 7q, 5q–, 11q23 cytogenetic abnormalities, or FLT 3 mutations with ITD.

EryilmazE, Canpolat C: Novel agents for the treatment of childhood leukemia: an update. Onco Targets Ther 2017 Jul 4;10:3299–3306 [PMID: 28740405].

Klein K, de Haas V, Kapers GJL: Clinical challenges in de novo pediatric acute myeloid leukemia. Expert Rev Anticancer Ther 2018 Mar;18(3):277–293 [PMID: 29338495].

Meshinchi S, Arceci RJ: Prognostic factors and risk-based therapy in pediatric acute myeloid leukemia. Oncologist 2007;12:341 [PMID: 17405900].

Rubnitz JE. Current management of childhood acute myeloid leukemia. Paediatr Drugs 2017 Feb;19(1):1–10 [PMID: 27785777].

Vardiman J et al: The 2008 revision of the World Health Organization (WHO) classification of myeloid neoplasms and acute leukemia: rationale and important changes. Blood 2009;114:937 [PMID: 19357394].

MYELOPROLIFERATIVE DISEASES

Myeloproliferative diseases in children are relatively rare. They are characterized by ineffective hematopoiesis that results in excessive peripheral blood counts. The three most important types are chronic myelogenous leukemia (CML), which accounts for less than 5% of the childhood leukemias, transient myeloproliferative disorder in children with Down syndrome, and juvenile myelomonocytic leukemia (Table 31–2).

1. Chronic Myelogenous Leukemia

General Considerations

Chronic myelogenous leukemia (CML) with translocation of chromosomes 9 and 22 (the Philadelphia chromosome, Ph+) is identical to adult Ph+CML. Translocation 9;22 results in the fusion of the *BCR* gene on chromosome 22 and the *ABL* gene on chromosome 9. The resulting fusion protein is a constitutively active tyrosine kinase that interacts with a variety of effector proteins and allows for deregulated cellular proliferation, decreased adherence of cells to the bone marrow extracellular matrix, and resistance to apoptosis. The disease usually progresses within 3 years to an accelerated phase and

Table 31–2. Comparison of JMML, CML, and TMD.

	CML	TMD	JMML
Age at onset	> 3 y	< 3 mo	< 2 y
Clinical presentation	Nonspecific constitutional complaints, massive splenomegaly, variable hepatomegaly	DS features, often no or few symptoms; or hepatosplenomegaly, respiratory symptoms	Abrupt onset; eczematoid skin rash, marked lymphadenopathy, bleeding tendency, moderate hepatosplenomegaly, fever
Chromosomal alterations	t(9;22)	Constitutional trisomy 21, but usually no other abnormality	Monosomy or del (7q) in 20% of patients
Laboratory features	Marked leukocytosis (> 100,000/µL), normal to elevated platelet count, decreased to absent leukocyte alkaline phosphatase, usually normal muramidase	Variable leukocytosis, normal to high platelet count, large platelets, myeloblasts	Moderate leukocytosis (> 10,000/µL), thrombocytopenia, monocytosis (> 1000/µL), elevated fetal hemoglobin, normal to diminished leukocyte alkaline phosphatase, elevated muramidase

CML, chronic myelogenous leukemia; DS, Down syndrome; JMML, juvenile myelomonocytic leukemia; TMD, transient myeloproliferative disorder.

then to a blast crisis. It is generally accepted that Ph+ cells have an increased susceptibility to the acquisition of additional molecular changes that lead to the accelerated and blast phases of disease.

Clinical Findings

Patients with CML may present with nonspecific complaints similar to those of acute leukemia, including bone pain, fever, night sweats, and fatigue. However, patients can also be asymptomatic. Patients with a total WBC count of more than 100,000/μL may have symptoms of leukostasis, such as dyspnea, priapism, or neurologic abnormalities. Physical findings may include fever, pallor, ecchymoses, and hepatosplenomegaly. Anemia, thrombocytosis, and leukocytosis are frequent laboratory findings. The peripheral smear is usually diagnostic, with a characteristic predominance of myeloid cells in all stages of maturation, increased basophils and relatively few blasts but needs to be confirmed at a pediatric center with hematology/oncology expertise.

Treatment & Prognosis

Historically, hydroxyurea or busulfan has been used to reduce or eliminate Ph+ cells, and HSCT was the only consistently curative intervention. Reported survival rates for patients younger than 20 years transplanted in the chronic phase from matched-related donors are 70%–80%. Unrelated stem cell transplants result in survival rates of 50%–65%.

The understanding of the molecular mechanisms involved in the pathogenesis of CML has led to the rational design of molecularly targeted therapy. Imatinib mesylate (Gleevec) is a TKI that has had dramatic success in the treatment of CML, with most adults and children achieving cytogenetic remission. There are now newer, more targeted TKIs including dasatinib, erlotinib, nilotinib, and ponatinib. These medications in adults have an increased incidence of molecular remissions and may be all that is required for long-term survival in adults. The durability of the remission for children with TKIs therapy alone is unclear but is now the accepted upfront therapy.

2. Transient Myeloproliferative Disorder

Transient myeloproliferative disorder is unique to patients with trisomy 21 or mosaicism for trisomy 21. It is characterized by uncontrolled proliferation of blasts, usually of megakaryocytic origin, during early infancy and spontaneous resolution. The pathogenesis of this process is not well understood, although mutations in the *GATA1* gene have recently been implicated as initial events.

Although the true incidence is unknown, it is estimated to occur in up to 10% of patients with Down syndrome. Despite the fact that the process usually resolves by 3 months of age, organ infiltration may cause significant morbidity and mortality.

Patients can present with hydrops fetalis, pericardial or pleural effusions, or hepatic fibrosis. More frequently, they are asymptomatic or only minimally ill. Therefore, treatment is primarily supportive. Patients without symptoms are not treated, and those with organ dysfunction receive low doses of chemotherapy or leukapheresis (or both) to reduce peripheral blood blast counts. Although patients with transient myeloproliferative disorder have apparent resolution of the process, approximately 30% go on to develop acute megakaryoblastic leukemia within 3 years.

3. Juvenile Myelomonocytic Leukemia

Juvenile myelomonocytic leukemia (JMML) accounts for approximately one-third of the myelodysplastic and myeloproliferative disorders in childhood. Patients with neurofibromatosis type 1 (NF-1) are at higher risk of JMML than the general population. It typically occurs in infants and very young children and is occasionally associated with monosomy 7 or a deletion of the long arm of chromosome 7.

Patients with JMML present similarly to those with other hematopoietic malignancies, with lymphadenopathy, hepatosplenomegaly, skin rash, or respiratory symptoms. Patients may have stigmata of NF-1 with neurofibromas or café au lait spots. Laboratory findings include anemia, thrombocytopenia, leukocytosis with monocytosis, and elevated fetal hemoglobin.

The results of chemotherapy for children with JMML have been disappointing, with estimated survival rates of less than 30%. Approximately 40%–45% of patients are projected to survive long term using HSCT, although optimizing conditioning regimens and donor selection may improve these results.

Hasle H: Myelodysplastic and myeloproliferative disorders of childhood. Hematology Am Soc Hematol Educ Program 2016 Dec 2;2016(1):598–604 [PMID: 27913534].

Hijiya N, Millot F, Suttorp M: Chronic myeloid leukemia in children: clinical findings, management, and unanswered questions. Pediatr Clin North Am 2014 Feb;62(1):107–119 [PMID: 25435115].

Hijiya N, Suttorp M: How I treat chronic myeloid leukemia in children and adolescents. Blood 2019 May 30;133(22):2374–2384 [PMID: 30917954].

Niemeyer CM: JMML genomics and decisions. Hematology Am Soc Hematol Educ Program 2018 Nov 30;2018(1):307–312 [PMID: 30504325].

Tunstall O et al: Guidelines for the investigation and management of transient leukaemia of Down syndrome. Br J Haematol 2018;182:200–211 [PMID: 29916557].

BRAIN TUMORS

General Considerations

The classic triad of morning headache, vomiting, and papilledema is present in fewer than 30% of children at presentation. School failure and personality changes are more common in older children while irritability, failure to thrive, and delayed development are common in very young children with brain tumors. Recent-onset head tilt can result from a posterior fossa tumor.

Brain tumors are the most common solid tumors of childhood, accounting for 1500–2000 new malignancies in children each year in the United States and for 25%–30% of all childhood cancers. In general, children with brain tumors have a better prognosis than do adults. Favorable outcome occurs most commonly with low-grade and fully resectable tumors as well as with chemoradiation responsive tumors such as medulloblastoma. Unfortunately, cranial irradiation in young children can have significant neuropsychological, intellectual, and endocrinologic sequelae.

Brain tumors in childhood are biologically and histologically heterogeneous, ranging from low-grade localized lesions to high-grade tumors with neuraxis dissemination. High-dose systemic chemotherapy is used frequently, especially in young children with high-grade tumors, in an effort to delay, decrease, or completely avoid cranial irradiation. Such intensive treatment may be accompanied by autologous HSCT or peripheral stem cell reconstitution.

The causes of most pediatric brain tumors are unknown. The risk of developing astrocytomas is increased in children with NF or tuberous sclerosis. Several studies show that some childhood brain tumors occur in families with increased genetic susceptibility to childhood cancers in general, brain tumors, or leukemia and lymphoma. A higher incidence of seizures has been observed in relatives of children with astrocytoma. The risk of developing a brain tumor is increased in children who received cranial irradiation for treatment of meningeal leukemia. All children with gliomas and meningiomas should be screened for NF-1. In children with meningiomas, without the skin findings of NF-1, NF-2, and von Hippel-Lindau syndrome should be considered. Inherited germline mutations are possible in atypical teratoid/rhabdoid tumors (AT/RTs) and in choroid plexus carcinomas. The syndrome of constitutional mismatch repair deficiency (CMMRD) should be considered carefully in the child presenting with a glioma who has been previously diagnosed with leukemia/lymphoma. There are treatment implications in recognizing CMMRD as these patients require additional life-long screening and may have an improved response to immunotherapy. Careful family histories should be taken in these tumors and genetic counseling considered if this is indicative of CMMRD, familial polyposis, or Li-Fraumeni syndrome (LFS).

Because pediatric brain tumors are rare, they are often misdiagnosed or diagnosed late; most pediatricians see no more than two children with brain tumors during their careers.

▶ Clinical Findings

A. Symptoms and Signs

Clinical findings at presentation vary depending on the child's age and the tumor's location. Children younger than 2 years more commonly have infratentorial tumors. Children with such tumors usually present with nonspecific symptoms such as vomiting, unsteadiness, lethargy, and irritability. Signs may be surprisingly few or may include macrocephaly, ataxia, hyperreflexia, and cranial nerve palsies. Because the head can expand in young children, papilledema is often absent. Measuring head circumference and observing gait are essential in evaluating a child for possible brain tumor. Eye findings and apparent visual disturbances such as difficulty tracking can occur in association with optic pathway tumors such as optic glioma. Optic glioma occurring in a young child is often associated with NF. These eye and visual changes have some potential for improvement with therapy, although permanent loss of vision may occur with these tumors. These patients should be closely followed by ophthalmology for potential eye patching, eye muscle surgery, or specialty glasses with prisms to manage double vision and vision loss.

Older children more commonly have supratentorial tumors, which are associated with headache, visual symptoms, seizures, and focal neurologic deficits. Initial presenting features are often nonspecific. School failure and personality changes are common. Vaguely described visual disturbance is often present, but the child must be directly asked. Headaches are common, but they often will not be predominantly in the morning. The headaches may be confused with migraine. If neurologic symptoms are severe, persistent, or worsening with time, a magnetic resonance imaging (MRI) of the brain would be recommended. Focal neurologic deficits or the presence of any indications of increased intracranial pressure (ie, papilledema) should be investigated by an MRI or a computed tomography (CT) if MRI is not readily available.

Older children with infratentorial tumors characteristically present with symptoms and signs of hydrocephalus, which include progressively worsening morning headache and vomiting, gait unsteadiness, double vision, and papilledema. Cerebellar astrocytomas enlarge slowly, and symptoms may worsen over several months. Morning vomiting may be the only symptom of posterior fossa ependymomas, which originate in the floor of the fourth ventricle near the vomiting center. Children with brainstem tumors may present with facial and extraocular muscle palsies, ataxia, and hemiparesis; hydrocephalus occurs in approximately 25% of these patients at diagnosis.

B. Imaging and Staging

In addition to the tumor biopsy, neuraxis imaging studies are obtained to determine whether dissemination has occurred. It is unusual for brain tumors in children and adolescents to disseminate outside the CNS.

MRI has become the preferred diagnostic study for pediatric brain tumors. MRI provides better definition of the tumor and delineates indolent gliomas that may not be seen on CT scan. In contrast, a CT scan can be done in less than 10 minutes—as opposed to the 30 minutes or more required for an MRI scan—and is still useful if an urgent diagnostic study is necessary or to detect calcification of a tumor. Both scans are generally done with and without contrast enhancement. Contrast enhances regions where the blood-brain barrier is disrupted. Postoperative scans to document the extent of tumor resection should be obtained within 48 hours after surgery to avoid postsurgical enhancement.

Imaging of the entire neuraxis and CSF cytologic examination should be part of the diagnostic evaluation for patients with tumors such as medulloblastoma, ependymoma, and pineal region tumors. Diagnosis of neuraxis drop metastases (tumor spread along the neuraxis) can be accomplished by gadolinium-enhanced MRI incorporating sagittal and axial views. MRI of the spine should be obtained preoperatively in all children with midline tumors of the fourth ventricle or cerebellum. A CSF sample should be obtained during the diagnostic surgery or, if that is not possible, 7–10 days after the surgery. Lumbar CSF is preferred over ventricular CSF for cytologic examination. Levels of biomarkers in the blood and CSF, such as human chorionic gonadotropin and α-fetoprotein, may be helpful in diagnosis and follow-up. Both human chorionic gonadotropin and α-fetoprotein should be obtained from the blood preoperatively for all pineal and suprasellar tumors, and if positive, the need for an operation should be discussed with a neuro-oncologist.

Except in emergencies, it is recommended that the neurosurgeon discuss staging and sample collection with an oncologist before surgery in a child newly presenting with a scan suggestive of brain tumor.

C. Classification

About 50% of the common pediatric brain tumors occur above the tentorium and 50% in the posterior fossa. In the very young child, posterior fossa tumors are more common. Most childhood brain tumors can be divided into two categories according to the cell of origin: (1) glial tumors, such as astrocytomas and ependymomas, or (2) embryonal tumors, such as medulloblastoma and AT/teratoid tumors. Some tumors contain both glial and neural elements (eg, ganglioglioma). A group of less common CNS tumors does not fit into either category (ie, craniopharyngiomas, germ cell tumors, choroid plexus tumors, and meningiomas). Low- and high-grade tumors are found in most categories. Table 31–3 lists the locations and frequencies of the common pediatric brain tumors.

Astrocytoma is the most common brain tumor of childhood. Most are juvenile pilocytic astrocytoma (WHO grade I) found in the posterior fossa with a bland cellular morphology and few or no mitotic figures. Low-grade astrocytomas occur in many cases, especially in the cerebellum

Table 31–3. Location and frequency of common pediatric brain tumors.

Location	Frequency of Occurrence (%)
Hemispheric	**37**
Low-grade astrocytoma	23
High-grade astrocytoma	11
Other	3
Posterior fossa	**49**
Medulloblastoma	15
Cerebellar astrocytoma	15
Brainstem glioma	15
Ependymoma	4
Midline	**14**
Craniopharyngioma	8
Chiasmal glioma	4
Pineal region tumor	2

curable by complete surgical excision alone. Upfront chemotherapy may be effective alone in about 40%–50% of low-grade astrocytomas but many will need to be treated multiple times. The recent advent of targeted therapy for mutations common in these tumors offers the potential for better outcomes.

Medulloblastoma are the most common high-grade brain tumors in children. These tumors usually occur in the first decade of life, with a peak incidence between ages 5 and 10 years and a female-male ratio of 2.1:1.3. The tumors typically arise in the midline cerebellar vermis, with variable extension into the fourth ventricle. Neuraxis dissemination at diagnosis affects from 10% to 46% of patients. Prognostic factors are outlined in Table 31–4. Determination of risk to date has largely used histology, age, and stage, but molecular classifications will be increasingly used to determine therapy.

Table 31–4. Prognostic factors in children with medulloblastoma.

Factor	Favorable	Unfavorable
Extent of disease	Nondisseminated	Disseminated
Histologic features	Undifferentiated, desmoplastic	Large cell, anaplastic
Age	≥ 4 y	< 4 y
Molecular tumor characteristics	WNT, young patients with SHH	MYC, MYCN

Brainstem tumors are third in frequency of occurrence in children. They are frequently of astrocytic origin and often are high grade. Children with tumors that diffusely infiltrate the brainstem and involve primarily the pons (diffuse intrinsic pontine gliomas) have a long-term survival rate of less than 5%. There has been considerable biologic discovery, largely from autopsy samples, in diffuse pontine gliomas in the very recent past. The discovery that most pontine gliomas have the histone mutation *H3 K27M* and that these diffuse gliomas can occur anywhere in the midline has led to a change in their classification. Diffuse pontine intrinsic gliomas are now largely subsumed, depending on mutational status in the new classification of diffuse midline glioma *H3 K27M*. It is hoped that the understanding of the mutational drivers in this tumor will result in improved therapy. Brainstem tumors that occur above or below the pons grow in an eccentric or cystic manner and do not have the K27M mutation have a somewhat better outcome. Exophytic tumors in this location may be amenable to surgery. Generally, brainstem tumors are treated without a tissue diagnosis although improved safety in the biopsy of brainstem tumors is increasing diagnostic sampling of these patients.

Other brain tumors such as ependymomas, germ cell tumors, choroid plexus tumors, and craniopharyngiomas are less common, and each is associated with unique diagnostic and therapeutic challenges.

▶ **Treatment**

A. Supportive Care

Dexamethasone should be started prior to initial surgery to help relieve symptoms. There is little proof that very high doses of dexamethasone have any advantage and we have now adopted dosages of 4 mg every 6 hours in those children greater than 4 years and 2 mg every 6 hours in those less than 4. Anticonvulsants should be started if the child has had a seizure or if the surgical approach is likely to induce seizures. Levetiracetam (Keppra) is now the preferred anticonvulsant in this population as it does not induce liver enzymes. Because postoperative treatment of young children with high-grade brain tumors incorporates increasingly more intensive systemic chemotherapy, consideration should also be given to the use of prophylaxis for *Pneumocystis* infection. Dexamethasone potentially reduces the effectiveness of chemotherapy and should be discontinued as soon after surgery as possible.

Optimum care for the pediatric patient with a brain tumor requires a multidisciplinary team including subspecialists in pediatric neurosurgery, neuro-oncology, neurology, endocrinology, neuropsychology, radiation therapy, and rehabilitation medicine, as well as highly specialized nurses, social workers, and staff in physical therapy, occupational therapy, and speech and language science.

B. Specific Therapy

The goal of treatment is to eradicate the tumor with the least short- and long-term morbidity. Long-term neuropsychological morbidity becomes an especially important issue related to deficits caused by the tumor itself and the sequelae of treatment. Meticulous surgical removal of as much tumor as possible is generally the preferred initial approach. Technologic advances in the operating microscope, the ultrasonic tissue aspirator, and the CO_2 laser (which is less commonly used in pediatric brain tumor surgery); the accuracy of computerized stereotactic resection; and the availability of intraoperative monitoring techniques such as evoked potentials and electrocorticography have increased the feasibility and safety of surgical resection of many pediatric brain tumors. Second-look surgery after chemotherapy is increasingly being used when tumors are incompletely resected at initial surgery.

Radiation therapy for pediatric brain tumors is in a state of evolution. For tumors with a high probability of neuraxis dissemination (eg, medulloblastoma), craniospinal irradiation is still standard therapy in children older than 3 years. Attempts at elimination of craniospinal radiation for certain types of intracranial germ-cell tumors and further reduction of craniospinal radiation dosing in medulloblastoma have not been successful. In others (eg, ependymoma), craniospinal irradiation has been abandoned because neuraxis dissemination at first relapse is rare. Conformal radiation and the use of three-dimensional treatment planning are now in routine. Proton beam radiation has become routine in some centers although safety studies in comparison to photon radiation are lacking in childhood.

Chemotherapy is effective in treating low-grade and malignant astrocytomas and medulloblastomas. Intensive chemotherapy is effective in a minority of children AT/RTs. The utility of chemotherapy in ependymoma is being reexplored in national trials. A series of brain tumor protocols for children younger than 3 years involved administering intensive chemotherapy after tumor resection and delaying or omitting radiation therapy. The results of these trials have generally continued to be disappointing but have taught valuable lessons regarding the varying responses to chemotherapy of different tumor types. Superior results seem to have been obtained in the very young with high-dose chemotherapy strategies with stem cell rescue often followed by conformal radiotherapy. Conformal techniques allow the delivery of radiation to strictly defined fields and may limit side effects.

Perhaps the most exciting development in pediatric neuro-oncology is the development of biologically and clinically relevant subclassifications in both medulloblastoma and ependymoma. This development will drive a new generation of targeted therapy aimed at these biologically defined groups. The consensus definition of four biologically defined entities in medulloblastoma, including the Wnt and SHH groups, is the best example of this. New studies based on this new-defined biology are ongoing.

In older children with malignant glioma, the current approach is surgical resection of the tumor and combined-modality treatment with irradiation and intensive chemotherapy. It has recently been realized there is considerable heterogeneity in pediatric high-grade gliomas. Some, such as the congenital tumors, may do well with relatively modest therapy. Others, such as epithelioid glioblastomas, may harbor *BRAF* mutations and may be targetable with specific agents. Generally, however, the prognosis is poor for children with high-grade gliomas, and there has been little progress in finding better chemotherapeutic agents and strategies for most children with these devastating tumors.

The treatment of low-grade astrocytomas with chemotherapy has likewise shown only disappointing progress. However, there are potentially exciting targeted agents in ongoing, and completed but unreported, low-grade astrocytoma trials that have the potential to greatly improve outcomes for these patients.

▶ Prognosis

Despite improvements in surgery and radiation therapy, the outlook for cure remains poor for children with high-grade glial tumors. For children with high-grade gliomas, an early CCG study showed a 45% progression-free survival rate for children who received radiation therapy and chemotherapy, but this may have been due to the inclusion of low-grade patients. More recent studies would suggest survival rate of less than 10%. The major exception to this is congenital glioblastomas that appear to have a much more favorable prognosis. Biologic factors that may affect survival are being increasingly recognized. The prognosis for diffuse pontine gliomas remains very poor, with the standard therapy of radiation alone, being only palliative.

The 5- and even 10-year survival rate for low-grade astrocytomas of childhood is 60%–90%. However, prognosis depends on both site and grade and, as it is increasingly realized, on biology. A child with a pilocytic astrocytoma of the cerebellum has a considerably better prognosis than a child with a fibrillary astrocytoma of the cerebral cortex. For recurrent or progressive low-grade astrocytoma of childhood, relatively moderate chemotherapy may improve the likelihood of survival.

Conventional craniospinal irradiation for children with low-stage medulloblastoma results in survival rates of 60%–90%. Ten-year survival rates are lower (40%–60%). Chemotherapy allows a reduction in the craniospinal radiation dose while improving survival rates for average-risk patients (86% survival at 5 years on the most recent COG average-risk protocol). However, even reduced-dose craniospinal irradiation has an adverse effect on intellect, especially in children younger than 7 years. Five-year survival rates for high-risk medulloblastoma have been 25%–40%, but this may be improved with the introduction of more chemotherapy during radiation although this still awaits the reporting of formal trials.

The previously poor prognosis for children with AT/RTs seems improved by intensive multimodality therapy in a national study.

Major challenges remain in treating brain tumors in children younger than 3 years and in treating diffuse midline glioma K27M and malignant gliomas. Given the inadequate results for treatment of childhood brain tumors, reduction of therapy trials should be fully evaluated and considered in the context of recent treatment failures using reduced therapy regimens. The increasing emphasis is on the quality of life of survivors, not just the survival rate.

Buczkowicz P et al: Genomic analysis of diffuse intrinsic pontine gliomas identifies three molecular subgroups and recurrent activating ACVR1 mutations. Nat Genet 2014;46(5):451–456 [PMID: 24705254].

Chi SN et al: Intensive multimodality treatment for children with newly diagnosed CNS atypical teratoid rhabdoid tumor. J Clin Oncol 2009;20:385 [PMID: 19064966].

Gajjar A et al; COG Brain Tumor Committee: Children's Oncology Group's 2013 blueprint for research: central nervous system tumors. Pediatr Blood Cancer 2013 Jun;60(6):1022–1026 [PMID: 23255213].

Jakacki R et al: Outcome for metastatic (M+) medulloblastoma (MB) treated with carboplatin during craniospinal radiotherapy (CSRT) followed by cyclophosphamide (CPM) and vincristine: preliminary results of COG 99701. J Clin Oncol 2007;25:A2017.

Korshunov A et al: Molecular staging of intracranial ependymoma in children and adults. J Clin Oncol 2010;28:3182 [PMID: 20516456].

Macy ME et al: Clinical and molecular characteristics of congenital glioblastoma. Neuro Oncol 2012;14:931 [PMID: 22711608].

Northcott PA et al: Medulloblastoma comprises four distinct molecular variants. J Clin Oncol 2011;29:1408 [PMID: 20823417].

Packer RJ et al: Phase III study of craniospinal radiation therapy followed by adjuvant chemotherapy for newly diagnosed average-risk medulloblastoma. J Clin Oncol 2006;24:4202 [PMID: 16943538].

LYMPHOMAS & LYMPHOPROLIFERATIVE DISORDERS

The term *lymphoma* refers to a malignant proliferation of lymphoid cells, usually in association with and arising from lymphoid tissues (ie, lymph nodes, thymus, spleen). In contrast, the term *leukemia* refers to a malignancy arising from the bone marrow, which may include lymphoid cells. Because lymphomas can involve the bone marrow, the distinction between the two can be confusing. The diagnosis of lymphoma is a common one among childhood cancers, accounting for 10%–15% of all malignancies. The most common form is Hodgkin disease, which represents nearly one-half of all cases. The remaining subtypes, referred to collectively as non-Hodgkin lymphoma (NHL), are divided into four main groups: lymphoblastic lymphoma (LL), small non-cleaved cell lymphoma, large B-cell lymphoma (LBCL), and anaplastic large cell lymphoma (ALCL).

In contrast to lymphomas, lymphoproliferative disorders (LPDs) are quite rare in the general population. Most are polyclonal, nonmalignant (though often life-threatening) accumulations of lymphocytes that occur when the immune system fails to control virally transformed lymphocytes. However, a malignant monoclonal proliferation can also arise. The posttransplant LPDs arise in patients who are immunosuppressed to prevent solid organ or bone marrow transplant rejection, particularly liver and heart transplant patients. Spontaneous LPDs occur in immunodeficient individuals and, less commonly, in immunocompetent persons.

1. Hodgkin Lymphoma

▶ General Considerations

Children with Hodgkin lymphoma have a better response to treatment than do adults, with greater than 90% 5- to 10-year overall survival rate when all stages are evaluated. Although adult therapies are applicable, the management of Hodgkin lymphoma in children younger than 18 years frequently differs. Because excellent disease control can result from several different therapeutic approaches, selection of staging procedures (radiographic, surgical, or other procedures to determine additional locations of disease) and treatment are often based on the potential long-term toxicity associated with the intervention.

Although Hodgkin lymphoma represents 50% of the lymphomas of childhood, only 15% of all cases occur in children aged 16 years or younger. Children younger than 5 years account for 3% of childhood cases. There is a 4:1 male predominance in the first decade. Notably, in underdeveloped countries the age distribution is quite different, with a peak incidence in younger children.

Hodgkin disease is subdivided into four histologic groups, and the distribution in children parallels that in adults: lymphocyte-predominant (10%–20%); nodular sclerosing (40%–60%) (increases with age); mixed cellularity (20%–40%); and lymphocyte-depleted (5%–10%). Prognosis is independent of subclassification, with appropriate therapy based on stage (see section Staging).

▶ Clinical Findings

A. Symptoms and Signs

Children with Hodgkin lymphoma usually present with painless cervical adenopathy. The lymph nodes often feel firmer than inflammatory nodes and have a rubbery texture. They may be discrete or matted together and are not fixed to surrounding tissue. The growth rate is variable, and involved nodes may wax and wane in size over weeks to months.

As Hodgkin lymphoma nearly always arises in lymph nodes and spreads to contiguous nodal groups, a detailed examination of all nodal sites is mandatory. Lymphadenopathy is common in children, so the decision to perform biopsy is often difficult or delayed for a prolonged period. Indications for consideration of early lymph node biopsy include lack of identifiable infection in the region drained by the enlarged node, a node greater than 2 cm in size, supraclavicular adenopathy or abnormal chest radiograph, and lymphadenopathy increasing in size after 2 weeks or failing to resolve within 4–8 weeks.

Constitutional symptoms occur in about one-third of children at presentation. Symptoms of fever greater than 38.0°C, weight loss of 10% in the previous 6 months, and drenching night sweats are defined by the Ann Arbor staging criteria as B symptoms. The A designation refers to the absence of these symptoms. B symptoms are of prognostic value, and more aggressive therapy is usually required for cure. Generalized pruritus and pain with alcohol ingestion may also occur.

One-half of patients have asymptomatic mediastinal disease (adenopathy or anterior mediastinal mass), although symptoms due to compression of vital structures in the thorax may occur. A chest radiograph should be obtained when lymphoma is being considered. The mediastinum must be evaluated thoroughly before any surgical procedure is undertaken to avoid airway obstruction or cardiovascular collapse during anesthesia and possible death. Splenomegaly or hepatomegaly is generally associated with advanced disease.

B. Laboratory Findings

The CBC is usually normal, although anemia, neutrophilia, eosinophilia, and thrombocytosis may be present. The erythrocyte sedimentation rate (ESR) and other acute-phase reactants are often elevated and can serve as markers of disease activity. Immunologic abnormalities occur, particularly in cell-mediated immunity, and anergy is common in patients with advanced-stage disease at diagnosis. Autoantibody phenomena such as hemolytic anemia and an idiopathic thrombocytopenic purpura–like picture have been reported.

C. Staging

Staging of Hodgkin lymphoma determines treatment and prognosis. The most common staging system is the Ann Arbor classification that describes extent of disease by I–IV and symptoms by an A or a B suffix (eg, stage IIIB). A systematic search for disease includes chest radiography; CT scan of the chest, abdomen, and pelvis; and bilateral bone marrow aspirates and biopsies. In recent years, positron emission tomography (PET) is increasingly used in the staging and follow-up of patients with Hodgkin disease.

D. Pathologic Findings

The diagnosis of Hodgkin lymphoma requires the histologic presence of the Reed-Sternberg cell or its variants in tissue. Reed-Sternberg cells are germinal-center B cells that have undergone malignant transformation. Nearly 20% of these tumors in developed countries are positive for EBV. EBV has been linked to Hodgkin disease, and the large portion of Hodgkin patients with increased EBV titers suggests that EBV activation may contribute to the onset of Hodgkin lymphoma.

▶ Treatment & Prognosis

Treatment decisions are based on presence of B symptoms, stage, tumor bulk, and number of involved nodal regions. To achieve long-term disease-free survival while minimizing treatment toxicity, Hodgkin disease is increasingly treated by chemotherapy alone—and less often by radiation therapy.

Several combinations of chemotherapeutic agents are effective, and treatment times are relatively short compared with pediatric oncology protocols for leukemia. Clinical trials have shown that only 9 weeks of therapy with AV-PC (Adriamycin [doxorubicin], vincristine, prednisone, and cyclophosphamide) is sufficient to induce a complete response in patients with low-risk Hodgkin lymphoma. Two additional drugs, bleomycin and etoposide, are currently added in the treatment of intermediate-risk patients for a total of 4–6 months of therapy for patients with intermediate-risk disease. The removal of involved field irradiation in patients with intermediate-risk Hodgkin lymphoma who respond early to chemotherapy has been shown to maintain excellent outcomes. Combined-modality therapy with chemotherapy and irradiation is used in advanced disease.

Current treatment gives an overall 5-year survival of 90–95% to children with stages I and II Hodgkin lymphoma. Two-thirds of all relapses occur within 2 years after diagnosis, and relapse rarely occurs beyond 4 years. Although patients with advanced disease (stages III and IV) have slightly lower overall survival, more patients are becoming long-term survivors of Hodgkin disease. As a result, the risk of secondary malignancies, both leukemias and solid tumors, is becoming more apparent and is higher in patients receiving radiation therapy. Therefore, elucidating the optimal treatment strategy that minimizes such risk should be the goal of future studies.

Relapsed Hodgkin lymphoma remains responsive to treatment with chemotherapy and radiation therapy. Autologous HSCT after remission is achieved is used as consolidative therapy to minimize the risk of subsequent relapse. Allogeneic HSCT is reserved for second or greater relapse as it carries increased risks of complications and may not offer added survival benefit.

Targeted therapies are being tested for children with high-risk Hodgkin lymphoma, including antibody conjugates targeting CD30, a transmembrane receptor highly expressed in Hodgkin lymphoma. A current COG trial is investigating if an anti-CD30 murine/human chimeric monoclonal antibody linked to monomethyl auristatin E is able to target the Reed-Stenberg cell in newly diagnosed high-risk Hodgkin lymphoma. Checkpoint inhibitors pembrolizumab and nivolumab that block PD-1 have recently been approved for recurrent Hodgkin lymphoma, as the tumor cells consistently express their target PDL-1 and PDL-2.

Friedman DL et al: Dose-intensive response-based chemotherapy and radiation therapy for children and adolescents with newly diagnosed intermediate-risk Hodgkin lymphoma: a report from the Children's Oncology Group Study AHOD0031. J Clin Oncol 2014;32:3561 [PMID: 25311218].

Jachimowicz RD et al: The challenging aspects of managing adolescents and young adults with Hodgkin's lymphoma. JAMA Acta Haematol 2014;132:274 [PMID: 2522855].

Mauz-Körholz C et al: Pediatric Hodgkin lymphoma. J Clin Oncol 2015 Sep 20;33(27):2975–2985. doi: 10.1200/JCO.2014.59.4853. Epub 2015 Aug 24 [PMID: 26304892].

Younes A, Ansell SM: Novel agents in the treatment of Hodgkin lymphoma: biological basis and clinical results. Semin Hematol 2016 Jul;53(3):186–189 [PMID: 27496310].

2. Non-Hodgkin Lymphoma

▶ General Considerations

Non-Hodgkin lymphomas (NHLs) are a diverse group of cancers accounting for 5%–10% of malignancies in children younger than 15 years. About 500 new cases arise per year in the United States. The incidence of NHLs increases with age. Children aged 15 years or younger account for only 3% of all cases of NHLs, and the disease is uncommon before age 5 years. There is a male predominance of approximately 3:1. In equatorial Africa, NHLs cause almost 50% of pediatric malignancies due to EBV and the associated Burkitt lymphoma (BL).

Most children who develop NHL are immunologically normal. However, children with congenital or acquired immune deficiencies (eg, Wiskott-Aldrich syndrome, severe combined immunodeficiency syndrome, X-linked lymphoproliferative syndrome, human immunodeficiency virus [HIV] infection, immunosuppressive therapy following solid-organ or marrow transplantation) have an increased risk of developing NHLs. It has been estimated that their risk is 100–10,000 times that of age-matched control subjects.

Animal models suggest a viral contribution to the pathogenesis of NHL, and there is evidence of viral involvement in human NHL as well. In equatorial Africa, 95% of BLs contain DNA from the EBV. But in North America, less than 20% of Burkitt tumors contain the EBV genome. The role of other viruses (eg, human herpes viruses 6 and 8), disturbances in host immunologic defenses, chronic immunostimulation, and specific chromosomal rearrangements as potential triggers in the development of NHL are under investigation.

Table 31–5. Comparison of pediatric non-Hodgkin lymphomas.

	Lymphoblastic Lymphoma	Small Noncleaved Cell Lymphoma (BL and BLL)	Large B-Cell Lymphoma	Anaplastic Large Cell Lymphoma
Incidence (%)	30–40	35–50	10–15	10–15
Histopathologic features	Indistinguishable from ALL lymphoblasts	Large nucleus with prominent nucleoli surrounded by very basophilic cytoplasm that contains lipid vacuoles	Large cells with cleaved or noncleaved nuclei	Large pleomorphic cells
Immunopheno-type	Immature T cell	B cell	B cell	T cell or null cell
Cytogenetic markers	Translocations involving chromosome 14q11 and chromosome 7; interstitial deletions of chromosome 1	t(8;14), t(8;22), t(2;8)	Many	t(2;5)
Clinical presentation	Intrathoracic tumor, mediastinal mass (50%–70%), lymphadenopathy above diaphragm (50%–80%)	Intra-abdominal tumor (90%), jaw involvement (10%–20% sporadic BL, 70% endemic BL), bone marrow involvement	Abdominal tumor most common; unusual sites: lung, face, brain, bone, testes, muscle	Lymphadenopathy, fever, weight loss, night sweats, extranodal sites including viscera and skin
Treatment	Similar to ALL therapy; 24 mo duration	Intensive administration of alkylating agents and methotrexate; CNS prophylaxis; 3–9 mo duration	Similar to therapy for BL/BLL	Similar to therapy for lymphoblastic lymphoma or BL/BLL

ALL, acute lymphoblastic leukemia; BL, Burkitt lymphoma; BLL, Burkitt-like lymphoma; CNS, central nervous system.

Unlike adult NHL, virtually all childhood NHLs are rapidly proliferating, high-grade, diffuse malignancies. These tumors exhibit aggressive behavior but are usually very responsive to treatment. Nearly all pediatric NHLs are histologically classified into four main groups: LL, small noncleaved cell lymphoma (BL and Burkitt-like lymphoma [BLL]), LBCL, and ALCL. Immunophenotyping and cytogenetic features, in addition to clinical presentation, are increasingly important in the classification, pathogenesis, and treatment of NHLs. Comparisons of pediatric NHLs are summarized in Table 31–5.

▶ **Clinical Findings**

A. Symptoms and Signs

Childhood NHLs can arise in any site of lymphoid tissue, including the lymph nodes, thymus, liver, and spleen. Common extra-lymphatic sites include bone, bone marrow, CNS, skin, and testes. Signs and symptoms at presentation are determined by the location of lesions and the degree of dissemination. Because NHL usually progresses very rapidly, the duration of symptoms is quite brief, from days to a few weeks. Nevertheless, children present with a limited number of syndromes, most of which correlate with cell type.

Children with LL often present with symptoms of airway compression (cough, dyspnea, orthopnea) or superior vena cava obstruction (facial edema, chemosis, plethora, venous engorgement), which are a result of mediastinal disease. *These symptoms are a true emergency necessitating rapid diagnosis and treatment.* Pleural or pericardial effusions may further compromise the patient's respiratory and cardiovascular status. CNS and bone marrow involvement are not common at diagnosis. When bone marrow contains more than 25% lymphoblasts, patients are diagnosed with ALL.

Most patients with BL and BLL present with abdominal disease. Abdominal pain, distention, a right lower quadrant mass, or intussusception in a child older than 5 years suggests the diagnosis of BL. Bone marrow involvement is common (~ 65% of patients). BL is the most rapidly proliferating tumor known and has a high rate of spontaneous cell death as it outgrows its blood supply. Consequently, children presenting with massive abdominal disease frequently have tumor lysis syndrome (hyperuricemia, hyperphosphatemia, and hyperkalemia). These abnormalities can be aggravated by tumor infiltration of the kidney or urinary obstruction by tumor. Although similar histologically, numerous differences exist between cases of BL occurring in endemic areas

Table 31–6. Comparison of endemic and sporadic Burkitt lymphoma.

	Endemic	Sporadic
Incidence	10 per 100,000	0.9 per 100,000
Cytogenetics	Chromosome 8 breakpoint upstream of c-*myc* locus	Chromosome 8 breakpoint within c-*myc* locus
EBV association	≥ 95%	≤ 20%
Disease sites at presentation	Jaw (58%), abdomen (58%), CNS (19%), orbit (11%), marrow (7%)	Jaw (7%), abdomen (91%), CNS (14%), orbit (1%), marrow (20%)

CNS, central nervous system; EBV, Epstein-Barr virus.

of equatorial Africa and the sporadic cases of North America (Table 31–6).

Large cell lymphomas are similar clinically to the small noncleaved cell lymphomas, although unusual sites of involvement are quite common, particularly with ALCL. Skin lesions, focal neurologic deficits, and pleural or peritoneal effusions without an obvious associated mass are frequently seen. With improved diagnostic techniques, new categories of LBCLs including primary mediastinal B-cell lymphoma and gray zone lymphomas have been identified. The distinction is an important one as the approach to therapy differs significantly.

B. Diagnostic Evaluation

Diagnosis is made by biopsy of involved tissue with histology, immunophenotyping, and cytogenetic studies. If mediastinal disease is present, general anesthesia must be avoided if the airway or vena cava is compromised by tumor. In these cases samples of pleural or ascitic fluid, bone marrow, or peripheral nodes obtained under local anesthesia (in the presence of an anesthesiologist) may confirm the diagnosis. Major abdominal surgery and intestinal resection should be avoided in patients with an abdominal mass that is likely to be BL, as the tumor will regress rapidly with the initiation of chemotherapy. The rapid growth of these tumors and the associated life-threatening complications demand that further studies be done expeditiously so that specific therapy is not delayed.

After a thorough physical examination, a CBC, liver function tests, and a biochemical profile (electrolytes, calcium, phosphorus, uric acid, renal function) should be obtained. An elevated LDH reflects tumor burden and can serve as a marker of disease activity. Imaging studies should include a chest radiograph and CT scans of the neck, chest, abdomen and pelvis, and a PET scan. Bone marrow and CSF examinations are also essential.

▶ **Treatment**

A. Supportive Care

The management of life-threatening problems at presentation is critical. The most common complications are superior mediastinal syndrome and acute tumor lysis syndrome. Patients with airway compromise require prompt initiation of specific therapy. Because of the risk of general anesthesia in these patients, it is occasionally necessary to initiate corticosteroids or low-dose emergency radiation therapy until the mass is small enough for a biopsy to be undertaken safely. Response to steroids and radiation therapy is usually prompt (12–24 hours).

Tumor lysis syndrome should be anticipated in all patients who have NHL with a large tumor burden. Maintaining a brisk urine output (> 5 mL/kg/h) with intravenous fluids and diuretics is the key to management. Allopurinol will reduce serum uric acid. Rasburicase is an effective intravenous alternative to allopurinol and is increasingly used for patients with high risk of tumor lysis based on tumor burden or in patients who do not have an optimal response to allopurinol. Renal dialysis is occasionally necessary to control metabolic abnormalities. Every attempt should be made to correct or minimize metabolic abnormalities before initiating chemotherapy; however, this period of stabilization should not exceed 24–48 hours.

B. Specific Therapy

Systemic chemotherapy is the mainstay of therapy for NHLs. Nearly all patients with NHL require intensive intrathecal chemotherapy for CNS prophylaxis. Surgical resection is not indicated unless the entire tumor can be resected safely, which is rare. Partial resection or debulking surgery has no role. Radiation therapy does not improve outcome, so its use is confined to exceptional circumstances.

Therapy for LL is generally based on treatment protocols designed for ALL and involves dose-intensive, multiagent chemotherapy. Current trials are testing whether the addition of bortezomib to the current multiagent chemotherapy regimen will decrease the risk of relapse for patients with T-cell LL. The duration of therapy is 2 years. Treatment of BL and BLL consists of alkylating agents and intermediate- to high-dose methotrexate administered intensively, but for a relatively short time it produces the highest cure rates. LBCLs are treated similarly, whereas ALCL has been treated with both BL and LL protocols. Dose-adjusted EPOCH-R has demonstrated improved outcomes in adults with primary mediastinal B-cell lymphoma and gray zone lymphomas. Clinical trials utilizing this regimen are ongoing in children with these rare NHLs.

Monoclonal antibodies such as rituximab (anti-CD20) allow for more targeted therapy of lymphomas and have been successful in improving outcomes in adults. Recent studies in children with high-risk mature B-cell lymphomas demonstrated improved outcomes with the addition of rituximab to conventional chemotherapy regimens. Additionally, oral small molecule inhibitors against the ALK oncogene are being explored as novel therapy for specific subsets of patients with ALCL. The ALK oncogene is activated by a 2;5 translocation leading to juxtaposition of NPM N-terminal region to the intracellular part of ALK and is the defining genetic lesions in ALK-positive ALCL. ALCL often express CD30 and studies are ongoing combining brentuximab vedotin and ALK inhibitors.

▶ Prognosis

A major predictor of outcome in NHL is the extent of disease at diagnosis. Ninety percent of patients with localized disease can expect long-term, disease-free survival. Patients with extensive disease on both sides of the diaphragm, CNS involvement, or bone marrow involvement in addition to a primary site have a 70%–80% failure-free survival (FFS) rate. Relapses occur early in NHL; patients with LL rarely have recurrences after 30 months from diagnosis, whereas patients with BL and BLL very rarely have recurrences beyond 1 year. The cure rate for patients with relapsed T-cell lymphoblastic leukemia/lymphoma is particularly poor (3-year EFS rates < 20%). Patients who experience relapse may have a chance for cure by autologous or allogeneic HSCT.

Goldman et al: Rituximab and FAB/LMB 96 chemotherapy in children with stage III/IV B-cell non-Hodgkin lymphoma: a Children's Oncology Group report. Leukemia 2013;27:1174 [PMID: 22940833].

Lange J et al: Treatment of adolescents with aggressive B-cell malignancies: the pediatric experience. Curr Hematol Malig Rep 2013;8:226 [PMID: 23812872].

Wolach O et al: Adolescents and young adults with non-Hodgkin's lymphoma: slipping between the cracks. Acta Haematol 2014;132:279 [PMID: 25228553].

Worch J et al: Mature B-cell lymphoma and leukemia in children and adolescents—review of standard chemotherapy regimen and perspectives. Pediatr Hematol Oncol 2013;30(6):465 [PMID: 23570584].

3. Lymphoproliferative Disorders

Lymphoproliferative disorders (LPDs) can be thought of as a part of a continuum with lymphomas. Whereas LPDs represent inappropriate, often polyclonal proliferations of nonmalignant lymphocytes, lymphomas represent the development of malignant clones, sometimes arising from recognized LPDs.

A. Posttransplantation Lymphoproliferative Disorders

Posttransplantation lymphoproliferative disorders (PTLDs) arise in patients who have received substantial immunosuppressive medications for solid organ or bone marrow transplantation. In these patients, reactivation of latent EBV infection in B cells drives a polyclonal proliferation of these cells that is fatal if not halted. Occasionally a true lymphoma develops, often bearing a chromosomal translocation.

LPDs are an increasingly common and significant complication of transplantation. The incidence of PTLD ranges from approximately 2% to 15% of transplant recipients, depending on the organ transplanted and the immunosuppressive regimen.

Treatment of these disorders is a challenge for transplant physicians and oncologists. The initial treatment is reduction in immunosuppression, which allows the patient's own immune cells to destroy the virally transformed lymphocytes. However, this is only effective in approximately half of the patients. For those patients who do not respond to reduced immune suppression, chemotherapy of various regimens may succeed. The use of anti–B-cell antibodies, such as rituximab (anti-CD20), for the treatment of PTLDs has been promising in clinical trials. More recently, T-cell–based immune therapies, such as donor lymphocyte infusions and adoptive transfer of EBV-specific cytotoxic T lymphocytes, have also been explored as novel approaches.

B. Spontaneous Lymphoproliferative Disease

Immunodeficiencies in which LPDs occur include Bloom syndrome, Chédiak-Higashi syndrome, ataxia-telangiectasia, Wiskott-Aldrich syndrome, X-linked lymphoproliferative syndrome, congenital T-cell immunodeficiencies, and HIV infection. Treatment depends on the circumstances, but unlike PTLD, few therapeutic options are often available. Castleman disease is an LPD occurring in pediatric patients without any apparent immunodeficiency. The autoimmune lymphoproliferative syndrome (ALPS) is characterized by widespread lymphadenopathy with hepatosplenomegaly, and autoimmune phenomena. ALPS results from mutations in the Fas ligand pathway that is critical in regulation of apoptosis.

Weintraub L et al: Identifying predictive factors for posttransplant lymphoproliferative disease in pediatric solid organ transplant recipients with Epstein-Barr virus viremia. J Pediatr Hematol Oncol 2014;36:e481 [PMID: 24878618].

Yang X et al: Lymphoproliferative disorders in immunocompromised individuals and therapeutic antibodies for treatment. Immunotherapy 2013;5:415 [PMID: 23557424].

NEUROBLASTOMA

▶ General Considerations

Neuroblastoma arises from neural crest tissue of the sympathetic ganglia or adrenal medulla. It is composed of small, uniform cells with scant cytoplasm and hyperchromatic nuclei that may form a rosette pattern. It must be differentiated from other "small, round, blue cell" malignancies of childhood, such as Ewing sarcoma, rhabdomyosarcoma (RMS), peripheral neuroectodermal tumor (PNET), and NHL.

Neuroblastoma accounts for 7%–10% of pediatric malignancies and is the most common solid neoplasm outside the CNS. Fifty percent of neuroblastomas are diagnosed before age 2 years and 90% before age 5 years. It is a biologically diverse disease with clinical behavior that can range from spontaneous regression to relentless progression despite aggressive therapy. Historically, cure rates for patients with high-risk neuroblastoma were very poor. With promising recent advances, however, cure rates have been steadily improving, albeit at the price of significant toxicity from treatment.

▶ Clinical Findings

A. Symptoms and Signs

Clinical manifestations vary based on tumor location and neuroendocrine function of the tumor. Many children present with constitutional symptoms such as fever, weight loss, and irritability. Bone pain suggests metastatic disease, which is present in 60% of children older than 1 year at diagnosis. Physical examination may reveal a firm, fixed, irregularly shaped midline abdominal mass. Although most children have an abdominal primary tumor (40% adrenal gland, 25% paraspinal ganglion), neuroblastoma can arise wherever there is sympathetic nervous tissue. In the posterior mediastinum, the tumor is usually asymptomatic and discovered incidentally on a chest radiograph. Patients with cervical neuroblastoma present with a neck mass, sometimes misdiagnosed as infection. Horner syndrome (unilateral ptosis, myosis, and anhidrosis) or heterochromia iridis (differently colored irises) may accompany cervical neuroblastoma. Paraspinous tumors can extend through the spinal foramen, causing cord compression and leading to paresis, paralysis, or bowel/bladder dysfunction.

The most common sites of metastases are bone, bone marrow, lymph nodes, liver, and subcutaneous tissue. Neuroblastoma has a predilection for metastasis to the skull, particularly the sphenoid bone and retrobulbar tissue, causing periorbital ecchymosis ("raccoon eyes") and proptosis. Liver metastasis, particularly in the newborn, can lead to massive hepatomegaly. Skin metastases can appear as bluish or purplish subcutaneous nodules ("blueberry muffin baby") and can be associated with an erythematous flush followed by blanching when compressed, probably due to catecholamine release.

Neuroblastoma can have paraneoplastic manifestations, the most striking example being opsoclonus-myoclonus-ataxia (OMA) syndrome ("dancing eyes/dancing feet"). This phenomenon is characterized by rapid and chaotic eye movements, myoclonic jerking of the limbs and trunk, ataxia, and behavioral disturbances. This process, which often persists after treatment of the neuroblastoma is complete, is due to cross-reacting anti-neuronal autoantibodies. Treatment is with immunosuppression. Intractable, watery diarrhea can occur due to secretion of vasoactive intestinal peptide (VIP) by the tumor. Interestingly, both of these paraneoplastic syndromes, despite their morbidity are associated with more favorable curative potential for the tumor itself.

B. Laboratory Findings

Anemia is present in 60% of children with neuroblastoma and can be due to chronic disease or marrow infiltration. Occasionally, thrombocytopenia is present, but thrombocytosis is a more common finding, even with metastatic disease in the marrow. Urinary catecholamines (vanillylmandelic acid [VMA] and homovanillic acid [HVA]) are elevated in at least 90% of patients at diagnosis and should be measured prior to surgery.

C. Imaging

Radiographs of the primary tumor may show stippled calcifications. Metastases to bone can appear irregular and lytic. Periosteal reaction and pathologic fractures may also be seen. CT scanning shows extent of the primary tumor, effects on surrounding structures, and the presence of metastatic disease. Classically, in tumors originating from the adrenal gland, the kidney is displaced inferolaterally, which helps to differentiate neuroblastoma from Wilms tumor. MRI is useful in determining the presence of spinal cord involvement in tumors that invade neural foramina.

I-123-Metaiodobenzylguanidine (MIBG), a radiolabeled compound that localizes to adrenal tissue, is used to detect and quantify the degree of metastatic disease at diagnosis and to track response to treatment. PET-CT can be utilized in patients whose tumors are MIBG non-avid (8.7% of cases). MIBG and PET-CT scanning have supplanted technetium-99m bone scanning for evaluation of bone metastases in neuroblastoma.

D. Staging

Staging of neuroblastoma is usually performed according to the International Neuroblastoma Staging System (INSS) (Table 31–7), though a newer, International Neuroblastoma Risk Group (INRG) staging system that incorporates image-defined risk factors as part of the staging process is being used more commonly. Biopsy of the tumor is essential to confirm the diagnosis and determine the biologic characteristics of the tumor. In addition, bilateral bone marrow aspirates and biopsies must be performed to evaluate for bone marrow involvement.

Tumors are classified as favorable or unfavorable based on histologic characteristics and the age of the patient at diagnosis, with younger age (<18 months) being associated with a

Table 31–7. International Neuroblastoma Staging System.

Stage	Description
1	Localized tumor with complete gross excision, with or without microscopic residual disease; representative ipsilateral lymph nodes negative for tumor microscopically.
2A	Localized tumor with incomplete gross excision; representative ipsilateral nonadherent lymph nodes negative for tumor microscopically.
2B	Localized tumor with or without complete gross excision, with ipsilateral nonadherent lymph nodes positive for tumor. Enlarged lymph nodes must be negative microscopically.
3	Unresectable unilateral tumor infiltrating across the midline, with or without regional lymph node involvement; or localized unilateral tumor with contralateral regional lymph node involvement; or midline tumor with bilateral extension by infiltration (unresectable) or by lymph node involvement. The midline is defined as the vertebral column. Tumors originating on one side and crossing the midline must infiltrate to or beyond the opposite side of the vertebral column.
4	Any primary tumor with dissemination to distant lymph nodes, bone, bone marrow, liver, skin, or other organs, except as defined for stage 4S.
4S	Localized primary tumor, as defined for stage 1, 2A, or 2B, with dissemination limited to skin, liver, or bone marrow, and limited to infants age < 1 y. Marrow involvement should be < 10% of nucleated cells.

more favorable prognosis. Amplification of the *MYCN* protooncogene is a reliable marker of aggressive clinical behavior. Tumor cell DNA content is also predictive of outcome. Hyperdiploidy is a favorable finding, whereas diploid DNA content is associated with a worse outcome. Loss of heterozygosity at chromosome bands 1p36 and 11q23 also confers a worse prognosis.

▶ Treatment & Prognosis

Patients are treated according to a risk stratification system that takes into account INSS or INRG stage, patient age, *MYCN* status, histology, cytogenetic findings, and DNA index. Based on these factors, patients are classified as having low-, intermediate-, or high-risk disease.

For low-risk disease (INSS stages 1 and 2, with favorable biologic features), surgical resection of more than 50% of the tumor is usually sufficient for cure. Aggressive surgery to remove the entire tumor at the expense of surrounding normal structures is not necessary and can lead to unnecessary morbidity. Infants younger than 6 months with small adrenal masses consistent radiographically with neuroblastoma can be treated with close observation alone, even in the absence of a biopsy. Survival rates for patients with low-risk neuroblastoma are more than 98%. Infants younger than 1 year with INSS stage 4S disease may need little if any therapy, with the disease regressing spontaneously, although chemotherapy may be initiated because of bulky disease (generally massive hepatomegaly) causing mechanical complications. Survival rates with 4S disease are more than 90%.

With intermediate-risk neuroblastoma (subsets of patients with INSS stages 3 and 4 disease), the primary treatment approach is surgery combined with chemotherapy. The size or location of the tumor often makes primary resection impossible. Under these circumstances, a biopsy alone is performed to make a definitive diagnosis and evaluate biologic characteristics. Shrinkage of the tumor with chemotherapy often allows a second surgery with more complete tumor resection. Chemotherapeutic agents typically used include carboplatin, etoposide, cyclophosphamide, vincristine, and doxorubicin. The number of cycles used (usually 2–8) depends on the multiple factors, including the age of the patient, the INSS stage, biologic features of the tumor, and response to treatment. Radiation therapy is rarely necessary. Survival rates for intermediate risk neuroblastoma are 90–95%.

High-risk patients (the majority with INSS stages 3 and 4 disease, generally with older age and unfavorable tumor biology) require intensive, multimodal therapy including chemotherapy, surgery, autologous HSCT, irradiation, biologic therapy, and immunotherapy. Several cycles of intensive chemotherapy are followed by resection of as much of the tumor as possible. Following this induction phase, tandem (two sequential) autologous HSCTs are performed as consolidative therapy. Following the HSCTs, the site of the primary tumor and any areas with evidence of active disease prior to transplant are irradiated. At this point, patients have reached a state of MRD. To reduce the risk of recurrence, a maintenance phase follows. Patients receive immunotherapy with an antibody directed against the GD2 antigen expressed on the surface of the neuroblastoma cells together with or GM-CSF to enhance immune-mediated cell killing. These treatments are alternated with treatments with 13-*cis*-retinoic acid, an agent that induces terminal differentiation of neuroblastoma cells. Results of recent studies incorporating all of these treatment modalities are encouraging, with 5-year EFS rates of 56% and overall survival rates of 73%. An upcoming COG treatment study will be looking at the incorporation of therapeutic radioactive I-121-MIBG into the upfront treatment regimen. Also, use of targeted therapies, such as ALK inhibition in patients whose tumors express ALK mutations, are being investigated. Despite advancements, high risk neuroblastoma remains a challenging disease, and much work remains to improve cure rates while minimizing the toxicity of treatment.

George RE et al: Hyperdiploidy plus nonamplified *MYCN* confers a favorable prognosis in children 12–18 months old with disseminated neuroblastoma: a Pediatric Oncology Group Study. J Clin Oncol 2005;23:6466 [PMID: 16116152].

London WB et al: Evidence for an age cutoff greater than 365 days for neuroblastoma risk group stratification in the Children's Oncology Group. J Clin Oncol 2005;23:6459 [PMID: 16116153].

Maris JM: Recent advances in neuroblastoma. N Engl J Med 2010;362:2202–2211 [PMID: 20558371].

Matthay KK et al: Long-term results for children with high-risk neuroblastoma treated on a randomized trial of myeloablative therapy followed by 13-*cis*-retinoic acid: a Children's Oncology Group study. J Clin Oncol 2009;27:1007 [PMID: 19171716].

National Cancer Institute: http://www.cancer.gov/cancertopics/types/neuroblastoma.

Nuchtern JG et al: A prospective study of expectant observation as primary therapy for neuroblastoma in young infants: a Children's Oncology Group study. Ann Surg 2012;256:573–580 [PMID: 22964741].

Schmidt ML et al: Favorable prognosis for patients 12–18 months of age with stage 4 nonamplified *MYCN* neuroblastoma: a Children's Cancer Group Study. J Clin Oncol 2005;23:6474 [PMID: 16116154].

Yu AL et al: Anti-GD2 antibody with GM-CSF, IL2 and isotretinoin for neuroblastoma. New Engl J Med 2010;363(14):1324 [PMID: 20879881].

WILMS TUMOR (NEPHROBLASTOMA)

▶ General Considerations

Approximately 460 new cases of Wilms tumor occur annually in the United States, representing 5%–6% of cancers in children younger than 15 years. After neuroblastoma, this is the second most common abdominal tumor in children. The majority of Wilms tumors are of sporadic occurrence. However, in a few children, Wilms tumor occurs in the setting of associated malformations or syndromes, including aniridia, hemihypertrophy, genitourinary (GU) malformations (eg, cryptorchidism, hypospadias, gonadal dysgenesis, pseudohermaphroditism, and horseshoe kidney), Beckwith-Wiedemann syndrome, Denys-Drash syndrome, and WAGR syndrome (Wilms tumor, aniridia, ambiguous genitalia, mental retardation).

The median age at diagnosis is related both to gender and laterality, with bilateral tumors presenting at a younger age than unilateral tumors, and males being diagnosed earlier than females. Wilms tumor occurs most commonly between ages 2 and 5 years; it is unusual after age 6 years. The mean age at diagnosis is 4 years.

▶ Clinical Findings

A. Symptoms and Signs

Most children with Wilms tumor present with increasing size of the abdomen or an asymptomatic abdominal mass incidentally discovered by a parent and/or health care provider. The mass is usually smooth and firm, well demarcated, and rarely crosses the midline, though it can extend inferiorly into the pelvis. About 25% of patients are hypertensive at presentation. Gross hematuria is an uncommon presentation, although microscopic hematuria occurs in approximately 25% of patients.

B. Laboratory Findings

The CBC is usually normal, but some patients have anemia secondary to hemorrhage into the tumor. Blood urea nitrogen and serum creatinine are usually normal. Urinalysis may show some blood or leukocytes.

C. Imaging and Staging

Ultrasonography or CT of the abdomen should establish the presence of an intrarenal mass. It is also essential to evaluate the contralateral kidney for presence and function as well as synchronous Wilms tumor. The inferior vena cava needs to be evaluated by ultrasonography with Doppler flow for the presence and extent of tumor propagation. The liver should be imaged for the presence of metastatic disease. Chest CT scan should be obtained to determine whether pulmonary metastases are present. Approximately 10% of patients will have metastatic disease at diagnosis. Of these, 80% will have pulmonary disease and 15% liver metastases. Bone and brain metastases are extremely uncommon and usually associated with the rarer, more aggressive renal tumor types, such as clear cell sarcoma or rhabdoid tumor; hence, bone scans and brain imaging are not routinely performed. The clinical stage is ultimately decided at surgery and confirmed by the pathologist.

▶ Treatment & Prognosis

In the United States, treatment of Wilms tumor begins with surgical exploration of the abdomen via an anterior surgical approach to allow for inspection and palpation of the contralateral kidney. The liver and lymph nodes are inspected and suspicious areas biopsied or excised. En bloc resection of the tumor is performed. Every attempt is made to avoid tumor spillage at surgery as this may increase the staging and treatment. Because therapy is tailored to tumor stage, it is imperative that a surgeon familiar with the staging requirements perform the operation.

In addition to the staging, the histologic type has implications for therapy and prognosis. Favorable histology (FH; see later discussion) refers to the classic triphasic Wilms tumor and its variants. Unfavorable histology (UH) refers to the presence of diffuse anaplasia (extreme nuclear atypia) and is present in 5% of Wilms tumors. Only a few small foci of anaplasia in a Wilms tumor give a worse prognosis to patients with stage II, III, or IV tumors. Loss of heterozygosity of chromosomes 1p and 16q are adverse prognostic

Table 31–8. Treatment of Wilms tumor.

Stage/Histologic Subtype	Treatment
I–II FH and I UH	18 wk (dactinomycin and vincristine)
III–IV FH and II–IV focal anaplasia	24 wk (dactinomycin, vincristine, and doxorubicin) with radiation
II–IV UH (diffuse anaplasia)	24 wk (vincristine, doxorubicin, etoposide, and cyclophosphamide) with radiation

FH, favorable histology; UH, unfavorable histology.

factors in those with favorable histology. Following excision and pathologic examination, the patient is assigned a stage that defines further therapy.

Improvement in the treatment of Wilms tumor has resulted in an overall cure rate of approximately 90%. The National Wilms' Tumor Study Group's fourth study (NWTS-4) demonstrated that survival rates were improved by intensifying therapy during the initial treatment phase while shortening overall treatment duration (24 vs 60 weeks of treatment).

Table 31–8 provides an overview of the current treatment recommendations in NWTS-5. Patients with stage III or IV Wilms tumor require radiation therapy to the tumor bed and to sites of metastatic disease. Chemotherapy is optimally begun within 5 days after surgery, whereas radiation therapy should be started within 10 days. Stage V (bilateral Wilms tumor) disease dictates a different approach, consisting of possible bilateral renal biopsies followed by chemotherapy and second-look renal-sparing surgery. Radiation therapy may also be necessary.

Using these approaches, 4-year overall survival rates through NWTS-4 are as follows: stage I FH, 96%; stages II–IV FH, 82%–92%; stages I–III UH (diffuse anaplasia), 56%–70%; and stage IV UH, 17%. Patients with recurrent Wilms tumor have a salvage rate of approximately 50% with surgery, radiation therapy, and chemotherapy (singly or in combination). HSCT is also being explored as a way to improve the chances of survival after relapse.

► Future Considerations

Although progress in the treatment of Wilms tumor has been extraordinary, important questions remain to be answered. Questions have been raised regarding the role of prenephrectomy chemotherapy in the treatment of Wilms tumor. Presurgical chemotherapy seems to decrease tumor rupture at resection but may unfavorably affect outcome by changing staging. Future studies will be directed at minimizing acute and long-term toxicities for those with low-risk disease and improving outcomes for those with high-risk and recurrent disease.

Aldrink JH et al: Update on Wilms tumor. J Pediatr Surg 2019 Mar;54(3):390–397 [PMID: 30270120].

Buckley KS: Pediatric genitourinary tumors. Curr Opin Oncol 2010;23(3):297 [PMID: 21460723].

Caldwell BT, Wilcox DT, Cost NG: Current management of pediatric urologic oncology. Adv Pediatr. 2017 Aug;64(1):191–223 [PMID: 28688589].

Lopes RF, Lorenza A: Recent advanced in the management of Wilms' tumor. F1000Res. 2017 May 12;6:670. doi: 10.12688/f1000research.10760.1. eCollection 2017 [PMID: 28620463].

Oostveen RM, Pritchard-Jones K: Pharmacotherapeutic management of Wilms tumor: an update. Paediatr Drugs 2019 Feb;21(1):1–13 [PMID: 30604241].

Sadak KT, Ritchey ML, Dome JS: Paediatric genitourinary cancers and late effects of treatment. Nat Rev Urol 2013 Jan;10(1):15–25 [PMID: 19657990].

Wilms Tumor and Other Childhood Kidney Tumors Treatment (PDQ®): Health Professional Version. PDQ Pediatric Treatment Editorial Board. PDQ Cancer Information Summaries [Internet]. Bethesda, MD: National Cancer Institute (US); 2002–2019 Jun 13 [PMID: 26389282].

BONE TUMORS

Primary malignant bone tumors are uncommon in childhood with only 650–700 new cases per year. Osteosarcoma accounts for 60% of cases and occurs mostly in adolescents and young adults. Ewing sarcoma is the second most common malignant tumor of bony origin and occurs in toddlers to young adults. Both tumors have a male predominance.

The cardinal signs of bone tumor are pain at the site of involvement, often following slight trauma, mass formation, and fracture through an area of cortical bone destruction.

1. Osteosarcoma

► General Considerations

Although osteosarcoma is the sixth most common malignancy in childhood, it ranks third among adolescents and young adults. This peak occurrence during the adolescent growth spurt suggests a causal relationship between rapid bone growth and malignant transformation. Further evidence for this relationship is found in epidemiologic data showing patients with osteosarcoma to be taller than their peers, osteosarcoma occurring most frequently at sites where the greatest increase in length and size of bone occurs, and osteosarcoma occurring at an earlier age in girls than boys, corresponding to their earlier growth spurt. The metaphyses of long tubular bones are primarily affected. The distal femur accounts for more than 40% of cases, with the proximal tibia, proximal humerus, and mid and proximal femur following in frequency.

Clinical Findings

A. Symptoms and Signs

Pain over the involved area is the usual presenting symptom with or without an associated soft tissue mass. Patients generally have symptoms for several months prior to diagnosis. Systemic symptoms (fever, weight loss) are rare. Laboratory evaluation may reveal elevated serum alkaline phosphatase or LDH levels.

B. Imaging and Staging

Radiographic findings show permeative ("moth-eaten" appearance) destruction of the normal bony trabecular pattern with indistinct margins. In addition, periosteal new bone formation and lifting of the bony cortex may create a Codman triangle. A soft tissue mass plus calcifications in a radial or sunburst pattern are frequently noted. MRI is more sensitive in defining the extent of the primary tumor and has mostly replaced CT scanning. The most common sites of metastases are the lung (≤ 20% of newly diagnosed cases) and the additional boney sites (10%). CT scan of the chest and bone scan are essential for detecting metastatic disease. PET-CT may be a consideration in monitoring response to therapy. Bone marrow aspirates and biopsies are not indicated.

Despite the rather characteristic radiographic appearance, a tissue sample is needed to confirm the diagnosis. Placement of the incision for biopsy is of critical importance. A misplaced incision could preclude a limb salvage procedure and necessitate amputation. The surgeon who will carry out the definitive surgical procedure should perform the biopsy. A staging system for osteosarcoma based on local tumor extent and presence or absence of distant metastasis has been proposed, but it has not been validated.

Treatment & Prognosis

Historical studies showed that over 50% of patients receiving surgery alone developed pulmonary metastases within 6 months after surgery. This suggests the presence of micrometastatic disease at diagnosis. Adjuvant chemotherapy trials showed improved disease-free survival rates of 55%–85% in patients followed for 3–10 years.

Osteosarcomas are highly radioresistant lesions; for this reason, radiation therapy has no role in its primary management. Chemotherapy is often administered prior to definitive surgery (neoadjuvant chemotherapy). This permits an early attack on micrometastatic disease and may also shrink the tumor, facilitating a limb salvage procedure. Preoperative chemotherapy also makes detailed histologic evaluation of tumor response to the chemotherapy agents possible. If the histologic response is poor (> 10% viable tumor tissue), postoperative chemotherapy can be changed accordingly, but a recently completed COG Group study showed increased toxicity with no additional benefit.

Chemotherapy may be administered intra-arterially or intravenously, although the benefits of intra-arterial chemotherapy (IAC) are disputed. Agents having efficacy in the treatment of osteosarcoma include doxorubicin, cisplatin, high-dose methotrexate, ifosfamide, and etoposide.

Definitive cure requires en bloc surgical resection of the tumor with a margin of uninvolved tissue. Amputation, limb salvage, and rotationplasty (Van Ness rotation) are equally effective in achieving local control of osteosarcoma. Contraindications to limb-sparing surgery include major involvement of the neurovascular bundle by tumor; immature skeletal age, particularly for lower extremity tumors; infection in the region of the tumor; inappropriate biopsy site; and extensive muscle involvement that would result in a poor functional outcome.

Postsurgical chemotherapy is generally continued until the patient has received 1 year of treatment. Relapses are unusual beyond 3 years, but late relapses do occur. Histologic response to neoadjuvant chemotherapy is an excellent predictor of outcome. Patients with localized disease having 90% or greater tumor necrosis have a 70%–75% long-term, disease-free survival rate. Other favorable prognostic factors include distal skeletal lesions, longer duration of symptoms, age older than 20 years, female gender, and near-diploid tumor DNA index. Patients with metastatic disease at diagnosis or multifocal bone lesions do not fair well, despite advances in chemotherapy and surgical techniques.

2. Ewing Sarcoma

General Considerations

Ewing sarcoma accounts for only 30% of primary malignant bone tumors; fewer than 200 new cases occur each year in the United States. It is a disease primarily of white males, almost never affects blacks, and occurs mostly in the second decade of life. Ewing sarcoma is considered a "small, round, blue cell" malignancy. The differential diagnosis includes RMS, lymphoma, and neuroblastoma. Although most commonly a tumor of bone, it may also occur in soft tissue (extraosseous Ewing sarcoma or PNET).

Clinical Findings

A. Symptoms and Signs

Pain at the site of the primary tumor is the most common presenting sign, with or without swelling and erythema. No specific laboratory findings are characteristic of Ewing sarcoma, but an elevated LDH may be present and is of prognostic significance. Associated symptoms include fevers and weight loss.

B. Imaging and Staging

The radiographic appearance of Ewing sarcoma overlaps with osteosarcoma, although Ewing sarcoma usually involves the diaphyses of long bones. The central axial skeleton gives rise to 40% of Ewing tumors. Evaluation of a patient diagnosed as having Ewing sarcoma should include an MRI of the primary lesion to define the extent of local disease as precisely as possible. This is imperative for planning future surgical procedures or radiation therapy. Metastatic disease is present in 25% of patients at diagnosis. The lung (38%), bone (particularly the spine) (31%), and the bone marrow (11%) are the most common sites for metastasis. CT scan of the chest, bone scan, and bilateral bone marrow aspirates and biopsies are all essential to the staging workup. PET-CT may be considered to help monitor therapy response.

A biopsy is essential to establishing the diagnosis. Histologically, Ewing sarcoma consists of sheets of undifferentiated cells with hyperchromatic nuclei, well-defined cell borders, and scanty cytoplasm. Necrosis is common. Electron microscopy, immunocytochemistry, and cytogenetics may be necessary to confirm the diagnosis. A generous tissue biopsy specimen is often necessary for diagnosis but should not delay starting chemotherapy.

A consistent cytogenetic abnormality, t(11;22), has been identified in Ewing sarcoma and PNET and is present in 85%–90% of tumors. These tumors also express the protooncogene c-myc, which may be helpful in differentiating Ewing sarcoma from neuroblastoma, in which c-myc is not expressed.

▶ Treatment & Prognosis

Therapy usually commences with the administration of chemotherapy after biopsy and is followed by local control measures. Depending on many factors, including the primary site of the tumor and the response to chemotherapy, local control can be achieved by surgery, radiation therapy, or a combination of these methods. Following local control, chemotherapy continues for approximately 6 months. Effective treatment for Ewing sarcoma uses combinations of dactinomycin, vincristine, doxorubicin, cyclophosphamide, etoposide, and ifosfamide. Recent data showed that giving chemotherapy every 2 weeks, rather than every 3 weeks, improved the EFS for localized Ewing sarcoma. The current COG nonmetastatic Ewing sarcoma study is looking at whether the addition of topotecan to the present five-drug regimen will improve survival.

Patients with small localized primary tumors have a 70%–75% long-term, disease-free survival rate. For patients with metastatic disease, survival is poor. Autologous HSCT may be considered as part of the treatment of these high-risk patients. Patients with pelvic tumors have an intermediate prognosis of around 50% long-term, disease-free survival.

Geller DS, Gorlick R: Osteosarcoma: a review of diagnosis, management and treatment strategies. Clin Adv Hematol Oncol 2010;8(10):705 [PMID: 2137869].

Harrison DJ, Geller DS, Gill JD, Lewis VO, Gorlick R: Current and future therapeutic approaches for osteosarcoma. Expert Rev Anticancer Ther 2018 Jan;18(1):39–50 [PMID: 29210294].

Jackson TM, Bittman M, Granowetter L: Pediatric malignant bone tumors: a review and update on current challenges, and emerging drug targets. Curr Probl Pediatr Adolesc Health Care 2016 Jul;46(7):213–228 [PMID: 27265835].

Moore DD et al: Ewing sarcoma of bone. Cancer Treat Res 2014;162:93 [PMID: 25070232].

Womer R et al: Randomized controlled trial of interval-compressed chemotherapy for the treatment of localized Ewing sarcoma: a report from the Children's Oncology Group. J Clin Oncol 2012;30(33):41–48 [PMID: 23091096].

RHABDOMYOSARCOMA

▶ General Considerations

Rhabdomyosarcoma (RMS) is the most common soft tissue sarcoma of childhood and accounts for 10% of childhood solid tumors. The peak incidence is at age 2–5 years. A second, smaller peak is seen in adolescents with extremity tumors. Males are affected more commonly than females. Seventy percent of children with RMS are diagnosed before age 10 years.

RMS can occur anywhere in the body. When it imitates striated muscle and cross-striations are seen by light microscopy, the diagnosis is straightforward. Immunohistochemistry looking for expression of myogenic regulatory factors such as myoD and myogenin can support the diagnosis. Electron microscopy and chromosomal analysis are also helpful diagnostic tools. RMS is classified into subtypes based on pathologic features: embryonal RMS (ERMS), including the botryoid variant (so named because of its gross appearance similar to a bunch of grapes), makes up approximately 70% of childhood RMS. It tends to occur in the GU tract and the head and neck, particularly the orbit, and is typically seen in young children. Alveolar RMS (ARMS) makes up most of the remaining cases. It tends to occur in the trunk or extremities in older children and adolescents and has a worse prognosis than ERMS. Two characteristic chromosomal translocations, t(2;13) and t(1;13), are seen in 80% of cases of ARMS, leading to fusion of the FOXO1 transcription factor gene on chromosome 13 to the PAX3 or PAX7 gene on chromosome 2 or 1, respectively. Some studies suggest that patients with t(2;13) have a poorer outcome than patients with t(1;13), particularly when there is metastatic disease at diagnosis. Sclerosing/spindle cell RMS (SRMS) is a less common subtype that tends to occur in the paratesticular and head and neck regions and behaves similarly to ERMS. Pleomorphic RMS (PRMS) is rare and occurs mostly in adults.

In young children with RMS, the possibility that they may harbor an underlying cancer predisposition syndrome should be considered. LFS is an inherited mutation of the p53 tumor suppressor gene that results in a high risk of bone and soft tissue sarcomas, including RMS, in childhood as well as breast cancer and other malignant neoplasms in adulthood. RMS in children with LFS typically exhibits anaplasia. In a patient with RMS with anaplasia, LFS should be strongly considered as a predisposing cause. Patients with NF-1 are also predisposed to develop RMS, typically ERMS involving the GU tract.

▶ Clinical Findings

A. Symptoms and Signs

The presenting symptoms and signs of RMS result from disturbances of normal body function due to tumor growth (Table 31–9). For example, patients with orbital RMS present with proptosis, whereas patients with RMS of the bladder can present with hematuria, urinary obstruction, or a pelvic mass.

B. Staging

A CT and/or MRI scan should be obtained to determine the extent of the primary tumor and to assess regional lymph nodes. A CT scan of the chest is used to assess for pulmonary metastasis, the most common site of metastatic disease at diagnosis. A bone scan screens for bony metastases. PET-CT is another useful imaging modality when evaluating for metastatic disease, though its role in the management of RMS continues to be studied. Bilateral bone marrow biopsies and aspirates are obtained to look for bone marrow involvement. Additional studies may occasionally be warranted. For example, for parameningeal primary tumors, a lumbar puncture is performed to evaluate for CNS involvement. Also, sentinel node biopsy for extremity ARMS or biopsy of any suspicious lymph nodes is important for staging and treatment planning.

▶ Treatment

Optimal treatment of RMS is complex and requires combined modality therapy delivered by a multidisciplinary team, including oncologists, surgeons, and radiation oncologists. When feasible, the tumor should be completely excised with clear margins at diagnosis, but this is frequently not possible because of the site of origin and size of the tumor. When only partial tumor resection is feasible, the operative procedure is usually limited to biopsy and sampling of lymph nodes. Chemotherapy can often convert an inoperable tumor to a resectable one. Radiation therapy is effective for local tumor control with both microscopic and gross residual disease. Most patients end up receiving radiation, the exception being those with a localized tumor that has been completely resected. All patients with RMS receive chemotherapy, even when the tumor is fully resected at diagnosis. The exact regimen and duration of chemotherapy are determined by the histologic subtype, age at diagnosis, the primary site, the TNM (tumor-lymph node-metastasis) staging classification, and the grouping classification (disease extent after initial surgery). Based on these factors, patients are categorized into low risk, with an FFS of approximately 90%, intermediate risk, with an FFS of 60%–70%, and high risk, with an FFS of less than 20%.

The combination of vincristine, dactinomycin, and cyclophosphamide (VAC) has shown the greatest efficacy in the treatment of RMS. For low-risk patients, recent COG studies have focused on reducing the amount of cyclophosphamide to minimize late effects such as infertility and secondary cancers while maintaining high cure rates. For intermediate-risk patients, current studies are looking at incorporating irinotecan into treatment and adding a maintenance phase that includes cyclophosphamide and vinorelbine. High-risk

Table 31–9. Characteristics of rhabdomyosarcoma.

Primary Site	Frequency (%)	Symptoms and Signs	Predominant Pathologic Subtype
Head and neck	35		Embryonal
Orbit	9	Proptosis	
Parameningeal	16	Cranial nerve palsies; aural or sinus obstruction with or without drainage	
Other	10	Painless, progressively enlarging mass	
Genitourinary	22		Embryonal (botryoid variant in bladder and vagina)
Bladder and prostate	13	Hematuria, urinary obstruction	
Vagina and uterus	2	Pelvic mass, vaginal discharge	
Paratesticular	7	Painless mass	
Extremities	18	Adolescents, swelling of affected body part	Alveolar (50%), undifferentiated
Other	25	Mass	Alveolar, undifferentiated

(metastatic) RMS remains a major therapeutic challenge. For high-risk patients, several treatment strategies have been attempted. The most recent COG high-risk RMS study added several agents (irinotecan, ifosfamide, etoposide, doxorubicin) to standard VAC therapy. It also compressed the timing of some of the cycles from every 3 weeks to every 2 weeks. Early results showed improvement in survival, but with longer follow-up most patients eventually relapsed, and survival rates were no better than what was seen historically. Clearly, new strategies are needed. A recent study treating patients with relapsed or refractory RMS with a combination of temsirolimus, vinorelbine, and cyclophosphamide showed promising results, prompting consideration of this drug combination for upfront treatment regimens. Agents targeting the insulin-like growth factor (IGF) pathway are also being investigated.

El Demellawy D et al: Update on molecular findings in rhabdomyosarcoma. Pathology 2017;49(3):238–246 [PMID: 28469406].

Harrison DJ et al: The role of 18F-FDG-PET/CT in pediatric sarcoma. Semin Nucl Med 2017;47(3):229–241 [PMID: 28476026].

Hawkins DS et al: What is new in the biology and treatment of pediatric rhabdomyosarcoma? Curr Opin Pediatr 2014;26(1):50 [PMID: 24326270].

Hayes-Jordan A, Andrassy R: Rhabdomyosarcoma in children. Curr Opin Pediatr 2009;21(3):373 [PMID: 19448544].

Malempati S, Hawkins DS: Rhabdomyosarcoma: review of the Children's Oncology Group (COG) soft-tissue sarcoma committee experience and rationale for current COG studies. Pediatr Blood Cancer 2012;59(1):5–10 [PMID: 22378628].

Martins AS et al: Targeting the insulin-like growth factor pathway in rhabdomyosarcomas: rationale and future perspectives. Sarcoma 2011;2011:209736 [PMID: 21437217].

National Cancer Institute: http://www.cancer.gov/cancertopics/types/childrhabdomyosarcoma.

Rodeberg D, Paidas C: Childhood rhabdomyosarcoma. Semin Pediatr Surg 2006;15(1):57 [PMID: 16458847].

Rudzinski ER et al: The World Health Organization classification of skeletal muscle tumors in pediatric rhabdomyosarcoma: a report from the Children's Oncology Group. Arch Pathol Lab Med 2015;139(10):1281–1287 [PMID: 25989287].

RETINOBLASTOMA

▶ General Considerations

Retinoblastoma is a neuroectodermal malignancy arising from embryonic retinal cells. It is rare, accounting for 3% of cases of childhood cancer. It is the most common intraocular tumor in children and causes 5% of cases of childhood blindness. In the United States, 200–300 new cases are diagnosed yearly. This is a malignancy of early childhood, with 90% of the tumors diagnosed before age 5 years. Retinoblastoma is the prototypic heritable cancer.

In almost all cases, retinoblastoma is caused by loss of function of *RB1*, a tumor suppressor gene located on the long arm of chromosome 13 (13q14). This gene encodes a protein that regulates progression through the cell cycle. When the gene is lost or inactivated, uncontrolled cell growth leads to tumor formation. Each cell carries two copies of *RB1*, one from each parent, and both copies must be lost or inactivated for tumor formation to occur.

Retinoblastoma exists in both a heritable and nonheritable form. The heritable form (30%–40% of cases) tends to have multiple tumors, is usually bilateral, and tends to occur at a younger age (median 14 months) while the nonheritable form is unilateral and tends to occur at an older median age (23 months). Based on these observations, Alfred Knudson proposed a "two-hit" hypothesis for retinoblastoma tumor development. He postulated that for a cell to become tumorigenic, it had to lose function of both copies of a tumor suppressor gene (later identified as *RB1*). In heritable cases, the first mutation is either inherited from a parent (10% of cases) or occurs very early in development (90% of cases), with the progeny of that cell all carrying the same mutation. In someone with germline loss of one allele, loss of function of the second *RB1* allele in a retinal cell is a likely event, occurring in 90% of persons who carry the germline mutation. Most will have multiple tumors and most will have bilateral disease. In nonheritable cases, both mutations must arise spontaneously in the same somatic cell, a much less likely event. Therefore, nonheritable cases are unilateral, single tumors. Because of the implications for both the patient and the patient's family, genetic counseling and *RB1* mutational analysis are essential for all patients diagnosed with retinoblastoma.

▶ Clinical Findings

A. Symptoms and Signs

Children with retinoblastoma in the United States generally come to medical attention while the tumor is still confined to the globe. Although sometimes present at birth, retinoblastoma is not usually detected until it has grown to a considerable size. Leukocoria (white pupillary reflex) is the most common sign (found in 60% of patients). Parents may note an unusual appearance of the eye or asymmetry of the eyes in a photograph. The differential diagnosis of leukocoria includes *Toxocara canis* granuloma, astrocytic hamartoma, retinopathy of prematurity, Coats disease, and persistent hyperplastic primary vitreous. Strabismus (in 20% of patients) is seen when the tumor involves the macula and central vision is lost. Rarely (in 7% of patients), a painful red eye with glaucoma, hyphema, or proptosis is the initial manifestation. A single focus or multiple foci of tumor may be seen in one or both eyes at diagnosis.

B. Diagnostic Evaluation

Suspected retinoblastoma requires a detailed ophthalmologic examination under general anesthesia. An ophthalmologist makes the diagnosis based on the appearance of the tumor within the eye, without pathologic confirmation. A white to creamy pink mass protruding into the vitreous matter suggests the diagnosis. Intraocular calcifications and vitreous seeding are virtually pathognomonic findings. A CT scan of the orbits and MRI of the orbits and brain detect intraocular calcification, evaluate the optic nerve for tumor infiltration, and detect extraocular extension of tumor or involvement of the pineal gland (trilateral retinoblastoma). Metastatic disease to the marrow or meninges can be detected with bilateral bone marrow aspirates and biopsies and CSF cytology, respectively.

▶ Treatment

The first goal of treatment is prevention of metastatic disease. While cure rates for retinoblastoma confined to the orbit are excellent, survival rates decrease precipitously once the disease has spread beyond the orbit. An important secondary goal is preservation of the eye and of useful vision, and a third goal is prevention of late effects of therapy. Each eye is treated according to its potential for useful vision, and every attempt is made to preserve vision. The choice of therapy depends on the size, location, and number of intraocular lesions as well as if the disease is unilateral or bilateral.

Children with retinoblastoma confined to the retina (whether unilateral or bilateral) have an excellent prognosis, with 5-year survival rates greater than 95% in the United States. Small lesions may be amenable to local therapies such as cryotherapy or laser therapy, or, depending on the location, placement of a radioactive plaque outside of the globe to provide localized radiation therapy. Larger tumors may require use of systemic chemotherapy to shrink the tumors and allow local therapies to be used in conjunction. The most commonly used agents are vincristine, etoposide, and carboplatin (VEC). For large intraocular tumors, a therapy that has been gaining in popularity is intra-arterial chemotherapy, where a catheter is threaded into the ophthalmic artery so that chemotherapy can be injected directly into the blood supply to the tumor. IAC is generally done in conjunction with other local therapies. Intravitreal injection of chemotherapy, usually melphalan, can be a particularly useful adjunctive therapy for treatment of vitreal tumor seeds. With use of these treatment modalities, many more eyes have been able to be saved and useful vision preserved.

Sometimes, enucleation of the eye is the best option. Absolute indications for enucleation include no salvageable vision, neovascular glaucoma, inability to examine the treated eye, suspicion of extraocular extension of tumor, and inability to control tumor growth with conservative treatment. Once the eye is removed, it is examined histopathologically to see if there are any high-risk features such as tumor invasion posterior to the lamina cribrosa of the optic nerve or extensive choroidal invasion by the tumor. In those situations, systemic chemotherapy is given to decrease risk of metastatic recurrence. Extraocular spread along the optic nerve or within the orbit requires treatment with systemic chemotherapy and external beam radiation. With proper treatment, cure rates remain good. With metastatic spread of disease outside of the orbit, however, cure rates are much poorer, with few patients cured of their disease. Treatment usually involves intensive chemotherapy followed by autologous HSCT. External beam irradiation was formerly a mainstay of therapy but now is used only in very select cases or with extraocular spread. Radiation leads to risk for significant late effects, including hypoplasia of the orbit and a greatly increased risk for secondary malignancies within the radiation field, particularly in patients with germline RB mutation.

Patients with the germline *RB1* mutation (heritable form) have a significant risk of developing second primary tumors. Osteosarcomas account for 40% of such tumors. The 30-year cumulative incidence for a second neoplasm is 35% in patients who received radiation therapy and 6% in those who did not receive radiation therapy. The risk continues to increase over time. Although radiation contributes to the risk, it is the presence of the retinoblastoma gene itself that is responsible for the development of nonocular tumors in these patients.

Dimaras H et al: Retinoblastoma. Nat Rev Dis Primers 2015;1:1–22 [PMID: 27189421].

Kiss S, Leiderman YI, Mukai S: Diagnosis, classification and treatment of retinoblastoma. Int Ophthalmol Clin 2008;48(2):135 [PMID: 18427266].

Lin P, O'Brien JM: Frontiers in the management of retinoblastoma. Am J Ophthalmol 2009;148(2):192 [PMID: 19477707].

Rodriguez-Galindo C et al: Treatment of intraocular retinoblastoma with vincristine and carboplatin. J Clin Oncol 2003;15:2019 [PMID: 12743157].

Sastre X et al: Proceedings of the consensus meetings from the International Retinoblastoma Staging Working Group on the pathology guidelines for the examination of enucleated eyes and evaluation of prognostic risk factors in retinoblastoma. Arch Pathol Lab Med 2009;133(8):1199 [PMID: 19653709].

Shields C et al: Targeted retinoblastoma management: when to use intravenous, intra-arterial, periocular, and intravitreal chemotherapy. Curr Opin Ophthalmol 2014;25(5):374–385 [PMID: 25014750].

Shinohara ET et al: Subsequent malignancies and their effect on survival in patients with retinoblastoma. Pediatr Blood Cancer 2014;61:116–119 [PMID: 23918737].

HEPATIC TUMORS (SEE ALSO CHAPTER 22)

Two-thirds of liver masses found in childhood are malignant. Ninety percent of hepatic malignancies are either hepatoblastoma or hepatocellular carcinoma. Hepatoblastoma accounts for the vast majority of liver tumors in children younger than 5 years, hepatocellular carcinoma for the majority in children aged 15–19 years. The features of these hepatic malignancies are compared in Table 31–10. Of the benign tumors, 60%

Table 31–10. Comparison of hepatoblastoma and hepatocellular carcinoma in childhood.

	Hepatoblastoma	Hepatocellular Carcinoma
Median age at presentation	1 y (0–3 y)	12 y (5–18 y)
Male-female ratio	1.7:1	1.4:1
Associated conditions	Hemihypertrophy, Beckwith-Wiedemann syndrome, prematurity, Gardner syndrome	Hepatitis B virus infection, hereditary tyrosinemia, biliary cirrhosis, α_1-antitrypsin deficiency
Pathologic features	Fetal or embryonal cells; mesenchymal component (30%)	Large pleomorphic tumor cells and tumor giant cells
Solitary hepatic lesion	80%	20%–50%
Unique features at diagnosis	Osteopenia (20%–30%), isosexual precocity (3%)	Hemoperitoneum, polycythemia
Laboratory features		
Hyperbilirubinemia	5%	25%
Elevated AFP	> 90%	50%
Abnormal liver function tests	15%–30%	> 30%–50%

AFP, α-fetoprotein.

are hamartomas or vascular tumors such as hemangiomas. There is mounting evidence for a strong association between prematurity and the risk of hepatoblastoma.

Children with hepatic tumors usually come to medical attention because of an enlarging abdomen. Approximately 10% of hepatoblastomas are first discovered on routine examination. Anorexia, weight loss, vomiting, and abdominal pain are associated more commonly with hepatocellular carcinoma. Serum α-fetoprotein is often elevated and is an excellent marker for response to treatment.

Imaging studies should include abdominal ultrasound, CT scan, or MRI. Malignant tumors have a diffuse hyperechoic pattern on ultrasonography, whereas benign tumors are usually poorly echoic. Vascular lesions contain areas with varying degrees of echogenicity. Ultrasound is also useful for imaging the hepatic veins, portal veins, and inferior vena cava. CT scanning and, in particular, MRI are important for defining the extent of tumor within the liver. CT scanning of the chest should be obtained to evaluate for metastatic spread. Because bone marrow involvement is extremely rare, bone marrow aspirates and biopsies are not indicated.

The prognosis for children with hepatic malignancies depends on the tumor type and the resectability of the tumor. Complete resectability is essential for survival. Chemotherapy can decrease the size of most hepatoblastomas. Following biopsy of the lesion, neoadjuvant chemotherapy is administered prior to attempting complete surgical resection. Monitoring the rate of decline of the α-fetoprotein levels can help indicate favorable versus poor responders to chemotherapy. Chemotherapy can often convert an inoperable tumor to a completely resectable one and can also eradicate metastatic disease. Approximately 50%–60% of

hepatoblastomas are fully resectable, following preoperative chemotherapy, whereas only one-third of hepatocellular carcinomas can be completely removed. Even with complete resection, only one-third of patients with hepatocellular carcinoma are long-term survivors. A recent CCG/Pediatric Oncology Group trial has shown cisplatin, fluorouracil, and vincristine to be as effective as but less toxic than cisplatin and doxorubicin in treating hepatoblastoma. The current open COG trial is using cisplatin, fluorouracil, vincristine, and doxorubicin along with the cardioprotectant dexrazoxane in intermediate-risk patients with the addition of temsirolimus in high-risk patients. Other drug combinations that have demonstrated benefit include carboplatin plus etoposide and doxorubicin plus ifosfamide. Liver transplantation has been shown to be a successful surgical option in patients whose tumors are considered to be unresectable.

Allen-Rhoades W, Whittle SB, Rainusso N: Pediatric solid tumors of infancy: an overview. Pediatr Rev 2018 Feb;39(2):57–67 [PMID: 29437125].

Czauderna P, Lopez-Terrada D, Hiyama E, Häberle B, Malogolowkin MH, Meyers RL: Hepatoblastoma state of the art: pathology, genetics, risk stratification and chemotherapy. Curr Opin Pediatr 2014 Feb;26(1):19–28 [PMID: 24322718].

Khaden S et al: Role of liver transplantation in the management of hepatoblastoma in the pediatric population. World J Transplant 2014;4(4):294 [PMID: 25540737].

Khan AS et al: Liver transplantation for malignant primary hepatic tumors. J Am Coll Surg 2017 Jul;225(1):103–113 [PMID: 28232059].

Trobaugh-Lotrario AD, Katzenstein HM: Chemotherapeutic approaches for newly diagnosed hepatoblastoma: past, present, and future strategies. Pediatr Blood Cancer 2012 Nov;59(5):809–812 [PMID: 22648979].

LANGERHANS CELL HISTIOCYTOSIS

▶ General Considerations

Langerhans cell histiocytosis (LCH) used to be called histiocytosis X, a name that highlighted its mysterious nature. It was long debated whether LCH was a dysregulation of the immune system or a neoplastic disorder. Our understanding of the biology of LCH has dramatically improved in recent years as we have learned more about the origin and genetics of the LCH cell. The discovery that most cases of LCH involve a V600E mutation of the *BRAF* gene or mutation of other genes in the RAS-RAF-MEK-ERK pathway has led us to view LCH as a neoplastic disorder, albeit one that does not typically behave in a malignant fashion. Studies on the origin of the LCH cell show that it is derived from a myeloid cell precursor rather than a mature Langerhans cell, placing it in the category of a myeloproliferative neoplasm. These discoveries have helped us to better understand the biology of LCH so that targeted treatments can be developed.

The distinctive pathologic feature of LCH is proliferation of abnormal histiocytes in an inflammatory background of eosinophils, neutrophils, macrophages, and lymphocytes. On light microscopy, the nuclei are deeply indented and elongated ("coffee bean–shaped"), and the cytoplasm is pale and abundant. Additional diagnostic characteristics include expression of CD1a, S-100, and CD207 (langerin), as detected by immunostaining, and the presence of Birbeck granules, recognizable by their tennis racquet appearance with electron microscopy.

▶ Clinical Findings

LCH can present as a wide spectrum of disease, ranging from an isolated bone lesion or chronic skin rash to a multisystem, life-threatening illness. Historically, LCH was classified into different descriptive categories, including eosinophilic granuloma (single or multiple lytic bone lesions, usually seen in older children and adolescents), Hand-Schüller-Christian disease (lytic bone lesions, exophthalmos, and diabetes insipidus [DI], typically in younger children), Letterer-Siwe disease (a severe, multisystem disorder involving the liver, spleen, lung, skin, and bone marrow, typically in infants aged < 2 years) and Hashimoto-Pritzker disease (also known as congenital self-healing reticulohistiocytosis, a cutaneous form of LCH in neonates that self-resolves during the first months of life). More recently, this terminology has been set aside in favor of a classification scheme based on site of disease, number of sites/organs involved, and the involvement of risk organs (bone marrow, liver, spleen), indicative of more aggressive disease, or CNS-risk lesions, indicative of an increased risk of development of neurodegenerative complications and DI.

The most common sites of disease are bone (80%), skin (33%), and the pituitary (25%). Bone lesions can be single or multiple and can occur anywhere in the skeleton, most commonly the skull. The lesions are usually painful. On plain film, a well-demarcated lytic bone lesion is seen. Vertebral lesions can present as vertebra plana. Lesions of the jaw can lead to loose or missing teeth. The skin rash can resemble seborrheic dermatitis, manifesting as a chronic rash resistant to treatment, or as a scattered papular rash. Involvement of the ear canal can lead to chronic ear drainage. Involvement of the pituitary most often manifests as DI. An MRI scan will show a thickened pituitary stalk and disappearance of the posterior pituitary bright spot on T1-weighted imaging, indicative of loss of vasopressin-containing granules. Other hormones produced by the anterior pituitary, such as growth hormone, can also be affected, leading to other endocrinopathies. Neurodegenerative LCH, manifested as neuromuscular, cognitive, and behavioral changes, is a rare but devastating complication of LCH. Liver, spleen, and bone marrow involvement are less common, though they indicate higher-risk disease. Lung involvement can be seen in young children with multisystem disease or in adults, usually associated with cigarette smoking. CT imaging of the lungs shows a reticulonodular pattern and bullae formation, with risk for spontaneous pneumothorax.

Diagnosis is confirmed by biopsy. Additional workup includes a CBC with differential, ESR, coagulation studies (PT/INR, PTT, fibrinogen), and liver and kidney function studies to screen for multisystem involvement. Measurement of urine osmolality from a first-morning void is a useful screen for DI. Chest x-ray (CXR) screens for pulmonary involvement, skeletal survey evaluates for multifocal bone involvement, and abdominal ultrasound assesses hepatosplenomegaly. PET-CT or technetium-99m bone scan can be used to evaluate extent of disease. PET-CT is particularly helpful in identifying active LCH lesions and monitoring response to therapy. Brain MRI should be obtained with suspicion of pituitary or CNS involvement.

▶ Treatment & Prognosis

Because LCH is a rare disorder with a wide clinical spectrum, it has been difficult to develop standardized diagnostic criteria and treatment regimens. The Histiocyte Society was founded in 1985 to advance knowledge of the disease and develop effective treatments through international collaboration. The society is currently supporting its fourth prospective trial, LCH-IV. The North American Consortium for Histiocytosis (NACHO) has also recently been formed to advance treatment for LCH refractory to standard treatments.

Treatment is based on the location and extent of disease. Isolated lytic bone lesions are generally treated with biopsy and curettage, which leads to healing and resolution of the lesion. Low-dose radiation is effective, though it is avoided in children due to concern for late effects. A study is underway to see if isolated skull lesions can be managed without biopsy and with observation alone if the lesion has a classic appearance by imaging. Isolated skin rashes can be observed and can resolve spontaneously or can be treated with topical steroids or nitrogen mustard. Young patients with isolated skin LCH need to be followed closely, since a significant percentage of them can progress to multisystem disease. Isolated lung LCH in adult smokers will often resolve with smoking cessation.

Multifocal bone disease, multisystem disease, disease involving CNS-risk sites (bones of the skull base and face, which have increased risk for development of DI or neurodegenerative LCH), disease involving risk organs, and disease that involves "special sites" (lesions that risk organ function and are not amenable to surgical treatment, such as vertebral lesions with soft tissue intraspinal extension) are all indications for systemic treatment. First-line treatment is usually with vinblastine and prednisone. The LCH-III study showed that treatment for 1 year led to reduced risk for disease recurrence compared with treatment for 6 months, so 1 year of treatment is currently the standard. LCH-IV is comparing 2 years of treatment with 1 year. Patients with multisystem disease with risk organ involvement also receive 6-mercaptopurine. For adolescent and young adult patients who may not tolerate the side effects of this regimen, single-agent treatment with cytarabine is effective and can be considered.

Multiple other options exist for disease that is recurrent or resistant to first-line treatments. A combination of vincristine and cytarabine is being studied as a second-line treatment in the LCH-IV study. Clofarabine or cladribine (2-Cda) used as single agents can be effective. Other effective agents include methotrexate and indomethacin. A combination of high-dose cytarabine and cladribine is being studied in patients with high-risk disease that fails first-line therapy, a patient population that has a particularly poor prognosis. Allogeneic bone marrow transplant may also be indicated in high-risk patients who fail other therapies.

The discovery of the role of *BRAF* mutations and the ERK pathway in the pathogenesis of LCH has led to the investigation of the use of kinase inhibitors such as vemurafenib (a BRAF kinase inhibitor) and trametinib (a MEK kinase inhibitor) in treatment of refractory disease. Early results are promising, and studies are ongoing.

In most cases, prognosis for LCH is excellent, though late effects can be problematic. If DI develops, it is usually permanent, requiring lifelong treatment. Late neurodegenerative changes can lead to severe disability or death. A major focus of current research is development of strategies to prevent these complications.

Allen CE, Ladisch S, McClain KL: How I treat Langerhans cell histiocytosis. Blood 2015;126(1):26–35 [PMID: 25827831].

Allen CE, Merad M, McClain KL: Langerhans-cell histiocytosis. N Engl J Med 2018;379:856–868 [PMID: 30157397].

Badalian-Very G et al: Recurrent *BRAF* mutations in Langerhans cell histiocytosis. Blood 2010;116(11):1919–1923 [PMID: 20519626].

Delprat C, Arico M: Blood spotlight on Langerhans cell histiocytosis. Blood 2014;124(6):867 [PMID: 24894775].

Emil JF et al: Revised classification of histiocytoses and neoplasms of the macrophage-dendritic cell lineages. Blood 2016;127(22):2672–2681 [PMID: 26966089].

Haroche J et al: Dramatic efficacy of vemurafenib in both multisystemic and refractory Erdheim-Chester disease and Langerhans cell histiocytosis harboring the *BRAF* V600E mutation. Blood 2013;121(9):1495–1500 [PMID: 23258922].

Haupt R et al: Langerhans cell histiocytosis (LCH): guidelines for diagnosis, clinical work-up, and treatment for patients till the age of 18 years. Pediatr Blood Cancer 2013;60:175–184 [PMID: 23109216].

Minkov M et al: Histiocyte Society Evaluation and Treatment Guidelines. https://histiocytesociety.org/document.doc?id=290. April 2009.

Monsereenusorn C, Rodriguez-Galindo C: Clinical characteristics and treatment of Langerhans cell histiocytosis. Hematol Oncol Clin N Am 2015;29:853–873 [PMID: 26461147].

Simko SJ et al: Clofarabine salvage therapy in refractory multifocal histiocytic disorders, including Langerhans cell histiocytosis, juvenile xanthogranuloma and Rosai-Dorfman disease. Pediatr Blood Cancer 2014;61:479–487 [PMID: 24106153].

Vaiselbuhh SR et al: Updates on histiocytic disorders. Pediatr Blood Cancer 2014;61(7):1329 [PMID: 24610771].

Weitzman S, Egeler RM: Langerhans cell histiocytosis: update for the pediatrician. Curr Opin Pediatr 2008;20(1):23 [PMID: 18197035].

BLOOD & MARROW TRANSPLANT & CELLULAR THERAPEUTICS

GENERAL CONSIDERATIONS

Blood and marrow transplant (BMT) is considered standard therapy for a variety of pediatric disorders including malignancies, hematologic disorders (bone marrow failure syndromes, aplastic anemia, hemoglobinopathies), inborn errors of metabolism, and severe immunodeficiencies. Autologous transplantation, often referred to as "stem cell rescue," is infusion of the patient's own hematopoietic stem cells. This is restricted to the treatment of certain pediatric malignancies, including neuroblastoma, lymphoma, selected brain tumors, germ cell tumors, and Ewing sarcoma. In contrast, allogeneic transplantation rescues hematopoiesis with stem cells from either a related family member or an unrelated individual from a volunteer bank. The selection of a suitable donor who matches the recipient most closely at key HLA loci, HLA-A, B, C, and DR, is critical, as disparities mediate graft rejection and graft-versus-host disease (GVHD). Every child expresses one set of paternal and one set of maternal HLA antigens. Thus, the probability of one child fully matching another full sibling is one in four. When selecting a donor, a fully matched sibling is preferred, assuming they do not have the same underlying disease as the recipient. If a matched sibling is unavailable, alternative donor sources include a matched unrelated donor, umbilical cord blood, or a haploidentical (half-matched) family member, each with their own unique risk/benefit profile. Large worldwide registries of unrelated bone marrow and umbilical cord blood donors have been developed. Unfortunately, identification of a closely matched unrelated donor can be challenging, especially for underrepresented minorities, making haploidentical transplant an important option.

In most instances, high doses of chemotherapy and/or radiation are given to the BMT patient for myeloablation prior to infusion of stem cells that rescue hematopoietic and lymphoid function. In patients with nonmalignant conditions, allogeneic donor stem cells replace the absent or defective hematopoietic or lymphoid elements of the recipient, curing the underlying disease. For children with oncologic disorders, high doses of chemotherapy and/or radiation are used to optimize tumor cell kill by overcoming cancer cell resistance. Additionally, in allogeneic BMT, the donor lymphoid cells may recognize the cancer as foreign and provide an immunologic attack on the malignancy, a concept known as graft-versus-leukemia (GVL).

BMT COMPLICATIONS

Supportive care after BMT includes management of chemotherapy side effects, nutritional support, prevention and treatment of infection, and the use of immunosuppressive medications to reduce the risk of GVHD in allogeneic BMT recipients. For the first several weeks, until the newly transplanted cells engraft, patients are most often pancytopenic and require frequent blood product support. These blood products should be leukocyte reduced to decrease the risk of CMV transmission and irradiated to prevent GVHD from residual lymphocytes that remain even in leukocyte-reduced blood products.

For many months following transplant, patients are profoundly immunocompromised. Infections from bacteria, viruses, fungi, and protozoa account for significant morbidity and mortality, and therefore routine prophylaxis and close surveillance are warranted. During profoundly neutropenic periods, patients often receive empiric coverage with broad-spectrum antibiotics to prevent bacteremia. Acyclovir prophylaxis is used to prevent the reactivation of herpes simplex virus that may occur early in up to 70% of seropositive patients as well as varicella zoster reactivation. Antifungal agents are routinely used to prevent infections from *Candida* and *Aspergillus* (Figure 31–1). Trimethoprim-sulfamethoxazole (or equivalent) is used to reduce the risk of *P jirovecii* pneumonia. While transplant patients will frequently recover neutrophil function within the first few weeks, they remain very lymphopenic for many months, requiring ongoing infectious prophylaxis and prevention often thru the first year or more post-transplant. Despite prophylaxis,

overwhelming illness from viral pathogens still occurs. CMV reactivation or de novo infection is relatively common and can result in retinitis, enteritis, and pneumonia. Treatment is usually successful if CMV infection is recognized early therefore routine surveillance is recommended. Common community-acquired viruses can also be life threatening, so prevention is critical. The use of frequent hand washing, contact restriction, and early treatment with available antiviral therapies, such as ribavirin and oseltamivir, can be lifesaving in this population.

GVHD occurs after allogeneic BMT when donor lymphocytes recognize the recipient tissues as foreign and mount an immunologic attack. Despite the use of immunosuppressive agents, anti–T-cell antibodies, and T-cell depletion of the donor graft, 20%–70% of allogeneic BMT patients experience some degree of acute GVHD. Factors influencing GVHD risk include the degree of HLA match, stem cell source, patient age, and donor sex. Acute GVHD generally occurs within the first 100 days after transplant but, on occasion, may occur later. Acute GVHD typically presents with a maculopapular skin rash, secretory diarrhea, and/or cholestatic jaundice. Chronic GVHD generally occurs after day 100 and may involve multiple organ systems; sclerotic skin, malabsorption, weight loss, keratoconjunctivitis sicca, oral mucositis, chronic lung disease, and cholestatic jaundice are common manifestations. Prevention and treatment of GVHD involves use of immunosuppressive agents. Patients on immunosuppressive treatment for GVHD have an increased and protracted risk of all types of infections.

Long-term follow-up of HSCT patients is essential. Patients are at risk for numerous complications, including pulmonary disease, cataracts, endocrine dysfunction affecting growth and fertility, cardiac dysfunction, avascular necrosis of bone, developmental delay, and second malignancies. Although HSCT has many challenges, it represents an important advance in curative treatment for a variety of serious pediatric illnesses.

CELLULAR THERAPEUTICS

Cellular therapy is the transfusion of cells designed to treat or to cure an underlying disease process, such as cancer or a viral infection. To date, the majority of cellular therapy has been administered to patients through clinical research trials. However, in 2017 the FDA approved the first cellular therapy known as CAR T cells for the treatment of pediatric ALL. This therapy involves collection of the patient's own T cells, which are then genetically engineered to produce chimeric antigen receptors (CARs) expressed on the cell surface. These receptors allow the T cells to recognize an antigen on the tumor cells. In the case of pediatric ALL, this receptor is CD19. After the T cells are engineered to express the CAR, they are expanded in the lab prior to infusion back into the patient. If successful, these T cells expand within the patient

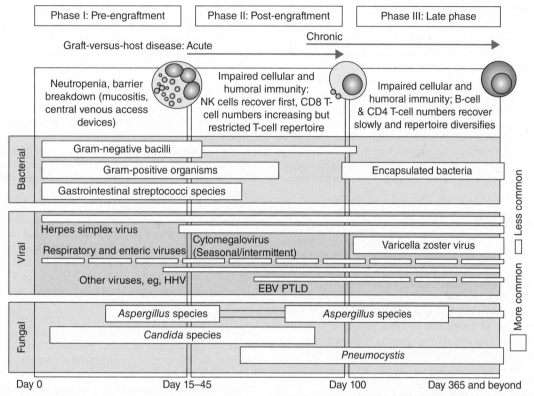

▲ **Figure 31–1.** Phases of opportunistic infections among allogeneic HCT recipients. EBV, Epstein-Barr virus; HHV6, human herpesvirus 6; PTLD, posttransplant lymphoproliferative disease. (Reproduced with permission from Tomblyn M, Chiller T, Einsele H, et al: Guidelines for preventing infectious complications among hematopoietic cell transplantation recipients: a global perspective. Biol Blood Marrow Transplant 2009 Oct;15(10):1143–1238.)

and eradicate any cells expressing the antigen the CAR T cells are designed to recognize. Development of CAR T cells against many other tumor antigens is ongoing. Similarly, T cells with activity against specific viruses such as CMV, EBV, and adenovirus can also be selected and expanded ex vivo and then infused into a patient with a known infection. These viral-specific T cells can be obtained from third-party donor banks or, after BMT, can be collected from the stem cell donor. Currently, all administration of viral-specific T cells is done on clinical research trials.

Ardura MI: Overview of infections complicating pediatric hematopoietic cell transplantation. Infect Dis Clin North Am 2018 Mar;32(1):237–252 [PMID: 29406976.

Chow EJ et al: Late effects surveillance recommendations among survivors of childhood hematopoietic cell transplantation: a Children's Oncology Group report. Biol Blood Marrow Transplant 2016 May;22(5):782–795 [PMID: 26802323.

Malhi K et al: Hematopoietic cell transplantation and cellular therapeutics in the treatment of childhood malignancies. Pediatr Clin North Am 2015 Feb;62(1):257–273 [PMID: 25435122.

Rocha V: Umbilical cord blood cells from unrelated donor as an alternative source of hematopoietic stem cells for transplantation in children and adults. Semin Hematol 2016 Oct;53(4): 237–245 [PMID: 27788761].

Sermer D, Brentjens R: CAR T-cell therapy: Full speed ahead. Heamtol Oncol 2019 Jun;37(S1):95–100 [PMID: 31187533].

Shenoy S, Boelens JJ: Advances in unrelated and alternative donor hematopoietic cell transplantation for nonmalignant disorders. Curr Opin Pediatr 2015 Feb;27(1):9–17 [PMID: 25565572].

Weisdorf D: can haploidentical transplantation meet all patients' needs? Best Pract Clin Haematol 2018 Dec;31(4):410–413 [PMID: 30466758].

LATE EFFECTS OF PEDIATRIC CANCER THERAPY

Late effects of treatment by surgery, radiation, and chemotherapy have been identified in survivors of pediatric cancer. Current estimates are that 1 in every 640 adults between the ages of 20 and 39 years is a pediatric cancer survivor. Recently it was reported that the prevalence of poor health status in this group is higher among adult survivors of pediatric cancer than siblings and increases rapidly with age, particularly among female survivors. One recent study found that 60% of survivors of pediatric cancer diagnosed between 1970 and 1986 have at least one chronic condition. Virtually any organ system can demonstrate sequelae related to previous cancer therapy. This has necessitated the creation of specialized oncology clinics whose function is to identify and provide treatment to these patients.

The Childhood Cancer Survivor Study, a pediatric multi-institutional collaborative project, was designed to investigate the various aspects of late effects of pediatric cancer therapy in a cohort of over 13,000 survivors of childhood cancer.

GROWTH COMPLICATIONS

Children who have received cranial irradiation are at highest risk of developing growth complications. Growth complications of cancer therapy in the pediatric survivor are generally secondary to direct damage to the pituitary gland, resulting in growth hormone deficiency. However, new evidence in children treated for ALL suggests that chemotherapy alone may result in an attenuation of linear growth without evidence of catch-up growth once therapy is discontinued. Up to 90% of patients who receive more than 30 Gy of radiation to the CNS will show evidence of growth hormone deficiency within 2 years. Approximately 50% of children receiving 24 Gy will have growth hormone problems. The effects of cranial irradiation appear to be age-related, with children younger than 5 years at the time of therapy being particularly vulnerable. These patients usually benefit from growth hormone therapy. Currently, there is no evidence that such therapy causes a recurrence of cancer.

Spinal irradiation inhibits vertebral body growth. In 30% of treated children, standing heights may be less than the fifth percentile. Asymmetrical exposure of the spine to radiation may result in scoliosis.

Growth should be monitored closely, particularly in young survivors of childhood cancer. Obesity may become an issue for selected survivors who are young at diagnosis and have received whole brain radiation. Follow-up studies should include height, weight, growth velocity, scoliosis examination, and, when indicated, growth hormone testing.

ENDOCRINE COMPLICATIONS

Thyroid dysfunction, manifesting as hypothyroidism, is common in children who received total body irradiation, cranial irradiation, or local radiation therapy to the neck and/or mediastinum. Particularly at risk are children with brain tumors who received more than 3000 cGy and those who received more than 4000 cGy to the neck region. The average time to develop thyroid dysfunction is 12 months after exposure, but the range is wide. Therefore, individuals at risk should be monitored yearly for at least 7 years from the completion of therapy. Although signs and symptoms of hypothyroidism may be present, most patients will have a normal thyroxine level with an elevated thyroid-stimulating hormone level. These individuals should be given thyroid hormone replacement because persistent stimulation of the thyroid from an elevated thyroid-stimulating hormone level may predispose to thyroid nodules and carcinomas. In a recent report from the Childhood Cancer Survivor Study, thyroid cancer occurred at 18 times the expected rate for the general population in pediatric cancer survivors who received radiation to the neck region. Hyperthyroidism, although rare, also occurs in patients who have received neck irradiation.

Precocious puberty, delayed puberty, and infertility are all potential consequences of cancer therapy. Precocious puberty, more common in girls, is usually a result of cranial irradiation causing premature activation of the hypothalamic-pituitary axis. This results in premature closure of the epiphysis and decreased adult height. Luteinizing hormone (LH) analogue and growth hormone are used to halt early puberty and facilitate continued growth.

Gonadal dysfunction in males is usually the result of radiation to the testes. Patients who receive testicular irradiation as part of their therapy for ALL, abdominal irradiation for Hodgkin disease, or total body irradiation for HSCT are at highest risk. Radiation damages both the germinal epithelium (producing azoospermia) and Leydig cells (causing low testosterone levels and delayed puberty). Alkylating agents such as ifosfamide and cyclophosphamide can also interfere with male gonadal function, resulting in oligospermia or azoospermia, low testosterone levels, and abnormal follicle-stimulating hormone (FSH) and LH levels. Determination of testicular size, semen analysis, and measurement of testosterone, FSH, and LH levels will help identify abnormalities in patients at risk. When therapy is expected to result in gonadal dysfunction, pretherapy sperm banking should be offered to adolescent males.

Exposure of the ovaries to abdominal radiation may result in delayed puberty with a resultant increase in FSH and LH and a decrease in estrogen. Girls receiving total body irradiation as preparation for HSCT and those receiving craniospinal irradiation are at particularly high risk for delayed puberty as well as premature menopause. In patients at high risk for development of gonadal complications, a detailed menstrual history should be obtained, and LH, FSH, and estrogen levels should be monitored if indicated.

No studies to date have confirmed an increased risk of spontaneous abortions, stillbirths, premature births, congenital malformations, or genetic diseases in the offspring of childhood cancer survivors. Women who have received abdominal irradiation may develop uterine vascular insufficiency or fibrosis of the abdominal and pelvic musculature or uterus, and their pregnancies should be considered high risk.

CARDIOPULMONARY COMPLICATIONS

Pulmonary dysfunction generally manifests as pulmonary fibrosis. Therapy-related factors known to cause pulmonary toxicities include certain chemotherapeutic agents, such as bleomycin, the nitrosoureas, and busulfan, as well as lung or total body irradiation. Pulmonary toxicity due to chemotherapy is related to the total cumulative dose received. Pulmonary function tests in patients with therapy-induced toxicity show restrictive lung disease, with decreased carbon monoxide diffusion and small lung volumes. Individuals exposed to these risk factors should be counseled to refrain from smoking and to give proper notification of the treatment history if they should require general anesthesia.

Cardiac complications usually result from exposure to anthracyclines (daunorubicin, doxorubicin, and mitoxantrone), which destroy myocytes and lead to inadequate myocardial growth as the child ages, and eventually result in congestive heart failure. The incidence of anthracycline cardiomyopathy increases in a dose-dependent fashion. A recent report indicates that survivors receiving cumulative doses larger than 360 mg/m^2 were more than 40 times more likely to die of cardiac disease. In a recent study, complications from these agents appeared 6–19 years following administration of the drugs. Pregnant women who have received anthracyclines should be followed closely for signs and symptoms of congestive heart failure, as peripartum cardiomyopathy has been reported.

Radiation therapy to the mediastinal region, which is a common component of therapy for Hodgkin disease, has been linked to an increased risk of coronary artery disease; chronic restrictive pericarditis may also occur in these patients.

Current recommendations include an echocardiogram and electrocardiogram every 1–5 years, depending on the age at therapy, total cumulative dose received, and presence or absence of mediastinal irradiation. Selective monitoring with various modalities is indicated for those who were treated with anthracyclines when they were younger than 4 years or received more than 500 mg/m^2 of these drugs. Biomarkers such as cardiac troponins and brain natriuretic peptides may be useful in assessing cardiotoxicity of anthracyclines.

RENAL COMPLICATIONS

Long-term renal side effects stem from therapy with cisplatin, alkylating agents (ifosfamide and cyclophosphamide), or pelvic irradiation. Patients who have received cisplatin may develop abnormal creatinine clearance, which may or may not be accompanied by abnormal serum creatinine levels, as well as persistent tubular dysfunction with hypomagnesemia. Alkylating agents can cause hemorrhagic cystitis, which may continue after chemotherapy has been terminated and has been associated with the development of bladder carcinoma. Ifosfamide can also cause Fanconi syndrome, which may result in clinical rickets if adequate phosphate replacement is not provided. Pelvic irradiation may result in abnormal bladder function with dribbling, frequency, and enuresis.

Patients seen in long-term follow-up who have received nephrotoxic agents should be monitored with urinalysis, appropriate electrolyte profiles, and blood pressure. Urine collection for creatinine clearance or renal ultrasound may be indicated in individuals with suspected renal toxicity.

NEUROPSYCHOLOGICAL COMPLICATIONS

Pediatric cancer survivors who have received cranial irradiation for ALL or brain tumors appear to be at greatest risk for neuropsychological sequelae. The severity of cranial irradiation effects varies among individual patients and depends on the dose and dose schedule, the size and location of the radiation field, the amount of time elapsed after treatment, the child's age at therapy, and the child's gender. Girls may be more susceptible than boys to CNS toxicity because of more rapid brain growth and development during childhood.

Auditory complications can be seen in childhood cancer survivors exposed to platinum-based chemotherapy and/or temporal or posterior fossa radiation. Difficulty hearing sounds, tinnitus, or hearing loss requiring an aid have been reported.

The main effects of CNS irradiation appear to be related to attention capacities, ability with nonverbal tasks and mathematics, and short-term memory. Recent studies support the association between treatment with high-dose systemic methotrexate, triple intrathecal chemotherapy, and, more recently, dexamethasone and more significant cognitive impairment.

Additionally, pediatric cancer patients have been reported as having more behavior problems and as being less socially competent than a sibling control group. Adolescent survivors of cancer demonstrate an increased sense of physical fragility and vulnerability manifested as hypochondriasis or phobic behaviors.

A recent report from Childhood Cancer Survivor Study noted that when compared to population norms, childhood cancer survivors and siblings report positive psychological health, good health-related quality of life, and life satisfaction. There are, however, subgroups that could be targeted for intervention.

SECOND MALIGNANCIES

Approximately 3%–12% of children receiving cancer treatment will develop a new cancer within 20 years of their first diagnosis. This is a 10-fold increased incidence when compared with age-matched control subjects. Particular risk factors include exposure to alkylating agents, epipodophyllotoxins (etoposide), and radiation therapy, primary diagnosis of retinoblastoma or Hodgkin disease, or the presence of an inherited genetic susceptibility syndrome (LFS or NF). In a recent report, the cumulative estimated incidence of second malignant neoplasms for the cohort of the Childhood Cancer Survivor Study was 3.2% at 20 years from diagnosis.

Second hematopoietic malignancies (acute myelogenous leukemia) occur as a result of therapy with epipodophyllo-toxins or alkylating agents. The schedule of drug adminis-tration (etoposide) and the total dose may be related to the development of this secondary leukemia.

Children receiving radiation therapy are at risk for devel-oping second malignancies, such as sarcomas, carcinomas, or brain tumors, in the field of radiation. A recent report examin-ing the incidence of second neoplasms in a cohort of pediatric Hodgkin disease patients showed the cumulative risk of a sec-ond neoplasm to be as high as 8% at 15 years from diagnosis. The most common solid tumor was breast cancer (the major-ity located within the radiation field) followed by thyroid cancer. Girls aged 10–16 years when they received radiation therapy were at highest risk and had an actuarial incidence that approached 35% by age 40 years. Secondary gastroines-tinal cancer is also increased in pediatric cancer survivors and is related to radiation exposure as well as to certain types of chemotherapeutic agents (procarbazine, platinum).

Bates JE et al: Therapy-related cardiac risk in childhood cancer survivors: an analysis of the Childhood Cancer Survivor Study. J Clin Oncol 2019 May 1;37(13):1090–1101 [PMID: 30860946].

Chow EJ et al: Decreased adult height in survivors of childhood acute lymphoblastic leukemia: a report from the Childhood Cancer Survivor Study. J Pediatr 2007;150:370 [PMID: 17382112].

Fidler MM, Frobisher C, Hawkins MM, Nathan PC: Challenges and opportunities in the care of survivors of adolescent and young adult cancers. Pediatr Blood Cancer 2019 Jun;66(6):e27668. [PMID: 30815985].

Gibson TM et al: Temporal patterns in the risk of chronic health conditions in survivors of childhood cancer diagnosed 1970–99: a report from the Childhood Cancer Survivor Study cohort. Lancet Oncol 2018 Dec;19(12):1590–1601 [PMID: 30416076].

Green DM et al: Risk factors for obesity in adult survivors of child-hood cancer: a report from the Childhood Cancer Survivor Study. J Clin Oncol 2012;30(3):246 [PMID: 22184380].

Henderson TO et al: Secondary gastrointestinal cancer in child-hood cancer survivors: a cohort study. Ann Intern Med 2012;156(11):757 [PMID: 22665813].

Hudson MM et al: Approach for classification and severity grading of long-term and late-onset health events among childhood cancer survivors in the St. Jude lifetime cohort. Cancer Epidemiol Bio-markers Prev 2017 May;26(5):666–674 [PMID: 28035022].

Late Effects of Treatment for Childhood Cancer (PDQ®): Health Professional Version. PDQ Pediatric Treatment Editorial Board. PDQ Cancer Information Summaries [Internet]. Bethesda, MD: National Cancer Institute (US); 2002–2019 Jun 12 [PMID: 26389273].

Whelan K et al: Auditory complications in childhood cancer survivors: a report from the Childhood Cancer Survivor Study. Pediatr Blood Cancer 2011;57:126 [PMID: 21328523].

Pain Management & Pediatric Palliative & End-of-Life Care

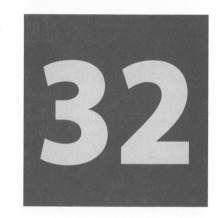

32

Brian S. Greffe, MD

Jeffrey L. Galinkin, MD

Nancy A. King, MSN, RN, CPNP

INTRODUCTION

Children experience pain to at least the same level as adults. Multiple studies have shown that neonates and infants perceive pain and have memory of these painful experiences. Frequently, children are underprescribed and underdosed for opioid and nonopioid analgesics due to excessive concerns of respiratory depression and/or poor understanding of the need for pain medications in children. Few data are available to guide the dosing of many pain medications, and the majority of pain medications available on the market today are unlabeled for use in pediatric patients.

Birnie KA, et al: Hospitalized children continue to report undertreated and preventable pain. Pain Res Manag 2014 Jul–Aug;19(4): 198–204. Epub 2014 May 7 [PMID: 24809068].

Taddio A, Katz J: The effects of early pain experience in neonates on pain responses in infancy and childhood. Pediatr Drugs 2005;7:245–257 [PMID: 16118561].

PAIN ASSESSMENT

Standardizing pain measurements require the use of appropriate pain scales. At most institutions, pain scales are stratified by age (Table 32–1) and are used throughout the institution from operating room to medical floor to clinic, creating a common language around a patient's pain. Pain assessment by scales has become the "5th vital sign" in hospital settings and is documented at least as frequently as heart rate and blood pressure at many pediatric centers around the world. There are many pain scales available, all of which have advantages and disadvantages (eg, Figures 32–1 and 32–2, and Table 32–2). It is less important what type of scale is used, but that they are used on a consistent and continuous basis.

Special Populations

Noncommunicative patients such as neonates and children with cognitive impairment are often difficult to assess for pain.

For these patients using an appropriate assessment tool (see Table 32–1) on a frequent basis (every 1–2 hours) is essential in ensuring adequate pain control. For these populations, increasing pain score trends are often a sign of discomfort.

Bieri D et al: The Faces Pain Scale for the self-assessment of the severity of pain experienced by children: development, initial validation, and preliminary investigation for ratio scale properties. Pain 1990;41:139–150 [PMID: 2367140].

Merkel SI et al: The FLACC: a behavioral scale for scoring postoperative pain in young children. Pediatr Nurs 1997;23:293–297 [PMID: 9220806].

Wong DL, Baker CM: Smiling faces as anchor for pain intensity scales. Pain 2001;89:295–300 [PMID: 11291631].

ACUTE PAIN

▶ Definition Etiology

Acute pain is caused by an identifiable source. In most cases, it is self-limiting and treatment is a reflection of severity and type of injury. In children, the majority of acute pain is caused by trauma or, if in a hospital setting, an iatrogenic source such as surgery.

▶ Treatment

Treatment of acute pain is dependent on the disposition of the individual patient. For outpatient care the mainstay of treatment is nonsteroidal anti-inflammatory drugs (NSAIDs) (Table 32–3). Acetaminophen is the most commonly used NSAID. Acetaminophen is administered via the oral or rectal routes. Acetaminophen is more predictable in its effects as an oral dose. It has also been found that round-the-clock administration (oral 10–15 mg/kg, rectal 20 mg/kg) is better than PRN dosing for both minor pain or as an adjunct for major pain. The toxicity of acetaminophen is low in clinically used doses. However, the use of acetaminophen combined with many over-the-counter and prescription

Table 32–1. Pain scales—description and age-appropriate use.

Name of Scale	Type	Description	Age Group
Numeric	Self-report	Verbal 0–10 scale; 0 = no pain, 10 = worst pain you could ever imagine	Children who understand the concept of numbers, rank, and order; approximately > 8 y
Bieri and Wong-Baker scales	Self-report	Six faces that range from no pain to the worst pain you can imagine	Younger children who have difficulty with numeric scale; cognitive age 3–7 y
FLACC	Behavioral observer	Five categories: face, legs, activity, cry, and consolability; range of total score is 0–10; score ≤ 7 is severe pain. Figures 32–1 and 32–2 and Table 32–2	Nonverbal children > 1 y
CRIES, NIPS, PIPP	Behavioral observer	Rates a set of standard criteria and gives a score	Nonverbal infant < 1 y

CRIES, **C**rying **R**equires O$_2$ saturation, **I**ncreased vital signs, **E**xpression, and **S**leeplessness; FLACC, **F**ace, **L**egs, **A**ctivity, **C**rying, **C**onsolability; NIPS, **N**eonatal **I**nfant **P**ain **S**cale; PIPP, **P**remature **I**nfant **P**ain **P**rofile.
Reproduced with permission from Motoyama EK, Davis PJ: *Smith's Anesthesia for Infants and Children*, 7th ed. St. Louis, MO: Mosby/Elsevier; 2006.

combination products has been a frequent cause of toxicity. Liver damage or failure can occur with doses exceeding 200 mg/kg/day. Other oral analgesics available in suspension are ibuprofen (10–15 mg/kg) and naproxen (10–20 mg/kg).

Motoyama EK, Davis PJ: *Smith's Anesthesia for Infants and Children*. 7th ed. St. Louis, MO: Mosby Elsevier; 2006:436–458.

When pain is more severe, oral opioids can be added for short-term use (Table 32–4). Many of these opioids come formulated with an NSAID, that is, oxycodone/acetaminophen (Percocet) and hydrocodone/acetaminophen (Lortab). When using these combination drugs, the dose of drug is based on the opioid component. Other concomitantly administered similar NSAIDs should be discontinued. The most commonly used oral opioids are oxycodone, hydrocodone, and codeine. The use of codeine is least recommended due to its metabolism. Codeine is metabolized to morphine via the cytochrome P-450 2D4 isoenzyme. From 1% to 10% people (Asians 1%–2%, African Americans 1%–3%, Caucasians 5%–10%) are poor metabolizers as a result of a genetic polymorphism. Thus, patients with this defect get no effect from this drug. A very small percentage of patients (primarily from East Africa) are ultrarapid metabolizers. These patients convert 10–15 times the amount of parent drug to active compound which can result in clinical toxicity. Morphine, oxycodone, and hydrocodone are all available as suspensions, are active as administered, and are metabolized by multiple routes.

Long-acting or extended-release preparations are available for morphine and oxycodone. These drugs are not recommended for acute pain management in children. They should be prescribed with great caution and only under close monitoring. Due to the high incidence of diversion and adulteration of these drugs for abuse, the Federal Drug Administration and manufactures of these products have worked together to develop abuse deterrent formulations of the extended-release products. When extended-release opioids are prescribed, it is prudent to administer an opioid risk assessment tool such as the CRAFFT assessment tool to assess the risk of potential opioid misuse (Box 32–1).

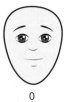 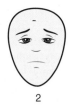 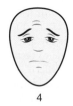 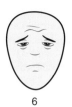 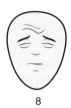 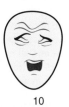

| 0 | 2 | 4 | 6 | 8 | 10 |

▲ **Figure 32–1.** Bieri Faces Pain Scale, revised. (Reproduced with permission from Hicks CL, von Baeyer CL, Spafford PA, et al: The Faces Pain Scale–Revised: toward a common metric in pediatric pain measurement. Pain 2001 Aug;93(2):173–183.)

Box 32–1. Opiod risk tool.

The CRAAFT assessment asks the following six yes or no questions:

- "Have you ever ridden in a car driven by someone (including your-self) who was high or had been using alcohol or drugs?"
- "Do you ever use alcohol or drugs to relax, feel better about your-self, or fit in?"
- "Do you ever use alcohol or drugs while you are by yourself (alone)?"
- "Do you forget things you did while using alcohol or drugs?"
- "Does your family or friends ever tell you that you should cut down on your drinking or drug use?"
- "Have you ever gotten into trouble while you were using alcohol or drugs?"

A score of 2 or higher on this scale for adolescents is associated with a higher risk of opioid misuse.

For severe pain not amenable to oral analgesics, an intra-venous opioid can be titrated to effect; options for pain relief are dependent on severity and location of pain and age. Intravenous opioids used as bolus dose, continuous infusion, and as part of a Patient-Controlled Analgesia (PCA) infusion have a long track record of both safe and efficacious use in children. Often the NSAID ketorolac 0.5–1.0 mg/kg is used as an adjunct for severe pain. Side effects of ketorolac are the same as for adults: renal insufficiency, gastric irritability, and prolonged bleeding times due to decreased platelet adhe-siveness. Patients with bleeding concerns should not receive ketorolac.

PCA pumps can be used in children as young as 6 years with proper instruction, frequent reminders and coach-ing (Table 32–5). Morphine and hydromorphone are the most commonly used drugs for PCA management in the United States. Whenever PCA is used, it is imperative to assess patients frequently (at least hourly) to ensure ade-quate pain relief.

Andersson T et al: Drug-metabolizing enzymes: evidence for clinical utility of pharmacogenomic tests. Clin Pharmacol Ther 2005;78:559–581 [PMID: 16338273].

Berde CB, Sethna N: Analgesics for the treatment of pain in children. N Engl J Med 2002 Oct 3;347(14):1094–1103 [PMID: 12362012].

McCabe SE, West BT, Teter CJ, Cranford JA, Ross-Durow PL, Boyd CJ: Adolescent nonmedical users of prescription opioids: brief screening and substance use disorders. Addict Behav 2012 May;37(5):651–656 [PMID: 22366397].

CHRONIC PAIN MANAGEMENT

▶ Assessment

Chronic pain is a pain that persists past the usual course of an acute illness or beyond the time that is expected for an acute injury. In children this is an increasingly recognized problem. It is estimated that chronic pain may affect as much as 10%–15% of the population. The most common prob-lems include headache, chronic abdominal pain, myofascial pain, fibromyalgia, juvenile rheumatoid arthritis, complex regional pain syndrome, phantom limb pain, and pain associated with cancer. Chronic pain in children often has multiple other contributing factors, including psychological issues, psychosocial factors, sociologic factors, and family dynamics. Associating pain with a single physical cause can lead the physician to investigate the patient with repeated invasive testing, laboratory tests, and procedures and to overprescribe medications. A multidimensional assessment to chronic pain is optimal and often required.

McGrath PA, Ruskin DA: Caring for children with chronic pain: ethical considerations. Paediatr Anaesth 2007 Jun;17(6):505–508 [PMID: 17498011].

Weisman SJ, Rusy LM: Pain management in infants and children. In: Motoyama EK, Davis PJ (eds): *Smith's Anesthesia for Infants and Children.* 7th ed. Mosby Elsevier; 2006:436–458.

▶ Treatment

When possible, a multidisciplinary team approach is stan-dard of care for treating chronic pain in children. All children

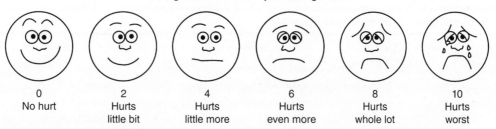

Wong-Bakers FACES® pain rating scale

0	2	4	6	8	10
No hurt	Hurts little bit	Hurts little more	Hurts even more	Hurts whole lot	Hurts worst

▲ **Figure 32–2.** Wong-Baker Pain Scale. Wong-Baker FACES Foundation (2019). Wong-Baker FACES® Pain Rating Scale. Retrieved [Date] with permission from http://www.WongBakerFACES.org. Originally published in Whaley & Wong's Nursing Care of Infants and Children. © Elsevier Inc.

Table 32–2. FLACC pain assessment tool.

Categories	Score 0	Score 1	Score 2
Face	No particular expression or smile	Occasional grimace or frown, withdrawn, disinterested	Frequent to constant frown, clenched jaw, quivering chin
Legs	Normal position or relaxed	Uneasy, restless, tense	Kicking, or legs drawn up
Activity	Lying quietly, normal position, moves easily	Squirming, shifting back and forth, tense	Arched, rigid, or jerking
Cry	No cry (awake or asleep)	Moans or whimpers, occasional complaint	Crying steadily, screams or sobs, frequent complaints
Consolability	Content, relaxed	Reassured by occasional touching, hugging, or being talked to, distractible	Difficult to console or comfort

evaluated for chronic pain should be seen on their initial visit by all primary members of the team to establish a management strategy. Team members should include a pain physician, a pediatric psychologist and/or a psychiatrist, occupational and physical therapists (OT/PT), advanced pain nurses (APNs), and a social worker. The majority of pediatric chronic pain management programs in the United States base their approach on combined intensive rehabilitation and intensive psychotherapy relying minimally on invasive procedures and pharmacotherapy.

A. Tolerance, Dependence, and Addiction

Physiologic and psychological responses to opioids are similar between adults and children. A consensus paper by the American Academy of Pain Medicine, American Pain Society, and American Society of Addiction Medicine defined important differences between normal and pathologic responses to opioids. The definitions of tolerance dependence and addiction are listed as follows.

1. Tolerance—A state of adaptation in which exposure to a drug induces changes that result in a diminution of one or more of the drug's effects over time. Tolerance develops at different rates for different opioid effects, that is, tolerance to

sleepiness and respiratory depression occurs earlier than that to constipation and analgesia.

2. Dependence—A state of adaptation that is manifested by a drug class-specific **withdrawal** syndrome that can be produced by abrupt cessation, rapid dose reduction, decreasing blood level of the drug, and/or administration of an antagonist.

3. Addiction—A primary, chronic, neurobiologic disease, with genetic, psychosocial, and environmental factors influencing its development and manifestations. It is characterized by behaviors that include one or more of the following:

- Loss of **C**ontrol over use of drug
- **C**raving and **C**ompulsive use of drug
- Use despite adverse **C**onsequences

Addiction is rare when opioids are used appropriately for acute pain on both inpatient and outpatient settings. It should be emphasized that tolerance and dependence do not equal addiction.

Heit HA: Addiction, physical dependence, and tolerance: precise definitions to help clinicians evaluate and treat chronic pain patients. J Pain Palliat Care Pharmacother 2003;17:15–29 [PMID: 14640337].

Table 32–3. Suggested doses for nonopioid analgesics.

	Route	Dosage Guidelines	Half-Life	Duration
Acetaminophen	PO	10–15 mg/kg/dose every 4–6 h, maximum dose 4000 mg/day	Neonates: 2–5 h	4 h
	PR	40 mg/kg loading dose, followed by 10–20 mg/kg/dose every 6 h	Adults: 2–3 h	
Ibuprofen	PO	4–10 mg/kg/dose every 6–8 h, maximum dose 40 mg/kg/day, no > 2400 mg/day	Children: 1–7 y: 1–2 h	6–8 h
			Adults: 2–4 h	
Ketorolac	IV	0.5 mg/kg/dose every 6 h, maximum of 30 mg/dose, maximum course of eight doses	Children: ~ 6 h	4–6 h
			Adults: ~ 5 h	

Table 32–4. Suggested doses of oral and intravenous opioids in infants and children.

Opioid Drug	Route	Dosage Guidelines	Onset	Duration
Fentanyl	IV intermittent	0.5–1 mcg/kg/dose (best for intermittent short duration analgesia; titrate to effect)	1–3 min	30–60 min
Hydromorphone	IV	Children: 0.015 mg/kg/dose every 3–6 h Adolescent: 1–4 mg every 3–6 h	15 min	4–5 h
Methadone	IV	0.1 mg/kg/dose every 4 h for two to three doses, then every 6–12 h	10–20 min	6–8 h (22–48 h after repeated doses)
Morphine	IV intermittent	0.05–0.1 mg/kg/dose every 2–4 h	Neonates: 7–8 h 1–3 mo: 6 h 6 mo–2.5 y: 3 h 3–19 y: 1–2 h Adults: 2–4 h	2–4 h
Codeine	PO	0.5–1 mg/kg/dose every 4–6 h, maximum of 60 mg/dose	30–60 min	4–6 h
Hydromorphone	PO	Children: 0.03–0.1 mg/kg/dose every 4–6 h Adolescents: 1–4 mg every 3–4 h	15–30 min	4–5 h
Hydrocodone (in Vicodin, Lortab elixir)	PO	Children: 0.15–0.2 mg/kg/dose every 4–6 h Adolescents: 1–2 tabs every 4–6 h (limited due to acetaminophen content; see acetaminophen recommendations in text)	10–20 min	3–6 h
Methadone	PO	0.1 mg/kg/dose every 4–6 h for two to three doses, then every 6–12 h	30–60 min	6–8 h (22–48 h after repeated doses)
Morphine	PO-IR PO-ER	0.2–0.5 mg/kg/dose every 4–6 h 0.3–0.6 mg/kg/dose every 12 h	15–60 min 1–2 h	3–5 h 8–12 h
Oxycodone	PO-IR PO-ER	0.05–0.15 mg/kg/dose every 6 h 0.2 mg/kg/dose every 12 h[a]	10–30 min 1 hour	3–6 h 12 h

[a]Approved for children 11 years of age and older.

Data from Perkins RM, Swift JD, Newton DA: *Pediatric Hospital Medicine,* 2nd ed. Philadelphia, PA: Lippincott Williams and Wilkins; 2008.

B. Withdrawal

1. Recognition—Withdrawal symptoms can be expected to occur for all patients after 1 week of opioid treatment. Signs of withdrawal in older children include agitation, irritability, dysphoria, tachycardia, tachypnea, nasal congestion, temperature instability, and feeding intolerance. In neonates with withdrawal (neonatal abstinence syndrome), common symptoms include neurologic excitability, gastrointestinal dysfunction, autonomic signs (increased sweating, nasal stuffiness, fever, mottling, poor weight gain), and skin excoriation secondary to excessive rubbing.

Table 32–5. PCA dosing recommendations.

	Morphine	Fentanyl	Hydromorphone
Solution	1 mg/mL	Solution 10 mcg/mL	0.1 mg/mL or 1 mg/mL
Initial dose	15–20 mcg/kg (max 1.5 mg)	0.25 mcg/kg	3–4 mcg/kg (max 0.3 mg)
Lockout time	8–10 min	8–10 min	8–10 min
Basal infusion	0–20 mcg/kg/h	0–1 mcg/kg/h	0–4 mcg/kg/h
Maximum starting dose (for nonopioid tolerant patients)	100 mcg/kg/h	1–2 mcg/kg/h	20 mcg/kg/h

2. Treatment

- Make a schedule/plan in conjunction with patient and family.

- Factor in duration of time on opioid.

- Consider switching to once-a-day opioid (see methadone dosing in Table 32–4).

- Decrease the dose by 10%–25% every 1–2 days.

- Look for signs of withdrawal.

- Consider adding lorazepam 0.05–0.1 mg/kg every 6–8 hours.

- Consider adding clonidine patch 0.1 mg/day (changed every fifth day).

Richard J et al: A prospective evaluation of opioid weaning in opioid-dependent pediatric critical care patients. Anesth Analg 2006;102:1045–1050 [PMID: 16551896].

▼ PEDIATRIC PALLIATIVE & END-OF-LIFE CARE

INTRODUCTION

It has been estimated that almost 55,000 children die each year in the United States. At least 50% of these children die during the newborn period or within the first year of life. Many of these children, particularly those older than 1 year of age, suffer from illnesses that are clearly life-limiting. Thousands more children are diagnosed with life-limiting illnesses, resulting in a chronic condition that may last for many years, even decades. Furthermore, children who are diagnosed with life-threatening illnesses that may be curable, such as cancer, continue to live with the potential of a recurrence of their malignancy for many years. The above populations are those where palliative and end-of-life care could play an important role during the illness of these patients.

It is estimated that over 8 million children worldwide are in need of specialized palliative care. For example, the estimated need for pediatric palliative care ranges from 120 per 10,000 children (Zimbabwe) to 20 per 10,000 children (United Kingdom). Early data regarding the impact of palliative care programs on resource utilization support a trend toward fewer hospital admissions and shorter durations of admissions, but no change in utilization of emergency and outpatient care. Many children still die in a hospital setting, but those who have had involvement with pediatric palliative care have less aggressive end of life care.

Although commonly used interchangeably, *palliative care* and *end-of-life care* are not synonymous terms. Palliative care aims to prevent, relieve, reduce, or soothe the symptoms produced by potential life-limiting illnesses or their treatments and to maintain the patient's quality of life along the entire continuum of treatment. Provision of palliative care does not imply imminent death nor does it prohibit aggressive curative treatment modalities. Rather, it acknowledges the uncertainty and potential for suffering inherent in a potentially life-limiting condition such as cancer. Understanding how a family defines quality of life and suffering for their child is imperative and provides a framework for decision-making between care provider and the family throughout treatment.

While a child is doing well with treatment, the primary focus will be on achieving cure or stabilization of the disease. Palliative care goals at this time focus on promoting quality of life in preparation for survivorship in the face of a potentially life-limiting illness. Some of these goals include helping a family come to terms with the diagnosis, addressing issues of treatment-related pain and distress, facilitating reintegration into the social realms of school and community, and promoting as much normalcy in the child's life as possible. When it becomes clear that the chances for cure are poor or present an unreasonable cost to the child's quality of life, the goals of palliative care will shift toward end-of-life care. The focus will still be on promoting quality of life but now in preparation for a comfortable and dignified end of life with increasingly less attention given to the treatment or cure of the disease itself.

Palliative care not only comprises support in the pain and symptom management of the disease but also addresses equally the psychosocial, emotional, and spiritual needs of the patient with a potential life-limiting illness and their family.

CHILDREN WHO MAY BENEFIT FROM PALLIATIVE CARE INTERVENTIONS

In a review by Himelstein et al, conditions that are appropriate for palliative care were divided into four groups as follows:

- Conditions for which curative treatment is possible but may fail such as advanced or progressive cancer and complex and severe congenital or acquired heart disease

- Conditions requiring intensive long-term treatment aimed at maintaining the quality of life such as HIV/AIDS, cystic fibrosis, and muscular dystrophy

- Progressive conditions in which treatment is exclusively palliative after diagnosis such as progressive metabolic disorders and certain chromosomal abnormalities

- Conditions involving severe, nonprogressive disability, causing extreme vulnerability to health complications such as severe cerebral palsy and anoxic brain injury

The United States Congress mandated in 2010 that palliative care will be covered concurrently with curative therapies for children with terminal conditions who are receiving Medicaid. Based on the *Patient Protection and Affordable Care Act*, a voluntary election to receive hospice care for a child does not constitute a waiver of any rights of the child to be provided with, or to have payments made for services that are related to the treatment of the child's condition. This significant milestone in pediatric palliative care should open the door to concurrent care being covered by private insurance companies in the future.

PAIN MANAGEMENT IN PEDIATRIC PALLIATIVE CARE

Optimal pain management is critical when providing pediatric palliative care. (See the section on Pain Management earlier for definitions and guidelines for treatment.) As end of life approaches, dosing of comfort medications may eventually exceed normally prescribed doses. The goal at all times must be to achieve and maintain comfort. When pain management at the end of life is provided with this goal at the forefront and in concert with careful ongoing assessment and documentation of the child's symptoms, there should be no reason to fear that this action is tantamount to euthanasia which is a conscious action intended to hasten death.

QUALITY-OF-LIFE ADJUNCTS & SYMPTOM MANAGEMENT IN PEDIATRIC PALLIATIVE CARE

When offering treatment to children with a life-limiting illness particularly at the end of life, certain nonpain symptoms and signs may develop more quickly in children when compared to the adult population. A thorough and complete history and physical examination should be obtained. It is critical to determine how much distress the symptom causes the child and how much it interferes with child and his/her family's routine when deciding upon treatment. Areas of management should include supportive treatment, including comfort medications, nursing care, and psychosocial support. Symptoms that commonly occur during disease progression and at the end of life in children with a life-limiting condition are listed in Table 32–6, with suggestions for management.

Complementary & Alternative Modalities

It is not unusual for families to seek complementary or alternative modalities (CAM) for their child when mainstream treatment has failed or is unavailable. Children with chronic conditions such as cancer, asthma, sickle cell disease, and epilepsy have a higher incidence of CAM usage compared to the general pediatric population (Post-White, 2009). The use of CAM in children is influenced primarily by parental use and acceptance of CAM. Culturally accepted beliefs and practices also play an important role. In Asia, the use of meditation and prayer as a method to control pain is well supported by the medical community. In Europe, whether the use of homeopathic remedies is commonplace as children approach end of life, many families opt to try some form of CAM. Most often, these treatments are aimed at improving physical or spiritual quality of life. Sometimes the goal is a desperate hope to find a treatment when other options have failed or an attempt to find something perceived as less toxic than mainstream treatments to induce remission, support the child's ability to fight the disease, or prolong life. Parents report using CAM gives them a sense of control and hope. The most common modalities reported in pediatrics are prayer/meditation, relaxation techniques, massage, chiropractic care including acupuncture, and nutritional supplements (Post-White et al, 2009).

Studies of the effectiveness of CAM use in children have been small and the data are often conflicting. There is generally an acceptance for the lack of harm associated with mind-body techniques such as prayer, meditation, touch and sensory modalities, and relaxation. Acupuncture and acupressure are gaining more acceptance in the Western medical community and may be beneficial in some children for relief of pain, nausea, and other symptoms. Touch and sensory modalities such as massage, healing touch, and aromatherapy can induce a relaxation response in some children which can be very helpful. The use of supplements including botanicals and vitamins has been of more concern due to the lack of dosing information for pediatrics, lack of standardization of products, and the potential for serious drug interactions and toxicities. Treatments touted as alternative "cures" are likely not beneficial and can have very dangerous consequences. Increasing numbers of parents are considering the use of cannabinoids due to increased availability and purported claims of symptom relief (nausea, pain, anxiety) or as a cure for their child's condition. There is currently no data on dosing or efficacy for children, nor for potential risks. The cost of CAM, particularly botanicals and alternative medicine treatments, can be prohibitive and the cost is rarely covered by insurance. Hospice providers frequently incorporate relaxation and mind/body/spirit modalities into their programs.

It is important for the health care provider to ask parents and adolescents about CAM usage and to be open to discussion with the family about modalities they are using or may wish to consider. Parents consistently have reported in studies their desire to inform and discuss CAM with their health care provider, but may be reluctant to do so if they are unsure what response they will get from the provider. Providing families with clear information about the treatment they are considering or using and any contraindications is key. In some cases, recommendation of complementary techniques such as massage, mind/body modalities, and acupuncture/acupressure may be appropriate.

PSYCHOSOCIAL ASPECTS OF PEDIATRIC PALLIATIVE CARE

Pediatric palliative care is unique in that caregivers must be familiar with children's normal emotional and spiritual development. Working with a child at his or her level of development through the use of both oral and expressive communication will allow the child to be more open with respect to hopes, dreams, and fears. A child's understanding

Table 32–6. Symptom management in pediatric palliative care.

Symptom	Etiology	Management
Nausea and vomiting	Chemotherapy, narcotics, metabolic	Diphenhydramine, hydroxyzine, 5-HT$_3$ inhibitors, prokinetic agents for GI motility
Anorexia	Cancer, pain, abnormal taste, GI alterations, metabolic changes, drugs, psychological factors	Treat underlying condition, exercise, dietary consultation, appetite stimulants (dronabinol, megestrol, steroid)
Constipation/diarrhea	Narcotics, chemotherapy, malabsorption, drug related	Laxatives (must be initiated whenever starting narcotics), loperamide for diarrhea, peripheral opioid antagonists (methylnaltrexone, alvimopan)
Dyspnea	Airway obstruction; decrease in functional lung tissue due to effusion, infection, metastases; impaired chest wall movement; anemia	Treatment of specific cause (surgery to alleviate obstruction, red blood cell transfusion, chemotherapy/radiation therapy for metastatic disease), nonpharmacologic management (reassurance, position of comfort, improvement of air circulation using electric fan, oxygen, and relaxation therapy), pharmacologic management with opioids given IV/SQ as continuous infusion, nebulized morphine in older patients, concomitant use of anxiolytics (lorazepam, midazolam) if agitation
Terminal respiratory congestion	Airway/oral secretions at the end of life, resulting in rattling, noisy, gurgling breath sounds	Repositioning, anticholinergics such as hyoscine IV/SQ/PO or transdermal scopolamine
Pressure sores	Direct tissue damage, tissue fragility, immobility, diminished response to pain or irritation	Prevention (avoidance of trauma, relieve pressure, good hygiene), treatment with local hygiene, debridement, use of appropriate wound dressings, antibiotics, analgesics
Bone pain	Bony metastases, leukemic infiltration of bone marrow	Palliative radiation, bone-seeking isotopes, bisphosphonates, chemotherapy, analgesics
Agitation	Present in conjunction with pain, dyspnea, terminal phase of illness	Benzodiazepines (midazolam), barbiturates to achieve complete sedation in terminal restlessness
Pruritus	Urticaria, postherpetic neuralgia, cholestasis, uremia, opioids	Antihistamines (cholestasis, uremia, opioids), 5-HT$_3$ receptor antagonists (cholestasis, opioids)
Hematologic	Marrow infiltration by malignant cells (leukemia)	Transfusions (red blood cells, platelets) to relieve symptoms, hemostatics (aminocaproic acid)
	Coagulopathy Bleeding from erosive or ulcerative processes	Dark bath towel (black, burgundy, or dark purple) to help absorb and camouflage blood
Intractable pain	Various	Chronic pain team consult; consider palliative sedation in very selected cases

of death will depend also on his or her stage of development. Children understand death as a changed state by 3 years of age, universality (death happens to all living things) by 5–6 years of age, and personal mortality by 8–9 years of age. Table 32–7 gives a broad overview of children's concepts of death and offers some helpful interventions.

CHILDREN'S CONCEPT OF DEATH

As end of life approaches, psychosocial support is invaluable to the child and family. Children may need someone to talk to outside of the family unit who can respond to their questions and concerns openly and honestly. Parents may need guidance and support in initiating discussions with or responding

to questions from their child about death and dying. Children and adolescents may have specific tasks they wish to complete before they die. Some want to have input into funeral and memorial service plans and disposition of their body. Parents often need support in making funeral arrangements, handling financial concerns, talking with siblings and other family members, and coping with their own grief.

It is important to recognize that grief is not an illness but a normal, multidimensional, unique, dynamic process presenting as pervasive distress due to a perceived loss. Once parents have accepted the reality of the loss of the child, they must then complete the other tasks of grief such as experiencing the pain of their loss and adjusting to an environment without their child in order to move on with their lives.

Table 32–7. Children's concepts of death.

Age Group and Cognitive Development	Cognitive Understanding of Death	Response to Stress	Helpful Interventions
Infancy: Sense of self is directly related to having needs met	None	Lethargy, irritability, failure to thrive	Maintain routines Prompt response to physical and emotional caretaking needs Cuddling, holding, rocking
Toddler: Egocentric, concrete thinking; see objects and events in relationship to their usefulness to self	None but beginning to perceive implications of separation	Irritability, change in sleepwake patterns, clinginess, regression, tantrums	Maintain routines Keep familiar people and objects at hand Prompt response to physical and emotional caretaking needs Accept need for increased physical and emotional comfort but continue to encourage acquisition of developmental skills
Preschool: Beginning to understand concept of time but limited sense of time permanence, curious, still quite concrete in thinking	View death as deliberately caused Magical thinking about causes of illness and death Death is not a permanent state	Oppositional behaviors, regression, sleep-wake changes, nightmares, somatic complaints Beginning to identify meaning and context of emotions	Simple, concrete explanations to questions—find out what it is they want to know Reassurance that death and illness are not the result of their thoughts or wishes Keep familiar people and objects at hand Play is a powerful tool to help children process events and emotions and as distraction from stressful situations
School age: Beginning of ability to apply logic; accept points of view other than their own	Death is seen in context of experience (pets, grandparents, what is seen on TV or in movies) Can understand that death is permanent	Oppositional behaviors, nightmares, sleep disruption, withdrawal, sadness Can verbally identify own feelings of fear, sadness, happiness	Ascertain how they perceive and understand what is happening and respond accordingly to their questions Acknowledge that feelings of sadness, fear, and anger are normal Allow age-appropriate control whenever possible Maintain as much normalcy in routine as possible Play is very important for expression of emotions and release of stress, amenable to directed play
Preadolescence and adolescence: Gaining mastery over themselves as individuals by exploring their own moral, ethical, and spiritual beliefs; increased reliance on peers for emotional support and information	Adult awareness of death but still may be highly experiential in understanding	Anger, withdrawal, sadness, depression, somatic complaints May have difficulty asking for emotional help	Set the tone for open, honest communication Allow the young person as much control as possible in decisions about his or her own health care Be willing to discuss and respect wishes and desires for disposition of belongings, funeral planning, what happens to his or her body Assist the young person in accomplishing important life tasks and activities that gives meaning to his or her existence or leaves behind a legacy

Parents who lose a child are at high risk for complicated grief reactions such as absent grief, delayed grief, and prolonged or unresolved grief. Siblings are also at risk for complicated grief and require special attention.

SPIRITUAL & CULTURAL SUPPORT

Health care decisions are often intertwined with a family's culture and belief system. Understanding the influences of a family's beliefs and culture allows the practitioner to provide sensitive, appropriate care, particularly at the end of life. Interaction with members of the family's faith and cultural communities can often be instrumental in helping both the care team and the community support of the family. Allowance for specific prayers, rituals, or other activities may help facilitate procedures and discussions.

Families who speak a foreign language probably suffer from inadequate support the most. Every effort should be made to find and utilize a qualified interpreter, particularly for any discussion that involves delivering difficult news or making critical decisions. Many times, the role of interpreter is imposed upon a bilingual family member or friend who may not understand medical terminology well enough to translate clearly or who may deliberately translate the information inaccurately in an attempt to protect the family.

The American Academy of Pediatrics has many resources listed on its website to help children, siblings, and parents at www.aap.org.

WITHDRAWAL OF MEDICAL LIFE SUPPORT

Medical technology has enabled many children with serious health conditions to enjoy a good quality of life. When technological support no longer enables a child's quality and enjoyment of life or there are no viable options to restore quality of life to the child, it may be appropriate to discontinue it. Feeding tubes, ventilators, dialysis, parenteral nutrition, and implanted cardiac pacemakers are examples of medical modalities that may need to be re-evaluated when a child's condition deteriorates or in the case of a catastrophic injury.

There are five circumstances in which withdrawal of medical support and technology can be considered in children (Tournay, 2000). (See the following table.)

Brain death	All reversible causes excluded, meets established criteria for determination of brain death
Persistent vegetative state (PVS)	Child totally dependent for all cares, has no ability to interact meaningfully with his environment. Lack of cortical peaks in the somatosensory evoked potential may be helpful in making prognosis of PVS
Treatment will delay death without significantly relieving the suffering caused by the condition	No chance for cure, invasiveness of the treatment may prolong life but does not diminish or increases suffering
Child's life may be saved, but at the cost of physical and mental impairment that makes life intolerable for the child	Important to understand how child and family defines "intolerable life"
Additional treatment with potential benefit will cause further suffering	Burden of suffering outweighs the potential for benefit

Helping families identify and define what quality of life means to their child and to the family and what would be an intolerable life for the child is important. It is critical to present in a clear and understandable format the child's medical condition, test results, and the treatments that have been tried, what the expectations are for the child's ability to survive or function and interact with his environment, and

why it is believed that current or additional interventions will be futile or induce further suffering. These discussions should be conducted with sensitivity and without need for an immediate answer from the parents. It often takes several such discussions for families to come to a decision that they themselves will be able to live with and families should not be rushed into decision-making. The family may request additional testing or retesting to assure themselves they are making the right decision for their child. When feasible, these requests should be honored. Spiritual support may be very helpful to families during this process and should be offered.

Once the family has made the decision to withdraw support, it is helpful to explain what the anticipated course will be following withdrawal, what the child will likely look like during that time and what the plan of care will be to ensure comfort. Create a plan with the family for time and place of withdrawal, who they would like to be there with them, any specific requests for environment such as music, a favorite movie playing, or a book being read, and who they would like to perform the withdrawal. Offering the opportunity for rituals, prayer, or private time prior to or during the withdrawal is appropriate. If death is anticipated to happen quickly after withdrawal, any specific religious requirements for the body after death should be arranged in advance. In all cases of withdrawal, the family should be offered support during the process and after the death occurs.

ADVANCE CARE PLANNING

Advance care planning allows patients and families to make known their wishes about what to do in case of serious or life-threatening problems. Himelstein et al describe advance care planning as a four-step process. First, those individuals considered decision makers are identified and included in the process. Second, an assessment of the patient's and family's understanding of the illness and prognosis is made and the impending death is described in terms that the child and family can understand. Third, on the basis of their understanding of the illness and prognosis, the goals of care are determined regarding current and future intervention—curative, uncertain, or primarily focused on providing comfort. Finally, shared decisions about the current and future use or abandonment of life-sustaining techniques and aggressive medical interventions are made. In the event of a disagreement between parents or parents and their patient regarding these techniques or interventions, it may be prudent to involve the hospital's ethics committee in order to resolve these issues.

Some states permit parents to sign an advanced directive that asserts their decision not to have resuscitative attempts made in the event of a cardiac or respiratory arrest outside of the hospital. When an advanced directive is in place, emergency responders are not required to provide cardiopulmonary resuscitation (CPR) if called to the scene. Some school districts will respect an advanced directive on school property, many will not. If a child with an advanced directive in place wishes to go to school, a discussion between the medical team and school officials should be arranged to determine the best plan should the child have a cardiac or respiratory arrest at school.

Parents and, occasionally, the child may bring up the possibility of donating organs or body tissues after death. Although the tissues that may be donated by a child may be limited in some instances by the type of disease (eg, cancer), some parents find immense comfort in knowing their child was able to benefit another. If the parents have not discussed donation with the physician by the time of death and donation is possible, the physician should offer the opportunity to the family.

Autopsy is another subject many physicians find difficult to approach with a family, but it is an important option to discuss. In cases of anticipated death from natural causes, autopsies are generally not mandatory; however, information obtained from an autopsy may be useful for parental peace of mind or medical research. If death at home is to be followed by an autopsy, special arrangements for transporting and receiving the body will need to be made with the mortuary or the coroner.

REFERENCES

Amano K et al: Association between early palliative care referrals, inpatient hospice utilization, and aggressiveness of care at the end of life. J Palliat Med 2015 Mar;18(3);270–273 [PMID: 25210851].

Becker G, Blum HE: Novel opioid antagonists for opioid-induced bowel dysfunction and postoperative ileus. Lancet 2009; 373:1198 [PMID: 19217656].

Conner SC: Estimating the global need for palliative care for children: a cross-sectional analysis. J Pain Symptom Manage 2017 Feb; 53(2):171 [PMID: 27765706].

Goldman A et al (eds): Oxford Textbook of Palliative Care for Children. Oxford University Press; 2006.

Hanny C: Complementary and alternative medicine use in pediatric hematology/oncology patients at the University of Mississippi Medical Center. J Altern Complement Med 2015 Nov 11; 21:660–666.

Himelstein B et al: Pediatric palliative care. N Engl J Med 2004; 350:1752 [PMID: 15103002].

Kang T, Munson D, Klick J (eds): Pediatric palliative care. Pediatr Clin North Am 2007;54(5).

Knapp C, Thompson L: Factors associated with perceived barriers to pediatric palliative care: a survey of pediatricians in Florida and California. Palliat Med 2012;26(3);268–274 [PMID: 21680751].

Lindenfelser KJ, Hense C, McFerran K: Music therapy in pediatric palliative care: family-centered care to enhance quality of life. Am J Hosp Palliat Care 2012;29(3):219–226 [PMID: 22144660].

October T et al: The parent perspective: "Being a good parent" when making critical decisions in the PICU. Pediatr Crit Care Med 2014;15:291–298 [PMID: 24583502].

O'Shea ER, Kanarek RB: Understanding pediatric palliative care: what it is and what it should be. J Pediatr Oncol Nurs 2013;(30)1:34–44 [PMID: 23372039].

Ott M: Mind-body therapies for the pediatric oncology patient: matching the right therapy with the right patient. J Pediatr Oncol Nurs 2006;223(5):254–257 [PMID: 16902078].

Pirie A: Pediatric palliative care communication: resources for the clinical nurse specialist. Clin Nurse Spec 2012;26(4):212–215 [PMID: 22678187].

Post-White J, Fitzgerald M, Hageness S, Sencer S: Complementary and alternative medicine use in children with cancer and general and specialty pediatrics. J Pediatr Oncol Nurs 2009;26(1):715 [PMID: 18936292].

Thompson LA et al: Pediatricians' perceptions of and preferred timing for pediatric palliative care. Pediatrics 2009;123:e777 [PMID: 19403469].

Tomlinson D et al: Chemotherapy versus supportive care alone in pediatric palliative care for cancer: comparing the preferences of parents and health care professionals. CMAJ 2011;183(17): E1252–E1258 [PMID: 22007121].

Tournay AE: Withdrawal of medical treatment in children. West J Med 2000;173:407–411 [PMID: 11112760].

Weaver MS et al: Establishing psychosocial palliative care standards for children and adolescents with cancer and their families: an integrative review. Palliat Med 2016 Mar;30(3): 212–223 [PMID: 25921709].

Weigand D: In their own time: the family experience during the process of withdrawal of life-sustaining therapy. J Palliat Med 2008 Nov 8;11:1115–1121 [PMID: 18980452].

Widger K, Picot C: Parents' perceptions of the quality of pediatric and perinatal end-of-life care. Pediatr Nurs 2008;34(1):53–58 [PMID: 18361087].

Woodruff R (ed): Palliative Medicine. Oxford University Press; 2005.

Youngblut JM, Brooten D: Perinatal and pediatric issues in palliative and end-of-life care from the 2011 Summit on the Science of Compassion. Nurs Outlook 2012;60(6):343–350 [PMID: 23036690].

Web Resources

Education on Palliative and End of Life Care (EPEC; adult focused): www.epec.net.

End of Life Nursing Education Consortium (ELNEC): http://www. aacn.nche.edu/elnec.

Initiative for Pediatric Palliative Care (IPPC): www.ippcweb.org.

National Hospice and Palliative Care Organization (NHPCO)—Children's Project on Palliative/Hospice Services (ChiPPs): www.nhpco.org.

Immunodeficiency

Jordan K. Abbott, MD, MA

Pia J. Hauk, MD

INTRODUCTION

Immune deficiencies that present in childhood comprise rare disorders that have been characterized by a combination of clinical patterns, immunologic laboratory tests, and often molecular identification of the mutant gene. Children with Primary Immunodeficiency (PID) commonly present with recurrent and/or severe bacterial infections, failure to thrive, and/or developmental delay as a result of infection. Immunodeficiency should be considered when infections are recurrent, severe, persistent, resistant to standard treatment, or caused by opportunistic organisms. Because delayed diagnosis of PIDs is common, heightened diagnostic suspicion is warranted.

The human immune system consists of the phylogenetically more primitive innate immune system and the adaptive immune system. For the purpose of clinical categorization, PIDs are commonly divided into four main groups: antibody deficiencies, combined T- and B-cell immunodeficiencies, phagocyte disorders, and other deficiencies of the innate immunity, which include complement deficiencies. Understanding the role each part of the immune system plays in host defense allows critical evaluation for possible immunodeficiency as the cause of recurrent infections and immune dysregulation, which can lead to associated autoimmunity and chronic inflammation.

Picard C et al: International Union of Immunological Societies: 2017 Primary Immunodeficiency Diseases Committee Report on Inborn Errors of Immunity. J Clin Immunol 2018;38(1):96–128 [PMID: 29226302].

IMMUNODEFICIENCY EVALUATION: PRIMARY CONSIDERATIONS

When evaluating for a possible PID, other conditions that increase susceptibility to infections have to be considered, such as allergic rhinitis, asthma, cystic fibrosis, foreign body aspiration, and conditions that interfere with skin barrier function. Common causes of secondary or acquired immunodeficiency need to be excluded. These include malnutrition, aging, certain drugs (chemotherapy, immunosuppressive medications, glucocorticoids, disease-modifying antirheumatic drugs, rituximab), protein loss via gastroenteropathy or kidney disease, and other diseases associated with impaired immunity (bone marrow and blood cell malignancies, and certain chronic infections, including AIDS). If a single site is involved, anatomic defects and foreign bodies may be present. Figure 33–1 outlines when PIDs should be considered.

Key clinical patterns can indicate the presence of a PID and the category of immune impairment. PID should be considered in patients with frequent, severe, or unusual infections. When the infection history suggests PID, the type of infections can help guide the initial workup. Antibody, complement, and phagocyte defects predispose mainly to bacterial infections, but diarrhea, superficial candidiasis, opportunistic infections, and severe herpesvirus infections are more characteristic of T-lymphocyte immunodeficiency. Location of infection can provide important clues. Additional features such as the presence of autoimmunity, poor wound healing, lymphoproliferative disease, age of disease onset, and failure to thrive can help further categorize the PID. Table 33–1 classifies PID into four main host immunity categories based on age of onset, infections with specific pathogens, affected organs, and other special features.

Initial laboratory investigation should be directed by the clinical presentation and the suspected category of host immunity impairment. If antibody deficiency is suspected, a complete blood cell (CBC) count with cell differential and measurement of quantitative immunoglobulins (Igs) will identify most patients. If T-cell deficiency is suspected, lymphocyte phenotyping to quantify blood T cells, B cells, and natural killer (NK) cells should be sent. For phagocyte defects, testing of oxidative burst in stimulated granulocytes

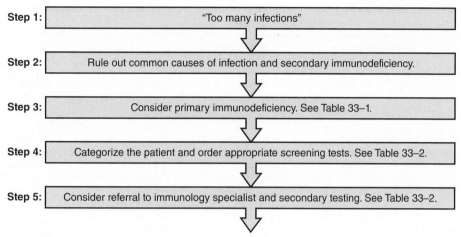

Step 1:	"Too many infections"
Step 2:	Rule out common causes of infection and secondary immunodeficiency.
Step 3:	Consider primary immunodeficiency. See Table 33–1.
Step 4:	Categorize the patient and order appropriate screening tests. See Table 33–2.
Step 5:	Consider referral to immunology specialist and secondary testing. See Table 33–2.

▲ **Figure 33–1.** General approach to primary immunodeficiencies.

should be performed. For complement deficiency, testing of the function of the classical and alternative pathway should be performed. Table 33–2 summarizes the approach to laboratory evaluation of PID.

Antibodies & Immunoglobulins

The initial laboratory screening for antibody deficiency includes the measurement of serum Igs: IgG, IgM, IgA, and IgE, which have age-dependent normal ranges (Table 33–3). By default, naïve B cells produce IgM, and production of the other isotypes requires further B-cell differentiation. When IgM but not other isotypes are present, a problem in B-cell differentiation is likely. When all Ig isotypes are decreased, an earlier defect in B-cell development should be suspected. Normal IgG, IgM, and IgA, and increased IgE levels usually indicate atopy. Elevated immunoglobulin levels are often seen in autoimmunity.

Some patients may have normal Ig levels but fail to make protective antibodies. Assessing the immunologic response to vaccination is therefore recommended. Specific IgG antibodies to protein antigens (tetanus, diphtheria, rubella, mumps) and protein-conjugated polysaccharide antigens (*Streptococcus pneumoniae, Haemophilus influenzae*) can be measured after routine immunization. To test the response to pure polysaccharide vaccine, Pneumovax®23 or Typhim Vi® can be administered. The response to polysaccharide antigens develops during the second year of life, but protein-conjugated vaccines elicit an earlier response in immunocompetent children. The gold standard is comparison of pre- and postimmunization titers.

If an initial screen reveals very low concentrations of Ig isotypes, further studies are aimed at identifying the cause of immunoglobulin deficiency. Certain types of hypogammaglobulinemia are characterized by low levels of

or absent B lymphocytes, such as X-linked Bruton agammaglobulinemia. Serum albumin should be measured in patients with hypogammaglobulinemia to exclude secondary deficiencies due to protein loss through bowel or kidneys. IgG or IgA subclass measurements may be abnormal in patients with varied immunodeficiency syndromes and malignancies but they are rarely helpful in an initial evaluation.

T Lymphocytes

The initial laboratory screening for a T-lymphocyte deficiency includes a CBC with cell differential to evaluate for a decreased absolute lymphocyte count (< 1000/μL) and enumeration of absolute numbers of T cells and their subsets, B cells, and NK cells (see Table 33–2). T-cell function can be analyzed by in vitro lymphocyte proliferation. Borderline function must be interpreted based on clinical correlation. T-lymphocyte function is often also studied in vivo by delayed hypersensitivity skin tests to specific antigens, including *Candida albicans*, tetanus, or mumps, but a negative result is not helpful, as it may be due to young age, chronic illness, vitamin D deficiency, or poor test technique. T-lymphocyte deficiencies will often not manifest as skin-test anergy until the impairment is severe, for example, as in AIDS. It is important to evaluate a patient's specific antibody production because proper B-lymphocyte function and antibody production are dependent on adequate T-lymphocyte function. Therefore, most T-lymphocyte deficiencies manifest as combined T- and B-lymphocyte deficiencies.

Phagocyte Immunity

Phagocyte defects typically involve reduction in phagocyte numbers or defects in phagocyte function. The initial laboratory screening for phagocyte disorders, mainly impaired

Table 33–1. Clinical features of primary immunodeficiencies.

Characteristic	Combined Deficiency (T- and B-Lymphocyte Defect)	Antibody Deficiency (B-Lymphocyte Defect)	Phagocyte Defect	Complement Defect
Age at onset of infections	Early onset, usually before 6 mo	Onset after maternal antibodies decline, usually after 3–6 mo; some later in childhood or adults	Early onset	Any age
Specific pathogens	**Bacteria:** *Streptococcus pneumoniae, Campylobacter fetus, Staphylococcus aureus, Haemophilus influenzae, Pseudomonas aeruginosa, Mycoplasma hominis, Ureaplasma urealyticum, Listeria monocytogenes, Salmonella* spp, enteric flora, atypical mycobacteria, and BCG **Viruses:** CMV, EBV, varicella, RSV, enterovirus, rotavirus **Fungi/protozoa:** *Candida albicans, Aspergillus fumigatus, Toxoplasma gondii* **Other:** *Pneumocystis carinii, Cryptosporidium*	**Bacteria:** *S pneumoniae, C fetus, H influenzae, P aeruginosa, U urealyticum, S aureus, M hominis* **Viruses:** Enteroviruses **Fungi/protozoa:** *Giardia lamblia*	**Bacteria:** *S aureus,* enteric flora, *Burkholderia* spp, *Aspergillus* spp, *P aeruginosa, Salmonella* spp, *Serratia* spp, *Nocardia asteroides, Klebsiella* spp, nontuberculous mycobacteria, and BCG **Viruses:** None **Fungi/protozoa:** *C albicans, A fumigatus*	**Bacteria:** *Neisseria meningitidis* and *gonorrhoeae, S pneumoniae, S aureus, P aeruginosa, H influenzae* **Viruses:** None **Fungi/protozoa:** None Common
Affected organs and infections	**General:** Failure to thrive **Infections:** Severe infections (meningitis, septicemia, sinopulmonary), recurrent candidiasis, protracted diarrhea	**Infections:** Recurrent sinopulmonary, pneumonia, meningitis **GI:** Chronic malabsorption, IBD-like symptoms **Other:** Arthritis	**Skin:** Dermatitis, abscesses, cellulitis **Lymph nodes:** Suppurative adenitis **Oral cavity:** Periodontitis, ulcers **Lungs:** Pneumonia, abscesses **Other:** Liver and brain abscesses, osteomyelitis	**Infections:** Meningitis, disseminated gonococcal infection, septicemia, pneumonia
Special features	GVHD from maternal T cells or blood product transfusion Disseminated infection after BCG or live polio immunization Absent lymphoid tissue Absent thymic shadow on chest radiograph	Autoimmunity Lymphoreticular malignancy Postvaccination polio Chronic enteroviral encephalitis	Poor wound healing Pyloric and urethral stenosis, IBD	**Autoimmune disorders:** SLE, vasculitis, dermatomyositis, scleroderma, glomerulonephritis **Other:** Hereditary angioedema, aHUS

aHUS, atypical hemolytic uremic syndrome; BCG, bacille Calmette-Guérin; CMV, cytomegalovirus; EBV, Epstein-Barr virus; GVHD, graft-versus-host disease; IBD, inflammatory bowel disease; RSV, respiratory syncytial virus; SLE, systemic lupus erythematosus.

neutrophil function, should include a CBC and cell differential to look for neutropenia. A blood smear can detect Howell-Jolly bodies in erythrocytes, indicative of asplenia, and abnormalities in lysosomal granules in neutrophils. An abnormality of the neutrophil respiratory burst, which would lead to impaired neutrophil bactericidal activity, can be tested by flow cytometric analysis of stimulated neutrophils pre-loaded with dihydrorhodamine (DHR). Leukocyte adhesion molecules can be studied by flow cytometry. Assays to study neutrophil phagocytosis of bacteria and phagocytic

microbicidal activity are available in specialized laboratories. The clinical symptom pattern that suggests a possible defect of phagocytic cell function should dictate which tests are used.

Complement Pathways (Figure 33–2)

Testing for total hemolytic complement activity with the CH50 assay screens for most diseases of the complement system that increase susceptibility to infection. A normal

Table 33–2. Laboratory evaluation for primary immunodeficiency.

Suspected Defect	Screening Evaluation	Specialist Evaluation
B lymphocyte	• CBC with differential • Quantitative immunoglobulins	• T-cell, B-cell, and NK-cell enumeration • Extended phenotyping of B cells • IgG levels to immunization antigens • DNA analysis for specific genetic mutations
T lymphocyte	• CBC with differential • Quantitative immunoglobulins • T-cell, B-cell, and NK-cell enumeration	• Extended phenotyping of T cells • Lymphocyte proliferation to mitogens and antigens • Delayed-type hypersensitivity skin test • Cytotoxicity studies • ADA or PNP levels of RBC • DNA analysis for specific genetic mutations
Phagocyte	• CBC with differential	• DHR flow cytometry assay • Nitroblue tetrazolium reduction assay • Bactericidal assays • CD11/18 analysis • Chemotaxis assay
Complement	• CH50 • AH50	• Complement component levels • Complement component function • Complement antibodies

ADA, adenosine deaminase; CBC, complete blood cell count; CD, cluster of differentiation; DHR, dihydrorhodamine; HIV, human immunodeficiency virus; NK, natural killer; PNP, purine nucleoside phosphorylase; RBC, red blood cell; WBC, white blood cell.
Adapted with permission from Cunningham-Rundles C: Immune deficiency: office evaluation and treatment. Allergy Asthma Proc 2003 Nov-Dec;24(6):409–415.

Table 33–3. Normal values for immunoglobulins by age.

Age	IgG (mg/dL)	IgM (mg/dL)	IgA (mg/dL)
Newborn	1031 ± 200	11 ± 7	2 ± 3
1–3 mo	430 ± 119	30 ± 11	21 ± 13
4–6 mo	427 ± 186	43 ± 17	28 ± 18
7–12 mo	661 ± 219	55 ± 23	37 ± 18
13–24 mo	762 ± 209	58 ± 23	50 ± 24
25–36 mo	892 ± 183	61 ± 19	71 ± 34
3–5 y	929 ± 228	56 ± 18	93 ± 27
6–8 y	923 ± 256	65 ± 25	124 ± 45
9–11 y	1124 ± 235	79 ± 33	131 ± 60
12–16 y	946 ± 124	59 ± 20	148 ± 63
Adults	1158 ± 305	99 ± 27	200 ± 61

Adapted with permission from Stiehm ER, Ochs HD, Winklestein JA, et al: *Immunologic Disorders of Infants and Children,* 5th ed. St. Louis, MO: Elsevier; 2004.

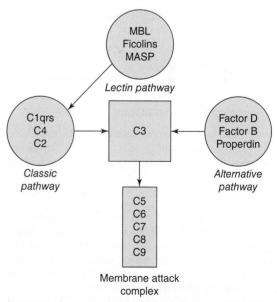

▲ **Figure 33–2.** Pathways of complement activation and the central functional role of C3. MASP, MBL-associated serine protease; MBL, mannose-binding lectin.

CH50 titer depends on the ability of all 11 components of the classic pathway and membrane attack complex to interact and then lyse antibody-coated sheep erythrocytes. Alternative complement pathway deficiencies are identified by subnormal lysis of rabbit erythrocytes in the AH50 assay. For both assays, the patient's serum must be separated and frozen at −70°C within 30–60 minutes after collection to prevent loss of activity. Measuring levels of individual components is not necessary when both CH50 and AH50 are normal. If both the CH50 and AH50 are low, a deficiency in their shared terminal pathway (C3, C5, C6, C7, C8, or C9) would be the most common explanation. If the CH50 is low but the AH50 is normal, the deficiency must affect C1, C4, or C2. If the AH50 is low but the CH50 is normal, a deficiency in factor D or B or properdin should be suspected. Most quantitative deficiencies of complement components result from pathway activation and resultant consumption. It is therefore essential that complement activation be ruled out prior to diagnosing an inherited complement deficiency.

SEVERE COMBINED IMMUNODEFICIENCY DISEASES

ESSENTIALS OF DIAGNOSIS & TYPICAL FEATURES

► Onset in first year of life.
► Recurrent infections caused by bacteria, viruses, fungi, and opportunistic pathogens.
► Chronic diarrhea and failure to thrive.
► Absent lymphoid tissue.

► General Considerations

Severe combined immunodeficiency disease (SCID) is a group of rare immunologic disorders with the defining characteristic of severe deficiency of T-cell function and/or number. Due to the centrality of T cells in the immune system, the severity of T-cell deficit results in widespread immunologic dysfunction and broad susceptibility to infection. Left untreated, SCID uniformly results in death before the first year of life. The treatment approach varies depending on the underlying molecular defect, but for the majority of patients with SCID, the optimal treatment is hematopoietic stem cell transplantation (HSCT). Transplant outcomes are favorable if performed within the first 3 months of life, or if performed prior to the onset of SCID-associated chronic infections. Newborn screening of dried blood spots for evidence of T-cell deficiency occurs universally in the United States and internationally to identify and treat these patients soon after birth. Suspected SCID is a medical emergency,

and both the necessary steps to confirm diagnosis and the initiation of treatment must be performed rapidly.

► Clinical Findings

A. Symptoms and Signs

SCID frequently presents with opportunistic, unusual, and persistent infection. Common organisms include but are not limited to *Pneumocystis jirovecii*, candidiasis, and cytomegalovirus. In the absence of an identified microorganism, SCID may present with any combination of the following: failure to thrive, chronic diarrhea, or unexplained chronic respiratory illness. Physical examination is notable for a lack of lymphoid tissue, including tonsils and lymph nodes. A chest radiograph usually demonstrates an absent thymic shadow.

B. Laboratory Findings

The characteristic feature of SCID is the deficiency in production of T cells by the host. Endogenous production of T cells can be verified by quantifying T-cell receptor rearrangement excision circles (TRECs) in blood or by measuring the expression of CD31 on peripheral blood T cells. The presence of normal numbers of lymphocytes in a CBC or even normal numbers of CD3 T cells does not rule out SCID because of the possibility of either maternally derived T-cell populations or abnormally expanded endogenous T-cell populations with severely limited diversity. Associated laboratory findings can include decreases in numbers of NK cells and B cells, poor lymphocyte proliferative response to mitogens, and low immunoglobulin levels. Genetic testing should be pursued to confirm the diagnosis; although, treatment should not be delayed while awaiting results of genetic testing. Known genetic etiologies of SCID are listed in Table 33–4.

► Differential Diagnosis

The differential diagnosis of SCID must be carefully considered as misdiagnosis could potentially result in unwarranted HSCT. Disorders that result in either the abnormal loss or the compartmentalization of lymphatic fluid such as chylothorax, lymphangiectasia, gastroschisis, and omphalocele can result in the apparent absence of endogenously generated T cells even though they are actually being normally produced. HIV disease can result in severe deficiency of CD4 T cells and the same infections seen in SCID. Prematurity can be associated with abnormally low TREC levels but these levels ultimately increase with increasing gestational age.

► Treatment

A variety of therapies are used in the treatment of SCID. These therapies include HSCT, gene therapy, thymus transplant, and enzyme replacement. Choice of therapy

Table 33–4. Severe combined immunodeficiency classification.

	Genes Containing Defects	Likely Etiology	Characteristic Features
Defective T-cell development			
• **Defective IL7R signaling**	*IL2RG, IL7RA, JAK3*	IL-7 signaling is essential for T-cell development.	• *IL2RG-* and *JAK3*-deficiency have associated absence of NK cells and functional B-cell deficiency.
• **Defective T-cell receptor (TCR) signaling**	*ZAP70, PTPRC, CD3D, CD3G, CD3E*	TCR signaling is essential for T-cell development.	• *ZAP70* has apparent deficiency of only CD8 T cells but CD4 T cells are also nonfunctional. • B cells are not affected.
• **RAG-recombination defect**	*RAG1, RAG2*	Functional TCR is not formed.	• Both B and T cells are deficient. NK cells are unaffected.
• **NHEJ-recombination defect**	*LIG4, NHEJ1, DCLRE1C, PRKDC*	Functional TCR is not formed.	• Both B and T cells are deficient. NK cells are unaffected. • Body wide sensitivity to radiation toxicity • Can be associated with microcephaly and other syndromic features
• **Absent thymus function**	22q11 deletion, CHARGE syndrome, *FOXN1*	Thymus is essential for T-cell development.	• B cell counts generally are not affected. • *FOXN1* deficiency is associated with nail dysplasia.
Impaired T-cell survival			
• **Impaired purine salvage**	*ADA, PNP*	Toxic metabolites	• B cell, T cell, and NK cells deficient
• **Dyskeratosis congenita** (Hoyeraal-Hreidarsson Syndrome)	*DKC1, ACD* (TPP1), *TINF2, TERT, RTEL1*	Telomere maintenance is severely defective.	• Associated IUGR and cerebellar hypoplasia
• **Reticular dysgenesis**	*AK2*	Possible cellular energy imbalance	• Associated with agranulocytosis and deficiency of all lymphocytes, but normal erythrocyte and platelet formation
• **One-carbon pathway**	*TCN2, MTHFD1*	Unclear	• Associated neurodegenerative defect • Megaloblastic anemia • Patients improve with adequate supplementation
• **Ribosomal defect**	*RMRP*	Unclear	• Associated with short-limb dwarfism
Impaired T-cell function			
• **Ca²⁺-signaling defect**	*STIM1, ORAI1*	IL-7 signaling is essential for T-cell development	• *IL2RG-* and *JAK3*-deficiency have associated absence of NK cells and functional B-cell deficiency.
• **Antigens to cells**	*CD3G, CD3E*	Impaired T-cell development and signal transduction	• B cells are not affected.

depends upon the specific genetic defect, age at diagnosis, access to a suitable HSCT donor, and comorbidities. To optimize the outcome of any chosen definitive therapy, concerted effort must be made to prevent clinical deterioration in the waiting period. Antimicrobial prophylaxis should be initiated with the aim of preventing pulmonary infection with *Pneumocystis*, as well as other fungal pathogens. Antiviral prophylaxis can be considered as well. Replacement Ig therapy should be initiated. Patients with suspected SCID should only be transfused with CMV-negative, irradiated blood products, and they should not receive any live vaccines. If the patient has received BCG vaccination, specific therapy should be considered. Isolation precautions should be initiated. Until we understand more about CMV-transmission in CMV-positive mothers, breast-feeding should be discouraged. Additional precautions can be tailored based on the individual risk factor of the patient.

Kelty WJ et al: The role of breast-feeding in cytomegalovirus transmission and hematopoietic stem cell transplant outcomes in infants with severe combined immunodeficiency. J Allergy Clin Immunol Pract 2019 Jun 5;7(8):2863–2865.e3. doi: 10.1016/j.jaip.2019.05.041 [PMID: 31326381].

SCID CLASSIFICATION

▶ Defective T-Cell Development

T cells develop in a multiple-stage process fostered by supporting cells and directive cytokines. Problems with the production or sensing of these developmental signals can result in a severe deficit of T-cell number.

Deficiency in the formation of a functionally rearranged T-cell receptor and DNA repair mechanisms results in absence of T cells, the latter also being associated with radiation sensitivity. Primary absence of the thymus prevents development of mature T cells in severe presentations of 22q11 deletion syndrome, CHARGE syndrome, and deficiency of *FOXN1*.

▶ Impaired T-Cell Survival

Impaired T-cell survival is seen in deficiency of both adenosine deaminase (ADA) and purine nucleoside phosphorylase (PNP), as well as reticular dysgenesis and dyskeratosis congenita. ADA and PNP are components of purine salvage in lymphocytes, and loss of these enzymes results in buildup of toxic purine by-products. Dyskeratosis congenita results from abnormal telomere maintenance and results in survival defects in hematologic cells. Reticular dysgenesis is possibly the most severe form of combined immunodeficiency as a result of increased apoptosis of myeloid and lymphoid precursors. It is associated with sensorineural deafness. Defects in the one-carbon pathway can also result in severe deficiency of hematopoietic cells.

▶ Impaired T-Cell Function

Few syndromes have been identified where T cells mature normally despite a residual impairment in T-cell receptor (TCR) signaling that results in susceptibility to infections typically seen in T-cell deficiency syndromes. In *STIM1* and *ORAI1* deficiency, defective mobilization of store-operated calcium channels results in inadequate activation of peripheral T cells despite normal numbers. In MHC Class II deficiency, normal T cells are unable to respond to antigen because it is not presented by antigen presenting cells.

Omenn Syndrome

Omenn syndrome is a presentation of SCID caused by residual autoreactive T cells in the absence of T-cell immune competence. The syndrome can include severe rash, failure to thrive, splenomegaly, diarrhea, eosinophilia, and elevated IgE in association with typical infections seen in conventional SCID. T-cell numbers are elevated, but detailed phenotyping reveals the majority of T cells to have a memory phenotype (CD45RO-positive). Omenn syndrome has been tied to mutations in genes known to cause conventional SCID,

arising in part due to mutation-specific factors and partly due to the individual susceptibility of the patient. A similar clinical presentation occurs in SCID patients who have engrafted maternal T cells.

OTHER COMBINED IMMUNODEFICIENCIES

ESSENTIALS OF DIAGNOSIS & TYPICAL FEATURES

▶ Varying severity of immunodeficiency.
▶ Onset of signs and symptoms of immunodeficiency may be delayed.
▶ Often associated with defined genetic syndromes.

▶ General Considerations

Combined immunodeficiencies include all defects that directly impair both T and B lymphocytes, as well as T lymphocyte-specific defects that affect B-lymphocyte function and antibody production. In contrast to SCID, the severity of the immunodeficiency varies, depending on the underlying cause. Several described genetic syndromes have associated combined immunodeficiency that is often identified after the syndrome has been diagnosed. In some cases, the immune defect may not be the major presenting clinical problem. Examples of well-described syndromes with combined immunodeficiencies are described below.

1. **DiGeorge syndrome or 22q11.2 deletion syndrome** is an AD syndrome, resulting in defective development of the third and fourth pharyngeal pouches. There is considerable variability in phenotype based on the location and extent of the deletion, but deletions that include the *TBX1* gene appear relevant. Overlapping syndromes include velocardiofacial syndrome and Shprintzen syndrome. The incidence is about 1:4000 births, and the abnormal chromosome is usually inherited from the mother. The associated immunodeficiency is secondary to the aplastic or hypoplastic thymus, where T-lymphocyte maturation occurs. Surprisingly, most patients have no or only mild immune defects. The term *partial DiGeorge syndrome* is commonly applied to these patients with impaired rather than absent thymic function. Clinical characteristics include congenital heart defects, hypocalcemia due to hypoparathyroidism, distinctive craniofacial features, renal anomalies, and thymic hypoplasia. Presentation usually results from cardiac failure or hypocalcemia 24–48 hours postpartum. The diagnosis is sometimes made during the course of cardiac surgery when no thymus is found

in the mediastinum. Infections commonly present as recurrent ENT (ear-nose-throat) infections. Additional important clinical issues include delayed speech, cognitive impairment, and behavioral problems. Patients have an increased risk to develop schizophrenia and autoimmune disorders. Laboratory evaluation typically reveals normal to decreased numbers of T lymphocytes with preserved T-lymphocyte function and normal B-lymphocyte function. In the rare patient with absent or dysfunctional T lymphocytes, B-lymphocyte function and antibody production may be abnormal. Over time, T-lymphocyte numbers normalize in the majority of patients who have low numbers of T lymphocytes at initial presentation. The diagnosis is confirmed via fluorescence in situ hybridization (FISH) chromosomal analysis for the microdeletion on chromosome 22, or microarray-based comparative genomic hybridization. Treatment of the 22q11.2 deletion syndrome may require surgery for cardiac defects, and vitamin D, calcium, or parathyroid hormone replacement to correct hypocalcemia and treat seizures. Transfusion products should be irradiated. Both thymic grafts and BMT have been used successfully in patients with absent T-lymphocyte immunity. Prior to giving live vaccines, T-cell numbers and function should be assessed if not done earlier, to prevent vaccine-related side effects.

2. **Ataxia telangiectasia (AT)** is a rare, neurodegenerative, AR-inherited disorder caused by mutations in the ataxia-telangiectasia–mutated (*ATM*) gene located on chromosome 11q22–23 that encodes the ATM protein, a protein kinase involved in repair of double-stranded DNA and cell cycle regulation. AT is characterized by progressive cerebellar ataxia, telangiectasia, and variable immunodeficiency. Children usually present as toddlers with slurred speech and balance problems, and also with sinus and pulmonary infections. Telangiectasias of the conjunctivae and exposed areas (eg, nose, ears, and shoulders) follow later during childhood. Respiratory tract infections promoted by respiratory muscle weakness, swallowing dysfunction and recurrent aspirations, and malignancies, including carcinomas and lymphomas, are the major causes of death between the second and fourth decade of life. Abnormal findings in AT include elevated serum α-fetoprotein levels that increase over time and are used diagnostically; immunoglobulin deficiencies, including low levels of IgA, IgE, or IgG; and defective ability to repair radiation-induced DNA fragmentation. There is no definitive treatment, although Ig replacement and aggressive antibiotics have been used with limited success. Heterozygotes have an increased risk for breast cancer. Similarly to AT, the **Nijmegen breakage** syndrome is a disorder associated with impaired DNA repair and mutations in the *NBS1* gene that shows more severe clinical features, including microcephaly and facial dysmorphisms, small stature, immunodeficiency, and increased risk for lymphoid malignancies.

3. **Immunodeficiency due to mutations in the gene for nuclear factor-κB (NF-κB)–essential modulator (NEMO; *IKBKG* gene)** is an XL syndrome in which male patients manifest ectodermal dysplasia (abnormal, conical teeth, fine sparse hair, and abnormal or absent sweat glands) and defects of T and B lymphocytes. NF-κB is involved in signaling through CD40 on B cells, and NEMO mutations result in abnormal immune-receptor signaling. Many mutations are fatal in utero for male infants. Female carriers may have incontinentia pigmenti. Surviving males present with early serious infections, including opportunistic infections with *P jirovecii* and atypical mycobacteria. Laboratory evaluation reveals hypogammaglobulinemia that may present as HIGM syndrome and poor specific antibody production, but normal numbers of T and B lymphocytes. Functional evaluation of lymphocytes demonstrates variable response. Because patients with confirmed NEMO mutations are quite rare, the best treatment course is unknown, but aggressive antibiotic therapy in combination with Ig replacement as well as HSCT has been used. The prognosis is dependent on the severity of immunodeficiency, with most deaths due to infection. Mutations in the *NF-κBIA* gene that encodes IκBα (nuclear factor of kappa light polypeptide gene enhancer in B-cell inhibitor alpha) result in an AD-inherited defect with similar clinical presentation.

4. **Major histocompatibility complex class I and II (MHC I, MHC II) deficiency or bare lymphocyte syndrome** are AR-combined immunodeficiencies. Patients with MHC I deficiency have abnormal expression of the transporter associated with antigen processing (TAP). TAP proteins are important for intracellular transport and expression of MHC I on cell surfaces. Patients with bare lymphocyte syndrome type I present with recurrent sinus and pulmonary as well as skin infections. The diagnosis is confirmed by demonstrating an absence of MHC I expression. In MHC II deficiency, cells lack MHC II expression due to mutations in *CIITA*, *RFX-5*, *RFXAP*, or *RFXANK* genes. Clinical presentation includes recurrent viral, bacterial, and fungal infections. Patients with bare lymphocyte syndrome type II have normal numbers of T and B lymphocytes, but low CD4+ lymphocyte numbers, abnormal lymphocyte function, and hypogammaglobulinemia. They also have a high incidence of sclerosing cholangitis. When this diagnosis is suspected, demonstration of absent MHC II molecules confirms the disorder. Severe cases are fatal without

HSCT, but milder phenotypes may be managed with Ig replacement and aggressive use of antibiotics.

5. **Cartilage-hair hypoplasia** is an AR form of chondrodysplasia manifesting with short-limbed short stature, hypoplastic hair, defective immunity, and poor erythrogenesis. The immune defect is characterized by mild to moderate lymphopenia and abnormal lymphocyte function, but normal antibody function. Affected patients have increased susceptibility to infections and increased risk of lymphoma. The disorder results from mutation in the *RMRP* gene that encodes the RNA component of an RNase MRP complex. BMT can restore cell-mediated immunity but does not correct the cartilage or hair abnormalities.

6. **WHIM (Warts, Hypogammaglobulinemia, Infection, Myelokathexis) syndrome** is a rare AD immunodeficiency caused by gain-of-function mutations in the gene encoding the chemokine receptor CXCR4. Patients have an increased susceptibility to viral infections (including HPV, EBV, and HSV) and recurrent bacterial infections. Laboratory evaluation reveals peripheral blood neutropenia with bone marrow hypercellularity, decreased B-cell numbers and hypogammaglobulinemia, and T-cell lymphopenia with normal CD4$^+$/CD8$^+$ ratio.

7. **Bloom syndrome** is characterized by growth retardation, microcephaly, sun-sensitive rashes, and telangiectasias of the face. The syndrome results from mutations in the *Blm* gene that encodes a RecQ-helicase involved in DNA repair.

8. **Immunodeficiency, centromeric instability, facial anomalies (ICF) syndrome** is a rare AR condition caused by abnormal DNA methyltransferase. In half of the patients, a mutation can be detected in the *DNMT3B* gene. Affected patients have severe respiratory, gastrointestinal, and skin infections due to low or absent immunoglobulins and abnormal T-lymphocyte numbers and function.

9. **Trisomy 21** or **Down syndrome** is associated with increased susceptibility to respiratory infection. Immunodeficiency is variable, and abnormal numbers and function of T and B lymphocytes have been reported. Additionally, patients have an increased incidence of autoimmune diseases.

10. **Turner syndrome** (partial or complete absence of one X chromosome) is associated with increased risk of otitis media, respiratory infections, and malignancies. Immune defects are variable but may include abnormal T-lymphocyte numbers and function and hypogammaglobulinemia.

11. Characterized by partial albinism, neutropenia, thrombocytopenia, and lymphohistiocytosis, **Griscelli syndrome** is a rare AR syndrome resulting from mutations in the myosin *VA* gene. Affected patients have recurrent and serious infections caused by fungi, viruses, and bacteria. Immunologic evaluation demonstrates variable immunoglobulin levels and antibody function with impaired T-lymphocyte function. BMT can correct the immunodeficiency.

12. **Hyper-IgE Syndrome (HIES)**, also known as *Job syndrome*, is a rare PID characterized by elevated levels of IgE (> 2000 IU/mL), neonatal eczematoid rash, recurrent infections with *Staphylococcus aureus*, recurrent pneumonia with pneumatocele formation, and typical facies. Mutations in a specific transcription factor, signal transducer and activator of transcription 3 (*STAT3*), underlie sporadic and AD forms of HIES. Additional clinical findings of HIES include retained primary teeth, scoliosis, hyperextensibility, high palate, and osteoporosis. In addition to staphylococcal infections, affected patients also have increased incidence of infections due to *Streptococcus* spp, *Pseudomonas* spp, *C albicans*, and even opportunistic infections with *P jirovecii*. AR HIES is associated with mutations in dedicator of cytokinesis 8 (*DOCK8*) and tyrosine kinase 2 (*TYK2*) genes. Patients with AR HIES have an increased susceptibility to viral infections, including recurrent molluscum contagiosum, warts, and herpes simplex infections. Increased susceptibility to mycobacterial infections is found in patients with *TYK2* mutations. Laboratory evaluation reveals normal to profoundly elevated levels of IgE and occasionally eosinophilia. However, atopic dermatitis and parasite infection are much more common causes of elevated IgE. Diagnosis is often difficult due to variable presentation, which may become progressively severe with increasing age, but genetic testing for *STAT3*, *DOCK8*, and *TYK2* mutations will help confirm the diagnosis of HIES particularly at a young age. All patients with HIES have impaired T$_H$17 cell function, and measurement of T$_H$17+ cells in the peripheral blood can be used as screening test if HIES is suspected. The mainstay of treatment is prophylactic and symptomatic antibiotic use in combination with good skin care. Ig replacement has been used with some success to decrease infections and possibly modify IgE levels. Successful stem cell transplants have been conducted in DOCK8 deficiency.

Abolhassani H et al: Clinical, immunologic, and genetic spectrum of 696 patients with combined immunodeficiency. *J Allergy Clin Immunol* 2018;141(4):1450–1458 [PMID: 28916186].

Puck JM: Newborn screening for severe combined immunodeficiency and T-cell lymphopenia. Immunol Rev 2019;287(1): 241–252 [PMID: 30565242].

ANTIBODY DEFICIENCY SYNDROMES

ESSENTIALS OF DIAGNOSIS & TYPICAL FEATURES

▶ Recurrent bacterial infections, typically due to encapsulated pyogenic bacteria.

▶ Low immunoglobulin levels.

▶ Inability to make specific antibodies to vaccine antigens or infections.

▶ General Considerations

Antibody deficiency syndromes include both congenital and acquired forms of hypogammaglobulinemia with low levels of one or more of the immunoglobulins IgM, IgG, and IgA. As a group, antibody deficiencies represent nearly half of all PIDs. They can be divided into (1) defects of B-cell development, (2) defects in Ig class switching, and (3) functional B-cell deficiency. Table 33–5 outlines primary antibody deficiency syndromes, laboratory findings, and genetic inheritance in these disorders.

▶ Clinical Findings

A. Symptoms and Signs

For patients with antibody deficiency, specific infectious susceptibility and other features of immune dysregulation are dependent upon the specific cause of antibody deficiency. In isolated early B-cell development defects, such as X-linked agammaglobulinemia, infections are limited to encapsulated bacteria, mycoplasma species, and enterovirus species. In the class-switching defect caused by defective CD40L, infectious susceptibility can include *Pneumocystis* and *Cryptosporidium*, whereas class-switching defects caused by absence of AICDA or UNG can include lymphoproliferation and autoimmunity. Functional defects in B cells or B-cell activation, such as in combined immunodeficiency syndromes or common variable immunodeficiency (CVID) syndromes will include infectious susceptibility dependent on the underlying molecular defect. Antibody deficiency therefore represents a broad and somewhat heterogeneous grouping whose individual features depend on the root cause of immune abnormality.

Independent of underlying cause, untreated antibody deficiency results in typical infections. Pulmonary infection can be severe and chronic, resulting in bronchiectasis or other permanent lung damage. Severe pulmonary infections are generally preceded by chronic, recurrent middle ear and sinus infections. Additional infections can include bacteremia, bacterial meningitis, skin infection, and joint infection.

Other sites of infection can arise depending on the underlying genetic defect.

B. Laboratory Findings

Numerous blood tests are available for the investigation of antibody production. Serum immunoglobulin levels are routinely tested and reference values are widely accessible. Antibodies to a particular antigen are measured to ensure that antibody production is specific. For instance, the amount of antibody to tetanus toxoid is frequently measured because the tetanus toxoid vaccine is routinely administered in developed countries. Vaccine titers to pneumococcal serotypes are frequently measured following vaccination with the unconjugated polysaccharide *S pneumoniae* vaccine. The increase in titers represents the ability of B cells to form antibodies in the absence of T-cell costimulation. Production of allo-specific IgM to red-cell antigens is also a measure of T-cell–independent antibody formation. When abnormalities are detected in immunoglobulin levels or antibody production, lymphocyte surface phenotyping may reveal additional aspects of the underlying abnormality, such as B- or T-cell deficiency.

The characteristic feature of antibody deficiency is the absence or severe deficiency of one of the three predominant immunoglobulins found in blood, IgG, IgA, or IgM. All three immunoglobulin isotypes are severely reduced in early B-cell development defects; although, IgG deficiency is rarely seen in children younger than 4 months due to the presence of placentally transferred maternal IgG. In class switching defects, IgM production can be normal or elevated, whereas production of IgG and IgA is deficient. In functional B-cell deficiencies, a combination of antibody production abnormalities may be detected. For instance, CVID is defined by the combination of poor vaccine response and a decrease in blood levels of IgG in conjunction with a severe decrease in levels of either IgM or IgA, or a decrease of both.

Blood cell abnormalities also vary according to the underlying cause of antibody deficiency. Many early B-cell development defects are limited to the B-cell compartment, and as a result, B-cell numbers are severely reduced, but levels of other blood cells are usually within normal limits. In class switching defects, peripheral B-cell numbers will also approach normal levels. On the other hand, functional antibody deficiency can arise in any combination of deficiency of specific lymphocyte subsets and other blood cells. For these deficiencies, the underlying genetic abnormality is most relevant to understand the resulting hematologic abnormality.

▶ Differential Diagnosis

The differential diagnosis of antibody deficiency includes secondary causes of decreased amount of immunoglobulin in the peripheral blood. Several medications are known to

Table 33–5. Antibody deficiency disorders.

	Genes Containing Defects	Likely Etiology	Characteristic Features
Defects in B-cell development			
• Defect in developmental signal	*TCF3, IKZF1, LRRC8A*	Commitment to B-cell lineage affected	• Peripheral B cells < 2% of lymphocyte count
• Defect in pre–B-cell receptor (BCR)	*IGHM, IGLL1, CD79A, CD79B,*	B-cell development requires functional pre-BCR.	• Peripheral B cells < 2% of lymphocyte count
• Defect in pre-BCR downstream signaling	*BLNK, BTK*	Pre-BCR signaling inadequate to support further development	• Peripheral B cells < 2% of lymphocyte count
• Block at Transitional B-cell stage	*CARD11*	Unclear	• Normal total B-cell numbers with decreased maturation beyond the transitional B-cell stage • Regulatory T-cell numbers reduced
Class-switching defects			
• Defect in CD40L-CD40 interaction	*CD40L, CD40*	CD40L signal initiates class switching	• Typically high IgM levels • No germinal centers • Susceptible to some typical T-cell deficiency-associated infections such as pneumocystis pneumonia and cryptosporidial infection • Associated with biliary malignancy possibly from chronic infection
• Defect in genomic rearrangement	*AICDA, UNG*	Rearrangement of the IgH constant region is defective	• Normal B-cell numbers • Associated with significant autoimmunity • Large germinal center reactions because proliferative signaling remains intact
• Varied	*IKBKG, IKBA, PIK3CD*	Unclear	• Usually associated with predominant T-cell abnormalities
Functional antibody deficiency			
• Common variable immunodeficiency (CVID)	Unknown	Heterogeneous	• Normal or low IgM, low IgG, low IgA, poor specific antibody production
• Monogenetic syndromes previously characterized as CVID	*ICOS, CD19, TNFRSF13B, TNFRSF13C, CD20, CD81, CD225*	Impaired signaling through B-cell coreceptors	• Normal or low IgM, low IgG, low IgA, poor specific antibody production
• Combined immunodeficiency syndromes	*CD21, CD27, PIK3D* gain of function	Impaired signaling through molecules present in B and T cells	• Normal or low IgM, low IgG, low IgA, poor specific antibody production • T-cell dysfunction
Selective immunoglobulin deficiencies			
• IgG subclass deficiency	*IGHG1, IGHG2, IGHG3, IGHG4*	Defects of isotype differentiation	• Decrease in one or more IgG isotypes
• IgA deficiency	*IGAD1*	Defect in IgA production	• Decrease or absent IgA
• Specific antibody deficiency	Unknown	Unclear	• Deficient antibody response to polysaccharide antigens

specifically decrease immunoglobulin levels in the blood. For some of these medications, the mechanism is idiosyncratic. For others, low immunoglobulin levels result from inhibition of normal B-cell development processes, such as in chronic prednisone use, or they result from direct effects on the B-cell compartment, such as with rituximab therapy. Additional secondary causes of low immunoglobulin include protein-losing states, malnutrition, and autoimmune conditions.

Treatment

Treatment of antibody syndromes is primarily directed at preventing bacterial infection. The primary intervention in achieving this goal is replacing deficient IgG. There are no formulations of isolated IgM or IgA used in clinical practice. Some treatment centers advocate the use of prophylactic antibiotic therapy. In combined immunodeficiency or antibody deficiency syndromes with associated autoimmunity, immunosuppressive therapy or even HSCT may be required.

Antibody Deficiency Classification

Defective B-Cell Development

Aborted B-cell development can occur at multiple developmental stages. Initially, B cells develop from precursors in the bone marrow in a process that is dependent on the generation of a functioning rearranged B-cell receptor. In the absence of the ability to transmit signals through a B-cell receptor, B cells do not continue development. Consistent with this model of B-cell development, congenital defects in several of the proteins essential for the formation and signaling of the B-cell receptor have been identified as causes of severe B-cell deficiency. Additional blocks in B-cell development have been identified prior to the expression of the B-cell receptor and also later in development as cells approach the naïve B-cell stage.

Patients with defects in B-cell development are generally immunologically normal with the exception of a severe reduction of B cells in the blood and infections that result from their absence. Patients with early defects have little detectable lymphoid tissue, and upon physical examination, one may find an absence of tonsils or palpable lymph nodes. Patients with later defects may have palpable lymphoid tissue. In both groups, the spleen is generally normal in size.

Class Switching Defects

Normal immunoglobulin isotype class switching occurs in germinal centers in response to antigenic and T-cell costimulatory signals, and the class switching defects involve severe dysfunction of this process. Defects in either T-cell surface CD40L or B-cell surface CD40 impair the initial step in the class-switching cascade, and as a result, no class switching occurs. Further downstream, defects in either AICDA or UNG impair class switching by preventing the formation of double-stranded breaks that are essential for the genomic rearrangement required to switch isotypes. Additional defects in class switching can be seen with genetic abnormalities in the NF-κB and also PIK3D activating mutations, but in either case, the class switching phenotype can be variable. Consultation of an immunologist will help determine where the class switching defect is located and direct clinical care.

Class switching presents with various associated features depending on the genetic cause. Defects in CD40L and CD40 can have risk of associated opportunistic infection with *Pneumocystis* and *Cryptosporidium*, the latter increasing the risk for sclerosing cholangitis, and they have hypoplastic lymphoid tissue. Patients with defective AICDA can have associated autoimmunity, including ITP, hemolytic anemia, autoimmune hepatitis, inflammatory bowel disease, arthritis, and interstitial lung disease. Both AICDA- and UNG-deficient patients suffer from lymphoid hyperplasia.

Transient Hypogammaglobulinemia

Serum IgG levels normally decrease during an infant's first 4–6 months of life as maternal IgG transmitted in utero is metabolized. Transient hypogammaglobulinemia represents a delay in the onset of immunoglobulin synthesis that results in a prolonged nadir. Symptomatic patients present with recurrent infections, including upper respiratory tract infections, otitis, and sinusitis. The diagnosis is suspected in infants and young children with low levels of IgG and IgA (usually two standard deviations below normal for age), but normal levels of IgM and normal numbers of circulating B lymphocytes. Most affected children have normal specific antibody responses and T-lymphocyte function. Apart from appropriate antibiotics, no treatment is required. Infants with severe infections and hypogammaglobulinemia could be given Ig replacement, but benefits and risk must be considered and this is rarely necessary. Recovery occurs between 18 and 30 months of age, and the prognosis for affected children is excellent provided infections are treated promptly and appropriately.

Functional Antibody Deficiency

The group of functional antibody deficiency disorders includes any disorder in which a persistent deficiency in immunoglobulin production has been identified, and the deficiency is not the result of a secondary cause. This group includes genetic syndromes, combined immunodeficiency syndromes, CVID, and monogenetic syndromes previously classified as CVID. As expected, this group contains highly variable phenotypes, in part due to the variety of associated non-B–cell immune abnormalities, and also due to modifying factors in the individual. If possible, understanding the underlying genetic defect of the individual syndrome dramatically improves the ability to anticipate additional complications and decide on treatment approaches. Even the need for immunoglobulin G replacement therapy will vary from individual to individual.

▶ Monogenetic Causes of Functional Antibody Deficiency

A number of monogenetic causes of functional antibody deficiency have been identified in scattered individuals that had previously been diagnosed with CVID. These syndromes encompass the range of phenotypes conventionally included in the broad category of CVID. Severe defects in the classic B-cell coreceptor complex, including CD19, CD21, CD81, and CD225, have been identified in individuals mainly with poor antibody response and infections that would be expected to follow. These defects presumably arise from an impaired germinal center reaction to foreign antigens in lymph nodes. Similar phenotypes were shown to result both with defects in other B-cell coreceptors such as BAFFR or TACI and also with defects in molecules that signal through these receptors such as ICOS. Additional syndromes that include involvement of T-cell dysfunction as well as functional antibody deficiency have been identified in molecules that function in both cell types. These syndromes include, but are not limited to, CD27 deficiency, PIK3D gain of function, and IL-21 deficiency. Additional syndromes with predominant features outside of functional antibody deficiency are discussed later in the chapter.

▶ CVID

Common variable immunodeficiency is a heterogeneous category of functional antibody deficiencies in which no other more appropriate classification is available. CVID is defined by the combination of poor vaccine response and a decrease in blood levels of IgG in conjunction with a severe decrease in levels of either IgM or IgA, or a decrease of both (see Table 33–5). Associated cellular abnormalities can include reduced numbers of memory B-cell subsets in the blood, as well as T-cell lymphopenia. Patients have recurrent infections, most often of the sinus and pulmonary tract, but chronic gastrointestinal infections may manifest with recurrent diarrhea. Patients with CVID are at risk for developing bronchiectasis, autoimmune diseases (idiopathic thrombocytopenic purpura, autoimmune hemolytic anemia, rheumatoid arthritis, and inflammatory bowel disease), and malignancies (especially gastric carcinoma and lymphoma).

Selective Immunoglobulin Deficiencies

Deficiency of an IgA or an IgG subclass can be seen in the presence of both recurrent infections and other immune abnormalities; however, these deficiencies are often seen in the absence of any other identifiable immune abnormality. With an incidence of 1:700, isolated IgA deficiency is a common laboratory finding. The majority of patients with isolated IgA deficiency are asymptomatic, but associations also exist with inflammatory bowel disease, allergic disease, asthma, and autoimmune disorders (thyroiditis, arthritis, vitiligo, thrombocytopenia, and diabetes). Deficiency of IgG subclasses 2–4 can be identified in the absence of other laboratory immune abnormalities; whereas, severe deficiency of IgG1 universally presents with an overall decrease in total IgG levels because it makes up the majority of IgG detectable in the blood. Deficiency of IgG2 can be seen in association with decreased IgA, and in that context, it is suggestive of an underlying functional antibody deficiency with a possibly identifiable genetic cause. IgG3 and IgG4 make up the smallest fraction of the total IgG pool, and in the absence of any other immune abnormality, deficiency of either of these IgG subclasses is generally not considered to cause increased susceptibility to infection. IgG replacement is not indicated in either IgA deficiency or IgG subclass deficiency when no other quantitative or functional immune abnormality has been identified. When other immune abnormalities are seen, antibody deficiency syndromes listed elsewhere in this chapter should be considered.

Durandy A, Kracker S, Fischer A: Primary antibody deficiencies. Nat Rev Immunol 2013;13:519033 [PMID: 23830147].

PHAGOCYTE DISORDERS

Phagocyte defects include abnormalities of both numbers (neutropenia) and function of polymorphonuclear neutrophils. Functional defects consist of impairments in adhesion, chemotaxis, bacterial killing, or, less often, of combinations of these.

1. Neutropenia

The presence of neutropenia should be considered when evaluating recurrent infections. The diagnosis and treatment of neutropenia is discussed in Chapter 30. Additionally, some PID syndromes are associated with neutropenia (eg, XLA).

2. Chronic Granulomatous Disease

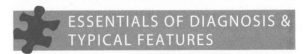
ESSENTIALS OF DIAGNOSIS & TYPICAL FEATURES

▶ Recurrent infections with catalase-positive bacteria and fungi.

▶ XL and AR forms.

▶ Caused by abnormal phagocytosis-associated generation of microbicidal oxygen metabolites (respiratory burst) by neutrophils, monocytes, and macrophages.

General Considerations

Chronic granulomatous disease (CGD) is caused by a defect in any of several genes encoding proteins in the enzyme complex nicotinamide adenine dinucleotide phosphate (NADPH) oxidase, which results in defective superoxide and hydrogen peroxide generation during ingestion of microbes. Most cases in the United States and Europe (probably 75%) are inherited as an XL recessive trait; however, in regions with widespread consanguineous mating, AR inheritance is seen with equal frequency.

Clinical Findings

A. Symptoms and Signs

The typical clinical presentation is characterized by recurrent abscess formation in subcutaneous tissue, lymph nodes, lungs, and liver, and by pneumonia and eczematous and purulent skin rashes. Infecting organisms are typically catalase-positive bacteria, which can break down their own hydrogen peroxide and thus avoid death when captured in a CGD phagocytic vacuole. Aspergillosis is also common and a frequent cause of death. Granulomatous inflammation can narrow the outlet of the stomach or bladder in these patients, leading to vomiting or urinary obstruction.

B. Laboratory Findings

Patients typically present with serious infection, positive microbial cultures, and neutrophilia. The most common infecting organisms are *S aureus*, *Aspergillus* species, *Burkholderia cepacia*, and *Serratia marcescens*. (Culture of either of the last two should suggest this diagnosis.) Patients also present with granulomas of lymph nodes, skin, liver, and genitourinary tract. The diagnosis is confirmed by demonstrating lack of hydrogen peroxide production using the DHR flow cytometry assay or lack of superoxide production using the NBT test. Both tests can demonstrate carrier status of an XL mutation.

Differential Diagnosis

The differential diagnosis includes other phagocyte abnormalities or deficiencies described in this section, as well as the rare neutrophil granule deficiency. Other immunodeficient states leading to severe bacterial or fungal infections should be considered.

Treatment

Daily intake of an antimicrobial agent such as trimethoprim-sulfamethoxazole is indicated in all patients; an oral antifungal agent like itraconazole and regular subcutaneous injections of interferon-γ can greatly reduce the risk of severe infections. BMT has been successful in some cases, but the risk of death is high unless the patient's condition is stable.

Gastric or GU obstruction can be relieved by short-term steroid therapy.

3. Leukocyte Adhesion Defects Types I & II

► Recurrent serious infections.

► "Cold" abscesses (those without pus formation).

► Poor wound healing.

► Gingival or periodontal disease (or both).

General Considerations

The ability of phagocytic cells to enter peripheral sites of infection is critical for effective host defense. In leukocyte adhesion defect (LAD), defects in proteins required for leukocyte adherence to and migration through blood vessel walls prevent these cells from arriving at the sites of infection. LAD I is an AR disease caused by mutations in the common chain of the β_2 integrin family (CD18) located on chromosome 21q22.3. These mutations result in impaired neutrophil migration, adherence, and antibody-dependent phagocytosis. LAD II is a rare AR disease caused by an inborn error in fucose metabolism that results in abnormal expression of leukocyte Sialyl-Lewis X (CD15s), which binds to selectins on the vessel endothelium. The resulting phenotype is similar to LAD I, with recurrent infections, lack of pus formation, poor wound healing, and periodontal disease. LAD II patients also have developmental delays, short stature, dysmorphic facies, and the Bombay (hh) blood group.

Clinical Findings

A. Symptoms and Signs

Patients present with variably severe phenotypes, including recurrent serious infections, lack of pus formation, poor wound healing, and gingival and periodontal disease. The hallmark is little inflammation and absent neutrophils on histopathologic evaluation of infected sites (ie, "cold" abscesses), especially when concurrent with neutrophilia, and expression of poor adherence to vessel walls. The most severe phenotype manifests with infections in the neonatal period, including delayed separation of the umbilical cord with associated omphalitis.

B. Laboratory Findings

Laboratory evaluation often demonstrates a striking neutrophilia. Diagnosis of suspected cases is confirmed by flow cytometry analysis for CD18 (LAD I) or CD15s (LAD II).

▶ Treatment

Treatment includes aggressive antibiotic therapy. Fucose supplementation in LAD II has been reported with some success.

Marciano BE et al: Common severe infections in chronic granulomatous disease. Clin Infect Dis 2015;60:1176–1183 [PMID: 25537876].

DEFICIENCIES OF THE INNATE IMMUNE SYSTEM

▶ General Considerations

Deficiencies in the innate immune response comprise defects that are not the result of an impaired adaptive T- and B-cell response. Besides impaired neutrophil function, they include deficiencies in complement function and other components of the innate immunity.

1. Complement Deficiencies

Complement contributes to innate immunity and facilitates antibody-mediated immunity through opsonization, lysis of target cells, and recruitment of phagocytic cells. The complement system includes three interactive pathways of enzymatic reactions: classic, alternative, and lectin (see Figure 33–2). All three pathways generate cleavage of C3 and result in promotion of inflammation, elimination of pathogens, and enhancement of the immune response. Activation of the complement system occurs through microbial products, tissue enzymes, and surface-bound IgG and IgM antibodies or pentraxins, for example, C-reactive protein.

▶ Complement Component Deficiencies

Deficiencies of individual complement components (C1–C9) are inherited as autosomal codominant traits, each parent contributing one null gene. Serum levels of the deficient component are about half normal in the parents and zero or almost zero in the patients. Deficiencies of C1, C2, or C4 predispose to increased infections but are particularly associated with autoimmune disorders such as systemic lupus erythematosus. Patients with homozygous C2 deficiency can present at any age in childhood with bacteremia or meningitis due to S pneumoniae or H influenzae. Primary C3 deficiency presents with severe pyogenic infections since C3 is critical for opsonization in both the classic and alternative pathways. Deficiency of the control protein factor I, which acts to break up the C3-cleaving complex formed in the classic or alternative pathway, leads to unbridled consumption of C3 and, thereby, severe bacterial infections. Deficiency of a terminal complement component in the membrane attack complex (C5, C6, C7, C8, and C9) or of properdin (an XL alternative pathway control protein) results in recurrent neisserial meningitidis or disseminated gonococcal infection. Survivors of either of these serious neisserial infections should be screened for complement deficiency, first with a CH50.

2. Pattern-Recognition Receptor Defects

Pattern-recognition receptor (PRR) defects are associated with altered cytokine production and increased susceptibility to specific microbes. The clinical presentation of affected patients is most severe during infancy and early childhood with improvement of infections while patients get older, suggesting that adaptive immune responses compensate for defects in innate immunity. TLRs and members of the interleukin-1 receptor (IL-1R) family signal through IL-1R–associated kinases (IRAK) 1 and 4 while using the adaptor molecule MyD88, leading to activation of NF-κB and inflammatory cytokine production. Patients with AR deficiencies in MyD88 and IRAK-4 are predisposed to severe bacterial infections that are not associated with a high fever or significant increase in C-reactive protein at the beginning of infection. Laboratory results may reveal a decreased antibody response to polysaccharide antigens, increased IgG and IgG$_4$ concentrations, and decreased IL-6 production upon whole blood stimulation through most TLR and IL-1R agonists. TLR3 deficiency increases susceptibility to infections with herpes simplex infections, while polymorphisms of TLR5 predispose to legionella pneumonia infections. Chronic mucocutaneous fungal infections have been linked to defects in the dectin-1/CARD9 pathway. Bacterial infections, specifically with *Neisseria meningitidis*, but also viral and fungal infections can occur in context of mannose-binding lectin deficiency.

3. Mendelian Susceptibility to Mycobacterial Disease

IFN-γ is critical for macrophage activation and resistance to mycobacterial infections. Mutations that cause deficiency or reduced function of proteins that participate in IFN-γ signaling result in Mendelian susceptibility to mycobacterial disease (MSMD). Thus far, 11 genes are known to harbor such mutations in affected individuals: *IL12B, IL12RB1, ISG15, TYK2, IRF8, SPPL2A, CYBB, IFNGR1, IFNGR2, STAT1, and NEMO*. The infection susceptibility seen in patients with these mutations includes infection with typically nonpathogenic mycobacteria such as *Mycobacterium avium* complex or bacille Calmette-Guérin (BCG), with some also demonstrating susceptibility to salmonellosis and candida infection. Treatment with supplemental IFN-γ is effective unless the IFN-γ receptor is not functional. Long-term mycobacterial prophylaxis should be considered in these individuals.

4. MonoMAC Syndrome

Disseminated infection by nontuberculous mycobacteria, viruses (ie, HPV), and fungi were recently described in association with

GATA2 mutations or MonoMAC (sporadic monocytopenia and mycobacterial infection) syndrome. Patients usually become symptomatic during adulthood, but younger patients may also be affected. Patients have peripheral blood monocytopenia, but presence of macrophages at sites of infections. B-lymphocyte and NK cell numbers are reported low with variable T-cell numbers. This is an autosomal-dominant inherited disease with an increased risk for malignancies, especially myelodysplasia and leukemia.

Degn SE, Jensenius JC, Thiel S: Disease-causing mutations in genes of the complement system. Am J Hum Genet 2011;88:689–705 [PMID: 21871896].

Netea MG, van der Meer JWM: Immunodeficiency and genetic defects of pattern-recognition receptors. N Engl J Med 2011;364:1–69 [PMID: 21208109].

Picard C et al: Infectious diseases in patients with IRAK-4, MyD88, NEMO, or IkBa deficiency. Clin Microbiol Rev 2011;24: 490–497 [PMID: 21734245].

Rosain J et al: Mendelian susceptibility to mycobacterial disease: 2014-2018 update. Immunol Cell Biol 2019 Apr;97(4):360–367 [PMID: 30264912].

IMMUNODEFICIENCY DISEASES THAT PRESENT WITH AUTOIMMUNITY

▶ General Considerations

Aberrant development of the immune system predisposes not only to a defective host immune response. Autoimmunity, chronic inflammation, and features of atopy may occur concurrently. Mechanisms contributing to autoimmunity include impaired development and function of regulatory T and B cells, production of autoantibodies often seen with B-cell defects affecting immunoglobulin class switching, and clearance of apoptotic cells. States of immune dysregulation can be associated with lymphoproliferation and enhanced inflammation.

1. Immune Dysregulation, Polyendocrinopathy, Enteropathy, X-Linked Syndrome

Immune dysregulation, polyendocrinopathy, enteropathy, X-linked (IPEX) syndrome is a rare disease that usually manifests with severe diarrhea and insulin-dependent diabetes mellitus within the first months of life. Affected males also have severe eczema, food allergy, autoimmune cytopenias, lymphadenopathy, splenomegaly, and recurrent infections. Most die before 2 years of age due to malnutrition or sepsis. IPEX syndrome results from mutations in the *FOXP3* gene that encodes a protein essential for developing regulatory T lymphocytes. Leukocyte counts and immunoglobulin levels are generally normal. Immunosuppression and nutritional supplementation produce temporary improvements, but the prognosis is poor and most cases result in early death. HSCT has been attempted with variable success. IPEX-like

syndromes have been described as associated with mutations of the gene encoding CD25, the high-affinity IL-2 receptor (IL2R) which is constitutively expressed on regulatory T cells, signal transducer and activator of transcription (STAT) 1, STAT3, STAT5 b, and ITCH. If IPEX or IPEX-like syndromes are suspected, the presence of FOXP3+/CD25+ regulatory T cells should be assessed not only in affected boys but also in girls. Genetic testing for FOXP3 or other suspected mutations will be helpful to identify affected patients and carriers of the gene mutation. In addition to IPEX syndrome, early onset pediatric inflammatory bowel disease has been described as a consequence of loss-of-function mutations in IL-10 and IL-10 receptor (encoded by *IL10RA* and *IL10RB*).

2. Autoimmune Polyendocrinopathy, Candidiasis, Ectodermal Dysplasia Syndrome

Autoimmune polyendocrinopathy, candidiasis, ectodermal dysplasia (APECED) syndrome is characterized by autoimmune endocrinopathies, ectodermal dystrophies, and recurrent *Candida* infections as a result of an abnormal T-lymphocyte response to *Candida*. Generalized lymphoproliferation is absent. APECED is caused by AR mutations in the gene for an important transcription regulator protein called *autoimmune regulator* (*AIRE*) that is critical for normal thymocyte development. In APECED, autoantibodies against IL17A and IL17F impair the T_H17 response and contribute to chronic mucocutaneous candidiasis (CMC). Several other gene defects have been associated with chronic CMC, a disorder characterized by isolated candidal infections of the skin, nails, and mucous membranes. Systemic disease is not characteristic, but case reports of intracranial mycotic aneurysms exist. Primary CMC most commonly occurs as an isolated syndrome, but it can be associated with endocrine or autoimmune disorders as in APECED syndrome. Mutations in the signal transducer and activator of transcription 3 (*STAT3*) gene and gain-of-function mutations in *STAT1* can lead to defective T_H17 responses, susceptibility to CMC, and *S aureus* infections. Mutations in *IL17F* and *IL17R*, C-type lectin–associated 7 (*CLEC7A* or *DECTIN1*) or caspase recruitment domain-containing protein 9 (*CARD9*) cells have also been associated with CMC. Treatment of CMC includes antifungal therapy in combination with therapy for associated endocrinopathies.

3. Autoimmune Lymphoproliferative Syndrome

Autoimmune lymphoproliferative syndrome (ALPS) results from mutations of genes important for regulating programmed lymphocyte death (apoptosis). Most commonly, the defect is in Fas (CD95) or Fas ligand, but other defects in the Fas pathway have also been described (eg, caspase 10).

Clinical presentation includes lymphadenopathy, spleno-megaly, and autoimmune disorders (autoimmune hemolytic anemia, neutropenia, thrombocytopenia, and sometimes arthritis). Occasionally, patients have frequent infections. The diagnosis is suspected when T-lymphocyte subsets by flow cytometry demonstrate elevated numbers of $CD3^+CD4^-CD8^-$ (double negative) T lymphocytes. Several different types of ALPS are distinguished by the response of lymphocytes to Fas-induced apoptosis. Patients are often heterozygous, and inheritance is mostly autosomal dominant. Treatment with prednisone often controls the lymph-adenopathy. Infections should be treated appropriately. In some cases, BMT has been curative. Affected patients are also at risk for lymphoma. Mutations affecting another apoptosis-related protein, caspase 8, cause an ALPS variant syndrome in which the susceptibility to infection by herpes simplex virus also increases.

4. Other Lymphoproliferative Syndromes

X-linked lymphoproliferative syndrome is an immuno-deficiency that usually develops following EBV infection. Affected males develop fulminant infectious mononucleo-sis with hemophagocytic syndrome, multiple organ system failure, and bone marrow aplasia. The mutated gene (*SH2D1A/SAP/DSHP*) encodes a signaling protein used by T lymphocytes and NK cells called *SLAM-adapter protein* (SAP). Affected boys are immunologically normal prior to EBV infection and during acute infection, they produce antibody to EBV. In most instances, infection with EBV is fatal. Patients who survive the initial episode or who are never infected with EBV in childhood develop lymphomas, vasculitis, hypogammaglobulinemias (with elevated IgM), or CVID in later life. Genetic analysis for a mutation of the SAP (*SH2D1A*) gene and testing for SAP protein expression are available. Mutations in the genes encoding for the X-linked inhibitor of apoptosis (XIAP), a potent regulator of lymphocyte homeostasis, and for IL-2–inducible T-cell kinase (ITK) have been described to present as an XLP-like syndrome. Testing for mutations of the gene encoding for XIAP (*BIRC4*) and XIAP protein expression will help establish the diagnosis. A decreased number of naïve, $CD45RA^+$ T cells are indicative of ITK deficiency, and further genetic analysis can establish the diagnosis.

5. Abnormal Responses to Cellular Debris

Large numbers of cells undergo programmed cell death (apoptosis) and need to be cleared daily. Apoptotic cells are being recognized by phagocytes either directly by scavenger receptors or after opsonization by early complement components through binding to complement receptors. Defective clearance of apoptotic cells leads to accumulation of cell debris, which can, similarly to debris from pathogens, trigger

inflammation with increased production of type I interferons (IFNs) and a shift to autoimmunity. This has been associated with the high incidence of systemic lupus in patients with C1q deficiency and discoid lupus in female carriers of CGD. Accumulation of nucleic acid debris due to decreased break-down caused by loss-of-function mutations of endonucleases, for example DNAse I and TREX1, and gain-of-function mutations in intracellular nucleic acid sensors, for example IFIH1 and STING, also contribute to an increased IFN I signature seen in a variety of autoimmune manifestations.

Allenspach E, Torgerson T: Autoimmunity and primary immuno-deficiency disorders. J Clin Immunol 2016;36:S57–S67 [PMID: 27210535].

Azizi G et al: Cellular and molecular mechanisms of immune dys-regulation and autoimmunity. Cell Immunol 2016;310:14–26 [PMID: 27614846].

IMMUNODEFICIENCY DISEASES THAT OVERLAP WITH ALLERGY

ESSENTIALS OF DIAGNOSIS & TYPICAL FEATURES

▶ Severe manifestations.

▶ Associated nonimmune features.

▶ Atypical manifestations.

▶ General Considerations

Some have incorrectly assumed that the state of immune deficiency is not compatible with allergy because allergy requires a coordinated allergen-specific immune response. To the contrary, several genetically defined immune deficiencies are known to associate with allergic diseases ranging from allergic rhinitis to food allergy and eczema. Still several more immune deficiencies are highly likely to manifest clinically with symptoms not necessarily the result of a specific allergy, but nonetheless likely to fall under the purview of allergy, such as urticaria and eczema-like rash. Some of these diseases are reviewed later.

▶ Clinical Findings

A. Symptoms and Signs

Immunodeficiencies that associate with allergic disease have varied clinical manifestations. In some cases, such as in DOCK8 deficiency, patients have severe allergic disease and recurrent infection without any accompanying non-immune features. In other syndromes, patients develop allergy in addition to other immune-related problems.

In immunodysregulation polyendocrinopathy X-linked (IPEX), patients develop autoimmune disease in addition to eczema and allergy. In other diseases, patients present with nonimmune features. For example, in Wiskott-Aldrich syndrome, patients present with eczema and bleeding as a result of platelet abnormalities. In PGM3 deficiency, patients have motor and cognitive impairment. Patients with Comel-Netherton syndrome have distinct structural abnormalities of the hair shaft. As can be seen in these examples, the association between allergic disease and immunodeficiency is not uncommon and results from various forms of genetic impairment.

B. Laboratory Findings

It is often difficult to use laboratory testing to distinguish an immunodeficiency that associates with allergy from severe allergy without immunodeficiency. While the finding on CBC of thrombocytopenia and small platelets assists in diagnosing Wiskott-Aldrich syndrome, the majority of immunodeficiency-allergy-overlap diseases lack distinguishing laboratory features. In light of a dearth of specific laboratory findings that indicate a patient's allergy is related to a more significant immune deficiency, the authors recommend that any severe abnormality discovered in routine hematologic

testing be viewed with suspicion in allergic patients. For example, a peripheral eosinophil count persistently above 1500/μL should raise concern for additional immune processes. Likewise, the finding of low levels of serum immunoglobulins could be the first clue to an underlying immune process.

C. Differential Diagnosis

If immune deficiency is suspected in an allergic patient, secondary causes of immune dysfunction should be considered. Hypogammaglobulinemia can result from protein loss through the GI tract or as the result of nutritional deficiency. Additional consideration should be made for the patient's home environment. Severe allergic sequelae are often the result of chronic exposure to an offending allergen, such as a pet in the house.

D. Treatment

Treatment of allergic symptoms in patients for which there is a suspected immune deficiency parallels treatment for immunocompetent patients with allergy except for the use of systemic immunosuppressants. For patients with cellular immunodeficiency that presents with allergy, the use of corticosteroids and perhaps other systemic immunosuppressants

Table 33–6. Allergy and immunodeficiency overlap diseases.

	Genes Containing Defects	Likely Etiology	Characteristic Features
Job syndrome (STAT3 deficiency)	Not increased	Elevated IgE	Cutaneous abscess, facial appearance, pulmonary, vascular
Netherton syndrome (SPINK5 deficiency)	Increased	Severe eczema	Cutaneous abscess, respiratory infection, abnormal hair
DOCK8 deficiency	Increased	Eczema, food allergy, eosinophilia	Vasculopathy
Wiskott-Aldrich syndrome (WASp deficiency)	Increased	Eczema, food allergy	Thrombocytopenia, autoimmunity, neutropenia
IPEX (FOXP3 deficiency)	Increased	Eczema, food allergy	Autoimmunity, enteropathy
Phosphoglucomutase 3 (PGM3) **deficiency**	Increased	Eczema, food allergy	Dysmorphism, skeletal abnormality, cognitive impairment, neutropenia, recurrent infection
Severe dermatitis, allergy, and metabolic wasting (SAM) **syndrome** (Desmoglein 1 deficiency)	Increased	Eczema, ichthyosis, food allergy	Palmoplantar keratoderma, nail abnormality, failure to thrive
PLCG2 associated antibody deficiency and immune dysregulation (PLAID)	Not increased	Cold-induced urticaria	Skin granuloma, low immunoglobulins, recurrent infection
FCAS, MWS, NOMID (associated with NLRP3 genetic variants)	Not increased	Cold-induced urticaria	Fever, arthralgia, conjunctivitis

DOCK8 (Dedicator of cytokinesis 8); FOXP3, Forkhead box protein P3; *IPEX*, Immune Polyendocrinopathy X-Linked; NLRP3, NACHT, LRR, and PYD domains-containing protein 3; SPINK5, Serine protease inhibitor Kazal-type 5.

can increase the risk of reactivation of latent viruses either from past infection or even past vaccination. In one report, use of corticosteroids in a patient with DOCK8 deficiency was associated with reactivation of vaccine strain varicella and the development of vasculopathy. Considering this additional risk, the authors recommend diagnostic re-evaluation when considering the use of systemic immunosuppressants for severe or unusual allergic manifestations. When severe immunodeficiency is identified in an allergic patient, treatment is dependent on the underlying diagnosis. Several of the diseases listed in Table 33–6 can be corrected through allogeneic HSCT, whereas others may respond better to replacement immunoglobulin, prophylactic antimicrobials, or immunosuppressive therapy.

Endocrine Disorders

Sarah Bartz, MD   Melanie Cree-Green, MD, PhD

Christina Chambers, MD   Shanlee Davis, MD, MSCS

Christine M. Chan, MD   Stephanie Hsu, MD, PhD

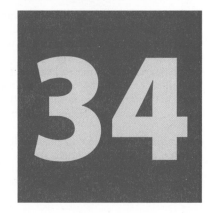

▼ GENERAL CONCEPTS

The classic concept that *endocrine* effects are the result of substances secreted into the blood with effects on a distant target cell has been updated to account for other ways in which hormonal effects occur. Specifically, some hormone systems involve the stimulation or inhibition of metabolic processes in neighboring cells (eg, within the pancreatic islets or cartilage). This phenomenon is termed *paracrine*. Other hormone effects reflect the action of hormones on the same cells that produced them. This action is termed *autocrine*. The discoveries of local production of ghrelin, somatostatin, cholecystokinin, incretins, and many other hormones in the brain and gut support the concept of paracrine and autocrine processes in these tissues.

Another significant discovery in endocrine physiology was an appreciation of the role of specific hormone receptors in target tissues, without which the hormonal effects cannot occur. For example, in nephrogenic diabetes insipidus (DI), affected children have defective vasopressin or receptor function, and show the metabolic effects of DI despite more-than-adequate vasopressin secretion. Alternatively, abnormal activation of a hormone receptor leads to the effects of the hormone without its abnormal secretion. Examples of this phenomenon include McCune-Albright syndrome (precocious puberty and hyperthyroidism), testotoxicosis (familial male precocious puberty), and hypercalciuric hypocalcemia.

HORMONE TYPES

Hormones are of three main chemical types: peptides and proteins, steroids, and amines. The peptide hormones include the releasing factors secreted by the hypothalamus; the hormones of the anterior and posterior pituitary gland; pancreatic islet cells; parathyroid glands, lung (angiotensin II), heart, and brain (atrial and brain natriuretic hormones); and local growth factors such as insulin-like growth factor 1 (IGF-1). Steroid hormones are secreted primarily by the adrenal cortex, gonads, and kidney (active vitamin D [$1,25(OH)_2$ D3]). The amine hormones are secreted by the adrenal medulla (epinephrine) and the thyroid gland (triiodothyronine [T_3] and thyroxine [T_4]).

Peptide hormones and epinephrine act through cell surface receptors. The metabolic effects of these hormones are usually stimulation or inhibition of the activity of pre-existing enzymes or transport proteins (posttranslational effects). The steroid hormones, thyroid hormone, and active vitamin D, in contrast, act more slowly and bind to cytoplasmic receptors inside the target cell and subsequently to specific regions on nuclear DNA. Their metabolic effects are generally caused by stimulating or inhibiting the synthesis of new enzymes or transport proteins (transcriptional effects).

Metabolic processes that require rapid response, such as blood glucose or calcium homeostasis, are usually controlled by peptide hormones and epinephrine, while processes that respond more slowly, such as pubertal development and metabolic rate, are controlled by steroid hormones and thyroid hormone. The control of electrolyte homeostasis is intermediate and is regulated by a combination of peptide and steroid hormones (Table 34–1).

FEEDBACK CONTROL OF HORMONE SECRETION

Hormone secretion is regulated by feedback in response to changes in the internal environment. When the metabolic imbalance is corrected, stimulation of the hormone secretion ceases and may even be inhibited. Overcorrection of the imbalance stimulates secretion of a counterbalancing hormone or hormones so that homeostasis is maintained within relatively narrow limits.

Hypothalamic-pituitary control of hormonal secretion is regulated by feedback. End-organ failure (endocrine gland insufficiency) leads to decreased circulating concentrations of endocrine gland hormones and increased secretion of the respective hypothalamic releasing and pituitary hormones (see Table 34–1; Figure 34–1). If restoration of normal circulating concentration of hormones occurs, feedback inhibition at the pituitary and hypothalamus results in cessation of the previously stimulated secretion of releasing and pituitary hormones and restoration of their circulating concentrations to normal.

Similarly, if there is autonomous endocrine gland hyperfunction (eg, McCune-Albright syndrome, Graves disease, or adrenal tumor), the specific hypothalamic releasing and pituitary hormones are suppressed (see Figure 34–1).

Bethin K, Fuqua JS: General concepts and physiology. In: Kappy MS, Allen DB, Geffner ME (eds): *Pediatric Practice-Endocrinology*. McGraw Hill; 2010:1–22.

▼ DISTURBANCES OF GROWTH

Disturbances of growth and development are the most common problems evaluated by a pediatric endocrinologist. While most cases represent normal developmental variants, it is critical to identify abnormal growth patterns, as deviations from the norm can be the first or only manifestation of an endocrine disorder. Height velocity is the most critical parameter in evaluating a child's growth.

Table 34–1. Hormonal regulation of metabolic processes.

Rapid Response, Most Direct			
Metabolite or Other Parameter	**Stimulus**	**Endocrine Gland**	**Hormone**
Glucose	Hyperglycemia	Pancreatic beta cell	Insulin
Glucose	Hypoglycemia	Pancreatic alpha cell	Glucagon
Glucose	Hypoglycemia	Adrenal medulla	Epinephrine
Calcium	Hypercalcemia	Thyroid C cell	Calcitonin
Calcium	Hypocalcemia	Parathyroid	PTH
Sodium/plasma osmolality	Hypernatremia/hyperosmolality	Hypothalamus with posterior pituitary gland as reservoir	ADH
Plasma volume	Hypervolemia	Heart	ANH
Intermediate Response, Multiple Intermediaries			
Metabolite or Other Parameter	**Abnormality**	**Endocrine Gland**	**Hormone**
Sodium/potassium	Hyponatremia	Kidney	Renin (an enzyme)
	Hyperkalemia	Liver and others	Angiotensin I
	Hypovolemia	Lung	Angiotensin II
		Adrenal cortex	Aldosterone
Slow Response, Longer Acting Processes			
Hypothalamic-Releasing Hormone	**Trophic Hormone (Pituitary Gland)**	**Endocrine Target Tissue**	**Endocrine Gland Hormone**
CRH	ACTH	Adrenal cortex	Cortisol
GHRH	GH	Liver and other tissues	IGF-1
GnRH	LH	Testis	Testosterone
GnRH	FSH/LH	Ovary	Estradiol/progesterone
TRH	TSH	Thyroid gland	T_4 and T_3

ACTH, adrenocorticotropic hormone; ADH, antidiuretic hormone; ANH, atrial natriuretic hormone; CRH, corticotropin-releasing hormone; FSH, follicle-stimulating hormone; GH, growth hormone; GHRH, growth hormone releasing hormone; GnRH, gonadotropin-releasing hormone; IGF-1, insulin-like growth factor 1; LH, luteinizing hormone; PTH, parathyroid hormone; T_3, triiodothyronine; T_4, thyroxine; TRH, thyrotropin-releasing hormone; TSH, thyroid-stimulating hormone.

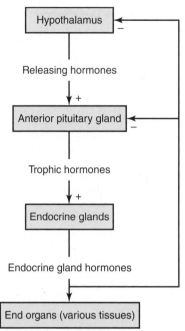

▲ **Figure 34–1.** General scheme of the hypothalamus-pituitary-endocrine gland axis. Releasing hormones synthesized in the hypothalamus are secreted into the hypophyseal portal circulation. Trophic hormones are secreted by the pituitary gland in response, and they in turn act on specific endocrine glands to stimulate the secretion of their respective hormones. The endocrine gland hormones exert their respective effects on various target tissues (end organs) and exert a negative feedback (feedback inhibition) on their own secretion by acting at the level of the pituitary and hypothalamus. This system is characteristic of those hormones listed in Table 34–1 (third level).

A persistent increase or decrease in height percentiles between age 2 years and the onset of puberty always warrants evaluation. Similarly, substantial deviations from target (midparental) height may be indications of underlying endocrine or skeletal disorders. It is more difficult to distinguish normal from abnormal growth in the first 2 years of life, as infants may have catch-up or catch-down growth during this period. Similarly, the variable timing of the onset of puberty makes early adolescence another period during which evaluation of growth abnormalities may require careful consideration.

Appropriate standards must be used to evaluate growth. The National Center for Health Statistics provides standard cross-sectional growth charts for North American children (see Chapter 9) and the World Health Organization (WHO) growth charts use an ethnically more diverse sample. Normal growth standards may vary with country of origin. Growth charts are available for some ethnic groups in North America and for some syndromes with specific growth disturbance such as Turner or Down syndromes. Current treatment practices for patients with Turner and Down syndrome (including the use of growth hormone in Turner syndrome) can cause children to grow differently than reflected in their specific growth charts.

TARGET HEIGHT & SKELETAL MATURATION

A child's height potential is determined largely by genetic factors. The target height of a child is calculated from the mean parental height plus 6.5 cm for boys or minus 6.5 cm for girls. This calculation helps identify a child's genetic growth potential. Most children achieve an adult height within 10 cm of the target height. Another parameter that determines growth potential is skeletal maturation or bone age. Beyond the neonatal period, bone age is evaluated by comparing a radiograph of the child's left hand and wrist with the standards of Greulich and Pyle. Delayed or advanced bone age is not diagnostic of any specific disease, but the extent of skeletal maturation allows determination of remaining growth potential as a percentage of total height and allows prediction of ultimate height. Additionally, the bone age delay or advancement can change over time. For example, children with a previously delayed bone age may develop a bone age closer to their chronological age closer to the time of puberty.

SHORT STATURE

It is important to distinguish normal variants of growth (familial short stature and constitutional growth delay) from pathologic conditions (Table 34–2). Pathologic short stature is more likely in children who have a low growth velocity (crossing major height percentiles on the growth curve, < 4 cm/y) or who are significantly short for their family. Children with chronic illness or nutritional deficiencies may have poor linear growth, and this can be associated with inadequate weight gain and low body mass index (BMI). In contrast, endocrine causes of short stature are usually associated with maintenance or increase in BMI percentiles. Subtypes of short stature are discussed next.

1. Familial Short Stature & Constitutional Growth Delay

Children with familial short stature typically have normal birth weight and length. In the first 2 years of life, their linear growth velocity decelerates as they near their genetically determined percentile. Once the target percentile is reached, the child resumes normal linear growth parallel to the growth

Table 34–2. Causes of short stature.

NORMAL
A. Genetic-familial short stature
B. Constitutional growth delay
PATHOLOGICAL
C. Endocrine disturbances
   1. Growth hormone (GH) deficiency
      a. Hereditary
      b. Idiopathic—with and without associated abnormalities of midline structures of the central nervous system
      c. Acquired
         (1) Transient (eg, psychosocial short stature)
         (2) Organic—tumor, irradiation of the central nervous system, infection, or trauma
   2. GH resistance/insulin-like growth factor 1 (IGF-1) deficiency
   3. Hypothyroidism
   4. Excess cortisol—Cushing disease and Cushing syndrome
   5. Diabetes mellitus (poorly controlled)
   6. Pseudohypoparathyroidism
   7. Rickets
D. Intrauterine growth restriction
   1. Intrinsic fetal abnormalities—chromosomal disorders
   2. Syndromes (eg, Russell-Silver, Noonan, Bloom, de Lange, Cockayne)
   3. Congenital infections
   4. Placental abnormalities
   5. Maternal abnormalities during pregnancy
E. Inborn errors of metabolism
F. Intrinsic diseases of bone
   1. Defects of growth of tubular bones or spine (skeletal dysplasias)
   2. Disorganized development of cartilage and fibrous components of the skeleton
G. Short stature associated with chromosomal defects
   1. Autosomal (eg, Down syndrome, Prader-Willi syndrome)
   2. Sex chromosomal (eg, Turner syndrome–XO)
H. Chronic systemic diseases, congenital defects, and cancers
I. Psychosocial short stature (deprivation dwarfism)

curve, usually between 2 and 3 years of age. Skeletal maturation and timing of puberty are consistent with chronologic age. The child grows along his/her own growth percentile and the final height is short but appropriate for the family (Figure 34–2).

Children with constitutional growth delay do not necessarily have short parents but have a growth pattern similar to those with familial short stature with a decline in linear growth velocity between ages 2 and 3 years and then maintenance of a normal growth velocity prior to puberty. The difference is that children with constitutional growth delay have a delay in skeletal maturation and a delay in the onset of puberty. In these children, growth continues beyond the time the average child stops growing, and final height is appropriate for target height (Figure 34–3).

2. Growth Hormone Deficiency

Human growth hormone (GH) is produced by the anterior pituitary gland. Secretion is stimulated by growth hormone-releasing hormone (GHRH) and inhibited by somatostatin. GH is secreted in a pulsatile pattern, and has direct growth-promoting and metabolic effects (Figure 34–4). GH also promotes growth indirectly by stimulating production of insulin-like growth factors, primarily IGF-1.

Growth hormone deficiency (GHD) is characterized by decreased growth velocity and delayed skeletal maturation in the absence of other explanations (Figure 34–5). Because GH promotes lipolysis, many GH-deficient children have excess truncal adiposity. GHD may be isolated or coexist with other pituitary hormone deficiencies and may be congenital (septo-optic dysplasia or ectopic posterior pituitary), genetic (GH or GHRH gene mutation), or acquired (craniopharyngioma, germinoma, histiocytosis, or cranial irradiation). Idiopathic GHD is the most common deficiency state with an incidence of about 1:4000 children. Patients have also been described with congenital GH-resistance syndromes. The presentation of GH resistance is similar to that of GHD, but short stature is often severe, with little or no response to GH therapy and may be accompanied by dysmorphic features.

Features of infantile GHD include normal birth weight and slightly reduced length, hypoglycemia (if accompanied by adrenal insufficiency), micropenis (if accompanied by gonadotropin deficiency), and conjugated hyperbilirubinemia (if other pituitary hormone deficiencies present). Growth retardation in isolated GHD and hypopituitarism may not present until late in infancy or childhood.

Laboratory tests to assess GH status may be difficult to interpret because there is significant overlap in GH secretion between normal and GH-deficient children. GH secretion is pulsatile, so random samples for measurement of serum GH are of no value in the diagnosis of GHD outside of the first week of life. Serum concentrations of IGF-1 give reasonable estimations of GH secretion and action in the adequately nourished child (see Figure 34–4), and are often used as a first step in the evaluation for GHD. IGF-binding protein 3 (IGFBP-3) is a much less sensitive marker of GH deficiency, but may be useful in the underweight child or in children younger than 4 years, since it is less affected by age or nutritional status. Provocative studies using such agents as insulin, arginine, levodopa, clonidine, or glucagon are traditionally done to clarify GH secretion, but are not physiologic and are often poorly reproducible, ultimately limiting their value in the clarification of GH secretion. The diagnosis of GHD is often a compilation of clinical and laboratory evidence and must be approached with care. All patients diagnosed with GHD should have an MRI of the hypothalamus and pituitary gland to evaluate for a tumor prior to starting therapy.

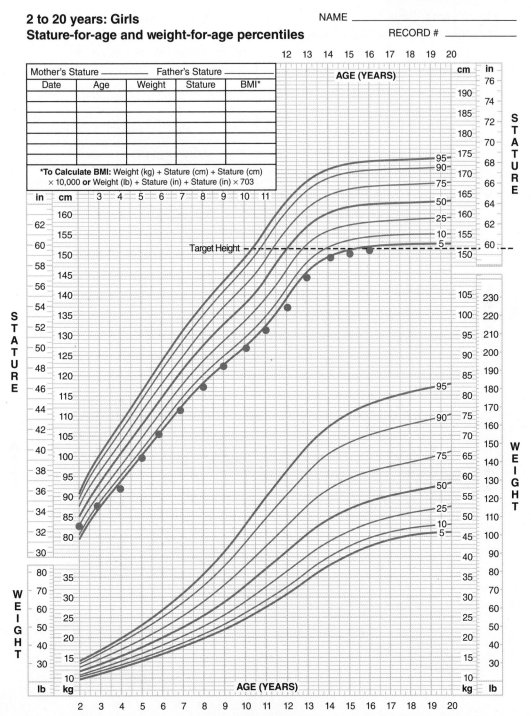

2 to 20 years: Girls
Stature-for-age and weight-for-age percentiles

NAME _____

RECORD # _____

*To Calculate BMI: Weight (kg) + Stature (cm) + Stature (cm) × 10,000 or Weight (lb) + Stature (in) + Stature (in) × 703

▲ **Figure 34–2.** Typical pattern of growth in a child with familial short stature. After attaining an appropriate percentile during the first 2 years of life, the child will have normal linear growth parallel to the growth curve. Skeletal maturation and the timing of puberty are consistent with chronologic age. The height percentile the child has been following is maintained, and final height is short but appropriate for the family.

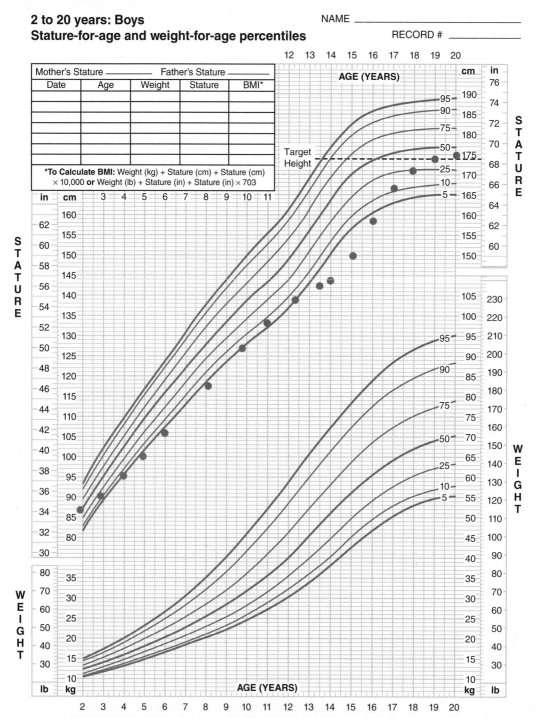

2 to 20 years: Boys
Stature-for-age and weight-for-age percentiles

NAME _____

RECORD # _____

Date	Age	Weight	Stature	BMI*

Mother's Stature _____ Father's Stature _____

*To Calculate BMI: Weight (kg) ÷ Stature (cm) ÷ Stature (cm)
× 10,000 **or** Weight (lb) ÷ Stature (in) ÷ Stature (in) × 703

▲ **Figure 34–3.** Typical pattern of growth in a child with constitutional growth delay. Growth slows during the first 2 years of life, similarly to children with familial short stature. Subsequently the child will have normal linear growth parallel to the growth curve. However, skeletal maturation and the onset of puberty are delayed. Growth continues beyond the time the average child has stopped growing, and final height is appropriate for target height.

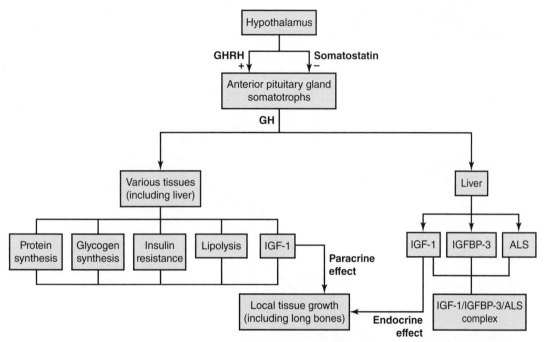

▲ **Figure 34–4.** The GHRH/GH/IGF-1 system. The effects of growth hormone (GH) on growth are partly due to its direct anabolic effects in the muscle, liver, and bone. In addition, GH stimulates many tissues to produce insulin-like growth factor 1 (IGF-1) locally, which stimulates the growth of the tissue itself (paracrine effect of IGF-1). The action of GH on the liver results in the secretion of IGF-1 (circulating IGF-1), which stimulates growth in other tissues (endocrine effect of IGF-1). The action of growth hormone on the liver also enhances the secretion of IGF-binding protein 3 (IGFBP-3) and acid-labile subunit (ALS), which form a high-molecular-weight complex with IGF-1. The function of this complex is to transport IGF-1 to its target tissues, but the complex also serves as a reservoir and possible inhibitor of IGF-1 action. In various chronic illnesses, the direct metabolic effects of GH are inhibited; the secretion of IGF-1 in response to GH is blunted, and in some cases IGFBP-3 synthesis is enhanced, resulting in marked inhibition in the growth of the child. GHRH, growth hormone-releasing hormone.

3. Small for Gestational Age/Intrauterine Growth Restriction

Small for gestational age (SGA) infants have a birth weight and/or length below the 3rd percentile for the population's birth weight–gestational age relationship. SGA infants include constitutionally small infants and infants with intrauterine growth restriction (IUGR). Many children with mild SGA/IUGR and no intrinsic fetal abnormalities exhibit catch-up growth during the first 3 years, but 15%–20% remain short throughout life. Catch-up growth may also be inadequate in preterm SGA/IUGR infants with poor postnatal nutrition. Children who do not show catch-up growth may have normal growth velocity but follow a lower height percentile than expected for the family. In contrast to children with constitutional growth delay, those with SGA/IUGR have skeletal maturation that corresponds to chronologic age or is only mildly delayed. GH therapy for SGA/IUGR children with growth delay is FDA-approved and appears to increase growth velocity and final adult height.

4. Disproportionate Short Stature

There are more than 200 sporadic and genetic skeletal dysplasias that may cause disproportionate short stature. Measurements of arm span and upper-to-lower body segment ratio are helpful in determining whether a child has normal body proportions. If disproportionate short stature is found, a skeletal survey may be useful to detect specific radiographic features characteristic of some disorders. The effect of GH on most of these rare disorders is unknown.

5. Short Stature Associated With Syndromes

Short stature is associated with many genetic syndromes, including Turner, Down, Noonan, and Prader-Willi. Girls with Turner syndrome often have recognizable features

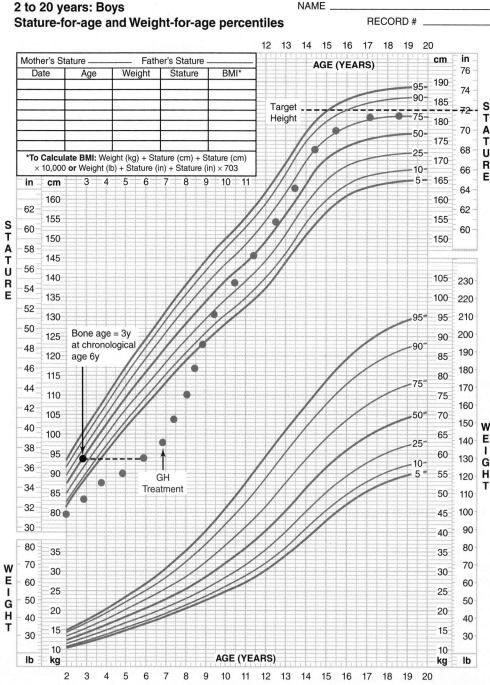

2 to 20 years: Boys
Stature-for-age and Weight-for-age percentiles

NAME _____

RECORD # _____

▲ **Figure 34–5.** Typical pattern of growth in a child with acquired growth hormone deficiency (GHD). Children with acquired GHD have an abnormal growth velocity and fail to maintain height percentile during childhood. Other phenotypic features (central adiposity and immaturity of facies) may be present. Children with congenital GHD will cross percentiles during the first 2 years of life, similarly to the pattern seen in familial short stature and constitutional delay, but will fail to attain a steady height percentile subsequently.

such as micrognathia, webbed neck, low posterior hairline, edema of hands and feet, multiple pigmented nevi, and an increased carrying angle. However, short stature can be the only obvious manifestation of Turner syndrome. Consequently, any girl with unexplained short stature for family warrants a chromosomal evaluation. Although girls with Turner syndrome are not usually GH deficient, GH therapy can improve final height by an average of 6 cm. Duration of GH therapy is a significant predictor of long-term height gain; consequently, it is important that Turner syndrome be diagnosed early and GH started as soon as possible if the family desires to maximize height.

GH is approved for treatment of growth failure in Prader-Willi syndrome–associated GHD. GH improves growth, body composition, and physical activity. A few deaths have been reported in Prader-Willi children receiving GH, all of which occurred in very obese children, children with respiratory impairments, sleep apnea, or possibly unidentified respiratory infections. The role of GH in these deaths is unknown, but it is recommended that all patients with Prader-Willi syndrome be evaluated for upper airway obstruction and sleep apnea prior to starting GH therapy.

Children with Down syndrome should be evaluated for GHD only if their linear growth is abnormal compared with the Down syndrome growth chart. Given their increased malignancy risk, some families may be wary of adding GH therapy.

6. Psychosocial Short Stature (Psychosocial Dwarfism)

Psychosocial short stature refers to growth retardation associated with emotional deprivation. Undernutrition probably contributes to growth retardation in some of these children. Other symptoms include unusual eating and drinking habits, bowel and bladder incontinence, social withdrawal, and delayed speech. GH secretion in children with psychosocial short stature is diminished, but GH therapy is usually not beneficial. A change in the psychological environment at home usually results in improved growth and improvement of GH secretion, personality, and eating behaviors.

▶ Clinical Evaluation

Laboratory investigation should be guided by the history and physical examination, including history of chronic illness and medications, birth weight and height, pattern of growth since birth, familial growth patterns, pubertal stage, dysmorphic features, body segment proportion, and psychological health. In a child with poor weight gain as the primary disturbance, a nutritional assessment is indicated. The following laboratory tests may be useful as guided by history and clinical judgment: (1) radiograph of left hand and wrist for bone age; (2) karyotype (girls) and/or Noonan syndrome testing; (3) thyroid function tests: thyroxine (T_4) and thyroid-stimulating hormone (TSH); (4) IGF-1 and/or IGFBP-3 in

children younger than 4 years or in malnourished individuals; (5) complete blood count (to detect chronic anemia or leukocyte markers of infection); (6) erythrocyte sedimentation rate (often elevated in collagen-vascular disease, cancer, chronic infection, and inflammatory bowel disease); (7) urinalysis, blood urea nitrogen, and serum creatinine (occult renal disease); (8) serum electrolytes, calcium, and phosphorus (renal tubular disease and metabolic bone disease); (9) stool examination for fat, or measurement of serum tissue transglutaminase (malabsorption or celiac disease).

▶ Growth Hormone Therapy

GH therapy is approved by the U.S. Food and Drug Administration (FDA) in children for GHD; growth restriction associated with chronic renal failure; Turner, Prader-Willi, and Noonan syndromes; children born small for gestational age (SGA) who fail to demonstrate catch-up growth by age 2; and SHOX gene mutations. GH therapy has also been approved for children with idiopathic short stature whose current height is more than 2.25 standard deviations below the normal range for age. With GH treatment, final height may be 5–7 cm taller in this population. The role of GH for idiopathic short stature is still unclear, especially due to the expense, long duration of treatment, and unclear psychological consequences. Side effects of recombinant GH are uncommon but include intracranial hypertension and slipped capital femoral epiphysis. With early diagnosis and treatment, children with GH deficiency reach normal or near-normal adult height. Recombinant IGF-1 injections may be used to treat children with GH resistance or IGF-1 deficiency, but improvements in growth may not be as substantial as seen with GH therapy for GH deficiency. Currently, the recommended schedule for GH therapy is subcutaneous recombinant GH given subcutaneously 6 or 7 days per week with total weekly dose of 0.15–0.47 mg/kg.

Altzoglou KS et al: Isolated growth hormone deficiency (GHD) in childhood and adolescence: recent advances. Endocr Rev 2014;35:376–432 [PMID: 24450934].

Cohen LE: Idiopathic short stature: a clinical review. JAMA 2014;311:1787–1796 [PMID: 24794372].

Loche S et al: Growth hormone treatment in non-growth hormone-deficiency children. Ann Pediatr Endocrinol Metab 2014;19:1–7 [PMID: 24926456].

Rogol AD, Hayden GF: Etiologies and early diagnosis of short stature and growth failure in children and adolescents. J Pediatr 2014 May;164(5 Suppl):S1–14.e6 [PMID: 24731744].

TALL STATURE

Although growth disturbances are usually associated with short stature, potentially serious pathologic conditions may also be associated with tall stature and excessive growth (Table 34–3). Excessive GH secretion is rare, particularly in

Table 34–3. Causes of tall stature.

A. Constitutional (familial)
B. Endocrine causes
   1. Growth hormone excess (pituitary gigantism)
   2. Precocious puberty
   3. Hypogonadism
C. Nonendocrine causes
   1. Klinefelter syndrome
   2. XYY males
   3. Marfan syndrome
   4. Cerebral gigantism (Sotos syndrome)
   5. Homocystinuria

children, and generally associated with a functioning pituitary adenoma. GH excess leads to gigantism if the epiphyses are open and to acromegaly if the epiphyses are closed. The diagnosis is confirmed by finding elevated random GH and IGF-1 levels and failure of GH suppression during an oral glucose tolerance test. Precocious puberty can also cause tall stature for age or rapid growth, but would be associated with early signs of puberty and an advanced bone age. Obese youth are also often tall for age, but they do not achieve a taller final height.

Davies JH, Cheetham T: Investigation and management of tall stature. Arch Dis Child 2014;99:772–777 [PMID: 24833789].

▼ DISORDERS OF THE POSTERIOR PITUITARY GLAND

The posterior pituitary (neurohypophysis) is an extension of the ventral hypothalamus. Its two principal hormones—oxytocin and arginine vasopressin—are synthesized in the supraoptic and paraventricular nuclei of the ventral hypothalamus. These peptide hormones are packaged in granules with specific neurophysins and transported via the axons to their storage site in the posterior pituitary. Vasopressin is essential for water balance; it acts primarily on the kidney to promote reabsorption of water from urine. Oxytocin is most active during parturition and breast feeding and is not discussed further here.

ARGININE VASOPRESSIN (ANTIDIURETIC HORMONE) PHYSIOLOGY

Vasopressin release is controlled primarily by serum osmolality and intravascular volume. Release is stimulated by minor increases in plasma osmolality (detected by osmoreceptors in the anterolateral hypothalamus) and large decreases in intravascular volume (detected by baroreceptors in the cardiac atria). Disorders of vasopressin release and action include: (1) central (neurogenic) DI, (2) nephrogenic DI (see Chapter 24), and (3) the syndrome of inappropriate secretion of antidiuretic hormone (SIADH).

CENTRAL DIABETES INSIPIDUS

 ESSENTIALS OF DIAGNOSIS & TYPICAL FEATURES

▶ Polydipsia, polyuria (> 2 L/m²/day), nocturia, dehydration, and hypernatremia.

▶ Inability to concentrate urine after fluid restriction (urine specific gravity < 1.010; urine osmolality < 300 mOsm/kg).

▶ Plasma osmolality greater than 300 mOsm/kg with urine osmolality less than 600 mOsm/kg.

▶ Low plasma vasopressin with antidiuretic response to exogenous vasopressin.

▶ General Considerations

Central diabetes insipidus (DI) is an inability to synthesize and release vasopressin. Without vasopressin, the kidneys cannot concentrate urine, causing excessive urinary water loss. Genetic causes of central DI are rare and include mutations in the vasopressin gene and the *WFS1* gene that causes DI, diabetes mellitus, optic atrophy, and deafness (Wolfram or DIDMOAD syndrome). The most common causes of pediatric central DI are midline defects (septo-optic dysplasia, holoprosencephaly); trauma (surgery, injury); infiltrative/neoplastic disease (tumors such as craniopharyngioma, germinoma, Langerhans cell histiocytosis, sarcoidosis); infectious (meningitis); and idiopathic.

Traumatic DI often has three phases. Initially, transient DI is caused by edema in the hypothalamus or pituitary area. In 2–5 days, unregulated release of vasopressin from dying neurons causes the SIADH. Finally, permanent DI occurs if a sufficient number of vasopressin neurons are destroyed.

▶ Clinical Findings

Onset of DI is characterized by polyuria, nocturia, enuresis, and intense thirst, usually with a preference for cold water. Hypernatremia, hyperosmolality, and dehydration occur if insufficient fluid intake does not keep up with urinary losses. In infants, symptoms may also include failure to thrive, vomiting, constipation, and unexplained fevers. Some infants may present with severe dehydration, circulatory collapse, and seizures. Vasopressin deficiency may be masked in patients with panhypopituitarism due to the impaired excretion of free water associated with ACTH insufficiency; treatment with glucocorticoids may unmask DI in these patients.

DI is confirmed when serum hyperosmolality is associated with urine hypo-osmolality. If the history indicates that the child can go through the night comfortably without drinking, outpatient testing is appropriate. Oral fluid intake is prohibited after midnight. Osmolality, sodium, and specific gravity of the first morning void are obtained. This can also be done as a water deprivation test in the hospital if screening results are unclear or if symptoms preclude safely withholding fluids at home. See "Essentials" box for diagnostic criteria. Children with central DI should have an MRI of the head with contrast to look for tumors or infiltrative processes.

Primary polydipsia must be distinguished from DI. Children with primary polydipsia tend to have lower serum sodium levels and usually can concentrate their urine with overnight fluid deprivation. Some may have secondary nephrogenic DI due to dilution of the renal medullary interstitium and decreased renal concentrating ability, but this resolves with restriction of fluid intake.

▶ Treatment

Central DI is treated with oral or intranasal desmopressin acetate (DDAVP). The aim of therapy is to provide antidiuresis that allows uninterrupted sleep. Breakthrough urination should occur before the next dose. It is important to note that postsurgical DI can be associated with disruption of thirst mechanism, and for these patients, a prescribed volume of fluid intake needs to be determined. Children hospitalized with acute-onset DI can be managed with intravenous or subcutaneous vasopressin. Due to the amount of antidiuresis, electrolytes should be closely monitored to avoid water intoxication. Infants with DI should not be treated with DDAVP, since their primary source of nutrition is through liquid calories and this combination can result in water intoxication. For this reason, infants are treated with extra free water to maintain normal hydration. A formula with a low renal solute load and chlorothiazides may be helpful in infants with central DI.

Di Iorgi N et al: Diabetes insipidus—diagnosis and management. Horm Res Paediatr 2012;77:69 [PMID: 22433947].

Rivkees SA et al: The management of central diabetes insipidus in infancy: desmopressin, low renal solute load formula, thiazide diuretics. J Pediatr Endocrinol Metab 2007;20:459 [PMID: 17550208].

Wise-Faberowski L et al: Perioperative management of diabetes insipidus in children. J Neurosurg Anesthesiol 2004;16:14 [PMID: 14676564].

▼ THYROID GLAND

FETAL DEVELOPMENT OF THE THYROID

As early as the 10th week of gestation, the fetal thyroid synthesizes thyroid hormone, which appears in the fetal serum by the 11th week of gestation and progressively increases throughout gestation. The fetal pituitary-thyroid axis functions largely independently of the maternal pituitary-thyroid axis because maternal TSH cannot cross the placenta. However, maternal thyroid hormone can cross the placenta in limited amounts.

At birth, there is a TSH surge peaking at about 70 mU/L within 30–60 minutes. Thyroid hormone serum level increases rapidly during the first days of life in response to this TSH surge. The TSH level decreases to childhood levels within a few weeks. The physiologic neonatal TSH surge can produce a false-positive newborn screen for hypothyroidism (ie, high TSH) if the blood sample for the screen is collected on the first day of life.

PHYSIOLOGY

Hypothalamic thyrotropin-releasing hormone (TRH) stimulates the anterior pituitary gland to release TSH. In turn, TSH stimulates the thyroid gland to take up iodine and synthesize and release T_4 and T_3. This process is regulated by negative feedback involving the hypothalamus, pituitary, and thyroid (see Figure 34–1).

T_4 is the predominant thyroid hormone secreted by the thyroid gland. Most circulating T_3 and T_4 are bound to thyroxine-binding globulin (TBG), albumin, and prealbumin. Less than 1% of thyroxine exists in the free form. T_4 is deiodinated in the tissues to T_3, which binds to high-affinity nuclear thyroid hormone receptors in the cytoplasm and translocates to the nucleus, exerting its biologic effects by modifying gene expression. Causes of low T_4 are hypothyroidism (central or primary), prematurity, malnutrition and severe illness, and following therapy with T_3.

Total T_4 is also low in situations that decrease TBG, such as familial TBG deficiency, cirrhosis, or renal failure and in patients receiving glucocorticoids or androgens. Since these effects primarily involve TBG, TSH, and free T_4 (FT_4) levels remain in the normal range. Conversely, total T_3 and T_4 levels may be elevated in conditions associated with increased TBG levels (congenital TBG excess, pregnancy, estrogen therapy) and increased thyroid hormone binding to transport proteins. Again, patients are clinically euthyroid in this circumstance. A T3 resin uptake can help differentiate between binding protein problems and true hypo- or hyperthyroidism.

HYPOTHYROIDISM (CONGENITAL & ACQUIRED)

ESSENTIALS OF DIAGNOSIS & TYPICAL FEATURES

▶ Growth retardation, decreased physical activity, weight gain, constipation, dry skin, cold intolerance, and delayed puberty.

▶ Untreated congenital hypothyroidism: thick tongue, large fontanels, poor muscle tone, hoarseness, umbilical hernia, jaundice, and intellectual retardation.

▶ T_4, FT_4, and T_3 resin uptake are low; TSH levels are elevated in primary hypothyroidism.

General Considerations

Thyroid hormone deficiency may be congenital or acquired (Table 34–4). It can be due to defects in the thyroid gland (primary hypothyroidism) or in the hypothalamus or pituitary (central hypothyroidism).

Congenital hypothyroidism occurs in about 1:3000–1:4000 infants. Untreated, it causes severe neurocognitive impairment. Most cases are sporadic resulting from hypoplasia or aplasia of the thyroid gland or failure of the gland to migrate to its normal anatomic location (ie, lingual or sublingual thyroid gland). Other causes are listed in Table 34–4. In severe maternal iodine deficiency, both the fetus and the mother are T_4-deficient, with irreversible brain damage to the fetus. Acquired hypothyroidism, particularly if goiter is present, is usually a result of chronic lymphocytic (Hashimoto) thyroiditis.

Several hundred patients with resistance to thyroid hormone have been described and present with elevations in T_4 and/or FT_4, with normal TSH. There is often a family history of the disorder. Clinical manifestations are highly variable due to differential expression of thyroid hormone receptor isoforms in different tissues.

Table 34–4. Causes of hypothyroidism.

A. Congenital
  1. Aplasia, hypoplasia, or maldescent of thyroid
  2. Inborn errors of thyroid hormone synthesis, secretion, or recycling
  3. Maternal antibody-mediated (inhibit TSH binding to receptor)
  4. TSH receptor defect
  5. Thyroid hormone receptor defect
  6. In utero exposures
     a. Radioiodine therapy
     b. Goitrogens (propylthiouracil, methimazole)
     c. Iodine excess
  7. Iodide deficiency
B. Acquired (juvenile hypothyroidism)
  1. Autoimmune (lymphocytic) thyroiditis
  2. Thyroidectomy or radioiodine therapy
  3. Irradiation to the thyroid
  4. Thyrotropin deficiency
  5. TRH deficiency due to hypothalamic injury or disease
  6. Medications
     a. Iodides
        (1) Excess (eg, amiodarone)
        (2) Deficiency
     b. Lithium
     c. Cobalt
  7. Large hemangiomas
  8. Idiopathic

T_3, triiodothyronine; T_4, thyroxine; TRH, thyrotropin-releasing hormone; TSH, thyroid-stimulating hormone.

Clinical Findings

A. Symptoms and Signs

Even when the thyroid gland is completely absent, most newborns with congenital hypothyroidism appear normal. However, because congenital hypothyroidism is associated with intellectual impairment, thyroid testing is included in the newborn screen and treatment must be initiated as early as possible. Jaundice associated with an unconjugated hyperbilirubinemia may be present in newborns with congenital hypothyroidism.

Features of juvenile hypothyroidism include poor linear growth; delayed bone age and retarded dental eruption; skin changes (dry, thick, scaly, coarse, pale, cool, or sallow); hair changes (dry, coarse, or brittle), hair loss; lateral thinning of the eyebrows; musculoskeletal findings (hypotonia and a slow relaxation component of deep tendon reflexes); physical and mental sluggishness; nonpitting myxedema; constipation; cold temperature intolerance; bradycardia; delayed puberty; occasional pseudopuberty (secondary to weak FSH activity of marked elevated TSH levels).

In hypothyroidism resulting from enzymatic defects, ingestion of goitrogens, or chronic lymphocytic thyroiditis, the thyroid gland may be enlarged. Thyroid enlargement in children is usually symmetrical, and the gland is moderately firm and not nodular. In chronic lymphocytic thyroiditis, however, the thyroid frequently has a cobblestone surface (see the following text).

B. Laboratory Findings

In primary hypothyroidism, the total T_4 and FT_4 may be normal or decreased and the serum TSH is elevated. Circulating autoantibodies to thyroid peroxidase and thyroglobulin may be present. In central hypothyroidism, the TSH is usually inappropriately normal and associated with a low total T_4 and FT_4. Serum prolactin may be elevated, resulting in galactorrhea. Other pituitary deficiencies may be present, as central hypothyroidism may be associated with congenital or acquired disorders of the hypothalamus or pituitary gland.

C. Imaging

Thyroid imaging, while helpful in establishing the cause of congenital hypothyroidism, does not affect the treatment plan and is not necessary. Bone age is delayed. Cardiomegaly is common. Long-standing primary hypothyroidism may be associated with thyrotrophic hyperplasia characterized by an enlarged sella or pituitary gland.

D. Screening Programs for Neonatal Hypothyroidism

All newborns should be screened for congenital hypothyroidism shortly after birth. Depending on the state, the newborn screen measures either the total T_4 or TSH level. Abnormal newborn screening results should be confirmed immediately with a venous T_4 and TSH level. Treatment should be started as soon as possible. Initiation of treatment in the first month of life and good compliance during infancy usually results in a normal neurocognitive outcome.

▶ Treatment

Levothyroxine (75–100 mcg/m²/day) is the drug of choice for acquired hypothyroidism. In neonates with congenital hypothyroidism, the recommended initial dose is 10–15 mcg/kg/day. Serum total T_4 or FT_4 concentrations are used to monitor the adequacy of initial therapy because the high neonatal TSH may not normalize for weeks. Subsequently, T_4 and TSH are monitored in combination.

Kaplowitz, P: Neonatal thyroid disease: testing and management. Pediatr Clin North Am 2019; 66(2):343–352 [PMID: 30819341].

Léger J et al: European Society for Paediatric Endocrinology consensus guidelines on screening, diagnosis, and management of congenital hypothyroidism. J Clin Endocrinol Metab 2014; 99(2):363–384 [PMID: 24446653].

van der Sluijs Veer L et al: Evaluation of cognitive and motor development in toddlers with congenital hypothyroidism diagnosed by neonatal screening. J Dev Behav Pediatr 2012;33: 633–640 [PMID: 23027136].

THYROIDITIS

1. Chronic Lymphocytic Thyroiditis (Chronic Autoimmune Thyroiditis, Hashimoto Thyroiditis)

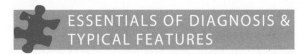

ESSENTIALS OF DIAGNOSIS &
TYPICAL FEATURES

▶ Firm, freely movable, nontender, diffusely enlarged thyroid gland.

▶ Thyroid function is usually normal but may be elevated or decreased depending on the stage of the disease.

▶ General Considerations

Chronic lymphocytic thyroiditis is the most common cause of goiter and acquired hypothyroidism in childhood. It is more common in girls, and the incidence peaks during puberty. The disease is caused by an autoimmune attack on the thyroid. Increased risk of thyroid autoimmunity (and other endocrine autoimmune disorders) is associated with certain histocompatibility alleles. The following conditions are

associated with increased risk for autoimmune (Hashimoto) thyroiditis: Down syndrome, Turner syndrome, celiac disease, vitiligo, alopecia, and type 1 diabetes.

▶ Clinical Findings

A. Symptoms and Signs

The thyroid is characteristically enlarged, firm, freely movable, nontender, and symmetrical. It may be nodular. Onset is usually insidious. Occasionally, patients note a sensation of tracheal compression or fullness, hoarseness, and dysphagia. No local signs of inflammation or systemic infection are present. Most patients are euthyroid. Some patients are symptomatically hypothyroid, and few patients are symptomatically hyperthyroid. A detailed family history may reveal the presence of multiple autoimmune diseases in family members. Individuals at a high risk based on a chromosomal disorder or other autoimmune disease benefit from careful monitoring of growth and development, routine screening (in the case of Down syndrome, Turner syndrome, and type 1 diabetes), and a low threshold for measurement of thyroid function.

B. Laboratory Findings

Laboratory findings vary. Serum concentrations of TSH, T_4, and FT_4 are usually normal. Some patients are hypothyroid with an elevated TSH and low thyroid hormone levels. A few patients are hyperthyroid with a suppressed TSH and elevated thyroid hormone levels. Thyroid antibodies (antithyroglobulin, antithyroid peroxidase) are frequently elevated.

C. Imaging

Routine thyroid ultrasound is not indicated unless focal nodule or mass is palpated. Thyroid uptake scan adds little to the diagnosis. Surgical or needle biopsy is diagnostic but seldom necessary.

▶ Treatment

There is controversy about the need to treat chronic lymphocytic thyroiditis with normal thyroid function. Full replacement doses of thyroid hormone may decrease the size of the thyroid, but may also result in hyperthyroidism. Hypothyroidism commonly develops over time. Consequently, patients require lifelong surveillance. Children with documented hypothyroidism should receive thyroid hormone replacement.

2. Acute (Suppurative) Thyroiditis

Acute thyroiditis is rare. The most common causes are group A streptococci, pneumococci, *Staphylococcus aureus*, and anaerobes. Thyroid abscesses may form. The patient is toxic with fever and chills. The thyroid gland is enlarged and exquisitely tender with associated erythema, hoarseness, and dysphagia. Thyroid function tests are typically normal. Patients have a leukocytosis, "left shift," and elevated erythrocyte sedimentation rate. Antibiotic therapy is required.

3. Subacute (Nonsuppurative) Thyroiditis

Subacute thyroiditis (de Quervain thyroiditis) is rare. It is thought to be caused by viral infection with mumps, influenza, echovirus, coxsackievirus, Epstein-Barr virus, or adenovirus. Presenting features are similar to acute thyroiditis—fever, malaise, sore throat, dysphagia, and thyroid pain that may radiate to the ear. The thyroid is firm and enlarged. Sedimentation rate is elevated. In contrast to acute thyroiditis, the onset is generally insidious and serum thyroid hormone concentrations may be elevated.

HYPERTHYROIDISM

ESSENTIALS OF DIAGNOSIS & TYPICAL FEATURES

▶ Nervousness, emotional lability, hyperactivity, fatigue, tremor, palpitations, excessive appetite, weight loss, increased perspiration, and heat intolerance.

▶ Goiter, exophthalmos, tachycardia, widened pulse pressure, systolic hypertension, weakness, and smooth, moist, warm skin.

▶ TSH is suppressed. Thyroid hormone levels (T_4, FT_4, T_3, T_3 resin uptake [T_3RU]) are elevated.

▶ General Considerations

In children, most cases of hyperthyroidism are due to Graves disease, caused by antibodies directed at the TSH receptor that stimulate thyroid hormone production. Other causes include thyroiditis (acute, subacute, or chronic); autonomous functioning thyroid nodules; tumors producing TSH; McCune-Albright syndrome; exogenous thyroid hormone excess; and acute iodine exposure.

▶ Clinical Findings

A. Symptoms and Signs

Hyperthyroidism is more common in females than males. In children, it most frequently occurs during adolescence. The course of hyperthyroidism may be cyclic, with spontaneous remissions and exacerbations. Symptoms include poor concentration, hyperactivity, fatigue, emotional lability, personality disturbance/unmasking of underlying psychosis, insomnia, weight loss (despite increased appetite), palpitations, heat intolerance, increased perspiration, increased stool frequency, polyuria, and irregular menses. Signs include tachycardia, systolic hypertension, increased pulse pressure, tremor, proximal muscle weakness, and moist, warm, skin. Accelerated growth and development may occur. Thyroid storm is a rare condition characterized by fever, cardiac failure, emesis, and delirium that can result in coma or death. Most cases of Graves disease are associated with a diffuse firm goiter. A thyroid bruit and thrill may be present. Many cases are associated with exophthalmos.

B. Laboratory Findings

TSH is suppressed. T_4, FT_4, T_3, and free T_3 (FT_3) are elevated except in rare cases in which only the serum T_3 is elevated (T_3 thyrotoxicosis). The presence of thyroid-stimulating immunoglobulin (TSI) or thyroid eye disease confirms the diagnosis of Graves disease. TSH receptor-binding antibodies (TRAb) are usually elevated.

C. Imaging

Radioactive iodine uptake by the thyroid is increased in Graves disease, whereas in subacute and chronic thyroiditis it is decreased. An autonomous hyperfunctioning nodule takes up iodine and appears as a "hot nodule" while the surrounding tissue has decreased iodine uptake. In children with hyperthyroidism, bone age may be advanced. In infants, accelerated skeletal maturation may be associated with premature fusion of the cranial sutures. Long-standing hyperthyroidism causes osteoporosis.

▶ Treatment

A. General Measures

Strenuous physical activity should be avoided in untreated hyperthyroidism.

B. Medical Treatment

1. β-Adrenergic blocking agents—These are adjuncts to therapy. They can rapidly ameliorate symptoms and are indicated in severe disease with tachycardia and hypertension. $β_1$-Specific agents such as atenolol are preferred because they are more cardioselective. Propranolol also decreases conversion of T_4 to active T_3, so is preferred in severe cases/thyrotoxicosis.

2. Antithyroid agents (methimazole)—Antithyroid agents are frequently used in the initial treatment of childhood hyperthyroidism. These drugs interfere with thyroid hormone synthesis, and usually take a few weeks to produce a clinical response. Adequate control is usually achieved within a few months. If medical therapy is unsuccessful, more definitive therapy, such as radioablation of the thyroid or thyroidectomy, should be considered. Propylthiouracil (PTU) is rarely utilized because of reports of severe hepatotoxicity.

A. INITIAL DOSAGE—Methimazole is initiated at a dose of 10–60 mg/day (0.5–1 mg/kg/day) given once a day. Initial dosing is continued until FT_4 or T_4 have normalized and signs and symptoms have subsided.

B. MAINTENANCE—The optimal dose of antithyroid agent for maintenance treatment remains unclear. Recent studies suggest that 10–15 mg/day of methimazole provides adequate long-term control in most patients with a minimum of side effects. If the TSH becomes elevated, many providers decrease the dose of the antithyroid agent; others continue the same dose of antithyroid agent and add exogenous thyroid hormone replacement. Treatment usually continues for 2 years with the goal of inducing remission. If thyroid hormone levels are stable at that point, a trial off medication could be considered.

C. TOXICITY—If vasculitis, arthralgia, arthritis, granulocytopenia, or hepatitis occur, the drug must be discontinued. Urticarial rash can sometimes be treated symptomatically.

3. Iodide—Large doses of iodide usually produce a rapid but short-lived blockade of thyroid hormone synthesis and release. This approach is recommended only for acute management of severely thyrotoxic patients or in preparation for thyroidectomy.

C. Radiation Therapy

Radioactive iodine ablation of the thyroid is usually reserved for children with Graves disease who do not respond to antithyroid agents, develop adverse effects from the antithyroid agents, fail to achieve remission after several years of medical therapy, or have poor medication adherence. Antithyroid agents should be discontinued 4–7 days prior to radioiodine treatment to allow radioiodine uptake by the thyroid. ^{131}I is administered orally, concentrating in the thyroid and resulting in decreased thyroid activity. In the first 2 weeks following radioiodine treatment, hyperthyroidism may worsen as thyroid tissue is destroyed and thyroid hormone is released and temporary therapy with a β-adrenergic antagonist or methimazole may be necessary. In most cases, hypothyroidism develops and thyroid hormone replacement is needed. Long-term follow-up studies have not shown any increased incidence of thyroid cancer, leukemia, infertility, or birth defects when ablative doses of ^{131}I were used.

D. Surgical Treatment

Subtotal and total thyroidectomies may also be considered in children with Graves disease. Surgery is indicated for extremely large goiters, goiters with a suspicious nodule, very young or pregnant patients, or patients refusing radioiodine ablation. Before surgery, a β-adrenergic blocking agent is given to treat symptoms, and antithyroid agents are given for several weeks to minimize the surgical risks associated with hyperthyroidism. Iodide (eg, Lugol solution, one drop every 8 hours, or saturated solution of potassium iodide, one to two drops three times per day) can be given for 1–2 weeks prior to surgery to reduce thyroid vascularity and inhibit release of thyroid hormone. Surgical complications include hypocalcemia due to hypoparathyroidism and recurrent laryngeal nerve damage. An experienced thyroid surgeon is crucial to good surgical outcome. After thyroidectomy, patients become hypothyroid and need thyroid hormone replacement.

▶ Course & Prognosis

Partial remissions and exacerbations may continue for several years. Treatment with an antithyroid agent results in prolonged remissions in one-third to two-thirds of children.

Bauer AJ: Approach to the pediatric patient with Graves' disease: when is definitive therapy warranted? J Clin Endocrinol Metab 2011;96:580–588 [PMID: 21378220].

Rivkees SA: Pediatric Graves' disease: management in the post-propylthiouracil. Era Int J Pediatrc Endocrinol 2014; 2014(1): 10 [PMID: 25089127].

Yuan L, Yang J: Radioiodine treatment in pediatric Graves' disease and thyroid carcinoma. J Pediatr Endocrinol Metab 2011;24: 877–883 [PMID: 22308835].

▶ Neonatal Graves Disease

Transient congenital hyperthyroidism (neonatal Graves disease) occurs in about 1% of infants born to mothers with Graves disease. It occurs when maternal TSH receptor antibodies cross the placenta and stimulate excess thyroid hormone production in the fetus and newborn. Neonatal Graves disease can be associated with irritability, intrauterine growth retardation (IUGR), poor weight gain, flushing, jaundice, hepatosplenomegaly, and thrombocytopenia. Severe cases may result in cardiac failure and death. Hyperthyroidism may develop several days after birth. In high-risk neonates, TSH receptor antibody (TRAb) level should be obtained at birth and free T4 and TSH obtained day of life 3–5. Immediate management should focus on the cardiac manifestations. Temporary treatment may be necessary with iodide, antithyroid agents, β-adrenergic antagonists, or corticosteroids. Hyperthyroidism gradually resolves over 1–3 months as maternal antibodies decline. As TRAbs may still be present in the serum of previously hyperthyroid mothers after thyroidectomy or radioablation, neonatal Graves disease should be considered in all infants of mothers with a history of hyperthyroidism.

Léger J, Carel JC: Hyperthyroidism in childhood: causes, when, and how to treat. J Clin Res Pediatr Endocrinol 2013;5(Suppl 1): 50–56 [PMID: 23154161].

Lewis KA et al: Neonatal Graves disease associated with severe metabolic abnormalities. Pediatrics 2011;128(1):e232–e236 [PMID: 21646263].

van der Kaay et al: Management of neonates born to mothers with Graves' disease. Pediatrics 2016;137(4):e20151878 [PMID: 26980880].

THYROID CANCER

Thyroid cancer is rare in childhood. Children usually present with a thyroid nodule or an asymptomatic asymmetrical neck mass. Dysphagia and hoarseness are unusual symptoms. Thyroid function tests are usually normal. A "cold" nodule is often seen on a technetium or radioiodine uptake scan of the thyroid. Fine-needle aspiration biopsy of the nodule assists in the diagnosis.

The most common thyroid cancer is papillary thyroid carcinoma, a well-differentiated carcinoma arising from the thyroid follicular cell. Children frequently present with local metastases to the cervical lymph nodes and occasionally with pulmonary metastases. Despite its aggressive presentation, children with papillary thyroid carcinoma have a relatively good prognosis, with a 20-year survival rate greater than 90%. Treatment consists of total thyroidectomy and removal of all involved lymph nodes, usually followed by radioiodine ablation to destroy residual thyroid remnant and metastatic tissue left behind after surgery. Thyroid hormone replacement is started to suppress TSH stimulation of residual thyroid tissue and to treat the hypothyroidism that results from surgical removal of the thyroid gland. Since papillary thyroid carcinoma in children is associated with a high recurrence rate, regular follow-up with serum thyroglobulin levels (a tumor marker), neck ultrasound, and radioiodine whole body scan are required.

Follicular thyroid carcinoma, medullary thyroid carcinoma, anaplastic carcinoma, and lymphoma are less common thyroid malignancies. Medullary thyroid carcinoma, due to autosomal dominant mutations in the RET protooncogene, arises from the thyroid C cells, which secrete calcitonin, and it is associated with elevated serum calcitonin levels. It can occur sporadically or be inherited in multiple endocrine neoplasia (MEN) type 2 and familial medullary thyroid carcinoma. In affected families, all members should be screened for the mutation, and those identified with the mutation should be treated with prophylactic thyroidectomy in early childhood.

Chan et al: Pediatric thyroid cancer. Adv Pediatr 2017;64(1): 171–190 [PMID: 28688588].

Francis GL et al: Management guidelines for children with thyroid nodules and differentiated thyroid cancer. Thyroid 2015;25(7):716–759 [PMID: 25900731].

Waguespack SG et al: Management of medullary thyroid carcinoma and MEN2 syndromes in childhood. Nat Rev Endocrinol 2011;23(7):596–607 [PMID: 21862994].

Wells SA Jr, et al: Revised American Thyroid Association guidelines for the management of medullary thyroid carcinoma. Thyroid 2015;25(6):567–610 [PMID: 25810047].

▼ DISORDERS OF CALCIUM & PHOSPHORUS METABOLISM

Serum calcium concentration is tightly regulated by the coordinated actions of the parathyroid glands, kidney, liver, and small intestine. Low serum calcium concentrations, detected by calcium-sensing receptors on the surface of parathyroid cells, stimulate parathyroid hormone (PTH) release. PTH in turn promotes release of calcium and phosphorus from the bone, reabsorption of calcium from the urinary filtrate, and excretion of phosphorus in the urine. Another essential cofactor in calcium homeostasis is 1,25-dihydroxy vitamin D (calcitriol). The first step in production of this active form of vitamin D occurs in the liver where dietary vitamin D is hydroxylated to 25-hydroxy vitamin D. The final step in formation of calcitriol is 1-hydroxylation, which takes place in the kidney under control of PTH. The primary effect of calcitriol is to promote the absorption of calcium from the intestines. In concert with PTH, however, it also facilitates calcium and phosphorus mobilization from bones. Deficiencies or excesses of PTH or calcitriol, abnormalities in their receptors, or abnormalities of vitamin D metabolism lead to clinically significant aberrations in calcium homeostasis. Although calcitonin, released from the thyroid gland C cells, also reduces serum calcium concentration, changes in its serum concentration rarely cause clinically relevant disease.

HYPOCALCEMIC DISORDERS

A normal serum calcium concentration is approximately 8.9–10.2 mg/dL. The normal concentration of ionized calcium is approximately 1.1–1.3 mmol/L. Serum calcium levels in newborns, which are slightly lower than in older children and adults, may be as low as 7 mg/dL in premature infants. Fifty to sixty percent of calcium in the serum is protein-bound and metabolically inactive. Thus, measurement of ionized serum calcium, the metabolically active form, is helpful if serum proteins are low or in conditions such as acidosis that cause abnormal calcium binding to protein.

ESSENTIALS OF DIAGNOSIS & TYPICAL FEATURES

▶ Tetany with facial and extremity numbness, tingling, cramps, spontaneous muscle contractures, carpopedal spasm, positive Trousseau and Chvostek signs, loss of consciousness, and convulsions.

▶ Diarrhea, prolongation of electrical systole (QT interval), and laryngospasm.

▶ In hypoparathyroidism or pseudohypoparathyroidism (PHP): defective nails and teeth, cataracts, and ectopic calcification in the subcutaneous tissues and basal ganglia.

▶ General Considerations

Hypocalcemia is a consistent feature of conditions such as hypoparathyroidism, PHP, transient neonatal hypoparathyroidism, and severe vitamin D deficiency rickets, and may be present in rare disorders of vitamin D action

(receptor defects, Malloy 2010). Causes of rickets are outlined in Table 34–5. Other causes of hypocalcemia include the following:

- Intestinal malabsorption of calcium (may be exacerbated by malabsorption of vitamin D and/or magnesium)
- Chronic renal disease
- Tumor lysis syndrome, rhabdomyolysis (due to cellular destruction that liberates large amounts of intracellular phosphate that complex with serum calcium)
- Activating mutation in the calcium-sensing receptor of the parathyroid glands and kidneys (hypercalciuric hypocalcemia, Hendy 2009)
- Hypoparathyroidism, including typically transient hypoparathyroidism following thyroidectomy

Deficient PTH *secretion* may be due to deficient parathyroid tissue (DiGeorge syndrome), autoimmunity, or sometimes, magnesium deficiency. Decreased PTH action may be due to magnesium deficiency, vitamin D deficiency, or defects in the PTH receptor (PHP). Occasionally, PTH deficiency is idiopathic. Table 34–6 summarizes the clinical

Table 34–5. Hypocalcemia associated with rickets.

Condition	Pathogenesis	Disease States/ Inheritance	Clinical Features	Initial Biochemical Findings			
				Serum Calcium	Serum Phosphorus	Serum Alkaline Phosphatase	Other
Vitamin D-deficiency rickets	Deficient dietary vitamin D, vitamin D malabsorption; other risk factors include dark skin and lack of sunlight exposure	May cluster in families due to shared risk factors	Characteristic skeletal changes appear early, poor growth, symptomatic hypocalcemia is a late finding	Normal until late in course	Low or normal	Elevated	Elevated PTH levels, low 25-OH vitamin D
Vitamin D 1α-hydroxylase deficiency	Mutation in 1-hydroxylase enzyme required for synthesis of fully active 1,25-OH vitamin D	Autosomal recessive inheritance	Skeletal changes of rickets, symptomatic hypocalcemia	Low	Low or normal	Elevated	Elevated PTH, low 1,25-OH vitamin D
Vitamin D resistance	Mutation in 1,25-OH vitamin D receptor	Autosomal recessive inheritance	Severe skeletal changes of rickets, total alopecia, symptomatic hypocalcemia	Low	Low or normal	Elevated	Elevated PTH, elevated 1,25-OH vitamin D
Hypophosphatemic rickets	Excessive loss of phosphate in the urine Decreased fibroblast growth factor 23 (FGF23) activity	X-linked dominant due to PHEX activation or autosomal dominant due to FGF23 mutations	Skeletal changes primarily in the lower extremities—genu varum or valgus, short stature	Normal or low	Very low	Usually high	Normal PTH levels initially, abnormally high urinary phosphate excretion

Table 34–6. Hypocalcemia associated with disorders of parathyroid hormone secretion or action.

Condition	Pathogenesis	Inheritance Pattern	Clinical Features	Initial Biochemical Findings[a]			
				Serum Calcium	Serum Phosphorus	Serum Alkaline Phosphatase	Serum PTH
Acquired isolated hypoparathyroidism	Trauma, surgical destruction, iron overload, isolated autoimmune destruction	None known	Symptoms of hypocalcemia	Low	High	Normal or low	Low, low 1,25-OH vitamin D
Familial Isolated hypoparathyroidism	Mutations in GCMB, PTH gene, preproPTH gene	Autosomal recessive (GCMB, PTH gene) or Autosomal dominant (preproPTH gene)	Symptoms of hypocalcemia	Low	High	Normal or low	Low, low 1,25-OH vitamin D
DiGeorge-syndrome	Deletion in chromosome 22	Majority represent new mutations	Symptoms of hypocalcemia, cardiac anomalies, immune disorder	Low	High	Normal or low	Low, low 1,25-OH vitamin D
APS type 1	Autoimmune destruction	Autosomal recessive	Mucocutaneous candidiasis, Addison disease; potential for autoimmune destruction in other endocrine glands	Low	High	Normal or low	Low, low 1,25-OH vitamin D
PHP type IA	Mutation in stimulatory G protein; resistance to PTH action	Autosomal dominant	AHO phenotype, short stature, variable hypocalcemia, may have resistance to other hormones using G protein signaling	Low or normal	Elevated or normal	Variable	Very elevated, low 1,25-OH vitamin D
PPHP	Mutation in stimulatory G protein	Autosomal dominant—frequently found within same families with PHP type IA	AHO phenotype, biochemical parameters are normal	Normal	Normal	Normal	Normal
Transient neonatal hypoparathyroidism—early	Deficiency in PTH secretion or action	Sporadic—associated with birth asphyxia, infants of diabetic mothers, or maternal hyperparathyroidism	Onset of symptoms of hypocalcemia within 2 wk of birth	Low	Normal or low	Normal or low	Normal or low, low 1,25-OH vitamin D
Transient neonatal hypoparathyroidism—late onset	Deficiency in PTH secretion or action	Sporadic—associated with infant formulas that have a high phosphate content	Onset of symptoms of hypocalcemia after 2 wk of age	Low	Normal or low	Normal or low	Normal or low, low 1,25-OH vitamin D
Familial hypercalciuric hypocalcemia	Gain of functional mutation of calcium-sensing receptor	Autosomal dominant	Symptoms of hypocalcemia, family history	Low	High	Normal or low	Low, low 1,25-OH vitamin D

AHO, Albright hereditary osteodystrophy; APS, autoimmune polyglandular syndrome; PHP, pseudohypoparathyroidism; PPHP, pseudo-pseudohypoparathyroidism; PTH, parathyroid hormone.
[a]Urinary calcium excretion (calcium-creatinine ratio) is low in all but familial hypercalciuric hypocalcemia.

and laboratory characteristics of disorders of PTH secretion and action.

Autoimmune parathyroid destruction with subsequent hypoparathyroidism may be isolated, or associated with other autoimmune disorders in the APECED (autoimmune polyendocrinopathy-candidiasis-ectodermal dystrophy, or APS-1) syndrome. Hypoparathyroidism may also be secondary to manipulation of the blood supply of the parathyroid glands or removal of the parathyroid glands during thyroidectomy. Autosomal dominant hypocalcemia, also called familial hypercalciuric hypocalcemia, is associated with a gain-of-function mutation in the calcium-sensing receptor, which causes a low serum PTH despite hypocalcemia, and excessive urinary loss of calcium. A family history of hypocalcemia may be the clue that differentiates this condition from other causes of hypocalcemia.

Transient neonatal hypoparathyroidism is caused both by a relative deficiency of PTH secretion and PTH action (see Table 34–6). In the early form, associated hypomagnesemia often aggravates hypoparathyroidism due to magnesium's role in facilitating PTH secretion. The late form of neonatal hypoparathyroidism (after 2 weeks of age) occurs in infants receiving high-phosphate formulas (whole cow's milk is a well-known example) due to intestinal calcium-phosphate binding, resulting in decreased absorption of intestinal calcium.

Rickets describes characteristic clinical and bony radiologic features associated with hypophosphatemia (see Chapter 11). Vitamin D deficiency, caused by lack of sunlight exposure or dietary deficiency, is the most common cause of rickets. Recently, high rates of occult vitamin D deficiency have formed the basis for the 2008 recommendation by the American Academy of Pediatrics that breastfed infants receive vitamin D supplementation of at least 400 IU/day. See Table 34–5 for features of other causes of rickets.

Familial hypophosphatemic rickets occurs due to abnormal renal phosphate loss related to abnormal fibroblast growth factor 23 (FGF23) regulation.

▶ Clinical Findings

A. Symptoms and Signs

Prolonged hypocalcemia from any cause is associated with tetany, photophobia, blepharospasm, and diarrhea. Symptoms of tetany include numbness, muscle cramps, twitching of the extremities, carpopedal spasm, and laryngospasm. Tapping the face in front of the ear causes facial spasms (Chvostek sign) and inflation of a sphygmomanometer above systolic blood pressure causes a carpal spasm (Trousseau's sign). Some patients with hypocalcemia exhibit bizarre behavior, irritability, loss of consciousness, and convulsions. Electrocardiogram may demonstrate prolonged QTc. Headache, vomiting, increased intracranial pressure,

and papilledema may occur. In early infancy, respiratory distress may be a presenting finding.

B. Laboratory Findings

Tables 34–5 and 34–6 outline the specific laboratory findings in various causes of hypocalcemia (Shaw, 2009). Magnesium levels may also be low. Measurement of urinary excretion of calcium (calcium-creatinine ratio) can assist in diagnosis and monitoring of therapy in children on calcitriol therapy.

C. Imaging

Soft tissue and basal ganglia calcification may occur in idiopathic hypoparathyroidism and PHP. Various skeletal changes are associated with rickets, including cupped and irregular long bone metaphyses. Torsional deformities can result in genu varum (bowleg). Accentuation of the costochondral junction gives the rachitic rosary appearance seen on the chest wall.

▶ Differential Diagnosis

Tables 34–5 and 34–6 outline the features of disorders associated with hypocalcemia. In individuals with hypoalbuminemia, the total serum calcium may be low and yet the functional serum ionized calcium is normal. Ionized calcium is the test of choice for hypocalcemia in patients with low serum albumin.

▶ Treatment

A. Acute or Severe Tetany

Symptoms are treated acutely by administration of intravenous calcium gluconate or calcium chloride at a dose of 10 mg/kg. Intravenous calcium infusions should not exceed 50 mg/min because of possible cardiac arrhythmia. Cardiac monitoring should be performed during calcium infusion. Rise in serum calcium is limited to about 2–3 hours after an intravenous calcium bolus infusion, therefore the bolus will need to be followed by oral or continuous calcium infusions if hypocalcemia persists.

B. Maintenance Management of Hypoparathyroidism or Chronic Hypocalcemia

The objective of treatment is to maintain the serum calcium and phosphate at near-normal levels without excess urinary calcium excretion.

1. Diet—Calcium supplementation should start at a dose of 50–75 mg of elemental calcium per kilogram per day divided in three to four doses. Supplemental calcium can often be discontinued in patients with rickets after vitamin D therapy has stabilized.

2. Vitamin D supplementation—Ergocalciferol (vitamin D_2) and cholecalciferol (vitamin D_3) are the most commonly used oral vitamin D preparations. Cholecalciferol is slightly more active than ergocalciferol. Calcitriol (1,25-dihydroxy vitamin D_3) supplementation is recommended for impaired metabolism of dietary vitamin D to 25-OH vitamin D as seen in hepatic dysfunction, or to its active end product, 1,25-dihydroxy vitamin D, or impaired PTH function. Selection and dosage of vitamin D supplements varies with the underlying condition and the response to therapy.

3. Monitoring—Dosage of calcium and vitamin D must be tailored for each patient. Monitoring serum calcium, urine calcium, and serum alkaline phosphatase levels at 1- to 3-month intervals is necessary to ensure adequate therapy and to prevent hypercalcemia, hypercalciuria/ nephrocalcinosis and vitamin D toxicity.

The major goals of monitoring in vitamin D deficiency are to ensure: (1) maintenance of serum calcium and phosphorus concentrations within normal ranges, (2) normalization of alkaline phosphatase activity for age, (3) regression of skeletal changes, and (4) maintenance of an age-appropriate urine calcium-creatinine ratio. The urine-creatinine ratio should be less than 0.8 in newborns, 0.3–0.6 in children, and less than 0.25 in adolescents (when using creatinine and calcium measured in milligrams per deciliter).

Monitoring goals are somewhat different in hypophosphatemic rickets. Serum calcium and alkaline phosphatase, and urinary calcium to creatinine ratio should be maintained within normal limits. Monitoring of serum PTH is necessary to ensure that secondary hyperparathyroidism does not develop from excessive phosphate treatment or inadequate calcitriol replacement.

PSEUDOHYPOPARATHYROIDISM (RESISTANCE TO PARATHYROID HORMONE ACTION)

In PHP, PTH production is adequate, but target organs (renal tubule, bone, or both) fail to respond because of receptor resistance. Resistance to PTH action is due to a heterozygous inactivating mutation in the stimulatory G protein subunit associated with the PTH receptor, which leads to impaired signaling. Resistance to other G protein-dependent hormones, such as TSH, GHRH, and follicle-stimulating hormone (FSH)/luteinizing hormone (LH), may also be present.

There are several types of PHP with variable biochemical and phenotypic features (see Table 34–6). Biochemical abnormalities in PHP (hypocalcemia and hyperphosphatemia) are similar to those seen in hypoparathyroidism, but the PTH levels are elevated. PHP may be accompanied by a characteristic phenotype known as Albright hereditary osteodystrophy (AHO), which includes short stature; round, full facies; irregularly shortened fourth metacarpal; a short, thick-set body; delayed and defective dentition; and mild intellectual disability. Corneal and lenticular opacities and

ectopic calcification of the basal ganglia and subcutaneous tissues (osteoma cutis) may occur with or without abnormal serum calcium levels. Treatment is the same as for hypoparathyroidism.

Pseudo-pseudohypoparathyroidism (PPHP) describes individuals with the AHO phenotype, but normal calcium homeostasis. PHP and PPHP can occur in the same cohort. Genomic imprinting is probably responsible for the different phenotypic expression of disease. Heterozygous loss of the maternal allele causes PHP while heterozygous loss of the paternal allele causes PPHP.

Elder CJ, Bishop NJ: Rickets [Review]. Lancet 2014;383:1665–1676 [PMID: 24412049].

Hendy GN, Guarnieri V, Canaff L: Calcium-sensing receptor and associated diseases [Review]. Prog Mol Biol Transl Sci 2009;89:31–95 [Epub 2009 Oct 7] [PMID: 20374733].

Lee JY, Imel EA: The changing face of hypophosphatemic disorders in the FGF-23 era [Review]. Pediatr Endocrinol Rev 2013;10(Suppl 2):367–379 [PMID: 23858620].

Malloy PJ, Feldman D: Genetic disorders and defects in vitamin D action. Endocrinol Metab Clin North Am 2010 Jun;39(2): 333–346 [PMID: 20511055].

Shaw N: A practical approach to hypocalcaemia in children [Review]. Endocr Dev 2009;16:73–92 [PMID: 19494662].

HYPERCALCEMIC STATES

Hypercalcemia is defined as a serum calcium level greater than 11 mg/dL. Severe hypercalcemia is a level greater than 13.5 mg/dL.

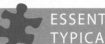

ESSENTIALS OF DIAGNOSIS & TYPICAL FEATURES

▶ Abdominal pain, polyuria, polydipsia, hypertension, nephrocalcinosis, failure to thrive, renal stones, intractable peptic ulcer, constipation, uremia, and pancreatitis.

▶ Bone pain or pathologic fractures, subperiosteal bone resorption, renal parenchymal calcification or stones, and osteitis fibrosa cystica.

▶ Impaired concentration, altered mental status, mood swings, and coma.

▶ General Considerations

Hypercalcemia is less common in children than in adults and etiology varies by age (McNeilly, 2016). Table 34–7 summarizes the differential diagnosis of childhood hypercalcemia (Lietman 2010).

Hyperparathyroidism is rare in childhood and may be primary or secondary (Belcher, 2013). The most common cause

Table 34–7. Hypercalcemic states.

A. Primary hyperparathyroidism
1. Parathyroid hyperplasia
2. Parathyroid adenoma
3. Familial, including MEN types 1 and 2
4. Ectopic PTH secretion
5. Maternal hypoparathyroidism
B. Other hypercalcemic states resulting from increased intestinal or renal absorption of calcium
1. Hypervitaminosis D (including idiopathic hypercalcemia of infancy)
2. Familial hypocalciuric hypercalcemia
3. Lithium therapy
4. Sarcoidosis
5. Phosphate depletion
6. Aluminum intoxication
7. Subcutaneous fat necrosis (due to vitamin D activation)
8. Premature infant on human milk or standard formula
C. Other hypercalcemic states
1. Hyperthyroidism
2. Immobilization
3. Lithium and Thiazides
4. Vitamin A intoxication
5. Adrenal insufficiency
6. Hypophosphatasia
7. Genetic syndromes
   a. William syndrome
   b. IMAGe syndrome
   c. Blue diaper syndrome
   d. Jansen metaphyseal chondrodysplasia
8. Malignant neoplasms
   a. Ectopic PTH secretion or PTH-related protein (PTHRP)
   b. Prostaglandin-secreting tumors
   c. Tumors metastatic to bone
   d. Myeloma

MEN, multiple endocrine neoplasia; PTH, parathyroid hormone.

of primary hyperparathyroidism is due to a single parathyroid adenoma. Familial hyperparathyroidism may be an isolated disease, or it may be associated with MEN type 1, or rarely type 2A (Iqbal, 2009). Hypercalcemia of malignancy is associated with solid and hematologic malignancies and is due either to local destruction of bone by tumor or to ectopic secretion of PTH-related protein. When ectopic PTH-related protein is present, calcium is elevated, serum PTH is suppressed, and serum PTH-related protein is elevated. Chronic renal disease with impaired phosphate excretion is the most common secondary cause of hyperparathyroidism (Kemper, 2014).

Belcher R, Metrailer AM, Bodenner DL, Stack BC Jr: Characterization of hyperparathyroidism in youth and adolescents: a literature review [Review]. Int J Pediatr Otorhinolaryngol 2013 Mar;77(3):318–322 [PMID: 23313432].

Iqbal CW, Wahoff DC: Diagnosis and management of pediatric endocrine neoplasms [Review]. Curr Opin Pediatr 2009 Jun;21(3):379–385 [PMID: 19421059].

Kemper MJ, vanHusen M: Renal osteodystrophy in children: pathogenesis, diagnosis and treatment [Review]. Curr Opin Pediatr 2014 Apr;26(2);180–186 [PMID: 24553631].

Lietman SA, Germain-Lee EL, Levine MA: Hypercalcemia in children and adolescents [Review]. Curr Opin Pediatr 2010 Aug;22(4):508–515 [PMID 20601885].

McNeilly JD, Boal R, Shaikh MG, Ahmed SF: Frequency and aetiology of hypercalcemia [Review]. Arch Dis Child 2016 Apr;101(4):344–347 [PMID: 26903499].

▶ **Clinical Findings**

A. Symptoms and Signs

1. Due to hypercalcemia—Manifestations include hypotonicity and muscle weakness; apathy, mood swings, and bizarre behavior; nausea, vomiting, abdominal pain, constipation, and weight loss; hyperextensibility of joints; and hypertension, cardiac irregularities, bradycardia, and shortening of the QT interval. Coma occurs rarely. Calcium deposits occur in the cornea or conjunctiva (band keratopathy) and are detected by slit-lamp examination. Intractable peptic ulcer and pancreatitis occur in adults but rarely in children.

2. Due to Increased calcium and phosphate excretion—Loss of renal concentrating ability causes polyuria, polydipsia, and calcium phosphate deposition in renal parenchyma or as urinary calculi with progressive renal damage.

3. Due to changes in the skeleton—Initial findings include bone pain, osteitis fibrosa cystica, subperiosteal bone absorption in the distal clavicles and phalanges, absence of lamina dura around the teeth, spontaneous fractures, and moth-eaten appearance of the skull on radiographs. Later, there is generalized demineralization.

B. Imaging

Bone changes may be subtle in children. Technetium sestamibi scintigraphy is preferred over conventional procedures (ultrasound, computed tomography, and MRI) for localizing parathyroid tumors.

▶ **Treatment**

A. Symptomatic

Initial management is vigorous hydration with normal saline and forced calcium diuresis with a loop diuretic such as furosemide (1 mg/kg given every 6 hours). If response is inadequate, glucocorticoids or calcitonin may be used. Bisphosphonates, standard agents for the management of acute hypercalcemia in adults, are being used more often in refractory pediatric hypercalcemia.

B. Chronic

Treatment options vary with the underlying cause. Resection of parathyroid adenoma or subtotal removal of hyperplastic parathyroid glands is the preferred treatment. Postoperatively, hypocalcemia due to the rapid remineralization of chronically calcium-deprived bones may occur. A diet high in calcium and vitamin D is recommended immediately postoperatively and is continued until serum calcium concentrations are normal and stable. Treatment of secondary hyperparathyroidism from chronic renal disease is primarily directed at controlling serum phosphorus levels with phosphate binders and pharmacologic doses of calcitriol are used to suppress PTH secretion. Long-term therapy for hypercalcemia of malignancy is the treatment of the underlying disorder. There has been an increasing role for bisphosphonates in treatment of chronic hypercalcemia, particularly in children with hypercalcemia of immobilization.

FAMILIAL HYPOCALCIURIC HYPERCALCEMIA (FAMILIAL BENIGN HYPERCALCEMIA)

Familial hypocalciuric hypercalcemia is distinguished by low urinary calcium excretion as a result of high renal reabsorption of calcium (Varghese, 2011). PTH is normal or slightly elevated. In most cases, the genetic defect is an inactivating mutation in the membrane-bound calcium-sensing receptor expressed on parathyroid and renal tubule cells. It is inherited as an autosomal dominant trait with high penetrance. There is a low rate of new mutations. Most patients are asymptomatic, and treatment is unnecessary. However, a severe form of symptomatic neonatal hyperparathyroidism may occur in infants homozygous for the receptor mutation.

HYPERVITAMINOSIS D

Vitamin D intoxication is almost always the result of ingestion of excessive amounts of vitamin D (Lietman, 2010). Signs and symptoms of vitamin D-induced hypercalcemia are the same as those in other hypercalcemic conditions. Treatment depends on the severity of hypercalcemia and initial treatment is similar to other hypercalcemic states. However, due to the storage of vitamin D in the adipose tissue, several months of a low-calcium, low-vitamin D diet may also be required.

WILLIAMS SYNDROME

Williams syndrome is an uncommon disorder of infancy characterized by elfin-appearing facies and hypercalcemia in infancy (Lietman, 2010). Other features include failure to thrive, mental and motor retardation, cardiovascular abnormalities (primarily supravalvular aortic stenosis), irritability, purposeless movements, constipation, hypotonia, polyuria, polydipsia, and hypertension. A gregarious and affectionate personality is the rule in children with the syndrome. Hypercalcemia may not appear until several months after birth. Treatment consists of restriction of dietary calcium and vitamin D (Calcilo formula) and, in severe cases, moderate doses of glucocorticoids or even bisphosphonates.

A defect in the metabolism of, or responsiveness to, vitamin D is postulated as the cause of Williams syndrome. Elastin deletions localized to chromosome 7 have been identified in more than 90% of patients and is generally identified by fluorescent in situ hybridization (FISH) analysis. The risk of hypercalcemia generally resolves by age 4.

IMMOBILIZATION HYPERCALCEMIA

Abrupt immobilization, particularly in a rapidly growing adolescent, may cause hypercalcemia and hypercalciuria (Lietman, 2010). Abnormalities often appear 1–3 weeks after immobilization. Medical or dietary intervention may be required in severe cases.

HYPOPHOSPHATASIA

Hypophosphatasia is a rare autosomal recessive condition characterized by deficiency of alkaline phosphatase activity in serum, bone, and tissues, resulting from mutations in the gene for tissue-nonspecific isozyme of alkaline phosphatase (TNSALP) (Whyte, 2012). Enzyme deficiency leads to poor skeletal mineralization with clinical and radiographic features similar to rickets. Severity ranges from severe skeletal deformity and perinatal death to milder skeletal findings (including craniosynostosis), reduced bone mineral density, and motor delays. Serum calcium levels may be elevated. The diagnosis of hypophosphatasia is made by demonstrating elevated urinary phosphoethanolamine associated with low serum alkaline phosphatase. Standard therapy is supportive care; enzyme-replacement therapy shows promise for improved prognosis.

Baroncelli GI, Bertolloni S: The use of bisphosphonates in pediatrics [Review]. Horm Res Paediatr 2014;82(5):290–301 [PMID: 25376487].

Lietman SA, Germain-Lee EL, Levine MA: Hypercalcemia in children and adolescents [Review]. Curr Opin Pediatr 2010 Aug;22(4):508–515 [PMID: 20601885].

Varghese J, Rich T, Jimenez C: Benign familial hypocalciuric hypercalcemia [Review]. Endocr Pract 2011 Mar–Apr;17(Suppl 1): 13–17 [PMID: 21478088].

Whyte MP et al: Enzyme-replacement therapy in life-threatening hypophosphatasia. N Engl J Med 2012 Mar 8;366(10):904–913 [PMID: 22397652].

GONADS (OVARIES & TESTES)

DEVELOPMENT

Sex development is a complex process beginning with the differentiation of the bipotential gonad into either a testis or ovary. In an infant with a Y chromosome, expression of the transcription factor *SRY* initiates a cascade of gene expression that directs the formation of testes. Without expression of *SRY*, ovaries develop; however, a 46,XX complement of chromosomes, in addition to several unique genes, is necessary for the development of normal ovaries. Secretion of testosterone and antimüllerian hormone (AMH) by the testes results in the development of male internal ducts (epididymis, seminal vesicle, and vas deferens) and regression of the müllerian ducts, which are the precursors of the female internal genital structures (fallopian tubes, uterus, and vagina) (Figure 34–6).

The external genitalia develop from sexually indifferent structures called the genital tubercle, the urethral folds, and the labioscrotal swellings (Figure 34–7). Development of typical male external genitalia depends on an adequate circulating concentration of testosterone and its metabolite dihydrotestosterone (DHT). Sexual differentiation of the external genitalia is completed at about 12 weeks of gestation.

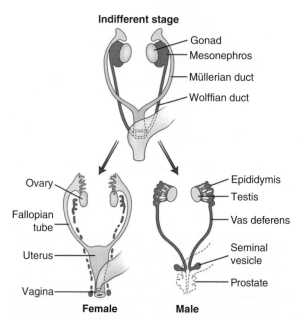

Indifferent stage

- Gonad
- Mesonephros
- Müllerian duct
- Wolffian duct

Female
- Ovary
- Fallopian tube
- Uterus
- Vagina

Male
- Epididymis
- Testis
- Vas deferens
- Seminal vesicle
- Prostate

▲ **Figure 34–6.** Differentiation of internal reproductive ducts. (Reproduced with permission from Kronenberg H: *Williams Textbook of Endocrinology*, 11th ed. Philadelphia, PA: Saunders/Elsevier; 2008.)

DISORDERS OF SEXUAL DEVELOPMENT

Disorders of sex development (DSD) can arise from alterations in three main processes: gonadal differentiation, steroidogenesis, or androgen action. Many DSDs will be evident in the newborn period, but some will not manifest until later with abnormal pubertal development. In disorders of gonadal differentiation, the testes or ovaries do not develop normally, which results in either ambiguous genitalia or sex reversal. As an example, individuals with 46,XY complete gonadal dysgenesis do not develop normal gonadal tissue (ie, have streak gonads), and this results in typical female internal and external reproductive structures. XY partial gonadal dysgenesis is associated with incomplete testes development and usually results in a phenotype of ambiguous genitalia. Mutations in genes important for gonadal differentiation have been demonstrated in many patients with both complete and partial gonadal dysgenesis. Mixed gonadal dysgenesis is usually due to presence of both 45,XO and 46,XY cell lines in the same individual. There is typically a testis on one side and a streak gonad on the contralateral side. Ovotesticular DSD occurs when there is both ovarian and testicular tissue. Steroidogenesis refers to steroid hormone biosynthesis and depends on the function of multiple enzymes (Figure 34–8). Enzymatic defects in this pathway can result in decreased or absent testosterone synthesis and in affected XY individuals, there will be reduced or lack of androgen effects resulting in ambiguous genitalia. Since the gonad and adrenal gland share common enzymes of steroid hormone production, some of the enzymatic defects associated with male undervirilization may also affect production of cortisol and aldosterone, leading to cortisol deficiency and salt wasting. Deficiency of 21-hydroxylase, an enzyme in the cortisol and aldosterone pathways, leads to overproduction of adrenal androgens and the most common form of congenital adrenal hyperplasia. In the classic salt-losing form of this disorder, 46,XX infants present with genital ambiguity due to the excess of adrenal androgen production, but have normal uterus and ovaries.

Disorders of androgen action include the diagnosis of androgen insensitivity syndrome (AIS) which is caused by an inactivating mutation in the androgen receptor gene located on the proximal long arm of the X chromosome. In complete AIS (CAIS), there is no androgen action; thus, 46,XY affected individuals have normal appearing female external genitalia with a short vagina, absent müllerian structures and absence or rudimentary wolffian structures. Gonads are located either intra-abdominally or in the inguinal canal. Many of these individuals present when surgery for an inguinal hernia reveals a testis in the hernia sack. With partial AIS (PAIS), the degree of virilization and ambiguity depends on the degree of abnormality in androgen binding.

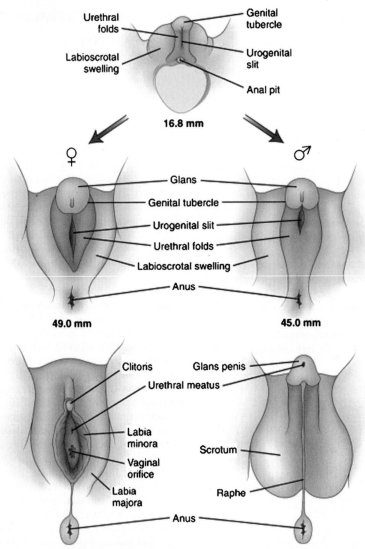

▲ **Figure 34–7.** Differentiation of external genitalia ducts. (Adapted with permission from Spaulding MH: The development of the external genitalia in the human embryo. Contrib Embryol 1921;13:69–88.)

Evaluation

On physical examination, dysmorphic features and other congenital anomalies should be noted. The genital examination should include measuring the width and length of the stretched phallus and noting the position of the urethral meatus as well as degree of labioscrotal fusion. The normal stretched penile length (SPL) is greater than 2.0 cm in term male infants. The labioscrotal and inguinal regions should be palpated for presence of gonads. Since ovaries and streak

gonads do not typically descend, the presence of a palpable gonad is suggestive of a 46,XY or 45X/46,XY karyotype. In all these infants, laboratory studies should be done within the first 24 hours of life and include a FISH for SRY/X-centromere, chromosomal analysis or microarray, electrolytes, LH, FSH, testosterone, and 17-hydroxyprogesterone. Additional laboratory evaluation is usually based on these results. A pelvic ultrasound can be helpful to evaluate for the presence of a uterus; however, ultrasound findings can be unreliable so should be done in an institution which has

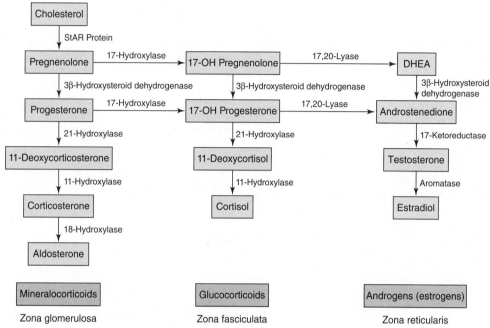

▲ **Figure 34–8.** The corticosteroid hormone synthetic pathway. The pathways illustrated are present in differing amounts in the steroid-producing tissues: adrenal glands, ovaries, and testes. In the adrenal glands, mineralocorticoids from the zona glomerulosa, glucocorticoids from the zona fasciculata, and androgens (and estrogens) from the zona reticularis are produced. The major adrenal androgen is androstenedione, because the activity of 17-ketoreductase is relatively low. The adrenal gland does secrete some testosterone and estrogen, however. The pathways leading to the synthesis of mineralocorticoids and glucocorticoids are not present to any significant degree in the gonads; however, the testes and ovaries each produce both androgens and estrogens. Further metabolism of testosterone to dihydrotestosterone occurs in target tissues of the action of the enzyme 5α-reductase. DHEA, dehydroepiandrosterone.

expertise in pediatric imaging. Many times, laparoscopic examination is necessary to delineate internal structures. It is important that gender assignment be avoided until expert evaluation by a multidisciplinary team is performed. Ideally this team includes pediatric specialists from endocrinology, urology, gynecology, genetics, psychology, and nursing. The team should develop a plan for diagnosis, gender assignment, and treatment options before making any recommendations. Open communications with the parents is essential and their participation in decision-making encouraged.

Arboleda VA, Sandberg DE, Vilain E: DSDs: genetics, underlying pathologies and psychosocial differentiation. Nat Rev Endocrinol 2014:10(10):603–615 [PMID: 25091731].

Lambert SM, Vilain EJ, Kolon TF: A practical approach to ambiguous genitalia in the newborn period. Urol Clin N Am 2010;37(2):195–205 [PMID: 20569798].

Ostrer H: Disorders of sex development (DSDs): an update. J Clin Endocrinol Metab 2014;99:1503–1509 [PMID: 24758178].

▼ ABNORMALITIES IN FEMALE PUBERTAL DEVELOPMENT & OVARIAN FUNCTION

1. Precocious Puberty in Girls

Precocious puberty is defined as pubertal development occurring below the age limit set for normal onset of puberty. Puberty is considered precocious in girls if the onset of secondary sexual characteristics occurs before age 8 years in Caucasian girls and 7 years for African-American and Hispanic girls. Precocious puberty is more common in girls than in boys. Many girls showing signs of puberty between 6 and 8 years of age have a benign, slowly progressing form that requires no intervention. The age of pubertal onset may be advanced by obesity.

Central (gonadotropin-releasing hormone [GnRH]-dependent) precocious puberty involves activation of the hypothalamic GnRH pulse generator, an increase in gonadotropin secretion, and a resultant increase in production of sex steroids (Table 34–8). The sequence of hormonal and

Table 34–8. Causes of precocious pubertal development.

A. Central (GnRH-dependent) precocious puberty
  1. Idiopathic
  2. Central nervous system abnormalities
     a. Acquired—abscess, chemotherapy, radiation, surgical trauma
     b. Congenital—arachnoid cyst, hydrocephalus, hypothalamic hamartoma, septo-optic dysplasia, suprasellar cyst
     c. Tumors—astrocytoma, craniopharyngioma, glioma
B. Peripheral (GnRH-independent) precocious puberty
  1. Congenital adrenal hyperplasia
  2. Adrenal tumors
  3. McCune-Albright syndrome
  4. Familial male-limited gonadotropin independent precocious puberty
  5. Gonadal tumors
  6. Exogenous estrogen—oral (contraceptive pills) or topical
  7. Ovarian cysts (females)
  8. HCG-secreting tumors (eg, hepatoblastomas, choriocarcinomas) (males)

GnRH, gonadotropin-releasing hormone; HCG, human chorionic gonadotropin.

physical events in central precocious puberty is identical to that of normal puberty. Central precocious puberty in girls is generally idiopathic but may be secondary to a central nervous system (CNS) abnormality that disrupts the prepubertal restraint on the GnRH pulse generator. Such CNS abnormalities include, but are not limited to, hypothalamic hamartomas, CNS tumors, cranial irradiation, hydrocephalus, and trauma. Peripheral precocious puberty (GnRH-independent) occurs independent of gonadotropin secretion. In girls, peripheral precocious puberty can be caused by ovarian or adrenal tumors, ovarian cysts, late-onset congenital adrenal hyperplasia, McCune-Albright syndrome, or exposure to exogenous estrogen.

▶ Clinical Findings

A. Symptoms and Signs

Female central precocious puberty usually starts with breast development, followed by pubic hair growth and menarche. However, the order may vary and girls younger than 5 years may not have pubic hair development. Girls with ovarian cysts or tumors generally have signs of estrogen excess such as breast development and possibly vaginal bleeding. Adrenal tumors and CAH produce signs of androgen excess which include pubic hair, axillary hair, acne, and increased body odor. Children with precocious puberty usually have accelerated growth and skeletal maturation, and may temporarily be tall for age. However, because skeletal maturation advances at a more rapid rate than linear growth, final adult stature may be compromised.

B. Laboratory Findings

If the bone age is advanced, further laboratory evaluation is warranted. In central precocious puberty, random FSH and LH concentrations may still be in the prepubertal range. If so, documentation of the maturity of the hypothalamic-pituitary axis depends on demonstrating a pubertal LH response after stimulation with a GnRH agonist. In peripheral precocious puberty, the LH response to GnRH stimulation is suppressed by feedback inhibition of the hypothalamic-pituitary axis by the autonomously secreted gonadal steroids (see Figure 34–1). In girls with an ovarian cyst or tumor, estradiol levels will be markedly elevated. In girls who present with pubic and/or axillary hair but no breast development, androgen levels (testosterone, androstenedione, dehydroepiandrosterone sulfate) and 17-hydroxyprogesterone should be measured.

C. Imaging

One of the first steps in evaluating a child with early pubertal development is obtaining a radiograph of the left hand and wrist to determine skeletal maturity (bone age). When a diagnosis of central precocious puberty is made, an MRI of the brain should be done to evaluate for CNS lesions. In girls whose laboratory tests suggest peripheral precocious puberty, an ultrasound of the ovaries and/or adrenal gland may be indicated.

▶ Treatment

Girls with central precocious puberty can be treated with GnRH analogues that downregulate pituitary GnRH receptors and thus decrease gonadotropin secretion. Currently, the two most common GnRH analogues used are (1) leuprolide, which is given as a monthly intramuscular injection or (2) histrelin subdermal implant, which is replaced annually. With treatment, physical changes of puberty regress or cease to progress and linear growth slows to a prepubertal rate. Projected final heights often increase as a result of slowing of skeletal maturation. After stopping therapy, pubertal progression resumes, and ovulation and pregnancy have been documented.

Treatment of peripheral precocious puberty is dependent on the underlying cause. In a girl with an ovarian cyst, intervention is generally not necessary, as the cyst usually regresses spontaneously. Serial ultrasounds are recommended to document this regression. Surgical resection and possibly chemotherapy are indicated for the rare adrenal or ovarian tumor. Regardless of the cause of precocious puberty or the medical therapy selected, attention to the psychological needs of the patient and family is essential.

2. Benign Variants of Precocious Puberty

Benign premature thelarche (benign early breast development) occurs most commonly in girls younger than 2 years of age. Girls present with isolated breast development without other signs of puberty such as linear growth acceleration and pubic hair development. The breast development is typically present since birth and often waxes and wanes in size. It may be unilateral or bilateral. Treatment is parental reassurance regarding the self-limited nature of the condition. Observation of the child every few months is indicated. Onset of the-larche after age 36 months or in association with other signs of puberty requires evaluation.

Benign premature adrenarche (benign early adrenal maturation) is manifested by early development of pubic hair, axillary hair, acne, and/or body odor. Benign premature adrenarche is characterized by normal linear growth and no or minimal bone age advancement. Laboratory tests (see earlier discussion) will differentiate benign premature adrenarche from late-onset CAH and adrenal tumors. It is recognized that approximately 15% of girls with benign premature adrenarche will go on to develop polycystic ovarian syndrome.

Fuqua J: Treatment and outcomes of precocious puberty: an update. J Clin Endocrinol Metab 2013;98(6):2198–2207 [PMID: 23515450].

Latronico AC, Brito VN, Carel JC: Causes, diagnosis, and treatment of central precocious puberty. Lancet Diabetes Endocrinol 2016;4(3):265–274 [PMID: 26852255].

Utriainen P et al: Premature adrenarche—a common condition with variable presentation. Horm Res Paediatr 2015;83(4): 221–231 [PMID: 25676474].

3. Delayed Puberty

Delayed puberty in girls should be evaluated if there are no pubertal signs by age 13 years or menarche by 16 years. Primary amenorrhea refers to the absence of menarche, and secondary amenorrhea refers to the absence of menses for at least 6 months after regular menses have been established. The most common cause of delayed puberty is constitutional growth delay (Table 34–9). This growth pattern, characterized by short stature, normal growth velocity, and a delay in skeletal maturation, is described in detail earlier in this chapter. The timing of puberty in children with constitutional growth delay is commensurate to the bone age, not the chronologic age. Girls may also have delayed puberty from any condition that delays growth and skeletal maturation, such as hypothyroidism and GHD.

Primary hypogonadism in girls refers to a primary abnormality of the ovaries. The most common diagnosis in this category is Turner syndrome, in which the lack of or an abnormal second X chromosome leads to early loss of oocytes and accelerated stromal fibrosis. Other types of primary ovarian insufficiency include 46,XY gonadal dysgenesis and 46,XX gonadal dysgenesis, galactosemia, autoimmune ovarian failure, radiation, and chemotherapy. Premutation carriers for fragile X syndrome are also at increased risk of premature ovarian failure.

Table 34–9. Causes of delayed puberty or amenorrhea.

A. Constitutional growth delay
B. Hypogonadism
  1. Primary ovarian insufficiency
    a. Gonadal dysgenesis (Turner syndrome, true gonadal dysgenesis)
    b. Premature ovarian failure
      (1) Autoimmune disease
      (2) Surgery, radiation, chemotherapy
    c. Galactosemia
  2. Central hypogonadism
    a. Hypothalamic or pituitary tumor, infection, irradiation
    b. Congenital hypopituitarism
    c. Kallmann syndrome (hypogonadism plus anosmia)
    d. Hyperprolactinemia, Cushing's syndrome, hypothyroidism
    e. Functional (chronic illness, undernutrition, exercise, hyperprolactinemia)
C. Anatomic
  1. Müllerian agenesis (Mayer-Rokitansky-Küster-Hauser syndrome)
  2. Complete androgen resistance

Central hypogonadism refers to a hypothalamic or pituitary deficiency of GnRH or FSH/LH, respectively. Central hypogonadism can be functional (reversible), caused by stress, undernutrition, prolactinemia, excessive exercise, or chronic illness. Permanent central hypogonadism is typically associated with conditions that cause multiple pituitary hormone deficiencies, such as congenital hypopituitarism, CNS tumors, or cranial irradiation. Isolated gonadotropin deficiency is rare but may occur in Kallmann syndrome, which is also characterized by hyposmia or anosmia. There are many genes that have been implicated in both isolated gonadotropin deficiency and Kallmann syndrome. In either primary or central hypogonadism, signs of adrenarche are generally present.

Delayed menarche or secondary amenorrhea may result from primary ovarian failure or central hypogonadism, or may be the consequence of hyperandrogenism, anatomic obstruction precluding menstrual outflow, or müllerian agenesis.

▶ Clinical Evaluation

The history should ascertain whether and when puberty commenced, level of exercise, nutritional intake, stressors, sense of smell, symptoms of chronic illness, and family history of delayed puberty. Past growth records should be assessed to determine if height and weight velocity have been appropriate. Physical examination includes body proportions, breast and genital development, and stigmata of Turner syndrome. Pelvic examination or pelvic ultrasonography should be considered, especially in girls with primary amenorrhea.

A bone age radiograph should be obtained first. If the bone age is lower than that consistent with pubertal onset (< 12 years in girls), evaluations should focus on finding the cause of the bone age delay. If short stature and normal growth velocity are present, constitutional growth delay is likely. If growth rate is abnormal, evaluation for causes of growth delay is warranted. Measurement of FSH and LH may not be helpful in the setting of delayed bone age since prepubertal levels are normally low.

If the patient has attained a bone age of more than 12 years and there are minimal or no signs of puberty on physical examination, FSH and LH levels will distinguish between primary ovarian failure (elevated FSH/LH) and central hypogonadism (low FSH/LH). If gonadotropins are elevated, a karyotype should be performed to evaluate for Turner syndrome. Central hypogonadism is characterized by low gonadotropin levels, and evaluation is geared toward determining if the hypogonadism is functional or permanent. Laboratory tests should be directed toward identifying chronic disease and hyperprolactinemia. Cranial MRI may be helpful.

In girls with adequate breast development and amenorrhea, a progesterone challenge may be helpful to determine if sufficient estrogen is being produced and to evaluate for anatomical defects. Girls who are producing estrogen have a withdrawal bleed after 5–10 days of oral progesterone, whereas those who are estrogen-deficient or have an anatomical defect have little or no bleeding. The most common cause of amenorrhea in girls with sufficient estrogen is polycystic ovarian syndrome. Girls who are estrogen-deficient should be evaluated similarly to those who have delayed puberty.

▶ Treatment

Replacement therapy in hypogonadal girls begins with estrogen alone at the lowest available dosage. Oral preparations such as estradiol or topical estrogen patches are used. Estrogen doses are gradually increased every 6 months and then 18–24 months later, progesterone is added either cyclically or continuously. Eventually, the patient may change over to an estrogen-progestin combined pill or patch if desired. Progesterone therapy is needed to counteract the effects of estrogen on the uterus, as unopposed estrogen promotes endometrial hyperplasia. Estrogen is also necessary to promote bone mineralization and prevent osteoporosis.

Nelson LM: Clinical practice: primary ovarian insufficiency. N Engl J Med 2009;360:606 [PMID: 19196677].

Silvereira LF, Latronico AC: Approach to the patient with hypogonadotropic hypogonadism. J Clin Endocrinol Metab 2013;98:1781–1788 [PMID: 23650335].

Villanueva C, Argente J: Pathology or normal variant: what constitutes a delay in puberty? Horm Res Paediatr 2014;82:213–221 [PMID: 25011467].

4. Secondary Amenorrhea

See discussion of amenorrhea in Chapter 4.

▼ POLYCYSTIC OVARIAN SYNDROME

ESSENTIALS OF DIAGNOSIS & TYPICAL FEATURES

▶ Oligomenorrhea or amenorrhea and clinical or laboratory signs of hyperandrogenism.

▶ Diagnosis of exclusion and other causes of menstrual dysfunction or elevated androgens need to be ruled out.

▶ Increased risk of many comorbidities including metabolic syndrome, depression, and obstructive sleep apnea.

1. General Considerations

Polycystic ovarian syndrome (PCOS) is one of the most common menstrual disorders in women, estimated to affect 10%–15% of all reproductive age women. The underlying pathology of PCOS is not well understood. Many girls with PCOS will have a history of early adrenarche. The diagnosis cannot formally be made until at least 1 year post-menarche or with primary amenorrhea, due to the normal duration of time required for girls to establish regular menstrual cycles. Many girls with PCOS are obese, and this is contributing to an increased prevalence of the disease, but PCOS is also present in girls without obesity. Adolescents with PCOS typically present for cosmetic concerns or menstrual irregularities. However, PCOS is associated with many comorbidities and it is important to provide comprehensive screening and care.

2. Clinical Findings

PCOS should be considered in adolescents who have (1) menstrual abnormalities including: (a) oligomenorrhea of < 8 menses a year 2 years following menarche, (b) severe oligomenorrhea: > 90 days between cycle at least a year post-menarche, (c) primary amenorrhea ≥ 15 years, or (d) primary amenorrhea ≥ 2 years after breast development; and (2) clinical signs and symptoms of hyperandrogenism such as hirsutism, cystic acne, androgenic alopecia, and/or biochemical hyperandrogenism. PCOS is a diagnosis of exclusion and other causes of irregular menses such a primary ovarian failure, prolactinoma, thyroid dysfunction, hypothalamic hypogonadotropic hypogonadism as seen in those who are underweight, ovarian tumor or pituitary mass and causes of hyperandrogenism such as adrenal tumors, ovarian tumors, or congenital adrenal hyperplasia should be ruled out with laboratory testing. The physical exam should be comprehensive and assess for severity of acne, hirsutism as scored by the Ferriman-Gallwey scale, alopecia, acanthosis nigricans, skin tags, pilonidal cysts, hidradenitis, thyroid size, airway and tonsil size, liver size, peripheral edema, striea size, and color and clitoral enlargement. Ovarian ultrasound is currently not recommended for the diagnosis of PCOS until 8 years post-menarche due to the large variability of normal ovaries in adolescent girls. Uterine ultrasound can be used to determine structural abnormalities causing amenorrhea, thickness of the endometrium in cases of failure to initiate a menstrual bleed following a short course of Provera or to monitor for large cysts causing ovarian pain.

Once a diagnosis of PCOS is established, girls also need to be screened for associated co-morbidities. Adolescents with PCOS have an increased risk of developing insulin resistance and type 2 diabetes, and a 75 g 2 hour oral glucose tolerance should be performed, or alternatively a hemoglobin A1C test at diagnosis and then every 1–2 years. Fasting lipids should be measured at diagnosis and then per American Academy of Pediatrics guidelines. Up to 50% of obese girls with PCOS have nonalcoholic fatty liver disease, and transaminases should be checked at diagnosis, and liver size assessed by exam. The risk of hypertension is increased, and blood pressure should be checked at every appointment with an appropriate sized cuff. If symptoms of obstructive sleep apnea are present, overnight polysomnography should be performed. All girls should be screened for anxiety and depression on a routine basis.

3. Treatment

The treatment for PCOS should be comprehensive, personalized for each individual, and ideally delivered via a coordinated multidisciplinary approach. All girls, even those of normal weight are encouraged to maintain a healthy lifestyle, with moderate to vigorous activity 3–5 days a week and a healthy diet. To induce weight loss, diets may need to be very low calorie (1200–1500 kcal/day) and exercise may need to be daily. Monophasic combined oral contraceptives, with 30–35 mcg of estradiol and a third- or fourth-generation nonandrogenic progestin are used to regulate menses, decrease acne, hirsutism, and alopecia. Other methods of delivery including combined estradiol and progesterone patches or vaginal rings can also be used, although they are less reliable for contraception in individuals greater than 200 pounds. Implantable and uterine progestins can be utilized to prevent endometrial hyperplasia, although due to the risk of weight gain and depression, injectable progesterone should be avoided. Cyclic oral progesterone, at a dose of 10 mg daily for 10 days can be utilized to initiate menses every 3 months in those that do not desire to take oral contraceptives. Metformin, at a dose of 1000 mg twice a day can be used to treat

insulin resistance and hyperglycemia, and can induce modest improvements in menstrual regularity. The extended release form can be prescribed at 2000 mg once a day in those with gastric intolerance to the regular formulation. Typical acne treatments should be used, and for hirsutism treatments include spironolactone up to 200 mg a day, eflornithine cream, electrolysis, and laser hair treatment. Topical minoxidil can reduce androgenic alopecia. Standard therapies for obstructive sleep apnea, hyperlipidemia, hypertension, and psychological disturbances should be utilized as needed. The use of weight loss medications should be considered in older obese adolescents in conjunction with lifestyle therapies. Patients should be seen every 3–6 months, pending the complexity of their medical needs.

Legro RS et al: Diagnosis and treatment of polycystic ovary syndrome: an endocrine society clinical practice guideline. J Clin Endocrinol Metab 2013;98:4565–4592 [PMID: 24151290].

Teede HJ et al: Recommendations from the international evidence-based guideline for the assessment and management of polycystic ovary syndrome. Hum Reprod 2018;33:1602–1618 [PMID: 30052961].

Witchel SF et al: The diagnosis of polycystic ovary syndrome during adolescence. Horm Res Paediatr 2015;83:376–389 [PMID: 25833060].

ABNORMALITIES IN MALE PUBERTAL DEVELOPMENT & TESTICULAR FUNCTION

1. Precocious Puberty in Boys

Puberty is considered precocious in boys if secondary sexual characteristics appear before age 9 years. While the frequency of central precocious puberty is much lower in boys than girls, boys are much more likely to have an associated CNS abnormality (see Table 34–8) and require medical evaluation. In addition, several types of gonadotropin-independent (peripheral) precocious puberty occur in boys (see Table 34–8).

▶ Clinical Findings

A. Symptoms and Signs

Appearance of pubic hair is the most common presenting sign of puberty in boys, since increased growth velocity occurs later in the process than in girls. Examination of the testes is a critical component of the evaluation of a boy with suspected precocious puberty. Testicular size differentiates central precocity, in which the testes enlarge (> 2 cm in the longitudinal axis or > 4 mL using Prader beads), from gonadotropin-independent causes, in which the testes usually remain small. In some cases of gonadotropin-independent precocious puberty, such as familial male precocious puberty and HCG-mediated precocious puberty, there may be some testicular enlargement, but usually less than expected for the degree of virilization. Tumors of the testis are associated with either asymmetrical or unilateral testicular enlargement.

B. Laboratory Findings

Testosterone concentrations are usually elevated in precocious puberty but do not differentiate the source. Basal high-sensitivity serum LH and FSH concentrations will be in the pubertal range in boys with central precocious puberty, but suppressed in peripheral, gonadotropin-independent precocity. GnRH-analogue (leuprolide) stimulation testing can also distinguish central from gonadotropin-independent puberty, but is often not needed in boys because increased testicular volume is usually a reliable physical sign of central puberty. In boys with peripheral precocious puberty caused by congenital adrenal hyperplasia (CAH) plasma adrenal androgens and 17-hydroxyprogesterone will be elevated. Serum β-HCG concentrations signify the presence of an HCG-producing tumor (eg, CNS dysgerminoma or hepatoma) in boys who present with precocious puberty and testicular enlargement but suppressed gonadotropins. Genetic testing may be helpful in diagnosing CAH or familial male precocious puberty (due to mutations in the LH receptor).

C. Imaging

A radiograph of the left hand to assess epiphyseal maturation (bone age) is often useful in evaluating precocious puberty. In all boys with central precocious puberty, cranial MRI should be obtained to evaluate for a CNS abnormality. If testing suggests peripheral precocious puberty and laboratory studies are not consistent with CAH, imaging may be useful to detect hepatic, adrenal, and testicular tumors.

▶ Treatment

Treatment of central precocious puberty in boys entails treatment of the underlying cause and the use of GnRH analogues. Boys with McCune-Albright syndrome or familial male precocious puberty are treated with agents that block steroid synthesis (eg, ketoconazole) or with a combination of antiandrogens (eg, spironolactone) and aromatase inhibitors (eg, anastrozole or letrozole) that block the conversion of testosterone to estrogen.

2. Delayed Puberty

Boys should be evaluated for delayed puberty if they have no secondary sexual characteristics by 14 years of age or if more than 5 years have elapsed since the first signs of puberty without completion of genital growth.

By far the most common cause of delayed puberty in boys is constitutional growth delay, a normal variant of growth described in detail earlier in this chapter. True hypogonadism in boys may be primary due to absence, malfunction, or destruction of testicular tissue; or central, due to pituitary or hypothalamic insufficiency.

Primary testicular insufficiency may be due to anorchia; Klinefelter syndrome (47,XXY) or other sex chromosome anomalies; enzymatic defects in testosterone synthesis; or inflammation or destruction of the testes following infection (eg, mumps), autoimmune disorders, radiation, trauma, or tumor.

Central hypogonadism may accompany multiple pituitary hormone deficiency or may be due to isolated or complete gonadotropin deficiency. The etiologies of central hypogonadism in boys is the same as girls (see Table 34–9).

▶ Clinical Evaluation

The history should focus on whether and when puberty started, history of cryptorchidism, hypospadias, or micropenis, growth pattern, symptoms of chronic illness, sense of smell, and family history of delayed puberty. Physical examination should include growth parameters, pubertal stage, and testicular location, size, and consistency. Testes less than 2 cm in length, or less than 4 mL using Prader beads, are prepubertal; symmetric testes more than 2.5 cm or more than 4 mL indicate onset of puberty.

A radiograph of the left hand and wrist to assess bone age should be the first step in evaluating delayed puberty. If bone age is delayed relative to chronological age and growth velocity is normal for a prepubertal boy, constitutional growth delay is the most likely diagnosis.

Laboratory evaluation may include measurement of LH and FSH levels (if bone age is > 12 years) with elevated gonadotropins indicating primary hypogonadism or testicular failure. Low gonadotropins are not specific but may suggest the possibility of central hypogonadism and further evaluation look for pituitary hormone deficiencies, chronic disease, undernutrition, hyperprolactinemia, or CNS abnormalities. Inhibin B is sometimes useful in differentiating between constitutional delay (normal concentrations) and idiopathic hypogonadotropic hypogonadism (lower concentrations), although there can be significant overlap in these conditions.

▶ Treatment

Boys with delayed puberty who are troubled by their stature and/or prepubertal appearance may be offered a 4- to 6-month course of low-dose depot testosterone (50–100 mg/mo given intramuscularly) to promote virilization and possibly "jump-start" their endogenous development. In adolescent boys with permanent hypogonadism, testosterone treatment will need to be gradually increased over 3–4 years to adult dosing. Topical testosterone gel applied daily is an alternative to injections but often is too potent in commercially available concentrations to use in early puberty. Other formulations of testosterone are not widely used in adolescents.

3. Cryptorchidism

Cryptorchidism (undescended testis) affects 2%–4% of full-term male newborns and up to 30% of premature infants. Cryptorchidism can occur in an isolated fashion or associated with other findings. Often the cause is unknown, however abnormalities in the hypothalamic-pituitary-gonadal axis, intrinsic testicular development defects, and androgen biosynthesis or receptor defects can result in cryptorchidism.

Infertility and testicular malignancy are major risks of untreated cryptorchidism. Histologic changes occur as early as age 6 months in children with undescended testes. Fertility is impaired by approximately 33% and 66% after unilateral and bilateral cryptorchidism, respectively. The cancer risk for adults after cryptorchidism in childhood is reported to be 5–10 times greater than normal. After 6 months of age, spontaneous descent occurs only very rarely. Consequently, intervention is typically considered beginning at this time.

▶ Clinical Findings

Exam should focus on whether testes can be palpated in the scrotum or inguinal canal, appearance of the genitalia, and any midline defects. To prevent retraction of the testis during exam, two hands are required. One hand milks the testes from the deep inguinal ring to the scrotum. The second hand lies over the scrotum to hold the testis. Examination in the squatting position for older children or in a warm bath can be helpful. Ultrasonography, CT, and MRI may detect testes in the inguinal region, but these studies are not completely reliable in finding abdominal testes.

In the mini-puberty period of infancy between 1 and 4 months of age, measurement of LH, FSH, and testosterone can assess the HPG axis. After this time, inhibin B and/or an HCG stimulation test can be done to confirm the presence or absence of functional abdominal testes.

▶ Differential Diagnosis

Various disorders of sexual development can present with cryptorchidism. A karyotype can identify a virilized 46,XX individual (CAH), mixed gonadal dysgenesis (45,X/46,XY), and 47,XXY/Klinefelter syndrome, all of which can be associated with unilateral or bilateral cryptorchidism. The diagnosis of bilateral cryptorchidism in an apparently normal male newborn should never be made until the possibility that the child is a fully virilized female with potentially fatal salt-losing CAH has been considered.

▶ Treatment

Surgical orchidopexy should be performed if descent has not occurred by 6–12 months of age. The recommended timing of surgical intervention is based on the assumption that early surgery will allow normal germ cell development and decrease the risk for future infertility and cancer. However, in some cases, a primary abnormality of the testis may be responsible for both the undescent and future risks. Therapy with HCG 250–1000 IU twice weekly for 5 weeks has been used to induce descent of the testis but has a low success rate.

4. Gynecomastia

Gynecomastia is a common, self-limited condition that occurs in up to 75% of normal pubertal boys. Adolescent gynecomastia typically resolves within 2 years but may not totally resolve if the degree of gynecomastia is extreme (> 2 cm of tissue). Gynecomastia is more common in obese boys, possibly due to adipose aromatization of testosterone to estrogen. Gynecomastia may also occur in male hypogonadism, such as Klinefelter syndrome, and as a side effect of some medications. Medical therapy using antiestrogens and/or aromatase inhibitors may be beneficial if initiated early when there is active stimulation of the mammary glands, but given most pubertal gynecomastia will self-resolve pharmacologic management is rarely pursued. Surgical intervention should be considered for prolonged and/or severe cases (see Chapter 4).

Hutson JM, Thorup J: Evaluation and management of the infant with cryptorchidism. Curr Opin Pediatr 2015 Aug;27(4):520–524 [PMID: 26087417].

Latronico AC, Brito VN, Carel JC: Causes, diagnosis, and treatment of central precocious puberty. Lancet Diabetes Endocrinol 2016 Mar;4(3):265–274. [PMID: 26852255].

Wei C, Crowne EC: Recent advances in the understanding and management of delayed puberty. Arch Dis Child 2016 May;101(5):481–488 [PMID: 26353794].

▼ ADRENAL CORTEX

The adult adrenal cortex consists of three zones responsible for synthesis of different steroids from the precursor, cholesterol (see Figure 34–8):

- Outermost zona glomerulosa—aldosterone.
- Middle zona fasciculata—cortisol and small amounts of mineralocorticoids.
- Innermost zona reticularis—androgens.

The predominant regulator of mineralocorticoid (primarily aldosterone) production and secretion is the volume- and sodium-sensitive renin-angiotensin-aldosterone system. Mineralocorticoids promote sodium retention and stimulate potassium excretion in the distal renal tubule.

Glucocorticoid production, primarily cortisol, is under the control of pituitary adrenocorticotropic hormone (ACTH; see Figure 34–1 and Table 34–1), which is in turn regulated by hypothalamic corticotropin-releasing hormone (CRH). ACTH concentration is greatest during the early morning hours with a smaller peak in the late afternoon and a nadir at night. The pattern of serum cortisol concentration follows this pattern with a lag of a few hours. In the absence of cortisol feedback, there is dramatic CRH and ACTH hypersecretion.

Glucocorticoids are critical for gene expression in a many cell types. Glucocorticoids also help maintain blood pressure by promoting peripheral vascular tone and sodium and water retention. In excess, glucocorticoids are both catabolic and antianabolic; they promote the release of amino acids from muscle and increase gluconeogenesis while decreasing incorporation of amino acids into muscle protein. They also antagonize insulin activity and facilitate lipolysis.

At the onset of puberty, production of androgens (dehydroepiandrosterone and androstenedione) increases and is an important contributor to pubertal development in both sexes. The adrenal gland is the major source of androgen in females.

ADRENOCORTICAL INSUFFICIENCY

Adrenal insufficiency may be primary—due to disorders of the adrenal gland itself, or central/secondary—due to disorders of CRH and/or ACTH secretion. Primary adrenal insufficiency impairs the production of all adrenal steroids, whereas secondary adrenal insufficiency should not affect production of mineralocorticoids or androgens as these are not regulated by ACTH. The causes of primary and secondary adrenal insufficiency are listed in Table 34–10.

Secondary adrenal insufficiency may be isolated ACTH deficiency or combined with other pituitary hormone deficiencies.

Table 34–10. Causes of adrenal insufficiency.

A. Primary adrenal insufficiency
  a. Congenital adrenal hyperplasia (enzyme defect)
  b. Addison disease (autoimmune)
  c. Hemorrhage (Waterhouse-Friderichsen syndrome)
  d. Tumor, calcification, or infection in the gland
  e. X-linked adrenal hypoplasia congenita (DAX1 mutation or deletion)
  f. Adrenoleukodystrophy
B. Secondary adrenal insufficiency
  a. Congenital hypopituitarism secondary to transcription factor mutations or structural defects of the hypothalamus or pituitary; sometimes associated with other midline defects or optic nerve hypoplasia sequence
  b. Congenital absence of transcription factors
  c. Intracranial tumor
  d. Surgery or radiation of the hypothalamus or pituitary gland

▶ Clinical Findings

A. Symptoms and Signs

1. Acute form (adrenal crisis)—Nausea, vomiting, abdominal pain; dehydration; fever (sometimes followed by hypothermia); weakness; hypoglycemia; hypotension and circulatory collapse; confusion and coma. Hyponatremia and hyperkalemia are seen in primary adrenal insufficiency. Acute illness, surgery, trauma, or hyperthermia may precipitate an adrenal crisis in patients with adrenal insufficiency.

2. Chronic form—Fatigue, hypotension, weakness, weight loss or failure to gain weight, vomiting and dehydration, recurrent hypoglycemia. In primary adrenal insufficiency, salt craving and hyponatremia and/or hyperkalemia can be seen. Diffuse tanning occurs with increased pigmentation over pressure points, scars, and mucous membranes in primary adrenal insufficiency due to melanocyte-stimulating activity of alternate products of hypersecreted proopiomelanocortin, the parent molecule of ACTH.

B. Laboratory Findings

1. Suggestive of adrenocortical insufficiency

- Primary adrenal insufficiency

  - Decreased—serum sodium, serum bicarbonate, serum glucose, blood pH, and blood volume.

  - Increased—serum potassium, urea nitrogen levels.

  - Urinary sodium and the ratio of urinary sodium to potassium inappropriate for the degree of hyponatremia.

- Central adrenal insufficiency—serum sodium levels may be mildly decreased as a result of impaired water excretion but true salt-wasting is not present (mineralocorticoid function should remain intact).

- Eosinophilia and moderate lymphopenia occur in both forms of insufficiency.

2. Confirmatory tests

A. ACTH (COSYNTROPIN) STIMULATION TEST

- Primary adrenal insufficiency—plasma cortisol less than 18 mcg/dL 30 and 60 minutes after 250 mcg of cosyntropin (high-dose stimulation test) given intravenously and failure of aldosterone to rise above baseline

- Central adrenal insufficiency—plasma cortisol less than 18 mcg/dL 30 and 60 minutes after 1 mcg of cosyntropin given intravenously (low-dose stimulation)

B. BASELINE SERUM ACTH CONCENTRATION—Elevated in primary adrenal failure and low/low-normal in central adrenal insufficiency

C. URINARY FREE CORTISOL—Decreased

D. CRH TEST—After administration of ovine CRH, serum concentrations of ACTH and cortisol are measured. Localization of the site of impairment is possible based on careful interpretation of results. The CRH test has not been widely used in pediatrics.

▶ Differential Diagnosis

Acute adrenal insufficiency must be differentiated from sepsis, diabetic coma, CNS disturbances, dehydration and acute poisoning. In the neonatal period, adrenal insufficiency may be clinically indistinguishable from respiratory distress, intracranial hemorrhage, or sepsis. Chronic adrenocortical insufficiency must be differentiated from anorexia nervosa, depression, certain muscular disorders (myasthenia gravis), salt-losing nephropathy, and chronic debilitating infections.

▶ Treatment

A. Acute Insufficiency (Adrenal Crisis)

1. Hydrocortisone sodium succinate—Hydrocortisone sodium succinate (50 mg/m^2 intravenously over 2–5 minutes or intramuscularly) is given initially followed by 12.5 mg/m^2, every 4–6 hours until stabilization is achieved and oral therapy can be tolerated. Cortisol replacement is critical because pressor agents may be ineffective with cortisol insufficiency.

2. Fluids and electrolytes—In primary adrenal insufficiency, 5%–10% glucose in normal saline, 10–20 mL/kg intravenously, is given over the first hour and repeated if necessary to reestablish vascular volume. Normal saline is continued thereafter at 1.5–2 times maintenance fluid requirements until volume and electrolytes have normalized. In central adrenal insufficiency, routine fluid management is generally adequate after initial restoration of vascular volume and institution of cortisol replacement.

3. Fludrocortisone—Treatment with fludrocortisone, a mineralocorticoid agonist, is not required acutely, as hydrocortisone in stress doses has adequate mineralocorticoid action. When oral intake is tolerated, fludrocortisone, is started, 0.05–0.15 mg daily, and continued every 12–24 hours for primary adrenal insufficiency.

B. Maintenance Therapy

1. Glucocorticoids—A maintenance dosage of 6–10 mg/m^2/day of hydrocortisone (or equivalent) is given orally in two or three divided doses. To prevent acute adrenal crises, the dosage of all glucocorticoids is increased to 30–50 mg/m^2/day during intercurrent illnesses or other times of stress (fever > 101.5°F, trauma, surgery, or systemic illness) and should also be increased during significant diarrhea due to reduced absorption. Families should be encouraged to give stress doses of hydrocortisone if they have concerns, as brief exposure to stress doses of hydrocortisone will not have adverse effects. Rarely, families become overly anxious and give stress doses frequently. This should be avoided as it can contribute to obesity, growth retardation, and other cushingoid features.

2. Mineralocorticoids—In primary adrenal insufficiency, fludrocortisone is given, 0.05–0.15 mg orally daily as a single dose or in two divided doses. Periodic monitoring of blood pressure is recommended to avoid overdosing.

3. Salt—Children should be given ready access to table salt. In the infant, supplementation of breast milk or formula with 3–5 mEq Na$^+$/kg/day is generally required until table foods are introduced.

▶ Course & Prognosis

If treated appropriately, the prognosis of adrenal insufficiency is good however spontaneous recovery is unlikely unless the etiology was transient (exogenous glucocorticoid exposure, eg). If adrenal crisis is not recognized and promptly treated with pharmacologic glucocorticoids, the course of acute adrenal insufficiency is rapid and death may occur within a few hours, particularly in infants. Regular care with an endocrinologist is required to evaluate management and adjust dosing to ensure adequate replacement while avoiding overdosing that could lead to impaired growth, hypertension, and Cushingoid features.

Park J, Didi M, Blair J: The diagnosis and treatment of adrenal insufficiency during childhood and adolescence. Arch Dis Child 2016 Sep;101(9):860–865 [PMID: 27083756].
Tucci V, Sokari T: The clinical manifestations, diagnosis, and treatment of adrenal emergencies. Emerg Med Clin North Am 2014 May;32(2):367–378 [PMID: 24766938].

CONGENITAL ADRENAL HYPERPLASIAS

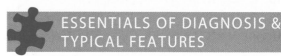

ESSENTIALS OF DIAGNOSIS & TYPICAL FEATURES

- ▶ Genital virilization in females, with labial fusion, urogenital sinus, enlargement of the clitoris, or other evidence of androgen action in the most common form.

- ▶ Increased linear growth and advanced skeletal maturation.

- ▶ Elevation of plasma 17-hydroxyprogesterone concentrations in the most common form; may be associated with hyponatremia, hyperkalemia, and metabolic acidosis if mineralocorticoid deficiency included.

General Considerations

Autosomal recessive mutations in the enzymes of adrenal steroidogenesis cause impaired cortisol biosynthesis with increased ACTH secretion. ACTH excess subsequently results in adrenal hyperplasia with increased production of adrenal hormone precursors that are metabolized through the unblocked androgen pathway. Increased pigmentation, especially of the scrotum, labia majora, and nipples, is common due to excessive ACTH secretion. CAH is most commonly (> 90% of patients) the result of homozygous or compound heterozygous mutations in the cytochrome P-450 C21 (CYP21A2) gene causing 21-hydroxylase deficiency (see Figure 34–8). The defective gene is present in 1:250–1:100 people and the worldwide incidence of the disorder is 1:15,000, with increased incidence in certain ethnic groups. In its severe form, excess adrenal androgen production starting in the first trimester of fetal development causes virilization of the female fetus and life-threatening hypovolemic, hyponatremic shock (adrenal crisis) in the newborn, if untreated. There are also other enzyme defects that less commonly result in CAH. The clinical syndromes associated with these defects are shown in Figure 34–8 and Table 34–11.

Prenatal diagnosis is now possible and newborn screening by measurement of serum 17-hydroxyprogesterone has been established in all 50 US states and many other countries worldwide.

In nonclassic presentations of 21-hydroxylase deficiency, affected individuals have a normal phenotype at birth but develop virilization during later childhood, adolescence, or early adulthood. Hormonal studies are characteristic of 21-hydroxylase deficiency, with cosyntropin stimulated 17-OHP levels intermediate between those of nonaffected individuals and those with the classic form of the disease. Individuals with the nonclassic form of the disease may be asymptomatic or only mildly symptomatic, but they can carry a severe CYP21A2 mutation resulting in offspring with the classic form.

Clinical Findings in 21-Hydroxylase Deficiency

A. Symptoms and Signs

1. In females—Abnormality of the external genitalia varies from mild enlargement of the clitoris to complete fusion of the labioscrotal folds, forming an empty scrotum, a penile urethra, a penile shaft, and clitoral enlargement sufficient to form a normal-sized glans (see Figure 34–7). Signs of adrenal insufficiency (salt loss) typically appear 5–14 days after birth. With milder enzyme defects, clinically apparent salt loss may not occur and virilization predominates with accelerated growth and skeletal maturation. Pubic hair appears early, acne may be excessive, and the voice may deepen. Excessive pigmentation may develop. Isosexual central precocious

Table 34–11. Clinical and laboratory findings in adrenal enzyme defects resulting in congenital adrenal hyperplasia.

Enzyme Deficiency[a]	Elevated Plasma Metabolite	Plasma Androgens	Aldosterone	Hypertension/ Salt Loss	External Genitalia
StAR protein	–	↓↓↓	↓↓↓	–/+	Males: ambiguous Females: normal
3β-Hydroxysteroid dehydrogenase	17-OH pregnenolone (DHEA)	↑ (DHEA)	↓↓↓	–/+	Males: ambiguous Females: possibly virilized
17α-Hydroxylase/17–20 lyase	Progesterone	↓↓	(↑ DOC)	+/–	Males: ambiguous Females: normal, absent puberty
21-Hydroxylase[a]	17-OHP	↑↑	↓↓	–/+	Males: normal Females: virilized
11β-Hydroxylase	11-Deoxycortisol, DOC	↑↑	(↑ DOC)	+/–	Males: normal Females: virilized
P450 oxidoreductase	17-OHP (mild elevation)	↓↓	Normal or mildly elevated	+/–	Males: ambiguous Females: ambiguous

DHEA, dehydroepiandrosterone; DOC, deoxycorticosterone; 17-OHP, 17-hydroxyprogestrone.
[a]Children with "simple virilizing (non–salt-wasting)" forms of 21-hydroxylase deficiency congenital adrenal hyperplasia (CAH) may have normal aldosterone production and serum electrolytes, but some children have normal aldosterone production and serum electrolytes at the expense of elevated plasma renin activity and are, by definition, compensated salt-wasters. These children usually receive mineralocorticoid as well as glucocorticoid treatment. Children with 21-hydroxylase deficiency CAH should therefore have documented normal plasma renin activity in addition to normal serum electrolytes before they are considered non–salt-wasters.

puberty may occur if treatment is not initiated before the bone age is significantly advanced. Final adult height is often compromised.

2. In males—The male infant usually appears normal at birth but may present with salt-losing crisis in the first weeks of life if treatment is not initiated. In milder forms, salt-losing crises may not occur and virilization predominates, with enlargement of the penis and increased pigmentation, as well as other symptoms and signs similar to those of affected females. The testes are not enlarged unless there are rare adrenal rests in the testes producing asymmetrical enlargement. In some rare enzyme defects, ambiguous genitalia may be present due to impaired androgen production (see Table 34–11).

B. Laboratory Findings

1. Blood—Hormonal studies are essential for accurate diagnosis. Findings characteristic of the enzyme deficiencies are shown in Table 34–11.

2. Genetic studies—Rapid assessment of genetic sex should be obtained in any newborn with ambiguous genitalia since 21-hydroxylase deficiency is the most common cause of ambiguity in females.

C. Imaging

Imaging is generally not required to make the diagnosis of CAH. Ultrasonography, CT scanning, and MRI may be useful in defining pelvic anatomy or to exclude an adrenal tumor.

▶ Treatment

A. Medical Treatment

Treatment goals in CAH are to provide the smallest dose of glucocorticoid that will adequately suppress excess androgen precursors and produce normalization of growth velocity and skeletal maturation; excessive glucocorticoids cause the undesirable side effects of Cushing syndrome. Mineralocorticoid replacement sustains normal electrolyte homeostasis, but excessive mineralocorticoids cause hypertension and hypokalemia.

1. Glucocorticoids—Supraphysiologic doses of hydrocortisone are often needed to suppress androgen excess in CAH. Initially, parenteral or oral hydrocortisone ($30–50 \text{ mg/m}^2$/day) is provided until suppression of abnormal adrenal steroidogenesis has been accomplished, as evidenced by normalization of serum 17-hydroxyprogesterone. Subsequently, patients are placed on maintenance doses of $10–15 \text{ mg/m}^2$/day in three divided doses. Dosage is adjusted to maintain normal growth rate and skeletal maturation. Serum 17-hydroxyprogesterone and androstenedione are usually used to monitor therapy; however, no one test is universally accepted.

2. Mineralocorticoids—Fludrocortisone, 0.05–0.15 mg/day, is given orally once a day or in two divided doses. Periodic monitoring of blood pressure and plasma renin activity are recommended to avoid overdosing.

B. Surgical Treatment

For affected females, consultation with a urologist or gynecologist experienced in female genital reconstruction should be arranged as soon as possible during infancy.

▶ Course & Prognosis

When initiated in early infancy, treatment with glucocorticoids permits normal growth, development, and sexual maturation. If not adequately controlled, CAH results in sexual precocity and masculinization throughout childhood. Affected individuals will be tall as children but short as adults because of rapid skeletal maturation and premature closure of the epiphyses. If treatment is delayed or inadequate, true central precocious puberty may occur in males and females.

Patient education stressing lifelong therapy is important to ensure compliance in adolescence and later life. Virilization and multiple surgical genital reconstructions may be associated with risk of psychosexual disturbances in female patients and ongoing psychological evaluation and support is a critical component of care.

Merke DP and Poppas DP: Management of adolescents with congenital adrenal hyperplasia. Lancet Diabetes Endocrinol 2013 Dec;1(4):341–52. [PMID: 24622419].

Speiser PW et al: Congenital adrenal hyperplasia due to steroid 21-hydroxylase deficiency: an Endocrine Society clinical practice guideline. J Clin Endocrinol Metab. 2010 Sep;95(9):4133–60. [PMID: 20823466].

Speiser PW et al: Congenital adrenal hyperplasia due to steroid 21-hydroxylase deficiency: an endocrine society clinical practice guideline. J Clin Endocrinol Metab 2018; 103(11):4043 [PMID: 30272171].

ADRENOCORTICAL HYPERFUNCTION

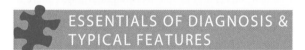

ESSENTIALS OF DIAGNOSIS & TYPICAL FEATURES

- ▶ Truncal adiposity, thin extremities, moon facies, muscle wasting, weakness, plethora, easy bruising, purple striae, decreased growth rate, and delayed skeletal maturation.
- ▶ Hypertension, osteoporosis, and glycosuria.
- ▶ Elevated 24-hour urinary free cortisol, elevated midnight salivary cortisol, failed low-dose dexamethasone suppression test.

▶ General Considerations

Cushing syndrome may result from excessive autonomous secretion of adrenal steroids (adrenal adenoma or carcinoma), excess pituitary ACTH secretion (Cushing disease), ectopic ACTH or CRH secretion, or chronic exposure to exogenous glucocorticoids. In children younger than 12 years, Cushing syndrome is usually iatrogenic. It is less commonly due to adrenal tumor, adrenal hyperplasia, pituitary adenoma, or extrapituitary ACTH-producing tumor.

▶ Clinical Findings

A. Symptoms and Signs

1. Excess glucocorticoid—Adiposity, most marked on the face, neck, and trunk—a fat pad (buffalo hump) in the interscapular area is characteristic but not diagnostic; fatigue; plethoric facies; purplish striae; easy bruising; osteoporosis and back pain; hypertension and glucose intolerance; proximal muscle wasting and weakness; retardation of growth and skeletal maturation.

2. Excess mineralocorticoid—Hypokalemia and mild hypernatremia, increased blood volume, edema, hypertension.

3. Excess androgen—Hirsutism, acne, virilization, and menstrual irregularities.

B. Diagnosis of Cushing Syndrome

1. Salivary cortisol—Elevated salivary cortisol obtained at midnight is a noninvasive and highly specific and sensitive test for hypercortisolism.

2. 24-Hour urinary-free cortisol excretion—Elevated 24-hour urinary free cortisol/creatinine suggests Cushing Syndrome.

3. Low-dose (15 mcg/kg) dexamethasone suppression test—Dexamethasone (15mcg/kg, max 1mg) is given at midnight followed by measurement of fasting plasma cortisol and ACTH at 8 AM the following morning. Failure to suppress cortisol < 1.8 ug/dL suggests Cushing Syndrome.

C. Establishing the Cause of Cushing Syndrome

1. ACTH concentration—Decreased ACTH values (< 5pg/mL) suggest an adrenal cause. Intermediate ACTH values (5–29 pg/mL) are indeterminant and warrant further investigation. Elevated ACTH values (> 29 pg/mL) suggest an ACTH-dependent (pituitary or ectopic) cause. ACTH.

2. High-dose (8 mg) dexamethasone testing—High-dose dexamethasone testing may help to determine ACTH-dependent Cushing syndrome from ACTH-independent Cushing syndrome.

D. Imaging

Pituitary imaging may demonstrate a pituitary adenoma. Adrenal imaging by CT scan may demonstrate adenoma or bilateral hyperplasia. MRI and nuclear medicine studies of the adrenals may be useful in complex cases. Skeletal maturation is usually delayed.

▶ Differential Diagnosis

Children with exogenous obesity accompanied by striae and hypertension are often suspected of having Cushing syndrome. However, children with Cushing syndrome have a poor growth velocity, relatively short stature, and delayed skeletal maturation, while those with exogenous obesity usually have a normal or slightly increased growth velocity, normal to tall stature, and advanced skeletal maturation. The color of the striae (purplish in Cushing syndrome, pink in obesity) and the distribution of the obesity may assist in differentiation. The urinary-free cortisol excretion (in milligrams per gram of creatinine) may be mildly elevated in obesity, but midnight salivary cortisol is normal and cortisol secretion is suppressed by low-dose dexamethasone suppression test.

▶ Treatment

In all cases of primary adrenal hyperfunction due to tumor, surgical removal is indicated if possible. Glucocorticoids should be administered parenterally in pharmacologic doses during and after surgery until the patient is stable. Supplemental oral glucocorticoids, potassium, salt, and mineralocorticoids may be necessary until the suppressed contralateral adrenal gland recovers, sometimes over a period of several months. Similarly, pituitary adenomas and ectopic sources of ACTH or CRH are generally treated surgically. Recurrent adenomas may respond to irradiation.

Stratakis CA: Diagnosis and clinical genetics of Cushing syndrome in pediatrics. Endocrinol Metab Clin North Am 2016 Jun;45(2):311–328 [PMID: 27241967].

PRIMARY HYPERALDOSTERONISM

Primary hyperaldosteronism may be caused by an adrenal adenoma or adrenal hyperplasia. It is characterized by paresthesias, tetany, weakness, periodic paralysis; nocturnal enuresis; hypokalemia, hypernatremia, metabolic alkalosis; hypertension; glucose intolerance; elevated plasma and urinary aldosterone; and suppressed plasma renin activity.

Primary hyperaldosteronism is rare in pediatrics. However, there are three recognized genetic causes (types I–III). Type I (glucocorticoid remediable hyperaldosteronism) is due to a hybrid of the genes encoding 11β-hydroxylase and aldosterone synthase. Type III results from mutations in the KCNJ5 gene encoding a K+ channel. Somatic mutations of this gene are also seen in later onset hyperaldosteronism. The cause for type II is unknown.

Treatment is with glucocorticoids (type I), spironolactone (type II), or subtotal or total adrenalectomy for hyperplasia or tumor.

Funder JW et al: The management of primary aldosteronism: case detection, diagnosis, and treatment: an Endocrine Society Clinical Practice Guideline. J Clin Endocrinol Metab 2016 May;101(5):1889–1916 [PMID: 26934393].

USES OF GLUCOCORTICOIDS & ADRENOCORTICOTROPIC HORMONE IN TREATMENT OF NONENDOCRINE DISEASES

Glucocorticoids are used for their anti-inflammatory and immunosuppressive properties in a variety of conditions in childhood. Pharmacologic doses are necessary to achieve these effects, and side effects are common. Numerous synthetic preparations possessing variable ratios of glucocorticoid to mineralocorticoid activity are available (Table 34–12).

When prolonged use of pharmacologic doses of glucocorticoids is necessary, clinical manifestations of Cushing syndrome are common. Side effects may occur with the use of synthetic exogenous agents by any route, including inhalation and topical administration, or with the use of ACTH. Alternate-day therapy lessens the incidence and severity of some of the side effects (Table 34–13).

► Tapering of Pharmacologic Doses of Steroids

Prolonged use of pharmacologic doses of glucocorticoids causes suppression of ACTH secretion and consequent adrenal atrophy; the abrupt discontinuation of glucocorticoids may result in adrenal insufficiency. ACTH secretion generally does not restart until the administered steroid has been given in subphysiologic doses (< 6 mg/m²/day orally) for several weeks.

If pharmacologic glucocorticoid therapy has been given for less than 10–14 days, the drug can be discontinued abruptly because adrenal suppression will be short-lived. However, it is advisable to educate the patient and family about the signs and symptoms of adrenal insufficiency in case problems arise.

If tapering is not required for the underlying disease, the dosage can be safely decreased to the physiologic range. Although a rapid decrease in dose to the physiologic range will not lead to frank adrenal insufficiency (because adequate exogenous cortisol is being provided), some patients may experience a steroid withdrawal syndrome, characterized by malaise, insomnia, fatigue, and loss of appetite. These symptoms may necessitate a two- or three-step decrease in dose to the physiologic range.

Once a physiologic equivalent dose (8–10 mg/m²/day hydrocortisone or equivalent) is achieved and the patient's underlying disease is stable, the dose can continue to be tapered. There is no clinical evidence to support any particular regimen of glucocorticoid tapering. Patient age, frailty, concomitant illness, and duration of glucocorticoid should all be taken into account when creating a taper regimen. If patients become symptomatic during the taper, the dose

Table 34–12. Potency equivalents for adrenocorticosteroids.

Adrenocorticosteroid	Trade Names	Potency/mg Compared With Cortisol (Glucocorticoid Effect)	Potency/mg Compared With Cortisol (Sodium-Retaining Effect)
Glucocorticoids			
Hydrocortisone (cortisol)	Cortef	1	1
Cortisone	Cortone Acetate	0.8	1
Prednisone	Meticorten, others	4–5	0.8
Methylprednisolone	Medrol, Meprolone	5–6	Minimal
Triamcinolone	Aristocort, Kenalog Kenacort, Atolone	5–6	Minimal
Dexamethasone	Decadron, others	25–40	Minimal
Betamethasone	Celestone	25	Minimal
Mineralocorticoid			
Fludrocortisone	Florinef	15–20	300–400

Table 34–13. Side effects of glucocorticoid use.

A. Endocrine and metabolic effects
1. Hyperglycemia and glycosuria (chemical diabetes)
2. Cushing syndrome
3. Persistent suppression of pituitary-adrenal responsiveness to stress with resultant hypoadrenocorticism

B. Effects on electrolytes and minerals
1. Marked retention of sodium and water, producing edema, increased blood volume, and hypertension (more common in endogenous hyperadrenal states)
2. Potassium loss with symptoms of hypokalemia
3. Hypocalcemia, tetany

C. Effects on protein metabolism and skeletal maturation
1. Negative nitrogen balance, with loss of body protein and bone protein, resulting in osteoporosis, pathologic fractures, and aseptic bone necrosis
2. Suppression of growth, retarded skeletal maturation
3. Muscular weakness and wasting
4. Osteoporosis
5. Avascular necrosis

D. Effects on the gastrointestinal tract
1. Excessive appetite and intake of food
2. Activation or production of peptic ulcer
3. Gastrointestinal bleeding from ulceration or from unknown cause (particularly in children with hepatic disease)
4. Fatty liver with embolism, pancreatitis, nodular panniculitis

E. Lowering of resistance to infectious agents; silent infection; decreased inflammatory reaction
1. Susceptibility to bacterial, fungal, and parasitic infections
2. Activation of tuberculosis; false-negative tuberculin reaction
3. Reactivation and poor containment of herpesviruses

F. Neuropsychiatric effects
1. Euphoria, excitability, psychotic behavior, and status epilepticus with electroencephalographic changes
2. Increased intracranial pressure with pseudotumor cerebri syndrome

G. Hematologic and vascular effects
1. Bleeding into the skin as a result of increased capillary fragility
2. Thrombosis, thrombophlebitis, cerebral hemorrhage

H. Miscellaneous effects
1. Myocarditis, pleuritis, and arteritis following abrupt cessation of therapy
2. Cardiomegaly
3. Nephrosclerosis, proteinuria
4. Acne (in older children), hirsutism, amenorrhea, irregular menses
5. Posterior subcapsular cataracts; glaucoma

should be increased back to the last asymptomatic dose and maintain that dose for two to four weeks. Then the taper can continue.

It is advisable to continue giving stress doses of glucocorticoids when appropriate until recovery of the response to stress has been documented. After basal physiologic adrenal function returns, the adrenal reserve or capacity to respond to stress and infection can be estimated by the low-dose ACTH stimulation test, in which 1 mcg of synthetic ACTH (cosyntropin) is administered intravenously. Plasma cortisol is measured 30 and 60 minutes after the infusion. A plasma cortisol concentration greater than 18 mg/dL indicates a satisfactory adrenal reserve. Even if the results of testing are normal, careful monitoring and the use of stress doses of glucocorticoids should be considered during severe illnesses and surgery.

Wildi-Runge S et al: A search for variables predicting cortisol response to low-dose corticotropin stimulation following supraphysiological doses of glucocorticoids. J Pediatr 2013 Aug;163(2):484–488 [PMID: 23414662].

ADRENAL MEDULLA PHEOCHROMOCYTOMA

Pheochromocytoma is an uncommon tumor, but up to 10% of reported cases occur in pediatric patients. The tumor can be located wherever chromaffin tissue (adrenal medulla, sympathetic ganglia, or carotid body) is present. It may be multiple, recurrent, and sometimes malignant. Familial forms include pheochromocytomas associated with the dominantly inherited neurofibromatosis type 1, MEN type 2, and von Hippel-Lindau syndromes, as well as mutations of the succinate dehydrogenase genes. Neuroblastomas, ganglioneuromas, and other neural crest tumors, as well as carcinoid tumors, may secrete pressor amines and mimic pheochromocytoma.

The symptoms of pheochromocytoma are caused by excessive secretion of epinephrine or norepinephrine: headache; sweating; tachycardia, hypertension, vasomotor instability (flushing and postural hypotension); anxiety; dizziness, weakness; nausea, vomiting, diarrhea; dilated pupils; blurred vision; abdominal and precordial pain.

Laboratory diagnosis is possible in more than 90% of cases. Serum and urine catecholamines are elevated, but abnormalities may be limited to periods of symptomatology or paroxysm. Plasma-free metanephrine is the most sensitive and specific test, though phenoxybenzamine, tricyclic antidepressants, and β-adrenoreceptor blockers can cause false-positive results. A level three times the normal range is diagnostic. Intermediate values may require additional testing with serum and urine catecholamines. After demonstrating a tumor biochemically, imaging methods including CT or MRI are used to localize the tumor and nuclear medicine using functional ligands such as (123)I-MIBG, [18F]DA positron emission tomography scanning, and somatostatin receptor scintigraphy (with either [123I]Tyr3-octreotide or [111In] DTPA-octreotide) are useful in further diagnostic evaluation.

Laparoscopic tumor removal is the treatment of choice; however, the procedure must be undertaken with great caution and with the patient properly stabilized. Oral phenoxybenzamine or intravenous phentolamine is used preoperatively. Profound hypotension may occur as the tumor is removed but may be controlled with an infusion of norepinephrine, which may have to be continued for 1–2 days.

Unless irreversible secondary vascular changes have occurred, complete relief of symptoms is to be expected after recovery from removal of a benign tumor.

However, prognosis is poor in patients with metastases, which occur more commonly with large, extra-adrenal pheochromocytomas.

Waguespack SG et al: A current review of the etiology, diagnosis, and treatment of pediatric pheochromocytoma and paraganglioma. J Clin Endocrinol Metab 2010;95(5):2023–2037 [PMID: 20215394].

Diabetes Mellitus

Brigitte I. Frohnert, MD, PhD

Peter H. Chase, MD

Marian Rewers, MD, PhD

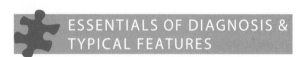

ESSENTIALS OF DIAGNOSIS & TYPICAL FEATURES

▶ Polyuria, polydipsia, and weight loss; respiratory distress, heavy diapers in infants.

▶ Hyperglycemia and glucosuria, often with ketonemia/ketonuria at presentation.

▶ Epidemiology & Description

A. Type 1 Diabetes

Type 1 diabetes (T1D) is the most common type of diabetes mellitus in people younger than 20 years, but it can develop at any age and most cases are diagnosed after age 20. The classical presentation includes increased thirst (polydipsia), increased urination (polyuria), and weight loss; however, the patient may be overweight or even obese. T1D is further divided into T1a (autoimmune) (~ 95% of the cases) and T1b (idiopathic) diabetes. T1b is more common in individuals of African or Asian ancestry. In the United States, T1D affects an estimated 1.5 million people, including more than 200,000 patients younger than 20 (~ 25,000 diagnosed annually).

T1D incidence is the highest in children of European ancestry, followed by African Americans and Hispanics; rates are low in Asians and Native Americans. About 6% of siblings or offspring of persons with T1D also develop diabetes (compared with prevalence in the general population of 0.2%–0.3%). However, fewer than 10% of children newly diagnosed with T1D have a parent or sibling with the disease.

B. Type 2 Diabetes

Type 2 diabetes (T2D) is a heterogeneous phenotype diagnosed most often in persons older than 40 who are usually obese and initially not insulin dependent. T2D is rare before age 10; however, puberty is a time of heightened risk for development of T2D in susceptible individuals. Due to the epidemic of childhood obesity, T2D has increased in frequency in older children. T2D is more common in youth of ethnic and racial minorities, particularly the native American population. Other risk factors include female sex, poor diet and sleep, and low socioeconomic status. The vast majority of the 30 million patients with diabetes in the United States have T2D, but less than 20,000 patients are younger than 20 (~ 5000 diagnosed annually).

C. Monogenic Forms of Diabetes

Monogenic forms of diabetes can be diagnosed at any age. They account for less than 1% of childhood diabetes, but form the majority of cases diagnosed before the ninth month of life. Neonatal diabetes is transient in about one-half of the cases; if persistent, it presents a significant clinical challenge and requires subspecialty care. Some infants respond better to sulfonylurea than insulin. Maturity-onset diabetes of the young (MODY) presents as a nonketotic and usually non–insulin-dependent diabetes in the absence of obesity or islet autoantibodies. A strong family history of early-onset diabetes is common. The most frequent forms are due to mutations in glucokinase or hepatic nuclear factor 1 or 2 genes. Glucokinase mutations rarely require therapy; other forms respond to oral hypoglycemic agents or insulin. Commercial and research-oriented genotyping services are available to aid correct diagnosis.

D. Cystic Fibrosis-Related Diabetes

Cystic fibrosis-related diabetes (CFRD) occurs in about 20% of adolescents with cystic fibrosis (CF) and is the most common comorbidity in CF (for more information, see Chapter 19). The primary defect is insulin insufficiency, exacerbated by insulin resistance especially in times of illness or with glucocorticoid therapy. The presence of CFRD is associated with worse

Table 35–1. Stages of type 1 diabetes.

Stage 1	Stage 2	Stage 3
Multiple islet autoantibodies	Multiple islet autoantibodies	Islet autoimmunity
Normoglycemia	Dysglycemia (see Table 35–2)[a]	Diabetes by standard criteria (see Table 35–2)
Asymptomatic	Asymptomatic	Clinical symptoms

[a]Additional proposed criteria for dysglycemia: ≥ 10% increase in HbA_{1C} from previous visit or ≥ 200 mg/dL (11.1 mmol/L) at an intermediate time point during oral glucose tolerance test (OGTT) (30, 60, or 90 minutes).

nutritional status, more severe lung disease, and greater mortality. Patients with CF should be routinely screened beginning by age 10, and treatment has been shown to improve outcomes.

▶ Pathogenesis

A. Type 1 Diabetes

T1D is caused by a combination of genetic factors and unknown environmental factors. The resulting autoimmune destruction of the insulin-producing β cells of the pancreatic islets is marked by the presence of autoantibodies to islet cell autoantigens (insulin, GAD65, IA-2, and ZnT8) that can be measured in the blood. The persistence of two or more islet autoantibodies is highly predictive of development of symptomatic diabetes. Thus, in 2015 a new staging definition of T1D was adopted with multiple islet autoimmunity being defined as stage 1 T1D (Table 35–1). Ongoing β-cell destruction occurs over months or years, leading first to asymptomatic dysglycemia (stage 2) and later to symptomatic T1D (stage 3) when most of the pancreatic β cells have been destroyed. Insulin production, measured by fasting or stimulated C-peptide levels, is usually low at diagnosis but may increase after initiation of insulin therapy ("honeymoon period") and persist for weeks or months until eventual total or near-complete loss of β-cell function.

More than 90% of children with T1D carry at least one of the two high-risk HLA haplotypes—DR4/DQ8 or DR3/DQ2—and 40% of US children diagnosed before age of 10 years have both (one from each parent), compared with only 2.5% of the general population. Over 50 non-HLA genetic variants have also been implicated.

B. Type 2 Diabetes

T2D has a strong genetic component, although the inherited defects of insulin secretion vary in different families. There is evidence to suggest that T2D progresses differently in youth compared to adults with more rapid decline in β-cell function and greater risk for early development of complications.

Obesity, particularly central, and lack of exercise do contribute but are rarely sufficient alone to cause diabetes in youth. T2D and associated insulin resistance adversely affect long-term cardiovascular health.

▶ Prevention

A. Type 1 Diabetes

Since the 1950s, the incidence of T1D has increased worldwide, doubling every 20 years. Despite much research on early childhood infections and diet, the environmental factor(s) responsible for this epidemic are poorly defined.

Islet autoantibodies do not mediate β-cell destruction but offer a useful screening tool as they are usually present for years prior to diagnosis. It has been shown that intensive follow-up of individuals with multiple islet autoantibodies (stage 1 T1D) reduces the severity of the presentation. Antibody screening is not yet standard of care but is available in the research setting for children with a first- or second-degree relative with T1D (www.trialnet.org) or in general population children living in Colorado (www.askhealth.org) or Bavaria, Germany (www.typ1diabetes-frueherkennung.de).

As β-cell damage is mediated by T lymphocytes, immunosuppression at different checkpoints of the autoimmune process can slow down β-cell loss. Immunomodulation, including induction of tolerance to islet autoantigens, with or without immunosuppression, is an area of intensive research. Various immunotherapies have shown promising effects in prolonging β-cell function ("honeymoon") in newly diagnosed individuals (stage 3 T1D). Recent stage II trials of teplizumab, an Fc receptor–nonbinding anti-CD3 monoclonal antibody, demonstrated for the first time delayed progression from stage 2 to 3 T1D. Identification of individuals with early-stage T1D is likely to play an important role in efforts to modify disease trajectory in the future.

B. Type 2 Diabetes

The Diabetes Prevention Program study done in adults with impaired glucose tolerance (IGT) found that 30 minutes of exercise per day (5 days/wk) and a low-fat diet reduced the risk of diabetes by 58%. In adults, taking metformin also reduced the risk of T2D by 31%. There is less data in youth; however, an intensive 12-month intensive behavior modification intervention resulted in reduced lipids, body mass index (BMI), and insulin resistance in obese youth without diabetes and improved glycemic profile in youth with prediabetes.

▶ Clinical Findings

A. Symptoms and Signs

A combination of polyuria, polydipsia, and weight loss in a child is unique to diabetes. Unfortunately, these symptoms are often missed by parents and primary care providers. The frequency of diabetic ketoacidosis (DKA) in US children with newly diagnosed T1D has not decreased in the past 20 years and is approximately 40%, a sign of poor provider and community awareness. More than one-half of DKA patients were seen by a provider in the days preceding diagnosis, and obvious symptoms and signs were missed. The correct diagnosis could be improved with better history-taking and point-of-care blood or urine analysis. Initial diagnosis can be easily confirmed by blood glucose and ketone measurements using widely available and inexpensive meters.

The clinical presentation of DKA includes abdominal pain, nausea, and vomiting that can mimic the flu, gastroenteritis or an acute abdomen. Patients are mildly to moderately dehydrated (5%–10%), may have Kussmaul respiration, and become progressively somnolent and obtunded. While the majority of diagnoses occur in older children, the distribution has shifted to include younger ages; infants, toddlers, and preschool age children. They often have symptoms of minor infection or gastrointestinal upset. A heavy diaper in a dehydrated child without diarrhea should always raise alarm. A blood or urine glucose test could be lifesaving.

B. Laboratory Findings

Laboratory findings diagnostic of diabetes are shown in Table 35–2.

It should be noted that while hemoglobin A_{1C} (HbA_{1C}) can be used for diagnosis of diabetes, most clinical laboratories do not perform HbA_{1C} assays that meet diagnostic criteria (ie, NGSP certified and standardized to the Diabetes Control and Complications Trial reference assay). For this reason, HbA_{1C} measurements are prone to error and must be interpreted with caution, especially in the absence of other signs or symptoms of diabetes. Additionally, the HbA_{1C} is less sensitive than blood glucose-based criteria and may underestimate dysglycemia in young children

whose progression to T1D can be especially rapid. Children with impaired fasting glucose (IFG) or IGT and no islet autoantibodies are at high risk of T2D and require careful follow-up and lifestyle modification with weight loss, if obese.

Blood glucose higher than 200 mg/dL in a child is always abnormal and must be promptly and meticulously followed in consultation with a pediatric endocrinology service. If there are significant ketones in urine or blood, treatment is urgent. Conversely, if the presentation is mild and an outpatient diabetes education service is available, hospitalization is often not necessary.

▶ Differential Diagnosis

A combination of polyuria, polydipsia, and weight loss in a child is unique to diabetes. Of note, not all hyperglycemia in children is diabetes; transient, "stress-" or steroid-induced hyperglycemia can occur with illness or trauma. In an asymptomatic, well child, the diagnosis must not be based on a single plasma glucose test or a borderline result obtained using a glucose meter.

The differentiation between type of diabetes can have important implications for management and education. Testing children for islet autoantibodies can be helpful to establish ongoing islet autoimmunity (T1D). The absence of the three most available autoantibodies (to insulin, GAD, and IA-2) provides 80% negative predictive value, and other causes of diabetes should be assessed. Monogenic diabetes should be considered in a child with an autosomal dominant family history of diabetes, presentation before 12 months of age, mild fasting hyperglycemia, a prolonged period of persistent insulin production ("honeymoon") over 1 year, or associated conditions such as syndromic features, deafness or optic atrophy. All children diagnosed with diabetes in the first 6 months of life should have genetic screening for neonatal diabetes.

Table 35–2. Laboratory values defining dysglycemia/prediabetes and diagnostic criteria for diabetes.

	Measure	Normal	Dysglycemia/Prediabetes	Diabetes
A.	Fasting plasma glucose (no intake for at least 8 h)	< 100 mg/dL (5.6 mmol/L)	IFG:100–125 mg/dL (5.6–6.9 mmol/L)	≥ 126 mg/dL (7.0 mmol/L)
B.	2-h plasma glucose during OGTT	< 140 mg/dL (7.8 mmol/L)	IGT: 140–199 mg/dL (7.8–11.0 mmol/L)	≥ 200 mg/dL (11.1 mmol/L)
C.	Hemoglobin A_{1C}[a]	< 5.7% (39 mmol/mol)	5.7–6.4% (39–47 mmol/mol)	≥ 6.5 (48 mmol/mol)
D.	Random plasma glucose (in patient with hyperglycemic crisis or classic symptoms of hyperglycemia):			≥ 200 mg/dL (11.1 mmol/L)

Note: For diagnosis of diabetes, any criteria A–D may be used; however, in the absence of symptoms, measures A–C must be repeated.
IFG, impaired fasting glucose; IGT, impaired glucose tolerance; OGTT, oral glucose tolerance test (performed as described by the World Health Organization [1.75 g glucose/kg up to a maximum of 75 g]).
[a]With laboratory method that is NGSP certified and standardized to the Diabetes Control and Complications Trial (DCCT) assay.

If HbA_{1C} is normal, home monitoring of blood glucose for several days, including fasting and 2-hour postprandial measurement, can be helpful to establish the glycemic profile. In children progressing to overt diabetes, hyperglycemia after meals is usually the initial abnormality, while fasting hyperglycemia develops much later.

In the era of increasing prevalence of childhood obesity, it is nonetheless important to note that T1D is still much more common in children overall, particularly those who are younger than 10 or prepubertal, regardless of weight status. Factors lending credence to a diagnosis of T2D include a strong family history, ethnic/racial minority status, central obesity, and pubertal status. Acanthosis nigricans, a thickening and darkening of the skin over the posterior neck, armpits, or elbows, is a sign of insulin resistance and may increase suspicion for T2D. It should be noted, however, that it is present in many obese children and is not specific for the diagnosis of T2D.

While DKA is more common at presentation of T1D, approximately 6% of children with T2D present in DKA.

▶ Treatment

Treatment of both T1D and T2D should take a holistic approach to the child in the context of family and greater environment. There are many common themes to management of diabetes in the pediatric patient, regardless of pathogenesis. Effective diabetes management requires access to a multidisciplinary diabetes team including a physician, diabetes nurse educator, registered dietician, and psychologist or social worker.

A. General Principles for Diabetes Management

1. Treatment goals—The HbA_{1C} level reflects the average blood glucose levels over the previous 3 months. The overarching goals of therapy in diabetes include prevention of acute and long-term complications by reducing chronic hyperglycemia while maximizing the quality of life. In T1D, these goals must be tempered by preventing frequent or prolonged hypoglycemia and associated morbidities. Each child should have targets individually determined to aim for the lowest HbA_{1C} that can be sustained without severe hypoglycemia or frequent moderate hypoglycemia (see Quality Assessment & Outcomes Metrics). In T2D, addressing obesity and associated comorbidities, when present, is also a major focus in maximizing health outcomes (see Chapters 4 and 11).

2. Patient and family education—All caregivers need to learn about diabetes, how to give insulin via injections or insulin pump, perform home blood glucose monitoring, and handle acute complications. While teenagers can be taught to perform many of the tasks of diabetes management, they do better when supportive, not overbearing, parents continue to be involved in management of their disease. The use of educational books (see below) can be very helpful to the family.

3. Psychological care—The diagnosis of diabetes changes lives of the affected families and brings on relentless challenges. It is impossible to take a "vacation" from diabetes without some unpleasant consequences. The stress imposed on the family around the time of initial diagnosis may lead to feelings of shock, denial, sadness, anger, fear, and guilt. Meeting with a counselor to express these feelings at the time of diagnosis helps with long-term adaptation. Persistent adjustment problems may indicate underlying dysfunction of the family or psychopathology of the child or caregiver. Young people with T1D are more frequently diagnosed with and treated for psychiatric disorders, disordered eating, neurocognitive learning problems, and poor coping skills than the general population. In T2D, socioeconomic status and obesity are both risk factors for the disease as well as for psychological stress, depression, and other mental illness.

Routine assessment should be made of developmental adjustment to and understanding of diabetes management, including diabetes-related knowledge, insulin adjustment skills, goal setting, problem-solving abilities, regimen adherence, and self-care autonomy and competence. This is especially important during late childhood and prior to adolescence. General and diabetes-related family functioning such as communication, parental involvement and support, and roles and responsibilities for self-care behaviors need to be assessed. Teaching parents effective behavior management skills, especially at diagnosis and prior to adolescence, emphasizes involvement and support, effective problem-solving, self-management skills, and realistic expectations. Adolescents should be encouraged to assume increased responsibility for diabetes management, but with continued, mutually agreed parental involvement and support. The transition to adult diabetes care should be negotiated and planned between adolescents, their parents, and the diabetes team well in advance of the actual transfer.

4. Diet and exercise—A thorough dietary history should be obtained including the family's dietary habits and traditions, the child's typical meal times, and patterns of food intake. At least 60 minutes of daily aerobic exercise is important for children with diabetes. Exercise fosters a sense of well-being; helps increase insulin sensitivity (a drop in glycemia in response to insulin); and helps maintain proper weight, blood pressure, and high-density lipoprotein (HDL)-cholesterol levels.

B. Treatment of Type 1 Diabetes

1. Home blood glucose monitoring—All families must be able to monitor blood glucose levels at least four times daily; however, 7–10 checks per day are typically needed for optimal diabetes management. Higher frequency of self-monitoring of blood glucose and/or use of continuous glucose monitoring (CGM) have been associated with improved HbA_{1C}.

CGM is now routinely available and can significantly improve diabetes management if used most of the time. Subcutaneous glucose levels are obtained every 1–5 minutes from a sensor placed under the skin. The sensor must be replaced every 6–10 days. A transmitter sends glucose levels from the sensor to a receiver that can be inside an insulin pump, smartphone, or separate receiver device. Low and high blood glucose alarms can be set. As with insulin pump therapy (see below), intensive education and follow-up are required, usually at a specialty diabetes center. The user is trained on how to keep the real-time displayed blood glucose "between the lines," that is, in the target range.

The Food and Drug Administration (FDA) has now approved insulin dosing based on the Dexcom G5 and G6 CGM glucose values, which reduces the need for fingersticks, particularly in the school setting. As subcutaneous glucose levels can lag behind blood glucose levels in times of rapid change, finger stick blood glucose is still recommended for treatment and monitoring of recovery from hypoglycemic or significant hyperglycemic events.

In some systems CGM data may be used to automatically change insulin pump delivery rate (see section "Artificial Pancreas" Systems).

Regular evaluation of blood glucose results or CGM data by the family helps to identify patterns of changing insulin needs, especially when combined with logs of insulin dosage and significant events (eg, illness, parties, exercise, menses, and episodes of hypoglycemia or ketonuria/ketosis). If more than 30% of the values are above the desired range for age or more than 15% below the desired range, the insulin dosage needs to be adjusted.

Some families are able to make these changes independently, whereas others need help from the health care provider to optimize insulin dose between visits. Children with diabetes should be evaluated by a diabetes provider every 3 months to check compliance, adjust insulin dose according to growth, measure HbA_{1C}, and review blood glucose patterns, as well as for routine review of systems, physical examination, and laboratory tests.

2. Nutritional management—Nutritional management in children with T1D does not require a restrictive diet, just a healthy dietary regimen from which both children and their families can benefit. Insulin pump and multiple daily injection (MDI) therapy utilize carbohydrate counting in which the grams of carbohydrate to be eaten are counted and a matching dose of insulin is administered. This plan allows for the most freedom and flexibility in food choices, but it requires expert education and commitment and may not be suitable for many families or situations, such as for school lunches and teenagers. As an alternative to precise carb counting, "exchanges" may be taught to estimate 10- or 15-g servings of carbohydrate.

3. Insulin—Insulin has three key functions: (1) it allows glucose to pass into the cell for oxidative utilization; (2) it decreases the physiologic production of glucose, particularly in the liver; and (3) it turns off lipolysis and ketone production.

A. INSULIN TREATMENT OF NEW-ONSET TYPE 1 DIABETES— In children who present without DKA and who have adequate oral intake, the initial insulin dose can be administered subcutaneously. Typically, 0.2–0.3 U/kg of long-acting insulin analog—glargine (Lantus or Basaglar), detemir (Levemir), or degludec (Tresiba)—can be administered subcutaneously to provide the "basal" level of insulin. Additionally, a small amount of short-acting insulin (regular) or, preferentially, rapid-acting analog: lispro (Humalog), aspart (NovoLog), or glulisine (Apidra) can be used for correction and mealtime dosing. This usually suffices for the initial 12–24 hours preceding systematic diabetes education.

The dose is adjusted with each injection during the first week. The rule of thumb is to start insulin at the low end of the estimated daily requirement and titrate it up based on frequent blood-glucose monitoring or CGM glucose levels. The initial daily dose of insulin is higher in the presence of ketosis, infection, obesity, or steroid treatment. It also varies with age, pubertal status and severity of onset. A total subcutaneous daily dose of 0.3–0.7 U/kg/day may suffice in prepubertal children, while pubertal or overweight children and those with initial HbA_{1C} greater than 12% commonly require 1.0–1.5 U/kg/day of insulin during the initial week of treatment. Children younger than 12 years cannot reliably administer insulin without adult supervision because they may lack fine motor control and/or may not understand the importance of accurate dosage.

The insulin dose peaks about 1 week after diagnosis and decreases slightly with the waning of glucotoxicity and voracious appetite. Approximately 3–6 weeks after diagnosis, most school children and adolescents experience a partial remission or "honeymoon period." Temporary decrease in the insulin dose during this period is necessary to avoid severe hypoglycemia. The remission tends to last longer in older children but is rarely complete and never permanent. Other types of diabetes should be considered in patients with unusually low insulin requirements.

B. LONG-TERM INSULIN DOSAGE—Children usually receive a rapid-acting insulin to cover food intake or correct high blood glucose and a long-acting insulin to suppress endogenous hepatic glucose production. This is achieved by combining insulins with the desired properties. Understanding the onset, peak, and duration of insulin activity is essential (Table 35–3).

Nearly all children diagnosed with T1D at our center receive insulin from a pump or through basal-bolus MDI. This usually consists of three to four injections (boluses) of rapid-acting analog before meals and one to two injections of long-acting analog insulin. The dose of premeal rapid-acting insulin is calculated based on anticipated carbohydrate

Table 35–3. Types of insulin and kinetics of action.[a]

Type of Insulin	Begins Working	Peak Effect	All Gone
Rapid-acting			
Insulin aspart (Fiasp)	< 5 min	60–70 min	5–7 h
Insulin aspart (NovoLog)	10–15 min	30–90 min	3–5 h
Insulin glulisine (Apidra)	15–30 min	30–90 min	3–5 h
Insulin lispro (Humalog, Admelog)	10–15 min	30–90 min	3–5 h
Inhaled insulin (Afrezza) (NOT approved for those aged < 18 y)	20 min	30–60 min	1–5 h
Short-acting			
Regular (Humulin R, Novolin R)	30–60 min	2–4 h	6–10 h
Intermediate-acting			
NPH (neutral protamine Hagedorn) (Humulin N, Novolin N)	1–4 h	4–12 h	8–18 h (usually ~ 12 h)
Long-acting			
Insulin degludec (Tresiba)	1–2 h	No peak	24–40 h
Insulin detemir (Levemir)	1–2 h	No peak	6–24 h
Insulin glargine (Lantus, Basaglar, Toujeo)	1–2 h	No peak	18–26 h
Premixed (available in various combinations)			
Humulin 70/30 or Novolin 70/30 (70% NPH + 30% regular)	30 min	Dual peak	10–18 h
NovoLog Mix 70/30 (70% NPH + 30% aspart) or Humalog Mix 75/25 (75% NPH + 25% lispro)	15 min	Dual peak	10–18 h

[a]Insulin action may vary between individuals or within individual.

content of the meal and additional insulin to correct for high blood glucose, if needed. Sliding scales for dosing of rapid-acting insulin (based only on current blood glucose level) are helpful initially, while families learn carbohydrate counting. This shortcut assumes that the content of carbohydrates, for example in dinner, does not vary from day to day; therefore, this may lead to significant under- and overdosing.

Children younger than 4 years usually need 0.5–2 units of rapid-acting insulin to cover carbohydrate intake. Children aged 4–10 years may require up to 4 units of rapid-acting insulin to cover breakfast and dinner, whereas 4–10 units of rapid-acting insulin are used in older children. These estimates do not include correction for high blood glucose.

Families gradually learn to make small weekly adjustments in insulin dosage based on home blood glucose testing or CGM values. Rapid-acting analog insulin is given 10–20 minutes before eating to account for delay in insulin action. If slower human regular insulin is used, the injections should be given 30–60 minutes before meals—rarely a practical option. In young children who eat unpredictably, it may be necessary to wait until after the meal to decide on the appropriate dose of rapid-acting insulin, which is a compromise between avoiding hypoglycemia and tolerating hyperglycemia after meals.

A long-acting analog insulin glargine (Lantus or Basaglar) or detemir (Levemir) is given once or twice a day to maintain basal insulin levels between meals. Degludec (Tresiba) is administered once daily, whenever convenient. Daily adjustments in long-acting insulin dose usually are not needed. However, decreases should be made for heavy activity (eg, sports, hikes) or overnight events.

In the past, most children would receive two injections per day of rapid-acting insulin and an intermediate-acting insulin (NPH), often mixed just before injection. About two-thirds of the total dosage would be given before breakfast and the remainder before dinner. This regimen has been shown to be inferior in achieving recommended HbA$_{1C}$ levels and avoiding hypoglycemia, compared with the basal-bolus regimen described above. When changing a patient from NPH insulin to an analog, initially only 50% of the daily units of long-acting insulin is recommended.

c. Insulin pump treatment—Continuous subcutaneous insulin infusion (insulin pump) therapy is currently the best way to restore the body's physiologic insulin profile. The standard insulin pump delivers a variable programmed basal rate that corresponds to the diurnal variation in insulin needs. Prepubertal children require higher basal rate in the early part of night, while postpubertal patients who experience the "dawn phenomenon" require higher rates in the morning. Lower rates are set for periods of vigorous activity. The user initiates bolus doses before meals and to correct hyperglycemia. Most pumps can receive wireless transmission of test results from glucose meters, but the patient or caregiver must still manually enter the amount of carbohydrate being consumed. The pump calculates the amount of insulin needed for a meal or correction based on previously entered parameters that include insulin-to-carbohydrate ratios, insulin sensitivity (or correction) factor, glycemic target, and duration of insulin action (set at 2–3 hours to protect from accumulating too much insulin). The user may override the suggestion or press a button to initiate the bolus.

Most clinical trials have demonstrated better HbA_{1C} and less severe hypoglycemia with pump therapy, compared to MDI. Pump therapy can improve the quality of life in children who have trouble with or fear of injections or who desire greater flexibility in their lifestyle, for example with sleeping in, sports, or irregular eating. Insulin pumps can be particularly helpful in young children or infants who have multiple meals and snacks and require multiple small doses of rapid-acting insulin. The newer generation of insulin pumps can deliver as little as 0.025 U/h, but higher rates using diluted insulin may be needed for uninterrupted flow.

Compliance problems include infrequent blood glucose testing, not changing pump infusion sets on a timely basis, not reacting to elevated blood glucose, incorrect carbohydrate counting, or missing mealtime boluses altogether. Side effects of insulin pump treatment include failures of insulin delivery because of a displaced or obstructed infusion set. Insulin pump treatment is significantly more expensive than regimens based on injections. For some patients, pumps may be too difficult to operate; some cannot comply with the multiple testing and carbohydrate counting requirements, or the pump is unacceptable because of body image issues or extreme physical activity (swimming, contact sports).

d. "Artificial pancreas" systems—The newest generation of insulin pumps receive CGM sensor input that leads to automatic changes in insulin infusion. The simplest system available features sensor-initiated automatic suspension of insulin delivery at a predetermined low-glucose level and automatic resumption of the delivery after glucose levels rise. Other systems react to predicted, rather than current, low or high blood glucose levels. The first hybrid closed-loop system, the Medtronic 670G, became available in 2017. The Tandem Control-IQ system was approved in 2020, and there are more systems in active development. The hybrid closed loop replaces a programmed basal rate with variable basal dosing determined automatically in response to CGM input. All current "artificial pancreas" systems still require the wearer to give boluses before meals based on carbohydrate consumption.

4. Exercise—Hypoglycemia during exercise or in the 2–12 hours after exercise can be prevented by (1) careful monitoring of blood glucose before, during, and after exercise; (2) reducing the dosage of the insulin active at the time of (or after) the exercise, including reducing or temporarily stopping the basal rate on an insulin pump; and (3) providing extra snacks. Fifteen grams of glucose usually covers about 30 minutes of exercise. The use of drinks containing 5%–10% dextrose, such as Gatorade, during the period of exercise is often beneficial. Insulin dose for meals as well as the basal insulin pump rate should be reduced before, during, and sometimes after the exercise; the longer and more vigorous the activity, the greater the reduction in insulin dose.

5. Sick day management—Families must be educated to check blood or urine ketone levels during any illness, when a fasting blood/CGM glucose level is above 240 mg/dL (13.3 mmol/L), or a randomly measured glucose level is above 300 mg/dL (16.6 mmol/L). The health care provider should be called in the presence of moderate or significant ketonuria or ketonemia (blood β-hydroxybutyrate > 1.0 mmol/L, by Precision Xtra meter). Usually 10%–20% of the total daily insulin dosage is given subcutaneously as rapid-acting analog or regular insulin every 2–3 hours until blood glucose normalizes. This prevents progression to ketoacidosis and allows most patients to receive treatment at home. Water is the oral fluid of choice if blood/CGM glucose is more than 250 mg/dL; at lower levels of glycemia, one should switch to Gatorade/Powerade or other glucose-containing beverages.

C. Treatment of Type 2 Diabetes

Treatment of T2D in children varies with the severity of the disease.

1. Lifestyle management—If the HbA_{1C} is still near normal, family-centered modification of lifestyle is the first line of therapy. Lifestyle interventions have mixed results in the pediatric population, compared to adults, possibly reflecting the complex family and environmental context for T2D in youth. Interventions should emphasize eating a balanced diet, achieving and maintaining a healthy weight and regular exercise. Dietary intervention should be culturally appropriate and recognize limitations in family resources.

2. Medications—Pharmacologic therapy has been historically limited to two approved medications: metformin and insulin; however, in 2019, for the first time in almost 20 years, an additional medication, liraglutide (Victoza), was approved for youth with T2D age 10 and older.

With HbA_{1C} less than 8.5% and no symptoms or ketosis, metformin is usually started at a dose of 500 mg daily with dose increased weekly to a maximum dose of 1000 mg twice daily. If the presentation is more severe, with ketosis, HbA_{1C} 8.5% or greater, random blood glucose levels 250 mg/dL or greater, or uncertainty regarding the distinction between T1D and T2D, initial treatment should include insulin. An initial basal insulin dose of 0.25–0.5 U/kg is typically effective. Metformin can be initiated after ketosis has resolved. An attempt to wean insulin can be started after 2–6 weeks, once fasting and postprandial glucose levels have reached normal or near-normal levels. If target HbA_{1C} of less than 7% (47.5 mmol/mol) is not achieved within 4 months on metformin alone, basal insulin should be considered up to 1.5 U/kg/day. If target is not reached on combination metformin and basal insulin, prandial insulin should be started (MDI or insulin pump).

If glycemic targets are not met with metformin (with or without basal insulin), liraglutide should be considered in those 10 years of age or greater. Personal or family history or medullary thyroid carcinoma or multiple endocrine neoplasia type 2 are contraindications. Liraglutide is given by once-daily injection and results in higher levels of glucagon-like peptide-1 (GLP-1) that increases insulin production, reduces glucagon levels, delays gastric emptying, and decreases appetite. When combined with either metformin alone or metformin and insulin, liraglutide reduced HbA_{1C} by 0.64%. Similar to adults, youth experienced gastrointestinal side effects (nausea, vomiting and diarrhea); this can be minimized with low initial dose and gradual increase. Of note, youth on liraglutide improved weight loss relative to placebo at 1 year of treatment.

Clinical trials are underway examining the safety and efficacy of additional pharmacologic therapies.

3. Home glucose monitoring—Home blood glucose monitoring is typically less frequent in youth who are treated with metformin or lifestyle alone (eg, first morning and 2-hour postprandial test on 3 days per week); however, those taking insulin may require more frequent testing depending on the dose and type of insulin used.

Copeland KC et al: Management of newly diagnosed type 2-diabetes mellitus (t2dm) in children and adolescents. Pediatrics 2013 Feb 1;131(2):364–382 [PMID: 23359574].

Nadeau KJ et al: Youth-onset type 2 diabetes consensus report: current status, challenges, and priorities. Diabetes Care 2016; 39:1635–1642 [PMID: 27486237].

Springer SC et al: Management of type 2 diabetes mellitus in children and adolescents. Pediatrics 2013 Feb 1;131(2):e648–e664 [PMID: 23359584].

QUALITY ASSESSMENT & OUTCOMES METRICS

Recommendations for the medical care of children and adolescents with diabetes and assessment of outcomes are summarized yearly in the American Diabetes Association's position statement, Standards of Medical Care in Diabetes, as well as the International Society for Pediatric and Adolescent Diabetes (ISPAD) Clinical Practice Consensus Guidelines (available online references in the following text).

In the seminal DCCT trial, HbA_{1C} values of 7%, compared to 9%, resulted in greater than 50% reductions in the eye, kidney, cardiovascular, and neurologic complications of T1D. Unfortunately less than 30% of the US children and youth with T1D have HbA_{1C} of less than 7.5%. At present, the ADA and ISPAD recommend individualized goals for children and adolescents with diabetes. All children should have a target HbA_{1C} of less than 7.5%. In patients with access to comprehensive diabetes care with analog insulins, insulin pump technology and the ability closely monitor glucose via frequent fingersticks or use of CGM, ISPAD recommends a target HbA_{1C} of less than 7.0%. A goal of HbA_{1C} less than 7.5% may be more appropriate for those with resource-limited environments, a history of severe hypoglycemia, an inability to articulate symptoms of hypoglycemia (eg, young children), or hypoglycemia unawareness. A more stringent target of less than 6.5% (48 mmol/mol) may be appropriate in selected patients, particularly those with residual β-cell function, if this can be achieved without significant hypoglycemia. CGM time in range (time with sensor values between 70 and 180 mg/dL [3.9–10.0 mmol/L]) is becoming a useful measure of diabetes control in those using these devices. Recommended goals for blood glucose and CGM values to reach HbA_{1C} targets are shown in Table 35–4.

Table 35–4. Blood glucose and CGM goals.

	All Children HbA_{1C} < 7.5%	Low Hypoglycemia Risk[a] HbA_{1C} < 7.0%
Targets for self-monitor blood glucose		
Premeal (≥ 2 h fast)	90–130 mg/dL (5.0–7.2 mmol/L)	70–130 mg/dL (3.9–7.2 mmol/L)
Postmeal		90–180 mg/dL (5.0–10.0 mmol/L)
Prebed/Overnight	90–150 mg/dL (5.0–8.3 mmol/L)	80–140 mg/dL (5.0–10.0 mmol/L)
Targets for CGM		
Time in range 70–180 mg/dL (3.9–10.0 mmol/L)	> 60%	> 70%

CGM, continuous glucose monitor; HbA_{1C}, hemoglobin A_{1C}. Goals are for general reference only. ADA guidelines recommend all targets should be individualized to patient.

[a]Low hypoglycemia risk includes children with access to optimal diabetes care (analog insulin, CGM, pumps), ability to recognize and communicate symptoms of hypoglycemia, and no history of severe hypoglycemic events.

International Society for Pediatric and Adolescent Diabetes (ISPAD) Clinical Practice Consensus Guidelines 2018. Pediatric Diabetes 2018;19 S27:5–338.
www.ispad.org/general/custom.asp?page=ISPADGuidelines2018
Standards of Medical Care in Diabetes—2020. Diabetes Care 2020 Jan;43(Suppl 1):S1–S212 [PMID: 30559224]. https://care.diabetesjournals.org/content/43/Supplement_1

▶ Complications

A. Diabetic Ketoacidosis (DKA)

Ketoacidosis (venous blood pH < 7.30 or bicarbonate < 15 mEq/L) is unfortunately still a frequent acute complication in patients with newly diagnosed T1D.

In established T1D, DKA may occur in those who miss insulin injections, do not check blood or urine ketone levels, or fail to seek help when ketones are elevated. Repeated episodes of DKA signify that counseling may be indicated, and that a responsible adult must take over the diabetes management. If, for any reason, this is not possible, a change in the child's living situation may be necessary.

Treatment of DKA is based on four physiologic principles: (1) restoration of fluid volume; (2) intravenous insulin to inhibit lipolysis and return to glucose utilization; (3) replacement of electrolytes; and (4) correction of acidosis. Mild DKA is defined as a venous blood pH of 7.2–7.3; moderate DKA, a pH of 7.10–7.19; and severe DKA, a pH below 7.10. Patients with severe DKA should be hospitalized in a pediatric intensive care unit, if available. Laboratory tests at the start of treatment should include venous blood pH, glucose, and an electrolyte panel. More severe cases may benefit from determination of blood osmolality, calcium, phosphorus, and urea nitrogen levels. Severe and moderate episodes of DKA generally require hourly determinations of serum glucose, electrolytes, and venous pH levels, whereas these parameters can be measured every 2 hours if the pH level is 7.20–7.30.

1. Restoration of fluid volume—Dehydration is judged by estimated loss of body weight, dryness of oral mucous membranes, low blood pressure, and tachycardia. Initial treatment is with normal saline (0.9%), 10–20 mL/kg during the first hour (can be repeated in severely dehydrated patients during the second hour). The total volume of fluid in the first 4 hours of treatment should not exceed 20–40 mL/kg because of the danger of cerebral edema. After initial expansion, 0.45%–0.9% saline is given at 1.5 times maintenance to replace losses over 24–36 hours. When blood glucose level falls below 250 mg/dL (13.9 mmol/L), 5% dextrose is added to the intravenous fluids. If blood glucose level falls below 120 mg/dL (6.6 mmol/L), 10% dextrose can be added.

2. Inhibition of lipolysis and return to glucose utilization—Insulin turns off fat breakdown and ketone formation. After initial fluid bolus, regular insulin is given as a continuous drip at a rate of 0.05–0.1 U/kg/h to achieve drop in blood glucose of approximately 100 mg/dL/h. An IV insulin bolus is not recommended as it may increase the risk of brain edema. Insulin should be delayed pending potassium replacement if the patient is hypokalemic (see below). If necessary to address rapid fall in glucose or hypokalemia, the insulin dosage can be reduced, but it should not be discontinued before the venous blood pH reaches 7.30. Intravenous insulin should be continued for at least 30 minutes after the initial subcutaneous injection of both a long- and short-acting insulin to prevent rebound ketosis.

3. Replacement of electrolytes—In patients with DKA, both sodium and potassium are depleted. Serum sodium concentrations may be corrected for hyperglycemia. Sodium is usually replaced adequately by the use of 0.45%–0.9% saline in the rehydration fluids.

Although total body potassium is often depleted, serum potassium levels may be elevated initially because of inability of potassium to stay in the cell in the presence of acidosis. Potassium should not be added to IV fluids until the serum potassium level is known to be less than 5.0 mEq/L and urine output is confirmed. It is then usually given in replacement fluid at a concentration of 40 mEq/L, with half of the potassium (20 mEq/L) either as potassium acetate or potassium chloride and the other half as potassium phosphate (20 mEq/L). Hypocalcemia can occur if all of the potassium is given as the phosphate salt; hypophosphatemia may occur if none of the potassium is the phosphate salt.

If initial potassium is low, potassium replacement should be started at the time of initial fluid bolus and *before* initiation of insulin. Failure to adequately replace potassium before starting insulin can lead to life-threatening cardiac complications.

4. Correction of acidosis—Acidosis corrects spontaneously as the fluid volume is restored and insulin facilitates aerobic glycolysis and inhibits ketogenesis. Bicarbonate is generally not recommended as it may increase risk of cerebral edema.

5. Management of cerebral edema—Some degree of cerebral edema has been shown by computed tomography scan to occur commonly in DKA. Associated clinical symptoms are rare, unpredictable, and may be associated with demise. Cerebral edema may be related to the degree of dehydration, cerebral hypoperfusion, acidosis, and hyperventilation at the time of presentation. In general, it is recommended that no more than 40 mL/kg of fluids be given in the first 4 hours of treatment and that subsequent fluid replacement does not exceed 1.5 times maintenance. Cerebral edema is more common when the serum sodium is noted to be falling rather than rising. Early neurologic signs may include headache, excessive drowsiness, and dilated pupils. Prompt initiation of therapy should include elevation of the head of the bed, mannitol (1 g/kg over 30 minutes), and fluid restriction. Hypertonic saline (3%) at 2.5–5 mL/kg over 10–15 minutes may be used as an alternative to mannitol or in addition to mannitol if there has been no response to initial bolus. If the cerebral edema is not recognized and treated early, over 50% of patients will die or have permanent brain damage.

B. Hyperosmolar Hyperglycemic State

Hyperosmolar hyperglycemic state (HHS) is rare but a severe metabolic decompensation in an individual with some level of insulin production. It is associated with hyperglycemia (plasma glucose > 600 mg/dL/ 33.3 mmol/L) and hyperosmolarity above 320 mOsm/kg. There is typically little to no ketosis (negative or "trace" urine dipstick) or acidosis (bicarbonate > 15 mEq/L, venous pH > 7.25). HHS can often go unrecognized until a profound level of dehydration occurs, up to twice the fluid loss seen in DKA. Presentation frequently includes profound mental status changes, ranging from combativeness to coma. Complications of HHS most often relate to thromboembolic events. Rhabdomyolysis may also occur, with associated muscle swelling, kidney failure, and electrolyte disturbances including hypokalemia and hypocalcemia with cardiac arrhythmia or arrest leading to compartment syndrome. There are several reports of a malignant hyperthermia-like syndrome of unclear cause, and treatment with dantrolene should be initiated early in children with fever associated with a rise in creatine kinase. While HHS would be suspected to have a risk of cerebral edema similar to DKA, this complication has been reported exceedingly rarely. Similar to reports in adults, HHS in the pediatric population is more common in obese, male African Americans. The adult literature describes HHS as a complication of T2D; however, in the pediatric population, it has been reported in individuals with both T1D and T2D.

Children with HHS should be managed in an intensive care unit with cardiac monitoring and hourly evaluation of serum glucose, vital signs, and hydration status as well as close monitoring of electrolytes, kidney function, osmolality, and creatine kinase (to evaluate for evolving rhabdomyolysis). Cornerstones of care include restoration of fluid volume, avoidance of overly rapid decline in blood glucose, and replacement of electrolytes.

Zeitler P, Zeitler P, Haqq A, Rosenbloom A, Glaser N; Drugs and Therapeutics Committee of the Lawson Wilkins Pediatric Endocrine Society: Hyperglycemic hyperosmolar syndrome in children: pathophysiologic considerations and suggested guidelines for treatment. J Pediatr 2011 Jan;158(1):9–14 [PMID: 21035820].

C. Hypoglycemia

Hypoglycemia (or "insulin reaction") is the most common acute complication of T1D and is defined as a blood glucose level below 60 mg/dL (3.3 mmol/L). For preschool children, values below 70 mg/dL (3.9 mmol/L) should be cause for concern. The common symptoms of hypoglycemia are hunger, weakness, shakiness, sweating, drowsiness (at an unusual time), headache, and behavioral changes. If low blood glucose is not treated immediately with simple sugar, hypoglycemia may result in loss of consciousness and seizures; brain damage or death can occur with prolonged hypoglycemia. Severe hypoglycemic episodes (loss of consciousness or seizure) occur at a rate of about 3–7 events per 100 patient-years.

Children learn to recognize hypoglycemia at different ages but can often report "feeling funny" as young as age 4–5 years. School personnel, sports coaches, and babysitters must be trained to recognize and treat hypoglycemia. Consistency in daily routine, correct insulin dosage, regular blood glucose monitoring, controlled snacking, compliance of patients and parents, and good education are all important in preventing severe hypoglycemia. In addition, insulin should not be injected prior to getting into a hot tub, bath, or shower as the heat may cause more rapid insulin uptake. The use of insulin analogs as well as technologies including insulin pumps, CGM and "artificial pancreas" systems that use CGM input to control insulin output (see Treatment section) have all helped to reduce the occurrence of hypoglycemia.

The treatment of mild hypoglycemia involves giving 4 oz of juice; a sugar-containing soda drink, or milk; and waiting 10–15 minutes. If the blood glucose level is still below 60 mg/dL (3.3 mmol/L), the liquids are repeated. If the glucose level is above 60 mg/dL, solid foods are given. Moderate hypoglycemia, in which the person is conscious but incoherent, can be treated by squeezing one-half tube of concentrated glucose (eg, Insta-Glucose or cake frosting) between the gums and lips and stroking the throat to encourage swallowing.

Families are advised to have glucagon in the home and in their travel pack to treat severe hypoglycemia by giving subcutaneous or intramuscular injections of 0.3 mL (30 units in an insulin syringe) for children younger than 5 years; 0.5 mL (50 units) to those older than 5 years; and 1 mL (100 units) to those heavier than 100 lb. Smaller doses of glucagon (2 units + number of units equal to the age of the child, eg, 2 + 10 = 12 units in a 10-year-old) up to a maximum of 15 units can be used to prevent severe hypoglycemia during nondiabetic illness (gastroenteritis, respiratory infections). Nasal glucagon, when available, is as effective as injected glucagon for resolution of hypoglycemia.

Some patients fail to recognize the symptoms of low blood glucose (hypoglycemic unawareness), often after a history of at least 10 years of diabetes or frequent hypoglycemic events. For these individuals, use of CGM with hypoglycemia alarms or artificial pancreas technologies should be considered.

D. Long-Term Complications

Table 35–5 summarizes routine tests helpful in assessing for and preventing long-term complications.

1. Hypertension—Elevated blood pressure is prevalent among children with diabetes and strongly predicts

Table 35–5. Checklist of good diabetes management in children and adolescents.

	Evaluation	Frequency	Assessment/Measure
Glycemic management	Hemoglobin A$_{1C}$ Glucose	Quarterly	See Table 35–4
	Glucose (glucometer or CGM download)	Quarterly	See Table 35–4
Cardiovascular risk	Blood pressure	Quarterly *If high-normal or hypertension, confirm on 3 separate days.	Target: < 95th percentile for age, sex, and height High-normal*: ≥ 90th percentile for age, sex, and height Hypertension*: ≥ 95th percentile for age, sex, and height
	Blood lipid panel (nonfasting)	T1D: Soon after diagnosis in those ≥ 2 y. If LDL ≤ 100 mg/dL, screen again at 9–11 years of age and every 3 years thereafter. T2D: At diagnosis; if normal repeat q5y	LDL (target: < 100 mg/dL [2.6 mmol/L]) HDL (target: > 35 mg/dL [0.91 mmol/L]) Triglycerides (target: < 150 mg/dL [1.7 mmol/L])
	Smoking	Screen at diagnosis and follow-up visits	
Microvascular complications	Nephropathy (Urine microalbumin)	T1D: Annually after 2–5 y of diabetes (Starting age > 10 y or puberty if earlier) T2D: At onset, then annually	ACR (nl: < 30 mg/g) First AM urine sample preferred Need 2 of 3 samples abnormal to confirm microalbuminuria
	Retinopathy	T1D: Annually after 2–5 y of diabetes (age ≥ 10 y) T2D: At onset, then annually	Ophthalmology referral for fundal photography or dilated ophthalmoscopy
	Neuropathy	T1D: Annually after 2–5 y of diabetes (age ≥ 10 y or puberty if earlier) T2D: At onset, then annually	Comprehensive foot exam: sensation, pulses, vibration and reflexes
Psychosocial	Psychosocial comorbidities	At diagnosis and routinely thereafter	Assess for depression, anxiety, poor diabetes adjustment, and disordered eating
Autoimmune conditions (for T1D only)	Autoimmune thyroid disease	Screen at diagnosis (TSH, TPO, and antithyroglobulin antibodies) Recheck TSH every 1–2 y; check sooner if suggestive signs or symptoms, thyromegaly, growth concerns or unexplained glycemic variability	TSH (nl: 0.5–5.0 IU/mL) T$_4$ (nl: 4.5–10 mcg/dL) TPO Ab antithyroglobulin Ab TRAb (TSI)
	Celiac disease	Screen at diagnosis (tTG IgA, total IgA) Repeat within 2 y after diagnosis and again after 5 y Consider more frequent screening if first-degree relative with celiac disease or suggestive signs/symptoms	tTG IgA Ab If IgA deficiency: tTG IgG or IgG-deamidated gliadin peptide Ab
	Addison disease	Quarterly: Assess for signs and symptoms of adrenal insufficiency. Consider lab evaluation if concerns.	21-hydroxylase Ab, ACTH, fasting AM cortisol, electrolytes, plasma renin
Obesity-associated comorbidities (typically T2D)	Nonalcoholic fatty liver disease	At diagnosis of T2D and annually thereafter.	AST ALT
	Sleep apnea	At diagnosis of T2D and routinely thereafter.	Assess for snoring, apnea, poor sleep quality, daytime sleepiness, morning headaches, and enuresis
	PCOS	For females at diagnosis of T2D and routinely thereafter	Assess for menstrual irregularities and signs/symptoms of hyperandrogenism

Ab, antibody; ACR, albumin/creatinine ratio; ACTH, adrenocorticotropic hormone; ALT, alanine aminotransferase; AST, aspartate aminotransferase; CGM, continuous glucose monitor; HDL, high-density lipoprotein; IgA, immunoglobulin A; IgG, immunoglobulin G; LDL, low-density lipoprotein; nl, normal range; T$_4$, thyroxine; T1D, type 1 diabetes; T2D, type 2 diabetes; TPO, thyroid peroxidase autoantibodies; TSH, thyroid-stimulating hormone; tTG: tissue transglutaminase.

micro- and macrovascular complications. Blood pressure should be evaluated at each clinic visit. If hypertension or high-normal blood pressure is confirmed, nondiabetic causes should first be excluded (see Chapter 20). High-normal blood pressure may be first addressed with dietary modification and exercise aimed at weight control, if appropriate, for 3–6 months before consideration of pharmacologic intervention. For confirmed hypertension, angiotensin-converting enzyme inhibitors are the first-line agents; if not tolerated well, angiotensin II receptor blockers can be used. Goal of therapy is blood pressure consistently below the 90th percentile for age, sex, and height. (The Fourth Report on the Diagnosis, Evaluation, and Treatment of High Blood Pressure in Children and Adolescents https://www.nhlbi.nih.gov/files/docs/resources/heart/hbp_ped.pdf.)

2. Lipid abnormalities—Lipid profiles are generally favorable in children with T1D, but dyslipidemia is more common in children with T2D. Good glycemic control should be established in newly diagnosed patients prior to screening, but screening should not be delayed more than 1 year after diagnosis. Abnormal results from a random lipid panel should be confirmed with a fasting lipid panel. Initial therapy includes optimizing glycemic control, increasing physical activity, and decreasing the amount of saturated fat in the diet using a step 2 American Heart Association diet. If lifestyle changes and improved diabetes management fail after 6 months, statin therapy should be considered. Criteria for considering stating therapy in T1D are age more than 10 years with low-density lipoprotein (LDL) levels greater than 160 mg/dL (4.1 mmol/L) or those with LDL greater than 130 mg/dL (3.4 mmol/L) and one or more cardiovascular disease risk factors. Criterion for statin therapy in youth with T2D is persistent LDL greater than 130 mg/dL (3.4 mmol/L). The treatment goals are LDL less than 100 mg/dL (2.6 mmol/L). Statins are teratogenic; therefore, prevention of unplanned pregnancies is critically important in postpubertal girls.

For youth with T2D and hypertriglyceridemia (fasting triglycerides > 400 mg/dL [5.6 mmol/L] or nonfasting > 1000 mg/dL [11.3 mmol/L]), beyond lifestyle modifications and promotion of weight loss, some studies have shown efficacy of omega-3 fatty acid supplementation at a dose of 2–4 g per day.

3. Nephropathy—Rapid decline of the glomerular filtration rate (GFR) is the first clinical manifestation of diabetic kidney disease and may be reversible with diligent glycemic and blood pressure control. Microalbuminuria is an established risk factor, defined as urinary albumin excretion rate between 20 and 200 mcg/min or urinary albumin/creatinine ratio 2.5–25 mg/mmol in males and 3.5–25 mg/mmol in females or 30–300 mg/g (spot urine). The diagnosis of microalbuminuria requires documentation of two out of three abnormal samples over a period of 3–6 months. Once persistent microalbuminuria is confirmed, nondiabetic causes of

renal disease should be excluded. Following this evaluation, treatment with an ACE inhibitor should be started, even if the blood pressure is normal. Patients should be counseled about the importance of glycemic and blood pressure control and smoking cessation, if applicable. Patients with T2D should have microalbuminuria assessed soon after diagnosis and then annually.

4. Retinopathy—While rare in children, proliferative retinopathy does occur in adolescents with long duration and poor control of diabetes. Laser treatment to coagulate proliferating capillaries prevents bleeding and leakage of blood into the vitreous fluid or behind the retina. This treatment preserves useful vision.

5. Neuropathy—Annual comprehensive foot examination should include inspection; palpation of dorsalis pedis and posterior tibial pulses; evaluation of patellar and Achilles reflexes; and determination of proprioception, vibration, and monofilament sensation.

ASSOCIATED AUTOIMMUNE DISEASES IN TYPE 1 DIABETES

Table 35–5 summarizes recommended screening for autoimmune diseases in T1D.

While Hashimoto thyroiditis is the most common autoimmune thyroid disorder in children with T1D, Graves disease can also occur. Thyroid peroxidase autoantibody (TPO) is usually the first test to become abnormal in the autoimmune thyroiditis affecting up to 20% of individuals with T1D. If TPO is positive, screening with TSH is recommended every 6–12 months (for management of thyroid disease, see Chapter 34).

Transglutaminase autoantibodies offer a sensitive and specific screening test for celiac disease affecting up to 10% of children with T1D with the highest risk in those diagnosed with T1D before age 5. Risk of celiac disease is most strongly associated with the HLA-DR3-DQ2 haplotype. Signs and symptoms suggestive of celiac include poor growth or poor weight gain, abdominal pain, signs of malabsorption, frequent unexplained hypoglycemia, or deteriorating glycemic control. About one-half of celiac disease cases develop several years after diagnosis of T1D. Most of the biopsy-confirmed children are "asymptomatic," but report improved health status upon initiation of gluten-free diet. Untreated celiac disease may lead to severe hypoglycemia, increased bone turnover, and decreased bone mineralization, among many other long-term complications (see Chapter 21).

The 21-hydroxylase autoantibody, a marker of increased risk of Addison disease, is present in approximately 1% of patients with T1D, although Addison disease develops (usually slowly) in only about one-third of these antibody-positive individuals (see Chapter 34 for further information).

Other less common autoimmune disorders include rheumatoid arthritis, lupus, psoriasis, scleroderma, vitiligo, dermatomyositis, autoimmune hepatitis, autoimmune gastritis, pernicious anemia, and myasthenia gravis.

ASSOCIATED CONDITIONS WITH TYPE 2 DIABETES

At the time of diagnosis of T2D, comorbidities such as hypertension, dyslipidemia, nephropathy, and retinopathy may already be present and therefore should be evaluated within initial visits followed by ongoing screening (see Table 35–5). As T2D in youth frequently occurs in the setting of obesity, associated comorbidities should be assessed including hepatic steatosis, sleep apnea, and orthopedic complications (see Chapters 4 and 11 for discussion). In female adolescents with T2D, assessment for polycystic ovary syndrome (PCOS) should also be considered (see Chapter 4).

Nadeau KJ et al: Youth-Onset Type 2 Diabetes Consensus Report: current status, challenges, and priorities. Diabetes Care 2016 Sep 1;39(9):1635–1642 [PMID: 27486237].

Zeitler P, Haqq A, Rosenbloom A, Glaser N; Drugs and Therapeutics Committee of the Lawson Wilkins Pediatric Endocrine Society: Hyperglycemic hyperosmolar syndrome in children: pathophysiological considerations and suggested guidelines for treatment. J Pediatr 2011 Jan;158(1):9–14, 14.e–2 [PMID: 21035820].

▶ Prognosis

The long-term prognosis of children diagnosed with T1D has improved significantly over the past 20 years, primarily due to better control of blood glucose and blood pressure. While life expectancy is now only slightly shorter in these patients compared to the general population, the risk of cardiovascular disease in later adulthood is still 4–10 times higher, especially in women with diabetes. Observation of teenagers and young adults who had been diagnosed with diabetes during childhood or adolescence showed that youth with T2D had a significantly higher prevalence of complications compared to those with T1D.

Modern diabetes care generally leads to excellent health outcomes. Tremendous progress in biotechnology—insulin analogs, insulin pumps, continuous glucose sensing, as well as the artificial pancreas—has reduced risk acute and long-term complications. However, comprehensive and continuing education of patients and their families remains the foundation of a healthy and quality life with diabetes.

REFERENCES

Understanding Diabetes and by H. Peter Chase et al: https://www.childrensdiabetesfoundation.org/books/.

Understanding Insulin Pumps, Continuous Glucose Monitors and the Artificial Pancreas by H. Peter Chase et al: https://www.childrensdiabetesfoundation.org/books/.

Inborn Errors of Metabolism

Janet A. Thomas, MD

Johan L. K. Van Hove, MD, PhD, MBA

Austin A. Larson, MD

Peter R. Baker II, MD

INTRODUCTION

Disorders in which single-gene defects cause clinically significant blocks in metabolic pathways are called *inborn errors of metabolism*. Once considered rare, the number of recognized inborn errors has increased dramatically, and they are now recognized to affect 1:1500 children. Many of these disorders can be treated effectively. Even when treatment is not available, correct diagnosis permits parents to make informed decisions about future offspring.

Pathology in metabolic disorders usually results from accumulation of enzyme substrate behind a metabolic block, or from deficiency of a reaction product. In some cases, the accumulated enzyme substrate is diffusible and has adverse effects on distant organs; in other cases, as in lysosomal storage diseases, the substrate primarily accumulates locally. The clinical manifestations of inborn errors vary widely with both mild and severe forms of virtually every disorder. Phenotypes vary from classic to more rare clinical presentations based on residual enzyme activity, which is in large part determined by specific mutations in a common gene.

A first treatment strategy is to enhance the reduced enzyme activity. Gene replacement is a long-term goal. Previous problems with gene delivery to target organs and control of gene action made this clinically unavailable; however, numerous clinical research trials are now occurring and offer hope for success. Enzyme-replacement therapies using intravenously, intrathecally, or intraventricularly administered recombinant enzymes have been developed as effective strategies in many lysosomal storage disorders and more continue to be developed. Subcutaneous enzyme replacement therapy is also under development. Enzyme substitution therapy via subcutaneous injection with a modified bacterial enzyme is also now available for at least one disorder. Organ transplantation (liver, kidney, heart, or bone marrow) can provide a source of enzyme for some conditions. Pharmacologic doses of a cofactor such as a vitamin can

sometimes be effective in restoring enzyme activity. Residual activity can be increased by pharmacologically promoting transcription (transcriptional upregulation) or by stabilizing the protein product through therapy with chaperones. Alternatively, some strategies are designed to cope with the consequences of enzyme deficiency. Strategies used to avoid substrate accumulation include restriction of precursor in the diet (eg, low-phenylalanine diet for phenylketonuria), avoidance of catabolism (fasting or vomiting illnesses), inhibition of an enzyme in the synthesis of the precursor (eg, the NTBC enzyme in tyrosinemia type I) (see section Hereditary Tyrosinemia), or removal of accumulated substrate pharmacologically (eg, glycine therapy for isovaleric acidemia) or by dialysis. An inadequately produced metabolite can also be supplemented (eg, glucose administration for glycogen storage disease type I).

Inborn errors can manifest at any age, affect any organ system, and mimic many common pediatric problems. This chapter focuses on when to consider a metabolic disorder in the differential diagnosis of common pediatric problems. A few of the more important disorders are then discussed in detail.

DIAGNOSIS

SUSPECTING INBORN ERRORS

Inborn errors must be considered in the differential diagnosis of critically ill newborns, children with seizures, neurodegeneration, recurrent vomiting, Reye-like syndrome, parenchymal liver disease, cardiomyopathy, rhabdomyolysis, renal insufficiency, unexplained metabolic acidosis, hyperammonemia, and hypoglycemia. Intellectual disability, developmental delay, and failure to thrive are often present but have little specificity. Inborn errors should be suspected when (1) degree of illness appears out of proportion to history, (2) symptoms accompany changes in diet, (3) the child's development regresses, (4) the child shows specific food preferences or aversions, or (5) the family has a history of parental consanguinity or problems suggestive of inborn error such as intellectual disability or unexplained deaths in first- and second-degree relatives.

Physical findings associated with inborn errors include alopecia or abnormal hair, retinal cherry-red spot or retinitis pigmentosa, optic atrophy, cataracts or corneal opacity, hepatomegaly or splenomegaly, coarse features, skeletal changes (including gibbus), neurologic regression, progressive changes in white matter, and intermittent or progressive ataxia or dystonia. Other features that may be important in the context of a suspicious history include failure to thrive, microcephaly, rash, jaundice, hypotonia, and hypertonia. Finally, more common clinical presentations that appear to be nonaccidental trauma or poison ingestion may actually be inborn errors such as glutaric acidemia type 1 or methylmalonic acidemia, respectively.

LABORATORY STUDIES

Laboratory studies are almost always needed for the diagnosis of inborn errors. Serum electrolytes and pH should be used to estimate anion gap and acid-base status. Urine ketones and blood glucose values are readily available at the bedside. Serum lactate, pyruvate, and ammonia levels are available in most hospitals, but care is needed in obtaining samples appropriately. Amino acid, acylcarnitine, and organic acid studies must be performed at specialized facilities to ensure accurate analysis and interpretation. An increasing number of inborn errors are diagnosed with DNA sequencing, but interpretation of private mutations, that is, mutations only seen in a single family, can be problematic. Knowing the causative mutation in the family allows prenatal diagnosis to be done by molecular analysis. This can be done on any material that contains fetal DNA such as chorionic villi, amniotic cells, or fetal blood obtained through umbilical cord blood sampling. Large-scale next-generation sequencing such as exome or genome sequencing has been very useful in identifying disorders with nonspecific symptoms that are not readily recognized by routine metabolite screening. Specific metabolite or enzyme assays are used for confirmation.

The physician should know what conditions a test can detect and when it can detect them. For example, urine organic acids may be normal in patients with medium-chain acyl-CoA dehydrogenase deficiency or biotinidase deficiency; glycine may be elevated only in cerebrospinal fluid (CSF) in patients with nonketotic hyperglycinemia. A result that is normal in one physiologic state may be abnormal in another. For instance, ketone production (identified easily in urine) in a child who is hypoglycemic is expected. The absence of ketones in such a child would suggest a defect in fatty acid oxidation. Conversely, a newborn does not naturally have the capacity to produce ketones. Neonatal ketosis suggests an organic acidemia.

Samples used to diagnose metabolic disease may be obtained at autopsy. Samples must be obtained in a timely fashion and may be analyzed directly or stored frozen until a particular analysis is justified by the results of postmortem examination, new clinical information, or developments in the field. Studies of other family members may help establish the diagnosis of a deceased patient. It may be possible to demonstrate that parents are heterozygous carriers of a specific disorder or that a sibling has the condition.

COMMON CLINICAL SITUATIONS

1. Intellectual Disability

Some inborn errors can cause intellectual disability without other distinguishing characteristics. Measurements of plasma amino acids, urine organic acids, and serum uric acid should be obtained in every patient with nonspecific intellectual disability. Urine screens for mucopolysaccharides and succinylpurines and serum testing for carbohydrate-deficient glycoproteins are useful because these disorders do not always have specific physical findings. Absent speech can point to disorders of creatine metabolism and transport. Abnormalities of the brain detected by magnetic resonance imaging (MRI) can suggest specific groups of disorders (eg, cortical migrational abnormalities in peroxisomal biogenesis disorders).

2. Acute Presentation in the Neonate

Acute metabolic disease in the neonate is most often a result of disorders of energy metabolism and may be clinically indistinguishable from sepsis. Prominent symptoms include poor feeding, vomiting, altered mental status or muscle tone, jitteriness, seizures, and jaundice. Acidosis, alkalosis, or altered mental status out of proportion to systemic symptoms should increase suspicion of a metabolic disorder. Laboratory measurements should include electrolytes, ammonia, lactate, glucose, blood pH, urine ketones, and urine carbohydrate analysis. Amino acids in CSF should be measured if nonketotic hyperglycinemia is suspected. Plasma and urine amino acid, urine organic acid, and serum acylcarnitine analysis should be performed urgently. Neonatal cardiomyopathy or ventricular arrhythmias should be investigated with serum acylcarnitine analysis and carnitine levels.

3. Vomiting & Encephalopathy in the Infant or Older Child

Electrolytes, ammonia, glucose, urine pH, urine carbohydrate analysis, and urine ketones should be measured in all patients with vomiting and encephalopathy before any treatment affects the results. Samples for plasma amino acids, serum acylcarnitine profile, and urine organic acid analysis should be obtained early. In the presentation of a Reye-like syndrome (ie, vomiting, encephalopathy, and hepatomegaly), amino acids, acylcarnitines, carnitine levels, and organic acids should be assessed immediately. Hypoglycemia with inappropriately low urine or quantitative serum ketones suggests the diagnosis of fatty acid oxidation or ketogenesis defects.

4. Hypoglycemia

Duration of fasting, presence or absence of hepatomegaly, and Kussmaul breathing provide clues to the differential diagnosis of hypoglycemia. Serum insulin, cortisol, and growth hormone should be obtained on presentation. Urine ketones, urine organic acids, plasma lactate, serum acylcarnitine profile, carnitine levels, ammonia, triglycerides, and uric acid should be measured. Ketone body production is usually not efficient in the neonate, and ketonuria in a hypoglycemic or acidotic neonate suggests an organic acidemia. In the older child, inappropriately low urine ketone levels suggest an inborn error of fatty acid oxidation. Assessment of ketone generation requires simultaneous measurements of quantitative serum 3-hydroxybutyrate, acetoacetate, and free fatty acids in relation to a sufficient duration of fasting and age. Metabolites obtained during the acute episode can be very helpful and avoid the need for a formal fasting test.

5. Hyperammonemia

Symptoms of hyperammonemia may appear and progress rapidly or insidiously. Decreased appetite, irritability, and behavioral changes appear first with vomiting, ataxia, lethargy, seizures, and coma appearing as ammonia levels increase. Tachypnea inducing respiratory alkalosis due to a direct effect on respiratory drive is characteristic. Respiratory alkalosis is usually present in urea cycle defects and transient hyperammonemia of the newborn, while acidosis is characteristic of hyperammonemia due to organic acidemias. Physical examination cannot exclude the presence of hyperammonemia, and serum ammonia should be measured whenever hyperammonemia is possible. Severe hyperammonemia may be due to urea cycle disorders, organic acidemias, or fatty acid oxidation disorders (such as carnitine-acylcarnitine translocase deficiency). Hyperammonemia may also present as transient hyperammonemia of the newborn in the premature infant, or as valproate toxicity in an older child. Genetic etiologies can usually be suggested by measuring quantitative plasma amino acids (eg, citrulline), plasma carnitine and acylcarnitine esters, and urine organic acids and orotic acid.

6. Acidosis

Inborn errors may cause chronic or acute acidosis at any age, with or without an increased anion gap. Inborn errors should be considered when acidosis occurs with recurrent vomiting or hyperammonemia and when acidosis is out of proportion to the clinical status. Acidosis due to an inborn error can be difficult to correct, while physiologic ketoacidosis in fasting is appropriate and corrects readily. The main causes of anion gap metabolic acidosis are lactic acidosis, ketoacidosis (including abnormal ketone body production such as in β-ketothiolase deficiency), methylmalonic aciduria or other organic acidurias, intoxication (ethanol, methanol, ethylene glycol, and salicylate), and uremia. Causes of non-anion gap metabolic acidosis include loss of base in diarrhea or renal tubular acidosis (isolated renal tubular acidosis or renal Fanconi syndrome). If renal bicarbonate loss is found, a distinction must be made between isolated renal tubular acidosis and a more generalized renal tubular disorder or renal Fanconi syndrome by testing for renal losses of phosphorus and amino acids. Inborn errors associated with renal tubular acidosis or renal Fanconi syndrome include cystinosis, tyrosinemia type I, carnitine palmitoyltransferase I, galactosemia, hereditary fructose intolerance (HFI), Lowe syndrome, lysinuric protein intolerance, and mitochondrial diseases. Tests indicated for anion gap metabolic acidosis include urine organic acids, serum lactate and pyruvate, serum 3-hydroxybutyrate and acetoacetate, and plasma amino acids, in addition to a toxicology screen.

▼ MANAGEMENT OF METABOLIC EMERGENCIES

Patients with severe acidosis, hypoglycemia, and hyperammonemia may be very ill; initially mild symptoms may worsen quickly, and coma and death may ensue within hours. With prompt and vigorous treatment, however, patients can recover completely, even from deep coma. All oral intakes should be stopped. Sufficient glucose should be given intravenously to avoid or minimize catabolism in a patient with a known inborn error who is at risk for crisis. Most conditions respond favorably to glucose administration, although a few (eg, primary lactic acidosis due to pyruvate dehydrogenase deficiency) do not. After exclusion of fatty acid oxidation disorders, immediate institution of intravenous fat emulsions (eg, intralipid) can provide crucial caloric input. Severe or increasing hyperammonemia should be treated pharmacologically or with dialysis (see section Disorders of the Urea Cycle), and severe acidosis should be treated with bicarbonate. More specific measures can be instituted when a diagnosis is established.

▼ NEWBORN SCREENING

Criteria for screening newborns for a disorder include its frequency, its consequences if untreated, the ability of therapy to mitigate consequences, the cost of testing, and the cost of treatment. With the availability of tandem mass spectrometry, newborn screening has expanded greatly to now include 35 core conditions and multiple secondary conditions screened by most states. In general, amino acidopathies, organic acidurias, and disorders of fatty acid oxidation are the disorders for which screening now occurs. Most states also screen for hypothyroidism, congenital adrenal hyperplasia, hemoglobinopathies, biotinidase deficiency, galactosemia, cystic fibrosis, and severe combined immune deficiency. Point-of-care screening occurs for hearing loss and congenital heart disease. An increasing number of states have begun screening for some of the lysosomal and peroxisomal disorders, and a few states have begun screening for spinal muscular atrophy (SMA). The Recommended Uniform Screening Panel (RUSP) from the Secretary of the Department of Health and Human Services provides guidance for the addition of new disorders to state newborn screening panels. Screening should occur for all infants between 24 and 72 hours of life or before hospital discharge.

Some screening tests measure a metabolite (eg, phenylalanine) that becomes abnormal with time and exposure to diet. In such instances, the disease cannot be detected reliably until intake of the substrate is established. Other tests measure enzyme activity and can be performed at any time (eg, biotinidase deficiency). Transfusions may cause false-negative results in this instance, and exposure of the sample to heat may cause false-positive results. False positives also result from prematurity, parenteral nutrition, hyperbilirubinemia, and liver or renal disease. Technologic advances have extended the power of newborn screening but have brought additional challenges. For example, although tandem mass spectrometry can detect many more disorders in the newborn period, consensus on diagnosis and treatment for some conditions is still under development.

Screening tests are not diagnostic, and diagnostic tests must be undertaken when an abnormal screening result is obtained. Because false-negative results occur, a normal newborn screening test does not rule out a condition, and some common disorders (eg, ornithine transcarbamylase deficiency) are not detectable in the screening tests performed in every state.

The appropriate response to an abnormal screening test depends on the condition in question and the predictive value of the test. For example, when screening for galactosemia by enzyme assay, complete absence of enzyme activity is highly predictive of classic galactosemia. Failure to treat may rapidly lead to death. In this case, treatment must be initiated immediately while diagnostic studies are pending. In phenylketonuria, however, a diet restricted in phenylalanine is harmful to the infant whose screening test is a false-positive, while diet therapy produces an excellent outcome in the truly affected infant if treatment is established within the first weeks of life. Therefore, treatment for phenylketonuria should only be instituted when the diagnosis is confirmed.

Physicians should review American College of Medical Genetics and Genomics recommendations, state laws, and regulations, and consult with their local metabolic center to arrive at appropriate strategies for each hospital and practice.

Agana M. Frueh J, Kamboj M, Patel DR, Kanungo S: Common metabolic disorder (inborn errors of metabolism) concerns in primary care pediatrics. Ann Transl Med 2018;6(24):469–476 [PMID: 30740400].

MacNeill EC, Walker CP: Inborn errors of metabolism in the emergency department (undiagnosed and management of the known). Emerg Med Clin North Am 2018;36(2):369–385 [PMID: 29622328].

Rajabi F: Updates in newborn screening. Pediatr Ann 2018;47(5): e187–e190 [PMID: 29750285].

Saudubray JM, Garcia-Cazorla A: Inborn errors of metabolism overview: pathophysiology, manifestations, evaluation, and management. Pediatr Clin North Am 2018;65(2):179–208 [PMID: 29502909].

▼ DISORDERS OF CARBOHYDRATE METABOLISM

GLYCOGEN STORAGE DISEASES

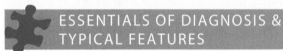

ESSENTIALS OF DIAGNOSIS & TYPICAL FEATURES

► Types 0, I, III, VI, and IX manifest with hypoglycemia in infants.

► Types II, V, and VII manifest with rhabdomyolysis or muscle weakness.

► Types IV and IX manifest with hepatic cirrhosis.

Glycogen is a highly branched polymer of glucose that is stored in the liver and muscle. Different enzyme defects affect its biosynthesis and degradation. The hepatic forms of the glycogenoses cause growth failure, hepatomegaly, and severe fasting hypoglycemia. They include glucose-6-phosphatase deficiency (type I; von Gierke disease), debrancher enzyme deficiency (type III), hepatic phosphorylase deficiency (type VI), and phosphorylase kinase deficiency (type IX), which normally regulates hepatic phosphorylase activity. Glycogen synthase deficiency (type 0) causes hypoglycemia, usually after about 12 hours of fasting, and can cause mild postprandial hyperglycemia and hyperlactatemia. There are two forms of glucose-6-phosphatase deficiency: In type Ia, the catalytic glucose-6-phosphatase is deficient, and there is pronounced lactic acidosis, hyperuricemia, and hyperlipidemia in addition to hypoglycemia, and in type Ib, the glucose-6-phosphate transporter is deficient and neutropenia also occurs. Glycogenosis type IV, brancher enzyme deficiency, usually presents with progressive liver cirrhosis, as do some rare forms of phosphorylase kinase deficiency. The gluconeogenesis disorder fructose-1,6-bisphosphatase deficiency presents with major lactic acidosis and delayed hypoglycemia on fasting.

The myopathic forms of glycogenosis affect skeletal muscle. Skeletal myopathy with weakness or rhabdomyolysis may be seen in muscle phosphorylase deficiency (type V), phosphofructokinase deficiency (type VII), and acid maltase deficiency (type II; Pompe disease). The infantile form of Pompe disease also has hypertrophic cardiomyopathy and macroglossia.

► Diagnosis

Initial tests include glucose, lactate, triglycerides, cholesterol, uric acid, transaminases, and creatine kinase. Functional testing includes responsiveness of blood glucose and lactate to fasting; for myopathic forms, an ischemic or nonischemic exercise test is helpful. Most glycogenoses can now be diagnosed by molecular analysis, including next-generation panels. Other diagnostic studies include enzyme assays of leukocytes, fibroblasts, liver, or muscle. Disorders diagnosable from analysis of red blood cells include deficiency of phosphorylase kinase (type IX) in half the cases. Pompe disease can usually be diagnosed by assaying acid maltase in a blood spot with confirmation in fibroblasts.

► Treatment

Treatment is designed to prevent hypoglycemia and avoid secondary metabolite accumulations such as elevated lactate in glycogenosis type I. In GSD1, the special diet must be strictly monitored with restriction of free sugars and measured amounts of uncooked cornstarch, which slowly releases glucose in the intestinal lumen. Good results have been reported following continuous nighttime carbohydrate feeding or uncooked cornstarch therapy. Late complications even after years of treatment include focal segmental glomerulosclerosis, hepatic adenoma or carcinoma, and gout. Enzyme-replacement therapy in Pompe disease corrects the cardiomyopathy, but the response in skeletal myopathy is variable with optimal results seen in patients treated early and who have mutations that allow formation of some residual protein which is detected as cross-reacting material on Western blotting. Immunomodulation is used for patients whose treatment response declines due to antibodies to the recombinant enzyme. In glycogen storage diseases with intact gluconeogenesis (GSD III, VI, IX), a high-protein diet improves glucose control and reduces late complications.

Kishnani PS et al: Diagnosis and management of glycogen storage disease type 1: a practice guideline of the American College of Medical Genetics and Genomics. Genet Med 2014;Nov 6. doi: 10.1038/gim.2014.128 [PMID: 25356975].

Patient and parent support group website with useful information for families: http://www.agsdus.org.
Tarnopolsky M et al: Pompe disease: diagnosis and management. Evidence-based guidelines from a Canadian expert panel. Can J Neurol Sci 2016;43(4):472–485 [PMID: 27055517].
Weinstein DA, Steuerwald U, De Souza CFM, Derks TGJ: Inborn errors of metabolism with hypoglycemia: glycogen storage diseases and inherited disorders of gluconeogenesis. Pediatr Clinic North Am 2018;65(2):247–265 [PMID: 29502912].

GALACTOSEMIA

ESSENTIALS OF DIAGNOSIS & TYPICAL FEATURES

► Severely deficient neonates present with vomiting, jaundice, and hepatomegaly on initiation of lactose-containing feedings.

► Renal Fanconi syndrome, cataracts of the ocular lens, hepatic cirrhosis, and sepsis occur in untreated children.

► Delayed, apraxic speech and ovarian failure occur frequently even with treatment. Developmental delay, tremor, and ataxia occur less frequently.

Classic galactosemia is caused by almost total deficiency of galactose-1-phosphate uridyltransferase. Accumulation of galactose-1-phosphate causes hepatic parenchymal disease and renal Fanconi syndrome. Onset of the severe disease is marked in the neonate by vomiting, jaundice (both direct and indirect), hepatomegaly, and rapid onset of liver insufficiency after initiation of milk feeding. Hepatic cirrhosis is progressive. Without treatment, death frequently occurs within 1 month, often from *Escherichia coli* sepsis. Cataracts usually develop within 2 months in untreated cases but usually reverse with treatment. With prompt institution of a galactose-free diet, the prognosis for survival without liver disease is excellent. Even when dietary restriction is instituted early, patients with galactosemia are at increased risk for speech and language deficits and ovarian failure. Some patients develop progressive intellectual disability, tremor, and ataxia. Milder variants of galactosemia with better prognosis exist.

The disorder is autosomal recessive with an incidence of approximately 1:40,000 live births.

► Diagnosis

In infants receiving foods containing galactose, laboratory findings include liver dysfunction, particularly PT prolongation, together with proteinuria and aminoaciduria. Galactose-1-phosphate is elevated in red blood cells.

When the diagnosis is suspected, galactose-1-phosphate uridyltransferase should be assayed in erythrocytes or *GALT* sequencing pursued. Blood transfusions give false-negative results and sample deterioration false-positive results.

Newborn screening by demonstrating enzyme deficiency in red cells or by demonstrating increased serum galactose allows timely institution of treatment. Some patients identified on newborn screening have a genotype that results in sufficient residual activity (Duarte allele) and treatment is not always required.

▶ Treatment

A galactose-free diet should be instituted as soon as the diagnosis is made or suspected. Compliance with the diet can be monitored by following galactose-1-phosphate levels in red blood cells or urinary galactitol levels. Appropriate diet management requires not only the exclusion of milk but also an understanding of the galactose content of foods. Avoidance of galactose should be lifelong with appropriate calcium and vitamin D replacement, intake of which tends to be low due to the restriction of dairy products. Dual-energy X-ray absorptiometry (DEXA) scans are recommended for monitoring of bone health. All children should be monitored for appropriate development with special attention to speech and language development, and girls should routinely be screened for hypergonadotropic hypogonadism during adolescence.

Carlock G et al: Developmental outcomes in Duarte galactosemia. Pediatrics 2019;143(1): e20182516 [PMID: 30593450].

Demirbas D, Brucker WJ, Berry GT: Inborn errors of metabolism with hepatopathy: metabolism defects of galactose, fructose, and tyrosine. Pediatr Clin North Am 2018;65(2):337–352 [PMID: 29502917].

Demirbas D, Coelho AI, Rubio-Gozalbo ME, Berry GT: Hereditary galactosemia. Metabolism 2018;83:188–196 [PMID: 29409891].

Patient and parent support group website with useful information for families: http://www.galactosemia.org.

Welling L et al: International clinical guideline for the management of classical galactosemia: diagnosis, treatment, and follow-up. J Inherit Metab Dis 2017;40:171–176 [PMID: 27858262].

HEREDITARY FRUCTOSE INTOLERANCE

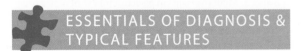

ESSENTIALS OF DIAGNOSIS & TYPICAL FEATURES

▶ Consider diagnosis in the setting of postprandial hypoglycemia and self-restriction of or aversion to sweets.

▶ Primary presentation outside of infancy includes poor growth and combined liver and kidney disease with lactic acidosis.

Hereditary fructose intolerance (HFI) is an autosomal recessive disorder in which deficient activity of fructose-1-phosphate aldolase (aldolase B) causes hypoglycemia and tissue accumulation of fructose-1-phosphate with fructose ingestion. This is genetically and clinically different from fructose malabsorption or "dietary fructose intolerance," which is similar in mechanism to lactose intolerance. Onset of HFI is typically in infancy when solid foods are introduced, but the disorder may go undiagnosed for years despite recurrent vomiting symptoms. Other abnormalities include failure to thrive, vomiting, jaundice, hepatomegaly, acute liver failure, proteinuria, renal Fanconi syndrome, and acute renal failure. Hypoglycemia directly follows fructose ingestion, and lactic acidosis, hypophosphatemia, and hyperuricemia may be significant. The untreated condition can progress to death from liver failure. Acute infusion of fructose may also result in death. Chronic liver disease, and more rarely chronic kidney disease, may occur even after treatment is implemented and strictly followed.

▶ Diagnosis

The diagnosis is suggested by finding fructosuria or an abnormal transferrin glycoform in the untreated patient. Although targeted testing of common mutations is available, diagnosis is best made by full sequencing of *ALDOB*. Alternatively, enzyme assay in liver tissue is available.

▶ Treatment

Treatment consists of strict dietary avoidance of fructose, sucrose, sorbitol, and related sugars. Vitamin supplementation is usually needed. Drugs and vitamins dispensed in a sucrose base should be avoided. Treatment monitoring can be done with transferrin glycoform analysis. If diet compliance is poor, physical growth retardation may occur. Growth should resume when more stringent dietary restrictions are reinstituted. If the disorder is recognized early, the prospects for normal development and life expectancy are good. As affected individuals grow up, intentional avoidance of fructose-containing foods, and resultantly good dentition, is common.

Baker P, II, Ayres L, Gaughan S, Weisfeld-Adams J: Hereditary fructose intolerance. In: Pagon RA et al (eds): *GeneReviews®*. Seattle, WA: University of Washington; 2015 [PMID: 26677512].

Patient and parent support group website with useful information for families: http://www.bu.edu/aldolase.

▼ DISORDERS OF ENERGY METABOLISM

The most common disorders of central mitochondrial energy metabolism are pyruvate dehydrogenase deficiency and deficiencies of respiratory chain components. Disorders of the Krebs cycle include deficiencies in fumarase, 2-ketoglutarate dehydrogenase, malate dehydrogenase, aconitase, and succinyl-CoA ligase. In many, but not in all, patients lactate is elevated in either blood or CSF. In pyruvate dehydrogenase deficiency, the lactate-pyruvate ratio is normal, whereas in respiratory chain disorders the ratio is often increased. Care must be taken to distinguish an elevated lactate level that is due to these conditions (called *primary lactic acidoses*) from elevated lactate that is a consequence of hypoxia, ischemia, or sampling problems. GDF15 is a recently described improved biomarker of mitochondrial diseases.

Patients with a defect in the pyruvate dehydrogenase complex often have agenesis of the corpus callosum or Leigh syndrome (lesions in the basal ganglia, dentate nucleus, and periaqueductal gray matter). They can have mild facial dysmorphism. Recurrent altered mental status, recurrent ataxia, and recurrent acidosis are typical of many disturbances of pyruvate metabolism. The most common genetic defect is in the X-linked $E_1\alpha$ component, with males carrying milder mutations and females carrying severe mutations leading to periventricular cystic brain lesions. The molecular heterogeneity is large as defects in each of the subunits, in the synthesis of the cofactors lipoate and thiamine, and in the transporters for thiamine and pyruvate are described.

The respiratory chain disorders are frequent (1:5000) and involve a heterogenous group of genetic defects that produce a variety of clinical syndromes (now > 50) of varying severity and presentation. The disorders can affect multiple organs. The following set of symptoms (not intended as a comprehensive listing) can indicate a respiratory chain disorder:

1. General: Failure to thrive
2. Brain: Progressive neurodegeneration, Leigh syndrome, myoclonic seizures, brain atrophy, movement disorders, cerebellar atrophy, and leukodystrophy
3. Eye: Optic neuropathy, retinitis pigmentosa, progressive external ophthalmoplegia, and cataracts
4. Ears: Sensorineural hearing loss
5. Muscle: Myopathy with decreased endurance or rhabdomyolysis
6. Kidney: Renal Fanconi syndrome, proteinuria (in coenzyme Q deficiency)
7. Endocrine: Diabetes mellitus and hypoparathyroidism
8. Intestinal: Pancreatic or liver insufficiency, or intestinal pseudoobstruction
9. Heart: Cardiomyopathy, conduction defects, and arrhythmias

Respiratory chain disorders are among the more common causes of progressive neurodevelopmental problems in children. Patients may present with nonspecific findings such as hypotonia, failure to thrive, or renal tubular acidosis, or with more specific features such as ophthalmoplegia or cardiomyopathy. Symptoms are often combined in recognizable clinical syndromes with ties to specific genetic causes (Table 36–1). Thirteen of the more than 100 genes that

Table 36–1. Clinical syndromes of mitochondrial diseases that present in childhood.

Leigh syndrome
Fatal infantile lactic acidosis and cardiomyopathy; isolated cardiomyopathy
Mitochondrial encephalomyopathy with lactic acidosis and stroke-like episodes (MELAS) (*MT-TL* m.3243A>G)
Myoclonic epilepsy and ragged red fibers (MERRF) (*MT-TK* m.8344A>G)
Progressive external ophthalmoplegia (PEO) or Kearns-Sayre -syndrome (mtDNA deletion, POLG, TWNKLE, RRM2B)
Alpers syndrome or hepatocerebral syndrome (*POLG, DGUOK*)
Leber hereditary optic neuropathy (LHON) (m.11778T>G, m.14484T>C, m.3460G>A, OPA1)
Myoneurogastrointestinal syndrome (MNGIE) (*TYMP*)
Neuropathy, ataxia, and retinitis pigmentosa (NARP) (*MT-ATP6/8* m.8993T>C and m.8993T>G)
Barth syndrome (*TAZ*)
Sensory ataxia, neuropathy, dysarthria, and ophthalmoparesis (SANDO) (*POLG, TWNKL*)
Myopathy, encephalomyopathy, reversible infantile myopathy
Leukoencephalopathy
Diabetes and deafness (*MT-TL* m.3243A>G)
Pearson syndrome (exocrine pancreatic and bone marrow failure) (mtDNA deletion)
Multisystem presentation

control activity of the respiratory chain are part of the mitochondrial genome. Therefore, inheritance of defects in the respiratory chain may be maternal as well as Mendelian. The genetic cause of mitochondrial disease is extremely heterogenous, and over 200 different genetic causes have already been described. Mitochondrial biology is a complex system involving the maintenance of mitochondrial DNA and its transcription and translation machinery, the assembly of the complexes including cofactors, the import and processing of nuclear encoded components and the maintenance of the mitochondrial membrane and structural environment, with defects described at every step (Figure 36–1). Some clinical presentations such as MNGIE have a specific genetic cause, but other clinical presentations such as Leigh disease and multisystem presentation have many causes.

Diagnosis

Pyruvate dehydrogenase deficiency is diagnosed by enzyme assay in leukocytes or fibroblasts. Confirmation can be obtained by molecular analysis. Diagnosis of respiratory chain disorders is based on a convergence of clinical, biochemical, morphologic, enzymatic, and molecular data. Classic pathologic features of mitochondrial disorders are the accumulation of mitochondria, which produces ragged red fibers in skeletal muscle biopsy, and abnormal mitochondrial shapes and inclusions inside mitochondria on electron

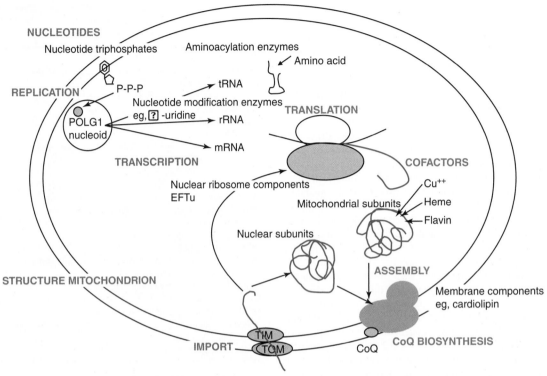

▲ **Figure 36–1.** Steps in mitochondrial biogenesis.

microscopy. However, these findings are only present in 5% of children.

Sometimes a clinical presentation is associated with a specific genetic cause (eg, Alpers syndrome caused by mutations in *POLG*), and directed genetic testing is possible. Most commonly, genetic testing starts with sequencing of mitochondrial DNA. Mitochondrial DNA abnormalities decrease in blood with age, and sometimes tissue samples (muscle) are needed. Next, large-scale genetic testing using either a large next-gen panel or whole exome sequencing is usually used.

Functional testing such as enzyme assays, nondenaturing blue native gel assays to analyze the assembly of complexes, and oxygen consumption-based tests in relevant tissues such as muscle and liver remain important for patients with genetic variants of unknown significance or for those where genetic testing did not yield a diagnosis. Tissue heterogeneity of expression of the functional defect may require the analysis of multiple tissues, and an overlap between normal and affected ranges makes interpretation often complex. Diagnostic criteria aid in appropriate clinical recognition. Advances in diagnostics now allow clinical diagnosis with a genetic cause to be ascertained in most cases. In some instances, the genetics and prognosis may be clear, but in other cases neither prognosis nor genetic risk can be predicted. Because of the high complexity of this group of

disorders, many patients require a high degree of expertise and multiple studies to arrive at a final diagnosis.

▶ **Treatment**

A consensus statement on the treatment of mitochondrial diseases from the Mitochondrial Medicine Society has been published. Patients should first avoid situations that further compromise mitochondrial capacity. Medications that impair mitochondrial translation (eg, certain antibiotics) or mitochondrial replication (eg, AZT/zidovudine) or exhibit mitochondrial toxicity (eg, valproate and propofol) should be avoided where possible. Catabolism due to prolonged fasting should be avoided by provision of sufficient calories. The best evidence for improvement in mitochondrial function is for a regimen of regular exercise (eg, 20 minutes of exercise daily). Certain conditions have specific treatments. A ketogenic diet is effective in pyruvate dehydrogenase deficiency for Leigh disease presentation. Coenzyme Q treatment is very effective in patients with primary coenzyme Q deficiency. A few conditions are responsive to riboflavin (*ACAD9*) or thiamin (*TPK, SLC19A3*). Stroke-like episodes in the MELAS syndrome should be treated with acute intravenous arginine, and either oral arginine or citrulline can be used for prevention of stroke-like episodes. Treatment with taurine improves the tRNA biochemistry in the m.3243A>G mutation and reduces stroke-like episodes. Liver transplantation has been important in the treatment of disorders with biochemical imbalance causing mitochondrial diseases such as ETHF1 and MNGIE. Other treatments are of theoretical value, with little data on efficacy. Antioxidants such as coenzyme Q are often used. Clinical trials of new, improved medications affecting mitochondrial function such as next-generation antioxidants, mitochondrial biogenesis upregulators, and molecular protectors offer new hope for defining proven therapeutic interventions.

Lake NJ, Compton AG, Rahman S, Thorburn DR: Leigh syndrome: one disorder, more than 75 monogenic causes. Ann Neurol 79(2):190–203 [PMID: 26506407].

Parikh S et al: Diagnosis and management of mitochondrial disease: a consensus statement from the Mitochondrial Medicine Society. Genet Med 2015;17(9):689–701 [PMID: 25503498].

Patient and parent support group website with useful information for families: http://www.umdf.org.

Wortmann SB, Koolen DA, Smeithink JA, van den Heuvel L, Rodenburg RJ: Whole exome sequencing of suspected mitochondrial patients in clinical practice. J Inherit Metab Dis 2015;38(3):437–443 [PMID: 25735936].

DISORDERS OF AMINO ACID METABOLISM

DISORDERS OF THE UREA CYCLE

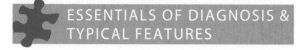

ESSENTIALS OF DIAGNOSIS & TYPICAL FEATURES

▶ Typical presentation is infantile encephalopathy; later onset presentations are common with cyclic vomiting or encephalopathy with illness or protein load.

▶ Diagnosis possibly suspected with the finding of hyperammonemia frequently with minimal other laboratory findings.

Ammonia is derived from the catabolism of amino acids and is converted to an amino group in urea by enzymes of the urea cycle. Patients with severe defects (often those enzymes early in the urea cycle such as ornithine transcarbamylase or argininosuccinic acid synthetase deficiency [citrullinemia]) usually present in infancy with severe hyperammonemia, vomiting, and encephalopathy, which is rapidly fatal. Patients with milder genetic defects may present with vomiting, encephalopathy, or liver failure after increased protein ingestion or infection. Although late defects such as deficiency in argininosuccinic acid lyase (argininosuccinic acidemia) or arginase may cause severe hyperammonemia in infancy, the usual clinical course is chronic with intellectual disability

without hyperammonemia. Ornithine transcarbamylase deficiency is X-linked; the others are autosomal recessive. Age at onset of symptoms varies with residual enzyme activity, protein intake, growth, and stressors such as infection. Even within a family, patients with ornithine transcarbamylase deficiency may differ by decades in the age of symptom onset. Many female carriers of ornithine transcarbamylase deficiency have protein intolerance. Some develop migraine-like symptoms after protein loads, and others develop potentially fatal episodes of vomiting and encephalopathy after protein ingestion, infections, or in the postpartum period. Trichorrhexis nodosa is common in patients with argininosuccinic aciduria. Arginase deficiency usually presents with spastic diplegia rather than hyperammonemia.

▶ Diagnosis

Blood ammonia should be measured in any acutely ill newborn in whom a cause is not obvious and any child with unexplained encephalopathy. In urea cycle defects, early hyperammonemia is associated with hyperventilation and respiratory alkalosis. Plasma citrulline is low or undetectable in carbamoyl phosphate synthetase and ornithine transcarbamylase deficiency, high in argininosuccinic acidemia, and very high in citrullinemia. Large amounts of argininosuccinic acid are found in the urine of patients with argininosuccinic acidemia. Urine orotic acid is increased in infants with ornithine transcarbamylase deficiency. Prenatal diagnosis is most commonly done by molecular methods. Other causes of severe neonatal hyperammonemia, which have a different prognosis and treatment, include liver failure; blood shunting to bypass the liver as seen in transient hyperammonemia of the neonate; and the metabolic disorders pyruvate carboxylase deficiency and mitochondrial carbonic anhydrase deficiency.

▶ Treatment

During treatment of acute hyperammonemic crisis, protein intake should be stopped, and glucose and lipids should be given to reduce endogenous protein breakdown from catabolism. Careful administration of essential amino acids facilitates protein anabolism. Arginine is given intravenously (except in arginase deficiency). It is an essential amino acid for patients with urea cycle defects and increases the excretion of waste nitrogen in citrullinemia and argininosuccinic acidemia. Sodium benzoate and phenylacetate are given intravenously to increase excretion of nitrogen as hippurate and phenylacetylglutamine. Additionally, hemodialysis or hemofiltration is indicated for severe or persistent hyperammonemia, as is usually the case in the newborn. Peritoneal dialysis and exchange transfusion are ineffective. Long-term treatment includes low-protein diet, oral administration of arginine or citrulline, and sodium benzoate or sodium phenylbutyrate (a prodrug of sodium phenylacetate). Symptomatic heterozygous female carriers of ornithine transcarbamylase deficiency should also receive such treatment. Liver transplantation may be curative and is indicated for patients with severe disorders. For arginase deficiency, enzyme replacement therapy is being developed to normalize arginine levels. Treatment with carbamylglutamate is effective for *N*-acetylglutamate synthase deficiency and, to some extent, mitochondrial carbonic anhydrase deficiency.

The outcome of urea cycle disorders depends on the genetic severity of the condition (residual activity) and the severity and prompt treatment of hyperammonemic episodes. Brain damage depends on the duration and the degree of elevation of ammonia and glutamine. Prolonged hyperammonemia causes permanent neurologic and intellectual impairments, with cortical atrophy and ventricular dilation seen on brain imaging. Rapid identification and treatment of the initial hyperammonemic episode is critical in improving outcome, and hyperammonemia constitutes a metabolic emergency.

Patient and parent support group website with useful information for families: http://www.nucdf.org.

Summar ML, Mew NA: Inborn errors of metabolism with hyperammonemia: urea cycle defects and related disorders. Pediatr Clin North Am 2018;65(2):231–246 [PMID: 29502911].

Urea Cycle Disorders Consortium: http://rarediseasesnetwork.epi.usf.edu/ucdc/about/index.htm.

PHENYLKETONURIA & THE HYPERPHENYLALANINEMIAS

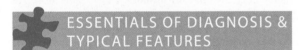

ESSENTIALS OF DIAGNOSIS & TYPICAL FEATURES

► Intellectual disability, hyperactivity, seizures, light complexion, and eczema characterize untreated patients.

► Newborn screening for elevated plasma phenylalanine identifies most infants.

► Disorders of cofactor metabolism also produce elevated plasma phenylalanine level.

► Early diagnosis and treatment with phenylalanine-restricted diet prevent intellectual disability.

Probably the best-known disorder of amino acid metabolism is the classic form of phenylketonuria caused by decreased activity of phenylalanine hydroxylase, the enzyme that converts phenylalanine to tyrosine. In classic phenylketonuria, there is little or no phenylalanine hydroxylase activity. In less severe hyperphenylalaninemia there may be significant residual activity. Rare variants can be due to deficiency of dihydropteridine reductase, defects in biopterin synthesis, or mutations in *DNAJC12*.

Phenylketonuria is an autosomal recessive trait, with an incidence in Caucasians of approximately 1:10,000 live births.

On a normal neonatal diet, affected patients develop elevated phenylalanine levels (hyperphenylalaninemia). Patients with untreated phenylketonuria exhibit severe intellectual disability, hyperactivity, seizures, a light complexion, and eczema.

Success in preventing severe intellectual disability in children with phenylketonuria by restricting phenylalanine starting in early infancy led to screening programs to detect the disease early. Because the outcome is best when treatment is begun in the first month of life, infants should be screened during the first few days. A second test is necessary when newborn screening is done before 24 hours of age, and should be completed by the second week of life.

► Diagnosis & Treatment

The diagnosis of phenylketonuria is based on finding elevated plasma phenylalanine and an elevated phenylalanine/tyrosine ratio in a child on a normal diet. The condition must be differentiated from other causes of hyperphenylalaninemia by examining pterins in urine and dihydropteridine reductase activity in blood. The diagnosis of hyperphenylalaninemia secondary to mutations in *DNAJC12* can only be made by molecular analysis. Determination of carrier status and prenatal diagnosis of phenylketonuria or pterin defects is possible using molecular methods.

A. Phenylalanine Hydroxylase Deficiency: Classic Phenylketonuria and Hyperphenylalaninemia

In phenylketonuria, plasma phenylalanine levels are persistently elevated above 1200 μM (20 mg/dL) on a regular diet, with normal or low plasma levels of tyrosine, and normal pterins. Poor phenylalanine tolerance persists throughout life. Treatment to decrease phenylalanine levels is always indicated. Hyperphenylalaninemia is diagnosed in infants whose plasma phenylalanine levels are usually 240–1200 μM (4–20 mg/dL), and pterins are normal while receiving a normal protein intake. Treatment to reduce phenylalanine levels is indicated if phenylalanine levels consistently exceed 360 μM (6 mg/dL). In contrast, in the rare case of transient hyperphenylalaninemia, plasma phenylalanine levels are elevated early but progressively decline toward normal. Dietary restriction is only temporary, if required at all.

Treatment of all forms of phenylketonuria is aimed at maintaining phenylalanine levels less than 360 μM (6 mg/dL). Treatment can consist of dietary restriction of phenylalanine, increasing enzyme activity with pharmacologic doses of R-tetrahydrobiopterin, or new methods to interfere with phenylalanine absorption or to breakdown phenylalanine.

Dietary restriction of phenylalanine intake to amounts that permit normal growth and development is the most common therapy and results in good outcome if instituted in the first weeks of life and carefully maintained. Metabolic formulas deficient in phenylalanine are available but must be supplemented with normal milk and other foods to supply enough phenylalanine to permit normal growth and development. Plasma phenylalanine concentrations must be monitored frequently while ensuring that growth, development, and nutrition are adequate. This monitoring is best done in experienced clinics. Children with classic phenylketonuria who receive treatment promptly after birth and achieve phenylalanine and tyrosine homeostasis will develop well physically and can be expected to have normal or near-normal intellectual development. Subtle changes in executive function may be apparent.

Phenylalanine restriction should continue throughout life. Patients who discontinued diet after treatment for several years have developed subtle changes in intellect and behavior, and risk neurologic damage. Counseling should be given during adolescence particularly to girls about the risk of maternal phenylketonuria (see as follows), and women's diets should be monitored closely prior to conception and throughout pregnancy. Late treatment may still be of benefit in reversing behaviors such as hyperactivity, irritability, and distractibility, but it does not reverse the intellectual disability.

Treatment with R-tetrahydrobiopterin results in improved phenylalanine tolerance in up to 50% of patients with a deficiency in phenylalanine hydroxylase. The best results and the most frequent responsiveness are seen in patients with hyperphenylalaninemia. Provision of high doses of large neutral amino acids results in a moderate reduction in phenylalanine and is used as an adjunctive treatment in some adults with phenylketonuria. Treatment with subcutaneous administration of pegylated phenylalanine ammonia lyase to decrease phenylalanine levels has recently been approved for adults with phenylketonuria.

B. Biopterin Defects: Dihydropteridine Reductase Deficiency and Defects in Biopterin Biosynthesis

In these patients, plasma phenylalanine levels vary. The pattern of pterin metabolites is abnormal. Clinical findings include myoclonus, tetraplegia, dystonia, oculogyric crises, and other movement disorders. Seizures and psychomotor regression occur even with diet therapy, probably because the enzyme defect also causes neuronal deficiency of serotonin and dopamine.

These deficiencies require treatment with levodopa, carbidopa, 5-hydroxytryptophan, and folinic acid. Tetrahydrobiopterin may be added for some biopterin synthesis defects.

C. Tyrosinemia of the Newborn

Plasma phenylalanine levels are lower than those associated with phenylketonuria and are accompanied by marked hypertyrosinemia. Tyrosinemia of the newborn usually occurs in premature infants and is due to immaturity of 4-hydroxyphenylpyruvic acid oxidase, resulting in increase in tyrosine and its precursor phenylalanine. The condition resolves spontaneously within 3 months, almost always without sequelae.

D. Maternal Phenylketonuria

Offspring of mothers with phenylketonuria may have transient hyperphenylalaninemia at birth. Elevated maternal phenylalanine during pregnancy causes intellectual disability, microcephaly, growth retardation, and often congenital heart disease or other malformations in the offspring. The risk to the fetus is lessened considerably by maternal phenylalanine restriction with maintenance of phenylalanine levels below 360 μM (6 mg/dL) throughout pregnancy and optimally started before conception.

E. Hyperphenylalaninemia due to *DNAJC12* Mutations

Mild, non–tetrahydrobiopterin-deficient hyperphenylalaninemia due to mutations in the gene *DNAJC12* is a recently reported autosomal recessive neurotransmitter disorder. DNAJC12 functions as a co-chaperone to prevent the misfolding of proteins and interacts with neuronal phenylalanine, tyrosine, and tryptophan hydroxylases. The clinical phenotype continues to be defined but appears heterogeneous and ranges from normal to intellectual disability, autism spectrum disorder, hyperactivity, dystonia, and parkinsonism. Laboratory studies typically reveal mild, BH4-responsive hyperphenylalaninemia (< 600 mmol/L) and low CSF homovanillic acid and 5-hydoxyindolacetic acid. Urine pterin profile and dihydropteridine reductase activity are normal. Some, but not all, patients may have an abnormal newborn screen suggestive of phenylketonuria. Therapy consists of sapropterin dihydrochloride with L-dopa/carbidopa, with or without 5-hydroxytryptophan, and should be started as early as possible for best outcome. Subjective improvement in cognitive and motor function has been noted even with later therapy. All children with mild hyperphenylalaninemia and global developmental delay warrant targeted testing for *DNAJC12* mutations.

Blau N, Martinez A, Hoffmann GF, Thony B: DNAJC12 deficiency: a new strategy in the diagnosis of hyperphenylalaninemia. Mol Genet Metab 2018;123(1):1–5 [PMID: 29174366].

Kure S, Shintaku H: Tetrahydrobiopterin-responsive phenylalanine hydroxylase deficiency. J Hum Genet 2019;64(2):67–71 [PMID: 30504912].

Levy HL, Sarkissian CN, Scriver CR: Phenylalanine ammonia lyase (PAL): from discovery to enzyme substitution therapy for phenylketonuria. Mol Genet Metab 2018;124(4):223–229 [PMID: 29941359].

Patient and parent support group websites with useful information for families: http://www.pkunews.org, www.pkunetwork.org, and www.npkua.org.

Prick BW, Hop WC, Duvekot JJ: Maternal phenylketonuria and hyperphenylalaninemia in pregnancy: pregnancy complications and neonatal sequelae in untreated and treated pregnancies. Am J Clin Nutr 2012;95(2):374 [PMID: 22205310].

Van Wegberg AMJ et al: The complete European guidelines on phenylketonuria: diagnosis and treatment. Orphanet J Rare Dis 2017;12(1):162 [PMID: 29025426].

HEREDITARY TYROSINEMIA

ESSENTIALS OF DIAGNOSIS & TYPICAL FEATURES

▶ Consider in a child presenting with liver disease with or without accompanying renal disease or bone disease.

▶ Elevated urinary succinylacetone is diagnostic of tyrosinemia, type 1.

Hereditary tyrosinemia type I is an autosomal recessive condition caused by deficiency of fumarylacetoacetase (*FAH*). It presents with acute or progressive hepatic parenchymal damage with elevated α-fetoprotein, renal tubular dysfunction with generalized aminoaciduria, hypophosphatemic rickets, or neuronopathic crises. Patients may also have impaired cognition. Tyrosine and methionine are increased in blood and tyrosine metabolites and δ-aminolevulinic acid in urine. The key diagnostic metabolite is elevated succinylacetone in blood or urine. Liver failure may be rapidly fatal in infancy or more chronic, with a high incidence of liver cell carcinoma in long-term survivors. Tyrosinemia type II (*TAT*) presents with corneal ulcers, palmar/plantar keratosis, neurologic dysfunction, and very high plasma tyrosine levels (> 600 μM). Patients with tyrosinemia type III (*HPD*) can also have developmental delay and ataxia.

▶ Diagnosis

Similar clinical and biochemical findings may occur in other liver diseases such as galactosemia and HFI. Increased succinylacetone occurs only in fumarylacetoacetase deficiency; an elevated level is diagnostic and is detected in newborn screening. Diagnosis is confirmed by mutation analysis or by enzyme assay in liver tissue. Prenatal diagnosis is possible. Tyrosinemia types II and III are diagnosed by gene sequencing.

▶ Treatment

A diet low in phenylalanine and tyrosine ameliorates liver disease. Pharmacologic therapy to inhibit the upstream enzyme 4-hydroxyphenylpyruvate dehydrogenase using 2-(2-nitro-4-trifluoromethylbenzoyl)-1,3-cyclohexanedione (NTBC) decreases the production of toxic metabolites, maleylacetoacetate and fumarylacetoacetate. It improves the liver disease and renal disease, prevents acute neuronopathic attacks, and greatly reduces the risk of hepatocellular carcinoma. Liver transplantation is effective therapy. Treatment

following diagnosis by newborn screen has an excellent outcome, but cognitive dysfunction is increasingly recognized. Tyrosinemia types II and III respond well to dietary tyrosine restriction.

Chinsky JM et al: Diagnosis and treatment of tyrosinemia type 1: a US and Canadian consensus group review and recommendations. Genet Med 2017;19(12): Epub 2017 Aug 3 [PMID: 28771246].

MAPLE SYRUP URINE DISEASE (BRANCHED-CHAIN KETOACIDURIA)

ESSENTIALS OF DIAGNOSIS & TYPICAL FEATURES

▶ Typical presentation is infantile encephalopathy.

▶ Diagnosis is suspected with elevated plasma branched-chain amino acids plus alloisoleucine.

Maple syrup urine disease is due to deficiency of the enzyme complex that catalyzes the oxidative decarboxylation of the branched-chain ketoacid derivatives of leucine, isoleucine, and valine. The complex is made up of three genetically distinct subunits. Accumulated ketoacids of leucine and isoleucine, which are converted to a compound sotolone, cause the characteristic sweet odor which may be detectable in cerumen as early as day of life 1. Only leucine and its corresponding ketoacid have been implicated in causing central nervous system (CNS) dysfunction. Many variants of this disorder have been described, including mild, intermittent, and thiamine-dependent forms. All are autosomal recessive.

Patients with classic maple syrup urine disease are normal at birth but shortly (day of life 2–3) develop irritability and feeding issues, and within 1 week progress to seizures and coma. Unless diagnosis is made and dietary restriction of branched-chain amino acids is begun, most will die in the first month of life. Nearly normal growth and development may be achieved if treatment is begun before 10 days of life, which is facilitated by newborn screening.

▶ Diagnosis

Amino acid analysis shows marked elevation of branched-chain amino acids including alloisoleucine, a diagnostic transamination product of the ketoacid of isoleucine. Urine organic acids demonstrate the characteristic ketoacids. The magnitude and consistency of metabolite changes are altered in mild and intermittent forms. A genetic testing panel that includes the multiple subunit genes can confirm the diagnosis and allows prenatal diagnosis by molecular analysis once the mutation in a family is known.

Treatment

Dietary leucine restriction and avoidance of catabolism are the cornerstones of treatment. Infant formulas deficient in branched-chain amino acids must be supplemented with normal foods to supply enough branched-chain amino acids to permit normal growth. Plasma levels of branched-chain amino acids must be monitored frequently to deal with changing protein requirements. Acute episodes of metabolic decompensation must be aggressively treated to prevent catabolism and negative nitrogen balance. Very high leucine levels require hemodialysis. Liver transplantation corrects the disorder, and the Maple Syrup Urine Disease affected liver may then safely be used for an unaffected recipient in a "domino" transplant because the recipient has enough whole body residual enzyme activity to metabolize branched-chain amino acids.

Burrage LC, Nagamani SC, Campeau PM, Lee BH: Branched-chain amino acid metabolism: from rare Mendelian diseases to more common disorders. Hum Mol Genet 2014;23:R1–R8 [PMID: 24651065].

Mohan N, Karkra S, Rastogi A, Vohra V, Soin AS: Living donor liver transplantation in maple syrup urine disease–case series and world's youngest domino liver donor and recipient. Pediatr Transplant 2016;20:395–400 [PMID: 26869348].

Patient and parent support group website with useful information for families: http://www.msud-support.org.

HOMOCYSTINURIA

ESSENTIALS OF DIAGNOSIS & TYPICAL FEATURES

▶ Consider in a child of any age with a marfanoid habitus, dislocated lenses, or thrombosis.

▶ Diagnosis is suggested by elevated total homocysteine and methionine.

▶ Newborn screening allows early diagnosis and treatment resulting in a normal outcome.

Homocystinuria is most often due to deficiency of cystathionine β-synthase (CBS) but may also be due to remethylation defects such as deficiency of methylenetetrahydrofolate reductase (MTHFR) or defects in the biosynthesis of methyl-cobalamin (vitamin B_{12}), the coenzyme for methionine synthase. Classic homocystinuria and most forms of inherited methyl-B_{12} deficiency are autosomal recessive. About 50% of patients with untreated CBS deficiency have intellectual disability, and most have arachnodactyly, osteoporosis, and a tendency to develop dislocated lenses and thromboembolic phenomena. Mild variants of CBS deficiency present with thromboembolic events.

Patients with severe remethylation defects usually exhibit failure to thrive and a variety of neurologic symptoms, including brain atrophy, microcephaly, hydrocephalus, and seizures in infancy and early childhood.

Diagnosis

Diagnosis is made by demonstrating elevated total serum homocysteine or by identifying homocystinuria in a patient who is not severely deficient in vitamin B_{12}. Plasma methionine levels are usually high in patients with CBS deficiency and often low in patients with inherited methyl-B_{12} deficiency. Cystathionine levels are low in CBS deficiency. In inherited methyl-B_{12} deficiency, megaloblastic anemia or hemolytic uremic syndrome may be present and an associated deficiency of adenosyl-B_{12} may cause methylmalonic aciduria. Mutation analysis or studies of cultured fibroblasts can make a specific diagnosis.

Treatment

About 50% of patients with CBS deficiency respond to large oral doses of pyridoxine. Pyridoxine nonresponders are treated with dietary methionine restriction and oral administration of betaine, which increases methylation of homocysteine to methionine and improves neurologic function. Early treatment prevents intellectual disability, lens dislocation, and thromboembolic manifestations, which justifies the screening of newborn infants. Large doses of vitamin B_{12} (eg, 1–5 mg hydroxocobalamin administered daily intramuscularly or subcutaneously) are indicated in some patients with defects in cobalamin metabolism. In remethylation defects methionine may be low, requiring oral supplementation.

Huemer M et al: Guidelines for diagnosis and management of the cobalamin-related remethylation disorders cblC, cblD, cblE, cblF, cblG, cblJ and MTHFR deficiency. J Inherit Metab Dis 2017;40(1):21–48 [PMID: 27905001].

Morris AA, et al: Guidelines for the diagnosis and management of cystathionine beta-synthase deficiency. J Inherit Metab Dis 2017;40(1):49–74 [PMID: 27778219].

NONKETOTIC HYPERGLYCINEMIA

ESSENTIALS OF DIAGNOSIS & TYPICAL FEATURES

▶ Severely affected newborns present with apnea, hypotonia, lethargy, myoclonic seizures, and hiccups, and develop severe mental and motor retardation.

▶ Mildly affected children have developmental delay, hyperactivity, mild chorea, and seizures.

▶ CSF glycine is elevated.

Inherited deficiency of protein subunits of the glycine cleavage enzyme causes classic nonketotic hyperglycinemia, and deficiency of the cofactor lipoate causes variant nonketotic hyperglycinemia. These defects and a defect in the glycine transporter *GLYT1* constitute the glycine encephalopathies. The pathophysiology of these disorders is poorly understood, but glycine accumulation in the brain may disturb neurotransmission of the glycinergic receptors and the *N*-methyl-D-aspartate type of glutamate receptor. The severe form of classic nonketotic hyperglycinemia presents in the newborn as hypotonia, lethargy proceeding to coma, myoclonic seizures, and hiccups, with a burst suppression pattern on EEG. Respiratory depression may require ventilator assistance in the first 2 weeks, followed by spontaneous recovery. Patients develop severe intellectual disability and recalcitrant seizures. Some patients have a small corpus callosum or may develop hydrocephalus. All patients have restricted diffusion on MRI in the already myelinated long tracts at birth. Patients with an attenuated form present with treatable seizures, varying developmental delay, and chorea, and one-half of these may present later in infancy or in childhood. All forms of the condition are autosomal recessive.

▶ Diagnosis

Nonketotic hyperglycinemia should be suspected in any neonate or infant with seizures, particularly those with burst suppression pattern on EEG. Diagnosis is confirmed by demonstrating a large increase in glycine in nonbloody CSF, with an abnormally high ratio of CSF glycine to plasma glycine. Combined sequencing and exonic copy number analysis of *GLDC* and *AMT* is diagnostic in more than 98% of cases. Defects in biosynthesis of the cofactors lipoate or pyridoxal phosphate also present with epileptic encephalopathy with elevated CSF glycine. Prenatal diagnosis is possible by molecular analysis.

▶ Treatment

In patients with mild disease, treatment with sodium benzoate (to normalize plasma glycine levels) and dextromethorphan or ketamine (to block *N*-methyl-D-aspartate type of glutamate receptors) controls seizures and improves neurodevelopmental outcome. Treatment of severely affected patients is generally unsuccessful. High-dose benzoate therapy can aid in seizure control but does not prevent severe intellectual disability. Ketogenic diet reduces glycine levels, but the impact on outcome is very limited.

Coughlin II C et al: The genetic basis of classic nonketotic hyperglycinemia due to mutations in *GLDC* and *AMT*. Genet Med 2017;19:104–111 [PMID: 27362913].

Patient and parent support group website with useful information for families: http://www.nkh-network.org.

Swanson MA et al: Biochemical and molecular predictors of prognosis in nonketotic hyperglycinemia. Ann Neurol 2015;78:606–618 [PMID: 26179960].

▼ ORGANIC ACIDEMIAS

ESSENTIALS OF DIAGNOSIS & TYPICAL FEATURES

▶ Consider in any child presenting with metabolic acidosis and ketosis in early infancy.

▶ Urine organic acid analysis is usually diagnostic.

Organic acidemias are disorders of amino and fatty acid metabolism in which nonamino organic acids accumulate in serum and urine. These conditions are usually diagnosed by examining organic acids in urine, a study usually performed only in specialized laboratories. Table 36–2 lists the clinical features of organic acidemias, together with the urine organic acid patterns typical of each. Additional details about some of the more important organic acidemias are provided in the sections that follow.

PROPIONIC & METHYLMALONIC ACIDEMIA (KETOTIC HYPERGLYCINEMIAS)

The oxidation of valine, odd chain length fatty acids, methionine, isoleucine, and threonine results in propionyl-CoA, which is converted into L-methylmalonyl-CoA by propionyl-CoA carboxylase, and then metabolized to succinyl-CoA via methylmalonyl-CoA mutase for entry into the tricarboxylic acid (Krebs) cycle. Gut bacteria also substantially contribute to propionyl-CoA production. Propionic acidemia is due to a defect in the biotin-containing enzyme propionyl-CoA carboxylase, and methylmalonic acidemia is due to a defect in methylmalonyl-CoA mutase, in either the mutase apoenzyme or in defects of synthesis of its cofactor, adenosyl-B_{12}. Some disorders of vitamin B_{12} metabolism affect only the synthesis of adenosyl-B_{12} (Cbl A or B), whereas in others (Cbl C, D, F, J, X), the synthesis of methyl-B_{12} is also blocked leading to elevated homocysteine in addition to methylmalonic acid (see Homocystinuria).

Clinical symptoms vary according to the location and severity of the enzyme block. Children with severe blocks present with acute, life-threatening metabolic ketoacidosis, hyperammonemia, coma, and bone marrow depression in early infancy or with metabolic acidosis, vomiting, and failure to thrive during the first few months of life. Most patients with severe disease have mild or moderate intellectual disability. Other complications include pancreatitis, basal ganglia stroke, cardiomyopathy (more in propionic), and interstitial nephritis and chronic kidney disease (more in methylmalonic).

All forms of propionic and methylmalonic acidemia are autosomal recessive traits (except for X-linked Cbl X) and can be diagnosed *in utero*.

Table 36–2. Clinical and laboratory features of organic acidemias.

Disorder	Enzyme Defect	Clinical and Laboratory Features
Isovaleric acidemia	Isovaleryl-CoA dehydrogenase	Acidosis and odor of sweaty feet in infancy, or growth retardation and episodes of vomiting, lethargy, and acidosis. Some forms mild. Persistent isovalerylglycine and intermittent 3-hydroxyisovaleric acid in urine.
3-Methylcrotonyl-CoA carboxylase deficiency	3-Methylcrotonyl-CoA carboxylase	Usually asymptomatic. Acidosis and feeding problems in infancy, or Reye-like episodes in older child. 3-Methylcrotonylglycine and 3-hydroxyisovaleric acid in urine.
Combined -carboxylase deficiency	Holocarboxylase synthetase	Hypotonia and lactic acidosis in infancy. 3-Hydroxyisovaleric acid in urine, often with small amounts of 3-hydroxypropionic and methylcitric acids. Often biotin responsive.
Biotinidase deficiency	Biotinidase	Alopecia, seborrheic rash, seizures, and ataxia in infancy or childhood. Urine organic acids as above. Always biotin responsive.
3-Hydroxy-3-methylglutaric acidemia	3-Hydroxy-3-methylglutaryl-CoA lyase	Hypoglycemia and acidosis in infancy; Reye-like episodes with nonketotic hypoglycemia or leukodystrophy in older children. 3-Hydroxy-3-methylglutaric, 3-methylglutaconic, and 3-hydroxyisovaleric acids in urine.
3-Ketothiolase deficiency	3-Ketothiolase	Episodes of vomiting, severe metabolic acidosis (hyperketosis), and encephalopathy. 2-Methyl-3-hydroxybutyric and 2-methylacetoacetic acids and tiglylglycine in urine, especially after isoleucine load.
Propionic acidemia	Propionyl-CoA carboxylase	Hyperammonemia and metabolic acidosis in infancy; ketotic hyperglycinemia syndrome later. 3-Hydroxypropionic and methylcitric acids in urine, with 3-hydroxy- and 3-ketovaleric acids during ketotic episodes.
Methylmalonic acidemia	Methylmalonyl-CoA mutase	Clinical features same as in propionic acidemia. Methylmalonic acid in urine, often with 3-hydroxypropionic and methylcitric acids.
	Defects in vitamin B_{12} biosynthesis	Clinical features same as above when adenosyl-B_{12} synthesis is decreased; early neurologic features prominent when accompanied by decreased synthesis of methyl-B_{12}. In latter instance, hypomethioninemia and homocystinuria accompany methylmalonic aciduria.
Pyroglutamic acidemia	Glutathione synthetase	Acidosis and hemolytic anemia in infancy; chronic acidosis later. Pyroglutamic acid in urine.
Glutaric acidemia type I	Glutaryl-CoA dehydrogenase	Progressive extrapyramidal movement disorder in childhood, with episodes of acidosis, vomiting, and encephalopathy. Risk window birth through 6 years. Glutaric acid and 3-hydroxyglutaric acid in serum and urine.
Glutaric acidemia type II	ETF:ubiquinone oxidoreductase (ETF dehydrogenase) and ETF	Hypoglycemia, acidosis, hyperammonemia, and odor of sweaty feet in infancy, often with polycystic and dysplastic kidneys. Severe neonatal onset is life limiting due to cardiac complications. Later onset may be with episodes of hypoketotic hypoglycemia, liver dysfunction, or slowly progressive skeletal myopathy. Glutaric, ethylmalonic, 3-hydroxyisovaleric, isovalerylglycine, and 2-hydroxyglutaric acids in urine, often with sarcosine in serum.
4-Hydroxybutyric acidemia	Succinic semialdehyde dehydrogenase	Seizures, ataxia, and developmental retardation. 4-Hydroxybutyric acid in urine.

CoA, coenzyme A; ETF, electron transfer flavoprotein.

Diagnosis

Laboratory findings consist of increases in urinary organic acids derived from propionyl-CoA or methylmalonic acid (see Table 36–2), and elevated propionylcarnitine (easily detected by the newborn screen). Hyperglycinemia and ketosis can be present, especially in acute illness. In some forms of abnormal vitamin B_{12} metabolism, homocysteine can be elevated. Confirmation is by molecular analysis and/or by assays in fibroblasts or lymphocytes (propionic only).

Treatment

Patients with enzyme blocks in B_{12} metabolism usually respond to pharmacologic doses of vitamin B_{12} (hydroxocobalamin) given subcutaneously or intramuscularly.

Vitamin B_{12} nonresponsive methylmalonic acidemia and propionic acidemia require amino acid restriction, strict prevention of catabolism, and carnitine supplementation to enhance propionylcarnitine excretion. Intermittent metronidazole can help reduce the propionate load from the gut. In the acute setting, hemodialysis or hemofiltration may be needed. Liver transplant, or combined liver-renal transplantation, is an option in severe forms of these disorders.

Critelli K et al: Liver transplantation for propionic acidemia and methylmalonic acidemia: perioperative management and clinical outcomes. Liver Transpl 2018;24(9):1260–1270 [PMID: 30080956].

Fraser JL, Venditti CP: Methylmalonic and propionic acidemias: clinical management update. Curr Opin Pediatr. 2016 Dec;28(6):682–693 [PMID: 27653704].

Manoli I, Sloan JL, Venditti CP: Isolated methylmalonic acidemia. In: Pagon RA et al (eds): *GeneReviews®*. Seattle, WA: University of Washington; 2016 [PMID: 20301409].

Patient and parent support group websites with useful information for families: www.oaanews.org and www.pafoundation.com.

Schillaci LP et al: Inborn errors of metabolism with acidosis: organic acidemias and defects of pyruvate and ketone body metabolism. Pediatr Clin North Am 2018;65(2):209–230 [PMID: 29502910].

CARBOXYLASE DEFICIENCY

Isolated pyruvate carboxylase deficiency presents with lactic acidosis and hyperammonemia in early infancy. Even if biochemically stabilized, the neurologic outcome is poor. Isolated 3-methylcrotonyl-CoA carboxylase deficiency is frequently recognized on newborn screening using acylcarnitine analysis. It is usually a benign condition that sometimes causes symptoms of acidosis and neurologic depression. All carboxylases require biotin as a cofactor. Holocarboxylase synthetase covalently binds biotin to the apocarboxylases for pyruvate, 3-methylcrotonyl-CoA, and propionyl-CoA; biotinidase releases biotin from these proteins and from proteins in the diet. Recessively inherited deficiency of either enzyme causes deficiency of all three carboxylases (ie, multiple carboxylase deficiency). Patients with holocarboxylase synthetase deficiency usually present as neonates with hypotonia, skin problems, and severe acidosis. Those with biotinidase deficiency present later with a syndrome of ataxia, seizures, seborrhea, and alopecia. Untreated patients can develop intellectual disability, hearing loss, and optic nerve atrophy. The sequelae of the disorder in many patients are preventable if treated early.

▶ Diagnosis

This diagnosis should be considered in patients with typical symptoms or in those with primary lactic acidosis. Urine organic acids are usually, but not always, abnormal (see Table 36–2). Diagnosis is made by enzyme assay of carboxylase activities in fibroblasts or leucocytes. Biotinidase can be assayed in serum, and holocarboxylase synthetase in leukocytes or fibroblasts. Nearly all children with the condition are now diagnosed with the newborn screen.

▶ Treatment

Isolated carboxylase deficiencies are often unresponsive to biotin supplementation. In biotinidase deficiency and holocarboxylase deficiencies, oral administration of pharmacologic doses of biotin reverses the organic aciduria within days and the clinical symptoms within days to weeks. Hearing loss can occur in patients with profound biotinidase deficiency despite treatment.

Donti TR, Blackburn PR, Atwal PS: Holocarboxylase synthetase deficiency pre and post newborn screening. Mol Genet Metab Rep 2016;7:40–44 [PMID: 27114915].

Wolf B: Biotinidase deficiency. In: Pagon RA et al (eds): *GeneReviews®*. Seattle, WA: University of Washington; 2016 [PMID: 20301497].

GLUTARIC ACIDEMIA TYPE I

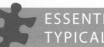

ESSENTIALS OF DIAGNOSIS & TYPICAL FEATURES

▶ Suspect in children with acute basal ganglia necrosis, macrocephaly with subdural bleeds, and acute or progressive dystonia.

▶ Presymptomatic diagnosis by newborn screening and treatment reduces the incidence of acute encephalopathic crises.

Glutaric acidemia type I occurs due to deficiency of glutaryl-CoA dehydrogenase. Patients have frontotemporal atrophy with enlarged sylvian fissures and macrocephaly. Sudden or chronic neuronal degeneration in the caudate and putamen causes an extrapyramidal movement disorder in childhood with dystonia and athetosis. Children with glutaric acidemia type I may present with retinal hemorrhages and intracranial bleeding, and may thus be falsely considered victims of child abuse. This is a disorder that primarily affects the central nervous system, and does not present with systemic acidosis, hypoglycemia, or primary end-organ damage elsewhere. Initial symptoms have only been reported in the first 6 years of life, which represents the vulnerable period. The condition is autosomal recessive and prenatal diagnosis is possible.

▶ Diagnosis

Glutaric acidemia type I should be suspected in patients with acute or progressive dystonia in the first 6 years of life.

MRI of the brain is highly suggestive. The diagnosis is supported by finding glutaric, 3-hydroxyglutaric acid, and glutarylcarnitine in urine or serum or by finding two mutations in the *GCDH* gene. Demonstration of deficiency of glutaryl-CoA dehydrogenase in fibroblasts can confirm the diagnosis. Prenatal diagnosis is by mutation analysis, enzyme assay, or quantitative metabolite analysis in amniotic fluid. This condition is detected on the newborn screen.

▶ Treatment

Strict prevention of catabolism in fasting or illness is critically important. Supplementation with carnitine and provision of a lysine and tryptophan restricted diet reduces the risk of degeneration of the basal ganglia. Benefit of arginine supplementation is controversial. Early diagnosis does not prevent neurologic disease in all patients, but it reduces the risk, warranting newborn screening. Despite treatment, affected individuals may have deficiencies in speech and fine motor skills. Neurologic symptoms, once present, do not typically resolve. Symptomatic treatment of severe dystonia is important for affected patients.

Boy N et al: Proposed recommendations for diagnosing and managing individuals with glutaric aciduria type I: second revision. J Inherit Metab Dis 2017;40:75–101 [PMID: 27853989].

Zielonka M, Braun K, Bengel A, Seitz A, Kolker S, Boy N: Severe acute subdural hemorrhage in a patient with glutaric aciduria type I after minor head trauma: a case report. J Child Neurol 2015;30:1065–1069 [PMID: 25038128].

▼ DISORDERS OF FATTY ACID OXIDATION & CARNITINE

FATTY ACID OXIDATION DISORDERS

ESSENTIALS OF DIAGNOSIS & TYPICAL FEATURES

▶ Obtain an acylcarnitine profile for children with hypoglycemia, rhabdomyolysis, hepatic encephalopathy, or cardiomyopathy to evaluate for a fatty acid oxidation defect.

▶ Early diagnosis and treatment can prevent morbidity and mortality in affected children, and avoidance of prolonged fasting is of paramount importance for long-term management.

Fatty acid oxidation disorders are disorders of the transport and catabolism of fatty acids in the mitochondria. In general, fatty acid oxidation disorders present with hypoketotic hypoglycemia and, depending on the specific disorder, may include mild hyperammonemia, hepatopathy,

encephalopathy, and/or skeletal myopathy or cardiomyopathy. The long-chain defects, which include very-long-chain acyl-CoA dehydrogenase (VLCAD), long-chain 3-hydroxyacyl-CoA dehydrogenase (LCHAD), carnitine palmitoyltransferase deficiency I and II, and carnitine-acylcarnitine translocase deficiency, cause episodic rhabdomyolysis, cardiomyopathy, and ventricular arrhythmias. Deficiencies of VLCAD and LCHAD cause hepatic encephalopathy (Reye-like) episodes. Sudden death in infancy is a less common presentation. Symptoms specific to LCHAD deficiency include progressive liver cirrhosis, peripheral neuropathy, and retinitis pigmentosa, and a higher than expected incidence of acute fatty liver of pregnancy and HELLP syndrome (hemolysis, elevated liver enzymes, and low platelets) during pregnancy in carrier mothers of affected infants.

Medium-chain acyl-CoA dehydrogenase (MCAD) deficiency is the most common fatty acid oxidation disorder, occurring in perhaps 1:9000 live births. Reye-like episodes, which historically have been largely caused by undiagnosed MCAD deficiency, may be fatal or cause residual neurologic damage. Episodes tend to become less frequent and severe with time. After the diagnosis is made and treatment instituted, morbidity decreases and mortality is avoided in MCAD deficiency.

Short-chain acyl-CoA dehydrogenase (SCAD) deficiency is characterized by the presence of ethylmalonic acid in the urine. Patients are generally asymptomatic; whether this deficiency is an actual clinical disease entity is increasingly being reconsidered. Glutaric acidemia type II (or multiple acyl-CoA dehydrogenase deficiency) results from defects in the flavin-mediated transfer of electrons from fatty acid oxidation and some amino acid oxidation into the respiratory chain. Some patients with glutaric acidemia type II have a clinical presentation resembling MCAD deficiency. Patients with a severe neonatal presentation may also have renal cystic disease, dysmorphic features, and profound cardiomyopathy. The least affected patients can present with late-onset myopathy and be riboflavin responsive. Some develop cardiomyopathy or leukodystrophy. Deficiency of the ketogenic enzymes 3-hydroxymethylglutaryl-CoA synthase and lyase present with hypoketotic hypoglycemia. These conditions are all autosomal recessive. Disorders of cytoplasmic fatty acid metabolism are being newly recognized. Deficiency of lipin 1, a cytoplasmic triglyceride lipase, causes severe episodes of rhabdomyolysis starting at a very early age.

▶ Diagnosis

All disorders of fatty acid oxidation have reduced ketogenesis in response to fasting. The analysis of acylcarnitine esters (via an acylcarnitine profile) is a first-line diagnostic test used in newborn screening because it reveals diagnostic metabolites regardless of clinical status. A typical pattern can be recognized for each disorder; for instance, MCAD deficiency is characterized by elevated octanoylcarnitine. Some disorders have elevated acylglycine esters which can be identified in urine organic acid analysis or on specific quantitative acyl-glycine analysis. Further confirmation can be obtained from targeted gene sequencing or analysis of fatty acid oxidation in fibroblasts; enzyme assays are only rarely available.

▶ Treatment

Management of all disorders of fatty acid oxidation involves prevention of hypoglycemia by avoiding prolonged fasting (> 8–12 hours). This includes vigorous treatment of fasting associated with illness with glucose. Because fatty acid oxidation can be compromised by associated carnitine deficiency, young patients with MCAD deficiency usually receive oral carnitine when carnitine levels are low. Restriction of dietary long-chain fats is not necessary in MCAD deficiency but is required for severe VLCAD and LCHAD deficiencies. Medium-chain triglycerides are contraindicated in MCAD deficiency but are a potential energy source for patients with severe VLCAD and LCHAD deficiencies or carnitine-acylcarnitine translocase deficiency. Other potential alternative fuel sources include protein and triheptanoin. Riboflavin may be beneficial in some patients with glutaric acidemia type II. Outcome in MCAD deficiency is excellent but is more guarded in patients with the other disorders.

Matern D, Rinaldo P: Medium-chain acyl-coenzyme A dehydrogenase deficiency. In: Pagon RA et al (eds): *GeneReviews®*. Seattle, WA: University of Washington; 2015 [PMID: 20301597].

Merritt JL 2nd et al: Fatty acid oxidation disorders. Ann Transl Med 2018 Dec;6(24):473 [PMID: 30740404].

Patient and parent support group website with useful information for families: http://www.fodsupport.org.

Wieser T: Carnitine palmitoyl transferase type 2 deficiency. In: Pagon RA et al (eds): *GeneReviews®*. Seattle, WA: University of Washington; 2019 [PMID: 20301431].

CARNITINE

ESSENTIALS OF DIAGNOSIS & TYPICAL FEATURES

▶ Primary carnitine deficiency manifests as cardiac disease including cardiomyopathy and sudden death, as hypo-ketotic hypoglycemia, or as exercise intolerance.

▶ Treatment of primary carnitine deficiency with carnitine improves outcome and prognosis.

▶ There are many causes of secondary carnitine deficiency.

Carnitine is an essential nutrient found in highest concentration in red meat. Its primary function is to transport long-chain fatty acids into mitochondria for oxidation. Primary carnitine uptake deficiency may manifest as hepatic encephalopathy (Reye-like syndrome), cardiomyopathy, or skeletal myopathy with hypotonia. These disorders are rare compared with secondary carnitine deficiency, which may be due to diet (vegan diet, intravenous alimentation, or keto-genic diet), renal losses, drug therapy (especially valproic acid), and other metabolic disorders (especially organic acidemias). The prognosis depends on the cause of the carnitine abnormality. Primary carnitine deficiency is one of the most treatable causes of dilated cardiomyopathy in children.

Free and esterified carnitine can be measured in blood. If carnitine insufficiency is suspected, the patient should be evaluated to rule out disorders that might cause secondary carnitine deficiency.

Oral or intravenous L-carnitine is used in carnitine deficiency or insufficiency in doses of 25–100 mg/kg/day or higher. Treatment is aimed at maintaining normal carnitine levels. Carnitine supplementation in patients with some disorders of fatty acid oxidation and organic acidurias may also augment excretion of accumulated metabolites, although supplementation may not prevent metabolic crises in such patients.

Longo N: Primary carnitine deficiency and newborn screening for disorders of the carnitine cycle. Ann Nutr Metab 2016;68 Suppl 3:5–9 [PMID: 27931018].

Longo N, Frigeni M, Pasquali M: Carnitine transport and fatty acid oxidation. Biochim Biophys Acta 2016;1863:2422–2435 [PMID: 26828774].

▼ PURINE METABOLISM DISORDERS

ESSENTIALS OF DIAGNOSIS & TYPICAL FEATURES

▶ Lesch-Nyhan syndrome is classically described in boys with spasticity, dystonia, and self-mutilating behaviors.

▶ Urinary uric acid to creatinine ratio or urine succinylpurines are useful screening tests.

Hypoxanthine-guanine phosphoribosyltransferase is an enzyme that recycles the purine bases hypoxanthine and guanine to inosine monophosphate and guanosine monophosphate, respectively. Hypoxanthine-guanine phosphoribosyltransferase deficiency (Lesch-Nyhan syndrome) is an X-linked recessive disorder. The complete deficiency is characterized by CNS dysfunction, purine wasting with compensatory increase in purine synthesis, and xanthine and hypoxanthine overproduction resulting in hyperuricemia and hyperuricosuria. Depending on the residual activity of the mutant enzyme, male hemizygous individuals may be severely disabled by choreoathetosis, spasticity, and compulsive, mutilating lip and finger biting, or they may have only gouty arthritis and urate ureterolithiasis. Adenylosuccinate lyase deficiency involves a defect in the synthesis of purines. Patients present with static intellectual disability, hypotonia, and seizures.

▶ Diagnosis

Diagnosis of Lesch-Nyhan syndrome is made by demonstrating an elevated uric acid:creatinine ratio in urine, followed by demonstration of enzyme deficiency in red blood cells or fibroblasts or by molecular analysis. Screening for adenylosuccinate lyase deficiency is by measurement of urine succinylpurines, with confirmation by further metabolite and molecular assays.

▶ Treatment

Hyperhydration and alkalinization are essential to prevent kidney stones and urate nephropathy. Allopurinol and probenecid may be given to reduce hyperuricemia and prevent gout but do not affect the neurologic status. Physical restraints are often more effective than neurologic medications for self-mutilation. No effective treatment exists for adenylosuccinate lyase deficiency.

Jurecka A, Zikanova M, Kmoch S, Tylki-Szymanska A: Adenylosuccinate lyase deficiency. J Inherit Metab Dis 2015;38:231–242 [PMID: 25112391].

Nyhan WL, O'Neill JP, Jinnah HA, Harris JC: Lesch-Nyhan syndrome. In: Pagon RA et al (eds): *GeneReviews®*. Seattle, WA: University of Washington; 2014 [PMID: 20301328].

Patient and parent support group websites with useful information for families: http://lndnet.ning.com and http://www.lesch-nyhan.org.

▼ LYSOSOMAL DISEASES

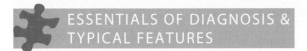

ESSENTIALS OF DIAGNOSIS & TYPICAL FEATURES

▶ Lysosomal storage disorders may present clinically with multisystem involvement including hepatosplenomegaly, cardiac disease, and skeletal features, with or without neurologic involvement.

▶ Brain imaging, skeletal survey, and urinary mucopolysaccharide or oligosaccharide analyses may be helpful in initial screening studies; most diagnoses are made by enzyme assay.

▶ Therapy may be available for many of these previously untreatable disorders.

Lysosomes are cellular organelles in which complex macromolecules are degraded by specific acid hydrolases. Deficiency of a lysosomal enzyme causes its substrate to accumulate in the lysosomes, resulting in a characteristic clinical picture. These lysosomal storage disorders are classified as mucopolysaccharidoses, lipidoses, or oligosaccharidoses, depending on the nature of the stored material. Two additional disorders, cystinosis and Salla disease, are caused by defects in lysosomal proteins that normally transport material from the lysosome to the cytoplasm. Table 36–3 lists clinical and laboratory features of these conditions. Most are inherited as autosomal recessive traits, and all can be diagnosed *in utero*.

▶ Diagnosis

The diagnosis of mucopolysaccharidosis is suggested by certain clinical and radiologic findings (dysostosis multiplex, which includes enlarged sella turcica, scaphocephaly, broad ribs, hook-shaped vertebrae [L1 and L2 most affected], and prominent pointing of the metacarpals and broad phalanges). Urine screening tests can detect increased mucopolysaccharides and oligosaccharides, and further identify which specific species are present. Diagnosis must be confirmed by enzyme assays using leukocytes or cultured fibroblasts. Lipidoses present with visceral symptoms or neurodegeneration. The pattern of the leukodystrophy associated with many lipidoses can indicate a specific condition. Diagnosis is made by appropriate enzyme assays of peripheral leukocytes or cultured skin fibroblasts. Molecular analysis is also available for most conditions.

▶ Treatment

Most conditions cannot be treated effectively, but new avenues have given hope in many conditions. Hematopoietic stem cell transplantation (HSCT) can greatly improve the course of some lysosomal diseases and is first-line treatment in some, such as infantile Hurler syndrome. Several disorders are treated with infusions of recombinant modified enzyme. Infusions are typically given intravenously; however, use of intrathecal infusion can allow for more effective treatment of neurologic symptoms. Treatment of Gaucher disease is very effective, and long-term data suggest excellent outcome. Similar treatments have been developed for Fabry disease, several mucopolysaccharidoses, Wolman, and Pompe disease. Substantial improvements in these conditions have been reported but with limitations. New avenues for treatment through substrate inhibition and chaperone therapy are being developed. Treatment of cystinosis with cysteamine results in depletion of stored cystine and prevention of complications including renal disease. Niemann-Pick C is being more effectively treated with cyclodextrin.

Table 36–3. Clinical and laboratory features of lysosomal storage diseases.

Disorder	Enzyme Defect	Clinical and Laboratory Features	Available Therapies
I. Mucopolysaccharidoses			
Hurler syndrome	α-Iduronidase	Autosomal recessive. ID, hepatomegaly, umbilical hernia, coarse facies, corneal clouding, dorsolumbar gibbus, severe heart disease. Heparan sulfate and dermatan sulfate in urine.	HSCT ERT
Scheie syndrome	α-Iduronidase (incomplete)	Autosomal recessive. Corneal clouding, stiff joints, normal intellect. Clinical types intermediate between Hurler and Scheie common. Heparan sulfate and dermatan sulfate in urine.	ERT
Hunter syndrome	Sulfoiduronate sulfatase	X-linked recessive. Coarse facies, hepatomegaly, ID variable. Corneal clouding and gibbus not present. Heparan sulfate and dermatan sulfate in urine.	HSCT ERT
Sanfilippo syndrome: Type A Type B Type C Type D	Sulfamidase α-N-Acetylglucosaminidase Acetyl-CoA: α-glucosaminide-N-acetyltransferase α-N-acetylglucosamine-6-sulfatase	Autosomal recessive. Severe ID and hyperactivity, with comparatively mild skeletal changes, visceromegaly, and facial coarseness. Types cannot be differentiated clinically. Heparan sulfate in urine.	
Morquio syndrome	N-Acetylgalactosamine-6-sulfatase	Autosomal recessive. Severe skeletal changes, platyspondylisis, corneal clouding. Keratan sulfate in urine.	ERT
Maroteaux-Lamy syndrome	N-Acetylgalactosamine-4-sulfatase	Autosomal recessive. Coarse facies, growth retardation, dorsolumbar gibbus, corneal clouding, hepatosplenomegaly, normal intellect. Dermatan sulfate in urine.	HSCT ERT
B-Glucuronidase deficiency	β-Glucuronidase	Autosomal recessive. Variable ID, dorsolumbar gibbus, corneal clouding, and hepatosplenomegaly to mild facial coarseness, retardation, and loose joints. Hearing loss common. Dermatan sulfate or heparan sulfate in urine.	HSCT
II. Oligosaccharidoses			
Mannosidosis	α-Mannosidase	Autosomal recessive. Variable ID, coarse facies, short stature, skeletal changes, and hepatosplenomegaly to mild facial coarseness and loose joints. Hearing loss common. Abnormal oligosaccharides in urine.	HSCT
Fucosidosis	α-Fucosidase	Autosomal recessive. Variable ID, coarse facies, skeletal changes, hepatosplenomegaly, occasional angiokeratomas. Abnormal oligosaccharides in urine.	HSCT
I-cell disease (mucolipidosis II)	N-Acetylglucosaminylphosphotransferase	Autosomal recessive; severe and mild forms known. Very short stature, ID, early facial coarsening, clear cornea, and stiffness of joints. Increased lysosomal enzymes in serum. Abnormal Sialyl oligosaccharides in urine.	HSCT
Sialidosis	Neuraminidase (sialidase)	Autosomal recessive. ID, coarse facies, skeletal dysplasia, myoclonic seizures, macular cherry-red spot. Abnormal Sialyl oligosaccharides in urine.	
III. Lipidoses			
Niemann-Pick disease	Sphingomyelinase	Autosomal recessive. Acute and chronic forms known. Acute neuronopathic form common in Eastern European Jewish ancestry. Accumulation of sphingomyelin in lysosomes of RE system and CNS. Hepatosplenomegaly, developmental retardation, macular cherry-red spot. Death by 1–4 y in severe type A; mild type B develops respiratory insufficiency usually in adulthood.	HSCT[a]

(Continued)

Table 36–3. Clinical and laboratory features of lysosomal storage diseases. (*Continued*)

Disorder	Enzyme Defect	Clinical and Laboratory Features	Available Therapies
Metachromatic leukodystrophy	Arylsulfatase A	Autosomal recessive. Late infantile form, with onset at 1–4 y, most common. Accumulation of sulfatide in white matter with central leukodystrophy and peripheral neuropathy. Gait disturbances (ataxia), motor incoordination, absent deep tendon reflexes, and dementia. Death usually in first decade.	HSCT[a]
Krabbe disease (globoid cell leukodystrophy)	Galactocerebroside α-galactosidase	Autosomal recessive. Globoid cells in white matter. Onset at 3–6 mo with seizures, irritability, retardation, and leukodystrophy. Death by 1–2 y. Juvenile and adult forms are rare.	HSCT[a]
Fabry disease	α-Galactosidase A	X-linked recessive. Storage of trihexosylceramide in endothelial cells. Pain in extremities, angiokeratoma and (later) poor vision, hypertension, and renal failure.	ERT, CT
Farber disease	Ceramidase	Autosomal recessive. Storage of ceramide in tissues. Subcutaneous nodules, arthropathy with deformed and painful joints, and poor growth and development. Death within first year.	HSCT[a]
Gaucher disease	Glucocerebroside β-glucosidase	Autosomal recessive. Accumulation of glucocerebroside in lysosomes of RE system and CNS. Acute neuronopathic form: ID, hepatosplenomegaly, macular cherry-red spot, and Gaucher cells in bone marrow. Death by 1–2 y. Chronic form common in Eastern European Jewish ancestry. Hepatosplenomegaly and flask-shaped osteolytic bone lesions. Consistent with normal life expectancy.	ERT SIT
G_{M1} gangliosidosis	G_{M1} ganglioside β-galactosidase	Autosomal recessive. Accumulation of G_{M1} ganglioside in lysosomes of RE system and CNS. Infantile form: abnormalities at birth with dysostosis multiplex, hepatosplenomegaly, macular cherry-red spot, and death by 2 y. Juvenile form: normal development to 1 y of age, then ataxia, weakness, dementia, and death by 4–5 y. Occasional inferior beaking of vertebral bodies of L1 and L2.	HSCT[a]
G_{M2} gangliosidoses Tay-Sachs disease Sandhoff disease	β-*N*-Acetylhexosaminidase A β-*N*-Acetylhexosaminidase A and B	Autosomal recessive. Tay-Sachs disease common in Eastern European Jewish ancestry; Sandhoff disease is pan-ethnic. Clinical phenotypes are identical, with accumulation of G_{M2} ganglioside in lysosomes of CNS. Onset at age 3–6 mo, with hypotonia, hyperacusis, ID, and macular cherry-red spot. Death by 2–3 y. Juvenile- and adult-onset forms of Tay-Sachs disease are rare.	
Wolman disease	Acid lipase	Autosomal recessive. Accumulation of cholesterol esters and triglycerides in lysosomes of reticuloendothelial system. Onset in infancy with gastrointestinal symptoms and hepatosplenomegaly, and death in the first year. Adrenals commonly enlarged and calcified.	HSCT ERT
Niemann-Pick disease type C	*NPC1* gene (95%), *NPC2* gene (5%)	Autosomal recessive. Blocked transport of lipids and cholesterol from late endosomes to lysosomes. Infantile cholestatic liver disease or later neurodegeneration with vertical supranuclear gaze palsy, ataxia, gelastic cataplexy, seizures, spasticity and loss of speech. Some have splenomegaly.	SIT

CNS, central nervous system; CT, Chaperone therapy; ERT, enzyme-replacement therapy; HSCT, hematopoietic stem cell transplantation; ID, intellectual disability; RE, reticuloendothelial; SIT, substrate inhibition therapy.
[a]May be useful in selected patients.

Elmonem MA, Veys KR, Soliman NA, van Dyck M, van den Heuvel LP, Levtchenko E: Cystinosis: a review. Orphanet J Rare Dis 2016; 11:47 [PMID: 27102039].

Hoffman EP, Barr ML, Giovanni MA, Murray MF: Lysosomal acid lipase deficiency. In: Pagon RA et al (eds): *GeneReviews®*. Seattle, WA: University of Washington; 2016 [PMID: 26225414].

James RA, Singh-Grewal D, Lee SJ, McGill J, Adib N; Australian Paediatric Rheumatology G: Lysosomal storage disorders: a review of the musculoskeletal features. J Paediatr Child Health 2016;52:262–271 [PMID: 27124840].

Khan S et al: Mucopolysaccharidosis IVA and glycosaminoglycans. Mol Genet Metab 2017;120:78–95 [PMID: 27979613].

Mole SE, Cotman SL: Genetics of the neuronal ceroid lipofuscinoses (Batten disease). Biochim Biophys Acta 2015;1852: 2237–2241 [PMID: 26026925].

Nalysnyk L, Rotella P, Simeone JC, Hamed A, Weinreb N: Gaucher disease epidemiology and natural history: a comprehensive review of the literature. Hematology 2017;22:65–73 [PMID: 27762169].

Patient and parent support group websites with useful information for families: http://www.mpssociety.org, www.ulf.org, www.lysosomallearning.com, www.fabry.org, www.gaucherdisease.org www.ntsad.org.

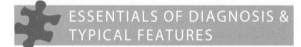 PEROXISOMAL DISEASES

ESSENTIALS OF DIAGNOSIS & TYPICAL FEATURES

▶ Dysmorphic features, hypotonia, hearing loss, seizures, cataracts, retinopathy, liver disease and renal disease are characteristic findings of severe peroxisomal disease.

▶ Change in behavior or school failure in a young boy may suggest X-linked adrenoleukodystrophy (X-ALD) and warrants a brain MRI with contrast.

▶ Very-long-chain fatty acid (VLCFA) analysis is a good screening test for most, but not all, peroxisomal disorders.

Peroxisomes are intracellular organelles that contain a large number (> 70) of enzymes. The enzyme systems in peroxisomes participate in metabolism of VLCFAs, branched chain fatty acids (phytanic and pristanic acid), bile acids, some amino acids, oxalate and plasmalogens.

In peroxisomal biogenesis disorders, multiple enzymes are deficient due to global peroxisomal dysfunction. The clinical presentations are termed Zellweger spectrum disorders. Patients present as neonates or infants with seizures, hypotonia, characteristic facies with a large forehead and fontanel, hepatopathy, feeding difficulties, retinal dystrophy, and hearing loss. At autopsy, renal cysts, brain neuronal migration abnormalities, and absent or empty peroxisomes are seen. Patients with a milder biochemical and clinical phenotype have ataxia, developmental delay, retinopathy, and hearing loss.

In other peroxisomal diseases, only a single enzyme is deficient. Patients with D-bifunctional protein deficiency or acyl-CoA oxidase deficiency have a Zellweger-like phenotype. Primary hyperoxaluria (alanine-glyoxylate aminotransferase deficiency) causes renal stones and nephropathy. Mutations in the X-linked VLCFA transporter gene, *ABCD1*, cause either a rapidly progressive and fatal leukodystrophy (X-linked adrenoleukodystrophy [X-ALD]) or a slowly progressive spasticity and neuropathy (adrenomyeloneuropathy). Adrenal insufficiency usually accompanies either neurologic presentation. Defective phytanic acid oxidation causes adult Refsum disease, with symptoms of ataxia, leukodystrophy, cardiomyopathy, neuropathy, and retinal dystrophy. Defects of plasmalogen synthesis cause rhizomelic chondrodysplasia punctata, with symptoms of skeletal dysplasia and neurologic disease. Except for X-ALD, all peroxisomal diseases have recessive inheritance.

▶ Diagnosis

The best initial test for Zellweger spectrum disorders and X-ALD is assessment of VLCFA levels in plasma. Measurements of phytanic acid, pristanic acid, pipecolic acid, bile acid intermediates, and plasmalogens are also appropriate for evaluation of some peroxisome disorders. Increasingly, peroxisomal disorders are identified with genetic testing. Several states test for X-ALD with newborn screening.

▶ Treatment

Treatment for most peroxisomal disorders is symptomatic and supportive. HSCT may be an effective treatment at the early stages of X-ALD, and close monitoring of affected males is necessary to determine optimal timing of HSCT. Corticosteroid treatment is necessary for any patients with adrenal insufficiency. Dietary treatment for avoidance of phytanic acid (mainly present in meat and dairy) is effective for adult Refsum disease. Liver transplantation is an effective treatment for primary hyperoxaluria.

Braverman NE et al: Peroxisome biogenesis disorders in the Zellweger spectrum: an overview of current diagnosis, clinical manifestations, and treatment guidelines. Mol Genet Metab 2016;117(3):313–321 [PMID: 26750748].

Patient and parent support group website with useful information for families: http://www.thegfpd.org.

Raymond GV, Moser AB, Fatemi A: X-linked adrenoleukodystrophy. *GeneReviews®* [Internet]. Seattle, WA: University of Washington; 2018. https://www.ncbi.nlm.nih.gov/books/NBK1315/.

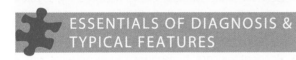

CONGENITAL DISORDERS OF GLYCOSYLATION

ESSENTIALS OF DIAGNOSIS & TYPICAL FEATURES

▶ Analysis of glycosylation patterns of marker glycoproteins such as transferrin (N-linked glycosylation) and apolipoprotein C (O-linked glycosylation) is an initial screening test for these broad-spectrum, multisystem disorders.

Many proteins, especially extracellular and lysosomal proteins, require glycosylation for normal function. The congenital disorders of glycosylation (CDGs) are a family of over 100 different disorders that result from defects in the synthesis of glycans or in the attachment of glycans (polysaccharides) to proteins as a post-translational modification. The most common CDG is phosphomannomutase-2 deficiency (PMM2-CDG). Children with PMM2-CDG may present with diarrhea, developmental delay, abnormal subcutaneous fat distribution, inverted nipples, strabismus, cerebellar hypoplasia, liver disease, cardiomyopathy and pericardial effusions, endocrine abnormalities, and peripheral neuropathy. Patients with phosphomannose isomerase deficiency (PMI-CDG) have a combination of hepatopathy, protein-losing enteropathy, and hyperinsulinemic hypoglycemia. Glycosylation defects have also been found to underlie syndromes such as multiple exostoses syndrome, Walker-Warburg syndrome, muscle-eye-brain disease, and dystroglycan-related muscular dystrophies.

Defects in the glycosylphosphatidylinositol anchor system cause neurologic symptoms such as epilepsy, hypotonia, brain abnormalities, and other organ dysfunction with characteristically elevated alkaline phosphatase due to lack of anchoring of the enzyme to the endothelial cell wall. Combined deficiencies are present in Golgi disorders such as abnormalities in the COG complex that moves glycoproteins; these present with variable combinations of liver disease, neurologic symptoms, recurrent infections and hyperthermia, cardiac defects, and cutis laxa. Phosphoglucoisomerase deficiency (PGM1-CDG) causes both a glycogen storage disease (type XIV) with hypoglycemia, but also malformations such as cleft palate and liver, cardiac, and endocrine abnormalities. Finally, N-glycanase-1 (NGLY1) is the first described disorder of deglycosylation and presents with developmental delays, elevated transaminases, chorea, and alacrima.

▶ Diagnosis

Diagnosis may be suspected in the setting of altered levels of glycosylated proteins such as transferrin, thyroxine-binding globulin, lysosomal enzymes, and clotting factors (IX, XI, antithrombin III, and proteins C and S). Diagnosis is confirmed by finding patterns of abnormal glycosylation of selected proteins. Most diagnostic laboratories examine serum transferrin to screen for N-linked CDGs and apo-CIII for O-linked CDGs. In some cases, muscle biopsy with immunohistochemistry may be a diagnostic test. CDG diagnosis may be further confirmed by assaying enzyme activity in some cases. Increasingly, broad genetic testing is the initial diagnostic modality that suggests a CDG.

▶ Treatment

Treatment is supportive, including monitoring and providing early treatment for expected clinical features. Mannose treatment is curative for patients with PMI-CDG, and galactose treatment is important for patients with PGM1-CDG, making timely recognition of these disorders important.

Sparks SE, Krasnewich DM: Congenital disorders of N-linked glycosylation and multiple pathway overview. *GeneReviews*® [Internet]. Seattle, WA: University of Washington; 2017. https://www.ncbi.nlm.nih.gov/books/NBK1332/.

Ng BG, Freeze HH: Perspectives on glycosylation and its congenital disorders. Trends Genet 2018;34(6):466–476 [PMID: 29606283].

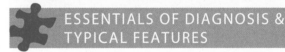

SMITH-LEMLI-OPITZ SYNDROME & DISORDERS OF CHOLESTEROL SYNTHESIS

ESSENTIALS OF DIAGNOSIS & TYPICAL FEATURES

▶ Elevated 7- and 8-dehydrocholesterol in serum is diagnostic in Smith-Lemli-Opitz (SLO) syndrome, which presents with developmental delay and malformations.

▶ Cerebrotendinous xanthomatosis (CTX) presents with cataracts and progressive neurologic symptoms. Treatment with chenodeoxycholic acid improves progression of disease.

Several defects of cholesterol synthesis are associated with malformations and neurodevelopmental disability. Smith-Lemli-Opitz (SLO) syndrome is an autosomal recessive disorder caused by a deficiency of the enzyme 7-dehydrocholesterol Δ7-reductase. It is characterized by microcephaly, poor growth, intellectual disability, typical dysmorphic features of face and extremities (particularly two- to three-toe syndactyly), and often malformations of the heart and genitourinary system. It is further described in Chapter 37. Conradi-Hünermann syndrome is characterized by chondrodysplasia punctata and atrophic skin. Defects in the metabolism of cholesterol to bile acids usually cause cholestatic liver disease and failure to thrive. Cerebrotendinous xanthomatosis (CTX) manifests with progressive ataxia, spastic paraparesis, cataracts, cognitive decline, and, later, xanthomatous eruptions of the skin. Some patients with CTX may initially present with cholestatic liver disease or chronic diarrhea in infancy.

▶ Diagnosis

In SLO, elevated 7- and 8-dehydrocholesterol in serum or amniotic fluid is diagnostic. Serum cholesterol levels may be low or in the normal range. Enzymes of cholesterol synthesis may be assayed in cultured fibroblasts or amniocytes, and mutation analysis is possible. CTX is diagnosed by detection of characteristic abnormalities of bile acids in blood and urine as well as elevated cholestanol.

▶ Treatment

Although postnatal treatment does not resolve prenatal injury, supplementation with cholesterol in SLO may improve growth and behavior. The role of supplemental bile acids is controversial. CTX responds to treatment with chenodeoxycholic acid, which inhibits the formation of bile alcohols by suppressing the first-step cholesterol 7α-hydroxylase, with substantial functional recovery.

Bianconi SE et al: Pathogenesis, epidemiology, diagnosis and clinical aspects of Smith–Lemli–Opitz syndrome. Expert Opin Orphan Drugs 2015;3(3):267–280 [PMID: 25734025].

Federico A, Dotti MT, Gallus GN: Cerebrotendinous xanthomatosis. 2003 Jul 16 [Updated 2016 Apr 14]. In: Adam MP et al (eds): *GeneReviews*® [Internet]. Seattle, WA: University of Washington; 1993–2019. https://www.ncbi.nlm.nih.gov/books/NBK1409/.

Patient and parent support group website with useful information for families: http://www.smithlemliopitz.org.

▼ DISORDERS OF BRAIN SPECIFIC METABOLISM: NEUROTRANSMITTERS, SYNTHESIS OF AMINO ACIDS & GLUCOSE TRANSPORT

🧩 ESSENTIALS OF DIAGNOSIS & TYPICAL FEATURES

▶ Consider in children with movement disorders, especially dystonia and oculogyric crises.

▶ Severe seizures, abnormal tone, ataxia, intellectual disability, and autonomic instability occur in severely affected infants.

▶ Mildly affected patients have dopa-responsive dystonia with diurnal variability.

▶ Deficient serine synthesis causes microcephaly, seizures, and failure of myelination in neonates, whereas deficiency of glutamine or asparagine synthesis causes severe microcephaly, intractable epilepsy, and brain malformations.

▶ Deficient glucose transporter causes seizures and a movement disorder. Identifiable on CSF analysis and treatable with a ketogenic diet.

▶ Pyridoxine-dependent epilepsy causes neonatal seizures and developmental delays and should always be biochemically evaluated because it can be effectively treated with pyridoxine and a lysine-restricted diet.

Abnormalities of neurotransmitter metabolism are increasingly recognized as causes of significant neurodevelopmental disabilities. These disorders impact the synthesis of the neurotransmitters dopamine and serotonin. Affected patients may present with movement disorders (especially dystonia and oculogyric crises), seizures, abnormal tone, or intellectual disability, and may initially be diagnosed with cerebral palsy. Patients may be mildly affected (eg, dopa-responsive dystonia with diurnal variation) or severely affected (eg, intractable seizures with profound intellectual disability).

Pyridoxine-dependent epilepsy manifests as a seizure disorder in the neonatal or early infantile period that responds to high doses of pyridoxine. The disorder is caused by deficient activity of the enzyme α-amino adipic semialdehyde dehydrogenase resulting from mutations in the antiquitin (*ALDH7A1*) gene. The enzyme is involved in lysine catabolism and dietary lysine restriction aids in treatment. Pyridoxal-phosphate–responsive encephalopathy manifests as a severe seizure disorder in infancy that responds to pyridoxal-phosphate supplementation. This disorder is caused by mutations in the *PNPO* gene encoding pyridox(am)ine oxidase, which is necessary for activation of pyridoxine.

Deficient serine synthesis leads to congenital microcephaly, infantile seizures, and failure of myelination. The most severe disorder of serine synthesis is Neu-Laxova syndrome, characterized by premature birth with microcephaly, skeletal abnormalities and early lethality. Classic serine deficiency presents with microcephaly, refractory epilepsy, and hypomyelination. Defects in all four genes involved in serine synthesis and transport (*PHGDH, PSAT1, PSPH, SLC4A1*) occur in an autosomal recessive pattern. Defects in asparagine synthase and glutamine synthase result in severe microcephaly, underdevelopment of the brain with gyral simplification, and refractory epilepsy.

Glut1 deficiency syndrome results from mutations in *SLC2A1*, which act in a dominant fashion. The resultant CSF glucose deficiency causes seizures as well as dystonia and other movement disorders.

Diagnosis

Although some disorders can be diagnosed by examining plasma amino acids or urine organic acids (eg, 4-hydroxybutyric aciduria), in most cases, diagnosis requires analysis of CSF. Spinal fluid samples for neurotransmitter analysis require special collection and handling, as the neurotransmitter levels are graduated along the axis of the CNS. A phenylalanine loading test can be diagnostic for mild defects in GTP-cyclohydrolase deficiency, in which neurotransmitter analysis may be insufficiently sensitive. Analysis of CSF shows elevated threonine and decreased pyridoxal-phosphate in pyridoxal-phosphate–responsive disease, and decreased serine and glycine in serine biosynthetic defects. Urine or plasma α-aminoadipic acid and piperideine-6-carboxylate best identifies infants with pyridoxine-dependent seizures. CSF analysis of serine, asparagine, or glutamine detects deficiencies in these amino acids most effectively. Glut1 deficiency syndrome can be diagnosed by demonstrating low glucose and lactate in CSF.

Treatment

Biosynthesis defects of dopamine and serotonin are usually treated with a combination of levodopa, 5-hydroxytryptophan, and carbidopa. Pyridoxine-dependent epilepsy is treated with pyridoxine in high doses and a lysine-restricted diet, whereas pyridoxal-phosphate–responsive encephalopathy requires pyridoxal-phosphate supplementation. Supplementation with serine and glycine can improve outcomes in serine deficiency. Glut1 deficiency syndrome is treatable with a ketogenic diet. For several conditions, such as pyridoxine-responsive seizures, pyridoxal-phosphate–responsive encephalopathy, or dopa-responsive dystonia, response to treatment is dramatic.

Coughlin CR II et al: Triple therapy with pyridoxine, arginine supplementation and dietary lysine restriction in pyridoxine-dependent epilepsy: neurodevelopmental outcome. Mol Genet Metab 2015;116:35–43 [PMID: 26026794].

El-Hattab AW: Serine biosynthesis and transport defects. Mol Genet Metab 2016;118(3):153–159 [PMID: 27161889].

Furukawa Y: GTP cyclohydrolase 1-deficient dopa-responsive dystonia. 2002 Feb 21 [Updated 2019 Jan 24]. In: Adam MP et al (eds): *GeneReviews*® [Internet]. Seattle, WA: University of Washington; 1993–2019.

Ng J, Papandreou A, Heales SJ, Kurian MA: Monoamine neurotransmitter disorders—clinical advances and future perspectives. Nat Rev Neurol 2015;11(10):567–584 [PMID: 26392380].

Patient and parent support group websites with useful information for families: http://www.pndassoc.org.

Wang D, Pascual JM, De Vivo D: Glucose transporter type 1 deficiency syndrome. *GeneReviews*® [Internet]. Seattle, WA: University of Washington; 2018. https://www.ncbi.nlm.nih.gov/books/NBK1430/.

▼ CREATINE SYNTHESIS DISORDERS

ESSENTIALS OF DIAGNOSIS & TYPICAL FEATURES

► Consider in children with seizures, movement disorders, autistic features, and developmental delay especially with severe expressive language delay.

► Early recognition and treatment of guanidinoacetate methyltransferase (GAMT) deficiency result in normal outcome.

Creatine is essential for storage and transmission of phosphate-bound energy in muscle and brain. The disorders arginine:glycine amidinotransferase (AGAT) deficiency and guanidinoacetate methyltransferase (GAMT) deficiency are autosomal recessive, whereas creatine transporter (CrT1) deficiency is X-linked. Patients demonstrate developmental delay, seizures, and severe expressive language delay (particularly in CrT1 deficiency). Patients may also show developmental regression and brain atrophy. Patients with GAMT deficiency have more severe seizures and an extrapyramidal movement disorder. The seizure disorder is milder in male CrT1-deficient patients. Some female heterozygotes may show learning disabilities.

Diagnosis

Creatine and guanidinoacetate levels may be measured in blood or urine and are typically the initial diagnostic study. Creatine transporter deficiency is detected using the urine creatine:creatinine ratio. Magnetic resonance spectroscopy may demonstrate decreased creatine concentration in the brain. Sequencing of *SLC6A8*, *GATM*, and *AGAT* as part of a broad genetic testing approach may be the initial diagnostic study for those patients with nonspecific presentations. Pilot studies of newborn screening for some creatine deficiency syndromes are underway.

Treatment

Treatment with oral creatine supplementation is partially successful in GAMT and AGAT deficiencies. Treatment with combined arginine restriction and ornithine supplementation in GAMT deficiency can decrease guanidinoacetate concentrations and improve the clinical course. Early treatment from infancy greatly improves outcomes in GAMT. Combined therapy using arginine, glycine, and creatine supplementation in CrT1 deficiency has been tried with variable efficacy.

Fons C, Campistol J: Creatine defects and central nervous system. Semin Pediatr Neurol 2016;23(4):285–289 [PMID: 28284390].

Miller JS et al: Early indicators of creatine transporter deficiency. J Pediatr 2019;206:283–285 [PMID: 30579583].

Stockler-Ipsiroglu S et al: Guanidinoacetate methyltransferase (GAMT) deficiency: outcomes in 48 individuals and recommendations for diagnosis, treatment and monitoring. Mol Genet Metab 2014;111(1):16 [PMID: 24268530].

QUALITY INITIATIVES IN THE FIELD OF METABOLIC DISEASE

Expanded newborn screening has had a large impact on the field of metabolic disorders. Patients are being diagnosed earlier, and for some patients, this dramatically reduces the disease burden. Expanded newborn screening has also revealed unexpected consequences. For example, the clinical spectrum of many disorders is being expanded to include mildly affected or asymptomatic patients. Gradually, a more refined therapeutic approach is being developed for the more mildly affected patients; for some patients on the milder end of a disease spectrum who would have never become symptomatic, therapy is not needed at all. In addition, newborn screening for several conditions detects maternal disease such as maternal vitamin B_{12} deficiency and maternal carnitine uptake deficiency; this poses new management and risk questions for this largely asymptomatic or presymptomatic population. Further, limitations in diagnostic testing create difficulty in discriminating carriers from patients affected with mild disease manifestations that still pose health risks (eg VLCAD deficiency and glutaric aciduria type I) and may detect the presence of pseudodeficiency alleles that show biochemical but not clinical enzymatic deficiency (eg, Hurler and Pompe disease). These diagnostic challenges not only add to parental anxiety, but treatment of an unaffected child may entail risk to the child or to family dynamics.

Continuous improvements in newborn screening have resulted in the addition of screening for several new conditions such as severe combined immunodeficiency (SCID) and peroxisomal and lysosomal storage disorders. Many more disorders will be considered candidates for newborn screening in the near future. Careful consideration will need to be given to the risks and benefits to screening for such conditions. The U.S. Secretary for Health and Human Services' Advisory Committee on Heritable Disorders in Newborns and Children has established a rigorous process for review before recommending a disorder be considered for nationwide screening. Despite approval through this rigorous process, many states are struggling with implementation of new screening tests.

Kelly N, Makaram DC, Wasserstein MP: Screening of newborns for disorders with high benefit-risk ratios should be mandatory. J Law Med Ethics 2016;44(2):231–240 [PMID: 27338599].

Kemper AR et al: Decision-making process for conditions nominated to the recommended uniform screening panel: statement of the US Department of Health and Human Services Secretary's Advisory Committee on Heritable Disorders in Newborns and Children. Genet Med 2014;16(2):183–187 [PMID: 23907646].

Genetics & Dysmorphology

Naomi J. L. Meeks, MD

Margarita Saenz, MD

Anne Chun-Hui Tsai, MD, MSc

Ellen R. Elias, MD

▼ FOUNDATIONS OF GENETIC DIAGNOSIS

CYTOGENETICS

Cytogenetics is the study of genetics at the chromosome level. Chromosomal anomalies occur in 0.4% of all live births and are a common cause of intellectual disabilities and congenital anomalies. The prevalence of chromosomal anomalies is much higher among spontaneous abortions and stillbirths.

Chromosomes

Human chromosomes consist of DNA (the blueprint of genetic material), specific proteins forming the backbone of the chromosome (called histones), and other chromatin structural and interactive proteins. Chromosomes contain most of the genetic information necessary for growth and differentiation. The nuclei of all normal human cells, with the exception of gametes, contain 46 chromosomes, consisting of 23 pairs (Figure 37–1). Of these, 22 pairs are called autosomes. They are numbered according to their size; chromosome 1 is the largest and chromosome 22 the smallest. In addition, there are two sex chromosomes: two X chromosomes in females and one X and one Y chromosome in males. The two members of a chromosome pair are called homologous chromosomes. One homolog of each chromosome pair is maternal in origin; the second is paternal. The egg and sperm each contain 23 chromosomes (haploid cells). During formation of the zygote, they fuse into a cell with 46 chromosomes (diploid cell).

Karyotype

A karyotype is the arrangement of chromosomes in homologous pairs in numerical order. There is a characteristic-banding pattern that is reproducible for each chromosome, allowing the chromosomes to be identified. High-resolution chromosome analysis is the study of more elongated chromosomes and can detect smaller imbalances than routine chromosome analysis (see Figure 37–1). Although the bands can be visualized in greater detail, subtle chromosomal rearrangements less than 5 million base pairs (5 Mb) can still be missed.

Fluorescence in situ hybridization (FISH) is a powerful technique that labels a known chromosome sequence with DNA probes attached to fluorescent dyes, thus enabling visualization of specific regions of chromosomes by fluorescent microscopy. FISH can detect submicroscopic structural rearrangements undetectable by classic cytogenetic techniques and can identify marker chromosomes. (For pictures of FISH studies, go to http://www.pathology.washington.edu/galleries/Cytogallery/main.php?file=fish_examples.)

Interphase FISH allows noncultured cells (lymphocytes, amniocytes) to be rapidly screened for numerical abnormalities such as trisomy 13, 18, or 21, and sex chromosome anomalies. However, because of the possible background or contamination of the signal, the abnormality must be confirmed by conventional chromosome analysis. Two hundred-cell FISH can also be used to ascertain mosaicism.

Chromosomal Microarray Analysis or Array Comparative Genomic Hybridization

Advances in technology and bioinformatics have led to the development of genetic testing using comparative genomic hybridization with microarray technique (aCGH). This technique allows detection of small genetic imbalances in the genome. It is used to detect interstitial and submicroscopic imbalances, to characterize their size at the molecular level, and to define the breakpoints of translocations. This test has replaced high-resolution chromosomes as the first-line test in evaluating children with developmental delays

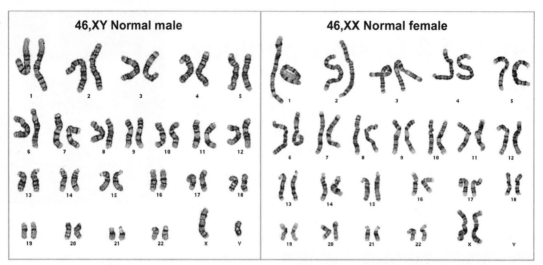

▲ **Figure 37–1.** Normal male and female human karyotype. (Used with permission from Colorado Genetics Laboratory.)

and multiple congenital anomalies. The principle behind aCGH is comparison of a patient's genome at hundreds of thousands of locations against a reference genome. Current aCGH are designed to screen the entire genome using single-nucleotide polymorphisms (SNPs), and these are particularly targeted toward known disease-causing regions. In some cases, the resolution in disease-related genes may be as small as several hundred base pairs. However, this technology is not able to detect very small deletions, duplications, or single-nucleotide changes. This technology can also identify cases of uniparental disomy (UPD) or consanguinity.

> Wiszneiwska J et al: Combined array CGH plus SNP genome analyses in a single assay for optimized clinical testing. Eur J Hum Genet 2014 Jan;22(1):79–87 [PMID: 23695279].

Chromosome Nomenclature

Visible under the microscope is a constriction site on the chromosome called the centromere, which separates the chromosome into two arms: p, for petite, refers to the short arm, and q, the letter following p, refers to the long arm. Each arm is further subdivided into numbered bands visible using different staining techniques. The use of named chromosome arms and bands provides a universal method of chromosome description. Common symbols include *del* (deletion), *dup* (duplication), *inv* (inversion), *ish* (in situ hybridization), *i* (isochromosome), *pat* (paternal origin), *mat* (maternal origin), and *r* (ring chromosome).

Chromosomal Abnormalities

There are two types of chromosomal anomalies: numerical and structural.

A. Abnormalities of Chromosomal Number

When a human cell has 23 chromosomes, such as human ova or sperm, it is in the haploid state (n). After conception, in cells other than the reproductive cells, 46 chromosomes are present in the diploid state (2n). Cells deviating from the multiple of the haploid number are called aneuploid, indicating an abnormal number of chromosomes. Trisomy, an example of aneuploidy, is the presence of three of a particular chromosome rather than two. It results from unequal division, called nondisjunction, of chromosomes into daughter cells. Trisomies are the most common numerical chromosomal anomalies found in humans (eg, trisomy 21 [Down syndrome], trisomy 18, and trisomy 13). Monosomies, the presence of only one member of a chromosome pair, may be complete or partial. All complete autosomal monosomies appear to be lethal early in development and only survive in mosaic forms. Sex chromosome monosomy, however, can be viable.

B. Abnormalities of Chromosomal Structure

Many different types of structural chromosomal anomalies exist. Figure 37–2 displays the formal nomenclature as well as the ideogram demonstrating chromosomal anomalies. In clinical context, the sign (+) or (−) *preceding* the chromosome number indicates increased or decreased number, respectively, of that particular whole chromosome in a cell. For example, 47, XY+21 designates a male with three copies of chromosome 21. The sign (+) or (−) *after* the chromosome number signifies extra material or missing material, respectively, on one of the arms of the chromosome. For example, 46, XX, 8q− denotes a deletion on the long arm of chromosome 8. Detailed nomenclature, such as 8q11, is required to

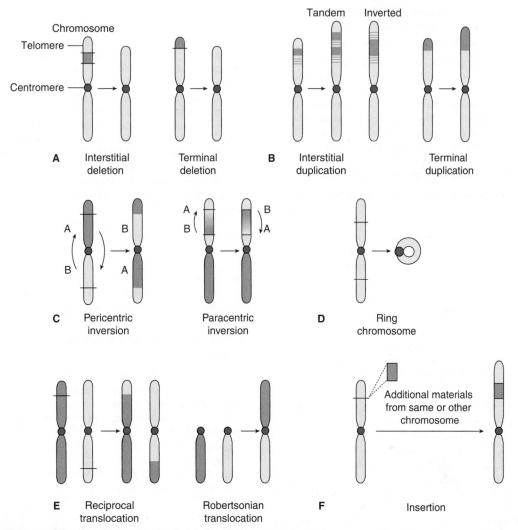

▲ **Figure 37–2.** Examples of structural chromosomal abnormalities: deletion, duplication, inversion, ring chromosome, translocation, and insertion.

further demonstrate a specific missing region so that genetic counseling can be provided.

1. Deletion (del) (see Figure 37–2A)—This refers to an absence of normal chromosomal material. It may be terminal (at the end of a chromosome) or interstitial (within a chromosome). The missing part is described using the code "del," followed by the number of the chromosome involved in parentheses, and a description of the missing region of that chromosome, also in parentheses, for example, 46, XX, del(1) (p36.3). This chromosome nomenclature describes the loss of genetic material from band 36.3 of the short arm of chromosome 1, which results in 1p36.3 deletion syndrome.

2. Duplication (dup) (see Figure 37–2B)—An extra copy of a chromosomal segment can be in tandem (genetic material present in the original direction) or inverted (genetic material present in the opposite direction). A well-described duplication of chromosome 22q11 causes Cat eye syndrome, resulting in iris coloboma and anal or ear anomalies.

3. Inversion (inv) (see Figure 37–2C)—In this aberration, a rearranged section of a chromosome is inverted. It can be paracentric (not involving the centromere) or pericentric (involving the centromere).

4. Ring chromosome (r) (see Figure 37–2D)—Deletion of the normal telomeres (and possibly other subtelomeric sequences) leads to subsequent fusion of both ends to form a circular chromosome. Ring chromosomal anomalies often cause growth retardation and intellectual disability.

5. Translocation (trans) (see Figure 37–2E)—This interchromosomal rearrangement of genetic material may be balanced (the cell has a normal content of genetic material arranged in a structurally abnormal way) or unbalanced (the cell has gained or lost genetic material as a result of chromosomal interchange). Balanced translocations may further be described as reciprocal, the exchange of genetic material between two nonhomologous chromosomes, or Robertsonian, the fusion of two acrocentric chromosomes.

6. Insertion (ins) (see Figure 37–2F)—Breakage within a chromosome at two points and incorporation of another piece of chromosomal material is called insertion. This may occur between two chromosomes or within the same chromosome. The clinical presentation or phenotype depends on the origin of the inserted materials as well as what material is disrupted.

C. Sex Chromosomal Anomalies

Abnormalities involving sex chromosomes, including aneuploidy and mosaicism, are relatively common in the general population. The most common sex chromosome anomalies include 45,X (Turner syndrome), 47,XXX,47,XXY (Klinefelter syndrome), 47,XYY, and different mosaic states.

D. Mosaicism

Mosaicism is the presence of two or more different chromosome constitutions in different cells of the same individual. For example, a patient may have some cells with 47 chromosomes and others with 46 chromosomes (46,XX/47,XX,+21 indicates mosaicism for trisomy 21; similarly, 45,X/46,XX/47,XXX indicates mosaicism for a monosomy and a trisomy X). Mosaicism should be suspected if clinical signs are milder than expected in a nonmosaic patient with the same chromosomal abnormality, or if the patient's skin shows unusual pigmentation. The prognosis can be better for a patient with mosaicism than for one with a corresponding chromosomal abnormality without mosaicism. In general, the smaller the proportion of the abnormal cell line, the better the prognosis. In the same patient, however, the proportion of normal and abnormal cells in various tissues, such as skin, brain, internal organs, and peripheral blood, may be significantly different. Therefore, the prognosis for a patient with chromosomal mosaicism can seldom be assessed reliably based on the karyotype in peripheral blood cells alone.

E. Uniparental Disomy

Under normal circumstances, one member of each homologous pair of chromosomes is of maternal origin from the egg and the other is of paternal origin from the sperm (Figure 37–3A). In UPD, both copies of a particular chromosome pair originate from the same parent. If UPD is caused by an error in the first meiotic division, both homologous chromosomes of that parent will be present in the gamete—a phenomenon called heterodisomy (Figure 37–3B). If the disomy is caused by an error in the second meiotic division, two copies of the same chromosome will be present through the mechanism of rescue, duplication, and complementation (Figure 37–3C through 37–3E)—a phenomenon called isodisomy. Isodisomy may also occur as a postfertilization error (Figure 37–3F).

Possible mechanisms for the adverse effects of UPD include homozygosity for deleterious recessive genes and the consequences of imprinting. It is suspected that UPD of some chromosomes is lethal.

UPD can cause a clinical phenotype when it occurs in certain human chromosomes, including chromosomes 6, 7, 11, 14, 15, and X. It has been found in patients with Prader-Willi, Angelman, and Beckwith-Wiedemann syndromes (BWS). On other chromosomes, by itself, it does not produce clinical features. Problems arise if it unmasks an underlying autosomal recessive condition in the case of isodisomy.

F. Microdeletion and Microduplication Syndromes

Microdeletion and microduplication syndromes result when there is a loss or gain of small regions of a chromosome. These are frequently referred to as copy number variants (CNVs). These may include one gene, multiple genes, or noncoding regions of the genome. Though high-resolution chromosomes can detect some CNVs, most are detected or confirmed by FISH or chromosomal microarray (CMA). These CNVs may be familial (passed on by a parent) or may occur *de novo*. Many CNVs are now known to be associated with specific syndromes. Generally, CNVs larger than 5–10 Megabases (Mb) have some sort of clinical impact. However some are not totally understood and may be classified as a variant of uncertain significance (VUS), or may be benign changes. Therefore, special caution and parental studies are often required in interpreting the results of genetic testing.

H. Chromosomal Abnormalities in Cancer

Numerical and structural chromosomal abnormalities are often identified in hematopoietic and solid-tumor neoplasms in individuals with otherwise normal chromosomes. These cytogenetic abnormalities have been categorized as primary and secondary. In primary abnormalities, their presence is necessary for initiation of the cancer; an example is 13q− in retinoblastoma. Secondary abnormalities appear de novo in somatic cells only after the cancer has developed, for example, Philadelphia chromosome, t(9;22)(q34;q11), in acute and chronic myeloid leukemia. Primary and secondary

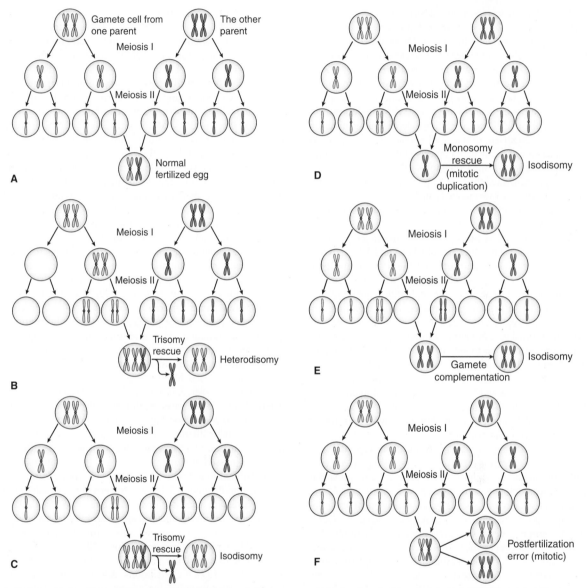

▲ **Figure 37-3.** The assortment of homologous chromosomes during normal gametogenesis and uniparental disomy. **A:** Fertilization of normal gametes. **B:** Heterodisomy by trisomy rescue. **C:** Isodisomy by trisomy rescue. **D:** Isodisomy by monosomy rescue (mitotic duplication). **E:** Gamete complementation. **F:** Postfertilization error.

chromosomal abnormalities are specific for particular neoplasms and can be used for diagnosis or prognosis. For example, the presence of the Philadelphia chromosome is a good prognostic sign in chronic myelogenous leukemia, but indicates a poor prognosis in acute lymphoblastic leukemia. The sites of chromosome breaks coincide with the known loci of oncogenes and tumor suppressor genes.

MOLECULAR GENETICS

Advances in molecular biology have revolutionized human genetics, as they allow for the localization, isolation, and characterization of genes that encode protein sequences. Molecular genetics can help explain the complex underlying biology involved in many human diseases.

Molecular diagnosis on a clinical basis can be achieved using many technologies. The **polymerase chain reaction (PCR)** replicates fragments of DNA between predetermined primers so that sufficient DNA is obtained for characterization or sequencing in the space of a few hours. **DNA sequencing** is the process of determining the nucleotide order of a given DNA fragment. **aCGH** can also be used to look for small deletions or duplications (as small as one exon) on the gene level. **Methylation** analysis can look for UPD or imprinting defects. **Next-generation sequencing (NextGen)** or massively parallel sequencing allows the sequencing of many genes quickly and accurately, and for less expense per gene than traditional DNA sequencing. This technology has allowed the screening of hundreds or thousands of genes at one time with targeted panel testing. This technology is also being used to perform **whole exome sequencing (WES)** or whole genome sequencing (WGS).

WES allows for sequencing of all known genes in the human genome. Difficulties in both WES and WGS involve limitations in the ability to interpret the result. Only about 25% of the genes contained within the human genome have a known function. Likewise, variations identified outside of coding regions of the genome (introns, regulatory regions) often have uncertain significance. Despite these limitations, WES or WGS performed in commercial laboratories has a meaningful diagnostic result in up to 40% of cases. NGS is changing the paradigm in Clinical Genetics. Rather than performing multiple single-gene tests, many geneticists are performing one or two screening tests and if testing is negative, moving toward WES or WGS to save time and limit costs. With improved technology, WES and WGS will allow not only for detection of sequence variants but eventually will be able to provide information related to CNVs as well as trinucleotide repeats.

Despite the advances in technology, there is significant variability in laboratories' ability to detect genetic changes as well as in their methodology for interpretation of results. Clinical laboratories must maintain rigorous quality management programs and undergo routine inspection by regulatory agencies (CLIA, CAP) to ensure generation of precise and accurate results. The American College of Medical Genetics and Genomics has partnered with the Association of Molecular Pathology to develop a set of guidelines to standardize laboratory interpretation practices. Variants may be classified as Pathogenic or Likely Pathogenic, Benign or Likely Benign, or of Uncertain Significance. Pathogenic and Likely Pathogenic variants are interpreted to mean disease causing whereas benign and likely benign are not. Variants of Uncertain Significance are variants for which there is not enough information published in the scientific literature to interpret the meaning. Parental testing or re-evaluation of variants over time may result in reclassification.

Genetics & Its Clinical Applications

There are multiple reasons a patient may undergo genetic testing. It's important for families to receive genetic counseling prior to testing to understand how that result may impact the patient and other family members.

Patients are often referred for genetic testing if they present with specific features of a known condition, if they have clinical characteristics but an unknown cause for those characteristics or because of a family history of a specific genetic condition. Genetic testing may confirm or identify a specific diagnosis, which can then be used to target specific treatments or interventions. Many families also feel a pressing need to know "why" a child has the condition they do; in some cases this may help alleviate feelings of guilt experienced by parents worrying there may have been something they did to cause a condition in their child. Even in cases where a genetic diagnosis does not alter treatments and interventions, some patients or families are seeking information about recurrence risks or information to allow prenatal or preimplantation genetic diagnosis.

In some genetic diagnoses, confirmation of a specific diagnosis results in additional recommendations for screening (laboratory and/or imaging studies) for additional medical complications. This can be seen in 22q11.2 Deletion Syndrome where those children are at risk for developmental delays, speech and palate problems, cardiac malformations, immune dysfunction, hormone imbalances, and growth delays/short stature among many others. In other diagnoses, specific medical treatments are indicated which do not impact the gene itself, but are designed to minimize complications of the disorder. An example of this is Marfan syndrome where diagnosis indicates treatment with beta blockers or an angiotensin-receptor blocker to prevent complications related to aortic dilation. In some inborn errors of metabolism, organ transplant can treat the disorder if the affected gene is expressed primarily in one organ (ie, liver transplantation in ornithine transcarbamylase deficiency). Finally, in rare genetic diagnoses, trials are underway to actually alter gene expression itself to ameliorate effects of the disease. An example of this is spinal muscular atrophy (SMA) where treatment to preserve a skipped exon in the gene has recently received Federal Drug Administration (FDA) approval.

Genetic testing allows practitioners to test patients for a wide variety of genetic conditions. Advances in this area of medicine have included the advent of parents requesting testing for adult onset disease, carrier status, and disease susceptibility in their children. There are significant ethical and legal issues surrounding this topic. The American College of Medical Genetics and Genomics and American Society of Human Genetics formed a consensus statement on the topic that educates families and health care providers on the potential negative impacts of such testing. In the face of whole exome or genome sequencing, single-gene analysis, and microarray analysis, carrier status for conditions may be revealed and this requires detailed genetic counseling. The decision-making capacity of the minor should also be taken into account where applicable.

Personalized medicine (precision medicine) is an advancing field of medicine that offers increased precision and effectiveness than traditional medicine. As opposed to the current paradigm where genetic testing is performed due to the presence of specific clinical signs or to diagnose rare disease, precision genetic testing may be ordered preemptively to better understand an individual's health risks or response to interventions. Pharmacogenomics offers enormous promise for predicting drug response in patients. For example, with DNA analysis of two specific genes, *CYP2C9* and *VKORC1*, it is now possible to predict response to warfarin anticoagulation therapy and to individualize the dose, saving the patient multiple blood tests and dosage adjustments.

Anderson JA et al: Predictive genetic testing for adult-onset disorders in minors: a critical analysis of the arguments for and against the 2013 ACMG guidelines. Clin Genet 2015 Apr;87(4):301–310 [PMID: 25046648].

Dickmann LJ, Ware JA: Pharmacogenomics in the age of personalized medicine. Drug Discov Today Technol 2016 Sep–Dec; 21–22:11–16 [PMID: 27978982].

Hammond SM et al: Systemic peptide-mediated oligonucleotide therapy improves long-term survival in spinal muscular atrophy. Proc Natl Acad Sci USA 2016 Sept 27;113(39):10962–10967 [PMID: 27621445].

Lionel AC et al: Improved diagnostic yield compared with targeted gene sequencing panels suggests a role for whole-genome sequencing as a first-tier genetic test. Genet Med 2018 Apr; 20 (4): 435–443 [PMID: 28771251].

Richards S et al: Standards and guidelines for the interpretation of sequence variants: a joint consensus recommendation of the American College of Medical Genetics and Genomics and the Association for Molecular Pathology. Genet Med 2015 May;17(5):405–424 [PMID: 25741868].

Trujillano D et al: Clinical exome sequencing: results from 2819 samples reflecting 1000 families. Eur J Hum Genet 2017;25: 176–182 [PMID: 27848944].

▼ PRINCIPLES OF INHERITED HUMAN DISORDERS

MENDELIAN INHERITANCE

Traditionally, autosomal single-gene disorders follow the principles explained by Gregor Mendel's observations. The inheritance of genetic traits through generations relies on segregation and independent assortment. **Segregation** is the process through which gene pairs are separated during gamete formation. **Independent assortment** refers to the segregation of different alleles independently.

Victor McKusick's catalog, *Mendelian Inheritance in Man*, lists more than 10,000 entries in which the mode of inheritance is presumed to be autosomal dominant, autosomal recessive, X-linked dominant, X-linked recessive, and Y-linked. Single genes at specific loci on one or a pair of chromosomes cause these disorders. An understanding of inheritance terminology is helpful in approaching Mendelian disorders. Analysis of the pedigree and the pattern of transmission in the family, identification of a specific condition, and knowledge of that condition's mode of inheritance usually allow for explanation of the inheritance pattern.

Terminology

The following terms are important in understanding heredity patterns:

1. Dominant and recessive—Concepts for dominant and recessive refer to the **phenotypic expression** of alleles and are not intrinsic characteristics of gene loci. Therefore, it is inappropriate to discuss "a dominant locus."

2. Genotype—Genotype means the genetic status, that is, the alleles an individual carries.

3. Phenotype—Phenotype is the expression of an individual's genotype, including appearance, physical features, organ structure, and biochemical and physiologic nature. It may be modified by environment.

4. Pleiotropy—Pleiotropy refers to the phenomenon whereby a single mutant allele can have widespread effects or expression in different tissues or organ systems. In other words, an allele may produce more than one effect on the phenotype. For example, Marfan syndrome has manifestations in different organ systems (skeletal, cardiac, ophthalmologic, etc) due to a single mutation within the *fibrillin* gene.

5. Penetrance—Penetrance refers to the proportion of individuals with a particular genotype that express the same phenotype. Penetrance is a proportion that ranges between 0 and 1 (or 0% and 100%). When 100% of mutant individuals express the phenotype, penetrance is **complete**. If some mutant individuals do not express the phenotype, penetrance is said to be **incomplete**, or **reduced**. Dominant conditions with incomplete penetrance, therefore, are characterized by "skipped" generations with unaffected, obligate gene carriers.

6. Expressivity—Expressivity refers to the variability in degree of phenotypic expression (severity) seen in different individuals with the same mutant genotype. Expressivity may be extremely variable or fairly consistent, both within and between families. Intrafamilial variability of expression may be due to factors such as epistasis, environment, genetic anticipation, presence of phenocopies, mosaicism, and chance (stochastic factors). Interfamilial variability of expression may be due to the previously mentioned factors, but may also be due to allelic or locus genetic heterogeneity. Expansion of this concept is frequently seen in newly described microdeletion and microduplication syndromes.

7. Genetic heterogeneity—Several different genetic mutations may produce phenotypes that are identical or similar enough to have been traditionally considered as one diagnosis. "Anemia" or "intellectual disability" are examples of this. There are two types of genetic heterogeneity, locus heterogeneity, and allelic heterogeneity.

A. **LOCUS HETEROGENEITY**—Locus heterogeneity describes a phenotype caused by mutations at more than one genetic locus; that is, mutations at different loci cause the same phenotype or a group of phenotypes that appear similar enough to have been previously classified as a single disease, clinical "entity," or diagnostic spectrum. An example would be Sanfilippo syndrome (mucopolysaccharidosis types IIIA, B, C, and D), in which the same phenotype is produced by four different enzyme deficiencies.

B. **ALLELIC HETEROGENEITY**—A phenotype causing different mutations at a single-gene locus. As an example, cystic fibrosis may be caused by many different genetic changes, such as homozygosity for the common Δ*F508* mutation, or Δ*F508* and an *R117H* mutation. The latter example represents **compound heterozygosity**.

8. Phenotypic heterogeneity or "clinical heterogeneity"—This term describes the situation in which more than one phenotype is caused by different allelic mutations at a single locus. For example, different mutations in the *FGFR2* gene can cause different craniosynostosis disorders, including Crouzon syndrome, Jackson-Weiss syndrome, Pfeiffer syndrome, and Apert syndrome. These syndromes are clinically distinguishable and are due to the presence of a variety of genetic mutations within single genes.

9. Homozygous—A cell or organism that has identical alleles at a particular locus is said to be homozygous. For example, a cystic fibrosis patient with a Δ*F508* mutation on both alleles would be called homozygous for that mutation.

10. Heterozygous—A cell or organism that has nonidentical alleles at a genetic locus is said to be heterozygous. In autosomal dominant conditions, a mutation of only one copy of the gene pair is all that is necessary to result in a disease state. However, an individual who is heterozygous for a recessive disorder will not manifest symptoms (see the next section).

Hereditary Patterns

A. Autosomal Dominant Inheritance

Autosomal dominant inheritance has the following characteristics:

1. If a parent is affected, the risk for each offspring of inheriting the abnormal dominant gene is 50%, or 1:2. This is true whether the gene is penetrant or not in the parent.

2. Both males and females can pass on the abnormal gene to children of either sex, although the manifestations may vary according to sex.

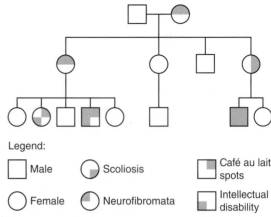

Legend:
□ Male ◑ Scoliosis ▣ Café au lait spots
○ Female ◑ Neurofibromata ▣ Intellectual disability

▲ **Figure 37–4.** Autosomal dominant inheritance. Variable expressivity in Neurofibromatosis type 1.

3. Dominant inheritance is typically said to be vertical, that is, the condition passes from one generation to the next in a vertical fashion (Figure 37–4).

4. Explanations for a negative family history include the following:

a. Nonpaternity/nonmaternity.

b. Decreased penetrance or mild manifestations in one of the parents.

c. Germline mosaicism (ie, mosaicism in the germ cell line of either parent). Germline mosaicism may mimic autosomal recessive inheritance, because it leads to situations in which two children of completely normal parents are affected with a genetic disorder. Recurrence risks are in the range of 1%–7%.

d. The abnormality present in the patient may be a phenocopy, or it may be a similar but genetically different abnormality with a different mode of inheritance.

e. De novo mutation.

B. Autosomal Recessive Inheritance

Autosomal recessive inheritance also has some distinctive characteristics:

1. The recurrence risk for parents of an affected child is 25%, or 1:4 for each pregnancy. The gene carrier frequency in the general population is used to assess the risk of having an affected child with a new partner, for unaffected siblings, and for the affected individuals themselves.

2. Parents are most often obligate carriers and are clinically unaffected. (Exceptions to this rule exist: Carriers of sickle cell trait may become symptomatic if they become hypoxic.)

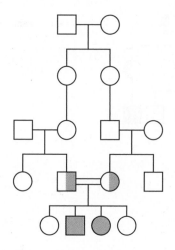

Legend:

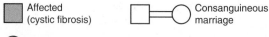

■ Affected (cystic fibrosis)

◻═○ Consanguineous marriage

◖ Carrier

▲ **Figure 37–5.** Autosomal recessive inheritance: cystic fibrosis.

3. Males and females are affected equally.

4. Inheritance is horizontal; siblings may be affected (Figure 37–5).

5. The family history is usually negative, with the exception of siblings.

6. In rare instances, a child with a recessive disorder may have inherited both copies of the abnormal gene from one parent and none from the other (UPD).

C. X-Linked Inheritance

When a gene for a specific disorder is on the X chromosome, the condition is said to be X-linked. Females may be either homozygous or heterozygous, because they have two X chromosomes. Males have only one X, and are hemizygous for any gene on their X chromosome. The severity of any X-linked disorder is generally greater in males than in females (within a specific family). According to the Lyon hypothesis, because one of the two X chromosomes in each cell is inactivated, and this inactivation is random, the clinical picture in females depends on the percentage of genetically altered versus normal alleles inactivated. The X chromosome is not activated until about 14 days of gestation, and parts of the short arm remain active throughout life.

1. X-linked recessive inheritance—The following features are characteristic of X-linked recessive inheritance:

a. Males are affected, and heterozygous females are either normal or have mild manifestations.

b. Inheritance is diagonal through the maternal side of the family (Figure 37–6A).

c. A female carrier has a 50% chance that each daughter will be a carrier and a 50% chance that each son will be affected.

d. All of the daughters of an affected male are carriers, and none of his sons are affected.

e. Occasionally a female may be fully affected. Several possible mechanisms may account for a fully affected female: (aa.) skewed X-inactivation; (bb.) 45,X karyotype; (cc.) homozygosity for the abnormal gene; (dd.) an X-autosome translocation, or other structural abnormality of one X chromosome, in which the X chromosome of normal structure is preferentially inactivated; (ee.) UPD; and (ff.) nonrandom inactivation, which may be controlled by an autosomal gene.

2. X-linked dominant inheritance—The X-linked dominant inheritance pattern is less common than the X-linked recessive type. Examples include incontinentia pigmenti and hypophosphatemic or vitamin D-resistant rickets. The following features are characteristic of X-linked dominant inheritance:

a. The heterozygous female is symptomatic, and the disease is twice as common in females because they have two X chromosomes that can have the mutation.

b. Clinical manifestations are more variable in females than in males.

c. The risk for the offspring of heterozygous females to be affected is 50% regardless of sex.

d. All of the daughters but none of the sons of affected males will have the disorder (Figure 37–6B).

e. Although a homozygous female is possible (particularly in an inbred population), she would be severely involved. All of her children would also be affected but more mildly.

f. Some disorders (eg, incontinentia pigmenti) are lethal in males (and in homozygous females). Affected women have twice as many daughters as sons and an increased incidence of miscarriages, because affected males will be spontaneously aborted. A 47,XXY karyotype has allowed affected males to survive.

D. Y-Linked Inheritance

In Y-linked inheritance, also known as "holandric" inheritance, a disorder is caused by genes located on the Y chromosome. These conditions are relatively rare. Male-to-male transmission is seen in this category, with all sons of affected males being affected and no daughters or females being affected.

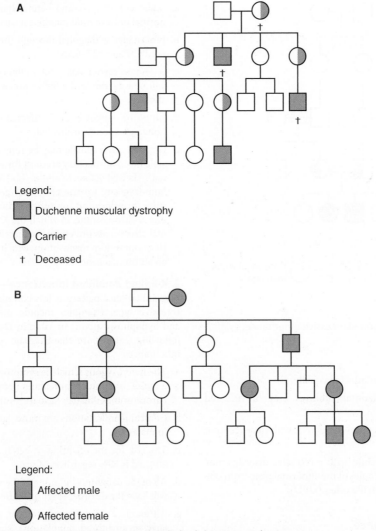

Legend:

■ Duchenne muscular dystrophy

◐ Carrier

† Deceased

Legend:

■ Affected male

● Affected female

▲ **Figure 37–6. A:** X-linked recessive inheritance. **B:** X-linked dominant inheritance.

MULTIFACTORIAL INHERITANCE

Many common attributes, such as height, are familial, and are the result of the actions of multiple rather than single genes. Inheritance of these traits is described as **polygenic** or **multifactorial**. The latter term recognizes that environmental factors such as diet also contribute to these traits. Targeted genetic testing for these conditions is not available.

Many disorders and congenital abnormalities that are clearly familial but do not segregate as Mendelian traits (eg, autosomal dominant, recessive) show polygenic inheritance. Generally speaking, these conditions become manifest when thresholds of additive gene actions or contributing environmental factors are exceeded. Many common disorders ranging from hypertension, stroke, and alcoholism demonstrate multifactorial (polygenic) inheritance. Some common birth defects, including isolated congenital heart disease, cleft lip and palate, and neural tube defects, also demonstrate polygenic inheritance. Polygenic or multifactorial inheritance has several distinctive characteristics:

1. The risk for relatives of affected persons is increased. The risk is higher for first-degree relatives (those who have 50% of their genes in common) and lower for more distant relations, although the risk for the latter is higher than for the general population (Table 37–1).

Table 37–1. Empiric risks for some congenital disorders.

Anencephaly and spina bifida: incidence (average) 1:1000
One affected child: 2%–3%
Two affected children: 10%–12%
One affected parent: 4%–5%
Hydrocephalus: incidence 1:2000 newborns
Occasional X-linked recessive
Often associated with neural tube defect
Some environmental etiologies (eg, toxoplasmosis)
Recurrence risk, one affected child
Hydrocephalus: 1%
Some central nervous system abnormality: 3%
Nonsyndromic cleft lip and/or palate: incidence (average) 1:1000
One affected child: 2%–4%
One affected parent: 2%–4%
Two affected children: 10%
One affected parent, one affected child: 10%–20%
Nonsyndromic cleft palate: incidence 1:2000
One affected child: 2%
Two affected children: 6%–8%
One affected parent: 4%–6%
One affected parent, one affected child: 15%–20%
Congenital heart disease: incidence 8:1000
One affected child: 2%–3%
One affected parent, one affected child: 10%
Clubfoot: incidence 1:1000 (male:female = 2:1)
One affected child: 2%–3%
Congenital dislocated hip: incidence 1:1000
(female > male) with marked regional variation
One child affected: 2%–14%

Pyloric stenosis: Incidence, males: 1:200; females: 1:1000

Male index patient	
Brothers	3.2%
Sons	6.8%
Sisters	3.0%
Daughters	1.2%
Female index patient	
Brothers	13.2%
Sons	20.5%
Sisters	2.5%
Daughters	11.1%

2. The risk is higher if the defect is more severe. In Hirschsprung disease, the longer the aganglionic segment, the higher is the recurrence risk.

3. Sex ratios may not be equal. If a marked discrepancy exists, the recurrence risk is higher if a child of the less commonly affected sex has the disorder. This assumes that more genetic factors are required to raise the more resistant sex above the threshold. For example, pyloric stenosis is more common in males. If the first affected child is a female, the recurrence risk is higher than if the child is a male.

4. The risk for the offspring of an affected person is approximately the same as the risk for siblings, assuming that the spouse of the affected person has a negative family history. For many conditions, however, assortative mating, "like marrying like," adds to risks in offspring.

NONMENDELIAN INHERITANCE

Epigenetic Regulation

Although development is regulated by genes, it is initiated and sustained by nongenetic processes. Epigenetic events are functionally relevant changes to the genome that are independent of changes in the primary DNA sequence. Genetic imprinting and DNA methylation are examples of epigenetic processes that affect expression. Certain genes important in regulation of growth and differentiation are themselves regulated by chemical modification that occurs in specific patterns in gametes. Certain techniques developed to assist infertile couples (advanced reproductive technology) may affect epigenetic processes and contribute to genetic disorders in the offspring conceived via these methods.

Storey KB: Regulation of hypometabolism: insights into epigenetic controls. J Exp Biol 2015 Jan 1;218(Pt 1):150–159 [PMID: 25568462].

Imprinting

The parental origin of chromosome pairs affects which genes are transcribed and which are inactivated. The term *imprinting* refers to the process by which preferential transcription of certain genes takes place. Various chromosomes, particularly chromosome X, 15, 11, and 7, have imprinted regions where some genes are only read from one homolog (ie, either the maternal or paternal allele). Under typical circumstances, the gene on the other parental homolog is typically inactivated. Errors in imprinting may arise because of UPD (in which a copy from one parent is missing), chromosomal deletion causing loss of the gene normally transcribed, mutations in the imprinting genes that normally code for transcription, or inactivation of other genes downstream. A good example of how imprinting may affect human disease is Beckwith-Wiedemann Syndrome; the locus is located on chromosome band 11p15.

Cohen JL: Diagnosis and management of the phenotypic spectrum of twins with Beckwith-Wiedemann syndrome. Am J Med Genet A 2019 May 8 [PMID: 31067005].

Genetic Anticipation

Anticipation is a pattern of inheritance in which symptoms became manifest at earlier ages and with increasing severity as traits are passed to subsequent generations. Associated repeat sequences of DNA at disease loci are not stable when passed through meiosis. Repeated DNA sequences, in particular triplets (eg, CGG and CAG), tend to increase their copy number. As these runs of triplets expand, they eventually affect the expression of genes and produce symptoms. Disorders undergoing triplet repeat expansion detected thus far produce primarily neurologic symptoms. Most conditions are progressive. The size of the triplet expansion is roughly correlated with the timing and severity of symptoms.

Autosomal dominant disorders include several spinal cerebellar atrophies, Huntington disease, and myotonic dystrophy. Unstable triplet repeat expansion contributes to at least one autosomal recessive disorder, Friedreich ataxia. The most common X-linked disorder demonstrating triplet repeat instability and expansion is Fragile X syndrome.

Mitochondrial Inheritance

Mitochondrial disorders can be caused by both nuclear and mitochondrial genes. Mitochondrial DNA (mtDNA) is double-stranded, 16,569 base pairs in length, circular, smaller than nuclear DNA, and is inherited maternally. It codes for 13 gene products involved in oxidative phosphorylation and electron transport.

MtDNA can sustain pathogenic point mutations, deletions, or duplications. However, there is a threshold effect depending on the heteroplasmy (cells contain both normal and abnormal mtDNA, Figure 37–7). Due to the difficulty in diagnosing mitochondrial DNA disorders, and the variability of the clinical course, it is often difficult to calculate specific recurrence risks. Further details are found in Chapter 36 Inborn Errors of Metabolism.

Copeland WC, Longley MJ: Mitochondrial genome maintenance in health and disease. DNA Repair (Amst) 2014 Jul;19:190–198 [PMID: 24780559].
Dimmock DP, Lawlor MW: Presentation and diagnostic evaluation of mitochondrial disease. Pediatr Clin North Am 2017 Feb; 64(1):161–171. doi: 10.1016/j.pcl.2016.08.011. Review. [PMID: 27894442].

FAMILY HISTORY & PEDIGREE

Critical in the evaluation of a potential genetic condition is the construction of a family tree, also known as a pedigree. Underused by most medical personnel, the pedigree is a valuable record of genetic and medical information, which

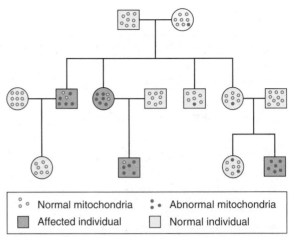

▲ **Figure 37–7.** Mitochondrial inheritance. Mutations are transmitted through the maternal line.

is much more useful in visual form than in list form. Tips for pedigree preparation include the following:

- Start with the proband—the patient's siblings and parents, and obtain a three-generational history at minimum, as possible.
- Always ask about consanguinity.
- Obtain data from both sides of the family.
- Ask about spontaneous abortions, stillbirths, infertility, children relinquished for adoption, and deceased individuals.

In the course of taking the family history, one may find information that is not relevant in elucidating the cause of the patients' problem but may indicate a risk for other important health concerns. Conditions unrelated to the chief complaint should be directed for follow-up care. Examples of the latter scenario include an overwhelming family history of early-onset breast and ovarian cancer, or multiple pregnancy losses noted in a pediatric genetic intake evaluation.

Bennett RL et al: Standardized human pedigree nomenclature: update and assessment of the recommendations of the National Society of genetic counselors. J Genet Couns 2008;17:424–433 [PMID: 18792771].
He D et al: IPED2X: a robust pedigree reconstruction algorithm for complicated pedigrees. J Bioinform Comput Biol 2014 Dec;12(6):1442007 [PMID: 25553812].

▼ DYSMORPHOLOGY & HUMAN EMBRYOLOGY

Birth defects are the leading cause of death in the first year of life. They are evident in 2%–3% of newborn infants and in up to 7% of adults. Many are detected by prenatal ultrasound. Clinical investigation of the causes and consequences of congenital structural defects is called dysmorphology.

MECHANISMS

Developmental Biology

Cell proliferation and programmed cell death (apoptosis) both contribute to embryonic structural formation. Products of other genes establish regulatory pathways in which positive and negative signaling loops initiate and maintain cell differentiation with precise timing. Further understanding of these mechanisms may lead to interventions that could prevent birth defects or potentially provide treatment prenatally. An example of the evolution of the aforementioned process is fetal surgery for neural tube defects.

Cellular Interactions

There is a hierarchy of gene expression during development. Morphogenesis begins with expression of genes encoding transcription factors. These proteins bind to DNA in undifferentiated embryonic cells and recruit them into developmental fields. Spatial relationships are established orientation of cells that occurs with respect to their neighbors. As fields differentiate into identifiable tissues (eg, ectoderm, mesoderm, and endoderm), cellular proliferation, migration, and further differentiation are mediated through genes encoding cell signaling proteins.

Signaling proteins include growth factors and their receptors, cellular adhesion molecules, and extracellular matrix proteins that both provide structure and position signals to developing tissues. Genetic mutations that alter these pathways can yield genetic disease.

Environmental Factors

The effects of exogenous agents during development are also mediated through genetically regulated pathways. At the cellular level, xenobiotics (compounds foreign to nature) cause birth defects either because they disrupt cell signaling and thereby misdirect morphogenesis, or because they are cytotoxic and lead to cell death in excess of the usual developmental program.

In general, drug receptors expressed in embryos and fetuses are the same molecules that mediate pharmacologic effects in adults. Over-the-counter, prescribed inhalants, and schedule I and II drugs that are pharmacologically active in mothers will be active across the placenta. Exposure to agents achieving cytotoxic levels in adults are likely to be teratogenic (ie, cause birth defects). Abused substances such as alcohol that are toxic to adults are predictably toxic to embryos and fetuses.

Transplacental pharmacologic effects can be therapeutic. The potential for embryonic and fetal drug therapies during pregnancy is increasing. Folic acid supplementation can lower risks for birth defects such as spina bifida, and maternally administered corticosteroids can induce fetal synthesis and secretion of pulmonary surfactants prior to delivery.

Mechanical Factors

Much of embryonic development and all of fetal growth occurs normally within the low pressure and space provided by amniotic fluid. Loss or inadequate production of amniotic fluid can have disastrous effects, as can disruption of placental membranes.

Lung and kidney development are particularly sensitive to mechanical forces. Constriction of the chest through malformation of the ribs, lack of surrounding amniotic fluid, or lack of movement (fetal breathing) leads to varying degrees of pulmonary hypoplasia in which lungs are smaller than normal and develop fewer alveoli. The presentation at birth is respiratory distress and may be lethal. This can be seen in conditions that cause renal malformations or agenesis such as 22q11.2 deletion syndrome.

Uteropelvic junction (UPJ) is frequently associated with obstruction of ureters or bladder outflow. As pressure within obstructed renal collecting systems increases, it distorts cell interactions and alters histogenesis. Developing kidneys exposed to increased internal pressures for long periods eventually become nonfunctional.

CLINICAL DYSMORPHOLOGY

An important task for the clinician presented with an infant with a birth defect is to determine whether the problem is isolated or part of a larger embryopathy (or syndrome).

Terminology

Classification of dysmorphic features strives to reflect mechanisms of abnormal development. Birth defects are referred to as **malformations** when they result from altered genetic or developmental processes such as Dandy Walker malformation. **Deformations** are mainly structural defects caused by a mechanical force, such as positional clubfeet. The term **dysplasia** is used to denote abnormal development or growth of a group of tissues, organs, or cells, such as skeletal dysplasia. When physical forces interrupt or distort morphogenesis, their effects are termed **disruptions**, such as seen in amniotic bands. Those in which the chronological order of abnormal development is understood may be referred to as sequences, such as Robin sequence (or Pierre Robin anomaly) which describes a U-shaped cleft palate that occurs secondary to jaw underdevelopment (retrognathia), subsequently displacing the tongue and preventing posterior closure of the palate. However, not all birth defects and dysmorphic features result from a single mechanism; Prune Belly syndrome is caused by urinary tract malformations that result in over extension of the abdominal muscles.

Malformations classified by pattern include syndrome and association. **Syndromes** are defined as a cluster of malformations that occurs in a recognizable pattern with a known genetic cause. Those malformations that are well known to co-occur are classified as **associations, such as VACTERL association**. Association should be used as a diagnosis of exclusion. When a unifying cause can be identified, such as a chromosomal anomaly or a pathogenic mutation of a single gene, a more precise diagnosis should replace "association."

Evaluation of the Dysmorphic Infant

History and physical examinations provide most of the clues to diagnosis. Special aspects of these procedures in a clinical genetics setting are outlined in the following sections. The extent of an infant's abnormalities may not be immediately apparent, and parents who feel grief and guilt are often desperate for information.

A. History

Pregnancy histories are a critical part of the history intake. Review of gestational age, intrauterine drug exposure, prenatal complications, and prenatal testing is important. Family histories are preferred in pedigree formation. Environmental histories should include descriptions of parental habits and work settings. Targeted histories, based on chief complaint should be obtained with past medical and surgical histories, developmental history, and review of systems.

B. Physical Examination

Meticulous physical examination is crucial for accurate diagnosis in dysmorphic infants and children. In addition to the routine procedures described in Chapter 2, special attention should be paid to the neonate's physical measurements. Photographs are helpful and should include a consistent method of measurement for reference.

C. Imaging and Laboratory Studies

Radiologic investigation is fundamental in the assessment and management of dysmorphic patients. A series of nine plain radiographs, called a skeletal survey, is useful in the evaluation of patients with suspected skeletal dysplasia. Magnetic resonance imaging (MRI), with or without angiogram, venogram, or spectroscopy, contributes to diagnostic evaluation when clinically indicated. Computed tomography (CT) is useful for bony structure assessment, but less so for deep tissue evaluation in comparison to MRI. Ultrasonography also has case-dependent utility for noninvasive imaging. Consultation with a radiologist is encouraged if there is any question about which imaging modality would serve the patient best.

Traditional cytogenetic analysis provides specific diagnoses in approximately 5% of dysmorphic infants who survive the neonatal period. Chromosomal abnormalities are recognized in 10%–15% of infants who die. The chromosomal microarray increases the diagnostic yield by 10%–15%. Of note, many copy number variations (CNVs) exist in different individuals; therefore, interpretation is sometimes difficult and may require parental samples for clarification. Common disorders such as trisomies 21, 13, and 18 can be determined

rapidly (48–72 hours) through use of FISH, but this technique should be accompanied by a complete karyotype. As a rule, a normal karyotype does not rule out the presence of significant genetic disease. Any case requiring rapid diagnosis should be discussed with an experienced clinical geneticist. The WES approach is also being used clinically to look for causal mutations across a patient's entire exome. The diagnostic yield of WES in a clinical laboratory setting for patients with a broad range of phenotypes is about 25% in pediatrics and 17% in adults.

Benachi A, Sarnacki S: Prenatal counseling and the role of the paediatric surgeon. Semin Pediatr Surg 2014 Oct;23(5):240–243 [PMID: 25459006].

Posey JE, Rosenfeld JA: Molecular diagnostic experience of whole-exome sequencing in adult patients. Genet Med 2016 Jul;18(7):678–685 [PMID: 26633545].

▼ CHROMOSOMAL DISORDERS: ABNORMAL NUMBER

TRISOMIES

1. Trisomy 21 (Down Syndrome)

ESSENTIALS OF DIAGNOSIS & TYPICAL FEATURES

- ▶ Characteristic features include upslanting palpebral fissures, epicanthal folds, midface hypoplasia, and small, dysplastic pinnae.
- ▶ Generalized hypotonia.
- ▶ Cognitive disabilities (usually mild to moderate).
- ▶ Associated with congenital heart disease and gastrointestinal anomalies.

Down syndrome occurs in about 1:700 newborns. Cognitive disabilities in the mild/moderate range are characteristic of Down syndrome, as is generalized hypotonia. The affected newborn may have prolonged physiologic jaundice, and transient blood count abnormalities. Feeding problems and constipation are common during infancy. Problems which may develop during childhood include thyroid dysfunction, visual issues, hearing loss, obstructive sleep apnea, celiac disease, atlanto-occipital instability, and autism. Leukemia is 12–20 times more common in patients with Down syndrome.

▶ Clinical Findings

The principal physical findings include a flattened occiput, characteristic facies (upslanting palpebral fissures, epicanthal folds, midface hypoplasia, and small, dysplastic pinnae), and minor limb abnormalities. About one-third to one-half of children with Down syndrome have congenital heart disease, most often endocardial cushion defects or other septal defects. Anomalies of the gastrointestinal tract, including esophageal and duodenal atresias, are seen in about 15% of cases.

Information regarding healthcare guidelines for patients with Down syndrome. https://www.healthychildren.org/English/health-issues/conditions/developmental-disabilities/Documents/Health_Care_Information_for_Families_of_Children_with_Down_Syndrome.pdf.

Marilyn Bull and the Committee on Genetics: Clinical report: health supervision for children with Down syndrome. Pediatrics 2011;128:393–406 [PMID: 21788214].

2. Trisomy 18 Syndrome

The incidence of trisomy 18 syndrome is about 1:4000 live births, and the ratio of affected males to females is approximately 1:3. Trisomy 18 is characterized by prenatal and postnatal growth retardation, which is often severe, and hypertonicity. Complications are related to associated anomalies. Death is often caused by heart failure or pneumonia and usually occurs in infancy or early childhood, although a small percentage of patients reach adulthood. Surviving children show severe cognitive disabilities with limited abilities to communicate and ambulate.

▶ Clinical Findings

Infants with trisomy 18 are often small for gestational age and have dysmorphic features including a characteristic facies and extremities (overlapping fingers and rocker-bottom feet) and congenital heart disease (often ventricular septal defect or patent ductus arteriosus). To see clinical pictures of patients with trisomy 18, visit the following website: http://medgen.genetics.utah.edu/photographs/pages/trisomy_18.htm.

3. Trisomy 13 Syndrome

The incidence of trisomy 13 is about 1 per 12,000 live births, and 60% of affected individuals are female. Most infants with trisomy 13 have congenital anomalies that are incompatible with survival. Surviving children demonstrate failure to thrive, cognitive disabilities, apneic spells, seizures, and deafness. Death usually occurs in early infancy or by the second year of life, commonly as a result of heart failure or infection.

▶ Clinical Findings

The symptoms and signs include characteristic features, often a normal birth weight, CNS malformations, eye malformations, cleft lip and palate, polydactyly or syndactyly, and congenital heart disease. The facies of an infant with trisomy 13 can be viewed at the following website: http://medgen.genetics.utah.edu/photographs/pages/trisomy_13.htm.

▶ Treatment of Trisomies

A. Medical Therapy

Trisomy 21: Interventions for specific issues such as surgical intervention for cardiac and GI anomalies, screening for autoimmune disorders such as hypothyroidism and celiac disease, developmental supports such as infant stimulation programs, special education, and physical, occupational, and speech therapies are all indicated. The goal of treatment is to help affected children develop to their full potential. Parents' participation in support groups such as the local chapter of the National Down Syndrome Congress should be encouraged. See the following website: http://www.ndss.org/.

There is no treatment other than general supportive care for trisomy 13 or 18. Rapid confirmation of suspected trisomy 13 or 18 can be made by FISH. A support group for families of children with trisomies 13 and 18 who survive beyond infancy is called SOFT. See the following website: http://www.trisomy.org/.

B. Genetic Counseling

Trisomy arises from errors of nondisjunction. Most parents of trisomic infants have normal karyotypes. The risk of having a child affected with a trisomy increases with maternal age. The recurrence risk for trisomy in future pregnancies is equal to 1 per 100 plus the age-specific maternal risk.

If the child has a trisomy resulting from a translocation, and the parent has an abnormal karyotype, the risks are increased. When the mother is the carrier of a balanced Robertsonian translocation, there is a 10%–15% chance that the child will be affected and a 33% chance that the child will be a balanced translocation carrier. When the father is the carrier, there is a smaller than 0.5% chance of having another affected child. If the child has a 21/21 translocation and one parent has the translocation, the recurrence risk is 100%.

SEX CHROMOSOME ABNORMALITIES

1. Turner Syndrome (Monosomy X)

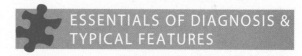

ESSENTIALS OF DIAGNOSIS & TYPICAL FEATURES

▶ Webbed neck, triangular facies, short stature, wide-set nipples, amenorrhea, and absence of secondary sex characteristics.

▶ Associated with coarctation of the aorta and genitourinary malformations.

▶ IQ is usually normal but learning disabilities are common.

▶ Mosaic individuals may manifest only short stature and amenorrhea.

The incidence of Turner syndrome is 1 per 10,000 females. However, it is estimated that 95% of conceptuses with monosomy X are miscarried and only 5% are liveborn.

▶ Clinical Findings

Newborns with Turner syndrome may have webbed neck, edema of the hands and feet, coarctation of the aorta, and a characteristic triangular facies. Other findings in older girls may include short stature, a shield chest with wide-set nipples, streak ovaries, amenorrhea, absence of secondary sex characteristics, and infertility. Some affected girls, particularly those with mosaicism, have only short stature and amenorrhea, without dysmorphic features. Learning disabilities are common, secondary to difficulties in perceptual motor integration.

▶ Treatment

Academic supports for learning issues perceptual difficulties are important. Hormonal treatment includes estrogen therapy, which permits development of secondary sex characteristics and normal menstruation, and prevents osteoporosis. Growth hormone therapy is also used to increase the height of affected girls. Females with 45,X or 45,X mosaicism have a low fertility rate, and those who become pregnant have a high risk of fetal death (spontaneous miscarriage, ~30%; stillbirth, 6%–10%). Furthermore, their liveborn offspring have an increased frequency of chromosomal abnormalities involving either sex chromosomes or autosomes and congenital malformations. Thus, prenatal ultrasonography and chromosome analysis are indicated for the offspring of females with sex chromosome abnormalities.

2. Klinefelter Syndrome (XXY)

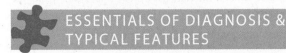

ESSENTIALS OF DIAGNOSIS & TYPICAL FEATURES

- ▶ Diagnosis is rarely made before puberty.
- ▶ Key findings include microorchidism; lack of libido; minimal facial hair; and tall, eunuchoid build.
- ▶ IQ can vary (normal to borderline with a small percentage showing cognitive disabilities).

The incidence of Klinefelter syndrome in the newborn population is roughly 1 per 1000, but it is about 1% among intellectual disabilities males and about 3% among males seen at infertility clinics. The maternal age at birth is often advanced. Unlike Turner syndrome, Klinefelter syndrome is rarely the cause of spontaneous abortions. The diagnosis is seldom made before puberty except as a result of prenatal diagnosis, because prepubertal boys have a normal phenotype.

▶ Clinical Findings

The characteristic findings after puberty include small testicles associated with otherwise normal external genitalia, azoospermia, sterility, gynecomastia, normal to borderline IQ, diminished facial hair, and a tall, eunuchoid build. In chromosome variants with three or four X chromosomes (XXXY and XXXXY), intellectual disabilities may be severe, and skeletal and genital anomalies may be present. In general, the physical and mental abnormalities associated with Klinefelter syndrome increase as the number of sex chromosomes increases.

▶ Treatment

Males with Klinefelter syndrome require testosterone replacement therapy. The presence of the extra X chromosome may allow expression of what might normally be a lethal X-linked disorder to occur.

3. XYY Syndrome

Newborns with XYY syndrome in general are normal. Affected individuals may on occasion exhibit an abnormal behavior pattern from early childhood and may have mild intellectual disabilities. Fertility may be normal. Many males with an XYY karyotype are normal. There is no treatment.

4. XXX Syndrome

The incidence of females with an XXX karyotype is approximately 1 per 1000. Females with XXX are phenotypically normal. However, they tend to be taller than usual and to have lower IQs than their normal siblings. Learning and behavioral issues are relatively common. This is in contrast to individuals with XXXX, a much more rare condition causing more severe developmental issues, and a dysmorphic phenotype reminiscent of Down syndrome.

Jones KL: *Smith's Recognizable Patterns of Human Malformation.* 7th ed. Philadelphia, PA: Elsevier; 2013.

▼ CHROMOSOMAL ABNORMALITIES: ABNORMAL STRUCTURE

Chromosomal abnormalities most often present in newborns as multiple congenital anomalies in association with intrauterine growth retardation. In addition to trisomies as just described, other more subtle chromosomal abnormalities are also common. In some cases, a chromosomal rearrangement is too subtle to be detected by karyotype. The current technology, comparative genomic hybridization array (microarray), enables screening for multiple submicroscopic chromosomal abnormalities simultaneously, and is a very helpful tool in evaluating the child with a suspected chromosomal abnormality.

Although most cases of severe chromosomal abnormality such as trisomy are lethal, some individuals may survive if the abnormality exists in mosaic form. Two examples of this include trisomy 8 and Cat eye syndrome, caused by extra genetic material, which is derived from a portion of chromosome 22.

Moeschler JB, Shevell M; Committee on Genetics: Comprehensive evaluation of the child with intellectual disability or global developmental delays. Pediatrics 2014 Sep;134(3):e903–e918 [PMID: 25157020].

CHROMOSOME DELETION DISORDERS

Three common chromosomal deletion disorders that were previously detected on routine karyotype analysis, and confirmed via FISH assay, but are now detected with microarray, are 1p36– syndrome, Wolf-Hirschhorn syndrome (4p–), and cri du chat syndrome (5p–). Microdeletion or contiguous gene syndrome are referring to those small deletion not readily picked up by karyotype but detected by microarray or FISH.

1. Deletion 1p36 Syndrome

Microcephaly and a large anterior fontanelle are characteristic features of 1p36– syndrome. Cardiac defects are common, and dilated cardiomyopathy may present in infancy. Intellectual disability, hypotonia, hearing loss, and seizures are usually seen.

2. Wolf-Hirschhorn Syndrome

Also known as 4p– (deletion of 4p16), this syndrome is characterized by microcephaly and unusual development of the nose and orbits that produces an appearance suggesting an ancient Greek warrior's helmet. Other anomalies commonly seen include cleft lip and palate and cardiac and renal defects. Seizure disorders are common, and the majority of patients have severe intellectual disability.

3. Cri du Chat Syndrome

Also known as 5p– (deletion of terminal chromosome 5p), this disorder is characterized by unique facial features, growth retardation, and microcephaly. Patients have an unusual catlike cry. Most patients have major organ anomalies and significant intellectual disability.

CONTIGUOUS GENE DISORDERS

Contiguous gene disorders are conditions caused by deletion or duplication of genetic material involving multiple genes. Three common contiguous gene disorders diagnosed by microarray are Williams syndrome, Smith-Magenis syndrome, and 22q11.2 deletion syndrome.

1. Williams Syndrome

Williams syndrome is a contiguous gene disorder that deletes the gene for elastin and other neighboring genes at 7q11.2. It is characterized by short stature; congenital heart disease (supravalvular aortic or pulmonic stenosis); coarse, elfin-like facies with prominent lips; hypercalcemia or hypercalciuria in infancy; developmental delay; and neonatal irritability evolving into an overly friendly personality. Calcium restriction may be necessary in early childhood to prevent nephrocalcinosis. The hypercalcemia often resolves during the first year of life. The natural history includes progression of cardiac disease and predisposition to hypertension and spinal osteoarthritis in adults. Most patients have mild to moderate intellectual deficits.

Duplication of chromosome 7q11.2 results in a syndrome that includes speech delay, and features of autistic spectrum disorders. Physical features are less consistent than in Williams syndrome.

2. Smith-Magenis Syndrome

This syndrome is associated with a microdeletion of 17p11 and is characterized by prominent forehead, deep-set eyes, cupid-shaped upper lip, self-mutilating behavior, sleep disturbance, and intellectual disabilities. Some patients also have seizure disorders, hearing loss, thyroid disease, and immunological and lipid abnormalities.

Duplication of 17p11 produces Potocki-Lupski syndrome that is characterized by growth failure, variable levels of cognitive deficiencies, autistic features, and, occasionally, structural abnormalities of the heart.

Neira-Fresneda J, Potocki L: Neurodevelopmental disorders associated with abnormal gene dosage: Smith-Magenis and Potocki-Lupski syndromes. J Pediatr Genet 2015 Sep;4(3):159–167 [PMID: 27617127].

3. 22q11.2 Deletion Syndrome (Velocardiofacial Syndrome or DiGeorge Syndrome)

This condition was originally described in newborns presenting with cyanotic congenital heart disease, usually involving great vessel abnormalities; thymic hypoplasia leading to immunodeficiency; and hypocalcemia due to absent parathyroid glands. This phenotype is highly variable. Other characteristics have also been described including mild microcephaly, hypothyroidism, kidney and cervical spine malformations, palatal clefting, velopharyngeal insufficiency, speech and language delays, congenital heart disease (great vessel abnormalities, tetralogy of Fallot, and a variety of other abnormalities), psychiatric diagnoses such as attention-deficit hyperactivity disorder, anxiety, psychoses and in about 25% of cases, schizophrenia.

Duplication of the 22q11 region produces a mild and highly variable phenotype that ranges from developmental delays and learning disabilities to functionally normal.

Chen CP et al: Chromosome 22q11.2 deletion syndrome: prenatal diagnosis, array comparative genomic hybridization characterization using uncultured amniocytes and literature review. Gene 2013 Sep 15;527(1):405–409 [PMID: 23791650].

▼ MENDELIAN DISORDERS

AUTOSOMAL DOMINANT DISORDERS

Neurofibromatosis, Marfan syndrome, achondroplasia, osteogenesis imperfecta, and the craniosynostoses are among the most well-known autosomal dominant disorders. There are many other common autosomal dominant disorders, including Treacher Collins syndrome, associated with a distinct craniofacial phenotype including malar and mandibular hypoplasia, and Noonan syndrome, which has a phenotype similar to Turner syndrome with characterization of short stature and nuchal redundancy. CHARGE syndrome and Cornelia de Lange syndrome are not infrequently encountered and have fairly consistent classic presentations.

1. Neurofibromatosis Type 1

Neurofibromatosis type 1 (NF-1) is one of the most common autosomal dominant disorders, occurring in 1 per 3000 births and seen in all races and ethnic groups. In general, the disorder is progressive, with new manifestations appearing over time. Neurofibromatosis type 2 (NF-2), characterized by bilateral acoustic neuromas with minimal or no skin manifestations, is a different disease caused by a different gene.

The gene for NF-1 is on the long arm of chromosome 17 and seems to code for a protein similar to a tumor suppresser factor. NF results from many different mutations of this gene. Approximately half of all NF cases are caused by new mutations. Careful evaluation of the parents is necessary to provide accurate genetic counseling. Recent evidence suggests that penetrance is close to 100% in those who carry a gene variant if individuals are examined carefully.

Café au lait (hyperpigmented), light brown macules may be present at birth, and the majority of individuals with NF-1 will have more than six by age 1 year. Neurocutaneous findings are declarative by age 8 years. Neurofibromas are benign tumors consisting of Schwann cells, nerve fibers, and fibroblasts; they may be discrete or plexiform. The incidence of Lisch nodules, which can be seen with a slit lamp, also increases with age. Affected individuals commonly have a large head, bony abnormalities on radiographic studies, scoliosis, and a wide spectrum of developmental problems. Half

of NF-1 patients will experience some form of intellectual delay. (For more details of medical evaluation and treatment, see Chapter 25 of this book.) Useful information is provided on the following website: http://www.nfinc.org.

Hyperpigmented macules can occur in other conditions such as McCune-Albright, Noonan, Leopard, and Bannayan-Riley-Ruvalcaba (BRR) syndromes reflective of typical wide differential diagnosis for a single physical attribute. The genes for NF-1, Noonan, and Leopard syndromes are molecules which control cell cycling through the RAS-MAPK signal transduction pathways; therefore, it is not surprising that some features can be shared.

2. Marfan Syndrome

ESSENTIALS OF DIAGNOSIS & TYPICAL FEATURES

► Skeletal abnormalities (Ghent criteria).
► Lens dislocation (ectopia lentis).
► Dilation of the aortic root.
► Dural ectasia.
► Positive family history in some cases.

▶ Clinical Findings

Genetic testing is available for mutations causing Marfan syndrome, but the diagnosis remains largely clinical and is based on the Ghent criteria (available at: https://www.marfan.org/dx/rules). Children can present with a positive family history, suspicious skeletal findings, or ophthalmologic complications. Motor milestones are frequently delayed due to joint laxity. Adolescents are prone to spontaneous pneumothorax. Dysrhythmias may be present. Aortic and valvular complications are not common in children but are more likely in sporadic cases. The characteristic facies is long and thin, with down-slanting palpebral fissures, malar flattening, and retrognathia. The palate is high arched, and dentition is often crowded. Mutations in the gene for fibrillin-1 (*FBN1*), an extracellular matrix protein (ECM), are causative.

▶ Differential Diagnosis

Homocystinuria should be excluded through metabolic testing in all individuals with marfanoid skeletal features. An X-linked recessive disorder, **Lujan syndrome**, combines marfanoid habitus with cognitive disability. Other connective tissue disorders including but not limited to: **Ehlers-Danlos syndrome** and **Stickler syndrome** may also be considered.

Mutations in the gene for fibrillin-2 (*FBN2*) and in transforming growth factor β (TGFβ) pathway can also produce phenotypes that fit in the criteria for clinical diagnosis of Marfan syndrome. Beals syndrome (FBN2), Shprintzen-Goldberg syndrome (SKI1), aneurysm-osteoarthritis syndrome, syndromic thoracic aortic aneurysms, and Loeys-Dietz syndromes (TGFβ pathway) are distinct connective tissue disorders with different medical management and prognostic implications. The reader is referred to reviews available at http://www .genereviews.org for descriptions of these disorders.

Complications

The skeletal problems including scoliosis are progressive. Astigmatism and myopia are very common and surveillance for lens dislocation is necessary.

The most serious associated medical problems involve the cardiovascular system. Although many patients with Marfan syndrome have mitral valve prolapse, the most serious concern is progressive aortic root dilation, which may lead to aneurysmal rupture and death, and progressive or acute valvular (aortic more frequently than mitral) incompetency.

Families and practitioners seeking additional information about Marfan syndrome can be referred to the National Marfan Foundation (http://www.marfan.org).

Treatment

A. Medical Therapy

Medical treatment for patients with Marfan syndrome includes surveillance for and appropriate management of the ophthalmologic, orthopedic, and cardiac issues. Serial echocardiograms are indicated to diagnose and follow the degree of aortic root enlargement, which can be managed medically or surgically, in more severe cases. Prophylactic β-adrenergic blockade or angiotensin II receptor antagonists can slow the rate of aortic dilation and reduce the development of aortic complications.

B. Genetic Counseling

Genetic testing for mutations in genes associated with aortopathy in patients with arterial dilatation should be considered in all individuals with Marfan syndrome as penetrance is variable and apparently unaffected family members can carry and pass on mutations.

Kumar A, Agarwal S: Marfan syndrome: an eyesight of syndrome. Meta Gene 2014 Jan 14;2:96–105 [PMID: 25606393].

3. Achondroplasia

Achondroplasia, the most common form of skeletal dysplasia, is caused by a mutation in *FGFR3*.

Clinical Findings

The classic phenotype includes relative macrocephaly, midface hypoplasia, short-limbed dwarfism, and trident-shaped hands. The phenotype is apparent at birth. Individuals with achondroplasia are cognitively normal.

Treatment

A. Medical Therapy

Orthopedic intervention is necessary for spinal problems including severe lumbar lordosis and gibbus deformity. Long bone lengthening surgery may help to improve upper extremity function.

Head circumference during infancy must be closely monitored and plotted on a diagnosis-specific head circumference chart. Bony overgrowth at the level of the foramen magnum may lead to progressive hydrocephalus and brainstem compression, and may warrant neurosurgical intervention.

Many patients find support through organizations such as the Little People of America, at the following website: http://www.lpaonline.org.

B. Genetic Counseling

The vast majority of cases (approximately 90%) represent a new mutation. Two heterozygous parents with achondroplasia have a 25% risk of having a child homozygous for *FGFR3* mutations, which is a lethal disorder.

4. Osteogenesis Imperfecta

Osteogenesis imperfecta (OI), or brittle bone disease, is a relatively common disorder. More than 85% of cases are caused by dominant mutations affecting COL1A1 and COL1A2. Rarer forms of OI are caused by mutations in other genes and may be inherited as autosomal.

Clinical Findings

The four most common forms of OI are the following:

1. Type I, a mild form, with bony fractures after birth and blue sclerae.

2. Type II, usually lethal in the newborn period with multiple congenital fractures and severe lung disease.

3. Type III, a severe form causing significant bony deformity secondary to multiple fractures (which are both congenital and after birth), blue sclerae, short stature, and mild restrictive lung disease.

4. Type IV, another mild form with increased incidence of fracturing after birth; dentinogenesis imperfecta is common.

Treatment

A. Medical Therapy

Geneticists and Endocrinologists are now treating OI patients with different forms of bisphosphonate compounds, which can reduce incidence of fracture and improve bone density. Patients should also be followed by an experienced orthopedist, as rodding of long bones and surgery to correct scoliosis are often required. Hearing assessments are indicated, because of the association between OI and deafness, as is close follow-up for dentinogenesis imperfecta.

B. Genetic Counseling

DNA analysis in blood can confirm mutations in the COL1A1 or COL1A2 genes which cause OI. The milder forms are often inherited as a dominant trait, while the more severe forms of OI generally result from new mutations.

5. Craniosynostosis Syndromes

The craniosynostosis disorders are common dominant disorders associated with premature fusion of cranial sutures. This class of disorders is usually caused by mutations in FGFR genes.

Crouzon syndrome is the most common of these disorders and is associated with multiple suture fusions, but with normal limbs. Other craniosynostosis disorders have limb as well as craniofacial anomalies, and include Pfeiffer, Apert, Jackson-Weiss, and Saethre-Chotzen syndromes.

Patients with craniosynostosis often have shallow orbits, midface narrowing that may result in upper airway obstruction, and hydrocephalus that may require shunting. Children with craniosynostosis may require multiple-staged craniofacial and neurosurgical procedures to address these issues, but usually have normal intelligence.

6. CHARGE Syndrome

CHARGE syndrome is a common genetic disorder presenting with unusual features, birth defects, intellectual disabilities, and abnormalities in vision and hearing. The acronym CHARGE serves as a mnemonic for associated abnormalities that include Colobomas, congenital Heart disease, choanal Atresia, growth Retardation, Genital abnormalities (hypogenitalism), and Ear abnormalities, with deafness. Facial asymmetry is a common finding. CHARGE is caused by mutations in the CHD7 gene on chromosome 8q. A website with information on CHARGE syndrome is available at http://www.chargesyndrome.org/.

Pauli S et al: CHD7 mutations causing CHARGE syndrome are predominantly of paternal origin. Clin Genet 2012;81:234–239 [PMID: 21554267].

7. Cornelia de Lange Syndrome

Cornelia de Lange syndrome is characterized by severe growth retardation; limb, especially hand, reduction defects (50%); congenital heart disease (25%); and stereotypical facies with hirsutism, medial fusion of eyebrows (synophrys), and thin, down-turned lips. The course and severity are variable, and milder presentations may be inherited as a dominant trait.

Heterozygous mutations in the cohesin regulator, NIPBL, or the cohesin structural components SMC1A and SMC3, have been identified in approximately 65% of individuals with CdLS. Cohesin regulates sister chromatid cohesion during mitosis and meiosis. In addition, cohesin has been demonstrated to play a critical role in the regulation of gene expression. Furthermore, multiple proteins in the cohesin pathway are also involved in additional fundamental biological events such as double-stranded DNA break repair, chromatin remodeling, and maintaining genomic stability.

Huisman et al: High rate of mosaicism in individuals with Cornelia de Lange syndrome. J Med Genet 2013;50:299–344 [PMID: 23505322].
Jones KL: *Recognizable Patterns of Human Malformation*. 6th ed. Philadelphia, PA: Elsevier; 2013.

8. Noonan Syndrome

Noonan syndrome is a common autosomal dominant disorder characterized by short stature, congenital heart disease, and mildly dysmoprhic features. Feeding problems may result in failure to thrive. Mild developmental delays are often present, but intelligence may be normal. Noonan syndrome and Noonan-like disorders are caused by mutations in the RAS-mitogen-activated protein kinase (MAPK) pathway, and thus are often called as "RASopathies." Noonan syndrome is the most common of these disorders, usually caused by mutations in PTPN11. Other related disorders include Cardiofacial Cutaneous syndrome and Costello syndromes. A DNA panel that screens for multiple genes in this pathway can help confirm a diagnosis. Because mutations in NF-1 causing neurofibromatosis also affect RAS proto-oncogene signaling, it is not surprising that there is an NF-1 subtype with an associated Noonan phenotype.

Roberts et al: Noonan syndrome. Lancet 2013;381(9863):333–342 [PMID: 23312968].

AUTOSOMAL RECESSIVE DISORDERS

1. Cystic Fibrosis

The gene for cystic fibrosis, CFTR, is found on the long arm of chromosome 7. Approximately 1 in 22 persons are carriers. Many different mutations have been identified; the most common mutation in the Caucasian population is known as Δ F508.

(For more details on medical management of cystic fibrosis, see Chapters 19 and 22.)

2. Smith-Lemli-Opitz Syndrome

Smith-Lemli-Opitz syndrome is a metabolic disorder in the final step of cholesterol production, resulting in low cholesterol levels and accumulation of the precursor 7-dehydrocholesterol (7-DHC). Because cholesterol is a necessary precursor for sterol hormones, and CNS myelin, and cholesterol content is crucial for the integrity of all cell membranes, the medical consequences of both cholesterol deficiency and 7-DHC accumulation are complex and severe. Also, 7-DHC is oxidized into substances called oxysterols, which are toxic to the retinal and brain.

▶ Clinical Findings

Patients with Smith-Lemli-Opitz syndrome present with a characteristic phenotype, including dysmorphic facial features (Figure 37–8), multiple congenital anomalies, hypotonia, growth failure, and intellectual disability. Mild cases may present with autism and 2–3 toe syndactyly. The diagnosis

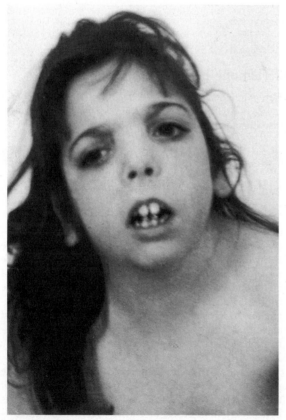

▲ **Figure 37–8.** Child with Smith-Lemli-Opitz syndrome, featuring bitemporal narrowing, upturned nares, ptosis, and small chin.

can be confirmed via a blood test looking for the presence of the precursor, 7-DHC. DNA analysis of mutations in the *DHCR7* gene is also available, as is prenatal testing.

▶ Treatment

Treatment with cholesterol can ameliorate the growth failure and lead to improvement in medical issues, although treatment does not cure this complex disorder. Antioxidant treatment is being used to prevent progressive retinal degeneration caused by oxysterol accumulation.

3. Sensorineural Hearing Loss

Although there is marked genetic heterogeneity in causes of sensorineural hearing loss, including dominant, recessive, and X-linked patterns, nonsyndromic, recessively inherited deafness is the predominant form of severe inherited childhood deafness. Several hundred genes are known to cause hereditary hearing loss and deafness. The hearing loss may be conductive, sensorineural, or a combination of both; syndromic or nonsyndromic; and prelingual (before language develops) or postlingual (after language develops). The genetic forms of hearing loss are diagnosed by otologic, audiologic, and physical examination; family history; ancillary testing (such as petrous Brain MRI to examine the inner ear and temporal bone); and molecular genetic testing. Panels screening for more than 100 genetic forms of hearing loss are available for many types of syndromic and nonsyndromic deafness.

Sartorato EL, Friderici K, Del Castillo I: Genetics of deafness. Genet Res Int 2012;2012:562848. doi: 10.1155/2012/562848 [PMID: 22567392].

4. Spinal Muscular Atrophy

Spinal muscular atrophy (SMA) is an autosomal recessive neuromuscular disorder in which anterior horn cells in the spinal cord degenerate. The mechanism for the loss of cells appears to involve apoptosis of neurons in the absence of the product of the *SMN1* (survival motor neuron) gene located on chromosome 5q. Loss of anterior horn cells leads to progressive atrophy of skeletal muscle. The disorder has an incidence of approximately 1 in 12,000, with the majority of the cases presenting in infancy. Carrier frequencies approach 1 in 40 in populations with European ancestry.

▶ Clinical Findings

Five clinical subtypes are recognized based on age of onset and rate of progression. SMA 0, which has prenatal onset, is the most devastating with profound hypotonia and respiratory failure at birth. SMA I presents with mild weakness at birth but is clearly evident by 3 months and is accompanied by loss of reflexes and fasciculations in affected muscles. Progression of the disorder leads to eventual respiratory failure, usually by age 1 year. Symptoms of SMA II begin later, with weakness and decreased reflexes generally apparent by age 2 years. Children affected with SMA III begin to become weak as they approach adolescence. SMA IV presents with onset of muscle weakness in the second or third decades with a normal life span.

Homozygous deletion of exon 7 of *SMN1* is detectable in approximately 95%–98% of cases of all types of SMA and confirms the diagnosis. The *SMN1* region on chromosome 5q is complex and variability in presentation of the disorder involves expression of up to three copies of the neighboring *SMN2* gene. More severe phenotypes have fewer *SMN2* copies. Approximately 2%–5% of patients affected with SMA will be compound heterozygotes in whom there is one copy of *SMN1* with exon 7 deleted and a second copy with a point mutation.

Prenatal diagnosis is available through genetic testing, but careful molecular analysis of the proband and demonstration of carrier status in parents is advised since, in addition to the problem of potential compound heterozygosity, 2% of cases occur as a result of a de novo mutation in one *SMN1* allele. In this case, one of the parents is not a carrier and recurrence risks are low. Carrier testing is further complicated by a duplication of *SMN1* in 4% of the population that results in there being two *SMN1* genes on one of their chromosomes. Hence, reproductive risk assessment, carrier testing, and prenatal diagnosis of SMA are best undertaken in the context of careful genetic counseling. In recent years, two different gene therapies have achieved FDA approval for the treatment of SMA. Both require immediate treatment in affected individuals raising the potential benefit of newborn screening for SMA.

X-LINKED DISORDERS

1. Duchenne & Becker Muscular Dystrophies

Duchenne muscular dystrophy (DMD) results from failure of synthesis of the muscle cytoskeletal protein dystrophin. The gene is located on the X chromosome, at position *Xp12*. Approximately 1 in 4000 male children is affected. Mutations in the same gene that result in partial expression of the dystrophin protein produce a less severe phenotype, Becker muscular dystrophy (BMD). In both DMD and BMD, progressive degeneration of skeletal and cardiac muscle occurs. Boys with DMD exhibit proximal muscle weakness and pseudohypertrophy of calf muscles by age 5–6 years. Patients become nonambulatory by their early teens. Serum creatine kinase levels are markedly elevated. Boys with DMD frequently die in their twenties of respiratory failure and cardiac dysfunction. The prognosis for BMD is more variable. Although corticosteroids are useful in maintaining strength, they do not slow progression of the disorder. Evolution of

the natural history of dystrophinopathies in females is demonstrating an increased incidence of serious cardiovascular disease, including cardiomyopathy and arrhythmias.

The gene for dystrophin is very large and a common target for mutation. Large deletions or duplications can be detected in the gene for dystrophin in 65% of cases. Molecular analysis has largely replaced muscle biopsy for diagnostic purposes.

One-third of DMD cases presenting with a negative family history are likely to be new mutations. Germline mosaicism for mutations in the dystrophin gene occur in approximately 15%–20% of families, which is among the highest rates for this otherwise rare phenomenon. GC is recommended for all sisters of affected boys. Since mutations are now detected in the great majority of DMD cases, we can offer more accurate recurrence risk and treatment in specific kind of gene changes. Exon skipping therapy has been applied in DMD: In molecular biology, exon skipping is a form of RNA splicing used to cause cells to "skip" over faulty or misaligned sections of genetic code, leading to a truncated but still functional protein despite the genetic mutation.

Echevarria L et al: Exon-skipping advances for Duchenne muscular dystrophy. Human Mol Genet 2019 Aug 1;27(R2): R163–R172 [PMID: 29771317].

2. Hemophilia

Hemophilia A is an X-linked, recessive, bleeding disorder caused by a deficiency in the activity of coagulation factor VIII. (See Chapter 30 for additional discussion.)

▼ NONMENDELIAN DISORDERS

DISORDERS OF IMPRINTING

1. Beckwith-Wiedemann Syndrome

The association of macrosomia (enlarged body size), macroglossia (enlarged tongue), and omphalocele constitutes the Beckwith-Wiedemann syndrome (BWS), now known to be related to abnormal expression of imprinted genes located on chromosome 11p15. Other associated findings include hypertelorism, unusual ear creases, infantile hypoglycemia due to transient hyperinsulinemia, multiple congenital anomalies (cleft palate and genitourinary anomalies common), and increased risk for certain malignancies, especially Wilms tumor (7%–10%).

Chromosomal abnormalities such as duplication of the paternal 11p15 region, or paternal UPD, or mutations of the CDKN1C gene are associated with BWS. Most patients have methylation errors of DMR1 (differentially methylated region1, *H19*, 5%), and DMR2 (LIT1, 50%). H19 is a long noncoding RNA with a role in the negative regulation of cell proliferation. Isolated hemihyperplasia can be a mild form of BWS. The main difference between the two is the relatively mosaic methylation pattern of the specific area of tissue. Children affected with BWS should undergo tumor surveillance protocols, including serum AFP levels every 3 months until they reach age 4 and an abdominal ultrasound every 3 months until they reach age 8. Recent guidelines have modified the tumor surveillance based on the specific molecular cause of BWS.

2. Prader-Willi Syndrome

Prader-Willi syndrome results from lack of expression of several imprinted genes, including *SNRPN*, located on chromosome 15q11. Clinical characteristics include severe hypotonia in infancy, often necessitating placement of a feeding gastrostomy tube. In older children, characteristic features include almond-shaped eyes, and strabismus. Obstructive sleep apnea is common as are short stature, obesity, hypogenitalism, and small hands and feet. Growth hormone treatment is now offered to PWS patients, which improves the above symptoms. Obsessive hyperphagia (usual onset 3–4 years) is the hallmark of this disorder. However, obesity can be prevented with use of growth hormone as well as family support and strict diet control if instituted early in life. Genetic testing for BWS includes methylation analysis, which can detect 99% of the cases which include paternally inherited deletions (~70%), maternal UPD (20%–30%), imprinting defects, imprinting center deletions, and unbalanced chromosome rearrangement. Of note, a SNP array can detect up to 90% of Prader-Willi patients.

3. Angelman Syndrome

Angelman syndrome also involves imprinting and results from a variety of mutations that inactivate a ubiquitin-protein ligase gene, *UBE3A*, located in the same region of chromosome 15 as *SNRPN*, the gene involved in Prader-Willi syndrome. The classic phenotype includes severe intellectual disability with prognathism, seizures, and marked delay in motor milestones, abnormal gait and posturing, poor language development, autism, and paroxysmal laughter and tongue thrusting.

Angelman syndrome is caused by deletions of the maternal allele at 15q11 (68%), UPD of the paternal allele (8%), and imprinting center deletions (3%). Mutations in *UBE3A* cause the disorder in about 11% of cases. Imprinting errors, such as those causing Angelman Syndrome, may be associated with advanced reproductive techniques. Methylation studies can detect 80% of patients and should be the first screening test.

Dagli AI, Mueller J, Williams CA: Angelman syndrome. 1998 Sep 15 [Updated 2015 May 14]. In: Pagon RA et al (eds): *GeneReviews®* [Internet]. Seattle, WA: University of Washington; 1993–2017. Available from: https://www.ncbi.nlm.nih.gov/books/NBK1144/ [PMID: 20301323].

Driscoll DJ et al: Prader-Willi syndrome. 1998 Oct 6 [updated 2017 Dec 14]. In: Adam MP et al (eds): GeneReviews® [Internet]. Seattle (WA): University of Washington, Seattle; 1993–2017. Available from: https://www.ncbi.nlm.nih.gov/books/NBK1330/.

DISORDERS ASSOCIATED WITH ANTICIPATION

Anticipation is the phenomenon where a genetic condition is passed from one generation to another and typically becomes more severe with each subsequent generation. Molecularly, anticipation is caused by an expansion of the size of a tri (or tetra) nucleotide repeat (eg, CTG).

1. Myotonic Dystrophy (Autosomal Dominant)

Myotonic dystrophy is an autosomal dominant condition characterized by muscle weakness and tonic muscle spasms (myotonia). Additional features include hypogonadism, frontal balding, cardiac conduction abnormalities, and cataracts. This disorder occurs when a CTG repeat in the *DMPK* gene on chromosome 19 expands to 50 or more copies. Normal individuals have from 5 to 35 CTG repeat copies. Individuals carrying 35–49 repeats are generally asymptomatic, but repeat copies greater than 35 are meiotically unstable and tend to further expand when passed to subsequent generations. Individuals with 50–100 copies may be only mildly affected (eg, cataracts). Most individuals with repeat copies greater than 100 will have symptoms or electrical myotonia as adults.

CTG repeat sizes in the 100–1000 range usually develop classic DM1 with muscle weakness and wasting, myotonia, cataracts, and often cardiac conduction abnormalities. Expansion from greater than 1000 copies often present as congenital DM: infantile hypotonia, respiratory deficits, and intellectual disability. This occurs most frequently when the unstable repeats are passed through an affected mother. Therefore, an important component in the workup of the floppy or weak infant is a careful neurologic assessment of both parents for evidence of weakness or myotonia. Molecular testing that measures the number of CTG repeats is diagnostic clinically and prenatally. (See Chapter 25 for additional discussion.) The detection rate of a CCTG expansion of CNBP causing Type 2 is more than 99%. Anticipation is less prominent in Type 2 myotonic dystrophy and the clinical presentation is usually milder.

2. Friedreich Ataxia (Autosomal Recessive)

Symptoms of Friedreich ataxia include dysarthria, muscle weakness, lower limb spasticity, bladder dysfunction, and absent lower limb reflexes. Both motor and sensory findings begin in preadolescence and typically progress through the teenage years. The presentation can be variable. FA results from an abnormally expanded GAA repeat in intron 1 of *FXN*. Unaffected individuals typically carry 7–33 GAA repeats at this locus. Close to 96% of affected patients are homozygous for repeat expansions that exceed 66 copies. Point mutations in the gene also occur. However, anticipation is not observed because the disease is typically not observed in more than one generation. Molecular diagnostic testing requires careful interpretation with respect to prognosis and reproductive risks. (See Chapter 25 for additional discussion.)

3. Fragile X Syndrome (X-Linked)

Fragile X syndrome, present in approximately 1 in 1000 males, is the most common cause of cognitive disabilities in males. The responsible gene is *FMR1*, which has unstable CGG repeats at the 5′ end. Normal individuals have up to 50 CGG repeats. Individuals with 51–200 CGG repeats have a premutation and may manifest symptoms including mild developmental disabilities and behavioral traits; premature ovarian failure in a subset of females; and a progressive, neurologic deterioration in older males called FXTAS (Fragile X-associated tremor-ataxia syndrome). Affected individuals with Fragile X syndrome (full mutation) have more than 200 CGG repeats and also have hypermethylation of both the CGG expansion and an adjacent CpG island. This methylation turns off the *FMR1* gene. DNA analysis, rather than cytogenetic testing, is the method of choice for confirming the diagnosis of Fragile X syndrome.

▶ Clinical Features

Most males with Fragile X syndrome present with intellectual disabilities, oblong facies with large ears, and large testicles after puberty. Other physical signs include hyperextensible joints and mitral valve prolapse. Many affected individuals are hyperactive and exhibit behaviors along the autism spectrum.

Unlike other X-linked disorders where female heterozygotes are asymptomatic, females with a full mutation may exhibit a phenotype ranging from normal IQ to intellectual disability, and may show behaviors along the autism spectrum.

Clinical expression of Fragile X differs in male and female offspring depending on which parent is transmitting the gene. The premutation can change into the full mutation only when passed through a female. DNA analysis is a reliable test for prenatal and postnatal diagnosis of Fragile X syndrome and facilitates genetic counseling. (Management considerations for patients with Fragile X syndrome are described in Chapter 3.)

Hersh JH, Saul RA; Committee on Genetics: Health supervision for children with Fragile X syndrome. Pediatrics 2011 May;127(5):994–1006 [PMID: 21518720].

DISORDERS OF MULTIFACTORIAL INHERITANCE

Multifactorial inheritance is a type of hereditary pattern seen when there is more than one genetic factors involved and, sometimes, when there are also environmental factors and stochastic events participating in the causation and presentation of a condition. Examples include the following:

CLEFT LIP & CLEFT PALATE

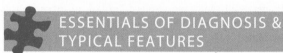

ESSENTIALS OF DIAGNOSIS & TYPICAL FEATURES

▶ Cleft lip is more common in males, cleft palate in females.

▶ Cleft lip and palate may be isolated defects (nonsyndromic) or associated with other anomalies as part of a genetic disorder (syndromic).

▶ General Considerations

From a genetic standpoint, cleft lip with or without cleft palate is distinct from isolated cleft palate. Although both can occur in a single family, particularly in association with certain syndromes, this pattern is unusual. Racial background is a factor in the incidence of facial clefting. The prevalence of facial clefting per 10,000 births is 10.2 in the United States, 12.1 in Western Europe and 20.0 in Japan. Some in utero exposures may cause cleft lip and palate such as anti-seizure medications, acne drugs containing Accutane and methotrexate.

▶ Findings

A cleft lip may be unilateral or bilateral and complete or incomplete. It may occur with a cleft of the entire palate or just the primary (anterior and gingival ridge) or secondary (posterior) palate. An isolated cleft palate can involve only the soft palate or both the soft and hard palates. It can be a V-shaped or a U-shaped cleft. When the cleft palate is associated with micrognathia and glossoptosis (a tongue that falls back and causes respiratory or feeding problems), it is called the **Pierre Robin sequence.** Among individuals with central clefts—more commonly those with isolated cleft palate—the incidence of other congenital abnormalities is increased, with up to a 60% association with other anomalies or syndromes.

▶ Differential Diagnosis

A facial cleft may occur in many different circumstances. It may be an isolated abnormality or part of a more generalized syndrome. Prognosis, management, and accurate determination of recurrence risks all depend on accurate diagnosis.

In evaluating a child with a facial cleft, the physician must determine if the cleft is nonsyndromic or syndromic.

A. Nonsyndromic

In the past, nonsyndromic cleft lip or cleft palate was considered a classic example of polygenic or multifactorial inheritance. Several recent studies have suggested that one or more major autosomal loci, both recessive and dominant may be involved. Empirically, however, the recurrence risk is still in the range of 2%–3% because of nonpenetrance or the presence of other contributing genes.

B. Syndromic

Cleft lip, with or without cleft palate, and isolated cleft palate may occur in a variety of syndromes that may be environmental, chromosomal, single gene, or of unknown origin (Table 37–2). Prognosis and accurate recurrence risks depend on the correct diagnosis.

▶ Complications

Problems associated with facial clefts include early feeding difficulties, which may be severe; airway obstruction necessitating tracheostomy; recurrent serous otitis media associated with fluctuating hearing and language delays; speech problems, including language delay, hypernasality, and articulation errors; and dental and orthodontic complications.

A. Medical Therapy

Long-term management ideally should be provided through a multidisciplinary cleft palate clinic to include otolaryngologists, audiologists, social work, speech therapist, dentists and genetic professionals.

Table 37–2. Syndromic isolated cleft palate (CP) and cleft lip with or without cleft palate (CL/CP).

Environmental
Maternal seizures, anticonvulsant usage (CL/CP or CP)
Fetal alcohol syndrome (CP)
Amniotic band syndrome (CL/CP)
Chromosomal
Trisomies 13 and 18 (CL/CP)
Wolf-Hirschhorn or 4p– syndrome (CL/CP)
Shprintzen or 22q11.2 deletion syndrome (CP)
Single-gene disorders
Treacher-Collins syndrome, AD (CP)
Stickler syndrome, AD (CP—particularly Pierre-Robin)
Smith-Lemli-Opitz, AR (CP)
Unknown cause
Moebius syndrome (CP)

AD, autosomal dominant; AR, autosomal recessive.

B. Genetic Counseling

Accurate counseling depends on accurate diagnosis and the differentiation of syndromic from nonsyndromic clefts. A complete family history must be taken, and the patient and both parents must be examined. The choice of laboratory studies is guided by the presence of other abnormalities and clinical suspicions, and may include microarray analysis and metabolic and DNA studies. Clefts of both the lip and the palate can be detected on detailed prenatal ultrasound.

Watkins SE, Meyer RE, Strauss RP, Aylsworth AS: Classification, epidemiology and genetics of orofacial clefts. Clin Plast Surg 2014 Apr;41(2):149–163 [PMID: 24607185].

NEURAL TUBE DEFECTS

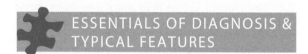

ESSENTIALS OF DIAGNOSIS & TYPICAL FEATURES

▶ Various defects, ranging from anencephaly to open or skin-covered lesions of the spinal cord, may occur in isolation or as part of a syndrome.

▶ Myelomeningocele is usually associated with hydrocephalus, Arnold-Chiari II malformation, neurogenic bladder and bowel, and congenital paralysis in the lower extremities.

▶ Anomalies of the CNS, heart, and kidneys may also be seen.

▶ MRI helps determine the extent of the anatomic defect in skin-covered lesions.

▶ General Considerations

Neural tube defects comprise a variety of malformations, including anencephaly, encephalocele, spina bifida (-myelomeningocele), sacral agenesis, and other spinal dysraphisms. Evidence suggests that the neural tube develops via closure at multiple closure sites and that each closure site is mediated by different genes and affected by different teratogens. Hydrocephalus associated with the Arnold-Chiari type II malformation commonly occurs with myelomeningocele. Sacral agenesis, also called the caudal regression syndrome, occurs more frequently in infants of diabetic mothers.

▶ Clinical Findings

At birth, neural tube defects can present as an obvious open lesion, or as a more subtle skin-covered lesion. In the latter case, MRI should be conducted to better define the anatomic defect. The extent of neurologic deficit depends on the level of the lesion and may include clubfeet, dislocated hips, neurogenic bowel and bladder, and total flaccid paralysis below the level of the lesion. Hydrocephalus may be apparent prenatally, or may develop after birth.

▶ **Differential Diagnosis**

Neural tube defects may occur in isolation (nonsyndromic) or as part of a genetic syndrome. Any infant with dysmorphic features or other major anomalies in addition to a neural tube defect should be evaluated by a geneticist, and a microarray analysis should be performed.

▶ **Treatment**

A. Neurosurgical Measures

Prenatal interventions including fetal surgery to correct an open neural tube defect are now much more common. After birth, infants with an open neural tube defect should be placed in prone position, and the lesion kept moist with sterile dressing. Neurosurgical closure should occur within 24–48 hours after birth to reduce risk of infection. Shunts are required in about 85% of cases of myelomeningocele and are associated with complications including malfunction and infection. Symptoms of the Arnold-Chiari II malformation include feeding dysfunction, abducens nerve palsy, vocal cord paralysis with stridor, and apnea. Shunt malfunction may cause an acute worsening of Arnold-Chiari symptoms that may be life-threatening.

B. Orthopedic Measures

Children with low lumbar and sacral lesions walk with minimal support, while those with high lumbar and thoracic lesions are rarely functional walkers. Orthopedic input is necessary to address foot deformities and scoliosis. Physical therapy services are indicated.

C. Urologic Measures

Neurogenic bladders require urological consultations. Continence may be achieved by the use of medications, clean intermittent catheterization, and a variety of urologic procedures. Renal function should be monitored regularly, and an ultrasound examination should be periodically repeated. Symptomatic infections should be treated.

Neurogenic bowel is managed with a combination of dietary modifications and medications. A surgical procedure called ACE (ante-grade continence enema) may be recommended for patients with severe constipation.

D. Genetic Counseling

Most isolated neural tube defects are polygenic, with a recurrence risk of 2%–3% in future pregnancies and a recurrence risk of 1%–2% for siblings. A patient with spina bifida has a 5% chance of having an affected child. Prenatal diagnosis is possible including maternal serum screening and prenatal ultrasound.

Prophylactic folic acid can significantly lower the incidence and recurrence rate of neural tube defects, if the intake of the folic acid starts at least 3 months prior to conception and continued for the first month of pregnancy. Folic acid supplementation prior to conception may also lower the incidence of other congenital malformations such as heart defects.

▶ **Special Issues & Prognosis**

All children requiring multiple surgical procedures (ie, patients with spina bifida or urinary tract anomalies) have a significant risk for developing hypersensitivity type I (IgE-mediated) allergic reactions to latex. For this reason, non-latex medical products are now routinely used when caring for patients with neural tube defects.

Most individuals with myelomeningocele are cognitively normal, but learning disabilities are common. Individuals with encephalocele or other CNS malformations have a much poorer intellectual prognosis. Individuals with neural tube defects have lifelong medical issues, requiring the input of a multidisciplinary medical team. A good support for families is the Spina Bifida Association, at the following website: https://www.spinabifidaassociation.org/.

▼ **COMMON RECOGNIZABLE DISORDERS WITH VARIABLE OR UNKNOWN CAUSE**

The text that follows describes several important and common human malformation syndromes. Good illustrations of these syndromes are found in *Smith's Recognizable Patterns of Human Malformation*. An excellent Internet site at the University of Kansas Medical Center can be consulted for further information: http://www.kumc.edu/gec/support.

1. Arthrogryposis Multiplex

The term *arthrogryposis* describes multiple congenital contractures that affect two or more different areas of the body. Arthrogryposis is not a specific diagnosis, but rather a clinical finding and it is a characteristic of more than 300 different disorders. Causes most often involve constraint, CNS malformation or injury, and neuromuscular disorders. Polyhydramnios is often present as a result of lack of fetal swallowing. Pulmonary hypoplasia may also be present, reflecting lack of fetal breathing. The initial workup includes brain imaging, consideration of metabolic disease, neurologic consultation, and in some cases, electrophysiologic studies and/or muscle biopsy. Consider parental evaluation to determine if they also have symptoms demonstrating an inherited cause.

Family history review for findings such as muscle weakness or cramping, cataracts, and early-onset heart disease that indicate myotonic dystrophy is important. Mutations in at least five genes (*TNNI2, TNNT3, TPM2, MYH3,* and *MYH8*) that encode components of the contractile apparatus of fast-twitch myofibers can cause distal arthrogryposis.

2. Goldenhar Syndrome

Goldenhar syndrome, also known as ocular-auriculo-vertebral (OAV) syndrome, is an association of multiple anomalies involving the head and neck. The classic phenotype includes hemifacial microsomia (one side of the face smaller than the other), and abnormalities of the pinna on the same side with associated deafness. Ear anomalies may be quite severe and include anotia and/or microtia. A characteristic benign fatty tumor in the outer eye, called an epibulbar dermoid, is frequently present, as are preauricular ear tags. Vertebral anomalies, particularly of the cervical vertebrae, are common. The Arnold-Chiari type I malformation (herniation of the cerebellum into the cervical spinal canal) is a common associated anomaly. Cardiac anomalies and hydrocephalus are seen in more severe cases. Most patients with Goldenhar syndrome have typical intelligence. The cause is unknown and some believe it is a blastocyst developmental field defect. Goldenhar is seen more frequently in infants of a diabetic mother. (See Craniofacial Microsomia Overview, GeneReviews, www.genereviews.org for an excellent discussion and differential diagnosis.)

3. Oligohydramnios Sequence (Potter Sequence)

This condition presents in newborns as severe respiratory distress due to pulmonary hypoplasia in association with positional deformities of the extremities, usually bilateral clubfeet, and typical facies consisting of suborbital creases, depressed nasal tip and low-set ears, and retrognathia. The sequence may be due to prolonged lack of amniotic fluid. Most often it is due to leakage of amniotic fluid, renal agenesis, or severe obstructive uropathy.

4. Overgrowth Syndromes

Overgrowth typically present at birth and is characterized by macrocephaly, motor delays (cerebral hypotonia), and occasional asymmetry of extremities. Bone age may be advanced and diagnosed in the older child. The most common single gene overgrowth syndrome is **Sotos syndrome**. Patients with Sotos syndrome have a characteristic facies with a prominent forehead, elongated nasal bridge and down-slanting palpebral features. Mutations in *NSD1* cause Sotos syndrome. Patients have a small but increased risk of cancer.

Golabi-Behmel syndrome, Bannayan-Riley-Ruvalcaba (BRR) syndrome, Weaver syndrome, and Sotos syndrome are often mistaken for one another due to their significant phenotypic overlap and similarities. A common cause for Weaver syndrome is mutations in the *EZH2* gene on chromosome 7q36. *EZH2* is the second histone methyltransferase associated with human overgrowth. Patients with **Simpson-Golabi-Behmel syndrome** exhibit a BWS-like phenotype, but with additional anomalies, including polydactyly and more severe facial dysmorphism and cognitive impairment. It is inherited as an X-linked disorder.

Some overgrowth syndromes may present with "somatic" and mosaic changes, such as the Megalencephaly-capillary malformation syndrome (MCAP) due to *PIK3CA* mutations and Proteus syndrome, caused by mosaic AKT-1 mutations are part of the PIK3CA-related overgrowth syndrome (PROS) spectrum. The **PI3K/AKT/mTOR pathway** is critical in regulating cellular proliferation, muscle development and thus mobility, and survival. Variation in genes of this pathway can result in several disorders characterized by a wide range of phenotypes including MCAP. MCAP is defined by the following characteristics: megalencephaly or hemimegalencephaly, hypotonia, seizures, intellectual disability, and cutaneous capillary malformations with focal or generalized somatic overgrowth. Cortical malformations are seen. Molecular analysis is most successful in affected tissue samples versus buccal swab or blood sample.

Keppler-Noreuil KM et al: Clinical delineation and natural history of the PIK3CA-related overgrowth spectrum. Am J Med Genet A 2014 Jul;164(7):1713–1733 [PMID: 24782230].

5. Syndromic Short Stature

Short stature is an important component of numerous syndromes, or it may be an isolated finding. In the absence of nutritional deficiencies, endocrine abnormalities, evidence of skeletal dysplasia (disproportionate growth with abnormal skeletal films), or a positive family history, intrinsic short stature can be due to UPD. The phenotype of Russell-Silver syndrome—short stature with normal head growth, typical development, and minor dysmorphic features (especially fifth finger clinodactyly)—has been associated in some cases with maternal UPD7 and hypomethylation of H19, which is the opposite molecular mechanism seen in BWS. The diagnostic pearl for this condition is prenatal onset IUGR with spared head circumference. Short stature in girls may also be caused by Turner syndrome or a *SHOX* deletion.

6. VACTERL Association

VACTERL is sporadic and some of the defects may be life-threatening. The prognosis for typical development is good. The cause is unknown, but a high association with monozygotic twinning suggests a mechanism dating back to events perhaps as early as blastogenesis.

Careful examination and follow-up are important, because numerous other syndromes have overlapping features. Microarray studies and genetic consultation are warranted. VACTERL is a diagnosis of exclusion.

ESSENTIALS OF DIAGNOSIS & TYPICAL FEATURES

VACTERL association is described by an acronym denoting the association of the following:

▶ Vertebral defects (segmentation anomalies).

▶ Imperforate anus.

▶ Cardiac malformation (most often ventricular septal defect).

▶ Tracheoesophageal fistula.

▶ Renal anomalies.

▶ Limb (most often radial ray) anomalies.

7. Kabuki Syndrome

Kabuki syndrome (KS) is characterized by typical facial features (elongated palpebral fissures with eversion of the lateral third of the lower eyelid; arched and broad eyebrows; short columella with depressed nasal tip; large, prominent, or cupped ears), minor skeletal anomalies, persistence of fetal fingertip pads, mild-to-moderate intellectual disability, and postnatal growth deficiency. Other findings may include congenital heart defects, genitourinary anomalies, cleft lip and/or palate, gastrointestinal anomalies, including anal atresia, ptosis and strabismus, and widely spaced teeth and hypodontia. Functional differences can include increased susceptibility to infections and autoimmune disorders, seizures, endocrinologic abnormalities including isolated premature thelarche in females, feeding problems, and hearing loss. Molecular genetic testing for *MLL2* and *KMT2D*, the only genes in which mutations are known to cause KS, are available on a clinical basis.

▼ GENETIC EVALUATION OF THE CHILD WITH DEVELOPMENTAL DISABILITIES

Cognitive disabilities or developmental delays affect 8% of the population. There are thousands of genes associated with developmental and intellectual disabilities, and determining an underlying genetic diagnosis may require consultation with a geneticist. Table 37–3 lists the main features of developmental delay, emphasizing the major clinical and genetic considerations. (See Chapter 3 for additional information about developmental delay and intellectual disability.)

Obtaining a detailed history, including pertinent prenatal and perinatal events, is critical. Feeding issues and slow growth velocity are seen in many genetic disorders causing developmental delay. Rate of developmental progress and particularly a history of loss of skills are important clues, as the latter might suggest a metabolic disorder with a neurodegenerative component. Family history can provide clues to suggest possible genetic etiologies, particularly if there is a history of consanguinity, which suggests recessive inheritance or a family pattern of other affected individuals.

Physical examination provides helpful clues. Referral to a clinical geneticist is indicated whenever unusual features are encountered. Neurologic, ophthalmologic, and audiologic consultation should be sought when indicated. Brain imaging (MRI) should be requested in cases involving unexplained deviations from normal head growth. Neuroimaging and skeletal studies may also be indicated when dysmorphic features are present.

Metabolic and genetic testing procedures other than those listed in the Table 37–3 may also be indicated.

Interpretation & Follow-Up

Clinical experience indicates that specific diagnoses can be made in approximately half of patients evaluated according to the protocol presented here. With specific diagnosis comes prognosis, ideas for management, and insight into recurrence risks.

Follow-up is important both for patients in whom diagnoses have been made and for those patients initially lacking a diagnosis. Genetic testing is advancing rapidly and can be translated into new diagnoses and better understanding with periodic review of clinical cases.

Adam MP et al: Kabuki syndrome. GeneReviews www.ncbi.nlm.nih.gov/books/ [PMID: 21882399].

Moeschler JB, Scevell M; Committee on Genetics: Comprehensive evaluation of the child with intellectual disability or global developmental delay. Pediatrics 2014;134:e903 [PMID: 25157020].

Autism

Autism is a developmental disorder comprising abnormal function in three domains: language development, social development, and behavior. Many patients with autism also have cognitive disabilities and might be appropriately evaluated according to the recommendations above. However, given the enormous increase in prevalence of autism in the past decade (1 in 68 children per latest CDC report), it is worth discussing the genetic evaluation of autism separately.

There are over 2000 genes associated with autism. Advances in molecular diagnosis, understanding of metabolic derangements, and technologies, such as microarray and Next-Generation Sequencing, are allowing more patients with autism to be identified with specific genetic disorders. This allows more accurate genetic counseling for recurrence risk, as well as diagnosis-specific interventions, which may improve prognosis.

Recommendations for the genetic evaluation of a child with autism include the following:

Table 37–3. Evaluation of the child with developmental delay.

History
  Pregnancy history
  Growth parameters at birth
  Neonatal complications
  Feeding history
  History of somatic growth
  Motor, language, and psychosocial milestones
  Seizures
  Loss of skills
  Abnormal movements
  Results of previous tests and examinations
Family history
  Developmental and educational histories
  Psychiatric disorders
  Pregnancy outcomes
  Medical history
  Consanguinity
Physical examination
  General pediatric examination, including growth parameters
  Focused dysmorphologic evaluation including measurement
    of facial features and limbs
  Complete neurologic examination
  Parental growth parameters (especially head circumferences)
    and dysmorphic features should also be assessed
Imaging studies
  See text
Laboratory assessment
  Microarray analysis (this has replaced chromosome analysis
    and FISH testing in most cases)
  Fragile X testing (analysis of FMR1 gene for triplet repeats)
  Other blood analyses: comprehensive metabolic panel,
    acylcarnitine profile, creatinine kinase (CK), lactate, pyruvate
    (this testing is helpful in the case of hypotonia)
  Other metabolic tests may be helpful as second tier tests,
    including:
    Serum amino acid analysis
    Urine amino and organic acid analysis
    Urine analysis for mucopolysaccharides (if coarse features
      and organomegaly)

1. Genetic referral if dysmorphic features or cutaneous abnormalities are present (ie, hypopigmented spots such as those seen in patients with **tuberous sclerosis**).

2. Laboratory testing to include the following:

   a. Microarray.

   b. Molecular testing for **Fragile X syndrome**.

   c. Methylation testing for UPD15 if phenotype is suggestive of **Angelman syndrome**.

   d. Measurement of cholesterol and 7-DHC if syndactyly is present between the second and third toes, to rule out a mild form of **Smith-Lemli-Opitz syndrome**.

   e. *MECP2* testing if clinical course is suggestive of **Rett syndrome** (ie, neurodegenerative course, progressive microcephaly, and seizures in a female patient).

   f. *PTEN* molecular testing if the head circumference is greater than two standard deviations above the mean, plus evidence of penile freckling, lipomatous lesions, or a strong family history of certain malignancies.

Autism spectrum disorders are discussed in more detail in Chapter 3.

Christensen DL; CDC: Prevalence of autism spectrum disorder among children aged 8 years—autism and developmental disabilities monitoring network, 11 Sites, United States, 2010. MMWR Surveill Summ 2016 Apr 1;65(3):1–23; (http://www.cdc.gov/mmwr) [PMID: 27031587].

▼ PERINATAL GENETICS

TERATOGENS

1. Drug Abuse & Fetal Alcohol Syndrome

Fetal alcohol syndrome (FAS) results from excessive exposure to alcohol during gestation and affects 30%–40% of offspring of mothers whose daily intake of alcohol exceeds 3 oz. Features of the syndrome include short stature, poor head growth (may be postnatal in onset), developmental delay, and midface hypoplasia characterized by a poorly developed philtrum, thin upper lip, narrow palpebral fissures, and short nose with anteverted nares. Facial findings may be subtle, but careful measurements and comparisons with standards are helpful. Structural abnormalities occur in half of affected children. Cardiac anomalies, genitourinary tract anomalies, and neural tube defects are commonly seen.

Alcohol exposure does not always result in classic FAS. In fact, facial and physical features are more related to the timing of exposure during the fetal development and do not necessarily correlate with neurological outcome. Alcohol-related neurodevelopmental disorder (ARND) describes the cognitive impairments linked to prenatal alcohol exposure including neurological deficits such as poor motor skills and hand-eye coordination. Individuals with ARND may also have a complex pattern of behavioral and learning problems, including difficulties with memory, attention, and judgment. One of the most challenging aspects in evaluating these children is the lack of a blood test to confirm or rule out this diagnosis; it is strictly based on maternal history and clinical findings.

Maternal abuse of psychoactive substances also is associated with increased risks for adverse perinatal outcomes including miscarriage, preterm delivery, growth restriction, and increased risk for injury to the developing CNS.

Methamphetamine exposure also has been found in limited studies to cause impairment in executive function. Maternal abuse of inhalants, such as glue, appears to be associated with findings similar to those of FAS.

Careful evaluation for other syndromes and chromosomal disorders should be included in the workup of exposed infants. Behavioral abnormalities in older children may be the result of maternally abused substances and poor early social circumstances but they may also reflect evolving psychiatric disorders. Psychiatric disorders, many recognized as heritable, affect large numbers of men and women with substance abuse problems. Fetal alcohol spectrum disorders are discussed in more detail in Chapter 3.

2. Maternal Anticonvulsant Effects

Anticonvulsant exposure during pregnancy is associated with adverse outcomes in approximately 10% of children born to women treated with these agents. A syndrome characterized by small head circumference, anteverted nares, cleft lip and palate (occasionally), and distal digital hypoplasia was first described in association with maternal use of phenytoin, but also occurs with other anticonvulsants. Risks for spina bifida are increased especially in pregnancies exposed to valproic acid.

3. Retinoic Acid Embryopathy

Vitamin A and its analogs have considerable teratogenic potential. Developmental toxicity occurs in approximately one-third of pregnancies exposed in the first trimester to the synthetic retinoid, isotretinoin, commonly prescribed to treat acne. Exposure produces CNS malformation, especially of the posterior fossa; ear anomalies (often absence of pinnae); congenital heart disease (great vessel anomalies); and tracheoesophageal fistula. It is now recognized that vitamin A itself, when taken as active retinoic acid in doses exceeding 25,000 IU/day during pregnancy, can produce similar fetal anomalies. Vitamin A intake is limited to 10,000 IU/day of retinoic acid. Maternal ingestion of large amounts of vitamin A taken as retinol during pregnancy, however, does not usually increase risks, because conversion of this precursor to active retinoic acid is internally regulated.

ASSISTED REPRODUCTION

Assisted reproductive technologies including in vitro fertilization are now used in a significant number of pregnancies. Although healthy live births are accepted as the usual outcomes resulting from successful application of these procedures, the actual number of viable embryos is limited and questions about the risks of adverse effects continue to be raised. Increased rates of twinning, both monozygotic and dizygotic, are well recognized while the possibility of increased rates of birth defects remains controversial.

Abnormal genetic imprinting appears to be associated with in vitro fertilization. Evidence supports increased prevalence of Beckwith-Wiedemann and Angelman syndromes among offspring of in vitro pregnancies.

PRENATAL DIAGNOSIS

Prenatal screening for birth defects is now routinely offered to pregnant women of all ages. Prenatal diagnosis introduces options for management.

Prenatal assessment of the fetus includes techniques that screen maternal blood, fetal imaging by ultrasound or MRI, fetal DNA analysis via maternal blood samples, and samples of fetal and placental tissues.

▶ Maternal Blood Analysis

Several options now exist to evaluate the fetus and pregnancy by obtaining a maternal blood sample. In the first trimester, measurements of PAPA (pregnancy-associated plasma protein A) and the free β-subunit of human chorionic gonadotropin (hCG) screen for trisomies 21 and 18. In the second trimester maternal α-fetoprotein (AFP), hCG, unconjugated estradiol, and inhibin ("quad screen") combine to estimate risks for trisomies 21 and 18. Low estradiol levels can also predict cases of Smith-Lemli-Opitz syndrome. Noninvasive prenatal testing using NextGen sequencing, via maternal blood sample (also known as cell free fetal DNA), can detect specific chromosome imbalances and typically tests for the presence of sex chromosomes as well as trisomies 13, 18, and 21. Some newer test platforms are starting to look for common microdeletion syndromes as well. It is important to note that this testing is a screening test and diagnoses always need to be confirmed by another method as described in the next section.

▶ Analysis of Fetal Samples

A. Amniocentesis

Amniocentesis samples fluid surrounding the fetus and is performed in the early second trimester (around 15–16 weeks' gestation). The cells obtained are cultured for cytogenetic, molecular, or metabolic analyses. α-Fetoprotein and other chemical markers can also be measured. This is a safe procedure with a complication rate (primarily for miscarriage) of less than 0.01% in experienced hands.

B. Chorionic Villus Sampling (Placental)

Chorionic villus sampling is generally performed at 11–12 weeks' gestation. Tissue obtained by chorionic villus sampling provides DNA for molecular analysis and contains dividing cells that can be rapidly evaluated by FISH. However, direct cytogenetic preparations may be of poor quality and placental fibroblasts must be routinely grown and analyzed. In addition, chromosomal abnormalities detected by this technique may be confined to the placenta (**confined placental mosaicism**) and be less informative than amniocentesis.

C. Fetal Blood and Tissue

Fetal blood can be sampled directly in late gestation through ultrasound-guided percutaneous umbilical blood sampling (PUBS). A wide range of diagnostic tests ranging from biochemical to aCGH can be applied. Fetal urine sampled from the bladder or dilated proximal structures can provide important information about fetal renal function.

It is occasionally necessary to obtain biopsy specimens of fetal tissues such as liver or muscle for accurate prenatal diagnosis. These procedures are available in only a few perinatal centers.

D. Preimplantation Genetic Diagnosis

With the advent of single-cell PCR techniques as well as interphase FISH it is now possible to make genetic diagnoses in pre-implantation human embryos by removing and analyzing blastocyst cells. Using this procedure parents can now consider selecting pregnancies for positive attributes such as becoming donors for transplantation of tissues to siblings affected by genetic disorders.

▶ Fetal Imaging

Fetal ultrasonography has become routine and MRI imaging is becoming increasingly common during pregnancy, while fetal x-rays are rarely employed. Ultrasonography has joined maternal blood sampling as a screening technique for common chromosomal aneuploidies, neural tube defects, and other structural anomalies. Pregnancies at increased risk for CNS anomalies, skeletal dysplasias, and structural defects of the heart and kidneys should be monitored by careful ultrasound examinations. Fetal MRI has become routine in the workup of suspected fetal CNS abnormalities as well as in an increasing number of other fetal anomalies.

Iwarsson E, Jacobsson B: Analysis of cell-free fetal DNA in maternal blood for detection of trisomy 21, 18 and 13 in a general pregnant population and in a high-risk population—a systematic review and meta-analysis. Acta Obstet Gynecol Scand 2017 Jan;96(1):7–18 [PMID: 27779757].

Liao GJ, Gronowski AM, Zhao Z: Non-invasive prenatal testing using cell-free fetal DNA in maternal circulation. Clin Chim Acta 2014 Jan 20;428:44–50 [PMID: 24482806].

Allergic Disorders

Ronina A. Covar, MD

David M. Fleischer, MD

Christine Cho, MD

Mark Boguniewicz, MD

INTRODUCTION

Allergic disorders are among the most common problems seen by pediatricians and primary care physicians, affecting over 25% of the population in developed countries. In the most recent National Health and Nutrition Examination Survey, 54% of the population had positive test responses to one or more allergens. According to a recent National Center for Health Statistics survey, the prevalence of food and skin allergies has increased over the past decade; with prevalence in 2015 of 5.7% and 12%, respectively. While the prevalence of respiratory allergies has been stable, it is still the highest among children (10.1%). In children, asthma, allergic rhinitis, and atopic dermatitis have been accompanied by significant morbidity and school absenteeism, with adverse consequences for school performance and quality of life, as well as economic burden measured in billions of dollars. In this chapter, atopy refers to a genetically determined predisposition to develop IgE antibodies found in patients with asthma, allergic rhinitis, and atopic dermatitis.

ASTHMA

ESSENTIALS OF DIAGNOSIS & TYPICAL FEATURES

▶ The diagnosis of asthma is based on recurrent episodes of cough, wheezing, dyspnea, or chest tightness, with various triggers, most commonly respiratory infections, exercise, aeroallergens, cold air, and irritants. At least 80% of children with asthma have an allergic predisposition.

▶ Chronic airway inflammation, variable expiratory airflow limitation, and bronchial reactivity characterize the disease, but presentation is heterogeneous, and course

over time, especially in children, is variable as well. The clinical course can be subtle for some children, but the risk of a severe, even life-threatening, asthma-related event is present.

▶ Assessment of severity can be challenging particularly if comorbidities and adverse effects of chronic disease and medications are present. Hence assessment of control is helpful when treatment changes are being made.

▶ The mainstay of asthma management involves targeting the inflammatory response and bronchoconstriction, avoidance of known triggers, identification of early warning signs, and creating an appropriate action plan. Regular assessment of response and control is necessary to prevent consequences of either poor disease control and medication side effects.

▶ Biologic therapy modulating T2 immune responses can be helpful at reducing morbidity in a subgroup of children with asthma.

The Global Strategy for Asthma Management and Prevention (www.ginasthma.org) report gives a definition of asthma as "a heterogeneous disease, usually characterized by chronic airway inflammation. It is defined by the history of respiratory symptoms such as wheeze, shortness of breath, chest tightness, and cough that vary over time and in intensity, together with variable expiratory limitation."

Asthma is the most common chronic disease of childhood, affecting 6.2 million children in the United States. While current prevalence rates for asthma had increased in the past decade, there has been an indication of a decrease in prevalence since 2011 (most recent estimate in children < 18 years is 8.4%). At least one-half of persons with current asthma reported having had an asthma attack in the past year. Gender, race, and socioeconomic disparities in the prevalence of asthma exist: (1) More boys than girls are affected in childhood; (2) higher percentage affected among black children compared to Hispanic and non-Hispanic white children; (3) children belonging to poor families are more likely to be affected.

There is still a disproportionately higher health care utilization for asthma among children compared to adults affected by this disease. Asthma accounts for almost 50% of the emergency department (ED) visits and one-third of the hospitalizations in children younger than 18 years. The ED visit rate due to asthma was the highest for children aged 0–4 years (20.8 visits per 100 persons with asthma). Children aged 0–17 years had a higher ED visit rate compared with adults (10.7 compared with 7.0 per 100 persons with asthma). Annual asthma hospitalizations rates were similar between children and adults. Still almost 140,000 children were hospitalized for asthma in 1 year. Hospitalizations and ED or urgent ambulatory or office visits, all indicators of asthma severity, impose significant costs to the health care system and to families, caretakers, schools, and parents' employers. About one-half of children with asthma report one or more asthma-related missed school days. Indirect costs primarily from loss of productivity due to school/work absences are harder to measure, yet considerable, and are estimated to be three times the direct costs. Asthma remains a potentially life-threatening disease for children; among children, the population-based rate of asthma deaths per million was 2.8 in 2009, and the at-risk based rate of asthma deaths per 10,000 children with asthma was 0.3. Similar to disparities in prevalence, morbidity and mortality rates for asthma are higher among minority and inner city populations. The reasons for this are unclear but may be related to a combination of more severe disease, poor access to health care, lack of asthma education, delay in use of appropriate controller therapy, and environmental factors (eg, irritants including smoke and air pollutants, and perennial allergen exposure).

Up to 80% of children with asthma develop symptoms before their fifth birthday. Atopy (personal or familial) is the strongest identifiable predisposing factor. Sensitization to inhalant allergens increases over time and is found in the majority of children with asthma. The principal allergens associated with asthma are perennial aeroallergens such as dust mite, animal dander, cockroach, and *Alternaria* (a soil mold). Rarely, foods may provoke isolated asthma symptoms.

About 40% of infants and young children who have wheezing with viral infections in the first few years of life will have continuing asthma through childhood. Viral infections (eg, respiratory syncytial virus [RSV], rhinovirus, parainfluenza and influenza viruses, metapneumovirus) are associated with wheezing episodes in young children. RSV may be the predominant pathogen of wheezing infants in the emergency room setting, but rhinovirus can be detected in the majority of older wheezing children. It is uncertain if these viruses contribute to the development of chronic asthma, independent of atopy. Severe RSV bronchiolitis in infancy has been linked to asthma and allergy in childhood. Although speculative, individuals with lower airways vulnerability to common respiratory viral pathogens may be at risk for persistent asthma.

In addition to atopy and infections being associated with the development of asthma, observational studies have also demonstrated an increased risk of asthma attributed to acetaminophen exposure during prenatal periods, infancy, childhood, and even adulthood. Acetaminophen is the most commonly used antipyretic medication for children in the United States. There is evidence from secondary analyses suggesting that acetaminophen exposure increases the risk for subsequent asthma exacerbations or wheeze compared to ibuprofen; and that a dose-dependent elevated risk of asthma symptoms could be found.

There are several mechanisms that have been proposed: acetaminophen interfering with glutathione (a tripeptide antioxidant that is involved in free radical scavenging and xenobiotic detoxification) pathway and impairing respiratory antioxidant defenses; presence of genetic polymorphisms in the glutathione pathway that are associated with increased susceptibility to asthma; and acetaminophen causing a switch to a TH2 from a TH1 response. However, a recent double-blind placebo-controlled trial study comparing acetaminophen and ibuprofen used for fever or pain in preschool-aged children with persistent asthma did not show increased asthma worsening with use of either drug.

Exposure to tobacco smoke is also a risk factor and a trigger for asthma. Other triggers include exercise, cold air, pollutants, strong chemical odors, and rapid changes in barometric pressure. Aspirin sensitivity is uncommon in children. There are data suggesting that microbiome may also play a role in the development of asthma and allergy. Psychological factors may precipitate asthma exacerbations and place the patient at high risk from the disease.

Pathologic features of asthma include shedding of airway epithelium, edema, mucus plug formation, mast cell activation, and collagen deposition beneath the basement membrane. The inflammatory cell infiltrate includes eosinophils, lymphocytes, and neutrophils, especially in fatal asthma exacerbations. Airway inflammation contributes to bronchial hyperresponsiveness, airflow limitation, and disease chronicity. Persistent airway inflammation can lead to airway wall remodeling and irreversible changes.

▶ Clinical Findings

A. Symptoms and Signs

The diagnosis of asthma in children, especially among preschool aged, is based largely on clinical judgment and an assessment of symptoms, activity limitation, and quality of life. For example, if a child with asthma refrains from participating in physical activities so as not to trigger asthma symptoms, their asthma would be inadequately controlled but not detected by the standard questions.

Wheezing is the most characteristic sign of asthma, although some children may have recurrent cough and shortness of breath. Complaints may include "chest congestion," prolonged cough, exercise intolerance, dyspnea, and recurrent bronchitis or pneumonia. Chest auscultation during forced expiration may reveal prolongation of the expiratory phase and wheezing. As the obstruction becomes more severe, wheezes become more high-pitched and breath sounds diminished. With severe obstruction, wheezes may not be heard because of poor air movement. Flaring of nostrils, intercostal and suprasternal retractions, and use of accessory muscles of respiration are signs of severe obstruction. Cyanosis of the lips and nail beds may be seen with underlying hypoxia. Tachycardia and pulsus paradoxus also occur. Agitation and lethargy may be signs of impending respiratory failure.

B. Laboratory Findings

The importance of confirming the diagnosis of asthma cannot be overemphasized, as there can be as many as 30% of people in whom the diagnosis cannot be confirmed. Bronchial hyperresponsiveness, reversible airflow limitation, and airway inflammation are key features of asthma. Documentation of all these components is not always necessary, unless the presentation is rather atypical.

Bronchial hyperresponsiveness to various stimuli is a hallmark of asthma. These stimuli include inhaled pharmacologic agents such as histamine, methacholine, and mannitol, as well as physical stimuli such as exercise and cold air. Mannitol (Aridol) bronchoprovocation has been approved by the US Food and Drug Administration (FDA) and is simpler and easier to administer in the office. It is available as a dry powder inhalation kit and takes less time to complete. Unlike methacholine and histamine challenges and similar to exercise challenge, it is considered an indirect challenge; that is, it simulates airway responses to specific physiologic situations, by creating an osmotic effect within the airway that subsequently leads to an inflammatory response. Airways may exhibit hyperresponsiveness or twitchiness even when baseline pulmonary function tests are normal. Giving increasing concentrations of a bronchoconstrictive agent to induce a decrease in lung function (usually a 20% drop in forced expiratory volume in 1 second [FEV_1] for histamine and methacholine and a 15% reduction for mannitol) and doing an exercise challenge are ways to determine airway responsiveness. Hyperresponsiveness in normal children younger than 5 years is greater than in older children. Bronchoprovocation challenges are not always available in a clinical setting, but they help to establish a diagnosis of asthma when the history, examination, and pulmonary function tests are not definitive.

The National Asthma Education and Prevention Program Expert Panel Report 3 (NAEPP3) reinforces the use of spirometry over peak expiratory flow rate (PEFR) measurements in the evaluation of airflow limitation in asthma. This can be measured by reduction in FEV_1 and FEV_1/FVC (forced vital capacity) values compared to reference or predicted values. By itself, it is not adequate in establishing a diagnosis, but it can be an important parameter to monitor asthma activity and treatment response. In children, FEV_1 may be normal, despite frequent symptoms. Spirometric measures of airflow limitation can be associated with symptom severity, likelihood of exacerbation, hospitalization, or respiratory compromise. Regular monitoring of prebronchodilator (and ideally postbronchodilator) FEV_1 can be used to track lung growth patterns over time. During acute asthma exacerbations, FEV_1 is diminished and the flow-volume curve shows a "scooping out" of the distal portion of the expiratory portion of the loop (Figure 38–1).

In addition to the importance placed on documentation of airflow limitation at any time during the diagnostic process, the GINA global strategy puts an emphasis on documenting excessive variability in lung function. This can be gleaned from any of the following:

- Bronchodilator reversibility: increase in FEV_1 greater than 12% predicted
- Excessive variability in twice-daily peak flow readings over 2 weeks: average daily diurnal PEF variability greater than 13% ([day's highest PEF minus day's lowest PEF]/mean of day's highest and lowest), averaged over 1 week
- Significant increase in lung function after 4 weeks of anti-inflammatory treatment (FEV_1 > 12% and 200 mL (or PEF > 20%)
- (+) Exercise challenge test: fall in FEV_1 greater than 12% predicted or PEF greater than 15%
- (+) Bronchoprovocation challenge test
- Excessive variation in lung function between visits: variation in FEV_1 of 12% or PEF greater than 15%

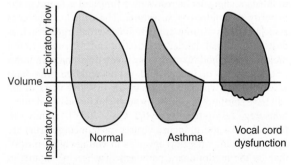

▲ **Figure 38–1.** Representative flow-volume loops in persons with normal lung function, asthma, and inducible laryngeal obstruction.

PEFR monitoring can be a simple and reproducible tool to assess asthma activity in children with moderate or severe asthma, a history of severe exacerbations, or poor perception of airflow limitation or worsening condition. Significant changes in PEFR may occur before symptoms become evident. In more severe cases, PEFR monitoring enables earlier recognition of suboptimal asthma control.

Lung function assessment using body box plethysmography to determine lung volume measurements can also be informative. The residual volume, functional residual capacity, and total lung capacity are usually increased, while the vital capacity is decreased. Reversal or significant improvement of these abnormalities in response to inhaled bronchodilator therapy or with anti-inflammatory therapy can be observed.

Infant pulmonary function can be measured in sedated children with compression techniques. The forced oscillation technique can be used to measure peripheral airway resistance even in younger children.

Hypoxemia is present early with a normal or low PCO_2 level and respiratory alkalosis. Hypoxemia may be aggravated during treatment with a β_2-agonist due to ventilation-perfusion mismatch. Oxygen saturation less than 91% is indicative of significant obstruction. Respiratory acidosis and increasing CO_2 tension may ensue with further airflow obstruction and signal impending respiratory failure. Hypercapnia is usually not seen until the FEV_1 falls below 20% of predicted value. Metabolic acidosis has also been noted in combination with respiratory acidosis in children with severe asthma and indicates imminent respiratory failure. Pao_2 less than 60 mm Hg despite oxygen therapy and $Paco_2$ over 60 mm Hg and rising more than 5 mm Hg/h are relative indications for mechanical ventilation in a child in status asthmaticus.

Pulsus paradoxus may be present with moderate or severe asthma exacerbation. In moderate asthma exacerbation in a child, this may be between 10 and 25 mm Hg, and in severe asthma exacerbation between 20 and 40 mm Hg. Absence of pulsus paradoxus in a child with severe asthma exacerbation may signal respiratory muscle fatigue.

Clumps of eosinophils on sputum smear and blood eosinophilia are findings in a subset of children with asthma. Their presence tends to reflect a specific phenotype and does not necessarily mean that allergic factors are involved. Leukocytosis is common in acute severe asthma without evidence of bacterial infection and may be more pronounced after epinephrine administration. Hematocrit can be elevated with dehydration during prolonged exacerbations or in severe chronic disease. Noninvasive measures of airway inflammation include exhaled nitric oxide concentrations, serum eosinophil cationic protein levels, serum total (and specific) IgE, and induced sputum. Some of these biomarkers can identify children who can benefit from certain interventions, and some, like exhaled nitric oxide, can be used to adjust treatment and reduce exacerbations of asthma.

C. Imaging

Evaluation of asthma usually does not need chest radiographs (posteroanterior and lateral views) since they often appear normal, although subtle and nonspecific findings of hyperinflation (flattening of the diaphragms), peribronchial thickening, prominence of the pulmonary arteries, and areas of patchy atelectasis may be present. Atelectasis may be misinterpreted as the infiltrates of pneumonia. Some lung abnormalities, such as bronchiectasis, which may point to a different diagnosis implicating an asthma masquerader, such as cystic fibrosis, allergic bronchopulmonary mycoses (aspergillosis), ciliary dyskinesias, immune deficiencies, or even aspiration, can be better appreciated with high-resolution, thin-section chest computed tomography (high-resolution computed tomography [HRCT]) scans. It is primarily useful clinically in ruling out certain diagnoses in patients with difficult to manage asthma but radiation exposure should be considered when ordering HRCT, especially done serially. However, algorithms used in newer scanners allow for much reduced radiation exposure.

Allergy testing is discussed in the section General Measures under Treatment, Chronic Asthma.

▶ Differential Diagnosis

Diseases that may be mistaken for asthma are often related to the patient's age (Table 38–1). Congenital abnormalities must be excluded in infants and young children. Asthma can be confused with croup, acute bronchiolitis, pneumonia, and pertussis. Immunodeficiency may be associated with cough and wheezing. Foreign bodies in the airway may cause dyspnea or wheezing of sudden onset, and on auscultation, wheezing may be unilateral. Asymmetry of the lungs

Table 38–1. Differential diagnosis of asthma in infants and children.

Viral bronchiolitis
Aspiration
Laryngotracheomalacia
Vascular rings
Airway stenosis or web
Enlarged lymph nodes
Mediastinal mass
Foreign body
Bronchopulmonary dysplasia
Obliterative bronchiolitis
Cystic fibrosis
Vocal cord dysfunction
Cardiovascular disease

secondary to air trapping may be seen on a chest radiograph, especially with forced expiration. Cystic fibrosis can be associated with or mistaken for asthma.

Inducible laryngeal obstruction (previously recognized as vocal cord dysfunction) is an important masquerader of asthma, although the two can coexist. It is characterized by the paradoxical closure of the vocal cords that can result in difficulty breathing commonly on inspiration, throat tightness, and even wheezing. In normal individuals, the vocal cords abduct during inspiration and may adduct slightly during expiration. Asthmatic patients may have narrowing of the glottis during expiration as a physiologic adaptation to airway obstruction. In contrast, patients with isolated inducible laryngeal obstruction typically show adduction of the anterior two-thirds of their vocal cords during inspiration, with a small diamond-shaped aperture posteriorly. Because this abnormal vocal cord pattern may be intermittently present, a normal examination does not exclude the diagnosis. Bronchial challenges preferably exercise can precipitate symptoms of inducible laryngeal obstruction. The flow-volume loop may provide additional clues to the diagnosis of inducible laryngeal obstruction. Truncation of the inspiratory portion can be demonstrated in most patients during an acute episode, and some patients continue to show this pattern even when they are asymptomatic (see Figure 38–1). Children with inducible laryngeal obstruction, especially adolescents, tend to be overly competitive, primarily in athletics and scholastics. A psychiatric consultation may help define underlying psychological issues and provide appropriate therapy. Treatment of isolated inducible laryngeal obstruction includes education regarding the condition, appropriate breathing exercises, and therapeutic continuous laryngoscopy. Biofeedback, psychotherapy, and even hypnosis have been effective for some patients.

Conditions That May Increase Asthma Severity

Chronic hyperplastic sinusitis is frequently found in association with asthma. Upper airway inflammation has been shown to contribute to the pathogenesis of asthma, and asthma may improve after treatment of sinusitis. However, sinus surgery is usually not indicated for initial treatment of chronic mucosal disease associated with allergy. In older children, rarely, hyperplastic sinusitis and polyposis and severe refractory asthma can be associated with aspirin sensitivity, known as aspirin-exacerbated respiratory disease (AERD).

A significant correlation has been observed between nocturnal asthma and gastroesophageal reflux. Patients may not complain of burning epigastric pain or have other reflux symptoms—cough may be the only sign. For patients with poorly controlled asthma, particularly with a nocturnal

component, investigation for gastroesophageal reflux may be warranted even in the absence of suggestive symptoms.

Population studies have demonstrated associations between obesity and asthma. Obesity has been linked not only to the development of asthma but also with asthma control and severity. What contributes to these associations or to what extent inflammation or physiologic impairment relates to both obesity and asthma is less established. It becomes difficult to determine if a child's trouble breathing is a result of obesity itself, its comorbidities (eg, gastroesophageal reflux or obstructive sleep apnea), and/or asthma. A management approach targeting weight reduction in obese children is encouraged to improve asthma control or its assessment.

The risk factors for death from asthma include psychological and sociologic factors. They are probably related to the consequences of illness denial, poor coping or self-management skills, as well as to nonadherence with prescribed therapy. Recent studies have shown that less than 50% of inhaled asthma medications are taken as prescribed and that compliance does not improve with increasing severity of illness. Moreover, children requiring hospitalization for asthma, or their caregivers, have often failed to institute appropriate home treatment.

Complications

With acute asthma, complications are primarily related to hypoxemia and acidosis and can include generalized seizures. Pneumomediastinum or pneumothorax can be a complication in status asthmaticus. With chronic asthma, recent studies point to airway wall remodeling and loss of pulmonary function with persistent airway inflammation. Childhood asthma independent of any corticosteroid therapy has been shown to be associated with delayed maturation and slowing of prepubertal growth velocity.

Treatment

A. Chronic Asthma

1. General measures—The NAEPP EPR3 and the GINA global strategy offer slightly different management approaches. The NAEPP EPR 3 was last published over 10 years ago, while GINA is updated about every 1–2 years based on new studies, with the most recent one from 2019 Both guideline approaches include an assessment and regular monitoring of disease activity, education and partnership to improve the child's and his/her family's knowledge and skills for self-management, identification, and management of triggers and conditions that may worsen asthma, and appropriate medications selected to address the patient's needs. The objective of asthma management is the attainment of the best possible asthma control.

2. Assessment of severity and control—The NAEPP EPR3 stepwise approach is based on an assessment of severity and control. An assessment of asthma severity (ie, the intrinsic intensity of disease) is generally most accurate in patients not receiving controller therapy. Hence, assessing asthma severity directs the level of initial therapy. For those already on treatment, asthma severity can be classified according to the level of medication requirement to maintain adequate asthma control. The two general categories are intermittent and persistent asthma; the latter is further subdivided into mild, moderate, and severe (Table 38–2). In contrast, asthma control refers to the degree to which symptoms, ongoing functional impairments, and risk of adverse events are minimized and goals of therapy are met. Assessment of asthma

Table 38–2. Assessing severity and initiating treatment for patients who are not currently taking long-term control medications.

		Classification of Asthma Severity			
			Persistent		
Components of Severity		**Intermittent**	**Mild**	**Moderate**	**Severe**
Impairment	Daytime symptoms	≤ 2 days/wk	> 2 days/wk but not daily	Daily	Throughout the day
	Nighttime awakenings				
	Age 0–4 y	0	1–2 ×/mo	3–4 ×/mo	> 1 ×/wk
	Age ≥ 5 y	≤ 2 ×/mo	3–4 ×/mo	> 1 ×/wk but not nightly	Often 7 ×/wk
	SABA use for symptoms (not prevention of EIB)	≤ 2 days/wk	> 2 days/wk but not daily, and not more than 1 × on any day	Daily	Several times per day
	Interference with normal activity	None	Minor limitation	Some limitation	Extremely limited
	Lung function				
	FEV$_1$% predicted	Normal FEV$_1$ between exacerbations			
	Age ≥ 5 y	> 80% predicted	≥ 80% predicted	60%–80% predicted	< 60% predicted
	FEV$_1$/FVC ratio				
Normal FEV$_1$/ FVC: 8–19 y,	Age 5–11 y	> 85%	> 80%	75%–80%	< 75%
85% 20–39 y, 80%	Age ≥ 12 y	Normal	Normal	Reduced 5%	Reduced > 5%
Risk	Exacerbations requiring systemic corticosteroids				
	Age 0–4 y	0–1/y (see *Notes*)	≥ 2 exacerbations in 6 mo requiring systemic corticosteroids OR ≥ 4 wheezing episodes/year lasting > 1 day and risk factors for persistent asthma		
	Age ≥ 5 y	0–1/y (see *Notes*)	≥ 2/y (see *Notes*)		
		Consider severity and interval since last exacerbation. Frequency and severity may fluctuate over time for patients in any severity category. Relative annual risk of exacerbations may be related to FEV$_1$.			

(Continued)

Table 38–2. Assessing severity and initiating treatment for patients who are not currently taking long-term control medications. (*Continued*)

	Classification of Asthma Severity			
			Persistent	
Components of Severity	**Intermittent**	**Mild**	**Moderate**	**Severe**
Recommended step for initiating therapy	Step 1	Step 2	Age 0–4 y	
			Step 3	Step 3
			Age 5–11 y	
			Step 3, medium-dose ICS option	Step 3, medium-dose ICS option, OR step 4
			Age ≥ 12 y	
			Step 3	Step 4 or 5
			Consider a short course of systemic corticosteroids	
	In 2–6 wk, evaluate level of asthma control that is achieved and adjust therapy accordingly. If no clear benefit is observed within 4–6 wk, consider adjusting therapy or alternative diagnoses.			

EIB, exercise-induced bronchospasm; FEV_1, forced expiratory volume in 1 second; FVC, forced vital capacity; ICS, inhaled corticosteroids; SABA, short-acting β_2-agonist.

Notes:

- The stepwise approach is meant to assist, not replace, the clinical decision making required to meet individual patient needs.
- Level of severity is determined by both impairment and risk. Assess impairment domain by patient's/caregiver's recall of previous 2–4 weeks. Symptom assessment for longer periods should reflect a global assessment such as inquiring whether a patient's asthma is better or worse since the last visit. Assign severity to the most severe category in which any feature occurs.
- At present, there are inadequate data to correspond frequencies of exacerbations with different levels of asthma severity. For treatment purposes, patients who had ≥ 2 exacerbations requiring oral systemic corticosteroids in the past 6 months, or ≥ 4 wheezing episodes in the past year, and who have risk factors for persistent asthma may be considered the same as patients who have persistent asthma, even in the absence of impairment levels consistent with persistent asthma.

Adapted with permission from Expert Panel Report 3 (EPR-3): Guidelines for the Diagnosis and Management of Asthma-Summary Report 2007. National Asthma Education and Prevention Program. J Allergy Clin Immunol. 2007 Nov;120(5 Suppl):S94-S138.

control should be done at every visit as this is important in adjusting therapy. It is categorized as "well controlled," "not well controlled," and "very poorly controlled" (Table 38–3). Responsiveness to therapy is the ease with which asthma control is attained by treatment. It can also encompass monitoring for adverse effects related to medication use.

The NAEPP EPR3 classification of either asthma severity or control is based on the domains of current *impairment* and *risk*, recognizing that these domains may respond differently to treatment. The level of asthma severity or control is established upon the most severe component of impairment or risk. Generally, the assessment of impairment is symptom based, except for the use of lung function for school-aged children and youths. Impairment includes an assessment of the patient's recent symptom frequency and intensity and functional limitations (ie, daytime symptoms, nighttime awakenings, need for short-acting β_2-agonists [SABA] for quick relief, work or school days missed, ability

to engage in normal or desired activities, and quality-of-life assessments) and airflow compromise preferably using spirometry. Numerous validated instruments and questionnaires for assessing health-related quality of life and asthma control have been developed. The Asthma Control Test (ACT, www.asthmacontrol.com), the Asthma Control Questionnaire (ACQ, www.qoltech.co.uk/Asthma1.htm), and the Asthma Therapy Assessment Questionnaire (ATAQ, www.ataqinstrument.com) for children 12 years of age and older and the Childhood ACT for children 4–11 years of age are examples of self-administered questionnaires that have been developed with the objective of addressing multiple aspects of asthma control such as frequency of daytime and nocturnal symptoms, use of reliever medications, functional status, missed school or work, and so on. A five-item caregiver-administered instrument, the Test for Respiratory and Asthma Control in Kids (TRACK), has been validated as a tool to assess both impairment and risk presented in the

Table 38–3. Assessing asthma control and adjusting therapy in children.

Components of Control		Classification of Asthma Control		
		Well Controlled	**Not Well Controlled**	**Very Poorly Controlled**
Impairment	Symptoms	≤ 2 days/wk but not more than once on each day	> 2 days/wk or multiple times on ≤ 2 days/wk	Throughout the day
	Nighttime awakenings			
	Age 0–4 y	≤ 1 × /mo	> 1 × /mo	> 1 × /wk
	Age 5–11 y	≤ 1 × /mo	≥ 2 × /mo	≥ 2 × /wk
	Age ≥ 12 y	≤ 2 × /mo	1–3 × /wk	≥ 4 × /wk
	SABA use for symptoms (not EIB pretreatment)	≤ 2 days/wk	> 2 days/wk	Several times per day
	Interference with normal activity	None	Some limitation	Extremely limited
	Lung function			
	Age 5–11 y			
	FEV$_1$% predicted or peak flow	> 80% predicted or personal best	60%–80% predicted or personal best	< 60% predicted or personal best
	FEV$_1$/FVC	> 80%	75%–80%	< 75%
	Age ≥ 12 y			
	FEV$_1$% predicted or peak flow	> 80% predicted or personal best	60%–80% predicted or personal best	< 60% predicted or personal best
	Validated questionnaires			
	Age ≥ 12 y			
	ATAQ	0	1–2	3–4
	ACQ	≤ 0.75[a]	≥ 1.5	N/A
	ACT	≥ 20	16–19	≤ 15
Risk	Exacerbations requiring systemic corticosteroids			
	Age 0–4 y	0–1 y	2–3/y	> 3/y
	Age ≥ 5 y	0–1 y	≥ 2/y (see *Notes*)	
	Consider severity and interval since last exacerbation.			
	Treatment-related adverse effects.	Medication side effects can vary in intensity from none to very troublesome and worrisome. The level of intensity does not correlate to specific levels of control but should be considered in the overall assessment of risk.		
	Reduction in lung growth or progressive loss of lung function.	Evaluation requires long-term follow-up care.		

(Continued)

Table 38–3. Assessing asthma control and adjusting therapy in children. (*Continued*)

Components of Control	Classification of Asthma Control		
	Well Controlled	**Not Well Controlled**	**Very Poorly Controlled**
Recommended action for treatment.	• Maintain current step. • Regular follow-up every 1–6 mo to maintain control. • Consider step-down if well controlled for at least 3 mo.	• Step up (1 step). • Reevaluate in 2–6 wk. • If no clear benefit in 4–6 wk, consider alternative diagnoses or adjusting therapy. • For side effects, consider alternative options.	• Consider short course of oral corticosteroids. • Step up (1–2 steps). • Reevaluate in 2 wk. • If no clear benefit in 4–6 wk, consider alternative diagnoses or adjusting therapy. • For side effects, consider alternative options.

EIB, exercise-induced bronchospasm; FEV_1, forced expiratory volume in 1 second; FVC, forced vital capacity; SABA, short-acting β_2-agonist.
Notes:
- The stepwise approach is meant to assist, not replace, the clinical decision making required to meet individual patient needs.
- The level of control is based on the most severe impairment or risk category. Assess impairment domain by caregiver's recall of previous 2–4 weeks. Symptom assessment for longer periods should reflect a global assessment such as inquiring whether the patient's asthma is better or worse since the last visit.
- At present, there are inadequate data to correspond frequencies of exacerbations with different levels of asthma control. In general, more frequent and intense exacerbations (eg, requiring urgent, unscheduled care, hospitalization, or ICU admission) indicate poorer disease control. For treatment purposes, patients who had ≥ 2 exacerbations requiring oral systemic corticosteroids in the past year may be considered the same as patients who have not–well-controlled asthma, even in the absence of impairment levels consistent with not–well-controlled asthma.
- Validated questionnaires for the impairment domain (the questionnaires do not assess lung function or the risk domain):
  a. ATAQ = Asthma Therapy Assessment Questionnaire
  b. ACQ = Asthma Control Questionnaire
  c. ACT = Asthma Control Test
  d. Minimal Important Difference: 1.0 for ATAQ; 0.5 for the ACQ; not determined for ACT; [a]ACQ values of 0.76–1.40 are indeterminate regarding well-controlled asthma.
- Before step-up therapy:
  a. Review adherence to medications, inhaler technique, and environmental control.
  b. If alternative treatment option was used in a step, discontinue it and use preferred treatment for that step.
Adapted with permission from Expert Panel Report 3 (EPR-3): Guidelines for the Diagnosis and Management of Asthma-Summary Report 2007. National Asthma Education and Prevention Program. J Allergy Clin Immunol. 2007 Nov;120(5 Suppl):S94-S138.

NAEPP Expert Panel Report 3 (EPR3) guidelines in young children with recurrent wheezing or respiratory symptoms consistent with asthma.

3. Risk assessment—"Risk" refers to an evaluation of the patient's likelihood of developing asthma exacerbations, reduced lung growth in children (or progressive decline in lung function in adults), or risk of untoward effects from medications. The GINA 2019 strategy also cites risk factors for poor asthma outcomes (ie, exacerbations, persistent airflow limitation, and medication side effects). Having uncontrolled asthma symptoms is a risk factor for exacerbations. In those with infrequent symptoms, the following are considered modifiable risk factors for flare-ups: excessive SABA use (> 1 200-dose canister/month); inadequate inhaled corticosteroid (ICS) (from lack of prescription, poor adherence, or incorrect inhaler technique); low FEV_1, especially if less than 60% predicted; major psychological or socioeconomic problems; presence of smoking or allergen exposure (if sensitized); having comorbidities (obesity, rhinosinusitis, confirmed food allergy); sputum or blood eosinophilia; elevated exhaled nitric oxide (in allergic asthmatics on an ICS), and pregnancy. Considered major independent risk factors for flare-ups are history of intubation or ICU admission for asthma and one or more severe exacerbations in past 12 months. Risk factors for developing persistent airflow limitation are preterm birth (or low birth weight and greater infant weight gain), lack of ICS treatment; exposures to tobacco smoke, noxious chemicals, occupational exposures; low initial FEV_1; and chronic mucus hypersecretion, sputum or blood eosinophilia. Frequent oral corticosteroid use, long-term high-dose and/or potent ICS, and intake of P450 inhibitors are risk factors for systemic medication side effects, while high-dose or potent ICS and poor inhaler technique are also risk factors for local side effects.

4. Education—Education is important and partnership with the child's family is a key component in the management to improve adherence and outcomes. The patient and family must understand the role of asthma triggers, the importance of disease activity even without obvious symptoms, how to use objective measures to gauge disease activity, and the importance of airway inflammation—and they must learn to recognize the warning signs of worsening asthma, allowing for early intervention. A stepwise care plan should be developed for all patients with asthma. Providing asthma action plans is currently a requirement that is tracked by many hospitals and others to document that educational instruction for chronic disease management has been given. Asthma action plans should be provided to school personnel and all those who care for children with asthma.

Because the degree of airflow limitation is poorly perceived by many patients, peak flow meters can aid in the assessment of airflow obstruction and day-to-day disease activity if used correctly and regularly, peak flow rates may provide early warning of worsening asthma. They are also helpful in monitoring the effects of medication changes. Spacer devices optimize delivery of medication from metered-dose inhalers (MDIs) to the lungs and, with inhaled steroids, minimize side effects. Large-volume spacers are preferred. Poor understanding by patients and families of proper device use can lead to inadequate delivery and treatment with inhaled medications, especially inhaled controllers. Short instructive videos for device use can be provided to educate families and other caregivers (http://www.thechildrenshospital.org/conditions/lung/asthmavideos.aspx).

5. Exposures—Patients should avoid exposure to tobacco smoke and allergens to which they are sensitized, exertion outdoors when levels of air pollution are high, β-blockers, and sulfite-containing foods. Patients with persistent asthma should be given the inactivated influenza vaccine yearly unless they have a contraindication.

For patients with persistent asthma, the clinician should use the patient's history to assess sensitivity to seasonal allergens and *Alternaria* mold and in vitro testing (either by skin or blood test) to assess sensitivity to perennial indoor allergens, to assess the significance of positive tests in the context of the patient's history, and to identify relevant allergen exposures. For dust mite–allergic children, important environmental control measures include encasing the pillow and mattress in an allergen-impermeable cover and washing the sheets and blankets on the patient's bed weekly in hot water. Other measures include keeping indoor humidity below 50%, minimizing the number of stuffed toys, and washing such toys weekly in hot water. Children allergic to furred animals or feathers should avoid indoor exposure to pets, especially for prolonged periods of time. If removal of the pet is not possible, the animal should be kept out of the bedroom with the door closed. Carpeting and upholstered furniture should be removed. While a high-efficiency particle-arresting filter unit in the bedroom may reduce allergen levels, symptoms may persist if the pet remains indoors. For cockroach-allergic children, control measures need to be instituted when infestation is present in the home. Poison baits, boric acid, and traps are preferred to chemical agents, which can be irritating if inhaled by asthmatic individuals. Indoor molds are especially prominent in humid or damp environments. Measures to control dampness or fungal growth in the home may be of benefit. Patients can reduce exposure to outdoor allergens by staying in an air-conditioned environment. Allergen immunotherapy may be useful for implicated aeroallergens that cannot be avoided. However, it should be administered only in facilities staffed and equipped to treat life-threatening reactions.

Patients should be treated for rhinitis, sinusitis, or gastroesophageal reflux, if present. Treatment of upper respiratory tract symptoms is an integral part of asthma management. Intranasal corticosteroids are recommended to treat chronic rhinosinusitis in patients with persistent asthma because they reduce lower airway hyperresponsiveness and asthma symptoms. Intranasal cromolyn reduces asthma symptoms during the ragweed season but less so than intranasal corticosteroids. Treatment of rhinosinusitis includes medical measures to promote drainage and the use of antibiotics for acute bacterial infections (see Chapter 18). Medical management of gastroesophageal reflux includes avoiding eating or drinking 2 hours before bedtime, elevating the head of the bed with 6- to 8-in blocks, and using appropriate pharmacologic therapy.

6. Pharmacologic therapy—A revised stepwise approach to pharmacologic therapy, broken down by age categories, is recommended in the NAEPP EPR3 (http://www.nhlbi.nih.gov) (Table 38–4). This approach is based on the concepts of asthma severity and asthma control. A separate set of recommendations for younger children is provided given the lack of tools which can be used to assess lung function and quality of life otherwise available for older children. Treatment recommendations for older children and adults are better supported by stronger evidence from available clinical trials, whereas those for younger children have been extrapolated from studies in older children and adults.

The choice of initial therapy is based on assessment of asthma severity. For patients who are already on controller therapy, treatment can be adjusted based on assessment of asthma control and responsiveness to therapy. The goals of therapy are to reduce the components of both impairment (eg, preventing chronic and troublesome symptoms, allowing infrequent need of quick-relief medications, maintaining "normal" lung function, maintaining normal activity levels including physical activity and school attendance, meeting families' expectations and satisfaction with asthma care) and

Table 38–4. Stepwise approach for managing asthma in children.

	Intermittent[a]	Persistent Asthma: Daily Medication					
Age 0–4 y	Step 1 *Preferred* SABA PRN	Step 2 *Preferred* Low-dose ICS *Alternative* Cromolyn or montelukast	Step 3 *Preferred* Medium-dose ICS	Step 4 *Preferred* Medium-dose ICS + either LABA or LTRA	Step 5 *Preferred* High-dose ICS + either LABA or LTRA	Step 6 *Preferred* High-dose ICS + either LABA or LTRA AND oral corticosteroid	
Age 5–11 y	*Preferred* SABA PRN	*Preferred* Low-dose ICS *Alternative* Cromolyn, LTRA, nedocromil, or theophylline	*Preferred* EITHER Low-dose ICS + either LABA, LTRA, or theophylline OR medium-dose ICS	*Preferred* Medium-dose ICS + LABA *Alternative* Medium-dose ICS + either LTRA or theophylline	*Preferred* High-dose ICS + LABA *Alternative* High-dose ICS + either LTRA or theophylline	*Preferred* High-dose ICS + LABA AND oral corticosteroid *Alternative* High-dose ICS + either LTRA or theophylline AND oral corticosteroid	Step down if possible (and asthma is well controlled at least 3 mo) **Assess Control** Step up if needed (first check inhaler technique, adherence, environmental control, and comorbid condition)
Age ≥ 12 y	*Preferred* SABA PRN	*Preferred* Low-dose ICS *Alternative* Cromolyn, LTRA, nedocromil, or theophylline	*Preferred* Low-dose ICS + LABA OR medium-dose ICS *Alternative* Low-dose ICS + either LTRA, theophylline, or zileuton	*Preferred* Medium-dose ICS + LABA *Alternative* Medium-dose ICS + either LTRA or theophylline or zileuton	*Preferred* High-dose ICS + LABA AND consider omalizumab for patients with allergies	*Preferred* High-dose ICS + LABA + oral corticosteroid AND consider omalizumab for patients with allergies	

Each step: Patient education, environmental control, and management of comorbidities.

Age ≥ 5 y: Steps 2–4: Consider subcutaneous allergen immunotherapy for patients who have allergic asthma.

Quick-Relief Medication for All Patients

- SABA as needed for symptoms. Intensity of treatment depends on severity of symptoms: up to three treatments at 20-min intervals as needed. Short course of oral systemic corticosteroids may be needed.
- Caution: Use of SABA > 2 days/wk for symptom relief (not prevention of EIB) generally indicates inadequate control and the need to step up treatment.
- For ages 0–4 y: With viral respiratory infection: SABA q4-6h up to 24 h (longer with physician consult). Consider short course of systemic corticosteroids if exacerbation is severe or patient has history of previous severe exacerbations.

ICS, inhaled corticosteroid; LABA, inhaled long-acting β$_2$-agonist; LTRA, leukotriene receptor antagonist; prn, as needed; SABA, inhaled short-acting β$_2$-agonist.

[a]Alphabetical order is used when more than one treatment option is listed within either preferred or alternative therapy.

Table 38–4. Stepwise approach for managing asthma in children. (*Continued*)

Intermittent[a]	Persistent Asthma: Daily Medication	

Notes:
- The stepwise approach is meant to assist, not replace, the clinical decision making required to meet individual patient needs.
- If alternative treatment is used and response is inadequate, discontinue it and use the preferred treatment before stepping up.
- If clear benefit is not observed within 4–6 weeks and patient/family medication technique and adherence are satisfactory, consider adjusting therapy or alternative diagnosis.
- Studies on children aged 0–4 years are limited. Step 2 therapy is based on Evidence A. All other recommendations are based on expert opinion and extrapolation from studies in older children.
- For age 5–11 years, steps 1 and 2 medications are based on Evidence A. Step 3 ICS + adjunctive therapy and ICS are based on Evidence B for efficacy of each treatment and extrapolation from comparator trials in older children and adults—comparator trials are not available for this age group; steps 4–6 are based on expert opinion and extrapolation from studies in older children and adults.
- For ages ≥ 12 years, steps 1, 2, and 3 preferred therapies are based on Evidence A; step 3 alternative therapy is based on Evidence A for LTRA, Evidence B for theophylline, and Evidence D for zileuton. Step 4 preferred therapy is based on Evidence B, and alternative therapy is based on Evidence B for LTRA and theophylline and Evidence D for zileuton. Step 5 preferred therapy is based on Evidence B. Step 6 preferred therapy is based on (EPR-1 1997) and Evidence B for omalizumab. In step 6, before oral systemic corticosteroids are introduced, a trial of high-dose ICS + LABA + either LTRA, theophylline, or zileuton may be considered, although this approach has not been studied in clinical trials.
- Clinicians who administer immunotherapy or omalizumab should be prepared and equipped to identify and treat anaphylaxis that may occur.
- Theophylline is a less desirable alternative due to the need to monitor serum concentration levels.
- Zileuton is less desirable alternative due to limited studies as adjunctive therapy and the need to monitor liver function.
- Immunotherapy for steps 2–4 is based on Evidence B for house dust mites, animal danders, and pollens; evidence is weak or lacking for molds and cockroaches. Evidence is strongest for immunotherapy with single allergens. The role of allergy in asthma is greater in children than in adults.

Adapted with permission from Expert Panel Report 3 (EPR-3): Guidelines for the Diagnosis and Management of Asthma-Summary Report 2007. National Asthma Education and Prevention Program. J Allergy Clin Immunol. 2007 Nov;120(5 Suppl):S94-S138.

risk (eg, preventing recurrent exacerbations, reduced lung growth, and medication adverse effects).

1. The stepwise approach is meant to assist, not replace, the clinical decision making required to meet individual patient needs.

2. In the absence of persistent symptoms, the new clinical guidelines recommend considering initiation of long-term controller therapy for infants and younger children who have risk factors for asthma (ie, modified asthma predictive index: parental history of asthma, physician-diagnosed atopic dermatitis, or sensitization to aeroallergens or two of the following: wheezing apart from colds, sensitization to foods, or peripheral eosinophilia) and four or more episodes of wheezing over the past year that lasted longer than 1 day and affected sleep or two or more exacerbations in 6 months requiring systemic corticosteroids.

3. ICS, either as monotherapy or in combination with adjunctive therapy, are preferred treatment for all levels of persistent asthma.

4. Along with medium-dose ICS, combination therapy with ICS plus any of the following adjunctive therapies—long-acting inhaled β₂-agonists (LABAs), leukotriene modifying agents, cromones, and theophylline—is recommended as step 3 treatment for moderate persistent asthma, or as step-up therapy for uncontrolled persistent asthma for school-aged children and youths. In children aged 0–4 years, medium-dose ICS as monotherapy remain the step 3 therapy, and combination therapy to be initiated only as a step 4 treatment. A rescue course of systemic corticosteroids may be necessary at any step.

The revised GINA global strategy has a very different set of recommending options for initiation of controller therapy (Table 38–5). *In their stepwise approach (Table 38–6), emphasis on maximizing benefit from available medications, inhaler technique, and adherence, and treatment of risk factors and comorbidities before step-up treatment are pursued.*

Asthma medications are classified as long-term controller medications and quick-relief medications. The former includes anti-inflammatory agents (ICS and leukotriene modifiers), long-acting bronchodilators (LABAs and long-acting antimuscarinic agents [LAMAs]), and biologics (omalizumab, mepolizumab, benralizumab, reslizumab, and dupilumab). Although LABAs (salmeterol, formoterol, and vilanterol) are β-agonists, they are considered to be daily controller medications, but unlike the other asthma controller medications with primarily anti-inflammatory properties, LABAs cannot be administered as monotherapy. In contrast, conventionally, ICS-LABAs are considered long-term controller medications, and GINA strategy now recommends them as as-needed, relief medications. Bronchial thermoplasty is also an option that can be considered for some adult patients with severe asthma.

Table 38–5. Initial asthma treatment-recommended options for adults and adolescents.

Presenting Symptoms	Preferred Initial Treatment
All patients	SABA-only treatment (without ICS) is not recommended
Infrequent asthma symptoms, eg, less than twice a month	• As-needed low-dose ICS-formoterol Other options include taking ICS whenever SABA is taken, in combination or separate inhalers
Asthma symptoms or need for reliever twice a month or more	• Low-dose ICS[a] with as needed SABA, *or* • As needed low-dose ICS-formoterol Other options include LTRA (less effective than ICS) or ICS whenever SABA is taken either in combination or separate inhalers. Consider likely adherence with controller if reliever is SABA.
Troublesome asthma symptoms most days; or waking due to asthma ≥ 1 a wk, especially if any risk factors exist	• Low-dose ICS-LABA[b] as maintenance and reliever therapy with ICS-formoterol,[c] or as conventional maintenance treatment with as-needed SABA, *or* • Medium-dose ICS with as-needed SABA
Initial asthma presentation is with severely uncontrolled asthma or with an acute exacerbation	• Short course of OCS *and* start regular controller treatment with high-dose ICS or medium-dose ICS-LABA[a]

Before starting initial controller treatment

- Record evidence for diagnosis of asthma, if possible
- Record the patient's level of symptom control and risk factors, including lung function
- Consider factors influencing choice between available treatment options
- Ensure that the patient can use the inhaler correctly
- Schedule an appointment for a follow-up visit

After starting initial controller treatment

- Review patient's response after 2–3 mo or earlier depending on clinical urgency
- See Table 38–6 for recommendations for ongoing treatment and other key management issues
- Step-down treatment once good control has been maintained for 3 mo

ICS, inhaled corticosteroids; LABA, long-acting β_2-agonist; LTRA, leukotriene-receptor antagonist; OCS: oral corticosteroids; SABA: short-acting β_2-agonist.
[a]Corresponds to starting at Step 2 in Table 38-6.
[b]Corresponds to starting at Step 3 in Table 38-6.
[c]Not recommended for initial treatment in children aged 6–11 years.
This table is based on evidence from available studies and consensus, including considerations of cost.

1. Inhaled corticosteroids (ICS)—ICS are the most potent inhaled anti-inflammatory agents currently available. Although recommended as daily controller therapy, studies have shown their efficacy even for intermittent use for rescue or at the onset of acute respiratory illnesses. GINA strategy recommends inhaled steroids for all steps of asthma care. Different ICS are not equivalent on a per puff or microgram basis (Table 38–7). For most patients, low-dose ICS can provide adequate control, although some patients may need higher doses due to variable ICS responsiveness. High doses are associated with increased risk of local and systemic adverse effects. Early intervention with ICS can improve asthma control and prevent exacerbations during treatment, but they do not prevent the development of persistent asthma nor do they alter its natural history. Long-term ICS may be associated with early slowing of growth velocity in children, and although this can impact the final adult height by a minimum degree, it is not a cumulative effect. Possible risks from ICS need to be weighed against the risks from undertreated asthma. The adverse effects from ICS are generally dose and duration dependent, so that greater risks for systemic adverse effects are expected with high doses. The various ICS are delivered in different devices such as MDI (beclomethasone, ciclesonide, fluticasone propionate, flunisolide, mometasone, and triamcinolone), dry powder inhaler (DPI) (fluticasone propionate [Diskus], fluticasone furoate [Ellipta], budesonide [Flexhaler], and mometasone [Twisthaler]), and nebulized aerosol suspensions (budesonide respules). Inhaled medications delivered in MDI now use the more ozone-friendly hydrofluoroalkane (HFA) propellant, which has replaced chlorofluorocarbons (CFC). See instructions for different device use at

Table 38–6. Asthma medication options (adapted from GINA 2019).

A. Children 6–11 y

	Step 1	Step 2 Daily low-dose inhaled corticosteroid (ICS)	Step 3 Low-dose ICS-LABA (long-acting β₂-agonist) or medium-dose ICS	Step 4 Medium-dose ICS-LABA Refer for expert advice	Step 5 Refer for phenotypic assessment ± add-on therapy, eg, anti-IgE
PREFERRED CONTROLLER to prevent exacerbations and control symptoms					
Other controller options	Low-dose ICS taken whenever SABA taken,[a] or daily low-dose ICS	Leukotriene-receptor antagonist (LTRA), or low-dose ICS taken when SABA taken[a]	Low-dose ICS+LTRA	High-dose ICS-LABA, or add-on tiotropium, or add-on LTRA	Add-on anti-IL5, or add-on low-dose oral corticosteroid (OCS), but consider side effects
RELIEVER	As-needed short-acting β₂-agonist (SABA)				

[a]Off-label; separate ICS and SABA inhalers; only one study in children.

B. Adolescents and adults

	Step 1 As-needed low-dose ICS-formoterol*	Step 2 Daily low-dose ICS or as-needed low-dose ICS-formoterol[a]	Step 3 Low-dose ICS-LABA	Step 4 Medium-dose ICS-LABA	Step 5 High-dose ICS-LABA Refer for phenotypic assessment ± add-on therapy, eg, tiotropium, anti-IgE, anti-IL5/5R, anti-IL4R
PREFERRED CONTROLLER to prevent exacerbations and control symptoms					
Other controller options	Low-dose ICS taken whenever SABA taken[b]	LTRA or low-dose ICS taken when SABA taken[b]	Medium-dose ICS or low-dose ICS + LTRA[d]	High-dose ICS, add-on tiotropium, or add-on LTRA[d]	Add low-dose OCS, but consider side effects
PREFERRED RELIEVER	As needed low dose ICS-formoterol[a]		As needed low dose ICS-formoterol for patients prescribed maintenance and reliever therapy[c]		
Other reliever options	As-needed short-acting β₂-agonist (SABA)				

[a]Off-label; data only with budesonide-formoterol (bud-form).
[b]Off-label, separate or combination ICS and SABA inhalers.
[c]Low-dose ICS-formoterol is the reliever for patients prescribed budesonide-formoterol or beclomethasone-formoterol maintenance and reliever therapy.
[d]Consider adding house dust mite sublingual immunotherapy for sensitized patients with allergic rhinitis and FEV1> 70% predicted.

the following URL: http://www.thechildrenshospital.org/conditions/lung/-asthmavideos.aspx.

Only ICS have been shown to be effective in long-term clinical studies for infants. Nebulized budesonide is approved for children as young as 12 months. The suspension (available in quantities of 0.25 mg/2 mL, 0.5 mg/2 mL, and 1.0 mg/2 mL) is usually administered either once or twice daily in divided doses. For effective drug delivery, it is critical that the child has a mask secured on the face for the entire treatment, as blowing it in the face is not effective and yet a common practice by parents. Notably, this drug should not be given by ultrasonic nebulizer. Limited data suggest that ICS may be effective even in very young children when delivered by MDI with a spacer and mask. Low daily dose in mcg (defined as a dose that has not been

associated with adverse effects in trials that evaluated safety measures) for various ICS for children 5 years and younger is as follows: beclomethasone dipropionate (HFA) 100 mcg; budesonide pMDI + spacer 200 mcg; budesonide nebulized 500 mcg; fluticasone propionate (HFA) 100 mcg; and ciclesonide 160 mcg.

2. Combination of inhaled steroid and long-acting bronchodilator—For school-aged children whose asthma is uncontrolled on low-dose ICS (ie, requiring step 3 guidelines therapy), majority are likely to respond to a step-up combination therapy with a LABA bronchodilator (eg, salmeterol and formoterol), although some respond best either to an increased dose of ICS or to an addition of a leukotriene-receptor antagonist (LTRA). Salmeterol is available

Table 38–7. Estimated comparative inhaled corticosteroid doses.

Drug	Low Daily Dose			Medium Daily Dose			High Daily Dose		
	0–4 y	5–11 y	≥12 y	0–4 y	5–11 y	≥12 y	0–4 y	5–11 y	≥12 y
Beclomethasone HFA, 40 or 80 mcg/puff	NA	80–160 mcg	80–240 mcg	NA	> 160–320 mcg	> 240–480 mcg	NA	> 320 mcg	> 480 mcg
Budesonide DPI 90, 80, or 200 mcg/inhalation	NA	180–400 mcg	180–600 mcg	NA	> 400–800 mcg	> 600–1200 mcg	NA	> 800 mcg	> 1200 mcg
Budesonide inhaled suspension for nebulization, 0.25-, 0.5-, and 1.0-mg dose	0.25–0.5 mg	0.5 mg	NA	> 0.5–1.0 mg	1.0 mg	NA	> 1.0 mg	2.0 mg	NA
Flunisolide, 250 mcg/puff	NA	500–750 mcg	500–1000 mcg	NA	1000–1250 mcg	> 1000–2000 mcg	NA	> 1250 mcg	> 2000 mcg
Flunisolide HFA, 80 mcg/puff	NA	160 mcg	320 mcg	NA	320 mcg	> 320–640 mcg	NA	≥ 640 mcg	> 640 mcg
Fluticasone HFA/MDI, 44, 110, or 220 mcg/puff	176 mcg	88–176 mcg	88–264 mcg	> 176–352 mcg	> 176–352 mcg	> 264–440 mcg	> 352 mcg	> 352 mcg	> 440 mcg
Fluticasone DPI, 50, 100, or 250 mcg/inhalation	NA	100–200 mcg	100–300 mcg	NA	> 200–400 mcg	> 300–500 mcg	NA	> 400 mcg	> 500 mcg
Mometasone DPI, 220 mcg/inhalation	NA	NA	220 mcg	NA	NA	440 mcg	NA	NA	> 440 mcg
Triamcinolone acetonide, 75 mcg/puff	NA	300–600 mcg	300–750 mcg	NA	> 600–900 mcg	> 750–1500 mcg	NA	> 900 mcg	> 1500 mcg

DPI, dry powder inhaler; HFA, hydrofluoroalkane; MDI, metered-dose inhaler; NA, not approved and no data available for this age group.
Data from Expert Panel Report 3 (EPR-3): Guidelines for the Diagnosis and Management of Asthma–Summary Report 2007. National Asthma Education and Prevention Program.
J Allergy Clin Immunol. 2007 Nov;120(5 Suppl):S94-S138.

as an inhalation powder (one inhalation twice daily). It is also available combined with fluticasone (50 mcg salmeterol with 100, 250, or 500 mcg fluticasone *or* 14 mcg salmeterol with 55, 113, and 232 mcg fluticasone in a DPI and 21 mcg salmeterol with 45, 115, or 230 mcg fluticasone in an MDI). For children 12 years and older, one inhalation DPI or two inhalations MDI can be taken twice daily. (*Note:* The 100/50 fluticasone/salmeterol combination is approved in children aged 4 and older.) Salmeterol can also be used 30 minutes before exercise (but not in addition to regularly used LABAs). Formoterol has a more rapid onset of action and is available singly either as a DPI (Aerolizer, 12 mcg) or a nebulized solution approved only for chronic obstructive pulmonary disease (COPD, Perforomist); or combined with an inhaled steroid (formoterol fumarate, either 4.5 mcg with budesonide [80 or 160 mcg] or 5 mcg with mometasone [100 or 200 mcg], in an MDI). The combination product is approved for children 6 years and older, two inhalations twice daily. For long-term control, formoterol should be used in combination with an anti-inflammatory agent. It can be used for exercise-induced bronchospasm in patients 5 years and older, one inhalation at least 15 minutes before exercise (but not in addition to regularly used LABAs). An even longer-acting LABA, vilanterol, with a 24-hour activity, combined with fluticasone furoate (Breo) is approved for asthma in patients 18 years and older. Of note, FDA had requested the manufacturers of Advair Diskus and HFA (salmeterol and fluticasone), Serevent Diskus (salmeterol xinafoate), Foradil Aerolizer (formoterol fumarate), Symbicort HFA, and Brovana (arformoterol tartrate inhalation solution, a LABA approved for COPD) to update their product information warning sections regarding an increase in severe asthma episodes associated with these agents. This action was in response to data showing an increased number of asthma-related deaths in patients receiving LABA therapy in addition to their usual asthma care as compared with patients not receiving LABAs. This notice was also intended to reinforce the appropriate use of LABAs in the management of asthma. Specifically, LABA products should not be initiated as first-line asthma therapy, used with worsening wheezing, or used for acute control of bronchospasm. No data are available regarding safety concerns in patients using these products for exercise-induced bronchoconstriction. Additional information, including copies of the Patient and Healthcare Professional information sheets, can be found at: http://www.fda.gov/cder/drug/infopage/LABA/default.htm. In 2010, the FDA requested the four manufacturers of LABAs to conduct a prospective trial to evaluate whether a LABA added to an ICS would be noninferior to an ICS alone with regard to the risk of serious asthma related event (hospitalization, endotracheal intubation, or death). One study, focused on the safety of LABAs in children 4–11 years of age, found that there was no excess risk of serious asthma related event associated with fluticasone propionate-salmeterol combination compared to fluticasone

alone. Similar findings were found in two other trials that enrolled adults and adolescents, that LABAs in fixed-dose combination with an ICS was associated with the risk of serious asthma-related event comparable to the risk with the ICS alone. Although not recommended in the United States and is still an off-label indication in other countries, GINA offers ICS-LABA (specifically low-dose beclomethasone/formoterol or budesonide/formoterol) as both maintenance and reliever treatment at steps 3–5 for adults and adolescents. In addition, for mild asthma as preferred controller for steps 1 and 2, GINA also now recommends symptom driven (as needed) or before exercise use of low-dose ICS-formoterol for adults and adolescents, instead of SABA alone. This option using ICS-LABA as reliever has been found to significantly reduce exacerbations and provide control at relatively low-maintenance ICS dose requirement. Patients prescribed as needed ICS-formoterol should seek medical attention if they consume 72 mcg formoterol in a day.

3. Leukotriene antagonists—Montelukast and zafirlukast are LTRAs available in oral formulations. Montelukast is given once daily and has been approved for treatment of chronic asthma in children aged 1 year and older, as an alternative step 2 monotherapy and add-on therapy for steps 3–6. It is also indicated for seasonal allergic rhinitis in patients 2 years and older, and for perennial allergic rhinitis in patients 6 months and older. To date, no drug interactions have been noted. The dosage is 4 mg for children 1–5 years (oral granules are available for children aged 12–23 months), 5 mg for children aged 6–14 years, and 10 mg for those aged 15 years and older. The drug is given without regard to mealtimes, preferably in the evening. Zafirlukast is approved for patients aged 5 years and older. The dose is 10 mg twice daily for those 5–11 years and 20 mg twice daily for those 12 years and older. It should be taken 1 hour before or 2 hours after meals. Zileuton is a 5-lipoxygenase inhibitor indicated for chronic treatment in children 12 years of age and older, available in regular 600 mg dose tablet four times a day or extended-release 600 mg dose tablet, two tablets twice a day. Patients need to have hepatic transaminase levels evaluated at initiation of therapy, then once a month for the first 3 months, every 2–3 months for the remainder of the first year, and periodically thereafter if receiving long-term zileuton therapy. Rare cases of Churg-Strauss syndrome have been reported in adult patients with severe asthma whose steroid dosage was being tapered during concomitant treatment with LTRAs (as well as ICS), but no causal link has been established. Both zafirlukast and zileuton are microsomal P-450 enzyme inhibitors that can inhibit the metabolism of drugs such as warfarin and theophylline. The FDA has requested that manufacturers include a precaution in the drug prescribing information (drug labeling) regarding neuropsychiatric events (agitation, aggression, anxiousness, dream abnormalities and hallucinations, depression, insomnia, irritability, restlessness, suicidal thinking and behavior, and tremor) based on postmarket reports of patients taking leukotriene-modifying agents. Of note, in a study of children with mild to moderate persistent asthma that looked at whether responses to an ICS and a LTRA were concordant for individuals or whether asthmatic patients who did not respond to one medication responded to the other, responses to fluticasone and montelukast were found to vary considerably. Children with low pulmonary function or high levels of markers associated with allergic inflammation responded better to the ICS.

Children with persistent asthma who remain uncontrolled on ICS monotherapy are more likely to respond to a combination treatment of an ICS and a LABA; however, there are children who can respond best to a higher dose of ICS, or even a low-dose ICS plus montelukast. It has not been definitely determined what clinical features would be helpful in selecting the most appropriate medication for any one patient.

4. Long-acting antimuscarinics—The LAMA, tiotropium (Spiriva Respimat [1.25 mcg] has now been approved as once-daily maintenance treatment for asthma in patients 6 years and older, as an add-on therapy to ICS. GINA 2019 recommends tiotropium by mist inhaler as an add-on "other" controller option for step 4 and "preferred" controller option for step 5 treatment for with a history of exacerbations. Tiotropium by mist inhaler (particularly at 5 mcg daily dose) improves lung function and time to severe exacerbation.

5. Other treatment options—Biologics: Anti-IgE (omalizumab) is a recombinant DNA-derived humanized IgG_1 monoclonal antibody that selectively binds to human IgE. It inhibits the binding of IgE to the high-affinity IgE receptor (FcεRI) on the surface of mast cells and basophils. Reduction in surface-bound IgE on FcεRI-bearing cells limits the degree of release of mediators of the allergic response. Treatment with omalizumab also reduces the number of FcεRI receptors on basophils in atopic patients. Omalizumab is now indicated for children as young as 6 years with moderate to severe persistent asthma who have a positive skin test or in vitro reactivity to a perennial aeroallergen with total serum IgE of 30–1300 IU/mL for children 6–11 years (30–700 IU/mL for adolescents), and whose symptoms are inadequately controlled with medium- to high-dose ICS. Omalizumab has been shown to decrease the incidence of asthma exacerbations and improve asthma control. Dosing is based on the patient's weight and serum IgE level and is given subcutaneously every 2–4 weeks. The FDA has ordered a black box warning to the label because of new reports of serious and life-threatening anaphylactic reactions (bronchospasm, hypotension, syncope, urticaria, and angioedema of the throat or tongue) in patients after treatment with omalizumab (Xolair®). Based on premarketing clinical trials in patients with asthma, anaphylaxis occurred with 0.1% of patients; in postmarketing spontaneous reports based on an estimated exposure of about 57,300 patients

from June 2003 through December 2006, the frequency of anaphylaxis attributed to Xolair® use was estimated to be at least 0.2% of patients. From a case-control study, patients with a history of anaphylaxis from whatever cause considered at increased risk of anaphylaxis with Xolair®, compared to those with no prior history of anaphylaxis. Although these reactions occurred within 2 hours of receiving a omalizumab subcutaneous injection, they also included reports of serious delayed reactions 2–24 hours or even longer after receiving the injections. Anaphylaxis occurred after any dose of omalizumab (including the first dose), even in patients with no allergic reaction to previous doses. Omalizumab-treated patients should be observed in the facility for an extended period after the drug is given, and medical providers who administer the injection should be prepared to manage life-threatening anaphylactic reactions. Patients who receive omalizumab should be fully informed about the signs and symptoms of anaphylaxis, their chance of developing delayed anaphylaxis following each injection, and how to treat it, including the use of autoinjectable epinephrine. Malignancy (eg, breast, non-melanoma skin, prostate, melanoma, and parotid, etc) was observed in 20 of 4127 (0.5%) Xolair-treated patients compared with 5 of 2236 (0.2%) control patients in clinical studies of adults and adolescents with asthma and other allergies. A more recent observational study of 5007 Xolair®-treated and 2829 non-Xolair®-treated patients with moderate to severe persistent allergic asthma followed for up to 5 years showed similar incidence rates (per/1000 patient years) of primary malignancies among Xolair®-treated (12.3) and non-Xolair®-treated patients (13.0).

In addition to omalizumab, new biologics or immunomodulators directed against specific T2 airway inflammation have been studied to target the inflammatory component of asthma. The US FDA has recommended approval of mepolizumab (Nucala, monoclonal antibody IgG1K, administered 100 mg subcutaneously every 4 weeks) for patients 12 years and older; reslizumab (Cinqair™, monoclonal antibody IgG4K, given 3 mg/kg intravenously monthly) for adult patients aged 18 years and older; and benralizumab (Fasenra™, humanized monoclonal antibody directed against the alpha subunit of the IL-5 receptor, subcutaneous injection 30 mg every 4 weeks for the first 3 doses, then 30 mg every 8 weeks thereafter), for aged 12 years and older, as add-on maintenance treatment of patients with severe asthma and with an eosinophilic phenotype. Dupilumab, (Dupixent®) a monoclonal antibody directed against the IL4 receptor alpha, is the first FDA approved biologic for asthma which can be self-administered subcutaneously every 2 weeks, for patients aged 12 years and older with eosinophilic moderate to severe asthma or oral-corticosteroid dependent asthma. These drugs have been shown to be effective at reducing exacerbations, improving lung function and symptom control, and decreasing oral corticosteroid use. A simple algorithm to

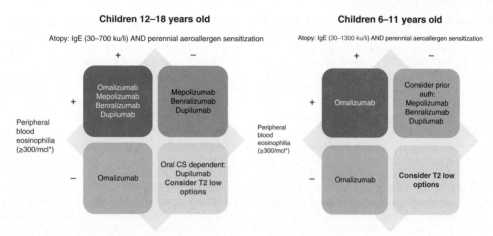

Children 12–18 years old

Atopy: IgE (30–700 ku/li) AND perennial aeroallergen sensitization

Children 6–11 years old

Atopy: IgE (30–1300 ku/li) AND perennial aeroallergen sensitization

*Cut off blood eosinophils ≥150/mcl for mepolizumab

▲ **Figure 38–2.** Biologic therapy options for children and adolescents.

direct specialists to biological therapy using available bio-markers is proposed, as shown in Figure 38–2.

Immunotherapy (discussed in more detail in section Immunotherapy) can be considered for children 5 years and older with allergic asthma. GINA recommends adding house dust mite sublingual immunotherapy for adults and adolescents on steps 3 or 4 who are sensitized with allergic rhinitis and FEV_1 more than 70% predicted.

Chronic azithromycin therapy is another off-label add-on option for patients with symptomatic asthma despite moderate to high-dose ICS/LABA combination.

Theophylline is rarely used and is no longer mentioned in the GINA guidelines. Sustained-release theophylline, an alternative long-term control medication for older children, may have particular risks of adverse effects in infants, who frequently have febrile illnesses that increase theophylline concentrations. Hence, if theophylline is used, it requires monitoring of serum concentration to prevent numerous dose-related acute toxicities.

Oral corticosteroids (low dose) are only recommended as "other" controller option for step 5 therapy in the GINA guidelines, because of adverse effects. They are recommended in NAEPP EPR step 6 therapy.

6. Monitoring and management—Continual monitoring is necessary to ensure that control of asthma is achieved and sustained. Once control is established, gradual reduction in therapy is appropriate and may help determine the minimum amount of medication necessary to maintain control. Regular follow-up visits with the clinician are important to assess the degree of control and consider appropriate adjustments in therapy. At each step, patients should be instructed to avoid or control exposure to allergens, irritants, or other factors that contribute to asthma severity.

Referral to an asthma specialist for consultation or co-management is recommended if there are difficulties in achieving or maintaining control. For children younger than 5 years, referral is recommended for moderate persistent asthma or if the patient requires step 3 or 4 care and should be considered if the patient requires step 2 care. For children 5 years and older, consultation with a specialist is recommended if the patient requires step 4 care or higher and should be considered at step 3. Referral is also recommended if allergen immunotherapy or a biologic is being considered.

Quick-relief medications include inhaled SABAs such as albuterol, levalbuterol, pirbuterol, or terbutaline. Albuterol can be given by nebulizer, 0.05 mg/kg (with a minimal dose of 0.63 mg and a maximum of 5 mg) in 2–3 mL saline (although it is also available in a 2.5 mg/3 mL single vial or 5 mg/mL concentrated solution) or by MDI (90 mcg/actuation) or by breath-actuated DPI (Respiclick). It is better to use SABAs as needed rather than on a regular basis. Increasing use, including more than one canister per month, may signify inadequate asthma control and the need to step up or revise controller therapy. Levalbuterol, the (R)-enantiomer of racemic albuterol, is available in solution for nebulization in patients aged 6–11 years, 0.31 mg every 8 hours, and in patients 12 years and older, 0.63–1.25 mg every 8 hours. It has recently become available in an HFA formulation for children 4 years and older, two inhalations (90 mcg) every 4–6 hours as needed. Anticholinergic agents such as ipratropium, one to three puffs or 0.25–0.5 mg by nebulizer every 6 hours may provide additive benefit when used together with an inhaled SABA. Systemic corticosteroids such as prednisone, prednisolone, and methylprednisolone can be given in a dosage of 1–2 mg/kg, usually up to 60 mg/day in single or divided doses for 3–10 days. There is no evidence that tapering the dose following a "burst" prevents relapse.

7. Exercise-induced bronchospasm—Exercise-induced bronchospasm should be anticipated in all asthma patients. It typically occurs during or minutes after vigorous activity, reaches its peak 5–10 minutes after stopping the activity, and usually resolves over the next 20–30 minutes. Participation in physical activity should be encouraged in children with asthma, although the choice of activity may need to be modified based on the severity of illness, presence of other triggers such as cold air, and, rarely, confounding factors such as osteoporosis. Poor endurance or exercise-induced bronchospasm can be an indication of poorly controlled persistent asthma. If symptoms occur during usual play activities, either initiation of or a step-up in long-term therapy is warranted. However, for those with exercise-induced bronchospasm as the only manifestation of asthma despite otherwise being "well-controlled," treatment immediately prior to vigorous activity or exercise is usually effective. SABAs, LTRAs, cromolyn, or nedocromil can be used before exercise. The combination of a SABA with either cromolyn or nedocromil is more effective than either drug alone. Salmeterol and formoterol may block exercise-induced bronchospasm for up to 12 hours (as discussed earlier). However, decreased duration of protection against exercise-induced bronchospasm can be expected with regular use. Montelukast may be effective up to 24 hours. An extended warm-up period may induce a refractory state, allowing patients to exercise without a need for repeat medications.

B. Acute Asthma

1. General measures—The most effective strategy in managing asthma exacerbations involves early recognition of warning signs and early treatment. For patients with moderate or severe persistent asthma or a history of severe exacerbations, this should include a written action plan. The latter usually defines the patient's green, yellow, and red zones based on symptoms (and PEFR for patients with poor symptom perception) with corresponding measures to take according to the state the patient is in. PEFR cutoff values are conventionally set as more than 80% (green), 50%–80% (yellow), and less than 50% (red) of the child's personal best. Prompt communication with the clinician is indicated with severe symptoms or a drop in peak flow or with decreased response to SABAs. At such times, intensification of therapy may include a short course of oral corticosteroids. The child should be removed from exposure to any irritants or allergens that could be contributing to the exacerbation.

2. Management at home—Early treatment of asthma exacerbations may prevent hospitalization and a life-threatening event. Initial treatment should be with a SABA such as albuterol or levalbuterol; two to six puffs from an MDI can be given every 20 minutes up to three times, or a single treatment can be given by nebulizer (0.05 mg/kg [minimum dose, 1.25 mg; maximum, 2.5 mg] of 0.5% solution of albuterol in 2–3 mL saline; or 0.075 mg/kg [minimum dose, 1.25 mg; maximum, 5 mg] of levalbuterol). If the response is good as assessed by sustained symptom relief or improvement in PEFR to over 80% of the patient's best, the SABA can be continued every 3–4 hours for 24–48 hours. Patients should be advised to seek medical care once excessive doses of bronchodilator therapy are used or for prolonged periods (eg, > 12 puffs/day for > 24 hours). Doubling the dose of ICS is not proven sufficient to prevent worsening of exacerbations; and a recent study in children with mild persistent asthma also demonstrated lack of benefit of quintupling low-dose ICS as a yellow zone action plan. If the patient does not completely improve from the initial therapy or PEFR falls between 50% and 80% predicted or personal best, the SABA should be continued, an oral corticosteroid should be added, and the patient should contact the physician urgently. If the child experiences marked distress or if PEFR persists at 50% or less, the patient should repeat the SABA immediately and go to the ED or call 911 or another emergency number for assistance.

3. Management in the office or emergency department—Functional assessment of the patient includes obtaining objective measures of airflow limitation with PEFR or FEV_1 and monitoring the patient's response to treatment; however, very severe exacerbations and respiratory distress may prevent the execution of lung function measurements using maximal expiratory maneuver. When possible flow-volume loops should be obtained to differentiate upper and lower airway obstruction, especially in patients with atypical presentation. Other tests should include oxygen saturation and if concerning then blood gases. Chest radiographs are not recommended routinely but should be considered to rule out pneumothorax, pneumomediastinum, pneumonia, or lobar atelectasis. If the initial FEV_1 or PEFR is over 40%, initial treatment can be with a SABA by inhaler (albuterol, four to eight puffs) or nebulizer (0.15 mg/kg of albuterol 0.5% solution; minimum dose, 2.5 mg), up to three doses in the first hour. Oxygen should be given to maintain oxygen saturation at greater than 90%. Oral corticosteroids (1–2 mg/kg/day in divided doses; maximum of 60 mg/day for children aged ≤ 12 years and 80 mg/day for those > 12 years) should be instituted if the patient responds poorly to therapy or if the patient has recently been on oral corticosteroids. Sensitivity to adrenergic drugs may improve after initiation of corticosteroids. For severe exacerbations or if the initial FEV_1 or PEFR is under 40%, initial treatment should be with a high-dose SABA plus ipratropium bromide, 1.5–3 mL every 20 minutes for three doses (each 3 mL vial contains 0.5 mg ipratropium bromide and 2.5 mg albuterol), then as needed by nebulizer. Continuous albuterol nebulized treatments (0.5 mg/kg/h for small and 10–15 mg/h for older children) can be administered for evidence of persistent obstruction. Oxygen should be given to maintain oxygen saturation at greater than 90%, and systemic corticosteroids should be administered. For patients with severe exacerbation having no response to initial aerosolized therapy, or for those who cannot cooperate with or who resist inhalation therapy, adjunctive therapies such as intravenous magnesium sulfate (25–75 mg/kg up to 2 g in children) and heliox-driven albuterol nebulization should be considered. There is an ongoing trial evaluating the efficacy of magnesium nebulization in the emergency room in preventing a hospital admission for asthma in children. Epinephrine 1:1000 or terbutaline 1 mg/mL (both 0.01 mg/kg up to 0.3–0.5 mg) may be administered subcutaneously every 20 minutes for three doses, although the use of intravenous β_2-agonists is still unproven. For impending or ongoing respiratory arrest, patients should be intubated and ventilated with 100% oxygen, given intravenous corticosteroids, and admitted to an intensive care unit (ICU). Potential indications for ICU admission also include any FEV_1 or PEFR less than 25% of predicted that improves less than 10% after treatment or values that fluctuate widely. (See asthma [life-threatening] in Chapter 14.) Further treatment is based on clinical response and objective laboratory findings. Hospitalization should be considered strongly for any patient with a history of respiratory failure.

4. Hospital management—For patients who do not respond to outpatient and ED treatment, admission to the hospital becomes necessary for more aggressive care and support. The decision to hospitalize should also be based on presence of risk factors for mortality from asthma, duration and severity of symptoms, severity of airflow limitation, course and severity of previous exacerbations, medication use at the time of the exacerbation, access to medical care, and home and psychosocial conditions. Fluids should be given at maintenance requirements unless the patient has poor oral intake secondary to respiratory distress or vomiting, because overhydration may contribute to pulmonary edema associated with high intrapleural pressures generated in severe asthma. Potassium requirements should be kept in mind because both corticosteroids and β_2-agonists can cause potassium loss. Moisturized oxygen should be titrated by oximetry to maintain oxygen saturation above 90%. Inhaled β_2-agonist should be continued by nebulization in single doses as needed or by continuous therapy, along with systemic corticosteroids (as discussed earlier). Ipratropium is no longer recommended during hospitalization. In addition, the role of methylxanthines in hospitalized children remains controversial. Antibiotics may be necessary to treat coexisting bacterial infection. Sedatives and anxiolytic agents are contraindicated in severely ill patients owing to their depressant effects on respiration. Chest physiotherapy is usually not recommended for acute exacerbations.

5. Patient discharge—Criteria for discharging patients home from the office or ED should include a sustained response of at least 1 hour to bronchodilator therapy with FEV_1 or PEFR greater than 70% of predicted or personal best and oxygen saturation greater than 90% in room air. Prior to discharge, the patient's or caregiver's ability to continue therapy and assess symptoms appropriately needs to be considered. Patients should be given an action plan for management of recurrent symptoms or exacerbations, and instructions about medications should be reviewed. The inhaled SABA as needed and oral corticosteroids should be continued, the latter for 3–10 days. Finally, the patient or caregiver should be instructed about the follow-up visit, recommended to happen within 2 days after an ED visit or hospitalization. Hospitalized patients should receive more intensive education prior to discharge. Referral to an asthma specialist should be considered for all children with severe exacerbations or multiple ED visits or hospitalizations.

▶ Prognosis

Since the 1970s, morbidity rates for asthma have increased, but mortality rates may have stabilized. Mortality statistics indicate that a high percentage of deaths have resulted from underrecognition of asthma severity and undertreatment, particularly in labile asthmatic patients and in asthmatic patients whose perception of pulmonary obstruction is poor. Long-term outcome studies suggest that children with mild symptoms generally outgrow their asthma, while patients with more severe symptoms, marked airway hyperresponsiveness, and a greater degree of atopy tend to have persistent disease. Data from an unselected birth cohort from New Zealand showed more than one in four children had wheezing that persisted from childhood to adulthood or that relapsed after remission. Recent evidence suggests that early intervention with anti-inflammatory therapy does not alter the development of persistent asthma, and it is also unclear if such intervention or environmental control measures influence the natural history of childhood asthma. Nonetheless, the pediatrician or primary care provider together with the asthma specialist has the responsibility to optimize control and, it is hoped, reduce the severity of asthma in children. Interventions that can have long-term effects such as halting progression or inducing remission are necessary to decrease the public health burden of this common condition.

Resources for health care providers, patients, and families include the following:

- Asthma and Allergy Foundation of America
- 1233 20th St NW, Suite 402
- Washington, DC 20036; (800) 7-ASTHMA
- http://www.aafa.org/
- Asthma and Allergy Network/Mothers of Asthmatics
- 2751 Prosperity Avenue, Suite 150
- Fairfax, VA 22031; (800) 878-4403
- http://www.aanma.org/

- Asthma Device Training: http://www.thechildrenshospital.org/conditions/lung/asthmavideos.aspx
- Global Initiative for Asthma 2019 (www.ginasthma.org)

Akinbami LJ, Simon AE, Rossen LM: Changing trends in asthma prevalence among children. Pediatrics 2016;137:2015–2354 [PMID: 26712860].

Centers for Disease Control and Prevention: National Center for Health Statistics. Health Data Interactive. Summary Health Statistics for U.S. Children: National Health Interview Survey, 2015. https://www.cdc.gov/nchs/fastats/asthma.htm. Accessed January 16, 2018.

Global Initiative for Asthma: http://www.nhlbi.nih.gov/guidelines/asthma/asthgdln.htm.

Global strategy for asthma management and prevention: Updated 2019. http://ginasthma.org/2019-gina-report-global-strategy-for-asthma-management-and-prevention/. Accessed June 30, 2019.

National Asthma Education and Prevention Program: Expert Panel Report 3 (EPR 3): Guidelines for the Diagnosis and Management of Asthma—Summary Report 2007. J Allergy Clin Immunol 2007;120(5 Suppl):S94 [PMID: 17983880].

ALLERGIC RHINOCONJUNCTIVITIS

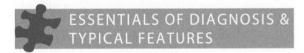

ESSENTIALS OF DIAGNOSIS & TYPICAL FEATURES

▶ Exposure to environmental allergens can affect primarily the nose and eyes, as they are major entry points, causing pruritus, mucus secretion or discharge, sneezing, irritation, and swelling.

▶ Although there is less threat of an acute major event, as seen with asthma and food- or drug-related reactions, the consequences of allergic rhino-conjunctivitis are certainly not trivial, especially when the symptoms occur chronically: sleep disturbance, poor school performance, uncontrolled asthma, sinusitis, and impaired quality of life.

▶ Similar to any allergic condition, avoidance of known triggers (determined from allergy skin testing or specific IgE antibody tests) is key. Pharmacologic chronic management can include systemic and topical antihistamines, mast cell stabilizers, topical corticosteroids, and LTRA.

▶ Immunotherapy, subcutaneous or oral, is recommended for more difficult to control disease.

Allergic rhinoconjunctivitis is the most common allergic disease and significantly affects quality of life as well as school performance and attendance. It frequently coexists with asthma, can impact asthma control, and is a risk factor for subsequent development of asthma. Over 80% of patients with asthma have rhinitis and 10%–14% of patients with rhinitis have asthma. About 80% of individuals with allergic rhinitis develop their symptoms before age 20 years. It is estimated that 13% of children have a physician diagnosis of allergic rhinitis. Prevalence of this disease increases during childhood, peaking at 15% in the post adolescent years. Although allergic rhinoconjunctivitis is more common in boys during early childhood, there is little difference in incidence between the sexes after adolescence. Race and socioeconomic status are not considered to be important factors.

The pathologic changes in allergic rhinoconjunctivitis are chiefly hyperemia, edema, and increased serous and mucoid secretions caused by mediator release, all of which lead to variable degrees of nasal obstruction and conjunctival injection, nasal and ocular pruritus, or nasal and ocular discharge. Ocular allergies can occur in isolation, but more commonly, they are in conjunction with nasal symptoms. This process may involve other structures, including the sinuses and possibly the middle ear. Inhalant allergens are primarily responsible for symptoms, but food allergens can cause symptoms as well. Children with allergic rhinitis seem to be more susceptible to—or at least may experience more symptoms from—upper respiratory infections, which, in turn, may aggravate the allergic rhinitis.

Allergic rhinoconjunctivitis has been classified as perennial (usually caused by indoor allergens such as house dust mites, molds, cockroaches, and animal dander), seasonal (hay fever most frequently caused by outdoor allergens such as pollens and molds)), or episodic; however, there are areas where pollens and soil molds may be present year round while exposure to typical perennial allergens such as indoor furred animals may be intermittent. For this reason, the preferred terms are *intermittent* (ie, symptoms present < 4 days a week or for < 4 weeks) and *persistent* (ie, symptoms present > 4 days a week and for > 4 weeks). In addition, severity should be noted as *mild* (ie, without impairment or disturbance of sleep, daily activities, leisure, sport, school, or work, or without troublesome symptoms) or *moderate-severe* (ie, presence of one or more of the aforementioned). The major pollen groups in the temperate zones include trees (late winter to early spring), grasses (late spring to early summer), and weeds (late summer to early fall), but seasons can vary significantly in different parts of the country. Mold spores also cause seasonal allergic rhinitis, principally in the summer and fall. Seasonal allergy symptoms may be aggravated by coincident exposure to perennial allergens.

▶ Clinical Findings

A. Symptoms and Signs

Patients may complain of itching of the nose, eyes, palate, or pharynx and loss of smell or taste. Nasal itching can cause paroxysmal sneezing and epistaxis. Repeated rubbing of the nose (so-called allergic salute) may lead to a horizontal crease across the lower third of the nose. Nasal obstruction is associated with mouth breathing, nasal speech, allergic salute, and snoring. Nasal turbinates may appear pale blue and swollen with dimpling or injected with minimal edema. Typically, clear and thin nasal secretions are increased, with anterior rhinorrhea, sniffling, postnasal drip, and congested cough. Nasal secretions often cause poor appetite, fatigue, and pharyngeal irritation. Conjunctival injection, tearing, periorbital edema, and infraorbital cyanosis (so-called allergic shiners) are frequently observed. Increased pharyngeal lymphoid tissue ("cobblestoning") from chronic drainage and enlarged tonsillar and adenoidal tissue may be present.

B. Laboratory Findings

Eosinophilia often can be demonstrated on smears of nasal secretions or blood. This is a frequent but nonspecific finding and may occur in nonallergic conditions. Although serum IgE may be elevated, measurement of total IgE is a poor screening tool owing to the wide overlap between atopic and nonatopic subjects. Skin testing to identify allergen-specific IgE is the most sensitive and specific test for inhalant allergies; alternatively, the Phadia ImmunoCAP assay, radioallergosorbent test (RAST), or other in vitro tests can be done for suspected allergens.

▶ Differential Diagnosis

Disorders that need to be differentiated from allergic rhinitis include infectious rhinosinusitis. Foreign bodies and structural abnormalities such as choanal atresia, marked septal deviation, nasal polyps, and adenoidal hypertrophy may cause chronic symptoms. Overuse of topical nasal decongestants may result in rhinitis medicamentosa (rebound congestion). Use of medications such as propranolol, clonidine, and some psychoactive drugs may cause nasal congestion. Illicit drugs such as cocaine can cause rhinorrhea. Spicy or hot foods may cause gustatory rhinitis. Nonallergic rhinitis with eosinophilia syndrome is usually not seen in young children. Vasomotor rhinitis is associated with persistent symptoms but without allergen exposure. Less common causes of symptoms that may be confused with allergic rhinitis include pregnancy, congenital syphilis, hypothyroidism, tumors, and cerebrospinal fluid rhinorrhea.

As in the differential diagnoses for allergic rhinitis, infectious conjunctivitis (secondary to viral, bacterial, or chlamydial etiology) can mimic allergic eye disorders. In this case, it typically develops in one eye first, and symptoms include stinging or burning sensation (rather than pruritus) with a foreign-body sensation and eye discharge (watery, mucoid, or purulent). Nasolacrimal duct obstruction, foreign body, blepharoconjunctivitis, dry eye, uveitis, and trauma are other masqueraders of ocular allergy.

The other conditions that comprise allergic eye diseases, presenting with bilateral conjunctivitis, include atopic keratoconjunctivitis, vernal conjunctivitis, and giant papillary conjunctivitis. Except for giant papillary conjunctivitis, the three (allergic conjunctivitis, atopic keratoconjunctivitis, and vernal conjunctivitis) are associated with allergic sensitization. Atopic keratoconjunctivitis and vernal conjunctivitis are both vision threatening. Atopic keratoconjunctivitis is rarely seen before late adolescence, and it most commonly involves the lower tarsal conjunctiva. Ocular symptoms (itching, burning, and tearing) are more severe than in allergic conjunctivitis and persist all year round, with accompanying eyelid eczema with erythema and thick, dry scaling skin, which can extend to the periorbital skin and cheeks. Vernal conjunctivitis is characterized by giant papillae, described as cobblestoning, seen in the upper tarsal conjunctiva. It affects boys more often than girls, and patients of Asian and African descent are more predisposed. It affects individuals in temperate areas, with exacerbations in the spring and summer months. In addition to severe pruritus that can be exacerbated by exposure to irritants, light, or perspiration, other accompanying signs and symptoms include photophobia, foreign body sensation, lacrimation, and presence of stringy or thick, ropey discharge, transient yellow-white points in the limbus (Trantas dots) and conjunctiva (Horner points), corneal "shield" ulcers, Dennie lines (prominent skin folds that extend in an arc form from the inner canthus beneath and parallel to the lower lid margin), and prominently long eyelashes. Giant papillary conjunctivitis is associated with exposure to foreign bodies such as contact lenses, ocular prostheses, and sutures. It is characterized by mild ocular itching, tearing, and mucoid discharge especially on awakening. Trantas dots, limbal infiltration, bulbar injection, and edema may also be found. One eye condition, contact allergy, which can also involve the conjunctivae especially when associated with use of topical medications, contact lens solutions, and preservatives, typically affects the eyelids.

▶ Complications

Sinusitis may accompany allergic rhinitis. Allergic mucosal swelling of the sinus ostia can obstruct sinus drainage, interfering with normal sinus function, and predisposing to chronic mucosal disease. Nasal polyps due to allergy are unusual in children, and cystic fibrosis should be considered if they are present. Unlike vision-threatening complications associated with atopic keratoconjunctivitis and vernal conjunctivitis, allergic conjunctivitis manifests primarily with significant pruritus and discomfort affecting the patients' quality of life.

▶ Treatment

A. General Measures

The value of identification and avoidance of causative allergens cannot be overstated. Reducing indoor allergens through environmental control measures as discussed in the section on asthma can be very effective. Nasal saline irrigation may be useful. For ocular allergies, cold compresses and lubrication are also important.

B. Pharmacologic Therapy

Evidence-based clinical practice guidelines such as the Allergic Rhinitis and its Impact on Asthma (ARIA) that include the pharmacologic management of allergic rhinitis have been developed based on the Grading of Recommendations Assessment, Development and Evaluation (GRADE) approach. While ARIA recommends the use of intranasal corticosteroids for adults with allergic rhinitis, the use of the topical corticosteroids over oral antihistamines for children is suggested.

The treatment of mild intermittent rhinitis includes oral or intranasal H_1-antihistamines and intranasal decongestants (for < 10 days and not to be repeated more than twice a month). Oral decongestants are not usually recommended in children. Options for moderate-severe intermittent rhinitis are oral or intranasal antihistamines, oral H_1-antihistamines and decongestants, intranasal corticosteroids, and cromones. The same medication options are available for persistent rhinitis, but a stepwise approach is proposed both for treatment of mild and moderate-severe persistent rhinitis. For mild persistent rhinitis, reassessment after 2–4 weeks is recommended and treatment should be continued, with a possible reduction in intranasal corticosteroids, even if the symptoms have abated. If, however, the patient has persistent mild symptoms while on H_1-antihistamines or cromones, an intranasal corticosteroid is appropriate. For moderate-severe persistent disease, use of intranasal corticosteroids as first-line therapy is recommended. For severe nasal congestion, either a short 1- to 2-week course of an oral corticosteroid or an intranasal decongestant for less than 10 days may be added. If the patient improves, the treatment should last for at least 3 months or until the pollen season is over. If the patient does not improve within 2–4 weeks despite adequate compliance and use of medications, comorbidities such as nasal polyps, sinusitis, and significant allergen exposure should be considered, as well as the possibility of misdiagnosis. Once these are ruled out, options include increasing the dose of the intranasal corticosteroid, combination therapy with an H_1-antihistamine (particularly if major symptoms are sneezing, itching, or rhinorrhea), ipratropium bromide (if major symptom is rhinorrhea), or an oral H_1-antihistamine and decongestant. Referral to a specialist may be considered if the treatment is not sufficient.

The recent ARIA update addressed several questions about comparative treatments for allergic rhinitis, based on a review of new pieces of evidence, albeit obtained mostly from adult patients. The recommendations on these questions are mostly considered conditional, based on low to at best moderate certainty of evidence. One question is whether to use combination antihistamine and nasal steroid spray compared to nasal steroid spray alone for the treatment of allergic rhinitis. Either option is appropriate for seasonal allergic rhinitis, while nasal steroid spray alone may be adequate for perennial allergic rhinitis. With regard to the use of nasal steroid with or without an intranasal antihistamine, either option for seasonal and perennial allergic rhinitis is also recommended. However, the combination of nasal steroid spray and intranasal antihistamine compared to intranasal antihistamine alone for seasonal rhinitis is favored. The use of a nasal steroid spray is favored over an intranasal antihistamine for both seasonal and perennial allergic rhinitis.

The preference of a LTRA versus an oral antihistamine was also evaluated. Either option is recommended for seasonal allergic rhinitis, while an oral antihistamine is suggested for perennial allergic rhinitis. Last, either intranasal or oral antihistamine for patients with seasonal or perennial allergic rhinitis can be used.

With most of these, patient preferences, cost, and local availability are determinants of choice of medications.

For allergic rhinoconjunctivitis, topical nasal corticosteroids also reduce ocular symptoms, presumably through a naso-ocular reflex. For ocular allergies that persist or occur independent of rhinitis, pharmacologic treatment includes use of oral or topical antihistamines, topical decongestants, mast cell stabilizers, and anti-inflammatory agents. In general, topical ophthalmic drops should not be used with contact lenses. Topical decongestants relieve erythema, congestion, and edema but do not affect the allergic response. Combined therapy with an antihistamine and a vasoconstrictive agent is more effective than either agent alone. Topical medications with both antihistamine and mast cell blocking properties provide the most benefits that incorporate fast-acting symptom relief and anti-inflammatory action. Refrigerating ophthalmic drops before use can provide soothing relief as well. However, children can get wary of eye drops and prefer oral preparations. Avoiding contamination by preventing the applicator tip from touching the eye or eyelid is important. Severe ocular allergy can be treated with topical, or rarely, oral corticosteroids. In such a case, a referral to an ophthalmologist is warranted, as these treatments can be associated with elevation of the intraocular pressure, viral infections, and cataract formation.

Allergen immunotherapy can be very effective in allergic rhinoconjunctivitis and may decrease the requirement for medications to control the symptoms in the long term.

1. Antihistamines—Antihistamines help control itching, sneezing, and rhinorrhea. Sedating antihistamines include diphenhydramine, chlorpheniramine, hydroxyzine, and clemastine. Sedating antihistamines may cause daytime somnolence and negatively affect school performance and other activities, especially driving. Second-generation antihistamines include loratadine, desloratadine, cetirizine, and fexofenadine. Cetirizine is approved for use in children aged 6–23 months (2.5 mg daily), 2–5 years (2.5–5.0 mg/day or

2.5 mg twice a day), and 6 years or older (5–10 mg/day). It is now available without a prescription. Loratadine is approved for use in children aged 2–5 years (5 mg/day) and 6 years or older (10 mg/day), and is available without prescription in tablet, rapidly disintegrating tablet, and liquid formulations. Desloratadine is approved for use in children aged 6–11 months (1 mg/day), 1–5 years (1.25 mg/day), and for 12 years and older (5 mg/day). Fexofenadine is approved for children aged 6–23 months (15 mg twice a day), 2–11 years (30 mg twice a day), and 12 years or older (60 mg twice a day or 180 mg once daily), and is also now available without a prescription. Levocetirizine (5 mg/day) is approved for children aged 6 years and older. Loratadine, fexofenadine, and cetirizine are available in combination with pseudoephedrine for patients aged 12 years or older, although regular use of these combination products is not recommended. Azelastine is available in nasal and ophthalmic formulations. Levocabastine and emedastine are available as ophthalmic preparations. They should not be used for treatment of contact lens–related irritation, and caution should be implemented with concomitant use of soft contact lenses.

2. Mast cell stabilizers—Intranasal ipratropium can be used as adjunctive therapy for rhinorrhea. Intranasal cromolyn may be used alone or in conjunction with oral antihistamines and decongestants. It is most effective when used prophylactically, one to two sprays per nostril, four times a day. This dose may be tapered if symptom control is achieved. Rarely, patients complain of nasal irritation or burning. Most patients find complying with four times–daily dosing difficult. Cromolyn is also available in an ophthalmic solution. It can be used to treat giant papillary and vernal conjunctivitis. Other ophthalmic mast cell stabilizers include lodoxamide 0.1% solution (can be used for vernal keratoconjunctivitis as well), one to two drops four times a day; nedocromil sodium 2%, one to two drops two times a day; and pemirolast potassium 0.1%, one to two drops four times a day.

3. Decongestants and vasoconstrictor agents—Nasal α-adrenergic agents help to relieve nasal congestion, and ophthalmic vasoconstrictors relieve ocular erythema, edema, and congestion. Topical nasal decongestants such as phenylephrine and oxymetazoline should not be used for more than 4 days for severe episodes because prolonged use may be associated with rhinitis medicamentosa. As with nasal decongestants, a rebound phenomenon (ie, conjunctivitis medicamentosa with hyperemia and stinging/burning) can occur with chronic use of ophthalmic vasoconstrictive agents such as naphazoline and tetrahydrozoline. Oral decongestants, including pseudoephedrine, phenylephrine, and phenylpropanolamine, are often combined with antihistamines or expectorants and cough suppressants in over-the-counter (OTC) cold medications, but there are no convincing data to support the use of oral decongestants for upper respiratory illnesses in children nor for regular use in patients with allergic rhinitis. They may cause insomnia, agitation, tachycardia, and, rarely, cardiac arrhythmias. Of note, the FDA has recommended the removal of phenylpropanolamine from all drug products due to a public health advisory concerning the risk of hemorrhagic stroke associated with its use.

4. Corticosteroids—Intranasal corticosteroid sprays are effective in controlling allergic rhinitis if used chronically. They are minimally absorbed in usual doses and are available in pressurized nasal inhalers and aqueous sprays. Mometasone and fluticasone furoate nasal sprays have been approved for use in children as young as age 2 years (one spray in each nostril once daily) and in children 12 years or older (two sprays/nostril once daily). Fluticasone propionate nasal spray is approved for children 4 years or older, and budesonide and triamcinolone nasal sprays are approved for those 6 years or older (one to two sprays/nostril once daily). Flunisolide is approved for ages 6–14 years (one spray/nostril three times a day or two sprays/nostril twice a day). Ciclesonide is approved for seasonal allergic rhinitis in children 6 years and older and those with perennial allergic rhinitis for children 12 years and older, two sprays in each nostril once daily. Side effects include nasal irritation, soreness, and bleeding, although epistaxis occurs commonly in patients with allergic rhinitis if corticosteroids are used chronically. Rarely, these drugs can cause septal perforation. Excessive doses may produce systemic effects, especially if used together with orally inhaled steroids for asthma. Onset of action is within hours, although clinical benefit is usually not observed for a week or more. They may be effective alone or together with antihistamines. A combination nasal corticosteroid-antihistamine formulation spray has been found to be better than either agent alone in alleviating symptoms for moderate to severe seasonal allergic rhinitis.

Use of oral or topical (eg, loteprednol etabonate) corticosteroids for the treatment of ocular allergy should be worked out in conjunction with an ophthalmologist due to potential complications mentioned in the preceding section.

5. Other pharmacologic agents—Montelukast is approved for perennial allergic rhinitis in children aged 6 months and older (4 mg/day for ages 6–23 months) and seasonal allergic rhinitis in children 2 years and older in doses as discussed in section Pharmacologic Therapy under Treatment, Chronic Asthma. Oral antihistamines are also available in combination with a decongestant. Ketorolac, a nonsteroidal anti-inflammatory drug (NSAID), is available as an ophthalmic solution but should be avoided in patients with aspirin or NSAID sensitivity and should be used with caution in those with complicated eye surgeries, corneal denervation or epithelial defects, ocular surface diseases, diabetes mellitus, or rheumatoid arthritis. Combination ophthalmic preparations are available. Both antazoline and pheniramine are antihistamine/vasoconstrictor formulations. Olopatadine 0.1%, epinastine 0.05%, and ketotifen 0.025% ophthalmic solutions have antihistamine and mast cell–stabilizing actions and can be given to children older than 3 years as one drop twice a day (8 hours apart) for olopatadine and every 8–12 hours for ketotifen, respectively. Ketotifen fumarate 0.025% is now available as an OTC ophthalmic medication. Olopatadine 0.2% is the first once-daily ophthalmic medication available for the treatment of ocular pruritus associated with allergic conjunctivitis.

C. Surgical Therapy

Surgical procedures, including turbinectomy, polypectomy, and functional endoscopic sinus surgery, are rarely indicated in allergic rhinitis or chronic hyperplastic sinusitis.

D. Immunotherapy

Allergen immunotherapy should be considered when symptoms are severe and due to unavoidable exposure to inhalant allergens, especially if symptomatic measures have failed. Immunotherapy is the only form of therapy that may alter the course of the disease. It should not be prescribed by sending the patient's serum to a laboratory where extracts based on in vitro tests are prepared for the patient (ie, the remote practice of allergy). Subcutaneous immunotherapy should be done in a facility where a physician prepared to treat anaphylaxis is present. Patients with concomitant asthma should not receive an injection if their asthma is not under good control (ie, peak flows preinjection are below 80% of personal best), and the patient should wait for 25–30 minutes after an injection before leaving the facility. Outcomes with single allergen immunotherapy show success rates of approximately 80%. The optimal duration of therapy is unknown, but data suggest that immunotherapy for 3–5 years may have lasting benefit.

Sublingual immunotherapy has been developed for treatment of allergic rhinitis caused by pollens in both adults and children and for allergic rhinitis caused by dust mites only in adults (in other countries). A recent specific SLIT practice parameter emphasized that this mode of immunotherapy may not be appropriate for patients with certain medical conditions, such as eosinophilic esophagitis and those that may hamper the patient's ability to deal with a systemic reaction or the treatment of the severe reaction.

There are no FDA-approved study indications for SLIT for oral allergy syndrome, food allergy, latex allergy, atopic dermatitis, or venom allergy. This mode of immunotherapy is attractive for pediatric patients because of convenience and ease. While there are off label SLIT preparations (eg, liquid SCIT extract delivered sublingually, sublingual drops), there are only three FDA approved sublingual immunotherapy tablets, all using a single allergen SLIT, as there are still no studies showing efficacy of multiple allergens in a mixture: Grastek, Ragwitek, and Oralair. Grastek may be prescribed for children (as young as 5 years) and adults who are allergic to timothy grass and cross-reactive pollens, while Ragwitek

may be prescribed for persons 18 through 65 years of age who are allergic to ragweed pollen. Oralair is indicated for the treatment of grass pollen-induced allergic rhinitis with or without conjunctivitis, for any of five grass species: sweet vernal, orchard, perennial rye, timothy, and Kentucky blue grass, in patients 10–65 years old. They are recommended to be taken daily for about 12 weeks before and throughout the grass or ragweed pollens season, respectively, over a period of at least 3 years for sustained effects. Both timothy grass SLIT and 5-grass tablets have shown benefits beginning in the first year of treatment.

The first dose of SLIT should be in a supervised medical setting with much experience in the diagnosis and management of anaphylaxis, where patients can be observed closely for 30 minutes after taking the dose. Most systemic allergic reactions have been found to be with the first dose. Nevertheless, epinephrine should still be prescribed to patients receiving SLIT, and they should be trained when and how to use the device. Patients on SLIT should see an allergy specialist regularly for monitoring.

▶ Prognosis

Allergic rhinoconjunctivitis associated with sensitization to indoor allergens tends to be protracted unless specific allergens can be identified and eliminated from the environment. In seasonal allergic rhinoconjunctivitis, symptoms are usually most severe from adolescence through mid-adult life. After moving to a region devoid of problem allergens, patients may be symptom free for several years, but they can develop new sensitivities to local aeroallergens.

Brozek JL et al: Allergic Rhinitis and its Impact on Asthma (ARIA) guidelines—2016 revision. J Allergy Clin Immunol 2017 Oct;140:950–958 [PMID: 28602936].

Cox L et al: Allergen immunotherapy: a practice parameter third update. J Allergy Clin Immunol 2011;127:S1 [PMID: 21122901].

Greenhawt M et al: Sublingual immunotherapy: a focused allergen immunotherapy practice parameter update. Ann Allergy Asthma Immunol 2017;118:276–282 [PMID: 28284533].

ATOPIC DERMATITIS

ESSENTIALS OF DIAGNOSIS & TYPICAL FEATURES

▶ Diagnosis of atopic dermatitis is based on the clinical features, including severe pruritus, a chronically relapsing course, and typical morphology and distribution of skin lesions.

▶ Patients with atopic dermatitis have increased susceptibility to infection or colonization with a variety of microbial organisms including *Staphylococcus aureus* and herpes simplex virus.

- ▶ Basics of skin care include avoidance of irritants and proven allergens along with appropriate skin hydration and use of a good-quality moisturizer.
- ▶ Topical corticosteroids are used as first-line therapy in patients requiring more than moisturizer with topical calcineurin inhibitors and topical phosphodiesterase 4 inhibitor approved in patients 2 years or older as second-line treatment.
- ▶ Dupilumab, a biologic systemic therapy has been approved for patients with moderate-to-severe atopic dermatitis ages 12 years and older.

Atopic dermatitis is a chronically relapsing inflammatory skin disease that typically presents in early childhood. Over one-third of patients with atopic dermatitis will develop asthma and/or allergic rhinitis. A subset of patients with atopic dermatitis has been shown to have mutations in the gene encoding filaggrin, a protein essential for normal epidermal barrier function. These patients have early-onset, more severe, and persistent disease. Mutations in filaggrin have also been associated with allergic sensitization as well as increased risk for asthma, but only in patients with atopic dermatitis. Atopic dermatitis may result in significant morbidity, leading to school absenteeism, occupational disability, and emotional stress.

▶ Clinical Findings

A. Symptoms and Signs

Atopic dermatitis has no pathognomonic skin lesions or laboratory parameters. Diagnosis is based on the clinical features, including severe pruritus, a chronically relapsing course, and typical morphology and distribution of the skin lesions. Acute atopic dermatitis is characterized by intensely pruritic, erythematous papules associated with excoriations, vesiculations, and serous exudate; subacute atopic dermatitis by erythematous, excoriated, scaling papules; and chronic atopic dermatitis by thickened skin with accentuated markings (lichenification) and fibrotic papules. Patients with chronic atopic dermatitis may have all three types of lesions present concurrently. In skin of color, it may be difficult to appreciate erythema and associated inflammation. Patients usually have dry, xerotic skin. During infancy, atopic dermatitis involves primarily the face, scalp, and extensor surfaces of the extremities. The diaper area is usually spared. In older patients with long-standing disease, the flexural folds of the extremities are the predominant location of lesions, although this distribution can be seen even in infants.

B. Laboratory Findings

In patients with persistent disease despite appropriate treatment, consideration should be given for irritant, allergic, or infectious triggers. Elevated serum IgE levels can be demonstrated in 80%–85% of patients with atopic dermatitis but have little clinical utility, although they may be helpful in interpreting specific IgE tests. Identification of allergens involves taking a careful history and performing selective immediate hypersensitivity skin tests or in vitro tests when appropriate. Negative skin tests with proper controls have a high predictive value for ruling out a suspected allergen. Positive skin tests have a lower correlation with clinical symptoms in suspected food allergen–induced atopic dermatitis and should be confirmed with food challenges unless there is a coincidental history of anaphylaxis to the suspected food. Specific IgE levels determine probability of reaction, but not type of reaction or severity. Clinicians should avoid extensive testing, as results may reflect elevated total serum IgE with no clinical significance.

Exacerbation of atopic dermatitis can occur with exposure to aeroallergens such as house dust mites, and environmental control measures have been shown to result in clinical improvement. Patients can make specific IgE directed at S aureus toxins secreted on the skin. Peripheral blood eosinophilia is a common finding. Routine skin biopsy does not differentiate atopic dermatitis from other eczematous processes but may be helpful in atypical cases. Tests for the most common filaggrin gene mutations may identify patients who would be at increased risk for more severe, persistent atopic dermatitis and be more likely to develop allergic sensitizations and asthma. However, filaggrin gene mutations occur in individuals without atopic dermatitis.

▶ Differential Diagnosis

Scabies can present as a pruritic skin disease. However, distribution in the genital and axillary areas and the presence of linear lesions as well as skin scrapings may help to distinguish it from atopic dermatitis. Seborrheic dermatitis may be distinguished by a lack of significant pruritus, its predilection for the scalp (so-called cradle cap), and its coarse, yellowish scales. Allergic contact dermatitis may be suggested by the distribution of lesions with a greater demarcation of dermatitis than in atopic dermatitis. Allergic contact dermatitis superimposed on atopic dermatitis may appear as an acute flare of the underlying disease. Nummular eczema is characterized by coin-shaped plaques. Although unusual in children, mycosis fungoides or cutaneous T-cell lymphoma has been described and is diagnosed by skin biopsy. Eczematous rash has been reported in patients with human immunodeficiency virus (HIV) infection. Other disorders that may resemble atopic dermatitis include Wiskott-Aldrich syndrome, severe combined immunodeficiency disease, hyper-IgE syndrome, immunodeficiency with DOCK8 mutations, IPEX (immune dysregulation, polyendocrinopathy, enteropathy, X-linked) syndrome, zinc deficiency, phenylketonuria, and Letterer-Siwe disease (see Chapter 33).

► Complications

Ocular complications associated with atopic dermatitis can lead to significant morbidity. Atopic keratoconjunctivitis is always bilateral, and symptoms include itching, burning, tearing, and copious mucoid discharge. It is frequently associated with eyelid dermatitis and chronic blepharitis and may result in visual impairment from corneal scarring (see Chapter 16). Keratoconus in atopic dermatitis is believed to result from persistent rubbing of the eyes in patients with atopic dermatitis and allergic rhinitis. Anterior subcapsular cataracts may develop during adolescence or early adult life.

Patients with atopic dermatitis have increased susceptibility to infection or colonization with a variety of organisms. These include viral infections with herpes simplex, molluscum contagiosum, and human papillomavirus. Of note, even a past history of atopic dermatitis is considered a contraindication for receiving the current smallpox (vaccinia) vaccine. Superimposed dermatophytosis may cause atopic dermatitis to flare. *S aureus* can be cultured from the skin of more than 90% of patients with atopic dermatitis, compared with only 5% of normal subjects. *S aureus* toxins can act as superantigens, contributing to persistent inflammation or exacerbations of atopic dermatitis. Community-acquired methicillin-resistant *S aureus* (MRSA) has become an increasing problem, especially in patients treated with frequent antibiotics. Although recurrent staphylococcal pustulosis can be a significant problem in atopic dermatitis, invasive *S aureus* infections occur rarely and should raise the possibility of an immunodeficiency.

Patients with atopic dermatitis often have nonspecific hand dermatitis. This is frequently irritant in nature and aggravated by repeated wetting.

Nutritional disturbances may result from unwarranted and extensive dietary restrictions imposed by providers or parents.

Poor academic performance and behavioral disturbances may be associated with uncontrolled itching, sleep loss, and poor self-image. Severe disease may lead to problems with social interactions and self-esteem.

► Treatment

A. General Measures

Avoidance of irritants such as detergents, chemicals, and abrasive materials as well as extremes of temperature and humidity is important. New clothing should be washed to reduce the content of formaldehyde and other chemicals. Because residual laundry detergent in clothing may be irritating, using a liquid rather than a powder detergent and adding an extra rinse cycle can be beneficial. Occlusive clothing should be avoided in favor of cotton or cotton blends. Temperature in the home should be controlled to minimize sweating. Swimming is usually well tolerated; however,

patients should shower and use a mild cleanser to remove chemicals such as chlorine, and then apply a moisturizer. Sunlight may be beneficial in moderation, but nonsensitizing sunscreens should be used to avoid sunburn.

Avoidance of foods implicated in controlled challenges can lead to clinical improvement. Extensive elimination diets are almost never warranted. In addition, elimination of foods that a child is tolerating may result in immediate-type allergic reactions with future reintroduction. Environmental control measures (eg, dust mite–proof covers) in sensitized patients may improve atopic dermatitis.

Evaluation by a behavioral health clinician may be of benefit when dealing with a pruritic, relapsing disease. Relaxation, behavioral modification, or biofeedback training may help patients with habitual scratching. Patients with severe or disfiguring disease may require psychotherapy.

Clinicians should provide the patient and family with both general information and specific written skin care recommendations. The patient or parent should demonstrate an appropriate level of understanding to help ensure a good outcome. Educational pamphlets and a video about atopic dermatitis can be obtained from the National Eczema Association, a national nonprofit, patient-oriented organization, at: http://www.nationaleczema.org.

B. Hydration

Patients with atopic dermatitis have evaporative losses due to a defective skin barrier, so soaking the affected area or bathing for approximately 10 minutes in warm (not lukewarm) water, then applying an occlusive agent to retain the absorbed water, is an essential component of therapy. Oatmeal or baking soda added to the bath may feel soothing to certain patients but does not improve water absorption. Atopic dermatitis of the face or neck can be treated by applying a wet facecloth or towel to the involved area. The washcloth may be more readily accepted by a child if it is turned into a mask and also allows the older patient to remain functional (eg, reading during bath). Lesions limited to the hands or feet can be treated by soaking in a basin. Daily baths may be needed and increased to several times daily during flares of atopic dermatitis, while showers may be adequate for patients with mild disease. It is important to apply a topical moisturizer or medication within a few minutes after soaking the skin to prevent evaporation, which is both drying and irritating.

C. Moisturizers and Occlusives

An effective moisturizer combined with hydration therapy will help skin healing and can reduce the need for topical medications. Moisturizers are available as lotions, creams, and ointments. Lotions can be drying because of their evaporative effect, especially in a nonhumid climate. Preservatives and fragrances in lotions and creams may cause skin irritation. Moisturizers often need to be applied several times daily on a long-term basis and should be obtained in the largest size available. Crisco shortening can be substituted as an inexpensive alternative. Petroleum jelly (Vaseline) is an effective occlusive agent when used to seal in water after bathing. There are several topical nonsteroidal creams (eg, EpiCeram) approved as medical devices (thus, currently requiring prescriptions) for relief and management of signs and symptoms of dermatoses. Their potential benefits need to be weighed against their cost.

D. Corticosteroids

Corticosteroids reduce the inflammation and pruritus in atopic dermatitis. Topical corticosteroids can decrease S aureus colonization. Systemic corticosteroids, including oral prednisone, should be avoided in the management of this chronic relapsing disease as the rapid clinical improvement may be associated with an equally dramatic disease flaring following discontinuation. Topical corticosteroids are available in a variety of formulations and range in potency, ranging from extremely high- to low-potency preparations (see Table 15–2). Choice of a particular product depends on the severity and distribution of skin lesions. Patients need to be counseled regarding the potency of their corticosteroid preparation and its potential side effects. In general, the least potent agent that is effective should be used. However, choosing a preparation that is too weak may result in persistence or worsening of the atopic dermatitis. Side effects include thinning of the skin, telangiectasias, bruising, hypopigmentation, acne, and striae, although these occur infrequently when low- to medium-potency topical corticosteroids are used appropriately. In contrast, use of potent topical corticosteroids for prolonged periods—especially under occlusion—may result in atrophic changes or rarely systemic side effects. The face (especially the eyelids) and intertriginous areas are especially sensitive to corticosteroid side effects, and only low-potency preparations should be used routinely on these areas. Perioral dermatitis may occasionally be worsened by use of topical steroids. Because topical corticosteroids are commercially available in a variety of bases, including ointments, creams, lotions, oil, solutions, gels, foams, and even tape, there is no need to compound them. Ointments are most occlusive and, in general, provide better delivery of the medication while preventing evaporative losses. However, in a humid environment, creams may be better tolerated than ointments because the increased occlusion may cause itching or even folliculitis. Lotions, while easier to spread, can contribute to skin dryness and irritation. Solutions can be used on the scalp and hirsute areas, although they can sting or be irritating, especially to open lesions so an oil or foam base may be preferred. With clinical improvement, a less potent corticosteroid should be prescribed and the frequency of use decreased. Topical corticosteroids can be discontinued when inflammation resolves, but hydration and moisturizers need to be continued. In patients with a relapsing course,

twice-weekly treatment to previously involved, clear or almost clear skin can be done as proactive therapy (off-label). Several topical steroids including alclometasone 0.05%, desonide 0.05% hydrogel, and fluticasone 0.05% cream have been approved in infants as young as 3 months of age for up to 28 days. Undertreatment remains a common problem due to caregiver concerns about potential side effects of topical corticosteroids along with inadequate prescription size.

E. Topical Calcineurin Inhibitors

Tacrolimus and pimecrolimus are nonsteroidal immunomodulatory agents that are available in topical formulations. Tacrolimus ointment—0.03% for children 2–15 years of age and 0.1% for older patients—is approved for twice-daily short-term and intermittent long-term use in moderate to severe atopic dermatitis. Pimecrolimus 1% cream is approved for patients 2 years of age or older who have mild to moderate atopic dermatitis. Local burning at the site of application, which occurs more frequently with tacrolimus ointment, has been the most common side effect, although this is usually a transient problem. As a precaution, patients should wear sunscreen with these medications drugs. In Europe, tacrolimus ointment is approved as twice-weekly maintenance therapy for patients 2 years and older with a relapsing course after clearing up eczema with reevaluation of need for continued therapy after 12 months.

Although there is no evidence of a causal link between the use of topical calcineurin inhibitors and malignancy, in 2006, the FDA issued a boxed warning for these medications because of a lack of long-term safety data (see US package inserts for Elidel [Valeant] and Protopic [Leo]). The labeling states that these drugs are recommended as second-line treatment for short-term and noncontinuous chronic treatment and that their use in children younger than 2 years is currently not recommended. Long-term surveillance registries have been established for pediatric patients who had been treated with both topical tacrolimus and pimecrolimus.

F. PDE4 Inhibitors

Crisaborole 2% ointment has been approved in patients 2 years or older for mild-moderate atopic dermatitis.

G. Systemic Biologic

Dupilumab is a fully human monoclonal antibody that blocks interleukin 4 receptor alpha through which both IL-4 and IL-13, two key type 2 cytokines, signal. It is approved for patients 12 years and older with moderate to severe atopic dermatitis not adequately controlled with topical medications or when those are not appropriate. In patients 12–17 years, dosing is weight based with patients less than 60 kg receiving an initial dose of 400 mg, then 200 mg every 2 weeks by subcutaneous injection and patients 60 kg or more,

600 mg initial dose, then 300 mg every 2 weeks. Injections can be self-administered at home and currently, and there is no requirement for any laboratory monitoring. Injection site reactions and conjunctivitis have been the most commonly reported adverse events.

H. Anti-Infective Therapy

Systemic antibiotic therapy may be important when treating atopic dermatitis secondarily infected with *S aureus*. For limited areas of involvement, a topical antibiotic such as mupirocin or retapamulin ointment may be effective. A first- or second-generation cephalosporin or semisynthetic penicillin is usually the first choice for oral therapy, as erythromycin-resistant organisms are fairly common. Overuse may result in colonization by MRSA. Dilute bleach baths (6% sodium hypochlorite, ½ cup in a full tub of water) two times per week may be helpful for patients with atopic dermatitis, especially those with recurrent skin infections, although some patients find this treatment irritating.

Disseminated eczema herpeticum usually requires treatment with systemic antiviral. Patients with recurrent cutaneous herpetic lesions can be given prophylactic oral acyclovir or valacyclovir. Superficial dermatophytosis and Malassezia sympodialis infection can be treated with topical or (rarely) systemic antifungal agents.

I. Antipruritic Agents

Pruritus is usually the least well-tolerated symptom of atopic dermatitis. Oral antihistamines and anxiolytics may be effective owing to their tranquilizing and sedating effects and can be taken primarily at bedtime to avoid daytime somnolence. Nonsedating antihistamines may be helpful for associated allergic symptoms but are not usually effective in treating pruritus. Use of topical antihistamines and local anesthetics should be avoided because of potential sensitization.

J. Recalcitrant Disease

Patients who are erythrodermic may need to be hospitalized. Hospitalization may also be appropriate for those with severe disease failing outpatient management. Marked clinical improvement often occurs when the patient is removed from environmental allergens or stressors. In the hospital, adherence to therapy can be monitored, the patient and family can receive in-depth hands-on education, and controlled challenges can be conducted to help identify triggering factors.

Wet wrap therapy has been shown to be beneficial in severe atopic dermatitis. It can serve as an effective barrier against the persistent scratching that often undermines therapy. A layer of wet clothing (eg, pajamas, long underwear, tube socks) with dry layer on top (pajamas or a sweat suit, tube socks) over topical corticosteroid can be used for severely involved areas. Alternatively, wet gauze with a layer of dry gauze over it can be used and secured in place with an elastic bandage. Wet wraps can be removed when they dry out, usually after several hours, and are often best tolerated at bedtime. They should be considered an acute, not chronic intervention as overuse can result in chilling, skin maceration, or secondary infection.

Systemic immunosuppressive drugs including cyclosporine, methotrexate, mycophenolate, and azathioprine have been used in recalcitrant disease but are not approved for treatment of children with atopic dermatitis. Limited published data are available on use of cyclosporine in children treated with both continuous and intermittent therapy (5 mg/kg daily) for up to 1 year. Patients treated with this agent should have their dose titrated to the lowest effective dose after the disease is brought under control with appropriate monitoring, under the care of a specialist familiar with the drug. Ultraviolet light therapy approved for patients 12 years or older can be useful in a subset of patients under the supervision of a dermatologist.

K. Experimental and Unproved Therapies

Subcutaneous desensitization to dust mite allergen has been shown to improve atopic dermatitis in adult patients and sublingual desensitization in dust mite allergic children showed benefit in mild-moderate atopic dermatitis; however, further controlled trials are needed before this form of therapy can be recommended for atopic dermatitis in children. Treatment of atopic dermatitis with omalizumab and high-dose intravenous immunoglobulin has not shown consistent benefit. Although disturbances in the metabolism of essential fatty acids have been reported in patients with atopic dermatitis, controlled trials with fish oil and evening primrose have shown no clinical benefit.

L. Prevention

Studies of different hydrolyzed formulas, probiotics and prebiotics have yielded inconsistent results. While preliminary studies suggested a beneficial effect with application of a moisturizer in high-risk infants from birth, recent large-scale studies did not show this benefit.

▶ Prognosis

While many children, especially those with mild disease will outgrow their atopic dermatitis, patients with filaggrin gene mutations are more likely to have more persistent and severe disease. In addition, these patients appear to be the ones at greater risk for developing asthma and allergic sensitizations.

Boguniewicz M et al: Atopic dermatitis yardstick: practical recommendations for an evolving therapeutic landscape. Ann Allergy Asthma Immunol 2018;120:10.e2 [PMID: 29273118].

Brar KK et al: Strategies for successful management of severe atopic dermatitis. J Allergy Clin Immunol Pract 2019;7:1 [PMID: 30598172].

URTICARIA & ANGIOEDEMA

ESSENTIALS OF DIAGNOSIS & TYPICAL FEATURES

▶ Urticaria and angioedema are caused by mast cell degranulation in the skin.

▶ The acute form (< 6 weeks duration) is most commonly caused by viral infections in children. Allergies to foods or drugs are other causes.

▶ Types of chronic urticaria (> 6 weeks duration) include chronic spontaneous urticaria, physical/inducible urticaria, and autoimmune urticaria.

▶ Allergy testing or testing for physical triggers can be performed if guided by history.

▶ First-line treatment is the use of second-generation oral antihistamines, given up to four times the standard dose.

▶ Omalizumab has been effective for antihistamine-refractory urticaria.

Urticaria and angioedema are common dermatologic conditions, with an incidence of 3%–6% in children. Urticarial lesions are arbitrarily designated as acute, lasting less than 6 weeks, or chronic, lasting more than 6 weeks. It is also classified by trigger: allergic, physical/inducible, infectious, autoimmune, or spontaneous/idiopathic. Note that bradykinin-mediated hereditary angioedema is discussed in the immunodeficiency chapter (see Chapter 33).

Mast cells are thought to play a critical role in the pathogenesis of urticaria or angioedema through release of a variety of vasoactive mediators. Mast cell activation and degranulation can be triggered by different stimuli, including cross-linking of Fc receptor–bound IgE by allergens or anti-FcεRI antibodies. Non–IgE-mediated mechanisms have also been identified, including complement anaphylatoxins (C3a, C5a), radiocontrast dyes, and physical stimuli.

Viral infections are identified as the cause of acute urticaria in over one-half of pediatric patients, while in chronic urticaria, infections are considered an exacerbating factor. Infectious organisms associated with urticaria include streptococci, mycoplasmas, hepatitis B virus, *Helicobacter pylori*, and Epstein-Barr virus. Allergies to foods, latex, drugs, or insect venoms, immune complex formation with complement activation from blood products, and triggering of mast cells by anaphylatoxins can cause acute urticaria or angioedema. Opiate analgesics, polymyxin B, tubocurarine, and radiocontrast media can induce acute urticaria by direct mast cell activation. Urticaria and angioedema can also occur following ingestion of aspirin or nonsteroidal anti-inflammatory agents (see section Adverse Reactions to Drugs & Biologicals).

Inducible (physical) urticarias represent a heterogeneous group of disorders in which urticaria or angioedema is triggered by physical stimuli, including friction, radiation (solar), pressure, cold, heat, sweat, water, or vibrations. Dermatographism is the most common form of physical urticaria, affecting up to 4% of the population and occurring at skin sites subjected to mechanical stimuli. Physical urticarias are usually rapid in onset, with resolution within hours. However, symptoms can recur for months to years.

The cause of chronic spontaneous urticaria is usually not due to allergies and typically cannot be determined. It can be associated with autoimmunity, such as autoimmune thyroid disease, or the presence of basophil-activating IgG autoantibodies directed at the high-affinity receptor for IgE or at IgE.

▶ Clinical Findings

A. Symptoms and Signs

Urticaria manifests as wheals with reflex erythema that are pruritic and transient. They resolve after hours without any change to the skin. Angioedema is rapid erythematous or skin-colored swelling that is associated with burning or pain more than pruritus. Cold-induced urticaria or angioedema can occur within minutes of exposure to a decreased ambient temperature or as the skin is warmed following direct cold contact. Systemic features include headache, wheezing, and syncope. If the entire body is cooled, as may occur during swimming, hypotension and collapse can occur. In solar urticaria, which occurs within minutes after exposure to light of appropriate wavelength, pruritus is followed by morbilliform erythema and urticaria. Cholinergic urticaria occurs after increases in core body and skin temperatures, and typically develops after a warm bath or shower, exercise, or episodes of fever. The eruption appears as small punctate wheals surrounded by extensive areas of erythema. Rarely, the urticarial lesions become confluent and angioedema develops. Associated features can include the following: headache, syncope, bronchospasm, abdominal pain, vomiting, and diarrhea. In severe cases, systemic anaphylaxis may develop. In pressure urticaria or angioedema, red, deep, painful swelling occurs immediately or 4–6 hours after the skin has been exposed to pressure. The immediate form is often associated with dermatographism. The delayed form, which may be associated with fever, chills, and arthralgias, may be accompanied by elevated erythrocyte sedimentation rate and leukocytosis. Lesions are frequently diffuse, tender, and painful rather than pruritic. They typically resolve within 48 hours.

B. Laboratory Findings

Laboratory tests are selected on the basis of the history and physical findings. Testing for specific IgE antibody to food or inhalant allergens or infections may be helpful in implicating a potential cause in acute urticaria particularly if the history is suggestive. Specific tests for inducible urticarias, such as an ice cube test or a pressure test, may be indicated. Intradermal injection of methacholine reproduces clinical symptoms locally in about one-third of patients with cholinergic urticaria. In chronic spontaneous urticaria, evaluation has rarely been helpful in management; therefore, diagnostic tests should be limited and guided by the history. Evaluation for underlying disease may be indicated, including a complete blood count, erythrocyte sedimentation rate, biochemistry panel, or antithyroid antibodies. Intradermal testing with the patient's serum has been suggested as a method of detecting histamine-releasing activity, including autoantibodies (autologous serum skin test). In patients with well-characterized autoimmune urticaria, donor basophil and mast cell activation markers including CD63 and CD203c have been shown to be upregulated in patient serum. If the history or appearance of the urticarial lesions suggests vasculitis, a skin biopsy for immunofluorescence is indicated.

▶ Differential Diagnosis

Urticarial lesions are usually easily recognized—the major dilemma is the etiologic diagnosis. Lesions of urticarial vasculitis typically last for more than 24 hours. "Papular urticaria" is a term used to characterize multiple papules from insect bites, found especially on the extremities, and is not true urticaria. Angioedema can be distinguished from other forms of edema because it is transient, asymmetrical, and nonpitting and does not occur predominantly in dependent areas. Hereditary angioedema is a rare autosomal dominant disorder caused by a quantitative or functional deficiency of C1-esterase inhibitor and characterized by episodic, frequently severe, nonpruritic angioedema of the skin, gastrointestinal tract, or upper respiratory tract (discussed in Chapter 33). Rare autoinflammatory disorders with urticaria or urticaria-vasculitic-like lesions include cold-induced autoinflammatory syndrome, Muckle-Wells syndrome, and Schnitzler syndrome.

▶ Complications

In severe cases of cholinergic urticaria, systemic anaphylaxis may develop. In cold-induced disease, sudden cooling of the entire body as can occur with swimming can result in hypotension and collapse.

▶ Treatment

A. General Measures

The most effective treatment is identification and avoidance of the triggering agent. Underlying infection should be treated appropriately. Patients with inducible urticarias should avoid the relevant physical stimulus. Patients with cold urticaria should be counseled not to swim alone and prescribed autoinjectable epinephrine in case of generalized

mast cell degranulation with immersion in cold water or other widespread cold exposures. Epinephrine autoinjectors should also be considered for those with severe cholinergic urticaria because of the risk of anaphylaxis.

B. Antihistamines

For the majority of patients, H_1-antihistamines given orally or systemically are the mainstay of therapy. Antihistamines are more effective when given on an ongoing basis rather than after lesions appear. Second-generation H_1-antihistamines (discussed previously under Allergic Rhinoconjunctivitis) are long acting, show good tissue levels, are non- or minimally sedating at usual dosing levels, and lack anticholinergic effects. They are the preferred first-line treatment for urticaria. If refractory at the recommended dose, second-line treatment is increasing the dose up to fourfold.

C. Other Pharmacologic Agents

Third-line treatment for chronic spontaneous urticaria is the addition of omalizumab. Omalizumab has been demonstrated to be effective in antihistamine resistant urticaria in a double-blind placebo-controlled trial and in case series in patients younger than 12 years. It obtained FDA approval for chronic urticaria in patients 12 years old or older in 2014. Dosing is 150 mg or 300 mg subcutaneously every 4 weeks. Oral steroid courses tapered for up to 10 days can be considered for acute urticaria or acute exacerbations of chronic spontaneous urticaria but should not be given chronically. Addition of a LTRA and/or H_2-antihistamines has not been shown to be as effective as omalizumab, but the cost and safety profiles of these medications may be favorable to trial. In the case of omalizumab failure, treatment of chronic spontaneous urticaria with cyclosporine, hydroxychloroquine, azathioprine, tacrolimus, sulfasalazine, dapsone, and vitamin D can be considered.

▶ Prognosis

Spontaneous remission of urticaria and angioedema is typical, but some patients have a prolonged course, especially those with inducible urticaria. Reassurance is important, because this disorder can cause significant frustration. Periodic follow-up is indicated, particularly for patients with development of noncutaneous symptoms, to monitor for possible underlying cause.

Al-Shaikhly T et al: Omalizumab for chronic urticaria in children less than 12 years of age: a systematic review. Ann Allergy Asthma Immunol 2019;135:67–75 [PMID: 31082483].

Zuberbier T et al: The EAACI/GA2LEN/EDF/WAO guideline for the definition, classification, diagnosis, and management of urticaria. Allergy 2018;73(7):1393–1414 [PMID: 29336054].

ANAPHYLAXIS

ESSENTIALS OF DIAGNOSIS & TYPICAL FEATURES

▶ A clinical history of rapid onset of skin-mucosal tissue (urticaria, angioedema), respiratory compromise, hypotension, and/or GI symptoms after exposure to a common trigger is the key for proper diagnosis.

▶ Epinephrine is the treatment of choice for anaphylaxis, along with other secondary life-supportive measures.

▶ Prevention of future episodes of anaphylaxis by strict avoidance of known triggers, along with education regarding carrying and proper usage of an epinephrine autoinjector, is essential for patient management.

▶ Considerations

Anaphylaxis is an acute life-threatening clinical syndrome that occurs when large quantities of inflammatory mediators are rapidly released from mast cells and basophils after exposure to an allergen in a previously sensitized patient. Anaphylactoid reactions mimic anaphylaxis but are not mediated by IgE antibodies. They may be mediated by anaphylatoxins such as C3a or C5a or through nonimmune mast cell degranulating agents. Some of the common causes of anaphylaxis or anaphylactoid reactions are listed in Table 38–8. Idiopathic anaphylaxis by definition has no

Table 38–8. Common causes of systemic allergic and pseudoallergic reactions.

Causes of anaphylaxis
Drugs
Antibiotics
Anesthetic agents
Foods
Peanuts, tree nuts, shellfish, and others
Biologicals
Latex
Insulin
Allergen extracts
Antisera
Blood products
Enzymes
Monoclonal antibodies (eg, omalizumab)
Insect venoms
Radiocontrast media
Aspirin and other nonsteroidal anti-inflammatory drugs
Anesthetic agents
Idiopathic

recognized external cause. The clinical history is the most important tool in making the diagnosis of anaphylaxis.

▶ Clinical Findings

A. Symptoms and Signs

The history is the most important tool to determine whether a patient has had anaphylaxis. The symptoms and signs of anaphylaxis depend on the organs affected. Onset typically occurs within minutes after exposure to the offending agent and can be short-lived, protracted, or biphasic, with recurrence after several hours despite treatment.

Anaphylaxis is highly likely when any one of the following three criteria is fulfilled:

1. Acute onset of an illness (minutes to several hours) with involvement of the skin, mucosal tissue, or both (eg, generalized hives, pruritus or flushing, swollen lips-tongue-uvula) *and at least one of the following*:

   a. Respiratory compromise (eg, dyspnea, wheeze, bronchospasm, stridor, reduced peak expiratory flow, hypoxemia)

   b. Reduced blood pressure or associated symptoms of end-organ dysfunction (eg, hypotonia [collapse], syncope, incontinence)

2. Two or more of the following that occur rapidly after exposure to a *likely* allergen for that patient (minutes to several hours):

   a. Involvement of the skin-mucosal tissue (eg, generalized urticaria, itch-flush, swollen lips-tongue-uvula)

   b. Respiratory compromise (eg, dyspnea, wheeze, bronchospasm, stridor, reduced PEFR, hypoxemia)

   c. Reduced blood pressure or associated symptoms (eg, hypotonia [collapse], syncope, incontinence)

   d. Persistent gastrointestinal symptoms (eg, crampy abdominal pain, vomiting)

3. Reduced blood pressure after exposure to a *known* allergen for that patient (minutes to several hours):

   a. Infants and children: low systolic blood pressure (age specific) or greater than 30% decrease in systolic pressure

   b. Low systolic blood pressure in children, defined as less than 70 mm Hg in those aged from 1 month to 1 year, less than (70 mm Hg + [2 × age]) in those 1–10 years of age, and less than 90 mm Hg in those 11–17 years

B. Laboratory Findings

An absence of laboratory findings does not rule out anaphylaxis. Tryptase released by mast cells can be measured in the serum within 3 hours of onset of the reaction and may be helpful when the diagnosis of anaphylaxis is in question.

However, tryptase levels are often normal, particularly in individuals with food-induced anaphylaxis. Electrocardiographic abnormalities may include ST-wave depression, bundle branch block, and various arrhythmias. Arterial blood gases may show hypoxemia, hypercapnia, and acidosis. The chest radiograph may show hyperinflation.

Differential Diagnosis

Although shock may be the only sign of anaphylaxis, other diagnoses should be considered, especially in the setting of sudden collapse without typical allergic findings. Other causes of shock along with cardiac arrhythmias must be ruled out (see Chapters 12 and 14). Respiratory failure associated with asthma may be confused with anaphylaxis. Mastocytosis, hereditary angioedema, scombroid fish poisoning, vasovagal reactions, inducible laryngeal obstruction, and anxiety attacks may cause symptoms mistaken for anaphylaxis.

Complications

Depending on the organs involved and the severity of the reaction, complications may vary from none to aspiration pneumonitis, acute tubular necrosis, bleeding diathesis, or sloughing of the intestinal mucosa. With irreversible shock, heart and brain damage can be terminal. Risk factors for fatal or near-fatal anaphylaxis include age (adolescents and young adults), reactions to peanut or tree nuts, associated asthma, strenuous exercise, and use of medications such as β-blockers.

Prevention

Strict avoidance of the causative agent is extremely important, and effort to determine its cause should be made, beginning with a thorough history. Typically, there is a strong temporal relationship between exposure and onset of symptoms. With exercise-induced anaphylaxis, patients should be instructed to exercise with another person and to stop exercising at the first sign of symptoms. If prior ingestion of food has been implicated, eating within 4 hours—perhaps up to 12 hours—before exercise should be avoided. Patients with a history of anaphylaxis should carry epinephrine for self-administration, preferably in the form of an autoinjector (eg, Auvi-Q or EpiPen in 0.15- and 0.3-mg doses), and they and all caregivers should be instructed on its use. They should also carry an oral antihistamine such as diphenhydramine or cetirizine, preferably in liquid or chewable preparation to hasten absorption, but epinephrine should be considered as the first-line treatment of anaphylaxis. Patients with idiopathic anaphylaxis may require prolonged treatment with oral corticosteroids. Specific measures for dealing with food, drug, latex, and insect venom allergies as well as radiocontrast media reactions are discussed in the next sections.

Treatment

A. General Measures

Anaphylaxis is a medical emergency that requires rapid assessment and treatment. Exposure to the triggering agent should be discontinued. Airway patency should be maintained and blood pressure and pulse monitored. Simultaneously and promptly, emergency medical services or a call for help to a resuscitation team should be made. The patient should be placed in a supine position with the legs elevated unless precluded by shortness of breath or emesis. Oxygen should be delivered by mask or nasal cannula with pulse oximetry monitoring. If the reaction is secondary to a sting or injection into an extremity, a tourniquet may be applied proximal to the site, briefly releasing it every 10–15 minutes.

B. Epinephrine

Epinephrine is the treatment of choice for anaphylaxis. Epinephrine 1:1000, 0.01 mg/kg to a maximum of 0.5 mg in adults and 0.3 mg in children, should be injected intramuscularly in the midanterolateral thigh without delay. This dose may be repeated at intervals of 5–15 minutes as necessary for controlling symptoms and maintaining blood pressure. There is no precisely established dosing regimen for intravenous epinephrine in anaphylaxis, but a 5–10 mcg intravenous bolus for hypotension and 0.1–0.5 mg intravenously for cardiovascular collapse have been suggested.

C. Antihistamines

Diphenhydramine, an H_1-blocker, 1–2 mg/kg up to 50 mg, can be given orally, intramuscularly or intravenously. Intravenous antihistamines should be infused over a period of 5–10 minutes to avoid inducing hypotension. Alternatively in young patients, cetirizine 0.25 mg/kg to a maximum dose of 10 mg could be given orally, as it was shown to have a longer duration of action and reduced sedation profile. Addition of ranitidine, an H_2-blocker, 1 mg/kg up to 50 mg intravenously, may be more effective than an H_1-blocker alone, especially for hypotension, but histamine blockers should be considered second-line treatment for anaphylaxis.

D. Fluids

Treatment of persistent hypotension despite epinephrine requires restoration of intravascular volume by fluid replacement, initially with a crystalloid solution, 20–30 mL/kg in the first hour.

E. Bronchodilators

Nebulized β_2-agonists such as albuterol 0.5% solution, 2.5 mg (0.5 mL) diluted in 2–3 mL saline, or levalbuterol, 0.63 mg or

1.25 mg, may be useful for reversing bronchospasm. Intravenous methylxanthines are generally not recommended because they provide little benefit over inhaled β_2-agonists and may contribute to toxicity.

F. Corticosteroids

Although corticosteroids do not provide immediate benefit, when given early they may prevent protracted or biphasic anaphylaxis, although data are limited regarding this. Intravenous methylprednisolone, 50–100 mg (adult) or 1 mg/kg, maximum 50 mg (child), can be given every 4–6 hours. Oral prednisone, 1 mg/kg up to 50 mg, might be sufficient for less severe episodes.

G. Vasopressors

Hypotension refractory to epinephrine and fluids should be treated with intravenous vasopressors such as noradrenaline, vasopressin, or dopamine (see Chapter 14).

H. Observation

The patient should be monitored after the initial symptoms have subsided, because biphasic or protracted anaphylaxis can occur despite ongoing therapy. Biphasic reactions occur in 1%–20% of anaphylactic reactions, but no reliable clinical predictors have been identified. Observation periods should be individualized based on the severity of the initial reaction, but a reasonable time for observation is 4–6 hours in most patients, with prolonged observation or admission for severe or refractory symptoms.

▶ Prognosis

Anaphylaxis can be fatal. The prognosis, however, is good when signs and symptoms are recognized promptly and treated aggressively, and the offending agent is subsequently avoided. Exercise-induced and idiopathic anaphylaxis may be recurrent. Because accidental exposure to the causative agent may occur, patients, parents, and caregivers must be prepared to recognize and treat anaphylaxis (have an anaphylaxis action plan and epinephrine readily available). Resources for anaphylaxis can be found by entering the term anaphylaxis in the search boxes at the websites for the national allergy and immunology academic societies: https://www.aaaai.org and https://acaai.org.

▶ Special Considerations: Infant Anaphylaxis

The recognition, diagnosis and management of anaphylaxis in infants/toddlers are associated with unique challenges given their nonverbal nature. Food allergy is the most common cause of anaphylaxis in this group. Guidance for the diagnosis and management of anaphylaxis in infants was recently published (see reference below). The FDA also approved an epinephrine autoinjector for infants and toddlers weighing between 7.5 and 15 kg (Auvi-Q 0.1 mg).

Greenhawt et al: Guiding principles for the recognition, diagnosis, and management of infants with anaphylaxis: an expert panel consensus. J Allergy Clin Immunol Pract 2019;7:1148–1156 [PMID: 30737191].

Lieberman P et al. Anaphylaxis—a practice parameter update 2015. Ann Allergy Asthma Immunol 2015;115:341–384 [PMID: 26505932].

Simons FE et al: International consensus on (ICON) anaphylaxis. World Allergy Organ J 2014;7:9 [PMID: 24920969].

ADVERSE REACTIONS TO DRUGS & BIOLOGICALS

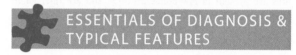

ESSENTIALS OF DIAGNOSIS & TYPICAL FEATURES

▶ Allergic or hypersensitivity drug reactions are adverse reactions involving immune mechanisms, accounting for only 5%–10% of all adverse drug reactions.

▶ Skin testing for immediate reactions to penicillin is the most validated form of drug testing available.

▶ Allergy to latex is seen in children with spina bifida or health care workers, although the incidence has decreased with decreased use of latex-containing medical equipment and gloves.

▶ Drug challenges can be performed for further evaluation of drug reactions, although they are contraindicated with history of severe, delayed-type reactions such as serum sickness, severe cutaneous reactions (TEN/SJS), or drug reaction with eosinophilia and systemic symptoms (DRESS) syndrome.

▶ Desensitization can be performed if drug allergy is suspected, and there is no other reasonable alternative for the drug. Desensitization causes temporary tolerance of the medication.

Adverse drug reactions are any undesirable and unintended response elicited by a drug. Allergic or hypersensitivity drug reactions are adverse reactions involving immune mechanisms. Although hypersensitivity reactions account for only 5%–10% of all adverse drug reactions, they are the most serious, with 1:10,000 resulting in death. Other causes of adverse drug reactions include idiosyncratic reactions, overdosage, pharmacologic side effects, nonspecific release of pharmacologic effector molecules, or drug interactions. Clinicians can report adverse drug reactions and get updated information on drugs, vaccines, and biologics at the FDA's MedWatch website.

1. Antibiotics

Antibiotics constitute the most frequent cause of allergic drug reactions. Amoxicillin, trimethoprim-sulfamethoxazole, and ampicillin are the most common causes of cutaneous drug reactions. It is important but challenging to help families understand that some antibiotics can cause a rash in the setting of infections, but this is not necessarily a true allergy to the medication.

The penicillins and other β-lactam antibiotics, including cephalosporins, carbacephems, carbapenems, and monobactams, share a common β-lactam ring structure and a marked propensity to couple to carrier proteins. Penicilloyl is the predominant allergenic metabolite of penicillin and is called the major determinant. The other penicillin metabolites are present in low concentrations and are referred to as minor determinants. Regarding cross-reactivity between penicillins and cephalosporins, the R-side chains of the penicillins and cephalosporins have been implicated in most allergic reactions to both of these medications.

Sulfonamide reactions are mediated presumably by a reactive metabolite (hydroxylamine) produced by cytochrome P-450 oxidative metabolism. Slow acetylators appear to be at increased risk. Other risk factors for drug reactions include previous exposure, previous reaction, age (20–49 years), route (parenteral), and dose of administration (high, intermittent). Atopy does not predispose to development of a reaction, but atopic individuals have more severe reactions.

Immunopathologic reactions to antibiotics include type I (IgE-mediated) reactions, type II (cytotoxic) reactions such as drug-induced hemolytic anemia or thrombocytopenia, type III (immune complex) reactions such as serum sickness, and type IV (T-cell–mediated) reactions such as allergic contact dermatitis. Immunopathologic reactions not fitting into the types I–IV classification include interstitial nephritis, pneumonitis, hepatitis, eosinophilia, fixed-drug eruption, acute generalized exanthematous pustulosis (AGEP), Stevens-Johnson syndrome, exfoliative dermatitis, and maculopapular exanthemas. The prevalence of morbilliform rashes in patients given ampicillin increases significantly during Epstein-Barr virus and cytomegalovirus infections or with acute lymphoblastic anemia, 69%–100% compared to 5%–9%. Serum sickness–like reactions resemble type III reactions, although immune complexes are not documented; β-lactams, especially cefaclor, and sulfonamides have been implicated most often. The incidence of "allergic" cutaneous reactions to trimethoprim-sulfamethoxazole in patients with AIDS has been reported to be as high as 70%. The mechanism is thought to relate to severe immune dysregulation, although it may be due to glutathione deficiency resulting in toxic metabolites.

2. Latex Allergy

Allergy to latex and rubber products was common among health care workers and children with spina bifida, but less so with the decreased use of latex equipment and gloves. The combination of atopy and frequent exposure seems to synergistically increase the risk of latex hypersensitivity. Nonmedical sources of latex are also common and include balloons, toys, rubber bands, erasers, condoms, and shoe soles. Pacifiers and bottle nipples have also been implicated as sources of latex allergen, although these products are molded rather than dipped, and allergic reactions to molded products are less common.

3. Vaccines

Mumps-measles-rubella (MMR) and the influenza vaccines have been shown to be safe in egg-allergic patients (although rare reactions to gelatin or neomycin can occur). Post-vaccination observation periods are no longer recommended. Local reactions are not associated with a higher rate of systemic allergic reactions. Skin testing can be performed if an IgE-mediated allergy to the vaccine is suspected.

4. Antiepileptic Drugs

Aromatic antiepileptic drugs (AEDs) have been most commonly implicated in drug hypersensitivity reactions to AEDs, which can be severe. This class of medications is one of the most common causes of drug rash with eosinophilia and systemic symptoms (DRESS) syndrome in children. This causes high fever, facial edema, morbilliform/confluent rash, eosinophilia, lymphadenopathy, and, most commonly, hepatic involvement 2–8 weeks after drug initiation. It can progress even with withdrawal of the offending medication and can last for months.

5. Radiocontrast Media

Non–IgE-mediated anaphylactoid reactions may occur with radiocontrast media with up to a 30% reaction rate on reexposure. Management involves using a low-molarity agent and premedication with prednisone, diphenhydramine, and, possibly, an H_2-blocker.

6. Insulin

Approximately 50% of patients receiving insulin have positive skin tests, but IgE-mediated reactions are rare. Insulin resistance is mediated by IgG. If less than 24 hours has elapsed after an allergic reaction to insulin, do not discontinue insulin but rather reduce the dose by one-third, then increase by 2–5 units per injection. Skin testing and desensitization are necessary if the interval between the allergic reaction and subsequent dose is greater than 24 hours.

7. Local Anesthetics

Less than 1% of reactions to local anesthetics are IgE-mediated. Management involves selecting a local anesthetic from another class. Esters of benzoic acid include benzocaine and procaine; amides include lidocaine and mepivacaine. Alternatively, the patient can be skin-tested with the suspected agent, followed by a provocative challenge.

8. Aspirin & Other Nonsteroidal Anti-Inflammatory Drugs

Adverse reactions to aspirin and NSAIDs include urticaria and angioedema; rhinosinusitis, nasal polyps, and asthma (AERD); anaphylactoid reactions; and NSAID-related hypersensitivity pneumonitis. All NSAIDs inhibiting cyclooxygenase (COX) cross-react with aspirin; patients with AERD and urticaria/angioedema will react to all. Fewer patients will react to only one NSAID. Cross-reactivity between aspirin and tartrazine (yellow dye No. 5) has not been substantiated in controlled trials. No skin test or in vitro test is available to diagnose aspirin sensitivity; the gold standard is a drug challenge. Aspirin desensitization can be performed to ameliorate the symptoms of AERD. LTRAs or 5-lipoxygenase inhibitors attenuate the reaction to aspirin challenge and may be beneficial adjunct treatment in AERD patients. COX-2 inhibitors are tolerated by patients with AERD.

9. Biological Agents

In recent years, a growing number of biological agents have become available for the treatment of autoimmune, neoplastic, cardiovascular, infectious, and allergic diseases, among others. Their use may be associated with a variety of adverse reactions, including increased risk of infections, neurologic defects, autoimmune syndromes, cardiovascular effects, and hypersensitivity reactions. Desensitization may be possible if there is no other good alternative in those patients who have developed an allergy to these medications.

10. Hypersensitivity to Retroviral Agents

Adverse drug reactions are being reported with increasing frequency to antiretroviral agents, including reverse transcriptase inhibitors, protease inhibitors, and fusion inhibitors. Hypersensitivity to abacavir is a well-described, multiorgan, potentially life-threatening reaction that occurs in HIV-infected children. The reaction is independent of dose with onset generally within 9–11 days of initiation of drug therapy. Susceptibility appears to be conferred by the HLA-B*5701 allele with a positive predictive value of more than 70% and negative predictive value of 95%–98%. Genetic screening would be cost-effective in Caucasians, but not in African or Asian populations as their HLA-B*5701 allele frequency is less than 1%.

11. Adverse Reactions to Chemotherapeutic Agents

A number of chemotherapeutic agents, including monoclonal antibodies, have been implicated in hypersensitivity reactions. Skin testing can be performed to platinum agents. Rapid desensitization to unrelated agents, including carboplatin, paclitaxel, and rituximab, has been reported. This 12-step protocol appeared to be successful in both IgE- and non–IgE-mediated reactions.

▶ Clinical Findings

A. Symptoms and Signs

Rash is the most common symptom of a hypersensitivity drug reaction in children. IgE-mediated reactions can cause pruritus, erythema, urticaria, angioedema, bronchospasm, or anaphylaxis within 1 hour of the dose. Delayed reactions can occur hours to weeks after the onset of a medication. Serum sickness is characterized by fever, rash, lymphadenopathy, myalgias, and arthralgias. Cytotoxic drug reactions can result in symptoms and signs associated with the underlying anemia or thrombocytopenia. Delayed-type hypersensitivity may cause contact dermatitis that appears 24–72 hours after contact.

B. Laboratory Findings

Skin testing is useful for evaluation of IgE-mediated drug allergies, particularly of β-lactam antibiotics where it has been most validated. Approximately 80% of patients with a history of penicillin allergy will have negative skin tests. Use of both the major determinants, Pre-Pen (penicilloyl-polylysine) and penicillin G or suspect penicillin, increases sensitivity to about 95%. Not using the minor determinant mixture, which is not commercially available, in skin testing can result in failure to predict potential anaphylactic reactions in up to 20% of those who test negative to both. Solid-phase in vitro immunoassays for IgE to penicillins are available for identification of IgE to penicilloyl but are considerably less sensitive than skin testing and the predictive values are not known. If skin testing is negative, drug provocation test should be performed for the final diagnosis.

Skin testing for non–β-lactam antibiotics is less reliable, because the relevant degradation products are for the most part unknown or multivalent reagents are unavailable.

For nonimmediate reactions, skin testing can be performed, but this is not validated and is controversial.

Patch testing with standardized Thin-Layer Rapid Use Epicutaneous Patch Test (T.R.U.E.) Test® or other sources of antigens can be performed when allergic contact dermatitis is suspected.

▶ Differential Diagnosis

Differential diagnosis for drug allergy includes other types of adverse drug reactions related to drug toxicity, drug interactions, idiosyncratic reactions, or pseudoallergic reactions. As infections commonly cause exanthems or urticaria, these are often confused with drug reactions when the patient is placed on antibiotics.

Treatment

A. General Measures

Withdrawal of the implicated drug is usually a central component of management. Acute IgE-mediated reactions such as anaphylaxis, urticaria, and angioedema are treated according to established therapeutic guidelines that include the use of epinephrine, H_1- and H_2-receptor blocking agents, volume replacement, and systemic corticosteroids. Antibiotic-induced immune cytopenias can be managed by withdrawal of the offending agent or reduction in dose. Drug-induced serum sickness can be suppressed by drug withdrawal, antihistamines, and corticosteroids. Contact allergy can be managed by avoidance and treatment with antihistamines and topical corticosteroids. Reactions such as toxic epidermal necrolysis and Stevens-Johnson syndrome require immediate drug withdrawal and supportive care.

B. Alternative Therapy

If possible, subsequent therapy should be with an alternative drug that has therapeutic actions similar to the drug in question but with no immunologic cross-reactivity.

C. Desensitization

Administering gradually increasing doses of the drug either orally or parentally over a period of hours to days may be considered if alternative therapy is not acceptable. This should be done only by a physician familiar with desensitization, typically in an intensive care setting. Of note, desensitization is only effective for the course of therapy for which the patient was desensitized, unless maintained on a chronic prophylactic dose of the medication as patients revert from a desensitized to allergic state after the drug is discontinued. In addition, desensitization does not reduce or prevent non–IgE-mediated reactions. Patients with Stevens-Johnson syndrome, DRESS, or serum sickness should not be desensitized because of the high morbidity and mortality rate.

Prognosis

The prognosis is good when drug allergens are identified early and avoided. Stevens-Johnson syndrome, toxic epidermal necrolysis, and DRESS syndrome may be associated with a high mortality rate.

Blumenthal KG et al: Antibiotic allergy. Lancet 2019;393:183–198 [PMID: 30558872].

FDA MedWatch: http://www.fda.gov/medwatch/index.html. Accessed June 10, 2019.

Kidon M et al: Diagnosis and management of drug-induced anaphylaxis in children: An EAACI position paper. Pediatr Allergy Immunol 2019;30:269–276 [PMID: 30734362].

Phillips EJ et al: Controversies in drug allergy: testing for delayed reactions. J Allergy Clin Immunol 2019;143:66–73 [PMID: 30573342].

FOOD ALLERGY

ESSENTIALS OF DIAGNOSIS & TYPICAL FEATURES

▶ Diagnosis of food allergy is made by a clinical history consistent with an immune-mediated reaction to a food, either IgE- or non–IgE-mediated.

▶ Treatment for food allergy includes avoidance of that food and providing education on how to treat an allergic reaction after an accidental exposure; consultation with an allergist and with a dietitian is recommended.

▶ New food allergy treatments using oral and epicutaneous immunotherapy may soon be available, and introduction of highly allergenic foods (eg, peanut, egg, milk) early into an infant's diet may prevent the development of allergy to those foods.

General Considerations

Food allergy is defined as an adverse health effect arising from a specific immune response that occurs reproducibly on exposure to a given food. Food allergy affects approximately 8% of young children and 3%–4% of adults. The most common IgE-associated food allergens in children are milk egg, peanut, soy, wheat, tree nuts, fish, and shellfish. In older patients, fish, shellfish, peanut, and tree nuts are most often involved in allergic reactions and are usually lifelong allergies. Food allergy can be caused by non–IgE-mediated mechanisms, in conditions such as food protein–induced enterocolitis (FPIES) or proctocolitis. It can also be caused by mixed IgE- and non–IgE-mediated mechanisms, as in eosinophilic esophagitis and gastroenteritis (Table 38–9).

Some adverse reactions diagnosed by patients or physicians as food allergy involve non–immune-mediated mechanisms, such as pharmacologic and metabolic mechanisms, reactions to food toxins, or intolerances (eg, lactose intolerance). These will not be covered in this chapter.

Clinical Findings

A. Symptoms and Signs

A thorough medical history is crucial to identifying symptoms associated with potential food allergy; a history of a temporal relationship between the ingestion of a suspected food and onset of a reaction—as well as the nature and

Table 38–9. Food allergy disorders.

IgE-mediated
  Gastrointestinal: Pollen-food allergy syndrome, immediate GI anaphylaxis
  Cutaneous: Urticaria, angioedema, morbilliform rashes, and flushing
  Respiratory: Acute rhinoconjunctivitis, acute wheezing
  Generalized: Anaphylactic shock
Mixed IgE- and non–IgE-mediated
  Gastrointestinal: Eosinophilic esophagitis/gastroenteritis/colitis
  Cutaneous: Atopic dermatitis
  Respiratory: Asthma
Non–IgE-mediated
  Gastrointestinal: Food protein–induced enterocolitis, proctocolitis, and enteropathy syndromes; celiac disease
  Cutaneous: Contact dermatitis, dermatitis herpetiformis
  Respiratory: Food-induced pulmonary hemosiderosis (Heiner syndrome)

duration of symptoms observed—is important in establishing the diagnosis. For all IgE-mediated reactions, reactions to foods occur within minutes and up to 2 hours after ingestion. Hives, flushing, facial angioedema, and mouth or throat itching are common. In severe cases, angioedema of the tongue, uvula, pharynx, or upper airway can occur. Gastrointestinal symptoms include abdominal discomfort or pain, nausea, vomiting, and diarrhea. Children with food allergy may occasionally have isolated rhinoconjunctivitis or wheezing. Rarely, anaphylaxis to food may involve only cardiovascular collapse.

In patients with IgE antibodies to galactose-a-1,3-galactose (a-Gal), delayed anaphylaxis, urticaria, and angioedema can occur up to 4–6 hours after ingestion of mammalian meats. For non–IgE-mediated and mixed disorders, reactions can be delayed in onset for more than several hours, such as in FPIES, to possibly days later with onset of vomiting or an eczema flare after food exposure due to eosinophilic esophagitis or atopic dermatitis, respectively.

B. Laboratory Findings

Typically, fewer than 50% of histories of adverse reactions to foods will be confirmed as food allergy by blinded food challenge (although this percentage is much higher in food-induced anaphylaxis). Prick skin testing is useful to rule out a suspected food allergen because the predictive value is high for a properly performed negative test with an extract of good quality (negative predictive accuracy of > 95%). In contrast, the predictive value for a positive skin test is approximately 50%. Serum food-specific IgE tests have lower specificity and positive predictive values; therefore, doing serum IgE food panels is not recommended, with referral to an allergist preferred to obtain a detailed clinical history and selective testing, if necessary. A list of nonstandardized and unproven procedures for the diagnosis of food allergy includes the

measurement of allergen-specific IgG, lymphocyte stimulation, cytotoxic assays, applied kinesiology, and provocation neutralization, to name a few.

The double-blind, placebo-controlled food challenge is considered the gold standard for diagnosing food allergy, except in severe reactions. If there is high suspicion of possible allergic reactivity to a food with a negative skin test or an undetectable serum IgE level (or both), a food challenge may be necessary to confirm the presence or absence of allergy. Even when multiple food allergies are suspected, most patients will test positive to only three or fewer foods on blinded challenge. Therefore, extensive elimination diets are almost never indicated, and an evaluation by an allergist is preferred before multiple foods are eliminated from the diet unnecessarily. Elimination diets and food challenges may be the only tools for evaluation of suspected non–IgE-mediated food reactions.

▶ **Differential Diagnosis**

Repeated vomiting in infancy may be due to pyloric stenosis or gastroesophageal reflux. With chronic gastrointestinal symptoms, enzyme deficiency (eg, lactase), cystic fibrosis, celiac disease, chronic intestinal infections, gastrointestinal malformations, and irritable bowel syndrome should be considered.

▶ **Treatment**

Treatment consists of eliminating and avoiding foods that have been documented to cause allergic reactions. This involves educating the patient, parent/caregivers and systems such as child care and schools regarding hidden food allergens, the necessity for reading labels, and the signs and symptoms of food allergy and its appropriate management (anaphylaxis action plan; a copy of this plan can be obtained from the references). Consultation with a dietitian familiar with food allergy may be helpful, especially when common foods such as milk, egg, peanut, soy, or wheat are involved. All patients with a history of IgE-mediated food allergy should carry self-injectable epinephrine (eg, Auvi-Q or Epipen) and a fast-acting antihistamine, have an anaphylaxis action plan, and consider wearing medical identification jewelry. Clinical trials of oral and epicutaneous immunotherapy are under investigation as potential future treatments of food allergy, currently in phase III for peanut and with possible FDA approval by 2020. However, diets containing extensively heated (baked) milk and egg are potential alternative approaches to food oral immunotherapy and are changing the previous standard of strict avoidance diets for patients with allergy to these foods.

▶ **Prognosis**

The prognosis is good if the offending food can be identified and avoided. Unfortunately, accidental exposure to food allergens in severely allergic patients can result in death. Most children outgrow food allergies to milk, egg, wheat, and soy but not to peanut or tree nuts (only 20% and 10% of children may outgrow peanut and tree nut allergy, respectively). The natural history of food allergy can be followed by measuring food-specific IgE levels and performing food challenges when indicated. Approximately 3%–4% of children will have food allergy as adults. Resources for food-allergic patients include the Food Allergy Research & Education: www.foodallergy.org; the Food Allergy & Anaphylaxis Connection Team: www.foodallergyawareness.org; and the Consortium of Food Allergy Research: www.cofargroup.org.

▶ Prevention

Recently, multiple randomized controlled trials (RCTs) and a meta-analysis have shown that there appears to be no benefit with respect to food allergy prevention in delaying the introduction of any major food allergen into an infant's diet. Specific guidelines for the prevention of peanut allergy have been published that provide recommendations and instructions on how and when to introduce peanut into an infant's diet (https://www.niaid.nih.gov/diseases-conditions/guidelines-clinicians-and-patients-food-allergy).

Boyce JA et al: Guidelines for the diagnosis and management of food allergy in the United States: report of the NIAID-sponsored expert panel. J Allergy Clin Immunol 2010;126(Suppl 1):158 [PMID: 21134576].

Fleischer DM et al: Effect of epicutaneous immunotherapy vs placebo on reaction to peanut protein ingestion among children with peanut allergy: the PEPITES randomized clinical trial. JAMA 2019;321(10):946–955 [PMID: 30794314].

Sampson HA et al: Food allergy: a practice parameter update-2014. J Allergy Clin Immunol 2014;134:1016–1025 [PMID: 25174862].

Vickery BP et al: AR101 oral immunotherapy for peanut allergy. N Engl J Med 2018;379:1991–2001 [PMID: 30449234].

INSECT ALLERGY

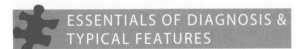

ESSENTIALS OF DIAGNOSIS & TYPICAL FEATURES

▶ Insect bites or stings can cause local or systemic reactions that can range from mild to fatal in susceptible individuals.

▶ Skin testing is indicated for children with systemic reactions to insect stings.

▶ Children who have had anaphylactic reactions to hymenoptera stings should have autoinjectable epinephrine and wear a medical alert bracelet.

▶ Patients who experience severe systemic reactions and have a positive skin test should receive venom immunotherapy.

Allergic reactions to insects include symptoms of respiratory allergy as a result of inhalation of particulate matter of insect origin, local cutaneous reactions to insect bites, and anaphylactic reactions to stings. The latter almost exclusively caused by Hymenoptera includes honeybees, yellow jackets, yellow hornets, white-faced hornets, wasps, and fire ants. Africanized honeybees, also known as killer bees, are a concern because of their aggressive behavior and excessive swarming, not because their venom is more toxic. Rarely, patients sensitized to reduviid bugs (also known as kissing bugs) may have episodes of nocturnal anaphylaxis. Lepidopterism refers to adverse effects secondary to contact with larval or adult butterflies and moths. Salivary gland antigens are responsible for immediate and delayed skin reactions in mosquito-sensitive patients.

▶ Clinical Findings

A. Symptoms and Signs

Insect bites or stings can cause local or systemic reactions ranging from mild to fatal responses in susceptible persons. Local cutaneous reactions include urticaria as well as papulovesicular eruptions and lesions that resemble delayed hypersensitivity reactions. Papular urticaria is almost always the result of insect bites, especially of mosquitoes, fleas, and bedbugs. Toxic systemic reactions consisting of gastrointestinal symptoms, headache, vertigo, syncope, convulsions, or fever can occur following multiple stings. These reactions result from histamine-like substances in the venom. In children with hypersensitivity to fire ant venom, sterile pustules occur at sting sites on a nonimmunologic basis due to the inherent toxicity of piperidine alkaloids in the venom. Mild systemic reactions include itching, flushing, and urticaria. Severe systemic reactions may include dyspnea, wheezing, chest tightness, hoarseness, fullness in the throat, hypotension, loss of consciousness, incontinence, nausea, vomiting, and abdominal pain. Delayed systemic reactions occur from 2 hours to 3 weeks following the sting and include serum sickness, peripheral neuritis, allergic vasculitis, and coagulation defects.

B. Laboratory Findings

Skin testing is indicated for children with systemic reactions to insect stings. Venoms of honeybee, yellow jacket, yellow hornet, white-faced hornet, and wasp are available for skin testing and treatment. Fire ant venom is not yet commercially available, but an extract made from fire ant bodies appears adequate to establish the presence of IgE antibodies to fire ant venom. Importantly, venom skin tests can be negative in patients with systemic allergic reactions, especially in the first few weeks after a sting, and the tests may need to be repeated. The presence of a positive skin test denotes prior sensitization but does not predict whether a reaction will occur with the patient's next sting, nor does it differentiate between local and systemic reactions. It is common for children who have had an allergic reaction to have positive skin tests to more than one venom. This might reflect sensitization from prior stings that did not result in an allergic reaction or cross-reactivity between closely related venoms. In vitro testing (compared with skin testing) has not substantially improved the ability to predict anaphylaxis. With in vitro testing, there is a 15%–20% incidence of both false-positive and false-negative results. IgE to mosquito saliva antigen can be measured by in vitro assay.

▶ Complications

Secondary infection can complicate allergic reactions to insect bites or stings. Serum sickness, nephrotic syndrome, vasculitis, neuritis, and encephalopathy may be seen as late sequelae of reactions to stinging insects.

▶ Treatment

For cutaneous reactions caused by biting insects, symptomatic therapy includes cold compresses, antipruritics (including antihistamines), and, occasionally, potent topical corticosteroids. Treatment of stings includes careful removal of the stinger, if present, by flicking it away from the wound, not by grasping in order to prevent further envenomation. Topical application of monosodium glutamate, baking soda, or vinegar compresses is of questionable efficacy. Local reactions can be treated with ice, elevation of the affected extremity, oral antihistamines, and NSAIDs as well as potent topical corticosteroids. Large local reactions may require a short course of oral corticosteroids. Anaphylactic reactions following Hymenoptera stings should be managed as discussed above (see section on Anaphylaxis). Children who have had severe or anaphylactic reactions to Hymenoptera stings—or their parents and caregivers—should be instructed in the use of autoinjectable epinephrine. Patients at risk for anaphylaxis from an insect sting should also wear a medical alert bracelet indicating their allergy. Children at risk from insect stings should avoid wearing bright-colored clothing and perfumes when outdoors and should wear long pants and shoes when walking in the grass. Patients who experience severe systemic reactions and have a positive skin test should receive venom immunotherapy. Venom immunotherapy is not indicated for children with only urticarial or local reactions.

▶ Prognosis

Children generally have milder reactions than adults after insect stings, and fatal reactions are extremely rare. Patients aged 3–16 years with reactions limited to the skin, such as urticaria and angioedema, appear to be at low risk for more severe reactions with subsequent stings.

Albuhairi S et al: A twenty-two-year experience with Hymenoptera venom immunotherapy in a US pediatric tertiary care center 1996-2018. Ann Allergy Asthma Immunol 2018;121:722.e1 [PMID: 30102964].

Golden DB et al: Stinging insect hypersensitivity: a practice parameter update 2016. Ann Allergy Asthma Immunol 2017;118:28 [PMID: 28007086].

39

Antimicrobial Therapy

Sarah K. Parker, MD

Jason Child, PharmD

Christine E. MacBrayne, PharmD, MSC

Andrew Haynes, MD

Justin Searns, MD

PRINCIPLES OF ANTIMICROBIAL THERAPY

The discovery and rapid development of targeted antimicrobial agents, beginning in the 1930s, are among the most important scientific developments of 20th-century medicine. These drugs have forever changed the practice of medicine, and antimicrobials remain one of medicine's most effective and widely used interventions. However, despite the impact of these drugs, choosing an appropriate antimicrobial can be a complex and difficult task. Optimal antimicrobial use requires appreciation of the complicated interactions between host, organism, and drug. This decision-making process, summarized in Table 39–1, begins with an accurate working diagnosis, based on the patient's history, physical examination, exposure history, and initial laboratory tests. From this foundation, the clinician must consider the most likely organism(s) and that organism's likely pattern of antimicrobial susceptibility. This information is considered in the context of numerous patient-specific factors, including age, immune status, relevant comorbidities, site of infection, and microbiology of his or her prior infections. Empiric therapy should be changed to definitive therapy as the clinical course evolves and additional laboratory data are available. Obtaining appropriate microbiologic specimens helps facilitate this transition.

For example, age impacts the likely pathogens; neonates are generally predisposed to infection with *Escherichia coli* and group B *Streptococcus*, while in older children, infections with *Streptococcus pneumoniae* and *Staphylococcus aureus* predominate. Children with chronic illness may have significant exposure to antimicrobials, and the effect of this on their microbial flora should be considered. Different exposures, based on environment, travel, diet, animal contact, or ill family members or other close contacts, may suggest a greater likelihood of certain organisms. Another important consideration is the pace and seriousness of the illness. A rapidly progressive and severe illness should be treated initially with broad-spectrum antimicrobials until a specific etiologic diagnosis is made. A mildly ill ambulatory patient should receive treatment with narrow-spectrum antimicrobials, per national guidelines when available. These many and often interconnected factors make the choice of empiric treatment challenging.

Once an appropriate initial antimicrobial is chosen, the clinician must consider the proper dose, route of administration, duration of therapy, and whether additional drugs are needed. Antimicrobial susceptibility, antimicrobial families, and dosing recommendations are listed in Tables 39–3 to 39–5. The need to balance a treatment's efficacy with the toxicities and side effects inherent in the drugs chosen makes this process even more complex. Often, decisions of when not to use antimicrobials are important, as additional drugs and longer durations may harm patients.

CONCEPTS FOR JUDICIOUS USE OF ANTIMICROBIALS

Antimicrobials are the most commonly prescribed class of medication in both adults and children. Over 25% of pediatric outpatient visits result in an antimicrobial prescription, and nearly 60% of pediatric inpatients receive antimicrobials. Much of this use (up to 40%–60%) is inappropriate. We not only overprescribe but also choose unnecessarily broad agents, even though they are often less effective. For example, azithromycin and cefdinir are among the top prescribed antibiotics in outpatient pediatrics, despite that they are rarely first-line agents on pediatric national guidelines and often inferior to alternative oral agents.

Historically, overprescribing was viewed as an "insurance policy." This approach was considered a cheap, safe, and reliable intervention that providers could offer to parents beyond reassurance. This era is over for six reasons. First, overuse leads to antibiotic resistance at a patient, hospital, and community level. Resistance is now commonplace and

Table 39–1. Steps in decision making for use of antimicrobial agents.

Step	Action	Example
1	Determine diagnosis	Septic arthritis and osteomyelitis
2	Consider age, preexisting condition, antimicrobial penetration	Previously healthy 2-year-old child, bone and joint penetration desired
3	Consider common organisms (for age and site of infection)	*Staphylococcus aureus, Kingella kingae*
4	Consider organism susceptibility	Penicillin- or ampicillin-resistant; frequency of MRSA in community
5	Obtain proper cultures and gram stains if clinically possible. Particularly important if the organism or susceptibilities are unpredictable	Blood cultures, joint fluid, bone biopsy
6	Initiate empiric therapy based on above considerations, and guidelines if they exist	Cefazolin, add vancomycin to cefazolin if seriously ill or MRSA prevalent
7	Modify therapy based on culture results and patient response	*S aureus* isolated. Choose cefazolin or vancomycin based on susceptibility
8	Follow clinical response, consider laboratory responses	Interval physical examination, inflammatory markers
9	Change to oral therapy	Cephalexin if cefazolin susceptible, anti-MRSA drug if needed based on susceptibility (eg, clindamycin, trimethoprim/sulfamethoxazole, linezolid). Change when afebrile, clinically improving, falling inflammatory markers, able to tolerate oral medications
10	Stop therapy	Clinically improved or well, treated minimal duration based on standard of care/guidelines

Methicillin-resistant *Staphylococcus aureus.*

increasing to the point the efficacy of some antimicrobials may be limited or completely lacking for some infections. Second, overuse impacts the patient's normal flora and creates a microbial "void" that multidrug-resistant organisms, *Clostridioides difficile* (formerly *Clostridium difficile*), yeasts, and molds can enter and become a reservoir for disease. In the United States, there are approximately 478,000 cases of

C difficile colitis and 2 million antimicrobial resistant infections (with at least 23,000 deaths) per year. Third, patients experience adverse drug reactions regularly; an adverse reaction occurs in approximately 30% of antibiotic courses, resulting in over 150,000 unplanned pediatric medical visits per year. In many instances of inappropriate prescribing, more patients will experience harm from an antibiotic than will benefit from it—in other words, when the likelihood of benefit is low, the number needed to treat (NNT) to benefit a patient can be higher than the number needed to NNT to harm (NNH) a patient. Adverse events include device-related complications (such as infections and clots of central lines inserted for antimicrobial use, and intravenous extravasations) and drug adverse effects (such as fever, rash, hives, Stevens-Johnson syndrome, drug-induced hypersensitivity syndrome [DIHS], drug-induced lupus, antibiotic-associated diarrhea, neutropenia, thrombocytopenia, anemia, renal toxicity, and hepatitis). Fourth, the impact of overuse on a patient's microbiome has been linked to untoward health effects, such as obesity in children and graft-versus-host disease in transplant recipients. Fifth, the drugs and their health consequences are expensive; for example, an episode of in-hospital *C difficile* has an attributable cost of $93,000. Sixth, provider's perception that a parent wants an antibiotic for their child is often unfounded. Data indicate that instead of antibiotics, the majority of parents want reassurance that their concern for their child was justified, and they want guidance on what to do if their child becomes more ill or does not improve. This misconception is a main driver of overprescribing. Finally, many of these factors together may lead to poorer clinical outcomes.

To avoid complications and side effects, providers should use guideline-recommended drugs, for the shortest efficacious durations, stop drugs when infections are unlikely and cultures are negative, and choose oral therapies when possible. Many drugs including metronidazole, clindamycin, fluconazole, levofloxacin, rifampin, linezolid, and trimethoprim/sulfamethoxazole are more than 90% bioavailable orally (and ciprofloxacin is 80%) and thus can be used orally, with similar efficacy to IV therapy, if the gastrointestinal tract is intact. Even for drugs that are less bioavailable, transition to oral therapy is still appropriate as step-down therapy once the patient is clinically improved (eg, amoxicillin for pneumonia or cephalexin for osteomyelitis after initial inpatient IV therapy).

Because of the documented harms of unrestrained antimicrobial use, antimicrobial stewardship programs (ASPs) have been endorsed by the Infectious Disease Society of America, US News and World Report, Centers for Medicaid and Medicare Services, and some state legislatures. ASPs are effective at improving antimicrobial use in many hospitals, resulting in decreased use of antimicrobials, decreased drug-resistant infections, decreased *C difficile* colitis, decreased costs, and improved clinical outcomes. ASPs are typically collaborative and cross-disciplinary, involving infectious diseases physicians, pharmacists, data analysts, and multiple other stakeholders. ASP models vary by location, but they include local guideline and policy development, antibiotic use prior authorization programs (where a prescriber must seek permission to prescribe certain antimicrobials), post-prescriptive review programs (where stewards review use and intervene when there is a question on appropriateness), IV to oral switch policies, prescriber feedback programs (where prescribing habits are compared and contrasted to others on either a unit, practice, or provider level), and multiple other interventions.

SUSCEPTIBILITY TESTING & DRUG DOSING PROPERTIES

Cultures and other diagnostic material should be obtained prior to starting antimicrobial therapy. This is especially important for complicated situations, such as when the patient has a serious infection, is at risk for drug-resistant organisms, has failed prior treatment, has unusual exposures, or multiagent empiric therapy is anticipated. When cultures identify the causative organism, therapy should be tailored to susceptibility and an appropriate duration selected.

Clinical specimens for diagnostic testing should be evaluated in a laboratory using carefully defined procedures (as defined by the Clinical and Laboratory Standards Institute [CLSI] or European Committee on Antimicrobial Susceptibility Testing [EUCAST]). For most bacteria, growth in culture remains the gold standard for identification and susceptibility testing. Though laboratory techniques continue to improve, the growth rate of the organism remains a limiting factor—multiple days are often required for an organism to grow, be identified, and susceptibilities determined. Though traditional biochemical testing is still the mainstay for most organisms, there are now much more rapid methods, such as polymerase chain reaction (PCR) panels and mass spectrometry-based identification. For detection of some mechanisms of resistance, such as *mecA* detection indicating methicillin-resistant *S aureus* (MRSA), rapid PCR methods are available in many clinical laboratories. However, most antimicrobial susceptibility testing is still done by determination of the minimum inhibitory concentration (MIC) for the organism-drug pair (eg, *S pneumoniae* and penicillin) in a culture-based system. The MIC represents the amount of antibiotic (in mcg/mL) necessary to inhibit growth of the organism under specific laboratory conditions. The organism is then deemed susceptible, intermediate, or resistant based on CLSI or EUCAST published breakpoints. Breakpoints are determined based on achievable levels of drug in the serum at recommended dosing in healthy adults. In certain circumstances, the levels in other body fluids are considered, such as in cerebral spinal fluid (CSF, eg, *S pneumoniae*) or in urine. In general, however, breakpoints do not consider drug penetration into certain infected spaces (like bone, lung, kidney parenchyma), a particular dosing strategy, or a patient's immune status. Providers must interpret microbiologic data as these data pertain to a particular patient or clinical scenario. For example, for osteomyelitis higher doses of cephalexin are used (100–150 mg/kg/day divided in three to four doses) to achieve sufficiently high antibiotic levels within bone for extended periods. Conversely, many drugs are highly concentrated in urine and can be used to successfully treat some urinary pathogens that are classified as "resistant" per published breakpoints (eg, a patient may have a good clinical response to cephalexin for a urinary tract infection (UTI) with *E coli* determined to be cephalexin-resistant in the laboratory). Ultimately, the true test of therapeutic efficacy is patient response. Patients who do not respond to seemingly appropriate therapy require reassessment, including reconsideration of the diagnosis, repeat cultures, and consideration of surgical debulking of the infection. Thus, antimicrobial susceptibility testing, although an essential part of therapeutic decision making, must be considered in context with drug concentrations at the site of infection, immune status, patient age, comorbid conditions, and pharmacodynamics.

PHARMACODYNAMIC CONCEPTS

When considering efficacy of antibiotics, there are three pharmacodynamic/pharmacokinetic models used to predict cure (Figure 39–1). Common to all these concepts is that the concentration of drug in the space of the infection must exceed the MIC. If an isolate is available, the MIC may be exactly determined in the clinical laboratory. Alternatively, general knowledge of the likely MIC based on historical data for the pathogen can be used to choose an antimicrobial. Apart from simply exceeding the MIC, efficacy is then correlated with either the time that the MIC is exceeded (time over MIC), the peak concentration over the MIC (peak over MIC), or a combination of both, described as "the area under the curve" (AUC) over the MIC (see Figure 39–1). Time over the MIC, which applies to all β-lactams, is calculated as the percentage of a 24-hour day that the drug concentration exceeds the MIC. Time over MIC targets can range from 30% to 40% to more than 90%, depending on the severity and site of infection and the immune status of the host. The typical target for peak over MIC (applicable to aminoglycosides) is a peak of 8- to 10-fold greater than the MIC, though this is not always possible. Time-dependent drugs rapidly enter the microbe at high concentrations, and even when the drug is gone, the surviving microbes take hours to recover the ability to replicate. This is called postantibiotic effect (PAE) and allows dosing at extended intervals, such as once daily. For most other drugs, the AUC over the MIC is the best predictor of bacterial killing because it incorporates both this PAE and the required time above MIC. These efficacy parameters are

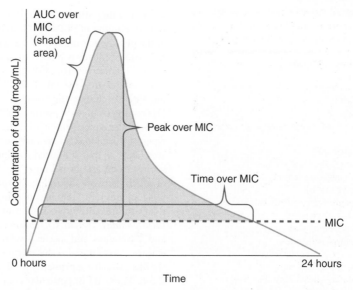

▲ **Figure 39–1.** Depiction of pharmacokinetic/pharmacodynamic parameters for antimicrobial efficacy.

affected by achievable drug concentrations, protein binding of the drug (protein-bound drug is not active), and the drug half-life. These parameters can be modified to increase efficacy by altering the dose, the route, or the interval.

Other patient factors affect dosing, most notably organ dysfunction, concomitant medications, obesity, and age. Drug metabolism (usually renal or hepatic), interactions, and side effects are addressed in the drug descriptions and tables in this chapter. Obesity affects drug distribution. For example, aminoglycosides do not rapidly distribute into fat, so an obese patient dosed by body weight may have supratherapeutic aminoglycoside levels. Age affects metabolism and excretion of all drugs, and absorption of oral drugs. Infants and toddlers may lack proteins necessary to transport drug, and their kidneys are relatively immature, both of which impact dosing.

USE OF ANTIMICROBIAL AGENTS TO PREVENT DISEASE

Antimicrobials are primarily used to treat active infections. However, they are also used to prevent new infections through preexposure prophylaxis (malaria prevention in travelers, dental prophylaxis to prevent endocarditis in patients with prosthetic valves, etc), postexposure prophylaxis (household meningococcal exposure, chlamydia disease in sexual partners, etc), and prophylaxis to prevent conversion of latent to active disease (latent *Mycobacterium tuberculosis* infection, recurrent herpes simplex virus [HSV] infection, etc). Surgical prophylaxis is another common use of antimicrobials, with

the goal to achieve high drug levels in the tissue at the time of incision and—along with good surgical technique—to minimize viable bacterial contamination of the wound. For most surgeries, a single dose is all that is necessary. A list of microbes and disease states for which prophylaxis may be considered is in Table 39–2.

CHOICE OF ANTIMICROBIAL AGENTS

Recommendations for choosing antibiotics for specific conditions are based on the patient's age, diagnosis, site of infection, severity of illness, local antimicrobial susceptibility patterns, antimicrobial susceptibility of patient-specific bacterial isolates (historical and current), history of drug allergy, and potential drug interactions and side effects, as discussed above. Tables 39–3 to 39–5 provide further information, including dosing. Always consult the package insert for detailed prescribing information. Empiric and definitive therapies for many particular clinical entities are addressed throughout this textbook and in Table 39–6. Mechanisms of action and efficacy parameters are noted later and indicated in Figure 39–2.

▼ SPECIFIC ANTIMICROBIAL AGENTS

β-LACTAM ANTIBIOTICS (STEP 1, FIGURE 39–2)

β-Lactam antimicrobials include the penicillins, cephalosporins, carbapenems, monobactams (step 1, Figure 39–2), and many β-lactamase inhibitors (step 3, Figure 39–2). They are

Table 39–2. Situations where prophylaxis (antimicrobials or immune globulin administration) may be indicated.[a]

Preexposure Prophylaxis May Be Indicated
Surgical site infection prevention
Bacterial endocarditis prevention during procedures (for selected patient with cardiac anomalies)
Malaria prophylaxis for travelers
Streptococcus pneumoniae (sickle cell disease, asplenia, complement deficiency)
Neisseria meningitides (eculizumab use)
Group A streptococcus (rheumatic fever)
Pneumocystis jirovecii (HIV [late stage and early perinatal diagnosis], some immunocompromised patients)
Mycobacterium avium-intracellulare complex (HIV [late stage], some immunocompromised patients)
Postexposure Prophylaxis May Be Indicated
Neisseria gonorrhoeae (ophthalmia neonatorum)
Bordetella pertussis (exposure to respiratory secretions)
Chlamydia trachomatis (sexual contact exposure)
Haemophilus influenzae type B (household exposure)
N meningitidis (household exposure)
N gonorrhoeae (sexual contact exposure)
Treponema pallidum (sexual contact exposure)
Pneumonic *Yersinia pestis* (exposure)
Francisella tularensis (aerosolized exposure)
HIV exposure (mother-to-child, or blood and body fluid exposures)
Raccoon feces exposure (Baylisascaris)
Monkey bite from Old World Macaque (herpes B)
Borrelia burgdorferi (tick bite from endemic area)
Rabies
Tetanus
Dog bite (not infected)
Hepatitis A
Hepatitis B
Varicella zoster virus
Measles
Influenza
Group B *Streptococcus* transmission (mother to child)
Mycobacterium tuberculosis (in exposed infants)
Prophylaxis Against Conversion From Latent Infection to Active Disease
Mycobacterium tuberculosis (latent infection)
HSV (to prevent recurrent outbreaks)
HSV/EBV/CMV (in some immunocompromised patients)

[a]For particular situations, choice, and dose of antimicrobials, refer to the Report of the Committee on Infectious Diseases (RedBook), particular society guidelines, or the Centers for Disease Control and Prevention website.

characterized by a four-member β-lactam ring, but otherwise they are structurally distinct, with differences in their ability to bind their target, the penicillin-binding proteins (PBPs, also called transpeptidases). Bacteria have a large variety and number of PBPs, so the spectrum of β-lactam activity is related to the binding affinity to the key PBPs in a given bacterial isolate. Binding of PBPs by β-lactams prevents cross-linking of the peptidoglycan layer of the cell wall, resulting in bacterial death. Efficacy is related to time over the MIC. Bacteria protect themselves from β-lactams mainly by (1) producing β-lactamases that hydrolyze the β-lactam ring, (2) altering the PBP to change the β-lactam–PBP-binding affinity, or (3) creating changes in porins or efflux pumps to decrease the intracellular concentration of drug. There are many different types of β-lactamases that vary from very narrow penicillinases (such as that produced routinely by *S aureus*) to more sophisticated and broad types produced by gram negatives, of which there are thousands. Among these are the inducible β-lactamases (IBL) that become clinically apparent only after β-lactam use. IBLs are common in some species of *Serratia, Pseudomonas, Proteus, Citrobacter, Enterobacter, Morganella,* and *Aeromonas,* and species-level lists can be found in the literature. There are also the extended spectrum β-lactamases (ESBLs), which are primarily produced by *Klebsiella* spp. and *E coli.* These are of particular concern because the plasmids (see Figure 39–2) encoding them are transmissible between organisms and often harbor other types of resistance. Of increasing concern are the plasmids encoding carbapenem resistance, because they often contain other types of resistance mutations and have the potential to lead to infections that are untreatable with current drugs.

Although allergy to β-lactam antimicrobials is reported commonly by parents, this history is not highly predictive of an allergic reaction. A history of anaphylactic-type reactions warrants caution or avoidance of cephalosporins and penicillins until evaluated by an allergist. However, because patients labeled with a penicillin allergy may receive inferior treatment strategies, confirming the details of the history is important. Patients unlikely to have a true allergy should be "de-labeled," and those with a history consistent with a concerning reaction should be referred for allergy testing.

β-LACTAM: PENICILLINS

Penicillins & Aminopenicillins

Penicillins, amoxicillin, and ampicillin are the drugs of choice to treat infections with most streptococci (including group A *Streptococcus*, group B *Streptococcus*, and *Pneumococcus*), most enterococci, *Treponema pallidum, Neisseria meningitides, Leptospira, Streptobacillus moniliformis* (rat-bite fever), *Actinomyces,* many oral anaerobes, and most *Clostridium* and *Bacillus* species. They are also used for prophylaxis in patients with rheumatic fever or asplenia. Amoxicillin and ampicillin are considered first line for community-acquired pneumonia and otitis media. They penetrate all tissues relatively well, and amoxicillin offers adequate oral bioavailability (it has the best bioavailability among β-lactams that,

Table 39–3. Susceptibility of some common pathogenic microorganisms to various antimicrobial drugs.

Organism	Potentially Useful Antibiotics	
Bacteria		
	First choice examples	Alternate choice examples
Anaerobic bacteria[a]	Metronidazole, cefoxitin	Clindamycin, penicillins with β-lactamase inhibitor, meropenem, ertapenem, imipenem, tigecycline
Bartonella henselae	Azithromycin	Ciprofloxacin, clarithromycin, doxycycline, erythromycin, rifampin
Bordetella pertussis	Azithromycin	Clarithromycin, erythromycin, trimethoprim/sulfamethoxazole
Campylobacter spp. (not fetus)	Azithromycin	Erythromycin, fluoroquinolones, doxycycline
Clostridium perfringens	Clindamycin, penicillin	Metronidazole, pipercillin/tazobactam, cephalosporins, doxycycline
Clostridioides difficile	Metronidazole, vancomycin (PO)	Vancomycin taper, fecal microbiota transplant
Corynebacterium diphtheriae	Erythromycin	Penicillin, clindamycin
Escherichia coli/Klebsiella sp.	Ampicillin/sulbactam, amoxicillin/clavulanate, cephalosporins	Aminoglycosides, aztreonam, fluoroquinolones
ESBL (*E coli/Klebsiella*)	Meropenem	Ceftolazone/tazobactam, aminoglycosides, fluoroquinolones, tigecycline
KPC (*E coli/Klebsiella*)	Ceftazidime/avibactam	Colistin, aminoglycosides, tigecycline
Enterococcus faecalis	Ampicillin, vancomycin, (± gentamicin),	Daptomycin, linezolid, carbapenems
Enterococcus faecium	vancomycin (± gentamicin)	Ampicillin, daptomycin, linezolid, tigecycline
Haemophilus influenzae	Amoxicillin/clavulanate, ampicillin (if β-lactamase–negative), ceftriaxone	Fluoroquinolones, cefuroxime (not meningitis)
Kingella kingae	Cefazolin, cephalexin	Nafcillin
Listeria monocytogenes	Ampicillin	Trimethoprim/sulfamethoxazole, vancomycin
Moraxella catarrhalis	Amoxicillin/clavulanate, ampicillin (if β-lactamase–negative)[b]	Cephalosporins (II and III), trimethoprim/sulfamethoxazole, macrolides, fluoroquinolones
Neisseria gonorrhoeae	Ceftriaxone	Azithromycin
Neisseria meningitidis	Ceftriaxone/cefotaxime	Ampicillin, penicillin
Nocardia asteroides	Trimethoprim/sulfamethoxazole (+ imipenem for severe infections)	Minocycline, (severe disease) linezolid + meropenem, imipenem + amikacin
Pasteurella multocida	Amoxicillin/clavulanate, ampicillin/sulbactam	Fluoroquinolones, cephalosporins, doxycycline, trimethoprim/sulfamethoxazole
Pseudomonas aeruginosa	Cefepime	Ciprofloxacin, anti-*Pseudomonas* penicillins, aminoglycosides, meropenem
Salmonella spp.	Azithromycin, ceftriaxone	Ampicillin, fluoroquinolones, trimethoprim/sulfamethoxazole
Shigella spp.	Fluoroquinolones	Azithromycin, ceftriaxone, trimethoprim/sulfamethoxazole
Staphylococcus aureus (MSSA)	Cefazolin, cephalexin, nafcillin, dicloxacillin	Clindamycin, trimethoprim/sulfamethoxazole, cefepime
S aureus (MRSA)	Vancomycin	Clindamycin, daptomycin, linezolid, trimethoprim/sulfamethoxazole, ceftaroline
Staphylococci (coagulase-negative)	Vancomycin	Cefazolin (if susceptible)[c], clindamycin, linezolid, trimethoprim/sulfamethoxazole

(Continued)

Table 39–3. Susceptibility of some common pathogenic microorganisms to various antimicrobial drugs. (*Continued*)

Organism	Potentially Useful Antibiotics	
Streptococci (groups A and B)	Penicillin, ampicillin, amoxicillin	Ceftriaxone, cefotaxime, clindamycin, levofloxacin, vancomycin
Streptococci (viridans and anginosus groups)	Ceftriaxone, vancomycin	Penicillins, clindamycin, daptomycin
Streptococcus pneumoniae[d]	Ampicillin, amoxicillin, ceftriaxone	Penicillins, cephalosporins, vancomycin, levofloxacin, meropenem
Atypical organisms		
Chlamydia spp.	Azithromycin	Clarithromycin, erythromycin, levofloxacin, ofloxacin, tetracyclines
Mycoplasma spp.	Azithromycin	Clarithromycin, erythromycin, fluoroquinolones, tetracyclines
Tick-borne illness		
Francisella tularensis (Tularemia)	Gentamicin	Streptomycin, ciprofloxacin, doxycycline
Borrelia burgdorferi (Lyme)	Doxycycline, amoxicillin, ceftriaxone	Cefuroxime, azithromycin
Borrelia hermsii (tick-borne relapsing fever)	Doxycycline	Erythromycin, ceftriaxone
Anaplasmosis/Ehrlichiosis/Rocky Mountain spotted fever	Doxycycline	
Babesiosis	Atovaquone + azithromycin	Clindamycin + quinine
Fungi		
Candida albicans	Fluconazole, echinocandins	Liposomal amphotericin B, azoles
Candida non-albicans	Echinocandins, fluconazole	Azoles, liposomal amphotericin B
Aspergillus spp.	Voriconazole, isavuconazole	Posaconazole, liposomal amphotericin B, echinocandins
Dimorphic fungi	Liposomal amphotericin B	Itraconazole, voriconazole, posaconazole, fluconazole
Mucormycosis	Liposomal amphotericin B (± echinocandin)	Posaconazole, isavuconazole
Scedosporium	Voriconazole (± echinocandin)	Posaconazole
Dermatophytes	Clotrimazole, econazole, fluconazole, griseofulvin, itraconazole, ketoconazole, miconazole, terbinafine, tolnaftate	Butenafine, ciclopirox olamine, naftifine, oxiconazole, sertaconazole, sulconazole,
Pneumocystis jirovecii	Trimethoprim/sulfamethoxazole	Clindamycin + primaquine, atovaquone
Viruses		
Herpes simplex	Acyclovir, valacyclovir	Famciclovir, (for resistant strains may use: ganciclovir, cidofovir, foscarnet) For ophthalmic use—idoxuridine,[e] trifluridine[e]
Human immunodeficiency virus	Six classes: (1) nucleoside reverse transcriptase inhibitors, (2) nonnucleoside reverse transcriptase inhibitors, (3) protease inhibitors, (4) fusion inhibitors, (5) integrase inhibitors, (6) CCR-5 coreceptor antagonists; combinations of 3 drugs from 2 different classes should be used (see Chapter 41)	Refer to Chapter 41 for more details. Refer to www.aidsinfo.nih.gov for current dosing information
Influenza virus	Oseltamivir, baloxavir (aged ≥ 12 y)	Peramivir, zanamivir
Respiratory syncytial virus	Ribavirin[f]	

(Continued)

Table 39–3. Susceptibility of some common pathogenic microorganisms to various antimicrobial drugs. (*Continued*)

Organism		Potentially Useful Antibiotics
Varicella-zoster virus	Acyclovir, valacyclovir	famciclovir (for resistant strains may use: ganciclovir, cidofovir, foscarnet)
Cytomegalovirus	Ganciclovir, valganciclovir	Foscarnet, cidofovir
Hepatitis B	Entecavir, tenofovir disoproxil fumarate, tenofovir alafenamide and interferon-α	Interferon-α, telbivudine, lamivudine, and adefovir
Hepatitis C	Peginterferon-α, ribavirin	Ledipasvir/sofosbuvir (aged ≥ 12 y)

[a]Species-dependent.
[b]Also applies to amoxicillin and related compounds.
[c]Only if the coagulase-negative *Staphylococcus* is also methicillin- or oxacillin-sensitive.
[d]Because of increasing frequency of *S pneumoniae* strains resistant to penicillin and cephalosporins, presumptive therapy for severe infections (eg, meningitis) should include vancomycin until susceptibility studies are available.
[e]Ophthalmic preparation.
[f]FDA approved for therapy of respiratory syncytial virus by aerosol, but clinical studies show variable efficacy.

Table 39–4. Guidelines for use of common antimicrobial agents in children age 1 month or older.

Agent	Treatment Category	Dose (mg/kg/day)	Maximum Daily Dose	Interval (h)	Adjustment	Other Considerations
β-Lactams						
Penicillin G	Mild, moderate Severe	100,000–150,000 U/kg 200,000–350,000 U/kg	24 million units	4–6	H, R	Thrombophlebitis May use as continuous infusion
Penicillin VK	Mild Moderate	25–50 25–50	2000 mg	12 6–8	H, R	Unpalatable (suspension) GI side effects
Ampicillin	Mild, moderate Severe	IV 100–200 200–400 PO	IV 12,000 mg PO	IV 4–6 PO	R	Short stability
Amoxicillin	Mild, moderate Severe	40–50 80–100	4000 mg	8–12 8	R	GI side effects
Ampicillin/sulbactam	Mild, moderate Severe	100–200 (ampicillin) 200–400 (ampicillin)	12,000 mg	4–6	R	Short stability
Amoxicillin/ clavulanate	Mild, moderate Severe	40–50 80–100	Based on formulation	8–12 8	R	GI side effects
Piperacillin/ tazobactam	Mild, moderate Severe	240 (piperacillin) 300 (piperacillin)	16,000 mg	4–6	R	Renal toxicity Neutropenia
Nafcillin	Moderate Severe	150 200	12,000 mg	4–6	H	Renal toxicity, venous irritant infuse through central line May use as continuous infusion

(*Continued*)

Table 39–4. Guidelines for use of common antimicrobial agents in children age 1 month or older. *(Continued)*

Agent	Treatment Category	Dose (mg/kg/day)	Maximum Daily Dose	Interval (h)	Adjustment	Other Considerations
Oxacillin	Moderate Severe	100 150-200	12,000 mg	4-6	R	GI side effects Neutropenia
Dicloxacillin	Mild, moderate Severe	25–50 50–100	2000 mg	6	R	GI side effects
Cefazolin	Mild, moderate Severe	50 100–150	8000 mg	8 6-8	R	Neutropenia
Cephalexin	Mild, moderate Severe	25–50 100–150	4000 mg	6	R	GI side effects
Cefadroxil	Mild, moderate Severe	30 150	1000 mg 2000 mg	12 8	R	GI side effects
Cefoxitin	Mild, moderate	80–160	12,000 mg	4–6	R	Neutropenia
Cefuroxime	Mild, moderate	100–150	6000 mg	8	R	Neutropenia
Cefuroxime axetil	Mild Severe	30–40 100	1000 mg	12	R	GI side effects Unpalatable (suspension)
Cefprozil	Mild	30	1000 mg	12	R	GI side effects
Cefpodoxime	Mild	10	400 mg	12	R	GI side effects
Ceftibuten	Mild	9	400 mg	24	R	GI side effects
Cefdinir	Mild	14–25	600 mg	12–24	R	GI side effects
Cefotaxime	Mild, moderate, severe	100–150 200–300	12,000 mg	6–8	R	Not readily available in the US
Ceftazidime	Mild, moderate, severe	100–150	6000 mg	8	R	Note does not cover *S. pneumoniae*
Ceftazidime/ avibactam	Moderate, severe	150	6000 mg (ceftazidime)	8	R	Infuse over 2 h
Ceftriaxone	Mild, moderate Severe	50–75 100	4000 mg/day (max 2000 mg in single dose)	12–24	R	Biliary sludging, bilirubin displacement, chelates with calcium Neutropenia
Cefepime	Mild, moderate Severe	100 150	6000 mg	8–12	R	Q12h dosing for UTI, systemic infection Q8h preferred
Ceftolozane/ tazobactam	Moderate Severe	60 120	6000 mg (ceftolozane)	8 8	R	Infuse over 60 min Anemia
Ceftaroline	Mild Moderate, Severe	24–36 30–45	1800 mg	8-12	R	Infuse over 2 h, positive Coombs w/wo hemolytic anemia, Q8h dosing recommended for pediatrics
Aztreonam	Moderate, severe Cystic fibrosis	90–120 150–300	8000 mg 12,000 mg	6–8	R	Neutropenia
Meropenem	Moderate Severe	60 120	6000 mg	8	R	Neutropenia

(Continued)

Table 39–4. Guidelines for use of common antimicrobial agents in children age 1 month or older. (*Continued*)

Agent	Treatment Category	Dose (mg/kg/day)	Maximum Daily Dose	Interval (h)	Adjustment	Other Considerations
Quinolones						
Ciprofloxacin (IV/PO)	Moderate Severe	20 30	1200 mg IV 1500 mg PO	8–12	R	Peripheral neuropathy Arthralgias Tendonitis/rupture Prolongs QTc
Levofloxacin (IV/PO)	Moderate, severe Moderate, severe Moderate, severe	< 5 y: 20 5–10 y: 14–16 >10 y: 10	750 mg	12 12 24	R	Peripheral neuropathy Arthralgias Tendonitis/rupture Prolongs QTc
Aminoglycosides						
Gentamicin	All infections	Empiric therapy max 3–7.5	Not applicable	8	R	Adjust based on levels Renal toxicity Ototoxicity
Tobramycin	All infections	Empiric therapy max 3–7.5	Not applicable	8	R	Adjust based on levels Renal toxicity Ototoxicity
Amikacin	All infections	Empiric therapy max 15–22.5	Not applicable	8	R	Adjust based on levels Renal toxicity Ototoxicity
Macrolides						
Erythromycin	Mild, moderate	20–50	4000 mg	6–12		GI side effects Prolongs QTc
Azithromycin (IV/PO)	Mild, moderate	10 × 1 then 5 12	1000 mg	24		GI side effects Prolongs QTc
Clarithromycin	Mild, moderate	15	1000 mg	12		GI side effects Prolongs QTc
Other						
Metronidazole (IV/PO)	Giardiasis C difficile, B fragilis Amebic	15 30 30–50	750 mg 1500 mg 2250 mg	8	H	May be administered once daily for appendicitis Neurotoxicity, metallic taste
Clindamycin (IV/PO)	Mild, moderate Severe	20–30 30–40	(IV) 2700 mg (PO) 1800 mg	6–8	H	GI side effects Pill formulations may cause esophagitis

(*Continued*)

Table 39–4. Guidelines for use of common antimicrobial agents in children age 1 month or older. (*Continued*)

Agent	Treatment Category	Dose (mg/kg/day)	Maximum Daily Dose	Interval (h)	Adjustment	Other Considerations
Vancomycin	Mild, moderate Severe	IV recommended starting dose 40–80 80 40–55 (as continuous infusion over 24 h)	(IV) 4000 mg	(IV) 6–8	R	Adjust based on levels Renal toxicity
	Clostridioides difficile	PO 40	(PO) 2000 mg	(PO) 6		PO Recommend 500 mg/day but may use higher dose for complicated disease
Linezolid (IV/PO)	Moderate, severe Moderate, severe	< 12 y: 30 ≥ 12 y: 20	1200–1800 mg 1200 mg	8 12	R	Thrombocytopenia Neutropenia
Trimethoprim/ sulfamethoxazole (IV/PO)	Mild, moderate Severe	8–12 (TMP) 15–20 (TMP)	320 mg (TMP) 640 mg (TMP)	6–12	R	Photosensitivity Stevens-Johnson syndrome No max for PCP tx
Rifampin (IV/PO)	Moderate, severe	10–20	600 mg	12–24	H	Red discoloration of secretions
Doxycycline (IV/PO)	Moderate, severe	2–4	200 mg	12	No data	Teeth staining < 8 y Photosensitivity, oral separate from dairy
Tetracycline[d]	Mild, moderate	25–50	2000 mg	6	R	Teeth staining < 8 y Separate from dairy Photosensitivity
Tigecycline	Moderate, severe	2.4	100 mg	12	H	Teeth staining < 8 y Photosensitivity, pancreatitis
Nitrofurantoin	Cystitis only	5–7	400 mg	6		Urine discoloration
Nitazoxanide	Giardiasis *C difficile*	1–3 y: 200 mg/day 4–11 y: 400 mg/day ≥ 12 y: 1000 mg/day	200 mg 400 mg 1000 mg	12		3 days treatment
Albendazole	Tapeworms Hookworms, roundworms Raccoon roundworm	15 ≤ 2 y 200 mg/day × 1 >2 y 400 mg/day × 1 25–50	800 mg 200 mg 400 mg 800 mg	12 Once Once 12–24		Max 800 mg/day
Mebendazole	Hookworms, roundworms	200 mg/day	200 mg	12	H	3 days treatment May crush or chew Hepatotoxicity
Praziquantel	Fish tape worm, flea tapeworm Schistosomiasis Liver fluke	5–10 60 75	No max	Once 8 8		Swallow whole tablet, bitter taste

(*Continued*)

Table 39–4. Guidelines for use of common antimicrobial agents in children age 1 month or older. (*Continued*)

Agent	Treatment Category	Dose (mg/kg/day)	Maximum Daily Dose	Interval (h)	Adjustment	Other Considerations
Antivirals						
Acyclovir	IV treatment HSV VZV	1 mo–3 mo: 60 > 3 mo: 30 All ages: 30 (or) All ages: 1500 mg/m^2/day		8 8 8 8	R	Renal toxicity, neutropenia Dose on ideal body weight
	Oral treatment HSV, VZV	≥ 2 y: 80 ≥ 12 y: 80	3200 mg 4000 mg	6–8 5 × daily		
	HSV suppression	1–7 mo: 900 mg/m^2/day 1–11 y: 60 ≥ 12 y: 60	N/A 1200 mg 800 mg	8 8 12		
Valacyclovir	Treatment VZV HSV	> 3 mo: 60 mg/kg/day > 3 mo: 40–60 mg/kg/day	3000 mg 2000–3000 mg (max 1000 mg in single dose)	8 8–12	R	Renal toxicity is a rare complication, neutropenia
	HSV suppression	≥ 3 mo: 40–60 ≥ 12 y: 40–60	1000 mg 1000 mg	8–12 12–24		
Ganciclovir	CMV treatment CMV suppression	10 5	Not applicable	12 24	R	Renal toxicity, neutropenia
Valganciclovir	CMV treatment CMV suppression	30–36 15–18	1800 mg 900 mg	12 24	R	Renal toxicity, neutropenia
Oseltamivir	Influenza treatment Influenza prophylaxis	6 3	150 mg 75 mg	12 24	R	Neuropsychiatric events
Baloxavir	Influenza treatment	≥ 12 y and ≥ 40 kg ≥ 80 kg	40 mg once 80 mg once	One-time dose	R	Diarrhea
Peramivir	Influenza treatment	≤ 30 days: 6 ≤ 90 days: 8 ≤ 180 days: 10 ≤ 5 y: 12 > 5 y: 10	600 mg	24	R	Nausea, vomiting, diarrhea, neutropenia
Zanamivir	Influenza treatment Influenza prophylaxis	≥ 7 y ≥ 5 y	2 inhalations 2 inhalations	12 24		Bronchospasm

(Continued)

Table 39–4. Guidelines for use of common antimicrobial agents in children age 1 month or older. (*Continued*)

Agent	Treatment Category	Dose (mg/kg/day)	Maximum Daily Dose	Interval (h)	Adjustment	Other Considerations
Antifungals						
Nystatin	Oral candidiasis	Infants: 400,000–800,000 U/day Children: 2,000,000–4,000,000 U/day		6		
Fluconazole (IV/PO)	Candidiasis Oral Esophageal Systemic	3 3–12 6–12	200 mg 400 mg 800 mg	24	R	QT prolongation Hepatotoxicity
Voriconazole (IV/PO)	All infections Dose adjustments indicated based on drug levels and organism MICs	Pediatric: 18 Adult: 12 × 1 day then 8 Pediatric: 18 Adult: 400 mg/day	 PO 700 mg	12 12 12 12	H H	Dosed on IBW Monitor trough concentrations Higher and more frequent dosing has been used to obtain target troughs Oral is 40%–60% bioavailable in pediatrics
Posaconazole (IV/PO)	All infections Dose adjustments indicated based on drug levels and organism MICs	IV 7–10 DR tab 7–10 Suspension 12–20	300 mg DR tab 300 mg Suspension 800 mg	24 24 6–12	H	Monitor trough concentrations Higher and more frequent dosing has been used to obtain target troughs for IV and DR tab Suspension–absorption is dose limiting Hepatotoxicity Poor CNS penetration
Micafungin	Prophylaxis Treatment	1–2 < 6 mo: 8–10 6 mo–6 y: 4 6–16 y: 2–3	Prophylaxis 50 mg Treatment 150 mg	24	H	Larger doses have been used in obese patients Hepatotoxicity Poor CNS penetration and poor urinary concentrations
Caspofungin	All infections	Loading dose 70 mg/m²/day Maintenance dose 50 mg/m²/day	Loading dose 70 mg Maintenance dose 50 mg	24	H	Poor CNS penetration and poor urinary concentrations
Amphotericin	All infections	0.5–1	N/A	24	R	Renal and hepatic toxicity
Liposomal amphotericin (AmBisome)	All infections	3–7.5	N/A	24	R	Renal and hepatic toxicity Doses as high as 10 mg/kg/dose have been used for CNS infections
Liposomal amphotericin (Abelcet)	All infections	3–5	N/A	24	R	Renal and hepatic toxicity Pulmonary edema and respiratory distress have been reported with infusions

Table 39–5. Guidelines for use of selected antimicrobial agents in newborns.

	Route	Body Weight (kg)	Dosage (mg/kg/day)				Other Considerations
			< 7 days	Interval (h)	8–30 days	Interval (h)	
β-Lactams							
Penicillin G[a]	IV	≤ 2	100,000	12	150,000	8	May use as continuous infusion
		> 2	150,000	8	200,000	6	
Ampicillin	IV, IM	≤ 2	50–200	12	75–400	6–8	Short stability
		> 2	75–300	8	100–400	6	
Ampicillin/ sulbactam	IV, IM	≤ 2	100	12	100	12	Short stability
		> 2	150	8	150	8	
Piperacillin/ tazobactam	IV, IM	≤ 2	300	8	320	6	Renal toxicity
		> 2	320	6	320	6	
Nafcillin	IV	≤ 2	50	12	75	8	Renal toxicity, venous irritant, infuse through central line
		> 2	75	8	150	6	May use as continuous infusion
Cefotaxime	IV, IM	≤ 2	100	12	150	8	
		> 2	100	12	150	8	
Ceftazidime	IV, IM	≤ 2	100	12	150	8	
		> 2	150	8	150	8	
Metronidazole	IV	≤ 2	15	12	15	12	
		> 2	22.5	8	30	8	
Other							
Erythromycin	PO	≤ 2	20	12	30	8	Prolongs QTc
		> 2	20	12	30	8	
Azithromycin	IV, PO		10	24	10	24	Prolongs QTc
Clindamycin	IV, IM	≤ 2	15	8	15	8	
		> 2	21	8	30	8	
Vancomycin[b]	IV	≤ 2	15	18	30	12	Renal toxicity
		> 2	30	12	45	8	
Antifungals							
Nystatin	PO		400,000–800,000 U/day	6	400,000–800,000 U/day	6	
fluconazole	IV, PO		3–12	24–72	3–12	24–72	
Antivirals							
Acyclovir	IV	≤ 2	40	12	60	8	Renal toxicity, neutropenia
		> 2	60	8	60	8	
Ganciclovir	IV		10	12	10	12	Renal toxicity, neutropenia
Valganciclovir	PO	> 1.8	32	12	32	12	Renal toxicity, neutropenia

(Continued)

Table 39–5. Guidelines for use of selected antimicrobial agents in newborns. *(Continued)*

Aminoglycosides	Route	Gestational Age/Postnatal Age	Dose (mg/kg/dose)	Interval (h)	Other Considerations
Amikacin[c]	IV, IM	GA: < 30 wk			Renal toxicity
		≤ 14 days	15	48	Ototoxicity
		> 14 days	15	24	
		GA: 30–34 wk	15	24	
		GA: ≥ 35 wk			
		≤ 7 days	15	24	
		> 7 days	17.5	24	
Gentamicin[c]	IV, IM	GA: < 30 wk	3	24	Renal toxicity
		GA: 30–34 wk	2.5	18	Ototoxicity
		GA: ≥ 35 wk			
		≤ 7 days	4	24	
		> 7 days	2.5	12	
Tobramycin[c]	IV, IM	GA: < 30 wk			Renal toxicity
		≤ 14 days	5	48	Ototoxicity
		> 14 days	5	36	
		GA: 30–34 wk			
		≤ 10 days	4.5	36	
		> 10 days	5	36	
		GA: ≥ 35 wk			
		≤ 7 days	4	24	
		> 7 days	5	24	

[a]Penicillin dosages are in U/kg/day. See specific diseases for dosage.
[b]Vancomycin dosing is dependent on gestational age and serum creatinine with monitoring of levels.
[c]Aminoglycoside dosing in neonates requires careful attention to changes in renal function and changes in the volume of distribution. For infants smaller than 1200 g, smaller doses may be needed.

as a class, are generally poorly absorbed). More time above the MIC is achieved with higher, more frequent dosing; for example, amoxicillin dosed 90 mg/kg divided three times daily for *S pneumoniae* (with MIC of 1–2 mcg/mL) will achieve 7–8 hours of time over the MIC, while if divided only two times a day, it will exceed the MIC for only 5–6 hours.

The common β-lactamase inhibitors are themselves β-lactams in structure (including sulbactam, clavulanic acid, and tazobactam, though not avibactam or vaborbactam), but they do not typically have antibacterial activity. Instead, they act as "decoys," binding bacterial β-lactamases so that their companion drug is free to bind the target PBP. They are available in combination aminopenicillins in amoxicillin-clavulanic acid (oral) and ampicillin/sulbactam (IV), offering expanded activity to methicillin-susceptible *S aureus* (MSSA), *Moraxella catarrhalis*, *Klebsiella* spp., and β-lactamase–producing gram negatives (such as some *Haemophilus influenzae*, *E coli*) and anaerobes (such as *Bacteroides fragilis* and *Fusobacteria* spp.). This makes them useful for treating mixed infections, for example dog bites or tonsillar and parapharyngeal abscesses, orbital cellulitis, step-down therapy

for ruptured appendicitis, and refractory sinusitis and otitis media. Notably, they offer no advantage in the treatment of *S pneumoniae* or other streptococci, as these organisms do not produce β-lactamases. Piperacillin/tazobactam similarly expands coverage, including possible coverage for *P aeruginosa*. This drug has a niche in complex abdominal infections and hospital-associated pneumonia, but it should be used sparingly due to its broad spectrum and risk of acute kidney injury (AKI), particularly if used with vancomycin. While the penetration of the penicillins and aminopenicillins is good into most spaces, the penetration of the β-lactamase inhibitors is poorly understood. Combinations of β-lactam with β-lactamase inhibitor are notorious for causing diarrhea, particularly amoxicillin/clavulanic acid, and care with dosing clavulanic acid is advised.

Penicillinase-Resistant Penicillins

The penicillinase-resistant penicillins were developed as anti-MSSA antibiotics to combat the narrow-spectrum β-lactamase (penicillinase) produced by nearly all MSSA.

Table 39–6. Empiric therapy for common clinical syndromes.[a]

Syndrome	Common Organisms (less common to consider)	Examples of Potentially Useful Empiric Antimicrobials (for specific bacteria, see Table 39–3)	Comments (relevant chapters/US guideline)
Fever in the normal newborn	Group B *Streptococcus* *Escherichia coli* *Enterococcus* (UTI) Other viral (enterovirus, parechovirus, RSV, rhinovirus) [*Meningococcus*] [HSV] [*Streptococcus pneumoniae*] [*Listeria* spp.]	IV: Age < 1 mo: • Ampicillin and gentamicin Age > 1 mo: • Ceftriaxone and vancomycin	Substitute cefotaxime for gentamicin if initial Gram stains (CSF, urine) concerning for gram-negative infection Consider HSV coverage (acyclovir) if clinical concern [see Newborn Infant and Infections: Bacterial and Spirochetal chapters]
Sepsis in previously healthy child	Neisseria meningitidis *Staphylococcus aureus* (MRSA or MSSA) GAS *S pneumoniae* [*Haemophilus influenzae* B]	IV: • Ceftriaxone or cefotaxime, and vancomycin	Consider protein synthesis inhibitor if toxic shock (clindamycin) Consider adding cefazolin if *Staphylococcus aureus* likely (better outcomes for MSSA than vancomycin) In many geographic areas, resistance to clindamycin among both MSSA and MRSA isolates is high. [see Infections: Bacterial and Spirochetal chapter]
Fever in patient with central venous access, not neutropenic	*Staphylococcus*, coagulase negative *S aureus* (MRSA or MSSA) Enteric gram negatives (particularly if GI compromise) *Enterococcus* spp. (particularly if GI compromise) [*Pseudomonas aeruginosa*] [Yeast]	IV: • Ceftriaxone or cefotaxime, and vancomycin	If recent history of resistant organism, add specific coverage GI/short gut patients higher risk for gram negatives If neutropenic, substitute cefepime for ceftriaxone/cefotaxime If high risk or not responding to antibiotics, consider coverage for yeast (fluconazole, micafungin) [see Infections: Bacterial and Spirochetal chapter]
Sepsis in a neutropenic child	*Pseudomonas aeruginosa* *Streptococcus viridans* *Staphylococcus*, coagulase negative *S aureus* (MRSA or MSSA) Enteric gram negatives [*Enterococcus* spp.] [Yeast]	IV: • Cefepime and vancomycin	If recent history of resistant organism, add specific coverage If high risk or not responding to antibiotics, consider coverage for yeast (micafungin) Consider adding ampicillin for *Enterococcus gallinarum* and *Enterococcus casseliflavus* or daptomycin for VRE depending on local epidemiology [see Infections: Bacterial and Spirochetal chapter]
Urinary tract infection/ pyelonephritis	*E coli* *Klebsiella* spp. *Enterococcus* spp. Other enteric gram negatives	Oral: • Cephalexin • Trimethoprim/ sulfamethoxaxole IV: • Ceftriaxone	Substitute amoxicillin/ampicillin for enterococcus [see Kidney and Urinary Tract and Infections: Bacterial and Spirochetal chapter, and US national guideline]

(Continued)

Table 39–6. Empiric therapy for common clinical syndromes.[a] (*Continued*)

Syndrome	Common Organisms (less common to consider)	Examples of Potentially Useful Empiric Antimicrobials (for specific bacteria, see Table 39–3)	Comments (relevant chapters/US guideline)
Acute suppurative otitis media	Virus *S pneumoniae* *H influenzae* *M catarrhalis*	Oral: • Amoxicillin (high dose) • Amoxicillin/clavulanic acid (if failed amoxicillin)	Antimicrobial therapy should be targeted toward *S pneumoniae*. As a large proportion of OM is viral, not all cases require treatment [see Ear, Nose and Throat and Infections: Bacterial and Spirochetal chapters, US national guideline]
Pharyngitis due to GAS	GAS	Oral: • Penicillin • Amoxicillin	Though other oral agents are active, they are broader than necessary and lead to resistance [see Ear, Nose and Throat and Infections: Bacterial and Spirochetal chapters, US national guideline]
Community-acquired pneumonia	Viruses *S pneumoniae* Mycoplasma [*S aureus* (MRSA or MSSA)] [GAS] [*H influenzae* (B or nontypable)] [*Moraxella catarrhalis*]	Oral: • Amoxicillin (high dose) IV: • Ampicillin	Antimicrobial therapy should be targeted toward *S pneumoniae*. For sicker inpatients, consider *S aureus* coverage. Coverage of penicillin-resistant gram negatives (*H influenzae, M catarrhalis*) uncommonly needed. Though mycoplasma is common, it is not clear that directed therapy improves outcomes; if coverage desired, azithromycin is drug of choice, but it does not provide *S pneumoniae* coverage. In many geographic areas, resistance to clindamycin among both MSSA and MRSA isolates is high. [see Respiratory Tract and Mediastinum, and Infections: Bacterial and Spirochetal chapters, US national guideline]
Skin and soft tissue infection	*S aureus* (MRSA or MSSA) GAS	Oral: • Cephalexin • Clindamycin • Trimethoprim/sulfamethoxazole	May require drainage Consider other organisms if history of bite or trauma In many geographic areas, resistance to clindamycin among both MSSA and MRSA isolates is high. In many geographic areas, resistance to trimethoprim/sulfamethoxazole among GAS isolates is high. [see Skin and Infections: Bacterial and Spirochetal chapters]
Acute suppurative adenitis	*S aureus* (MRSA or MSSA) GAS	Oral: • Cephalexin • Clindamycin IV: • Cefazolin • Clindamycin	May require drainage In many geographic areas, resistance to clindamycin among both MSSA and MRSA isolates is high. [see Ear, Nose and Throat and Infections: Bacterial and Spirochetal chapters]
Acute bacterial sinusitis	*S pneumoniae* *H influenzae* (B or nontypable) *M catarrhalis* *S aureus* (MRSA or MSSA) Anaerobic bacteria	Oral: • Amoxicillin (high dose) • Amoxicillin/clavulanic acid (high dose)	Therapy should be directed against *S pneumoniae* (amoxicillin); in severe sinusitis, expansion to other organisms reasonable. [see Ear, Nose and Throat and Infections: Bacterial and Spirochetal chapters, US national guideline]

(*Continued*)

Table 39–6. Empiric therapy for common clinical syndromes.[a] (*Continued*)

Syndrome	Common Organisms (less common to consider)	Examples of Potentially Useful Empiric Antimicrobials (for specific bacteria, see Table 39–3)	Comments (relevant chapters/US guideline)
Orbital cellulitis (sinusitis associated)	S pneumoniae S anginosus/viridans H influenzae (B or nontypable) M catarrhalis S aureus (MRSA or MSSA) Anaerobic bacteria	IV: • Ampicillin/sulbactam • Ceftriaxone + clindamycin	Consider addition of MRSA coverage (vancomycin) May require drainage In many geographic areas, resistance to clindamycin among both MSSA and MRSA isolates is high. [see Ear, Nose and Throat and Infections: Bacterial and Spirochetal chapters, US national guideline]
Acute suppurative mastoiditis	S pneumoniae GAS S aureus (MRSA or MSSA) [H influenzae (B or nontypable)] [Pseudomonas spp.]	IV: • Ampicillin/sulbactam • Ceftriaxone + clindamycin	May require drainage. In many geographic areas, resistance to clindamycin among both MSSA and MRSA isolates is high. [see Ear, Nose and Throat and Infections: Bacterial and Spirochetal chapters]
Brain abscess (sinusitis associated)	S anginosus/viridans S pneumoniae H influenzae (B or nontypable) M catarrhalis S aureus (MRSA or MSSA) Anaerobic bacteria	IV: • Vancomycin, ceftriaxone and metronidazole	May require drainage [see Ear, Nose and Throat and Infections: Bacterial and Spirochetal chapters]
Dental abscess	Polymicrobial mouth flora	Oral: • Penicillin • Clindamycin • Amoxicillin/clavulanic acid IV: • Ampicillin/sulbactam • Clindamycin	May require tooth extraction [see Oral Medicine and Dentistry and Infections: Bacterial and Spirochetal chapters]
Peritonsillar or parapharyngeal abscess	GAS S aureus (MRSA or MSSA) S anginosus/viridans Other oral flora	IV: • Ampicillin/sulbactam • Ceftriaxone +clindamycin	May require drainage In many geographic areas, resistance to clindamycin among both MSSA and MRSA isolates is high. [see Ear, Nose and Throat and Infections: Bacterial and Spirochetal chapters]
Infected dog and cat bites	Pasteurella spp. S aureus (MRSA or MSSA) GAS [Capnocytophaga canimorsus]	Oral: • Amoxicillin/clavulanic acid (high dose) • Clindamycin + FLQ IV: • Ampicillin/sulbactam • Ceftriaxone + clindamycin	Consider rabies and tetanus prophylaxis May require suture removal and/or drainage In many geographic areas, resistance to clindamycin among both MSSA and MRSA isolates is high. [see Emergencies and Injuries and Infections: Bacterial and Spirochetal chapters, US national guideline]

(Continued)

Table 39–6. Empiric therapy for common clinical syndromes.[a] *(Continued)*

Syndrome	Common Organisms (less common to consider)	Examples of Potentially Useful Empiric Antimicrobials (for specific bacteria, see Table 39–3)	Comments (relevant chapters/US guideline)
Acute hematogenous musculoskeletal infection	*S aureus* (MRSA or MSSA) *Kingella kingae* GAS [*S pneumoniae*] [*N meningitides*] [*Salmonella* spp.]	Oral: • Cephalexin • Clindamycin IV: • Cefazolin • Clindamycin • Vancomycin	In many geographic areas, resistance to clindamycin among both MSSA and MRSA is high. [see Orthopedic and Infections: Bacterial and Spirochetal chapters]
Acute endocarditis	*S viridans* *S aureus* (MRSA or MSSA) HACEK organisms	IV: • Ceftriaxone + vancomycin + gentamicin	Assure multiple blood cultures prior to antibiotics. Alter empiric coverage based on risk factors.
Acute traveler's diarrhea	*E coli* *Campylobacter* *Salmonella* spp. *Shigella* spp. Others	Oral: • Azithromycin • Rifaximin • Ciprofloxacin • Cefixime	Choice of agent tailored to resistance in area of travel (see CDC travel website)
Acute appendicitis	*E coli* *Bacteroides fragilis*	IV: • Ceftriaxone + metronidazole	Both ceftriaxone and metronidazole can be dosed once daily for appendicitis
Liver abscess	*S anginosus* *E coli* *Bacteroides fragilis* Other GI flora [*Entamoeba histolytica*]	IV: • Ceftriaxone + metronidazole	May require drainage Consider *E. histolytica* if drainage with few PMNs, "anchovy paste" appearance, epidemiology supports [see Infections: Bacterial and Spirochetal chapters]

CDC, Centers for Disease Control and Prevention; CSF, cerebrospinal fluid; FLQ, fluoroquinolone; GAS, group A *Streptococcus*; GI, gastrointestinal; HSV, herpes simplex virus; IV, intravenous; MRSA, methicillin-resistant *S aureus*; MSSA, methicillin-susceptible *S aureus*; PMN, polymorphonuclear neutrophils; RSV, respiratory syncytial virus; UTI, urinary tract infection.
Organisms [in brackets] are less likely, but need consideration in empiric choice of antimicrobials
[a]Empiric therapy should always be tailored to specific risk factors and clinical clues on a case by case basis. Antimicrobial choices populated on right of table do not necessarily cover all microbes listed to left, rather they are meant as one potential option for empiric coverage. Local susceptibility patterns should always be considered in choice of empiric therapy. Antimicrobials should be adjusted to organism and susceptibility once known.

These drugs, which include nafcillin, oxacillin, methicillin, and dicloxacillin, offer structural protection to the β-lactam ring so that it is unavailable to penicillinases. They are associated with renal and hepatic toxicity, which does limit their use. Drug fever, rashes, and neutropenia are also common. Oxacillin and methicillin are renally excreted, whereas nafcillin is excreted through the biliary tract. Nafcillin is a venous irritant, making it difficult to maintain peripheral intravenous access; it also causes damage with extravasation, so it is best used with large or central lines. Because of their expense and side-effect profiles, these drugs have largely been supplanted by cefazolin (IV) and cephalexin (oral), but the IV forms retain a niche in the treatment of endocarditis and central nervous system (CNS) infections caused by MSSA. Dicloxacillin is used as step-down oral therapy when appropriate and for outpatient treatment of skin/soft tissue infections (SSTI) in adults.

β-LACTAM: CEPHALOSPORINS

Cephalosporins are often categorized in "generations," which is not a chemical relationship, but rather represents similarity in antimicrobial spectra based on binding to various PBPs. All the resistance mechanisms mentioned above

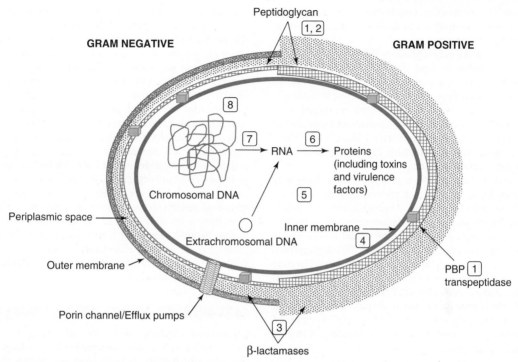

GRAM NEGATIVE

GRAM POSITIVE

Peptidoglycan

Chromosomal DNA

RNA → Proteins (including toxins and virulence factors)

Periplasmic space

Inner membrane

Extrachromosomal DNA

Outer membrane

PBP 1 transpeptidase

Porin channel/Efflux pumps

β-lactamases

▲ **Figure 39–2.** Simple schematic of bacterial cell with drug targets (numbers) and resistance mechanisms.

for β-lactams also apply to cephalosporins. Gram-negative organisms have an ever-expanding variety of β-lactamases, the most problematic of which in routine practice are the inducible and extended spectrum β-lactamases (IBLs and ESBLs). No cephalosporins approved for use in the United States have activity against enterococci.

The first-generation cephalosporins include cefazolin (IV) and cephalexin (oral), which are mainly used to treat infections with MSSA or as empiric therapy for UTIs. They are highly effective treatments for SSTI, as they also have activity against group A streptococci, and in initial and oral step-down treatment of musculoskeletal infections in children. Because of its high concentration in urine, cephalexin is considered first line for UTIs and often achieves adequate killing in organisms deemed "resistant." In the laboratory, cephalothin is commonly used as a surrogate for cefazolin/cephalexin susceptibility.

The second-generation cephalosporins include cefuroxime (IV) and cefprozil and cefuroxime (oral). These have somewhat reduced, but acceptable, activity against gram-positive cocci, and greater activity against some gram-negative rods compared with first-generation cephalosporins, but not as much as the third-generation cephalosporins described below. They are active against *H influenzae* and *M catarrhalis*, including strains that produce β-lactamases

capable of inactivating ampicillin. Cefoxitin and cefotetan, which are considered second generation, offer activity against anaerobes, making them potentially useful in the treatment of nonperforated appendicitis, pediatric cholangitis, and pelvic inflammatory disease; however, increasing resistance and short half-life (cefoxitin) are limitations.

Third-generation cephalosporins have substantially less activity against MSSA compared to first-generation cephalosporins, though notably increased activity against *S pneumoniae*. They also have increased activity against aerobic gram-negative bacteria that harbor narrow-spectrum β-lactamases. The most common intravenous forms are ceftriaxone and cefotaxime; due to production issues, availability of cefotaxime is currently limited. Ceftazidime provides similar coverage (with decreased *S pneumoniae* coverage compared to ceftriaxone) but provides some activity against *P aeruginosa*, though resistance may be induced quickly. These IV formulations have good CNS penetration. Cefpodoxime, cefixime, and cefdinir are oral options but are limited by low serum levels.

Cefepime is considered a fourth-generation cephalosporin. It retains considerable activity against MSSA while also being active against *P aeruginosa* and some other IBL producers, such as *Enterobacter* spp. It is a zwitterion and as such efficiently penetrates the gram-negative outer cell membrane. Despite its efficacy against IBL-producing organisms, cefepime is hydrolyzed by ESBLs so generally confers no advantage in that situation.

Ceftaroline is the only cephalosporin able to treat MRSA based on its ability to bind the PBP (PBP2a) in MRSA (encoded by *mecA*); it does not, however, have activity against *P aeruginosa*. Ceftaroline was recently approved in children.

There are now two cephalosporins combined with β-lactamase inhibitors, ceftazidime/avibactam (approved in pediatrics) and ceftolozane/tazobactam. These have activity against *P aeruginosa*, and variable coverage against many other highly resistant gram negatives.

The oral cephalosporins, except cephalexin, have very poor serum levels and may not achieve adequate time over the MIC for sufficient killing. In general, they are poorly absorbed, highly protein bound, often are given at ineffectively long intervals. In general, they should not be widely used. For organisms susceptible to amoxicillin, oral cephalosporins are pharmacokinetically inferior and should be used only to patients with penicillin allergy. For example, high-dose amoxicillin is more effective than cefdinir for infections where *S pneumoniae* is the most likely pathogen. In general, longer time above the MIC is achieved in the middle ear and urine compared to other locations for β-lactams, improving likelihood of cure in those locations.

β-LACTAM: MONOBACTAMS

Aztreonam is the only monobactam approved for use in the United States. Aztreonam is active against aerobic gram-negative rods, including *P aeruginosa*. Aztreonam has activity against *H influenzae* and *M catarrhalis*, including those that are β-lactamase producers. The most common uses of aztreonam are as an aerosol for therapy of *P aeruginosa* infection in patients with cystic fibrosis, and as an alternative therapy for severely β-lactam allergic patients, as there is little cross-reactivity between aztreonam and other β-lactams, except ceftazidime as they share a common side chain.

β-LACTAM: CARBAPENEMS

Meropenem, ertapenem, doripenem, and imipenem comprise the carbapenems, which are very broad antimicrobials effective against gram-negative aerobes, most anaerobes, and many gram-positive organisms. They have some activity against MSSA (but not MRSA), *S pneumoniae*, *E faecalis* (but not *E faecium*), and various other gram positives. Except for ertapenem, they have good activity against *P aeruginosa* and retain activity against many multidrug-resistant gram negatives, including and those with IBLs and ESBLs. Imipenem is sold in combination with cilastatin, which inhibits the metabolism of imipenem in the kidneys resulting in high serum and urine levels. An increased frequency of

seizures is encountered when CNS infections are treated with carbapenems, particularly imipenem; carbapenems also decrease valproic acid levels. Because carbapenems are active against so many species of bacteria, there is a strong temptation to use them as single-drug empiric therapy. However, overuse is linked to the development of multidrug resistance. Hospitals that use carbapenems heavily encounter resistance in many different species of gram-negative rods. This resistance can develop in a single patient within days due to bacteria developing a porin/efflux mechanism. Carbapenem use should therefore be reserved only for patients with confirmed (or at high risk for) infection due to highly resistant organisms. Bacteria with β-lactamases capable of attacking the carbapenems now exist and are spreading worldwide; organisms harboring these plasmids often have many resistance mechanisms and are susceptible to few (if any) remaining treatment options. To address some of these resistance mechanisms, meropenem is now available with a β-lactamase inhibitor, vaborbactam, though this is not yet approved in children.

GLYCOPEPTIDE AGENTS (STEP 2, FIGURE 39–2)

Glycopeptides include vancomycin, telavancin, oritavancin, and dalbavancin. They are characterized by their large molecular size, which prevents them from penetrating the outer membrane of gram-negative organisms. Like the β-lactams, they also are active on the cell wall, inhibiting peptidoglycan synthesis by preventing cross-linking at the terminal amino acids (D-alanine). It is debated if their efficacy is most related to time over the MIC or AUC over MIC. Bacteria protect themselves mainly through (1) changing the terminal amino acid to D-lactate so that vancomycin cannot bind or (2) thickening the cell wall (vancomycin-intermediate and resistant *S aureus*) such that the glycopeptide cannot bind a sufficient number of targets to prevent cross-linking. They have notable nephrotoxicity and are a common cause of drug-related AKI. Red-man syndrome (flushing and itching with infusion), which is not an allergic response, can be mitigated with slower infusions (over 2 hours) and premedication with diphenhydramine or hydrocortisone. All the glycopeptides have similar spectra of activity, including MRSA, coagulase negative staphylococci, ampicillin-resistant enterococci, and resistant *S pneumoniae*. Oral vancomycin is not systemically absorbed but effectively kills *C difficile* in the GI tract. IDSA guidelines recommend oral vancomycin preferentially over metronidazole for severe or recurrent *C difficile* enteritis in pediatrics and for all cases in adults. The glycopeptides differ in dosing strategies, with telavancin dosed once daily, and both dalbavancin and oritavancin dosed once weekly. These three drugs are not Food and Drug Administration (FDA) approved for use in children.

The empiric use of vancomycin has increased tremendously over the past decade. Thus, vancomycin-resistant enterococci

(VRE) are now problematic, particularly in inpatient units, intensive care units, and oncology wards. Vancomycin-intermediate and vancomycin-resistant *S aureus* exist, which is of concern because of the inherent virulence of many *S aureus* strains. Vancomycin use should be monitored carefully in hospitals and intensive care units. Vancomycin should not be used empirically when an infection is mild or when other antimicrobial agents are likely to be effective, and it should be stopped promptly if infection is caused by organisms susceptible to other antimicrobials. Attention to obtaining cultures prior to vancomycin initiation is required, as susceptibility to oral alternatives is not predictable.

Efficacy of vancomycin requires sufficient drug exposure (typically approximated by achieving trough levels of 15–20 mcg/mL for CNS infections, endocarditis, and bone infections, 10–15 mcg/mL for other infections); this can be difficult to achieve in some pediatric ages. Thus monitoring and dose adjustment are necessary. Continuous infusion can be used if sufficient levels are not achievable with every 6 hour dosing. The trough concentrations are usually drawn before the fourth dose but should be drawn sooner if the patient is at risk of AKI. A high trough can cause renal injury and will be observed when renal function is impaired. Serum creatinine should be checked in all patients administered vancomycin to monitor for AKI. Some experts argue that vancomycin should be dosed based on AUC (goal 400–600 mg*h/L), though in pediatrics this requires multiple serum drug levels and some dosing expertise, as trough levels may not be a good predictor of AUC. For patients receiving antimicrobials for weeks to months, weekly clinical and laboratory assessment, including drug levels, creatinine, and complete blood count will facilitate detection of toxicity.

DAPTOMYCIN (STEP 4, FIGURE 39–2)

Daptomycin is unique in being a lipopeptide that inserts into the lipid-rich cell inner membrane of gram-positive bacteria. This results in depolarization and cell death. It is unclear if efficacy correlates with the time that intracellular levels exceed the MIC or whether AUC over MIC is most important. Microbes protect themselves by changing the charge of their cell membranes, such that daptomycin cannot penetrate the inner membrane. Since daptomycin cannot penetrate the gram-negative outer cell membrane (envelope), it is only active against gram-positive organisms and has a clinical niche against MRSA and vancomycin-resistant *E faecium*. Daptomycin may insert itself into lipid layers of human cells, particularly muscle, causing creatinine phosphokinase (CPK) elevation. Rhabdomyolysis has been reported and monitoring of CPK in children is recommended. Because daptomycin is a lipid-like molecule, pulmonary surfactant envelops the drug rendering it inactive, so it is typically not used for lung infections.

TRIMETHOPRIM/SULFAMETHOXAZOLE (STEP 5, FIGURE 39–2)

Sulfonamides—the oldest class of antimicrobials—are usually used in a fixed combination with trimethoprim (TMP-SMX) to inhibit two steps in the folate synthesis pathway (which then inhibits DNA biosynthesis, step 8, Figure 39–2) for greater efficacy. AUC over MIC correlates with efficacy. Resistance is usually related to alterations in the binding targets or decreased drug concentrations due to efflux or decreased entry. TMP-SMX is particularly associated with drug hypersensitivity reactions and, more rarely, severe skin reactions such as Stevens-Johnson syndrome. It also may cause hematologic abnormalities that can be severe. It should not be used in patients with G6PD deficiency. TMP-SMX is most often used clinically to treat MRSA SSTIs, UTIs, and susceptible strains of *Haemophilus* spp., *Shigella* spp., or *Salmonella* spp. TMP-SMX is a mainstay in prophylaxis and treatment of *Pneumocystis jirovecii* infection, and in treatment of *Nocardia* spp., brucellosis, and *Stenotrophomonas maltophilia*. As an intravenous formulation, it requires large volume infusion over 2 hours every 6–12 hours, so is rarely given via this route (especially given its high oral bioavailability). Pathogens with significant resistance include group A *Streptococcus*, *S pneumoniae*, and various gram negatives.

METRONIDAZOLE (STEP 6, FIGURE 39–2)

Metronidazole is a prodrug that is only converted to its active form by anaerobic and amoebic and other protozoal organisms. It is unclear if these active intermediates bind DNA, RNA, or essential proteins that result in cell death. Effective killing is related to the AUC over MIC. It has a PAE and a long half-life so could be dosed less frequently than the current recommendation of three to four times daily. In pediatric appendicitis, it often is dosed once daily. Resistance mechanisms are not well investigated, but they likely relate to lack of conversion to active drug. It is most active against gram-negative and gram-positive anaerobic rods, such as *Bacteroides*, *Fusobacterium*, *Clostridium*, *Prevotella*, and *Porphyromonas*. Gram-positive anaerobic cocci such as *Peptococcus* and *Peptostreptococcus* are often more susceptible to penicillin or to clindamycin. Metronidazole is the drug of choice for bacterial vaginosis and among the recommended options for *C difficile* enterocolitis. It is active against many parasites, including *Giardia lamblia* and *Entamoeba histolytica*. Metronidazole is highly bioavailable and has excellent tissue penetration, including to the CNS.

MACROLIDES (STEP 6, FIGURE 39–2)

The macrolide antimicrobials in common use include erythromycin, azithromycin, and clarithromycin. They inhibit protein synthesis by blocking RNA translation and assembly of the 50S ribosomal subunit. Efficacy is related to AUC over MIC. Microbes protect themselves by altering the macrolide binding site with methylation or through efflux of the drug. Because of ease of dosing and tolerability, azithromycin is the most commonly prescribed macrolide worldwide, and is one of the most commonly prescribed antimicrobials in the United States. This likely indicates overuse, as macrolides are rarely considered first-line agents in national treatment guidelines, and high rates of resistance have developed among S pneumoniae, for which it is commonly prescribed. Gastrointestinal side effects are common with the macrolides, particularly with erythromycin, which is sometimes used as a promotility agent. Exposure to macrolides early in life is associated with infantile hypertrophic pyloric stenosis, though azithromycin is thought to pose a lower risk than erythromycin. They all prolong the QTc interval, a consideration in at-risk patients.

Azithromycin has a large volume of distribution and a long half-life; after a 5-day treatment course, intracellular drug is present for approximately 10 days. Azithromycin is used to treat Campylobacter, Shigella, and Salmonella infections, including typhoid fever resistant to ampicillin and TMP-SMX, and is thus used for presumed bacterial traveler's diarrhea. All macrolides are active against many bacteria that are intrinsically resistant to cell wall–active antimicrobials, and are the drugs of choice for Bordetella pertussis, Legionella pneumophila, Chlamydophila pneumoniae, Mycoplasma pneumoniae, and Chlamydia trachomatis infections. Azithromycin and clarithromycin also have activity against some mycobacteria. Resistance among other common pathogens, such as S pneumoniae, group A Streptococcus, S aureus, and Haemophilus spp., limits efficacy of azithromycin efficacy for otitis media, sinusitis, and community-acquired pneumonia (except for Mycoplasma).

LINCOSAMIDES (STEP 6, FIGURE 39–2)

Clindamycin targets protein synthesis through inhibiting peptidyl transferase at the 50S ribosomal subunit. Its efficacy is related to the AUC over MIC. Resistance, which is mediated by methylation of the binding site, may be constitutive or may be detected only after induction with erythromycin (using a D-test). Efflux of drug is another mechanism of resistance. Clindamycin is highly bioavailable and penetrates most body tissues well except for spinal fluid and urine; it should not be used for infection in those spaces. Though clindamycin is not used to treat CNS bacterial infections, it does achieve sufficient CNS levels to treat CNS toxoplasmosis (the parasiticidal concentration is 6 ng/mL), though it is not considered a first-line agent. It is active against many anaerobes and gram-positive aerobic organisms, including S pneumoniae, S pyogenes, and MRSA, though resistance is becoming more prevalent. It is not active against enterococci. Because of its unique spectrum of activity, it is often used to treat mixed aerobic gram-positive and anaerobic infections, such as sinusitis, dental, oral, and neck abscesses; pelvic inflammatory disease; and deep infections from pressure ulcers. Because it inhibits protein synthesis (and thus toxin production), it is often used as an adjunct to treat serious toxin-mediated diseases such as toxic shock syndrome. It also is considered to be more active than β-lactams against nonreplicating bacteria that may be present in undrained abscesses. Clindamycin is associated with C difficile–related pseudomembranous colitis in adults, but this relationship is uncommon in children, although diarrhea is a frequent side effect. Though clindamycin is an old drug, it is often more expensive than alternatives and has palatability issues.

OXAZOLIDINONES (STEP 6, FIGURE 39–2)

Linezolid is the first oxazolidinone in use. It targets the 50S-ribosomal RNA subunit to prevent initiation of protein synthesis. Cross-resistance with other ribosomally active antimicrobials is uncommon, though a unique mutation of the binding site has made resistance increasingly common. Efficacy is related to AUC over MIC. Linezolid has broad gram-positive activity, including some anaerobes, but it is typically reserved for particular drug-resistant organisms (eg, VRE) when first-line agents are contraindicated (eg, for MRSA when vancomycin is avoided due to significant renal insufficiency) or when oral therapy is desired and no other oral options are available. It has very limited gram-negative activity. Linezolid comes in an IV formulation, but it is highly bioavailable and is usually used orally. Linezolid is safe and well tolerated in children, but neutropenia and thrombocytopenia are common and frequently dose limiting. A complete blood count should be monitored in patients at increased risk for these problems and in patients receiving therapy for 2 weeks or longer. Linezolid is an inhibitor of monoamine oxidase (MAO) and should not be used in patients taking MAO inhibitors.

TETRACYCLINES (STEP 6, FIGURE 39–2)

Tetracyclines, including doxycycline, minocycline, tigecycline, and eravacycline, interact with transfer RNA (tRNA) at the 30S ribosomal subunit to prevent protein synthesis. Resistance occurs when the microbe develops proteins that protect the tRNA target or when it encodes efflux pumps to decrease intracellular drug concentrations. Efficacy is related to AUC over MIC. Tetracyclines are broadly effective but are most commonly used against B pertussis, many species of Rickettsia, Chlamydia/Chlamydophila, and Mycoplasma. Doxycycline can also be used for eradication of C trachomatis in pelvic inflammatory disease and nongonococcal urethritis. Among tetracyclines, doxycycline is often preferred because it is better tolerated than tetracycline, its twice-daily administration is convenient, and it can be taken with food.

Notable side effects of the tetracyclines are staining of permanent teeth, so long courses (longer than 21 days for doxycycline) are generally not given to children younger than 8 years if an alternative exists. However, a single course of a tetracycline does not pose a significant risk of tooth staining. Increased photosensitivity is a notable side effect, and minocycline (commonly used for acne) has a particular association with DIHS.

Doxycycline is used for therapy of Q fever and rickettsial infections (Rocky Mountain spotted fever, ehrlichiosis, anaplasmosis, rickettsialpox) and endemic and murine typhus. It is also first line for treatment of *Borrelia* spp. (Lyme disease, relapsing fever). Doxycycline can also be used as an alternative to macrolides for *M pneumoniae* and *C pneumoniae* infections and for treatment of psittacosis, brucellosis, and *P multocida* infection. Doxycycline also retains good activity against MRSA.

Tigecycline is a glycylcycline (an analogue of tetracycline) that is active against many gram-negative aerobes, anaerobes, and gram-positive cocci including MRSA and enterococci. Tigecycline is not active against *P aeruginosa* but is useful against VRE and resistant gram negatives other than *P aeruginosa*. It is inferior to other agents for bacteremia if the organism is susceptible to alternative antibiotics. It is approved for children over 8 years.

AMINOGLYCOSIDES (STEP 6, FIGURE 39–2)

The aminoglycosides include gentamicin, tobramycin, amikacin, and streptomycin. They bind to ribosomal RNA in the 30S subunit to inhibit protein synthesis. A high peak above MIC is required for efficacy. Because microbes will not replicate for a long time after aminoglycoside exposure (postantibiotic effect), aminoglycosides can be dosed once daily. However, once-daily dosing is still controversial in pediatrics due to faster clearance in children. Variation in dosing strategies exists due to lack of consensus. While efficacy is associated with an adequate peak to MIC ratio (with a goal peak of at least eight times the MIC to achieve a longer PAE), toxicity is associated with a high trough. Renal toxicity is most common, followed by ototoxicity. Bacteria gain resistance either through bacterial enzymatic modification of the aminoglycoside to limit binding to its target or through changes in drug entry due to alterations in porin channels. Aminoglycosides are active against gram-negative bacteria. When used together with β-lactams and vancomycin, which damage cell walls against some gram positives, there is a synergistic effect such that aminoglycosides enter bacteria more efficiently. Synergy is described for group B streptococci, enterococci, staphylococci, and *Listeria monocytogenes* at a low aminoglycoside dose. All aminoglycosides are active against pseudomonas, but especially tobramycin. Amikacin is less susceptible to microbial modification, so organisms resistant to other aminoglycosides may remain susceptible to amikacin. Addition of an aminoglycoside to another active agent, such as described for a β-lactam for gram-negative infections, such as for *P aeruginosa*, is generally considered to add more toxicity than benefit. However, this remains appropriate for empiric therapy in patients at risk for resistant gram-negative bacteria while awaiting speciation and susceptibilities. Tobramycin and amikacin have inhaled formulations, and though relative penetration to alveoli is not clear, they are used in patients with cystic fibrosis. Streptomycin is still used for tuberculosis in endemic areas of the world, but ototoxicity otherwise limits its usefulness. As a group, the aminoglycosides do not penetrate CSF well; thus, treatment with a third-generation cephalosporin is preferred for CNS infection. Aminoglycosides also are not active in acidic environments, rendering them less active in abscesses and bone.

Because of their renal and ototoxicity, creatinine measurement and therapeutic drug level monitoring is necessary. Drug levels are usually checked between the third and fourth doses, but sooner in children at high risk for renal impairment. Efficacy of gentamicin and tobramycin are correlated with a peak of 8–12 mcg/mL for dosing every 8 hours or 20–30 mcg/mL for once daily dosing. The goal is for trough levels less than 2 mcg/mL, which correlates with less toxicity. For amikacin, desired peak for every 8 hour dosing is 20–35 mcg/mL and a trough less than 10 mcg/mL. In children expected to receive long-term therapy, drug levels and creatinine should be checked weekly and hearing screening should be considered, especially for those with elevated trough levels.

RIFAMYCINS (STEP 7, FIGURE 39–2)

Rifamycins include rifampin, rifabutin, rifaximin, and rifamycin B. They are the only antimicrobial inhibitors of RNA polymerase. They are active against a wide variety of organisms, including many mycobacteria. Resistance develops quickly (usually via a mutation in RNA polymerase) so they should not be used as monotherapy, except in select circumstances. Rifampin monotherapy is used as prophylaxis against disease in those exposed to *H influenzae* or *N meningitides*, as well as to treat latent *M tuberculosis* infection. It is also used as combination therapy to penetrate bacterial biofilms for patients with prosthetic material in place. Rifampin and rifabutin are used in combination therapy for active tuberculosis; rifabutin is often preferred in patients co-infected with human immunodeficiency virus (HIV) as rifampin decreases levels of some HIV medications. Most rifamycins, rifampin in particular, induce P450 enzymes, lowering the concentrations of many other drugs, including birth control, opiates, immune-suppressive agents, HIV medications, some chemotherapy agents, and some anesthetics, and thus their possible benefit must be weighed against the dangers of lowering levels of these other drugs.

These drugs penetrate many tissue spaces and will turn body fluids such as tears, urine, and feces orange. This is an important and troubling side effect to warn patients about, and those with contact lenses should be counseled to wear glasses while on therapy to prevent staining. Oral preparations of rifamycins are highly bioavailable. Rifaximin, because it is nonabsorbable, avoids drug interactions or side effects and is used for the treatment and prevention of traveler's diarrhea in people older than 12 years, though this will predispose to the acquisition of drug-resistant organisms (as do all antibiotics used for these indications).

FLUOROQUINOLONES (STEP 8, FIGURE 39–2)

Fluoroquinolones include norfloxacin, ofloxacin, ciprofloxacin, levofloxacin, moxifloxacin, and gatifloxacin drops. They target bacterial topoisomerases, inhibiting DNA replication and repair. Efficacy is based on the AUC over MIC. Levofloxacin and ciprofloxacin are active against *P aeruginosa*, with moxifloxacin having reduced systemic activity against *P aeruginosa*. In addition to gram-negative activity, levofloxacin has activity against some strains of MRSA, *S pneumoniae*, and *Enterococcus faecalis* (not *E faecium*). They are also active against many atypical pathogens, such as *Mycoplasma*, *Chlamydophila*, and *Legionella*. Ofloxacin and levofloxacin are used for treatment of some cases of *M tuberculosis* and some atypical mycobacterial infections. Due to activity against *N meningitides* and *Yersinia pestis*, ciprofloxacin is an option for prophylaxis of exposed persons. Fluoroquinolones are often active against *N gonorrhea* (though increasing resistance described) and *C trachomatis*. They often are active against the common causes of traveler's diarrhea, though increasing resistance has removed them as first-line agents (in favor of azithromycin) in many geographic areas. Bacteria become resistant by mutating the targeted topoisomerases to avoid binding or by efflux of drug. This class of drugs is highly associated with bacterial resistance and secondary *C difficile* infection. When these organisms acquire mutations that encode resistance, they often are accompanied by genes encoding resistance to other classes of antimicrobials. They also select for hypervirulent, hyperspreading strains of *C difficile* that endanger not only the patient receiving the fluoroquinolone but other patients on the same unit to whom the strain may spread. When an outbreak of *C difficile* infection is present in a hospital setting, stopping use of these drugs is an appropriate intervention. They are also associated with tendon rupture in adults, leading to an FDA warning to limit use, and with arthropathy in children, and can prolong the QTc interval. These drugs are highly bioavailable and generally should be used orally. One caveat is that they are inactivated by divalent cations, so they cannot be given with multivitamins, dairy containing products, or infant formulas, making them difficult to administer to infants and children. Due to the issues mentioned above, fluoroquinolones should be used sparingly in pediatrics (and adults). They do have a place in the treatment of organisms resistant to other classes of drugs.

ANTIFUNGALS

The principles of antifungal therapy are similar to those of antibacterials, though there are fewer classes of agents. Amphotericin B is a polyene that interacts with ergosterol to disrupt the fungal cell membrane; ergosterol is not a component of mammalian cell membranes. Amphotericin B also inhibits fungal ATPase. It is available in deoxycholate or liposomal/lipid complex formulations, the latter of which has reduced side effects, including less renal toxicity. Lipid-based and conventional amphotericin are not interchangeable for dosing purposes. Its efficacy parameter is peak to MIC. Amphotericin is active against a broad range of yeasts and molds, with some rare but important exceptions. It is also a mainstay of treatment for some protozoal infections, for example *Leishmania* spp.

The azoles, which are another important class of antifungals, include ketoconazole, fluconazole, itraconazole, voriconazole, and posaconazole. The azole efficacy parameter is AUC over MIC. Azoles work through inhibition of the enzymes that convert lanosterol to ergosterol. Their spectra of activity, tissue penetration, side effects, drug interactions, and bioavailability vary, all of which should be considered when choosing an agent and route of administration. For some drugs, monitoring of serum levels is indicated.

The echinocandins (micafungin, caspofungin, anidulafungin) are a third class of antifungals for systemic use. These drugs, which have become a mainstay for the treatment of yeasts, work through inhibition of enzymes important to cell membrane integrity (β-(1-3)-D-glucan). They generally provide more rapid and reliable killing of yeasts (eg, *Candida* spp.) than of molds (eg, *Aspergillus* spp.); they have minimal activity against most molds other than *Aspergillus*. Echinocandins cannot be used reliably for CNS or urinary tract infections due to poor CSF and urine drug penetration. Their spectra of activity and side-effect profiles are generally similar. Last, flucytosine is a less commonly used antifungal that inhibits fungal protein synthesis. Its niche is only as an adjunctive agent for some fungal CNS infections due to its high CNS penetration. Its use is severely limited due to cost and the common occurrence of neutropenia. Combination therapy remains controversial, though it can be considered in the situation of unknown/unpredictable susceptibilities, unclear tissue penetration, or bridge to an oral agent (as therapeutic levels of voriconazole or posaconazole are often difficult to obtain in children). Additional detail on antifungals and some antiparasitics is available in Chapter 43, and limited information is included in Tables 39–3 through 39–5.

ANTIVIRALS

Antivirals are a complex group of agents that target various stages in the viral life cycle. This cycle occurs solely within a eukaryotic host cell, since viral replication depends on host cell machinery. Individual antiviral drugs may target viral entry into host cells, intracellular viral uncoating, integration, nucleic acid replication, assembly/packaging, and viral release from the host cell. Viral life cycles also vary, sometimes requiring infection of specific cell types, presence of certain host proteins, and/or incorporation into host DNA. Last, many viruses, especially RNA viruses, develop resistant mutants quickly, making the development of antivirals challenging. Anti-HIV agents are discussed in Chapter 41; anti-influenza and anti-herpes (HSV, cytomegalovirus [CMV], Epstein-Barr virus [EBV]) agents in Chapter 40; and antihepatitis virus agents in Chapter 22. Limited information is included in Tables 39–3 through 39–5.

REFERENCES

American Academy of Pediatrics. Committee on Infectious D, American Academy of Pediatrics. Committee on the Control of Infectious D. *Red book online.* 2018.

Barlam TF et al: Implementing an Antibiotic Stewardship Program: guidelines by the Infectious Diseases Society of America and the Society for Healthcare Epidemiology of America. Clin Infect Dis 2016;62(10):e51–e77.

Berrios-Torres SI et al: Centers for Disease Control and Prevention guideline for the prevention of surgical site infection, 2017. JAMA Surg 2017;152(8):784–791 [PMID: 28467526].

Bradley JS: *2019 Nelson's Pediatric Antimicrobial Therapy.* American Academy of Pediatrics; 2019.

King LM, Bartoces M, Fleming-Dutra KE, Roberts RM, Hicks LA: Changes in US outpatient antibiotic prescriptions from 2011–2016. Clin Infect Dis 2019 Mar 16. pii: ciz225 [PMID: 30882145].

The Sanford Guide to Antimicrobial Therapy. 50th ed. Sperryville, VA:: Antimicrobial Therapy; 2019.

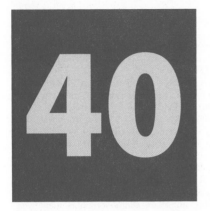

40

Infections: Viral & Rickettsial

Daniel Olson, MD

Myron J. Levin, MD

Edwin J. Asturias, MD

▼ VIRAL INFECTIONS

Viruses cause most pediatric infections. Mixed viral or viral-bacterial infections of the respiratory and intestinal tracts are common, as is prolonged asymptomatic shedding of many viruses in childhood, especially in young children. Thus, the detection of a virus is not always proof that it is the cause of a given illness. Viruses are often a predisposing factor for bacterial respiratory infections (eg, otitis, sinusitis, and pneumonia).

Many respiratory viruses and herpesviruses can now be detected within 24 through antigen or nucleic acid detection techniques. Polymerase chain reaction (PCR) amplification of viral genes has led to detection of previously unrecognized infections. It is now possible to detect multiple organisms causing the same syndrome (eg, respiratory, gastrointestinal, encephalitis/meningitis) within a single test system (multiplex assay). The available tests vary in format and turnaround time, and can include both viral and bacterial etiologies. New diagnostic tests have changed some basic concepts about viral diseases and made diagnosis of viral infections both more certain and more complex. Only laboratories with excellent quality-control procedures should be used. The availability of specific antiviral agents increases the value of early diagnosis for some serious viral infections. Table 40–1 lists diagnostic tests. The viral diagnostic laboratory should be contacted for details regarding specimen collection, handling, and shipping. Table 40–2 lists common causes of red rashes in children that should be considered in the differential diagnosis of certain viral illnesses.

▼ RESPIRATORY INFECTIONS

Many viral infections can cause either upper or lower respiratory tract signs and symptoms, sometimes both in the same patient. Many so-called respiratory viruses can also produce distinct nonrespiratory disease (eg, enteritis, cystitis or myocarditis caused by adenoviruses; parotitis caused by parainfluenza viruses). Respiratory viruses can cause disease in any area of the respiratory tree, although certain viruses tend to be closely associated with one anatomic area (eg, parainfluenza with croup, respiratory syncytial virus [RSV] with bronchiolitis) or with discrete epidemics (eg, influenza, RSV, parainfluenza). Thus, it is usually impossible on clinical grounds alone to be certain of the specific viral cause of an infection in a given child. The information provided by the virology laboratory is often important for epidemiologic, therapeutic, and preventive reasons. In immunocompromised patients, otherwise benign viruses can cause severe pneumonia.

VIRUSES CAUSING THE COMMON COLD

The common cold syndrome (also called upper respiratory infection) is characterized by combinations of runny nose, nasal congestion, sore throat, conjunctivitis, cough, and sneezing. Low-grade fever may be present. Rhinoviruses, which are the most common cause (30%–40%), are present throughout the year, but are more prevalent in the colder months in temperate climates. Adenoviruses also cause colds in all seasons and epidemics are common. RSV, parainfluenza viruses, human metapneumovirus (hMPV), and influenza viruses cause the cold syndrome during epidemics from late fall through winter. Multiple strains of coronaviruses account for 5%–10% of cold syndromes in winter. Often (25%–50%) more than one virus is detected during a common cold. The precise role of newly identified respiratory viruses, such as the human bocavirus (a parvovirus) and several polyomaviruses, are under study. Enteroviruses cause the "summer cold." The usual outcome of the common cold is morbidity continuing for 5–7 days. However, changes in the respiratory epithelium, local mucosal swelling, and altered local immunity may act as precursors to more severe bacterial illnesses, such as otitis media, pneumonia, and sinusitis.

Table 40–1. Diagnostic tests for viral infections.

Agent	Rapid Antigen Detection (Specimen)	Tissue Culture Mean Days to Positive (Range)	Serology Acute	Serology Paired	PCR	Comments
Adenovirus	+ (Respiratory, eye, and enteric)	10 (1–21)	–	+	+	"Enteric" strains detected by culture on special cell line, antigen detection, or PCR
Arboviruses	–	–	+	+	+	Acute serum (IgM) may diagnose many forms; these may be negative by day 7. May cross-react with other prior arbovirus infections; confirm by neutralization
Astrovirus	+ RL	–	–	–	+ RL	Diagnosis by electron microscopy
Calicivirus (norovirus)	RL	–	–	–	+	PCR generally available for norovirus; present in RL for others
Chikungunya virus	–	–	+	+	+	
Colorado tick virus	On RBC	–	–	RL, CDC	+	IgM may be positive as late as 2–3 wk
Coronavirus	–	RL	–	+	+	
Cytomegalovirus	+ (Tissue, urine, blood, respiratory secretions, saliva)	2 (2–28)	+	+	+	Diagnosis by presence of IgM antibody; rapid culture or PCR; low avidity antibody indicates recent infection
Dengue virus	+ (Days 1–6)	5 (RL)	+	+	+ (Days 1–5)	Serologic testing may cross-react with Zika and yellow fever viruses, so PCR or NS1 antigen detection during acute disease is preferred
Enterovirus	–	3 (2–8) Coxsackie A; difficult to culture		+	+	PCR more sensitive than culture; poliovirus also isolated in cultures and detected by PCR
Epstein-Barr virus	–	–	+	++	++	Single serologic panel defines infection status; heterophil antibodies less sensitive
Hantavirus	–	–	+	ND	RL (blood, not lavage fluid)	Diagnosis by presence of IgM antibody
Hepatitis A virus	–	–	+	ND	RL	Diagnosis by presence of IgM antibody
Hepatitis B virus	+ (Blood)	–	+	ND	+	Diagnosis by presence of hepatitis B surface antigen or IgM anticore antibody
Hepatitis C virus	–	–	+	ND	+	Positive serology suggests that hepatitis C could be the causative agent; PCR is confirmatory. PCR may be positive before serology
Hepatitis D			+		+	
Hepatitis E			+		+ (RL)	
Herpes simplex virus	+ (Mucosa, tissue, respiratory secretions, skin, blood, conjunctiva, CSF)	1 (1–5)	+	+	+	Serology rarely used for herpes simplex; IgM antibody used in selected cases
Human herpesvirus 6 and 7	–	2 (RL)	+	+	+	Roseola agent; type-specific serology available; PCR and serology may have low sensitivity

(Continued)

Table 40–1. Diagnostic tests for viral infections. (*Continued*)

Agent	Rapid Antigen Detection (Specimen)	Tissue Culture Mean Days to Positive (Range)	Serology Acute	Serology Paired	PCR	Comments
Human immunode-ficiency virus	+ (Blood) (acid dissociation of immune complexes); widely available as part of fourth-generation direct blood tests	15 (5–28)	+	ND	+	Antibody proves infection unless passively acquired (maternal antibody gone by age 15 mo); culture not widely available; PCR definitive for early diagnosis in infant (detect RNA or DNA)
Human papillomavirus					+	Cytology is frequently done
Human metapneu-movirus	+ (Respiratory secretions)	2	–	+	+	
Influenza virus	+ (Respiratory secretions)	2 (2–4)	–	+	+	Antigen detection 40%–90% sensitive (varies with virus strain) PCR preferable
Lymphocytic choriomeningitis virus	–	–	+	+	RL	Can be isolated in suckling mice
Measles virus	+ (Respiratory secretions)	–	+	+	+	Difficult to grow; IgM serology or PCR diagnostic
Mumps virus	–	> 5	+	+	+	IgM ELISA antibody may allow single-specimen diagnosis
Parvovirus B19	–	–	+	ND	+	Erythema infectiosum agent; IgM serology is often diagnostic but may be positive for a prolonged period
Poliovirus	+ RL				+	
Parainfluenza virus	+ (Respiratory secretions)	5 (4–7)	–	+	+	Serology rarely helpful
Rabies virus	+ (Skin, conjunctiva, suspected animal source)	rarely used	+		CDC	Usually diagnosed by antigen detection
Respiratory syncytial virus	+ (Respiratory secretions)	2 (1–5)	–	+ (rarely used)	+	Rapid antigen detection; 90% sensitive; PCR has excellent sensitivity
Rhinovirus	–	4 (2–7)	–	–	+	Too many strains to type serologically
Rotavirus	+ (Feces)	–	–	–	+	Rapid assay methods are usually reliable; can be positive in recent vaccinees
Rubella virus	–	> 10	+	+	+	Notify lab before culture; recommended that paired sera be tested simultaneously
Varicella-zoster virus	+ (Skin [vesicle] scraping, blood, CSF)	3 (3–21)	+	+	+	

(*Continued*)

Table 40–1. Diagnostic tests for viral infections. (*Continued*)

Agent	Rapid Antigen Detection (Specimen)	Tissue Culture Mean Days to Positive (Range)	Serology		PCR	Comments
			Acute	Paired		
West Nile virus	–	RL	+	+	+	IgM antibody usually detected by 1 wk; PCR is useful only on CSF
Zika virus	+	–	+	+	+	Serologic testing may cross-react with dengue virus, so PCR or NS1 antigen during acute disease is preferred

CSF, cerebrospinal fluid; ELISA, enzyme-linked immunosorbent assay; PCR, polymerase chain reaction; RBC, red blood cell. Plus signs signify commercially or widely available; minus signs signify not commercially available.
Note: Results from some commercial laboratories are unreliable. RL indicates research laboratory only; CDC: Specific antibody titers or PCR available by arrangement with individual research laboratories or the Centers for Disease Control and Prevention. ND: Not done.

During and following a cold, the bacterial flora changes and bacteria are found in normally sterile areas of the upper airway. Asthma attacks are frequently provoked by any of the viruses that cause the common cold. These "cold viruses" are also a common cause of lower respiratory tract infection in young children. There is no evidence that antibiotics will prevent complications of the common cold, and they do not limit the duration of purulent rhinitis.

In 5%–10% of children, symptoms from these virus infections persist for more than 10 days. Overlap with the symptoms of bacterial sinusitis presents a difficult problem for clinicians, especially because colds can produce sinuses abnormalities on computed tomography (CT) scan. Viruses that cause a minor illness in immunocompetent children, such as rhinoviruses, influenza, RSV, and metapneumovirus, can cause severe lower respiratory disease in immunologically or anatomically compromised children.

There is conflicting evidence that symptomatic relief for children can be achieved with oral antihistamines, decongestants, or cough suppressants. The FDA has recommended that such over-the-counter medications not be used in children less than 2 years old. Topical decongestants do not provide clinically important improvement in nasal symptoms. Vitamin C has not been shown to have a significant preventative or therapeutic role. Zinc therapy for the common cold and prevention with zinc may be effective in adults, but there is great uncertainty about dosing and some adverse effects. Humidified air and garlic do not alter the course of colds.

Deckx L et al: Nasal decongestants in monotherapy for the common cold. Cochrane Database Syst Rev 2016;CD0096 [PMID: 27748955].
DeSutter AI, Saraswat A, van Driel KL: Antihistamines for the common cold. Cochrane Database Syst Rev 2015;CD009345 [PMID: 26615034].
Tran DN et al: Human rhinovirus infection in hospitalized children: clinical, epidemiological and virological features. Epidemiol Infect 2016;144:346 [PMID: 26112743].

INFECTIONS DUE TO ADENOVIRUSES

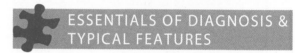

ESSENTIALS OF DIAGNOSIS & TYPICAL FEATURES

- ▶ Multiple syndromes, depending on the type of adenovirus.
- ▶ Upper respiratory infections; most notable is severe pharyngitis with tonsillitis and cervical adenopathy.
- ▶ Conjunctivitis.
- ▶ Pneumonia.
- ▶ Enteric adenoviruses cause mild diarrheal illnesses.
- ▶ Definitive diagnosis by antigen detection, PCR, or culture.

There are more than 50 types of adenoviruses, which account for 5%–15% of all respiratory illnesses in childhood, usually pharyngitis or tracheitis, but also including 5% of childhood lower respiratory tract infections. Adenoviral infections, which are common early in life (most < 2 years old), occur 3–10 days after exposure to respiratory droplets or fomites. Enteric adenoviruses are an important cause of childhood diarrhea, most often in children younger than 4 years. Epidemic respiratory disease from adenoviruses occurs in winter and spring, especially in closed environments such as day care centers and institutions. Because of latent infection in lymphoid tissue, asymptomatic shedding from the respiratory or intestinal tract is common.

Specific Adenoviral Syndromes

A. Pharyngitis

Pharyngitis is the most common adenoviral disease, and the most common viral cause of severe pharyngitis in children. Fever and adenopathy are common. Tonsillitis may

Table 40–2. Some red rashes in children.

Condition	Incubation Period (day)	Prodrome	Rash	Laboratory Tests	Comments, Other Diagnostic Features
Adenovirus	4–5	URI; cough; fever	Morbilliform (may be petechial)	Normal; may see leukopenia or lymphocytosis	Upper or lower respiratory symptoms are prominent. No Koplik spots. No desquamation. Hemorrhagic conjunctivitis.
Dengue virus	4–7	Usually none	Erythema early on; maculopapular or urticarial in febrile phase	Leukopenia, thrombocytopenia, elevated transaminases; PCR	Rash has been described as "islands of white on a sea of red."
Drug allergy	Any time post-exposure	None, or fever alone, or with myalgia, pruritus	Macular, maculopapular, urticarial, or erythroderma, target lesions	Leukopenia, eosinophilia	Rash variable. Severe reactions may resemble measles, scarlet fever; Kawasaki disease; marked toxicity possible.
Enterovirus	2–7	Variable fever, chills, myalgia, sore throat	Variable; usually macular, maculopapular on trunk or palms, soles; vesicles or petechiae also seen	PCR	Varied rashes may resemble those of many other infections. Pharyngeal or hand-foot-mouth vesicles may occur.
Ehrlichiosis (monocytic)	5–21	Fever; headache; flu-like; myalgia; GI symptoms	Variable; maculopapular, petechial, scarlatiniform, vasculitic	Leukopenia, thrombocytopenia, abnormal liver function. Serology for diagnosis; morulae in monocytes	Geographic distribution is a clue; seasonal; tick exposure; rash present in only 45%.
Erythema multiforme	—	Usually none or related to underlying cause	Discrete, red maculopapular lesions; symmetrical, distal, palms and soles; target lesions classic	Normal or eosinophilia	Reaction to drugs (especially sulfonamides), or infectious agents (*Mycoplasma*; herpes simplex virus). Urticaria, arthralgia also seen.
Infectious mononucleosis (EBV infection)	30–60	Fever, malaise	Macular, scarlatiniform, or urticarial in 5% to almost 100% who are on penicillins and related drugs (not a penicillin allergy)	Atypical lymphocytosis; heterophil antibodies; EBV-specific antibodies in an acute pattern EBV; abnormal liver function tests	Pharyngitis, lymphadenopathy, hepatosplenomegaly.
Juvenile rheumatoid arthritis (systemic; Still diseases)	—	High fever, malaise	Evanescent salmon-pink macules, especially in pressure areas (prominent when fever is present)	Increased inflammatory markers; leukocytosis; thrombocytosis	Oligo- or polyarticular arthritis; asymptomatic anterior uveitis.
Kawasaki disease	Unknown	Fever, cervical adenopathy, irritability	Polymorphous (may be erythroderma) on trunk and extremities; red palms and soles, conjunctiva, lips, tongue, pharynx. Late desquamation is common. Some of these findings may be absent with atypical disease	Leukocytosis, thrombocytosis, elevated ESR or CRP; pyuria; decreased albumin; negative cultures and streptococcal serology; resting tachycardia	Swollen hands, feet; prolonged illness; uveitis; aseptic meningitis; no response to antibiotics. Vasculitis and aneurysms of coronary and other arteries occur (cardiac ultrasound).
Leptospirosis	4–19	Fever (biphasic), myalgia, chills	Variable erythroderma	Leukocytosis; hematuria, proteinuria; hyperbilirubinemia	Conjunctivitis; hepatitis, aseptic meningitis may be seen. Rodent, dog contact.
Measles	9–14	Cough, rhinitis, conjunctivitis	Maculopapular; face to trunk; lasts 7–10 days; Koplik spots in mouth for 1–2 days	Leukopenia; anti-measles IgM	Toxic. Bright red rash becomes confluent, may desquamate. Fever falls after rash appears. Inadequate measles vaccination.

Disease	Incubation	Prodrome	Rash	Laboratory	Comments
Parvovirus (erythema infectiosum)	10–17 (rash)	Mild (flu-like)	Maculopapular on cheeks ("slapped cheek"), forehead, chin; then down limbs, trunk, buttocks; may fade and reappear for several weeks	IgM-EIA; PCR	Purpuric stocking-glove rash is rare, but distinctive; aplastic crisis in patients with chronic hemolytic anemia. May cause arthritis or arthralgia.
Rocky Mountain spotted fever	3–12	Headache (retro-orbital); toxic; GI symptoms; high fever; flu-like	Onset 2–6 days after fever; palpable maculopapular on palms, soles, extremities, with spread centrally; petechial	Leukopenia; thrombocytopenia; abnormal liver function; CSF pleocytosis; serology positive at 7–10 days of rash; biopsy will give earlier diagnosis	Eastern seaboard and southeastern United States; April–September; tick exposure.
Roseola (exanthem subitum) (HHV-6)	10–14	Fever (mean 4 days; 15 ≥ 6 days)	Pink, macular rash occurs at the end of febrile period; transient (only 20% get rash)	Normal; RT-PCR	Fever often high; disappears when rash develops; child appears well. Usually occurs in children 6 mo to 3 y of age. Seizures may complicate.
Rubella	14–21	Usually none	Mild maculopapular; rapid spread face to extremities; gone by day 4	Normal or leukopenia	Postauricular, occipital adenopathy common. Polyarthralgia in some older girls. Mild clinical illness. Inadequate rubella vaccination.
Staphylococcal scalded skin	Variable	Irritability, absent to low fever	Painful erythroderma, followed in 1–2 days by cracking around eyes, mouth; bullae form with friction (Nikolsky sign)	Normal if only colonized by staphylococci; leukocytosis and sometimes bacteremia if infected	Normal pharynx. Look for focal staphylococcal infection. Usually occurs in infants.
Staphylococcal scarlet fever	1–7	Variable fever	Diffuse erythroderma; resembles streptococcal scarlet fever except eyes may be hyperemic and no "strawberry" tongue; pharynx spared	Leukocytosis is common because of infected focus	Focal infection usually present.
Stevens-Johnson syndrome	—	Pharyngitis, conjunctivitis, fever, malaise	Bullous erythema multiforme; may slough in large areas; hemorrhagic lips; purulent conjunctivitis	Leukocytosis	Classic precipitants are drugs (especially sulfonamides); *Mycoplasma pneumoniae* and herpes simplex infections. Pneumonitis and urethritis also seen.
Streptococcal scarlet fever	1–7	Fever, abdominal pain, headache, sore throat	Diffuse erythema, "sandpaper" texture; neck, axillae, inguinal areas; spreads to rest of body; desquamates 7–14 days; eyes not red	Leukocytosis; positive group A *Streptococcus* culture of throat or wound; positive streptococcal antigen test in pharynx	Strawberry tongue, red pharynx with or without exudate. Eyes, perioral and periorbital area, palms, and soles spared. Pastia lines. Cervical adenopathy. Usually occurs in children 2–10 y of age.
Toxic shock syndrome	Variable	Fever, myalgia, headache, diarrhea, vomiting	Nontender erythroderma; red eyes, palms, soles, pharynx, lips	Leukocytosis; abnormal liver enzymes and coagulation tests; proteinuria	*Staphylococcus aureus* infection; toxin-mediated multiorgan involvement. Swollen hands, feet. Hypotension or shock.
Zika virus	3–7	Variable	Common; erythema, macular, or maculopapular; conjunctivitis	Leukocytosis, thrombocytopenia, elevated transaminases; PCR	Rash is common and variable in nature; often pruritic; petechiae are rare; conjunctivitis is common.

CRP, C-reactive protein; CSF, cerebrospinal fluid; EIA, enzyme immunoassay; ESR, erythrocyte sedimentation rate; GI, gastrointestinal; HHV-6, human herpesvirus 6; IFA, immunofluorescent assay; PCR, polymerase chain reaction; URI, upper respiratory infection.

be exudative. Rhinitis and an influenza-like systemic illness may be present. Laryngotracheitis or bronchitis may accompany pharyngitis.

B. Pharyngoconjunctival Fever

Conjunctivitis may occur alone and be prolonged, but most often is associated with preauricular adenopathy, fever, pharyngitis, and cervical adenopathy. Foreign body sensation in the eye and other symptoms last less than a week. Lower respiratory symptoms are uncommon.

C. Epidemic Keratoconjunctivitis

Symptoms include severe conjunctivitis with punctate keratitis and occasionally visual impairment. A foreign body sensation, photophobia, and swelling of conjunctiva and eyelids are characteristic. Preauricular adenopathy and subconjunctival hemorrhage are common.

D. Pneumonia

Severe pneumonia may occur at any age. It is especially common in young children (< 3 years). Chest radiographs show bilateral peribronchial and patchy ground-glass interstitial infiltrates in the lower lobes. Symptoms persist for 2–4 weeks. Adenoviral pneumonia can be necrotizing and cause permanent lung damage, such as bronchiectasis and bronchiolitis obliterans. A pertussis-like syndrome with typical cough and lymphocytosis can occur with lower respiratory tract infection. A new variant of adenovirus serotype 14 can cause unusually severe, sometimes fatal pneumonia in children and adults.

E. Rash

A diffuse morbilliform (rarely petechial) rash resembling measles, rubella, or roseola may occur alone or with respiratory symptoms. Koplik spots are absent.

F. Diarrhea

Enteric adenoviruses (types 40 and 41) cause 3%–5% of cases of short-lived diarrhea in afebrile children, especially in those younger than 4 years.

G. Mesenteric Lymphadenitis

Fever and abdominal pain may mimic appendicitis. Pharyngitis is often associated. Adenovirus-induced adenopathy may be a factor in appendicitis and intussusception.

H. Other Syndromes

Immunosuppressed patients, including neonates, may develop severe or fatal pulmonary or gastrointestinal

infections or multisystem disease. Hemorrhagic cystitis can be a serious problem in immunocompromised children. Other rare complications that can occur in the immunocompetent child include encephalitis, hepatitis, and myocarditis. Adenoviruses have been implicated in the syndrome of idiopathic myocardiopathy.

▶ Laboratory & Diagnostic Studies

PCR of respiratory specimens, conjunctival, or stool specimens is rapid, sensitive, and the preferred diagnostic method for adenovirus infections. Diagnosis can also be made by conventional culture, but several days to weeks are required. Viral culture using the rapid culture technique with immunodiagnostic reagents detects adenovirus in 48 hours. Adenovirus infection can also be diagnosed using these reagents directly on respiratory secretions. This is quicker, but less sensitive, than the culture methods. ELISA (enzyme-linked immunosorbent assay) tests rapidly detect enteric adenoviruses in diarrheal specimens. Respiratory adenovirus infections can be detected retrospectively by comparing acute and convalescent sera, but this is not helpful during an acute illness.

▶ Treatment

There is no specific treatment for adenovirus infections. Intravenous immunoglobulin (IVIG) may be tried in immunocompromised patients with severe pneumonia. Adoptive T-cell transfer has shown promising results in hematopoietic stem cell transplant recipients. There is some evidence of successful treatment of immunocompromised patients with cidofovir and, more recently, with brincidofovir, a cidofovir derivative with good oral bioavailability and less nephrotoxicity than the parent drug.

Lion T: Adenovirus infections in immune competent and immunocompromised patients. Clin Microbiol Rev 2014;27:441 [PMID: 24982316].

INFLUENZA

ESSENTIALS OF DIAGNOSIS & TYPICAL FEATURES

▶ Fever, cough, pharyngitis, malaise, congestion.

▶ Pneumonia.

▶ Encephalitis.

▶ Seasonal: late fall through mid-spring.

▶ Detection of virus, viral antigens, or nucleic acid in respiratory secretions.

Symptomatic infections are common in children because they lack immunologic experience with influenza viruses. Infection rates in children are greater than in adults and are instrumental in initiating community outbreaks. Epidemics occur in fall and winter. Three main types of influenza viruses (A/H1N1, A/H3N2, B) cause most human epidemics, with antigenic drift ensuring a supply of susceptible hosts of all ages. In recent years, avian influenza A/H5N1 and A/H7N9 caused isolated human outbreaks in Asia that were associated with high rates of hospitalization and death. A swine-origin influenza A/H1N1 caused a human pandemic in 2009 and 2010 and has since circulated with seasonal periodicity.

Clinical Findings

Spread of influenza occurs by way of airborne respiratory secretions. The incubation period is 2–7 days.

A. Symptoms and Signs

Influenza infection in older children and adults produces a characteristic syndrome of sudden onset of high fever, severe myalgia, headache, and chills. These symptoms overshadow the associated coryza, pharyngitis, and cough. Usually absent are rash, marked conjunctivitis, adenopathy, exudative pharyngitis, and dehydrating enteritis. Fever, diarrhea, vomiting, and abdominal pain are common in young children. Infants may develop a sepsis-like illness and apnea. Chest examination is usually unremarkable. Less frequent clinical findings include croup (most severe with type A influenza), exacerbation of asthma, myositis (especially calf muscles), myocarditis, parotitis, encephalopathy, nephritis, and a transient maculopapular rash. Acute illness lasts 2–5 days. Cough and fatigue may last several weeks. Viral shedding may persist for several weeks in young children.

B. Laboratory Findings

The leukocyte count is normal to low, with variable shift. Influenza infections may be more difficult to recognize in children than in adults even during epidemics, and therefore a specific laboratory test is highly recommended. The virus can be found in respiratory secretions by direct fluorescent antibody (DFA) staining of nasopharyngeal epithelial cells, ELISA, optic immunoassay (OIA), and PCR. PCR has the highest sensitivity and specificity (close to 100%) and has become the preferred test as the results can be available within several hours. Influenza virus can be cultured within 3–7 days from pharyngeal swabs or throat washings, but this is mainly of value for epidemiology and antiviral sensitivity testing. Some laboratories use the rapid culture technique by centrifuging specimens onto cultured cell layers and detecting viral antigen after 48 hours. Other body fluids or tissues (except lung) rarely yield the virus in culture and are more appropriately tested by PCR. A late diagnosis may be made with paired serology, using hemagglutination inhibition assays.

C. Imaging

The chest radiograph is nonspecific; it may show hyperaeration, peribronchial thickening, diffuse interstitial infiltrates, or bronchopneumonia in severe cases. Hilar nodes are not enlarged. Pleural effusion is rare in uncomplicated influenza.

Differential Diagnosis

The following may be considered: all other respiratory viruses, *Mycoplasma pneumoniae* or *Chlamydia pneumoniae* (longer incubation period, prolonged illness), streptococcal pharyngitis (pharyngeal exudate or petechiae, adenitis, no cough), bacterial sepsis (petechial or purpuric rash may occur), toxic shock syndrome (rash, hypotension), and rickettsial infections (rash, different season, insect exposure). High fever, the nature of preceding or concurrent illness in family members, and the presence of influenza in the community are distinguishing features from parainfluenza or RSV infections.

Complications & Sequelae

Lower respiratory tract symptoms are most common in children younger than 5 years. Hospitalization rates are highest in children younger than 2 years. Influenza can cause croup in these children. Secondary bacterial infections (classically staphylococcal) of the middle ear, sinuses, or lungs are common. Children with influenza who develop protracted vomiting or irrational behavior while on aspirin should be evaluated for Reye syndrome. Influenza can also cause viral or postviral encephalitis, with cerebral symptoms much more prominent than those of the accompanying respiratory infection. Although the myositis is usually mild and resolves promptly, severe rhabdomyolysis and renal failure have been reported.

Children with underlying obesity, cardiopulmonary, metabolic, neuromuscular, or immunosuppressive disease are at risk for severe disease.

Prevention

The trivalent and quadrivalent influenza vaccines are licensed as inactivated (IIV) or live attenuated (LAIV) and are moderately protective (see Chapter 10). Influenza vaccination should occur before onset of influenza activity in the community, though immunity may wane during a single season. For egg-allergic children, observation for 30 minutes postvaccination is now the only precaution, and those with a history of severe allergic reaction to egg (eg, any symptom other than hives) should be vaccinated in an inpatient or outpatient medical setting under the supervision of a health care provider. Prophylaxis with oseltamivir can be used in select cases for children older than 3 months (children < 15 kg, 30 mg daily; those 15–23 kg, 45 mg daily; those 23–40 kg, 60 mg daily; and those > 40 kg, 75 mg daily). Inhaled zanamivir can also be used in children older than 5 years, but avoid use in children with asthma or chronic pulmonary disease. Chemoprophylaxis may be considered during an epidemic for high-risk children who cannot be immunized or who have not yet developed immunity (about 6 weeks after primary vaccination or 2 weeks after a booster dose). For outbreak prophylaxis, therapy should be maintained for 2 weeks or more and for 1 week after the last case of influenza is diagnosed.

Treatment & Prognosis

Treatment consists of general support and management of pulmonary complications, especially bacterial superinfections. Antivirals are of benefit against seasonal influenza in immunocompetent hosts if begun within 48 hours after symptom onset. In hospitalized children, early antiviral treatment shortens the duration of hospitalization. Treatment duration is 5 days and the doses are twice those used for prophylaxis (see earlier). Studies in immunocompromised patients during the 2009/2010 pandemic showed that oseltamivir was useful even when initiated later than 2 days after the onset of disease. Peramivir, a neuraminidase inhibitor that is available for IV administration, is approved for treatment.

Recovery is usually complete unless severe cardiopulmonary or neurologic damage has occurred. Fatal cases occur in very young infants, immunodeficient and anatomically compromised children, pregnant women, including the first 2 weeks postpartum, and obese individuals. Effective treatment or prophylaxis of influenza in children markedly reduces the incidence of acute otitis media and antibiotic usage during the flu season.

Grohskopf LA et al: Prevention and control of seasonal influenza with vaccines: recommendations of the Advisory Committee on Immunization Practices—United States, 2018–19 influenza season. MMWR Recomm Rep 2018 Aug 24;67(3):1–20 [PMID: 30141464].

PARAINFLUENZA (CROUP)

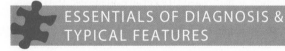

ESSENTIALS OF DIAGNOSIS & TYPICAL FEATURES

▶ Fever, nasal congestion, sore throat, cough.

▶ Croup and bronchiolitis.

▶ Detection of live virus, antigens, or nucleic acid in respiratory secretions.

Human parainfluenza viruses (HPIV) are the most important cause of croup in children. Four types of HPIV (1–4) are known. HPIV 1 and 2 cause most cases of croup, and infections occur during the first 5 years of life, usually during outbreaks in the fall. Most infants are infected with type 3 within the first 3 years of life, most often in the first year. HPIV 4 has year-round circulation and may be less pathogenic than other types.

Clinical Findings

A. Symptoms and Signs

The incubation period is 2–7 days. Clinical disease has an acute onset that includes febrile upper respiratory infection (especially in older children with re-exposure), laryngitis, tracheobronchitis, croup, and bronchiolitis (second most common cause after RSV). The relative incidence of these manifestations is type-specific. HPIVs (especially type 1) cause 65% of cases of croup in young children, 25% of tracheobronchitis, and 50% of laryngitis. Croup is characterized by a barking cough, inspiratory stridor, and hoarseness. HPIV can cause pneumonia in infants and immunodeficient children, and causes particularly high mortality among stem cell recipients.

B. Laboratory Findings

Diagnosis is often based on clinical findings. These viruses can be identified by PCR (< 24 hours), conventional or rapid culture techniques (48 hours), or by direct immunofluorescence on nasopharyngeal epithelial cells in respiratory secretions (< 3 hours).

Differential Diagnosis

HPIV-induced respiratory syndromes are difficult to distinguish from those caused by other respiratory viruses. Viral croup must be distinguished from epiglottitis caused by *Haemophilus influenzae* type b (if unimmunized) or other bacterial infections causing upper airway obstruction (eg, peritonsillar abscess).

Treatment

No specific therapy or vaccine is available. Croup management is discussed in Chapter 19. Ribavirin is active in vitro and has been used in immunocompromised children, but its efficacy is unproven.

Frost HM et al: Epidemiology and clinical presentation of parainfluenza type 4 in children: a 3-year comparative study to parainfluenza types 1-3. J Clin Infect Dis 2014;209:695 [PMID: 24133181].

RESPIRATORY SYNCYTIAL VIRUS DISEASE

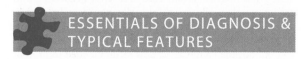

ESSENTIALS OF DIAGNOSIS & TYPICAL FEATURES

▶ Diffuse wheezing and tachypnea following upper respiratory symptoms in an infant (bronchiolitis).

▶ Epidemics in late fall to early spring (January–February peak).

▶ Hyperinflation on chest radiograph.

▶ Detection of RSV antigen or nucleic acid in nasal secretions.

▶ General Considerations

Respiratory syncytial virus (RSV) is the most important cause of lower respiratory tract illness in young children, accounting for more than 70% of cases of bronchiolitis and 40% of cases of pneumonia. RSV is very common in early childhood. Almost all children develop upper respiratory symptoms, and 20%–30% will manifest as lower respiratory infection. Outbreaks occur annually, and attack rates are high; 60% of children are infected in the first year of life, and 90% by age 2 years. During peak season (cold weather in temperate climates), the clinical diagnosis of RSV infection in infants with bronchiolitis is as accurate as most laboratory tests. Despite the presence of serum antibody, reinfection is common. Two distinct genotypes can cocirculate or one may predominate in a community. Yearly shift in prevalence of these genotypes is a partial explanation for reinfection. However, reinfection generally causes only upper respiratory symptoms in anatomically normal children. Immunosuppressed patients may develop progressive severe pneumonia. Children with congenital heart disease with increased pulmonary blood flow, children with chronic lung disease (eg, cystic fibrosis), and premature infants younger than 6 months (especially when they have chronic lung disease of prematurity) are also at higher risk for severe illness. No vaccine is available.

▶ Clinical Findings

A. Symptoms and Signs

Initial symptoms are those of upper respiratory infection. Low-grade fever may be present. The classic disease is bronchiolitis, characterized by diffuse wheezing, variable fever, cough, tachypnea, difficulty feeding, and in severe cases, cyanosis. Hyperinflation, crackles, prolonged expiration, wheezing, hypoxia, and retractions may be present. The liver and spleen may be palpable because of lung hyperinflation, but

are not enlarged. The disease usually lasts 3–7 days in previously healthy children. Fever is present for 2–4 days; it does not correlate with pulmonary symptoms and may be absent during the height of lung involvement.

Apnea, poor feeding, and lethargy may be presenting manifestations, especially in premature infants, in the first few months of life. Apnea usually resolves after a few days, often being replaced by obvious signs of bronchiolitis.

RSV infection in older children is more likely to cause tracheobronchitis or upper respiratory tract infection. Exceptions are immunocompromised children and those with severe chronic lung or heart disease, who may have especially severe or prolonged primary infections and are subject to additional attacks of severe pneumonitis.

B. Laboratory Findings

Rapid detection of RSV antigen in nasal or pulmonary secretions by fluorescent antibody staining or ELISA requires only several hours and is more than 90% sensitive and specific. Real-time PCR is more sensitive and expensive than antigen testing and is often multiplexed to detect additional respiratory pathogens in the same assay. Rapid tissue culture methods take 48 hours and have comparable sensitivity, but require a carefully collected and handled specimen.

C. Imaging

Diffuse hyperinflation and peribronchiolar thickening are most common; atelectasis and patchy infiltrates also occur in uncomplicated infection, but pleural effusions are rare. Consolidation (usually subsegmental) occurs in 25% of children with lower respiratory tract disease.

▶ Differential Diagnosis

Although almost all cases of bronchiolitis are due to RSV during an epidemic, parainfluenza, rhinovirus, and especially hMPV cannot be excluded. Mixed infections with other viruses or bacteria can occur. Wheezing may be due to asthma, a foreign body, or other airway obstruction. RSV infection may closely resemble *Mycoplasma* or chlamydial pneumonitis when fine crackles are present and fever and wheezing are not prominent. The two may also coexist. Cystic fibrosis may present with respiratory symptoms resembling RSV infection; a positive family history or failure to thrive associated with GI symptoms, hyponatremia or hypoalbuminemia should prompt a sweat chloride test. Pertussis should also be considered in this age group, especially if cough is prominent and the infant is younger than 6 months. A markedly elevated leukocyte count should suggest bacterial superinfection (neutrophilia) or pertussis (lymphocytosis).

Complications

RSV commonly infects the middle ear. Symptomatic otitis media is more likely when secondary bacterial infection is present (usually due to pneumococci or nontypable *H influenzae*). This is the most common complication (10%–20%) of RSV infection. Bacterial pneumonia complicates only 0.5%–1% of hospitalized patients. Sudden exacerbations of fever and leukocytosis should suggest bacterial infection. Respiratory failure or apnea may require mechanical ventilation, but occurs in less than 2% of hospitalized previously healthy full-term infants. Cardiac failure may occur as a complication of pulmonary disease or myocarditis. RSV commonly causes exacerbations of asthma. Nosocomial RSV infection is so common during outbreaks that elective hospitalization or surgery, especially for those with underlying illness, may be postponed. Well-designed hospital programs to prevent nosocomial spread are imperative (see the next section).

Prevention & Treatment

Oxygen therapy is only indicated in infants and children with oxyhemoglobin saturation less than 90%. Children who are very hypoxic or cannot feed because of respiratory distress must be hospitalized and given humidified oxygen as directed by oxygen saturation, and given tube or intravenous feedings. Antibiotics, decongestants, and expectorants are of no value in routine infections. RSV-infected children should be kept in respiratory isolation. Cohorting ill infants in respiratory isolation during peak season (with or without rapid diagnostic attempts) and emphasizing good hand washing should decrease nosocomial transmission.

Clinicians should not administer albuterol (or salbutamol) or epinephrine to infants and children with a diagnosis of bronchiolitis since this does not impact disease resolution, need for hospitalization, or length of stay. The use of systemic corticosteroids is also discouraged in RSV bronchiolitis, unless there are complicating features such as asthma and chronic lung disease of prematurity. A meta-analysis of numerous studies of corticosteroid therapy indicated a significant effect on hospital stay, especially in those most ill at the time of treatment, but use of a single dose of corticosteroids in an outpatient setting had no lasting effect on respiratory status and did not prevent hospitalization.

Ribavirin is the only licensed antiviral therapy used for RSV infection. It is given by continuous aerosolization. It is rarely used in infants without significant anatomic or immunologic defects. At best, there is a very modest effect on disease severity in immunocompetent infants with no underlying anatomic abnormality. Even in high-risk infants, a favorable clinical response to ribavirin therapy was not demonstrated in several studies, although some data suggest that it might be more efficacious if initiated early in the illness. Thus, ribavirin is only used in severely ill children who are immunologically or anatomically compromised and in those with severe cardiac disease.

Monthly intramuscular administration of humanized RSV monoclonal antibody is now recommended to prevent severe disease in selected high-risk patients during epidemic periods. Monthly administration should be considered during the RSV season for high-risk children (described in Chapter 10). Long-acting monoclonal antibodies are also under development. Use of passive immunization for immunocompromised children is logical but not established. RSV antibody is not effective for treatment of established infection.

Prognosis

Although mild bronchiolitis does not produce long-term problems, 30%–40% of patients hospitalized with this infection will wheeze later in childhood, and RSV infection in infancy may be an important precursor to asthma. Chronic restrictive lung disease and bronchiolitis obliterans are rare sequelae.

Geevarghese B, Simoes EA: Antibodies for prevention and treatment of respiratory syncytial virus infections in children. Antivir Ther 2012;17(1 Pt B):201 [PMID: 22311607].
Hall CB et al: The burden of respiratory syncytial virus infection in young children. N Engl J Med 2009 Feb 5;360(6):588–598 [PMID: 19196675].
Ralston SL et al; American Academy of Pediatrics: Clinical practice guidelines: the diagnosis, management, and prevention of bronchiolitis. Pediatrics 2014 Nov;134(5):e1474–e1502 [PMID: 25349312].

HUMAN METAPNEUMOVIRUS INFECTION

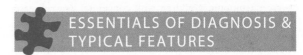

ESSENTIALS OF DIAGNOSIS & TYPICAL FEATURES

▶ Cough, coryza, sore throat.

▶ Bronchiolitis.

▶ Detection of viral antigens or nucleic acid in respiratory secretions.

General Considerations

Human metapneumovirus (hMPV) is a common agent of respiratory tract infections that is very similar to RSV in epidemiologic and clinical characteristics. Like RSV, parainfluenza, mumps, and measles, hMPV belongs to the paramyxovirus family. Humans are its only known reservoir. Seroepidemiologic surveys indicate that the virus has worldwide distribution. More than 90% of children contract hMPV infection by age 5 years, typically during late autumn through early spring outbreaks. hMPV accounts for 15%–25% of the cases of bronchiolitis and pneumonia in children younger than 2 years. Older children and adults can also develop symptomatic infection.

▶ Clinical Findings

A. Symptoms and Signs

The most common symptoms are fever, cough, rhinorrhea, and sore throat. Bronchiolitis and pneumonia occur in 40%–70% of the children who acquire hMPV before the age of 2 years. Asymptomatic infection is uncommon. Other manifestations include otitis, conjunctivitis, diarrhea, and myalgia. Acute wheezing has been associated with hMPV in children of all ages, raising the possibility that this virus, like RSV, might trigger reactive airway disease. Dual infection with hMPV and RSV or other respiratory viruses seems to be a common occurrence and may increase morbidity and mortality.

B. Laboratory Findings

The preferred method of diagnosis is PCR performed on respiratory specimens. Rapid shell vial culture is an acceptable, albeit less sensitive. Antibody tests are most appropriately used for epidemiologic studies.

C. Imaging

Lower respiratory tract infection frequently shows hyperinflation and patchy pneumonitis on chest radiographs.

▶ Treatment & Prognosis

No antiviral therapy is available to treat hMPV. Ribavirin has in vitro activity against hMPV, but there are no data to support its therapeutic value. Children with lower respiratory tract disease may require hospitalization and ventilatory support, but less frequently than with RSV-associated bronchiolitis. Duration of hospitalization in hMPV is typically shorter than in RSV. Infection of immune compromised children can lead to severe or fatal disease.

Esposito S, Masstrolia MV: Metapneumovirus infections and respiratory complications. Semin Respir Crit Care Med 2016;37:512 [PMID: 27486733].

Taylor S, Lopez P, Boria-Tabora C: Respiratory viruses and influenza-like illness: epidemiology and outcomes in children aged 6 months to 10 years in a multi-country population sample. J Infect 2017;29:74 [PMID: 27667752].

INFECTIONS DUE TO HUMAN CORONAVIRUSES

 ## ESSENTIALS OF DIAGNOSIS & TYPICAL FEATURES

▶ Common cold limited to upper respiratory signs and symptoms

▶ Lower respiratory tract disease and severe acute respiratory syndromes

▶ Pneumonia in immunocompromised children

▶ Definitive diagnosis by PCR

Human coronaviruses (HCoVs) are RNA viruses that can infect humans and various animals. They are transmitted via inoculation of the respiratory tract by droplets from the respiratory tract of infected individuals. The incubation period is 2-5 days for the non-severe infections and likely longer for severe acute respiratory syndromes. Infections from HCoVs, including strains OC43, NL63, HKU1, and 229E, manifest each year as the common cold and lower respiratory tract disease (LRTD). However, LRTD is more frequent and severe in immunocompromised children. Co-infections with other viruses occur in 10–40% of HCoV infections.

▶ HCoV Clinical Syndromes

A. Upper and Lower Respiratory Tract Infection

HCoVs 229E, OC43, NL63 and HKU1 are the second most common cause of the common cold after rhinoviruses and manifest with rhinorrhea, sore throat, cough, and occasionally fever. HCoVs may also present as acute otitis media or trigger asthma exacerbations. HCoV NL63 is the second most common cause of croup after parainfluenza 1. HCoV HKU1 also can present as acute gastroenteritis.

B. Severe Acute Respiratory Syndromes (SARS)

The three novel HCoVs causing severe symptoms are SARS-CoV, which emerged in 2002 in China. This had moderate infectivity, caused epidemics in several countries, and had a case fatality rate of ~10%. The Middle Eastern Respiratory Syndrome (MERS)-CoV appeared in 2012 in Saudi Arabia, was less infectious, but more severe clinically with a case fatality rate of ~30%. It is endemic in the Middle East and acquired by close contact with camels, although human-to-human spread also occurs. The SARS-CoV-2 virus originated in China in 2019 and resulted in worldwide spread. This virus appears to spread somewhat more readily than influenza virus. HCoVs that cause severe disease disproportionally affect immune- or anatomically-compromised adults and the elderly. Infected children are either asymptomatic or have typically milder symptoms that include fever, cough, myalgia, mild diarrhea, and abdominal pain. Complications including multiorgan dysfunction and death can occur in children with co-morbidities.

The recently emerged SARS-CoV-2 manifests as fever, cough, and less commonly with shortness of breath (COVID-19). Most children with pulmonary symptoms may have radiographic evidence of bilateral disease, including ground-glass opacities with surrounding halo sign and occasional small nodules. Young children shed SARS-CoV-2 for prolonged periods.

▶ Laboratory and Diagnostic Studies

Children infected with the novel SARS-CoV-2 have elevated procalcitonin in 80% of the symptomatic cases. The new multiple rt-PCR test for respiratory viruses may include detection of HCoVs 229E, OC43, NL54, and HKU1. Public health laboratories have added the capacity to diagnose novel coronaviruses causing severe disease, including the current pandemic SARS-CoV-2, by rt-PCR.

▶ Treatment and Prevention

Most common HCoVs cause mild, self-limited disease. For the novel coronavirus infections associated with severe disease, especially in immunocompromised children, type 1 interferon, ribavirin, and convalescent plasma have been used with anecdotal benefit. Antiviral drugs that are effective against HCoVs in vitro are in phase III trials and vaccines are rapidly under development in the SARS-CoV-2 pandemic. Appropriate hand hygiene, social distancing, and isolation precautions, including personal protective equipment for health care workers, are considered useful for limiting transmission. Contact tracing and quarantine were effective for SARS-CoV, but failed to stop the pandemic of SARS-CoV-2 in 2020.

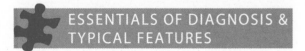

INFECTIONS DUE TO ENTEROVIRUSES & PARECHOVIRUSES

ESSENTIALS OF DIAGNOSIS & TYPICAL FEATURES

- ▶ Acute febrile illness with headache and sore throat.
- ▶ Summer-fall epidemics.
- ▶ Other common features: rash, nonexudative pharyngitis.
- ▶ Common cause of aseptic and viral meningitis.
- ▶ Complications: myocarditis, neurologic damage, life-threatening illness in newborns.

Enteroviruses (EV) are a major cause of acute febrile illness in young children. From the family of picornaviruses ("small"), antigenically they are divided into four groups: polioviruses (PV), coxsackieviruses A and B, and echoviruses. Their common RNA sequences and group antigens are the basis for diagnostic tests for enterovirus-specific nucleic acid and proteins. A PCR assay is available in many medical centers as a one-step test with results in a few hours. Cross-reactivity with rhinoviruses is common on the PCR respiratory panel. Viral cultures are more specific but take 2–5 days. PCR is now the diagnostic method of choice for meningoencephalitis and severe unexplained illness in neonates.

Parechoviruses (HPeV), also picornaviruses, are responsible for severe infections in young children including sepsis and meningitis. Some of the 15 types of parechoviruses infect almost every child before the age of 2 years; others before age 5 years.

Transmission of EV and HPeV is fecal-oral or from upper respiratory secretions. Multiple enteroviruses circulate in the community at any one time; summer-fall outbreaks are common in temperate climates, but infections are seen year-round. After poliovirus, coxsackie B virus is most virulent, followed by echovirus. Neurologic, cardiac, and overwhelming neonatal infections are the most severe forms of illness.

ACUTE FEBRILE ILLNESS

Accompanied by nonspecific upper respiratory or enteric symptoms, the sudden onset of fever and irritability in infants or young children is often enteroviral, especially in late summer and fall. More than 90% of enteroviral infections are not distinctive. Occasionally a petechial rash is seen; more often a diffuse maculopapular or morbilliform eruption (often prominent on palms and soles) occurs on the second to fourth day of fever. Rapid recovery is the rule. More than one febrile enteroviral illness can occur in a patient in one season. The leukocyte count is usually normal. Infants, because of fever and irritability, may undergo an evaluation for sepsis or meningitis and be hospitalized. Approximately half of these infants have aseptic meningitis. Duration of illness is 4–5 days.

Abedi GR et al: Picornavirus etiology of acute infections among hospitalized infants. J Clin Virol 2019;116:39–43. doi: 10.1016/j.jcv.2019.04.005 [PMID: 31100674].

RESPIRATORY TRACT ILLNESSES

1. Acute Febrile Pharyngitis

Sore throat, headache, myalgia, and abdominal discomfort lasting 3–4 days are common in older children. Vesicles or papules may be seen in the pharynx without exudate. Occasionally, enteroviruses are the cause of croup, bronchitis, or pneumonia. They may also exacerbate asthma as seen with the recent outbreaks of EV68.

2. Herpangina

Herpangina manifests as acute onset fever and posterior pharyngeal grayish white vesicles that quickly form ulcers (< 20 in number), linearly along the posterior palate, uvula, and tonsillar pillars. Bilateral facial ulcers may also be seen. Dysphagia, drooling, vomiting, abdominal pain, and anorexia also occur and, rarely, parotitis or vaginal ulcers. Symptoms disappear in 4–5 days. Coxsackievirus A10 has been associated with a sporadic febrile pharyngitis, called acute lymphonodular pharyngitis, which is characterized by nonulcerative yellow-white posterior pharyngeal papules in the same distribution as herpangina. The duration is 1–2 weeks. Therapy is supportive.

Primary herpes simplex gingivostomatitis (ulcers are more prominent anteriorly, and gingivitis is present), aphthous stomatitis (fever absent, recurrent episodes, anterior lesions), trauma, hand-foot-and-mouth disease (see discussion in section Rashes [Including Hand-Foot-&-Mouth Disease]), and Vincent angina (painful gingivitis spreading from the gum line; older child; underlying dental disease) should be in the differential diagnosis.

3. Pleurodynia (Bornholm Disease, Epidemic Myalgia)

Caused by coxsackie B virus (epidemic form) or many nonpolio enteroviruses (sporadic form), pleurodynia is associated with an abrupt onset of unilateral or bilateral spasmodic pain over the lower ribs or upper abdomen. Associated symptoms include headache, fever, vomiting, myalgias, and abdominal and neck pain. Physical findings include fever, chest muscle tenderness, decreased thoracic excursion, and occasionally a friction rub. The chest radiograph is normal. Hematologic tests are not diagnostic. The illness generally lasts less than 1 week.

This is a disease of muscles, but the differential diagnosis includes bacterial pneumonia, bacterial and tuberculous effusion, and endemic fungal infections (all excluded radiographically and by auscultation), costochondritis (no fever or other symptoms), and a variety of abdominal problems, especially those causing diaphragmatic irritation. Epidemics of acute myalgia have also been reported due to HPeV type 3 in Japan in children and adults. Potent analgesic agents and chest splinting alleviate the pain.

Lugo D, Krogstad P: Enteroviruses in the early 21st century: new manifestations and challenges. Curr Opin Pediatr 2016 Feb;28(1):107–113. doi: 10.1097/MOP.0000000000000303 [PMID: 26709690].

RASHES (INCLUDING HAND-FOOT-&-MOUTH DISEASE)

The EV rash can be macular, maculopapular, urticarial, scarlatiniform, petechial, or vesicular. One of the most characteristic is that of hand-foot-and-mouth disease (caused by coxsackieviruses, especially types A5, A10, and A16), in which vesicles or red papules are found on the tongue, oral mucosa, hands, and feet. Often, they appear near the nails and on the heels and may last up to 1–2 weeks. Associated fever, sore throat, and malaise are mild. The rash may appear when fever abates, simulating roseola.

Cardiac Involvement

Myocarditis and pericarditis can be caused by a number of nonpolio enteroviruses, particularly type B coxsackieviruses. Most commonly, upper respiratory symptoms are followed by substernal pain, dyspnea, and exercise intolerance. A friction rub or gallop may be detected. Ultrasound will define ventricular dysfunction or pericardial effusion, and electrocardiography may show pericarditis or ventricular irritability. Creatine phosphokinase may be elevated and troponin (hs-TnT) is highly sensitive for acute myocarditis. The disease may be mild or fatal; most children recover completely. In infants, other organs may be involved at the same time; in older patients, cardiac disease is usually the sole manifestation (see Chapter 20 for therapy). Enteroviral RNA is present in cardiac tissue in some cases of dilated cardiomyopathy or myocarditis; the significance of this finding is unknown. Epidemics of EV 71 in Asia, as well as sporadic cases in the United States, are associated with severe left ventricular dysfunction and pulmonary edema following typical mucocutaneous manifestations of enterovirus infection. Enterovirus 71 also can cause isolated severe neurologic disease or neurologic disease in combination with myocardial disease.

Esposito S, Principi N: Hand, foot and mouth disease: current knowledge on clinical manifestations, epidemiology, aetiology and prevention. Eur J Clin Microbiol Infect Dis 2018 Mar;37(3):391–398 [PMID: 29411190].

Noor A, Krilov LR: Enterovirus infections. Pediatr Rev 2016;37(12):505–515 [PMID: 27909105].

Severe Neonatal Infection

Neonatal EV infection is usually systemic and severe in otherwise normal newborns. Clinical manifestations include fever, rash, pneumonitis, meningo-encephalitis, hepatitis, gastroenteritis, myocarditis, pancreatitis, and myositis. Transplacental infections present within 1 week of birth as sepsis with cyanosis, dyspnea, and seizures. Nosocomial outbreaks are less common. The differential diagnosis includes bacterial and herpes simplex infections, necrotizing enterocolitis, other causes of heart or liver failure, and metabolic diseases. Diagnosis is suggested by the finding of cerebrospinal fluid (CSF) mononuclear pleocytosis and detection of EV RNA in stool or pharynx, and confirmed by PCR in CSF, blood, or urine. IVIG is often administered, but its value is still uncertain. Some investigational antivirals (eg, pleconaril, pocapavir) have shown promise. Passively acquired maternal antibody may protect newborns from severe disease. Parechovirus infection of neonates is similar to EV but occurs in older neonates, with almost half of infected newborns requiring ICU management.

CENTRAL NERVOUS SYSTEM ILLNESSES

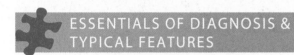

▶ Acute meningoencephalitis: headache, fever, meningismus.
▶ Asymmetrical, flaccid paralysis; muscle tenderness and hyperesthesia; intact sensation; late atrophy.

1. Poliomyelitis, Acute Flaccid Myelitis, & Acute Flaccid Paralysis

▶ General Considerations

Poliovirus infection is asymptomatic in 90%–95% of cases; presents as acute febrile illness in about 5% of cases or as aseptic meningitis, with or without paralysis, in 1%–3%. Polio has been eliminated from more than 99% of the world's population with the only endemic areas now in Nigeria, Pakistan, and Afghanistan. Most older children and adults are now protected due to vaccination or previous silent infection. Occasional cases in the United States have occurred in unvaccinated travelers to foreign countries or in populations with low polio vaccine coverage who come in contact with visitors from endemic areas. Vaccine-associated paralytic polio (VAPP) and vaccine-derived polio viruses (VDPV) are a consequence of oral polio vaccine (OPV) that has mutated and reverted to neurovirulent. The later has caused outbreaks of acute flaccid paralysis (AFP) similar to wild-type polio. Since 2000, inactivated poliovirus vaccine (IPV) has been the only polio vaccine in use in the United States, and since 2016, at least one dose of IPV along with bivalent OPV (types 1 and 3) is being given to children worldwide to prevent cVDPV (see Chapter 10). Other nonpolio EV can present as AFP, including EV71 in Asia and since 2014, EV-68 in Europe and the United States as acute flaccid myelitis (AFM).

▶ Clinical Findings

A. Symptoms and Signs

The initial symptoms of polioviruses as well as other neurotropic enteroviruses (EV71 and EV68) are fever, myalgia,

sore throat, and headache for 2–6 days. In less than 5% of infected children, symptom-free days are followed by recurrent fever and signs of aseptic meningitis: headache, nuchal rigidity, and nausea. Mild cases resolve completely. In 1%–2% of those infected, high fever, severe myalgia, and anxiety herald progression to loss of reflexes and subsequent acute flaccid asymmetrical paralysis. Proximal limb muscles are more often involved than distal, and lower limb involvement is more common than upper. Sensation remains intact, although hyperesthesia of skin overlying paralyzed muscles is common and pathognomonic.

Bulbar involvement affects swallowing, speech, and cardiorespiratory function and accounts for most deaths. Bladder distention and marked constipation characteristically accompany lower limb paralysis. Paralysis is usually complete by the time the temperature normalizes. Atrophy is usually apparent by 4–8 weeks. Most improvement of muscle paralysis occurs within 6 months.

B. Laboratory Findings

In patients with meningeal symptoms, the CSF shows a lymphocytic pleocytosis and a normal glucose with mildly elevated protein concentration. Poliovirus is easy to grow in cell culture and can be readily differentiated from other enteroviruses. It is rarely isolated from spinal fluid but is often present in the throat and stool for several weeks following infection. PCR is the method of choice for detection of polioviruses as well as other neurotropic enteroviruses.

▶ Differential Diagnosis

Aseptic meningitis due to poliovirus is indistinguishable from that due to other viruses. Paralytic disease in the United States is usually due to nonpolio enteroviruses (recently EV68). Polio and neurotropic EVs may resemble Guillain-Barré syndrome (minimal sensory loss, ascending symmetrical loss of function; minimal pleocytosis, high protein concentration in spinal fluid), polyneuritis (sensory loss), pseudoparalysis due to bone or joint problems (eg, trauma, infection), botulism, or tick paralysis. West Nile virus infection can present like AFP in children.

▶ Complications

Complications are the result of permanent destruction of anterior horn cells and paralysis. Respiratory, pharyngeal, bladder, and bowel malfunction are most critical. Death is usually the consequence of respiratory dysfunction. Limbs injured near the time of infection (by intramuscular injections, prior excessive prior, or trauma) tend to be most severely involved and have the worst prognosis for recovery (provocation paralysis).

Treatment & Prognosis

Therapy is supportive and although some antivirals are under investigation (eg, pocapavir), none are available for the treatment of enterovirus infections. Several potent antivirals are available to inhibit other positive-strand RNA viruses with a similar replication strategy. Bed rest, fever and pain control (heat therapy is helpful), and careful attention to progression of weakness (particularly of respiratory muscles) are important. Early or late corticosteroid treatment has been associated with increased mortality in children infected with EV-7, so they are not recommended. No intramuscular injections should be given during the acute phase. Intubation or tracheostomy for secretion control and ventilation, enteral feeding and catheter drainage of the bladder may be needed. Disease is worse in adults and pregnant women. Postpolio muscular atrophy occurs in 30%–40% of paralyzed limbs 20–30 years later, characterized by increasing weakness and fasciculations in previously affected, partially recovered limbs.

2. Nonpolio Viral Meningitis

Nonpolio enteroviruses cause over 80% of cases of aseptic meningitis at all ages, especially in the summer and fall. Nosocomial outbreaks also occur.

Clinical Findings

The usual EV incubation period is 4–6 days. Most EV infections are subclinical or not associated with central nervous system (CNS) symptoms; therefore, a history of a sick contact is unusual. Neonates may acquire infection from maternal blood, vaginal secretions, or feces at birth; occasionally the mother has had a febrile illness just prior to delivery.

A. Symptoms and Signs

Incidence is much greater in children younger than 1 year, and CSF pleocytosis is more frequent in very young children undergoing a septic work up during the summer and fall. Onset is usually acute with fever, marked irritability, and lethargy in infants. Older children also describe frontal headache, photophobia, and myalgia. Abdominal pain, diarrhea, and projectile vomiting may occur. The incidence of rash varies with the infecting strain. If rash occurs, it is usually seen after several days of illness and is diffuse, macular or maculopapular, occasionally petechial, but not purpuric. Oropharyngeal vesicles and rash on the palms and soles suggest an enterovirus. The anterior fontanel may be full and meningismus present. The illness may be biphasic, with nonspecific symptoms and signs preceding those related to the CNS. In older children, meningeal signs are more frequent, but seizures are unusual. Focal neurologic findings, which are

rare, should lead to a search for an alternative cause. Frank encephalitis, which is uncommon at any age, occurs most often in neonates. Because of the overall frequency of enteroviral disease in children, 5%–10% of all cases of encephalitis of proved viral origin are caused by enteroviruses. Enteroviruses tend to cause less severe encephalitis than other viruses. However, parechoviruses, which have recently been demonstrated to be a significant cause of aseptic meningitis, sometimes cause white matter changes.

Enterovirus 71 infections that begin with typical mucocutaneous manifestations of enteroviruses can be complicated by severe brainstem encephalitis. Outbreaks of respiratory disease with meningitis and acute paralysis due to EV68 have occurred in western United States and Europe. Enterovirus 70 outbreaks are characterized by hemorrhagic conjunctivitis together with paralytic poliomyelitis.

B. Laboratory Findings

Blood leukocyte counts are often normal. The spinal fluid leukocyte count is 100–1000/μL with polymorphonuclear cells predominating early and shifting to mononuclear cells within 8–36 hours. In about 95% of cases, spinal fluid parameters include a total leukocyte count less than 3000/μL, protein less than 80 mg/dL, and glucose more than 60% of serum values. Marked deviation from any of these findings should prompt consideration of another diagnosis (see following section).

Culture of CSF may yield an enterovirus within a few days (< 70%), but EV PCR is the most useful diagnostic method in many centers (sensitivity > 90%) and can give an answer within few hours. Parechoviruses will be detected by most PCR methods, but will be identified as "enterovirus." Virus may be detected even with no CSF pleocytosis. Detection of an enterovirus from throat or stool suggests, but does not prove, enteroviral meningitis. Vaccine-derived poliovirus present in feces in infants being evaluated for aseptic meningitis may confuse the diagnosis, but history of travel or exposure to OPV should help.

C. Imaging

Cerebral imaging is not often indicated; if done, it is usually normal. Subdural effusions, infarcts, edema, or focal abnormalities seen in bacterial meningitis are absent except for the rare case of focal encephalitis.

Differential Diagnosis

Enteroviral infections account for up to 90% of the cases of aseptic meningitis in which an etiologic agent is identified, especially in the summer and fall. Other causative viruses are mosquito-borne (flavivirus, bunyavirus) and are part of the investigation of encephalitis, but many of them are more likely to cause isolated meningitis. Primary herpes simplex infection can cause aseptic meningitis in adolescents who have a genital herpes infection. In neonates, early herpes simplex meningoencephalitis may mimic enteroviral disease (see section Infections Due to Herpesviruses) and if suspected urgent antiviral therapy is recommended. Lymphocytic choriomeningitis virus causes meningitis in children in contact with rodents (pet or environmental exposure). Meningitis occurs in some patients at the time of infection with human immunodeficiency virus (HIV).

Other causes of aseptic meningitis that may resemble enteroviral infection include partially treated bacterial meningitis (recent antibiotic treatment, CSF parameters resembling those seen in bacterial disease and bacterial antigen sometimes present); bacterial parameningeal foci such as brain abscess, subdural empyema, mastoiditis (predisposing factors, lower CSF glucose level, focal neurologic signs, and characteristic imaging); tumors or cysts (malignant cells on cytologic examination, higher protein or lower glucose levels in CSF); trauma (presence, without exception, of crenated red blood cells and fail to clear); tuberculous or fungal meningitis (see Chapters 42 and 43); cysticercosis; para and postinfectious encephalopathies (*M pneumoniae*, cat-scratch disease, influenza; leptospirosis; rickettsial diseases including Lyme; and acute demyelinating encephalomyelitis.

▶ Prevention & Treatment

No specific antiviral therapy exists. Infants are usually hospitalized, isolated, and treated with fluids and antipyretics. Moderately to severely ill infants are given empiric antibiotics for bacterial pathogens until cultures, or PCR, are negative. In children and infants at low risk of serious bacterial infection, antibiotics may be withheld and the child observed until PCR results are available. The illness usually lasts less than 1 week. Strong analgesics may be needed. With clinical deterioration, repeat lumbar puncture, cerebral imaging, neurologic consultation, and more aggressive diagnostic tests should be considered. Herpesvirus encephalitis is an important consideration in such cases, particularly in infants younger than 1 month, and often warrants empiric acyclovir until HSV infection can be ruled out.

▶ Prognosis

In general, enteroviral meningitis has no significant short-term neurologic or developmental sequelae. Developmental delay may follow severe neonatal infections. Unlike mumps, enterovirus infections rarely cause hearing loss.

de Crom SC, Rossen JW, van Furth AM, Obihara CC: Enterovirus and parechovirus infection in children: a brief overview. Eur J Pediatr 2016;175(8):1023–1029 [PMID: 27156106].

Messacar K, Abzug MJ, Dominguez SR: 2014 outbreak of enterovirus D68 in North America. J Med Virol 2016 May;88(5):739–745. doi: 10.1002/jmv.24410 [PMID: 26489019].

Messacar K et al: Enterovirus D68 and acute flaccid myelitis-evaluating the evidence for causality. Lancet Infect Dis 2018 Aug;18(8):e239–e247 [PMID: 29482893].

▼ INFECTIONS DUE TO HERPESVIRUSES

HERPES SIMPLEX INFECTIONS

ESSENTIALS OF DIAGNOSIS & TYPICAL FEATURES

▶ Grouped vesicles on an erythematous base, typically in or around the mouth or genitals.

▶ Fever, malaise, and tender regional adenopathy common with primary infection.

▶ Recurrent episodes.

▶ General Considerations

There are two types of herpes simplex virus (HSV). Type 1 (HSV-1) causes most cases of oral, perioral, skin, and cerebral disease in children, while type 2 (HSV-2) is now equally as common as HSV-1 as cause of genital and congenital HSV infections. Latent infection is routinely established in sensory ganglia during primary infection. Recurrences, due to reactivation of latent HSV, may be spontaneous or induced by external events (eg, fever, menstruation, or sunlight) or immunosuppression. Transmission is by direct contact with infected secretions.

Primary infection with HSV-1 often occurs early in childhood by contact with infected oral secretions of playmates or caretakers, with a second peak of infection later in life as a sexually transmitted disease. Primary infection with HSV-1 is subclinical in 80% of cases and causes gingivostomatitis or genital disease in the remainder. HSV-2, which is transmitted sexually, is also subclinical (65%) or produces mild, nonspecific symptoms. The source of primary infection is usually an asymptomatic excreter. Most previously infected individuals shed HSV at irregular intervals. At any one time (point prevalence), more than 5% of seropositive adults excrete HSV-1 in the saliva; the percentage is higher in recently infected children, and detection of viral DNA exceeds 12%. HSV-2 shedding in genital secretions occurs with a similar or higher point prevalence exceeding 15%, depending on the method of detection (viral isolation vs PCR) and the interval since the initial infection. A history of contact with clinically apparent HSV lesions is unusual. Infection with one type of HSV may prevent or attenuate clinically apparent infection with the other type, but individuals can be infected at different times with both HSV-1 and HSV-2.

▶ Clinical Findings

A. Symptoms and Signs

1. Gingivostomatitis—High fever, irritability, and drooling occur in infants. Multiple oral ulcers are seen on the tongue and on the buccal and gingival mucosa, occasionally extending to the pharynx. Pharyngeal ulcers may predominate in older children and adolescents. Diffusely swollen red gums that are friable and bleed easily are typical. Cervical nodes are swollen and tender. Duration is 7–14 days. Herpangina, aphthous stomatitis, thrush, and Vincent angina should be excluded.

2. Vulvovaginitis or urethritis (See Chapter 44)—Genital herpes (especially HSV-2) in a prepubertal child should suggest sexual abuse. In sexually adolescents, active vesicles or painful ulcers on the vulva, vagina, or penis and tender adenopathy are typical. Systemic symptoms (fever, flu-like illness, myalgia) are common with the initial episode. Painful urination is frequent, especially in females. Primary infection lasts 10–14 days before healing. Lesions may resemble trauma, syphilis (ulcers are painless), or chancroid (ulcers are painful and nodes are erythematous and fluctuant) in the adolescent, and bullous impetigo or severe chemical irritation in younger children.

3. Cutaneous infections—Direct inoculation onto cuts or abrasions may produce localized vesicles or ulcers. A deep HSV infection on the finger (called herpetic whitlow) may be mistaken for a bacterial felon or paronychia; surgical drainage is of no value and is contraindicated. HSV infection of eczematous skin may result in extensive areas of vesicles and shallow ulcers (eczema herpeticum), which may be mistaken for impetigo or varicella.

4. Recurrent mucocutaneous infection—Recurrent oral shedding is asymptomatic. Recurrent perioral lesions (sometimes perinasal) often begin with a prodrome of tingling or burning limited to the vermillion border, followed by vesiculation, scabbing, and crusting around the lips over 3–5 days. Recurrent intraoral lesions are rare. Fever, adenopathy, and other symptoms are absent. Recurrent cutaneous herpes most closely resembles impetigo, but the latter is often outside the perinasal and perioral region, recurs infrequently in the same area of skin, responds to antibiotics, yields a positive result on Gram stain, and *Streptococcus pyogenes* or *Staphylococcus aureus* can be isolated. Recurrent genital disease is common after the initial infection with HSV-2. Recurrent infection is shorter (5–7 days) and milder (mean, four lesions) than primary infection and is not associated with systemic symptoms. Recurrent genital disease, which may also recur on the thighs and buttocks, is also preceded by a cutaneous sensory prodrome. Recurrence of HSV-1 in the genital region is much less frequent than are HSV-2 recurrences.

5. Keratoconjunctivitis—Keratoconjunctivitis may be part of a primary infection due to spread from infected saliva. Most cases are caused by reactivation of virus latent in the ciliary ganglion. Keratoconjunctivitis produces photophobia, pain, and conjunctival irritation. Dendritic corneal ulcers may be demonstrable with fluorescein staining. Stromal invasion may occur. Corticosteroids should never be used for unilateral keratitis without ophthalmologic consultation. Other causes of these symptoms include trauma, bacterial infections, and other viral infections (especially adenovirus if pharyngitis is present; bilateral involvement makes HSV unlikely) (see Chapter 16).

6. Encephalitis—Although unusual in infants outside the neonatal period, encephalitis may occur at any age, usually without cutaneous herpes lesions. In older children, HSV encephalitis can follow a primary infection, but usually represents reactivation of latent virus. HSV is the most common identifiable cause of sporadic severe encephalitis. Diagnosis of HSV encephalitis is very important because it can be treated with specific antiviral therapy. Acute onset is associated with fever, headache, behavioral changes, and focal neurologic deficits and/or focal seizures. Mononuclear pleocytosis is typically present along with an elevated protein concentration. In older children, hypodense areas with a medial and inferior temporal lobe predilection are seen on CT scan, especially after 3–5 days, but the findings in infants may be more diffuse. Magnetic resonance imaging (MRI) is more sensitive and is positive sooner. Periodic focal epileptiform discharges are seen on electroencephalograms, but are not diagnostic of HSV infection. Viral cultures of CSF are rarely positive. The PCR assay to detect HSV DNA in CSF is a sensitive and specific rapid test. Without early antiviral therapy, the prognosis is poor. The differential diagnosis includes mosquito-borne and other viral encephalitides, parainfectious and postinfectious encephalopathy, brain abscess, acute demyelinating syndromes, and bacterial meningoencephalitis.

7. Neonatal infections—Infection is occasionally acquired by ascending spread prior to delivery (< 5% of cases), but most often occurs at the time of vaginal delivery from a mother with genital infection. Eight to fifteen percent of HSV-2–seropositive pregnant women at delivery have HSV-2 detected by PCR in the genital tract. However, in most cases this represents reactivation of infection acquired in the distant past. HSV-1 has now become a common cause of neonatal HSV infection. Neonatal infection is rarely acquired from mothers with reactivation disease, whereas it is frequently acquired during delivery of mothers with current or recent primary infection. This is because transplacentally acquired antibody is usually protective. Occasionally, the infection is acquired in the postpartum period from oral secretions of family members or hospital personnel. A history of genital herpes in the mother is often absent.

Within a few days and up to 6 weeks (most often within 4 weeks), skin vesicles appear (especially at sites of trauma, such as where scalp monitors were placed). Some infants (45%) have infection limited to the skin, eye, or mouth. Other infants are acutely ill, presenting with jaundice, shock, bleeding, or respiratory distress (25%). Some infants appear well initially, but dissemination of the infection to the brain or other organs becomes evident during the ensuing week. HSV infection (and empiric therapy) should be strongly considered in newborns with the sepsis syndrome that is unresponsive to antibiotic therapy and has negative bacterial cultures. A mononuclear pleocytosis in the CSF and suggestive skin lesions support this, although skin lesions may be absent at the time of presentation or may never develop. Some infected infants exhibit only neurologic symptoms at 2–3 weeks after delivery: apnea, lethargy, fever, poor feeding, or persistent seizures. The brain infection in these children is often diffuse and is best diagnosed by MRI. The skin lesions may resemble impetigo, bacterial scalp abscesses, or miliaria. Skin lesions may recur over weeks or months after recovery from the acute illness. Progressive culture-negative pneumonitis is another manifestation of neonatal HSV. Most cases of neonatal HSV infection are acquired from mothers with undiagnosed genital herpes, most of whom acquired the infection during the pregnancy—especially near term.

B. Laboratory Findings

Abnormalities in platelets, clotting factors, and liver function tests are often present in infants with multisystem disease. Lymphocytic pleocytosis and elevated CSF protein indicates viral meningitis or encephalitis. Virus may be cultured from infected epithelial sites (vesicles, ulcers, or conjunctival scrapings). Viral cultures of CSF yield positive results in about 50% of neonatal cases, but are uncommon in older children. HSV will be detected within 2 days by rapid tissue culture methods, but PCR is the preferred diagnostic method for all specimens. A positive test from skin, throat, eye, or stool of a newborn is diagnostic. Vaginal culture of the mother may offer circumstantial evidence for the diagnosis, but may be negative.

Rapid diagnostic tests include immunofluorescent stains or ELISA to detect viral antigen in skin or mucosal scrapings. The PCR assay for HSV DNA is positive (> 95%) in the CSF when there is brain involvement. HSV DNA is often present in the blood of patients with multisystem disease. Typing of genital HSV isolates from adolescents has prognostic value, since HSV-1 genital infection recurs much less frequently than genital HSV-2 infection.

▶ Complications, Sequelae, & Prognosis

Gingivostomatitis may result in dehydration due to dysphagia; severe chronic oral disease and esophageal involvement may occur in immunosuppressed patients. Primary vulvovaginitis may be associated with aseptic meningitis,

paresthesias, autonomic dysfunction due to neuritis (urinary retention, constipation), and secondary candidal infection. HIV transmission is facilitated from individuals who are also seropositive for HSV infection, and HIV acquisition is enhanced in HSV-infected contacts. Extensive cutaneous disease (as in eczema) may be associated with dissemination and bacterial superinfection. Keratitis may result in corneal opacification. Untreated encephalitis is fatal in 70% of patients and causes severe damage in most of the remainder. Even with early acyclovir treatment, 20% of patients die and 40% are neurologically impaired.

Disseminated neonatal infection is fatal for 30% of neonates in spite of therapy, and 20% of survivors are often impaired. Treated infants with CNS infection (30% of cases) have a 5% mortality and 70% of survivors are impaired; treated neonates with infection limited to skin, eye, and mouth survive without sequelae.

▶ Treatment

A. Specific Measures

HSV is sensitive to antiviral therapy.

1. Topical antivirals—Antiviral agents are effective for corneal disease and include 1% trifluridine and 0.15% ganciclovir (1–2 drops five times daily). These agents should be used with the guidance of an ophthalmologist and concurrently with oral antiviral therapy.

2. Mucocutaneous HSV infections—These infections respond to administration of oral nucleoside analogues (acyclovir, valacyclovir, or famciclovir). The main indications are severe genital HSV infection in adolescents (see Chapter 44; acyclovir, 400 mg three times daily for 7–10 days) and severe gingivostomatitis in young children. Antiviral therapy is beneficial for primary disease when begun early. Recurrent disease rarely requires therapy. Frequent genital recurrences may be suppressed by oral administration of nucleoside analogues (acyclovir, 400 mg twice daily), but this approach should be used sparingly. Other forms of severe cutaneous disease, such as eczema herpeticum, respond to antivirals. Intravenous acyclovir may be required when disease is extensive in immunocompromised children (10–15 mg/kg or 500 mg/m² every 8 hours for 14–21 days). Oral acyclovir, which is available in suspension, is also used within 72–96 hours for severe primary gingivostomatitis in immunocompetent young children (20 mg/kg per dose [maximum of 400 mg per dose] four times a day for 7 days). Antiviral therapy does not alter the incidence or severity of subsequent recurrences of oral or genital infection. Development of resistance to antivirals, which is very rare after treating immunocompetent patients, occurs in immunocompromised patients who receive frequent and prolonged therapy.

3. Encephalitis—Treatment consists of intravenous acyclovir, 20 mg/kg (500 mg/m²) every 8 hours for 21 days.

4. Neonatal infection—Newborns receive intravenous acyclovir, 20 mg/kg every 8 hours for 21 days (14 days if infection is limited to skin, eye, or mouth). Therapy should not be discontinued unless a repeat CSF HSV PCR assay is negative near the end of treatment. The outcome at 1 year is improved in infants that receive oral acyclovir (300 mg/m²/dose three times daily) for 6 months after completion of IV therapy.

B. General Measures

1. Gingivostomatitis—Gingivostomatitis is treated with pain relief and temperature control measures. Maintaining hydration is important because of the long duration of illness (7–14 days). Topical anesthetic agents (eg, viscous lidocaine or an equal mixture of kaolin–attapulgite [Kaopectate], diphenhydramine, and viscous lidocaine) may be used as a mouthwash for older children who will not swallow it; ingested lidocaine may be toxic to infants or may lead to aspiration. Antiviral therapy is indicated in normal hosts with severe disease.

2. Genital infections—Genital infections may require pain relief, assistance with voiding (warm baths, topical anesthetics, rarely catheterization), and psychological support. Lesions should be kept clean; drying may shorten the duration of symptoms. Sexual contact should be avoided during the interval from prodrome to crusting stages. Because of the frequency of asymptomatic shedding, the only effective way to prevent sexual transmission is the use of condoms. Candidal superinfection occurs in 10% of women with primary genital infections.

3. Cutaneous lesions—Skin lesions should be kept clean, dry, and covered if possible to prevent spread. Systemic analgesics may be helpful. Secondary bacterial infection is uncommon in patients with lesions on the mucosa or involving small areas, and with recurrences. Secondary infection should be considered and treated if necessary in patients with more extensive lesions.

4. Recurrent cutaneous disease—Recurrent disease is usually the cause of lesions. Sun block lip balm helps prevent labial recurrences that follow intense sun exposure. There is no evidence that the many popular topical or vitamin therapies are efficacious.

5. Keratoconjunctivitis—An ophthalmologist should be consulted regarding the use of cycloplegics, anti-inflammatory agents, local debridement, and other therapies.

6. Encephalitis—Extensive support will be required for obtunded or comatose patients. Rehabilitation and psychological support are often needed for survivors.

7. Neonatal infection—Infected infants should be isolated and given acyclovir. Cesarean delivery is indicated if the mother has obvious cervical or vaginal lesions, especially if these represent primary infection (35%–50% transmission rate). With infants born vaginally to mothers who have active lesions of recurrent genital herpes, appropriate cultures and PCR should be obtained at 24 hours after birth, and the infant evaluated thoroughly for possible HSV infection. If the results are positive or the infant has suggestive signs or symptoms preemptive therapy should be started. Treatment is given to infants whose culture results are positive or who appear ill. Infants born to mothers with obvious primary genital herpes should also be evaluated, but should then receive therapy before the culture or PCR results are known. For women with a history of genital herpes infection, but no genital lesions, vaginal delivery with peripartum cultures of maternal cervix is the standard. Clinical follow-up of the newborn is recommended when maternal culture results are positive. Repeated cervical cultures during pregnancy are not useful.

A challenging problem is the newborn, especially in the first 3 weeks of life, that presents with fever (or hypothermia) and a sepsis-like picture. This is further confounded in the late summer by the existence of circulating enteroviruses. These infants should be considered for empiric acyclovir therapy, pending results of PCR studies, given the poor outcome of disseminated herpes in the newborn. The index of suspicion is increased when there is a CSF pleocytosis, elevated hepatic transaminase levels, a very ill-appearing infant, rash, or respiratory distress.

Gnann JW Jr, Whitely RJ: Genital herpes. N Eng J Med 2016;375:666 [PMID: 27532632].

James SH, Kimberlin DW: Neonatal herpes simplex virus infection: epidemiology and treatment. Clin Perinatol 2015;427:4 [PMID: 25677996].

VARICELLA & HERPES ZOSTER

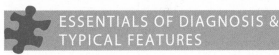

ESSENTIALS OF DIAGNOSIS & TYPICAL FEATURES

▶ Varicella (chickenpox):
- Follows exposure to varicella or herpes zoster 10–21 days previously; no prior history of varicella.
- Widely scattered red macules and papules concentrated on the face and trunk, rapidly progressing to clear vesicles on an erythematous base, pustules, and then crusts, over 5–6 days.
- Variable fever and nonspecific systemic symptoms.

▶ Herpes zoster (shingles):
- History of varicella.
- Dermatomal paresthesias and pain prior to eruption (more common in older children).
- Dermatomal distribution of grouped vesicles on an erythematous base; often accompanied by pain.

General Considerations

Primary infection with varicella-zoster virus results in vari-cella, which generally confers lifelong immunity, but the virus remains latent lifelong in sensory ganglia. Herpes zoster, which represents reactivation of this latent virus, occurs in 30% of individuals at some time in their life. The incidence of herpes zoster is highest in elderly individuals and in immunosuppressed patients, but herpes zoster occurs in immunocompetent children. Spread of varicella from a close contact is mainly by respiratory droplets or aerosols (occasionally direct contact) from vesicles or pustules, with an 85% infection rate in susceptible persons. Over 95% of young adults with a history of varicella are immune, as is 90% of native-born Americans who are unaware of having had varicella. Many individuals from tropical or subtropi-cal regions fail to develop varicella in their childhood and remain susceptible through early adulthood. Humans are the only reservoir.

Clinical Findings

Exposure to varicella or herpes zoster has usually occurred 14–16 days previously (range, 10–21 days). Contact may not be recognized, since the index case of varicella is infec-tious 1–2 days before rash appears. A 1- to 3-day prodrome of fever, malaise, respiratory symptoms, and headache may occur, especially in older children. The unilateral, dermato-mal vesicular rash and pain of herpes zoster is very distinc-tive. The preeruptive pain of herpes zoster may last several days and be mistaken for other illnesses.

A. Symptoms and Signs

1. Varicella—The usual case consists of mild systemic symptoms followed by crops of red macules that rap-idly become small vesicles with surrounding erythema (described as a "dew drop on a rose petal"), form pustules, become crusted, and then scab. Pruritus may be intense; scarring occurs, but it is not common. The rash appears predominantly on the trunk and face. Lesions occur in the scalp, and sometimes in the nose, mouth (where they are nonspecific ulcers), conjunctiva, and vagina. The magni-tude of systemic symptoms usually parallels skin involve-ment. Up to five crops of lesions may be seen. New crops stop forming after 5–7 days. Pruritus is often intense. If varicella occurs in the first few months of life (except for the early postpartum period), it is often mild as a result of transplacentally acquired maternal antibody. Once crust-ing begins, the patient is no longer contagious. A modified form of varicella occurs in about 15% of vaccinated chil-dren exposed to varicella, in spite of receiving a single dose of varicella vaccine. This is usually much milder than typi-cal varicella, with fewer lesions that heal rapidly. Cases of modified varicella are contagious.

2. Herpes zoster (shingles)—This eruption involves a single dermatome (thus unilateral and does not cross the midline), usually truncal or cranial; occasionally a contigu-ous dermatome is involved. Especially in older children this is preceded by neuropathic pain or itching in the same area (designated the "prodrome"). Ophthalmic zoster may be associated with corneal involvement. The closely grouped vesicles, which resemble a localized version of varicella or herpes simplex, often coalesce. Crusting occurs in 7–10 days. Postherpetic neuralgia is rare in children. Herpes zoster is a common problem in HIV-infected or other immunocom-promised children, and is also common in children who had varicella in early infancy (< 1–2 years old) or whose mothers had varicella during pregnancy. Herpes zoster can occur infrequently in children who received the varicella vaccine.

B. Laboratory Findings

Leukocyte counts are normal or low. Leukocytosis sug-gests secondary bacterial infection. Vesicular fluid or a scab can be used to identify the virus using PCR as the method of choice. DFA assay is less sensitive. Serum ami-notransferase levels may be modestly elevated during typical varicella.

C. Imaging

Varicella pneumonia classically produces numerous bilat-eral nodular densities and hyperinflation. This is very rare in immunocompetent children, but is seen more frequently in adults and immunocompromised children.

Differential Diagnosis

Varicella is usually distinctive. Similar rashes include those of coxsackievirus infection (fewer lesions, lack of crusting), impetigo (fewer lesions, smaller area, no classic vesicles, positive Gram stain, perioral or peripheral lesions), papu-lar urticaria (insect bite history, nonvesicular rash), scabies (burrows, no typical vesicles, failure to resolve), paraparaso-sis (rare in children < 10 years, chronic or recurrent, often a history of prior varicella), rickettsial pox (eschar where the mite bites, smaller lesions, no crusting), dermatitis herpeti-formis (chronic, urticaria, residual pigmentation), and fol-liculitis. Herpes zoster is sometimes confused with a linear eruption of herpes simplex or a contact dermatitis.

Complications & Sequelae

A. Varicella

Secondary bacterial infection with staphylococci or group A streptococci is most common, presenting as impetigo, cel-lulitis or fasciitis, abscesses, scarlet fever, or sepsis. Bacterial superinfection occurs in 2%–3% of children with varicella.

Before a vaccine became available, hospitalization rates associated with varicella were 1:750–1:1000 cases in children and 10-fold higher in adults.

Protracted vomiting or a change in sensorium suggests Reye syndrome or encephalitis. Because Reye syndrome usually occurs in patients who are also receiving salicylates, these should be avoided in patients with varicella. Encephalitis occurs in less than 0.1% of cases, usually in the first week of illness, and is usually limited to cerebellitis with ataxia, which resolves completely. Diffuse encephalitis can be severe.

Varicella pneumonia usually afflicts immunocompromised children (especially those receiving high doses of corticosteroids or chemotherapy) and adults. Cough, dyspnea, tachypnea, rales, and cyanosis occur several days after onset of rash. New lesions may erupt for an extended period, and varicella may be life-threatening in immunosuppressed patients. In addition to pneumonitis, their disease may be complicated by hepatitis and encephalitis. The acute illness in these children often begins with unexplained severe abdominal pain. Varicella exposure in varicella-naïve severely immunocompromised children must be evaluated immediately for postexposure prophylaxis (see Chapter 10).

Hemorrhagic varicella lesions may be seen without other complications. This is most often caused by autoimmune thrombocytopenia, but hemorrhagic lesions can occasionally represent idiopathic disseminated intravascular coagulation (purpura fulminans).

Neonates born to mothers who develop varicella from 5 days before to 2 days after delivery are at high risk for severe or fatal (5%) disease and must be given varicella-zoster immunoglobulin (VariZIG) and followed closely (see Chapter 10).

Varicella occurring during the first 20 weeks of pregnancy may cause (2% incidence) congenital infection associated with cicatricial skin lesions, associated limb anomalies, eye abnormalities, and cortical atrophy.

Unusual complications of varicella include optic neuritis, myocarditis, transverse myelitis, orchitis, and arthritis.

B. Herpes Zoster

Complications of herpes zoster include secondary bacterial infection, motor or cranial nerve paralysis, meningitis, encephalitis, keratitis and other ocular complications, and dissemination in immunosuppressed patients. These complications are rare in immunocompetent children. Postherpetic neuralgia occurs in immunocompromised children, but is rare in immunocompetent children.

▶ Prevention

Varicella-specific hyperimmune globulin is available for postexposure prevention of varicella in high-risk susceptible persons (see Chapter 10). In immunocompetent children, postexposure prophylaxis with acyclovir is effective when it is started at 7–9 days after exposure and is continued for 7 days, as is varicella vaccine when given within 3–5 days of the exposure.

Two doses of the live attenuated varicella vaccine provide close to 92% protection and are now part of routine childhood immunization. Catch-up immunization is recommended for all other susceptible children and adults.

▶ Treatment

A. General Measures

Supportive measures include maintenance of hydration, administration of acetaminophen for discomfort, cool soaks or antipruritics for itching (diphenhydramine, 1.25 mg/kg every 6 hours, or hydroxyzine, 0.5 mg/kg every 6 hours), and observance of general hygiene measures (keep nails trimmed and skin clean). Care must be taken to avoid overdosage with antihistaminic agents. Topical or systemic antibiotics may be needed for bacterial superinfection.

B. Specific Measures

Acyclovir is the preferred drug for varicella and herpes zoster infections. Recommended parenteral acyclovir dosage for severe disease is 10 mg/kg (500 mg/m^2) intravenously every 8 hours, each dose infused over 1 hour, for 7–10 days. Parenteral therapy should be started early in immunocompromised patients or high-risk infected neonates. Hyperimmune globulin is of no value for established disease. The effect of oral acyclovir (80 mg/kg/day, divided in four doses) on varicella in immunocompetent children is modestly beneficial and nontoxic, but only when administered within 24 hours after the onset of varicella. Valacyclovir (20 mg/kg [maximum 1 g] PO TID) may be preferable (≥ 2 years). Oral acyclovir should be used selectively in immunocompetent children. For example, when a significant concomitant or underlying illness is present or possibly when the index case is a sibling or when the patient is an adolescent, both of which are associated with more severe disease, and in children with a significant underlying chronic illness. Valacyclovir and famciclovir are superior antiviral agents because of better absorption; only acyclovir is available as a pediatric suspension. Herpes zoster in an immunocompromised child should be treated with intravenous acyclovir when it is severe, but oral valacyclovir or famciclovir can be used in immunocompromised children when the nature of the underlying illness and the immune status support this decision.

▶ Prognosis

Except for secondary bacterial infections, serious complications are rare and recovery complete in immunocompetent hosts. Complications are common in severely immune compromised children unless treated promptly.

Leung J, Harpaz R: Impact of the maturing varicella vaccination program on varicella and related outcomes in the United States: 1994–2012. J Ped Infect Dis Soc 2016;5:395 [PMID: 26407276].

Lopez AS, Zhang J, Marin M: Epidemiology of varicella during the 2-dose vaccination program—United States, 2005–2014. MMWR Morb Mortal Wkly Rep 2016;65:902 [PMID: 27584717].

ROSEOLA INFANTUM (EXANTHEM SUBITUM)

ESSENTIALS OF DIAGNOSIS & TYPICAL FEATURES

▶ High fever in a child aged 6–36 months.

▶ Minimal toxicity.

▶ Rose-pink maculopapular rash appears when fever subsides.

▶ General Considerations

Roseola infantum (also called exanthem subitum) is a benign illness caused by HHV-6 or HHV-7. HHV-6 is a major cause of acute febrile illness in young children. Its significance is that it may be confused with more serious causes of high fever and its role in inciting febrile seizures.

▶ Clinical Findings

The most prominent historical feature is the abrupt onset of fever, often reaching greater than 39.5°C, and lasting for 3–7 days (mean, 4 days; 15% ≥ 6 days) in an otherwise mildly ill child. The fever then ceases abruptly, and a characteristic rash may appear. Roseola occurs predominantly in children aged 6 months to 3 years, with 90% of cases occurring before the second year. HHV-7 infection tends to occur somewhat later in childhood. These viruses are the most common recognized cause of fever and rash in this age group and are responsible for 20% of emergency department visits by children aged 6–12 months.

A. Symptoms and Signs

Mild lethargy and irritability may be present, but generally there is dissociation between other systemic symptoms and the febrile course. The pharynx, tonsils, and tympanic membranes may be injected. Conjunctivitis and pharyngeal exudate are notably absent. Diarrhea and vomiting occur in one-third of patients. Adenopathy of the head (especially postoccipital) and neck often occurs. The anterior fontanelle is bulging in one-quarter of HHV-6–infected infants. If rash appears (20%–30% incidence), it coincides with lysis of fever and begins on the trunk and spreads to the face, neck, and extremities. Rose-pink macules or maculopapules, 2–3 mm in diameter, are nonpruritic, tend to coalesce, and disappear in 1–2 days without pigmentation or desquamation. Rash may occur without fever.

B. Laboratory Findings

Leukopenia and lymphocytopenia are present early. Laboratory evidence of hepatitis occurs in some patients, especially adults. Detection of HHV-6 and HHV-7 by PCR is available but rarely influences clinical management except in immunocompromised children. Some newly available multiplex CSF PCR includes HHV-6, but given the chromosomal integration of the virus, a positive result should be interpreted with caution in the presence of pleocytosis.

▶ Differential Diagnosis

The initial high fever may require exclusion of serious bacterial infection. The relative well-being of most children and the typical course and rash soon clarify the diagnosis. These distinguish roseola from measles, rubella, adenoviruses, enteroviruses, drug reactions, and scarlet fever. In a child with febrile seizures, exclusion of bacterial meningitis is important. The CSF is normal in children with roseola. In children who receive antibiotics or other medication at the beginning of the fever, the rash may be attributed incorrectly to drug allergy.

▶ Complications & Sequelae

Febrile seizures occur in up to 10% of patients (even higher percentages in those with HHV-7 infections); especially if less than 24 months old. There is evidence that HHV-6 can directly infect the CNS, causing meningoencephalitis. Multiorgan disease (pneumonia, hepatitis, bone marrow suppression, encephalitis) may occur in immunocompromised patients.

▶ Treatment & Prognosis

Fever is managed readily with acetaminophen and sponge baths. Fever control should be a major consideration in children with a history of febrile seizures. Roseola infantum is otherwise entirely benign. Systemic infection in immunocompromised children is treated with antiviral agents.

Mohammadpour Touserkani F, Gaínza-Lein M, Jafarpour S, Brinegar K, Kapur K, Loddenkemper T: HHV-6 and seizure: a systematic review and meta-analysis. J Med Virol 2017;89(1):161–169 [PMID: 27272972].

Tesini BL, Epstein LG, Casarti TM: Clinical impact of primary infection with roseola viruses. Curr Opin Virol 2014;9:91 [PMID: 25462439].

CYTOMEGALOVIRUS INFECTIONS

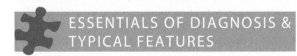

ESSENTIALS OF DIAGNOSIS & TYPICAL FEATURES

▶ Primary infection:
  • Asymptomatic or minor illness in young children.
  • Mononucleosis-like syndrome without pharyngitis in adolescents.
▶ Congenital infection:
  • Intrauterine growth retardation.
  • Microcephaly with intracerebral calcifications and seizures.
  • Retinitis and encephalitis.
  • Hepatosplenomegaly with thrombocytopenia.
  • "Blueberry muffin" small purpuric spots rash.
  • Sensorineural deafness.
▶ Immunocompromised hosts:
  • Retinitis and encephalitis.
  • Pneumonitis, enteritis, and hepatitis.
  • Bone marrow suppression.

▶ General Considerations

Cytomegalovirus (CMV) is a ubiquitous herpesvirus transmitted by many routes. It can be acquired in utero following maternal viremia or postpartum from birth canal secretions or maternal milk. Young children are infected by the saliva of playmates; older individuals are infected by sexual partners (eg, from saliva, vaginal secretions, or semen). Transfused blood products and transplanted organs can be a source of CMV infection. Clinical illness is determined largely by the patient's immune competence. Immunocompetent individuals usually develop a mild self-limited illness, whereas immunocompromised children can develop severe, progressive, often multiorgan disease. In utero infection can be teratogenic.

1. In Utero Cytomegalovirus Infection

Approximately 0.5%–1.5% of children are born with CMV infections acquired during maternal viremia. CMV infection is asymptomatic in over 90% of these children, who are usually born to mothers who had experienced reactivation of latent CMV infection during the pregnancy. Symptomatic infection occurs predominantly in infants born to mothers with primary CMV infection, but can also result from reinfection during pregnancy. Even when exposed to a primary maternal infection, less than 50% of fetuses are infected, and in only 10% of those infants is the infection symptomatic at birth. Primary infection in the first half of pregnancy poses the greatest risk for severe fetal damage.

▶ Clinical Findings

A. Symptoms and Signs

Severely affected infants are born ill; they are often small for gestational age, floppy, and lethargic. They feed poorly and have poor temperature control. Hepatosplenomegaly, jaundice, petechiae, seizures, and microcephaly are common. Characteristic signs are a distinctive chorioretinitis and periventricular calcification. A purpuric rash (so-called "blueberry muffin") similar to that seen with congenital rubella may be present, secondary to extramedullary hematopoiesis. The mortality rate is 10%–20%. Survivors usually have significant sequelae, especially mental retardation, neurologic deficits, retinopathy, and hearing loss. Isolated hepatosplenomegaly or thrombocytopenia may occur. Even mildly affected children may subsequently manifest mental retardation and psychomotor delay. Most infected infants (90%) are born to mothers with preexisting immunity who experienced a reactivation of latent CMV or reinfection during pregnancy. These children have no clinical manifestations at birth. Of these, 10%–15% develop sensorineural hearing loss, which is often bilateral and may appear several years after birth.

B. Laboratory Findings

In severely ill infants, anemia, thrombocytopenia, hyperbilirubinemia, and elevated aminotransferase levels are common. Lymphocytosis occurs occasionally. Pleocytosis and an elevated protein concentration are found in CSF. The diagnosis is readily confirmed by PCR or isolation of CMV from urine or saliva within 48 hours, using rapid culture methods combined with immunoassay. The presence in the infant of IgM-specific CMV antibodies suggests the diagnosis. Some commercial ELISA kits are 90% sensitive and specific for these antibodies. Universal screening of asymptomatic children using blood or saliva CMV PCR during the first weeks of life is useful for early detection of children at high risk of developing hearing loss. Retrospective diagnosis of congenital CMV following hearing loss identified later in infancy is difficult.

C. Imaging

Head radiologic examinations may show microcephaly, periventricular calcifications, and ventricular dilation. These findings strongly correlate with neurologic sequelae and retardation. Long bone radiographs may show the "celery stalk" pattern characteristic of congenital viral infections. Interstitial pneumonia may be present.

Differential Diagnosis

CMV infection should be considered in any newborn that is seriously ill shortly after birth, especially once bacterial sepsis, metabolic disease, intracranial bleeding, and cardiac disease have been excluded. Other congenital infections to be considered in the differential diagnosis include toxoplasmosis (more diffuse calcification of the CNS, specific type of retinitis, macrocephaly, serology), rubella (specific type of retinitis, cardiac lesions, eye abnormalities, serology), enteroviral infections (time of year, maternal illness, severe hepatitis, PCR), herpes simplex (skin lesions, cultures, severe hepatitis, PCR), Zika virus (exposure, microcephaly, PCR, serology), and syphilis (skin lesions, bone involvement, serology of both infant and mother).

Prevention & Treatment

Support is rarely required for anemia and thrombocytopenia. Most children with symptoms at birth have significant neurologic, intellectual, visual, or auditory impairment. Ganciclovir (6 mg/kg every 12 hours, for 6 weeks) has been recommended for children with severe, life- or sight-threatening disease, or if end-organ disease recurs or progresses. A recent randomized placebo-controlled study showed efficacy in reducing hearing loss using oral valganciclovir at 16 mg/kg twice daily for 6 months in children symptomatic at birth. Patients undergoing treatment should be monitored for neutropenia.

Recent developments in the diagnosis of primary CMV infection during pregnancy using anti-CMV IgM and low-avidity IgG assays followed by quantitative CMV PCR testing of the amniotic fluid at 20–24 weeks gestation have made possible the diagnosis of congenital CMV infection before birth. Many pregnant women elect to terminate gestation under these circumstances. Passive immunoprophylaxis with hyperimmune CMV IgG did not prevent development of congenital disease in a randomized placebo-controlled trial.

2. Perinatal Cytomegalovirus Infection

CMV infection can be acquired from birth canal secretions or shortly after birth from breast milk. In some socioeconomic groups, 10%–20% of infants are infected at birth and excrete CMV for many months. Infection can also be acquired in the postnatal period from unscreened transfused blood products.

Clinical Findings

A. Symptoms and Signs

Ninety percent of immunocompetent infants infected by their mothers at birth develop subclinical illness (ie, virus excretion only) or a minor illness within 1–3 months. The remainder develops an illness lasting several weeks characterized by hepatosplenomegaly, lymphadenopathy, and interstitial pneumonitis in various combinations. Very low birth weight and premature infants are at greater risk for severe disease. If they are born to CMV-negative mothers and subsequently receive CMV-containing blood or breast milk, they may develop severe infection and pneumonia after a 2- to 6-week incubation period.

B. Laboratory Findings

Lymphocytosis, atypical lymphocytes, anemia, and thrombocytopenia may be present, especially in premature infants. Liver function is abnormal. CMV is readily isolated from urine and saliva. Secretions obtained at bronchoscopy contain CMV and epithelial cells bearing CMV antigens. Serum levels of CMV antibody rise significantly.

C. Imaging

Chest radiographs may show a diffuse interstitial pneumonitis in severely affected infants.

Differential Diagnosis

CMV infection should be considered as a cause of any prolonged illness in early infancy, especially if hepatosplenomegaly, lymphadenopathy, or atypical lymphocytosis is present. This must be distinguished from granulomatous or malignant diseases and from congenital infections (syphilis, toxoplasmosis, hepatitis B, HIV) not previously diagnosed. Other viruses (Epstein-Barr virus [EBV], HIV, adenovirus) can cause this syndrome. CMV is a recognized cause of viral pneumonia in this age group. Because asymptomatic CMV excretion is common in early infancy, care must be taken to establish the diagnosis and to rule out concomitant pathogens such as *Chlamydia* and RSV. Severe CMV infection in early infancy may indicate that the child has a congenital or acquired immune deficiency.

Prevention & Treatment

The self-limited disease of normal infants requires no therapy. Severe pneumonitis in premature infants requires oxygen administration and often intubation. Very ill infants should receive ganciclovir (6 mg/kg every 12 hours). CMV infection acquired by transfusion can be prevented by excluding CMV-seropositive blood donors. Milk donors should also be screened for prior CMV infection. A common practice of freezing the milk prior to administration was shown to lack preventive effectiveness. It is likely that high-risk infants receiving large doses of IVIG for other reasons will be protected against severe CMV disease.

3. Cytomegalovirus Infection Acquired in Childhood & Adolescence

Young children are readily infected by playmates, especially because CMV continues to be excreted in saliva and urine for many months after infection. The cumulative annual incidence of CMV excretion by children in day care centers exceeds 75%. In fact, young children in a family are often the source of primary CMV infection of their mothers during subsequent pregnancies. An additional peak of CMV infection takes place when adolescents become sexually active. Sporadic acquisition of CMV occurs after blood transfusion and transplantation.

► Clinical Findings

A. Symptoms and Signs

Most young children who acquire CMV are asymptomatic or have a minor febrile illness, occasionally with adenopathy. They provide an important reservoir of virus shedders that facilitates spread of CMV. Occasionally a child may have prolonged fever with hepatosplenomegaly and adenopathy. Older children and adults, many of whom are infected during sexual activity, are more likely to be symptomatic and can present with a syndrome that mimics the infectious mononucleosis syndrome that follows EBV infection (1–2 weeks of fever, malaise, anorexia, splenomegaly, mild hepatitis, and some adenopathy; see the next section). This syndrome can also occur 2–4 weeks after transfusion of CMV-infected blood.

B. Laboratory Findings

In the CMV mononucleosis syndrome, lymphocytosis and atypical lymphocytes are common, as is a mild rise in aminotransferase levels. CMV is present in saliva and urine; CMV DNA can be uniformly detected in plasma or blood.

► Differential Diagnosis

In older children, CMV infection should be included as a possible cause of fever of unknown origin, especially when lymphocytosis and atypical lymphocytes are present. CMV infection is distinguished from EBV infection by the absence of pharyngitis, the relatively minor adenopathy, and the absence of serologic evidence of acute EBV infection. Mononucleosis syndromes also are caused by *Toxoplasma gondii*, rubella virus, adenovirus, hepatitis A virus, and HIV.

► Prevention

Screening of transfused blood or filtering blood (thus removing CMV-containing white blood cells) prevents cases related to this source.

4. Cytomegalovirus Infection in Immunocompromised Children

In addition to symptoms experienced during primary infection, immunocompromised hosts develop symptoms with reinfection or reactivation of latent CMV. This is clearly seen in children with acquired immunodeficiency syndrome (AIDS), after transplantation, or with congenital immunodeficiencies.

However, in most immunocompromised patients, primary infection is more likely to cause severe symptoms than is reactivation or reinfection. The severity of the resulting disease is generally proportionate to the degree of immunosuppression.

► Clinical Findings

A. Symptoms and Signs

A mild febrile illness with myalgia, malaise, and arthralgia may occur, especially with reactivation disease. Severe disease often includes subacute onset of dyspnea and cyanosis as manifestations of interstitial pneumonitis. Auscultation reveals only coarse breath sounds and scattered rales. A rapid respiratory rate may precede clinical or radiographic evidence of pneumonia. Hepatitis without jaundice and hepatomegaly are common. Diarrhea, which can be severe, occurs with CMV colitis, and CMV can cause esophagitis with symptoms of odynophagia or dysphagia. These enteropathies are most common in AIDS, as is the presence of a retinitis that often progresses to blindness, encephalitis, and polyradiculitis.

B. Laboratory Findings

Neutropenia and thrombocytopenia are common. Atypical lymphocytosis is infrequent. Serum aminotransferase levels are often elevated. The stools may contain occult blood if enteropathy is present. CMV is readily isolated from saliva, urine, buffy coat, and bronchial secretions. Results are available in 48 hours. Interpretation of positive cultures is made difficult by asymptomatic shedding of CMV in saliva and urine in many immunocompromised patients. CMV disease correlates more closely with the presence of CMV in the blood or lung lavage fluid. Monitoring for the appearance of CMV DNA in plasma or CMV antigen in blood mononuclear cells is used as a guide to early antiviral ("preemptive") therapy.

C. Imaging

Bilateral interstitial pneumonitis may be present on chest radiographs.

► Differential Diagnosis

The initial febrile illness must be distinguished from treatable bacterial or fungal infection. Similarly, the pulmonary disease must be distinguished from intrapulmonary hemorrhage; drug-induced or radiation pneumonitis; pulmonary edema; and bacterial, fungal, parasitic, or other viral infections. CMV infection causes bilateral and interstitial abnormalities on chest radiographs, cough is nonproductive, chest pain is absent, and the patient is not usually toxic. *Pneumocystis jiroveci* infection may have a similar presentation. These patients may have polymicrobial disease. It is suspected that bacterial and fungal infections are enhanced by the neutropenia that can accompany CMV infection. Infection of the gastrointestinal tract is diagnosed by endoscopy.

This will exclude candidal, adenoviral, and herpes simplex infections and allows tissue confirmation of CMV-induced mucosal ulcerations.

▶ Prevention & Treatment

Blood donors should be screened to exclude those with prior CMV infection, or blood should be filtered. Ideally, seronegative transplant recipients should receive organs from seronegative donors. Severe symptoms, most commonly pneumonitis, often respond to early therapy with intravenous ganciclovir (5 mg/kg every 12 hours for 14–21 days). Neutropenia is a frequent side effect of this therapy. Foscarnet and cidofovir are alternative therapeutic agents recommended for patients with ganciclovir-resistant virus. Prophylactic use of oral or intravenous ganciclovir or foscarnet may prevent CMV infections in organ transplant recipients. Preemptive therapy can be used in transplant recipients by monitoring CMV in blood by PCR and instituting therapy when the results reach a certain threshold regardless of clinical signs or symptoms.

Fowler KB, Boppana SB: Congenital cytomegalovirus infection. Semin Perinatol 2018 Apr;42(3):149–154 [PMID: 29503048]

Vora SB, Englund JA. Cytomegalovirus in immunocompromised children. Curr Opin Infect Dis 2015 Aug;28(4):323–329. doi: 10.1097/QCO.0000000000000174. Review [PMID: 26098503].

INFECTIOUS MONONUCLEOSIS (EPSTEIN-BARR VIRUS)

ESSENTIALS OF DIAGNOSIS & TYPICAL FEATURES

- ▶ Prolonged fever.
- ▶ Exudative pharyngitis.
- ▶ Generalized adenopathy.
- ▶ Hepatosplenomegaly.
- ▶ Atypical lymphocytes.
- ▶ Heterophil antibodies.

▶ General Considerations

Mononucleosis is the most characteristic syndrome produced by Epstein-Barr virus (EBV) infection. Young children infected with EBV have either no symptoms or a mild nonspecific febrile illness. As the age of the host increases, EBV infection is more likely to produce the typical mononucleosis syndrome reaching 20%–25% of infected adolescents. EBV is acquired by close contact from asymptomatic carriers (15%–20% of whom excrete the virus in saliva on any given

day) and from recently ill patients, who excrete virus for many months. Young children are infected from the saliva of playmates and family members. Adolescents contract the infection primarily by deep kissing. EBV can also be transmitted by blood transfusion and organ transplantation.

▶ Clinical Findings

A. Symptoms and Signs

After an incubation period of 32–49 days, a 2- to 3-day prodrome of malaise and anorexia yields, abruptly or insidiously, to a febrile illness with temperatures exceeding 39°C. The major complaint is pharyngitis, which is often (50%) exudative with transient petechiae. Lymph nodes are enlarged, firm, and mildly tender. Any area may be affected, but posterior and anterior cervical nodes are almost always enlarged. Splenomegaly is present in 50%–75% of patients. Hepatomegaly is common (30%), and the liver is frequently tender. Five percent of patients have a rash, which can be macular, scarlatiniform, or urticarial. Rash is almost universal in patients taking penicillin or ampicillin. Soft palate petechiae and eyelid edema are also observed.

B. Laboratory Findings

1. Peripheral blood—Leukopenia may occur early, but an atypical lymphocytosis (comprising over 10% of the total leukocytes at some time in the illness) is most notable. Lymphocyte count less than 4000 mm^3 has a 99% negative predictive value for infectious mononucleosis. Hematologic changes may not be seen until the third week of illness and may be entirely absent in some EBV syndromes (eg, neurologic).

2. Heterophile antibodies—These nonspecific antibodies appear in over 90% of older patients with mononucleosis, but in fewer than 50% of children younger than age 5 years. They may not be detectable until the second week of illness and may persist for up to 12 months after recovery. Rapid screening tests (slide agglutination) are usually positive if the titer is significant; a positive result strongly suggests but does not prove EBV infection.

3. Anti-EBV antibodies—Specific antibody titers have a 97% sensitivity and 94% specificity for diagnosis and are especially useful in children younger than 5 years. Acute EBV infection is established by detecting IgM antibody to the viral capsid antigen (VCA) or by detecting a fourfold or greater change of IgG anti-VCA titers (in normal hosts, IgG antibody peaks by the time symptoms appear; in immunocompromised hosts, the tempo of antibody production may be delayed). The absence of anti-EBV nuclear antigen (EBNA) antibodies, which are typically first detected at least 4 weeks after the initiation of symptoms, may also be used to diagnose acute infection in immunocompetent hosts. However, immunocompromised hosts may fail to develop anti-EBNA antibodies.

4. EBV PCR—Site-specific detection of EBV DNA is the method of choice for the diagnosis of CNS and ocular infections. Quantitative EBV PCR in peripheral blood mononuclear cells has been used to diagnose EBV-related lymphoproliferative disorders in transplant patients. EBV PCR is less useful than serology for diagnosis of acute EBV infection in immunocompetent hosts.

▶ Differential Diagnosis

Severe pharyngitis may suggest group A streptococcal infection. Enlargement of only the anterior cervical lymph nodes, a neutrophilic leukocytosis, and the absence of splenomegaly suggest bacterial infection. Although a child with a positive throat culture result for *Streptococcus* usually requires therapy, up to 10% of children with mononucleosis are asymptomatic streptococcal carriers. In this group, penicillin therapy is unnecessary and often causes a rash. Severe primary herpes simplex pharyngitis, occurring in adolescence, may also mimic infectious mononucleosis. With herpes simplex pharyngitis, some anterior mouth ulcerations should suggest the correct diagnosis. Adenoviruses are another cause of severe, often exudative pharyngitis. EBV infection should be considered in the differential diagnosis of any perplexing prolonged febrile illness. Similar illnesses that produce atypical lymphocytosis include rubella (pharyngitis not prominent, shorter illness, less adenopathy and splenomegaly), adenovirus (upper respiratory symptoms and cough, conjunctivitis, less adenopathy, fewer atypical lymphocytes), hepatitis A or B (more severe liver function abnormalities, no pharyngitis, no lymphadenopathy), and toxoplasmosis (negative heterophil test, less pharyngitis). Serum sickness-like drug reactions and leukemia (smear morphology is important) may be confused with infectious mononucleosis. CMV mononucleosis is a close mimic except for minimal pharyngitis and less adenopathy; it is much less common. Serologic tests for EBV and CMV should clarify the correct diagnosis. The acute initial manifestation of HIV infection can be a mononucleosis-like syndrome.

▶ Complications

Splenic rupture is a rare complication, which usually follows significant trauma. Hematologic complications, including hemolytic anemia, thrombocytopenia, and neutropenia, are more common. Neurologic involvement can include aseptic meningitis, encephalitis, isolated neuropathy such as Bell palsy, and Guillain-Barré syndrome. Any of these may appear prior to or in the absence of the more typical signs and symptoms of infectious mononucleosis. Rare complications include myocarditis, pericarditis, and atypical pneumonia. Recurrence or persistence of acute EBV-associated symptoms for 6 months or longer characterizes chronic active EBV. This uncommon presentation is due to continuous viral replication and warrants specific antiviral therapy. Rarely EBV infection becomes a progressive

lymphoproliferative disorder characterized by persistent fever, multiple organ involvement, neutropenia or pancytopenia, and agammaglobulinemia. Hemocytophagia is often present in the bone marrow. An X-linked genetic defect in immune response has been inferred for some patients (Duncan syndrome, X-linked lymphoproliferative disorder). Children with other congenital immunodeficiencies or chemotherapy-induced immunosuppression can also develop progressive EBV infection, EBV-associated lymphoproliferative disorder, lymphoma, and other malignancies.

▶ Treatment & Prognosis

Bed rest may be necessary in severe cases. Acetaminophen controls high fever. Potential airway obstruction due to swollen pharyngeal lymphoid tissue responds rapidly to systemic corticosteroids. Corticosteroids may also be given for hematologic and neurologic complications, although no controlled trials have proven their efficacy in these conditions. Fever and pharyngitis disappear spontaneously by 10–14 days. Adenopathy and splenomegaly can persist several weeks longer. Some patients complain of fatigue, malaise, or lack of well-being for several months. Although corticosteroids may shorten the duration of illness by 12 hours, there is no evidence that its use decreases the course or severity of the disease. Patients may return to contact sports after 4 weeks if they have had resolution of symptoms and no splenomegaly. Acyclovir, valacyclovir, penciclovir, ganciclovir, and foscarnet are active against EBV and are indicated in the treatment of chronic active EBV. Antiviral therapy in the immunocompetent child has not proven efficacious.

Management of EBV-related lymphoproliferative disorders relies primarily on decreasing the immunosuppression whenever possible. Adjunctive therapy with acyclovir, ganciclovir, or another antiviral active against EBV as well as γ globulin has been used without scientific evidence of efficacy.

Balfour HH Jr, Dunmire SK, Hogquist KA: Infectious mononucleosis. Clin Transl Immunology 2015 Feb 27;4(2):e33 [PMID: 25774295].

Marshall-Andon T, Heinz P. How to use … the Monospot and other heterophile antibody tests. Arch Dis Child Educ Pract Ed 2017;102(4):188–193 [PMID: 28130396].

Worth AJ, Houldcroft CJ, Booth C: Severe Epstein-Barr virus infection in primary immunodeficiency and the normal host. Br J Haematol 2016;175(4):559–576 [PMID: 27748521].

▼ VIRAL INFECTIONS SPREAD BY INSECT VECTORS

In the United States, mosquitoes are the most common insect vectors that spread viral infections (Table 40–3). As a consequence, these infections—and others that are spread by ticks—tend to occur as summer-fall epidemics that coincide with the seasonal breeding and feeding habits of the vector, and the

Table 40–3. Some insect-borne viral diseases occurring in the United States or in returning US travelers.

Disease	Natural Reservoir (Vector)	Geographic Distribution	Incubation Period	Clinical Presentations	Laboratory Findings	Complications, Sequelae	Diagnosis, Therapy, Comments
Flaviviruses							
St. Louis encephalitis (SLE)	Birds (*Culex* mosquitoes)	Southern Canada, central and southern United States, Texas, Caribbean, South America	2–5 days (up to 3 wk)	Second most common cause of arbovirus encephalitis in United States. Abrupt onset of fever, chills, headache, nausea, vomiting; may develop generalized weakness, seizures, coma, ataxia, cranial nerve palsies. Aseptic meningitis is common in children.	Modest leukocytosis, neutrophilia, elevated liver enzymes. CSF: 100–200 WBCs/µL; PMNs predominate early.	Mortality rate 2%–5% at age < 5 or > 50 y. Neurologic sequelae in 1%–20%.	~ 15 cases/y, < 2% symptomatic. (Worse in elderly.) Therapy: supportive. Diagnosis: serology. Specific antibody often present within 5 days.
Dengue	Humans (*Aedes* mosquitoes)	Asia, Africa, Central and South America, Caribbean; observed in Texas/Mexico border area and Florida	4–7 days (range, 3–14 days)	Only 25% symptomatic. Fever, headache, myalgia, joint and bone pain, retroocular pain, nausea and vomiting; maculopapular or petechial rash in 50%, sparing palms and soles. Encephalitis in 5%–10% of children.	Leukopenia, thrombocytopenia. CSF: 100–500 mononuclear cells/µL if neurologic sign11s are present.	Hemorrhagic fever, shock syndrome, prolonged weakness, encephalitis.	High infection rate in endemic areas. Therapy: supportive. Diagnosis: RT-PCR or NS1 antigen first 5 days or IgM-EIA antibody by day 5. IgM and IgG may crossreact with other flaviviruses (Zika, Japanese encephalitis), so should be confirmed with plaque reduction neutralization testing.
West Nile	Birds (*Culex* mosquitoes); small mammals	North Africa, Middle East, parts of Asia, Europe, continental United States	2–14 days	Abrupt onset of fever, headache, sore throat, myalgia, retroocular pain, conjunctivitis; 20%–50% with rash; adenopathy. Meningitis alone is most common in children. Encephalitis may be accompanied by muscle weakness, flaccid paralysis, or movement disorders.	Mild leukocytosis; 10%–15% lymphopenic or thrombocytopenic; CSF pleocytosis with < 500 cells; may be neutrophils early.	Mortality rate 10%, of those with CNS symptoms, but rare in children; weakness and myalgia may persist for an extended period.	Most important mosquitoborne encephalitis in the United States. (~ 150 cases reported each year.) Diagnosis: IgM-EIA serology; cross-reacts with St. Louis encephalitis; positive by 5–6 days after onset of CNS symptoms. Diagnosis by PCR is less sensitive. Therapy: supportive.

	Reservoir	Distribution	Incubation	Clinical Features	Laboratory Findings	Complications	Comments
Japanese encephalitis	Birds, large mammals; reptiles (*Culex* mosquitos)	SE Asia; Australia	5–14 days	Onset with fever, cough, coryza, headache. Aseptic meningitis is common in children.	CSF: 10–100 lymphocytes/µL; atypical lymphocytes may be present; protein may reach 200 mg/dL.	Seizures are common in children; when encephalitis occurs, it can result in lasting motor, learning, and behavioral abnormalities.	Vaccination is an important consideration for children visiting or residing in endemic areas. IgM and IgG may crossreact with other flaviviruses (dengue, Zika), so should be confirmed with PRNT.
Zika	Humans (*Aedes* mosquitoes)	Asia, Africa, Central and South America, Caribbean; cases in Texas border area and Florida	3–7 days	Only 20% symptomatic. Maculopapular rash, fever, conjunctivitis, arthralgia. Congenital Zika syndrome with vertical transmission during pregnancy	Leukopenia, thrombocytopenia, elevated liver transaminases	Congenital Zika syndrome with many sequelae (eg, microcephaly, seizures, arthrogryposis, hearing and vision problems). Increased risk for Guillain Barré syndrome	High infection rate during epidemics. Therapy: supportive. Diagnosis: RT-PCR or NS1 antigen first 14 days and/or IgM-EIA antibody by day 5. IgM and IgG may crossreact with other flaviviruses (dengue, Japanese encephalitis), so should be confirmed with PRNT.
Alpha toga viruses							
Chikungunya	Humans (*Aedes* mosquitoes)	Asia, Africa, Central and South America, Caribbean	3–7 days (range, 1–14 days)	Symptomatic in > 50%. Fever, headache, myalgia, conjunctivitis; arthralgia and/or arthritis in multiple joints, symmetric, mainly hands and feet; maculopapular rash in 30%–60%.	Leukopenia, thrombocytopenia, elevated creatinine and liver transaminases	Severe persistent arthralgia in adolescents and adults. Encephalitis, seizures, and bleeding in infants with risk of neurodevelopmental sequelae.	Therapy: supportive. Use NSAID for arthritis after dengue ruled out. Diagnosis: RT-PCR in first 7 days or IgM-EIA antibody after day 5 at CDC.
Eastern equine encephalitis	Birds (*Aedes*, *Coquillettidia*, and *Culex* mosquitoes)	Eastern seaboard United States, Caribbean, South America	2–5 days	Similar to that of St. Louis encephalitis, but more severe. Progresses rapidly in one-third to coma and death.	Leukocytosis with neutrophilia. CSF: 500–2000 WBCs/µL; PMNs predominate early.	Mortality rate 20%–50%; neurologic 50% of children.	< 10 cases/y usually. Only 3%–10% of cases are symptomatic, but sequelae are common in young children who develop symptoms. Therapy: supportive. Diagnosis: serology. Titers often positive in the first week. Equine deaths may signal an outbreak.

(Continued)

Table 40–3. Some insect-borne viral diseases occurring in the United States or in returning US travelers. (*Continued*)

Disease	Natural Reservoir (Vector)	Geographic Distribution	Incubation Period	Clinical Presentations	Laboratory Findings	Complications, Sequelae	Diagnosis, Therapy, Comments
Western equine encephalitis	Birds (mostly *Culex* mosquitoes)	Canada, Mexico, and United States west of Mississippi River	2–5 days	Similar to that of St. Louis encephalitis. Most infections are subclinical.	Variable white counts. CSF: 10–300 WBCs/µL.	Permanent brain damage, 10% overall; most severe in older adults.	No reported cases in the United States in recent years. Case/infection is 1:1000 for older adults and 1:1 for infants. Equine illness precedes human outbreaks. Diagnosis: IgM antibody in the first week. Therapy: supportive.
Venezuelan equine encephalitis	Horses (10 species of mosquitoes)	South and Central America, Texas	1–6 days	Similar to that of St. Louis encephalitis.	Lymphopenia, mild thrombocytopenia, abnormal liver function tests. CSF: 50–200 mononuclear cells/µL.	Severe disease more common in infants; 20% fatality rate for encephalitis.	Most infections do not cause encephalitis. No cases in the United States in recent years. Vaccination of horses will stop epidemic. Therapy: supportive. Diagnosis: IgM antibody (EIA).
Bunyavirus							
California encephalitis serogroup (LaCrosse, Jamestown Canyon, California)	Chipmunks and other small mammals (*Aedes* mosquitoes)	Northern and mid-central United States, southern Canada	3–7 days	Second most common arbovirus etiology, especially LaCrosse. Symptoms are similar to those of St. Louis encephalitis; sore throat and respiratory symptoms common; focal neurologic signs in up to 25%. Seizures prominent. Prepubertal children are most likely to have severe disease. Can mimic herpes simplex encephalitis.	Variable white counts. CSF: 30–200 up to 600 WBCs/µL; variable PMNs; protein often normal.	Mortality rate < 2%. Seizures may occur during acute illness.	~ 75 cases/y in the United States, 5% symptomatic. > 10% with sequelae. Therapy: supportive. Diagnosis: serology. Up to 90% have specific IgM antibody in the first week; 25% of population in certain regions has IgG antibody.
Coltivirus							
Colorado tick fever	Small mammals (*Dermacentor andersoni* or wood tick)	Rocky Mountain region of United States and Canada	3–4 days (range, 2–14 days)	Fever, chills, myalgia, conjunctivitis, headache, retro-orbital pain; rash in < 10%. No respiratory symptoms. Biphasic fever in 50%.	Leukopenia (maximum at 4–6 days), mild thrombocytopenia.	Rare encephalitis, coagulopathy.	Patient may have no known tick bite. Acute illness lasts 7–10 days; prolonged fatigue in adults. Therapy: supportive. Diagnosis: serology, direct FA staining of red cells for viral antigen, PCR.

CNS, central nervous system; CSF, cerebrospinal fluid; EIA, enzyme immunoassay; FA, fluorescent antibody; NSAID, nonsteroidal anti-inflammatory drug; PCR, polymerase chain reaction; PMN, polymorphonuclear neutrophil; WBC, white blood cell.

etiologic agent varies by region. Other insect-borne viral infections are seen in international travelers. Thus, a careful travel and exposure history is critical for correct diagnostic workup.

ENCEPHALITIS

ESSENTIALS OF DIAGNOSIS & TYPICAL FEATURES

▶ Fever and headache.

▶ Change in mental status and/or behavior, with or without focal neurologic deficits.

▶ Mononuclear cell pleocytosis, elevated protein level, and normal glucose level.

Encephalitis is a common severe manifestation of many infections spread by insects (see Table 40–3). With many viral pathogens, the infection is often subclinical, or includes mild CNS disease such as meningitis. These infections have some distinguishing features in terms of subclinical infection rate, unique neurologic syndromes, associated systemic symptoms, and prognosis. The diagnosis is generally made clinically during recognized outbreaks and is confirmed by virus-specific serology or PCR. Prevention consists of control of mosquito vectors and precautions with proper clothing and insect repellents to minimize mosquito and tick bites. It is essential before making the diagnosis of arboviral encephalitis, which is not treatable, to exclude herpes encephalitis, which warrants specific antiviral therapy. Delay in administering this therapy may have dire consequences.

▶ West Nile Virus Encephalitis

This flavivirus, primarily transmitted by *Culex* mosquitos, is the most important arbovirus infection in the United States. In 2003, there were more than 10,000 clinically apparent infections, more than 2900 nervous system infections, and 265 deaths in 47 states. In 2012, there was a resurgence to more than 5000 reported cases, of which approximately half were neuroinvasive; 240 were fatal. Other years typically have 1500–3000 reported cases. The reservoir of West Nile virus includes more than 160 species of birds whose migration explains the extent of endemic disease. Epidemics occur in summer-fall. Approximately 20% of infected individuals develop West Nile fever, characterized by fever, headache, retro-orbital pain, nausea, vomiting, lymphadenopathy, and a maculopapular rash (20%–50%). Less than 1% of infected patients develop meningitis or encephalitis, but 10% of these cases are fatal. The major risk factors for severe disease are age > 50 years and immune compromise. Symptomatic children usually manifest with West Nile fever and less than one-third will develop neuroinvasive disease, most likely limited to meningitis. Neurologic manifestations are most often those found with other meningoencephalitides, but some distinguishing features include polio-like acute flaccid paralysis, movement disorders (Parkinsonism, tremor, and myoclonus), brainstem symptoms, polyneuropathy, and optic neuritis. Muscle weakness, facial palsy, and hyporeflexia are common (20%). Recovery is slow and significant sequelae may persist in some severely affected patients. Diagnosis is best made by detecting IgM antibody (enzyme immunoassay) to the virus in CSF. This will be present by 5–6 days (95%) after onset. PCR is a specific diagnostic tool, but is less sensitive than antibody detection. Antibody rise in serum can also be used for diagnosis.

Treatment is supportive, although various antivirals and specific immunoglobulins are being studied. The infection is not spread between contacts, but can be spread by donated organs, blood, breast milk, and transplacentally.

Colpitts TM, Conway MJ, Montgomery RR, Fikrig E: West Nile virus: biology, transmission, and human infection. Clin Micro Rev 2012;25(4):635 [PMID: 20121004].

Gaensbauer JT, Lindsey NP, Messacar K, Staples JE, Fischer M: Neuroinvasive arboviral disease in the United States: 2003 to 2012. Pediatrics 2014;134(3):e642–e650 [PMID: 25113294].

DENGUE

ESSENTIALS OF DIAGNOSIS & TYPICAL FEATURES

▶ Travel or residence in an endemic area.

▶ First infection (first episode) is asymptomatic or may result in fever, rash, retro-orbital pain, severe myalgia, and/or arthralgia.

▶ Second infection with a different dengue serotype is more likely to result in severe dengue, which includes symptoms of plasma leakage, and may progress to dengue hemorrhagic fever (thrombocytopenia, bleeding) and dengue shock syndrome.

Dengue virus is responsible for an estimated 400 million infections and 100 million episodes of symptomatic dengue fever annually. Dengue is one of the most common cause of fever in returning travelers and occurs throughout Latin America, the Caribbean, Southeast Asia, Oceania, and Africa; sporadic outbreaks occur occasionally in the southern United States, and dengue is hyperendemic (≥ 2 serotypes) in Puerto Rico. The spread of dengue requires the *Aedes* mosquito (present in the southern United States), which transmits virus from a reservoir of viremic humans in endemic areas. Most symptomatic patients have mild disease, especially young children, who may have a nonspecific fever and rash. Severity is a function of age, and prior infection with other serotypes of dengue virus significantly increases the risk for severe complications.

Clinical Findings

A. Symptoms and Signs

Dengue fever begins abruptly 4–7 days after transmission (range, 3–14 days) with fever, chills, severe retro-orbital pain, severe muscle and joint pain ("breakbone fever"), nausea, and vomiting. Erythema of the face and torso may occur early. After 3–4 days, a centrifugal maculopapular rash appears in half of the patients described as "islands of white in a sea of red." The rash can become petechial, and mild hemorrhagic signs (epistaxis, gingival bleeding, microscopic blood in stool or urine) may be noted. The illness lasts 3–7 days, although rarely fever may reappear for several additional days. Fever may become relatively lower on the third day, only to become higher until defervescence. Since there are four serotypes of dengue virus, multiple sequential infections can occur.

B. Laboratory Findings

In most symptomatic cases, mild leukopenia and thrombocytopenia are common. Liver transaminases are usually normal. Diagnosis during acute infection (≤ 5 days of symptoms) is usually made by detection of viral antigenemia (NS1 antigen) or dengue virus reverse transcription polymerase chain reaction (RT-PCR) (80%–90% sensitive, 95% specific). After 5 days, dengue may be diagnosed by detection of IgM-specific antibodies (70%–80% sensitive by day 6, and increases thereafter) or a rise in type-specific antibody during convalescent testing (10–14 days later). Neutralizing antibodies against dengue virus are the most accurate serologic method, but they may cross-react with other flaviviruses (eg, Zika), especially with multiple prior dengue infections. Therefore, early testing by RT-PCR or NS1 antigen is preferable.

Differential Diagnosis

This diagnosis should be considered for any traveler to an endemic area who has symptoms suggestive of a systemic viral illness, although less than 1 in 1000 travelers to these areas develops dengue. Often the areas visited have other endogenous pathogens circulating (eg, malaria, typhoid fever, leptospirosis, rickettsial diseases, other endemic alphaviruses and flaviviruses, and measles). Chikungunya has a similar geographic distribution and also presents with fever and rash, but is more strongly associated with arthralgia/arthritis, which may persist for weeks to months. Zika is also clinically indistinguishable from dengue, though conjunctivitis may be more common with Zika. EBV, influenza, enteroviruses, and acute HIV infection may produce a similar illness. Dengue is not associated with sore throat or cough. An illness that starts 2 weeks after the trip ends or that lasts longer than 2 weeks is probably not dengue.

Complications

More common in endemic areas is the appearance of severe dengue, which typically occurs at the time of defervescence (day 3–7) and may include respiratory distress, circulatory shock (dengue septic shock), severe bleeding (dengue hemorrhagic fever), and end-organ damage. Severe dengue typically occurs during a second dengue episode as a consequence of pre-existing, non-neutralizing antibodies enhancing virus uptake into cells and leading to increased viremia and cytokine response (antibody-dependent enhancement). Warning signs for severe dengue that may be seen during the acute febrile phase of illness include abdominal pain, persistent vomiting, clinical fluid accumulation (eg, pleural effusion, ascites), mucosal bleeding, altered mental status, hepatomegaly, and hemoconcentration (hematocrit > 20% higher than baseline) with concurrent thrombocytopenia (< 100,000 cells/μL).

Prevention

Prevention of dengue fever involves avoiding high-risk areas and using conventional mosquito avoidance measures. The *Aedes* mosquito vector is a daytime feeder. Several dengue vaccines are under development, and one licensed vaccine demonstrated 60% efficacy in clinical trials, though it was associated with increased risk of subsequent severe dengue disease in children without prior immunity. No vaccines are currently recommended for travelers.

Treatment

Dengue fever is treated by oral rehydration and antipyretics, avoiding nonsteroidal anti-inflammatory agents that affect platelet function. Recovery is complete without sequelae. The hemorrhagic syndrome and shock require prompt fluid therapy with plasma expanders and isotonic saline along with close ICU monitoring.

Guzman MG, Harris E: Dengue. Lancet 2015;385(9966):453–465 [PMID: 25230594].
Simmons CP, Farrar JJ, van Vinh Chau N, Wills B: Dengue. N Engl J Med 2012;366(15):14–23 [PMID: 22494122].

CHIKUNGUNYA

ESSENTIALS OF DIAGNOSIS & TYPICAL FEATURES

- Same mosquito vector and geographic distribution as dengue and Zika viruses.
- Acute symptoms are similar to dengue and Zika virus (fever, rash, headache), but arthralgia and arthritis can be more severe and persist for weeks to months.
- Perinatal and neonatal infection can be severe and include bleeding and/or neurological disease, resulting in neurodevelopmental sequelae.

Chikungunya has been endemic in Africa and Asia for decades, but emerged in the Americas for the first time in 2013, leading to a widespread epidemic that included transmission within the southern United States. Chikungunya is transmitted by *Aedes* mosquitos and has a similar geographic distribution and acute clinical presentation to dengue and Zika. The name "chikungunya" means "that which bends up" in the Makonde language from where it was first described in Tanzania, referring to the debilitating musculoskeletal symptoms (eg, arthralgia, arthritis) associated with the disease.

Clinical Findings

A. Symptoms and Signs

After a 3–7 day incubation period (maximum 14 days), high-grade fever appears suddenly and lasts 3–5 days. Symptoms may include headache (15%) and a diffuse maculopapular rash (30%–60%). Myalgia, arthralgia, and arthritis are more common in adults (87%–99%) than in children (30%–50%), and can be debilitating. Young children and infants, especially those perinatally infected, are more likely to have neurologic symptoms (seizure, encephalitis), bleeding, and multiorgan failure.

B. Laboratory Findings

Leukopenia, thrombocytopenia, and elevated transaminases may be seen, especially in young infants. Elevated creatinine is also observed. In the first 5–7 days of infection, RT-PCR is the preferred diagnostic test. Chikungunya IgM antibodies appear around day 5, lasting for 1–3 months and sometimes longer in individuals with persistent joint disease; IgG antibodies appear by 2 weeks and persist for years. They do not cross-react with flaviviruses.

Differential Diagnosis

Chikungunya is clinically indistinguishable from dengue and Zika, which all demonstrate similar geographic distribution. Chikungunya is less likely than dengue to result in bleeding and shock (except in young infants), and Zika may be more likely to produce conjunctivitis. Other infections with similar clinical presentations include parvovirus, rubella, measles, leptospirosis, malaria, typhoid, *Rickettsia*, and influenza. A febrile illness that starts 2 weeks after the trip ends or that lasts longer than 2 weeks is probably not chikungunya.

Complications

Chronic musculoskeletal symptoms (arthritis, arthralgia, and tenosynovitis), though less common in children, may persist or relapse for months or even years following infection and can be severely debilitating. Affected individuals, especially young infants, may have long-term neurodevelopmental sequelae including hearing and vision impairment as well as cerebral disorders (eg, attention deficit hyperactivity disorder).

Prevention & Treatment

Prevention includes avoiding high-risk areas and using conventional mosquito avoidance measures. Treatment involves supportive care, including fluids and acetaminophen or nonsteroidal anti-inflammatory drugs (NSAIDs) for fever and pain, though NSAIDS should be avoided if dengue is a possibility or if the patient has thrombocytopenia or bleeding. Chronic symptoms may be treated with NSAIDs and physical therapy. Vaccines are under development.

Ritz N et al: Chikungunya in children. Pediatr Infect Dis J 2015;34(7):789–791 [PMID: 26069950].

Weaver SC, Lecuit M: Chikungunya virus and the global spread of a mosquito-borne disease. N Engl J Med 2015;372(13):1231–1239 [PMID: 25806915].

ZIKA

ESSENTIALS OF DIAGNOSIS & TYPICAL FEATURES

▶ Transmitted by *Aedes* mosquitos (same vector as dengue and chikungunya), sexual intercourse, and vertically (mother-to-child) during pregnancy.

▶ Acute symptoms are usually mild and similar to dengue and chikungunya (rash, fever, conjunctivitis).

▶ Vertical transmission to fetus during pregnancy may result in congenital Zika syndrome.

Zika virus has been endemic in Africa and Asia for decades but recently emerged in the Americas and resulted in a widespread epidemic, including endemic cases in the southern United States. Zika can be transmitted by *Aedes* mosquitos and sexually. Though most Zika infections are asymptomatic or benign, infection during pregnancy can result in vertical transmission and lead to severe neurodevelopmental sequelae in the infant, known as congenital Zika syndrome. Diagnosis is made difficult by similar geographic distribution and clinical presentation to dengue and chikungunya, as well as cross-reactivity of serologic testing with other flaviviruses such as dengue.

Clinical Findings

A. Symptoms and Signs

After a 3- to 7-day incubation period, most acute Zika infections are asymptomatic (up to 80%) or mild. Symptoms are similar to dengue and chikungunya and include maculopapular rash, low-grade fever, nonpurulent conjunctivitis, and arthralgia. The vast majority of infections resolve within 2–7 days.

Maternal infection during pregnancy, which may be symptomatic or subclinical, can result in vertical transmission and lead to congenital Zika syndrome (see Complications).

B. Laboratory Findings

Leukopenia, thrombocytopenia, and elevated liver transaminases may be seen during acute infection. In the first 14 days of infection, RT-PCR of blood or urine is usually obtained first, but a negative result does not rule out infection. IgM antibodies against Zika appear around day 4 and usually last around 3 months. Early testing by RT-PCR is preferable as Zika antibodies may cross-react with other flaviviruses (eg, dengue), making serologic diagnosis more difficult. Infants exposed in utero should undergo extensive diagnostic evaluation for infection according to the latest guidelines, which may include placental and umbilical cord tissue assessment by RT-PCR. Congenitally exposed infants should also undergo neurodevelopment, ophthalmologic, and audiometric evaluation.

C. Radiologic Findings

Radiologic imaging of the fetus or neonate with congenital Zika syndrome may demonstrate growth restriction, intracranial calcifications, ventriculomegaly, reduced brain volume, and other abnormalities.

▶ Differential Diagnosis

Zika is clinically indistinguishable from dengue and chikungunya, which are both transmitted by the same *Aedes* mosquito vectors. Unlike dengue, Zika does not lead to hemorrhage or shock. Unlike chikungunya, Zika does not lead to severe or persistent musculoskeletal symptoms. Other infections with similar acute presentations include parvovirus, rubella, measles, leptospirosis, malaria, typhoid, rickettsia, and influenza. Rubella, cytomegalovirus, toxoplasmosis, and other congenital infections should be considered in infants undergoing evaluation for congenital Zika syndrome. A febrile illness that starts 2 weeks after the trip ends or that lasts longer than 2 weeks is probably not Zika.

▶ Complications

Infants affected with congenital Zika syndrome may be small for gestational age and demonstrate neurodevelopmental sequelae, including microcephaly, seizures, irritability, spasticity, feeding difficulty, arthrogryposis, ocular findings, and sensorineural hearing loss. Additional sequelae may be described as more data become available and affected infants are followed into childhood, but preliminary data suggests 1%–13% of congenital infections

result in congenital Zika syndrome, with higher risk in the first trimester (but risk persists into the third trimester). There is an increased risk of Guillain-Barré syndrome following Zika infection.

Prevention and Treatment

Prevention, which is particularly important for pregnant women and those intending to conceive, involves avoiding high-risk areas, using conventional mosquito avoidance measures, and using a barrier method for sex with potentially infected individuals (Zika virus persists in the genital tract for weeks to months). Acute disease is treated with supportive care. Multiple vaccines are in clinical trials.

Adebanjo T: Update: Interim guidance for the diagnosis, evaluation, and management of infants with possible congenital Zika virus infection—United States, October 2017. MMWR Morb Mortal Wkly Rep 2017;66:1089–1099 [PMID: 29049277].

Muss D et al: Zika virus. Clin Microbial Rev 2016;29(3):487–524 [PMID: 27029595].

Read JS et al: Symptomatic Zika virus infection in infants, children, and adolescents living in Puerto Rico. JAMA Pediatr 2018 Jul 1;172(7):686–693 [PMID: 29813148].

COLORADO TICK FEVER

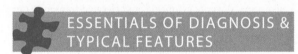

ESSENTIALS OF DIAGNOSIS & TYPICAL FEATURES

▶ Travel in endemic area; tick bite.

▶ Fever, chills, headache, retro-orbital pain, myalgia.

▶ Biphasic fever curve.

▶ Leukopenia early in the illness.

Colorado tick fever is endemic in the high plains and mountains of the central and northern Rocky Mountains and northern Pacific coast of the United States. The reservoir of the virus consists of squirrels and chipmunks. Many hundreds of cases of Colorado tick fever occur each year in visitors or laborers entering this region, primarily from May through July.

▶ Clinical Findings

A. Symptoms and Signs

After a 3- to 4-day incubation period (maximum, 14 days), fever begins suddenly together with chills, lethargy, headache, ocular pain, myalgia, abdominal pain, nausea, and vomiting. Conjunctivitis may be present. A nondistinctive maculopapular rash occurs in 5%–10% of patients. The illness lasts 7–10 days, and half of patients have a biphasic fever curve with several afebrile days in the midst of the illness.

B. Laboratory Findings

Leukopenia is characteristic early in the illness. Platelets are modestly decreased. Specific ELISA testing is available, but 2–3 weeks may elapse before seroconversion. Fluorescent antibody staining will detect virus-infected erythrocytes during the illness and for weeks after recovery. RT-PCR is available in some areas and will be positive within the first week of illness.

▶ Differential Diagnosis

Early findings, especially if rash is present, may suggest enterovirus, measles, or rubella infection. Enteric fever may be an early consideration because of the presence of leukopenia and thrombocytopenia. A history of tick bite, information about local risk, and the biphasic fever pattern will help with the diagnosis. Because of the wilderness exposure, diseases such as leptospirosis, borreliosis, tularemia, ehrlichiosis, and Rocky Mountain spotted fever will be considerations.

▶ Complications

Meningoencephalitis occurs in 3%–7% of patients. Cardiac and pulmonary complications are rare.

▶ Prevention & Treatment

Prevention involves avoiding endemic areas and using conventional means to avoid tick bite. Therapy is supportive. Do not use analgesics that modify platelet function.

Choi E, Piyzocha NJ, Mauver DM: Tick-borne illnesses. Curr Sports Med Rep 2016;15:98 [PMID: 26963018].
Yendell SJ et al: Colorado tick fever in the United States, 2002-2012. Vector Borne Zoonotic Dis 2015 May;15(5):311–316 [PMID: 25988440].

▼ OTHER MAJOR VIRAL CHILDHOOD EXANTHEMS

See section Infections Due to Herpesviruses for a discussion of varicella and roseola, the two other major childhood exanthems.

ERYTHEMA INFECTIOSUM

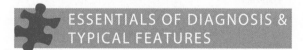

ESSENTIALS OF DIAGNOSIS & TYPICAL FEATURES

▶ Fever and rash with "slapped-cheek" appearance, followed by a symmetrical, full-body maculopapular rash.

▶ Arthritis in older children.

▶ Profound anemia in patients with impaired erythrocyte production.

▶ Nonimmune hydrops fetalis following infection of pregnant women.

▶ General Considerations

This benign exanthematous illness of school-aged children is caused by the human parvovirus B19. Spread is respiratory, occurring in winter-spring epidemics. A nonspecific mild flu-like illness may occur during the viremia at 7–10 days; the characteristic rash occurring at 10–17 days represents an immune response. The patient is viremic and contagious prior to—but not after—the onset of rash.

Approximately half of infected individuals have a subclinical illness. Most cases (60%) occur in children between ages 5 and 15 years, with an additional 40% occurring later in life. Forty percent of adults are seronegative. The secondary attack rate in a school or household setting is 50% among susceptible children and 20%–30% among susceptible adults.

▶ Clinical Findings

Owing to the nonspecific nature of the exanthem and the many subclinical cases, a history of contact with an infected individual is often absent or unreliable. Recognition of the illness is easier during outbreaks.

A. Symptoms and Signs

Typically, the first sign of illness is the rash, which begins as raised, fiery red maculopapular lesions on the cheeks that coalesce to give a "slapped-cheek" appearance. The lesions are warm, nontender, and sometimes pruritic. They may be scattered on the forehead, chin, and postauricular areas, but the circumoral region is spared. Within 1–2 days, similar lesions appear on the proximal extensor surfaces of the extremities and spread distally in a symmetrical fashion. Palms and soles are usually spared. The trunk, neck, and buttocks are also commonly involved. Central clearing of confluent lesions produces a characteristic lace-like pattern. The rash fades in days to several weeks, but frequently reappears in response to local irritation, heat (bathing), sunlight, and stress. Nearly 50% of infected children have some rash remaining (or recurring) for 10 days. Fine desquamation may be present. Mild low-grade fever, malaise, myalgia, sore throat, and coryza occur in up to 50% of children. These symptoms appear for 2–3 days followed by a week-long asymptomatic phase before the rashes appear.

Purpuric stocking-glove rashes, neurologic disease, and severe disorders resembling hemolytic-uremic syndrome have also been described in association with parvovirus B19.

B. Laboratory Findings

A mild leukopenia occurs early in some patients, followed by leukocytosis and lymphocytosis. Specific IgM and IgG serum antibody tests are available, but care must be used in choosing a reliable laboratory. IgM antibody is present in 90% of patients at the time of the rash. Nucleic acid detection tests are often definitive, but parvovirus DNA may be detectable in blood for prolonged periods. The disease is not diagnosed by routine viral culture.

▶ Differential Diagnosis

In children immunized against measles and rubella, parvovirus B19 is the most frequent agent of morbilliform and rubelliform rashes. The characteristic rash and the mild nature of the illness distinguish erythema infectiosum from other childhood exanthems. It lacks the prodromal symptoms of measles and the lymphadenopathy of rubella. Systemic symptoms and pharyngitis are more prominent with enteroviral infections and scarlet fever.

▶ Complications & Sequelae

A. Arthritis

Arthritis is more common in older patients, beginning with late adolescence. Approximately 10% of older children have severe joint symptoms. Girls are affected more commonly than boys. Pain and stiffness occur symmetrically in the peripheral joints. Arthritis usually follows the rash and may persist for 2–6 weeks, but resolves without permanent damage.

B. Aplastic Crisis and Other Hematologic Abnormalities

Parvovirus B19 may cause reticulocytopenia for approximately 1 week during the illness. This goes unnoticed in individuals with a normal erythrocyte half-life, but results in severe anemia in patients with chronic hemolytic anemia.

Pure red cell aplasia, leukopenia, pancytopenia, idiopathic thrombocytopenic purpura, and a hemophagocytic syndrome have been described. Patients with HIV infection and other immunosuppressive illnesses may develop prolonged anemia or pancytopenia. Patients with hemolytic anemia and aplastic crisis, or with immunosuppression, may be contagious and should be isolated while in the hospital.

C. Other End-Organ Infections

Parvovirus has been associated with neurologic syndromes, hepatitis, and suppression of bone marrow lineages. It is implicated as a cause of myocarditis.

D. In Utero Infections

Infection of susceptible pregnant women may produce fetal infection with hydrops fetalis. Fetal death occurs in about 6% of cases, most often in the first 20 weeks. This rate of fetal loss is higher than expected in typical pregnancies. Congenital anomalies have not been associated with parvovirus B19 infection during pregnancy.

▶ Treatment & Prognosis

Erythema infectiosum is a benign illness for immunocompetent individuals. Patients with aplastic crisis may require blood transfusions. It is unlikely that this complication can be prevented by quarantine measures because acute parvovirus infection in contacts is often unrecognized and is most contagious prior to the rash. Pregnant women who are exposed to erythema infectiosum or who work in a setting in which an epidemic occurs should be tested for evidence of prior infection. Susceptible pregnant women should then be followed up for evidence of parvovirus infection. Approximately 1.5% of women of childbearing age are infected during pregnancy. If maternal infection occurs, the fetus should be followed by ultrasonography for evidence of hydrops and distress. In utero transfusion or early delivery may salvage some fetuses. Pregnancies are typically not terminated because of parvovirus infection. The risk of fetal death among exposed pregnant women of unknown serologic status is less than 2.5%.

Intramuscular immunoglobulin is not protective. High-dose IVIG has stopped viremia and led to marrow recovery in some cases of prolonged aplasia. Its role in immunocompetent patients and pregnant women is unknown.

Qiu J, Soderland-Venemo M, Young NS: Human parvoviruses. Clin Microbiol Rev 2017;30:43 [PMID: 27806994].

Rogo LD, Maokhtari-Azad T, Kabir MH, Rezael F: Human parvovirus: a review. Acta Virol 2014;58:199 [PMID: 25283854].

MEASLES (RUBEOLA)

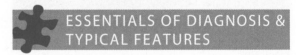

ESSENTIALS OF DIAGNOSIS & TYPICAL FEATURES

- ▶ Exposure to measles 9–14 days previously.
- ▶ Prodrome (2–3 days) of fever, cough, conjunctivitis, and coryza.
- ▶ Koplik spots (few to many small white papules on a diffusely red base on the buccal mucosa) 1–2 days prior to and after onset of rash.
- ▶ Maculopapular rash spreading from the face and hairline to the trunk over 3 days and later becoming confluent.
- ▶ Leukopenia.

General Considerations

Measles is one of the most contagious infectious diseases of childhood that presents as a febrile exanthema. The attack rate in susceptible individuals is extremely high; spread is via respiratory droplets. Considered eliminated from the United States in 2000, frequent outbreaks have occurred recently (including 1000 cases in the first half of 2019), mainly due to accumulation of susceptible individuals, low vaccination coverage, increasing vaccine hesitancy, and importation. It is recommended that all children receive two doses of measles vaccine prior to primary or secondary school entry (see Chapter 10). Morbidity and mortality rates in the developing world are substantial because of underlying malnutrition and secondary infections. Because humans are the sole reservoir of measles, there is the potential to eliminate this disease worldwide.

Clinical Findings

A history of contact with a suspected case may be absent because airborne spread is efficient and patients are contagious during the prodrome. Contact with an imported case may not be recognized. In temperate climates, epidemic measles is a winter-spring disease. Because measles is uncommon in the United States, a high index of suspicion is required during outbreaks.

A. Symptoms and Signs

After 2–3 days of a prodrome of sneezing, eyelid edema, tearing, copious coryza, photophobia, and harsh cough, high fever and lethargy become prominent. Koplik spots are white macular lesions on the buccal mucosa, typically opposite the lower molars that appear in the first 2–4 days of the illness. A discrete maculopapular rash begins when the respiratory symptoms and fever are maximal and spreads quickly from the face to the trunk, coalescing to a bright red. As it spreads to the extremities, the rash fades turning coppery from the face and is completely gone within 6 days; fine desquamation may occur. Diarrhea can occur in young children and lead to hospitalization; persistent fever and cough may signal pneumonia. Measles should be considered in any child with febrile rash illness, especially if recently traveled internationally or exposed to a person with febrile rash illness. Suspected measles cases should be reported to local health department within 24 hours.

B. Laboratory Findings

Lymphopenia is characteristic. The diagnosis is usually made by PCR testing of oropharyngeal secretions (or urine), which is extremely sensitive and specific and can detect infection up to 5 days before symptoms. Measles may be diagnosed serologically by IgM detection in serum at ≥3 days after the onset of rash (false negative may occur early in infection), or significant rise in IgG antibody between acute and convalescent samples.

C. Imaging

Chest radiographs often show hyperinflation, perihilar infiltrates, or parenchymal patchy, fluffy densities. Secondary consolidation or effusion may be visible.

Differential Diagnosis

Table 40–2 lists other illnesses that may resemble measles.

Complications & Sequelae

A. Respiratory Complications

These occur in up to 15% of patients. Bacterial superinfection of the lungs, middle ear, sinus, and cervical nodes are most common. Fever that persists after the third or fourth day of rash and/or leukocytosis suggests such a complication. Bronchospasm, severe croup, and progressive viral pneumonia or bronchiolitis (in infants) also occur. Immunosuppressed patients are at much greater risk for fatal pneumonia than are immunocompetent patients.

B. Cerebral Complications

Encephalitis occurs in 1 in 2000 cases. Onset is usually within a week after appearance of rash. Symptoms include combativeness, ataxia, vomiting, seizures, and coma. Lymphocytic pleocytosis and a mildly elevated protein concentration are usual CSF findings, but the fluid may be normal. Forty percent of patients so affected die or have severe neurologic sequelae.

Subacute sclerosing panencephalitis (SSPE) is a slow measles virus infection of the brain that becomes symptomatic years later in about 1 in 100,000 previously infected children. This progressive cerebral deterioration is associated with myoclonic jerks and a typical electroencephalographic pattern. It is fatal in 6–12 months. High titers of measles antibody are present in serum and CSF.

C. Other Complications

These include hemorrhagic measles (severe disease with multiorgan bleeding, fever, and cerebral symptoms), thrombocytopenia, appendicitis, keratitis, myocarditis, and premature delivery or stillbirth. Mild liver function test elevation is detected in up to 50% of cases in young adults; jaundice may also occur. Measles causes transient immunosuppression; thus, reactivation or progression of tuberculosis (including transient cutaneous anergy) can occur in children.

Prevention

The current two-dose active vaccination strategy provides more than 97% protection. Vaccine should not be withheld for concurrent mild acute illness, tuberculosis or positive tuberculin skin test, breast-feeding, or exposure to an immunodeficient contact. The vaccine is recommended for HIV-infected children without severe HIV complications, with CD4 cells ≥ 15%, and preferably receiving antiretroviral therapy.

Treatment & Prognosis

Vaccination prevents the disease in susceptible exposed individuals if given within 72 hours (see Chapter 10). Immunoglobulin (0.25 mL/kg intramuscularly; 0.5 mL/kg if immunocompromised) will prevent or modify measles if given within 6 days. Suspected cases should be diagnosed promptly and reported to the local health department.

Recovery generally occurs 7–10 days after onset of symptoms. Therapy is supportive: eye care, cough relief (avoid opioid suppressants in infants), and fever reduction (acetaminophen, lukewarm baths; avoid salicylates). Secondary bacterial infections should be treated promptly; antimicrobial prophylaxis is not indicated. Ribavirin is active in vitro and may be useful in infected immunocompromised children. In malnourished children, vitamin A supplementation should be given to avoid blindness and decrease mortality.

Mayo-Wilson E et al: Vitamin A supplementation for preventing mortality, illness, and blindness in children aged under 5: systematic review and meta-analysis. BMJ 2011;343:d5094 [PMID: 21868478].
Moss WJ: Measles. Lancet 2017 Dec 2;390(10111):2490–2502 [PMID: 28673424].

RUBELLA

ESSENTIALS OF DIAGNOSIS & TYPICAL FEATURES

► History of rubella vaccination usually absent.

► Fever with postauricular and occipital adenopathy.

► Maculopapular rash beginning on face, rapidly spreading to the entire body, and disappearing by fourth day.

► Congenital infection: delayed growth and development; cataracts, retinopathy; purpuric rash ("blueberry muffin") at birth; jaundice, thrombocytopenia; deafness, congenital heart defects.

General Considerations

Rubella is a togavirus that causes a mild, self-limited exanthema (> 80% of infections are subclinical), but infection during pregnancy leads to teratogenicity and miscarriage. Rubella is transmitted by aerosolized respiratory secretions. Patients are infectious 5 days before until 5 days after the rash. Endemic rubella is absent in the United States and the Americas, and congenital rubella in infants born to unimmunized women and the occasional woman who is reinfected in pregnancy, is now very rare. Sporadic cases occur in migrants to the United States from Asia and Africa.

Clinical Findings

The incubation period is 14–21 days. The nondistinctive signs may make exposure history unreliable. A history of immunization makes rubella unlikely but still possible. Congenital rubella usually follows maternal infection in the first trimester.

A. Symptoms and Signs

1. Infection in children—Young children may only have rash. Older patients often have a nonspecific prodrome of low-grade fever, ocular pain, sore throat, and myalgia. Postauricular and suboccipital adenopathy (sometimes generalized) is characteristic. The rash consists of erythematous discrete maculopapules beginning on the face and spreading to the trunk and extremities within 24 hours. Scarlatiniform, morbilliform, and erythema infectiosum-like rash variants may occur. The rash fades from the face to extremities by the third day. Enanthema is usually absent.

2. Congenital infection—More than 80% of women infected in the first 4 months of pregnancy (25% near the end of the second trimester) deliver an affected infant; congenital disease occurs in less than 5% of women infected later in pregnancy. Later infections can result in isolated defects, such as deafness. The main manifestations include the following: growth retardation (50%–85%), cardiac anomalies (pulmonary artery stenosis, patent ductus arteriosus, ventricular septal defects), ocular anomalies (cataracts, microphthalmia, glaucoma, retinitis), sensorineural hearing loss (> 50%), cerebral disorders (chronic encephalitis, developmental delay), hematologic disorders (thrombocytopenia, extramedullary "blueberry muffin" hematopoiesis, lymphopenia), and others (hepatitis, osteomyelitis, immune disorders, malabsorption, diabetes).

B. Laboratory Findings

Leukopenia is common, and platelet counts may be low. Congenital infection is associated with low platelet counts, abnormal liver function tests, hemolytic anemia, and CSF pleocytosis in the newborn period. Virus may be isolated from oral secretions or urine from 1 week before to 2 weeks after onset of rash. Children with congenital infection are infectious for months. PCR is very sensitive. Serologic immunoassay diagnosis is best made by demonstrating a fourfold rise in antibody titer between specimens drawn 1–2 weeks apart. The first should be drawn promptly, because titers increase rapidly after onset of rash; both specimens must be tested simultaneously by a single laboratory. Rubella IgM is present in 50% of patients at the onset of the rash, but in almost all by 5 days. Because the decision to terminate a pregnancy is usually based on serologic results, testing must be done carefully.

C. Imaging

Pneumonitis and bone metaphyseal longitudinal lucencies may be present in radiographs of children with congenital infection.

▶ Differential Diagnosis

Rubella may resemble infections due to measles, enterovirus, adenovirus, EBV, roseola, parvovirus, and *T gondii*. Drug reactions may also mimic rubella. Because public health implications are great, sporadic suspected cases should be confirmed serologically or virologically. Congenital rubella must be differentiated from congenital CMV infection, toxoplasmosis, Zika, and syphilis.

▶ Complications & Sequelae

A. Arthralgia and Arthritis

Both occur more often in adult women. Polyarticular involvement (fingers, knees, wrists) lasting a few days to weeks is typical. Frank arthritis occurs in a small percentage of patients. It may resemble acute rheumatoid arthritis.

B. Encephalitis

With an incidence of about 1:6000, this is a parainfectious encephalitis associated with a low mortality rate. A syndrome resembling SSPE (see section on Measles) has also been described in congenital rubella.

C. Rubella in Pregnancy

Infection in the mother as in older children is self-limited and not severe.

▶ Prevention

Rubella is one of the infections that could be eradicated through vaccination (see Chapter 10). Standard prenatal care should include rubella antibody testing. Seropositive mothers are at no risk; seronegative mothers are vaccinated after delivery.

A pregnant woman possibly exposed to rubella should be tested immediately; if seropositive, she is considered protected and without risk to the fetus. If she is seronegative, a second specimen should be drawn in 4 weeks, and both specimens should be tested simultaneously. Seroconversion

in the first trimester is associated with high fetal risk; such women require counseling regarding therapeutic abortion.

When pregnancy termination is not an option, some experts recommend intramuscular administration of immunoglobulin (up to 0.55 mL/kg IM) within 72 hours after exposure in an attempt to prevent infection. Only very small fractions of IgG are transferred to the fetus in early pregnancy and the efficacy of this practice is unknown.

▶ Treatment & Prognosis

Symptomatic therapy is sufficient. Arthritis may improve with administration of anti-inflammatory agents. The prognosis is poor in congenitally infected infants, in whom most defects are irreversible or progressive. The severe cognitive defects in these infants seem to correlate closely with the degree of growth failure.

Lambert N, Strebel P, Orensterin W, Icenogle J, Poland GA: Rubella. Lancet 2015 Jun 6;385(9984):2297–2307 [PMID: 25576992].

White SJ et al: Measles, mumps, and rubella. Clin Obstet Gynecol 2012;55(2):550 [PMID: 22510638].

▼ INFECTIONS DUE TO OTHER VIRUSES

HANTAVIRUS CARDIOPULMONARY SYNDROME

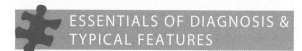

ESSENTIALS OF DIAGNOSIS & TYPICAL FEATURES

- ▶ Influenza-like prodrome for 3–7 days (fever, myalgia, headache, cough).
- ▶ Rapid onset of unexplained pulmonary edema and myocardiopathy.
- ▶ Residence or travel in endemic area; exposure to aerosols from mouse droppings or secretions.

▶ General Considerations

Hantavirus cardiopulmonary syndrome is the first native bunyavirus infection endemic in the United States. This syndrome is distinctly different in mode of spread (no arthropod vector) and clinical picture from other bunyavirus diseases.

▶ Clinical Findings

Hantavirus cardiopulmonary syndrome has been confirmed in more than 34 states and Canada that have the appropriate rodent reservoirs. Epidemics occur when environmental conditions favor large increases in the rodent population and increased prevalence of virus.

A. Symptoms and Signs

After an incubation period of 1–3 weeks, onset is sudden, with a nonspecific virus-like prodrome: fever; back, hip, and leg pain; chills; headache; and nausea and vomiting. Abdominal pain may be present. Sore throat, conjunctivitis, rash, and adenopathy are absent, and respiratory symptoms are absent or limited to a dry cough. After 3–7 days, dyspnea, tachypnea, and evidence of a pulmonary capillary leak syndrome appear. This often progresses rapidly over hours. Hypotension is common, not only from hypoxemia but also from myocardial dysfunction, which is different from septic shock. Copious, amber-colored, nonpurulent secretions are common. Decreased cardiac output due to myocardiopathy and elevated systemic vascular resistance distinguish this disease from early bacterial sepsis.

B. Laboratory Findings

The hemogram shows leukocytosis with a prominent left shift and immunoblasts, thrombocytopenia, and hemoconcentration. Lactate dehydrogenase (LDH) is elevated, as are liver function tests; serum albumin is low. Creatinine is elevated in some patients, and proteinuria is common. Lactic acidosis and low venous bicarbonate are poor prognostic signs. A serum IgM ELISA test is positive early in the illness. Otherwise, the diagnosis is made by PCR or specific staining of tissue at autopsy.

C. Imaging

Initial chest radiographs are normal. Subsequent radiographs show bilateral interstitial infiltrates with the typical butterfly pattern of acute pulmonary edema, bibasilar airspace disease, or both. Significant pleural effusions are often present. These findings contrast with those of other causes of acute respiratory distress syndrome.

D. Differential Diagnosis

In some geographic areas, plague and tularemia may be possibilities. Infections with viral respiratory pathogens and *Mycoplasma* have a slower progression, do not elevate the LDH, and do not cause the hematologic changes seen in this syndrome. Q fever, psittacosis, toxin exposure, legionellosis, and fungal infections are possibilities, but the history, tempo of the illness, and blood findings, as well as the exposure history, should be distinguishing features. Hantavirus cardiopulmonary syndrome is a consideration in previously healthy persons from a rural area or potential exposure to wild rodents, who have a febrile illness associated with unexplained pulmonary edema.

E. Treatment and Prognosis

There is no established antiviral therapy. Management should concentrate on oxygen therapy and mechanical ventilation as required. Because of capillary leakage, Swan-Ganz catheterization to monitor cardiac output and inotropic support—rather than fluid therapy—should be used to maintain perfusion. Venoarterial extracorporeal membrane oxygenation can provide short-term support for selected patients. The strains of virus present in North America are not spread by person-to-person contact. No isolation is required. The case fatality rate is 30%–40%. Guidelines are available for reduction of exposure to the infectious agent.

Avsic T, Saksida A, Korva M: Hantavirus infection. Clin Microbiol Infect 2015 June; 21S:e6–e16 [PMID: 24750436].

Sargianou M et al: Hantavirus infections for the clinician: from case presentation to diagnosis and treatment. Crit Rev Microbiol 2012;38(4):317 [PMID: 22553984].

MUMPS

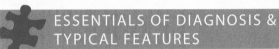

ESSENTIALS OF DIAGNOSIS & TYPICAL FEATURES

► No prior mumps immunization or waning vaccine immunity.

► Parotid gland swelling.

► Aseptic meningitis with or without parotitis.

► General Considerations

Mumps virus, a paramyxovirus, is spread by the respiratory route and attacks almost all nonprotected children (asymptomatically in 30%–40% of cases). As a result of prior clinical or subclinical infection, or childhood immunization, 95% of adults are immune, although immunity can wane in late adolescence. When the number of unprotected rises, epidemics (5833 cases in 2016 and 3176 at mid-2017) can occur, which are aborted by reimmunization of the at-risk population, especially college students. Infected patients are infectious from 2 days prior to 5 days after the onset of parotitis. The incubation period is 14–21 days. In an adequately immunized individual, parotitis is usually due to another cause. Two doses of the vaccine are 88% (range: 66%–95%) effective at protecting against mumps; one dose is 78% effective (range: 49%–92%). However, an outbreak in Guam occurred even when most children had two doses of vaccine, likely spread by crowding.

► Clinical Findings

A. Symptoms and Signs

1. Salivary gland disease—After a prodrome of fever, severe headache, arthralgia, and anorexia, tender swelling of parotid glands occurs (70%–80% bilateral). The ear is displaced upward and outward; the mandibular angle is obliterated. Parotid stimulation with sour foods may be quite painful. The orifice of the Stensen duct may be red and swollen; yellow secretions may be expressed, but pus is absent. Parotid swelling dissipates after 1 week.

2. Meningoencephalitis—Once the most common cause of aseptic meningitis, mumps meningitis was manifested by severe headache, vomiting, and/or asymptomatic mononuclear pleocytosis. Fewer than 10% of patients had clinical meningitis or encephalitis. Parotitis is present in only half of the cases of mumps meningoencephalitis. Although neck stiffness, nausea, and vomiting can occur, encephalitic symptoms are rare (1:4000 cases of mumps); recovery in 3–10 days is the rule.

3. Pancreatitis—Epigastric abdominal pain may represent transient pancreatitis. Because salivary gland disease may elevate serum amylase, specific markers of pancreatic function (lipase, amylase isoenzymes) are required for assessing pancreatic involvement.

4. Orchitis, oophoritis—Involvement of the gonads is associated with fever, local tenderness, and swelling and is second to parotitis as presentation of mumps in adolescents. Epididymitis is usually present. Most often unilateral, it resolves in 1–2 weeks. Although one-third of infected testes atrophy, bilateral involvement and sterility are rare.

5. Other—Thyroiditis, mastitis (especially in adolescent females), arthritis, and presternal edema (occasionally with dysphagia or hoarseness) may be seen.

B. Laboratory Findings

Peripheral blood leukocyte count is usually normal. CSF may contain a modest number of cells (~ 250 cells/μL, predominantly lymphocytes), with mildly elevated protein and normal to slightly decreased glucose. Viral PCR or culture of saliva, throat, urine, or spinal fluid may be positive for at least 1 week after onset. Paired sera assayed by ELISA or a single positive IgM antibody test may be used for diagnosis.

▶ Differential Diagnosis

A history of contact with a child with parotitis is not proof of mumps exposure. Mumps parotitis may resemble cervical adenitis (the jaw angle may be obliterated, but the ear does not usually protrude; the Stensen duct orifice is normal; leukocytosis and neutrophilia are observed), bacterial parotitis (pus in the Stensen duct, toxicity, exquisite tenderness), recurrent parotitis (idiopathic or associated with calculi), tumors or leukemia, and tooth infections. Many viruses, including parainfluenza, enteroviruses, EBV, CMV, and influenza, can cause parotitis. Parotid swelling in HIV infection is less painful and tends to be bilateral and chronic, but may occur.

Unless parotitis is present, mumps meningitis resembles that caused by enteroviruses or early bacterial infection. An elevated amylase level may be useful clue in this situation. Isolated pancreatitis is not distinguishable from many other causes of epigastric pain and vomiting. Mumps is a classic cause of orchitis, but torsion, bacterial or chlamydial epididymitis, *Mycoplasma* infection, other viral infections, hematomas, hernias, and tumors must also be considered.

▶ Complications

The major neurologic complication is nerve deafness (usually unilateral) which can result in inability to hear high tones. Although rare, occurring in less than 0.1% of cases of mumps, it may occur without meningitis. Aqueductal stenosis and hydrocephalus (especially following congenital infection), myocarditis, transverse myelitis, and facial paralysis are other rare complications.

▶ Treatment & Prognosis

Treatment is supportive and includes provision of fluids, analgesics, and scrotal support for orchitis. Systemic corticosteroids have been used for orchitis, but their value is anecdotal.

Rubin S, Kennedy R, Poland G: Emerging mumps infection. Pediatr Infect Dis J 2016 Jul;35(7):799–801 [PMID: 27097351].

RABIES

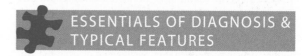

ESSENTIALS OF DIAGNOSIS & TYPICAL FEATURES

▶ History of animal bite 10 days to 1 year (usually < 90 days) previously.

▶ Paresthesias or hyperesthesia in bite area.

▶ Progressive limb and facial weakness in some patients (dumb rabies; 30%).

▶ Irritability followed by fever, confusion, combativeness, muscle spasms (especially pharyngeal with swallowing) in all patients (furious rabies).

▶ Rabies nucleic acid (RT-PCR) or antigen detected in corneal scrapings or tissue obtained by brain or skin biopsy; Negri bodies seen in brain tissue.

▶ General Considerations

Rabies is an acute progressive CNS viral zoonotic infection. It remains a serious public health problem wherever animal immunization is not widely practiced or when humans play or work in areas with sylvan rabies. Infection is almost invariably fatal and will occur in 40% after rabid animal bites. Any warm-blooded animal may be infected, but susceptibility and transmissibility vary with different species. Bats often carry and excrete the virus in saliva or feces for prolonged periods; they are the major cause of rabies in the United States. Dogs and cats, responsible for most rabies in the world, are usually clinically ill within 10 days after becoming contagious (the standard quarantine period for suspect animals). Valid quarantine periods or signs of illness are not fully known for many species. Rodents rarely transmit infection. Animal vaccines are very effective when properly administered, but a single inoculation may fail to produce immunity in up to 20% of dogs.

The risk is assessed according to the type of animal (high-risk animals include bats, raccoons, skunks, and foxes), wound extent and location (infection more common after head or hand bites, or if wounds have extensive salivary contamination and are not quickly and thoroughly cleaned), geographic area (urban rabies is rare to nonexistent in the United States; rural rabies is possible, especially outside the United States), and animal vaccination history (risk low if documented). Most rabies in the United States is caused by bat genotypes, yet a history of bat bite is often not obtained especially in young children. Aerosolized virus in caves inhabited by bats has caused infection.

Clinical Findings

A. Symptoms and Signs

Most cases occur within 3–12 weeks of exposure and may present with vague symptoms. Paresthesia at the bite site is usually the first symptom. Nonspecific anxiety, excitability, or depression follows, then muscle spasms, drooling, hydrophobia, delirium, and lethargy. Swallowing or even the sensation of air blown on the face may cause pharyngeal spasms. Seizures, fever, cranial nerve palsies, coma, and death follow within 7–14 days after onset. In a minority of patients, the spastic components are initially absent and the symptoms are primarily flaccid paralysis and cranial nerve defects. The furious components appear subsequently.

B. Laboratory Findings

Leukocytosis is common. CSF is usually normal, but may show elevation of protein and mononuclear cell pleocytosis. Cerebral imaging and electroencephalography are not diagnostic. Infection in an animal may be determined by PCR or fluorescent antibody test to examine brain tissue for antigen. Rabies virus is excreted in the saliva of infected humans, but the diagnosis is usually made by nucleic acid (RT-PCR) or antigen detection in scrapings or tissue samples of richly innervated epithelium, such as the cornea or the hairline of the neck. Classic Negri cytoplasmic inclusion bodies in brain tissue are not always present. Seroconversion measured by neutralizing antibody occurs after 7–10 days. Clinical recovery has been associated with detection of neutralizing antibody and clearance of infectious rabies virus in the CNS.

Differential Diagnosis

Failure to elicit the bite history in areas where rabies is rare may delay diagnosis. Other disorders to be considered include parainfectious encephalopathy; encephalitis due to herpes simplex, mosquito-borne viruses, or other causes of viral encephalitis or acute paralysis. However, classic furious rabies is not readily confused with these alternative diagnoses.

Prevention

See Chapter 10 for information regarding vaccination and postexposure prophylaxis. Rabies immunoglobulin and diploid cell vaccine have made prophylaxis more effective and minimally toxic. Because rabies is almost always fatal, presumed exposures must be managed carefully.

Treatment & Prognosis

Survival is very rare, but it has been reported in a very small number of patients receiving meticulous intensive care and protocols that focus on the altered CNS metabolic state (eg, Milwaukee protocol). Early diagnosis is important for the protection and postexposure prophylaxis of patient contacts.

Willoughby RE Jr: Rabies: rare human infection—common questions. Infect Dis Clin North Am 2015 Dec;29(4):637–650. doi: 10.1016/j.idc.2015.07.006 [PMID: 26384549].

▼ RICKETTSIAL INFECTIONS AND Q FEVER

Rickettsiae are pleomorphic, gram-negative coccobacilli that are obligate intracellular parasites. Rickettsial diseases are often included in the differential diagnosis of febrile rashes. Severe headache, myalgia, and pulmonary symptoms are prominent manifestations. The endothelium is the primary target tissue, and the ensuing vasculitis is responsible for severe illness.

All rickettsioses are transmitted by arthropod contact (ticks, fleas, lice—depending on the disease), either by bite or by contamination of skin breaks with vector feces. Except Rocky Mountain spotted fever and murine typhus, all other rickettsial diseases have a characteristic eschar at the bite site, called the *tache noire*. Evidence of arthropod contact by history or physical examination may be lacking, especially in young children. The geographic distribution of the vector is often the primary determinant for suspicion of these infections. Therapy often must be empiric. Many new broad-spectrum antimicrobials are inactive against these cell wall-deficient organisms; tetracyclines are usually effective.

Q fever, which is not a rickettsiae, is included here because it was long classified as such and, like rickettsiae, is an obligate intracellular bacterium. It is not transmitted by an insect vector and is not characterized by rash.

HUMAN EHRLICHIOSIS & ANAPLASMOSIS

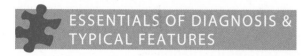

ESSENTIALS OF DIAGNOSIS & TYPICAL FEATURES

▶ Residing or travel in endemic area when ticks are active.

▶ Tick bite noted (~ 75%).

▶ Fever, headache, rash (~ 67%), gastrointestinal symptoms.

▶ Leukopenia, thrombocytopenia, elevated serum transaminases, hypoalbuminemia.

▶ Definitive diagnosis by specific serology.

In children, the major agent of North American human ehrlichiosis is *Ehrlichia chaffeensis*. The reservoir hosts are probably wild rodents, deer, and sheep; ticks are the vectors. Most cases caused by this agent are reported in the south-central, southeastern, and middle Atlantic states (Arkansas, Missouri, Oklahoma, Kentucky, Tennessee, and North Carolina are high-prevalence areas). Almost all cases occur between March and October, when ticks are active.

A second ehrlichiosis syndrome, seen in the upper Midwest and Northeast (Rhode Island, Connecticut, Wisconsin, Minnesota, and New York are high-prevalence areas), is caused by *Anaplasma phagocytophilum* and *Ehrlichia ewingii*. Anaplasmosis also occurs in the western United States.

E chaffeensis has a predilection for mononuclear cells, whereas *A phagocytophilum* and *E ewingii* infect and produce intracytoplasmic inclusions in granulocytes. Hence, diseases caused by these agents are referred to as human monocytic ehrlichiosis or human granulocytic ehrlichiosis, respectively. Ehrlichiosis, Lyme disease, and babesiosis share some tick vectors; thus, dual infections can occur and should be considered in patients who fail to respond to therapy.

Clinical Findings

In approximately 75% of patients, a history of tick bite can be elicited. The majority of the remaining patients report having been in a tick-infested area. The usual incubation period is 5–21 days.

A. Symptoms and Signs

Fever is universally present and headache is common (less so in children). Gastrointestinal symptoms (abdominal pain, anorexia, nausea, and vomiting) are reported in most pediatric patients. Distal limb edema may occur. Chills, photophobia, conjunctivitis, and myalgia occur in more than half

of patients. Rash occurs in ~ 50% of children with monocytic ehrlichiosis and is much less common in granulocytic ehrlichiosis. Rash may be erythematous, macular, papular, petechial, scarlatiniform, or vasculitic. Meningitis occurs, and altered mental status is common. Interstitial pneumonitis, acute respiratory distress syndrome, and renal failure occur in severe cases. Physical examination reveals rash (not usually palms and soles), mild adenopathy, and hepatomegaly. In children without a rash, infection may present as a fever of unknown origin.

B. Laboratory Findings

Laboratory abnormalities include leukopenia with left shift, lymphopenia, thrombocytopenia, elevated aminotransferase and LDH levels. Hypoalbuminemia and hyponatremia are common. Disseminated intravascular coagulation can occur. Anemia occurs in one-third of patients. CSF pleocytosis (mononuclear cells and increased protein) is common. The definitive diagnosis can be made by PCR or serologically, either by a single high titer or a fourfold rise in titer during acute and convalescent samples. The CDC uses an immunofluorescent antibody test to distinguish between the etiologic agents. Intracytoplasmic inclusions (morulae) may occasionally be observed in mononuclear cells in monocytic ehrlichiosis, and are usually observed in polymorphonuclear cells from the peripheral blood or bone marrow in granulocytic ehrlichiosis. PCR may be negative after 48 hours if patient is on appropriate antibiotics.

Differential Diagnosis

In regions where these infections exist, ehrlichiosis should be included in the differential diagnosis of children who present during tick season with fever, leukopenia or thrombocytopenia (or both), increased serum transaminase levels, and rash. The differential diagnosis includes septic or toxic shock, other rickettsial infections (especially Rocky Mountain spotted fever), Colorado tick fever, leptospirosis, Lyme borreliosis, relapsing fever, EBV, CMV, viral hepatitis and other viral infections, Kawasaki disease, systemic lupus erythematosus, and leukemia.

Treatment & Prognosis

Asymptomatic or clinically mild and undiagnosed infections are common in some endemic areas. The disease may last several weeks if untreated. One-quarter of hospitalized children require intensive care. Meningoencephalitis and persisting neurologic deficits occur in 5%–10% of patients. Doxycycline for 7–10 days is the treatment of choice. Patients with suspected disease must be treated preemptively concurrently with attempts to establish the diagnosis. Response to therapy should be evident in 24–48 hours. Deaths are uncommon in children. Immune compromise and asplenia are risk factors for severe disease.

Sanchez E, Vannier E, Wormser GP: Diagnosis, treatment and prevention of Lyme disease, human granulocytic anaplasmosis and babesiosis. JAMA 2016;315:1767 [PMID: 27115378].

Schultz GE, Buckingham SC, Marshall GS: Human monocytic ehrlichiosis in children. Pediatr Infect Dis J 2007;26:475 [PMID: 17529862].

ROCKY MOUNTAIN SPOTTED FEVER

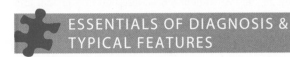

ESSENTIALS OF DIAGNOSIS & TYPICAL FEATURES

▶ Residing or travel in endemic area with ticks; tick bite reported for 50% only.

▶ Fever, rash (palms and soles), gastrointestinal symptoms, headache.

▶ Thrombocytopenia, hyponatremia, hypoalbuminemia.

▶ Begin treatment with doxycycline based on clinical suspicion.

Rickettsia rickettsii causes one of many similar tick-borne illnesses characterized by fever and rash that occur worldwide. Most are named after their geographic area. Dogs and rodents, as well as large mammals, are reservoirs of *R rickettsii*.

Rocky Mountain spotted fever is the most severe rickettsial infection and the most important (~ 2000 cases per year) in the United States. It occurs predominantly along the eastern seaboard; in the southeastern states; and in Arkansas, Missouri, and Oklahoma. It is much less common in the west. Most cases occur in children exposed in rural areas from April to September. Infection can be acquired from dog ticks.

▶ Clinical Findings

A. Symptoms and Signs

After the incubation period of 3–12 days (mean, 7 days), there is high fever (> 40°C), usually of abrupt onset, myalgia, severe and persistent headache (retro-orbital), toxicity, photophobia, vomiting, abdominal pain, and diarrhea. A rash occurs in more than 95% of patients and appears 2–6 days after fever onset as macules and papules; most characteristic (65%) is involvement of the palms, soles, and extremities; the face is spared. The rash becomes petechial and spreads centrally from the extremities. The rash reflects infection of endothelial cells, which also causes vascular leak and resulting edema, hypovolemia, and hypotension. Conjunctivitis, splenomegaly, pneumonitis, meningismus, and confusion may occur.

B. Laboratory Findings

Laboratory findings reflect diffuse vasculitis: thrombocytopenia, hyponatremia, early mild leukopenia, proteinuria, mildly abnormal liver function tests, hypoalbuminemia, and hematuria. CSF pleocytosis is common. Serologic diagnosis is achieved with indirect fluorescent or latex agglutination antibody methods, but generally is informative only 7–10 days after onset of the illness. Skin biopsy with specific fluorescent staining is a specific and moderately sensitive diagnostic method available during the first week of the illness.

▶ Differential Diagnosis

The differential diagnosis includes meningococcemia, measles, meningococcal meningitis, staphylococcal sepsis, EBV infection, enteroviral infection, leptospirosis, Colorado tick fever, scarlet fever, murine typhus, Kawasaki disease, and ehrlichiosis.

▶ Treatment & Prognosis

To be effective, therapy for Rocky Mountain spotted fever must be started early, most often on the basis of a high clinical suspicion prior to rash onset in endemic areas. Atypical presentations, such as the absence of pathognomonic rash, can lead to delay in appropriate therapy. Rash is rarely present during the first day of diagnosis and in 50% within 3 days of onset of fever. Doxycycline is the treatment of choice for children, regardless of age, and should be continued for 10 days and at least 2–3 days after resolution of fever for a full day.

Complications and death result from severe vasculitis, especially in the brain, heart, and lungs. The mortality rate is 5%–7%. Persistent neurologic deficits occur in 10%–15% of children who recover. Delay in therapy is an important determinant of sequelae and mortality.

Because tick attachment lasting 6 hours or longer is associated with transmission of the pathogen, frequent tick removal is a preventive measure.

Mukkada S, Buckingham SC: Recognition and prompt treatment for tick-born infection in children. Infect Dis Clin North Am 2015;29:539 [PMID: 26188606].

ENDEMIC TYPHUS (MURINE TYPHUS)

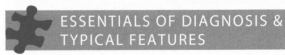

ESSENTIALS OF DIAGNOSIS & TYPICAL FEATURES

▶ Residing in endemic area.

▶ Fever for 10–14 days.

▶ Headache, chills, myalgia.

▶ Maculopapular rash spreading from trunk to extremities (not on palms and soles) 3–7 days after fever onset.

▶ Definitive diagnosis by serology.

Endemic typhus is present in the southern United States, mainly in southern Texas, southern California, and Hawaii. The disease is transmitted by fleas from infected rodents or inhalation of rodent feces. Domestic cats, dogs, and opossums may play a role in the transmission of suburban cases. The incubation period is 6–14 days. Headache, myalgia and arthralgia, and chills slowly worsen. Fever may last 10–14 days. After 3–7 days, a rash appears. Truncal macules and papules spread to the extremities; the rash is rarely petechial and resolves in < 5 days. The location of the rash in typhus, with sparing of the palms and soles, helps distinguish the disease from Rocky Mountain spotted fever. Rash may be absent in 20%–40% of patients. Hepatomegaly may be present. Intestinal and respiratory symptoms may occur. Mild thrombocytopenia and elevated liver enzymes may be present. Prolonged neurologic symptoms can occur. Clinicians in endemic areas should consider early treatment when presented with a child with protracted fever, rash, and headache. Doxycycline is the drug of choice, which should be continued for 3 days after evidence of clinical improvement. Fluorescent antibody and ELISA tests are available.

Liddel PW, Sparks MJ: Murine typhus: endemic *Rickettsia* in southwest Texas. Clin Lab Sci 2012;25(2):81 [PMID: 20120614].

Tsioutis C: Clinical and laboratory characteristics, epidemiology, and outcomes of murine typhus: a systematic review. Acta Trop 2017 Feb;166:16–24 [PMID: 27983969].

Q FEVER

ESSENTIALS OF DIAGNOSIS & TYPICAL FEATURES

▶ Exposure to farm animals (sheep, goats, cattle) and pets.

▶ Flu-like illness (fever, severe headache, myalgia).

▶ Cough; atypical pneumonia.

▶ Hepatomegaly and hepatitis.

▶ Diagnosis by serology.

Coxiella burnetii is transmitted by inhalation rather than by an arthropod bite. Q fever is also distinguished from rickettsial diseases by the infrequent occurrence of cutaneous manifestations and by the prominence of pulmonary disease. The birth tissues and excreta of domestic animals and of some rodents are major infectious sources. The organisms may be carried long distances in fine particle aerosols. Unpasteurized milk from infected animals may also transmit disease.

▶ Clinical Findings

A. Symptoms and Signs

Most patients have a self-limited flu-like syndrome of chills, fever, severe headache, and myalgia of abrupt onset occurring 10–25 days after exposure. Abdominal pain, vomiting, chest pain, and dry cough are prominent in children. Examination of the chest may yield few findings, as in other atypical pneumonias. Hepatosplenomegaly is common. The illness lasts 1–4 weeks and frequently is associated with weight loss. Only about 50% of infected patients develop significant symptoms.

B. Laboratory Findings

Leukopenia with left shift is characteristic. Thrombocytopenia is unusual, which is another distinction from rickettsial diseases. Aminotransferase and γ-glutamyl transferase levels are elevated, but significant bilirubin elevation is unusual. Diagnosis is made by positive PCR or serologic response (fourfold rise or single high titer in ELISA, IFA, or CF antibody assay) to the phase II organism. Chronic infection is indicated by antibody against the phase I organism. IgM ELISA tests are available.

C. Imaging

Pneumonitis occurs in 50% of patients. Multiple segmental infiltrates are common, but the radiographic appearance is not pathognomonic. Consolidation and pleural effusion are rare.

▶ Differential Diagnosis

In the appropriate epidemiologic setting, Q fever should be considered in evaluating causes of atypical pneumonias, such as *M pneumoniae*, viruses, *Legionella*, and *C pneumoniae*. It should also be included among the causes of mild to moderate hepatitis without rash or adenopathy in children with exposure to farm animals.

▶ Treatment & Prognosis

Typically the illness lasts 1–2 weeks without therapy. The course of the uncomplicated illness is shortened with doxycycline. Therapy is continued for several days after the patient becomes afebrile (usually 10–14 days). Quinolones are also effective.

One complication is chronic disease, which often implies myocarditis or granulomatous hepatitis. Meningoencephalitis is a rare complication. *C burnetii* is also one of the causes of "culture-negative" endocarditis. Coxiella endocarditis often occurs in the setting of valve abnormalities and is difficult to treat; mortality approaches 50%.

Eldin C, Melenotte C, Mediannikov O: From Q fever to *Coxiella burnetii* infection: a paradigm change. Clin Micro Rev 2017;30:115 [PMID: 27856520].

Human Immunodeficiency Virus Infection

Elizabeth J. McFarland, MD

PATHOGENESIS & EPIDEMIOLOGY

▶ Pathogenesis & Transmission

Human immunodeficiency virus (HIV) is a retrovirus that enters and then integrates its nucleic acid into the DNA of cells of the immune system, including helper T lymphocytes (CD4 T lymphocytes), monocytes, and macrophages. The function and number of CD4 T lymphocytes and other affected cells are diminished by HIV infection, resulting in profound defects in cell-mediated and humoral immunity. HIV is found in blood, semen, preseminal fluids, rectal fluids, vaginal fluids, and breast milk, with transmission occurring via sexual contact, sharing contaminated needles, and perinatal transmission (in utero, peripartum, breast-feeding). Rarely, infants have acquired HIV from food premasticated by a person with HIV. Casual, classroom, or household contact with an HIV-infected person poses no risk of transmission in the absence of contact with blood or bloody secretions. Exposure resulting from accidental needle sticks or, rarely, mucosal exposure to blood may occur, mainly in health care settings.

At the time of exposure, HIV migrates to regional lymph nodes, replicates, and spreads to lymphoid tissues throughout the body. Based on nonhuman primate models, replicating virus is disseminated by 48 hours postinfection. Approximately 2 weeks after exposure, a high level of virus is detected in the bloodstream. In adults without therapy, the level of viremia declines concurrent with the appearance of an HIV-specific host immune response, and plasma viremia usually reaches a steady-state level about 6 months after primary infection. An asymptomatic period usually follows, lasting from 1 year to more than 12 years. However, ongoing viremia and immune activation causes injury to the immune system and other organs.

Infants with perinatal HIV infection have viremia that rises steeply after birth, reaching a peak at 1–2 months of age. In contrast with adults, infants have a gradual decline in plasma viremia that extends to age 4–5 years. Without treatment, up to 50% of infants will have rapid disease progression to AIDS or death by age 2 years.

HIV infection, in the absence of treatment, causes progressive immune incompetence with the hallmark loss of CD4 T-lymphocyte numbers, leading to conditions that meet the definition of acquired immunodeficiency syndrome (AIDS) and, eventually, death. AIDS is diagnosed when an HIV-infected individual develops any of the stage 3 opportunistic illnesses or other conditions listed in Table 41–1. In adults and children older than 6 years, the criteria for a diagnosis of AIDS also include an absolute CD4 T-lymphocyte count of 200 cells/μL or less.

Antiretroviral treatment (ART) inhibits virus replication and permits immune reconstitution. Cells with latent HIV infection persist and viral replication recurs if ART is interrupted; thus, treatment must be lifelong. Even with effective viral suppression, ongoing immune activation results in end-organ (eg, cardiovascular and central nervous system) damage consistent with premature aging. Nevertheless, HIV infection, once a terminal disease, is now a chronic condition for people with access to treatment.

▶ Epidemiology

The World Health Organization (WHO) estimated in 2018 that there are 37.9 million adults and 1.7 million children living with HIV (https://www.who.int/hiv/data/2018_summary-global-hiv-epi.png?ua=1). Over 90% live in low- and middle-income countries, primarily sub-Saharan Africa and South and Southeast Asia. The annual number of new infections decreased by 36% between 2000 and 2017, but infection and mortality rates remain high. Among children younger than 15 years, there were 160,000 new infections and 100,000 deaths in 2018.

Table 41–1. HIV-related symptoms in children.

Mild symptoms	Severe (stage 3-defining) opportunistic illnesses and other conditions
Having two or more of the following conditions:	Bacterial infections, multiple or recurrent[a]
Lymphadenopathy	Candidiasis of bronchi, trachea, or lungs
Hepatomegaly	Candidiasis of esophagus
Splenomegaly	Cervical cancer, invasive[b]
Dermatitis	Coccidioidomycosis, disseminated or extrapulmonary
Parotitis	Cryptococcosis, extrapulmonary
Recurrent or persistent upper respiratory infection, sinusitis, or otitis media	Cryptosporidiosis, chronic intestinal (> 1 mo duration)
Moderate symptoms	Cytomegalovirus disease (other than liver, spleen, or nodes) with onset > age 1 mo
Anemia, neutropenia, thrombocytopenia	Cytomegalovirus retinitis (with loss of vision)
Bacterial meningitis, pneumonia, sepsis (single episode)	Encephalopathy attributed to HIV
Candidiasis, oropharyngeal, persisting > 2 mo, in a child > 6 mo of age	Herpes simplex virus: chronic oral lesions (> 1 mo), or bronchitis, pneumonitis, or esophagitis (onset at > age 1 mo)
Cardiomyopathy	Histoplasmosis, disseminated or extrapulmonary
Cytomegalovirus infection with onset < age 1 mo	Isosporiasis, chronic intestinal (> 1 mo duration)
Diarrhea, recurrent or chronic	Kaposi sarcoma
Hepatitis	Lymphoma: Burkitt, immunoblastic, or primary lesion in brain
Herpes simplex virus stomatitis (> 2 episodes in 1 y), bronchitis, pneumonitis, esophagitis at < 1 mo of age	*Mycobacterium avium* complex or *Mycobacterium kansasii*, disseminated or extrapulmonary
Herpes zoster, two or more episodes or more than one dermatome	*Mycobacterium tuberculosis* of any site, pulmonary,[b] disseminated, extrapulmonary
Leiomyosarcoma	Mycobacterium, other species or unidentified, disseminated or extrapulmonary
Lymphoid interstitial pneumonia	
Nephropathy	*Pneumocystis jiroveci* pneumonia
Nocardiosis	Pneumonia, recurrent[b]
Persistent fever (lasting > 1 mo)	Progressive multifocal leukoencephalopathy
Toxoplasmosis with onset < age 1 mo	*Salmonella* septicemia, recurrent
Varicella, complicated	Toxoplasmosis of the brain with onset > age 1 mo
	Wasting syndrome

[a]Only among children younger than 6 years.
[b]Only among adults, adolescents, and children older than or equal to 6 years.
Data from Centers for Disease Control and Prevention (CDC): Revised surveillance case definition for HIV infection—United States, 2014. MMWR Recomm Rep 2014 Apr 11;63(RR-03):1–10 and AIDS info Guidelines for the Use of Antiretroviral Agents in Pediatric HIV infection, 1/21/16.

Preventative measures can reduce the rate of perinatal transmission from 40% to less than 1%. New pediatric infections continue to occur in resource-limited settings due to inadequate access to care; approximately 80% of all pregnant women living with HIV globally received recommended treatment in 2017 (https://www.who.int/news-room/fact-sheets/detail/hiv-aids). In the United States, successful implementation of preventative interventions for perinatal HIV has made new perinatally acquired HIV cases rare (73 cases reported in 2017). In 2016, there were 2238 children younger than 13 years living with HIV in the United States, of whom the majority are foreign-born. Overall, there are approximately 10,000 people living with perinatally acquired HIV, some having reach their fourth decade as a result of highly effective treatment (https://www.cdc.gov/hiv/pdf/library/reports/surveillance/cdc-hiv-surveillance-report-2017-vol-29.pdf).

By contrast, adolescents and young adults in the United States continue to be at risk of HIV acquisition; youth aged 13–24 years accounted for 21% (8164) of the 38,739 new HIV infections in 2017. The primary HIV exposure was male-to-male sexual contact, with the majority (87%) of the infections among gay and bisexual men, predominantly African American (51%) and Hispanic (25%) (https://www.cdc.gov/hiv/group/age/youth/index.html).

Centers for Disease Control and Prevention: *HIV Surveillance Report, 2017.* Vol 29. http://www.cdc.gov/hiv/library/reports/hiv-surveillance.html. Published November 2018. Accessed May 25, 2019.
World Health Organization (WHO): HIV/AIDS Data and statistics. Available at: http://www.who.int/hiv/data/en/. Accessed May 25, 2019.

PREVENTION

ESSENTIALS OF DIAGNOSIS & TYPICAL FEATURES

▶ Prevention of mother-to-child transmission (PMTCT) is highly successful with timely use of antiretroviral drugs during pregnancy and breast-feeding.

▶ Prevention of sexual transmission can be accomplished through integrated biomedical and behavioral interventions, including antiretroviral drugs for pre- and postexposure prophylaxis (PEP) and condom use.

▶ Application of universal precautions (assumes all blood or bloody secretions are potentially infectious) prevents horizontal environmental transmission.

▶ Prevention of Perinatal HIV Transmission

Key to prevention of perinatal HIV transmission is identification of pregnant women with HIV infection. Standard pregnancy care should include routine HIV testing early in gestation for all pregnant women (and their partners) and repeat testing in the third trimester if there have been risk factors for HIV acquisition, an illness consistent with acute HIV infection, or HIV seroprevalence is high (≥ 1/1000) among women delivering at the facility. For woman presenting in labor without previously documented HIV testing, HIV testing is recommended using assays that yield results within 60 minutes or less so that antiretrovirals (ARV) can be initiated for the mother during labor and/or for the infant immediately postpartum.

Maternal ART started before or early in pregnancy, in combination with infant ARV prophylaxis for 4–6 weeks postpartum, reduces the risk of transmission from 25%–40% to less than 1% with optimal maternal viral suppression. The choice of optimal ART during pregnancy is complex, and guidelines are updated frequently by the U.S. Department of Health and Human Services (https://aidsinfo.nih.gov/guidelines/html/3/perinatal/0). In addition, a consult line is available 24/7 for questions about prevention of perinatal HIV transmission (http://nccc.ucsf.edu/clinician-consultation/perinatal-hiv-aids/, 888-448-8765). Elective C-section prior to labor will also reduce transmission risk for women who have plasma viral load greater than or equal to 1000 copies/mL. Even if diagnosis of HIV is late, ARV medications given to women in labor and/or to infants as late as 48 hours postpartum reduce transmission by as much as 50%.

In resource-limited settings, breast-feeding increases survival and, therefore, breast-feeding is usually preferred to formula-feeding. Continuation of maternal ART or extended ARV prophylaxis given to the infant for the duration of breast-feeding markedly reduces transmission resulting from breast milk. Breast-feeding is not recommended in the United States where access to safe formula is readily available. However, a minority of women may choose to breast-feed for cultural or other reasons. In this scenario, attention to maternal adherence to ART and frequent monitoring of the mother for detectable plasma virus and of the infant for transmission is recommended. Several cases of HIV transmission have resulted from HIV-infected caregivers feeding children premasticated food; hence, families should be advised against this practice.

▶ Prevention of Sexual Transmission

For individuals at risk of HIV acquisition through sexual contact, prevention efforts should integrate biomedical and behavioral methods. The FDA has approved the antiretroviral tenofovir/emtricitabine, a once daily, fixed-dose, single pill, for preexposure prophylaxis (PrEP) for adults and adolescents (https://www.cdc.gov/hiv/pdf/risk/prep/cdc-hiv-prep-guidelines-2017.pdf). Combination ARV is also effective as PEP (https://stacks.cdc.gov/view/cdc/38856). These regimens are described in Chapter 44. The CDC publishes a compendium of evidence-based behavioral interventions for safer sex practices (https://www.cdc.gov/hiv/research/interventionresearch/compendium/rr/index.html).

On a public health level, a high priority for HIV prevention is widespread diagnosis and treatment of people living with HIV. Treatment of partners with HIV resulted in a 96% reduction in transmission to uninfected partners. Thus, treatment benefits the health of the individual with HIV and reduces the risk of transmission to others. Large studies of partners discordant for HIV demonstrate that there is effectively no risk of sexual transmission of HIV when the partner living with HIV on ART has a durably undetectable viral load (https://www.niaid.nih.gov/news-events/undetectable-equals-untransmittable). Broad recognition of this concept (termed Undetectable = Untransmittable), partnered with effective treatment, has the potential to markedly reduce the stigma associated with an HIV diagnosis.

▶ Prevention Through Universal Precautions

Horizontal transmission (in the absence of sexual contact or injecting drug use) of HIV is exceedingly rare and is associated with exposure of nonintact skin or mucous membranes to HIV-infected blood or bloody secretions. Saliva, tears, urine, and stool are not infectious if they do not contain gross blood. Barrier protection (eg, latex or rubber gloves or thick pads of fabric or paper) should be used when possible contact with blood or bloody body fluids may occur. Objects that might be contaminated with blood, such as razors or toothbrushes, should not be shared. No special care is required for dishes, towels, toys, or bedclothes. Blood-soiled clothing may be washed routinely with hot water and detergent. Contaminated surfaces may be disinfected easily with a variety of agents, including household bleach (1:10 dilution), some commercial disinfectants (eg, Lysol), or 70% isopropyl alcohol.

The infant or child with HIV who is well enough to attend day care or school should not be treated differently from other children. The exception may be a toddler with uncontrollable biting behavior or bleeding lesions that cannot be covered adequately; in these situations, the child may be withheld from group day care. Families may choose to make the school health care provider and/or teacher aware of the diagnosis, but there is no legal requirement that any individual at the school or day care center be informed. The parents and child may prefer to keep the diagnosis confidential, because the stigma associated with HIV infection remains difficult to overcome. Because undiagnosed HIV-infected infants and children might be enrolled, all schools and day care centers should have policies with simple guidelines for using universal precautions to prevent transmission of HIV infection in these settings.

Centers for Disease Control and Prevention: US Public Health Service: Preexposure prophylaxis for the prevention of HIV infection in the United States—2017 Update: a clinical practice guideline. https://www.cdc.gov/hiv/pdf/risk/prep/cdc-hiv-prep-guidelines-2017.pdf. Published March 2018.

National Clinicians Consultation Center PrEPline. http://nccc.ucsf.edu/clinician-consultation/prep-pre-exposure-prophylaxis/.

Panel on Treatment of HIV-Infected Pregnant Women and Prevention of Perinatal Transmission. Recommendations for Use of Antiretroviral Drugs in Pregnant HIV-1-Infected Women for Maternal Health and Interventions to Reduce Perinatal HIV Transmission in the United States. Available at http://aidsinfo.nih.gov/contentfiles/lvguidelines/PerinatalGL.pdf. Accessed July 18, 2019.

PERINATALLY HIV-EXPOSED INFANT

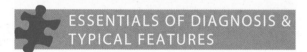

ESSENTIALS OF DIAGNOSIS & TYPICAL FEATURES

► HIV infection can be diagnosed or excluded with HIV nucleic acid testing (NAT) by age 3–4 months.

► Infection is typically asymptomatic at birth.

► Early diagnosis and treatment within a few weeks of birth reduce mortality.

Management of the Perinatally HIV-Exposed Infant

Infants with perinatal HIV exposure receive ARV prophylaxis for 4–6 weeks, whether or not they have breast milk exposure. For infants born to women with optimal ART during pregnancy, monotherapy with zidovudine or nevirapine is sufficient; for infants at higher risk of transmission, prophylaxis with two ARV or empiric treatment with three ARV is recommended (details of regimens are found at https://aidsinfo.nih.gov/guidelines/html/3/perinatal/187/antiretroviral-management-of-newborns-with-perinatal-hiv-exposure-or-perinatal-hiv). During the period of ARV prophylaxis, some infants have reversible anemia or neutropenia that is usually not clinically significant. Viral nucleic acid tests to detect HIV in blood allow for presumptive and definitive determination of HIV infection status by age 4 weeks and 4 months, respectively. Early infant diagnosis allows for early initiation of ART, which reduces the otherwise high rate of early mortality among infants with perinatal HIV. Infants with HIV have a high risk of *Pneumocystis jiroveci* pneumonia (PCP), with the peak incidence at age 2–6 months. Thus, prophylaxis for *P jiroveci* pneumonia is given to infants born to HIV-infected mothers beginning at age 4–6 weeks and continuing until HIV infection has been excluded or until age 12 months for infants found to have HIV infection. PCP prophylaxis may be avoided for infants with negative HIV NAT at 2 and 4 weeks of age. Infants with ongoing HIV exposure via breast-feeding are recommended to continue PCP prophylaxis, at least until HIV infection has been excluded after cessation of breast-feeding.

► Clinical Findings

Newborns with HIV infection rarely have symptoms or physical examination findings at birth or in the first months of life. However, 30%–80% of infected infants develop symptoms or signs within the first year of life. Hepatomegaly, splenomegaly, lymphadenopathy, parotitis, and recurrent respiratory tract infections are signs associated with slow progression. Severe bacterial infections, progressive neurologic disease, anemia, and fever are associated with rapid progression.

HIV-exposed but uninfected (HEU) infants are generally healthy, but a number of studies find higher morbidity and mortality compared with HIV-unexposed infants. Alterations in growth, neurocognitive development, immune function, and end-organ parameters are also reported in this population, although their clinical significance is under investigation. Some studies have found symptoms consistent with mitochondrial toxicity associated with perinatal ARV exposure; other studies have failed to confirm these findings. There is biological plausibility for this toxicity because the nucleoside analogue drugs used for PMTCT may cause mitochondrial toxicity. The benefit of prenatal and postnatal treatment to prevent HIV transmission outweighs the potential risk but ongoing studies are important to elucidate the effects of in utero and perinatal HIV and ARV exposure and to identify the safest regimens.

► Laboratory Diagnosis

Infants born to HIV-infected mothers will have transplacental maternal HIV antibody regardless of their infection status. The median time to seroreversion with current antibody assays in uninfected infants is 13.9 months, and most uninfected infants become antibody negative by 18 months; in a minority of infants (approximately 14%), however, maternal antibody is detected until age 24 months. Therefore, early infant diagnosis must be made by direct detection of viral nucleic acid, either DNA or RNA, in blood. A recommended schedule of HIV NAT and antibody testing for infants is outlined in Table 41–2. Positive HIV NAT at any age requires a subsequent sample for confirmation to rule out a false positive, particularly for a test with low RNA copy number (< 5000 copies/mL).

HIV NAT is positive in blood at birth for the fraction of infants infected in utero, but negative for infants who acquire infection at birth. Most infected infants with either in utero or peripartum acquisition will have detectable HIV NAT

by 2 weeks of life, over 95% will have detectable virus by 4 weeks, and virtually all by 4 months. Thus, infection can be "presumptively" excluded by negative HIV NAT at age 2 and 4 weeks. For the higher risk infant, receipt of combination ARV may inhibit detection of virus in blood and, hence, an additional NAT at age 8–10 weeks, 2–4 weeks after cessation of combination ARV, is performed for early identification of infection. Definitive evidence of absence of infection, if no breast-feeding, is defined by negative HIV NAT at age greater than or equal to 1 and 4 months (and at age 8–10 weeks if received combination ARV). Breast-fed infants may acquire HIV at any time until they are fully weaned, and virus may not be detected until several weeks or months after exposure. Therefore, breast milk-exposed infants should be tested at 6 weeks, 3 months, and 6 months after their last exposure.

For infants with negative NAT, many clinicians obtain HIV antibody testing at 12–24 months of age to demonstrate reversion to seronegative status. After age 24 months, diagnosis can be accomplished with the standard multitest algorithm used for adolescents and adults, screening with an HIV antibody/antigen test, with reactive tests followed by a confirmatory antibody test using a different detection platform.

Table 41–2. Age-specific laboratory diagnostic schedule for perinatal HIV.[a]

Age	Infant at Low Risk (ARV Single-Drug Prophylaxis)	Infant at Higher Risk (ARV Combination Prophylaxis)
Birth	Optional nucleic acid test[b]	Nucleic acid test
2–3 wk	Nucleic acid test	Nucleic acid test
4–8 wk	Nucleic acid test	Nucleic acid test
8–10 wk		Nucleic acid test[c]
4–6 mo	Nucleic acid test	Nucleic acid test
12–24 mo	HIV antibody[d]	HIV antibody[d]
Over 24 mo	HIV antibody[e]	

[a]Definitive infection requires two positives on two samples obtained on different dates.

[b]Some clinicians do not obtain birth testing since transmission is unlikely and therefore birth testing is low yield and does not contribute to excluding HIV infection.

[c]Nucleic acid testing (NAT) at 2–4 weeks after cessation of combination ARV but before definitive testing at older than 4 months allows for earlier detection of previously ARV-suppressed viremia.

[d]Although the majority of exposed infants are antibody negative by 18 months of age, in some studies, up to 14% of exposed children have detectable HIV antibodies until age 24 months. If needed, positive HIV NAT testing differentiates infection from persistent maternal antibodies.

[e]For children identified at risk of HIV at older than or equal to 24 months, a screening HIV antibody or antigen/antibody test, which if reactive, is followed with a confirmatory test on the same specimen using a different test principle, usually an HIV–1/2 differentiating test, to determine or exclude infection.

Centers for Disease Control and Prevention: Revised surveillance case definition for HIV infection—United States, 2014. MMWR Recomm Rep 2014;63(RR-03):1–10 [PMID: 24717910].

Panel on Antiretroviral Therapy and Medical Management of Children Living with HIV. Guidelines for the Use of Antiretroviral Agents in Pediatric HIV Infection. Available at http://aidsinfo.nih.gov/contentfiles/lvguidelines/pediatricguidelines.pdf. Accessed July 18, 2019, Diagnosis of HIV Infection in Infants and Children.

ADOLESCENTS & YOUTH WITH HIV EXPOSURE

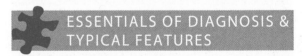

ESSENTIALS OF DIAGNOSIS & TYPICAL FEATURES

► Adolescent transmission occurs primarily through sexual contact and less commonly via contaminated needles.

► Nonspecific acute symptoms (fever, pharyngitis, adenopathy, rash) are common during primary infection.

► After primary infection, infected individuals are initially asymptomatic for years but have ongoing, active viral replication and potential to transmit HIV.

► HIV NAT is an important test for diagnosis during acute infection.

► HIV antibody/antigen testing is the primary test used for diagnosis of established infection.

Among adolescents and adults with primary HIV infection, nonspecific symptoms (eg, flu- or mild mononucleosis-like illness) beginning 2–4 weeks after exposure occur in 30%–90%, but they are frequently not severe enough to be brought to medical attention. This *acute retroviral syndrome* is described in more detail in Chapter 44. After acute infection, adolescents may be asymptomatic for several years, but during that time will have disease progression and the potential to transmit HIV to their sexual partners.

▶ Laboratory Diagnosis

In the early weeks after acute infection HIV antibody may be absent, but HIV RNA and DNA are usually detected within a week of infection. Therefore, if acute infection is suspected, HIV NAT should be obtained in addition to antibody/antigen-based testing.

Current laboratory-based screening tests detect HIV-1 and HIV-2 antibody and HIV-1 p24 antigen. These tests are more sensitive for acute/early infection than earlier generation antibody tests because antigen may be detected in advance of antibodies (however, these tests still may be negative very early after acute infection). A second antibody test on the same sample using a different methodology is conducted to confirm the presence of antibodies because rare individuals have cross-reacting antibodies which result in a false-positive antibody test. If the initial test used detects both HIV antigen and anti-HIV antibody and the confirmatory test that detects only antibody is nonreactive, HIV NAT testing is indicated if acute HIV infection is a possibility, as antigen detection may precede antibody formation. Definitive diagnosis of HIV infection requires a positive result on a second sample obtained on a different occasion. Most patients will seroconvert by 6 weeks after exposure, but occasionally seroconversion does not occur for 3–6 months. Additional information about the use of available HIV diagnostic tests for a range of settings (clinics, community-based or field locations, home testing) is found at https://www.cdc.gov/hiv/testing/index.html.

The Centers for Disease Control and Prevention (CDC) recommends that HIV screening tests be conducted in routine health care settings with patient knowledge and right of refusal for patients aged 13–64 years and that all adults should be tested at least once for HIV during their lives (https://www.cdc.gov/hiv/guidelines/testing.html). The American Academy of Pediatrics recommends at least one-time testing for 16- to 18-year-old adolescents living in areas of high (≥ 0.1%) or unknown seroprevalence, irrespective of individual risk factors. In areas of lower seroprevalence, testing is encouraged for all sexually active adolescents and those with other risk factors for HIV infection. Point-of-care HIV antibody testing performed in the community and home HIV testing kits are strategies to increase access to testing for those at risk.

CDC Recommended Laboratory HIV Testing Algorithm for Serum or Plasma Specimens. https://www.cdc.gov/hiv/pdf/guidelines_testing_recommendedlabtestingalgorithm.pdf.

Centers for Disease Control and Prevention; Association of Public Health Laboratories: Laboratory Testing for the Diagnosis of HIV Infection: Updated Recommendations. Available at http://dx.doi.org/10.15620/cdc.23447. Published June 27, 2014. Accessed May 29, 2017.

PROGRESSIVE HIV DISEASE

ESSENTIALS OF DIAGNOSIS & TYPICAL FEATURES

▶ Ongoing viral replication leads to cellular and humoral immunodeficiency and end-organ pathology.

▶ Immunodeficiency is staged by monitoring CD4 T-lymphocyte count decline.

▶ As immunodeficiency progresses, patients are at risk for bacteremia, infections by pathogens such as herpes zoster, *Mycobacterium tuberculosis*, and opportunistic infections such as *P jiroveci*, cytomegalovirus, and *Mycobacterium avium* complex (MAC) infection.

▶ Patients with progressive HIV disease are also at risk for encephalopathy, nephropathy, hepatitis, cardiomyopathy, chronic diarrhea, and pulmonary disease.

▶ HIV-infected individuals have higher rates of non-Hodgkin's lymphoma and cervical and anal neoplasia.

A. Clinical Findings

1. Disease staging—The CDC published revised disease staging for HIV-infected adults, adolescents, and children in 2014 (http://www.cdc.gov/mmwr/preview/mmwrhtml/rr6303a1.htm) (Tables 41–1 and 41–3). Stages 1, 2, and 3 are determined by categories of age-adjusted absolute CD4 T-lymphocyte counts and percentages that indicate progressively severe immune suppression; stage 3 is defined as AIDS (see Table 41–3). AIDS is also diagnosed in individuals having one or more of the severe opportunistic illnesses or other serious conditions listed in Table 41–1. An individual's staging may vary with time, improving or worsening depending on the outcome of the patient's treatment course. The WHO has established a clinical staging system that is used widely outside the United States (WHO Consolidated guidelines on antiretroviral drugs for treatment and preventing HIV, Annex 10, found at https://www.who.int/hiv/pub/arv/arv-2016/en/). Risk of progression to AIDS or death for a child at specific ages can be determined with CD4 parameters and

Table 41–3. HIV infection stage based on age-specific CD4 T-lymphocyte counts and percentages of total lymphocytes.

Stage	Age of Child					
	<1 y		1–5 y		≥6 y	
	Cells/μL	%	Cells/μL	%	Cells/μL	%
1	≥ 1500	≥ 34	≥ 1000	≥ 30	≥ 500	≥ 26
2	750–1499	26–33	500–999	22–29	200–499	14–25
3	< 750	< 26	< 500	< 22	< 200	< 14

Adapted with permission from Centers for Disease Control and Prevention (CDC): Revised surveillance case definition for HIV infection—United States, 2014. MMWR Recomm Rep 2014 Apr 11;63(RR-03):1–10.

HIV viral load (tables for risk calculation found at https://aidsinfo.nih.gov/guidelines/html/2/pediatric-arv/440/appendix-c-supplemental-information).

2. Infections related to immunodeficiency—Bacteremia, especially due to *Streptococcus pneumoniae*, occurs at rates of 3 per 100 child-years without ART and decreases to 0.36 per 100 child-years with ART, but this remains approximately ten times higher than in HIV-uninfected children. Infections with *M tuberculosis* are a major cause of morbidity in countries with high rates of endemic tuberculosis (TB). Given the frequency of coinfection, diagnosis of *M tuberculosis* in a child is an indication for HIV testing. Likewise, children with HIV infection and their family members should have annual TB testing if there is potential for *M tuberculosis* exposure. Herpes zoster (shingles) occurs 10 times more frequently among untreated HIV-infected children compared with age-matched healthy children.

Late-stage immunodeficiency is accompanied by susceptibility to a variety of opportunistic pathogens. Pneumonia caused by *P jiroveci* is a common AIDS-defining diagnosis in children with unrecognized HIV infection who, therefore, are not receiving PCP prophylaxis. Symptoms are difficult to distinguish from those of viral or atypical pneumonia (see Chapter 43). Persistent candida mucocutaneous infections (oral, cutaneous, and vaginal) are common. Candida esophagitis occurs with more advanced disease. Cytomegalovirus (CMV) infections may result in disseminated disease, hepatitis, gastroenteritis, retinitis, and encephalitis. Disseminated infection with MAC, presenting with fever, night sweats, weight loss, diarrhea, fatigue, lymphadenopathy, hepatomegaly, anemia, and granulocytopenia, may occur in those who have CD4 T-lymphocyte counts below 50–100/μL. A variety of diarrheal pathogens that cause mild, self-limited symptoms in healthy persons may result in severe, chronic diarrhea in HIV-infected persons. These include *Cryptosporidium parvum*, *Microsporidia*, *Cyclospora*, *Isospora belli*, *Giardia lamblia*, and bacterial

pathogens. Chronic parvovirus infection manifested by anemia can occur. In late-stage disease, prophylactic measures are recommended to prevent selected opportunistic infections (https://aidsinfo.nih.gov/guidelines/html/5/pediatric-oi-prevention-and-treatment-guidelines/0).

3. Organ system disease—HIV infection may directly affect a variety of organ systems and produce disease manifestations that include encephalopathy, pneumonitis, hepatitis, diarrhea, hematologic suppression, nephropathy, and cardiomyopathy. On average, HIV-infected children have lower than normal neuropsychological functioning which may not normalize when ART is started, despite suppression of viremia. Without ART, findings include acquired microcephaly, progressive motor deficit, ataxia, pseudobulbar palsy, and failure to attain (or loss of) developmental milestones.

Lymphoid interstitial pneumonitis, which is common in untreated children with HIV infection, is characterized by a diffuse peribronchial and interstitial infiltrate composed of lymphocytes and plasma cells. It may be asymptomatic or associated with dry cough, hypoxemia, dyspnea or wheezing on exertion, and clubbing of the digits. Children with this disorder frequently have enlargement of the parotid glands and generalized lymphadenopathy.

4. Malignancy—Children with HIV are at increased risk of malignancy. The most commonly occurring tumors are non-Hodgkin lymphomas, which may occur at unusual extranodal sites (central nervous system, bone, gastrointestinal tract, liver, or lungs). Human papillomavirus infection of the cervix is more likely to progress to neoplasia. Anal carcinoma due to human papillomavirus is also a concern. Kaposi sarcoma, a skin and mucous membrane malignancy that is common in HIV-infected men who have sex with men with advanced disease, is also observed among HIV-infected African children, but it is rare in children in the United States.

B. Laboratory Findings

The hallmark of HIV disease progression is decline in the absolute number and percentage of CD4 T lymphocytes and an increasing percentage of CD8 T lymphocytes. The CD4 T-lymphocyte values are predictive of the child's risk of opportunistic infections. Healthy infants and children have CD4 T-lymphocyte numbers that are much higher than in adults; these gradually decline to adult levels by age 5–6 years. Hence, age-adjusted values must be used when assessing a child's absolute CD4 T-lymphocyte count (see Table 41–3). CD4 T-lymphocyte percentage, which is less variable with age, is used when CD4 T-cell count is not available.

Hypergammaglobulinemia of IgG, IgA, and IgM is characteristic in untreated HIV. Late in the disease, some individuals may become hypogammaglobulinemic. Hematologic abnormalities (anemia, neutropenia, and thrombocytopenia) may occur due to effects of HIV disease or ART. Cerebrospinal fluid (CSF) may either be normal or may be associated with elevated protein and a mononuclear pleocytosis; HIV NAT may be positive in CSF.

C. Differential Diagnosis

HIV infection should be in the differential diagnosis for children being evaluated for immunodeficiency. Depending on the degree of immunosuppression, the presentation in HIV infection may be similar to that of B-cell (eg, hypogammaglobinemia), T-cell, or combined immunodeficiencies (eg, severe combined immunodeficiency) (see Chapter 33). HIV infection should also be considered in the evaluation of individuals with failure to thrive, developmental delay, chronic lung disease, and *M tuberculosis* infection. HIV infection presenting with generalized lymphadenopathy or hepatosplenomegaly may resemble infections with viruses such as Epstein-Barr virus or CMV in children or adolescents. Because blood tests are definitive for the diagnosis of HIV infection, the diagnosis can be readily established or excluded. In rare cases, HIV-infected people with hypogammaglobinemia have falsely negative antibody tests but may be diagnosed with a nucleic acid-based test. Because recognized maternal or behavioral risk factors may not always be elicited, testing for HIV should be performed if the patient has signs consistent with HIV-associated disease even when the history or maternal testing early in pregnancy does not suggest increased risk.

Panel on Opportunistic Infections in HIV-Exposed and HIV-Infected Children. Guidelines for the Prevention and Treatment of Opportunistic Infections in HIV-Exposed and HIV-Infected Children. Department of Health and Human Services. Available at http://aidsinfo.nih.gov/contentfiles/lvguidelines/oi_guidelines _pediatrics.pdf. Section accessed July 18, 2019.

TREATMENT

ESSENTIALS OF DIAGNOSIS & TYPICAL FEATURES

► ART suppresses viral replication and forestalls immunodeficiency.

► Early initiation of ART is recommended for all people living with HIV.

► Combinations of antiretroviral drugs are required to avoid induction of viral drug resistance.

► ART is lifelong due to inability to eradicate latent virus.

► Adherence support is critical for durable viral suppression.

► Complications of ART may include metabolic syndrome, decreased bone mineralization, renal dysfunction, lipodystrophy, and lactic acidosis.

A. Specific Measures

1. Principles of HIV treatment—Studies in young infants and adults support initiation of ART early after infection to prevent HIV progression, and current US and WHO guidelines recommend ART for all individuals soon after diagnosis. For children, initiation of ART is urgent for those with stage 3 clinical or CD4 T-cell parameters or younger than 12 months (irrespective of CD4 count). Older children with less advanced infection are also recommended to start treatment but with more time allowed to prepare the family for successful adherence to treatment. The goal of ART is suppression of viral replication (plasma virus < 20–75 copies/mL), resulting in an increase in CD4 T-lymphocyte count and reconstitution of immune function (or maintenance, if baseline parameters are within normal limits). HIV has a high spontaneous mutation rate allowing emergence of drug resistance with single-drug treatment; therefore, combinations of three drugs, including two drugs with different mechanisms of action, are standard. Optimally, children initiating ART will have laboratory monitoring at 2–4 weeks and then every 3–4 months to confirm viral suppression. If plasma virus becomes consistently detectable (> 200 copies/mL), the underlying cause must be determined (eg, poor adherence or viral resistance), and, if necessary, a change in the medication combination is made. Latent HIV persists in long-lived resting cells, the so-called viral reservoir, and cessation of ARV treatment results in resumption of viremia. Therefore, treatment for HIV with currently available modalities must be lifelong.

Strict adherence to the prescribed treatment is critical. A wide range of issues may impact adherence, including pill burden, dosing frequency, and tolerability, as well as psychosocial factors such as developmental stage, mental health of child and caregiver, HIV knowledge, and beliefs about treatment. Programs and services that enhance adherence are essential adjuncts of any HIV treatment regimen.

2. Antiretroviral medications—There are numerous ARV medications approved by the U.S. Food and Drug Administration (FDA) categorized into five different drug classes for the treatment of HIV. Many of the drugs have pediatric indications for older children, but pharmacokinetic data and administration forms appropriate for infants and toddlers are more limited. The drug classes and mechanism of action of each class are described briefly in Table 41–4. Recommended regimens vary by age but will generally include two nucleoside/nucleotide reverse transcriptase inhibitors (NRTIs) plus one drug from another class. Fixed dose formulations including two or three drugs at adult dosages in a single pill have become common and offer simplified regimens, often a once-daily pill, for adolescents. Guidelines for the treatment of HIV developed by US national working groups of pediatric HIV specialists are published and updated frequently at: http://www.aidsinfo .nih.gov and WHO recommendations are found at: http:// www.who.int/hiv/pub/guidelines/en/.

3. Complications of antiretroviral medications—ART may result in a range of adverse effects. Each medication has specific toxicities which are described in detail in the Guidelines for Use of ARV in Pediatric HIV Infection, Tables 15a–15k (found at https://www.aidsinfo.nih.gov/contentfiles/ lvguidelines/PedARV_TablesOnly.pdf). Common adverse events are gastrointestinal distress, hematologic toxicity (anemia, neutropenia), elevated liver enzymes, dyslipidemia (elevated LDL-cholesterol and triglycerides). Less common are glucose intolerance and abnormal fat distribution (lipodystrophy). Reduced bone mineral content and renal dysfunction may result from drug effects as well as from direct effects of HIV. Several drugs (eg, nevirapine, abacavir) have been associated with severe hepatitis, usually occurring in the first 6 weeks of treatment, and may occur in the context of a systemic hypersensitivity reaction. These events may be life-threatening if not identified early or upon rechallenge with the same medication. The nucleoside and nucleotide analogues have low-level affinity for the human mitochondrial DNA polymerase. Therefore, these analogues may be incorporated into mitochondrial DNA, which is one mechanism that may lead to adverse effects. Mitochondrial toxicity can result in lactic acidosis, a rare, but potentially fatal, complication. During the initial weeks of treatment, immune restoration may lead to worsening or unmasking of underlying infection with other organisms such as *M tuberculosis*, an event termed *immune reconstitution inflammatory syndrome* (IRIS).

Table 41–4. Antiretroviral drug class and mechanism of action.

Drug Class	Selected Antiretroviral Drugs	Mechanism of Action
Nucleoside/nucleotide reverse transcriptase inhibitors (NRTIs)	Abacavir Lamivudine Tenofovir alafenamide Zidovudine	Chain termination during reverse transcription of HIV DNA
Non-nucleoside reverse transcriptase inhibitors (NNRTIs)	Efavirenz Nevirapine	Viral reverse transcriptase inhibited to prevent transcription of HIV RNA to DNA
Integrase inhibitor (INSTIs, IIs)	Raltegravir Dolutegravir	Integration of HIV DNA in host genome prevented
Protease inhibitors (PIs)	Lopinavir/ ritonavir Atazanavir	Viral protease inhibited resulting in production of noninfectious virions
Viral entry inhibitors	Enfuvirtide	Inhibition of virus-cell membrane fusion
	Maraviroc	Blocking CCR5 co-receptor CD4 postattachment inhibitor

Panel on Antiretroviral Therapy and Medical Management of Children Living with HIV. Guidelines for the Use of Antiretroviral Agents in Pediatric HIV Infection. Available at http:// aidsinfo.nih.gov/contentfiles/lvguidelines/pediatricguidelines. pdf. Accessed July 18, 2019.

B. General Measures

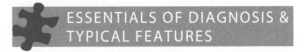

ESSENTIALS OF DIAGNOSIS & TYPICAL FEATURES

► Inactivated vaccines are recommended, and some require additional doses.

► Selected live attenuated vaccines (LAV) are recommended in the absence of severe immunosuppression.

► Prophylaxis for opportunistic infections is indicated for low CD4 lymphocyte counts.

► Higher rates of mental health disorders indicate the need for psychosocial support.

Table 41–5. Recommendations for routine vaccination of children with HIV.[a,b]

Vaccine	Recommendation
Hepatitis B vaccine	• Usual regimen for primary series and catchup. • Test for serum Hepatitis B surface antibody (anti-HepBs) after primary series; if < 10 mIU/mL, repeat the three-dose series and retest for anti-HepBs at 1–2 mo after 3rd dose. If still < 10 mIU/mL, child is considered at risk for Hep B acquisition. • A booster dose may be considered for those with ongoing Hep B exposure if annual testing identifies anti-HepBs < 10 mIU/mL.
Rotavirus vaccine	• Usual regimen if no severe immunosuppression.[c] Not recommended if severe immunosuppression.[c]
Vaccines with diphtheria toxoid, Tetanus toxoids, acellular Pertussis (DTaP, Tdap, Td)	• Usual regimen for primary series, catchup, and boosters.
Haemophilus influenza type b conjugate (Hib) vaccine	• Usual regimen for primary series and catchup prior to 12 mo. • Catchup regimen: Age 12–59 mo with ≤ 1 dose before age 12 mo, give two additional doses, 8 wk apart; if ≤ 2 doses before 12 mo, give 1 additional dose. • Age > 5 to 18 y and no prior Hib vaccine, administer one dose.
Pneumococcal conjugate vaccine (PCV13)	• Usual regimen for primary series and catchup prior to age 2 y. • Catchup regimen: Age 2–5 y administer 1 dose if any incomplete schedule of 3 doses; administer 2 doses separated by 8 wk if < 3 doses previously. Age 6–18 y administer 1 dose if no prior doses.
Pneumococcal polysaccharide vaccine 23 valent (PPSV23)	• Recommended at ≥ 8 wk after last dose of pneumococcal conjugate vaccine and age ≥ 2 y. • Second dose once at 5 y after the first dose.
Polio vaccine	• Usual regimen, inactivated polio vaccine; Oral polio vaccine not recommended.
Influenza vaccine	• Usual regimen, inactivated influenza vaccine; live attenuated influenza vaccine not recommended. • Immunize household contacts.
Measles, mumps, rubella vaccine (MMR)	• Usual regimen recommended if no severe immunosuppression.[c] Not recommended if severe immunosuppression.[c] • If immunized prior to ART, repeat the two-dose series after starting ART when CD4 percentage has been ≥ 15% and, for children ≥ 5 y, CD4 ≥ 15% and ≥ 200 lymphocytes/μL, for ≥ 6 mo.
Varicella-zoster vaccine (VAR)	• Usual regimen if no severe immunosuppression.[c] Not recommended if severe immunosuppression.[c]
Measles, mumps, rubella, varicella vaccine (MMRV)	• Not recommended; no safety or efficacy data.
Hepatitis A vaccine	• Usual regimen.
Meningococcal conjugate vaccine (MenACWY)[d]	• Primary series Age < 2 y: 4 doses of MenACWY-CRM at 2, 4, 6, and 12–16 mo.[e] Age > 2 y: 2 doses of MenACWY-CRM or MenACWY-D[d] separated by 8–12 wk. • Catchup Age ≥ 2 y with 1 prior dose of MenACWY should receive a second if at least 8 wk elapsed and then booster doses at intervals based on age. • Booster dose of MenACWY-CRM or MenACWY-D.[f] Age < 7 y at previous dose, booster dose at 3 y after last dose. Age ≥ 7 y at previous dose, booster dose at 5 y after last dose. For all ages after first booster dose, boosters repeated every 5 y thereafter.

(Continued)

Table 41–5. Recommendations for routine vaccination of children with HIV.[a,b] (*Continued*)

Vaccine	Recommendation
Meningococcus B vaccine[d]	• HIV infection alone is not included as a high-risk category for MenB. Follow usual recommendations if child has other risk factors (or clinical discretion if no risk factors).
Human papilloma vaccine (HPV)	• Three-dose schedule is recommended irrespective of age of first dose.

[a]Recommendations from https://www.cdc.gov/vaccines/schedules/downloads/child/0-18yrs-child-combined-schedule.pdf; Rubin LG et al: 2013 IDSA clinical practice guideline for vaccination of the immunocompromised host. Clin Infect Dis 2014;58(3):e44–e100; Centers for Disease Control and Prevention: A comprehensive immunization strategy to eliminate transmission of hepatitis B virus infection in the United States: recommendations of the Advisory Committee on Immunization Practices (ACIP); Part 1: Immunization of Infants, Children, and Adolescents. MMWR Recomm Rep 2005;54(No. RR-16); Center for Disease Control and Prevention: Recommendations for use of meningococcal conjugate vaccines in HIV-infected persons—Advisory Committee on Immunization Practices, MMWR Morb Mortal Wkly Rep 2016 *Weekly* / Nov 4, 2016 / 65(43);1189–1194.

[b]Travel vaccines not discussed.

[c]Severe immunosuppression defined as CD4 T-lymphocyte percentage < 15% for any age or CD4 T-lymphocyte count < 200 lymphocytes/μL for older than or equal to 5 years.

[d]For detailed recommendations see https://www.cdc.gov/mmwr/volumes/65/wr/mm6543a3.htm.

[e]For children age 7–23 months when starting immunization with MenACWY-CRM, give two doses separated by 12 weeks, with the second dose administered after their first birthday.

[f]MenACWY-D should be given after all PCV13 doses completed and should be given before or concurrent with DTaP.

1. Immunizations—Inactivated vaccines are recommended, as they are safe and generally immunogenic in HIV-infected children. The use of LAV depends on the child's immune stage and particular vaccine. Generally, LAV are not recommended for children with severe immunosuppression, defined as CD4 T-lymphocyte percentage less than 15% at any age and/or a CD4 T-lymphocyte count less than 200 cells/μL at age greater than or equal to 5 years. However, for children with CD4 T-lymphocyte parameters that exceed those values for at least the preceding 6 months, rotavirus, measles-mumps-rubella, and varicella-zoster virus LAV are recommended. Yellow fever vaccine may be given to stage 1 individuals and may also be considered for children in stage 2. Bacille Calmette-Guérin (BCG), oral polio, smallpox, and live typhoid vaccines should not be given to HIV-infected people, irrespective of stage. Based on studies demonstrating diminished magnitude or durability of vaccine-induced immune responses, additional doses are recommended for particular vaccines. Vaccine responses are more robust with higher CD4 T-lymphocyte counts and suppressed plasma virus. Therefore, for children who were immunized prior to establishment of effective ART, reimmunization should be considered and is specifically recommended for measles-mumps-rubella vaccine. Children with HIV have higher rates of disease from pneumococcus, *Haemophilus influenzae* type b, and meningococcus; therefore, recommendations for high-risk groups for these vaccines apply. Details of modified recommendations for children with HIV infection are provided in Table 41–5 (CDC guidance for vaccines indicated for children based on medical indications https://www.cdc.gov/vaccines/schedules/hcp/imz/child-indications.html).

2. Psychosocial support and mental health—Evaluation and support for psychosocial needs of HIV-affected families is imperative. As with other chronic illnesses, HIV infection affects all family members and also carries additional social stigma. Emotional concerns and financial needs, which are more prominent than medical needs at many stages of the disease process, influence the family's ability to comply with a medical treatment regimen. HIV-infected children often have comorbid mental health conditions. Rates of attention-deficit/hyperactivity disorder range from 20% to 50% in various studies. Hospital admissions for mental health disorders are more frequent among HIV-infected children. In one study, dual diagnosis of HIV and a mental health disorder occurred in 85% of adolescents who acquired HIV infection through high-risk behaviors. Ideally, care should be coordinated by a team of caregivers that is familiar with HIV disease and its comorbidities, newest therapies, and community resources.

QUALITY ASSURANCE & OUTCOME METRICS

Evidence-based care guidelines are published by the U.S. Department of Health and Human Services and are updated frequently (http://aidsinfo.nih.gov/). The guidelines establish best practices for prevention, initiation of treatment, choice of ARV, monitoring frequency, and prophylaxis for opportunistic infections, and the HIV/AIDS Bureau (HAB) of Human Resources and Services Administration has established quality performance measures based on these guidelines (http://hab.hrsa.gov/deliverhivaidscare/habperformmeasures.html).

In addition, a major quality emphasis is on monitoring success of the continuum care at local and national levels. This continuum describes the percentage of people living with HIV in a defined community who have completed the sequential stages in successful HIV care: (1) diagnosis, (2) linkage to care, (3) engagement and retention in care, (4) prescription of ART, and, finally, (5) viral suppression. Many countries have endorsed the UNAIDS goals that 90% of those living with HIV know their diagnosis, 90% of those diagnosed be engaged in care, and 90% of those engaged in care have a viral load below 200 copies/mL, the so-called 90 / 90 / 90 target. Several US national quality groups collect and publish data across clinics on these cascade outcomes, thereby setting national metrics and providing technical assistance to HIV programs (in+care Campaign at http://www.incarecampaign.org/; National Quality Center at https://targethiv.org/cqii).

Lally MA et al; Adolescent Medicine Trials Network for HIV/AIDS Interventions (ATN): HIV continuum of care for youth in the United States. J Acquir Immune Defic Syndr 2018 Jan 1; 77(1):110–117. doi: 10.1097/QAI.0000000000001563 [PMID: 28991884] [PMCID: PMC5774627].

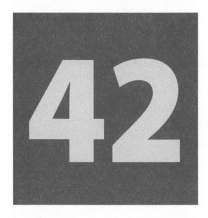

Infections: Bacterial & Spirochetal

James Gaensbauer, MD, MScPH

Yosuke Nomura, MD

John W. Ogle, MD

▼ BACTERIAL INFECTIONS

GROUP A STREPTOCOCCAL INFECTIONS

ESSENTIALS OF DIAGNOSIS & TYPICAL FEATURES

► Streptococcal pharyngitis:
  • Sore throat, purulent tonsillitis, tender cervical adenopathy, fever, and absence of viral respiratory symptoms.
  • Throat culture or rapid antigen detection test positive for group A streptococci (GAS).
► Impetigo:
  • Rapidly spreading, highly infectious skin rash.
  • Erythematous denuded areas and honey-colored crusts.
  • GAS are grown in culture from most (not all) cases.

▶ General Considerations

Group A streptococci (GAS) are common gram-positive bacteria producing a wide variety of clinical illnesses, including acute pharyngitis, impetigo, cellulitis, and scarlet fever. GAS can also cause pneumonia, septic arthritis, osteomyelitis, meningitis, and other less common infections. GAS infections may also produce postinfectious sequelae (rheumatic fever and acute glomerulonephritis [AGN]).

Almost all GAS are β-hemolytic. These organisms may be carried without symptoms on the skin and in the pharynx, rectum, and vagina. All GAS are sensitive to penicillin. Resistance to erythromycin is common in some countries and has increased in the United States.

▶ Prevention

GAS pharyngitis usually occurs after contact with respiratory secretions of a person infected with GAS. Crowding facilitates spread of GAS and outbreaks of pharyngitis and impetigo occur. Prompt recognition and institution of antibiotics may decrease spread. Treatment with antibiotics prevents acute rheumatic fever.

▶ Clinical Findings

A. Symptoms and Signs

1. Respiratory infections

A. INFANCY AND EARLY CHILDHOOD (AGE < 3 YEARS)—The onset is insidious, with mild symptoms (low-grade fever, serous nasal discharge, and pallor). Otitis media is common. Exudative pharyngitis and cervical adenitis are uncommon in this age group.

B. CHILDHOOD TYPE—Classic GAS pharyngitis presents with the sudden onset of fever, sore throat, malaise, and often vomiting. On examination, tonsillar exudate and tender anterior cervical adenopathy are usually noted. Petechiae are frequently seen on the soft palate. In **scarlet fever**, the skin is diffusely erythematous and appears sunburned and roughened (sandpaper rash); most intense in the axillae, groin, and on the abdomen and trunk. It blanches except in the skin folds, which do not blanch and are pigmented (Pastia sign). The rash usually appears 24 hours after the onset of fever and rapidly spreads over the next 1–2 days. Desquamation begins on the face at the end of the first week and becomes generalized by the third week. Early in the infection, there is circumoral pallor and the surface of the tongue is coated white, with the papillae enlarged and bright red (white strawberry tongue). Subsequently desquamation occurs, and the tongue appears beefy red (strawberry tongue). Petechiae may be seen on any mucosal surfaces.

2. Impetigo—Streptococcal impetigo begins as a papule that vesiculates and then breaks, leaving a denuded area covered by a honey-colored crust. Both *Staphylococcus aureus* and GAS are isolated in some cases. The lesions spread readily and diffusely. Local lymph nodes may become swollen and inflamed. Although the child often lacks systemic symptoms, a high fever and toxicity may be present. If flaccid bullae are noted, the disease is called bullous impetigo and is caused by an epidermolytic toxin-producing strain of *S aureus*.

3. Cellulitis—The portal of entry is often an insect bite or superficial abrasion. A diffuse, rapidly spreading cellulitis occurs that involves the subcutaneous tissues and extends along the lymphatic pathways with only minimal local suppuration. Local acute lymphadenitis occurs. The child is usually acutely ill, with fever and malaise. In classic erysipelas, the involved area is bright red, swollen, warm, and very tender. The infection may extend rapidly from the lymphatics to the bloodstream.

Streptococcal perianal cellulitis is an entity peculiar to young children. Pain with defecation often leads to constipation, which may be the presenting complaint. The child is afebrile and otherwise well. Perianal erythema, tenderness, and painful rectal examination are the only abnormal physical findings. Scant rectal bleeding with defecation may occur. A perianal swab culture usually yields heavy growth of GAS. A variant of this syndrome is streptococcal vaginitis in prepubertal girls. Symptoms are dysuria and pain; marked erythema and tenderness of the introitus and blood-tinged discharge are seen.

4. Necrotizing skin and soft tissue infection—This dangerous disease is reported sporadically and may occur as a complication of varicella infection. GAS is the most common cause of necrotizing skin and soft tissue infection in children, followed by *S aureus*. The disease is characterized by extensive necrosis of superficial fasciae, undermining of surrounding tissue, and usually systemic toxicity. Initially the skin overlying the infection is tender and pale red without distinct borders, resembling cellulitis. Blisters or bullae may appear. The color deepens to a distinct purple or in some cases becomes pale. Tenderness out of proportion to the clinical appearance, skin anesthesia (due to infarction of superficial nerves), or "woody" induration suggest necrotizing fasciitis. Involved areas may develop mild to massive edema. Early recognition and aggressive debridement of necrotic tissue are essential.

5. Group A streptococcal infections in newborn nurseries—GAS epidemics occur occasionally in nurseries. The organism may be introduced into the nursery from the vaginal tract of a mother or from the throat or nose of a mother or a staff member. The organism then spreads from infant to infant. The umbilical stump is colonized while the infant is in the nursery. Most often, a colonized infant develops a chronic oozing omphalitis days later. The organism may spread from the infant to other family members. Serious and even fatal infections may develop, including sepsis, meningitis, empyema, septic arthritis, and peritonitis.

6. Streptococcal sepsis—Sepsis frequently occurs in conjunction with a focal source of infection, but can also manifest as isolated bacteremia. Rash and scarlet fever may or may not be present. Prostration and shock result in high mortality rates. Pharyngitis is uncommon as an antecedent illness. Underlying disease is a predisposing factor.

7. Streptococcal toxic shock syndrome (STSS)—Toxic shock syndrome (TSS) can be caused by GAS and is typically more severe than *S aureus*–associated toxic shock; multiorgan system involvement is a prominent part of the illness. The diagnostic criteria include (1) isolation of GAS from a normally sterile site, (2) hypotension or shock, and (3) at least two of the following: renal impairment (creatinine more than two times the upper limit of normal for age), thrombocytopenia (< 100,000/mm^3) or coagulopathy, liver involvement (transaminases or bilirubin ≥ two times normal), acute respiratory distress syndrome, erythematous macular rash, or soft tissue necrosis (myositis, necrotizing fasciitis, gangrene). In cases that otherwise meet clinical criteria, isolation of GAS from a nonsterile site (throat, wound, or vagina) is indicative of a "probable case."

B. Laboratory Findings

Leukocytosis with a marked shift to the left is seen early. β-Hemolytic streptococci are cultured from the throat or site of infection. For suspected GAS pharyngitis, the throat should be swabbed and the specimen sent for GAS testing (rapid antigen detection tests and/or culture for GAS) because the clinical features of some viral infections may overlap with the clinical features of GAS. In children and adolescents, negative rapid antigen tests should be backed up by a culture. Patients with positive rapid strep antigen tests do not need a confirmation by throat culture, since the specificities of antigen tests are high. The Food and Drug Administration (FDA) has recently approved nucleic acid amplification tests (NAATs) for the detection of GAS from throat swab specimens. The organism may be cultured from the skin and by needle aspiration from subcutaneous tissues and other involved sites such as infected nodes. Occasionally blood cultures are positive.

Antistreptolysin O (ASO) titers rise about 150 units within 2 weeks after acute infection. Elevated ASO and anti-DNase B titers may be useful in documenting prior throat infections in cases of acute rheumatic fever, although they may remain elevated for several months and even years after the original infection.

Proteinuria, cylindruria, and minimal hematuria may be seen early in children with streptococcal infection. True poststreptococcal glomerulonephritis is seen 1–4 weeks after the respiratory or skin infection.

Differential Diagnosis

Streptococcal infection in early childhood must be differentiated from adenovirus and other respiratory virus infections. The pharyngitis in herpangina (coxsackievirus A) is vesicular or ulcerative. Herpes simplex also causes ulcerative lesions, which most commonly involve the anterior pharynx, tongue, and gums. In infectious mononucleosis, the pharyngitis is also exudative, but splenomegaly and generalized adenopathy are typical, and laboratory findings are often diagnostic (atypical lymphocytes, a positive heterophile, or other serologic test for mononucleosis). Uncomplicated streptococcal pharyngitis improves within 24–48 hours if penicillin is given and by 72–96 hours without antimicrobials.

Arcanobacterium hemolyticum may cause pharyngitis with scarlatina-like or maculopapular truncal rash. In diphtheria, systemic symptoms, vomiting, and fever are less marked; pharyngeal pseudomembrane is confluent and adherent; the throat is less red; and cervical adenopathy is prominent. Pharyngeal tularemia causes white rather than yellow exudate; there is little erythema; and cultures for β-hemolytic streptococci are negative. A history of exposure to rabbits and a failure to respond to antimicrobials may suggest the diagnosis. Oral gonococcal infection may also cause pharyngitis with tonsillar exudate. Leukemia and agranulocytosis may present with pharyngitis and are diagnosed by bone marrow examination.

Scarlet fever must be differentiated from other exanthematous diseases, erythema due to sunburn, drug reactions, Kawasaki disease, TSS, and staphylococcal scalded skin syndrome (see also Table 40–3).

Complications

Suppurative complications of GAS infections include sinusitis, otitis, mastoiditis, cervical lymphadenitis, pneumonia, empyema, septic arthritis, sepsis, and meningitis. Spread of streptococcal infection from the throat to other sites—principally the skin (impetigo) and vagina—is common and should be considered in every instance of chronic vaginal discharge or chronic skin infection, such as that complicating childhood eczema. Both acute rheumatic fever and AGN are nonsuppurative complications of GAS infections.

A. Acute Rheumatic Fever (See Chapter 20)

B. Acute Glomerulonephritis

Poststreptococcal glomerulonephritis (PSGN) can follow streptococcal infections of either the pharynx or the skin—in contrast to rheumatic fever, which follows pharyngeal infection (See Chapter 20). PSGN may occur at any age. The risk is higher in school-aged children and members of indigenous populations. In most reports of PSGN, males predominate by a ratio of 2:1. Rheumatic fever occurs with equal frequency in both sexes. Certain GAS strains are associated with PSGN (nephritogenic types).

The median period between infection and the development of glomerulonephritis is 10 days. In contrast, acute rheumatic fever occurs after a median of 18 days.

C. Poststreptococcal Reactive Arthritis

Following an episode of group A streptococcal (GAS) pharyngitis, reactive arthritis develops in some patients. This reactive arthritis is believed to be due to immune complex deposition and is seen about 1–2 weeks following the acute infection. Patients with poststreptococcal reactive arthritis do not have the full constellation of clinical and laboratory criteria needed to fulfill the Jones criteria for a diagnosis of acute rheumatic fever.

Treatment

A. Specific Measures

Treatment is directed toward both eradication of acute infection and prevention of rheumatic fever. In patients with pharyngitis, antibiotics should be started early to relieve symptoms and should be continued for 10 days to prevent rheumatic fever. Although early therapy has not been shown to prevent PSGN, it seems advisable to treat impetigo promptly in sibling contacts of patients with poststreptococcal nephritis. Neither sulfonamides nor trimethoprim-sulfamethoxazole (TMP-SMX) is effective in the treatment of streptococcal infections. Although topical therapy for impetigo with antimicrobial ointments (especially mupirocin) is as effective as systemic therapy, it does not eradicate pharyngeal carriage and is less practical for extensive disease.

1. Penicillin—For GAS pharyngitis, the following regimens can be used. Except for penicillin-allergic patients, penicillin V (phenoxymethyl penicillin) is the drug of choice. Penicillin resistance has never been documented. For children weighing less than 27 kg, the regimen is 250 mg, given orally two or three times a day for 10 days. For children or adults weighting more than 27 kg, 500 mg two or three times a day is recommended. Giving penicillin V twice daily is as effective as more frequent oral administration. Alternatively, amoxicillin 50 mg/kg/day as a single daily dose (maximum 1000 mg) can be used. Another alternative for treatment of pharyngitis and impetigo is a single dose of penicillin G benzathine given intramuscularly (600,000 units for children weighing ≤ 27 kg and 1.2 million units for children weighing > 27 kg). Intramuscular delivery ensures compliance, but is painful. Parenteral therapy is indicated if vomiting is present. Mild cellulitis due to GAS may be treated orally or intramuscularly. For severe or invasive GAS infections intravenous antibiotics are indicated.

GAS cellulitis requiring hospitalization can be treated with aqueous penicillin G (150,000 U/kg/day, given intravenously in four divided doses) or cefazolin (100 mg/kg/day, given intravenously in three divided doses) until there is marked improvement. Penicillin V (50 mg/kg/day in four divided doses) or cephalexin (50–75 mg/kg/day in four divided doses) may then be given orally to complete a 10-day course. Acute cervical lymphadenitis may require incision and drainage. Treatment of necrotizing fasciitis requires emergency surgical debridement followed by high-dose parenteral antibiotics appropriate to the organisms cultured.

2. Other antibiotics—Cephalexin and azithromycin are other effective oral antimicrobials. Clindamycin is also effective, but resistance is occasionally present (labs can check for susceptibility to clindamycin). For penicillin-allergic patients with pharyngitis or impetigo the following alternative regimens have been used: azithromycin (12 mg/kg/day on day 1 followed by 6 mg/kg/day for days 2–5; maximum 500 mg/day) or clindamycin (20–30 mg/kg/day in three divided doses; maximum 600 mg per dose) for 10 days. Patients with immediate, anaphylactic hypersensitivity to penicillin should not receive cephalosporins, because up to 15% will also be allergic to cephalosporins. Macrolide resistance rates vary and may be high in some areas of the world. In general, macrolide resistance rates in most areas of the United States are between 5% and 8%. In most studies, bacteriologic failures after cephalosporin therapy are less frequent than failures following penicillin. However, there are few conclusive data on the ability of these agents to prevent rheumatic fever. Therefore, penicillin remains the agent of choice for nonallergic patients. Many strains are resistant to tetracycline.

For serious infections requiring intravenous therapy, aqueous penicillin G (250,000 U/kg in six divided doses) given intravenously is usually the drug of choice. Cefazolin (100 mg/kg/day intravenously or intramuscularly in three divided doses), clindamycin (30–40 mg/kg/day intravenously in four divided doses), and vancomycin (40 mg/kg/day intravenously in four divided doses) are alternatives in penicillin-allergic pediatric patients. Clindamycin should not be used alone empirically for severe, suspected GAS infections because a small percentage of isolates in the United States are resistant.

3. Serious GAS disease—Serious GAS infections, such as pneumonia, osteomyelitis, septic arthritis, sepsis, endocarditis, meningitis, and STSS, require parenteral antimicrobial therapy. Penicillin G is the drug of choice for these invasive infections. Clindamycin, a protein synthesis inhibitor, is advocated by many experts for STSS or necrotizing fasciitis as a second agent along with penicillin G to inhibit toxin production. Necrotizing skin and soft tissue infection requires prompt surgical debridement. In STSS, volume status and blood pressure should be monitored and patients evaluated for a focus of infection, if not readily apparent. Intravenous immunoglobulin (in addition to antibiotics) has been used in severe cases.

4. Treatment failure—Even when compliance is perfect, organisms will be found in cultures in 5%–35% of children after cessation of therapy. Reculture is indicated only in patients with relapse or recrudescence of pharyngitis or those with a personal or family history of rheumatic fever. Repeat treatment at least once with an oral cephalosporin or clindamycin is indicated in patients with recurrent culture-positive pharyngitis.

5. Prevention of recurrences in patients with previous rheumatic fever—The preferred prophylaxis for rheumatic individuals is benzathine penicillin G, 1.2 million units (600,000 units for patients weighing < 27 kg) intramuscularly every 4 weeks. If the risk of streptococcal exposure is high, every 3-week dosing is preferred. One of the following alternative oral prophylactic regimens may be used: penicillin V, 250 mg twice daily; or sulfadiazine, 0.5 g once a day (if < 27 kg) or 1 g once a day (if > 27 kg). In patients allergic to both penicillin and sulfonamide drugs, erythromycin 250 mg twice daily orally can be used. If carditis is absent, continued prophylaxis is recommended for at least 5 years after the last episode of acute rheumatic fever or until 21 years of age (whichever is longer). Prophylaxis should be continued longer if the risk of contact with persons with GAS is high (eg, parents of school-aged children, pediatric nurses, and teachers). In the presence of carditis without residual heart or valvular disease, a minimum of 10 years after the last episode of acute rheumatic fever or until 21 years of age (whichever is longer) is the minimum duration. If the patient has residual valvular heart disease, many recommend lifelong prophylaxis. These patients should be at least 10 years from their last episode of rheumatic disease and at least 40 years of age before considering discontinuation of prophylaxis. Those with severe valvular heart disease or with risk of ongoing exposure to GAS may benefit from lifelong prophylaxis.

6. Poststreptococcal reactive arthritis—In contrast to rheumatic fever, nonsteroidal agents may not dramatically improve joint symptoms. However, like patients with rheumatic fever, some patients with poststreptococcal reactive arthritis have developed carditis several weeks to months after their arthritis symptoms began. Patients should be monitored for development of carditis for the next 1–2 years. Some experts recommend antibiotic prophylaxis of these patients (same prophylaxis regimens as in prevention of recurrences of acute rheumatic fever) for 1–2 years and monitoring for signs of carditis (see recommendations for prevention of recurrences of rheumatic fever, above). If carditis does not develop, prophylaxis could then be discontinued. If carditis develops, the patient should be considered to have acute rheumatic fever and prophylaxis continued as described above.

B. General Measures

Acetaminophen or ibuprofen is useful for pain or fever. Local treatment of impetigo may promote earlier healing. Crusts should first be soaked off. Areas beneath the crusts should then be washed with soap daily.

C. Treatment of Complications

Rheumatic fever is best prevented by early and adequate penicillin treatment of the streptococcal infection.

D. Treatment of Carriers

Identification and treatment of GAS carriers are difficult. There are no established clinical or serologic criteria for differentiating carriers from the truly infected. Up to 20% of school-aged children in some studies are asymptomatic pharyngeal carriers of GAS. Streptococcal carriers are individuals who do not mount an immune response to the organism and are therefore believed to be at low risk for nonsuppurative sequelae.

Some children receive multiple courses of antimicrobials, with persistence of GAS in the throat, leading to a "streptococcal neurosis" on the part of families.

In certain circumstances, eradication of carriage may be desirable: (1) when a family member has a history of rheumatic fever; (2) when an episode of STSS or necrotizing fasciitis has occurred in a household contact; (3) multiple, recurring, documented episodes of GAS in family members despite adequate therapy; and (4) during an outbreak of rheumatic fever or GAS-associated glomerulonephritis. Clindamycin (20–30 mg/kg/day, given orally in three divided doses; maximum dose 300 mg) or a combination of rifampin (20 mg/kg/day, given orally for 4 days) and penicillin in standard dosage given orally has been used to attempt eradication of carriage.

▶ Prognosis

Death is rare except in infants or young children with sepsis, necrotizing infection, or pneumonia. The febrile course is shortened, and complications are eliminated by early and adequate treatment with penicillin.

Centers for Disease Control and Prevention: https://www.cdc.gov/groupastrep/diseases-hcp/index.html. Accessed June 30, 2019.

Shulman ST et al: Clinical practice guideline for the diagnosis and management of group A streptococcal pharyngitis: 2012 update by the Infectious Diseases Society of America. Clin Infect Dis 2012;55(10):1279–1282. http://cid.oxfordjournals.org/content/early/2012/09/06/cid.cis629.full [PMID: 22965026].

GROUP B STREPTOCOCCAL INFECTIONS

ESSENTIALS OF DIAGNOSIS & TYPICAL FEATURES

▶ Early-onset disease:

- Newborn younger than 7 days, with rapidly progressing overwhelming sepsis, with or without meningitis.
- Pneumonia with respiratory failure is frequent; chest radiograph resembles that seen in hyaline membrane disease.
- Blood or cerebrospinal fluid (CSF) cultures growing group B streptococci (GBS).

▶ Late-onset disease:

- Meningitis, sepsis, or other focal infection in a child aged 7–89 days with blood or CSF cultures growing GBS.

▶ Prevention

Many women of childbearing age possess type-specific circulating antibody to the polysaccharide antigens for group B *Streptococcus* (GBS). These antibodies are transferred to the newborn via the placental circulation. GBS carriers delivering healthy infants have significant serum levels of IgG antibody to this antigen. In contrast, women delivering infants who develop either early- or late-onset GBS disease rarely have detectable antibody in their sera. There is no licensed vaccine for GBS disease prevention. Vaccines have been studied in pregnant women, and research is ongoing.

▶ CDC Recommendations for Prevention of Perinatal GBS Disease

1. Caregivers for pregnant women are referred to the Centers for Disease Control and Prevention (CDC) guidelines for screening of pregnant women for GBS and use of intrapartum antibiotic prophylaxis (IAP)—see CDC guidelines http://www.cdc.gov/mmwr/pdf/rr/rr5910.pdf and http://www.cdc.gov/groupbstrep/clinicians/obstetric-providers.html.

2. Indications and nonindications for IAP to prevent early-onset group B streptococcal (GBS) disease are given in Table 42–1.

3. Algorithm for secondary prevention of early-onset GBS disease among newborns (management of a newborn whose mother received IAP for prevention of GBS or suspected chorioamnionitis)—Figure 42–1.

Table 42–1. Indications and nonindications for intrapartum antibiotic prophylaxis to prevent early-onset group B streptococcal (GBS) disease.

Intrapartum GBS Prophylaxis Indicated	Intrapartum GBS Prophylaxis Not Indicated
Previous infant with invasive GBS disease	• Colonization with GBS during a previous pregnancy (unless an indication for GBS prophylaxis is present for current pregnancy)
• GBS bacteriuria during any trimester of the current pregnancy[a]	• GBS bacteriuria during previous pregnancy (unless an indication for GBS prophylaxis is present for current pregnancy)
• Positive GBS vaginal-rectal screening culture in late gestation[b] during current pregnancy[a]	• Negative vaginal and rectal GBS screening culture in late gestation[b] during the current pregnancy, regardless of intrapartum risk factors
• Unknown GBS status at the onset of labor (culture not done, incomplete, or results unknown) and any of the following: 　• Delivery at < 37 wk gestation[c] 　• Amniotic membrane rupture ≥ 18 h 　• Intrapartum temperature ≥ 100.4°F (≥ 38.0°C)[d] 　• Intrapartum NAAT[e] positive for GBS	• Cesarean delivery performed before onset of labor on a woman with intact amniotic membranes, regardless of GBS colonization status or gestational age

NAAT, nucleic acid amplification tests.

[a]Intrapartum antibiotic prophylaxis is not indicated in this circumstance if a cesarean delivery is performed before onset of labor on a woman with intact amniotic membranes.

[b]Optimal timing for prenatal GBS screening is at 35–37 weeks' gestation.

[c]Recommendations for the use of intrapartum antibiotics for prevention of early-onset GBS disease in the setting of threatened preterm delivery are presented in Figure 42–1.

[d]If amnionitis is suspected, broad-spectrum antibiotic therapy that includes an agent known to be active against GBS should replace GBS prophylaxis.

[e]NAAT testing for GBS is optional and might not be available in all settings. If intrapartum NAAT is negative for GBS but any other intrapartum risk factor (delivery at < 37 weeks' gestation, amniotic membrane rupture at ≥ 18 hours, or temperature ≥ 100.4°F [≥ 38.0°C]) is present, then intrapartum antibiotic prophylaxis is indicated.

Reproduced with permission from Verani JR, McGee L, Schrag SJ, et al: Prevention of perinatal group B streptococcal disease—revised guidelines from CDC, 2010. MMWR Recomm Rep 2010 Nov 19;59(RR-10):1–36.

▶ Clinical Findings

The incidence of perinatal GBS disease has declined dramatically since screening of pregnant mothers and provision of IAP began. Although most patients with GBS disease are infants younger than 3 months, cases are seen in infants aged 4–5 months. Serious GBS infection also occurs in women with puerperal sepsis, immunocompromised patients, patients with cirrhosis and spontaneous peritonitis, and diabetic patients with cellulitis. Two distinct clinical syndromes distinguished by differing perinatal event and age at onset occur in infants.

A. Early-Onset Disease

"Early-onset" disease is observed in newborns younger than 7 days. Risk factors for early-onset disease include maternal GBS colonization, gestational age less than 37 weeks, rupture of membranes more than 18 hours prior to presentation, young maternal age, history of a previous infant with invasive GBS disease, African American or Hispanic ethnicity, and low or absent maternal GBS anticapsular antibodies. The onset of symptoms in the majority of these infants is in the first 48 hours of life, and most are ill within 6 hours. Respiratory abnormalities, irritability, lethargy, temperature instability, or poor perfusion may be presenting signs. Sepsis, shock, meningitis, and pneumonia are the most common clinical presentations. Although premature infants are at increased risk for the disease, most infants with early-onset infections are full term. Newborns with early-onset infection acquire GBS in utero as an ascending infection or during passage through the birth canal.

B. Late-Onset Disease

"Late-onset" disease occurs in infants between ages 7 and 89 days (median age at onset is about 4 weeks). Maternal obstetric complications are not usually associated with late-onset disease. However, young maternal age and prematurity remain risk factors. Late-onset disease is not prevented by IAP. The most common presentation of late-onset disease is bacteremia without focus, and compared to early-onset disease, a higher proportion presents with meningitis. Pneumonia, septic arthritis and osteomyelitis, otitis media, ethmoiditis, conjunctivitis, cellulitis (particularly of the face

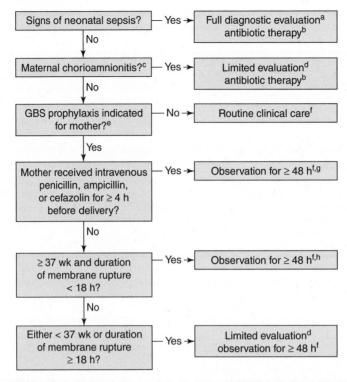

Signs of neonatal sepsis? — Yes → Full diagnostic evaluation[a] antibiotic therapy[b]

No

Maternal chorioamnionitis?[c] — Yes → Limited evaluation[d] antibiotic therapy[b]

No

GBS prophylaxis indicated for mother?[e] — No → Routine clinical care[f]

Yes

Mother received intravenous penicillin, ampicillin, or cefazolin for ≥ 4 h before delivery? — Yes → Observation for ≥ 48 h[f,g]

No

≥ 37 wk and duration of membrane rupture < 18 h? — Yes → Observation for ≥ 48 h[f,h]

No

Either < 37 wk or duration of membrane rupture ≥ 18 h? — Yes → Limited evaluation[d] observation for ≥ 48 h[f]

[a]Full diagnostic evaluation includes a blood culture, a complete blood count (CBC) including white blood cell differential and platelet counts, chest radiograph (if respiratory abnormalities are present), and lumbar puncture (if the patient is stable enough to tolerate procedure and sepsis is suspected).

[b]Antibiotic therapy should be directed toward the most common causes of neonatal sepsis, including intravenous ampicillin for GBS and coverage for other organisms (including *Escherichia coli* and other gram-negative pathogens) and should take into account local antibiotic-resistance patterns.

[c]Consultation with obstetric providers is important to determine the level of clinical suspicion for chorioamnionitis. Chorioamnionitis is diagnosed clinically, and some of the signs are nonspecific.

[d]Limited evaluation includes blood culture (at birth) and CBC with differential and platelets (at birth and/or at 6–12 hours of life).

[e]See Table 42–1 for indications for intrapartum GBS prophylaxis.

[f]If signs of sepsis develop, a full diagnostic evaluation should be conducted and antibiotic therapy initiated.

[g]If ≥ 37 weeks' gestation, observation may occur at home after 24 hours if other discharge criteria have been met, access to medical care is readily available, and a person who is able to comply fully with instructions for home observation will be present. If any of these conditions is not met, the infant should be observed in the hospital for at least 48 hours and until discharge criteria are achieved.

[h]Some experts recommend a CBC with differential and platelets at age 6–12 hours.

▲ **Figure 42–1.** Algorithm for secondary prevention of early-onset group B streptococcal (GBS) disease among newborns. (Reproduced with permission from Verani JR, McGee L, Schrag SJ, et al: Prevention of perinatal group B streptococcal disease—revised guidelines from CDC, 2010. MMWR Recomm Rep 2010 Nov 19;59(RR-10):1–36.)

or submandibular area), lymphadenitis, breast abscess, empyema, and impetigo have also been described. The exact mode of transmission of the organisms is not well defined.

C. Laboratory Findings

Culture of GBS from a normally sterile site such as blood, pleural fluid, or CSF provides proof of diagnosis.

▶ **Treatment**

Intravenous ampicillin and an aminoglycoside are the initial regimens of choice for newborns with presumptive invasive GBS disease. For neonates 7 days of age or younger with meningitis, the recommended ampicillin dosage is 200–300 mg/kg/day, given intravenously in three divided doses. For infants older than 7 days, the recommended ampicillin dosage is 300 mg/kg/day, given intravenously in four divided doses.

Penicillin G can be used alone once GBS is identified and clinical and microbiologic responses have occurred. GBS is less susceptible than other streptococci to penicillin, and high doses are recommended, especially for meningitis. In infants with meningitis, the recommended dosage of penicillin G varies with age: for infants 7 days or younger, 250,000–450,000 U/kg/day, given intravenously in three divided doses; for infants older than 7 days, 450,000–500,000 U/kg/day, given intravenously in four divided doses.

A second lumbar puncture after 24–48 hours of therapy is recommended by some experts to assess efficacy. Duration of therapy is 2 weeks for uncomplicated meningitis; at least 4 weeks for osteomyelitis, cerebritis, ventriculitis, or endocarditis, and 10 days for bacteremia. Therapy does not eradicate carriage of the organism.

Although streptococci have been universally susceptible to penicillins, increased minimum inhibitory concentrations (MICs) have been observed in some isolates. Resistance of isolates to clindamycin and erythromycin has increased significantly worldwide.

Infants diagnosed with GBS infection who are part of a multiple birth (twins, triplets, etc) define a risk for acquisition of invasive GBS disease in their siblings. Those siblings should be closely monitored and if signs of illness occur, promptly evaluated and antibiotics instituted for possible systemic infection.

Centers for disease control and prevention (CDC): prevention of perinatal group b streptococcal disease revised guidelines from CDC, 2010. MMWR 2010;59(RR-10):132. http://www.cdc.gov/mmwr/pdf/rr/rr5910.pdf.

STREPTOCOCCAL INFECTIONS WITH ORGANISMS OTHER THAN GROUP A OR B

General Considerations

Streptococci of groups other than A and B are part of the normal flora of humans and can occasionally cause disease. Group C or G organisms occasionally produce pharyngitis, but without risk of subsequent rheumatic fever. AGN may occasionally occur. Group D streptococci and *Enterococcus* species are normal inhabitants of the gastrointestinal tract and may produce urinary tract infections, meningitis, and sepsis in the newborn, as well as endocarditis.

Nosocomial infections caused by *Enterococcus* are frequent in neonatal and oncology units and in patients with central venous catheters. Nonhemolytic aerobic streptococci and β-hemolytic streptococci are normal flora of the mouth. They are involved in the production of dental plaque and probably dental caries and are the most common cause of subacute infective endocarditis. Finally, there are numerous anaerobic

and microaerophilic streptococci, normal flora of the mouth, skin, and gastrointestinal tract, which alone or in combination with other bacteria may cause sinusitis, dental abscesses, brain abscesses, and intra-abdominal or lung abscesses.

▶ Prevention

Streptococci (other than group A or B) are common normal flora in humans. Some disease caused by these organisms can be prevented by maintaining good oral hygiene. Spread of vancomycin-resistant enterococcal strains can be limited by good infection control practices in healthcare environments. Development of resistant strains can also be limited by antimicrobial stewardship. There are no vaccines that prevent infections with these organisms.

▶ Treatment

A. Enterococcal Infections

Enterococcus faecalis and *Enterococcus faecium* are the two most common and most important strains causing human infections. In general, *E faecalis* is more susceptible to antibiotics than *E faecium*, but antibiotic resistance is commonly seen with both species. Invasive enterococcal infections should be treated with ampicillin if the isolate is susceptible or vancomycin in combination with gentamicin. Gentamicin should be discontinued if susceptibility testing demonstrates high-level resistance to gentamicin. Isolates that are resistant to both ampicillin and vancomycin necessitate other therapeutic options.

1. Infections with ampicillin-susceptible enterococci— Lower tract urinary infections can be treated with oral amoxicillin. Pyelonephritis should be treated intravenously with ampicillin. Sepsis or meningitis in the newborn should be treated intravenously with a combination of ampicillin and gentamicin. Peak serum gentamicin levels of 3–5 mcg/mL are adequate as gentamicin is functioning as a synergistic agent. Consult the American Heart Association guidelines for treatment recommendations for infective endocarditis.

2. Infections with ampicillin-resistant- or vancomycin-resistant enterococci—Ampicillin-resistant enterococci are often susceptible to vancomycin. Vancomycin-resistant enterococci are usually also resistant to ampicillin. Linezolid is the only agent approved for use in children for vancomycin-resistant *E faecium* infections. Daptomycin and tigecycline have been used off-label for vancomycin-resistant enterococci; quinupristin-dalfopristin has been used to treat vancomycin-resistant *E faecium* but is not effective against *E faecalis*. Isolates resistant to linezolid, daptomycin, and quinupristin-dalfopristin have been reported. Infectious disease consultation is recommended when use of these drugs is entertained or when vancomycin-resistant enterococcal infections are identified.

B. Viridans Streptococci Infections (Subacute Infective Endocarditis)

It is important to determine the penicillin sensitivity of the infecting strain as early as possible in the treatment of viridans streptococcal endocarditis. Resistant organisms are most commonly seen in patients receiving penicillin prophylaxis for rheumatic heart disease. Treatment of endocarditis varies depending on whether the patient has native valves or prosthetic valves/material and whether the organism is penicillin susceptible. Refer to the American Heart Guidelines on Infective Endocarditis for a complete discussion and recommendations.

C. Other Viridans Streptococci–Related Infections

Viridans streptococci are normal flora of the gastrointestinal tract, respiratory tract, and the mouth. In many cases, isolation of viridans streptococci from a blood culture is considered to be a "contaminant" in the absence of signs or symptoms of endocarditis or other invasive disease. However, in children who are immunocompromised, have congenital or acquired valvular heart disease, or who have indwelling lines, viridans streptococci may be a cause of serious morbidity. About one-third of bacteremias in patients with malignancies may be due to bacteria from the *Streptococcus* viridans group. Mucositis and gastrointestinal toxicity from chemotherapy are risk factors for developing disease. Even in children with normal immune systems, viridans streptococci sometimes cause serious infections. For example, viridans streptococci isolated from an abdominal abscess after rupture of the appendix represents a true pathogen. *Streptococcus anginosus*, a member of the *Streptococcus* viridans group, can cause intracranial abscess (often as a complication of sinusitis) and abdominal abscesses. In patients with risk factors or signs/symptoms for subacute endocarditis, isolation of one of the members of the *Streptococcus* viridans group should prompt consideration and evaluation for possible endocarditis (see previous section).

Increasing prevalence of penicillin resistance has been seen in isolates of the streptococci viridans group. Penicillin resistance varies with geographic region, institution, and the populations tested, but ranges from 30% to 70% in oncology patients. Cephalosporin resistance is also relatively common. Therefore, it is important to obtain antibiotic susceptibilities to the organism to select effective therapy. Vancomycin, linezolid, and quinupristin-dalfopristin remain effective against most isolates.

Baltimore RS et al: Infective endocarditis in childhood: 2015 update: a scientific statement from the American Heart Association. Circulation 2015;132(15):1487–1515 [PMID: 26373317]. http://circ.ahajournals.org/content/132/15/1487.

Centers for Disease Control and Prevention: http://www.cdc.gov/hai/organisms/vre/vre.html. Accessed January 1, 2018.

PNEUMOCOCCAL INFECTIONS

ESSENTIALS OF DIAGNOSIS & TYPICAL FEATURES

▶ Bacteremia:
  • High fever (> 39.4°C).
  • Leukocytosis (> 15,000/μL).
▶ Pneumonia:
  • Fever, leukocytosis, and tachypnea.
  • Localized chest pain.
  • Localized or diffuse rales. Chest radiograph may show lobar infiltrate (with effusion).
▶ Meningitis:
  • Fever, leukocytosis.
  • Bulging fontanelle, neck stiffness.
  • Irritability and lethargy.
▶ All types:
  • Diagnosis confirmed by cultures of blood, CSF, pleural fluid, or other body fluid.

▶ General Considerations

Sepsis, sinusitis, otitis media, pneumonitis, meningitis, osteomyelitis, cellulitis, arthritis, vaginitis, and peritonitis are part of the spectrum of pneumococcal infection. Clinical findings that correlate with occult bacteremia in ambulatory patients include age (6–24 months), degree of temperature elevation (> 39.4°C), and leukocytosis (> 15,000/μL). Although each of these findings is in itself nonspecific, a combination of them should arouse suspicion.

Streptococcus pneumoniae is a common cause of acute purulent otitis media and is the organism responsible for most cases of acute bacterial pneumonia in children. Effusions are common, although frank empyema is less common. Abscesses also occasionally occur.

The incidence of pneumococcal meningitis has decreased since incorporation of the pneumococcal conjugate vaccine into the infant vaccine schedule; however, sporadic cases still occur. Pneumococcal meningitis, sometimes recurrent, may complicate serious head trauma, particularly if there is persistent leakage of CSF.

Children with sickle cell disease, other hemoglobinopathies, congenital or acquired asplenia, and some immunoglobulin and complement deficiencies are unusually susceptible to pneumococcal sepsis and meningitis. They often have a catastrophic illness with shock and disseminated intravascular coagulation (DIC). The spleen is important in the control of pneumococcal infection. Autosplenectomy may explain why children with sickle cell disease are at increased risk of developing serious pneumococcal infections. Children with cochlear implants are at higher risk for pneumococcal meningitis.

S pneumoniae rarely causes serious disease in the neonate. However, occasionally pneumonia, sepsis, or meningitis may occur and clinically is similar to GBS infection.

Historically, penicillin was the agent of choice for pneumococcal infections, and some strains are still highly susceptible to penicillin. However, pneumococci with moderately increased resistance to penicillin are found in most communities. There is some evidence that rates of antibiotic resistant pneumococcus are declining because non–vaccine-covered serotypes are less likely to be resistant. Nevertheless, empiric antibiotic coverage for suspected invasive pneumococcal disease should always account for the possibility of resistance.

▶ Prevention

Two pneumococcal vaccines are licensed for use in children in the United States: 13-valent pneumococcal conjugate vaccine (PCV13) and 23-valent pneumococcal polysaccharide vaccine (PPSV23). PCV13 was licensed in 2010 (replacing the 7-valent pneumococcal vaccine). It contains antigens from 13 pneumococcal serotypes and is currently recommended for routine use in the infant and childhood immunization schedule. These vaccines and indications for use (including use of pneumococcal vaccines in children at high risk for invasive pneumococcal disease) are discussed in detail in Chapter 10.

▶ Clinical Findings

A. Symptoms and Signs

In pneumococcal sepsis, fever usually appears abruptly, often accompanied by chills. There may be no respiratory symptoms. In infants and young children with pneumonia, fever, and tachypnea without auscultatory changes are the usual presenting signs. Respiratory distress is manifested by nasal flaring, chest retractions, and tachypnea. Abdominal pain is common. In older children, the adult form of pneumococcal pneumonia with signs of lobar consolidation may occur, but sputum is rarely bloody. Inspiratory pain (from pleural involvement) is sometimes present, but is less common in children. With involvement of the right hemidiaphragm, pain may be referred to the right lower quadrant, suggesting appendicitis. Vomiting is common at onset but seldom persists. Convulsions are relatively common at onset in infants.

Meningitis is characterized by fever, irritability, convulsions, and neck stiffness. The most important sign in very young infants is a tense, bulging anterior fontanelle. In older children, fever, chills, headache, and vomiting are common. Classic signs are nuchal rigidity associated with positive Brudzinski and Kernig signs. With progression of untreated disease, the child may develop opisthotonos, stupor, and coma.

B. Laboratory Findings

Leukocytosis is often pronounced (20,000–45,000/μL), with 80%–90% polymorphonuclear neutrophils and levels of C-reactive protein and procalcitonin are typically very elevated. Neutropenia may be seen early in very serious infections. The presence of pneumococci in the nasopharynx is not a helpful finding, because up to 40% of normal children carry pneumococci in the upper respiratory tract. Large numbers of organisms are seen on Gram-stained smears of endotracheal aspirates from patients with pneumonia. In meningitis, CSF usually shows an elevated white blood cell (WBC) count of several thousand, chiefly polymorphonuclear neutrophils, with decreased glucose and elevated protein levels. Gram-positive diplococci may be seen on some (but not all) stained smears of CSF sediment. Isolation of *S pneumoniae* from a normally sterile site (eg, blood, CSF, joint fluid, middle ear fluid) or from a suppurative focus confirms the diagnosis. The diagnosis can also be confirmed using as polymerase chain reaction (PCR)—often in the context of multiplex-PCR assays of positive blood culture samples or in CSF.

▶ Differential Diagnosis

There are many causes of high fever and leukocytosis in young infants other than invasive pneumococcal disease. The differential diagnosis includes viral infection, urinary tract infection, unrecognized focal infection elsewhere in the body, salmonellosis, or early acute shigellosis.

Staphylococcal pneumonia may be indistinguishable early in its course from pneumococcal pneumonia.

In primary pulmonary tuberculosis (TB), children do not have a toxic appearance, and radiographs show a primary focus associated with hilar adenopathy and often with pleural involvement. Miliary TB presents a classic radiographic appearance.

Pneumonia caused by *Mycoplasma pneumoniae* may result in a similar illness to pneumococcal disease, though onset is typically more insidious, with infrequent chills, low-grade fever, prominent headache and malaise, cough, and, often, striking radiographic changes. Marked leukocytosis (> 18,000/μL) is unusual.

Pneumococcal meningitis is diagnosed by lumbar puncture. Without a Gram-stained smear and culture of CSF, pneumococcal meningitis is not distinguishable from other types of acute bacterial meningitis.

▶ Complications

Complications of sepsis include meningitis and osteomyelitis; complications of pneumonia include empyema, parapneumonic effusion, and, rarely, lung abscess. Mastoiditis, subdural empyema, and brain abscess may follow untreated pneumococcal otitis media. Both pneumococcal meningitis and peritonitis are more likely to occur independently without coexisting pneumonia. Shock, DIC, and Waterhouse-Friderichsen syndrome resembling meningococcemia are occasionally seen in pneumococcal sepsis, particularly in asplenic patients. Hemolytic-uremic syndrome (HUS) may occur as a complication of pneumococcal pneumonia or sepsis.

▶ **Treatment**

A. Specific Measures

All *S pneumoniae* isolated from normally sterile sites should be tested for antimicrobial susceptibility. The term "nonsusceptible" is used to describe both intermediate and resistant isolates. Antimicrobial susceptibility breakpoints for *S pneumoniae* to penicillin and ceftriaxone are based on whether the patient has meningitis and the drug route (oral vs intravenous; Table 42–2). Therapy of meningitis, empyema, osteomyelitis, and endocarditis due to nonsusceptible *S pneumoniae* is challenging because penetration of antimicrobials to these sites is limited. Infectious disease consultation

Table 42–2. Penicillin breakpoints (minimum inhibitory concentrations [MIC]) for *Streptococcus pneumoniae* by susceptibility category—Clinical and Laboratory Standards Institute, 2008.

Drug	Clinical Syndrome and Drug Route	Susceptibility Category MIC (mcg/mL)		
		Susceptible	Intermediate	Resistant
Penicillin	Meningitis, intravenous penicillin	≤ 0.06	None[a]	≥ 0.12
	Nonmeningitis, intravenous penicillin	≤ 2	4	≥ 8
	Nonmeningitis, oral penicillin	≤ 0.06	0.12–1	≥ 2
Cefotaxime or ceftriaxone	Meningitis, intravenous cefotaxime or ceftriaxone	≤ 0.5	1	≥ 2
	Nonmeningitis, intravenous cefotaxime or ceftriaxone	≤ 1	2	≥ 4

[a]There is no intermediate category for meningitis.

Reproduced with permission from Centers for Disease Control and Prevention (CDC): Effects of new penicillin susceptibility breakpoints for *Streptococcus pneumoniae*—United States, 2006–2007. MMWR Morb Mortal Wkly Rep 2008 Dec 19;57(50):1353–1355.

is recommended for advice regarding these problems. For empiric therapy of serious or life-threatening infections pending susceptibility test results, vancomycin and ceftriaxone are recommended.

1. Bacteremia—Prior to routine childhood immunization with conjugated pneumococcal vaccine, 3%–5% of blood cultures in patients aged younger than 2 years yielded *S pneumoniae*, but these percentages decreased with the current vaccine schedule. Some children with positive blood cultures were well-appearing; such "occult bacteremias" were often managed with oral antibiotics. This clinical scenario has largely disappeared with pneumococcal conjugate vaccination. All children with blood cultures that grow pneumococci should be reexamined as soon as possible. The child who has a focal infection, such as meningitis, or who appears septic should be admitted to the hospital to receive parenteral antimicrobials. If the child is afebrile and appears well or mildly ill, outpatient management is appropriate. Severely ill or immunocompromised children, in whom invasive infection with *S pneumoniae* is suspected, should be empirically treated with vancomycin (in addition to other appropriate antibiotics to cover other suspected pathogens). If meningitis is also suspected, use ceftriaxone in addition to vancomycin until the susceptibilities of the organism are known.

2. Pneumonia—For infants (≥ 1 month of age) with susceptible organisms, appropriate regimens include ampicillin (150–200 mg/kg/day intravenously in four divided doses) or ceftriaxone (50 mg/kg intravenously every 24 hours). If susceptibilities are not known and the patient is severely ill or immunocompromised, vancomycin should be used as part of the regimen to provide coverage for penicillin- or cephalosporin-resistant pneumococcus. Once results of susceptibility testing are available, the regimen can be tailored. Mild pneumonia may be treated with amoxicillin (80–90 mg/kg/day) for 7–10 days. Oral cephalosporins are alternatives for penicillin allergic patients, but many (eg, cefdinir) have unfavorable pharmacokinetics for severe infection. Alternative regimens for penicillin and cephalosporin allergies include fluoroquinolones.

3. Otitis media—Most experts recommend oral amoxicillin (80–90 mg/kg/day, divided in two doses) as first-line therapy. Children younger than 2 years require 10 days of treatment. Shorter courses (5–7 days) may be adequate for older children with mild or moderate otitis. Treatment failures may be treated with amoxicillin-clavulanate (80–90 mg/kg/day of the amoxicillin component in the 14:1 formulation), though the addition of a β-lactamase inhibitor does not improve activity against pneumococcus. Intramuscular administration of ceftriaxone may be required for refractory cases of presumed pneumococcal acute otitis media (AOM).

4. Meningitis—Until bacteriologic confirmation and susceptibility testing are completed, patients should receive vancomycin (60 mg/kg/day, given intravenously in four divided doses) and ceftriaxone (100 mg/kg/day intravenously in two divided doses). Patients with serious hypersensitivity to β-lactam antibiotics (eg, penicillins, cephalosporins) can be treated with a combination of vancomycin (see previous dosage) and levofloxacin or meropenem. These regimens provide additional gram-negative coverage until culture and susceptibility results are obtained. Corticosteroids (dexamethasone, 0.6 mg/kg/day, in four divided doses for 4 days) are recommended by many experts as adjunctive therapy for pneumococcal meningitis. A repeat lumbar puncture at 24–48 hours should be considered to ensure sterility of the CSF if resistant pneumococci were initially isolated or if the patient is not demonstrating expected improvement after 24–48 hours on therapy.

If the isolate is penicillin-susceptible, aqueous penicillin G can be administered (300,000–400,000 U/kg/day intravenously in four to six divided doses for 10–14 days). Alternatively, use of ceftriaxone is an acceptable alternative therapy for penicillin- and cephalosporin-susceptible isolates. Consult an infectious disease specialist or the *Red Book* (American Academy of Pediatrics, 2018) for a complete discussion of pneumococcal meningitis and for therapeutic options for isolates that are nonsusceptible to penicillin or cephalosporins.

Prognosis

In children, case fatality rates of less than 1% should be achieved except for meningitis, where rates of 5%–20% still prevail. The presence of large numbers of organisms without a prominent CSF inflammatory response or meningitis due to a penicillin-resistant strain indicates a poor prognosis. Serious neurologic sequelae, particularly hearing loss, are frequent following pneumococcal meningitis.

Bradley JS et al: The management of community-acquired pneumonia in infants and children older than 3 months of age: clinical practice guidelines by the Pediatric Infectious Diseases Society and the Infectious Diseases Society of America. Clin Infect Dis 2011 Oct;53(7):617–630 [PMID: 21890766].

Centers for Disease Control and Prevention (CDC): Prevention of pneumococcal disease among infants and children—use of 13-valent pneumococcal conjugate vaccine and 23-valent pneumococcal polysaccharide vaccine—recommendations of the Advisory Committee on Immunization Practices (ACIP). MMWR Recomm Rep 2010 Dec 10;59(RR-11):118 [PMID: 21150868].

Pneumococcal infections. In: Kimberlin DW, Brady MT, Jackson MA, Long SS (eds): *Red Book: 2018 Report of the Committee on Infectious Diseases.* 31th ed. Elk Grove Village, IL: American Academy of Pediatrics; 2018;626–638.

STAPHYLOCOCCAL INFECTIONS

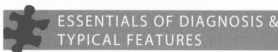

ESSENTIALS OF DIAGNOSIS & TYPICAL FEATURES

▶ Purulent infections at one or more sites.

▶ Toxin production causing shock or organ dysfunction.

▶ Positive culture of *Staphylococcus* from blood, purulent secretions, or mucosal sites.

General Considerations

Staphylococcal infections are common in childhood and range from mild localized infections to overwhelming systemic infections. Diseases caused by staphylococci include, but are not limited to, furuncles, carbuncles, scalded skin syndrome, osteomyelitis, pyomyositis, septic arthritis, pneumonia, bacteremia, endocarditis, meningitis, and TSS. Staphylococci are the major cause of skin, soft tissue, bone and joint infections, and are an uncommon but important cause of bacterial pneumonia. Staphylococci are frequent colonizers of the nasopharynx, and a common route of entry to the body is through disruptions in the skin.

S aureus is the most common pathogenic species and most *S aureus* strains produce coagulase. Staphylococci that do not produce the enzyme coagulase are termed *coagulase-negative staphylococci.* The latter rarely cause disease except in compromised hosts, the newborn, or patients with indwelling lines.

Most strains of *S aureus* elaborate β-lactamase that confers penicillin resistance. This can be overcome in clinical practice by the use of a cephalosporin or a penicillinase-resistant penicillin, such as oxacillin, nafcillin, cloxacillin, or dicloxacillin. Methicillin-resistant *S aureus* (MRSA) are resistant in vivo to all of these penicillinase-resistant penicillins and cephalosporins. MRSA has dramatically increased in prevalence globally as both a healthcare-associated and a community-associated pathogen. Health care–associated infections are likely to be multidrug resistant. Community-associated MRSA are most often susceptible to clindamycin and/or TMP-SMX, but resistance rates to these agents vary widely geographically. MRSA strains with intermediate susceptibility to vancomycin occur, and vancomycin-resistant strains have been isolated. The existence of such strains is of concern because of the inherent virulence of most strains of *S aureus* and limited choices for therapy.

S aureus produces a variety of exotoxins that contribute to specific disease manifestations. The exfoliatin toxin is largely responsible for bullous impetigo and scalded skin syndrome. Enterotoxin causes staphylococcal food poisoning. The exoprotein toxin most commonly associated with TSS has been termed TSST-1. Panton-Valentine leukocidin (PVL) is an exotoxin produced by some clinical isolates of methicillin-susceptible *S aureus* (MSSA) and MRSA strains. PVL is a virulence factor that causes leukocyte destruction and tissue necrosis. PVL-producing *S aureus* strains are often community-acquired and have most commonly produced boils and abscesses. However, they also have been associated with severe cellulitis, osteomyelitis, and deaths from necrotizing pneumonia.

▶ **Prevention**

No licensed vaccines are available. Patients with recurrent skin infections with *S aureus* should practice good skin hygiene to try to prevent recurrences. Weekly baths with bleach (1 tsp per gallon or ¼ cup per ½ tub [~20 gal]) or chlorhexidine 4% may decrease skin contamination. Household eradication regimens may also include treatment of the patient and family with intranasal antibiotics (eg, mupirocin) and hot water washing of clothes and linens. Keeping fingernails short, good skin hygiene, not sharing towels or other personal items, and use of a clean towel daily may also help prevent recurrences.

▶ **Clinical Findings**

A. Symptoms and Signs

1. Staphylococcal skin diseases—Dermal infection with MRSA and MSSA causes pustules, furuncles, carbuncles, or cellulitis. Skin lesions can be seen anywhere on the body but are commonly seen on the buttocks in infants and young children. Factors that facilitate transmission of MRSA or MSSA include crowding, compromised skin (eg, eczema), participation on contact sports teams, day care attendance, bare skin contact with surfaces used by others (exercise mats, sauna benches), and sharing towels or other personal items.

S aureus are often found along with streptococci in impetigo. If the strains produce exfoliatin, localized lesions become bullous (bullous impetigo).

Scalded skin syndrome is a toxin-mediated illness caused by exfoliative toxins A and B produced by certain strains of *S aureus*. The initial infection may begin at any site but occurs most frequently in the nasopharynx, a site that is frequently colonized by *S aureus*. Skin erythema, often beginning around the nose and mouth, is accompanied by fever and irritability. The involved skin becomes tender to touch. A day or so later, exfoliation begins, usually around the mouth. The inside of the mouth is red, and a peeling rash is present around the lips, often in a radial pattern. Generalized, painful peeling may follow, involving the limbs and trunk but often sparing the feet. If erythematous but unpeeled skin is rubbed, superficial epidermal layers separate from deeper ones and slough (Nikolsky sign). Generally, if secondary infection does not occur, there is healing without scarring.

In the newborn, the disease is termed *Ritter disease* and may be fulminant.

2. Osteomyelitis and septic arthritis—(See Chapter 26.) MRSA invasive disease including osteomyelitis and septic arthritis is increasingly common.

3. Staphylococcal pneumonia—Staphylococcal pneumonia is often characterized by a severe respiratory and systemic illness. In the lungs, the organism is necrotizing, producing bronchoalveolar destruction. Pneumatoceles, pyopneumothorax, and empyema are frequently encountered. Rapid progression of disease is characteristic. Purulent pericarditis occurs by direct extension in about 10% of cases, with or without empyema. MSSA and MRSA pneumonias are frequently encountered in the setting of a primary influenza infection, or in the context of a multifocal or disseminated staphylococcal infection associated with endovascular infection and persistent bacteremia.

Staphylococcal pneumonia can also occur in newborns, and though infection with coagulase-negative *Staphylococcus* is more common, infection with *S aureus* is more likely to result in a fulminant course. Most staphylococcal lung infections in newborns occur in susceptible infants with indwelling catheters, endotracheal tubes, and are part of a systemic infectious process.

4. Staphylococcal food poisoning—Staphylococcal food poisoning is a result of ingestion of preformed enterotoxin produced by staphylococci growing in undercooked or improperly stored food. The disease is characterized by vomiting, prostration, and diarrhea occurring 2–6 hours after ingestion of contaminated foods.

5. Endocarditis and endovascular infection—Although the presence of a damaged or artificial heart valve or endocardium in children with congenital or rheumatic heart disease predisposes to endocarditis, *S aureus* may also produce infection of normal heart valves. A major risk factor for pediatric staphylococcal endocarditis is the presence of intravascular foreign bodies, including indwelling central catheters. Recent studies have indicated that *S aureus* may now cause approximately 50% of all cases of endocarditis in children. Infection usually begins in an extracardiac focus, often the skin or a catheter insertion site. Involvement of the endocardium should be considered when blood cultures grow *S aureus*, particularly when cultures are persistently positive and/or in the presence of congenital heart disease.

The presenting symptoms in staphylococcal endocarditis are fever, weight loss, weakness, muscle pain or diffuse skeletal pain, poor feeding, pallor, and cardiac decompensation. Signs include splenomegaly, cardiomegaly, petechiae, hematuria, and a new or changing murmur. The course of *S aureus* endocarditis is rapid, although subacute disease occurs occasionally. Peripheral septic embolization and uncontrollable cardiac failure are common, even when optimal antibiotic therapy is administered and may be indications for surgical intervention (see section 5. Staphylococcal Endocarditis).

Septic thrombophlebitis can occur in the setting of localized primary infections such as osteomyelitis. Patients often progress to septic shock, respiratory failure, and multiorgan dysfunction due to persistent bacteremia and disseminated embolic foci. Imaging studies to identify infected thromboses should be considered in the presence of severe illness and persistent bacteremia.

6. Toxic shock syndrome—TSS is characterized by fever, blanching erythroderma, diarrhea, vomiting, myalgia, prostration, hypotension, and multiorgan dysfunction. It is due to *S aureus* focal infection, usually without bacteremia. Large numbers of cases have been described in menstruating adolescents using vaginal tampons. TSS has also been reported with focal staphylococcal infections and in individuals with wound infections due to *S aureus*. Additional clinical features include sudden onset; conjunctival suffusion; mucosal hyperemia; desquamation of skin on the palms, soles, fingers, and toes during convalescence; DIC in severe cases; renal and hepatic functional abnormalities; and myolysis. The mortality rate with early treatment is now less than 1%. Recurrences during subsequent menstrual periods are not unusual, occurring in as many as 60% of untreated women who continue to use tampons.

7. Coagulase-negative staphylococcal infections— Localized and systemic coagulase-negative staphylococcal infections occur primarily in immunocompromised patients, high-risk (especially premature) newborns, and patients with intravascular foreign bodies. Coagulase-negative staphylococci are the most common nosocomial pathogen in hospitalized low-birth-weight neonates in the United States. Intravenous administration of lipid emulsions and indwelling central venous catheters are risk factors contributing to coagulase-negative staphylococcal bacteremia in newborns. Coagulase-negative staphylococci are a common cause of bacteremia and sepsis in patients with an artificial heart valve, a Dacron patch, a ventriculoperitoneal shunt, or a central venous catheter, often necessitating removal of the foreign material and protracted antibiotic therapy. Coagulase-negative staphylococci are also normal skin flora and are thus a common cause of blood culture contamination.

B. Laboratory Findings

Moderate leukocytosis (15,000–20,000/μL) with a shift to the left is occasionally found, although normal counts are common, particularly in infants, and leukopenia (< 5000/μL) can occur in severe cases. Markers of inflammation, including the C-reactive protein, procalcitonin and sedimentation rate are frequently elevated except in localized mild infections. Blood cultures are frequently positive in systemic staphylococcal

disease and should always be obtained when it is suspected. Similarly, pus from sites of infection should always be aspirated or obtained surgically, examined with Gram stain, and cultured. This is particularly important when MRSA is a possible pathogen. There are no useful serologic tests for staphylococcal disease.

▶ Differential Diagnosis

Staphylococcal skin disease takes many forms; therefore, the differential list is long. Bullous impetigo must be differentiated from chemical or thermal burns, drug reactions, and, in the very young, from the various congenital epidermolytic syndromes or herpes simplex infections. Staphylococcal scalded skin syndrome may resemble scarlet fever, Kawasaki disease, Stevens-Johnson syndrome, erythema multiforme, and other drug reactions. A skin biopsy may be critical in establishing the diagnosis. Varicella lesions may become superinfected with exfoliatin-producing staphylococci and produce a combination of the two diseases (bullous varicella).

Severe, rapidly progressing pneumonia with formation of abscesses, pneumatoceles, and empyemas is typical of *S aureus* infection and group A *Streptococcus* (GAS), but may occasionally be produced by pneumococci, *Klebsiella pneumoniae* and *Haemophilus influenzae*.

Staphylococcal food poisoning often occurs in clusters associated with a single food source. It is differentiated from other common-source gastroenteritis syndromes (*Salmonella*, *Clostridium perfringens*, and *Vibrio parahaemolyticus*) by the short incubation period (2–6 hours), the prominence of vomiting (as opposed to diarrhea), and the absence of fever. Food poisoning from *Bacillus cereus* can result in a vomiting illness clinically indistinguishable from *S aureus*.

Endocarditis is suspected with *S aureus* bacteremia, particularly when a significant heart murmur or preexisting cardiac disease is present (see Chapter 20).

Neonatal infections with *S aureus* and coagulase-negative staphylococci can resemble infections with streptococci and a variety of gram-negative organisms. Umbilical and respiratory tract colonization occurs with many pathogenic organisms (GBS, *Escherichia coli*, and *Klebsiella*), and both skin and systemic infections occur with virtually all of these organisms.

TSS must be differentiated from Rocky Mountain spotted fever, leptospirosis, Kawasaki disease, drug reactions, adenovirus, and measles (see Table 40–2).

▶ Treatment

A. Specific Measures

The incidence of community-acquired MRSA isolates varies greatly geographically, but in many communities in the United States, MRSA is the most common pathogen isolated from skin and soft tissue infections. For empiric coverage of potentially life-threatening infections with suspected

S aureus (in which susceptibilities are not known), initial therapy should include vancomycin in combination with either nafcillin or oxacillin (in addition to appropriate antibiotic therapy for other suspected pathogens). Antibiotic therapy can then be adjusted based on identification of the organism and susceptibility results.

Currently, most community-acquired MRSA strains are susceptible to TMP-SMX, and many are susceptible to clindamycin, though this varies geographically. Knowledge of local MRSA susceptibility patterns is useful in guiding empiric therapy. Less serious infections in nontoxic patients may be initially treated using TMP-SMX or clindamycin, while awaiting cultures and susceptibility data, if community MRSA resistance to these agents is low.

For MSSA strains, a β-lactamase–resistant penicillin is the drug of choice (oxacillin or nafcillin) and is preferred over vancomycin. In serious systemic disease, in osteomyelitis, and in the treatment of large abscesses, intravenous therapy is indicated initially (oxacillin or nafcillin, 100–150 mg/kg/day in four divided doses). In serious or life-threatening illness, consultation with an infectious disease physician is recommended.

Many cephalosporins are active against MSSA. Cefazolin, 100–150 mg/kg/day, given intravenously in three divided doses, or cephalexin, 50–100 mg/kg/day, given orally in four divided doses, can be used once a child is able to take oral antibiotics. The third-generation cephalosporins should not generally be used for proven staphylococcal infections.

For serious *S aureus* infections, initial therapy with vancomycin (15 mg/kg/dose intravenously every 6 hours) plus nafcillin or oxacillin is recommended until susceptibilities are available. For nosocomially acquired MRSA infections, vancomycin should be used until results of susceptibility testing are available to guide therapy. Newer antistaphylococcal antibiotics with activity against MRSA include daptomycin, linezolid, and ceftaroline; these drugs and may be used for severe infections under the guidance of infectious disease specialists. To date there is little pediatric data for the use of novel long half-life lipoglycopeptides (eg, oritavancin, dalbavancin). Rifampin is used occasionally for adjunctive treatment of persistent staphylococcal infections, particularly in the presence of foreign material, but it should never be used as monotherapy.

1. Skin infections—Treatment of skin and soft tissue infections depends, in part, on the extent of the lesion, immunocompetence of the host, and the toxicity of the patient. Afebrile, well-appearing patients with small abscesses may do well with incision and drainage (with or without the addition of oral antimicrobials). More serious infections or infections in immunocompromised patients should be treated more aggressively. Hospitalization and intravenous antibiotics may be required. Culture and susceptibility testing will help guide therapy.

For patients who are not sick enough to require hospitalization or intravenous therapy, selection of the best empiric antimicrobial depends on local rates of MRSA and local susceptibilities. β-Lactam antibiotics, such as penicillins and cephalosporins, can no longer depend on as single agents for the majority of cases in communities with high MRSA rates, but may be considered as initial treatment in milder infections where good follow-up can be assured. TMP-SMX or clindamycin (depending on local susceptibility patterns) may be used for empiric staphylococcal coverage. However, GAS may be resistant to TMP-SMX, and not all MSSA or MRSA will be covered by clindamycin. Many clinicians empirically use a combination of TMP-SMX and cefazolin/cephalexin for empiric treatment of skin and soft tissue infections.

2. Osteomyelitis and septic arthritis—Treatment should be begun intravenously, with antibiotics selected to cover the most likely organisms (staphylococci in hematogenous osteomyelitis; meningococci, pneumococci, *Kingella kingae*, staphylococci in children aged < 3 years with septic arthritis; staphylococci and gonococci in older children with septic arthritis). Knowledge of local MRSA rates will help guide empiric therapy. Antibiotic levels should be kept high at all times.

Clinical studies support the use of intravenous treatment for osteomyelitis until fever and local symptoms and signs and inflammatory markers are subsiding—usually at least 3–5 days—followed by oral therapy. For both osteomyelitis and joint infections, good compliance with oral therapy is important for successful cure.

Nafcillin or cefazolin can be used for intravenous therapy of MSSA strains. Clindamycin is an alternative agent if the organism is susceptible, and the patient does not have a severe or life-threatening infection or ongoing bacteremia. Cephalexin 100–150 mg/kg/day in four divided doses can be used when the patient is ready for oral therapy.

Vancomycin can be used initially for MRSA osteomyelitis, while awaiting final susceptibilities. Antibiotic regimens for MRSA osteomyelitis should be based on susceptibility results; isolates may be susceptible to clindamycin or linezolid, but susceptibility patterns vary geographically.

The C-reactive protein (in the first or second week after therapy is started) and the erythrocyte sedimentation rate (ESR) (usually measured weekly) are good indicators of response to therapy. Duration of therapy is typically 3–4 weeks for septic arthritis and 4–6 weeks for acute osteomyelitis. Surgical drainage of osteomyelitis or septic arthritis is often required (see Chapter 26).

3. Staphylococcal pneumonia—For MSSA pneumonia, nafcillin and oxacillin are the usual drugs of choice. Vancomycin can be used empirically until results of cultures and susceptibility tests are obtained if community or hospital MRSA rates are high. In sicker patients, vancomycin plus nafcillin can be used (in addition to coverage of other pathogens) until the etiologic agent and susceptibilities are established. Linezolid has been reported to be as efficacious as vancomycin for the treatment of resistant gram-positive pneumonia and soft tissue infections.

Empyema and pyopneumothorax require drainage. The choice of chest tube versus thoracoscopic drainage depends on local institutional practice. If staphylococcal pneumonia is treated promptly and empyema drained, resolution in children often is complete.

4. Staphylococcal food poisoning—Therapy is supportive and usually not required except in severe cases or for small infants with marked dehydration.

5. Staphylococcal endocarditis—The treatment of staphylococcal endocarditis depends on whether the patient has a prosthetic valve or material in the heart and on the susceptibilities of the organism. Please see the American Heart Association's Guidelines on Infective Endocarditis: Diagnosis and Management, and consult an infectious disease physician for this serious and sometimes complicated problem. High-dose, prolonged parenteral treatment is indicated. Therapy lasts in all instances for at least 6 weeks.

Occasionally, medical treatment fails. Signs of treatment failure are: (1) recurrent fever without apparent treatable other cause (eg, thrombophlebitis, respiratory or urinary tract infection, drug fever), (2) persistently positive blood cultures, (3) intractable and progressive congestive heart failure, and (4) recurrent (septic) embolization. In such circumstances—particularly (2), (3), and (4)—evaluation for valve replacement becomes necessary. Antibiotics are continued for at least another 4 weeks after blood cultures are proven negative. Persistent or recurrent infection may require a second surgical procedure.

6. Toxic shock syndrome—Treatment is aimed at expanding blood volume, maintaining perfusion pressure with inotropic agents, ensuring prompt drainage of a focus of infection (or removal of tampons or foreign bodies), and giving intravenous antibiotics.

Vancomycin, in addition to a β-lactam antibiotic (oxacillin or nafcillin), can be used for empiric therapy because TSS can be challenging to discriminate from staphylococcal sepsis. Many experts also add clindamycin, since clindamycin is a protein synthesis inhibitor and may limit toxin production. Clindamycin should not be used empirically as a single agent until susceptibilities are known. Intravenous immunoglobulin has been used as adjunctive therapy for severe disease.

7. Vancomycin-resistant *S aureus* infections (VRSA)—Reports of VRSA isolates are rare but are likely to increase in frequency. Such isolates are sometimes susceptible to clindamycin or TMP-SMX. If not, therapeutic options include linezolid, ceftaroline or daptomycin, assuming the strain is susceptible to these agents. Consultation with an infectious disease specialist is recommended.

8. Coagulase-negative staphylococcal infections—Coagulase-negative staphylococci are frequently resistant to penicillins and cephalosporins. Bacteremia and other serious coagulase-negative staphylococcal infections are treated initially with vancomycin, with susceptibility results guiding subsequent therapy. Coagulase-negative staphylococci are uncommonly resistant to vancomycin (see Chapter 39 for dosing). Many drugs used for MRSA are also effective against these pathogens.

Baltimore RS: Infective endocarditis in childhood: 2015 update: a scientific statement from the American Heart Association. Circulation 2015 Oct 13;132(15):1487–1515. doi: 10.1161/CIR.0000000000000298 [PMID: 26373317].

DeRonde KJ et al: Management of pediatric acute hematogenous osteomyelitis, part II: a focus on methicillin-resistant *Staphylococcus aureus*, current and emerging therapies. Pharmacotherapy 2018 Oct;38(10):1021–1037. doi: 10.1002/phar.2164. Epub 2018 Sep 4 [PMID: 29989190].

MENINGOCOCCAL INFECTIONS

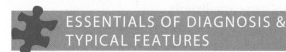

ESSENTIALS OF DIAGNOSIS & TYPICAL FEATURES

▶ Fever, headache, vomiting, convulsions, shock (meningitis).

▶ Fever, shock, petechial or purpuric skin rash (meningococcemia).

▶ Diagnosis confirmed by culture of normally sterile body fluids.

▶ General Considerations

Meningococci (*Neisseria meningitidis*) may be carried asymptomatically for months in the upper respiratory tract. Less than 1% of carriers develop disease. Meningitis and sepsis are the two most common forms of illness, but septic arthritis, pericarditis, pneumonia, chronic meningococcemia, otitis media, conjunctivitis, and vaginitis also occur. Meningococcal cases in the United States have continued to decline; currently there are an estimated 400–600 cases annually. The highest attack rate for meningococcal meningitis is in the first year of life, with a secondary peak during the teen years. The development of irreversible shock with multiorgan failure is a significant factor in the fatal outcome of acute meningococcal infections.

Meningococci are gram-negative organisms containing endotoxin in their cell walls. Endotoxins cause capillary vascular injury and leak as well as DIC. Meningococci are classified serologically into groups: A, B, C, Y, and W are the groups most commonly implicated in systemic disease. Currently in the United States, more than one-half of cases in infants, children, and adolescents are caused by serogroup B. Over the last few years, several outbreaks on college campus have been caused by serogroup B. Serogroup A causes epidemics in sub-Saharan Africa but rarely is associated with cases of meningococcal disease in the United States. *N meningitidis* with increased MICs to penicillin G are reported, but the clinical significance of this is unclear. A small number of these isolates are reported in the United States. Resistant isolates are susceptible to third-generation cephalosporins. Few isolates are resistant to rifampin. In recent years, fluoroquinolone-resistant *N meningitidis* has emerged.

Patients deficient in one of the late components of the complement pathway are uniquely susceptible to meningococcal infection. Deficiencies of early and alternative pathway complement components, anatomic or functional asplenia, eculizumab use, and human immunodeficiency virus (HIV) infection also are associated with increased susceptibility.

▶ Prevention

A. Chemoprophylaxis

Household contacts, day care center contacts, and hospital personnel directly exposed to the respiratory secretions of patients are at increased risk for developing meningococcal infection and should be given chemoprophylaxis. The secondary attack rate among household members is about 500–800 times the attack rate in the general population. Children between the ages of 3 months and 2 years are at greatest risk, presumably because they lack protective antibodies. Secondary cases may occur in day care centers and in classrooms. Hospital personnel are not at increased risk unless they have had contact with a patient's oral secretions, for example, during mouth-to-mouth resuscitation, intubation, or suctioning procedures. Approximately 50% of secondary cases in households have their onset within 24 hours of identification of the index case. Exposed contacts should be notified promptly. If they are febrile, they should be fully evaluated and given high doses of penicillin or another effective antimicrobial pending the results of blood cultures.

All high-risk contacts should receive chemoprophylaxis for meningococcal disease as soon as an index case is identified. High-risk contacts are defined as:

- All household contacts (especially children < 2 years of age)
- Persons with child care or preschool contact with the index patient at any time in the 7 days prior to illness onset
- Persons with direct exposure to index patients secretions (sharing of drinks, straws, cigarettes, toothbrushes, eating utensils, kissing) during the 7 days prior to illness onset

- Persons who have performed mouth-to-mouth resuscitation or performed unprotected endotracheal intubation of the index patient during the 7 days prior to illness onset
- Persons who have slept in the same dwelling as the index patient within 7 days of illness onset
- Passengers who were seated directly next to the index patient on a flight of more than 8 hours duration

The most commonly used agent for meningococcal chemoprophylaxis is oral rifampin given twice daily for 2 days (600 mg for adults; 15–20 mg/kg for children *older* than 1 month [maximum dosage 600 mg] and 5 mg/kg for infants *younger* than 1 month). Rifampin may stain a patient's tears (and contact lenses), sweat, and urine orange; it may also affect the reliability of oral contraceptives, and alternative contraceptive measures should therefore be employed when rifampin is administered. Rifampin should not be given to pregnant women. Instead, intramuscular ceftriaxone is the preferred agent: 125 mg given as a single dose if the patient is younger than 15 years; 250 mg given as a single dose if the patient is aged 15 years or older. Penicillin and most other antibiotics (even with parenteral administration) are not effective chemoprophylactic agents, because they do not eradicate upper respiratory tract carriage of meningococci. Ciprofloxacin (20 mg/kg as a single dose, maximum dose 500 mg) effectively eradicates nasopharyngeal carriage in adults and children but is not recommended in pregnant women or in communities where fluoroquinolone-resistant strains of *N meningitidis* have been identified. Throat cultures to identify carriers are not useful.

B. Vaccine

Several types of vaccines are currently licensed in the United States for meningococcal disease prevention; 2-quadrivalent meningococcal conjugate vaccines (see Chapter 10) that cover serogroups A, C, Y, and W are available in the United States. Two serogroup B vaccines are licensed for ages 10–25 years. (See Chapter 10 for a discussion on meningococcal vaccines.)

▶ Clinical Findings

A. Symptoms and Signs

Many children with clinical meningococcemia also have meningitis, and some have other foci of infection. All children with suspected meningococcemia should have a lumbar puncture.

1. Meningococcemia—A prodrome of upper respiratory infection is followed by high fever, headache, nausea, marked toxicity, and hypotension. Purpura, petechiae, and occasionally bright pink, tender macules or papules over the extremities, and trunk are seen. The rash usually progresses rapidly. Occasional cases lack rash. Fulminant meningococcemia is characterized by DIC, massive skin and mucosal hemorrhages, and shock. This syndrome also may be caused by *H influenzae*, *S pneumoniae*, or other bacteria. Chronic meningococcemia is a rare condition characterized by periodic bouts of fever, arthralgia or arthritis, and recurrent petechiae. Splenomegaly often is present. Patients may be free of symptoms between bouts. Chronic meningococcemia occurs primarily in adults and mimics Henoch-Schönlein purpura.

2. Meningitis—In many children, meningococcemia is followed within a few hours to several days by symptoms and signs of acute purulent meningitis, with severe headache, stiff neck, nausea, vomiting, and stupor. Children with meningitis generally fare better than children with meningococcemia alone, probably because they have survived long enough to develop clinical signs of meningitis.

B. Laboratory Findings

The peripheral WBC count may be either low or elevated. Thrombocytopenia may be present with or without DIC (see Chapter 30). If petechial or hemorrhagic lesions are present, meningococci can sometimes be seen microscopically in tissue fluid expressed from a punctured lesion. CSF is generally cloudy and contains more than 1000 WBCs/μL, with many polymorphonuclear neutrophils and gram-negative intracellular diplococci. A total hemolytic complement assay may reveal absence of late components as an underlying cause. PCR assays with high sensitivity and specificity are now available to detect *N meningitidis*, and can be useful, especially in cases where antibiotics were initiated before any cultures were obtained; however, culture remains the gold standard.

▶ Differential Diagnosis

The skin lesions of *H influenzae* or pneumococci, enterovirus infection, endocarditis, leptospirosis, Rocky Mountain spotted fever, other rickettsial diseases, Henoch-Schönlein purpura, and blood dyscrasias may be similar to meningococcemia. Severe *S aureus* sepsis has been reported in some patients to present with purpura. Other causes of sepsis and meningitis are distinguished by appropriate Gram stain and cultures.

▶ Complications

Meningitis may lead to permanent central nervous system (CNS) damage, with deafness, convulsions, paralysis, or impaired intellectual function. Hydrocephalus may develop and requires ventriculoperitoneal shunt. Subdural collections of fluid are common but usually resolve spontaneously. Extensive skin necrosis, loss of digits or extremities, intestinal hemorrhage, and late adrenal insufficiency may complicate fulminant meningococcemia.

▶ Treatment

Blood cultures should be obtained for all children with fever and purpura or other signs of meningococcemia, and antibiotics should be administered immediately as an emergency procedure.

Children with meningococcemia or meningococcal meningitis should be treated as though shock were imminent even if their vital signs are stable when they are first seen. If hypotension is present, supportive measures should be aggressive, because the prognosis is grave in such situations. Treatment should be started emergently in an intensive care setting, but should not be delayed while transporting the patient. Shock may worsen following antimicrobial therapy due to endotoxin release. To minimize the risk of nosocomial transmission, patients should be placed in respiratory isolation for the first 24 hours of antibiotic treatment.

A. Specific Measures

Antibiotics should be initiated promptly. Because other bacteria, such as *S pneumoniae*, *S aureus*, or other gram-negative organisms, can cause identical syndromes, initial therapy should be broad. Vancomycin and cefotaxime (or ceftriaxone) are preferred initial coverage. Once *N meningitidis* has been isolated, penicillin G, cefotaxime, or ceftriaxone intravenously for 7 days are the drugs of choice. Relative penicillin resistance is uncommon but has been reported in the United States.

B. General Measures

Blood cultures should be drawn prior to initiation of antibiotic therapy; however antibiotic therapy should not be delayed in order to obtain a lumbar puncture as prompt treatment portends better outcomes due to the aggressive nature of this infection. Supportive care includes early and aggressive fluid resuscitation and vasopressor initiation.

▶ Prognosis

Unfavorable prognostic features include shock, DIC, and extensive skin lesions. The case fatality rate in fulminant meningococcemia is over 30%. In uncomplicated meningococcal meningitis, the fatality rate is much lower (10%–20%). An invasive meningococcal infection may be the first indication of an underlying immunodeficiency, particularly defects in terminal complement function.

Centers for Disease Control and Prevention (CDC): Meningococcal disease. http://www.cdc.gov/meningococcal/clinical-info.html. Accessed July 3, 2019.

Cohn AC et al; Centers for Disease Control and Prevention (CDC): Prevention and control of meningococcal disease: recommendations of the Advisory Committee on Immunization Practices (ACIP). MMWR Recomm Rep 2013;62(RR-2):1 [PMID: 23515099]. http://www.cdc.gov/mmwr/preview/mmwrhtml/rr6202a1.htm.

GONOCOCCAL INFECTIONS

ESSENTIALS OF DIAGNOSIS & TYPICAL FEATURES

▶ Purulent urethral discharge with intracellular gram negative diplococci on smear in male patients (usually adolescents) (see Chapter 44).

▶ Purulent, edematous, sometimes hemorrhagic conjunctivitis with intracellular gram-negative diplococci in 2- to 4-day-old infants.

▶ Fever, arthritis (often polyarticular) or tenosynovitis, and maculopapular peripheral rash that may be vesiculopustular or hemorrhagic.

▶ Positive culture of blood, pharyngeal, or genital secretions.

▶ NAAT on urine or genital secretions.

▶ General Considerations

Neisseria gonorrhoeae is a gram-negative diplococcus. Although morphologically similar to other Neisseriae, it differs in its ability to grow on selective media and to ferment carbohydrates. The cell wall of *N gonorrhoeae* contains endotoxin, which is liberated when the organism dies and stimulates the production of a cellular exudate. The incubation period is short, usually 2–5 days.

Reported cases of gonorrhea exceeded 555,000 in the United States in 2017 and have continued to increase since reaching historic lows in 2009. Gonococcal disease in children may be transmitted sexually or nonsexually. Prepubertal gonococcal infection outside the neonatal period should be considered presumptive evidence of sexual contact or child abuse. Prepubertal girls usually manifest gonococcal vulvovaginitis without cervicitis because of the neutral to alkaline pH of the vagina and thin vaginal mucosa.

In the adolescent or adult, the workup of every case of gonorrhea should include a careful and accurate inquiry into the patient's sexual practices and appropriate cultures obtained, because pharyngeal and/or anorectal infections may be difficult to eradicate. Efforts should be made to identify and provide treatment to all sexual contacts. Programs of expedited partner treatment where prescriptions are provided without first examining the sexual contact increase successful treatment. Young women are at risk for serious health consequences including infertility due to gonococcal and chlamydia infection.

▶ Clinical Findings

A. Symptoms and Signs

1. Asymptomatic gonorrhea—The ratio of asymptomatic to symptomatic gonorrheal infections in adolescents and adults

is probably 3–4:1 in women and 0.5–1:1 in men. Asymptomatic infections are as infectious as symptomatic ones.

2. Uncomplicated genital gonorrhea

A. MALE WITH URETHRITIS/EPIDIDYMITIS—Urethral discharge is sometimes painful and bloody and may be white, yellow, or green. There may be associated dysuria. Epididymitis may present with acute scrotal swelling or pain. The patient usually is afebrile.

B. PREPUBERTAL FEMALE WITH VAGINITIS—The only clinical findings initially may be dysuria and polymorphonuclear neutrophils in the urine. Vulvitis characterized by erythema, edema, and excoriation accompanied by a purulent discharge may follow.

C. POSTPUBERTAL FEMALE WITH CERVICITIS—Symptomatic disease is characterized by a purulent, foul-smelling vaginal discharge, dysuria, and occasionally dyspareunia. Fever and abdominal pain are absent. The cervix is frequently hyperemic and tender when touched. This tenderness is not worsened by moving the cervix, nor is the adnexa tender to palpation.

D. RECTAL GONORRHEA—Rectal gonorrhea often is asymptomatic. There may be purulent discharge, edema, and pain during evacuation.

3. Pharyngeal gonorrhea—Pharyngeal infection usually is asymptomatic. There may be some sore throat and, rarely, acute exudative tonsillitis with bilateral cervical lymphadenopathy and fever.

4. Conjunctivitis and iridocyclitis—Copious, usually purulent exudate is characteristic of gonococcal conjunctivitis. Newborns are symptomatic on days 2–4 of life. In the adolescent or adult, infection probably is spread from infected genital secretions by the fingers.

5. Pelvic inflammatory disease (salpingitis)—The interval between initiation of genital infection and its ascent to the uterine tubes is variable and may range from days to months. Menses frequently are the initiating factor. With the onset of a menstrual period, gonococci invade the endometrium, causing transient endometritis. Subsequently salpingitis may occur, resulting in pyosalpinx or hydrosalpinx. Rarely infection progresses to peritonitis or perihepatitis. Gonococcal salpingitis occurs in an acute, subacute, or chronic form. All three forms have in common tenderness on gentle movement of the cervix and adnexal tenderness during pelvic examination.

Gonococci or *Chlamydia trachomatis* are the cause of about 50% of cases of pelvic inflammatory disease. A mixed infection caused by enteric bacilli, *Bacteroides fragilis*, or other anaerobes occurs in the other 50%.

6. Gonococcal perihepatitis (Fitz-Hugh-Curtis syndrome)— Typically the patient presents with right upper quadrant tenderness in association with signs of acute or subacute salpingitis. Pain may be pleuritic and referred to the shoulder. Hepatic friction rub is a valuable but inconstant sign.

7. Disseminated gonorrhea— Dissemination follows asymptomatic more often than symptomatic genital infection, often from gonococcal pharyngitis or anorectal gonorrhea. The most common form of disseminated gonorrhea is the triad of polyarthralgia, tenosynovitis, and dermatitis (also referred to as arthritis-dermatitis syndrome) although patients may not present with all three. Septic arthritis is less common, and gonococcal endocarditis and meningitis are rare.

A. ARTHRITIS-DERMATITIS SYNDROME—Disease usually begins with the simultaneous onset of low-grade fever, polyarthralgia, and malaise. After a day or so, joint symptoms become acute. Swelling, redness, and tenderness occur, frequently over the wrists, ankles, and knees but also in the fingers, feet, and other peripheral joints. The arthralgia may be migratory. Skin lesions may be noted at the same time. Discrete, tender, maculopapular lesions 5–8 mm in diameter appear that may become vesicular, pustular, and then hemorrhagic. They are few in number and noted on the fingers, palms, feet, and other distal surfaces. In patients with this form of the disease, blood cultures are often positive, but joint fluid rarely yields organisms. Skin lesions often are positive by Gram stain but rarely by culture. Genital, rectal, and pharyngeal cultures must be performed.

B. SEPTIC ARTHRITIS—In this less common form of disseminated gonorrhea, fever is often absent. Arthritis evolves in one or more joints. Dermatitis usually does not occur. Systemic symptoms are minimal. Blood cultures are negative, but joint aspirates may yield gonococci on smear and culture. Genital, rectal, and pharyngeal cultures must be performed.

B. Laboratory Findings

Demonstration of gram-negative, kidney-shaped diplococci in smears of urethral exudate in males is presumptive evidence of gonorrhea. Positive culture confirms the diagnosis. Negative smears do not rule out gonorrhea. Gram-stained smears of cervical or vaginal discharge in girls are more difficult to interpret because of normal gram-negative flora, but they may be useful when technical personnel are experienced. NAAT on urine or genital specimens enable detection of *N gonorrhoeae* and *C trachomatis*. These tests have excellent sensitivity and are replacing culture in many laboratories. All children or adolescents with a suspected or established diagnosis of gonorrhea should have serologic tests for syphilis and HIV.

If cultures are obtained, use of a selective chocolate agar–containing antibiotics (eg, Thayer-Martin agar) is needed to suppress normal flora. If bacteriologic diagnosis is critical, suspected material should be cultured on chocolate agar

as well. Because gonococci are labile, agar plates should be inoculated immediately and placed without delay in an atmosphere containing CO_2. When transport of specimens is necessary, material should be inoculated directly into an appropriate transport medium prior to shipment to the laboratory. In cases of possible sexual molestation, notify the laboratory that definite speciation is needed, because non-gonococcal *Neisseria* species can grow on the selective media.

▶ Differential Diagnosis

Urethritis in the male may be gonococcal or nongonococcal (NGU). NGU is a syndrome characterized by discharge (rarely painful), mild dysuria, and a subacute course. The discharge is usually scant or moderate and nonpurulent. *C trachomatis* is the most common cause of NGU. Doxycycline (100 mg orally twice a day for 7 days) is efficacious. Single-dose azithromycin, 1 g orally, may achieve better compliance. *C trachomatis* has been shown to cause epididymitis in males and salpingitis in females.

Vulvovaginitis in a prepubertal female may be due to infection caused by miscellaneous bacteria, including *Shigella*, GAS, *Candida*, and herpes simplex. Discharges may be caused by trichomonads, *Enterobius vermicularis* (pin-worm), candidiasis or foreign bodies. Symptom-free discharge (leukorrhea) normally accompanies rising estrogen levels.

Cervicitis in a postpubertal female, alone or in association with urethritis and involvement of Skene and Bartholin glands, may be due to infection caused by *Candida*, herpes simplex, *Trichomonas*, or discharge resulting from inflammation caused by foreign bodies (usually some form of contraceptive device). Leukorrhea may be associated with birth control pills.

Salpingitis may be due to infection with other organisms. The symptoms must be differentiated from those of appendicitis, urinary tract infection, ectopic pregnancy, endometriosis, or ovarian cysts or torsion.

Disseminated gonorrhea presents a differential diagnosis that includes meningococcemia, acute rheumatic fever, Henoch-Schönlein purpura, juvenile idiopathic arthritis, lupus erythematosus, leptospirosis, secondary syphilis, certain viral infections (particularly rubella, but also enteroviruses and parvovirus), serum sickness, type B hepatitis (in the prodromal phase), infective endocarditis, and even acute leukemia and other types of cancer.

▶ Prevention

Prevention of gonorrhea is principally a matter of sex education, condom use, and identification and treatment of contacts.

▶ Treatment

Antimicrobial-resistant gonococci are a serious problem. *N gonorrhoeae* infections resistant to tetracyclines, penicillins, and fluoroquinolones are common. In some cases, clinicians will have very limited choices for therapy. Many clinical laboratories do not routinely perform antimicrobial susceptibility tests on *N gonorrhoeae*, and many infections are documented by nonculture methods.

A. Uncomplicated Urogenital, Pharyngeal, or Rectal Gonococcal Infections in Adolescents

Ceftriaxone (250 mg intramuscularly in a single dose) and azithromycin (1 g orally in a single dose) is recommended. Fluoroquinolones are no longer recommended for therapy due to increasing rates of resistance. If ceftriaxone cannot be used, cefixime (400 mg orally in a single dose) and azithromycin (1 g orally in a single dose) is recommended. Doxycycline (100 mg orally twice daily for 7 days) can be used in place of azithromycin in these regimens, but azithromycin is preferred due to convenience and compliance advantages. Azithromycin (2 g orally once) in combination with either gemifloxacin (320 mg orally once) or gentamicin (240 mg intramuscularly once) can be used in cases of severe cephalosporin allergy.

A test-of-cure is not recommended for asymptomatic individuals who have received one of the recommended regimens for gonococcal infection. However, a patient receiving an alternative regimen for pharyngeal infection should be retested 14 days after completing treatment.

B. Disseminated Gonorrhea

Recommended regimens include ceftriaxone (1 g intramuscularly or intravenously once daily) plus azithromycin (1 g orally in a single dose). Alternative regimens include azithromycin (1 g orally in a single dose) plus either cefotaxime (1 g intravenously every 8 hours) or ceftizoxime (1 g intravenously every 8 hours). Oral therapy may follow parenteral therapy 24–48 hours after improvement. Recommended regimens include cefixime (400 mg) twice daily to complete 7 days of therapy. Fluoroquinolones are not recommended.

C. Pelvic Inflammatory Disease

Doxycycline (100 mg twice a day orally or intravenously) and either cefoxitin (2 g intravenously every 6 hours) or cefotetan (2 g intravenously every 12 hours) are given until the patient is clinically improved; then doxycycline is administered by mouth to complete 14 days of therapy. Clindamycin (900 mg intravenously every 8 hours) plus gentamicin (2 mg/kg loading dose intravenously or intramuscularly, followed by a maintenance dose 1.5 mg/kg every 8 hours) until the patient improves clinically may also be used. When tubo-ovarian abscess is present, either clindamycin (450 mg orally four times daily) or

metronidazole (500 mg orally twice daily) should be used in addition to doxycycline for at least 14 days in order to provide better anaerobic coverage. In women with mild to moderate PID, an intramuscular plus oral regimen can be considered—see the CDC STD Treatment Guidelines for further details.

D. Prepubertal Gonococcal Infections

1. Uncomplicated genitourinary, rectal, or pharyngeal infections—These infections may be treated with ceftriaxone (25–50 mg/kg to a maximum of 125 mg intramuscularly in a single dose) in prepubertal children who weigh less than 45 kg. Children who weigh 45 kg or greater and are older than 8 years should receive ceftriaxone (250 mg intramuscularly in a single dose) and azithromycin (1 g orally in a single dose). The physician should evaluate all children for evidence of sexual abuse and coinfection with syphilis, *Chlamydia*, and HIV.

2. Disseminated gonorrhea—Prepubertal children weighing less than 45 kg should be treated with ceftriaxone (50 mg/kg (max 1 g) once daily parenterally for 7 days. For prepubertal children who weigh 45 kg or greater, the regimen is the same as the adult regimen.

Gonococcal infections. In: Kimberlin DW, Brady MT, Jackson MA, Long SS (eds): *Red Book: 2018–2021 Report of the Committee on Infectious Diseases.* 31st ed. Itasca, IL: American Academy of Pediatrics; 2018:355–364.

Workowski KA, Berman GA; Centers for Disease Control and Prevention (CDC): Sexually transmitted diseases treatment guidelines, 2015. MMWR Recomm Rep 2015;64(RR-03):1–37 [PMID: 26042815].

BOTULISM

ESSENTIALS OF DIAGNOSIS & TYPICAL FEATURES

▶ Dry mucous membranes.

▶ Diplopia; dilated, unreactive pupils.

▶ Descending paralysis.

▶ Difficulty in swallowing and speaking within 12–36 hours after ingestion of toxin-contaminated food.

▶ Multiple cases in a family or group.

▶ Hypotonia and constipation in infants.

▶ Diagnosis by clinical findings and identification of toxin in blood, stool, or implicated food.

General Considerations

Botulism is a paralytic disease caused by *Clostridium botulinum*, an anaerobic, gram-positive, spore-forming bacillus normally found in soil. The organism produces an extremely potent neurotoxin. Of the seven types of toxin (A–G), types A, B, and E cause most human diseases. The toxin, a polypeptide, is so potent that 0.1 mg is lethal for humans.

Food-borne botulism usually results from ingestion of toxin-containing food. Preformed toxin is absorbed from the gut and produces paralysis by preventing acetylcholine release from cholinergic fibers at neuromuscular junctions. Virtually any food will support the growth of *C botulinum* spores into vegetative toxin-producing bacilli if an anaerobic, nonacid environment is provided. The food may not appear or taste spoiled. The toxin is heat-labile, but the spores are heat-resistant. Inadequate heating during processing (temperature < 115°C) allows the spores to survive and later resume toxin production.

Infant botulism occurs in infants younger than 12 months. The toxin is produced by ingested *C botulinum* spores that germinate and produce toxin in the gastrointestinal tract.

Annually, 10–15 cases of wound botulism are reported. Most cases occur in drug abusers with infection in intravenous or intramuscular injection sites.

Prevention

Infant botulism is acquired by ingestion of botulism spores that then sporulate into *C botulinum* organisms that form botulinum toxin. Honey can contain botulism spores so it is recommended that honey not be consumed by infants younger than 12 months.

Food-borne botulism is acquired by ingesting preformed botulism toxin in food. In the United States, food-borne botulism is most commonly seen with ingestion of home-canned foods of low acidity (ie, corn, asparagus, green beans, potatoes). However, other foods have been associated with botulism. Persons who eat home-canned foods should consider boiling foods for at least 10 minutes or heating to 80°F for 30 minutes (can destroy potential toxin). Safe food handling practices include keeping foods either refrigerated (< 45°F) or hot (> 185°F), and disposing of any cracked jars or bulging/dented cans.

Clinical Findings

A. Symptoms and Signs

The incubation period for food-borne botulism may range from 2 hours to 12 days. The initial symptoms are lethargy and headache. These are followed by double vision, dilated pupils, ptosis, and within a few hours, difficulty with swallowing and speech. The mucous membranes often are very dry. Descending skeletal muscle paralysis may be seen. Death usually results from respiratory failure.

Botulism patients present with a "classic triad": (1) afebrile; (2) symmetrical, flaccid, descending paralysis with prominent bulbar palsies; and (3) clear sensorium. Recognition of this triad is important in making the clinical diagnosis. Botulism is caused by a toxin; thus, there is no fever unless secondary infection (eg, aspiration pneumonia) occurs. Common bulbar palsies seen include dysphonia, dysphagia, dysarthria, and diplopia (four "Ds").

Infant botulism is seen in infants younger than 12 months (peak onset 2–8 months). Infants younger than 2 weeks rarely develop botulism. The initial symptoms are usually constipation and progressive, often severe, hypotonia. Clinical findings include loss of facial expression, constipation, weak suck and cry, pooled oral secretions, cranial nerve deficits, generalized weakness, and, on occasion, apnea.

B. Laboratory Findings

The diagnosis is made by demonstration of *C botulinum* toxin in stool, gastric aspirate or vomitus, or serum. Serum and stool samples can be sent for toxin confirmation (done by toxin neutralization mouse bioassay at CDC or state health departments). In infant botulism, serum assays for *C botulinum* toxin are usually negative. The tests take time, and therapy should not be withheld awaiting testing results. Foods that are suspected to be contaminated should be kept refrigerated and given to public health personnel for testing. Laboratory findings, including CSF examination, are usually normal. Electromyography suggests the diagnosis if the characteristic brief, small abundant motor-unit action potentials (BSAP) abnormalities are seen. A nondiagnostic electromyogram does not exclude the diagnosis.

Differential Diagnosis

Guillain-Barré syndrome is characterized by ascending paralysis, sensory deficits, and elevated CSF protein without pleocytosis.

Other illnesses that should be considered include poliomyelitis, acute flaccid myelitis, post diphtheritic polyneuritis, certain chemical intoxications, tick paralysis, and myasthenia gravis. The history and elevated CSF protein characterize postdiphtheritic polyneuritis. Tick paralysis presents with a flaccid ascending motor paralysis. An attached tick should be sought. Myasthenia gravis usually occurs in adolescent girls. It is characterized by ocular and bulbar symptoms, normal pupils, fluctuating weakness, absence of other neurologic signs, and clinical response to cholinesterase inhibitors.

Complications

Difficulty in swallowing leads to aspiration pneumonia. Serious respiratory paralysis may be fatal despite assisted ventilation and intensive supportive measures.

Treatment

A. Specific Measures

Patients with suspected botulism should be hospitalized and monitored closely for signs of impending respiratory failure and inability to manage secretions. Early treatment of botulism with antitoxin is beneficial. The type of antitoxin treatment recommended differs depending on the type of botulism. Treatment should begin as soon as the clinical diagnosis is suspected (prior to microbiologic or toxin confirmation). Contact your state health department's emergency 24-hour telephone number immediately when a case of botulism is suspected to assist in therapeutic decisions and to help obtain treatment product.

For treatment of suspected infant botulism, intravenous human botulism immunoglobulin (BabyBIG) is approved by the US FDA. BabyBIG contains neutralizing antibodies against types A and B toxin. A placebo-controlled clinical trial of BabyBIG use in infant botulism showed substantial reductions in the mean hospital stay, mechanical ventilation days, and intensive care days in the BabyBIG-treated group. BabyBIG is not indicated for use in any form of botulism (wound, food-borne) other than infant botulism. To obtain BabyBIG (in any state), contact the California Department of Public Health (24-hour telephone number: 510-231-7600; www.infantbotulism.org/). Antimicrobial agents are not recommended to treat infant botulism, except when bacterial complications occur (ie, pneumonia, line infection, etc).

For other types of botulism (noninfant botulism), patients should be treated with heptavalent botulinum antitoxin (HBAT), which was licensed by the FDA in 2013 for treatment of adult and pediatric botulism. HBAT is an equine-derived antitoxin that contains antibodies to all seven botulinum toxin types (A through G). The treatment protocol (available from the CDC) includes detailed instructions for intravenous administration of antitoxin. State health departments can assist practitioners in obtaining the antitoxin; if state health department officials are unavailable, the CDC (770-488-7100) can be contacted for help in obtaining the product and for consultation. In addition, epidemic assistance, and laboratory testing services are available from the CDC through state health departments. For wound botulism, penicillin or metronidazole can be considered, once HBAT has been given. Surgical debridement of involved tissue is recommended.

B. General Measures

General and supportive therapy consists of bed rest, ventilatory support (if necessary), fluid therapy, and enteral or parenteral nutrition. Aminoglycosides and clindamycin may exacerbate neuromuscular blockage and should be avoided.

Prognosis

The mortality rate has declined substantially in recent years and currently is about 3%–5%. The prospect for full recovery is good but may take weeks to months depending on the severity of the initial illness.

Botulism and infant botulism. In: Kimberlin DW, Brady MT, Jackson MA, Long SS, (eds): *Red Book: 2018–2021 Report of the Committee on Infectious Diseases.* 31st ed. Itasca, IL: American Academy of Pediatrics; 2018;283–285.

Centers for Disease Control and Prevention (CDC): Botulism. https://www.cdc.gov/botulism. Accessed July 3, 2019.

Chatham-Stephens K et al: Clinical features of foodborne and wound botulism: a systematic review of the literature, 1932–2015. Clin Infect Dis 2017 Dec 27;66(Suppl_1):S11–S16 [PMID: 29293923].

Long SS: Infant botulism and treatment with BIG-IV (BabyBIG). Pediatr Infect Dis J 2007;26:261 [PMID: 17484226].

Underwood K et al: Infant botulism: a 30-year experience spanning the introduction of botulism immune globulin intravenous in the intensive care unit at Children's Hospital Los Angeles. Pediatrics 2007;120(6):e1380–e1385 [PMID: 18055655].

TETANUS

ESSENTIALS OF DIAGNOSIS & TYPICAL FEATURES

▶ Nonimmunized or partially immunized patient.

▶ History of skin wound.

▶ Spasms of jaw muscles (trismus).

▶ Stiffness of neck, back, and abdominal muscles, with hyperirritability and hyperreflexia.

▶ Episodic, generalized muscle contractions.

▶ Diagnosis is based on clinical findings and the immunization history.

General Considerations

Tetanus is caused by *Clostridium tetani*, an anaerobic, gram-positive bacillus that produces a potent neurotoxin.

In unimmunized or incompletely immunized individuals, infection follows contamination of a wound by soil-containing clostridial spores from animal manure. The toxin reaches the CNS by retrograde axon transport, is bound to cerebral gangliosides, and increases reflex excitability in neurons of the spinal cord by blocking function of inhibitory synapses. Intense muscle spasms result. Two-thirds of cases in the United States follow minor puncture wounds of the hands or feet. In many cases, no history of a wound can be obtained. IV drug use and diabetes may be risk factors (in individuals who are not tetanus-immune). In the newborn, usually in underdeveloped countries, infection generally results from contamination of the umbilical cord. The incubation period typically is 3–21 days but may be longer. In the United States, cases in young children are due to inadequate immunization. Eighty-five percent of cases occur in adults older than 25 years.

Prevention

A. Tetanus Toxoid

Active immunization with tetanus toxoid prevents tetanus. Immunity is almost always achieved after the third dose of vaccine. Tetanus immunoglobulin (TIG) is an additional agent used to prevent tetanus in persons who have received less than three doses of tetanus toxoid or in immunocompromised patients who do not make sufficient antibody (ie, HIV infection; see Chapter 10). A tetanus toxoid booster at the time of injury is needed if none has been given in the past 10 years—or within 5 years for heavily contaminated wounds. Nearly all cases of tetanus (99%) in the United States are in nonimmunized or incompletely immunized individuals. Many adolescents and adults lack protective antibody.

B. Wound Care and Prophylaxis for Tetanus-Prone Wounds

Wounds that are contaminated with soil, debris, feces, or saliva are at increased risk for tetanus. Puncture wounds, crush injuries, avulsions, frostbite, burns, or other wounds that contain devitalized tissue are also at increased risk of infection with C tetani. All wounds should be adequately cleaned, foreign material removed, and debrided if necrotic or devitalized tissue or residual foreign matter is present. The decision to use tetanus toxoid–containing vaccine, human TIG, or both depends on the type of injury and the tetanus immunization status of the patient (see Chapter 10; Table 10–5). TIG should be used in children with fewer than three previous tetanus toxoid immunizations (DPT, DTaP, DT, Td, Tdap) who have tetanus-prone wounds and in immune compromised children, including those with HIV, who have tetanus-prone wounds, regardless of their immunization history. When TIG is indicated for wound prophylaxis 250 units are given intramuscularly regardless of age. If tetanus immunization is incomplete, a dose of age-appropriate vaccine should be given. When both are indicated, tetanus toxoid and TIG should be administered concurrently at different sites using different syringes (see Chapter 10).

Prophylactic antimicrobials are useful if the child is unimmunized and TIG is not available.

Clinical Findings

A. Symptoms and Signs

The first symptom often is mild pain at the site of the wound, followed by hypertonicity and spasm of the regional muscles. Characteristically, difficulty in opening the mouth (trismus) is evident within 48 hours. In newborns, the first signs are irritability and inability to nurse. The infant may then develop stiffness of the jaw and neck, increasing dysphagia, and generalized hyperreflexia with rigidity and spasms of all muscles of the abdomen and back (opisthotonos). The facial distortion resembles a grimace (risus sardonicus). Difficulty in swallowing and convulsions triggered by minimal stimuli such as sound, light, or movement may occur. Individual spasms may last seconds or minutes. Recurrent spasms are seen several times each hour, or they may be almost continuous. In most cases, the temperature is normal or only mildly elevated. A high or subnormal temperature is a bad prognostic sign. Patients are fully conscious and lucid. A profound circulatory disturbance associated with sympathetic overactivity (elevated blood pressure, tachycardia, arrhythmia) may occur on the second to fourth day, which may contribute to the mortality rate.

B. Laboratory Findings

The diagnosis is made on clinical grounds. There may be a mild polymorphonuclear leukocytosis. The CSF is normal with the exception of mild elevation of opening pressure. Serum muscle enzymes may be elevated. Anaerobic culture and microscopic examination of pus from the wound can be helpful, but C tetani is difficult to grow.

Differential Diagnosis

Poliomyelitis is characterized by asymmetrical flaccid paralysis in an incompletely immunized child. The history of an animal bite and the absence of trismus may suggest rabies. Local infections of the throat and jaw should be easily recognized. Bacterial meningitis, phenothiazine reactions, decerebrate posturing, narcotic withdrawal, spondylitis, and hypocalcemic tetany may be confused with tetanus.

Complications

Complications include sepsis, malnutrition, pneumonia, atelectasis, asphyxial spasms, decubitus ulcers, and fractures of the spine due to intense contractions. They can be prevented in part by skilled supportive care.

Treatment of Tetanus

A. Specific Measures

Human TIG in a single dose of 3000–6000 units, intramuscularly, is given to children and adults. Some experts suggest that a dose of 500 units is just as effective. Infiltration of part of the TIG dose around the wound is recommended. If TIG is indicated, but not available, intravenous immunoglobulin in a dose of 200–400 mg/kg intravenously can be infused over several hours (although it is not licensed for this indication; see package insert for infusion instructions). In countries where TIG or immunoglobulins are not available, equine tetanus antitoxin may be available. Surgical debridement of wounds is indicated, but more extensive surgery or amputation to eliminate the site of infection is not necessary. Antibiotics are given in an attempt to decrease the bacterial load and subsequent toxin production: oral or intravenous metronidazole (30 mg/kg/day in four divided doses; maximum 4 g/day) for 10–14 days is the preferred agent. Parenteral penicillin G (100,000 U/kg/day in four to six divided doses; maximum 12 million U/day) is an alternative regimen. An age-appropriate tetanus toxoid containing vaccine should be administered in a different limb from the TIG administration site.

B. General Measures

Treatment of tetanus is usually best accomplished in an intensive care unit. The patient is kept in a quiet room with minimal stimulation. Control of spasms and prevention of hypoxic episodes are crucial. Benzodiazepines can be used to help control spasms and provide some sedation. Mechanical ventilation and muscle paralysis are necessary in severe cases. Nasogastric or intravenous feedings should be used to limit stimulation of feedings and prevent aspiration.

Prognosis

The fatality rate in newborns and heroin-addicted individuals is high. The overall mortality rate in the United States is 8%. The fatality rate depends on the quality of supportive care, the patient's age, and the patient's vaccination history. Many deaths are due to pneumonia or respiratory failure. If the patient survives 1 week, recovery is likely.

Centers for Disease Control and Prevention (CDC): Clinical Information. http://www.cdc.gov/tetanus/clinicians.html. Accessed July 1, 2019.

Centers for Disease Control and Prevention (CDC): Tetanus. http://www.cdc.gov/vaccines/pubs/pinkbook/tetanus.html. Accessed July 1, 2019.

GAS GANGRENE

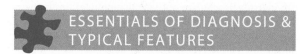

ESSENTIALS OF DIAGNOSIS & TYPICAL FEATURES

► Contamination of a wound with soil or feces.

► Massive edema, skin discoloration, bleb formation, and pain in an area of trauma.

► Serosanguineous exudate from wound.

► Crepitation of subcutaneous tissue.

► Rapid progression of signs and symptoms.

► Clostridia cultured or seen on stained smears.

General Considerations

Gas gangrene (clostridial myonecrosis) is a necrotizing infection that follows trauma or surgery and is caused by several anaerobic, gram-positive, spore-forming bacilli of the genus *Clostridium*. Occasionally the source is the gastrointestinal tract, and muscles are hematogenously seeded. The spores are found in soil, feces, and vaginal secretions. In devitalized tissue, the spores germinate into vegetative bacilli that proliferate and produce toxins, causing thrombosis, hemolysis, and tissue necrosis. *C perfringens*, the species causing approximately 80% of cases of gas gangrene, produces at least eight toxins. The areas involved most often are the extremities, abdomen, and uterus. *Clostridium septicum* may also cause myonecrosis and causes septicemia in patients with neutropenia. Nonclostridial infections with gas formation can mimic clostridial infections and are more common. Neutropenia is a risk factor for this severe infection.

Prevention

Gas gangrene can be prevented by the adequate cleansing and debridement of all wounds. It is essential that foreign bodies and dead tissue be removed. A clean wound does not provide a suitable anaerobic environment for the growth of clostridial species.

▶ Clinical Findings

A. Symptoms and Signs

The onset of gas gangrene usually is sudden, often 1 day after trauma or surgery, but can be delayed up to 20 days. Pain and swelling usually are intense. The skin around the wound becomes discolored (pale, red, or purple), with hemorrhagic bullae, serosanguineous exudate, and crepitus may be observed the subcutaneous tissues. The absence of crepitus does not rule out the diagnosis. Systemic illness appears early and progresses rapidly to intravascular hemolysis, jaundice, shock, toxic delirium, and renal failure.

B. Laboratory Findings

Isolation of the organism requires anaerobic cultures. The wound exudate, soft tissue, muscle and blood can be cultured. Gram-stained smears may demonstrate many gram-positive rods and few inflammatory cells.

C. Imaging

Radiographs may demonstrate gas in tissues, but this is a late finding and is also seen in infections with other gas-forming organisms or may be due to air introduced into tissues during trauma or surgery.

D. Operative Findings

Direct visualization of the muscle at surgery may be necessary to diagnose gas gangrene. Early, the muscle is pale and edematous and does not contract normally; later, the muscle may be frankly gangrenous.

▶ Differential Diagnosis

Gangrene and cellulitis caused by other organisms and clostridial cellulitis (not myonecrosis) must be distinguished. Necrotizing fasciitis may resemble gas gangrene.

▶ Treatment

A. Specific Measures

Penicillin G (300,000–400,000 U/kg/day intravenously in six divided doses) should be given. Clindamycin, metronidazole, meropenem, and ertapenem are alternatives for penicillin-allergic patients. Some experts recommend a combination of penicillin and clindamycin; clindamycin may inhibit toxin production.

B. Surgical Measures

Surgery should be prompt and extensive, with removal of all necrotic tissue. Compartment syndromes can occur even if there are few cutaneous findings. Checking compartment pressures in patients with severe pain and any signs of compartment syndrome is prudent.

C. Hyperbaric Oxygen

Hyperbaric oxygen therapy is controversial, but good outcomes have been reported in nonrandomized studies using hyperbaric oxygen in combination with surgery and antibiotics.

▶ Prognosis

Clostridial myonecrosis is fatal if untreated. With early diagnosis, antibiotics, and surgery, the mortality rate is 20%–60%. Involvement of the abdominal wall, leukopenia, intravascular hemolysis, renal failure, and shock are ominous prognostic signs.

Smith-Slatas CL et al: *Clostridium septicum* infections in children: a case report and review of the literature. Pediatrics 2006;117:e796 [PMID: 16567392].

Stevens DL et al: Practice guidelines for the diagnosis and management of skin and soft tissue infections: 2014 update by the Infectious Diseases Society of America. Clin Infect Dis 2014;59:e10 [PMID: 24973422].

DIPHTHERIA

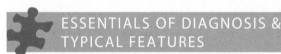

ESSENTIALS OF DIAGNOSIS & TYPICAL FEATURES

▶ Gray, adherent pseudomembrane, most often in the pharynx but also in the nasopharynx or trachea.

▶ Sore throat, serosanguineous nasal discharge, hoarseness, and fever in a nonimmunized child.

▶ Peripheral neuritis or myocarditis.

▶ Positive culture.

▶ Treatment should not be withheld pending culture results.

▶ General Considerations

Diphtheria is an acute infection of the upper respiratory tract or skin caused by toxin-producing *Corynebacterium diphtheriae*. Diphtheria in the United States is rare; between 2004 and 2017, two cases have been reported. However, significant numbers of elderly adults and unimmunized children are susceptible to infection. Diphtheria still occurs in epidemics in countries where immunization is not universal. Unimmunized travelers to these areas may acquire the disease.

Corynebacteria are gram-positive, club-shaped rods with a beaded appearance on Gram stain. The capacity to produce exotoxin is conferred by a lysogenic bacteriophage and is not present in all strains of *C diphtheriae*. In immunized communities, infection probably occurs through spread of the phage among carriers of susceptible *C diphtheriae* rather than through spread of phage-containing bacteria themselves. Diphtheria toxin kills susceptible cells by irreversible inhibition of protein synthesis.

The toxin is absorbed into the mucous membranes and causes destruction of epithelium and a superficial inflammatory response. The necrotic epithelium becomes embedded in exuded fibrin with WBCs and RBCs (red blood cells), forming a grayish pseudomembrane over the tonsils, pharynx, or larynx. Any attempt to remove the membrane exposes and tears the capillaries, resulting in bleeding. The diphtheria bacilli within the membrane continue to produce toxin, which is absorbed and may result in toxic injury to the heart muscle, liver, kidneys, and adrenals, and is sometimes accompanied by hemorrhage. The toxin also produces neuritis, resulting in paralysis of the soft palate, eye muscles, or extremities. Death may result from respiratory obstruction or toxemia and circulatory collapse. The patient may succumb after a somewhat longer time as a result of cardiac damage. The incubation period is 2–5 days.

▶ Clinical Findings

A. Symptoms and Signs

1. Pharyngeal diphtheria—Early manifestations of diphtheritic pharyngitis are mild sore throat, moderate fever, and malaise, followed fairly rapidly by prostration and circulatory collapse. The pulse is more rapid than the fever would seem to justify. A pharyngeal membrane forms and may spread into the nasopharynx or the trachea, producing respiratory obstruction. The membrane is tenacious and gray, and is surrounded by a narrow zone of erythema and a broader zone of edema. The cervical lymph nodes become swollen, which is associated with brawny edema of the neck (so-called bull neck). Laryngeal diphtheria presents with stridor, which can progress to airway obstruction.

2. Other forms—Cutaneous, vaginal, and wound diphtheria cases account for up to one-third and are characterized by ulcerative lesions with membrane formation.

B. Laboratory Findings

Diagnosis requires culture of *C. diphtheriae* obtained from the nose, throat, or skin lesions, if present. Specialized culture media is required so laboratory personnel should be notified if diphtheria is suspected. A toxigenicity test should be performed to differentiate toxigenic from nontoxigenic strains of *C. diphtheriae*. New non–culture-based methods such as PCR or matrix-assisted laser desorption/ionization

(MALDI-TOF) mass spectroscopy can be useful as cultures may be negative in individuals who have received antibiotics. The WBC count usually is normal, but hemolytic anemia and thrombocytopenia are frequent.

▶ Differential Diagnosis

Pharyngeal diphtheria resembles pharyngitis secondary to β-hemolytic *Streptococcus*, Epstein-Barr virus, or other viral respiratory pathogens. A nasal foreign body or purulent sinusitis may mimic nasal diphtheria. Other causes of laryngeal obstruction include epiglottitis and viral croup. Guillain-Barré syndrome, poliomyelitis, or acute poisoning may mimic the neuropathy of diphtheria.

▶ Complications

A. Myocarditis

Diphtheritic myocarditis is characterized by a rapid, thready pulse; indistinct heart sounds, ST-T-wave changes, conduction abnormalities, dysrhythmias, or cardiac failure; hepatomegaly; and fluid retention. Myocardial dysfunction may occur from 2 to 40 days after the onset of pharyngitis.

B. Polyneuritis

Neuritis of the palatal and pharyngeal nerves occurs during the first or second week. Nasal speech and regurgitation of food through the nose are seen. Diplopia and strabismus occur during the third week or later. Neuritis may also involve peripheral nerves supplying the intercostal muscles, diaphragm, and other muscle groups. Generalized paresis usually occurs after the fourth week.

C. Bronchopneumonia

Secondary pneumonia is common in fatal cases.

▶ Prevention

A. Immunization

Immunization with diphtheria toxoid combined with pertussis and tetanus toxoids (DTaP) should be used routinely for infants and children (see Chapter 10).

B. Care of Exposed Susceptibles

Children exposed to diphtheria should be examined, and nose and throat cultures obtained. Immunized asymptomatic individuals who have not received a diphtheria toxoid booster within 5 years and inadequately immunized individuals all should receive a diphtheroid toxoid vaccine. Regardless of immunization status, close contacts should receive either erythromycin orally (40 mg/kg/day in four divided doses) for 7–10 days or a single dose of benzathine penicillin G intramuscularly (600,000 units for children weighing < 30 kg, and 1.2 million units for children weighing ≥ 30 kg and for adults) and be closely observed.

▶ Treatment

A. Specific Measures

1. Antitoxin—Suspected diphtheria should be reported promptly to the Centers for Disease Control Emergency Center (770-488-7100) so diphtheria antitoxin can be obtained. Diphtheria antitoxin is no longer commercially available. To be effective, diphtheria antitoxin should be administered within 48 hours (see Chapter 9).

2. Antibiotics—Acceptable regimens include erythromycin (40 mg/kg/day, maximum 2g/day) given parenterally or orally, or procaine penicillin G intramuscularly (300,000 units every 12 hours for those weighing ≤ 10 kg, and 600,000 units every 12 hours for those weighing > 10 kg). Treatment should be given for 14 days.

B. General Measures

Patients should receive a diphtheria toxoid–containing vaccine during convalescence as infection does not confer immunity. Observation of patients in the hospital for 10–14 days is usually required. All patients must be strictly isolated for 1–7 days until respiratory secretions are noncontagious. Isolation may be discontinued when two successive nose and throat cultures at 24-hour intervals are negative. These cultures should not be taken until at least 24 hours have elapsed since the cessation of antibiotic treatment.

C. Treatment of Carriers

All carriers should receive either erythromycin (40 mg/kg/day orally in three or four divided doses) for 10–14 days or a single dose of benzathine penicillin G (600,000 units for children weighing < 30 kg, and 1.2 million units for children weighing ≥ 30 kg or for adults), and they must be quarantined. Before release from quarantine carriers must have two negative cultures of both the nose and the throat taken 24 hours apart and obtained at least 24 hours after the cessation of antibiotic therapy. If follow-up cultures remain positive, they should receive another 10 day course of erythromycin.

▶ Prognosis

Mortality varies from 3% to 25% and is particularly high in the presence of early myocarditis. Neuritis is reversible. Diphtheria is fatal if an intact airway and adequate respiration cannot be maintained. Permanent heart damage from myocarditis occurs rarely.

Centers for Disease Control and Prevention (CDC): Diphtheria. http://www.cdc.gov/diphtheria/clinicians.html.

Santos LS et al: Diphtheria outbreak in Maranhoa, Brazil: microbiological, clinical, and epidemiological aspects. Epidmiol Infect 2015;143(4):791 [PMID: 25703400].

INFECTIONS DUE TO ENTEROBACTERIACEAE

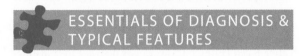

ESSENTIALS OF DIAGNOSIS & TYPICAL FEATURES

▶ Diarrhea by several different mechanisms due to *E coli*.

▶ Hemorrhagic colitis and HUS.

▶ Neonatal sepsis or meningitis.

▶ Urinary tract infection.

▶ Opportunistic infections.

▶ Diagnosis confirmed by culture or PCR.

▶ General Considerations

Enterobacteriaceae are a family of gram-negative bacilli that are normal flora in the gastrointestinal tract of people and animals that contaminate water and soil. They cause gastroenteritis, urinary tract infections, neonatal sepsis and meningitis, and opportunistic infections. *E coli* is the organism in this family that most commonly causes infection in children, but *Klebsiella*, *Morganella*, *Enterobacter*, *Serratia*, *Proteus*, and other genera are also important, particularly in hospitalized persons or immune compromised hosts. *Shigella* and *Salmonella* are discussed in separate sections.

E coli strains capable of causing diarrhea were originally termed *enteropathogenic E coli* (EPEC) and were recognized by serotype. It is now known that *E coli* may cause diarrhea by several distinct mechanisms. Classic EPEC strains cause a characteristic histologic injury in the small bowel termed adherence and effacement. Enterotoxigenic *E coli* (ETEC) causes a secretory, watery diarrhea. ETEC adheres to enterocytes and secretes one or more plasmid-encoded enterotoxins. One of these, heat-labile toxin, resembles cholera toxin in structure, function, and mechanism of action. Enteroinvasive *E coli* (EIEC) are very similar to *Shigella* in their pathogenetic mechanisms. Shigella-toxin producing *E coli* (STEC) cause hemorrhagic colitis and the HUS. The STEC serotype is O157:H7 that is particularly virulent, although several other serotypes cause the same syndrome. These strains elaborate one of several cytotoxins, closely related to Shiga toxin produced by *Shigella dysenteriae*. Outbreaks of HUS associated with STEC have followed consumption of inadequately cooked ground beef. Thorough heating to 71°C (160°F) is considered preventative. Unpasteurized fruit juice, various uncooked vegetables, flour, and contaminated water also have caused infections and epidemics. The common source for STEC in all of these foods and water is the feces of cattle or several other animals. Person-to-person spread including spread in day care centers by the fecal-oral route has been reported. Over 7000 cases of STEC were reported in the United States in 2016, although many more cases are estimated to have occurred. *E coli* defined by their tendency to aggregate on the surface of human epithelial cells in tissue culture are termed enteroaggregative *E coli* (EAEC). EAEC causes diarrhea by a distinct but unknown mechanism. Eighty percent of *E coli* strains causing neonatal meningitis possess a specific capsular polysaccharide (K1 antigen), which, alone or in association with specific somatic antigens, confers virulence.

Klebsiella, *Enterobacter*, *Serratia*, and *Morganella* are normally found in the gastrointestinal tract and in soil and water. *Klebsiella* may cause a bronchopneumonia with cavity formation. *Klebsiella*, *Enterobacter*, and *Serratia* are often hospital-acquired opportunists associated with antibiotic usage, debilitated states, and chronic respiratory conditions. They frequently cause urinary tract infection or sepsis. Many of these infections are difficult to treat because of antibiotic resistance. Carbapenem-resistant Enterobacteriaceae (CRE) are a serious concern due to limited options for therapy. Antibiotic susceptibility tests are necessary. Parenteral third-generation cephalosporins are usually more active than ampicillin, but resistance due to extended-spectrum β-lactamase (ESBL) may occur. Aminoglycoside antibiotics are usually effective but require monitoring of serum levels to ensure therapeutic and nontoxic levels.

▶ Clinical Findings

A. Symptoms and Signs

1. *E coli* gastroenteritis—*E coli* may cause diarrhea of varying types and severity. ETEC usually produce mild, self-limiting illness without significant fever or systemic toxicity, often known as traveler's diarrhea. However, diarrhea may be severe in newborns and infants, and occasionally an older child or adult will have a cholera-like syndrome. EIEC strains, which cause a shigellosis-like illness, characterized by fever, systemic symptoms, blood and mucus in the stool, are uncommon in the United States. STEC strains cause hemorrhagic colitis. Diarrhea initially is watery and fever usually is absent. Abdominal pain and cramping occur; diarrhea progresses to blood streaking or grossly bloody stools. HUS occurs within a few days of diarrhea in 2%–5% of children with STEC diarrhea, with a rate of 15% in children with O157:H7, and is characterized by microangiopathic

hemolytic anemia, thrombocytopenia, and renal failure (see Chapter 24). STEC encoding a gene for Shiga toxin 2 are more virulent than those with only Shiga toxin 1.

2. Neonatal sepsis—Findings include jaundice, hepatosplenomegaly, fever, temperature lability, apneic spells, irritability, and poor feeding. Respiratory distress develops when pneumonia occurs; it may appear indistinguishable from respiratory distress syndrome in preterm infants. Meningitis is associated with bacteremia in 25%–40% of cases. Other metastatic foci of infection may be present, including pneumonia and pyelonephritis. Sepsis may lead to severe metabolic acidosis, shock, DIC, and death.

3. Neonatal meningitis—Findings include high fever, full fontanelles, vomiting, coma, convulsions, pareses or paralyses, poor or absent Moro reflex, opisthotonos, and occasionally hypertonia or hypotonia. Sepsis coexists or precedes meningitis in most cases. Thus, signs of sepsis often accompany those of meningitis. CSF usually shows a cell count of over 1000 WBC/μL, mostly polymorphonuclear neutrophils, and bacteria on Gram stain. CSF glucose concentration is low (usually less than half that of blood), and the protein is elevated above the levels normally seen in newborns and premature infants (> 150 mg/dL).

4. Acute urinary tract infection—Symptoms include dysuria, increased urinary frequency, and fever in the older child. Nonspecific symptoms such as anorexia, vomiting, irritability, failure to thrive, and unexplained fever are seen in children younger than age 2 years. Young infants may present with jaundice. As many as 1%–3% of school-aged girls and 0.5% of boys have asymptomatic bacteriuria. Screening for and treatment of asymptomatic bacteriuria is not recommended.

B. Laboratory Findings

Because *E coli* are normal flora in the stool, a positive stool culture alone does not prove that the *E coli* in the stool are causing disease. Multiplex PCR tests are available to rapidly diagnose STEC and other enteropathogens. Rapid immunologic assays such as enzyme immunoassays (EIA) and immunochromatographic assays are available to detect Shiga toxin. Blood cultures are positive in neonatal sepsis. Cultures of CSF and urine should also be obtained. The diagnosis of urinary tract infections is discussed in Chapter 24.

▶ Differential Diagnosis

The clinical picture of *E coli* infection may resemble that of other enteric infections such as salmonellosis, shigellosis, or viral gastroenteritis. Neonatal sepsis and meningitis caused by *E coli* can be differentiated from other causes of neonatal infection only by blood and CSF culture.

▶ Treatment

A. Specific Measures

1. *E coli* gastroenteritis—Gastroenteritis seldom requires antimicrobial treatment. Fluid and electrolyte therapy, preferably given orally, may be required to avoid dehydration. Antibiotics are generally not recommended because of potential selection for resistant organisms, risks and side effects of antibiotics, and the fact that diarrhea will typically resolve spontaneously. Traveler's diarrhea may be treated with azithromycin in children and with fluoroquinolones in adults, although resistance to these drugs is increasing. The risk of HUS is not proven to be increased by antimicrobial therapy of STEC cases, but most experts recommend no antimicrobial treatment of suspected cases.

2. *E coli* sepsis and pneumonia—The drugs of choice are ampicillin (150–200 mg/kg/day intravenously or intramuscularly in divided doses every 4–6 hours), ceftriaxone (50–100 mg/kg/day parenterally as single dose or in two divided doses), and gentamicin (6–7.5 mg/kg/day intramuscularly or intravenously in divided doses every 8 hours). Initial therapy often includes at least two drugs until microbial etiology is established and susceptibility testing is completed. Treatment is continued for 10–14 days. Amikacin or tobramycin may be used instead of gentamicin if the strain is susceptible. Third-generation cephalosporins are often an attractive alternative as single-drug therapy and do not require monitoring for toxicity.

3. *E coli* meningitis—Third-generation cephalosporins such as ceftriaxone (100 mg/kg/day intravenously) are given for a minimum of 3 weeks. Ampicillin (300–400 mg/kg/day intravenously in four to six divided doses) and gentamicin (7.5 mg/kg/day intramuscularly or intravenously in three divided doses) also are effective for susceptible strains. Serum levels need to be monitored. Treatment with intrathecal and intraventricular aminoglycosides does not improve outcome.

4. Acute urinary tract infection—(See Chapter 24.)

▶ Prognosis

Death due to gastroenteritis leading to dehydration can be prevented by early fluid and electrolyte therapy. Effective treatment has reduced mortality from neonatal sepsis with meningitis to 10%–20%; however, many survivors have some degree of residual disability. Most children with recurrent urinary tract infections do well if they have no underlying anatomic defects. The mortality rate in opportunistic infections usually depends on the severity of infection and the underlying immune compromising condition.

Biondi E et al: Epidemiology of bacteremia in febrile infants in the United States. Pediatrics 2013:132(6):990 [PMID: 24218461].

Centers for Disease Control and Prevention (CDC): Diarrheagenic *Escherichia coli*. http://www.cdc.gov/ecoli/. Accessed July 4, 2019.

Denno DM et al: Diarrhea etiology in a pediatric emergency department: a case control study. Clin Infect Dis 2012;55(7):897 [PMID: 22700832].

Hsu JF et al: Predictors of clinical and microbiological treatment failure in neonatal bloodstream infections. Clin Microbiol Infect 2015;S1198:741 [PMID: 25749002].

Mody RK et al: Postdiarrheal hemolytic uremic syndrome in the United States children: clinical spectrum and predictors of in-hospital death. J Pediatr 2015 Apr;166(4):1022–1029 doi: 10.1016/j.jpeds.2014.12.064. Epub 2015 Feb 4 [PMID: 25661408].

Shane AL et al: 2017 Infectious Diseases Society of America clinical practice guidelines for the diagnosis and management of infectious diarrhea. Clin Infect Dis 2017;65(12):1963–1973 [PMID: 29194529].

Sodha SV et al: National patterns of *Escherichia coli* O157 infections, USA, 1996–2011. Epidemiol Infect 2015;143(2):267 [PMID: 24731294].

PSEUDOMONAS INFECTIONS

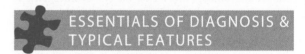

ESSENTIALS OF DIAGNOSIS & TYPICAL FEATURES

▶ Opportunistic infection.

▶ Confirmed by cultures.

▶ General Considerations

Pseudomonas aeruginosa is an aerobic gram-negative rod with versatile metabolic requirements. The organism may grow in distilled water and in commonly used disinfectants, complicating infection control in medical facilities. *P aeruginosa* is both invasive and destructive to tissue as well as toxigenic due to secreted exotoxins, all factors that contribute to virulence. Other genera previously classified as *Pseudomonas* frequently cause nosocomial infections and infections in immunocompromised children. *Stenotrophomonas maltophilia* (previously *Pseudomonas maltophilia*) and *Burkholderia cepacia* (previously *Pseudomonas cepacia*) are the most frequent.

P aeruginosa is an important cause of infection in children with cystic fibrosis, neoplastic disease, neutropenia, or extensive burns and in those receiving antibiotic therapy. Infections of the urinary and respiratory tracts, ears, mastoids, paranasal sinuses, eyes, skin, meninges, and bones are seen. *Pseudomonas* pneumonia is a common nosocomial infection in patients receiving assisted ventilation.

P aeruginosa sepsis may be accompanied by characteristic peripheral lesions called ecthyma gangrenosum. Ecthyma gangrenosum also may occur by direct invasion through intact skin in the groin, axilla, or other skinfolds. *P aeruginosa* is an infrequent cause of sepsis in previously healthy infants and may be the initial sign of underlying medical problems. Osteomyelitis of the calcaneus or other foot bones, which occurs after punctures such as stepping on a nail, is commonly due to *P aeruginosa*.

P aeruginosa is a frequent cause of malignant external otitis media and of chronic suppurative otitis media. Outbreaks of vesiculopustular skin rash have been associated with exposure to contaminated water in whirlpool baths and hot tubs.

P aeruginosa infects the tracheobronchial tree of nearly all patients with cystic fibrosis. Mucoid exopolysaccharide, an exuberant capsule, is characteristically overproduced by isolates from patients with cystic fibrosis. Although bacteremia seldom occurs, patients with cystic fibrosis often ultimately succumb to chronic lung infection with *P aeruginosa*. Infection due to *B cepacia* has caused a rapidly progressive pulmonary disease in some colonized patients and may be spread by close contact.

▶ Clinical Findings

The clinical findings depend on the site of infection and the patient's underlying disease. Sepsis with these organisms resembles gram-negative sepsis with other organisms, although the presence of ecthyma gangrenosum suggests the etiologic diagnosis. The diagnosis is made by culture. *Pseudomonas* infection should be suspected in neonates and neutropenic patients with clinical sepsis. A severe necrotizing pneumonia occurs in patients on ventilators.

Patients with cystic fibrosis have a persistent bronchitis that progresses to bronchiectasis and ultimately to respiratory failure. During exacerbations of illness, cough and sputum production increase along with low-grade fever, malaise, and diminished energy.

The purulent aural drainage without fever in patients with chronic suppurative otitis media is not distinguishable from that due to other causes.

▶ Prevention

A. Infections in Debilitated Patients

Colonization of extensive second- and third-degree burns by *P aeruginosa* can lead to fatal septicemia. Aggressive debridement and topical treatment with 0.5% silver nitrate solution, 10% mafenide cream, or silver sulfadiazine will greatly inhibit *P aeruginosa* contamination of burns. (See Chapter 12 for a discussion of burn wound infections and prevention.)

B. Nosocomial Infections

Faucet aerators, communal soap dispensers, disinfectants, improperly cleaned inhalation therapy equipment, infant incubators, and many other sources that usually are associated with wet or humid conditions all have been associated with *Pseudomonas* epidemics. Patient-to patient transmission by hospital staff carrying *Pseudomonas* on the hands occurs in some units where hand hygiene is inadequate. Careful maintenance of equipment and enforcement of infection control procedures are essential to minimize nosocomial transmission.

C. Patients with Cystic Fibrosis

Chronic infection of the lower respiratory tract occurs in nearly all patients with cystic fibrosis. The infecting organism is seldom cleared from the respiratory tract, even with intensive antimicrobial therapy, and the resultant injury to the lung eventually leads to pulmonary insufficiency. Treatment is aimed at controlling signs and symptoms of the infection.

▶ Treatment

P aeruginosa is inherently resistant to many antimicrobials and may develop resistance during therapy. Mortality rates in hospitalized patients exceed 50%, owing both to the severity of underlying illnesses in patients predisposed to *Pseudomonas* infection and to the limitations of therapy. Antibiotics effective against *Pseudomonas* include the aminoglycosides, ureidopenicillins (piperacillin), β-lactamase inhibitor with a ureidopenicillin (piperacillin-tazobactam), expanded-spectrum cephalosporins (ceftazidime and cefepime), monobactams (aztreonam), carbapenems (doripenem, meropenem), and fluoroquinolones (ciprofloxacin, levofloxacin). Aminoglycosides may be used as an adjunct to the above regimen, but not as monotherapy except in the case of urinary tract infections. Colistin has been used in some children with multidrug resistance. Antimicrobial susceptibility patterns vary from area to area, and sometimes by unit within a hospital. Resistance tends to appear as new drugs become popular. Treatment of infections is best guided by clinical response and susceptibility tests.

Gentamicin or tobramycin (5.0–7.5 mg/kg/day intramuscularly or intravenously in three divided doses) or amikacin (15–22 mg/kg/day in two or three divided doses) in combination with piperacillin (240–300 mg/kg/day intravenously in four to six divided doses) or with another antipseudomonal β-lactam antibiotic is recommended for treatment of serious *Pseudomonas* infections. Ceftazidime (150–200 mg/kg/day in four divided doses) or cefepime (150 mg/kg/day in three divided doses) has activity against susceptible strains. Treatment should be continued for 10–14 days. Treatment with two active drugs is recommended for all serious infections. Aerosolized antipseudomonal antibiotics, tobramycin, and aztreonam have been very useful adjunctive therapy for patients with cystic fibrosis.

Pseudomonas osteomyelitis due to punctures requires thorough surgical debridement and antimicrobial therapy. *Pseudomonas* folliculitis does not require antibiotic therapy.

Oral or intravenous ciprofloxacin is also effective against susceptible *P aeruginosa* but is not approved by the FDA for use in children except in the case of urinary tract infection. Nonetheless, in some circumstances of antimicrobial resistance, or when the benefits clearly outweigh the small risks, ciprofloxacin may be used.

Chronic suppurative otitis media may be treated with topical ofloxacin or ciprofloxacin and aural toilet. Failure of treatment with conservative measures may necessitate oral or parenteral antibiotic therapy guided by culture results. Swimmer's ear may be caused by *P aeruginosa* and responds well to topical drying agents (alcohol–vinegar mix) and cleansing.

▶ Prognosis

Because debilitated patients are most frequently affected, the mortality rate is high. These infections may have a protracted course, and eradication of the organisms may be difficult.

Biddeci G et al: Ecthyma gangrenosum of the check in a 6-month-old infant. Arch Dis Child 2015:100(1):55 [PMID: 25053733].

Dantas RC et al: *Pseudomonas aeruginosa* bacteraemia: independent risk factors for mortality and impact of resistance on outcome. J Med Microbiol 2014;63(Pt 12):1679 [PMID: 25261066].

Paksu MS et al: Old agent, new experience: colistin use in the paediatric intensive care unit—a multicentre study. Int J Antimicrob Agents 2012;40(2):140 [PMID: 22727770].

Tiddens HA et al: Open label study of inhaled aztreonam for *Pseudomonas* eradication in children with cystic fibrosis: the ALPINE study. J Cyst Fibros 2015;14(1):111 [PMID: 25091537].

SALMONELLA GASTROENTERITIS

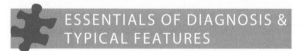

ESSENTIALS OF DIAGNOSIS & TYPICAL FEATURES

▶ Nausea, vomiting, headache, meningismus.

▶ Fever, diarrhea, abdominal pain.

▶ Culture or PCR of organism from stool, blood, or other specimens.

▶ General Considerations

Salmonellae are gram-negative rods that frequently cause food-borne gastroenteritis and occasionally bacteremic infection of bone, meninges, and other foci. Approximately 2400 serotypes of *Salmonella enterica* are recognized. *Salmonella*

typhimurium is the most frequently isolated serotype in most parts of the world. Although 51,400 cases were reported in 2014, it is estimated that more than 1 million cases occur yearly in the United States, as only a small percent of patients are cultured.

Salmonellae are able to penetrate the mucin layer of the small bowel and attach to epithelial cells. Organisms penetrate the epithelial cells and multiply in the submucosa. Infection results in fever, vomiting, and watery diarrhea; the diarrhea occasionally includes mucus and polymorphonuclear neutrophils in the stool. *Salmonella* infections in childhood occur in two major forms: (1) gastroenteritis (including food poisoning), which may be complicated by sepsis and focal suppurative complications; and (2) enteric fever (typhoid fever and paratyphoid fever) (see section Typhoid Fever & Paratyphoid Fever). Although the incidence of typhoid fever has decreased in the United States, the incidence of *Salmonella* gastroenteritis has greatly increased in the past 15–20 years. The highest attack rates occur in children younger than 6 years, with a peak in the age group from 6 months to 2 years.

Salmonellae are widespread in nature, infecting domestic and wild animals. Fowl and reptiles have a particularly high carriage rate. Outbreaks have been associated with petting zoos and keeping reptiles or backyard chickens as pets. Transmission occurs by the fecal-oral route via contaminated food, water, fomites, and sometimes person to person. Numerous foods, especially milk and egg products, are associated with outbreaks.

Because salmonellae are susceptible to gastric acidity, elderly, infants, and patients taking antacids or H_2-blocking drugs are at increased risk for infection. Most cases of *Salmonella* meningitis (80%) and bacteremia occur in infancy. Newborns may acquire the infection from their mothers during delivery and may precipitate outbreaks in nurseries. Newborns are at special risk for developing meningitis.

▶ Clinical Findings

A. Symptoms and Signs

There is a very wide range of severity of infection. Infants usually develop fever, vomiting, and diarrhea. The older child also may complain of headache, nausea, and abdominal pain. Stools are often watery or may contain mucus and, in some instances, blood, suggesting shigellosis. Drowsiness and disorientation may be associated with meningismus. Convulsions occur less frequently than with shigellosis. Splenomegaly occasionally occurs. In the usual case, diarrhea is moderate and subsides after 4–5 days, but it may be protracted.

B. Laboratory Findings

Diagnosis is made by isolation in culture or by PCR of the organism from stool, blood, or, in some cases from urine,

CSF, or pus from a suppurative lesion. The WBC count usually shows a polymorphonuclear leukocytosis but may show leukopenia. *Salmonella* isolates should be reported to public health authorities for epidemiologic purposes.

Differential Diagnosis

In staphylococcal food poisoning, the incubation period is shorter (2–4 hours) than in *Salmonella* food poisoning (12–24 hours), fever is absent, and vomiting rather than diarrhea is the main symptom. In shigellosis, many polymorphonuclear leukocytes usually are seen on a stained smear of stool, and the peripheral WBC count is more likely to slow a marked left shift, although some cases of salmonellosis are indistinguishable from shigellosis. *Campylobacter* gastroenteritis commonly resembles salmonellosis. Culture or PCR of stool is necessary to distinguish the causes of bacterial gastroenteritis.

Complications

Unlike most causes of infectious diarrhea, salmonellosis is frequently accompanied by bacteremia, especially in newborns and infants. Septicemia with extraintestinal infection is seen, most commonly with *Salmonella choleraesuis* but also with *S enterica, S typhimurium*, and *S paratyphi* serotypes. The organism may spread to any tissue and may cause arthritis, osteomyelitis, cholecystitis, endocarditis, meningitis, pericarditis, pneumonia, or pyelonephritis. Patients with sickle cell anemia or other hemoglobinopathies have a predilection for the development of osteomyelitis. Severe dehydration and shock are more likely to occur with shigellosis but may occur with *Salmonella* gastroenteritis.

Prevention

Measures for the prevention of *Salmonella* infections include thorough cooking of foodstuffs derived from contaminated sources, adequate refrigeration, control of infection among domestic animals, and meticulous meat and poultry inspections. Raw and undercooked fresh eggs or uncooked flour should be avoided. Food handlers and child care workers with salmonellosis should have three negative stool cultures before resuming work. Asymptomatic children, who have recovered from *Salmonella* infection, do not need school or day-care exclusion.

Treatment

A. Specific Measures

In uncomplicated *Salmonella* gastroenteritis, antibiotic treatment does not shorten the course of the clinical illness and may prolong convalescent carriage of the organism. Colitis or secretory diarrhea due to *Salmonella* may improve with antibiotic therapy. Azithromycin (10 mg/kg/day × 3 days) may be effective for moderate to severe colitis and is often used empirically for traveler's diarrhea.

Because of the higher risk of sepsis and focal disease, antibiotic treatment is recommended in infants younger than 3 months, in severely ill children, and in children with sickle cell disease, liver disease, recent gastrointestinal surgery, cancer, depressed immunity, or chronic renal or cardiac disease. Infants younger than 3 months with positive stool cultures or suspected salmonellosis sepsis should be admitted to the hospital, evaluated for focal infection including cultures of blood and CSF, and given treatment intravenously. A third-generation cephalosporin is usually recommended due to frequent resistance to ampicillin and TMP-SMX. Older patients developing bacteremia during the course of gastroenteritis should receive parenteral treatment initially, and a careful search should be made for additional foci of infection. After signs and symptoms subside, these patients should receive oral medication. Parenteral and oral treatment should last a total of 7–10 days. Longer treatment is indicated for specific complications. If susceptibility tests indicate resistance to ampicillin, third-generation cephalosporins or TMP-SMX should be given if susceptible. Fluoroquinolones or azithromycin are used for strains resistant to multiple other drugs.

Outbreaks on pediatric wards are difficult to control. Strict hand washing, cohorting of patients and personnel, and, ultimately, closure of the unit may be necessary.

B. Treatment of the Carrier State

About one-half of patients may have positive stool cultures after 4 weeks. Infants tend to remain convalescent carriers for up to 1 year. Antibiotic treatment of carriers is not effective.

C. General Measures

Careful attention must be given to maintaining fluid and electrolyte balance, especially in infants.

Prognosis

In gastroenteritis, the prognosis is good. In sepsis with focal suppurative complications, the prognosis is more guarded. The case fatality rate of *Salmonella* meningitis is high in infants. There is a tendency to relapse if treatment is not continued for at least 4 weeks.

Centers for Disease Control and Prevention (CDC): *Salmonella* infection (salmonellosis). http://www.cdc.gov/salmonella/. Accessed July 2, 2019.

Shane AL et al: 2017 Infectious Diseases Society of America clinical practice guidelines for the diagnosis and management of infectious diarrhea. Clin Infect Dis 2017 Dec 15;65(12):e45–e80 [PMID: 29053792].

Wen SC et al: Non-typhoidal *Salmonella* infections in children: review of literature and recommendations for management. J Paediatr Child Health 2017 Oct;53(10):936–941. doi: 10.1111/jpc.13585 [PMID: 28556448].

TYPHOID FEVER & PARATYPHOID FEVER

ESSENTIALS OF DIAGNOSIS & TYPICAL FEATURES

▶ Insidious or acute onset of headache, anorexia, vomiting, constipation or diarrhea, ileus, and high fever.

▶ Meningismus, splenomegaly, and rose spots.

▶ Leukopenia; positive blood, stool, bone marrow, and urine cultures.

▶ Fever in the returning traveler.

▶ General Considerations

Typhoid fever is caused by the gram-negative bacillus *S enterica* serotype typhi and paratyphi. Children have a shorter incubation period than do adults (usually 5–8 days instead of 8–14 days). The organism enters the body through the walls of the intestinal tract and, following a transient bacteremia, multiplies in the reticuloendothelial cells of the liver and spleen. Persistent bacteremia and symptoms then follow. Reinfection of the intestine occurs as organisms are excreted in the bile. Bacterial emboli produce the characteristic skin lesions (rose spots). Typhoid fever is transmitted by the fecal-oral route and by contamination of food or water. Unlike other *Salmonella* species, there are no animal reservoirs of *typhoid*; each case is the result of direct or indirect contact with the organism or with an individual who is actively infected or a chronic carrier.

About 300 cases per year were reported in the United States in 2015, 79% of which were acquired during foreign travel. Multidrug-resistant *S enterica* serotype *typhi* isolates are an increasing global problem.

▶ Clinical Findings

A. Symptoms and Signs

In children, the onset of typhoid fever usually is sudden rather than insidious, with malaise, headache, cough, crampy abdominal pains and distention, and sometimes constipation followed within 48 hours by diarrhea, high fever, and toxemia. An encephalopathy may be seen with irritability, confusion, delirium, and stupor. Vomiting and meningismus may be prominent in infants and young children. The classic lengthy three-stage disease seen in adult patients often is shortened in children. The prodrome may last only 2–4 days, the toxic stage only 2–3 days, and the defervescence stage 1–2 weeks.

During the prodromal stage, physical findings may be absent, but abdominal distention and tenderness, meningismus, mild hepatomegaly and splenomegaly may be present. The typical typhoidal rash (rose spots) is present in 10%–15% of children. It appears during the second week of the disease and may erupt in crops for the succeeding 10–14 days. Rose spots are erythematous maculopapular lesions 2–3 mm in diameter that blanch on pressure. They are found principally on the trunk and chest, and they generally disappear within 3–4 days. The lesions usually number fewer than 20.

B. Laboratory Findings

Typhoid bacilli can be isolated from many sites, including blood, stool, urine, and bone marrow. Blood cultures are positive in 50%–80% of cases during the first week and less often later in the illness. Stool cultures are positive in about 30% of cases after the first week. Urine and bone marrow cultures also are valuable. Most patients will have negative cultures (including stool) by the end of a 6-week period. Serologic tests (Widal reaction) are not as useful as cultures because both false-positive and false-negative results occur. Leukopenia is common in the second week of the disease, but in the first week, leukocytosis may be seen. Proteinuria, mild elevation of liver enzymes, thrombocytopenia, and DIC are common.

▶ Differential Diagnosis

Typhoid and paratyphoid fevers must be distinguished from other serious prolonged fevers. These include typhus, brucellosis, malaria, tularemia, TB, psittacosis, vasculitis, lymphoma, mononucleosis, and Kawasaki disease. Prolonged fever is a common presentation of typhoid in a returning traveler. The diagnosis of typhoid fever often is made clinically in developing countries, but the accuracy of clinical diagnosis is variable. In developed countries, where typhoid fever is uncommon and physicians are unfamiliar with the clinical picture, the diagnosis often is not suspected until late in the course. Positive cultures confirm the diagnosis.

▶ Complications

The most serious complications of typhoid fever are gastrointestinal hemorrhage (2%–10%) and perforation (1%–3%). They occur toward the end of the second week or during the third week of the disease.

Intestinal perforation is one of the principal causes of death. The site of perforation generally is the terminal ileum or cecum. The clinical manifestations are indistinguishable from those of acute appendicitis, with pain, tenderness, and rigidity in the right lower quadrant.

Bacterial pneumonia, meningitis, septic arthritis, abscesses, and osteomyelitis are uncommon complications, particularly if specific treatment is given promptly. Shock and electrolyte disturbances may lead to death.

About 1%–3% of patients become chronic typhoid carriers. Chronic carriage is defined as excretion of typhoid bacilli for more than a year, but carriage is often lifelong. Adults with underlying biliary or urinary tract disease are much more likely than children to become chronic carriers.

Prevention

Routine typhoid vaccine is not recommended in the United States but should be considered for foreign travel to endemic areas. An attenuated oral typhoid vaccine produced from strain Ty21a has better efficacy and causes minimal side effects but is not approved for children younger than 6 years. The vaccine is repeated after 5 years. A capsular polysaccharide vaccine (ViCPS) requires one intramuscular injection and may be given to children 2 years and older. (See Chapter 10.)

Treatment

A. Specific Measures

Third-generation cephalosporins such as ceftriaxone (50 mg/kg/dose every 24 hours), azithromycin (10 mg/kg on day 1, followed by 5 mg/kg on subsequent days), or a fluoroquinolone are used for presumptive therapy. Antimicrobial susceptibility testing and local experience are used to direct subsequent therapy. Typical courses of treatment are at least 7 days. Alternative regimens for susceptible strains include the following: TMP-SMX (10 mg/kg trimethoprim and 50 mg/kg sulfamethoxazole per day orally in two or three divided doses), amoxicillin (100 mg/kg/day orally in four divided doses), and ampicillin (100–200 mg/kg/day intravenously in four divided doses). These regimens generally require longer durations (14–21 days) than azithromycin or fluoroquinolone-based regimens. Aminoglycosides and first- and second-generation cephalosporins are clinically ineffective regardless of in vitro susceptibility results. Patients may remain febrile for 3–5 days even with appropriate therapy.

B. General Measures

General support of the patient is exceedingly important and includes rest, good nutrition and hydration, and careful observation, with particular regard to evidence of intestinal bleeding or perforation. Blood transfusions may be needed even in the absence of frank hemorrhage.

Prognosis

A prolonged convalescent carrier stage may occur in children. Three negative cultures after all antibiotics have been stopped are required before contact precautions are stopped. With early antibiotic therapy, the prognosis is excellent, and the mortality rate is less than 1%. Relapse occurs

1–3 weeks later in 10%–20% of patients despite appropriate antibiotic treatment.

Date KA et al: Typhoid fever surveillance and vaccine use—South-East Asia and Western Pacific regions, 2009–2013. MMWR Morb Mortal Wkly Rep 2014:63(39):855 [PMID: 25275329].

Halbert J et al: Fever in the returning child traveller: approach to diagnosis and management. Arch Dis Child 2014;99(10):938 [PMID: 24667950].

Kariuki S et al: Antimicrobial resistance and management of invasive *Salmonella* disease. Vaccine 2015 Jun 19;33 Suppl 3:C21–9. doi: 10.1016/j.vaccine.2015.03.102 [PMID: 25912288].

SHIGELLOSIS (BACILLARY DYSENTERY)

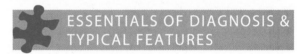

ESSENTIALS OF DIAGNOSIS & TYPICAL FEATURES

- ► Cramps and bloody diarrhea.
- ► High fever, malaise, convulsions.
- ► Pus and blood in diarrheal stools examined microscopically.
- ► Diagnosis confirmed by stool culture.

General Considerations

Shigellae are nonmotile gram-negative rods of the family Enterobacteriaceae that are closely related to *E coli*. The genus *Shigella* is divided into four species: *S dysenteriae*, *Shigella flexneri*, *Shigella boydii*, and *Shigella sonnei*. An estimated 500,000 cases of *Shigella* diarrhea occur every year in the United States. *S sonnei* followed by *S flexneri* are the most common isolates. *S dysenteriae*, which causes the most severe diarrhea of all species and the greatest number of extraintestinal complications, accounts for less than 1% of all *Shigella* infections in the United States.

Shigellosis may be a serious disease, particularly in young children, and without supportive treatment an appreciable mortality rate results. In older children and adults, the disease tends to be self-limited and milder. *Shigella* is usually transmitted by the fecal-oral route. Food- and water-borne outbreaks are increasing in occurrence, but are less important overall than person-to-person transmission. The disease is very communicable—as few as 200 bacteria can produce illness in an adult volunteer. The secondary attack rate in families is high, and shigellosis is a serious problem in day care centers and custodial institutions. *Shigella* organisms produce disease by invading the colonic mucosa, causing mucosal ulcerations and microabscesses.

Clinical Findings

A. Symptoms and Signs

The incubation period of shigellosis is usually 1–3 days. Onset is abrupt, with abdominal cramps, urgency, tenesmus, chills, fever, malaise, and diarrhea. Hallucinations and seizures sometimes accompany high fever. In severe forms, blood and mucus are seen in small stools. In older children, the disease may be mild and characterized by watery diarrhea without blood. In young children, a fever of 39.4°C–40°C is common. Rarely there is rectal prolapse. Symptoms generally last 3–7 days.

B. Laboratory Findings

The total WBC count varies, but often there is a marked left shift. The stool may contain gross blood and mucus, and many neutrophils are seen if mucus from the stool is examined microscopically. Stool cultures are usually positive; however, they may be negative because the organism is somewhat fragile and present in small numbers late in the disease. Multiplex PCR tests are available for rapid diagnosis of *Shigella* and other enteropathogens.

Differential Diagnosis

Usually children with viral gastroenteritis are not as febrile or toxic as those with shigellosis, and the stool does not contain gross blood or neutrophils. Intestinal infections caused by *Salmonella* or *Campylobacter* are differentiated by culture or PCR. Grossly bloody stools in a patient without fever or stool leukocytes suggest *E coli* O157:H7 infection. Amebic dysentery is diagnosed by antigen detection or microscopic examination of fresh stools or sigmoidoscopy specimens. Intussusception is characterized by an abdominal mass with so-called currant jelly stools without leukocytes, and by absence of initial fever. Mild shigellosis is not distinguishable clinically from other forms of infectious diarrhea.

Complications

Dehydration, acidosis, shock, and renal failure are the major complications. In some cases, a chronic form of dysentery occurs, characterized by mucoid stools and poor nutrition. Bacteremia and metastatic infections are rare but serious complications. Febrile seizures are common. Fulminating fatal dysentery and HUS occur rarely. Reactive arthritis may follow *Shigella* infection in patients with HLA-B27 genotype.

Treatment

A. Specific Measures

Milder infections may not require antibiotic treatment. Antibiotic resistance in *Shigella* is an increasing problem,

including to TMP-SMX, ampicillin and more recently to fluoroquinolones. Azithromycin (12 mg/kg/day on day 1, then 6 mg/kg/day for 2 days) is usually effective, as is ciprofloxacin, though the latter should not be used routinely in children. Parenteral ceftriaxone (50 mg/kg/day) is an option for severe infections. Successful treatment reduces the duration of fever, cramping, and diarrhea and terminates fecal excretion of *Shigella*. Presumptive therapy should be limited to children with classic shigellosis or known outbreaks.

B. General Measures

In severe cases, immediate rehydration is critical. A mild form of chronic malabsorption syndrome may supervene and require prolonged dietary control. Zinc supplementation may aid recovery in populations at risk of deficiency.

Prognosis

The prognosis is excellent if vascular collapse is prevented or treated promptly by adequate fluid therapy. The mortality rate is high in very young, malnourished infants who do not receive fluid and electrolyte therapy. Convalescent fecal excretion of *Shigella* lasts 1–4 weeks in patients not receiving antimicrobial therapy. Long-term carriers are rare.

Centers for Disease Control and Prevention (CDC): Shigellosis. www.cdc.gov/shigella/index.html. Accessed June 30, 2019.

Puzari M et al. Emergence of antibiotic resistant *Shigella* species: a matter of concern. J Infect Public Health 2018 Jul–Aug;11(4):451–454. doi: 10.1016/j.jiph.2017.09.025 [PMID: 29066021].

Shane AL et al: 2017 Infectious Diseases Society of America clinical practice guidelines for the diagnosis and management of infectious diarrhea. Clin Infect Dis 2017 Dec 15;65(12):e45–e80 [PMID: 29053792].

CHOLERA

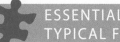

ESSENTIALS OF DIAGNOSIS & TYPICAL FEATURES

- ▶ Sudden onset of severe watery diarrhea.
- ▶ Persistent vomiting without nausea or fever.
- ▶ Extreme and rapid dehydration and electrolyte loss, with rapid development of vascular collapse.
- ▶ Contact with a case of cholera or with shellfish, or the presence of cholera in the community.
- ▶ Diagnosis confirmed by stool culture.

▶ General Considerations

Cholera is an acute diarrheal disease caused by the gram-negative organism *Vibrio cholerae*. It is transmitted by contaminated water or food, especially contaminated shellfish. Epidemics are common in impoverished areas where hygiene and safe water supply are limited. Typical disease is generally so dramatic that in endemic areas the diagnosis is obvious. Individuals with mild illness and young children may play an important role in transmission of the infection.

Asymptomatic infection is far more common than clinical disease. In endemic areas, rising titers of vibriocidal antibody are seen with increasing age. Infection occurs in individuals with low titers. The age-specific attack rate is highest in children younger than 5 years and declines with age. Cholera is unusual in infancy.

Cholera toxin is a protein enterotoxin that is responsible for symptoms. Cholera toxin binds to a regulatory subunit of adenylyl cyclase in enterocytes, causing increased cyclic adenosine monophosphate and an outpouring of NaCl and water into the lumen of the small bowel.

Nutritional status is an important factor determining the severity of the diarrhea. Duration of diarrhea is prolonged in adults and children with severe malnutrition.

Cholera is endemic in India and southern and Southeast Asia and in parts of Africa. The most recent pandemic, caused by the El Tor biotype of *V cholerae* 01, began in 1961 in Indonesia. Epidemic cholera spread in Central and South America, with a total of 1 million cases and 9500 deaths reported through 1994. A severe cholera outbreak in Haiti began in October 2010 and many cases continue to occur. A recent outbreak in Yemen demonstrates the vulnerability of populations to cholera emergence in conflict settings. Cholera in the United States occurs after foreign travel or rarely as a result of consumption of contaminated imported food.

V cholerae is a natural inhabitant of shellfish and copepods in estuarine environments. Seasonal multiplication of *V cholerae* may provide a source of outbreaks in endemic areas. Chronic cholera carriers are rare. The incubation period is short, usually 1–3 days.

▶ Clinical Findings

A. Symptoms and Signs

Many patients infected with *V cholerae* have mild disease, with 1%–2% developing severe diarrhea. During severe cholera, there is a sudden onset of massive, frequent, watery stools, generally light gray in color (so-called rice-water stools) and containing some mucus but no pus. Vomiting may be projectile and is not accompanied by nausea. Within 2–3 hours, the tremendous loss of fluids results in life-threatening dehydration, hypochloremia, and hypokalemia, with marked weakness and collapse. Renal failure and irreversible peripheral vascular collapse will occur if fluid

therapy is not administered. The illness lasts 1–7 days and is shortened by appropriate antibiotic therapy.

B. Laboratory Findings

Markedly elevated hemoglobin (20 g/dL) and marked acidosis, hypochloremia, and hyponatremia are seen. Culture confirmation requires specific media and takes 16–18 hours for a presumptive diagnosis and 36–48 hours for a definitive bacteriologic diagnosis.

▶ Prevention

A live attenuated oral cholera vaccine was approved in the United States in 2016 for adults traveling to cholera endemic areas. It is estimated to provide 80%–90% protection. Other cholera vaccines are available outside of the United States and provides 50%–75% efficacy. Protection lasts 3–6 months. Tourists visiting endemic areas are at little risk if they exercise caution in what they eat and drink and maintain good personal hygiene. In endemic areas, all water must be boiled, shellfish should be thoroughly cooked, food and drink protected from flies, and sanitary precautions observed. Foods should be promptly refrigerated whenever possible after meals. Simple filtration of water is highly effective in reducing cases. All patients with cholera should be isolated.

Chemoprophylaxis (tetracycline 500 mg/day for 5 days) can limit secondary cases in a household if administered rapidly. It should be initiated as soon as possible after the onset of the disease in the index patient. TMP-SMX may be substituted in children.

▶ Treatment

Replacement and maintenance of fluids and electrolytes hydration are the most important aspects of cholera treatment. Physiologic saline or lactated Ringer solution should be administered intravenously in large amounts to restore blood volume and urine output and to prevent irreversible shock. Potassium supplements are required. Sodium bicarbonate, given intravenously, also may be needed initially to overcome profound metabolic acidosis from bicarbonate loss in the stool. Moderate dehydration and acidosis can be corrected in 3–6 hours by oral therapy alone, because the active glucose transport system of the small bowel is normally functional. The optimal composition of the oral solution is described in Table 45–5.

Antibiotic treatment can also shorten the duration and decrease the severity of cholera. First-line treatment for children in the United States is doxycycline (4.4 mg/kg/day divided twice daily). Azithromycin (10 mg/kg/day in one dose for 1–5 days) is also effective. Antibiotic treatment prevents clinical relapse but is not as important as fluid and electrolyte therapy.

Prognosis

With early and rapid replacement of fluids and electrolytes, the case fatality rate is 1%–2% in children. If significant symptoms appear and no treatment is given, the mortality rate is over 50%.

Centers for Disease Control and Prevention: Cholera. www.cdc.gov/cholera/index.html. Accessed June 30, 2019.

Kuna A, Gajewski M: Cholera—the new strike of an old foe. Int Marit Health 2017;68(3):163–167. doi: 10.5603/IMH.2017.0029 [PMID: 28952662].

Leibovici-Weissman Y, Neuberger A, Bitterman R, Sinclair D, Salam MA, Paul M: Antimicrobial drugs for treating cholera. Cochrane Database Syst Rev 2014 Jun 19;(6):CD008625. doi: 10.1002/14651858.CD008625.pub2 [PMID: 24944120].

Wong KK et al: Recommendations of the Advisory Committee on Immunization Practices for Use of Cholera Vaccine. MMWR Morb Mortal Wkly Rep. 2017 May 12;66(18):482–485 [PMID: 28493859].

CAMPYLOBACTER INFECTION

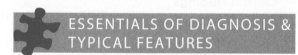

ESSENTIALS OF DIAGNOSIS & TYPICAL FEATURES

▶ Fever, vomiting, abdominal pain, diarrhea.

▶ Definitive diagnosis by stool culture or PCR.

General Considerations

Campylobacter species are small gram-negative, curved or spiral bacilli that are commensals or pathogens in many animals. *Campylobacter jejuni* frequently causes acute enteritis in humans. In the United States gastroenteritis due to *C jejuni* affects an estimated 1.3 million people annually and is more common than that due to *Salmonella* or *Shigella*. *Campylobacter fetus* causes bacteremia and meningitis in immunocompromised patients. *C fetus* may cause maternal fever, abortion, stillbirth, and severe neonatal infection.

Campylobacter colonizes domestic and wild animals, especially poultry. Numerous cases have been associated with sick puppies or other animal contacts. Contaminated food and water, undercooked poultry, and person-to-person spread by the fecal-oral route are common routes of transmission. Outbreaks associated with day care centers, contaminated water supplies, and raw milk have been reported. Newborns may acquire the organism from their mothers at delivery. *Campylobacter* is a major cause of diarrhea in travelers to low- and middle-income countries.

Clinical Findings

A. Symptoms and Signs

C jejuni enteritis can be mild or severe. In tropical countries, asymptomatic stool carriage is common. The incubation period is usually 1–7 days. The disease usually begins with sudden onset of high fever, malaise, headache, abdominal cramps, nausea, and vomiting. Diarrhea follows and may be watery or bile stained, mucoid, and bloody. The illness is self-limiting, lasting 2–7 days, but relapses may occur. Without antimicrobial treatment, the organism remains in the stool for 1–6 weeks. Immune compromised patients may suffer prolonged or relapsing disease or complications due to bacteremia.

B. Laboratory Findings

The peripheral WBC count generally is elevated, with many band forms. Microscopic examination of stool reveals erythrocytes and leukocytes.

Isolation of *C jejuni* from stool is not difficult but requires selective agar and incubation conditions. Multiplex PCR tests are available for rapid diagnosis of *Campylobacter* and other enteropathogens.

Differential Diagnosis

Campylobacter enteritis may resemble viral gastroenteritis, salmonellosis, shigellosis, amebiasis, or other infectious diarrheas. Because it also mimics ulcerative colitis, Crohn disease, intussusception, and appendicitis, mistaken diagnosis can lead to unnecessary diagnostic testing or surgery.

Complications

The most common complication is dehydration. Other uncommon complications include erythema nodosum, convulsions, reactive arthritis, bacteremia, urinary tract infection, and cholecystitis. *Campylobacter* is the most commonly identified cause of Guillain-Barré syndrome (estimated to occur in 1 in 1000 cases) that typically follows *C jejuni* infection by 1–3 weeks.

Prevention

No vaccine is available. Hand washing and adherence to basic food sanitation practices help prevent disease. Hand washing and cleaning of kitchen utensils after contact with raw poultry are important. Adequate cooking of poultry is important.

Treatment

Treatment of fluid and electrolyte disturbances is important and in milder cases is the only required intervention. Antimicrobial therapy given early in the course of the illness will shorten the duration of symptoms. Treatment with azithromycin (10 mg/kg/day orally once daily) for 3 days, or ciprofloxacin terminates fecal excretion and may limit spread in households. Fluoroquinolone-resistant *C jejuni* are now common worldwide.

▶ Prognosis

The outlook is excellent if dehydration is corrected, and misdiagnosis does not lead to inappropriate diagnostic or surgical procedures.

Centers for Disease Control and Prevention (CDC): *Campylobacter* infections. http://www.cdc.gov/nczved/divisions/dfbmd/diseases/campylobacter. Accessed June 30, 2019.

Ricotta EE et al: Epidemiology and antimicrobial resistance of international travel associated *Campylobacter* infections in the United States, 2005–2011. Am J Public Health 2014;104(7):e108–e114 [PMID: 24832415].

Shane AL et al: 2017 Infectious Diseases Society of America clinical practice guidelines for the diagnosis and management of infectious diarrhea. Clin Infect Dis 2017 Dec 15;65(12):e45–e80 [PMID: 29053792].

TULAREMIA

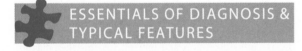

ESSENTIALS OF DIAGNOSIS & TYPICAL FEATURES

▶ A cutaneous or mucous membrane lesion at the site of inoculation and regional lymph node enlargement.

▶ Sudden onset of fever, chills, and prostration.

▶ History of contact with infected animals, principally wild rabbits, or tick or deer fly exposure.

▶ Positive culture, PCR or immunofluorescent staining of samples from mucocutaneous ulcer or regional lymph nodes.

▶ High serum antibody titer.

▶ General Considerations

Tularemia is caused by *Francisella tularensis*, a gram-negative organism usually acquired directly from infected animals or by the bite of an infected tick or deer fly. Occasionally infection is acquired from infected domestic dogs or cats; by contamination of the skin or mucous membranes with infected blood or tissues; by inhalation of infected material; or by ingestion of contaminated meat or water. The incubation period is short, usually 3–7 days, but may vary from 2 to 25 days. In the United States 239 cases of tularemia were reported in 2017.

Ticks (dog tick, wood tick, lone star tick) are important vectors of tularemia transmission and rabbits are the classic vector. It is important to seek a history of rabbit hunting, skinning, or food preparation in any patient who has a febrile illness with tender lymphadenopathy, often in the region of a draining skin ulcer.

▶ Prevention

Children should be protected from insect bites, especially those of ticks and deer flies, by the use of proper clothing and repellents. Because rabbits are the source of most human infections, the dressing and handling of such game should be performed with great care. Rubber gloves should be worn by hunters or food handlers when handling carcasses of wild rabbits. Care should be taken to avoid mowing over dead animals. If contact occurs, thorough washing with soap and water is indicated. For postexposure prophylaxis of *F tularensis* (such as might occur in a bioterrorism event), a 14-day course of doxycycline is recommended.

▶ Clinical Findings

A. Symptoms and Signs

Several clinical types of tularemia occur in children. Sixty percent of infections are of the ulceroglandular form that starts as a relatively nonpainful, reddened papule that may be pruritic and quickly ulcerates. Soon, the regional lymph nodes become large and tender. Fluctuance quickly follows. There may be marked systemic symptoms, including high fever, chills, weakness, and vomiting. Pneumonitis occasionally accompanies the ulceroglandular form or may be seen as the sole manifestation of infection (pneumonic form). A detectable skin lesion may be absent, and localized lymphoid enlargement may exist alone (glandular form). Oculoglandular and oropharyngeal forms also occur. The latter is characterized by tonsillitis, often with membrane formation, cervical adenopathy, and high fever. In the absence of a primary ulcer or localized lymphadenitis, a prolonged febrile disease reminiscent of typhoid fever can occur (typhoidal form). Splenomegaly is common in all forms.

B. Laboratory Findings

F tularensis can be recovered from ulcers, regional lymph nodes, blood, and sputum of patients with the pneumonic form. However, the organism grows only on an enriched medium (blood-cystine-glucose agar), and laboratory handling is dangerous owing to the risk of airborne transmission to laboratory personnel. PCR or immunofluorescent staining of biopsy material or aspirates of involved lymph nodes is diagnostic.

The WBC count is not remarkable. The diagnosis is typically confirmed with serologic testing. Antibodies are usually present during the second week of illness. In the absence of a positive culture, a tube agglutination antibody titer of 1:160 or greater or a microagglutination titer of 1:128 or greater is presumptively positive for the diagnosis of tularemia. Confirmation of disease is established by demonstration of a fourfold antibody titer rise between acute and convalescent serum samples. PCR of blood, lymph node aspirate, or tissue may be available through state health departments.

Differential Diagnosis

The typhoidal form of tularemia may mimic typhoid, brucellosis, miliary TB, Rocky Mountain spotted fever, and mononucleosis. Pneumonic tularemia resembles atypical pneumonia. The ulceroglandular type of tularemia resembles pyoderma caused by staphylococci or streptococci, plague, anthrax, and cat-scratch fever. The oropharyngeal type must be distinguished from streptococcal or diphtheritic pharyngitis, mononucleosis, herpangina, or other viral pharyngitides.

Treatment

A. Specific Measures

Historically, streptomycin was the drug of choice. However, gentamicin (5 mg/kg/day) is efficacious, more available, and familiar to clinicians. A 10-day course is usually sufficient, although more severe infections may need longer therapy. Ciprofloxacin also can be used in patients with less severe disease. Doxycycline is often effective but is a static (as opposed to cidal) agent and is associated with higher relapse rates.

B. General Measures

Antipyretics and analgesics may be given as necessary. Skin lesions are best left open. Glandular lesions occasionally require incision and drainage.

Prognosis

The prognosis is excellent in most cases of tularemia that are recognized early and treated appropriately.

Centers for Disease Control (CDC) and Prevention: Tularemia. http://www.cdc.gov/tularemia/clinicians/index.html. Accessed June 30, 2019.

Harik NS: Tularemia: epidemiology, diagnosis and treatment. Pediatr Ann 2013;42(7):288–292 [PMID: 23805970].

Pedati C et al: Notes from the field: increase in human cases of Tularemia—Colorado, Nebraska, South Dakota, and Wyoming, January–September 2015. 2015 Dec 4;64(47):1317–1318 [PMID: 26632662].

PLAGUE

ESSENTIALS OF DIAGNOSIS & TYPICAL FEATURES

▶ Sudden onset of fever, chills, and prostration.

▶ Regional lymphadenitis with suppuration of nodes (bubonic form).

▶ Hemorrhage into skin and mucous membranes and shock (septicemia).

▶ Cough, dyspnea, cyanosis, and hemoptysis (pneumonia).

▶ History of exposure to infected animals.

▶ Diagnosis is confirmed by positive culture, PCR, or immunofluorescent staining of culture material.

General Considerations

Plague is an extremely serious acute infection caused by a gram-negative bacillus, *Yersinia pestis*. It is a disease of rodents that is transmitted to humans by flea bites. Plague bacilli have been isolated from ground squirrels, prairie dogs, and other wild rodents in many of the western and southwestern states in the United States. Most cases have come from New Mexico, Arizona, Colorado, and California. Direct contact with rodents, rabbits, or domestic dogs and cats provides exposure to fleas infected with plague bacilli. Contact with an infected dog caused a cluster of four cases in 2014. Most cases occur from June through September. Human plague in the United States appears to occur in cycles that reflect cycles in wild animal reservoirs. On average, seven cases per year are reported in the United States.

Prevention

Proper disposal of household and commercial wastes and control of rats and other animals are basic elements of plague prevention. Flea control is also important. Children vacationing in remote areas should be warned not to handle dead or dying animals. Domestic cats that roam freely in suburban areas may contact infected wild animals and acquire infected fleas. There is no commercially available vaccine for plague.

All persons exposed to plague in the previous 6 days (via personal contact with an infected person, contact with plague infected fleas, or exposure to infected tissues) should be given antimicrobial prophylaxis or be instructed to report fever or other symptoms to their physician. Persons who have close personal contact (< 2 m) with a person with pneumonic plague should receive antimicrobial prophylaxis for 7 days from the last exposure. Doxycycline or ciprofloxacin are the recommended agents for prophylaxis. Patients on prophylaxis should still seek prompt medical care for onset of fever or other illness.

▶ Clinical Findings

A. Symptoms and Signs

Plague assumes several clinical forms; the two most common are bubonic and septicemic. Pneumonic plague is uncommon.

1. Bubonic plague—After an incubation period of 2–8 days, there is the sudden onset of high fever, chills, headache, vomiting, and marked delirium or clouding of consciousness. A less severe form also exists, with a less precipitous onset, but with progression over several days to severe symptoms. Although the flea bite is rarely seen, the regional lymph node, usually inguinal and unilateral, is/are painful and tender, 1–5 cm in diameter. The node usually suppurates and drains spontaneously after 1 week. Plague bacilli produce endotoxin that causes vascular necrosis. Bacilli may overwhelm regional lymph nodes and enter the circulation to produce septicemia. Severe vascular necrosis results in widely disseminated hemorrhage in skin, mucous membranes, liver, and spleen. Myocarditis and circulatory collapse may result from damage by the endotoxin. Plague meningitis or pneumonia may occur following bacteremic spread from an infected lymph node.

2. Septicemic plague—Plague may initially present as septicemia without evidence of lymphadenopathy. In some series, 25% of cases are initially septicemic. Septicemic plague carries a worse prognosis than bubonic plague, largely because it is not recognized and treated early. Patients may present with a nonspecific febrile illness characterized by fever, myalgia, chills, and anorexia. Septicemic plague may be complicated by secondary seeding of the lung causing plague pneumonia. Necrosis of distal body parts such as the fingers, toes, and nose tip may occur.

3. Primary pneumonic plague—Inhalation of *Y pestis* bacilli causes primary plague pneumonia. This form of plague is transmitted from human to human and to humans from cats or dogs with pneumonic plague and would be the form of plague most likely seen after aerosolized release of *Y pestis* in a bioterrorist incident. After an incubation of 1–6 days, the patient develops fever; cough; shortness of breath; and bloody, watery, or purulent sputum. Gastrointestinal symptoms are sometimes prominent. Because the initial focus of infection is the lung, buboes are usually absent; occasionally cervical buboes may be seen.

B. Laboratory Findings

Aspirate from a bubo contains bipolar-staining gram-negative bacilli. Pus, sputum, and blood all yield the organism. Rapid diagnosis can be made with fluorescent antibody detection or PCR on clinical specimens (available through state health departments). Confirmation is made by culture or serologic testing. Cultures are usually positive within 48 hours. Paired acute and convalescent sera may be tested for a fourfold antibody rise. Automated bacterial identification systems have been known to misidentify *Y pestis* and are unreliable.

▶ Differential Diagnosis

The septic phase of the disease may be confused with illnesses such as meningococcemia, sepsis caused by other bacteria, and rickettsioses. The bubonic form resembles tularemia, anthrax, cat-scratch fever, lymphadenitis, and cellulitis.

▶ Treatment

A. Specific Measures

Streptomycin or gentamicin for 10–14 days (or until several days after defervescence) is effective. For patients not requiring parenteral therapy, doxycycline, ciprofloxacin, TMP-SMX, or chloramphenicol may be given.

Every effort should be made to effect resolution of buboes without surgery. Pus from draining lymph nodes is infectious.

B. General Measures

State health officials should be notified immediately about suspected cases of plague. Pneumonic plague is highly infectious, and droplet isolation is required until the patient has been on effective antimicrobial therapy for 48 hours. Laboratory personnel should be notified if suspicion for plague exists in order to exercise precaution and prevent occupational acquisition.

▶ Prognosis

The mortality rate in untreated bubonic plague is about 50%. The mortality rate for treated pneumonic plague is 50%–60%. Recent mortality rates in New Mexico were 3% for bubonic plague and 71% for the septicemic form.

Centers for Disease Control and Prevention (CDC): Plague. http://www.cdc.gov/plague/healthcare/clinicians.html. Accessed July 4, 2019.

Kugeler KJ et al: Epidemiology of human plague in the United States, 1900–2012. Emerg Infect Dis 2015 Jan;21(1):16–22 [PMID: 25529546].

Prentice MB, Rahalison L: Plague. Lancet 2007;369:1196 [PMID: 17416264].

HAEMOPHILUS INFLUENZAE TYPE B INFECTIONS

ESSENTIALS OF DIAGNOSIS & TYPICAL FEATURES

▶ Purulent meningitis in children younger than 4 years with direct smears of CSF showing gram-negative pleomorphic rods.

▶ Acute epiglottitis: high fever, drooling, dysphagia, aphonia, and stridor.

▶ Septic arthritis: fever, local redness, swelling, heat, and pain with active or passive motion of the involved joint in a child 4 months to 4 years of age.

▶ Cellulitis: sudden onset of fever and distinctive cellulitis in an infant, often involving the cheek or periorbital area.

▶ In all cases, a positive culture from the blood, CSF, or aspirated pus confirms the diagnosis.

General Considerations

H influenzae is classified by its polysaccharide capsule into six serotypes (a–f), and those without a polysaccharide capsule are considered nontypeable. *H influenzae* type b (Hib) that was a common cause of invasive disease, such as meningitis, bacteremia, epiglottitis, septic arthritis, periorbital and facial cellulitis, pneumonia, and pericarditis, has become uncommon because of widespread immunization in early infancy. The 99% reduction in incidence seen in many parts of the United States is due to high rates of vaccine coverage and reduced nasopharyngeal carriage after vaccination. Now, non–type b and nontypeable *H influenzae* cause the majority of invasive disease. Non–type b serotypes may cause meningitis, bacteremia and other diseases previously caused by Hib.

Unencapsulated, nontypeable *H influenzae* frequently colonize the mucous membranes and cause otitis media, sinusitis, bronchitis, and pneumonia in children and adults. Unencapsulated, nontypeable *H influenzae* also cause invasive disease. Neonatal sepsis similar to early-onset GBS is recognized and is more common in preterm and low-birth-weight infants. Obstetric complications of chorioamnionitis and bacteremia are usually the source of neonatal cases.

Ampicillin resistance occurs in 25%–40% of nontypeable *H influenzae*. β-Lactamase-negative, ampicillin-resistant (BLNAR) *H influenzae* has emerged as a clinically important pathogen in Europe, Japan, and Canada. In the United States, the prevalence of BLNAR strains currently remains at around 3%.

Among children younger than 5 years, American Indian and Alaska Native children have a substantially higher incidence of invasive *H influenzae* disease, greater than five times the rate of other races.

▶ Prevention

Several carbohydrate protein conjugate Hib vaccines are currently available (see Chapter 10).

The risk of invasive Hib disease is highest in unimmunized, or partially immunized, household contacts of a Hib patient when the contact is younger than 4 years. The following situations require rifampin chemoprophylaxis of all household contacts (except pregnant women) to eradicate potential nasopharyngeal colonization with Hib and limit risk of invasive disease: (1) families where at least one household contact is younger than 4 years and either unimmunized or incompletely immunized against Hib; (2) an immunocompromised child (of any age or immunization status) resides in the household; or (3) a child younger than 12 months resides in the home and has not received the primary series of the Hib vaccine. Preschool and day care center contacts may need prophylaxis if more than one case has occurred in the center in the previous 60 days (discuss with state health officials). The index case also needs chemoprophylaxis if the patient is younger than 2 years or if the patient resides in a household with a household contact at risk of disease (as described above) *and* if treated with an antibiotic regimen *other than* ceftriaxone or cefotaxime (both are effective in eradication of Hib from the nasopharynx). Household contacts and index cases older than 1 month who need chemoprophylaxis should be given rifampin, 20 mg/kg per dose (maximum adult dose, 600 mg) orally, once daily for 4 successive days. Infants who are younger than 1 month should be given oral rifampin (10 mg/kg per dose once daily for 4 days). Rifampin should not be used in pregnant females. Chemoprophylaxis may be considered for household contacts of children with invasive disease caused by *H influenzae* type A. For other strains, including nontypeable *H influenzae*, chemoprophylaxis is generally not recommended because secondary cases are rare.

▶ Clinical Findings

A. Symptoms and Signs Hib and Non–Type B Invasive Disease

1. Meningitis—Infants usually present with fever, irritability, lethargy, poor feeding with or without vomiting, and a high-pitched cry.

2. Acute epiglottitis—The most useful clinical finding in the early diagnosis of *Haemophilus* epiglottitis is evidence of dysphagia, characterized by a refusal to eat or swallow saliva and by drooling. This finding, plus the presence of a high fever in a toxic child—even in the absence of a cherry-red epiglottis on direct examination—should strongly suggest the diagnosis and lead to prompt intubation. Stridor is a late sign (see Chapter 19).

3. Septic arthritis—In the prevaccine era, Hib was a common cause of septic arthritis in unimmunized children younger than 4 years in the United States. The child is febrile and refuses to move the involved joint and limb. Examination reveals swelling, warmth, redness, tenderness on palpation, and severe pain on attempted movement of the joint.

4. Cellulitis—Cellulitis due to *Hib* occurs almost exclusively in children between the ages of 3 months and 4 years but is now uncommon as a result of immunization. The cheek or periorbital (preseptal) area is often involved.

B. Laboratory Findings

The WBC count in Hib infections may be high or normal with a shift to the left. A positive culture of blood, CSF, aspirated pus, or fluid from the involved site proves the diagnosis. In untreated meningitis, CSF smear may show the characteristic pleomorphic gram-negative rods. Recently, the FDA approved a multiplex PCR test for CSF that includes *H influenzae* among the pathogens that can be detected.

C. Imaging

A lateral view of the neck may suggest the diagnosis in suspected acute epiglottitis, but misinterpretation is common. Intubation should not be delayed to obtain radiographs.

▶ Differential Diagnosis

A. Meningitis

Meningitis must be differentiated from head injury, brain abscess, tumor, lead encephalopathy, and other forms of meningoencephalitis, including mycobacterial, viral, fungal, and bacterial agents.

B. Acute Epiglottitis

In croup caused by viral agents (parainfluenza 1, 2, and 3, respiratory syncytial virus, influenza A, adenovirus), the child has more definite upper respiratory symptoms, cough, hoarseness, slower progression of obstructive signs, and lower fever. Spasmodic croup usually occurs at night in a child with a history of previous attacks. Sudden onset of choking and paroxysmal coughing suggests foreign-body aspiration. Retropharyngeal abscess may have to be differentiated from epiglottitis.

C. Septic Arthritis

Differential diagnosis includes acute osteomyelitis, prepatellar bursitis, cellulitis, rheumatic fever, and fractures and sprains.

D. Cellulitis

Erysipelas, streptococcal cellulitis, insect bites, and trauma (including popsicle panniculitis or other types of freezing injury) may mimic Hib cellulitis. Periorbital cellulitis must be differentiated from paranasal sinus disease without cellulitis, allergic inflammatory disease of the lids, conjunctivitis, and herpes zoster infection.

▶ Complications

A. Meningitis (See Chapter 25)

B. Acute Epiglottitis

The disease may rapidly progress to complete airway obstruction with complications owing to hypoxia (see Chapter 25). Mediastinal emphysema and pneumothorax may occur.

C. Septic Arthritis

Septic arthritis may result in rapid destruction of cartilage and ankylosis if diagnosis and treatment are delayed. Even with early treatment, the incidence of residual damage and disability after septic arthritis in weight-bearing joints may be as high as 25%.

D. Cellulitis

Bacteremia from a cutaneous source may lead to meningitis or pyarthrosis.

▶ Treatment

All patients with bacteremic or potentially bacteremic *H influenzae* diseases require hospitalization for treatment. The drug of choice in hospitalized patients is a third-generation cephalosporin (cefotaxime or ceftriaxone) until the sensitivity of the organism is known. Meropenem is an alternative choice. Persons with invasive Hib disease should be in droplet isolation for 24 hours after initiation of parenteral antibiotic therapy.

A. Meningitis

Therapy is begun as soon as bacterial meningitis is suspected. Empiric intravenous therapy recommended for meningitis (until organism identified) is vancomycin in combination with ceftriaxone. Once the organism has been identified as *H influenzae* and the susceptibilities are known, the antibiotic regimen can be tailored accordingly. Most isolates will be susceptible to ceftriaxone, and some to ampicillin. Therapy should be given intravenously for the entire course. Ceftriaxone may be given intramuscularly if venous access becomes difficult.

Duration of therapy is 10 days for uncomplicated meningitis. Longer treatment is reserved for children who respond slowly or have complications.

Dexamethasone given immediately after diagnosis and continued for up to 4 days may reduce the incidence of hearing loss in children with Hib meningitis. The use of dexamethasone is controversial, but when it is used, the dosage is 0.6 mg/kg/day in four divided doses for 2–4 days. Starting dexamethasone more than 6 hours after antibiotics have been initiated is unlikely to provide benefits.

Repeated lumbar punctures are usually not necessary in Hib meningitis. They should be obtained in the following circumstances: unsatisfactory or questionable clinical response, seizure occurring after several days of therapy, if the neurologic examination is abnormal or difficult to evaluate, or prolonged (7 days) or recurrent fever.

B. Acute Epiglottitis (See Chapter 19)

C. Septic Arthritis

Initial therapy should include an effective antistaphylococcal antibiotic and cefotaxime or ceftriaxone until identification of the organism is made and continued, once the isolate is known to be *Haemophilus* and susceptibilities are known (see Chapter 19). If a child is improved following initial intravenous therapy, the patient can be transitioned to oral therapy based on susceptibilities. Possible oral agents should be chosen based on susceptibilities but might include amoxicillin/clavulanate (90–100 mg/kg/day of amoxicillin component in four divided doses every 6 hours). Alternative agents include second- or third-generation cephalosporins. Antibiotics should be administered to complete a 2- to 4-week course (longer if complications or signs and symptoms are unresolved). Drainage of infected joint fluid is an essential part of treatment. In joints other than the hip, this can often be accomplished by one or more needle aspirations. In hip infections—and in arthritis of other joints when treatment is delayed or clinical response is slow—surgical drainage is advised.

D. Cellulitis, Including Orbital Cellulitis

Initial therapy for orbital cellulitis should be broad spectrum antibiotics. Once the organism is identified as *H influenzae* and susceptibilities are known, cefotaxime, ceftriaxone, or meropenem can be used depending on susceptibilities. Mixed infections are common and may require additional agents. Therapy is given parenterally for at least 3–7 days followed by oral treatment. There is usually marked improvement after 72 hours of treatment. The total antibiotic course will vary with the severity of the infection, response to therapy, the presence of an abscess, and whether drainage was performed. A minimum course of 21 days is reasonable in uncomplicated cases without abscess and good therapeutic response, assuming all signs of orbital cellulitis have completely resolved. In cases with severe ethmoid sinusitis and evidence of boney destruction at least a 4-week treatment course is advisable. Complicated cases may require longer treatment courses.

▶ Prognosis

The case fatality rate for invasive *H influenzae* is 15% but may be higher depending on the serotype. Young infants and older adults have the highest mortality rate. Hearing loss or other neurologic sequelae develop in 15%–30% of patients with Hib meningitis. Patients with Hib meningitis should have their hearing checked during the course of the illness or shortly after recovery. Children in whom invasive Hib infection develops despite appropriate immunization should have tests to investigate immune function and to rule out HIV. Deaths from epiglottitis are associated with bacteremia and the rapid development of airway obstruction. The prognosis for the other diseases requiring hospitalization is good with the early institution of adequate antibiotic therapy.

Briere EC, Rubin L, Moro PL, Cohn A, Clark T, Messonnier N; Division of Bacterial Diseases, National Center for Immunization and Respiratory Diseases, CDC: Prevention and control of *Haemophilus influenzae* type B disease: recommendations of the Advisory Committee on Immunization Practices (ACIP). MMWR Recomm Rep 2014;63(RR-01):114 [PMID: 24572654]. http://www.cdc.gov/mmwr/preview/mmwrhtml/rr6301a1.htm.

Centers for Disease Control and Prevention: Epidemiology and prevention of vaccine-preventable diseases. http://www.cdc.gov/vaccines/pubs/pinkbook/hib.html.

Soeters HM et al: Current epidemiology and trends in invasive *Haemophilus influenzae* disease—United States, 2009–2015. Clin Infect Dis 2018 Aug 31;67(6):881–889 [PMID: 29509834].

PERTUSSIS (WHOOPING COUGH)

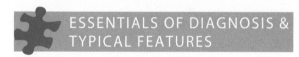

ESSENTIALS OF DIAGNOSIS & TYPICAL FEATURES

- ▶ Prodromal catarrhal stage (1–3 weeks) characterized by mild cough and coryza, but without fever.
- ▶ Persistent staccato, paroxysmal cough ending with a high-pitched inspiratory "whoop."
- ▶ Convalescent phase: slowly resolving cough over weeks to months.
- ▶ Leukocytosis with absolute lymphocytosis.
- ▶ Diagnosis confirmed by PCR of nasopharyngeal secretions.

▶ General Considerations

Pertussis is an acute, highly communicable infection of the respiratory tract caused by *Bordetella pertussis* that is characterized by severe bronchitis. Children usually acquire the disease from symptomatic family contacts. Adults and adolescents who have mild respiratory illness, not recognized as pertussis, frequently are the source of infection. Asymptomatic carriage of *B pertussis* has not been demonstrated. Infectivity is greatest during the catarrhal and early paroxysmal cough stage (for about 4 weeks after onset).

In the United States, more than 48,000 cases were reported in 2012, but rates in recent years have declined to approximately to 18,000—20,000/year; many cases go unreported. Pertussis is most severe in the very young. Fifty percent of children younger than 1 year with a diagnosis of pertussis are hospitalized. Fatality rates in infants younger than 2 months are approximately 2% and approximately 1% for infants in their first year of life.

The duration of immunity following natural pertussis is not known but is not lifelong. Reinfections are usually mild. Immunity following vaccination wanes in 5–10 years; thus the majority of young adults in the United States are susceptible to pertussis infection, and disease is probably common but unrecognized. Decreased efficacy of acellular vaccines (now standard in the United States) compared to whole-cell vaccines and low rates of immunization due to vaccine hesitancy in some communities have contributed significantly to pertussis epidemics in the United States.

Bordetella parapertussis and *Bordetella holmesii* cause a similar but milder syndrome.

B pertussis organisms attach to the ciliated respiratory epithelium and multiply there; deeper invasion does not occur. Disease is due to several bacterial toxins, the most potent of which is pertussis toxin, which is responsible for the typical lymphocytosis.

▶ Clinical Findings

A. Symptoms and Signs

The onset of pertussis is insidious, with catarrhal upper respiratory tract symptoms (rhinitis, sneezing, and an irritating cough). Fever above 38.3 is unusual and suggests an alternative diagnosis. After about 2 weeks, cough becomes paroxysmal, characterized by repeated forceful coughing ending with a loud inspiration (the whoop). Infants and adults with severe pertussis, as well as patients with milder pertussis, may lack the characteristic whoop. Vomiting commonly follows a paroxysm. Coughing may be accompanied by cyanosis, sweating, prostration, and exhaustion. Coughing fits occur more frequently at night. This stage lasts for 2–4 weeks, with gradual improvement. Paroxysmal coughing may continue for some months and may worsen with intercurrent viral respiratory infection. In adults, older children, and partially immunized individuals, symptoms may consist only of irritating cough lasting 1–2 weeks. Clinical pertussis is milder in immunized children.

B. Laboratory Findings

WBC counts of 20,000–30,000/μL with 70%–80% lymphocytes typically appear near the end of the catarrhal stage, and the degree of lymphocytosis correlates with the severity of disease. Severe pulmonary hypertension and hyperleukocytosis (> 70,000/μL) are associated with severe disease and death in young children with pertussis. The blood picture may resemble lymphocytic leukemia or leukemoid reactions. Many older children and adults with mild infections never demonstrate lymphocytosis.

The preferred method of diagnosis in most centers is identification of *B pertussis* by PCR from nasopharyngeal specimens. The organism may be found in the respiratory tract in diminishing numbers beginning in the catarrhal stage and ending about 2 weeks after the beginning of the paroxysmal stage. After several weeks of symptoms, PCR testing is frequently negative. Culture requires specialized media, careful attention to specimen collection and transport, and is now unavailable in many labs.

The chest radiograph reveals thickened bronchi and sometimes shows a "shaggy" heart border.

▶ Differential Diagnosis

In the catarrhal phase, pertussis is extremely difficult to discriminate from viral causes of upper respiratory infection. The differential diagnosis of pertussis includes bacterial (particularly *M pneumoniae*), tuberculous, chlamydial, and viral pneumonia. The absence of fever in pertussis differentiates this disease from most bacterial infections. Cystic fibrosis and foreign-body aspiration may be considerations with chronic cough. Adenoviruses and respiratory syncytial virus may cause paroxysmal coughing with an associated elevation of lymphocytes in the peripheral blood, mimicking pertussis.

▶ Complications

Bronchopneumonia due to superinfection is the most common serious complication. It is characterized by abrupt clinical deterioration during the paroxysmal stage, accompanied by high fever and sometimes a striking leukemoid reaction with a shift to predominantly polymorphonuclear neutrophils. Intercurrent viral respiratory infection is also a common complication and may provoke worsening or recurrence of paroxysmal coughing. Otitis media is common. Residual chronic bronchiectasis is an infrequent but serious complication. Apnea and sudden death may occur during a particularly severe paroxysm. Rib fractures may occur due to the force of coughing. Seizures complicate 1.5% of cases, and encephalopathy occurs in 0.1%. The encephalopathy frequently is fatal. Anoxic brain damage, cerebral hemorrhage, or pertussis neurotoxins are suggested contributors, but anoxia is most likely the cause. Epistaxis and subconjunctival hemorrhages are common. Rib fractures may occur due to forceful coughing.

In infants, choking, apnea, poor feeding, and failure to thrive are common.

Prevention

Active immunization (see Chapter 10) with DTaP (diphtheria, tetanus, and acellular pertussis) vaccine should be given in early infancy. The occurrence and increased recognition of disease in adolescents and adults contribute to the increasing number of cases. A booster dose of vaccine for adolescents between the ages of 11 and 18 years is recommended. Subsequent booster doses of Tdap are recommended for adults aged 18–60 years to replace Td boosters. Immunization of pregnant women in the last trimester prior to 36 weeks' gestation, new mothers, care givers of infants younger than 6 months, and health care workers of young children is also recommended.

Chemoprophylaxis with azithromycin should be considered for exposed family, household, and hospital contacts who are within 21 days since the onset of cough in the index case, particularly for pregnant women, children younger than 12 months, and people with chronic medical problems. Hospitalized children with pertussis should be isolated because of the great risk of transmission to patients and staff. Several large hospital outbreaks have been reported.

Treatment

A. Specific Measures

Antibiotics may ameliorate early infections (ie, in the catarrhal phase) but have no effect on clinical symptoms in the paroxysmal stage. Thus, treatment should be initiated as quickly as possible and should not wait for confirmatory testing in cases where the diagnosis is strongly suspected. Azithromycin (10 mg/kg/dose up to 500 mg on day 1, followed by 5 mg/kg/dose up to 250 mg daily for 4 more days) is the drug of choice because it promptly terminates respiratory tract carriage of *B pertussis*. Erythromycin given four times daily for 14 days is acceptable but not preferred. Resistance to macrolides has been rarely reported. TMP-SMX may also be used for erythromycin-intolerant patients. Erythromycin has been associated with pyloric stenosis in infants younger than 1 month, and azithromycin is preferred in this age. The risk of pyloric stenosis after azithromycin treatment is likely less, but cases have occurred. Parents of infants younger than 1 month who require treatment with azithromycin should be informed of this risk and counseled on the signs of pyloric stenosis.

B. General Measures

Nutritional support during the paroxysmal phase is important. Frequent small feedings, tube feeding, or parenteral fluid supplementation may be needed. Minimizing stimuli that trigger paroxysms is probably the best way of controlling cough. Though numerous medications have been proposed, including albuterol, corticosteroids, and diphenhydramine, there are no adequate clinical trials that identify an effective treatment for cough paroxysms.

C. Treatment of Complications

Respiratory insufficiency due to pneumonia or other pulmonary complications should be treated with oxygen and assisted ventilation if necessary. Convulsions are treated with appropriate supportive care and anticonvulsants. Bacterial pneumonia or otitis media may require additional antibiotics. Infants with an extremely high WBC count (> 70,000/μL) are at high risk of death and may benefit from extracorporeal membrane oxygenation (ECMO).

Prognosis

The prognosis for patients with pertussis has improved in recent years because of excellent nursing care, treatment of complications, attention to nutrition, and modern intensive care. However, the disease is still very serious in infants younger than 1 year; most deaths occur in this age group. Children with encephalopathy have a poor prognosis.

Atwell JE, Salmon DA: Pertussis resurgence and vaccine uptake: implications for reducing vaccine hesitancy. Pediatrics 2014;134(3):602 [PMID: 25116049].

Lumbreras AM et al. Antenatal vaccination to decrease pertussis in infants: safety, effectiveness, timing, and implementation. J Matern Fetal Neonatal Med 2019 May;32(9):1541–1546. doi: 10.1080/14767058.2017.1406475 [PMID: 29199493].

McGirr A, Fisman DN: Duration of pertussis immunity after DTaP immunization: a meta-analysis. Pediatrics 2015;135(2):331 [PMID: 25560446].

Wang K et al: Symptomatic treatment of the cough in whooping cough. Cochrane Database Syst Rev Sep 22, 2014;(9):CD003257. doi:10.1002/14651858.CD003257.pub5 [PMID: 25243777].

LISTERIOSIS

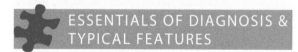

ESSENTIALS OF DIAGNOSIS & TYPICAL FEATURES

► Early-onset neonatal disease:
  • Signs of sepsis a few hours after birth in an infant born with fetal distress and hepatosplenomegaly; maternal fever.

► Late-onset neonatal disease:
  • Meningitis, sometimes with monocytosis in the CSF and peripheral blood.
  • Onset at age 9–30 days.

► Immunosuppressed patients:
  • Fever and meningitis.

General Considerations

Listeria monocytogenes is a gram-positive, non–spore-forming aerobic rod distributed widely in animals and in food, dust, and soil. It causes systemic infections in newborn infants and immunosuppressed older children. In pregnant women, infection is relatively mild, with fever, aches, and chills, but is accompanied by bacteremia and sometimes results in intrauterine or perinatal infection with grave consequences for the fetus or newborn. Pregnant women are particularly susceptible to listeriosis, and 20% of affected pregnancies end in stillbirth or neonatal death. In the United States, pregnant Hispanic women are 24 times more likely to contract listeriosis than the general population. Outbreaks of listeriosis have been associated with multiple foods, particularly unpasteurized dairy products including homemade Mexican-style cheese and prepared meats. Though cases have decreased since the adoption of strict regulations for ready-to-eat foods, outbreaks continue to occur in the United States; eight cases in four states associated with deli meats were reported by the CDC in 2019.

Clinical Findings

A. Symptoms and Signs

In the early neonatal form, symptoms of listeriosis usually appear on the first day of life and always by the third day. Fetal distress is common, and infants frequently have signs of severe disease at birth. Respiratory distress, diarrhea, and fever occur. On examination, hepatosplenomegaly and a papular rash are found. A history of maternal fever is common. Meningitis may accompany the septic course. The late neonatal form usually occurs after 9 days until as late as 5 weeks. Meningitis is common, characterized by irritability, fever, and poor feeding.

Listeria infections are rare in older children and usually are associated with immunodeficiency including treatment with tumor necrosis factor-α inhibitors. Signs and symptoms are those of meningitis or meningoencephalitis, often with insidious onset.

B. Laboratory Findings

In all patients except those receiving white cell depressant drugs, the WBC count is elevated, with 10%–20% monocytes. The characteristic CSF cell count in meningitis is high (> 500/μL) with a predominance of polymorphonuclear neutrophils, though monocytes may predominate in up to 30% of cases. *Listeria* are typically gram-positive rods, though they can be gram variable, and may be mistaken for "diphtheroids." Gram-stained smears of CSF are frequently negative. The chief pathologic feature in severe neonatal sepsis is miliary granulomatosis with microabscesses in the liver, spleen, CNS, lung, and bowel.

Culture results are frequently positive from multiple sites, including blood from the infant and the mother.

Differential Diagnosis

Early-onset neonatal disease resembles hemolytic disease of the newborn, GBS sepsis or severe cytomegalovirus infection or toxoplasmosis. Late-onset disease must be differentiated from meningitis due to echovirus and coxsackievirus, GBS, and gram-negative enteric bacteria.

Prevention

Immunosuppressed, pregnant, and elderly patients can decrease the risk of *Listeria* infection by avoiding soft unpasteurized cheeses, by thoroughly reheating or avoiding delicatessen and ready-to-eat foods, by avoiding raw meat and milk, and by thoroughly washing fresh vegetables.

Treatment

Ampicillin is the drug of choice in most cases of listeriosis. Gentamicin has a synergistic effect with ampicillin and should be given in serious infections and to patients with immune deficits; doses depend on age and birth weight. If ampicillin cannot be used, TMP-SMX is effective and achieves adequate levels in the CNS. Meropenem and linezolid are also active and may be used in certain scenarios. Vancomycin may be substituted for ampicillin when empirically treating meningitis. Cephalosporins are not active. Treatment of severe disease should continue for at least 2 weeks; meningitis is treated 21 days.

Controversy exists about the need for empiric *Listeria* coverage for a febrile neonate; factors such as disease severity, maternal illness, maternal risk factors (eg, exposure to unpasteurized cheese, early/severe onset of infection or suspected meningitis) make empiric coverage more prudent.

Prognosis

In a recent outbreak of early-onset neonatal disease, the mortality rate was 27% despite aggressive and appropriate management. Meningitis in older infants has a good prognosis.

Centers for Disease Control and Prevention (CDC): Listeriosis. http://www.cdc.gov/listeria/index.html. Accessed June 27, 2019.

Charlier C et al: Clinical features and prognostic factors of listeriosis: the MONOAISA national prospective cohort study. Lancet Infect Dis 2017;17(5):510–519 [PMID: 28139432].

McCollum JY et al: Multistate outbreak of listeriosis associated with cantaloupe. N Eng J Med 2013;369(10):944 [PMID: 24004121].

TUBERCULOSIS

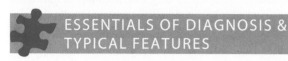

ESSENTIALS OF DIAGNOSIS & TYPICAL FEATURES

▶ All types: positive tuberculin test or interferon-γ release assay (IGRA) in patient or members of household, suggestive chest radiograph, history of contact, and demonstration of organism by stain and culture.

▶ Pulmonary: fatigue, irritability, weight loss, with or without fever and cough.

▶ Glandular: chronic cervical adenitis.

▶ Miliary: classic snowstorm appearance of chest radiograph.

▶ Meningitis: fever and manifestations of meningeal irritation and increased intracranial pressure, with characteristic CSF.

▶ General Considerations

Tuberculosis (TB) is a granulomatous disease caused by *Mycobacterium tuberculosis* (MTb). It is a leading cause of death throughout the world. Children younger than 5 years are most susceptible with highest risk in the first year of life. Primary infection occurs via the lungs with subsequent lymphohematogenous dissemination to extrapulmonary sites, including lymph nodes, the brain and meninges, bones and joints, kidneys, intestine, larynx, eyes, and skin. A greater proportion of pediatric TB disease is extrapulmonary compared to adults. Though TB is rare in many US communities, outbreaks in pediatric populations, particularly in schools do occur. Exposure to an infected adult is the most important risk factor for a pediatric patient. Groups at highest risk of TB infection are those who were born or lived in TB endemic countries and, to a lesser extent, US-born children with family members from endemic countries. Additional epidemiologic risk factors may include exposure to foreign-born persons, prisoners, residents of nursing homes, indigents, migrant workers, and health care providers. Rates of TB in American Indians, Asian, Hawaiian and Pacific Islanders, and Hispanic people are substantially greater than in Caucasians. Nationally about 1% if the TB cases are multiple drug resistant (MDR). HIV infection and other immune compromising diseases are important risk factors for both development and spread of disease.

An important distinction is the difference between TB infection and disease. In infection, there are no clinical or radiographic signs of active disease. This scenario is frequently referred to as latent tuberculosis infection (LTBI) and may affect up to one-quarter of the world population.

LTBI may progress (quickly in the very young, and often after decades of infection in older children and adults) to symptomatic disease that requires aggressive multidrug therapy.

Mycobacterium bovis infection is clinically identical to *M tuberculosis*, though extrapulmonary disease (particularly gastrointestinal) is more common with *M bovis*. *M bovis* may be acquired from unpasteurized dairy products obtained outside the United States.

▶ Clinical Findings

A. Symptoms and Signs

1. Latent Tuberculosis Infection—By definition, there are no symptoms or signs of LTBI, and diagnosis occurs in the context of a positive skin or blood test on TB screening.

2. Pulmonary—(See Chapter 19.)

3. Miliary—This manifestation of disseminated disease is common in young children and can be rapidly progressive. Affected children have fever, weight loss, or failure to thrive, and can become systemically unwell. Diagnosis is suggested by the classic "snowstorm" or "millet seed" appearance of lung fields on radiograph, although early in the course the chest radiograph may show only subtle abnormalities. Other tissues may be infected to produce osteomyelitis, arthritis, meningitis, tuberculomas of the brain, enteritis, or infection of the kidneys and liver.

4. Meningitis—Symptoms include fever, vomiting, headache, lethargy, and irritability, with signs of meningeal irritation and increased intracranial pressure, cranial nerve palsies, convulsions, and coma.

5. Lymphatic—Enlarged cervical lymph nodes usually present in a subacute manner. Involved nodes may become fixed to the overlying skin, suppurate, and drain.

B. Laboratory Findings

For decades, the tuberculin skin test (TST) has been the standard diagnostic tool for TB. However, the skin test has a number of disadvantages: Placement of TST can be difficult, measurement of induration can be subjective, it requires two health care visits to complete, the amount of induration that indicates a positive reaction varies with the epidemiologic risk and immune status of the patient (Table 42–3), and both false-positive and false-negative results occur. False-positive reactions are most common in children previously vaccinated with bacille Calmette-Guerin (BCG), though exposure to nontuberculous mycobacteria (NTM) can also lead to TST positivity. Approximately 75% of positive TSTs in BCG-vaccinated individuals (children and adults) may be due to the BCG rather than latent TB. This has significant implications for screening populations

Table 42–3. Interpretation of tuberculin skin test reactions.[a]

Degree of Risk	Risk Factors	Positive Reaction
High	Recent close contact with a case of active tuberculosis	≥ 5 mm induration
	Chest radiograph compatible with tuberculosis	
	Immune compromise; HIV infection	
Medium	Current or previous residence in high-prevalence area (Asia, Africa, Latin America)	≥ 10 mm induration
	Skin test converters within past 2 y	
	Intravenous drug use	
	Homeless or residence in a correctional institution	
	Recent weight loss or malnutrition	
	Leukemia, Hodgkin disease, or diabetes mellitus	
	Age < 4 y	
Low	Children ≥ 4 y without any risk factor	≥ 15 mm induration

[a]Standard intradermal Mantoux test, 5 test units. Measure perpendicular to the long axis of the arm. Induration only, not erythema, is measured.

from TB endemic countries where the majority of children receive BCG. False-negative reactions are also a concern, occurring in malnourished patients, those with overwhelming disease, and in 10% of children with isolated pulmonary disease. Temporary suppression of tuberculin reactivity may be seen with viral infections (eg, measles, influenza, varicella, and mumps), after live virus immunization, and during corticosteroid or other immunosuppressive drug therapy. For these reasons, a negative TST does not exclude the diagnosis of TB.

IGRAs measure in vitro release of interferon-γ from blood lymphocytes in response to TB-specific antigens. These assays, which have much higher specificity for MTb, do not react with antigens in BCG and the majority of NTM. IGRAs are done on blood obtained by venipuncture and require only a single visit. These tests are preferred in adults and BCG-immunized children older than 2 years. IGRAs are reported as positive, negative, or indeterminate.

Definitive diagnosis of TB disease requires microbiologic or molecular identification of *M tuberculosis*. However, children have pauci-bacillary disease and at young age are less able to produce sputa, even with induction. Cultures of pooled early morning gastric aspirates from 3 successive days will yield *M tuberculosis* in about 40% of cases, but smears

on gastric specimens are usually negative. Biopsy may be necessary to establish the diagnosis, but it may be difficult to justify invasive tests in mildly ill or asymptomatic children. Therapy should not be delayed in suspected cases. The CSF in tuberculous meningitis shows slight to moderate pleocytosis (50–300 WBCs/μL, predominantly lymphocytes), decreased glucose, and increased protein.

Acid-fast bacilli can be demonstrated on microscopy from patient samples. Culture for definitive identification and susceptibilities remains a mainstay of laboratory diagnosis, though nucleic amplification tests including the Xpert MTB/RIF are increasingly available and are able to rapidly identify *Mtb* genes associated with antimicrobial susceptibilities direct patient samples. Current World Health Organization (WHO) guidelines recommend utilization of Xpert testing on all sputa tested for TB.

C. Imaging

Chest radiograph should be obtained in all children with suspicion of TB at any site or with a positive TB test. Segmental consolidation with some volume loss and hilar adenopathy are common findings in children. Paratracheal adenopathy is a classic presentation. Pleural effusion also occurs with primary infection. Cavities and apical disease are unusual in children but are common in adolescents and adults. Computed tomography (CT) scanning more clearly demonstrates pathology in questionable cases but is unnecessary in the majority of cases.

▶ Differential Diagnosis

Pulmonary TB must be differentiated from fungal, parasitic, mycoplasmal, and bacterial pneumonias; lung abscess; foreign-body aspiration; lipoid pneumonia; sarcoidosis; and mediastinal cancer. Cervical lymphadenitis is most likely due to streptococcal or staphylococcal infections. Cat-scratch fever and infection with atypical mycobacteria may need to be distinguished from tuberculous lymphadenitis. Viral meningoencephalitis, head trauma (child abuse), lead poisoning, brain abscess, acute bacterial meningitis, brain tumor, and disseminated fungal infections must be excluded in tuberculous meningitis. A positive TST or IGRA in the patient or family contacts is frequently valuable in suggesting the diagnosis of TB. A negative TST or IGRA does not exclude TB.

▶ Prevention

A. BCG Vaccine

BCG vaccines are live-attenuated strains of *M bovis*. Although neonatal and childhood administration of BCG is carried out in countries with a high prevalence of TB, protective efficacy varies greatly with vaccine potency and method of delivery. BCG protects infants and toddlers against disseminated TB and meningitis but does not protect against pulmonary TB later in childhood or adolescence. In the United States where rates of

TB are low among US-born children, BCG vaccination is not recommended, in part because of challenges posed by potential false positive TST reactions in BCG-vaccinated children.

B. LTBI Treatment and Window Prophylaxis

Children with LTBI should be treated to prevent future development of TB disease. Traditionally, treatment with 9 months of isoniazid (9H) as been utilized, but shorter regimens of daily rifampin (15–20 mg/kg/day) for 4 months or once-weekly isoniazid/rifapentine (15 mg/kg/dose) are now preferred by many experts. These regimens have equal efficacy and better completion rates compared to 9H. Because it can take up to 8 weeks for IGRA or skin tests to convert after infection and disease can progress quickly in young children, exposed asymptomatic children younger than 5 years should receive treatment as for LTBI until repeat testing can be performed at least 8 weeks after the last exposure (window prophylaxis). If follow-up testing is positive, they can simply complete the LTBI treatment.

C. Other Measures

Prevention of TB in children requires identification and treatment of infectious adult cases in a community or within a household. Because children are not generally contagious, a pediatric case indicates an active adult case, often a family member in the household. Contact tracing through public health agencies and TB screening of high-risk individuals are the most effective ways to prevent pediatric TB cases. Routine TB testing is not recommended for children without risk factors who reside in communities with a low incidence of TB. Children with travel or immigration from a country with a high incidence of infection should be tested on entry to the United States or upon presentation to health care providers.

▶ Treatment

A. Specific Measures

Most children with suspected active TB do not require hospitalization. If the infecting organism has not been isolated from the presumed source (and therefore susceptibility testing is unavailable), reasonable attempts should be made to obtain it from the child using morning gastric aspirates, sputum, bronchoscopy, thoracentesis, or biopsy when appropriate. Unfortunately, cultures are frequently negative in children, and the risk of these procedures must be weighed against the yield.

Directly observed administration of all doses of antituberculosis therapy by a trained healthcare professional is essential to ensure compliance with therapy.

Most regimens for active TB infection begin with four drug therapy for the first 2 months. For example, children with active pulmonary disease receive isoniazid (10 mg/kg/day), rifampin (20 mg/kg/day), pyrazinamide (35 mg/kg/day),

and ethambutol (20 mg/kg/day) in single daily oral doses for 2 months, followed by isoniazid plus rifampin (either in a daily or thrice-weekly regimen) for 4 months. This is effective for eliminating isoniazid-susceptible organisms. For more severe disease, such as miliary or CNS infection, higher doses of drugs are used, and the duration of the two drug continuation phase is increased to 10 months or more. The duration of therapy is prolonged in immunocompromised children and if drug resistance necessitates alternative regimens and such patients should be managed in consultation with a TB specialist. TB meningitis is often treated with additional IV medications to achieve better CSF penetration, including levofloxacin, linezolid, and amikacin.

Drugs to treat TB are generally better tolerated in children than adults. Clinically significant hepatotoxicity is rare, and routine monitoring or liver function tests in otherwise healthy children is generally not required. Peripheral neuropathy associated with pyridoxine deficiency is rare in children, and it is not necessary to add pyridoxine unless significant malnutrition coexists or if the child is strictly breast-fed. Rifampin causes an orange color of urine and secretions, which is benign but may stain contact lenses or clothes. Rifampin alters the kinetics of many medications including some anticonvulsants and oral contraceptives.

Optic neuritis is the major side effect of ethambutol in adults; thus, there has been concern with use in children too young to screen for color discrimination. However, optic neuritis is rare and usually occurs in adults receiving more than the recommended dosage of 25 mg/kg/day. Since documentation of optic neuritis in children is lacking despite considerable worldwide experience, many four-drug regimens for children now include ethambutol.

B. Chemotherapy for Drug-Resistant Tuberculosis

The incidence of drug resistance is increasing and reaches 10%–20% in some areas of the United States. Transmission of MDR and extensively drug-resistant strains to contacts has occurred in some epidemics. Therapy should continue for 18 months or longer. Often, four to six first- and second-line medications including parenteral formulations are needed. Consultation with a local expert in treating TB is recommended.

C. General Measures

Corticosteroids may be used for suppressing inflammatory reactions in meningeal, pleural, and pericardial TB and for the relief of bronchial obstruction due to hilar adenopathy. Prednisone is given orally, 1 mg/kg/day for 2 weeks, with gradual withdrawal over the next 4–6 weeks. The use of corticosteroids may mask progression of disease. Accordingly, the clinician needs to be sure that an effective regimen is being used.

Prognosis

If bacteria are sensitive and treatment is completed, most children are cured with minimal sequelae. Repeat treatment is more difficult and less successful. Without treatment, the mortality rate in both miliary TB and tuberculous meningitis is almost 100%. In the latter form, about two-thirds of patients receiving treatment survive, but there may be a high incidence of neurologic abnormalities among survivors if treatment is started late.

Lewinsohn DM et al: Official ATS/CDC/IDSA clinical practice guidelines: diagnosis of tuberculosis in adults and children. Clin Infect Dis 2017;64(2):e1–e33 [PMID: 27932390].

Nahid P. et al. Official ATS/CDC/IDSA clinical practice guidelines: treatment of drug susceptible tuberculosis. Clin Infect Dis 2016;63(1 Oct):e147 [PMID: 31729908].

Starke JR: Improving tuberculosis care for children in high-burden settings. Pediatrics 2014;134(4):655 [PMID: 25266434].

Villarino ME et al: Treatment for preventing tuberculosis in children and adolescents: a randomized clinical trial of a 3-month, 12-dose regimen of a combination of rifapentine and isoniazid. JAMA Pediatr 2015 Mar;169(3):247–255. doi: 10.1001/jamapediatrics.2014.3158 [PMID: 25580725].

INFECTIONS WITH NONTUBERCULOUS MYCOBACTERIA

ESSENTIALS OF DIAGNOSIS & TYPICAL FEATURES

► Chronic unilateral cervical lymphadenitis.

► Granulomas of the skin.

► Chronic bone lesion with draining sinus (chronic osteomyelitis).

► TST of 5–8 mm, negative chest radiograph, and negative history of contact with TB.

► Diagnosis by positive culture.

► Disseminated infection in immunocompromised patients, particularly with AIDS.

General Considerations

More than 130 species of acid-fast mycobacteria other than *M tuberculosis* may cause subclinical infections and occasionally clinical disease resembling TB. Strains of NTM are common in soil, food, and water. Organisms enter the host by small abrasions in skin, oral mucosa, or gastrointestinal mucosa.

Mycobacterium avium complex (MAC), *Mycobacterium kansasii*, *Mycobacterium fortuitum*, *Mycobacterium abscessus*, *Mycobacterium marinum*, and *Mycobacterium chelonae* are most commonly encountered. *M fortuitum*, *M abscessus*, and *M chelonae* are "rapid growers" requiring 3–7 days for recovery in culture, whereas other mycobacteria require up to several weeks. After inoculation they form colonies closely resembling *M tuberculosis* morphologically.

Clinical Findings

A. Symptoms and Signs

1. Lymphadenitis—In children, the most common form of infection due to NTM is cervical lymphadenitis. In the United States MAC is the most common organism. A submandibular or cervical node swells slowly and is firm and initially somewhat tender. A purplish hue in the overlying skin is commonly noted. Low-grade fever may occur. Over time, the node may suppurate and drain chronically. Nodes in other areas of the head and neck and elsewhere are sometimes involved. Chronic intermittent drainage is common, but in many cases spontaneous healing occurs after 4–12 months.

2. Pulmonary disease—In the western United States, pulmonary disease is usually due to *M kansasii* or MAC. In the eastern United States and in other countries, disease is usually caused by MAC. In adults, there is usually underlying chronic pulmonary disease. Immune deficiency, particularly deficiency of cellular immunity, is commonly present. Presentation is clinically indistinguishable from that of TB. Adolescents with cystic fibrosis may be infected with NTM with resulting fever and declining pulmonary function.

3. Swimming pool granuloma—This is commonly due to *M marinum*. A solitary chronic granulomatous lesion with satellite lesions develops after minor trauma in infected swimming pools or other aquatic sources. Minor trauma during exposure to home aquariums or other aquatic environments may also lead to infection.

4. Chronic osteomyelitis—Osteomyelitis is caused by MAC, *M kansasii*, *M fortuitum*, or other rapid growers. Findings include swelling and pain over a distal extremity, radiolucent defects in bone, fever, and clinical and radiographic evidence of bronchopneumonia. Such cases are rare.

5. Disseminated infection—Disseminated infection occurs most often, though not exclusively, in children with immune deficiency. Children are ill, with fever and hepatosplenomegaly, and organisms are demonstrated in bone lesions, blood culture, lymph nodes, or liver. Chest radiographs are usually normal. Prior to antiretroviral therapy 60%–80% of patients with AIDS acquired disseminated MAC infection, characterized by fever, night sweats, weight loss, and diarrhea. Infection usually indicates severe immune dysfunction and is associated with CD4 lymphocyte counts less than 50/μL.

B. Laboratory Findings

In most cases, there is a negative or small reaction to TST (< 10 mm); larger reactions may be seen particularly with *M marinum* infection. IGRA tests are commonly negative although *M marinum, M kansasii*, and *M szulgai* may cause cross-reactions. The chest radiograph is negative, and there is no history of contact with a case of TB. Needle aspiration of the node excludes bacterial infection and may yield acid-fast bacilli on stain or culture. Fistulization should not be a problem because total excision is usually recommended for infection due to atypical mycobacteria. Cultures of any normally sterile body site may yield MAC in immunocompromised patients with disseminated disease. Blood cultures are frequently positive.

▶ Differential Diagnosis

See section on differential diagnosis in the previous discussion of TB and in Chapter 19.

▶ Treatment

A. Specific Measures

Medical therapy for NTM can be complex and it is prudent to obtain expert consultation for complicated, refractory or severe infections. The usual treatment of lymphadenitis is complete surgical excision after which antimicrobial therapy may be unnecessary. Conversely, many cases can be successfully treated nonsurgically. A typical regimen for cervical adenopathy involves multiple months of azithromycin, ethambutol, and/or rifampin. Susceptibility testing is useful to optimize therapy. More locally invasive or disseminated disease often requires a combination of three or more active drugs. A macrolide is typically a backbone of treatment, with addition of TMP-SMX, a rifamycin (eg, rifampin), ethambutol, an aminoglycoside (eg, amikacin), doxycycline, a fluoroquinolone (eg, ciprofloxacin), linezolid, or a carbapenem (eg, meropenem), depending on the infecting species and susceptibility patterns from culture. When *M tuberculosis* cannot be excluded, it is sometimes necessary to add a macrolide to typical four-drug MTb treatment regimens.

B. Chemoprophylaxis

Unsuccessfully treated children with HIV are given chemoprophylaxis with azithromycin to prevent disseminated MAC infection when CD4+ T-lymphocyte counts fall below age-specific levels. This is a rare scenario in the present era of highly active antiretroviral therapy.

C. General Measures

Isolation of the patient is usually not necessary. General supportive care is indicated for the child with disseminated disease.

▶ Prognosis

The prognosis is good for patients with localized disease, although fatalities occur in immunocompromised patients with disseminated disease.

Gallois Y et al: Nontuberculous mycobacterial lymphadenitis in children: what management strategy? Int J Pediatr Otorhinolaryngol 2019 Jul;122:196–202. doi: 10.1016/j.ijporl.2019.04.012 [PMID: 31039497].

Lopez-Varela E et al: Non-tuberculous mycobacteria in children: muddying the waters of tuberculosis diagnosis. Lancet Respir Med 2015;3(3):244 [PMID: 25773213].

LEGIONELLA INFECTION

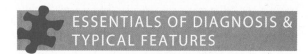

ESSENTIALS OF DIAGNOSIS & TYPICAL FEATURES

▶ Severe progressive pneumonia in a child with compromised immunity.

▶ Hospital-acquired infection can be due to contaminated water supply.

▶ Culture and urine antigen in suspected patients.

▶ General Considerations

Legionella pneumophila is a ubiquitous gram-negative bacillus that causes two distinct clinical syndromes: Legionnaires disease and Pontiac fever. *L pneumophila* causes most infections, though many other *Legionella* species can be pathogenic. *Legionella* is present in many natural water sources as well as domestic water supplies and fountains. In water, Legionella can reside inside amoebas, which may protect the organism from chlorination. Infection is thought to be acquired by inhalation of a contaminated aerosol. Contaminated cooling towers and heat exchangers have been implicated in several large institutional outbreaks, including health care facilities. Person-to-person transmission is extremely rare.

Legionella is rare in children. Most, but not all, cases occur in children with compromised cellular immunity, and neonates, particularly premature infants. In adults, risk factors include smoking, underlying cardiopulmonary or renal disease, alcoholism, and diabetes. Significant epidemiologic risk factors include travel (especially cruise ship) or a stay in a health care facility.

The bacteria are phagocytosed but proliferate within macrophages. Cell-mediated immunity is necessary to activate macrophages to kill intracellular bacteria.

Prevention

Ensuring proper disinfectant (eg, monochloramine rather than chlorine) and water temperature maintenance of building and municipal water systems is essential. Regular cleaning, attention to pH, and proper disinfectants in hot tubs are important.

Clinical Findings

A. Symptoms and Signs

Legionella can cause both community- and hospital-acquired pneumonia, often characterized by abrupt onset of fever, chills, anorexia, and headache. Pulmonary symptoms appear within 2–3 days and progress rapidly. The cough is nonproductive early. Purulent sputum occurs late. Hemoptysis, diarrhea, and neurologic signs (including lethargy, irritability, tremors, and delirium) are seen. Pontiac fever is a milder, self-limited flu-like illness not associated with pneumonia. In neonates infection can cause sepsis and cardiorespiratory failure.

B. Laboratory Findings

The WBC count is usually elevated with neutrophilia in Legionnaires disease. Chest radiographs show rapidly progressive patchy consolidation. Cavitation and large pleural effusions are uncommon. *Legionella* take up Gram stain poorly so may be observed during the initial microscopic examination of respiratory specimens. Cultures from sputum, tracheal aspirates, or bronchoscopic specimens, when grown on specialized media, are positive in 70%–80% of patients but can take up to 5 days to grow. Direct fluorescent antibody staining of sputum or other respiratory specimens is 95% specific but is only 25%–75% sensitive. A false-positive test can be seen in patients with tularemia. PCR detection of respiratory secretions for *Legionella* is available at some centers and is highly sensitive and specific. Urine antigen tests for *Legionella* antigen are rapid and highly specific but only detect *L pneumophila* serotype 1, which is the most common community-acquired *L pneumophila* infection. A positive urine antigen in a patient with pneumonia is strong evidence of the diagnosis.

Differential Diagnosis

Legionnaires disease is usually a rapidly progressive pneumonia in a patient who appears very ill with unremitting fevers, particularly those who have been hospitalized or who are immunodeficient. Other bacterial, viral, and fungal pathogens should be considered.

Complications

In sporadic untreated cases, mortality rates are 5%–25%. The mortality rate is less than 5% in normal hosts with early, appropriate therapy. In immunocompromised patients with untreated disease, mortality approaches 80%. Hematogenous dissemination may result in extrapulmonary foci of infection, including the pericardium, myocardium, and kidneys. *Legionella* may cause culture-negative endocarditis.

Treatment

Children with *Legionella* infection should be treated with levofloxacin (10 mg/kg/dose daily or BID depending on age, up to 750 mg) or azithromycin (10 mg/kg/day given as a once-daily dose up to 500 mg). Immunocompromised children should receive levofloxacin. Doxycycline and TMP-SMX are alternative agents. Duration of therapy is 5–10 days if azithromycin is used; for other antibiotics a 14- to 21-day course. Oral therapy may be substituted for intravenous therapy as the patient's condition improves. Pontiac fever does not require antibiotic treatment.

Prognosis

Mortality rate is high if treatment is delayed. Malaise, problems with memory, and fatigue are common after recovery.

Centers for Disease Control and Prevention: *Legionella*. http://www.cdc.gov/legionella/clinicians.html. Accessed June 27, 2019

Herwaldt LA et al: *Legionella*: a reemerging pathogen. Curr Opin Infect Dis 2018 Aug;31(4):325–333.

CHLAMYDOPHILA & CHLAMYDIA INFECTIONS (PSITTACOSIS, C PNEUMONIAE, & C TRACHOMATIS)

ESSENTIALS OF DIAGNOSIS & TYPICAL FEATURES

▶ Psittacosis:
- Fever, cough, malaise, chills, headache.
- Diffuse rales; no consolidation.
- Long-lasting radiographic findings of bronchopneumonia.
- Exposure to infected birds (ornithosis).

▶ Neonatal *Chlamydia* conjunctivitis:
- Watery, mucopurulent, to blood tinged discharge and conjunctival injection presenting from a few days of life until 16 weeks of age.
- May be associated with *Chlamydia* pneumonia.
- Identification of *Chlamydia* conjunctivitis or pneumonia in a neonate should prompt evaluation and treatment of the mother and her sexual partner.

▶ General Considerations

New taxonomic studies distinguish the genera *Chlamydophila* (*C psittaci, C pneumoniae*) and *Chlamydia* (*C trachomatis*) within the family Chlamydiaceae.

Psittacosis is a rare but potentially severe pulmonary infection caused by *Chlamydophila psittaci*, transmitted to humans from psittacine birds (parrots, parakeets, cockatoos, and budgerigars), as well as other avian species (eg, turkeys). Infections are rare in children, and human-to-human spread rarely occurs. The incubation period is 5–14 days. The bird from which the disease was transmitted may not be ill.

C pneumoniae (formerly *Chlamydia pneumoniae*) may cause atypical pneumonia similar to that due to *M pneumoniae*. Transmission is by respiratory spread. Lower respiratory tract infection due to *C pneumoniae* is uncommon in infants and young children and is most common in the second decade. *C pneumoniae* has been associated with acute chest syndrome in children with sickle cell disease.

C trachomatis causes urogenital infections in adults including asymptomatic infections, lymphogranuloma venereum, NGU, epididymitis, cervicitis, and pelvic inflammatory disease. Serovars D–K (and L1, L2, L3 in lymphogranuloma venereum) are responsible for most of these infections. Sexually transmitted urogenital infections caused by *C trachomatis* are discussed in Chapter 44. In infants born to infected mothers, *C trachomatis* infection can be acquired through exposure in the birth canal, causing neonatal conjunctivitis and/or pneumonia. The risk of acquisition for a baby born vaginally to an infected mother is as high as 30%.

Trachoma is a rare disease in the United States but is a major cause of disability in low-income countries. Trachoma is caused by certain *C trachomatis* serovars (A–C) that cause chronic keratoconjunctivitis that results in inflammation and neovascularization of the cornea, leading to corneal scarring and blindness. High rates of trachoma in a community are an indication for community antibiotic prophylaxis.

▶ Prevention

Care should be taken to avoid exposure to aerosolized *C psittaci* when handling birds and cleaning cages, particularly when the bird is sick. *C psittaci* is susceptible to a 1:100 dilution of household bleach. Sick birds should be evaluated by a veterinarian and treated with antimicrobials. *C pneumoniae* is transmitted person to person by infected respiratory tract secretions. Prevention involves avoidance of known infected persons, using good hand hygiene, and encouraging good respiratory hygiene (covering mouth with coughing, disposing of tissues contaminated with respiratory secretions).

The diagnosis and treatment of genital *Chlamydophila* (chlamydial) infections in pregnant women and their sexual partners is the most effective way to prevent neonatal conjunctivitis and pneumonia (see Chapter 44). Application of ocular prophylactic antibiotic after birth reduces gonococcal infection, but it is not effective at preventing *C trachomatis* infection.

▶ Clinical Findings

A. Symptoms and Signs

1. *C psittaci* pneumonia—The disease is extremely variable but tends to be mild in children. The onset is rapid or insidious, with fever, chills, headache, backache, malaise, myalgia, and dry cough. Signs include pneumonitis, altered percussion notes and breathe sounds, and rales. Pulmonary findings may be absent early. Dyspnea and cyanosis may occur later. Splenomegaly, epistaxis, prostration, and meningismus are occasionally seen. Delirium, constipation or diarrhea, and abdominal distress may occur.

2. *C pneumoniae* pneumonia—Clinically, *C pneumoniae* infection is similar to *M pneumoniae* infection. Most patients have mild upper respiratory symptoms. Lower respiratory tract infection is characterized by fever, sore throat, cough, and bilateral pulmonary findings and infiltrates. Many infections are mild and self-limited.

3. *C trachomatis* neonatal conjunctivitis and pneumonia—Neonatal conjunctivitis caused by *C trachomatis* can occur from a few days until 12–16 weeks after birth but is most common at 5–10 days (in contrast to gonococcal ophthalmia neonatorum which typically occurs before 5 days) (see Chapter 16). There may be mild to moderate swelling of the lids and watery or mucopurulent discharge. A pseudomembrane may be present, and the conjunctivae may be friable and there may be some bloody discharge. Pneumonia may occur in babies with or without neonatal conjunctivitis. Pneumonia is most commonly seen between 2 and 12 weeks of age. Most babies are afebrile, tachypneic, and have a staccato cough.

4. *C trachomatis* trachoma—Trachoma is seen in developing countries where poor hygienic conditions exist. It is the most common cause of acquired blindness worldwide. The peak incidence of trachoma is seen at 4–6 years of age, with scarring and eventual blindness occurring in adulthood. Infections occur from direct contact with infected secretions (eye, nose, throat) or by direct contact with contaminated objects (secretions on towels, washcloths, handkerchiefs).

B. Laboratory Findings

1. *C Psittaci*—In psittacosis, the WBC count is normal or decreased, often with a left shift. Proteinuria is common. Hepatitis is common in severe infections. *C psittaci* is present in the blood and sputum during the first 2 weeks of illness, but submitting cultures can represent a hazard to laboratory workers and should generally be avoided. Serologic testing is challenging and may be affected by antimicrobial treatment and cross-react with other chlamydial species. Acute and convalescent titers may help confirm infection but are impractical for therapeutic decisions; empiric treatment in the right clinical and exposure setting is common.

2. *C Pneumoniae*—Eosinophilia is sometimes present. PCR-based diagnosis from respiratory samples, which is increasingly available as part of a multiplex PCR platform, is rapidly replacing culture and serologic diagnostic methods.

3. *C trachomatis*—NAATs have largely replaced direct immunostaining methods for the diagnosis of chlamydia infections in children. In countries where the disease trachoma occurs, the diagnosis is often made clinically.

C. Imaging

The radiographic findings in psittacosis are those of central pneumonia that later becomes widespread or migratory. Psittacosis is indistinguishable from viral pneumonias by radiograph. Signs of pneumonitis may appear on radiograph in the absence of clinical suspicion of pulmonary involvement. Pneumonia from *C pneumoniae* produces variable radiographic findings including bilateral interstitial infiltrates or a unilateral subsegmental infiltrate. In neonatal pneumonia due to *C trachomatis*, infiltrates, and often hyperinflation, are seen.

▶ Differential Diagnosis

Psittacosis can be differentiated from viral or mycoplasmal pneumonias only by the history of contact with potentially infected birds. In severe or prolonged cases with extrapulmonary involvement the differential diagnosis is broad, including typhoid fever, brucellosis, and rheumatic fever.

C pneumoniae pneumonia is not distinguishable clinically from *Mycoplasma* or viral pneumonia.

C trachomatis conjunctivitis must be differentiated from gonococcal conjunctivitis, chemical conjunctivitis, or viral conjunctivitis. Gonococcal conjunctivitis is often severe, with purulent drainage. PCR of conjunctival discharge can aid in the diagnosis of gonococcal conjunctivitis.

▶ Complications

Complications of psittacosis include myocarditis, endocarditis, hepatitis, pancreatitis, and secondary bacterial pneumonia. *C pneumoniae* infection may be prolonged or may recur.

▶ Treatment

Psittacosis—Doxycycline is the preferred treatment and should be used for all critically ill children regardless of age. Alternatively, erythromycin or azithromycin may be used, though treatment failures with macrolides have been described.

Chlamydophila pneumonia—Many suspected atypical pneumonias are treated empirically. *C pneumoniae* responds to macrolides (azithromycin, 10 mg/kg/day on day 1, followed by 5 mg/kg/day on days 2–5). Doxycycline for 10–14 days is an alternative.

Neonatal conjunctivitis or pneumonia—Systemic antibiotic therapy is required for neonatal chlamydia infections, even when the only manifestation is conjunctivitis. Although the current consensus recommendation is a 10-day course of erythromycin base or ethylsuccinate (50 mg/kg/day given in four divided doses), treatment with azithromycin (20 mg/kg/day once daily for 3 days) appears effective and may increase compliance with treatment. Both erythromycin and azithromycin are associated with an increased risk of pyloric stenosis in infants and parents should be counseled to recognize the symptoms of this condition. The diagnosis of an infant with chlamydial conjunctivitis and/or pneumonia should prompt evaluation and treatment of the mother and her sexual partner for *Chlamydia* and other sexually transmitted diseases (see Chapter 44).

Trachoma is treated with a single dose of oral azithromycin (20 mg/kg/dose). Because trachoma is highly contagious, the WHO recommends community or regional mass treatment when the prevalence of trachoma among children exceeds 10%.

Centers for Disease Control and Prevention: Psittacosis. http://www.cdc.gov/pneumonia/atypical/psittacosis.html.

Pickering LK: American Academy of Pediatrics: chlamydial infections. *Red Book: 2018 Report of the Committee on Infectious Diseases.* 31st ed. Elk Grove Village, IL: American Academy of Pediatrics; 2015.

Zikic A et al: Treatment of neonatal chlamydial conjunctivitis: a systematic review and meta-analysis. J Pediatric Infect Dis Soc 2018 Aug 17;7(3):e107–e115 [PMID: 30007329].

CAT-SCRATCH DISEASE

ESSENTIALS OF DIAGNOSIS & TYPICAL FEATURES

▶ History of a cat scratch or cat contact.

▶ Primary lesion (papule, pustule, or conjunctivitis) at site of inoculation.

▶ Acute or subacute regional lymphadenopathy.

▶ Biopsy of node or papule showing histopathologic findings consistent with cat-scratch disease and occasionally characteristic bacilli on Warthin-Starry stain.

▶ Positive cat-scratch serology (antibody to *Bartonella henselae*).

General Considerations

The causative agent of cat-scratch disease is *B henselae*, a gram-negative bacillus that also causes bacillary angiomatosis. It is estimated that more than 20,000 cases per year occur in the United States, the majority of which are in the southeast. Children 5–9 years old have the highest incidence. Cat-scratch disease is usually a benign, self-limited form of lymphadenitis. Patients often report a cat scratch (67%), bite (less common), or contact with a cat or kitten (90%). The organism is transmitted among cats by fleas, and kittens are more likely to be bacteremic. Occasionally dogs can be infected and transmit disease.

Prevention

Cat-scratch disease can be largely prevented by avoiding cat scratches or bites, especially by kittens. Flea control of animals will reduce cat-to-cat transmission.

Clinical Findings

A. Symptoms and Signs

About 50% of patients with cat-scratch disease develop a primary lesion at the site of the wound. The lesion usually is a papule or pustule that appears 7–10 days after injury and is located most often on the arm or hand (50%), head or leg (30%), or trunk or neck (10%). The lesion may be conjunctival (10%). Regional lymphadenopathy appears 10–50 days later and may be accompanied by mild malaise, lassitude, headache, and fever. Multiple sites are seen in about 10% of cases. Involved nodes may be hard or soft and 1–6 cm in diameter. They are usually tender, warm, and erythematous and 10%–20% suppurate. Lymphadenopathy usually resolves in about 2 months but may persist for up to 8 months.

Unusual manifestations include erythema nodosum, thrombocytopenic purpura, conjunctivitis (Parinaud oculoglandular syndrome), parotid swelling, pneumonia, osteolytic lesions, mesenteric and mediastinal adenitis, neuroretinitis, peripheral neuritis, hepatitis, granulomata of the liver and spleen, and encephalopathy. Bartonella can cause a subacute endocarditis.

Immunocompetent patients may uncommonly develop a systemic form of cat-scratch disease. These patients have prolonged fever, fatigue, and malaise. Lymphadenopathy may be present. Hepatosplenomegaly or low-density hepatic or splenic lesions visualized by ultrasound or CT scan are seen in some patients.

Infection in immunocompromised individuals may take the form of bacillary angiomatosis, presenting as vascular tumors of the skin and subcutaneous tissues. Immunocompromised patients may also have bacteremia or infection of the liver (peliosis hepatis).

B. Laboratory Findings

Serologic evidence of *Bartonella* infection by indirect immunofluorescent antibody with IgG titer of more than 1:256 is strongly suggestive of recent infection. A positive IgM antibody is sometimes positive. Aspirated samples from infected lymph nodes can be tested for *Bartonella* by PCR. *Bartonella* is rarely isolated in culture.

Histopathologic examination of involved tissue may show pyogenic granulomas or bacillary forms demonstrated by Warthin-Starry silver stain (bacillary forms on stain are not specific for cat scratch disease). Later in the course necrotizing granulomas may be seen. In patients with CNS involvement, the CSF is usually normal but may show a slight pleocytosis and modest elevation of protein.

Differential Diagnosis

Cat-scratch disease must be distinguished from pyogenic adenitis, TB (typical and atypical), tularemia, brucellosis, lymphoma, primary toxoplasmosis, infectious mononucleosis, lymphogranuloma venereum, and fungal infections.

Treatment

Treatment of cat-scratch disease adenopathy is not always required because the disease typically resolves without therapy treatment. A 5-day course of azithromycin speeds resolution of lymphadenopathy. In one randomized placebo-controlled trial, lymph node volume decreased faster than placebo by 1 month, but there was no difference in long-term resolution in the azithromycin and placebo groups. In cases of nodal suppuration, needle aspiration under local anesthesia relieves the pain. Excision of the involved node is indicated in cases of chronic adenitis.

Immunocompromised patients with evidence of infection should be treated with antibiotics: long-term therapy (months) of these patients with azithromycin or doxycycline often is needed to prevent relapses. Immunocompetent patients with more severe disease or evidence of systemic infection (eg, hepatic or splenic lesions) should also be treated with antibiotics.

Prognosis

The prognosis is good if complications do not occur.

Angelakis E, Raoult D: Pathogenicity and treatment of *Bartonella* infections. Int J Antimicrob Agents 2014;44:16–25 [PMID: 24933445].

Centers for Disease Control and Prevention: Bartonella. http://www.cdc.gov/bartonella/clinicians/index.html. Accessed June 27, 2019.

Nelson CA, Saha S, Mead PS: Cat-scratch disease in the United States, 2005–2013. Emerg Infect Dis Oct 2016;22(10):1741–1746. doi: 10.3201/eid2210.160115 [PMID: 27648778].

▼ **SPIROCHETAL INFECTIONS**

SYPHILIS

 ESSENTIALS OF DIAGNOSIS & TYPICAL FEATURES

▶ Congenital:

- All types: history of untreated maternal syphilis, a positive serologic test, or a positive darkfield examination.
- Newborn: hepatosplenomegaly, characteristic radiographic bone changes, anemia, increased nucleated red cells, thrombocytopenia, abnormal spinal fluid, jaundice, edema.
- Young infant (3–12 weeks): snuffles, maculopapular skin rash, mucocutaneous lesions, pseudoparalysis (in addition to radiographic bone changes).
- Children: stigmata of early congenital syphilis, Hutchinson teeth, sensorineural hearing loss, interstitial keratitis, saber shins, gummas of nose and palate.

▶ Acquired:

- Chancre of genitals, lip, or anus in child or adolescent.
- History of sexual contact and a positive serologic test.

▶ **General Considerations**

Syphilis is a chronic, generalized infectious disease caused by a spirochete, *Treponema pallidum*. In the acquired form, the disease is transmitted by sexual contact. Primary syphilis is characterized by the presence of an indurated painless chancre, which heals in 7–10 days. A secondary eruption involving the skin and mucous membranes appears in 4–6 weeks. After a long latency period, late lesions of tertiary syphilis involve the eyes, skin, bones, viscera, CNS, and cardiovascular system.

Congenital syphilis results from transplacental infection. Infection may result in stillbirth or produce illness in the newborn, in early infancy, or later in childhood. Syphilis occurring in the newborn and young infant is comparable to secondary disease in the adult but is more severe and may be life threatening. Late congenital syphilis (developing in childhood) is comparable to tertiary disease.

The incidence of all forms of syphilis is increasing in the United States particularly among men who have sex with men. In 2017, there were over 900 cases of congenital syphilis and over 100,000 total reported cases.

▶ **Prevention**

A serologic test for syphilis should be performed at the initiation of prenatal care and should be repeated at delivery in women at increased risk for syphilis. Serologic tests may be negative on both the mother and infant at the time of birth if the mother acquires syphilis near term. Adequate treatment of mothers with secondary syphilis before the last month of pregnancy reduces the incidence of congenital syphilis from 90% to less than 2%. Examination and serologic testing of sexual partners and siblings should also be done.

▶ **Clinical Findings**

A. Symptoms and Signs

1. Congenital syphilis

A. NEWBORNS—Most newborns with congenital syphilis are asymptomatic. If infection is not detected and treated, symptoms develop within weeks to months. When clinical signs are present, they usually consist of jaundice, anemia with or without thrombocytopenia, increase in nucleated red blood cells, hepatosplenomegaly, and edema. Overt signs of meningitis (bulging fontanelle or opisthotonos) may be present, but subclinical infection with CSF abnormalities is more common.

B. YOUNG INFANTS (3–12 WEEKS)—The infant may appear normal for the first few weeks of life only to develop mucocutaneous lesions and pseudoparalysis of the arms or legs. Shotty lymphadenopathy may be felt. Hepatomegaly is universal, with splenomegaly in 50% of patients. Other signs of disease similar to those seen in the newborn may be present. Anemia has been reported as the only presenting manifestation of congenital syphilis in this age group. "Snuffles" (syphilitic rhinitis), characterized by a profuse mucopurulent discharge, is present in 15–25% of patients. A syphilitic rash is common on the palms and soles but may occur anywhere on the body. The rash consists of bright red, raised maculopapular lesions that gradually fade. Occasionally the rash is vesicular or bullous. Moist lesions occur at the mucocutaneous junctions (nose, mouth, anus, and genitals) and lead to fissuring and bleeding.

C. CHILDREN—Syphilis in later childhood may present with characteristic facial features such as rhagades (scars) around the mouth or nose, a depressed bridge of the nose (saddle nose), and a high forehead (secondary to mild hydrocephalus associated with low-grade meningitis and frontal periostitis). The permanent upper central incisors may be peg-shaped with a central notch (Hutchinson teeth), and the cusps of the sixth-year molars may have a lobulated mulberry appearance. Bilateral interstitial keratitis (at age 6–12 years) is characterized by photophobia, increased lacrimation, and vascularization of the cornea associated with exudation. Sensorineural hearing loss (at age 8–10 years), interstitial keratitis, and Hutchinson teeth comprise Hutchinson triad. Chorioretinitis and optic atrophy may also be seen. Meningovascular syphilis (at age 2–10 years) is usually slowly progressive, with mental retardation, spasticity, abnormal pupillary response, speech defects, and abnormal CSF. Thickening of the periosteum of the anterior tibias produces saber shins. A bilateral effusion in the knee joints may occur but is not associated with sequelae. Soft inflammatory growths called gummas may develop in the nasal septum, palate, long bones, and subcutaneous tissues.

2. Acquired syphilis—The primary chancre of the genitals, mouth, or anus may occur from genital, anal, or oral sexual contact. If the chancre is missed, signs of secondary syphilis, such as rash, fever, headache, and malaise, may be the first manifestations. Latent syphilis, by definition, lacks any clinical manifestations.

B. Laboratory Findings

1. Darkfield microscopy—Treponemes can be seen in scrapings from a chancre and from moist lesions, but darkfield examinations are not often available.

2. Serologic tests for syphilis—There are two general types of serologic tests for syphilis: treponemal and nontreponemal. The two nontreponemal tests, Venereal Disease Research Laboratory (VDRL) and the rapid plasma reagin (RPR), are useful for screening and may be quantitated to follow disease activity and adequacy of therapy. False-positive nontreponemal tests can occur in patient with measles, hepatitis, mononucleosis, lymphoma, TB, endocarditis, pregnancy, autoimmune diseases, and intravenous drug abuse. When evaluating a newborn for potential syphilis, umbilical cord blood specimens should not be used for nontreponemal tests: a false-positive test may result from Wharton jelly contamination of the sample. Conversely, a false-negative test may be seen in the setting where maternal infection occurred late in pregnancy.

Positive nontreponemal tests should be confirmed with a more specific treponemal test such as the fluorescent treponemal antibody absorbed (FTA-ABS) test or the *T pallidum* particle agglutination (TP-PA) test. False-positive FTA-ABS tests are uncommon except with other spirochetal diseases such as leptospirosis, rat bite fever, and Lyme disease.

One or two weeks after the onset of primary syphilis (chancre), the FTA-ABS test becomes positive. The nontreponemal tests usually turns positive a few days later. By the time the secondary stage has been reached, virtually all patients show both positive FTA-ABS and positive nontreponemal tests. During latent and tertiary syphilis, the VDRL may become negative, but the FTA-ABS test usually remains positive. The quantitative VDRL or RPR should be used to follow up treated cases (see following discussion).

EIA tests specific for *T pallidum* are available in many laboratories and are replacing FTA-ABS and TP-PA tests. As these are rapid, inexpensive tests with greater specificity, a "reverse" screening strategy is used by some laboratories. The initial screen is done with EIA test followed by the RPR or VDRL, if positive. If results are discordant, a third treponemal test such as the FTA-ABS or TP-PA may serve as a tie-breaker.

For evaluation of possible neurosyphilis, the CSF should be examined for cell count, glucose, protein, and a CSF VDRL. A negative CSF VDRL does not rule out neurosyphilis.

C. Imaging

Radiographic abnormalities are present in 90% of infants with symptoms of congenital syphilis and in 20% of asymptomatic infants. Metaphyseal lucent bands, periostitis, and a widened zone of provisional calcification may be present. Bilateral symmetrical osteomyelitis with pathologic fractures of the medial tibial metaphyses (Wimberger sign) is almost pathognomonic.

▶ Differential Diagnosis

A. Congenital Syphilis

1. Newborns—Sepsis, congestive heart failure, congenital rubella, toxoplasmosis, disseminated herpes simplex, cytomegalovirus infection, and hemolytic disease of the newborn have to be differentiated. A positive Coombs test and blood group incompatibility distinguish hemolytic disease.

2. Young infants—Injury to the brachial plexus, poliomyelitis, acute osteomyelitis, and septic arthritis must be differentiated from pseudoparalysis. Coryza due to viral infection often responds to symptomatic treatment. Rash (ammoniacal diaper rash) and scabies may be confused with a syphilitic eruption.

3. Children—Interstitial keratitis and bone lesions of TB are distinguished by positive tuberculin reaction and chest radiograph. Arthritis associated with syphilis is unaccompanied by systemic signs, and joints are nontender. Mental retardation, spasticity, and hyperactivity are shown to be of syphilitic origin by strongly positive serologic tests.

B. Acquired Syphilis

Herpes genitalis, traumatic lesions, and other venereal diseases must be differentiated from primary chancres.

▶ Treatment

A. Specific Measures

Penicillin is the drug of choice for *T pallidum* infection. If the patient is allergic to penicillin, desensitization should be attempted especially in neurosyphilis, congenital syphilis, syphilis during pregnancy, and with HIV infection. Azithromycin, ceftriaxone or one of the tetracyclines are alternative agents but are not proven efficacious.

1. Congenital syphilis

A. INITIAL EVALUATION AND TREATMENT—Newborns should not be discharged from the hospital until the mother's serologic status for syphilis has been determined. Infants born to seropositive mothers require careful examination and quantitative nontreponemal syphilis testing. The same quantitative nontreponemal test used in evaluating the mother should be used in the infant so the titers can be compared. Maternal records regarding any prior diagnosis of syphilis, treatment, and follow-up titers should be reviewed. Infants should be further evaluated for congenital syphilis in any of the following circumstances:

- The infant's titer is at least fourfold greater than the maternal titer.
- Signs of syphilis are found on examination.
- Maternal syphilis was not treated or was inadequately treated during pregnancy.
- Maternal syphilis was treated with a nonpenicillin regimen, or the regimen or dose of medication is undocumented.
- Maternal syphilis was treated during pregnancy, but therapy was completed less than 4 weeks prior to delivery.
- Maternal syphilis was treated appropriately during pregnancy, but without the appropriate decrease in maternal nontreponemal titers after treatment.

The complete evaluation of an infant for possible congenital syphilis includes complete blood count, liver function tests, long bone radiographs, CSF examination (cell counts, glucose, and protein), CSF VDRL, and quantitative serologic tests. In addition, the placenta and umbilical cord, if available, should be examined pathologically using fluorescent treponemal antibody. If clinically indicated, ophthalmologic examination, auditory brainstem response, chest radiograph, and cranial ultrasound may also be done.

Treatment for congenital syphilis is indicated for infants with consistent physical signs, umbilical cord or placenta positive for DFA-TP staining or darkfield examination, abnormal radiographs, elevated CSF protein or cell counts, reactive CSF VDRL, or serum quantitative nontreponemal titer that is more than fourfold higher than the maternal titer (using same test). Newborns with proven or highly probable congenital syphilis should receive (1) aqueous crystalline penicillin G, 50,000 U/kg per dose intravenously every 12 hours (if < 1 week old) or (2) every 8 hours (if 1–4 weeks old) for 10 days. Procaine

penicillin G, 50,000 U/kg in a single daily intramuscular dose for 10 days is an alternative if compliance is assured. All infants diagnosed after age 4 weeks should receive 50,000 U/kg per dose aqueous crystalline penicillin intravenously every 4–6 hours for 10 days.

Additionally, treatment should be given to infants whose mothers have inadequately treated syphilis, whose mothers received treatment less than 1 month before delivery, whose mothers have undocumented or inadequate serologic response to therapy, and whose mothers were given nonpenicillin drugs to treat syphilis. In these instances, if the infant is asymptomatic, has a normal physical examination, normal CSF parameters, nonreactive CSF VDRL, normal bone films, quantitative nontreponemal titer less than fourfold of the mother's titer, and good follow-up is certain, some experts would give a single dose of penicillin G benzathine, 50,000 U/kg intramuscularly. If there is any abnormality in the preceding evaluation or if the CSF testing is not interpretable, the full 10 days of intravenous penicillin should be given. Close clinical and serologic monthly follow-up is necessary.

Asymptomatic, seropositive infants with normal physical examinations born to mothers who received adequate syphilis treatment (completed > 4 weeks prior to delivery) and whose mothers have an appropriate serologic response (fourfold or greater decrease in titer) to treatment may be at lower risk for congenital syphilis. Some experts believe complete laboratory and radiographic evaluation in these infants (CSF and long bone films) is not necessary. Infants who meet the preceding criteria, who have nontreponemal titers less than fourfold higher than maternal titers, and for whom follow-ups are certain can be given benzathine penicillin G, 50,000 U/kg intramuscularly in a single dose. Infants should be followed with quantitative serologic tests and physical examinations until the nontreponemal serologic test is negative (see discussion of follow-up, next). Rising titers or clinical signs require a full evaluation (including CSF studies and long bone radiographs) and institution of intravenous penicillin therapy, even if previously treated.

B. FOLLOW-UP FOR CONGENITAL SYPHILIS—Children treated for congenital syphilis need both physical examinations and quantitative VDRL or RPR tests performed every 2–3 months until the tests become nonreactive. Repeat CSF examination, including a CSF VDRL test every 6 months until normal, is indicated for infants with an initial positive CSF VDRL reaction or with abnormal cell counts or protein in the CSF. A reactive CSF VDRL test or abnormal CSF indices at the 6-month interval is an indication for retreatment. Serum titers decline with treatment and are usually negative by 6 months. Repeat treatment is indicated for children with rising titers or stable serum titers that do not decline.

2. Acquired syphilis of less than 1 year's duration—
Benzathine penicillin G (50,000 U/kg, given intramuscularly, to a maximum of 2.4 million units) is given to adolescents with primary, secondary, or latent disease of less than 1 year's duration. All children with recently diagnosed or suspected syphilis should have a CSF examination (with CSF VDRL) prior to commencing therapy, to exclude neurosyphilis. Adolescents and adults need a CSF examination if clinical signs or symptoms suggest neurologic involvement or if they are HIV infected.

3. Syphilis of more than 1 year's duration (late latent disease)—Syphilis of more than 1 year's duration (without evidence of neurosyphilis) requires weekly intramuscular benzathine penicillin G therapy for 3 weeks. CSF examination and VDRL test should be done on all children and patients with coexisting HIV infection, or neurologic or ophthalmic symptoms, or evidence of active tertiary syphilis. In addition, patients who have failed treatment or who were previously treated with an agent other than penicillin need a CSF examination and CSF VDRL.

4. Neurosyphilis—Aqueous crystalline penicillin G is recommended, 50,000 U/kg/dose every 4–6 hours, given intravenously for 10–14 days. The maximum adult dose is 4 million units per dose. Some experts recommend following this regimen with an intramuscular course of benzathine G penicillin, 50,000 U/kg given once a week for 3 consecutive weeks, to a maximum dose of 2.4 million units.

B. General Measures

Penicillin treatment of early congenital, primary, or secondary syphilis may result in a dramatic systemic febrile illness termed the Jarisch-Herxheimer reaction. Treatment is symptomatic, with careful follow-up.

Prognosis

Severe disease, if undiagnosed, may be fatal in the newborn. Complete cure can be expected if the young infant is given penicillin. Serologic reversal usually occurs within 1 year. Treatment of primary syphilis with penicillin is curative. Permanent neurologic sequelae may occur in meningovascular syphilis.

Centers for Disease Control and Prevention: 2017 Sexually Transmitted Diseases Surveillance: syphilis. https://www.cdc.gov/std/stats17/Syphilis.html. Accessed July 24, 2018.

Syphilis. In: Kimberlin DW, Brady MT, Jackson MA, Long SS (eds): *Red Book: 2018–2021 Report of the Committee on Infectious Diseases.* 31st ed. Itasca, IL: American Academy of Pediatrics; 2018:773–787.

Workowski KA: Sexually transmitted diseases treatment guidelines, 2015. MMWR Recomm Rep 2015 Jun 5;64(RR-03):1137. Erratum in MMWR Recomm Rep 2015Aug 28;64(33):924 [PMID: 26042815].

RELAPSING FEVER

ESSENTIALS OF DIAGNOSIS & TYPICAL FEATURES

► Episodes of relapsing fever, chills, malaise.

► Occasional rash, arthritis, cough, hepatosplenomegaly, conjunctivitis.

► Diagnosis confirmed by direct microscopic identification of spirochetes in smears of peripheral blood.

General Considerations

Relapsing fever is a vector-borne disease caused by spirochetes of the genus *Borrelia*. There are two forms: Epidemic relapsing fever is transmitted to humans by body lice (*Pediculus humanus*) and endemic relapsing fever by soft-bodied ticks (genus *Ornithodoros*). Tick-borne relapsing fever, most commonly due to *Borrelia hermsii*, is endemic in the western United States, and infection is commonly associated with tick exposure in mountain cabins. Transmission usually takes place during the warm months, though winter cases occur in warmer climes and in cabins that have been heated. *Ornithodoros* ticks are nocturnal feeders and remain attached for only 5–20 minutes. Consequently, the patient seldom remembers a tick bite. As the adaptive immune system begins to produce antibodies, *B hermsii* uses genetic recombination to modify its surface antigens, resulting in relapse. Louse-borne relapsing fever was a cause of significant mortality in the early 20th century and World War I. It remains a major health problem among displaced and refugee populations.

Clinical Findings

A. Symptoms and Signs

The incubation period is 2–18 days. The attack is sudden, with high fever, chills, sweats, tachycardia, nausea and vomiting, headache, myalgia, and arthralgia. Febrile episodes classically last 3 days and end abruptly and dramatically (chill phase, flush phase). If untreated, relapses typically occur at 1-week intervals. The relapses duplicate the initial attack but become progressively less severe. In louse-borne relapsing fever, there is usually a single relapse. In tick-borne infection, 2–10 relapses occur.

Hepatomegaly, splenomegaly, pneumonitis, meningitis, and myocarditis may appear later in the course of the disease. An erythematous rash may be seen over the trunk and extremities, and petechiae may be present. Jaundice, iritis, conjunctivitis, cranial nerve palsies, and hemorrhage occur more commonly during relapses.

B. Laboratory Findings

During febrile episodes, the patient's urine contains protein, casts, and occasionally erythrocytes; a marked polymorphonuclear leukocytosis is present; about 25% of patients have a false-positive serologic test for syphilis. Spirochetes can be found in the peripheral blood by direct microscopy in approximately 70% of cases by darkfield examination or by Wright, Giemsa, or acridine orange staining of thick and thin smears. Spirochetes are not found during afebrile periods. Immunofluorescent antibody (or enzyme-linked immunosorbent assay [ELISA] confirmed by Western blot) can help establish the diagnosis serologically. However, high titers of *B hermsii* can cross-react with *Borrelia burgdorferi* (the agent in Lyme disease) or *Leptospira*. Serologic testing is available at laboratories in many western US state health departments or through the CDC.

Differential Diagnosis

Relapsing fever may be confused with malaria, leptospirosis, dengue, typhus, rat-bite fever, Colorado tick fever, Rocky Mountain spotted fever, and collagen-vascular disease.

Complications

Complications include facial paralysis, iridocyclitis, optic atrophy, hypochromic anemia, pneumonia, nephritis, myocarditis, endocarditis, and seizures. CNS involvement occurs in 10%–30% of patients.

Treatment

Doxycycline is the treatment of choice for children with tickborne relapsing fever, regardless of age. Severe disease has also been successfully treated with initial use of IV ceftriaxone or IV penicillin G. Louse-borne relapsing fever is most commonly treated with tetracycline or erythromycin.

Severely ill patients should be hospitalized. Patients may experience a Jarisch-Herxheimer reaction (usually noted in the first few hours after commencing antibiotics). Isolation precautions are not necessary for relapsing fever.

Prevention

Measures that decrease exposures to soft ticks and body lice will prevent most cases. Soft-bodied ticks often are found in rodent burrows or nests, so rodent (the tick reservoir host) control, particularly in mountain cabins, is important.

The mortality rate in treated cases of relapsing fever is very low, except in debilitated or very young children. With treatment, the initial attack is shortened and relapses are prevented.

Centers for Disease Control: Relapsing fever. http://www.cdc.gov/relapsing-fever/. Accessed June 28, 2019.

Forrester JD et al: Tickborne relapsing fever—United States, 1990–2011. MMWR Morb Mortal Wkly Rep 2015 Jan 30; 64(3):58–60 [PMID: 25632952].

Warrell DA: Louse-borne relapsing fever (*Borrelia recurrentis* infection). Epidemiol Infect 2019 Jan;147:e106 [PMID: 30869050].

LEPTOSPIROSIS

ESSENTIALS OF DIAGNOSIS & TYPICAL FEATURES

► Classic course is biphasic lasting 2–3 weeks.

► Initial phase: high fever, headache, myalgia, and conjunctivitis.

► Apparent recovery for 2–3 days.

► Return of fever associated with meningitis.

► Jaundice, hemorrhages, and renal insufficiency (severe cases).

► Positive leptospiral agglutination test.

General Considerations

Leptospirosis is a zoonosis caused by many antigenically distinct but morphologically similar spirochetes. The organism enters through the skin or respiratory tract after exposure to infectious animal urine or contaminated water or soil. A variety of animals (eg, dogs, rats, and cattle) may serve as reservoirs for pathogenic *Leptospira*, and severe disease may be caused by many different serogroups.

In the United States, leptospirosis usually occurs after contact with infected dogs. Cattle, swine, or rodents may transmit the organism. Sewer workers, farmers, slaughterhouse workers, animal handlers, and soldiers are at risk for occupational exposure. Outbreaks have resulted from swimming in contaminated streams and harvesting field crops. Floods and hurricanes can increase risk in affected populations. In the United States, about 100 cases are reported yearly, about one-third of them in children. The highest US rates of leptospirosis infection occur in Hawaii. Leptospirosis occurs throughout the developing world, particularly in the tropics. Leptospirosis is an important consideration in returned travelers with febrile illness, particularly if there is a history of fresh-water exposure.

Prevention

Preventive measures with endemic exposure include avoidance of contaminated water and soil—particularly with mucous membranes or nonintact skin, rodent control, immunization of dogs and other domestic animals and avoidance of contact with animal urine.

Clinical Findings

A. Symptoms and Signs

1. Initial phase—The incubation period is 4–19 days (mean, 10 days). Chills, fever, headache, myalgia (especially lumbar area and calves), conjunctivitis without exudate, photophobia, cervical lymphadenopathy, and pharyngitis commonly occur. The initial leptospiremic phase lasts for 3–7 days.

2. Phase of apparent recovery—Symptoms typically (but not always) subside for 2–3 days.

3. Systemic phase—Fever reappears and is associated with headache, muscular pain, tenderness in the abdomen and back, and nausea and vomiting. Conjunctivitis and uveitis are common. Lung, heart, and joint involvements occasionally occur. These manifestations are due to extensive vasculitis.

A. CNS INVOLVEMENT—The CNS is involved in 50%–90% of cases. Severe headache and mild nuchal rigidity are usual, but delirium, coma, and focal neurologic signs may be seen.

B. RENAL AND HEPATIC INVOLVEMENT (WEIL SYNDROME)—In about 50% of cases, the kidneys or liver is affected. Gross hematuria and oliguria or anuria is sometimes seen. Jaundice may be associated with an enlarged and tender liver.

C. GALLBLADDER INVOLVEMENT—Leptospirosis may cause acalculous cholecystitis in children, demonstrable by abdominal ultrasound as a dilated, nonfunctioning gallbladder. Pancreatitis is unusual.

D. HEMORRHAGE—Petechiae, ecchymoses, and gastrointestinal bleeding may be severe.

E. RASH—A rash is seen in 10%–30% of cases. It may be maculopapular and generalized or may be petechial or purpuric. Occasionally erythema nodosum is seen. Peripheral desquamation of the rash may occur. Gangrenous areas are sometimes noted over the distal extremities. In such cases, skin biopsy demonstrates the presence of severe vasculitis involving both the arterial and the venous circulations.

B. Laboratory Findings

Leptospires are present in the blood and CSF only during the first 10 days of illness. They appear in the urine during the second week, where they may persist for 30 days or longer. Culture is difficult and requires specialized media and conditions. The WBC count often is elevated, especially when there is liver involvement. Other liver function tests may be abnormal; the aspartate transaminase usually is only slightly elevated. An elevated serum creatine kinase is frequently found. CSF shows moderate pleocytosis (< 500/μL), predominantly mononuclear cells, increased protein (50–100 mg/dL), and normal glucose. Urine often shows microscopic pyuria, hematuria, and, less often, moderate proteinuria (or greater). The ESR is elevated markedly. Chest radiograph may show pneumonitis.

Serum antibodies measured by enzyme immunoassay may be demonstrated during or after the second week of illness. The confirmatory test is a microscopic agglutination test performed at the CDC. Leptospiral agglutinins generally reach peak levels by the third to fourth week. Fourfold or greater titer rise in acute and convalescent specimens is diagnostic. PCR-based assays are increasingly available at specialized research centers or through the CDC.

Differential Diagnosis

During the prodrome, malaria, typhoid fever, murine typhus, rheumatoid arthritis, brucellosis, and influenza may be suspected. Later, depending on the organ systems involved, a variety of other diseases need to be distinguished, including encephalitis, viral or tuberculous meningitis, viral hepatitis, glomerulonephritis, viral or bacterial pneumonia, rheumatic fever, subacute infective endocarditis, acute surgical abdomen, and Kawasaki disease (see Table 40–3).

Treatment

A. Specific Measures

Aqueous penicillin G (150,000 U/kg/day in four to six divided doses intravenously for 7–10 days) should be given when the diagnosis is suspected. Alternative agents include parenteral ceftriaxone or doxycycline. A Jarisch-Herxheimer reaction may occur. Oral doxycycline may be used for mildly ill patients.

B. General Measures

Symptomatic and supportive care, in addition to antibiotics, is indicated. Renal failure may require dialysis.

Prognosis

Leptospirosis is usually self-limiting and not characterized by jaundice. The disease usually lasts 1–3 weeks but may be more prolonged. Relapse may occur. There are usually no permanent sequelae associated with CNS infection, although headache may persist. The mortality rate in the United States is 5%, usually from renal failure. The mortality rate may reach 20% or more in elderly patients who have severe kidney and hepatic involvement.

Bourke DL, Vinetz JM: Illnesses associated with freshwater recreation during international travel. Curr Infect Dis Rep 2018 May 22;20(7):19 [PMID: 29789961].

Centers for Disease Control and Prevention: Leptospirosis. http://www.cdc.gov/leptospirosis/infection/index.html. Accessed June 28, 2019.

Haake DA et al: Leptospirosis in humans. Curr Top Microbiol Immunol 2015;387:65–97 [PMID: 25388133].

LYME DISEASE

ESSENTIALS OF DIAGNOSIS & TYPICAL FEATURES

▶ Early localized disease: characteristic skin lesion (erythema migrans [EM]) 3–30 days after tick bite.

▶ Early disseminated: multiple EM, constitutional symptoms, cranial nerve palsies, meningitis.

▶ Late disease: arthritis, usually pauciarticular, occurring about 4 weeks after appearance of skin lesion.

▶ Residence or travel in an endemic area during the late spring to early fall.

▶ General Considerations

Lyme disease is a subacute or chronic spirochetal infection caused by *B burgdorferi* that is transmitted by an infected deer tick (*Ixodes* species). The most prominent endemic areas in the United States include the Northeast and upper Midwest. Although both under- and overreporting occur, it is estimated that more than 300,000 cases per year occur in the United States. Knowledge of the local epidemiology is important as Lyme disease is common in certain areas of the United States, but very rare in others. Most cases with rash are recognized in spring and summer, when most tick bites occur; however, because the incubation period for joint and neurologic disease may be months, cases may present at any time. *Ixodes* ticks are very small, and their bite is often unrecognized.

▶ Clinical Findings

A. Symptoms and Signs

Early localized disease: Erythema migrans (EM), the most characteristic feature of Lyme disease, is recognized in 60%–80% of patients. Between 3 and 30 days after the bite, a ring of erythema develops at the site and spreads over days. It may attain a diameter of 20 cm. The center of the lesion may clear (resembling tinea corporis), remain red, or become raised (suggesting infectious cellulitis). Mild tenderness may occur. Most patients are otherwise asymptomatic, but mild constitutional symptoms may occur. Untreated, the rash lasts days to 3 weeks.

Early disseminated disease: Multiple satellite EM lesions, urticaria, or diffuse erythema may occur. Fever, headache, myalgias and constitutional symptoms are more common than in localized disease. Neurologic manifestations, which develop in up to 20% of untreated patients, commonly include Bell palsy, aseptic meningitis, or polyradiculitis, alone or in

various combinations. Peripheral neuritis, Guillain-Barré syndrome, encephalitis, ataxia, chorea, and other cranial neuropathies are less common. Seizures suggest another diagnosis. Untreated, the neurologic symptoms are usually self-limited but may be chronic or permanent. Self-limited heart block or myocardial dysfunction occurs in less than 5% of patients.

Late disease: In up to 50% of untreated patients, arthritis develops several weeks to months after the bite. Recurrent attacks of migratory, monoarticular, or pauciarticular arthritis involving the knees (90%) and other large joints occur. Pain is often less pronounced than swelling. Each attack lasts for days to a few weeks. Fever is common and may be high. Complete resolution between attacks is typical. Chronic arthritis develops in less than 10% of patients, more often in those with the DR4 haplotype. Neurologic manifestations of late disease are uncommon.

Although fatigue and nonspecific neurologic symptoms may be prolonged in a few patients, Lyme disease is not a cause of chronic fatigue syndrome. Persistence of symptoms of fatigue, myalgia, and arthralgia for greater than 6 months are termed posttreatment Lyme disease syndrome, but there is no evidence that chronic Lyme infection exists, nor is there any evidence of benefit from antibiotic therapy in patients properly treated for Lyme disease.

B. Laboratory Findings

Most patients with only rash have normal laboratory tests. Children with arthritis may have moderately elevated ESRs and WBC counts; the antinuclear antibodies and rheumatoid factor tests are negative or nonspecific; streptococcal antibodies are not elevated. Joint fluid may show up to 100,000 cells with a polymorphonuclear predominance, normal glucose, and elevated protein and immune complexes; Gram stain and culture are negative. In patients with CNS involvement, the CSF may show lymphocytic pleocytosis and elevated protein; the glucose and all cultures and stains are negative. Papilledema may be present on fundoscopic examination. Abnormal nerve conduction may be present with peripheral neuropathy. Electrocardiogram (ECG) may show carditis in early disseminated disease.

C. Diagnosis

Lyme disease is a clinical diagnosis. Local epidemiology, history of travel to endemic areas, physical examination, and laboratory features are important to consider. Serologic testing may support the clinical diagnosis. Serologic diagnosis of Lyme disease is based on a two-test approach: an antibody screen (IgM and/or IgG) with an immunoblot to confirm a positive or indeterminate screening test. Antibodies may not be detectable until several weeks after infection has occurred; therefore, serologic testing in children with a typical acute EM rash is not recommended. Therapy early in disease may blunt antibody titers. Serologic testing of patients with nonspecific complaints from low prevalence areas results in falsely positive tests, particularly when ordered through "specialty" labs. Sera from patients with syphilis, HIV, and leptospirosis may give false-positive results. Diagnosis of CNS disease requires objective abnormalities of the neurologic examination, laboratory or radiographic studies, and consistent positive serology.

Differential Diagnosis

EM rash may resemble pityriasis, erythema multiforme, a drug eruption, or erythema nodosum. Southern tick-associated rash illness (STARI) is an uncommon condition associated with a bite from the lone-star tick (*Amblyomma americanum*), which can result in a rash and clinical syndrome indistinguishable from acute Lyme infection. Lyme cases with more severe manifestations (especially hematologic or hepatic abnormalities) may represent co-infection with Anaplasma or Babesia. The arthritis may resemble juvenile rheumatoid arthritis, reactive arthritis, septic arthritis, rheumatic fever, poststreptococcal arthritis/acute rheumatic fever, systemic lupus erythematosus, and Henoch-Schönlein purpura. The neurologic signs may suggest idiopathic Bell palsy, viral or parainfectious meningitis or meningoencephalitis, lead poisoning, and psychosomatic illness.

Prevention

Prevention consists of avoidance of endemic areas or if in these areas wearing long sleeves and pants, frequent checks for ticks, and application of tick repellents. Ticks are attached for a minimum of 36–48 hours before transmission of Lyme disease occurs. Ticks should be removed with a tweezer by pulling gently without twisting or excessive squeezing of the tick. Permethrin sprayed on clothing decreases tick attachment. Repellents containing high concentrations of N,N-Diethyl-meta-toluamide (DEET) are also effective. Prophylactic antibiotics for tick bites in areas of high endemicity when the tick can be identified as *Ixodes scapularis*, has been attached for more than 36 hours (based on exposure or tick engorgement), and prophylaxis can be started within 72 hours of tick removal. There is no current Lyme vaccine.

Treatment

Antimicrobial therapy is beneficial in most cases of Lyme disease. It is most effective if started early. Prolonged treatment is important for all forms. Relapses occur in some patients on all regimens.

A. Rash, Early Infections

Doxycycline (2.2 mg/kg/dose max 100 mg/dose orally twice a day) for 10 days or amoxicillin (50 mg/kg/day orally in two divided doses, to a maximum of 2 g/day) for 14 days are the currently recommended treatments. Azithromycin or cefuroxime orally in two divided doses are used in children who cannot tolerate doxycycline or amoxicillin.

B. Arthritis

The amoxicillin or doxycycline regimen (same dosage as for the rash) should be used, but treatment should continue for 4 weeks. Parenteral ceftriaxone (50–75 mg/kg/day) is used for recurrent arthritis.

C. Bell Palsy

Doxycycline for 2 weeks is preferred.

D. Other Neurologic Disease or Cardiac Disease

Parenteral therapy with 14 days of ceftriaxone was traditionally used for meningitis, but recent evidence demonstrates that doxycycline orally for the same duration is equally effective. Both ceftriaxone and oral doxycycline are effective for Lyme carditis.

Centers for Disease Control and Prevention (CDC): Lyme disease. http://www.cdc.gov/lyme/. Accessed June 28, 2019.

Halperin JJ: Chronic Lyme disease: misconceptions and challenges for patient management. Infect Drug Resist 2015 May 15;8: 119–128 [PMID: 26028977].

Lopez SMC, Campfield BT, Nowalk AJ: Oral management for pediatric Lyme meningitis. J Pediatric Infect Dis Soc 2019 Jul 1;8(3):272–275 [PMID: 30169816].

Sood SK: Lyme disease in children. Infect Dis Clin North Am Jun 2015;29(2):281–294. doi: 10.1016/j.idc.2015.02.011 [PMID: 25999224].

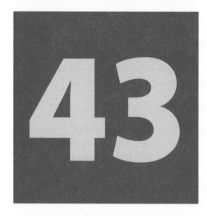

Infections: Parasitic & Mycotic

James Gaensbauer, MD, MScPH

Myron J. Levin, MD

The parasites that cause human disease represent a diverse, highly evolved and complex group of organisms. Parasitic diseases are a major cause of global pediatric morbidity and mortality, with the heaviest disease burden occurring in low- and middle-income countries. Though less common in industrialized nations, parasites represent an important class of pathogens to recognize in this setting, as both endemic and imported cases are frequently encountered in pediatric practice. Given the complexity of this category of pathogens, a framework to organize human parasites according to their major biologic classification and predominant site (intestinal vs blood/tissue) of human interaction can be useful to the learner (Table 43–1). Additionally, understanding organisms associated with potential clinical presentations of parasitic diseases can help focus the diagnostic process (Table 43–2).

Selection of Patients for Evaluation

The incidence of parasitic infections varies greatly with geographic area. Children who have traveled or lived in areas where parasitic infections are endemic are at risk for infection with a variety of intestinal and tissue parasites. Children who have resided only in developed countries are usually free of tissue parasites (with few exceptions, eg, *Toxocara, Toxoplasma*). Searching for intestinal parasites is expensive for the patient and time-consuming for the laboratory, and more than 90% of ova and parasite (O&P) examinations performed in the United States are negative. A frequent misperception is that intestinal helminths are common causes of diarrhea; with rare exception (eg, Trichuris dysentery syndrome) they are not. Parasitic diarrhea is almost exclusively caused by protozoa (*Giardia, Cryptosporidium, Entamoeba*) which are now commonly diagnosed with molecular methods. Thus, an O&P for a patient with diarrhea is rarely the correct test. It may also be more cost-effective to empirically treat symptomatic US immigrants with albendazole for common intestinal parasites and to investigate only those whose symptoms persist.

Immunodeficient children are very susceptible to protozoal intestinal infections. Multiple opportunistic pathogens are often identified, and the threshold for evaluation should be low for these children.

Laude A et al: Is real-time PCR-based diagnosis similar in performance to routine parasitological examination for the identification of Giardia intestinalis, *Cryptosporidium parvum/Cryptosporidium hominis* and *Entamoeba histolytica* from stool samples? Evaluation of a new commercial multiplex PCR assay and literature review. *Clin Microbiol Infect* 2016 Feb;22(2):190.e1–190.e8 [PMID: 26548509].

Specimen Processing

Many laboratories are now using PCR-based diagnostic assays for stool pathogens, which present fewer specimen handling challenges. Practitioners should contact the laboratory for proper collection procedures for diagnostic testing that requires microscopy, or a fresh sample to visualize viable parasites such as Giardia trophozoites. Many laboratories will reject formed stool samples submitted for parasites which cause diarrhea. The US Centers for Disease Control and Prevention (CDC) provide a website (http://dpd.cdc.gov/dpdx) to assist in the laboratory diagnosis of common parasitic diseases, including specimen collection and processing.

Eosinophilia & Parasitic Infections

Although certain parasites commonly cause eosinophilia, in developed countries other causes are much more common. These include allergies, drugs, and other infections. Nor do all parasitic infections result in eosinophilia. Eosinophilia due to parasitic infection is most common when multicellular

Table 43–1. Framework for conceptualization of human parasitic infections and examples of representative organisms.

Parasite Class	Prominent Site of Involvement	
	Intestinal	Tissue/Blood
Protozoa	*Entamoeba* *Giardia* *Cryptosporidium*	Malaria *Leishmania* *Naegleria* *Toxoplasma*
Platyhelminthes (flatworms) Cestodes	*Taenia* (ingested larvae) *Diphyllobothrium*	*Taenia*/cysticercosis (ingested eggs) *Echinococcus*
Trematodes (flukes)		*Schistosoma* *Fasciola* *Clonorchis*
Nematodes (roundworms)	*Ascaris* Hookworms *Strongyloides* *Trichuris*	*Trichinella* *Dracunculus* *Angiostrongylus* *Filaria*

organisms are migrating through host tissues (eg, lymphatic filariasis, hookworm). The unicellular protozoa (eg, malaria, leishmaniasis) rarely cause eosinophilia, even when infection is severe or invasive (eg, amebic liver abscess). Likewise eosinophilia is uncommon with parasites residing exclusively in the lumen of the intestinal tract.

The most common parasitic infection in the United States that causes significant eosinophilia with negative stool examination is toxocariasis. Trichinosis, which is a rare parasitic infection in the United States, causes marked eosinophilia. Strongyloidiasis is a cause of eosinophilia that may be difficult to diagnose with stool examinations. The differential diagnosis of eosinophilia is broad for patients who have been in developing countries (see Table 43–2).

▼ PROTOZOAL INFECTIONS

SYSTEMIC INFECTIONS

1. Malaria

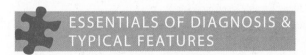

ESSENTIALS OF DIAGNOSIS & TYPICAL FEATURES

▶ Residence in or travel to an endemic area (fever in the returning traveler).

▶ Paroxysms of fever, chills, and intense sweating.

▶ Headache, backache, cough, abdominal pain, nausea, vomiting, diarrhea.

▶ Splenomegaly, anemia.

▶ Can progress to coma, seizures.

▶ Malaria parasites in peripheral blood smear.

▶ General Considerations

Malaria causes more than 400,000 deaths each year, over 80% of which occur in children younger than 5 years of age in sub-Saharan Africa and India. Global efforts toward malaria prevention and treatment have led to declining mortality and morbidity. Approximately 2000 imported cases are diagnosed in the United States each year. Human malaria is caused by five *Plasmodium* species—*Plasmodium vivax* (most common), *Plasmodium falciparum* (most virulent), *Plasmodium ovale* (similar to *P vivax*), *Plasmodium malariae*, and *Plasmodium knowlesi* (a primate parasite now recognized as a cause of falciparum-like malaria in humans).

The female *Anopheles* mosquito transmits the parasites. Infected mosquitoes inoculate sporozoites into the bloodstream of a susceptible host, resulting in infection of hepatocytes. In the hepatic phase, the parasites mature into schizonts, which rupture and release merozoites into the circulation. These infect and rupture red blood cells in the erythrocytic phase, as they mature from trophozoites to schizonts and release additional merozoites. In early stages of infection, asynchronous erythrocytic cycles of hemolysis commonly cause daily fevers. Eventually if untreated, synchronous erythrocytic cycles may begin as parasites rupture the infected cells at more regular 48- or 72-hour intervals, depending on the infecting species. A small percentage of trophozoites mature into the sexual form (gametocytes) which are taken up in a mosquito blood-meal, thus completing the cycle. Two species, *P vivax* and *P ovale*, can remain dormant in liver cells (hypnozoites) leading to recrudescence, months and even years after the acute infection.

Disease severity in malaria is closely linked with prior immunity. Thus, in areas where transmission is stable and frequent, older children and adults will generally develop milder illness with infection, though complete protective immunity rarely occurs. On the other hand, younger children, persons without prior exposure (eg, foreign travelers) or individuals living in areas where transmission is intermittent are at increased risk of severe disease. Additionally, young children, pregnant women, and persons with certain immune dysfunctions (eg, asplenia) are at higher risk of severe disease regardless of prior exposure.

Evidence of the central role malaria has played in human history can be found in the frequency of genetic mutations leading to altered red blood cell phenotypes, including

Table 43–2. Signs and symptoms of parasitic infection.

Sign/Symptom	Agent	Comments[a]
Abdominal pain	*Anisakis*	Shortly after raw fish ingestion.
	Ascaris	Heavy infection may obstruct bowel, biliary tract.
	Clonorchis	Heavy, early infection. Hepatomegaly later.
	Entamoeba histolytica	Hematochezia, variable fever, diarrhea.
	Fasciola hepatica	Diarrhea, vomiting.
	Hookworm	Iron deficiency anemia with heavy infection.
	Strongyloides	Eosinophilia, pruritus. May resemble peptic disease.
	Trichinella	Myalgia, periorbital edema, eosinophilia.
	Trichuris	Diarrhea, dysentery with heavy infection.
Cough	*Ascaris*	Wheezing, eosinophilia during migration phase.
	Paragonimus westermani	Hemoptysis; chronic. May mimic tuberculosis.
	Strongyloides	Wheezing, pruritus, eosinophilia during migration or dissemination.
	Toxocara	Affects ages 1–5 y; hepatosplenomegaly; eosinophilia.
	Tropical eosinophilia	Pulmonary infiltrates, eosinophilia.
Diarrhea	*Blastocystis*	Unclear significance as a diarrheal pathogen immunoefficiency may be a risk factor.
	Cyclospora	Watery; severe in immunosuppressed individuals.
	Cryptosporidium	Watery; chronic in immunosuppressed individuals.
	Dientamoeba fragilis	Only with heavy infection.
	E histolytica	Hematochezia, variable fever; no eosinophilia.
	Giardia	Afebrile, chronic; anorexia.
	Schistosoma	Chronic; hepatosplenomegaly (some types).
	Strongyloides	Abdominal pain; eosinophilia.
	Trichinella	Myalgia, periorbital edema, eosinophilia.
	Trichuris	With heavy infection.
Dysentery	*Balantidium coli*	Swine contact.
	E histolytica	Few to no leukocytes in stool; fever; hematochezia.
	Schistosoma	During acute infection.
	Trichuris	With heavy infection.
Dysuria	*Enterobius*	Usually girls with worms in urethra, bladder; nocturnal, perianal pruritus.
	Schistosoma (*S haematobium*)	Hematuria. Exclude bacteriuria, stones (some types).
Headache (and other cerebral symptoms)	*Angiostrongylus*	Eosinophilic meningitis.
	Baylisascaris procyonis	Eosinophilic meningitis.
	Gnathostoma	Eosinophilic meningitis.
	Naegleria	Freshwater swimming; rapidly progressive meningoencephalitis.
	Plasmodium	Fever, chills, jaundice, splenomegaly. Cerebral ischemia (with *P falciparum*).
	Taenia solium	Cysticercosis. Focal seizures, deficits; hydrocephalus, aseptic meningitis.
	Toxoplasma	Meningoencephalitis (especially in infants and the immunosuppressed); focal lesions in immunosuppressed; hydrocephalus in infants.
	Trypanosoma	African forms. Chronic lethargy (sleeping sickness).
Pruritus	*Ancylostoma braziliense*	Creeping eruption; dermal serpiginous burrow.
	Enterobius	Perianal, nocturnal.
	Filaria	Variable; seen in many filarial diseases; eosinophilia.
	Hookworm	Local at penetration site in heavy exposure.
	Strongyloides	Diffuse with migration; may be recurrent.
	Trypanosoma	African forms; one of many nonspecific symptoms.

(Continued)

Table 43–2. Signs and symptoms of parasitic infection. (*Continued*)

Sign/Symptom	Agent	Comments[a]
Rash	Hookworm	Pruritic, papulovesicular rash at site of penetration.
	Schistosoma	Maculopapular rash at site of penetration.
	Strongyloides	Pruritic rash at site of penetration.
	Toxoplasma	Maculopapular rash seen with congenital and sometimes acquired infection.
Anemia	*Diphyllobothrium*	Megaloblastic due to vitamin B_{12} deficiency; rare.
	Hookworm	Iron deficiency.
	L donovani	Fever, hepatosplenomegaly, leukopenia (kala-azar).
	Plasmodium	Hemolysis.
	Trichuris	Heavy infection; due to iron loss.
Eosinophilia	*Angiostrongylus*	Eosinophilic meningitis.
	Baylisascaris procyonis	Eosinophilic meningitis.
	Fasciola	Abdominal pain.
	Gnathostoma	Eosinophilic meningitis.
	Filaria	Microfilariae in blood; lymphadenopathy.
	Onchocerca	Skin nodules, keratitis.
	Schistosoma	Chronic; intestinal or genitourinary symptoms.
	Strongyloides	Abdominal pain, diarrhea.
	Toxocara	Hepatosplenomegaly, cough; affects ages 1–5 y.
	Trichinella	Myalgia, periorbital edema.
	Tropical pulmonary eosinophilia	Cough; pulmonary infiltrates.
	T solium (cysticercosis)	Eosinophils in CSF.
Hematuria	*Schistosoma*	*S haematobium.* Bladder, urethral granulomas. Exclude stones.
Hemoptysis	*P westermani*	Lung fluke. Variable chest pain; chronic.
Hepatomegaly	*Clonorchis*	Heavy infection. Tenderness early; cirrhosis late.
	Echinococcus	Chronic; cysts.
	E histolytica	Toxic hepatitis or abscess. No eosinophilia.
	L donovani	Splenomegaly, fever, pancytopenia.
	Schistosoma (not *haematobium*)	Chronic; hepatic fibrosis, splenomegaly (some types).
	Toxocara	Splenomegaly, eosinophilia, cough; no adenopathy.
Splenomegaly	*L donovani*	Hepatomegaly, fever, anemia.
	Plasmodium	Fever, chills, jaundice, headache.
	Schistosoma (not *haematobium*)	Hepatomegaly.
	Toxocara	Eosinophilia, hepatomegaly.
	Toxoplasma	Lymphadenopathy, other symptoms.
Lymphadenopathy	*Filaria*	Inguinal typical; chronic.
	L donovani	Hepatosplenomegaly, pancytopenia, fever.
	Schistosoma	Acute infection; fever, rash, arthralgia, hepatosplenomegaly.
	Toxoplasma	Cervical common; may involve single group of nodes; splenomegaly.
	Trypanosoma	Localized near bite or generalized; hepatosplenomegaly (Chagas disease); generalized (especially posterior cervical) in African forms.

[a]Symptoms usually related to degree of infestation. Infestation with small numbers of organisms is often asymptomatic.

hemoglobin S, hemoglobin F, the thalassemias, possibly glucose-6-phosphate dehydrogenase [G6PD] deficiency, and absent Duffy antigen on red blood cells (which confers protection against *P vivax*) that may confer partial protection against malaria among populations whose origins are from malaria endemic areas.

► Clinical Findings

A. Symptoms and Signs

Clinical manifestations vary according to infecting species and host immunity. The most common manifestations of acute malaria in children include fever, chills, malaise, and headache. Nausea, vomiting, and abdominal pain are common. Infants commonly present with recurrent fever, irritability, poor feeding, vomiting, jaundice, and splenomegaly. Rash is usually absent, which helps distinguish malaria from some viral infections in patients presenting with similar symptoms. In the classic descriptions of malaria, cyclic patterns of fever specific to the infecting species were noted. This finding can take many days to develop and is affected by numerous factors including prior immunity, multiple species infection and treatment, and is rarely useful diagnostically in current practice.

The clinician must be vigilant in monitoring patients with malaria for signs and symptoms of complicated or severe infection, including severe anemia and cerebral malaria, described later.

Infection during pregnancy often causes intrauterine growth restriction or premature delivery, but rarely true fetal infection.

Physical examination in patients with uncomplicated cases may show only mild splenomegaly and mild pallor.

B. Laboratory Findings

Because the manifestations of malaria overlap with a number of other common conditions, the diagnosis should always be confirmed with laboratory testing. The diagnosis relies on detection of one or more of the five human plasmodia in thick and thin blood smears. Three separate sets of thick and thin smears separated by 12–24 hours in a 72-hour period are recommended to rule out malaria infection. Thick smears are most sensitive for detection of small numbers of malaria parasites; thin smears allow identification of species and semiquantitative determination of percentage of parasitemia.

Most acute infections are caused by *P vivax*, *P ovale*, or *P falciparum*, although 5%–7% are due to multiple species. Identification of the *Plasmodium* species relies on morphologic criteria and requires an experienced observer. Bench aids to assist in the identification of *Plasmodium* species can be found at http://www.dpd.cdc.gov/dpdx/HTML/Malaria.htm. A U.S. Food and Drug Administration

(FDA)-approved antigen detection test is available and approved for rapid diagnostic testing of malaria. This test should be used in conjunction with microscopic examination to confirm diagnosis, look for mixed infection, and quantitate degree of parasitemia. The rapid antigen test has poor sensitivity for low levels of parasitemia. Up-to-date information on rapid diagnostic testing for malaria can be found at www.cdc.gov/malaria/diagnosis_treatment/index.html. Alternative techniques of similar or higher diagnostic accuracy for *P falciparum* include DNA hybridization and polymerase chain reaction (PCR), which are only available in research and reference laboratories and at CDC and some health departments.

Determining the degree of parasitemia (% of visualized erythrocytes that are infected) from thin smears is important because high levels (> 5%), most often seen in *P falciparum* malaria, are associated with increased morbidity and mortality and require hospitalization. Measurement over time (12–24 hours) can also be used to monitor treatment responses; the parasite burden should decrease over the first 24–48 hours.

Hemolytic anemia and thrombocytopenia are common; the incidence of leukocytosis is variable. In severe cases, metabolic acidosis, hypoglycemia, and azotemia may occur. The pathogenesis of cerebral malaria is microvascular obstruction. CSF analysis is typically normal.

► Differential Diagnosis

Clinical features may not reliably distinguish malaria from other infections in children, so a high index of suspicion in patients with exposure in endemic areas is necessary. The differential diagnosis of fever in a returning traveler should be based on diseases endemic to the region of travel and may include typhoid fever, tuberculosis, rickettsial disease, brucellosis, leptospirosis, yellow fever, dengue fever, chikungunya, and borreliosis. However, other common nontropical causes of fever such as influenza should be considered. Though CSF is typically normal in cerebral malaria, any child with suspected cerebral malaria should undergo lumbar puncture to exclude bacterial meningitis. Malaria may also coexist with other diseases.

► Complications & Sequelae

Severe complications, which occur most often in *P falciparum* and *P knowlesi* infection, result from hemolysis, microvascular obstruction, and tissue ischemia. The most common complications of malaria in children are cerebral malaria, respiratory distress, severe anemia, and/or hypoglycemia. Cerebral malaria, which is the most serious and life-threatening complication of malaria in children, may progress to seizures, coma, and death. Approximately 20% of children with cerebral malaria die and 10% have long-term neurologic sequelae. Signs of severe malaria in children include altered mental status, seizures, respiratory distress, hypoglycemia, acidosis, end-organ failure, extreme pallor, and parasitemia greater than 5%.

▶ Prevention

There are many strategies to prevent malaria transmission in a community. The most effective is widespread use of bed nets impregnated with long-acting insecticide, because the majority of *Anopheles* bites occur in evening or night. Mosquito larva control and indoor insecticide spraying are also widespread.

Strategies for personal protection against malaria (particularly for travelers to endemic areas) include use of bed nets, proper clothing, insect repellent, and malaria chemoprophylaxis. The most common medications for malaria prevention in travelers are mefloquine, atovaquone-proguanil, and doxycycline (see Chapter 45). Chloroquine is of limited utility due to widespread resistance. Factors impacting decisions regarding choice of medication include cost, side effects, drug interactions, and epidemiology and resistance patterns in the planned travel area. Specific requirements for starting medication before travel and continuing for a certain duration after travel depend on the medication.

No drug regimen guarantees protection against malaria. If fever develops within 1 year (particularly within 2 months) after travel to an endemic area, the possibility of malaria should be considered.

▶ Treatment

Choice of antimalarial treatment depends on the immune status of the person, plasmodium species, degree of parasitemia, and resistance patterns in the geographical region of acquisition. A description of the recommended antimalarial drugs available in the United States with updated treatment guidelines is available at https://www.cdc.gov/malaria/diagnosis_treatment/treatment.html. Atovaquone/proguanil and the artemisinin combination artemether/lumefantrine are first-line therapies for uncomplicated malaria in the United States. For severe malaria, intravenous artesunate is superior to quinidine and can result in rapid reduction in parasitemia, but must always be followed by an oral combination drug when the patient improves in order to prevent resistance. IV artesunate is available under an expanded access investigational new drug protocol through the CDC. Common treatments for infections with *P vivax* and *P ovale* include chloroquine plus either primaquine or the recently approved tafenoquine, which can eradicate liver stage malaria with a single dose. The CDC provides 24-hour telephone malaria hotline consultation for providers at (770) 488-7788.

Treatment for malaria includes a variety of supportive strategies in addition to the antimalarial drugs. It is advisable to hospitalize nonimmune patients infected with *P falciparum* and *P knowlesi* until a decrease in parasitemia

is demonstrated, indicating that treatment is effective and severe complications are unlikely to occur. Patients with signs of severe malaria (parasitemia > 5%, cerebral malaria, acidosis, hypoglycemia, shock) require intensive care and parenteral treatment. Hydration and treatment of hypoglycemia are of utmost importance. Anemia, seizures, pulmonary edema, and renal failure require conventional supportive management. Corticosteroids are contraindicated for cerebral malaria because of increased mortality. Exchange transfusion is no longer recommended for the treatment of severe malaria.

Partially immune patients with uncomplicated *P falciparum* and *P knowlesi* infection and nonimmune persons infected with *P vivax*, *P ovale*, or *P malariae* can receive outpatient treatment if follow-up is reliable.

Crawley J et al: Malaria in children. Lancet 2010;375:1468–1481 [PMID: 20417858].
Rodrigo C et al: Tafenoquine for primary and terminal prophylaxis of malaria in apparently healthy people: a systematic review. Trans R Soc Trop Med Hyg 2019 Jun 21. pii: trz052. doi: 10.1093/trstmh/trz052.
Sinclair D et al: Artesunate versus quinine for treating severe malaria. Cochrane Database Syst Rev 2012 Jun 13;(6):CD005967. https://doi.org/10.1002/14651858.CD005967.pub4. [PMID: 22696354]
http://www.cdc.gov/malaria/. Accessed June 25, 2019.
https://www.cdc.gov/dpdx/malaria/index.html. Accessed March 1, 2020.
https://www.cdc.gov/malaria/diagnosis_treatment/treatment.html. Accessed March 1, 2020.

2. Babesiosis

Babesia microti is a malaria-like protozoan that infects humans bitten by infected nymphal-stage *Ixodes scapularis* (deer tick). After inoculation, the protozoan penetrates erythrocytes and starts an asynchronous cycle that causes hemolysis. In the United States, the majority of cases occur in the Northeast and upper Midwest from May to October. Babesia infection is also a transfusion-transmissible disease.

▶ Clinical Findings

A. Symptoms and Signs

The incubation period is 1–4 weeks after tick bite, or 1–9 weeks after blood transfusion. The tick bite may go unnoticed as *Ixodes* nymphs are about the size of a poppy seed. Approximately half of infected children are asymptomatic. Symptoms are nonspecific and most commonly include sustained or cyclic high fever, rigors, and sweats. Other associated nonspecific symptoms include malaise, fatigue, anorexia, arthralgias, myalgias, and headache. Physical examination findings are usually minimal, but may include hepatosplenomegaly, jaundice, or dark urine. The disease is usually self-limited, causing symptoms for 1–2 weeks with fatigue that may persist for months. Severe cases have been described in asplenic patients, immunocompromised hosts, and elderly patients with comorbidities. Because *Babesia*, *Borrelia burgdorferi*, and *Anaplasma phagocytophilum* share a common vector, physicians should consider the possibility of coinfection in patients diagnosed with any of these pathogens.

B. Laboratory Findings

Anemia, thrombocytopenia, and evidence of renal insufficiency may be noted. Definitive diagnosis is made by identifying babesial parasites in blood by microscopic evaluation of thin or thick blood smears or by PCR amplification of babesial DNA in blood samples. *Babesia* parasites are intraerythrocytic organisms that resemble *P falciparum* ring forms. The tetrad form (Maltese cross), if visualized, is pathognomonic. Specific serologic tests are also available through the CDC.

▶ Treatment

Azithromycin (10 mg/kg up to 500 mg on the first day, followed by 5 mg/kg up to 250 mg/day) in combination with atovaquone (20 mg/kg, up to 750 mg, twice a day) for 7–10 days is the treatment of choice for mild-to-moderate disease. For severely ill patients, clindamycin (10 mg/kg, up to 600 mg, every 8 hours) in combination with quinine (8 mg/kg, up to 650 mg, every 8 hours) is standard of care. Longer courses of treatment may be needed in immunocompromised patients. Partial or complete RBC exchange transfusion is indicated for persons with severe babesiosis, as indicated by high-grade parasitemia ($\geq$ 10%); significant hemolysis; or renal, hepatic, or pulmonary compromise.

http://www.cdc.gov/parasites/babesiosis/. Accessed June 25, 2019.
http://www.dpd.cdc.gov/dpdx/HTML/Babesiosis.htm. Accessed June 25, 2019.
Krause PJ: Human babesiosis. Int J Parasitol 2019 Feb;49(2): 165–174. doi: 10.1016/j.ijpara.2018.11.007. [PMID: 18755385].

3. Toxoplasmosis

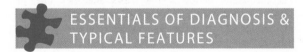

ESSENTIALS OF DIAGNOSIS & TYPICAL FEATURES

▶ *Congenital toxoplasmosis:* chorioretinitis, microphthalmia, strabismus, microcephaly, hydrocephaly, convulsions, psychomotor retardation, intracranial calcifications, jaundice, hepatosplenomegaly, abnormal blood cell counts.

▶ *Acquired toxoplasmosis in an immunocompetent host:* lymphadenopathy, hepatosplenomegaly, rash.

▶ *Acquired or reactivated toxoplasmosis in an immunocompromised host:* encephalitis, chorioretinitis, myocarditis, and pneumonitis.

▶ *Ocular toxoplasmosis:* chorioretinitis.

▶ Serologic evidence of infection with *Toxoplasma gondii* or demonstration of the agent in tissue or body fluids.

▶ General Considerations

T gondii is a worldwide parasite of animals and birds. Felines, the definitive hosts, excrete oocysts in their feces. Ingested mature oocysts or tissue cysts lead to tachyzoite invasion of intestinal cells. Intracellular replication of the tachyzoites causes cell lysis and spread of the infection to adjacent cells or to other tissues via the bloodstream. In chronic infection, *T gondii* appears as bradyzoite-containing tissue cysts that do not trigger an inflammatory reaction. In immunocompromised hosts, tachyzoites are released from cysts and begin a new cycle of infection.

The two major routes of *Toxoplasma* transmission to humans are oral and congenital. Oral infection occurs after ingestion of cysts from food, water, or soil contaminated with cat feces or from ingestion of undercooked meat or other food products that contain cysts. Oocysts survive up to 18 months in moist soil but survival is limited in dry, very cold, or very hot conditions and at high altitude, which probably accounts for the lower incidence of toxoplasmosis in these climatic regions. In the United States, less than 1% of cattle and 25% of sheep and pigs are infected with toxoplasmosis. In humans, depending on geographic area, seropositivity increases with age from 0% to 10% in children younger than 10 years to 3%–70% in adults.

Congenital transmission occurs during acute infection of pregnant women. Rarely, fetal infection has been documented in immunocompromised mothers who have chronic toxoplasmosis. Treatment during pregnancy decreases transmission by 60%.

▶ Clinical Findings

Clinical toxoplasmosis can be divided into four groups: (1) congenital infection, (2) infection acquired in the immunocompetent host, (3) infection acquired or reactivated in the immunocompromised host, and (4) ocular disease.

A. Congenital Toxoplasmosis

Congenital toxoplasmosis, which is the result of acute infection during pregnancy, occurs in 1 in 3000–10,000 live births in the United States. The rate of transmission and disease severity in the baby vary according to when in pregnancy the infection is acquired. First-trimester infections lead to congenital infections about 10%–20% of the time. Clinical disease that occurs at this time can be severe, with microcephaly or hydrocephaly, severe chorioretinitis, hearing loss, convulsions, abnormal cerebrospinal fluid (CSF) (xanthochromia and mononuclear pleocytosis), cerebral calcifications, and intellectual disability. Other findings include strabismus, maculopapular rash, pneumonitis, myocarditis, hepatosplenomegaly, jaundice, thrombocytopenia, lymphocytosis and monocytosis, and an erythroblastosis-like syndrome. Infection of a mother in the third trimester results in a 70%–90% rate of congenital infection, but most of these children are asymptomatic at birth, although they remain at risk of subsequent ocular disease and subtle neurologic deficits.

B. Acquired *Toxoplasma* Infection in the Immunocompetent Host

Typically, acquired infection in the immunocompetent host is asymptomatic. About 10%–20% of patients develop an infectious mononucleosis-like syndrome with lymphadenopathy and/or a flu-like illness. Affected nodes are discrete, variably tender, and do not suppurate. Cervical lymph nodes are most frequently involved, but any nodes may be enlarged. Less common findings include fever, malaise, myalgias, fatigue, hepatosplenomegaly, lymphopenia (usually < 10%), and liver enzyme elevations. Unilateral chorioretinitis may occur. Recovery typically occurs without any specific antiparasitic treatment, although lymph node enlargement may persist or wax and wane for a few months to 1 or more years. Animal and epidemiologic studies have suggested an association between toxoplasmosis infection and behavioral changes and mental illness (particularly schizophrenia) but these associations remain unproven.

C. Acute Toxoplasmosis in the Immunodeficient Host

Patients infected with human immunodeficiency virus (HIV), and those with lymphoma, leukemia, or transplantation, are at high risk for developing severe disease (most commonly central nervous system disease, but also chorioretinitis, myocarditis, or pneumonitis) following acute infection or reactivation. Toxoplasmic encephalitis is a common cause of mass lesions in the brains of persons with HIV/AIDS.

D. Ocular Toxoplasmosis

Ocular toxoplasmosis is an important cause of chorioretinitis in the United States. In children, it results most often from reactivation of congenital infection but can also follow acquired infection. Congenitally infected individuals are usually asymptomatic until the second or third decade of life

when symptomatic eye disease occurs due to the rupture of tissue cysts and the release of bradyzoites and tachyzoites into the retina. Typically, ocular toxoplasmosis presents as a focal necrotizing retinochoroiditis often associated with a preexistent chorioretinal scar, and variable involvement of the vitreous, retinal blood vessels, optic nerve, and anterior segment of the eye.

E. Diagnostic Findings

Serologic tests are the primary means of diagnosis, but results must be interpreted carefully, particularly in the evaluation of congenital toxoplasmosis. Active infection can also be diagnosed by PCR of blood or body fluids; by visualization of tachyzoites in histologic sections or cytology preparations, cysts in placenta or fetal tissues; or by characteristic lymph node histology. IgG antibodies become detectable 1–2 weeks after infection, peak at 1–2 months, and thereafter persist for life. IgM antibodies appear earlier and decline faster than IgG antibodies, but can last for 12–18 months after acute infection. Isolated IgM antibodies with negative IgG, should not be interpreted as positive due to poor specificity. A single positive titer determination is nondiagnostic; IgG seroconversion or a fourfold increase in titer from paired samples drawn at least 3 weeks apart are diagnostic in the right clinical scenario. Absence of both serum IgG and IgM in an immunocompetent individual virtually rules out the diagnosis of toxoplasmosis. In the immunocompromised host, serologic tests are not sensitive, and active infection is documented by PCR or finding tachyzoites by histologic examination.

The diagnosis of toxoplasmosis in the older child with visual complaints is usually made by finding *T gondii* IgG or IgM antibodies in the serum in the presence of a typical eye lesion. The diagnosis can be confirmed by detecting *T gondii* DNA by PCR in the aqueous humor, though this is rarely performed.

Congenital infection is confirmed by histologic or molecular identification of trophozoites in amniotic fluid, placenta, or infant tissue. Infant blood, CSF, and amniotic fluid specimens should be assayed by PCR. More often, diagnosis is established using a combination of serologic testing of mother and baby and clinical findings. Evaluation of a newborn should include *Toxoplasma*-specific IgG, IgM, IgA, and IgE of the newborn and mother in coordination with an experienced reference lab. A congenital infection is confirmed serologically by detecting persistent or increasing IgG antibody levels compared to the mother, persistently positive IgG antibodies beyond the first year of life, and/or a positive *T gondii*-specific IgM or IgA antibody test in the infant. In addition, the child should have thorough ophthalmologic, auditory, and neurologic evaluation; a lumbar puncture; and computed tomographic (CT) scan of the head (to detect CNS calcifications).

Differential Diagnosis

Congenital toxoplasmosis must be differentiated from infection with cytomegalovirus, rubella, herpes simplex, and syphilis. Acquired infection in immune competent host can mimic infectious mononucleosis, as well as viral, bacterial, or lymphoproliferative disorders. Ocular toxoplasmosis can mimic other infectious, noninfectious, and neoplastic ocular conditions.

Prevention

Primary prevention of toxoplasmosis in pregnant women (and immunocompromised patients) is an essential public health goal. Effective strategies to prevent food-borne transmission of toxoplasmosis include adequate cooking or prolonged precooking freezing of meats; washing of fruits, vegetables, and cooking surfaces; and avoidance of unpasteurized goat milk and uncooked crustaceans (oysters, clams, mussels), particularly during pregnancy. Exposure to potential environmental sources can be minimized by using gloves when gardening/handling soil that may have been contaminated by cat feces, covering sandboxes, and good hygiene. Pregnant women should not purchase a new kitten and avoid changing cat litter; if unavoidable, gloves and hand-hygiene are essential and litter should be changed regularly because oocysts require 48–72 hours to sporulate and become infectious. Though maternal treatment can prevent congenital transmission, implementation of serologic screening of pregnant women is challenging.

Treatment

The most common medications to treat toxoplasmosis are pyrimethamine (given with leucovorin to limit bone marrow toxicity) and sulfadiazine. Acute toxoplasmosis in the immunocompetent host does not require specific therapy, unless the infection occurs during pregnancy. In primary maternal infection during the first 18 weeks of pregnancy, spiramycin is recommended to attempt to prevent fetal infection. Spiramycin does not cross the placenta, so does not treat fetal infection once established. If fetal infection has been documented or if primary maternal infection occurs after the first 18 weeks of pregnancy, pyrimethamine, sulfadiazine, and leucovorin are recommended. Pyrimethamine is teratogenic and should not be used before 18 weeks of gestation.

Treatment of toxoplasmic chorioretinitis consists of oral pyrimethamine (2 mg/kg maximum, 200 mg loading dose followed by 1 mg/kg daily [maximum 75 mg]) plus sulfadiazine (100 mg/kg daily, maximum 1500 mg), given with leucovorin (10–20 mg three times a week). In addition, corticosteroids (prednisone 1 mg/kg daily) are given when lesions threaten vision. The duration of additional therapy should be guided by frequent ophthalmologic examinations. Pyrimethamine can cause gastrointestinal upset, leukopenia, thrombocytopenia, and rarely, agranulocytosis; weekly complete blood counts should be checked while on therapy.

A year of treatment is recommended for all congenitally infected infants. Children treated with pyrimethamine (loading dose 2 mg/kg daily for 2 days followed by 1 mg/kg daily for 6 months followed by 1 mg/kg every Monday, Wednesday, and Friday for 6 months) plus sulfadiazine (100 mg/kg divided twice daily for 12 months) plus leucovorin (10 mg three times a week) have better neurodevelopmental and visual outcomes than historical controls. While on therapy, infants should be monitored for bone marrow toxicity.

Fuglewicz AJ: Relationship between toxoplasmosis and schizophrenia: a review. Adv Clin Exp Med 2017 Sep;26(6): 1031–1036. doi: 10.17219/acem/61435 [PMID: 29068607].

http://www.cdc.gov/parasites/toxoplasmosis/. Accessed June 25, 2019.

Maldonado YA, Read JS; AAP Committee on Infectious Diseases: Diagnosis, treatment, and prevention of congenital toxoplasmosis in the United States. Pediatrics 2017;139(2):e20163860 [PMID: 28138010].

McAuley JB: Toxoplasmosis in children. Pediatr Infect Dis J 2008;27:161–162 [PMID: 18227714].

Robert-Gangneux F: It is not only the cat that did it: how to prevent and treat congenital toxoplasmosis. J Infect 2014 Jan;68 Suppl 1: S125–S133. doi: 10.1016/j.jinf.2013.09.023 [PMID: 24119928].

GASTROINTESTINAL INFECTIONS

1. Amebiasis

ESSENTIALS OF DIAGNOSIS & TYPICAL FEATURES

► Acute dysentery: diarrhea with blood and mucus, abdominal pain, tenesmus.

► Chronic nondysenteric diarrhea.

► Hepatic abscess.

► Amebas or cysts in stool or abscesses.

► Ameba antigen in stool.

► Serologic evidence of amebic infection.

General Considerations

Infection with *Entamoeba histolytica* occurs worldwide, but has a particularly high prevalence in areas with poor sanitation and socioeconomic conditions. In the United States, most infections are seen in travelers to, and emigrants from, endemic areas, but can occur without travel exposure. The majority of infections are asymptomatic (> 90%), but tissue invasion can result in amebic colitis, hepatic abscess, and hematogenous spread to other organs. Transmission is usually fecal-oral. Two *Entamoeba species, E dispar* and *E moshkovskii*, are morphologically indistinguishable from *E histolytica* and are much more commonly encountered in stool samples. Infections with these species are cause minimal (*E moshkovskii*) or no human disease (*E dispar*). Molecular techniques are likely to identify additional species in the future (eg, *E bangladeshi*).

▶ Clinical Findings

A. Symptoms and Signs

Patients with intestinal amebiasis can have asymptomatic cyst passage (> 90%), or be symptomatic with acute amebic proctocolitis, chronic nondysenteric colitis, or ameboma. Patients with acute amebic colitis typically have a 1- to 2-week history of loose stools containing blood and mucus, abdominal pain, and tenesmus. A minority of patients are febrile or dehydrated. Abdominal examination may reveal pain over the lower abdomen.

Fulminant colitis is an unusual complication of amebic dysentery that is associated with a grave prognosis (> 50% mortality), and is characterized by severe bloody diarrhea, fever, and diffuse abdominal pain. Children younger than age 2 years are at increased risk for this condition. Chronic amebic colitis causes recurrent episodes of bloody diarrhea over a period of years and is clinically indistinguishable from idiopathic inflammatory bowel disease. An ameboma is a localized amebic infection, usually in the cecum or ascending colon, which presents as a painful abdominal mass.

The most common complications of intestinal amebiasis are intestinal perforation, toxic megacolon, and peritonitis. Perianal ulcers, a less common complication, are painful, punched-out lesions that usually respond to medical therapy. Infrequently, colonic strictures may develop following colitis.

Patients with amebic liver abscess, the most common form of extraintestinal amebiasis, typically present with acute fever and right upper quadrant tenderness. The pain may be dull, pleuritic, or referred to the right shoulder. Physical examination reveals liver enlargement in fewer than 50% of affected patients. Some patients have a subacute presentation lasting 2 weeks to 6 months. In these patients, hepatomegaly, anemia, and weight loss are common findings, and fever is less common. Jaundice and diarrhea are rarely associated with an amebic liver abscess. In children with fever of unknown origin who live in, or travel to, endemic areas, amebic liver abscess should be considered in the differential diagnosis.

The most common complication of amebic liver abscess is pleuropulmonary amebiasis due to rupture of a right liver lobe abscess. Lung abscesses may occur from hematogenous spread. Cough, dyspnea, and pleuritic pain can be caused by the serous pleural effusions and atelectasis that frequently accompany amebic liver abscesses. Rupture of hepatic abscesses can lead to peritonitis and more rarely to pericarditis. Amebic brain or spinal cord abscess is an infrequent manifestation.

B. Diagnostic Findings

The differential diagnosis of acute amebic colitis includes bacterial (eg, *Salmonella* spp, *Shigella* spp, *E coli* spp, *Campylobacter* spp), parasitic (eg, *Balantidium coli*), and noninfectious (eg, inflammatory bowel disease, diverticulitis, ischemic colitis) causes of dysentery. Chronic amebic colitis has to be distinguished from inflammatory bowel disease and *Cyclospora*. Amebic liver abscess must be distinguished from an echinococcal hydatid cyst and abscesses caused by typical enteric bacteria. Occult blood is present in virtually all cases of amebic colitis and can be used as an inexpensive screening test. Fecal leukocytes are uncommon.

Intestinal amebiasis has been traditionally diagnosed by detecting the parasite on stool examination or mucosal biopsy. However, *E histolytica* is morphologically identical to nonpathogenic *E dispar* and *E moshkovskii*, and the majority of amebas diagnosed by microscopy are not *E histolytica* and cannot be easily differentiated by microscopy. Stool antigen detection tests are very sensitive and specific for *E histolytica*. Increasingly, diagnosis is confirmed using PCR, often in the context of a multiplex stool pathogen panel. Though these assays appear sensitive and specific for *E histolytica*, identification of multiple pathogens in a stool sample can present challenges in determining the actual cause of diarrhea. Colonoscopy and biopsy are most helpful when stool studies are nondiagnostic and other intestinal pathology (eg, Crohn's) are possible. Barium studies are contraindicated for patients with suspected acute amebic colitis due to risk of perforation.

Because extra-intestinal manifestations of *E histolitica* infection most commonly occur in individuals with negative stool testing, diagnosis in these settings often relies on serum specific antibody detection. ELISA assays are positive in approximately 95% of patients with extraintestinal amebiasis, 70% with intestinal *E histolytica* disease, and 10% of asymptomatic patients shedding *E histolytica* cysts. However, these antibodies persist for years, and a positive result does not distinguish between acute and past infection. Ultrasonographic examination and CT, which are sensitive techniques to detect hepatic abscesses, can be used to guide fine-needle aspiration to obtain specimens for definitive diagnosis. The classic appearance of drainage from a hepatic amebic abscess is described as "anchovy paste."

Prevention & Treatment

Travelers to endemic areas should drink bottled or boiled water and eat cooked or peeled vegetables and fruits to prevent enteric infection.

Treatment of amebic infection is complex because different agents are required for eradicating the parasite from the bowel or tissue (Table 43–3). Whether treatment of asymptomatic cyst passers is indicated is controversial. The prevalent opinion is that confirmed asymptomatic infection with *E histolytica* should be treated in nonendemic areas.

Asymptomatic *E histolytica* cyst excreters may be treated with paromomycin, a nonabsorbable intraluminal amebicide. Metronidazole is not effective against cysts.

Patients with symptomatic intestinal amebiasis or extraintestinal disease require treatment with an absorbable agent, such as metronidazole or tinidazole, followed by an intraluminal agent, even if the stool examination is negative. Tinidazole is a more effective treatment than metronidazole and is well tolerated in children. Metronidazole and paromomycin should not be given concurrently, because the diarrhea that is a common side effect of paromomycin may make it difficult to assess response to therapy. In most patients with amebic liver abscess, aspiration is unnecessary and does not speed recovery. Patients with large, thin-walled hepatic abscesses may need therapeutic aspiration to avoid abscess rupture. Drainage may also be considered when response to medical therapy is inadequate.

Table 43–3. Treatment of amebiasis.

Type of Infection	Drug of Choice	Dosage
Asymptomatic	Paromomycin	25–35 mg/kg/day in three doses for 7 day
	or	
	Iodoquinol	30–40 mg/kg/day (maximum, 2 g) in three doses for 20 days
	or	
	Diloxanide furoate[a]	20 mg/kg/day up to 1.5 g/day in three doses for 10 days
Intestinal disease and hepatic abscess[b]	Metronidazole	35–50 mg/kg/day up to 2.25 g/day in three doses for 10 days
	or	
	Tinidazole[c]	50 or 60 mg/kg up to 2 g/day for 3 days

[a]Diloxanide furoate is available from the CDC Drug Service: (404) 639–3670.
[b]Treatment should be followed by iodoquinol or paromomycin.
[c]Not marketed in the United States; higher dosage.

Buss SN et al: Multicenter evaluation of the BioFire FilmArray gastrointestinal panel for etiologic diagnosis of infectious gastroenteritis. J Clin Microbiol 2015 Mar;53(3):915–925. doi: 10.1128/JCM.02674-14. [PMID: 25588652].

Gonzales MLM et al: Antiamoebic drugs for treating amoebic colitis. Cochrane Database Syst Rev 2019 Jan 9;1:CD006085. doi: 10.1002/14651858.CD006085.pub3. [PMID: 30624763].

2. Giardiasis

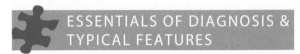

ESSENTIALS OF DIAGNOSIS & TYPICAL FEATURES

▶ Chronic relapsing diarrhea, flatulence, bloating, anorexia, poor weight gain.

▶ Absence of fever or hematochezia.

▶ Detection of trophozoites, cysts, or *Giardia* antigens in stool, or positive stool PCR.

General Considerations

Giardiasis, caused by *Giardia intestinalis*, is the most common intestinal protozoal infection in children in the United States and in most of the world. The infection is classically associated with drinking contaminated water, either in rural areas or in areas with faulty purification systems. Even ostensibly clean urban water supplies and pristine mountain streams can be contaminated intermittently, and infection has been acquired in swimming pools. Fecal-oral contamination allows person-to-person spread. Day care centers are a major source of infection. Food-borne outbreaks also occur. Giardiasis may occur at any age, although infection is rare in neonates. High rates of transmission occur among men who have sex with men. Domestic animals are rarely sources of human infection due to strain differences between humans and pets.

Clinical Findings

A. Symptoms and Signs

Giardia infection results in either asymptomatic cyst passage, acute self-limited diarrhea, or a chronic syndrome of diarrhea, malabsorption, and weight loss. Acute diarrhea occurs 1–2 weeks after infection and is characterized by abrupt onset of diarrhea with greasy, malodorous stools, malaise, flatulence, bloating, and nausea. Fever and vomiting are unusual. The disease has a protracted course (> 1 week) and frequently leads to weight loss. Patients who develop chronic diarrhea complain of profound malaise, lassitude, headache, and diffuse abdominal pain in association with bouts of diarrhea—most typically foul-smelling, greasy stools—intercalated with periods of constipation or normal bowel habits. This syndrome can persist for months until specific therapy is administered or until it subsides spontaneously. Chronic diarrhea frequently leads to malabsorption, steatorrhea, micronutrient deficiencies, and disaccharidase depletion. Lactose intolerance, which develops in 20%–40% of patients can persist for several weeks after treatment, and needs to be differentiated from relapsing giardiasis or reinfection.

B. Laboratory Findings

Increasingly, the diagnosis of giardiasis in the United States is made by stool PCR, often in the context of a multiplex stool pathogen panel. Though these assays appear sensitive and specific for *Giardia*, identification of multiple pathogens in a stool sample can present challenges in determining the actual cause of diarrhea, particularly in patients exposed in poor income countries where carriage of *Giardia* is extremely common. Alternative methods of diagnosis include *Giardia* antigen detection by means of ELISAs, nonenzymatic immunoassays, and direct fluorescence antibody tests. In areas without access to PCR or antigen tests, the diagnosis of giardiasis can be made by finding the parasite in stool. For O&P examination, a fresh stool provides the best results. Liquid stools have the highest yield of mobile trophozoites, which are more readily identified on wet mounts. With semiformed stools or those that cannot immediately be examined, the examiner should look for cysts in fresh or fixed specimens, preferably using a concentration technique.

▶ Prevention

The prevention of giardiasis requires proper treatment of water supplies and interruption of person-to-person transmission. Where water might be contaminated, travelers, campers, and hikers should use methods to make water safe for drinking. Boiling is the most reliable method; the necessary time of boiling (1–3 minute at sea level) will depend on the altitude. Chemical disinfection with iodine or chlorine and filtration are alternative methods of water treatment.

Interrupting fecal-oral transmission requires strict hand washing. However, outbreaks of diarrhea in day care centers might be particularly difficult to eradicate. Reinforcing hand washing and treating the disease in both symptomatic and asymptomatic carriers may be necessary.

▶ Treatment

Metronidazole, tinidazole, and nitazoxanide are the traditional drugs of choice for treatment of giardiasis. A recent meta-analysis concluded that single dose tinidazole (50 mg/kg; max 2 g) should be the preferred treatment based on both better efficacy and convenience compared to other treatments. There are fewer data on the use of tinidazole in children under 3 years. When given at 5 mg/kg (up to 250 mg) three times a day for 5–7 days, metronidazole has 80%–95% efficacy. Nitazoxanide (100 mg [5 mL] every 12 hours for children 12–47 months of age, 200 mg every 12 hours for 4- to 11-year-olds, and 500 mg every 12 hours for children 12 years or older) is available in liquid formulation and requires only 3 days of treatment. For patients who do not respond to therapy or are reinfected, a second course with the same drug or switching to another drug is equally effective. In cases of repeated treatment failure paromomycin or albendazole may be effective.

http://www.cdc.gov/parasites/giardia/. Accessed June 26, 2019.
Ordóñez-Mena JM et al: Comparative efficacy of drugs for treating giardiasis: a systematic update of the literature and network meta-analysis of randomized clinical trials. J Antimicrob Chemother 2018;73(3):596 [PMID: 29186570].

3. Cryptosporidiosis

The intracellular protozoa *Cryptosporidia* are the leading cause of recreational water-associated diarrheal outbreaks in the United States. *Cryptosporidia* may also cause severe and devastating diarrhea in patients with untreated acquired immunodeficiency syndrome (AIDS) and in other immunodeficient persons. This ubiquitous parasite infects and reproduces in the epithelial cell lining of the digestive and respiratory tracts of humans and most other vertebrate animals. Humans acquire the infection from contaminated drinking water, recreation water sources (including swimming pools, fountains, and lake water), or from close contact with infected humans or animals. Petting zoos and day care centers have been other sources of *Cryptosporidia* outbreaks. Most human infections are caused by *C parvum* or *C hominis*.

▶ Clinical Findings

A. Symptoms and Signs

Immunocompetent persons infected with *Cryptosporidium* usually develop self-limited diarrhea (2–26 days) with or without abdominal cramps. Diarrhea can be mild and intermittent or continuous, watery, and voluminous. Low-grade fever, nausea, vomiting, loss of appetite, and malaise may accompany the diarrhea. Children younger than 2 years are more susceptible to infection than older children. Immunocompromised patients (either cellular or humoral deficiency) tend to develop a severe, prolonged, chronic diarrhea which, despite treatment, can result in severe malnutrition and subside only after the immunodeficiency is corrected. Other clinical manifestations associated with cryptosporidiosis in immunocompromised hosts include cholecystitis, pancreatitis, hepatitis, biliary tree involvement, and respiratory symptoms.

B. Laboratory Findings

Though visualization of *Cryptosporidia* oocysts in concentrated stool samples is diagnostic, PCR—often in the context of a multiplex stool pathogen panel—is rapidly replacing diagnostic microscopy, and is highly sensitive and specific. Alternate tests include direct immunofluorescent antibody (DFA) of stool.

▶ Prevention & Treatment

Prevention of *Cryptosporidium* infection is limited by oocyst resistance to some of the standard water purification procedures (including chlorine) and common disinfectants. Enteric precautions are recommended for infected persons. Boiled or bottled drinking water may be considered for patients at high risk for developing chronic infection (eg, inadequately treated patients with AIDS). Infected persons should avoid swimming pools.

Many infections in immunocompetent individuals are self-limited, thus treatment is supportive and primarily directed at prevention of dehydration. Severe of prolonged cases in immunocompetent patients and some patients with immunodeficiencies respond to treatment with nitazoxanide, antidiarrheal agents, and hydration. Immunocompromised patients usually require more intense supportive care with parenteral nutrition in addition to hydration and nonspecific antidiarrheal agents. Recommended doses of nitazoxanide are 100 mg (5 mL) every 12 hours for children 12–47 months of age, 200 mg every 12 hours for 4–11 year olds, and 500 mg every 12 hours for children 12 years or older. For patients with advanced AIDS, antiparasitic therapy alone has not proven efficacious. Institution of effective antiretroviral therapy results in elimination of symptomatic cryptosporidiosis.

Davies AP et al: Cryptosporidiosis. BMJ 2009;399:963–967 [PMID: 19841008].

http://www.cdc.gov/parasites/crypto/. Accessed June 26, 2019.

Hussien SM: Comparative study between the effect of nitazoxanide and paromomycine in treatment of cryptosporidiosis in hospitalized children. J Egypt Soc Parasitol 2013 Aug;43(2):463–470 [PMID: 24260825].

4. Cyclosporiasis

Cyclospora spp are ubiquitous coccidian parasites that infect humans and a variety of animals worldwide. *Cyclospora cayetanensis* is the only species known to infect humans. Cyclosporiasis is seen in three main epidemiologic settings: sporadic cases in endemic areas, travelers to endemic areas, and in food- or water-borne outbreaks in nonendemic areas, particularly in relation to importation of fresh produce. The incubation period is approximately 7 days (range 2–14 days). Infection may be asymptomatic, cause mild-to-moderate self-limited diarrhea, or cause protracted or severe diarrhea. In the immunocompetent host, diarrhea usually lasts 10–25 days but may be followed by a relapsing pattern that can last several months. Diarrhea is frequent, watery, sometimes explosive, and often accompanied by nausea, vomiting, abdominal cramping, and bloating. Profound fatigue, anorexia, and myalgia have been reported. The infection can be unusually severe in immunocompromised patients, especially those with inadequately treated HIV/AIDS. Although the illness is self-limited, it may last for several weeks in the absence of treatment. Diagnosis is based on finding oocysts 8–10 mm in diameter on examination of stool specimens stained with acid-fast stain. PCR of stool is available at the CDC and some reference laboratories. Treatment is trimethoprim-sulfamethoxazole for 7 days; no other medication has proven effective.

Casillas S et al: Notes from the field: multiple cyclosporiasis outbreaks—United States, 2018. MMWR 2018 October 5; 67(39):1101–1102 [PMID: 30286055].

5. Free-Living Amebas

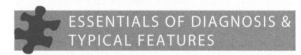

ESSENTIALS OF DIAGNOSIS & TYPICAL FEATURES

▶ Acute meningoencephalitis: fever, headache, meningism, acute mental deterioration.

▶ Swimming in warm, freshwater in an endemic area.

▶ Chronic granulomatous encephalitis: insidious onset of focal neurologic deficits.

▶ Keratitis: pain, photophobia, conjunctivitis, blurred vision.

▶ General Considerations

Infections with free-living amoebas are uncommon. *Naegleria* species, *Acanthamoeba* species, and *Balamuthia* amoebas have been associated with human disease, primarily infections of the central nervous system.

Acute meningoencephalitis, caused by *Naegleria fowleri*, occurs mostly in children and young adults. Patients present with abrupt fever, headache, nausea, and vomiting, disturbances in smell and taste, meningismus, and decreased mental status a few days to 2 weeks after exposure. Infection is often associated with swimming in warm freshwater lakes and using contaminated tap water for nasal irrigation. CNS invasion occurs after nasal inoculation of *N fowleri* which travel along the olfactory nerves via the cribiform plate to the brain.

The disease is rapidly progressive and nearly universally fatal within a week of symptom onset.

Chronic granulomatous encephalitis, caused by *Acanthamoeba* or *Balamuthia*, can occur in immunocompetent patients, but occurs more commonly in immunocompromised patients. There is no association with freshwater swimming. This disease has an insidious onset of focal neurologic deficits, and approximately 50% of patients present with headache. Skin, sinus, or lung infections with *Acanthamoeba* precede many of the CNS infections and may still be present at the onset of neurologic disease. Granulomatous encephalitis progresses to fatal outcome over a period of weeks to months (average 6 weeks).

Acanthamoeba keratitis is a corneal infection associated with minor trauma or use of soft contact lenses in otherwise healthy persons. Clinical findings of *Acanthamoeba* keratitis include radial keratoneuritis and stromal ring infiltrate. Amebic keratitis usually follows an indolent course and initially may resemble herpes simplex or bacterial keratitis; delay in diagnosis is associated with worse outcomes.

▶ Clinical Findings & Differential Diagnosis

Amebic encephalitis should be included in the differential diagnosis of acute meningoencephalitis in children with a history of recent freshwater swimming. The CSF is usually hemorrhagic, with leukocyte counts that may be normal early in the disease but later range from 400 to 2600/mL with neutrophil predominance, low to normal glucose, and elevated protein. The etiologic diagnosis relies on finding trophozoites on a wet mount of the CSF. Immunofluorescent and PCR-based diagnostic assays are available through the CDC.

Granulomatous encephalitis is diagnosed by brain biopsy of CT-identified nonenhancing lucent areas. The CSF of these patients is usually nondiagnostic with a lymphocytic pleocytosis, mild to severe elevation of protein (> 1000 mg/dL), and normal or low glucose. *Acanthamoeba* and *Balamuthia* amoebas have only rarely been found in the CSF; however, they can be visualized in brain biopsies or grown from brain or other infected tissues. Immunofluorescent and PCR-based diagnostic assays are available through the CDC.

Acanthamoeba keratitis is diagnosed by finding the trophozoites in corneal scrapings or by isolating the parasite from corneal specimens or contact lens cultures.

▶ Prevention

Because primary amebic meningitis occurs infrequently, active surveillance of lakes for *N fowleri* is not warranted. However, in the presence of a documented case, it is advisable to close the implicated lake to swimming. Sterile or boiled water should be used for nasal irrigation. *Acanthamoeba* keratitis can be prevented by heat disinfection of contact lenses, storage of lenses in sterile solutions, use of disposable daily lenses, and by not wearing lenses when swimming in freshwater or showering.

▶ Treatment

Treatment of amebic encephalitis is complex and frequently unsuccessful. Urgent consultation with the CDC is recommended for all cases (CDC Emergency Operations Center at 770-488-7100). Though treatment numbers are small, regimens containing miltefosine (an antiparasitic used for treatment of leishmania) may increase survival in *Balamuthia mandrillaris* and Acanthamoeba infections. A recent case demonstrated successful treatment of a 9-year-old with *Naegleria* meningoencephalitis using miltefosine in combination with amphotericin B, fluconazole, rifampin, azithromycin, dexamethasone, and whole-body cooling to 34°C.

Acanthamoeba keratitis responds well to surgical debridement followed by 3–4 weeks of topical 1% miconazole; 0.1% propamidine isethionate; and polymyxin B sulfate, neomycin, and bacitracin (Neosporin).

Cope J et al: Primary amebic meningoencephalitis: what have we learned in the last 5 years? Curr Infect Dis Rep 2016;18: 31. Doi: 10.1007/s11908-016-0539-4. [PMID: 27614893].

Heggie TW, Küpper T: Surviving *Naegleria fowleri* infections: a successful case report and novel therapeutic approach. Travel Med Infect Dis 2016 Dec 22. doi: 10.1016/j.tmaid.2016.12.005. [PMID: 28013053].

http://www.cdc.gov/parasites/acanthamoeba/. Accessed June 26, 2019.

http://www.cdc.gov/parasites/balamuthia/. Accessed June 26, 2019.

http://www.cdc.gov/parasites/naegleria/. Accessed June 26, 2019.

TRICHOMONIASIS

Trichomonas vaginalis infection is discussed in Chapter 44.

▼ METAZOAL INFECTIONS

NEMATODE INFECTIONS

1. Enterobiasis (Pinworms)

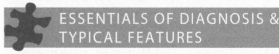

ESSENTIALS OF DIAGNOSIS & TYPICAL FEATURES

▶ Anal pruritus.
▶ Worms in the stool or eggs on perianal skin.

▶ General Considerations

This worldwide infection is caused by *Enterobius vermicularis*. The adult worms are about 5–10 mm long and live in the colon; females deposit eggs on the perianal area, primarily at night, which cause intense pruritus. Scratching contaminates the fingers and allows transmission back to the host (autoinfection) or to contacts through fecal-oral spread.

Clinical Findings

A. Symptoms and Signs

Pinworms are associated with intense localized pruritis of the anus and vulva. Adult worms may migrate within the colon or up the urethra or vagina in girls. They can be found within the bowel wall, in the lumen of the appendix (usually an incidental finding by the pathologist), in the bladder, and even in the peritoneal cavity of girls.

B. Laboratory Findings

The usual diagnostic test consists of pressing a piece of transparent tape on the child's anus in the morning prior to bathing, then placing it on a drop of xylene on a slide. Microscopic examination under low power usually demonstrates the ova. Scrapings from under fingernails may also be positive. Parents may visualize adult worms in the perianal region, often at nighttime while the child is asleep. Though stool testing for pinworm is typically negative, incidental identification of the flagellate parasite *Dientamoeba fragilis* in a stool O&P examination may suggest the presence of Enterobius, though the relationship between these two organisms is incompletely understood.

Differential Diagnosis

Nonspecific irritation or vaginitis, streptococcal perianal cellulitis (usually painful with marked erythema), and vaginal or urinary bacterial infections may at times resemble pinworm infection, although the symptoms of pinworms are often so suggestive that a therapeutic trial is justified without a confirmed diagnosis.

Treatment

A. Specific Measures

Treat all household members at the same time to prevent reinfections. Because the drugs are not active against the eggs, therapy should be repeated after 2 weeks to kill the recently hatched adults. Significant constipation may impair treatment responses.

Pyrantel pamoate, available without a prescription, is given as a single dose (11 mg/kg; maximum 1 g); it is safe, inexpensive and very effective. Albendazole (400 or 200 mg in children 1–2 years of age) in a single dose is also highly effective for all ages (though not approved by the US FDA). Ivermectin is also effective against pinworm.

B. General Measures

Personal hygiene must be emphasized. Nails should be kept short and clean. Children should wear undergarments in bed

to diminish contamination of fingers; bedclothes should be laundered frequently; infected persons should bathe in the morning, thereby removing a large proportion of eggs.

https://www.cdc.gov/parasites/pinworm/index.html. Accessed June 26, 2019.

2. Ascariasis

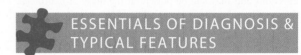

ESSENTIALS OF DIAGNOSIS & TYPICAL FEATURES

▶ Often asymptomatic but impacts micronutrient absorption.

▶ Abdominal cramps and discomfort.

▶ Large, white or reddish, round worms, or ova in the feces.

General Considerations

The whipworm, hookworms (see later), and *Ascaris* comprise the "soil-transmitted helminths." These parasites cause human infection through contact with eggs or larvae that thrive in the moist soil of the tropics and subtropics. Worldwide, more than a billion people are infected with at least one of these parasites, and, especially in less developed countries, it is not uncommon for children to be chronically and repeatedly infected with multiple worms. These parasites are strongly associated with poverty and lack of clean water and sanitation. Children infected with these worms are at increased risk for malnutrition, stunted growth, intellectual disability, and cognitive and education deficits. Together, the soil-transmitted helminths are one of the world's most important causes of physical and intellectual impairment, with the majority of this burden falling on children.

Ascaris lumbricoides is a worldwide human parasite. Ova passed by carriers may remain viable for months under the proper soil conditions. The ova contaminate food or fingers and are subsequently ingested by a new host. The larvae hatch, penetrate the intestinal wall, enter the venous system, reach the alveoli, are coughed up the trachea and swallowed, returning to the small intestine, where they mature. The female lays thousands of eggs daily.

Clinical Findings

A. Symptoms and Signs

The majority of infections with *A lumbricoides* are asymptomatic, although moderate to heavy infections are associated with abdominal pain, weight loss, anorexia, diarrhea, and vomiting, and may lead to malnutrition. During the larval migratory phase, an acute transient eosinophilic pneumonitis (Löffler syndrome) may occur. Acute intestinal obstruction has been associated with heavy infections, which is more common in children due to their smaller intestinal diameter and higher worm burden. Worm migration can cause appendicitis, common bile duct obstruction (resulting in biliary colic, cholangitis, or pancreatitis), or peritonitis.

B. Laboratory Findings

The diagnosis is made by observing the large roundworms (15–40 cm) in the stool or by microscopic detection of the ova on concentrated stool examination.

▶ Treatment

Ascaris is treated with albendazole (400 mg in a single dose, or 200 mg in children 1–2 years of age), mebendazole (100 mg twice a day for 3 days or 500 mg once), and ivermectin (150–200 mcg/kg orally once). Nitazoxizide is also effective. In cases of intestinal or biliary obstruction, piperazine (150 mg/kg initially, followed by six doses of 65 mg/kg every 12 hours by nasogastric tube) can be used to paralyze the worms and help relieve obstruction. However, surgical removal is occasionally required. Because reinfection is common in areas of high worm burden, regular deworming programs are employed to mitigate chronic nutritional and development impacts on children, though results have been disappointing in the setting of rapid reinfection.

http://www.cdc.gov/parasites/sth/. Accessed June 26, 2019.
http://www.who.int/intestinal_worms/. Accessed June 26, 2019.
World Health Organization. Eliminating soil-transmitted helminthiases as a public health problem in children: Progress report 2001–2010 and strategic plan 2011–2020. June 2012. ISBN: 978 92 4 150 312 9; WHO/HTM/NTD/PCT/2012.4

3. Trichuriasis (Whipworm)

Trichuris trichiura is a widespread human and animal parasite common in children living in warm, humid areas conducive to survival of the ova, and is one of the soil-transmitted helminths of major global health significance. Ingested infectious eggs hatch in the upper small intestine. The adult worms live in the cecum and colon; the ova are passed and become infectious after several weeks in the soil. Unlike *Ascaris*, *Trichuris* does not have a migratory tissue phase. Symptoms are not present unless the infection is severe, in which case pain, diarrhea, iron-deficiency anemia, and mild abdominal distention are present. Massive infections may also cause rectal prolapse and dysentery. Detection of the characteristic barrel-shaped ova in the feces confirms the diagnosis. Adult worms may be seen in the prolapsed rectum or at proctoscopy; their thin heads are buried in the mucosa, and the thicker posterior portions protrude. Mild-to-moderate eosinophilia may be present.

Treatment with mebendazole (100 mg orally twice a day for 3 days) or albendazole (400 mg in a single dose for 3 days, or 200 mg in children 1–2 years of age) tends to improve gastrointestinal symptoms when present. Combination therapy involving more than one drug may be more effective than single-drug therapy for refractory cases.

Adegnika AA et al: Update on treatment and resistance of human trichuriasis. Curr Trop Med Rep 2015 Dec; 2(4):218–223.
http://www.who.int/intestinal_worms/. Accessed June 26, 2019.
http://www.cdc.gov/parasites/sth/. Accessed June 26, 2019.

4. Hookworm

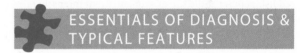

ESSENTIALS OF DIAGNOSIS & TYPICAL FEATURES

- ▶ Iron-deficiency anemia.
- ▶ Abdominal discomfort, weight loss, pruritic skin eruption.
- ▶ Ova in the feces.

▶ General Considerations

The common human hookworms are *Ancylostoma duodenale* and *Necator americanus*. Both are widespread in the tropics and subtropics, with an estimated 600–700 million people infected worldwide. The larger *A duodenale* is more pathogenic because it consumes more blood, up to 0.5 mL per worm per day.

The adults live in the jejunum. Eggs are passed in the feces and develop and hatch into infectious in warm, damp soil within 2 weeks. The larvae penetrate human skin on contact, enter the blood, reach the alveoli, are coughed up and swallowed, and develop into adults in the intestine. The adult worms attach to intestinal mucosa, from which they suck blood. Blood loss is the major sequela of infection; protein loss due to bleeding and disruption of the mucosal surface may also occur. Infection rates reach 90% in areas without sanitation.

Ancylostoma braziliense and *Ancylostoma caninum* (the dog and cat hookworm) cause cutaneous larva migrans, a creeping skin eruption in children and others who come in contact with soil contaminated with cat and dog feces. In the United States, the disease is most prevalent in the Southeast, but most cases are imported by travelers returning from tropical and subtropical areas.

Clinical Findings

A. Symptoms and Signs

Patients with hookworm infection usually are asymptomatic. Chronic hookworm infection leads to blood loss and iron-deficiency anemia. Heavy infection can cause hypoproteinemia with edema. Chronic hookworm infection in children may lead to growth delay, deficits in cognition, and developmental delay. The larvae usually penetrate the skin of the feet and cause a stinging or burning sensation, followed by an intense local itching (ground itch) and a papulovesicular rash that may persist for 1–2 weeks. Pneumonitis associated with migrating larvae is uncommon and usually mild, except during heavy infections. Colicky abdominal pain, nausea, and/or diarrhea and marked eosinophilia may be observed.

In cutaneous larva migrans, larvae produce pruritic, reddish papules at the site of skin entry and intensely pruritic, serpiginous tracks or bullae appear as they migrate through the skin, which is pathognomonic for this disease. Larvae can move up to a few centimeters a day and activity can continue for several weeks, but eventually the rash is self-limiting.

B. Laboratory Findings

The large ova of both species of hookworm are found in feces and are indistinguishable. Microcytic anemia, hypoalbuminemia, eosinophilia, and hematochezia occur in severe cases.

Prevention

Avoiding fecal contamination of soil and avoiding barefoot skin contact with potentially contaminated soil is recommended.

Treatment

A. Specific Measures

Albendazole (400 mg orally in a single dose, or 200 mg in children 1–2 years of age) is significantly more efficacious than mebendazole or pyrantel pamoate and is considered the drug of choice for treatment of hookworm infections.

B. General Measures

Iron therapy and vitamin A supplementation in conjunction with deworming programs may help mitigate some of the negative nutritional and micronutrient effects of infection with hookworm and the other soil-transmitted helminths, particularly in settings where reinfection occurs rapidly.

http://www.cdc.gov/parasites/sth/. Accessed June 26, 2019.
http://www.who.int/intestinal_worms/. Accessed June 26, 2019.
World Health Organization. Preventive chemotherapy to control soil-transmitted helminth infections in at-risk population groups. 2017. ISBN: 978 92 4 155011 6.

5. Strongyloidiasis

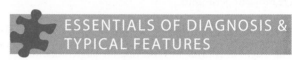

ESSENTIALS OF DIAGNOSIS & TYPICAL FEATURES

▶ Abdominal pain, diarrhea.

▶ Eosinophilia.

▶ Larvae in stools and duodenal aspirates.

▶ Serum antibodies.

General Considerations

Strongyloides stercoralis is unique in having both parasitic and free-living forms; the latter can survive in the soil for prolonged periods. The parasite is found in most tropical and subtropical regions of the world, including some areas of the southeastern United States. The adults live in the submucosal tissue of the duodenum and occasionally elsewhere in the intestines. Eggs deposited in the mucosa hatch rapidly and thus the first-stage (rhabditiform) larvae are the predominant form found in duodenal aspirates and feces, rather than eggs. The larvae mature rapidly to the tissue-penetrating filariform stage and initiate internal autoinfection within the intestine or in the perianal area. The filariform larvae passed in stool to the environment persist in soil and can penetrate the skin of another host, subsequently migrating into veins and pulmonary alveoli, reaching the intestine when coughed up and swallowed.

Older children and adults are infected more often than are young children. Immunosuppressed patients may develop fatal disseminated strongyloidiasis, known as the *hyperinfection syndrome*. Autoinfection can result in persistent infection for decades.

Clinical Findings

A. Symptoms and Signs

Chronic *S stercoralis* infections can be asymptomatic or cause cutaneous, gastrointestinal, and/or pulmonary symptoms. At the site of skin penetration, a pruritic rash may occur. Autoinfection from larvae present in stool may result in severe itching in the perianal area and a rapidly migrating rash called larva currens. Migrating larvae in the lungs can cause wheezing, cough, shortness of breath, and hemoptysis. Although intestinal infections are often asymptomatic, the most prominent features of clinical strongyloidiasis include abdominal pain, distention, diarrhea, vomiting, and occasionally malabsorption.

Patients with cellular immunodeficiencies and those on corticosteroids or chemotherapy may develop disseminated infection, sometimes many years after the last exposure (eg, in immigrants living for prolonged periods in the United States), involving the intestine, the lungs, and the meninges. Gram-negative sepsis may complicate disseminated strongyloidiasis.

B. Laboratory Findings

A marked eosinophilia is common in strongyloidiasis. Definitive diagnosis can be difficult because of low parasite load and irregular larval output in stool; a minimum of three stool samples should be examined. Finding larvae (not eggs) in the feces, duodenal aspirates, or sputum is diagnostic. IgG antibodies measured by ELISA or immunoblot are relatively sensitive (83%–93%). The presence of specific antibody does not distinguish between past and present infection. However, because prolonged, minimally symptomatic infections frequently occur, a person with a positive IgG test and no history of treatment should be considered infected. *Strongyloides* antibody assays can cross-react with other helminth infections. Patients with pulmonary symptoms with suspected *Strongyloides* infection should have sputum samples evaluated for the detection of *S stercoralis* in addition to antibody testing.

▶ Differential Diagnosis

Strongyloidiasis should be differentiated from peptic disease, celiac disease, regional or tuberculous enteritis, and hookworm infections. The pulmonary phase may mimic asthma or bronchopneumonia. Patients with severe infection can present with an acute abdomen.

▶ Prevention & Treatment

Ivermectin (two doses of 0.2 mg/kg given 1–14 days apart) is the drug of choice. Albendazole is an alternative treatment but appears to have lower efficacy. Relapses are common. In the hyperinfection syndrome, 1–3 weeks of therapy with ivermectin may be necessary and multiple follow-up stool studies for 2 weeks after therapy are indicated to ensure clearance of larvae. Patients from endemic areas should be serotested and treated at the time of immigration or before undergoing immunosuppression, including short courses of corticosteroid therapy for conditions such as asthma.

http://www.cdc.gov/parasites/strongyloides/. Accessed June 26, 2019.

Krolewiecki AJ et al: A public health response against *Strongyloides stercoralis*: time to look at soil-transmitted helminthiasis in full. PLoS Negl Trop Dis 2013 May 9;7(5):e2165 [PMID: 23675541].

Montes M et al: *Strongyloides stercoralis*: there but not seen. Curr Opin Infect Dis 2010;23:500–504 [PMID: 20733481].

Requena-Méndez A et al: Evidence-based guidelines for screening and management of strongyloidiasis in non-endemic countries. Am J Trop Med Hyg 2017 Sep 7; 97(3):645–652 [PMID: 28749768].

6. Visceral Larva Migrans (Toxocariasis)

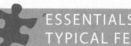

ESSENTIALS OF DIAGNOSIS & TYPICAL FEATURES

▶ Visceral involvement, including hepatomegaly, marked eosinophilia, and anemia.

▶ Posterior or peripheral ocular inflammatory mass.

▶ Elevated antibody titers in serum or aqueous fluid; demonstration of *Toxocara* larvae in biopsy specimen.

▶ General Considerations

Visceral larva migrans is a worldwide disease including all areas of the United States. The agent is the cosmopolitan intestinal ascarid of dogs and cats, *Toxocara canis* or *Toxocara cati*. The eggs passed by infected animals contaminate parks and other areas that young children frequent. Children with pica are at increased risk. In the United States, seropositivity ranges from 2.8% in unselected populations to 23% in southern states to 54% in rural areas. Ingested eggs hatch and penetrate the intestinal wall, then migrate to the liver. Most of the larvae are retained in the liver, but some may pass through the organ reaching the lungs, eyes, muscles, and/or the CNS, where they die and incite a granulomatous inflammatory reaction.

▶ Clinical Findings

A. Visceral Larva Migrans

Toxocariasis is usually asymptomatic, but young children (aged 1–5 years) sometimes present with anorexia, fever, fatigue, pallor, abdominal pain and distention, nausea, vomiting, and cough. Hepatomegaly is common, splenomegaly is unusual, and adenopathy is absent. Lung involvement, usually asymptomatic, can be demonstrated readily by radiologic examination. Seizures are common, but more severe neurologic abnormalities are infrequent. IgG antibody detection by ELISA is sensitive, specific, and useful in confirming the clinical diagnosis. Most patients recover spontaneously, but disease may last up to 6 months.

B. Ocular Larva Migrans

This condition occurs in older children and adults who present with a unilateral posterior or peripheral inflammatory eye mass. History of visceral larva migrans and eosinophilia are typically absent. Anti-*toxocara* antibody titers are low in the serum but may be elevated in vitreous and aqueous fluids.

C. Diagnostic Findings

Leukocytosis with marked eosinophilia, anemia, and elevated liver function tests are typical. Hypergamma-globulinemia may be present. The diagnosis can be confirmed by finding larvae in granulomatous lesions. More often, positive serology and the exclusion of other causes of hypereosinophilia provide a presumptive diagnosis in typical cases.

Differential Diagnosis

Diseases associated with hypereosinophilia must be considered. Other parasitic infections include trichinosis (enlarged liver not common; muscle tenderness common), *Baylisascaris* (racoon roundworm, also encountered in US children), *Ascaris*, and *strongyloides*. Noninfectious causes of significant eosinophilia in children include allergies and drug hypersensitivity syndromes, and rarely eosinophilic leukemia and collagen-vascular disease.

Prevention & Treatment

A. Specific Measures

Treatment with albendazole (400 mg twice a day for 5 days) or mebendazole (100–200 mg twice a day for 5 days) is recommended for visceral infection. Aggressive anti-inflammatory treatment with systemic corticosteroids should accompany anti-parasitic treatment for ocular larva migrans.

B. General Measures

Treating any cause of pica, such as iron deficiency, is important. Corticosteroids are used to treat marked inflammation of lungs, eyes, or other organs. Pets should be dewormed routinely.

Rubingsy-Elefant G et al: Human toxocariasis: diagnosis, worldwide seroprevalences and clinical expression of the systemic and ocular forms. Ann Trop Med Parasitol 2010;104:323 [PMID: 20149289].

Woodhall D et al: Toxocariasis: a review for pediatricians. J Pediatric Infect Dis Soc 2014 June; 3(2):154–159 [PMID: 26625368].

7. Trichinosis

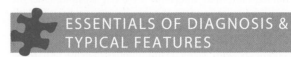

ESSENTIALS OF DIAGNOSIS & TYPICAL FEATURES

► Vomiting, diarrhea, and abdominal pain within 1 week of eating infected meat.
► Fever, periorbital edema, myalgia, and marked eosinophilia.

General Considerations

Trichinella are small roundworms that infest hogs and several other meat-eating animals. Currently, there are eight recognized *Trichinella* species, of which *Trichinella spiralis* is the most common human pathogen, and most adapted to domestic and wild swine. The most important source of human infection worldwide is the domestic pig. Cases and outbreaks have been associated with numerous game animals, particularly wild boar and bear, but also wild felines, fox, horse, seal, and walrus. The human cycle begins with ingestion of viable larvae in undercooked meat. In the small intestine, the larvae develop into adult worms that mate and produce larvae, which enter the bloodstream and migrate to the striated muscle where they continue to grow and eventually encyst. Symptoms are caused by the inflammatory response in the intestines or muscle.

Clinical Findings

A. Symptoms and Signs

Most infections are asymptomatic. The severity of clinical disease is strongly correlated with the number of ingested larvae. Infection can be divided into two phases: an intestinal phase (typically within 1–2 days of cyst ingestion) and a muscular or systemic phase (typically 2 weeks after infection). The initial bowel penetration may cause fever, headache, chills, and abdominal pain, nausea, vomiting, and diarrhea within 1 week after ingestion of contaminated meat. This may progress to the classic myopathic form, which consists of fever, eyelid or facial edema, myalgia, and weakness. Other signs may include maculopapular exanthem, subungual bleeding, conjunctivitis and subconjunctival hemorrhages, headaches, dry cough, and painful movement of the eye muscles. Rare complications include myocarditis, thromboembolic disease, and encephalitis. Severe cerebral involvement or myocarditis can be fatal. Symptoms usually peak after 2–3 weeks but may last for months. Children typically have milder clinical and laboratory findings than adults.

B. Diagnosis

The diagnosis of trichinosis is suggested by the constellation of typical clinical findings (fever; myalgias; eyelid and/or facial edema; gastrointestinal symptoms and subconjunctival, subungual, and retinal hemorrhages), history of potential exposure (particularly to wild game or undercooked pork), and nonspecific laboratory findings (particularly marked eosinophilia, elevated muscle enzymes). Confirmation can be challenging, and depends primarily on demonstration of *Trichinella*-specific IgG antibody. Sensitivity and specificity of serologic testing may be enhanced by serial testing to demonstrate a rise in titer. Muscle biopsy may demonstrate encysted larvae, which are diagnostic.

▶ Differential Diagnosis

Manifestations of the intestinal phase of trichinosis are similar to many acute gastrointestinal infections; obtaining a history of recent dietary exposure to a potential source of *Trichinella* is essential if the diagnosis is to be considered at this stage. The systemic phase may mimic the fever and myalgias of influenza. The classic symptoms are pathognomonic if one is aware of this disease. Facial swelling may mimic complicated sinusitis. Marked eosinophilia is seen in toxocariasis, strongyloidiasis, and schistosomiasis (travel history).

▶ Prevention

Because a microscopic examination must be performed, meat in the United States is not inspected for trichinosis. Although all states require the cooking of hog swill, hog-to-hog or hog-to-rat cycles may continue. All pork and sylvatic meat (eg, bear or walrus) should be cooked at least > 160°F followed by a 3 minute rest. Freezing meat to at least 5°F for 3 weeks may also prevent transmission. Animals used for food should not be fed or allowed access to raw meat. Careful cleaning and disinfection of meat-grinding equipment is essential, particularly after processing of wild game.

▶ Treatment

Albendazole (400 mg twice daily for 8–14 days) is the drug of choice for trichinosis. Concurrent corticosteroids (prednisone 30–60 mg/day for 10–15 days) are used for treatment of severe symptoms. Administration of analgesics is sometimes required. Relapses occur, particularly when treatment occurs late in the myopathic stage.

▶ Prognosis

Prognosis for severe cases with cardiac and cerebral complications is poor, with a mortality rate around 5%. In milder cases, prognosis is good, and most patients' symptoms disappear within 2–6 months.

Gottstein B et al: Epidemiology, diagnosis, treatment, and control of trichinellosis. Clin Micro Rev 2009;22:127–145 [PMID: 19136437].

http://www.cdc.gov/parasites/trichinellosis/. Accessed June 26, 2019.

Wilson D et al: Trichinellosis surveillance—United States, 2008–2012. MMWR Surveill Summ 2015 Jan 16;64(SS01):1–8 [PMID: 25590865].

8. Raccoon Roundworm Infections

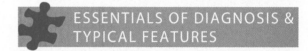

ESSENTIALS OF DIAGNOSIS & TYPICAL FEATURES

▶ Eosinophilic meningoencephalitis or encephalopathy.

▶ Ocular larva migrans.

▶ Contact with raccoons or raccoon feces.

▶ General Considerations

Human infections with *Baylisascaris procyonis*, the raccoon roundworm, though rare, may result in a severe and potentially fatal illness. Humans who ingest the eggs excreted in raccoon feces become accidental hosts when the larvae penetrate the gut and disseminate via the bloodstream to the brain, eyes, viscera, and muscles. Pica and exposure to raccoon latrines (location of communal raccoon defecation) represent the main risk factors. Most infections are asymptomatic, but cases of severe encephalitis (neural larva migrans), endophthalmitis (ocular larva migrans), and visceral larva migrans may occur. Symptoms typically begin 2–4 weeks after inoculation. CNS infections present as acute, rapidly progressive encephalitis with eosinophilic pleocytosis of the CSF (varies from 4% to 68% eosinophils in mild pleocytosis). Death or severe neurologic injuries are common. Both CNS and ocular infections resemble other larva migrans infections such as toxocariasis; therefore, *B procyonis* should be considered in the differential diagnosis of these infections when *Toxocara* serology is negative. The diagnosis of *B procyonis* is established by observing the larvae on examination of tissue biopsies or by serology (of serum or CSF), and should be considered in the differential diagnosis in anyone with CSF eosinophilia. Antihelmintic drugs have not been shown to have any beneficial effect for the treatment of baylisascariasis, since they lack larvicidal effects in human tissues. Nevertheless, albendazole (20–40 mg/kg/day for 1–4 weeks) has been used to treat most cases, together with anti-inflammatory drugs. Complete resolution of symptoms has not been achieved thus far. Immediate prophylactic treatment with albendazole (25 mg/kg daily for 20 days) should be considered for those with known ingestion of raccoon feces.

http://www.cdc.gov/parasites/baylisascaris/. Accessed June 26, 2019.
Sircar AD et al: Raccoon roundworm infection associated with central nervous system disease and ocular disease—six states, 2013-2015. MMWR 2016 Sep 9; 65(35):930–933. doi: 10.15585/mmwr.mm6535a2 [PMID: 27608169].

CESTODE INFECTIONS (FLUKES)

1. Taeniasis & Cysticercosis

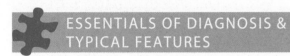

ESSENTIALS OF DIAGNOSIS & TYPICAL FEATURES

▶ Mild abdominal pain; passage of worm segments (taeniasis).

▶ Focal seizures, headaches (neurocysticercosis).

▶ Cysticerci present in biopsy specimens, on plain films (as calcified masses), or on CT scan or magnetic resonance imaging (MRI).

▶ Proglottids and eggs in feces; specific antibodies in serum or CSF.

▶ General Considerations

Cysticercosis affects as many as 100 million people globally, and is the leading cause of seizures in many developing countries. In the United States, cases are most often noted in individuals who have resided in Latin America. Pigs are the usual intermediate host of the tapeworm *Taenia solium*. Human cysticercosis occurs when the eggs, which are excreted in the feces of a human infected with the parasite, are ingested. Importantly, cysticercosis cannot be acquired by eating pork; rather, ingestion of pork may result in adult tapeworm infection (taeniasis) because infected pork contains the larval cysts that develop into the adult tapeworm but does not contain the eggs which cause cysticercosis. It is possible for an individual with taeniasis to auto-ingest eggs from their own intestinal tapeworm, and thus develop cysticercosis.

Larvae released from ingested eggs enter the circulation to encyst in a variety of tissues, especially muscle and brain (neurocysticercosis). Full larval maturation occurs in 2 months, but the cysts cause little inflammation until the larvae die months to years later. Inflammatory edema ensues with calcification or disappearance of the cyst. A slowly expanding mass of sterile cysts at the base of the brain may cause obstructive hydrocephalus (racemose cysticercosis).

T solium and the beef tapeworm (*Taenia saginata*), which can causes taeniasis but not cysticercosis, are distributed worldwide. Contamination of foods by eggs in human feces allows person-to-person spread without travel to endemic areas.

▶ Clinical Findings

A. Symptoms and Signs

1. Taeniasis—In most tapeworm infections, the only clinical manifestation is the passage of fecal proglottids, which are white, motile segments of tapeworm 1–2 cm in size. In contrast to the soil transmitted helminths (hookworms, ascaris) tapeworms are not associated with significant nutritional deficiencies. Children may harbor the adult worm for years and complain of abdominal pain, anorexia, and diarrhea. As they are often longer (up to 30 feet) *T saginata* may cause more symptoms than *T solium*.

2. Cysticercosis—In the parenchymatous form, the parasite lodges in tissue as a single or multiple cysts. Granuloma formation results with eventual pericystic inflammation, which is the cause of seizures in most patients. The initial stage of the cyst is viable, where the scolex exists within the cyst and there is minimal or no enhancement due to a limited host immune response. As the scolex dies, either due to the host immune response or cysticidal treatment there is a strong immune response, characterized by enhancement on CT or MRI. As the cyst further degenerates, it calcifies, leading to punctuate calcifications on CT scan. Brain cysts may remain silent or cause seizures, headache, hydrocephalus, and basilar meningitis. Rarely, the spinal cord is involved. Neurocysticercosis manifests an average of 5 years after exposure, but may cause symptoms in the first year of life. In the eyes, cysts cause bleeding, retinal detachment, and uveitis. Definitive diagnosis requires histologic demonstration of larvae or cyst membrane. Presumptive diagnosis is often made by the characteristics of the cysts seen on CT scan or MRI. The presence of *T solium* eggs in feces is uncommon with cysticercosis (see above) but can support the diagnosis.

B. Laboratory Findings

Neuroimaging is the mainstay of diagnosis of neurocysticercosis. The diagnosis should be suspected in any patient who has lived in an endemic area and presents with a compatible clinical picture and suggestive lesions on neuroimaging. In endemic areas it is not uncommon for lesions of cysticercosis to be noted incidentally on neuroimaging performed for other reasons (eg, trauma).

Eggs or proglottids may be found in feces or on the perianal skin (using the tape method employed for pinworms). Eggs of both *Taenia* species are identical. The species are identified by examination of proglottids.

Peripheral eosinophilia is minimal or absent. CSF eosinophilia is seen in 10%–75% of cases of neurocysticercosis; its presence supports an otherwise presumptive diagnosis.

Antibody testing of serum and CSF can strongly support the diagnosis when neuroimaging is abnormal. Titers are eventually positive in up to 98% of serum specimens and over 75% of CSF specimens from patients with neurocysticercosis. Solitary cysts are associated with seropositivity less often than are multiple cysts. High titers tend to correlate with more severe disease or more numerous encysted lesions. CSF titers are higher if cysts are near the meninges.

The differential diagnosis of neurocysticercosis includes tuberculous granuloma, microabscesses, arachnoid cyst, neoplasms, and vascular lesions.

► Treatment

A. Taeniasis

Oral praziquantel (5–10 mg/kg once) or niclosamide (50 mg/kg once, maximum 2 g) can be used for treatment of tapeworm carriers.

B. Cysticercosis

The treatment modalities for neurocysticercosis include cysticidal agents (to kill larvae), corticosteroids (to decrease or prevent the inflammatory reaction), antiepileptic drugs (to control seizures if present), and surgery (to remove cysts or for placement of a shunt for hydrocephalus). Most experts would recommend treatment with a cysticidal agent in most cases of neurocysticercosis, except in patients with inactive, calcified lesions. In patients with viable parenchymal cysts, cysticidal therapy decreases the burden of parasites and the number of seizures. Similarly, cysticidal therapy is associated with more complete and faster resolution on imaging and fewer seizures in patients with a single, small enhancing lesion. Ophthalmic examination should be conducted prior to cysticidal therapy to rule out intraocular cysts.

Albendazole, 15 mg/kg/day (maximum, 800 mg) divided in two doses daily for 8–15 days, is the treatment of choice. Larval death may result in clinical worsening because of inflammatory edema. A concurrent course of dexamethasone (0.1 mg/kg/day to a maximum of 6 mg/day) or prednisolone (1 mg/kg/day to a maximum of 40–60 mg) is recommended to decrease these symptoms. Corticosteroids are mandatory treatment for large intraventricular cysts and encephalitis (dexamethasone 0.1 mg/kg/day or prednisolone 1 mg/kg/day for as long as needed). Giant subarachnoidal cysts may require more than one cycle of therapy or surgery (or both). Minimally invasive neurosurgery (neuroendoscopic extraction) is the currently recommended management of intraventricular cysts. Follow-up scans every several months help assess the response to therapy.

► Prevention

Prevention of taeniasis requires proper cooking of meat. Neurocysticercosis is prevented by careful washing of raw vegetables and fruits, treating intestinal carriers, avoiding the use of human excrement for fertilizer, and providing proper sanitary facilities.

► Prognosis

The prognosis is good in intestinal taeniasis. Symptoms associated with a few cerebral cysts may disappear in a few months; heavy brain infections may cause death or chronic neurologic impairment. Seizures may persist even in those patients with only calcified lesions and anticonvulsants may be needed indefinitely.

Cantey P et al: Neglected parasitic infections in the United States: cysticercosis. Am J Trop Med Hyg 2014;90:805–809. doi:10.4269/ajtmh.13-0724 [PMID: 24808248].

Garcia HH et al: Cysticercosis of the central nervous system: how should it be managed? Curr Opin Infect Dis 2011;24:423–427 [PMID: 21788891].

http://www.cdc.gov/parasites/cysticercosis/. Accessed June 26, 2019.

2. Hymenolepiasis

Hymenolepis nana, or dwarf tapeworm, is a common parasite of children; *Hymenolepis diminuta*, the rat tapeworm, is rare. The former is capable of causing autoinfection. Larvae hatched from ingested eggs penetrate the intestinal wall and then reenter the lumen to mature into adults. Their eggs are immediately infectious for the same or a new host. The adult is only a few centimeters long. Finding the characteristic eggs in feces is diagnostic.

H diminuta has an intermediate stage in rat fleas and other insects; children are infected when they ingest these insects.

Light infections with either tapeworm are usually asymptomatic; heavy infection can cause diarrhea and abdominal pain. Therapy is with praziquantel (25 mg/kg once).

http://www.cdc.gov/parasites/hymenolepis/. Accessed June 26, 2019.

3. Echinococcosis

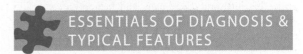

ESSENTIALS OF DIAGNOSIS & TYPICAL FEATURES

► Cystic tumors of the liver and lungs, rarely kidneys, bones, brain, and other organs.

► Eosinophilia.

► Urticaria and pruritus if cysts rupture.

► Protoscoleces or daughter cysts in the primary cyst.

► Positive serology.

► Epidemiologic evidence of exposure.

► General Considerations

Two species of *Echinococcus* can cause disease in humans, *E granulosus* and *E multilocularis*. The two forms of echinococcus, cystic and alveolar, cause significant morbidity and mortality worldwide; cystic echinococcus is endemic in many areas of the developing world, and alveolar echinococcus is typically found in far norther latitudes. Dogs and other canids are the definitive host for *E granulosis* and become infected through ingestion of infected organs of numerous herbivorous animals (especially sheep, but also goats, swine, horses, cattle, and camels) which serve as intermediate hosts. For *E multilocularis*, foxes are the principle definitive hosts and rodents are the intermediate hosts. Human infection occurs following incidental ingestion of eggs in canid stool. When ingested by humans, the eggs hatch, and the larvae penetrate the intestinal mucosa and disseminate via the bloodstream to produce cysts; the primary sites of involvement are the liver (60%–70%) and the lungs (20%–25%). A unilocular cyst is most common. Over time, the cyst may reach 25 cm in diameter, although most are much smaller. The cysts of *Echinococcus multilocularis* are multilocular and demonstrate more rapid growth.

► Clinical Findings

A. Symptoms and Signs

The clinical manifestations of echinococcosis are variable and depend primarily on the site, size, and condition of the cysts. The rates of growth of cysts are variable, and range between 1 and 5 cm in diameter per year. In cystic echinococcus, a slowly growing single cyst often goes unnoticed until it causes dysfunction due to its size. Hepatomegaly, right upper quadrant pain, nausea, and vomiting may occur. If a cyst ruptures, the sudden release of its contents can result in a severe allergic reaction. Cysts may cause biliary obstruction. Most hepatic cysts are in the right lobe. Alveolar echinococcus typically involves lung, and is characterized by a tumor-like lesion that can invade, necrose, and metastasize.

Rupture of a pulmonary cyst causes coughing, dyspnea, wheezing, urticaria, chest pain, and hemoptysis; cyst and worm remnants are found in sputum. Brain cysts may cause focal neurologic signs and convulsions; renal cysts cause pain and hematuria; bone cysts cause pain.

B. Laboratory Findings

Antibody assays are useful to support the diagnosis following identification of a cystic lesion on imaging, and currently available ELISA tests have high sensitivity. Immunoblot assays and direct parasitologic examination can confirm the presence of echinococcus from aspirated or resected samples. Eosinophilia is present in only about 25% of patients. Abnormal liver enzymes may suggest biliary obstruction.

C. Imaging

The presence of a cyst-like mass in a person with appropriate epidemiologic exposure supports the diagnosis. Visualization of daughter cysts (cysts within a larger cyst) is highly suggestive of echinococcosis. CT, MRI, and ultrasonography are useful for the diagnosis of deep-seated lesions. Abdominal ultrasonography is the most widely used diagnostic tool. Pulmonary or bone cysts may be visible on plain films.

► Differential Diagnosis

Tumors, bacterial or amebic abscess, cavitary pulmonary tuberculosis, mycoses, and benign cysts must be considered.

► Complications

Sudden cyst rupture with anaphylaxis and death is the worst complication. If the patient survives, secondary infections from seeding of daughter cysts may occur. Segmental lung collapse, secondary bacterial infections, effects of increased intracranial pressure, and severe liver or renal damage due to cysts are other potential complications.

► Treatment

There is no "best" treatment option for cystic echinococcus, and no clinical trial has compared all the different treatment modalities. Definitive therapy of *E multilocularis* requires meticulous surgical removal of the cysts. A surgeon familiar with this disease should be consulted. Albendazole chemotherapy should be initiated for several days prior to surgery. Chemotherapy alone cures about one-third of patients. Albendazole (15 mg/kg/day divided in two doses for 3 months, max 400 mg twice daily), sometimes with the addition of praziquantel, is the regimen of choice. A third treatment option is a four-step procedure (PAIR: puncture, aspiration, injection, and reaspiration). This procedure consists of (1) percutaneous puncture using ultrasound guidance, (2) aspiration of liquid contents, (3) injection of a protoscolicidal agents (95% ethanol or hypertonic saline for at least 15 minutes), and (4) reaspiration. PAIR is indicated for uncomplicated cases, or those not amenable to surgery. If the cyst leaks or ruptures during surgical or percutaneous drainage a severe, potentially life-threatening allergic reaction may occur. For alveolar echinococcus, radical surgery for complete resection of the cyst is the goal. In some patients (particularly in whom complete resection is not possible), lifetime chemotherapy may be required.

► Prognosis

Patients with large liver cysts may be asymptomatic for years. Surgery is often curative for lung and liver cysts, but not always for cysts in other locations.

http://www.cdc.gov/parasites/echinococcosis/. Accessed June 26, 2019.

McManus DP et al: Diagnosis, treatment, and management of echinococcosis. BMJ 2012;344:e3866 [PMID: 22689886].

Nasseri-Moghaddam S, Abrishami A, Taefi A, Malekzadeh R: Percutaneous needle aspiration, injection, and re-aspiration with or without benzimidazole coverage for uncomplicated hepatic hydatid cysts. Cochrane Database Syst Rev 2011 Jan 19; (1):CD003623. doi: 10.1002/14651858.CD003623.pub3 [PMID: 21249654].

TREMATODE INFECTIONS

Schistosomiasis

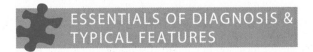

ESSENTIALS OF DIAGNOSIS & TYPICAL FEATURES

▶ Transient pruritic rash after exposure to freshwater.

▶ Fever, urticaria, arthralgias, cough, lymphadenitis, and eosinophilia.

▶ Weight loss, anorexia, hepatosplenomegaly, or hematuria.

▶ Eggs in stool, urine, or rectal biopsy specimens.

▶ General Considerations

One of the most common serious parasitic diseases, schistosomiasis, is caused by several species of *Schistosoma* flukes. *Schistosoma japonicum*, *Schistosoma mekongi*, and *Schistosoma mansoni* involve the intestines, and *Schistosoma haematobium* involves the urinary tract. The first two species are found in eastern and southeastern Asia; *S mansoni* in tropical Africa, the Caribbean, and parts of South America; and *S haematobium* in Africa. Important transmission sites include Lake Malawi and Lake Victoria in Africa, Poyang and Dongting Lakes in China, and along the Mekong River in Laos.

Infection is caused by free-swimming larvae (cercariae), which emerge from the intermediate hosts that are certain species of freshwater snails. The cercariae penetrate human skin, migrate to the liver, and mature into adults, which then migrate through the portal vein to lodge in the bladder veins (*S haematobium*), superior mesenteric veins (*S mekongi* and *S japonicum*), or inferior mesenteric veins (*S mansoni*). Clinical disease results primarily from inflammation caused by the many eggs that are laid in the perivascular tissues or that embolize to the liver. Escape of ova into bowel or bladder lumen allows microscopic visualization and diagnosis from stool or urine specimens, as well as contamination of freshwater and infection of the snail hosts that ingest them.

▶ Clinical Findings

Much of the population in endemic areas is infected but asymptomatic. Only heavy infections produce symptoms.

A. Symptoms and Signs

Schistosomiasis progresses in three distinct phases: acute, chronic, and advanced disease. The cercarial penetration may cause a maculopapular, pruritic rash, comprising discrete, erythematous, raised lesions that vary in size from 1 to 3 cm. The symptoms of acute schistosomiasis (Katayama syndrome) can last from days to weeks, and can include fever, malaise, cough, diarrhea, hematuria, and right upper quadrant pain. The chronic stages of gastrointestinal disease are characterized by hepatic fibrosis, portal hypertension, splenomegaly, ascites, and bleeding from esophageal varices. The chronic stages of genitourinary tract disease may result in obstructive uropathy, stones, infection, bladder cancer, fistulas, and anemia due to chronic hematuria. Terminal hematuria in children from an endemic region is a red flag for urinary schistosomiasis. Spinal cord granulomas and paraplegia due to egg embolization into the Batson plexus have been reported.

B. Laboratory Findings

The diagnosis is made by finding the species-specific eggs in feces (*S japonicum*, *S mekongi*, *S mansoni*, and occasionally *S haematobium*) or urine (*S haematobium* and occasionally *S mansoni*). If no eggs are found, concentration methods should be used. Because the shedding of eggs can vary, three specimens should be obtained. Urine specimens should be collected between 10 AM and 2 PM to coincide with the timing of maximal egg secretion. Testing should wait until 2 months after the last known freshwater contact as this is the time required for worms to start producing eggs following infection. Serological tests are also useful, especially for making the diagnosis in patients who are not excreting eggs. Peripheral eosinophilia is common, and eosinophils may be seen in urine.

▶ Prevention

The best prevention is to avoid contact with contaminated freshwater in endemic areas. Efforts to destroy the snail hosts have been successful in areas of accelerated economic development.

▶ Treatment

A. Specific Measures

Praziquantel is the treatment of choice for schistosomiasis. A dosage of 40 mg/kg/day in two divided doses (*S mansoni* or *S haematobium*) over 1 day or 20 mg/kg three times a day (*S japonicum* or *S mekongi*) over 1 day is very effective and nontoxic. Praziquantel has no effect on eggs and immature worms and therefore a repeat dose 4–6 weeks later is sometimes needed.

B. General Measures

The patient's urinary tract should be evaluated carefully in *S haematobium* infection; reconstructive surgery may be needed. Hepatic fibrosis requires careful evaluation of the portal venous system and surgical management of portal hypertension when appropriate.

▶ Prognosis

Therapy decreases the worm burden and liver size, despite continued exposure in endemic areas. Early disease responds well to therapy, but once significant scarring or severe inflammation has occurred, eradication of the parasites is of little benefit.

Colley DG et al: Human schistosomiasis. Lancet 2014 Jun 28; 383(9936):2253–2264 [PMID: 24698483].

http://www.cdc.gov/parasites/schistosomiasis/. Accessed June 26, 2019.

http://www.who.int/topics/schistosomiasis/. Accessed June 26, 2019.

Kramer CV et al: Drugs for treating urinary schistosomiasis. Cochrane Database Syst Rev 2014;8:CD000053. doi: 10.1002/14651858. CD000053.pub3 [PMID: 25099517].

▼ MYCOTIC INFECTIONS

Fungi can be classified as yeasts, which are unicellular and reproduce by budding; as molds, which are multicellular and consist of tubular structures (hyphae) and grow by elongation and branching; or as dimorphic fungi, which can exist either as yeasts or molds depending on environmental conditions. Categorization according to anatomic and epidemiologic features is shown in Table 43–4. Fungal cells are taxonomically distinct from plant and animal cells. These differences, especially cell wall and cell membrane components, are utilized for diagnosis and are the basis of specific therapy.

In the United States, systemic fungal disease in normal hosts is commonly caused by three endemic organisms— *Coccidioides*, *Histoplasma*, and *Blastomyces*—which are restricted to certain geographic areas. Prior residence in or travel to these areas, even for a brief time, is a prerequisite for inclusion in a differential diagnosis. Of these three, *Histoplasma* most often relapses years later in patients who are immunosuppressed.

Immunosuppression (especially depressed T-cell–mediated immunity), foreign bodies (eg, urinary and central catheters for Candida), ulceration of gastrointestinal and respiratory mucosa, severe burns, broad-spectrum antimicrobial therapy, malnutrition, HIV infection, and

Table 43–4. Pediatric fungal infections.

Type	Agents	Incidence	Diagnosis	Diagnostic Tests	Therapy	Prognosis
Superficial	Candida[a] Dermatophytes Malassezia	Very common	Simple	KOH prep	Topical/Oral	Good
Subcutaneous	Sporothrix[a]	Uncommon	Simple[b]	Culture	Oral	Good
Systemic: normal host (endemic)	Coccidioides Histoplasma Blastomyces	Common: regional	Often presumptive	Chest radiograph; serology, antigen detection; tissue biopsy, culture	None[c] or systemic	Good
Systemic: opportunistic infection	Candida[a] Pneumocystis[d] Aspergillus Mucorales Malassezia Pseudallescheria Cryptococcus[c]	Uncommon	Difficult[e]	Tissue biopsy, culture, antigen/ fungal product/ DNA detection and NMR for Candida	Systemic, prolonged	Poor if therapy is delayed and patient is severely immune compromised.

KOH, potassium hydroxide; NMR, nuclear magnetic resonance.
[a]*Candida* and *Sporothrix* in immunocompromised patients may cause severe, rapidly progressive disease and require systemic therapy.
[b]Sporotrichosis may require biopsy for diagnosis.
[c]Can be self-limited in normal host.
[d]Asymptomatically infects many normal hosts.
[e]Except *Cryptococcus*, which is often diagnosed by antigen detection.

neutropenia or neutrophil defects are major risk factors for fungal infections (termed "opportunistic fungal infections").

Laboratory diagnosis may be difficult because of the small number of fungi present in some lesions, slow growth of some organisms, and difficulty in distinguishing normal colonization of mucosal surfaces from infection. A tissue biopsy with fungal stains and culture is the best method for diagnosing some systemic fungal disease. Repeat blood cultures may be negative even in the presence of intravascular infections. Serologic tests are useful for diagnosing coccidioidomycosis and histoplasmosis, and antigen detection in urine and blood is useful for diagnosing blastomycosis, histoplasmosis, cryptococcosis, and aspergillosis.

The common superficial fungal infections of the hair and skin are discussed in Chapter 15.

Centers for Disease Control and Prevention. Fungal diseases. Available at https://www.cdc.gov/fungal/index.html. Accessed July 2, 2019.

Hage CA, Knox KS, Wheat LJ: Endemic mycoses: overlooked causes of community acquired pneumonia. Respir Med 2012;106(6):769 [PMID: 22386326].

Blastomycosis

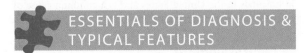

ESSENTIALS OF DIAGNOSIS & TYPICAL FEATURES

► Residence in, or travel to, an endemic area.

► In immunocompetent patients, most often a self-limited flu-like illness; acute pneumonia occurs in a minority of cases.

► Complications include progressive pneumonia and disseminated disease (CNS, skin, bone and joints, genitourinary tract).

► Diagnosis by culture of specimens from bronchoscopy, skin, or other tissue, or antigen detection.

▶ General Considerations

The causative fungus, *Blastomyces dermatitidis*, is found in soil primarily in the Mississippi and Ohio River valleys, additional southeastern and south central states, and the states bordering the Great Lakes. Transmission is by inhalation of spores. Subclinical disease is common. Infection rates are similar in both sexes in children, but severe disease is much more common in adults and males.

▶ Clinical Findings

A. Symptoms and Signs

Primary infection is often unrecognized (> 50%). Clinical disease typically includes cough with purulent sputum, chest pain, headache, weight loss, night sweats, and fever. These occur several weeks to months after inoculation. Infection is most often self-limited in immunocompetent patients, but in some patients an indolent progressive pulmonary disease occurs after an incubation period of 20–100 (median 45) days. Cutaneous lesions (20% of patients) usually represent disseminated disease. Skin lesions are slowly progressive and become ulcers with a sharp, heaped-up border or develop a verrucous appearance. Bone disease resembles other forms of chronic osteomyelitis. Lytic skull lesions in children are typical, but long bones, vertebrae, and the pelvis may be involved. Extrapulmonary disease occurs in 25%–40% of patients with progressive disease. A total body radiographic examination is advisable when blastomycosis is diagnosed in the skin or other extrapulmonary site.

B. Laboratory Findings

An initial suppurative response is followed by an increase in mononuclear cells and subsequent formation of noncaseating granulomas. Diagnosis requires isolation or visualization of the fungus. Pulmonary specimens (sputum, tracheal aspirates, or lung biopsy) may be positive using conventional or fungal cell wall stains. The budding yeasts have refractile thick walls and are very large and distinctive (figure-of-eight appearance). The fungus can be readily isolated in most laboratories, but a week is often required. Sputum specimens are positive in more than 80% of cases and in almost all bronchial washings, and skin lesions are positive in 80%–100%. Antibody tests are generally not helpful for diagnosis, but an ELISA antigen detection method, similar to that used for histoplasmosis, readily detects *Blastomyces* antigen in serum, urine, and lung lavage fluids. In this assay, there is cross-reactivity with histoplamosis. Methods based on detecting blastomyces DNA are now available.

C. Imaging

Radiographic lobar consolidation and fibronodular interstitial and patchy alveolar infiltrates are typical in cases with progressive pneumonia; effusions, hilar nodes, and cavities are less common. The paucity of cavitation and absence of hilar adenopathy distinguishes acute blastomycosis from histoplasmosis and tuberculosis. Miliary patterns also occur with acute infection. Chronic disease can develop in the upper lobes, with cavities and fibronodular infiltrations similar to those seen in tuberculosis. However, unlike tuberculosis or histoplasmosis, these lesions rarely caseate or calcify.

Differential Diagnosis

Primary pulmonary infection resembles acute viral, bacterial, or mycoplasmal infections and is generally confused with atypical community-acquired pneumonia. Blastomycosis should be considered when a significant pulmonary infection in an endemic area fails to respond to antibiotic therapy. Subacute infection mimics tuberculosis, histoplasmosis, and coccidioidomycosis. Chronic pulmonary or disseminated disease must be differentiated from cancer, tuberculosis, or other fungal infections.

Treatment

One view is that all children with proven blastomyces should receive antifungal therapy. Certainly any patient who is symptomatic at the time of diagnosis with moderately severe or life-threatening blastomycosis (especially if immuno-compromised), or has CNS infection, should have therapy initiated with the lipid formulation of amphotericin B (3–5 mg/kg intravenously) for 1–2 weeks or until improved. This is followed by oral itraconazole (5–10 mg/kg/day; divided into two doses [maximum = 400 mg]) for 6 months. Mild-to-moderate blastomycosis is often treated with oral itraconazole alone for 6–12 months. Bone disease may require a full year of itraconazole therapy. Surgical debridement is required for devitalized bone, drainage of large abscesses, and pulmonary lesions not responding to medical therapy.

Prognosis

Treatment with at least 1 g of amphotericin results in 75%–90% clearance without relapse. Patients initially treated with itraconazole have a 95% cure rate.

Castillo CG: Blastomycosis. Infect Dis Clin North Am 2016;30:247 [PMID: 26739607].

Frost HM, Anderson J, Ivacic L, Meece J: Blastomycosis in children: analysis of clinical, epidemiologic, and genetic features. J Ped Infect Dis Soc 2017;6:49 [PMID: 26703241].

Candidiasis

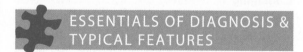

ESSENTIALS OF DIAGNOSIS & TYPICAL FEATURES

► In normal or immunosuppressed individuals: superficial infections (oral thrush or ulcerations, vulvovaginitis, erythematous intertriginous rash with satellite lesions); fungemia related to intravascular devices.

► In immunosuppressed individuals: systemic infections (candidemia with renal, hepatic, splenic, pulmonary, or cerebral abscesses); chorioretinitis; cutaneous nodules.

► In either patient population: budding yeast and pseudohyphae are seen in biopsy specimens, body fluids, or scrapings of lesions; positive culture, spectrophotometric, and PCR methods for diagnosing candida in body fluids.

General Considerations

Disease due to *Candida* is caused by *C albicans* in greater than 50% of cases in children; severe systemic infection may also be caused by *C tropicalis*, *C parapsilosis*, *C glabrata*, *C krusei*, and a few other *Candida* species. Infections with *C auris* have become a major global health threat. *C auris* is frequently highly drug-resistant and has been associated with several outbreaks in health care settings. Speciation is important because of differences in pathogenicity and response to antifungal therapy.

C albicans is ubiquitous, usually in small numbers, on skin, mucous membranes, or in the intestinal tract. Normal bacterial flora, intact epithelial barriers, neutrophils, and macrophages, in conjunction with antibody and complement and normal lymphocyte function, are factors in preventing invasion. Disseminated infection is almost always preceded by prolonged broad-spectrum antibiotic therapy, instrumentation (including intravascular catheters), and/or immunosuppression. Patients with diabetes mellitus are prone to superficial *Candida* infection; thrush and vaginitis are most common. *Candida* is the fourth most common blood isolate in hospitals in the United States and is a common cause of catheter-related urinary tract infection.

Clinical Findings

A. Symptoms and Signs

1. Oral candidiasis (Thrush)—Adherent creamy white plaques on the buccal, gingival, or lingual mucosa are seen. These may be painful. Lesions may be few and asymptomatic, or they may be extensive, extending into the esophagus. Thrush is very common in otherwise normal infants in the first weeks of life and may last weeks despite topical therapy. Spontaneous thrush in older children is unusual unless they have recently received antimicrobials. Corticosteroid inhalation for asthma predisposes patients to thrush. HIV infection or other immune deficiency should be considered if there is no other reason for oral thrush, especially when it is persistent or recurrent. Angular cheilitis is the name given to painful erythematous fissures caused by *Candida* at the corners of the mouth, occasionally in association with vitamin or iron deficiencies.

2. Vaginal infection—Vulvovaginitis occurs in sexually active girls, in diabetic patients, and in girls receiving antibiotics. Oral contraception and pregnancy are risk factors. Thick, odorless, cheesy discharge with intense pruritus is typical.

The vagina and labia are usually erythematous and swollen. Outbreaks are more frequent before menses.

3. Skin infection

A. DERMATITIS—Diaper dermatitis is often due entirely or partly to *Candida*. Pronounced erythema with a sharply defined margin and satellite lesions is typical. Pustules, vesicles, papules, or scales may be seen. Weeping, eroded lesions with a scalloped border are common. Any moist area, such as axillae, under breasts, and inguinal or neck folds, may be involved.

B. SCATTERED RED PAPULES OR NODULES—Such findings in immunocompromised patients may represent cutaneous dissemination.

C. PARONYCHIA AND ONYCHOMYCOSIS—These conditions occur in immunocompetent children but more commonly with immunosuppression, hypoparathyroidism, or adrenal insufficiency (*Candida* endocrinopathy syndrome). The selective absence of specific innate and T-cell responses to *Candida* can lead to marked, chronic skin and nail infections called *chronic mucocutaneous candidiasis.*

D. CHRONIC DRAINING OTITIS MEDIA—This may occur in patients who have received multiple courses of antibiotics and are superinfected with *Candida*.

4. Enteric infection

Esophageal involvement in immunocompromised patients is the most common enteric manifestation, resulting in substernal pain, dysphagia, and painful swallowing. Nausea and vomiting are common in young children. Most patients do not have thrush. Stomach or intestinal ulcers also occur. Candidal peritonitis can occur following intestinal perforation, particularly of the duodenum.

5. Pulmonary infection

Because the organism frequently colonizes the upper respiratory tract, it is commonly isolated from respiratory secretions. Thus, demonstration of tissue invasion is needed to diagnose *Candida* pneumonia or tracheitis. It is rare, seen mainly in immunosuppressed patients and patients intubated for long periods, usually while taking antibiotics. The infection may cause abscesses, nodular infiltrates, and effusion.

6. Renal infection

Candiduria may be the only manifestation of disseminated disease. Most often, candiduria is associated with instrumentation, an indwelling catheter, or anatomic abnormality of the urinary tract. Symptoms of cystitis may be present. Masses of *Candida* may obstruct ureters and cause obstructive nephropathy. *Candida* casts in the urine suggest renal tissue infection.

7. Other infections

Meningitis, and osteomyelitis usually occur only in immunocompromised patients or neonates, generally in those with high-grade candidemia. Endocarditis may occur on an artificial or abnormal heart valve, especially when an intravascular line is present.

8. Disseminated candidiasis

Skin and mucosal colonization precedes but does not predict dissemination. Too often, dissemination is confused with bacterial sepsis. This occurs in neonates—especially premature infants—in an intensive care unit setting and is recognized when a sick infant fails to respond to antibiotics or when candidemia is documented. Invasive disease can occur in greater than 50% of very low-birth-weight infants. These infants often have unexplained feeding intolerance, cardiovascular instability, apnea, new or worsening respiratory failure, glucose intolerance, thrombocytopenia, or hyperbilirubinemia. A careful search in immunocompromised patients should be carried out for lesions suggestive of disseminated *Candida* (retinal cotton-wool spots or chorioretinitis; nodular dermal abscesses). If these findings are absent, diagnosis is often based presumptively on the presence of a compatible illness in an immunocompromised patient; a burn patient; or a patient with prolonged postsurgical or intensive care unit course who has no other cause for symptoms and who fails to respond to antimicrobials. Such patients usually have *Candida* colonization of mucosal surfaces. Treatment for presumptive infection is often undertaken because candidemia is not identified antemortem in some such patients.

Hepatosplenic and renal candidiasis occurs in immunosuppressed patients. The typical case is a severely neutropenic patient who develops chronic fever, variable abdominal pain, and abnormal liver function tests. No causative bacterial pathogen is isolated, and there is no response to antimicrobials. Ultrasound or CT scan of the liver, spleen, and kidney demonstrates multiple round lesions. Biopsy is needed to confirm the diagnosis.

B. Laboratory Findings

Budding yeast cells are easily seen in scrapings or other samples. A wet mount preparation of vaginal secretions is 40%–50% sensitive; this is increased to 50%–70% with the addition of 10% potassium hydroxide to the sample. The use of a Gram-stained smear is 70%–100% sensitive. Stains for fungal cell walls will increase sensitivity. The presence of pseudohyphae suggests tissue invasion. Positive cultures from nonsterile sites may reflect colonization and need to be carefully evaluated, but *Candida* should never be considered a contaminant in cultures from normally sterile sites. *Candida* grows on routine media more slowly than many bacteria; growth is usually evident on agar after 2–3 days and in blood culture within 3 days, but cultures may remain negative (10%–40%) even with disseminated disease or endocarditis. The ability of yeast to form germ tubes when incubated in human serum gives a presumptive speciation for *C albicans*. However, newly available NMR (nuclear magnetic resonance) and PCR methods greatly shorten the delay in diagnosis and speciation. *Candida* in any number in appropriately collected urine suggests true infection.

Differential Diagnosis

Thrush may resemble milk or formula (which can be easily wiped away with a tongue blade or swab, revealing normal mucosa without underlying erythema or erosion), other types of ulcers (including herpes), or oral changes induced by chemotherapy. Skin lesions may resemble contact, allergic, chemical, or bacterial dermatitis; miliaria; folliculitis; or eczema. Vulvovaginitis needs to be distinguished from other causes of vaginal discharge and discomfort. Candidemia and systemic infection should be considered in any seriously ill patient with the risk factors previously mentioned.

Complications

Arthritis and meningitis occur more often in neonates than in older children, and abscesses can occur in any organ. The greater the length or extent of immunosuppression and the longer the delay before therapy, the more likely that complications will occur.

Treatment

A. Oral Candidiasis

In infants, oral nystatin suspension (100,000 units four to six times a day in the buccal fold after feeding for 2–3 days after resolution) usually suffices. Nystatin must come in contact with the lesions because it is not absorbed systemically. Older children may use it as a mouthwash (200,000–500,000 units five times a day), although it is poorly tolerated because of its taste. Clotrimazole troches (10 mg) four times a day are an alternative in older children. Prolonged therapy with either agent or more frequent dosing may be needed. Painting the lesions with a cotton swab dipped in gentian violet (0.5%–1%) is visually dramatic and messy but may help refractory cases. Eradication of *Candida* from pacifiers, bottle nipples, toys, or the mother's breasts (if the infant is breast-feeding and there is candidal infection of the nipples) may be helpful.

Oral azoles, such as fluconazole (6 mg/kg/day), are effective in older children with candidal infection refractory to nystatin. Discontinuation of antibiotics or corticosteroids is advised when possible. Esophageal candidiasis should be treated with systemic therapy as described later.

B. Skin Infection

Cutaneous infection usually responds to a cream or lotion containing nystatin, amphotericin B, or an imidazole (miconazole, clotrimazole, naftidene, and others). Associated inflammation such as severe diaper dermatitis is helped by concurrent use of a topical low concentration corticosteroid cream, such as 1% hydrocortisone. It may help to keep the involved area dry; a heat lamp and nystatin powder may be used. Suppression of intestinal *Candida* with nystatin and

eradicating thrush may speed recovery and prevent recurrence of diaper dermatitis.

C. Vaginal Infections

Vulvovaginal candidiasis (see Chapter 44) is treated with clotrimazole, miconazole, triazoles, or nystatin (cheapest if generic is used) suppositories or creams, usually applied once nightly for 3–7 days. A high-dose topical clotrimazole formulation can be given for only a single night. Oral azole therapy is equally effective. A single 150-mg oral dose of fluconazole is effective for vaginitis in older girls. It is more expensive but very convenient. *Candida* balanitis in sexual partners should be treated, but no controlled study has shown that treating colonization of male sexual partners prevents recurrence in females. Frequent recurrent infections (often with *C glabrata*) may require elimination of risk factors, the use of oral therapy, or some prophylactic antifungal therapy, such as a single dose of fluconazole weekly for 6 months.

D. Renal Infection

Candiduria in an immunocompetent host with a urinary catheter may respond to catheter removal. Candiduria is treated in all high-risk patients, usually with a 7- to 14-day course of fluconazole (3–6 mg/kg/day), which is concentrated in the urine. Amphotericin B is required for patients with fluconazole-resistant organisms. Renal abscesses or ureteral fungus balls require intravenous antifungal therapy. Removal of an indwelling catheter is imperative.

E. Systemic Infection

1. Disseminated *Candida* infection—Systemic infection is dangerous and resistant to therapy. Surgical drainage of abscesses and removal of all infected tissue (eg, a heart valve) are required for cure. An echinocandin is the preferred therapy. The initial dose and maintenance dosing varies with the drug chosen. Fluconazole may be substituted after 5–7 days if the response to therapy is satisfactory. Fluconazole as initial therapy is an alternative for selected patients who are not critically ill and who are likely to have a sensitive organism. Lipid formulations of amphotericin are alternatives when other drugs are not tolerated or when the isolate has an unfavorable resistance pattern. Hepatosplenic candidiasis should be treated until all lesions have disappeared or calcified.

Fluconazole and itraconazole (best absorbed from the liquid solution) and newer azole drugs, such as voriconazole and posaconazole, or echinocandins, are used interchangeably with or in conjunction with amphotericin. They are often preferred because they are less likely to be toxic than amphotericin. They are acceptable alternatives for serious *C albicans* infections in nonneutropenic patients and are often effective as first-line therapy in immunocompromised patients. The decision to use systemic azole therapy should include consideration of the local experience with azole-resistant *Candida* and if the patient had received prophylaxis or treatment with azoles. Fluconazole is well absorbed (oral and intravenous therapy are equivalent), reasonably nontoxic, and effective for a variety of *Candida* infections. Fluconazole dosage is 8–12 mg/kg/day in a single-daily dose for initial therapy of severely ill children. Selected patients with prolonged immunosuppression (eg, after hematopoietic stem cell transplantation) should receive prophylactic azole or echinocandin prophylaxis. Susceptibility testing for *Candida* species is available to guide this decision. *Candida glabrata* and *C krusei* are common isolates that may be resistant to fluconazole; these are often susceptible to the newer azoles and echinocandins. *Candida lusitaniae* is usually resistant to amphotericin. Many isolates of *C auris* are azole resistant; in the United States, most isolates remain susceptible to the echinocandins.

Correction of predisposing factors is important (eg, discontinuing antibiotics and immunosuppressives, improving control of diabetes, and removing infected devices and lines).

2. Candidemia—Infected central venous lines should be removed immediately; this alone often is curative. If the infection is considered limited to the line and environs, a 14-day course (after the last positive culture) of a systemic antifungal agent following line removal is recommended for nonneutropenic patients. An echinocandin is preferred, with completion of therapy with fluconazole when sensitivity is established. This is because of the late occurrence of focal *Candida* infection, especially retinal infection in some cases. Persistent fever and candidemia suggest infected thrombus, endocarditis, or tissue infection. All such patients should be examined by an ophthalmologist.

3. Very low-birth-weight infants—In many nurseries rates of severe *Candida* infection can exceed 5%–10%. Infected infants should receive intravenous amphotericin B (1 mg/kg/day) or fluconazole (12 mg/kg IV or PO) if no prior fluconazole. Treatment should continue until 2 weeks after the last positive culture. Lumbar puncture and eye examination should be performed. Prophylaxis in this setting is fluconazole (3 mg/kg twice weekly) for 6 weeks or until IV therapy is not needed.

▶ **Prognosis**

Superficial disease in normal hosts has a good prognosis; in abnormal hosts, it may be refractory to therapy. Early therapy of systemic disease is often curative if the underlying immune response is adequate. The outcome is poor when therapy is delayed or when host response is inadequate. Candidemia in the severely premature neonate increases the chance of death and poor neurodevelopmental outcome.

Barton M et al: Invasive candidiasis in low birth weight infants: risk factors, clinical course and outcome in a prospective multicenter study of cases and their matched controls. BMC Infect Dis 2014;14:327 [PMID: 24924877].

Bassett M: The current treatment landscape: candidiasis. J Antimicrob Therap Chemother 2016;71(suppl 2):ii13 [PMID: 27880665].

Forsberg K et al: Candida auris: the recent emergence of a multidrug-resistant fungal pathogen. Med Mycol 2019 Jan;57(1): 1–12 [PMID: 30715430].

Lollis TR, Bradshaw WT: Fungal prophylaxis in neonates: a review article. Adv Neonatal Care 2014;14(1):17 [PMID: 24472884].

Pappas PG, Kauffman CA, Andes DR: Executive summary: clinical practice guideline for the management of candidiasis: 2016 update by the Infectious Diseases Society of America. Clin Infect Dis 2016 Feb 15; 62(4):409–417 [PMID: 26810419].

Coccidioidomycosis

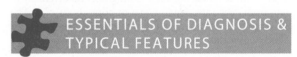

ESSENTIALS OF DIAGNOSIS & TYPICAL FEATURES

▶ Residence in, or travel to, an endemic area.

▶ Primary pulmonary form: fever, chest pain, cough, anorexia, weight loss, and often a macular rash; erythema nodosum or erythema multiforme occurs during the acute phase.

▶ Primary cutaneous form: skin trauma followed in 1–3 weeks by an ulcer and regional adenopathy.

▶ Spherules (endospores in tissue) seen in pus, sputum, CSF, joint fluid; positive culture.

▶ Appearance of precipitating (early) and complement-fixing antibodies (late).

▶ **General Considerations**

Coccidioidomycosis is caused by the dimorphic fungus *Coccidioides* (*immitis* or *posadasii*), which is endemic in the Sonoran Desert areas of western Texas, southern New Mexico and Arizona, southern California, northern Mexico, and South America. Infection results from inhalation or inoculation of arthrospores (highly contagious and readily airborne in the dry climate). Even brief travel in or through an endemic area, especially during windy seasons, may result in infection. Human-to-human transmission does not occur. More than 60% of infections are asymptomatic, and less than 5% are associated with significant pulmonary disease. Chronic pulmonary disease or dissemination occurs in less than 1% of cases.

▶ Clinical Findings

A. Symptoms and Signs

1. Primary disease—The incubation period is 10–16 days (range, 7–28 days). Symptoms vary from those of a mild fever and arthralgia to severe influenza-like illness with high fever, nonproductive cough, pleuritic chest pains, arthralgias, headache, and night sweats. Upper respiratory tract signs are uncommon. Most infections are self-limited or minimal in severity. Signs vary from none to rash, rales, pleural rubs, and signs of pulmonary consolidation. Weight loss may occur.

2. Skin disease—Up to 10% of children develop erythema nodosum or erythema multiforme. These manifestations imply a favorable host response to the organism. Less specific maculopapular eruptions occur in a larger number of children. Skin lesions can occur following fungemia. Primary skin inoculation sites develop indurated ulcers with local adenopathy. Contiguous involvement of skin from deep infection in nodes or bone also occurs. The presence of chronic skin lesions should lead to a search for internal infection.

3. Chronic pulmonary disease—This is uncommon in children. Chronic disease is manifested by chronic cough (occasionally with hemoptysis), weight loss, and radiologic abnormalities.

4. Disseminated disease—This is less common in children than adults, and is more common in infants, neonates, pregnant women (especially during the third trimester), African Americans, Filipinos, American Indians, and patients with HIV or other defective T-cell–mediated immunity. More than one organ may be involved. The most common extrapulmonary sites involved are bone or joint (usually a single bone or joint; subacute or chronic swelling, pain, redness), nodes, meninges (slowly progressive meningeal signs, ataxia, vomiting, headache, and cranial neuropathies), and kidneys (dysuria and urinary frequency). As with most fungal diseases, the evolution of the illness is usually slow.

B. Laboratory Findings

Direct examination of respiratory secretions, pus, CSF, or tissue may reveal large spherules (30–60 μm) containing endospores germinating in tissue. The organism is detected by using periodic acid–Schiff reagent, methenamine silver, and calcofluor stains. Characteristic colonies grow within 2–5 days on routine fungal and many other media. CSF cultures are often falsely negative.

The sedimentation rate is usually elevated. Eosinophilia may occur, particularly prior to dissemination, and is more common in coccidioidomycosis than in many other conditions with similar symptoms. Meningitis causes a mononuclear pleocytosis (70% contain eosinophils) with elevated protein and mild hypoglycorrhachia.

Antibodies consist of precipitins (usually measurable by 2–3 weeks in 90% of cases and gone by 12 weeks) and complement-fixing antibodies (delayed for several weeks; appear as the precipitins are falling and should disappear by 8 months). Thus, serum precipitins usually indicate acute infection. The extent of the complement-fixing antibody response reflects the severity of infection. Persistent high levels suggest dissemination. ELISA assays, which detect IgM and IgG antibodies against coccidioidal antigens, become positive as early as 1–3 weeks (90% of positive tests) after onset of symptoms. The presence of antibody in CSF indicates CNS infection; CSF and serum antibody titers correlate with disease progression and response to therapy.

Galactomannan antigen from *Coccidioides* is detected in urine and serum of patients. This occurs more frequently in severe disease compared to moderate disease. Testing both urine and serum should provide a diagnosis in more than 75% of patients.

A skin test with coccidioides antigen can provide evidence of prior infection and conversion implies recent infection. A positive test is a good prognostic sign. Detection of coccidioidal antigen in CSF is useful to establish CNS infection.

C. Imaging

Approximately half of symptomatic infections are associated with abnormal chest radiographs—usually infiltrates with hilar adenopathy. Pulmonary consolidation, effusion, and thin-walled cavities may be seen. About 5% of infected patients have asymptomatic nodules or cysts after recovery. Unlike tuberculosis reactivation, apical disease is not prominent. Bone infection causes osteolysis that enhances with technetium. Cerebral imaging may show hydrocephalus and meningitis; intracranial abscesses and calcifications are unusual. Radiographic evolution of lesions is slow.

▶ Differential Diagnosis

Primary pulmonary infection resembles acute viral, bacterial, or mycoplasmal infections; subacute presentation mimics tuberculosis, histoplasmosis, and blastomycosis. Chronic pulmonary or disseminated disease must be differentiated from cancer, tuberculosis, or other fungal infections.

▶ Complications

Dissemination of primary pulmonary disease is associated with permissive ethnic background, prolonged fever (> 1 month), a negative skin test, high complement-fixation antibody titer, and marked hilar adenopathy. Pulmonary complications include effusion, empyema, and pneumothorax. Cerebral infection can cause noncommunicating hydrocephalus due to basilar meningitis.

Treatment

A. Specific Measures

Mild pulmonary infections in most immune competent patients do not require therapy, although some experts argue for treatment of all infections. Untreated patients should be assessed for 1–2 years to document resolution and to identify any complications. Antifungal therapy is used for prolonged fever, weight loss (> 10%), prolonged duration of night sweats, severe pneumonitis (especially if persisting for 4–6 weeks), or any form of disseminated disease. Neonates, pregnant women, high-risk racial background, and patients with high antibody titers also receive treatment.

Lipid formulation of amphotericin B is used to treat extensive pulmonary or disseminated disease or disease in immunosuppressed patients (2–5 mg/kg/day). In general, the more rapidly progressive the infection, the more compelling the case for amphotericin B therapy. For less severe disease and for meningeal disease, fluconazole or itraconazole is preferred (duration of therapy is 3–6 months or is lifelong for meningeal disease). Measurement of serum levels is suggested to monitor therapy. Chronic fibrocavitary pneumonia is treated for at least 12 months. Itraconazole may be superior to fluconazole. Refractory infection often responds to voriconazle together with caspofungin, and refractory meningitis may require prolonged intrathecal or intraventricular amphotericin B therapy.

B. General Measures

Most pulmonary infections require only symptomatic therapy, self-limited activity, and good nutrition. Patients are not contagious.

C. Surgical Measures

Excision of chronic pulmonary cavities or abscesses may be needed. Infected nodes, sinus tracts, and bone are other operable lesions. Azole therapy should be given prior to surgery to prevent dissemination and should be continued for 4 weeks arbitrarily or until other criteria for cure are met.

Prognosis

Most patients recover. Even with amphotericin B, however, disseminated disease may be fatal, especially in those racially predisposed to severe disease (African American, Filipino). A negative skin test or a rising complement-fixing antibody titer is an ominous sign. Individuals who later in life undergo immunosuppressive therapy or develop HIV may experience reactivation of dormant disease. Thus, some transplant, rheumatology, and oncology programs determine prior infection by serology and either provide prophylaxis or observe patients closely during periods of intense immune suppression.

Dimitrova D, Ross L: Experience from a children's hospital in an area of endemicity. J Ped Infect Dis Soc 2014;5:89 [PMID: 26908496].

Stockamp NW, Thompson GR III: Coccidiodomycosis. Infect Dis Clin North Am 2016;30:229 [PMID: 26739609].

Cryptococcosis

ESSENTIALS OF DIAGNOSIS & TYPICAL FEATURES

▶ Acute pneumonitis in immunocompetent individuals.

▶ Immunosuppressed patients especially vulnerable to CNS infection (headache, vomiting, cranial nerve palsies, meningeal signs; mononuclear cell pleocytosis).

▶ Cryptococcal antigen detected in CSF; also in serum and urine in some patients.

▶ *Cryptococcus* is readily isolated on routine media.

General Considerations

Cryptococcus neoformans is a ubiquitous soil yeast. It survives best in soil contaminated with bird excrement. However, most infections in humans are not associated with a history of significant contact with birds. Inhalation is the presumed route of inoculation. Infections in children are rare, even in heavily immunocompromised patients such as those with HIV infection. Immunocompetent individuals can also be infected, especially by *Cryptococcus gattii*, which is an emerging pathogen in Canada and the Pacific Northwest. Asymptomatic carriage does not occur.

Clinical Findings

A. Symptoms and Signs

1. Pulmonary disease—Pulmonary infection precedes dissemination to other organs. It is frequently asymptomatic (many older children and adults have serologic evidence of prior infection) and often not clinically apparent. Pneumonia is the primary manifestation in one-third of patients; CNS disease is the primary manifestation in 50% of patients. Cryptococcal pneumonia may coexist with CNS involvement. Symptoms are nonspecific and subacute—cough, weight loss, and fatigue.

2. Meningitis—The most common clinical disease is meningitis, which follows hematogenous spread from a pulmonary focus. This is much more likely to occur in an immunosuppressed patient (especially HIV). Symptoms of headache, vomiting, and fever occur over days to months. Meningeal signs and papilledema are common. Cranial nerve dysfunction and seizures may occur.

3. Other forms—Cutaneous disease is usually secondary to dissemination. Papules, pustules, and ulcerating nodules are typical. Bones (rarely joints) may be infected; osteolytic areas are seen, and the process may resemble osteosarcoma. Many other organs, especially the eyes, can be involved with dissemination.

B. Laboratory Findings

The CSF usually has a lymphocytic pleocytosis; it may be completely normal in immunosuppressed patients with meningeal infection. Direct microscopy may reveal organisms in sputum, CSF, or other specimens. The capsular antigen can be detected by latex agglutination or ELISA, which are both sensitive (> 90%) and specific. False-negative CSF tests are rare. Serum, CSF, and urine should be tested when this infection is suspected. The serum may be negative if the only organ infected is the lung. The organism grows well after several days on many routine media. For optimal culture, collecting and concentrating a large volume of CSF (10 mL) is recommended because the number of organisms may be low. *Cryptococcus* is included in some multiplex PCR panels for meningitis.

C. Imaging

Radiographic findings are usually lower lobe infiltrates or nodular densities; less often effusions; and rarely cavitation, hilar adenopathy, or calcification. Single or multiple focal mass lesions (cryptococcoma) may be detected in the CNS on CT or MRI scan.

▶ Differential Diagnosis

Cryptococcal meningitis may mimic tuberculosis, viral meningoencephalitis, meningitis due to other fungi, or a space-occupying CNS lesion. Lung infection is difficult to differentiate from many causes of pneumonia.

▶ Complications

Hydrocephalus may be caused by chronic basilar meningitis. Symptomatic and recalcitrant intracranial hypertension is common. Significant pulmonary or osseous disease may accompany the primary infection or dissemination.

▶ Treatment

Patients with symptomatic pulmonary disease should receive fluconazole for 3–6 months. All immunocompromised patients with cryptococcal pulmonary disease should have a lumbar puncture to rule out CNS infection; this should also be done for immunocompetent patients with cryptococcal antigen in the serum. Severely ill patients should receive amphotericin B

deoxycholate (1.0 mg/kg/day); lipid or liposomal formulations of amphotericin B may be equally effective with fewer side effects. Meningitis is treated with liposomal amphotericin B (3 mg/kg/day) or amphotericin B lipid complex (5 mg/kg/day) and flucytosine (100 mg/kg/day divided into four doses). Fluconazole may be substituted for flucytosine. Induction therapy is continued for a minimum of 2 weeks for CNS infections. Transition to consolidation therapy after this point depends on clinical response and measurement of cryptococcal antigen in CSF. Consolidation is with fluconazole alone (5 mg/kg BID) for 8 weeks followed by a reduced dose (maintenance therapy) for an additional 6–12 months. Some evidence suggests that voriconazole or posaconazole may have greater anticryptococcal activity. Fluconazole remains the preferred maintenance therapy to prevent relapses in high-risk (eg, HIV) patients. Intracranial hypertension is treated by frequent spinal taps or a lumbar drain.

▶ Prognosis

Treatment failure, including death, is common in immunosuppressed patients, especially those with AIDS. Lifelong maintenance therapy may be required in these patients. Poor prognostic signs are the presence of extrameningeal disease, fewer than 20 cells/μL of initial CSF, and initial CSF antigen titer greater than 1:32.

Fisher JF: Pulmonary cryptococcosis in the immunocompetent patient—many questions, some answers. Open Forum Infect Dis 2016;3(3) [PMID: 27704021].

Perfect JR: Clinical practice guidelines for the management of cryptococcal disease: 2010 update by the infectious diseases society of America. Clin Infect Dis 2010;50(3):291–322 [PMID: 20047480].

Sun H et al: Lipid formulations of amphotericin B significantly improve outcome in solid organ transplant recipients with central nervous system cryptococcosis. Clin Infect Dis 2009;49(11):1721 [PMID: 19886800].

Histoplasmosis

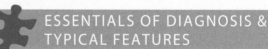

ESSENTIALS OF DIAGNOSIS & TYPICAL FEATURES

▶ Residence in or travel to an endemic area.

▶ Pneumonia with flu-like illness.

▶ If disseminated, hepatosplenomegaly, anemia, leukopenia.

▶ Histoplasmal antigen in urine, blood, bronchoalveolar lavage fluid or CSF.

▶ Detection by staining the organism in smears or tissue, or by culture.

General Considerations

The dimorphic fungus *Histoplasma capsulatum* is found in the central and eastern United States (Ohio, Mississippi, and Missouri River valleys), Mexico, and most of South America. Soil contamination is enhanced by the presence of bat or bird feces. Infection is acquired by inhaling spores that transform into the pathogenic yeast form in infected tissues, especially within macrophages. Infections in endemic areas are very common at all ages and are usually asymptomatic. Over two-thirds of children are infected in these areas. Reactivation is rare in children, but occurs after treatment with immune suppressive agents, such as biological response modifiers and chemotherapy, even years after primary infection. Reinfection also occurs. The extent of symptoms with primary infection or reinfection is influenced by the size of the infecting inoculum.

Clinical Findings

Human-to-human transmission does not occur. Infection implies environmental exposure in an endemic area—usually within prior weeks or months. Congenital infection does not occur.

A. Symptoms and Signs

1. Asymptomatic infection (90% of infections)— Asymptomatic histoplasmosis is usually diagnosed by the presence of scattered calcifications in lungs or spleen and a positive skin test or serology. The calcification may resemble that caused by tuberculosis, but may be more extensive than the typical Ghon complex.

2. Pneumonia—Approximately 5% of patients have mild-to-moderate disease. The cause of this illness is usually not recognized as being histoplasma. Acute pulmonary disease may resemble influenza: fever, malaise, myalgia, arthralgia, and nonproductive cough occur 1–3 weeks after a heavy exposure (may be longer with less intense exposure). The subacute form resembles infections such as tuberculosis with cough, weight loss, night sweats, and pleurisy. Chronic disease is unusual in children. Physical examination may be normal, or rales may be heard. A small number of patients may have immune-mediated signs such as arthritis, pericarditis, and erythema nodosum. The usual duration of the disease is less than 2 weeks, followed by complete resolution, but without treatment, symptoms may last several months.

3. Disseminated infection (5% of infections)—Fungemia during primary infection probably occurs in the first 2 weeks of all infections, including those with minimal symptoms. Transient hepatosplenomegaly may occur, but resolution is the rule in immunocompetent individuals. Heavy exposure, severe underlying pulmonary disease, and immunocompromise are risk factors for progressive infection characterized by anemia, fever, weight loss, organomegaly, CNS or bone marrow involvement, and death. Dissemination may occur in otherwise immunocompetent children; usually they are younger than 2 years.

4. Other forms—Ocular involvement consists of multifocal choroiditis. This usually occurs in immunocompetent adults with other evidence of disseminated disease. Brain, pericardium, intestine, and skin (oral ulcers and nodules) are other sites that can be involved. Adrenal gland involvement is common with systemic disease.

B. Laboratory Findings

Routine tests are normal or nonspecific in the benign forms. Pancytopenia is present in many patients with disseminated disease. The diagnosis can be made by demonstrating the organism by histology or culture. Tissue yeast forms are small and may be mistaken for artifact. They are usually found in macrophages, occasionally in peripheral blood leukocytes in severe disease, but infrequently in sputum, urine, or CSF. Cultures of infected fluids or tissues may yield the organism after 1–4 weeks of incubation on fungal media, but even cultures of bronchoalveolar lavage or transbronchial biopsy specimens in immunocompromised patients are often negative (15%). Thus, bone marrow and tissue specimens are needed. Detection of histoplasmal antigen in blood, urine, CSF, and bronchoalveolar lavage fluid is the most sensitive diagnostic test (90% positive in the urine with disseminated disease, 75% positive with acute pneumonia), but false-negative results may occur. Cross-reactions occur with other fungal infections. Both urine and serum should be tested for optimal results. The level of antigen correlates with the extent of the infection, and antigen levels can be used to follow the response to therapy and to indicate low-grade infection persisting after completion of therapy (eg, in a child with HIV infection).

Antibodies may be detected by immunodiffusion and complement fixation; the latter rises in the first 2–6 weeks of illness and falls thereafter unless dissemination occurs. Cross-reactions occur with some other endemic fungi. A single high titer or rising titer indicates a high likelihood of disease, but antigen detection has replaced serology as a rapid diagnostic test.

C. Imaging

Scattered pulmonary calcifications in a well-child are typical of past infection. Bronchopneumonia (focal mid-lung infiltrates) occurs with acute disease, often with hilar and mediastinal adenopathy, occasionally with nodules, but seldom with effusion. Localized or patchy infiltrates occur in subacute disease. Apical cavitation occurs with chronic infection, often on the background of preexisting pulmonary infection.

Differential Diagnosis

Pulmonary disease resembles viral infection, other causes of community-acquired pneumonia, tuberculosis, coccidioidomycosis, and blastomycosis. Systemic disease resembles disseminated fungal or mycobacterial infection, leukemia, histiocytosis, or cancer.

Treatment

Most patients with acute pulmonary disease will benefit from oral itraconazole. Those with subacute disease are generally better when the diagnosis is established, but if still symptomatic should receive oral therapy. Treatment with lipid formulation of amphotericin B (2–5 mg/kg/day) is indicated for severe pulmonary disease (diffuse radiographic involvement); disseminated disease; or when endovascular, CNS, or chronic pulmonary disease is present; and for children younger than 1 year. Disseminated disease in infants may respond to as few as 10 days of amphotericin B, although 4–6 weeks is usually recommended. Patients with severe disease (especially pulmonary) may benefit from a short course of corticosteroid therapy. Surgical excision of chronic pulmonary lesions is rarely required. Itraconazole (3–5 mg/kg/day for 6–12 weeks; achieve peak serum level of > 1.0 mcg/mL) appears to be equivalent to amphotericin B therapy for mild disease and can be substituted in severe disease after a favorable initial (2 weeks) response to amphotericin B. Chronic pulmonary, CNS, or disseminated disease should be treated for at least a year after switching to oral drug.

Quantitation of fungal antigen is useful for directing therapy, and should be monitored for 1 year after successful treatment of severe disease. Relapse may occur in up to 15% of patients with treated chronic disease. Histoplasmosis can reactivate in previously infected individuals who subsequently become immunosuppressed. Chronically immunosuppressed patients may require lifelong maintenance therapy with itraconazole.

Prognosis

Patients with mild and moderately severe infections have a good prognosis. With early diagnosis and treatment, infants with disseminated disease usually recover; the prognosis worsens if the immune response is poor.

Hage CA: Histoplasmosis: up-to-date evidence-based approach to diagnosis and management. Semin Respir Crit Care Med 2015;36(5):729–745 [PMID: 26398539].

Richer SM: Improved diagnosis of acute pulmonary histoplasmosis by combining antigen and antibody detection. Clin Infect Dis 2016;62(7):896–902 [PMID: 26797210].

Wheat LJ: Histoplasmosis. Infect Dis Clin North Am 2016;30(1):207–227 [PMID: 26897068].

Sporotrichosis

ESSENTIALS OF DIAGNOSIS & TYPICAL FEATURES

► Subacute cutaneous ulcers.
► New lesions appearing proximal to existing lesions along a draining lymphatic.
► Absence of systemic symptoms.
► Isolation of *Sporothrix schenckii* from wound drainage or biopsy.

General Considerations

Sporotrichosis is caused by *S schenckii*, a dimorphic fungus present as a mold in soil, plants, and plant products from most areas of North and South America. Spores of the fungus can cause infection when they breach the skin at areas of minor trauma. Sporotrichosis has been transmitted from cutaneous lesions of pets.

Clinical Findings

Cutaneous disease is by far the most common manifestation. Typically at the site of inapparent skin injury, an initial painless papular lesion will slowly become nodular and ulcerate. Subsequent new lesions develop in a similar fashion proximally along lymphatics draining the primary lesion. This sequence of developing painless, chronic ulcers in a linear pattern is strongly suggestive of the diagnosis. Solitary lesions may exist and some lesions may develop a verrucous character. Systemic symptoms are absent and laboratory evaluations are normal, except for acute-phase reactants. The fungus rarely disseminates in immunocompetent hosts. Cavitary pneumonia is a rare manifestation when patients inhale the spores. Immunocompromised patients, especially those with HIV infection, may develop disseminated skin lesions and multiorgan disease with extensive pneumonia.

Differential Diagnosis

The differential diagnosis of nodular lymphangitis (sporotrichoid infection) includes other endemic fungi and some bacteria, especially atypical mycobacteria and nocardiosis, pyoderma gangrenosum, and syphilis. Diagnosis is made by culture. Biopsy of skin lesions will demonstrate a suppurative response with granulomas and provides the best source for laboratory isolation. Occasionally, the characteristic yeast will be seen in the biopsy.

▶ Treatment & Prognosis

Treatment is with itraconazole (200 mg/day or 5 mg/kg/day divided BID) for 2–4 weeks after lesions heal, usually 3–6 months. Prognosis is excellent with lymphocutaneous disease in immunocompetent children. Pulmonary or osteoarticular disease, especially in immunocompromised individuals, requires longer therapy. Amphotericin B may be required for disseminated disease, CNS disease, and severe pulmonary disease. Surgical debridement may be required.

Orfino-Costa R et al: Sporotrichosis: an update on epidemiology, etiopathogenesis, laboratory and clinical therapeutics. An Bras Dermatol 2017 Sep-Oct;92(5):606–620 [PMID: 29166494].

PNEUMOCYSTIS & OTHER OPPORTUNISTIC FUNGAL INFECTIONS

The title of this section indicates that fungi that are normally not pathogenic, or do not cause severe disease, may do so when given the *opportunity* by changes in host defenses. They occur most commonly when patients are treated with corticosteroids, antineoplastic drugs, biological modifiers, or radiation, thereby reducing the number and function of neutrophils and B and T cells. Inborn errors in immune function (such as combined immunodeficiency or chronic granulomatous disease) may also be complicated by these fungal infections. Opportunistic infections are facilitated by altering the normal flora with antibiotics and by disruption of mucous membranes or skin with antineoplastic therapy or indwelling lines and tubes.

Table 43–5 indicates that filamentous fungi are prominent causes of severe systemic fungal disease in immunocompromised patients. *Aspergillus* species (usually *fumigatus*) and Zygomycetes (usually Mucorales) cause subacute pneumonia and sinusitis and should be considered when these conditions do not respond to antibiotics in immunocompromised patients. *Aspergillus* species also commonly cause invasive disease in patients with chronic granulomatous disease. Mucormycosis is especially likely to produce severe sinusitis in poorly controlled diabetics with acidosis. This fungus may invade the orbit and cause brain infection. Mucormycosis also occurs in patients receiving iron chelation therapy. These fungal infections may disseminate widely. Imaging procedures may suggest the etiology, but this is best diagnosed by aspiration or biopsy of infected tissues. A characteristic CT finding is the "halo sign," which is a ground-glass opacity surrounding a pulmonary nodule or mass. The "reversed halo sign" is a focal rounded ground-glass opacity surrounded by a crescent or complete ring of consolidation. Detection of galactomannose and β-D-glucan in blood and alveolar fluid may be useful for the diagnosis of presumptive of aspergillosis and other opportunistic fungal pathogens.

Although *Cryptococcus* can cause disease in the immunocompetent hosts, it is more likely to be clinically apparent or more severe in immunocompromised patients. This yeast causes pneumonia and is a prominent cause of fungal meningitis (see earlier section in this chapter). *Candida* species in these patients cause fungemia and multiorgan disease, with lungs, esophagus, liver, and spleen frequently affected (see the earlier section on Disseminated *Candida* infection).

Opportunistic fungal infections should always be included in the differential diagnosis of unexplained fever or pulmonary infiltrates in immunocompromised patients. These pathogens should be aggressively pursued with imaging studies and with tissue sampling when clues are available. *Cryptococcus* and *Aspergillus* may be demonstrated with specific antigen tests. Aspergillus and mucorales can be suspected by detecting fungal cell wall components or by PCR. Interpretation of these results may be difficult, with greater uncertainty in pediatric patients. Opportunistic infections are difficult to treat because of the deficiencies in host immune response. Treatment should be undertaken with consultants who are expert in managing these infections. Voriconazole is the drug of choice for many mold infections, but both echinocandins and amphotericin B formulations are good alternatives in certain scenarios. Serum levels of voriconazole should be determined to guide therapy. Combinations of current antifungal drugs are being tested to improve the outcome. Many children who will have depressed phagocytic and T-cell–mediated immune function for long periods (eg, after hematopoietic stem cell transplants) should receive antifungal prophylaxis during the period of severe immune suppression, most often with fluconazole or itraconazole. Very low-birth-weight infants, who are at high risk for systemic *Candida* infection, often receive similar prophylaxis for prolonged periods.

Malassezia furfur is a yeast that normally causes the superficial skin infection known as tinea versicolor (see Chapter 15). This organism is considered an opportunist when fungemia is associated with prolonged intravenous therapy, especially with central lines used for hyperalimentation. The yeast, which requires skin lipids for its growth, can infect lines when lipids are present in the infusate. Some species will grow in the absence of lipids. Unexplained fever and thrombocytopenia are common. Pulmonary infiltrates may be present. The diagnosis is facilitated by alerting the bacteriology laboratory to add olive oil to culture media. The infection will respond to removal of the line or the lipid supplement. Amphotericin B may hasten resolution.

Arvanitis M: Galactomannan and polymerase chain reaction-based screening for invasive aspergillosis among high-risk hematology patients: a diagnostic meta-analysis. Clin Infect Dis 2015;61(8):1263–1272 [PMID: 26157047].

Table 43–5. Unusual fungal infections in children.

Organism	Predisposing Factors	Route of Infection	Clinical Disease	Diagnostic Tests	Therapy and Comments
Aspergillus species	None	Inhalation of spores	Allergic bronchopulmonary aspergillosis; wheezing, cough, migratory infiltrates, eosinophilia.	Organisms in sputum; positive skin test; specific IgE antibody; elevated IgE levels.	Hypersensitivity to fungal antigens. Use steroids. Antifungals may not be needed.
	Immunosuppression	Inhalation of spores	Progressive pulmonary disease: consolidation, nodules, abscesses. Sinusitis	Disseminated disease: usually lung, brain; occasionally intestine, kidney, heart, bone. Invades blood vessels. Demonstrate fungus in tissues by stain or culture; septate hyphae branching at 45-degree angle; detecting antigen/fungal components in blood or respiratory samples may be useful; PCR available at some sites.	Amphotericin B, voriconazole, and oral caspofungin are equally effective; these can be used in combination.
Malassezia furfur, M pachydermatis	Central venous catheter, usually lipid infusion (can occur in the absence of lipid)	Line infection from skin colonization	Sepsis; pneumonitis, thrombocytopenia.	Culture of catheter or blood on lipid-enriched media (for *M furfur*; *M pachydermatis* does not need lipid). Fungus may be seen in buffy coat.	Discontinuation of lipid may be sufficient. Remove catheter. Short-term amphotericin B may be added. Organism ubiquitous on normal skin; requires long-chain fatty acids for growth.
Mucorales (*Mucor, Rhizopus, Absidia*)	Immunosuppression, diabetic acidosis, iron overload	Inhalation, mucosal colonization	Rhinocerebral: sinus, nose, necrotizing vasculitis; central nervous system spread. Pulmonary. Disseminated: any organ.	Demonstrate broad aseptate hyphae branching at 90-degree angles in tissues by stain. Culture: rapidly growing, fluffy fungus. Detecting antigen/fungal components in blood or respiratory samples may be useful.	Amphotericin B, surgical debridement; voriconazole and posaconazole also often effective or can be used as a second agent for combined therapy. Poor prognosis.
Scedosporium spp	Immunosuppression	Inhalation	Disseminated abscesses (lung, brain, liver, spleen, other).	Culture of pus or tissue. Yellow-white granules in pus. Culture.	Surgical drainage; voriconazole or caspofungin. Aggressive surgery.
	Minor trauma	Cutaneous	Mycetoma (most common).		
Candida and cruptococcus	See earlier in chapter				

Lehrnbecher T: Galactomannan, β-D-glucan, and polymerase chain reaction-based assays for the diagnosis of invasive fungal disease in pediatric cancer and hematopoietic stem cell transplantation: a systematic review and meta-analysis. Clin Infect Dis 2016;63(10):1340–1348 [PMID: 27567122].

Patterson TF: Practice guidelines for the diagnosis and management of aspergillosis: 2016 update by the Infectious Diseases Society of America. Clin Infect Dis 2016;63:e1–e60 [PMID: 27365388].

Riley TT: Breaking the mold: a review of mucormycosis and current pharmacological treatment options. Ann Pharmacother 2016;50(9):747–757 [PMID: 27307416].

Wattier RL: A prospective, international cohort study of invasive mold infections in children. J Pediatric Infect Dis Soc 2015;4(4):313–322 [PMID: 26582870].

PNEUMOCYSTIS JIROVECI INFECTION

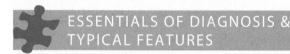

ESSENTIALS OF DIAGNOSIS & TYPICAL FEATURES

▶ Significant immunosuppression.

▶ Fever, tachypnea, cough, dyspnea.

▶ Hypoxemia; diffuse interstitial infiltrates.

▶ Detection of the organism in specimens of pulmonary origin.

▶ General Considerations

Although classified as a fungus on the basis of structural and nucleic acid characteristics, *Pneumocystis* responds readily to antiprotozoal drugs and antifolates. It is a ubiquitous pathogen. Initial infection is presumed to occur asymptomatically via inhalation, usually in early childhood, and to become a clinical problem upon reactivation associated with immune suppression. Person-to-person transmission may contribute to symptomatic disease in immunocompromised individuals. Clinical disease rarely occurs in the normal host. A syndrome of afebrile pneumonia similar to that caused by *Chlamydia trachomatis* in normal infants has been described, but its etiology is rarely appreciated. Whether by reactivation or new exposure, severe signs and symptoms occur chiefly in patients with abnormal T-cell function, such as hematologic malignancies and organ transplantation. *Pneumocystis* also causes severe pneumonia in patients with γ-globulin deficiency and is an AIDS-defining illness for children with advanced HIV infection. Prophylaxis usually prevents this infection (see Chapter 41).

Prolonged, high-dose corticosteroid therapy for any condition is a risk factor, with typical pneumonitis beginning as steroids are tapered.

Severely malnourished infants with no underlying illness may also develop this infection, as can those with congenital immunodeficiency. The incubation period is usually at least 1 month after onset of immunosuppressive therapy.

▶ Clinical Findings

A. Symptoms and Signs

In most patients, a gradual onset of fever, tachypnea, dyspnea, and mild, nonproductive cough occurs over 1–4 weeks. Initially the chest is clear, although retractions and nasal flaring are present. At this stage the illness is nonspecific. Hypoxemia out of proportion to the clinical and radiographic signs is an early finding; however, even minimally decreased arterial oxygen pressure values should suggest this diagnosis in immunosuppressed children. Tachypnea, nonproductive cough, and dyspnea progress. Respiratory failure and death occur without treatment. In some children with AIDS or severe immunosuppression from chemotherapy or organ transplantation, the onset may be abrupt and progression more rapid. Acute dyspnea with pleuritic pain may indicate the complication of pneumothorax.

The general examination is unremarkable except for tachypnea and tachycardia; rales may be absent. There are no upper respiratory signs, conjunctivitis, organomegaly, enanthem, or rash.

B. Laboratory Findings

Laboratory findings reflect the individual child's underlying illness and are not specific. Serum lactate dehydrogenase levels may be elevated markedly as a result of pulmonary damage. In moderately severe cases, the arterial oxygen pressure is less than 70 mm Hg or the alveolar-arterial gradient is less than 35 mm Hg.

C. Imaging

Early chest radiographs are normal. The classic pattern in later films is bilateral, interstitial, lower lobe alveolar disease starting in the perihilar regions, without effusion, consolidation, or hilar adenopathy. High-resolution CT scanning may reveal extensive ground-glass attenuation or cystic lesions. Older HIV-infected patients present with other patterns, including nodular infiltrates, lobar pneumonia, cavities, and upper lobe infiltrates.

D. Diagnostic Findings

Diagnosis requires finding characteristic round (6–8 mm) cysts in a lung biopsy specimen, bronchial brushings, alveolar washings, induced sputum, or tracheal aspirates. Tracheal aspirates are less sensitive, but are more rapidly and easily obtained. They are more often negative in children with leukemia compared with those with HIV infection; presumably, greater immunosuppression permits replication of a larger numbers of organisms. Because pneumonia in immunosuppressed patients may have many causes, negative results from tracheal secretions in suspected cases should prompt more aggressive diagnostic attempts. Bronchial washing using fiberoptic bronchoscopy is usually well tolerated and rapidly performed.

Several rapid stains—as well as the standard methenamine silver stain—are useful. The indirect fluorescent antibody method is most sensitive. These methods require competent laboratory evaluation, because few organisms may be present and many artifacts may be found. PCR methods are an important alternative.

▶ Differential Diagnosis

In immunocompetent infants, *C trachomatis* pneumonia is the most common cause of the afebrile pneumonia syndrome described for *Pneumocystis*. In older immunocompromised children, the differential diagnosis includes influenza, respiratory syncytial virus, cytomegalovirus, adenovirus, and other viral infections; bacterial and fungal pneumonia; pulmonary emboli or hemorrhage; congestive heart failure; and *Chlamydophila pneumoniae* and *Mycoplasma pneumoniae* infections. Lymphoid interstitial pneumonitis, which occurs in older infants with untreated HIV infection, is more indolent and the patient's lactate dehydrogenase level is normal (see Chapter 41). *Pneumocystis* pneumonia is rare in children who are complying with prophylactic regimens.

▶ Prevention

Children at high risk for developing *Pneumocystis* infection should receive prophylactic therapy. Children at risk include those with hematologic malignancies, children who for other reasons are receiving intensive chemotherapy or high-dose corticosteroids, and children with organ transplants or advanced HIV infection. All children born to HIV-infected mothers should receive prophylaxis against *Pneumocystis* starting at age 6 weeks unless HIV infection has been ruled out by tests for HIV in serum. HIV-infected infants often receive therapy for the first year of life, or until the patient's immunologic status is defined sufficiently to determine the need for additional prophylaxis (see Chapter 41). The prophylaxis of choice is trimethoprim-sulfamethoxazole (150 mg/m^2/day of trimethoprim and 750 mg/m^2/day of sulfamethoxazole) for 3 consecutive days of each week. Alternatives to this prophylaxis regimen for children who cannot tolerate trimethoprim-sulfamethoxazole include

atovaquone, dapsone, or aerosolized pentamidine (https://aidsinfo.nih.gov/guidelines/html/5/pediatric-oi-prevention-and-treatment-guidelines/415/pneumocystis-jirovecii-pneumonia).

▶ Treatment

A. General Measures

Supplemental oxygen and nutritional support may be needed. The patient should be in respiratory isolation.

B. Specific Measures

Trimethoprim-sulfamethoxazole (20 mg/kg/day of trimethoprim and 100 mg/kg/day of sulfamethoxazole in four divided doses intravenously or orally if well tolerated) is the treatment of choice. Improvement may not be seen for 3–5 days. Duration of treatment is 3 weeks in HIV-infected children. Methylprednisolone (2–4 mg/kg/day in four divided doses intravenously) should also be given to patients with moderate to severe infection (partial oxygen pressure < 70 mm Hg or alveolar-arterial gradient > 35) for the first 5 days of treatment. The dosage is reduced by 50% for the next 5 days and further by 50% until antibiotic treatment is completed. If trimethoprim-sulfamethoxazole is not tolerated or there is no clinical response in 5 days, pentamidine isethionate (4 mg/kg once daily by slow intravenous infusion) should be given. Clinical efficacy is similar with pentamidine, but adverse reactions are more common. These reactions include dysglycemia, pancreatitis, nephrotoxicity, and leukopenia. Other effective alternatives utilized in adults include atovaquone, trimethoprim plus dapsone, and primaquine plus clindamycin.

▶ Prognosis

The mortality rate is high in immunosuppressed patients who receive treatment late in the illness.

Avino LJ et al: *Pneumocystis jirovecii* pneumonia in the non-HIV-infected population. Ann Pharmacother 2016;50:673 [PMID: 27242349].

Ebner L: Clinical course, radiological manifestations, and outcome of *Pneumocystis jirovecii* pneumonia in HIV patients and renal transplant recipients. PLoS One 2016 Nov 8;11(11):e0164320 [PMID: 27824870].

Unnewehr M: High diagnostic value of a new real-time pneumocystis PCR from bronchoalveolar lavage in a real-life clinical setting. Respiration 2016;92(3):144–149 [PMID: 27595408].

Sexually Transmitted Infections

Daniel H. Reirden, MD

Ann-Christine Nyquist, MD, MSPH

INTRODUCTION

The rate of sexually transmitted infections (STIs) acquired during adolescence remains high despite widespread educational programs and increased access to health care. By senior year in high school, over half of youth will have had sexual intercourse. The highest age-specific rates for gonorrhea, chlamydia, and human papillomavirus (HPV) infection occur in adolescents and young adults (15–24 years of age). While this age group accounts for only 25% of the sexually active population, it accounts for almost half of the incident STIs. Adolescents contract STIs at a higher rate than adults because of sexual risk taking, age-related biologic factors, and barriers to health care access. In every state and the District of Columbia, adolescents can provide consent for the diagnosis and treatment of STIs without parental consent; 18 states allow for the disclosure to a parent. In many states, adolescents can also provide consent for human immunodeficiency virus (HIV) counseling and testing. Since individual state laws vary, health care providers should be knowledgeable about the legal definitions regarding age of consent and confidentiality requirements in their state.

Providers should screen sexually experienced adolescents for STIs and use this opportunity to discuss risk reduction. Since not all adolescents receive regular preventive care, providers should use acute care visits to offer screening and education. Health education counseling should be nonjudgmental and appropriate for the developmental level, yet sufficiently thorough to identify risk behaviors because many adolescents may not readily acknowledge engaging in these behaviors.

ADOLESCENT SEXUALITY

The spectrum of sexual behavior includes holding hands and kissing, touching, mutual masturbation, oral-genital contact, and vaginal and anal intercourse. Each has its associated risks. A small, but statistically significant, trend has occurred in the epidemiology of sexual risk taking toward less sexual involvement and later onset of vaginal intercourse. The most recent Youth Risk Behavior Survey (2017) reports that 40% of high school students have had sexual intercourse; 3.4% of teenagers initiated sex by age 13. Racial and gender differences exist; non-Hispanic black adolescents report a higher prevalence of sexual activity and an earlier age of initiation. Twenty-nine percent of students had sex in the 3 months prior to the survey—44% of twelfth-graders and 13% of ninth-graders. 10% of students reported having had four or more lifetime sexual intercourse partners. Among those youths currently sexually active, 54% reported that either they or their partner had used a condom during their last sexual intercourse. Paradoxically, condom use decreases with age—58% of tenth-graders reported condom use at their last intercourse compared with 50% of twelfth-graders. Substance use contributes to an increase in risky sexual activity; 19% of sexually active youth report that they used alcohol or drugs prior to their last intercourse.

Although there may be variations among groups of teens, oral sex is relatively common in adolescents with approximately two-thirds of 15–24-year-olds reporting oral sexual activity. Anal intercourse occurs in both hetero- and homosexual populations. Adolescent development is a time of exploration, including one's sexual orientation. Frequently, teenagers may not identify themselves as gay, lesbian, or bisexual; thus, sensitive, nonjudgmental history taking is necessary to elicit a history of same-sex partners. Adolescents struggling with their emerging sexual orientation and associated stigma may engage in sexual activity with partners of both sexes or may use substances to cope, thereby impairing their decision-making abilities.

Breuner CC, Mattson G; Committee on Adolescence; Committee on Psychosocial Aspects of Child and Family Health: Sexuality education for children and adolescents. Pediatrics 2016;138(2):e20161348 [PMID: 27432849].

https://www.guttmacher.org/united-states/teens. Accessed July 19, 2019.

Kann L et al: Youth risk behavior surveillance—United States, 2017. MMWR Surveill Summ 2018;67(8):1–114 [PMID: 29902162].

Marcell AV, Burstein GR, AAP Committee on Adolescence: Sexual and reproductive health care services in the pediatric setting. Pediatrics 2017;140(5):e20172858 [PMID: 29061870].

Pfeffer B, Ellsworth TR, Gold MA: Interviewing adolescents about sexual matters. Pediatr Clin N Am 2017;64:291–304 [PMID: 28292446].

RISK FACTORS

Certain behaviors and experiences are risk factors for an adolescent to develop STIs. These include early age at sexual debut, lack of condom use, multiple partners, prior STI, history of STI in a partner, and sex with a partner who is 3 or more years older. The type of sex affects risk as well, with intercourse being riskier than oral sex. Other risk factors associated with STIs in adolescents are smoking, alcohol use, drug use, dropping out of school, pregnancy, and depression.

The adolescent female is especially predisposed to chlamydia, gonorrhea, and HPV infection because the cervix during adolescence has an exposed squamocolumnar junction. The rapidly dividing cells in this area are especially susceptible to microorganism attachment and infection. During early to mid-puberty, this junction slowly invaginates as the uterus and cervix mature, and by the late teens to early 20s the squamocolumnar junction is inside the cervix.

PREVENTION OF SEXUALLY TRANSMITTED INFECTIONS

Efforts to reduce STI risk behavior should begin before the onset of sexual experimentation: first by helping youth personalize their risk for STIs and encouraging positive behaviors that minimize these risks, and then by enhancing communication skills with sexual partners about STI prevention, abstinence, and condom use.

Primary prevention focuses largely on education and risk-reduction techniques. It is essential to recognize that a key task of adolescence is developing a sexual identity. Teenagers are sexual beings that will decide if, when, and how they are going to initiate sexual involvement. Health care providers should routinely address sexuality as part of well-adolescent checkups. Being open and frank about the risks and benefits of each specific type of sexual activity will help youth think about their decision and the consequences. Although more than 90% of students have been taught about HIV infection and other STIs in school, adolescents still have a difficult time personalizing risk. Discussing prevalence, symptoms, and sequelae of STIs can raise awareness and help teenagers make informed decisions about initiating sexual activity and the use of safer sex techniques. Abstinence is theoretically an effective method of preventing STIs. However, many studies have failed to show sustainable protection. Making condoms available reiterates the message that safer sex is vital to health. Discussing condoms, dental dams, and the proper use of lubrication also facilitates safer sex practices. Condoms prevent infections with HIV, HPV, gonorrhea, *Chlamydia*, and herpes simplex virus (HSV). They are probably effective in preventing other STIs as well.

Secondary prevention requires identifying and treating STIs (see the next section Screening for Sexually Transmitted Infections) before infected individuals transmit infection to others. Access to confidential medical care is critical to this objective. Identifying and treating STIs in partners is essential to limit the spread of these infections. Cooperation with the state or county health departments is valuable, because these agencies assume responsibility for locating the contacts of infected persons and ensuring appropriate treatment.

Tertiary prevention is directed toward complications of a specific illness. Examples of tertiary prevention would be treating pelvic inflammatory disease (PID) before infertility develops, following the serologic response to syphilis to prevent late-stage syphilis, treating cervicitis to prevent PID, or treating a chlamydial infection before epididymitis ensues.

Finally, preexposure vaccination against hepatitis B, hepatitis A, and HPV reduces the risk of acquiring these preventable STIs. All adolescents should have prior or current immunization against hepatitis B (see Chapter 10). However, because hepatitis B infection is frequently sexually transmitted, this vaccine is especially critical for all unvaccinated patients being evaluated for an STI. Hepatitis A vaccination is recommended for all individuals. Preexposure vaccination for HPV will decrease the risk for cervical dysplasia and cervical cancer in females, and decreases the risk for genital warts and both anal and oropharyngeal cancers in males and females, which typically occur decades later (see Chapter 10).

SCREENING FOR SEXUALLY TRANSMITTED INFECTIONS

The ability of the health care provider to obtain an accurate sexual history is crucial in prevention and control efforts. Teenagers should be asked open-ended questions about their sexual experiences to assess their risk for STIs. Questions must be clear to the youth, so choose language that the adolescent will understand. If the adolescent has ever engaged in sexual activity, the provider needs to determine what kind of sexual activity (mutual masturbation or oral, anal, or vaginal sex); whether it has been opposite sex, same sex, or both; whether birth control and condoms were used; and whether it has been consensual or forced. During the interview, the clinician should take the opportunity to discuss risk-reduction techniques regardless of the history obtained from the youth.

A routine laboratory screening process is warranted if the patient has engaged in intercourse, presents with STI symptoms, or reports a partner with an STI. The availability of nucleic acid amplification tests (NAATs), primarily for *Chlamydia* and *Neisseria gonorrhoeae*, has changed the nature of STI screening and intervention. NAATs are more than 95% sensitive and more than 99% specific, using either urine or cervical/urethral or vaginal swabs. Annual screening of all sexually active females aged 25 years or younger is recommended for *Chlamydia trachomatis* and *N gonorrhoeae*. Routine chlamydial testing should be considered for all adolescent males, especially for males who have sex with men (MSM), have new or multiple sex partners, or are in correctional facilities. For men who have sex with men, consideration should be given to testing oropharyngeal and rectal sites, as asymptomatic infections are common. Use of NAAT is recommended for samples from these sites, but such tests are not currently FDA-approved and providers must locate a laboratory that has performed the necessary validation studies.

Initial screening for urethritis in males begins with a physical examination. A first-catch urine sample (the first 10–20 mL of voided urine collected after not voiding for 2 hours) should be sent for *Chlamydia* and *N gonorrhoeae* testing if there are no signs (urethral discharge or lesions) or symptoms. With signs or symptoms of urethritis, a urethral swab should be sent to test for both *N gonorrhoeae* and *Chlamydia*. A wet mount preparation should then be done on a spun urine sample or from urethral discharge, evaluating for the presence of *Trichomonas vaginalis*. Newer technologies, such as enzyme-linked immunoassays (EIA) and NAATs, allow greater sensitivity and specificity in making the diagnosis of *T vaginalis* in males and females.

Screening asymptomatic females is more complicated because a variety of approaches are available. Generally, either a first-void urine specimen, a cervical swab, or a vaginal swab is used to screen for *Chlamydia* and *N gonorrhoeae* by NAAT. Any vaginal discharge should be evaluated with a wet mount of vaginal secretions to check for bacterial vaginosis and trichomoniasis, and a potassium hydroxide (KOH) preparation to screen for yeast infections. The Papanicolaou (Pap) smear serves to evaluate the cervix for the presence of dysplasia. The first Pap smear should be performed at age 21 years and then every 3 years. HPV typing is not recommended before age 30.

In urban areas with a relatively high rate of syphilis and in MSM, a screening test should be drawn yearly or more frequently if higher risk encounters are more frequent. Rapid plasma reagin (RPR) antibody tests should be done in all individuals in whom a concomitant STI is present. HIV antibody testing is recommended at least once for all patients and repeat testing undertaken when an STI is present or the history includes multiple partners and high-risk behaviors.

Wangu Z, Burstein GR: Adolescent sexuality updates to the sexually transmitted infection guidelines. Pediatr Clin N Am 2017;64(2):389–411 [PMID: 28292454].

SIGNS & SYMPTOMS

The most common symptoms in males are dysuria and penile discharge resulting from urethral inflammation. However, providers should be aware that many urethral infections are asymptomatic. Less common symptoms are scrotal pain, hematuria, proctitis, and pruritus in the pubic region. Signs include epididymitis, orchitis, and urethral discharge. Rarely do males develop systemic symptoms. Acute HIV seroconversion illness should be considered in the differential diagnoses for any sexually active adolescent at risk for HIV infection who presents with nonspecific viral symptoms. This is especially true for MSM, for females, the most common symptoms are vaginal discharge and dysuria. Again, infection may be asymptomatic. Vaginal itching and irregular menses or spotting are also common. Abdominal pain, fever, and vomiting, although less common and specific, are signs of PID. Pain in the genital region and dyspareunia may be present.

Signs that can be found in both males and females with an STI include genital ulcerations, adenopathy, and genital warts.

▼ THE MOST COMMON ANTIBIOTIC-RESPONSIVE SEXUALLY TRANSMITTED INFECTIONS

CHLAMYDIA TRACHOMATIS INFECTION

▶ General Considerations

C trachomatis is the most common bacterial cause of STIs in the United States. In 2017, over 1.05 million cases in adolescents and young adults were reported to the CDC, representing 63% of reported chlamydia cases. *C trachomatis* is an obligate intracellular bacterium that replicates within the cytoplasm of host cells. Destruction of *Chlamydia*-infected cells is mediated by host immune responses.

▶ Clinical Findings

A. Symptoms and Signs

Clinical infection in females manifests as dysuria, urethritis, vaginal discharge, cervicitis, irregular vaginal bleeding, or PID. The presence of mucopus at the cervical os (mucopurulent cervicitis) is a sign of chlamydial infection or gonorrhea. Chlamydial infection is asymptomatic in 75% of females.

Chlamydial infection may be asymptomatic in 70% of males or manifest as dysuria, urethritis, or epididymitis. Some patients complain of urethral discharge. On clinical examination, a clear white discharge may be found after milking the penis. Proctitis or proctocolitis from *Chlamydia* may occur in adolescents practicing receptive anal intercourse.

B. Laboratory Findings

NAAT is the most sensitive (92%–99%) way to detect *Chlamydia*. Enzyme-linked immunosorbent assay (ELISA) or direct fluorescent antibody (DFA) tests are less sensitive, but may be the only testing option in some centers.

A cervical or vaginal swab, using the manufacturer's swab provided with the specific test, or first-void urine specimen, should be obtained. For urine screening, yields of testing are maximized when collecting between 10 and 20 mL of urine and ensuring that patient has not voided for 2 hours. Often a single swab can be used to collect both the *Chlamydia* and *N gonorrhoeae* specimen. To optimize detection of *Chlamydia* from the cervix, columnar cells need to be collected by inserting the swab in the os and rotating it 360 degrees. NAAT is not licensed for rectal samples but some laboratories have validated testing on rectal specimens for *C trachomatis*. Thus, when a rectal specimen is obtained, this must often be evaluated by less sensitive culture methods unless there is access to a laboratory that has validated *Chlamydia* NAAT for nongenital sites.

A first-void urine sample, or urethral swab for NAAT, should be obtained at least annually. Some studies suggest that more frequent screenings—every 6 months—in higher-prevalence populations will decrease endemic chlamydial infection. For both males and females, testing urine allows for more frequent screening and simplifies screening in large group settings, such as schools and correctional facilities.

▶ Complications

Epididymitis is a complication in males. Reiter syndrome occurs in association with chlamydial urethritis. This should be suspected in male patients who are sexually active and present with low back pain (sacroiliitis), arthritis (polyarticular), characteristic mucocutaneous lesions, and conjunctivitis. PID is an important complication in females.

▶ Treatment

Infected patients and their contacts, regardless of the extent of signs or symptoms, need to receive treatment (Table 44–1). Reinfection caused by failure of contacts to receive treatment or the initiation of sexual activity with a newly infected partner puts the adolescent at high risk of acquiring a repeat chlamydial infection within several months of the first infection. Because of this increased risk, all infected females and males should be retested approximately 3 months after treatment.

Wiesenfeld HC: Screening for *Chlamydia trachomatis* infections in women. N Engl J Med 2017;376(8):765–773 [PMID: 282225683].

NEISSERIA GONORRHOEAE INFECTION

▶ General Considerations

Gonorrhea is the second most prevalent bacterial STI in the United States, where over 556,000 new *N gonorrhoeae* infections were reported in 2017. Among 15–19-year-olds the rate of gonorrhea infections increased 15.5% in 2016–2017. During this same time rates increased 12.8% among those aged 20–24 years.

Sites of infection include the cervix, urethra, rectum, and pharynx. In addition, gonorrhea is a cause of PID. Humans are the natural reservoir. Gonococci are present in the exudate and secretions of infected mucous membranes.

▶ Clinical Findings

A. Symptoms and Signs

In uncomplicated gonococcal cervicitis, females are symptomatic 23%–57% of the time, presenting with vaginal discharge and dysuria. Urethritis and pyuria may also be present. Mucopurulent cervicitis with a yellowish discharge may be found, and the cervix may be edematous and friable. Other symptoms include abnormal menstrual periods and dyspareunia. Approximately 15% of females with endocervical gonorrhea have signs of involvement of the upper genital tract. Compared with chlamydial infection, pelvic inflammation with gonorrhea has a shorter duration, but an increased intensity of symptoms, and is more often associated with fever. Symptomatic males usually have a yellowish-green urethral discharge and burning on urination, but most males (55%–67%) with *N gonorrhoeae* are asymptomatic. Both males and females can develop gonococcal proctitis and pharyngitis after appropriate exposure.

B. Laboratory Findings

A first-void urine sample or cervical or vaginal swab from females should be sent for NAAT. Culture or NAAT for *N gonorrhoeae* in males can be achieved with a swab of the urethra or first-void urine. Urethral culture is less sensitive (85%) compared with the 95%–99% sensitivity using NAAT methods on either urethral or urine specimens. Gram stain of urethral discharge showing gram-negative intracellular diplococci indicates gonorrhea in a male.

If proctitis is present, appropriate cultures should be obtained and treatment for both gonorrhea and chlamydial infection given. If oral exposure to gonorrhea is suspected, cultures should be taken and the patient given empiric treatment. If there is access to a laboratory that has validated NAAT for oropharyngeal or rectal specimens, this will substantially increase detection over culture methods.

Table 44–1. Treatment regimens for sexually transmitted infections.

	Recommended Regimens	Pregnancy[a] [Category]
Pelvic inflammatory disease (PID)		
Parenteral therapy regimen A **Note:** Therapy should be continued for 24–48 h after patient has improved; therapy can then be switched to either oral regimen to complete a 14-day course	Cefotetan, 2 g IV every 12 h or Cefoxitin, 2 g IV every 6 h plus Doxycycline, 100 mg IV or orally every 12 h	Safe [B] Safe [B] Contraindicated [D]
Parenteral therapy regimen B **Note:** Once clinically improved for 48 h, patients can continue clindamycin, 100 mg PO bid for 14 days total[c]	Clindamycin, 900 mg IV every 8 h plus Gentamicin, 2 mg/kg IV/IM loading dose, then 1.5 mg/kg IV every 8 h[b]	Safe [B] Safe [B]
Alternative parenteral regimens	Ampicillin/sulbactam, 3 g IV every 6 h plus Doxycycline, 100 mg IV or orally every 12 h	Safe [A] Contraindicated [D]
Recommended outpatient regimen **Note:** Pregnant patients with PID and women with tubo-ovarian abscesses should be hospitalized and given parenteral antibiotics[c]	Ceftriaxone, 250 mg IM once or Cefoxitin, 2 g IM once plus probenecid, 1 g orally as a single dose or other parenteral third-generation cephalosporin (eg, ceftizoxime or cefotaxime) plus Doxycycline, 100 mg orally twice a day for 14 days with or without Metronidazole, 500 mg orally twice a day for 14 days	Safe [B], Safe [B], Safe [B] Contraindicated [D] Safe [B]
Cervicitis		
Chlamydia	Azithromycin, 1 g orally as single dose or Doxycycline, 100 mg orally twice a day for 7 days	Safe [B] Contraindicated [D]
Alternative regimens	Erythromycin base, 500 mg orally four times a day for 7 days or Erythromycin ethylsuccinate, 800 mg orally four times a day for 7 days or Levofloxacin, 500 mg orally once daily for 7 days or Ofloxacin, 300 mg orally twice a day for 7 days	Safe [B] Safe [B] Contraindicated [C] Contraindicated [C]
Gonorrhea, uncomplicated		
Cervicitis, urethritis, rectal, pharyngitis **Note:** Empiric combination treatment with azithromycin is recommended due improving treatment efficacy and potentially delaying the emergence and spread of resistance to cephalosporins	Ceftriaxone, 250 mg IM as single dose plus Azithromycin, 1 g orally as single dose	Safe [B] Safe [B]
Alternative oral regimen (if ceftriaxone is not available)	Cefixime, 400 mg orally as single dose or Cefixime suspension, 400 mg by suspension (200 mg/5 mL) orally as single dose plus Azithromycin, 1 g orally as single dose	Safe [B] Safe [B] Safe [B]
Gonorrhea, disseminated		
Note: Treat IV until clinically improved (usually 48 h; then switch to PO); complete at least a 7-day course	Ceftriaxone, 1 g IV or IM every 24 h plus Azithromycin, 1 g orally as single dose	Safe [B] Safe [B]

(Continued)

Table 44–1. Treatment regimens for sexually transmitted infections. (*Continued*)

	Recommended Regimens	Pregnancy[a] [Category]
Gonorrhea, disseminated (Cont.)		
Alternative regimens	Cefotaxime, 1 g IV every 8 h	Safe [B]
	or	
	Ceftizoxime, 1 g IV every 8 h	Safe [B]
	plus	
	Azithromycin, 1 g orally as single dose	Safe [B]
Nongonococcal, nonchlamydial urethritis		
	Azithromycin, 1 g orally as single dose	Safe [B]
	or	
	Doxycycline, 100 mg orally twice a day for 7 days	Contraindicated [D]
Alternative regimens	Erythromycin base, 500 mg orally four times a day for 7 days	Safe [B]
	or	
	Erythromycin ethylsuccinate, 800 mg orally four times a day for 7 days	Safe [B]
	or	
	Levofloxacin, 500 mg orally once daily for 7 days	Contraindicated [C]
	or	
	Ofloxacin, 300 mg orally twice a day for 7 days	Contraindicated [C]
Proctitis, proctocolitis, and enteritis		
	Ceftriaxone, 250 mg IM as single dose	Safe [B]
	plus	
	Doxycycline, 100 mg orally twice a day for 7 days	Contraindicated [D]
***Trichomonas vaginalis* vaginitis or urethritis**		
	Metronidazole, 2 g orally as single dose	Safe [B]
	or	
	Tinidazole, 2 g orally as single dose	Contraindicated [C]
Alternative regimen	Metronidazole, 500 mg orally twice a day for 7 days	Safe [B]
Bacterial vaginosis		
	Metronidazole, 500 mg orally twice a day for 7 days	Safe [B]
	or	
	Metronidazole, 0.75% gel, one applicator (5 g) intravaginally once daily for 5 days	Safe [B]
	or	
	Clindamycin cream, 2%, one applicator (5 g) intravaginally at bedtime for 7 days	Safe [B]
Alternative regimen	Clindamycin, 300 mg orally twice a day for 7 days	Safe [B]
	or	
	Clindamycin ovule, 100 mg intravaginally once at bedtime for 3 days	Safe [B]
	or	
	Tinidazole, 2 g orally once daily for 2 days	Contraindicated [C]
	or	
	Tinidazole, 1 g orally once daily for 5 days	Contraindicated [C]
Vulvovaginal candidiasis		
	Butoconazole, clotrimazole, miconazole, terconazole or tioconazole, intravaginally for 1, 3, or 7 days	Safe [B]
	or	
	Butoconazole sustained-release, 5 g once intravaginally	Safe [B]
	or	
	Fluconazole, 150 mg oral tablet, in single dose	Contraindicated [C]

(*Continued*)

Table 44–1. Treatment regimens for sexually transmitted infections. (*Continued*)

	Recommended Regimens	Pregnancy[a] [Category]
Syphilis		
Early (primary, secondary, or latent < 1 y)	Benzathine penicillin G, 2.4 million units IM (for patients > 40 kg) or	Safe [B]
	Benzathine penicillin G, 50,000 U/kg IM (for patients < 40 kg); up to 2.4 million units in one dose	Safe [B]
Late (> 1-y duration or of unknown duration)	Benzathine penicillin G, 7.2 million units total, administered as three doses of 2.4 million units IM each at 1-wk intervals or	Safe [B]
	Benzathine penicillin G, 50,000 U/kg IM (for patients < 40 kg) once a week for 3 consecutive wk; up to 2.4 million units in one dose	Safe [B]
Tertiary (with normal CSF examination)	Benzathine penicillin G, 7.2 million units total, administered as three doses of 2.4 million units IM each at 1-wk intervals or	Safe [B]
	Benzathine penicillin G, 50,000 U/kg IM (for patients < 40 kg) once a week for 3 consecutive wk; up to 2.4 million units in one dose	Safe [B]
Neurosyphilis		
	Aqueous crystalline penicillin G, 18–24 million U/day, administered as 3–4 million units IV every 4 h or continuous infusion for 10–14 days or	Safe [B]
Alternative regimen (if compliance can be assured)	Procaine penicillin, 2.4 million units IM once daily plus Probenecid 500 mg orally four times a day for 10–14 days	Safe [B] Safe [B]
Epididymitis		
Most likely caused by gonococcal or chlamydial infection	Ceftriaxone, 250 mg IM as single dose plus Doxycycline, 100 mg orally twice a day for 10 days	
Most likely caused by enteric organisms	Ceftriaxone, 250 mg IM as single dose plus Levofloxacin, 500 mg orally once daily for 10 days or Ofloxacin, 300 mg orally twice a day for 10 days	
C trachomatis infection		
Cervicitis or urethritis	Azithromycin, 1 g orally as single dose or	Safe [B]
	Doxycycline, 100 mg orally twice a day for 7 days	Contraindicated [D]
Alternative regimen[b]	Erythromycin, 500 mg orally four times a day for 7 days or	Safe [B]
	Erythromycin ethylsuccinate, 800 mg orally four times a day for 7 days or	Safe [B]
	Levofloxacin 500 mg orally once daily for 7 days or	Contraindicated [C]
	Ofloxacin, 300 mg orally twice a day for 7 days	Contraindicated [C]

(*Continued*)

Table 44–1. Treatment regimens for sexually transmitted infections. (*Continued*)

	Recommended Regimens	Pregnancy[a] [Category]
Granuloma inguinale		
	Azithromycin, 1 g orally once a week or 500 mg daily for at least 3 wk and until all lesions have completely healed	Safe [B]
Alternative regimen	Ciprofloxacin, 750 mg orally twice a day for at least 3 wk and until all lesions have completely healed	Contraindicated [C]
	or	
	Erythromycin base, 500 mg orally four times a day for at least 3 wk and until all lesions have completely healed	Safe [B]
	or	
	Doxycycline, 100 mg orally twice a day for 3 wk or and until all lesions have completely healed	Contraindicated [D]
	or	
	Trimethoprim–sulfamethoxazole, one double-strength tablet orally twice a day for at least 3 wk and until all lesions have completely healed	Contraindicated [C]
Lymphogranuloma venereum		
	Doxycycline, 100 mg orally twice a day for 21 days	Contraindicated [C]
Alternative regimen	Erythromycin, 500 mg orally four times a day for 21 days	Safe [B]
Herpes simplex infection		
First episode, genital	Acyclovir, 400 mg orally three times a day for 7–10 days	Safe [B]
	or	
	Acyclovir, 200 mg orally five times a day for 7–10 days	Safe [B]
	or	
	Famciclovir, 250 mg orally three times a day for 7–10 days	Safe [B]
	or	
	Valacyclovir, 1 g orally twice a day for 7–10 days	Safe [B]
Episodic therapy for recurrent genital herpes	Acyclovir, 400 mg orally three times a day for 5 days	Safe [B]
	or	
	Acyclovir, 800 mg orally twice a day for 5 days	Safe [B]
	or	
	Acyclovir, 800 mg orally three times a day for 2 days	Safe [B]
	or	
	Famciclovir, 125 mg orally twice a day for 5 days	Safe [B]
	or	
	Famciclovir, 1000 mg orally twice a day for 1 day	Safe [B]
	or	
	Famciclovir, 500 mg once orally, followed by 250 mg orally twice a day for 2 days	Safe [B]
	or	
	Valacyclovir, 500 mg orally twice a day for 3 days	Safe [B]
	or	
	Valacyclovir, 1 g orally once daily for 5 days	Safe [B]
Suppressive therapy for recurrent genital herpes	Acyclovir, 400 mg orally twice a day	Safe [B]
	or	
	Famciclovir, 250 mg orally twice a day	Safe [B]
	or	
	Valacyclovir, 500 mg orally daily (if < 10 recurrences per year; if ≥ 10 recurrences, use 1 g daily)	Safe [B]
Chancroid		
	Azithromycin, 1 g orally as single dose	Safe [B]
	or	
	Ceftriaxone, 250 mg IM once	Safe [B]
	or	
	Ciprofloxacin, 500 mg orally twice a day for 3 days	Contraindicated [D]
	or	
	Erythromycin base, 500 mg orally three times a day for 7 days	Safe [B]

(*Continued*)

Table 44–1. Treatment regimens for sexually transmitted infections. (*Continued*)

	Recommended Regimens	Pregnancy[a] [Category]
Human papillomavirus infection		
External lesions (patient-applied) **Note:** Topical therapies usually require weekly treatments for 4 consecutive weeks	Podofilox, 0.5% solution or gel; apply twice a day for 3 days; used by patient at home; practitioner needs to demonstrate how compound is applied (to be used only on external lesions)	Contraindicated [C]
	or	
	Imiquimod 5% cream, applied three times a week overnight (maximum of 16 wk)	Contraindicated [C]
	or	
	Imiquimod 3.75% cream, applied daily at bedtime (maximum of 16 wk)	Contraindicated [C]
	or	
	Sinecatechins 15% ointment, applied three times daily (maximum of 16 wk)	Unknown safety
External lesions (provider-applied)	Trichloroacetic acid (85%) or bichloracetic acid; apply directly to warts; wash off in 6–8 h; weekly	Safe
	or	
	Cryotherapy: liquid nitrogen, cryoprobe safe laser surgery	Safe
Ectoparasitic infections		
Pubic lice[d]	Permethrin 1% creme rinse: wash off after 10 min	Safe [B]
	or	
	Pyrethrins with piperonyl butoxide: apply, wash off after 10 min	Safe [B]
Alternative regimen	Malathion 0.5% lotion: wash off after 8–12 h	Safe [B]
	or	
	Ivermectin, 250 mcg/kg orally, repeated in 2 wk	Contraindicated [C]
Scabies[d]	Permethrin cream 5%: apply to entire body from the neck down, wash off after 8–14 h	Safe [B]
	or	
	Ivermectin, 200 mcg/kg orally, repeat in 7–14 days	Contraindicated [C]
Alternative regimen	Lindane (1%): apply to entire body from neck down, wash off after 8 h	Contraindicated [C]

IM, intramuscular; IV, intravenous; NAAT, nucleic acid amplification test.

[a]FDA use in pregnancy ratings: [A] *Controlled studies show no risk.* Adequate, well-controlled studies in pregnant women have failed to demonstrate a risk to the fetus in any trimester of pregnancy. [B] *No evidence of risk in humans.* Adequate, well-controlled studies in pregnant women have not shown increased risk of fetal abnormalities despite adverse findings in animals, in the absence of adequate human studies, animal studies show no fetal risk. The chance of fetal harm is remote but remains a possibility. [C] *Risk cannot be ruled out.* Adequate, well-controlled human studies are lacking, and animal studies have shown a risk to the fetus or are lacking as well. There is a chance of fetal harm if the drug is administered during pregnancy; but the potential benefits outweigh the potential risk. [D] *Positive evidence of risk.* Studies in humans, or investigational or postmarketing data, have demonstrated fetal risk. Nevertheless, potential benefits from the use of the drug may outweigh the potential risk. For example, the drug may be acceptable if needed in a life-threatening situation or serious disease for which safer drugs cannot be used or are ineffective. [X] *Contraindicated in pregnancy.* Studies in animals or humans, or despite adverse findings in animals, or investigational or postmarketing reports have demonstrated positive evidence of fetal abnormalities or risk that clearly outweighs any possible benefit to the patient.

[b]Single daily dose (3–5 mg/kg) IV can be substituted.

[c]Doxycycline is contraindicated in pregnancy. Alternative therapies during pregnancy which include erythromycin, azithromycin, and amoxicillin are not as effective, but are clinically useful if the recommended regimens cannot be used due to allergy or pregnancy.

[d]Bedding and clothing need to be decontaminated by washing in hot water or by dry cleaning. Regimen may be repeated in 1 week if complete response is not achieved.

▶ Differential Diagnosis

Gonococcal pharyngitis needs to be differentiated from pharyngitis caused by streptococcal infection, herpes simplex, adenovirus, and infectious mononucleosis (EBV). Chlamydial infection needs to be differentiated from gonococcal infection.

▶ Complications

Disseminated gonococcal infection occurs in a minority (0.5%–3%) of patients with untreated gonorrhea. Hematogenous spread most commonly causes arthritis and dermatitis. The joints most frequently involved are the wrist, metacarpophalangeal joints, knee, and ankle. Skin lesions are typically tender, with hemorrhagic or necrotic pustules or bullae on an erythematous base occurring on the distal extremities. Disseminated disease occurs more frequently in females than in males. Risk factors include pregnancy and gonococcal pharyngitis. Gonorrhea is complicated occasionally by perihepatitis.

▶ Treatment (see Table 44–1)

Since 2010, the CDC made two significant changes to gonorrhea treatment recommendations: dual treatment with azithromycin and ceftriaxone regardless of anatomic site involved and removal of the recommendation of oral cefixime treatment of gonorrhea. These changes reflect increasing resistance to cephalosporins, the frequency of coinfection with Chlamydia, and the need to increase consistency of treatment regimens.

CDC guidelines also state that *N gonorrhoeae* and *C trachomatis* do not require tests of cure when they are treated with first-line medications, unless the patient remains symptomatic. If retesting is indicated, it should be delayed for 1 month after completion of therapy if NAATs are used. Retesting might also be considered for sexually active adolescents likely to be reinfected. Due to increasing resistance of *N gonorrhoeae* to cephalosporins, providers considering treatment failure should also obtain a gonorrhea culture to assess for antibiotic resistance. Patients should be advised to abstain from sexual intercourse until both they and their partners have completed a course of treatment. Treatment for disseminated disease may require hospitalization. Quinolones should no longer be used to treat gonorrhea due to high levels of quinolone resistance in the United States. Failure of initial treatment should prompt reevaluation of the patient and consideration of retreatment with ceftriaxone.

Gonococcal Isolate Surveillance Project (GISP): https://www.cdc.gov/std/gisp/default.htm. Accessed July 19, 2019.

▼ THE SPECTRUM OF SIGNS & SYMPTOMS OF SEXUALLY TRANSMITTED INFECTIONS

The patient presenting with an STI usually has one or more of the signs or symptoms described in this section. Management considerations for STIs include assessing the patient's adherence to therapy and ensuring follow-up, treating STIs in partners, and determining pregnancy risk. Treatment of each STI is detailed in Table 44–1.

CERVICITIS

▶ General Considerations

In most cases of cervicitis no organism is isolated. The most common causes include *C trachomatis* or *N gonorrhoeae*. HSV, *T vaginalis*, and *Mycoplasma genitalium* are less common causes. Bacterial vaginosis is now recognized as a cause of cervicitis. Cervicitis can also be present without an STI.

▶ Clinical Findings

A. Symptoms and Signs

Two major diagnostic signs characterize cervicitis: (1) purulent or mucopurulent endocervical exudate visible in the endocervical canal or on an endocervical swab and (2) easily induced bleeding with the passage of a cotton swab through the cervical os. Cervicitis is often asymptomatic, but many patients with cervicitis have an abnormal vaginal discharge or postcoital bleeding.

B. Laboratory Findings

Although endocervical Gram stain may show an increased number of polymorphonuclear leukocytes, this finding has a low positive predictive value and is not recommended for diagnosis. Patients with cervicitis should be tested for *C trachomatis*, *N gonorrhoeae*, and trichomoniasis by using the most sensitive and specific tests available at the site.

▶ Complications

Persistent cervicitis is difficult to manage and requires reassessment of the initial diagnosis and reevaluation for possible re-exposure to an STI. Cervicitis can persist despite repeated courses of antimicrobial therapy. Presence of a large ectropion can contribute to persistent cervicitis.

▶ Treatment

Empiric treatment for both gonorrhea and chlamydial infection is recommended because coinfection is common. If the patient is asymptomatic except for cervicitis, then treatment may wait until diagnostic test results are available (see Table 44–1). Follow-up is recommended if symptoms persist. Patients should be instructed to abstain from sexual intercourse until they and their sex partners are cured and treatment is completed.

PELVIC INFLAMMATORY DISEASE

▶ General Considerations

Pelvic inflammatory disease (PID) is defined as inflammation of the upper female genital tract and may include endometritis, salpingitis, tubo-ovarian abscess, and pelvic peritonitis. It is the most common gynecologic disorder necessitating hospitalization for female patients of reproductive age in the United States. The incidence is highest in teenage girls. Those who are sexually active have a high risk (1 in 8) of developing PID, whereas women in their 20s have one-tenth the risk. Predisposing risk factors include multiple sexual partners, younger age of initiating sexual intercourse, prior history of PID, and lack of condom use. Lack of protective antibody from previous exposure to sexually transmitted organisms and cervical ectopy contribute to the development of PID. Many adolescents with subacute or asymptomatic PID are never identified.

PID is a polymicrobial infection. Causative agents include *N gonorrhoeae*, *C trachomatis*, anaerobic bacteria that reside in the vagina, and genital mycoplasmas. Vaginal douching and other mechanical factors such as intrauterine devices in place for multiple years or prior gynecologic surgery increase the risk of PID by providing access of lower genital tract organisms to pelvic organs. Recent menses and bacterial vaginosis have been associated with the development of PID.

▶ Clinical Findings

A. Symptoms and Signs

PID may be challenging to diagnose because of the wide variation in the symptoms and signs. No single historical, clinical, or laboratory finding has both high sensitivity and specificity for the diagnosis. Diagnosis of PID is usually made clinically (Table 44–2). Typical patients have lower abdominal pain, pelvic pain, or dyspareunia. Systemic symptoms such fever, nausea, or vomiting may be present. Vaginal discharge is variable. Cervical motion tenderness, uterine or adnexal tenderness, or signs of peritonitis are often present. Mucopurulent cervicitis is present in 50% of patients. Tubo-ovarian abscesses can often be detected by careful physical examination (feeling a mass or fullness in the adnexa).

B. Laboratory Findings

Laboratory findings may include elevated WBCs with a left shift and elevated acute-phase reactants (erythrocyte sedimentation rate or C-reactive protein). A positive test for *N gonorrhoeae* or *C trachomatis* is supportive, although 25% of the time neither of these bacteria is detected. Pregnancy

Table 44–2. Diagnostic criteria for pelvic inflammatory disease.

Minimum criteria
Empiric treatment of PID should be initiated in sexually active young women and others at risk for sexually transmitted infections if one or more of the following minimum criteria are present:
• They are experiencing pelvic or lower abdominal pain and no other cause(s) for the illness can be identified
• Cervical motion tenderness or uterine tenderness or adnexal tenderness
Additional supportive criteria
Oral temperature > 38.3°C (101°F)
Abnormal cervical or vaginal mucopurulent discharge or cervical friability
Presence of abundant white blood cells on microscopic evaluation of vaginal secretions diluted in saline
Elevated erythrocyte sedimentation rate or elevated C-reactive protein
Laboratory documentation of infection with *Neisseria gonorrhoeae* or *Chlamydia trachomatis*
Definitive criteria (selected cases)
Histopathologic evidence of endometritis on endometrial biopsy
Tubo-ovarian abscess on sonography or other radiologic tests
Laparoscopic abnormalities consistent with PID

Adapted with permission from Centers for Disease Control and Prevention: Sexually transmitted diseases treatment guidelines 2015.

needs to be ruled out, because patients with an ectopic pregnancy can present with abdominal pain and concomitant pregnancy will affect management.

C. Diagnostic Studies

Laparoscopy is the gold standard for detecting salpingitis. It is used if the diagnosis is in question or to help differentiate PID from an ectopic pregnancy, ovarian cysts, or adnexal torsion. Endometrial biopsy should be performed in women undergoing laparoscopy who do not have visual evidence of salpingitis because some women may have isolated endometritis. The clinical diagnosis of PID has a positive predictive value for salpingitis of 65%–90% in comparison with laparoscopy. Pelvic ultrasonography also is helpful in detecting tubo-ovarian abscesses, which are found in almost 20% of teens with PID. Transvaginal ultrasound is more sensitive than abdominal ultrasound. All women who have acute PID should be tested for *N gonorrhoeae* and *C trachomatis* and should be screened for HIV infection.

▶ Differential Diagnosis

Differential diagnosis includes other gynecologic illnesses (ectopic pregnancy, threatened or septic abortion, adnexal torsion, ruptured and hemorrhagic ovarian cysts, dysmenorrhea, endometriosis, or mittelschmerz), gastrointestinal illnesses (appendicitis, cholecystitis, hepatitis, gastroenteritis, or inflammatory bowel disease), and urinary tract illnesses (cystitis, pyelonephritis, or urinary calculi).

▶ Complications

Scarring of the fallopian tubes is one of the major sequelae of PID. After one episode of PID, 17% of patients become infertile, 17% develop chronic pelvic pain, and 10% will have an ectopic pregnancy. Infertility rates increase with each episode of PID; three episodes of PID result in a 73% infertility rate. Duration of symptoms appears to be the largest determinant of infertility. Hematogenous or lymphatic spread of organisms from the fallopian tubes rarely causes inflammation of the liver capsule (perihepatitis) resulting in symptoms of pleuritic right upper quadrant pain and elevation of liver function tests.

▶ Treatment

The objectives of treatment are both to achieve a clinical cure and to prevent long-term sequelae. There are no differences in short- and long-term clinical and microbiologic response rates resulting from parenteral or oral therapy. PID is frequently managed at the outpatient level, although some clinicians argue that all adolescents with PID should be hospitalized because of the frequency of complications. Severe systemic symptoms and toxicity, signs of peritonitis, inability to take fluids, pregnancy, nonresponse or intolerance of oral antimicrobial therapy, and tubo-ovarian abscess favor hospitalization. In addition, if the health care provider believes that the patient will not adhere to treatment, hospitalization is warranted. Pregnant women with PID should be admitted to hospital and treated with parental antibiotics to reduce the risk of increased morbidity. Surgical drainage may be required for adequate treatment of tubo-ovarian abscesses.

The broad-spectrum antibiotic regimens described in Table 44–1 cover the numerous microorganisms associated with PID. All treatment regimens should be effective against *N gonorrhoeae* and *C trachomatis* because negative endocervical screening tests do not rule out upper reproductive tract infection with these organisms. Outpatient treatment should be reserved for compliant patients who have classic signs of PID without systemic symptoms. Patients with PID who receive outpatient treatment should be reexamined within 24–48 hours, with phone contact in the interim, to assess persistent disease or treatment failure. Patients should have substantial improvement within 48–72 hours. An adolescent should be reexamined 7–10 days after the completion of therapy to ensure the resolution of symptoms.

Brunham RC, Gottlieb SL, Paavonen J: Pelvic inflammatory disease. N Engl J Med 2015;372(21):2039–2048 [PMID: 25992748].

URETHRITIS

▶ General Considerations

The most common bacterial causes of urethritis in males are *N gonorrhoeae* and *C trachomatis*. Additionally, *T vaginalis*, HSV, *Ureaplasma urealyticum*, and *M genitalium* cause urethritis. Approximately 15%–25% of nongonococcal, nonchlamydial urethritis can be attributed to either *M genitalium* or *U urealyticum*. Coliforms may cause urethritis in males practicing insertive anal intercourse. Mechanical manipulation or contact with irritants can also cause transient urethritis. It is important to recognize that urethritis in both males and females are frequently asymptomatic.

Females often present with symptoms of a urinary tract infection and "sterile pyuria" (no enteric bacterial pathogens isolated), which reflects urethritis caused by the organisms described above.

▶ Clinical Findings

A. Symptoms and Signs

If symptomatic, males present most commonly with a clear or purulent discharge from the urethra, dysuria, or urethral pruritus. Hematuria and inguinal adenopathy can occur. Most infections caused by *C trachomatis* and *T vaginalis* are asymptomatic, while 70% of males with *M genitalium* and 23%–90% with gonococcal urethritis are symptomatic.

B. Laboratory Findings

In a symptomatic male a positive leukocyte esterase test on first-void urine, or microscopic examination of first-void urine demonstrating more than 10 WBCs per high-power field, is suggestive of urethritis. Gram stain of urethral secretions demonstrating more than 5 WBCs per high-power field is also suggestive. Gonococcal urethritis is established by documenting the presence of WBCs containing intracellular gram-negative diplococci. Urethral swab or first-void urine for NAAT should be sent to the laboratory to detect *N gonorrhoeae* and *C trachomatis*. Evaluation for *T vaginalis* should be considered as newer technologies increase the sensitivity and specificity of detecting *T vaginalis* over wet mount. Microscopic examination of urethral discharge is not a sensitive test. Specific NAAT testing of urine is available for *Mycoplasma* and *Ureaplasma*, though it is not often clinically utilized.

▶ Complications

Complications include recurrent or persistent urethritis, epididymitis, prostatitis, or Reiter syndrome.

▶ Treatment (see Table 44–1)

Patients with objective evidence of urethritis should receive empiric treatment for gonorrhea and chlamydial infection, ideally directly observed in the office. Some data suggest better outcomes for treatment of *M genitalium* with azithromycin. If the infection is unresponsive to initial treatment and the infection is NAAT-negative, trichomoniasis should be ruled out and nongonococcal, nonchlamydial urethritis should be suspected and treated appropriately. Patients should be instructed to return for evaluation if symptoms persist or recur after completion of initial empiric therapy. Symptoms alone, without documentation of signs or laboratory evidence of urethral inflammation, are not a sufficient basis for retreatment. Sexual partners should either be evaluated or treated for gonorrhea and chlamydial infection.

EPIDIDYMITIS

▶ General Considerations

Epididymitis in a male who is sexually active is most often caused by *C trachomatis* or *N gonorrhoeae*. Epididymitis caused by *Escherichia coli* occurs among males who are the insertive partners during anal intercourse and in males who have urinary tract abnormalities.

▶ Clinical Findings

A. Symptoms and Signs

Epididymitis presents as a constellation of pain, swelling, and inflammation of the epididymis. In many cases, the testis is also involved.

B. Laboratory and Diagnostic Studies

Diagnosis is generally made clinically. Color Doppler ultrasound can help make the diagnosis. Although often not available, radionuclide scanning of the scrotum is the most accurate method of diagnosis. Laboratory evaluation is the same as for suspected urethritis and should include urine culture if NAAT is negative.

▶ Differential Diagnosis

Acute epididymitis must be distinguished from orchitis due to infarct, testicular torsion, or viral infection. Less common and more chronic illnesses include testicular cancer, tuberculosis, or fungal infection.

▶ Complications

Infertility is rare, and chronic local pain is uncommon.

▶ Treatment

Empiric therapy (see Table 44–1) is indicated before culture results are available. As an adjunct to therapy, bed rest, scrotal elevation, and analgesics are recommended until fever and local inflammation subside. Lack of improvement of swelling and tenderness within 3 days requires reevaluation of both the diagnosis and therapy. Sex partners should be evaluated and treated for gonorrhea and chlamydial infections.

PROCTITIS, PROCTOCOLITIS, & ENTERITIS

▶ General Considerations

Proctitis occurs predominantly among persons who participate in anal intercourse. Enteritis occurs among those whose sexual practices include oral-fecal contact. Proctocolitis can be acquired by either route depending on the pathogen. Common sexually transmitted pathogens causing proctitis or proctocolitis include *C trachomatis* (including lymphogranuloma venereum [LGV] serovars), *Treponema pallidum*, HSV, *N gonorrhoeae*, *Giardia lamblia*, and enteric organisms. As many as 85% of rectal infections with *N gonorrhoeae* and *C trachomatis* are asymptomatic. The presence of symptomatic or asymptomatic proctitis may facilitate the transmission of HIV infection.

▶ Clinical Findings

A. Symptoms and Signs

Proctitis, defined as inflammation limited to the distal 10–12 cm of the rectum, is associated with anorectal pain, tenesmus, and rectal discharge. Acute proctitis among persons who have recently practiced receptive anal intercourse is most often sexually transmitted. The symptoms of proctocolitis combine those of proctitis, plus diarrhea or abdominal cramps (or both), because of inflamed colonic mucosa more than 12 cm from the anus. Enteritis usually results in diarrhea and abdominal cramping without signs of proctitis or proctocolitis.

B. Laboratory and Diagnostic Studies

Evaluation may include anoscopy or sigmoidoscopy, stool examination, culture or NAAT for appropriate organisms, and serology for syphilis.

▶ Treatment

Management will be determined by the etiologic agent (see Table 44–1 and Chapter 42). Reinfection may be difficult to distinguish from treatment failure.

VAGINAL DISCHARGE

Adolescent girls may have a normal physiologic leukorrhea, secondary to turnover of vaginal epithelium. Infectious causes of discharge include *T vaginalis*, *C trachomatis*, *N gonorrhoeae*, and bacterial vaginosis pathogens. Candidiasis is a yeast infection that produces vaginal discharge, but is not usually sexually transmitted. Vaginitis in general may cause vaginal discharge, vulvar itching, and irritation. Discharge may be white, gray, or yellow. Physiologic leukorrhea is usually white, homogeneous, and not associated with itching, irritation, or foul odor. Mechanical, chemical, allergic, or other noninfectious irritants of the vagina may cause vaginal discharge.

1. Bacterial Vaginosis

▶ General Considerations

Bacterial vaginosis is a polymicrobial infection of the vagina caused by an imbalance of the normal bacterial vaginal flora. The altered flora has a paucity of hydrogen peroxide-producing lactobacilli and increased concentrations of anaerobic bacteria (*Prevotella* spp and *Mobiluncus* spp), *Gardnerella vaginalis, Ureaplasma,* and *Mycoplasma*. It is unclear whether bacterial vaginosis is sexually transmitted, but it is associated with having multiple sex partners and women with bacterial vaginosis are at increased risk for other STIs.

▶ Clinical Findings

A. Symptoms and signs

The most common symptom is a copious, malodorous, homogeneous thin gray-white vaginal discharge. Patients may report vaginal itching or dysuria. A fishy odor may be most noticeable after intercourse or during menses, when the high pH of blood or semen volatilizes the amines.

B. Laboratory Findings

Bacterial vaginosis is most often diagnosed by the use of clinical criteria, which include: (1) presence of thin, white discharge that smoothly coats the vaginal walls; (2) fishy (amine) odor before or after the addition of 10% KOH (whiff test); (3) pH of vaginal fluid greater than 4.5 determined with narrow-range pH paper; and (4) presence of "clue cells" on microscopic examination. Clue cells are squamous epithelial cells that have multiple bacteria adhering to them, making their borders irregular and giving them a speckled appearance. Diagnosis requires three out of four criteria, although many female patients who fulfill these criteria have no discharge or other symptoms.

▶ Complications

Bacterial vaginosis during pregnancy is associated with adverse outcomes such as premature labor, preterm delivery, intra-amniotic infection, and postpartum endometritis. In the nonpregnant individual, it may be associated with PID and urinary tract infections.

▶ Treatment

All female patients who have symptomatic disease should receive treatment to relieve vaginal symptoms and signs of infection (see Table 44–1). Pregnant patients should receive treatment to prevent adverse outcomes of pregnancy. Treatment for patients who do not complain of vaginal discharge or itching, but who demonstrate bacterial vaginosis on routine pelvic examination, is unclear. Because some studies associate bacterial vaginosis and PID, the recommendation is to have a low threshold for treating asymptomatic bacterial vaginosis. Follow-up visits are unnecessary if symptoms resolve. Recurrence of bacterial vaginosis is not unusual. Follow-up examination 1 month after treatment for high-risk pregnant patients is recommended.

Males do not develop infection equivalent to bacterial vaginosis and are often asymptomatic. Treatment of male partners has no effect on the course of infection in females but treatment is recommended for women who have sex with women.

Bradshaw CS, Sobel JD: Current treatment of bacterial vaginosis-limitations and need for innovation. J Infect Dis 2016;214 Suppl 1: S14–S20 [PMID: 27449869].

2. Trichomoniasis

▶ General Considerations

Trichomoniasis is caused by *T vaginalis*, a flagellated protozoan that infects 3.7 million people annually in the United States.

▶ Clinical Findings

A. Symptoms and Signs

Fifty percent of females with trichomoniasis develop a symptomatic vaginitis with vaginal itching, a green-gray malodorous frothy discharge, and dysuria. Occasionally postcoital bleeding and dyspareunia may be present. The vulva may be erythematous and the cervix friable.

B. Laboratory Findings

Mixing the discharge with normal saline facilitates detection of the flagellated protozoan on microscopic examination (wet preparation). This has a sensitivity of only 60%–70% even with immediate evaluation of the slide to achieve optimal results. Culture and NAAT testing are available when the diagnosis is unclear. NAAT tests are sensitive, but expensive, and not readily available. Two FDA-approved, point-of-care antigen-based detection assays for *T vaginalis* are available, but false positive results are problematic in low disease prevalence populations. Both antigen assays are performed on vaginal secretions and have a sensitivity greater than 83% and a specificity greater than 97%. Trichomonal urethritis frequently causes a positive urine leukocyte esterase test and WBCs on urethral smear.

Complications

Trichomonas infection in females has been associated with adverse pregnancy outcomes. Male partners of females diagnosed with trichomoniasis have a 22% chance of having trichomoniasis. Half of males with trichomoniasis will have urethritis. Male partners should receive empiric therapy for trichomoniasis. Rescreening for *T vaginalis* at 3 months following initial infection is recommended for women due to the high rate of reinfection.

Treatment

See Table 44–1 for treatment recommendations.

Meites E et al: A review of evidence-based care of symptomatic Trichomoniasis and Asymptomatic *Trichomonas vaginalis* infections. Clin Infect Dis 2015;61 suppl 8:S837–S848 [PMID: 26602621].

3. Vulvovaginal Candidiasis

General Considerations

Vulvovaginal candidiasis is caused by *Candida albicans* in 85%–90% of cases. Most females will have at least one episode of vulvovaginal candidiasis in their lifetime, and almost half will have two or more episodes. The highest incidence is between ages 16 and 30 years. Predisposing factors include recent use of antibiotics, diabetes, pregnancy, and HIV. Risk factors include vaginal intercourse, especially with a new sexual partner, use of oral contraceptives, and use of spermicide. This disease is usually caused by unrestrained growth of *Candida* that normally colonizes the vagina asymptomatically or is infected secondarily from *Candida* present in the GI tract. Recurrences reflect reactivation of colonization.

Clinical Findings

A. Symptoms and Signs

Typical symptoms include pruritus and a white, cottage cheese-like vaginal discharge without odor. The itching is more common midcycle and shortly after menses. Other symptoms include vaginal soreness, vulvar burning, vulvar edema and redness, dyspareunia, and dysuria (especially after intercourse).

B. Laboratory Findings

The diagnosis is usually made by visualizing yeast or pseudohyphae with 10% KOH (90% sensitive) or Gram stain (77% sensitive) in the vaginal discharge. Fungal culture can be used if symptoms and microscopy are not definitive or if disease is unresponsive or recurrent. However, culture is not very specific as colonization is common in asymptomatic females. Vaginal pH is normal with yeast infections.

Complications

The only complication of vulvovaginal candidiasis is recurrent infections. Most females with recurrent infection have no apparent predisposing or underlying conditions.

Treatment

Short-course topical formulations effectively treat uncomplicated vaginal yeast infections (see Table 44–1). The topically applied azole drugs are more effective than nystatin. Treatment with azoles results in relief of symptoms and negative cultures in 80%–90% of patients who complete therapy. Oral fluconazole as a one-time dose is an effective oral treatment. Patients should be instructed to return for follow-up visits only if symptoms persist or recur. Six-month prophylaxis regimens have been effective in many female patients with persistent or recurrent yeast infection. Recurrent disease is usually due to *C albicans* that remains susceptible to azoles, and should be treated for 14 days with oral azoles. Some nonalbicans *Candida* will respond to itraconazole or boric acid gelatin capsules (600 mg daily for 14 days) intravaginally. Treatment of sex partners is not recommended, but may be considered for females who have recurrent infection.

GENITAL ULCERATIONS

In the United States, young, sexually active patients who have genital ulcers have genital herpes or syphilis. The relative frequency of each disease differs by geographic area and patient population; however, in most areas, genital herpes is the most prevalent of these diseases. More than one of these diseases could be present in a patient with genital ulcers. All ulcerative diseases are associated with an increased risk for HIV infection. Primary HIV infection (acute retroviral syndrome) may present with oral and genital lesions. Less common causes of genital ulceration include chancroid and donovanosis.

Location of the ulcers is dependent on the specific type of sexual behavior. Ulcers may be vaginal, vulvar, cervical, penile, or rectal. Oral lesions may occur concomitantly with genital ulcerations. Each etiologic agent has specific characteristics that are described in the following sections. Lesion pain, inguinal lymphadenopathy, and urethritis may be found in association with the ulcers.

1. Herpes Simplex Virus Infection (See Also Chapter 40)

General Considerations

HSV is the most common cause of visible genital ulcers. HSV-1 is commonly associated with infections of the face, including the eyes, pharynx, and mouth. However, each serotype is capable of infecting either region. HSV-1 infections are frequently established in children by age 5 through oral acquisition; lower socioeconomic groups have higher infection rates. Both HSV-1 and HSV-2 cause STIs. The prevalence of both infections in the United States increases during teen years. In this age group and young adults, HSV-1 has become the predominant cause of genital infection. Rates of HSV-2 seroprevalence reach 20%–40% in 40-year-olds. HSV infections are lifelong as a result of latent infection of sensory ganglia, although many individuals infected with either type of HSV infection, may not be aware of their infection because of mild or nonspecific symptoms. Nevertheless, these individuals can still asymptomatically shed virus and thereby unknowingly transmit the infection, and they can reactivate the virus to cause clinical infection in themselves.

▶ Clinical Findings

A. Symptoms and Signs

Symptomatic initial genital HSV infection causes vesicles of the vulva, vagina, cervix, penis, rectum, or urethra, which are quickly followed by shallow, painful ulcerations. Atypical presentation of HSV infection includes vulvar erythema and fissures. Urethritis may occur. Initial infection can be severe, lasting up to 3 weeks, and be associated with fever and malaise, as well as localized tender adenopathy. The pain and dysuria can be extremely uncomfortable, requiring sitz baths, topical anesthetics, and occasionally catheterization for urinary retention.

Symptoms tend to be more severe in females. Recurrence in the genital area with HSV-2 is likely (65%–90%). Approximately 40% of individuals infected with HSV-2 will experience at least six recurrences per year in the early years after initial infection. Prodromal pain in the genital, buttock, or pelvic region is common prior to recurrences. Recurrent genital HSV is of shorter duration (5–7 days), with fewer lesions and usually no systemic symptoms. Commonly, the frequency of recurrences decreases over time, although approximately one-third of individuals fail to demonstrate this improvement. First-episode genital herpes infection caused by HSV-1 is usually the consequence of oral-genital sex. Primary HSV-1 infection generally is as severe as HSV-2 infection, and treatment is the same. Recurrence of genital HSV-1 is less frequent than genital HSV-2. Genital HSV-1 occurs in less than 50% of patients.

B. Laboratory Findings

Diagnosis of genital HSV infection is often made presumptively, but in one large series this diagnosis was incorrect for 20% of cases. Cell culture and PCR testing are the CDC's preferred methods of testing. NAAT is more sensitive. Direct immunofluorescence assays are available, but lack sensitivity.

▶ Differential Diagnosis

Genital HSV infections must be distinguished from other ulcerative STI lesions, including syphilis, chancroid, and lymphogranuloma venereum (LGV). Non-STIs might include herpes zoster, Behçet syndrome, or lichen sclerosis. (See next two sections Syphilis and Chancroid.)

▶ Complications

Complications, almost always only with the first episode of genital HSV infection, include viral meningitis, urinary retention, transmission to newborns at birth, and pharyngitis. Infection with genital HSV, whether active or not, greatly increases the likelihood of transmitting or acquiring HIV infection within couples discordant for HIV.

▶ Prevention

All patients with active lesions should be counseled to abstain from sexual contact. Almost all patients have very frequent periodic asymptomatic shedding of HSV, and most cases of genital HSV infection are transmitted by persons who are unaware that they have the infection or are asymptomatic when transmission occurs. Reactivation with asymptomatic shedding occurs even in individuals who were asymptomatically infected. Individuals with prior HSV infection should be encouraged to use condoms to protect susceptible partners. Antiviral prophylaxis of infected individuals reduces shedding and significantly reduces the chance of transmission to their sexual partners.

▶ Treatment

Antiviral drugs administered within the first 5 days of primary infection decrease the duration and severity of HSV infection (see Table 44–1). The effect of antivirals on the severity or duration of recurrent disease is limited. For best results with recurrent disease, therapy should be started with the prodrome or during the first day of the recurrence. Patients should have a prescription at home to initiate treatment. If recurrences are frequent and cause significant physical or emotional discomfort, patients may elect to take antiviral prophylaxis on a daily basis to reduce the frequency (70% decrease) and duration of recurrences. Treatment of first or subsequent attacks will not prevent future attacks.

2. Syphilis

▶ General Considerations

Syphilis is an acute and chronic STI caused by infection with *T pallidum*. The national rate of syphilis has increased annually since reaching an all-time low in 2000. Increases have been observed in both genders, but predominantly in MSM, who now account for 58% of primary and secondary cases reported to the CDC. In 2017, the CDC reported an increase of 21% in new cases of primary and secondary syphilis among women with subsequent increases in the rate of congenital syphilis. Men between the ages of 25 and 29 years have the highest rates of syphilis. Nearly 50% of the cases of syphilis in MSM in 2017 were also living with HIV.

▶ Clinical Findings

A. Symptoms and Signs

Skin and mucous membrane lesions characterize the acute phase of primary and secondary syphilis. Lesions of the bone, viscera, aorta, and central nervous system predominate in the chronic phase (tertiary syphilis) (see Chapter 42). Prevention of syphilis is also important because syphilitic mucosal lesions facilitate transmission of HIV.

Primary syphilis usually presents as a solitary chancre at the point of inoculation. Characteristically, the chancre presents as a painless, indurated, nonpurulent ulcer with a clean base and associated nontender, firm adenopathy. The chancre appears on average 21 days (range: 3–90 days) after exposure and resolves spontaneously 4–8 weeks later. Because it is painless, it may go undetected, especially if the lesion is within the vagina, oropharynx, urethra, or rectum. Chancres may occur on the genitalia, anus, or oropharynx. Secondary syphilis occurs 4–10 weeks after the chancre appears, with generalized malaise, painless adenopathy, and a nonpruritic maculopapular rash that often includes the palms and soles. Secondary syphilis resolves in 1–3 months, but can recur. Verrucous lesions known as condylomata lata may develop on the genitalia. These must be distinguished from genital warts.

B. Laboratory Findings

If the patient has a suspect primary lesion, is at high risk, is a contact, or may have secondary syphilis, a nontreponemal serum screen—either RPR or VDRL—should be performed. If the nontreponemal test is positive, then a specific treponemal test—a fluorescent treponemal antibody-absorbed (FTA-ABS) or microhemagglutination–*T pallidum* (MHA-TP) test—is done to confirm the diagnosis.

If a patient is engaging in high-risk sexual behavior or is living in an area in which syphilis is endemic, RPRs should be drawn yearly to screen for asymptomatic infection. Annual RPR testing among high-risk groups is essential to distinguish between early latent syphilis (1 year or less postinfection), late latent syphilis (> 1 year postinfection), or syphilis of unknown duration, as treatment recommendations vary. Syphilis is reportable to state health departments, and all sexual contacts need to be evaluated. Patients also need to be evaluated for other STIs, especially HIV. People with HIV have increased rates of failure with some treatment regimens and treatment of the HIV infection should occur as soon as indicated after diagnosis.

▶ Complications

Untreated syphilis can lead to tertiary complications with serious multiorgan involvement, including aortitis and neurosyphilis. Transmission to the fetus can occur from an untreated pregnant woman (see Chapters 2 and 42).

▶ Treatment

See Table 44–1 for treatment recommendations. Patients should be reexamined and serologically evaluated with nontreponemal tests at 6 and 12 months after treatment. If signs or symptoms persist or recur, or patients do not have a fourfold decrease in their nontreponemal test titer, they should be considered to have failed treatment or be reinfected and need retreatment.

3. Chancroid

▶ General Considerations

Chancroid is caused by *Haemophilus ducreyi*. It is relatively rare outside of the tropics and subtropics, but is endemic in some urban areas in the United States, and has been associated with HIV infection, drug use, and prostitution. Coinfection with syphilis or HSV occurs in as many as 17% of patients. A detailed history, including travel, may prove to be important in identifying this infection.

▶ Clinical Findings

A. Symptoms and Signs

The typical lesion begins as a papule that erodes after 24–48 hours into an ulcer. The ulcer is painful and has ragged, sharply demarcated edges and a purulent base (unlike syphilis). The ulcer is typically solitary and somewhat deeper than HSV infection. The lesions may occur anywhere on the genitals and are more common in men than in women. Tender, fluctuant (unlike syphilis and HSV) inguinal adenopathy is present in 50% of patients. A painful ulcer in combination with suppurative inguinal adenopathy is very often chancroid.

B. Laboratory Findings

Gram stain shows gram-positive cocci arranged in a boxcar formation. Culture, which has a sensitivity of less than 80%, can be performed on a special medium that is available in academic centers. NAAT testing may improve laboratory diagnosis in areas where such testing is available.

▶ Differential Diagnosis

Chancroid is distinguished from syphilis by the painful nature of the ulcer and the associated tender suppurative adenopathy. HSV vesicles often produce painful ulcers, but these are multiple, smaller, and shallower than chancroid ulcers. Adenopathy associated with initial HSV infection does not suppurate. A presumptive diagnosis of chancroid should be considered in a patient with typical painful genital ulcers and regional adenopathy when the test results for syphilis and HSV are negative.

▶ Treatment

Symptoms improve within 3 days after therapy (see Table 44–1). Most ulcers resolve in 7 days, although large ulcers may take 2 weeks to heal. All sexual contacts need to be examined and given treatment, even if asymptomatic. Individuals with HIV coinfection may have slower rates of healing or treatment failures.

4. Lymphogranuloma Venereum

▶ General Considerations

Lymphogranuloma venereum (LGV), caused by *C trachomatis* serovars L1, L2, or L3, is generally rare in the United States. The disease is endemic in Southeast Asia, the Caribbean, Latin America, and areas of Africa. Since 2003, an increased number of cases in the United States, Western Europe, and Canada have occurred primarily among MSM and has been associated with HIV coinfection.

▶ Clinical Findings

A. Symptoms and Signs

Patients with LGV present with a painless vesicle or ulcer that heals spontaneously, followed by the development of tender adenopathy that is typically unilateral. A classic finding is the groove sign—an inguinal crease created by concomitant involvement of inguinal and femoral nodes. These nodes become matted and fluctuant and may rupture. LGV can cause proctocolitis with rectal ulceration, purulent anal discharge, fever, tenesmus, and lower abdominal pain, primarily in MSM.

B. Laboratory Findings

Diagnosis of LGV can be difficult. It generally requires a clinical suspicion based on physical examination findings. Lesion swabs and lymph node aspirates can be tested for *Chlamydia* by culture, DFA, or NAAT. NAAT is not FDA cleared for rectal specimens. Additional genotyping is necessary to differentiate LGV from non-LGV serovars of *Chlamydia*. In the absence of laboratory testing to confirm the diagnosis, one should treat for LGV if clinical suspicion is high.

▶ Differential Diagnosis

Differential diagnosis during the adenopathy phase includes bacterial adenitis, lymphoma, and cat-scratch disease. Differential diagnosis during the ulcerative phase encompasses all causes of genital ulcers.

▶ Treatment

See Table 44–1 for treatment recommendations. Despite the effectiveness of azithromycin for non-LGV chlamydial infections, there have been no controlled treatment trials to recommend its use in LGV. HIV-infected individuals are treated the same as non–HIV-infected individuals, but should be monitored closely to assess response to treatment.

Stoner BP, Cohen SE: Lymphogranuloma venereum 2015: clinical presentation, diagnosis, and treatment. Clin Infect Dis 2015 Dec 15;61 Suppl 8:S865–S873. doi: 10.1093/cid/civ756 [PMID: 26602624].

5. Other Ulcerations

Granuloma inguinale, or donovanosis, is caused by *Klebsiella granulomatis*, a gram-negative bacillus that is rare in the United States, but is endemic in India, the Caribbean, and southern Africa. An indurated subcutaneous nodule erodes to form a painless, friable ulcer with granulation tissue. Diagnosis is based on clinical suspicion and supported by a Wright or Giemsa stain of the granulation tissue that reveals intracytoplasmic rods (Donovan bodies) in mononuclear cells. See Table 44–1 for treatment recommendations. Relapse may occur 6–18 months after apparently effective treatment with a 3-week course of doxycycline.

GENITAL WARTS & HUMAN PAPILLOMAVIRUS

▶ General Considerations

Condylomata acuminata, or genital warts, are caused by HPV, which can also cause cervical dysplasia and cervical cancer, and oropharyngeal and anal cancers. HPV is transmitted sexually. An estimated 20 million people in the United States are infected annually with HPV, including approximately more than 9 million sexually active adolescents and young adults 15–24 years of age. The majority (74%) of new HPV infections occurs among those 15–24 years of age; in females younger than age 25 years, the prevalence ranges between 28%

and 46%. It is estimated that 32%–50% of adolescent females having sexual intercourse in the United States have HPV infections, though only 1% may have visible lesions. Thirty to 60% of males whose partners have HPV have evidence of genital warts on examination. An estimated 1 million new cases of genital warts occur every year in the United States.

Although there are almost 100 serotypes of HPV, types 6 and 11 cause approximately 90% of genital warts, and HPV types 16 and 18 cause more than 70% of cervical dysplasia and cervical cancer. The infection is more common in persons with multiple partners and in those who initiate sexual intercourse at an early age.

Pap smears should be obtained starting at age 21 and then every 3 years. More frequent and earlier evaluations are recommended if there are additional risk factors such as coinfection with HIV.

Clinical Findings

A. Symptoms and Signs

For males, verrucous lesions are found on the shaft or corona of the penis. Lesions also may develop in the urethra or rectum. Lesions do not produce discomfort. They may be single or found in clusters. Females develop verrucous lesions on any genital mucosal surface, either internally or externally, and often develop perianal lesions.

B. Laboratory Findings

External, visible lesions have unique characteristics that make the diagnosis straightforward. Condylomata acuminata can be distinguished from condylomata lata (syphilis), skin tags, and molluscum contagiosum by application of 5% acetic acid solution. Blanching of skin or mucous membranes, after application of 3%–5% acetic acid solution, acetowhitening, is used to indicate the extent of cervical infection.

Pap smears detect cervical abnormalities. HPV infection is the most frequent cause of an abnormal smear. Pap smear findings are graded by the atypical nature of the cervical cells. These changes range from atypical squamous cells of undetermined significance (ASCUS) to low-grade squamous intraepithelial lesions (LSIL) and high-grade squamous intraepithelial lesions (HSIL). LSIL encompasses cellular changes associated with HPV and mild dysplasia. HSIL includes moderate dysplasia, severe dysplasia, and carcinoma in situ.

Follow-up for ASCUS is controversial, as only 25% progress to dysplasia, and the remainder is stable or regress. Updated recommendations prefer repeat cytology in 12 months with no HPV DNA testing. If a test for HPV DNA is performed and is positive, then repeat cytology in 12 months is recommended. If the grade of the atypical squamous cells remains uncertain or if there is HSIL, colposcopy is recommended. If LSIL is detected, colposcopy is not

needed, but a repeat Pap smear should be done in 1 year, and if LSIL or HSIL are subsequently detected, the patient should be referred for colposcopy for direct visualization or biopsy of the cervix (or both). If a Pap smear shows signs of inflammation only, and concomitant infection such as vaginitis or cervicitis is present, the smear should be repeated after the inflammation has cleared.

Differential Diagnosis

The differential diagnosis includes normal anatomic structures (pearly penile papules, vestibular papillae, and sebaceous glands), molluscum contagiosum, seborrheic keratosis, and syphilis.

Complications

Because genital warts can proliferate and become friable during pregnancy, many experts advocate their removal during pregnancy. HPV types 6 and 11 can cause laryngeal papillomatosis in infants and children. Complications of appropriate treatment include scarring with changes in skin pigmentation or pain at the treatment site. Pap smears with persistent or high-grade dysplasia require biopsy and/or resection, which may result in cervical abnormalities that complicate pregnancy. Cervical cancer is the most common and important sequelae of HPV and persistent cervical dysplasia.

Prevention

The use of condoms significantly reduces, but does not eliminate, the risk for transmission to uninfected partners. The 9-valent HPV vaccine is 96%–100% effective in preventing HPV-6 and 11-related genital warts and HPV-16 and 18-related cervical dysplasia and many of the cervical lesions caused by less common serotypes. It is recommended for females and males aged 9–26 years. Males are protected against genital warts and anal cancer, which has a significantly increased incidence in males who practice anal sex (see Chapter 10).

Treatment

Penile and external vaginal or vulvar lesions can be treated topically. Treatment may need to occur weekly for 4–6 weeks. An experienced practitioner should treat internal and cervical lesions (see Table 44–1). Treatment may clear the visible lesions, but not reduce the presence of virus, nor is it clear whether transmission of HPV is reduced by treatment.

Warts may resolve or remain unchanged if left untreated or they may increase in size or number. Treatment can induce wart-free periods in most patients. Most recurrences occur within the 3 months following completion of a treatment regimen. Appropriate follow-up of abnormal Pap smears is essential to detect any progression to malignancy.

ASCCP Consensus Guidelines for Management of Abnormal Cervical Cytology. Available at: http://www.asccp.org/management-guidelines. Accessed July 19, 2019.

Sawaya GF, Smith-McCune K, Kupperman M: Cervical cancer screening: more choices in 2019. JAMA 2019;321(20):2018–2019 [PMID: 31135834].

OTHER VIRAL INFECTIONS

1. Hepatitis (See also Chapter 22)

▶ **General Considerations**

In the United States, viral hepatitis is linked primarily to three viruses: hepatitis A (HAV), hepatitis B (HBV), and hepatitis C (HCV). Each virus has the potential to be spread through sexual activity. HAV is spread via fecal-oral transmission and oral-anal contact. Both HBV and HCV are spread through contact with blood or body fluids. Sexual transmission of HBV is believed to be much more efficient than that of HCV although recent data have suggested increased transmission of HCV in MSM.

Universal immunization recommendations for HAV and HBV have contributed to the decline in the prevalence of these diseases. However, individuals born before implementation of routine vaccination, especially those in high-risk groups (multiple sexual partners or MSM should receive vaccination).

2. Human Immunodeficiency Virus (See also Chapter 41)

▶ **General Considerations**

In 2017, 21% of new HIV infections in the United States occurred in youth and young adults aged 13–24 years. Data suggest that adolescents and young adults are less likely to be aware of their HIV infection than older individuals with HIV. Because of the long latency period between infection with HIV and progression to AIDS, it is felt that many HIV-positive young adults contracted HIV during adolescence. CDC incidence data indicate that young men who have sex with men continue to be the highest-risk group, particularly young men of color. Young women account for approximately 13% of the infections in this age group with black and Hispanic women bearing a disproportionate burden of the disease. Risk factors for contracting HIV include a prior STI, infrequent condom use, practicing insertive or receptive anal sex (both males and females), prior genital HSV infection, practicing survival sex (ie, trading sex for money or drugs), intravenous drug or crack cocaine or crystal methamphetamine use, homelessness, and being the victim of sexual abuse (males).

HIV infection should be considered in all sexually active youth, whether they have sex with males, females, or both.

The CDC and the United States Preventative Services Task Force recommend adolescents be offered HIV testing at least once. Individual risk factors should then be used to determine the frequency of repeat testing. Opportunities for HIV screening in adolescents should include STI screening or treatment, pregnancy testing, or routine health evaluations. Most states allow adolescents to consent to HIV testing and treatment, but providers should be aware of their particular State's laws.

▶ **Clinical Findings**

A. Symptoms and Signs

Adolescents may be asymptomatic with recent HIV infection or may present with the acute retroviral syndrome, which is evident 2–6 weeks after exposure. The acute clinical syndrome, which occurs in about 50% of patients, is generally indistinguishable from other viral illnesses with respect to fever, malaise, and upper respiratory symptoms. Distinguishing features include generalized lymphadenopathy, rash, oral and genital ulcerations, aseptic meningitis, and thrush. After the acute illness, signs and symptoms may be absent for many years.

B. Laboratory Findings

In 2014, the CDC updated its recommendations for HIV screening. The new recommendations are based on the availability of technologies that allow for earlier detection of HIV infection than offered by ELISA followed by Western Blot confirmation. The new testing algorithm for serum or plasma recommends the use of an HIV 1/2 antigen/antibody combination immunoassay for initial testing. This test detects antibodies to both HIV-1 and HIV-2 and the HIV-1 p24 antigen, which can occur approximately 3 weeks following HIV infection. This detects both established infections and more recent infections.

If acute HIV infection is suspected, HIV testing should be done by HIV RNA PCR testing or HIV DNA PCR testing. Routine serological testing may not be positive for 2–3 weeks or longer. Viral load values of less than 3000 copies/mL by RNA PCR may indicate a false positive in this setting and repeat testing would be indicated.

▶ **Treatment**

The most important aspect of identifying adolescents and young adults with HIV infection is linking them to care. Data support the treatment of youth with HIV infection in care settings that provide comprehensive, multidisciplinary care. These settings will be best equipped to provide emotional support, preventative care, risk reduction for contacts, access to research, and guidance on the appropriate timing of antiretroviral therapies.

Centers for Disease Control and Prevention: *HIV Surveillance Report, 2017*; vol. 29. http://www.cdc.gov/hiv/library/reports/hiv-surveillance.html. Published November 2018. Accessed July 20, 2019.

Centers for Disease Control and Prevention; Association of Public Health Laboratories: Laboratory Testing for the Diagnosis of HIV Infection: Updated Recommendations. Available at: http://dx.doi.org/10.15620/cdc.23447. Published June 27, 2014. Accessed July 19, 2019.

Moyer VA: Screening for HIV: U.S. Preventive Services Task Force recommendation statement. Ann Intern Med 2013;159(3):161–168 [PMID: 23698354].

3. HIV Postsexual Exposure Prophylaxis

Adolescents may present to health care providers seeking nonoccupational HIV postexposure prophylaxis (nPEP) following an assault or a high-risk sexual encounter. The risk of acquiring HIV infection through sexual assault or abuse is low but present. The risk for HIV transmission from a positive contact per episode of receptive penile-anal sexual exposure is estimated at 0.5%–3%; the risk per episode of receptive vaginal exposure is estimated at less than 0.1%–0.2%. HIV transmission also occurs from receptive oral exposure, but the risk is unknown. The risk of HIV transmission may be increased in certain conditions: traumatic vaginal, anal, or oral penetration; site of exposure to ejaculate; HIV viral load in ejaculate; duration of HIV infection in the assailant or partner; and presence of an STI, prior genital HSV infection or genital lesions in either partner. The risk is greatly reduced if the contact is successfully receiving antiretroviral therapy.

Health care providers that consider offering nPEP should take into account the likelihood that exposure to HIV occurred, the potential benefits and risks of such therapy, and the interval between the exposure and initiation of therapy. It will be helpful to know the HIV status of the sexual contact. The CDC provides an algorithm for consideration of nPEP. In general, nPEP is not recommended when more than 72 hours have passed since exposure. If the patient decides to take nPEP, clinical management should be implemented according to published CDC guidelines. Providers should be aware that structural barriers exist to obtaining nPEP, and that adolescent assault victims have a high discontinuation rate due to adverse effects from the medication.

Centers for Disease Control and Prevention: Updated Guidelines for Antiretroviral Postexposure Prophylaxis After Sexual, Injection Drug Use, or Other Nonoccupational Exposure to HIV— United States, 2016. https://www.cdc.gov/hiv/pdf/programresources/cdc-hiv-npep-guidelines.pdf. Accessed July 20, 2019.

4. HIV Preexposure Prophylaxis

In 2014, the U.S. Public Health Service released guidance on the use of preexposure prophylaxis (PrEP) in the United States. The guidance followed the Food and Drug Administration's approval of a coformulated HIV antiretroviral (tenofovir and emtricitabine [TDF-FTC]) for use as PrEP based on data from two large international trials. In 2018, the Food and Drug Administration approved TDF-FTC as PrEP for individuals greater than or equal to 35 kg, without renal impairment. Initial studies to determine safety and acceptability in younger individuals at high risk for HIV acquisition revealed high rates of acceptability but adherence dropped as intervals between study visits lengthened, suggesting that increased adherence support may be needed. Providers considering the use of PrEP in a minor at risk of infection should consult with an experienced prescriber and know the laws of their particular state with respect to providing preventive HIV medication without parental consent.

Centers for Disease Control and Prevention: US Public Health Service: Preexposure Prophylaxis for the Prevention of HIV Infection in the United States—2017 Update: A Clinical Practice Guideline. https://www.cdc.gov/hiv/pdf/risk/prep/cdc-hiv-prep-guidelines-2017.pdf. Published March 2018. Accessed July 20, 2019.

Hosek SG et al: An HIV Preexposure prophylaxis demonstration project and safety study for young MSM. J Acquir Immune Defic Syndr 2017;74(1):21–29 [PMID: 27632233].

ECTOPARASITIC INFECTIONS

1. Pubic Lice

Pthirus pubis, the pubic louse, lives in pubic hair. The louse or the nits can be transmitted by close contact from person to person. Patients complain of itching and may report having seen the insect. Examination of the pubic hair may reveal the louse crawling around or attached to the hair. Closer inspection may reveal the nit or sac of eggs, which is a gelatinous material (1–2 mm) stuck to the hair shaft. See Table 44–1 for treatment recommendations.

2. Scabies

Sarcoptes scabiei, the causative organism in scabies, is smaller than the louse. It can be identified by the classic burrow, which is created by the organism laying eggs and traveling just below the skin surface. Scabies can be sexually transmitted by close skin-to-skin contact and can be found in the pubic region, groin, lower abdomen, or upper thighs. The rash is intensely pruritic, especially at night, erythematous, and scaly. See Table 44–1 for treatment options. Ivermectin is an oral therapeutic option for scabies that may hold particular promise in the treatment of severe infestations or in epidemic situations. When treating with lotion or shampoo, the entire area needs to be covered for the time specified by the manufacturer. One treatment usually clears the infestation, although a second treatment may be necessary. Bed sheets and clothes must be washed in hot water. Both sexual and close personal or household contacts within the preceding month should be examined and treated.

Currie BJ, McCarthy JS: Permethrin and ivermectin for scabies. N Engl J Med 2010;362:717 [PMID: 20181973].

Leone PA: Scabies and pediculosis pubis: an update of treatment regimens and general review. Clin Infect Dis 2007;44:S153 [PMID: 17342668].

REFERENCES

Centers for Disease Control and Prevention: *Sexually Transmitted Disease Surveillance 2017*. Atlanta, GA: U.S. Department of Health and Human Services; 2018. Available at: https://www.cdc.gov/std/stats17/default.htm. Accessed July 19, 2019.

Snook ML et al: Adolescent gynecology: special considerations for special patients. Clin Obstet Gynecol 2012;55:651 [PMID: 22828097].

Workowski KA, Bolan GA: Sexually transmitted diseases treatment guidelines, 2015. MMWR 2015 Jun 5;64:1–137 [PMID: 26042815]. Available at: https://www.cdc.gov/std/tg2015/default.htm. Accessed July 19, 2019.

Travel Medicine

Suchitra Rao, MBBS, MSCS

INTRODUCTION

Twenty-seven million people from the United States travel internationally per year; one-third of them travel to developing nations. Approximately 50%–70% of travelers become ill during their travel overseas. The number of children traveling with families continues to increase. Children who travel are especially susceptible to infectious diseases, trauma, and other health problems, which vary with the destination. Preparation for travel with children and infants includes consideration of destination-specific risks, underlying medical problems, and administration of both routine and travel-related vaccines. Pretravel counseling should ideally take place at least 1 month prior to travel, given the need to develop an effective immune response from any travel-associated vaccinations. The physician involved in pretravel counseling should focus on the issues listed in Table 45–1.

PREPARING CHILDREN & INFANTS FOR TRAVEL

▶ Travel Plans

Parents and care providers should be advised that travel with children and infants is much more enjoyable when the number of journeys in a single trip is limited, travel time is kept relatively short, and travel delays are anticipated. Planning for delays and other problems should include bringing new or favorite toys or games for distraction and carrying extra food and drink, changes of clothing, and fever medications.

Medical Care During Travel

It is useful to obtain names and addresses of local health care providers at the family's destination. This is available from travel medicine practitioners or from the membership directory of the International Society of Travel Medicine. The International Association for Medical Assistance to Travelers website (www.iamat.org) is another useful resource with a worldwide

directory of providers proficient in English. Travel insurance, which is highly encouraged, should not only cover medical care at the destination but also provide 24-hour helplines with information regarding English-speaking physicians and hospitals, and arrange and pay for evacuation to a medical facility that provides necessary treatment that is not available locally. In emergencies, parents and caretakers should take their children to the largest medical facility in the area, which is more likely to have a pediatric unit and trauma services.

Trauma

Trauma is a common cause of morbidity and mortality in traveling children. Parents should rent larger, safer vehicles, and use car seats whenever possible. However, in many developing countries, car seats are not available, so caretakers may need to travel with their own. Taxis often do not have seatbelts, so it may be necessary to request taxis with seatbelts by calling in advance.

Air Travel

Healthy term infants can travel by commercial pressurized airplane. Children at higher risk during air travel may include premature infants and those with chronic cardiac or pulmonary disease, so appropriate counseling with their specialist is indicated. Many parents request advice regarding sedation of their child during travel. While this is not recommended, the most widely used agent is diphenhydramine. It is advisable to try a test dose prior to travel as idiosyncratic reactions and overdosing can lead to an anticholinergic syndrome or a paradoxical stimulating effect.

Ear Pain

Children and infants often have pain during ascent and descent of commercial airplanes due to changes in middle ear pressure causing retraction or protrusion of the tympanic membrane. Methods that can alleviate or minimize ear pain

Table 45–1. Preparing for travel—issues specific to travel as indicated.

Vaccinations (indications, safety, and tolerability)
Insect precautions (use of protective clothing, repellants, bed nets, insecticides)
Malaria chemoprophylaxis (benefits of a particular regimen vs potential adverse reactions)
Food and water precautions and environmental risks from waterborne disease
Traveler's diarrhea and self-treatment
Health insurance/evacuation insurance
Trauma prevention and car seats
Access to medical care during travel
Altitude sickness
Disease outbreaks in destination
Climate
Jetlag
Animal exposure, trauma from animals
General health and routine illness
Clothing and footwear
Copies of prescriptions, vaccination documentation, physician's letter, list of medications
Travel-specific medications
Safe sex counseling
First-aid kits
Crime and safety

during these times include chewing, swallowing, nursing, and bottle feeding.

Motion Sickness

Almost 60% of children will experience motion sickness during travel. While older children have symptoms similar to those in adults (such as nausea, epigastric discomfort, headache, general discomfort), children younger than 5 years may have gait abnormalities as the predominant symptom. Nonpharmacologic preventive strategies include eating a light meal at least 3 hours before travel; avoiding dairy products and foods high in calories, protein, and sodium before travel; sitting in the middle of the back seat or in the front seat if age-appropriate; focusing on a stable object or the horizon; avoiding reading or other visual stimuli; eye closure; fresh air; and limiting excessive head movement. Pharmacologic intervention has not been well studied in children, but if necessary, antihistamines such as diphenhydramine are recommended for children younger than 12 years and scopolamine is acceptable for children older than 12 years. These measures, however, are not evidence-based.

High Altitude

Acute mountain sickness is as common in children as in adults, but it may go unrecognized due to its subtle presentation, such as unexplained mental fussiness or change in appetite and sleep patterns. High-altitude pulmonary edema (HAPE) is seen in children traveling to high altitudes; it also occurs in children who live at high altitude, descend for an extended period, and return to altitude. Mild symptoms of altitude sickness can be treated with rest and hydration, or analgesics such as ibuprofen or acetaminophen. High-altitude sickness is milder and resolves much more quickly in children compared to adults, so prophylaxis is usually not required. Acetazolamide has not been studied in children for acute mountain sickness, but it is safe in this age group and has been used for both prophylaxis and treatment. The pediatric dose is 5 mg/kg/day (125 mg maximum) divided twice daily, starting 1 day before ascent, and continued for 2 days at high altitude.

Medications/First-Aid Kit

A small medical kit is useful when traveling. Included in this kit should be medications for illnesses that the child experiences at home, trip-specific items, and the usual first-aid kit items (Table 45–2). Medications should be purchased prior to travel, as those obtained at some destinations may be of poor quality or contain toxic substances.

Table 45–2. First-aid kit for international travel.

Medications
    Malaria prophylaxis
    Acetaminophen and ibuprofen
    Antibiotics
    Antihistamines
Topical formulations
    Hydrocortisone ointment
    Antibiotic and antifungal ointment
    Insect repellants
    Sunscreen
    Antibacterial soap/alcohol-based hand sanitizer
    Antiseptic wipes
Other
    Bed nets
    Thermometer
    Medicine spoon and cup
    Oral rehydration salts in powder form
    Sterile cotton balls, cotton tip applicators
    Tweezers, scissors, safety pins
    Water purification tablets
    Gauze bandages
    Tape—hypoallergenic, waterproof
    Triangular bandage/sling/splint
    Tongue depressor
    Adhesive bandages
    Flashlight
    First-aid book
    Copies of prescriptions, list of medications, copy of insurance coverage

Feja KN, Tolan RW Jr: Infections related to international travel and adoption. Adv Pediatr 2013;60(1):107–139 [PMID: 24007842].

Fhogartaigh CN, Sanford C, Behrens RH: Preparing young travelers for low resource destinations. BMJ 2012;345:e7179 [PMID: 23131670].

Leung DT, LaRocque RC, Ryan ET: Travel medicine. Ann Intern Med 2018 Jan 2;168(1):ITC1–ITC16 [PMID: 29297035].

Neumann K: Pediatric travel medicine: where we are and where we hope to go. J Travel Med 2012;19(3):137–139 [PMID: 22530818].

Stauffer W, Christenson JC, Fischer PR: Preparing children for international travel. Travel Med Infect Dis 2008;6(3):101–113 [PMID: 18486064].

VACCINATIONS—ROUTINE CHILDHOOD VACCINES MODIFIED FOR TRAVEL

Many vaccine-preventable diseases remain prevalent in developing countries, and outbreaks still occur in areas where these diseases are considered rare. The schedule for some vaccines may be accelerated for travel, and some vaccines can be given earlier than the recommended age. Vaccination pertaining to children traveling follows the routine vaccination schedule as outlined in Chapter 10. The recommended intervals balance the high-risk age for disease with infant immunologic responses. The recommended minimum interval between doses is listed in Table 45–3. Barriers to some early immunizations are antibody from the mother interfering with an infant's ability to mount an antibody response, particularly to live vaccines, and the lack of a T-cell–dependent immune response to certain immunogens in those younger than 2 years. Minor febrile illnesses are not a contraindication to routine or travel vaccines and should not lead to their postponement. Live vaccines should be given together or separated by 30 days or more.

Diphtheria-Tetanus-Acellular Pertussis Vaccine

Immunization is recommended prior to travel to developing countries because of the greater risk of disease from diphtheria, tetanus, and pertussis. Tetanus risk is high in several areas of the developing world where fecal contamination of soil is extensive. Infants should receive their first diphtheria-tetanus-acellular pertussis (DTaP) at 6 weeks of age for an adequate immune response, with a 4-week interval between the subsequent two doses. Adequate protection is achieved after the third dose. The fourth dose may be given 6–12 months after the third dose provided that the child is 12 months of age or older. Tdap is licensed for children at least 11 years of age. Adolescents and adult caretakers, who are prominent vectors in the spread of pertussis to young children, should receive a single Tdap booster. If more than 5 years have elapsed since the last dose, a booster should be considered for children and adolescents to minimize tetanus

Table 45–3. Accelerated vaccinations schedule.

Vaccine	Minimum Age for First Dose	Minimum Time to Second Dose (wk)	Minimum Time to Third Dose (wk)	Minimum Time for Fourth Dose (wk)
MMR	12 mo[a]	4	—	—
Hepatitis B	Birth	4	8[b]	—
DTaP	6 wk	4	4	6 mo
Hib	6 wk	4	4	8[c]
IPV	6 wk	4	4	6 mo[d]
MCV	6 wk[e]	8	[e]	[e]
MPS4	2 y[e]	5 y	[e]	[e]
PCV	4 wk	4	4	8
Varicella	12 mo	4	—	—
Rotavirus	4 wk[f]	4	4[g]	
Hepatitis A	1 y	6 mo	—	—

DTaP, diphtheria-tetanus-acellular pertussis; Hib, *Haemophilus influenzae* type b; IPV, inactivated polio vaccine; MCV, meningococcal conjugate vaccine; MMR, measles-mumps-rubella; MPS4, meningococcal polysaccharide; PCV, pneumococcal conjugate vaccine.

[a]Children traveling abroad may be vaccinated as early as 6 months of age. Before departure, children aged 6–11 months should receive the first dose of MMR vaccine. This will not count toward their series, and they will still require two doses after 12 months of age.

[b]The third dose should be given at least 4 months after the first dose and at a minimum of 6 months of age.

[c]If third dose is given after 4 years, the fourth dose is not required.

[d]Recommended at 6–18 months of age, minimum age 4 years for final dose.

[e]Minimum 6 weeks for Hib-MenCY, 9 months for Menactra (MCV4-D), 2 years for Menveo (MCV4-CRM). Repeat vaccination depends on host status and ongoing risk factors.

[f]This differs from the package insert but is validated by data held by the manufacturer.

[g]No third dose is required if Rotarix is given.

risk. Tdap is preferred to Td in children older than 11 years if they have not received Tdap previously.

Haemophilus influenzae Type b Vaccine

The indications for vaccination of *Haemophilus influenzae* type b (Hib) in children traveling are the same as for the US residents. If previously unvaccinated, infants younger than 15 months should receive at least two doses prior to travel. An accelerated schedule can start at a minimum of 6 weeks of age, with a 4-week interval between the first, second, and third doses, and at least 8 weeks between third and fourth doses.

Hepatitis A Vaccine

Hepatitis A is one of the most common vaccine-preventable illnesses globally, and vaccination should be provided prior to travel to developing countries. Hepatitis A is much less common in the developed world, so children from these areas are likely to be susceptible when traveling to high-risk areas. Although two doses of the vaccine are recommended 6–12 months apart, a single dose will provide protection during the trip if given at least 2 weeks prior to departure. The earliest age of administration is 1 year in the United States. If travel will occur within 2 weeks of travel consultation, immune globulin (IG) (0.1 mL/kg IM) can be given simultaneously with hepatitis A vaccine, or for protection of children younger than 1 year traveling for up to 1 month or 0.2 mL/kg if traveling up to 2 months. Additional doses can be given every 2 months (0.2 mL/kg) for ongoing travel in a high-risk setting until 1 year of age, after which time vaccination should be encouraged. IG interferes with measles-mumps-rubella (MMR) and varicella vaccination, so these vaccines should be given 2 weeks prior to immunoglobulin.

Hepatitis B Vaccine

Areas of high endemicity for hepatitis B include most of Asia, the Middle East, Africa, and the Amazon Basin. Unimmunized children are at risk if they receive blood transfusions that have not been screened for HBV surface antigen (HBsAg) or are exposed to unsterilized medical or dental equipment. Children traveling to developing countries should be vaccinated before departure. An accelerated schedule is possible, with the second dose given with a minimum 4-week interval and the third dose given at least 8 weeks after the second dose. The third dose should not be given before 24 weeks of age.

Influenza Vaccine

Children are at high risk of respiratory infection during travel. The influenza vaccine is recommended for travel during the influenza season, which is between September and March in the Northern Hemisphere, and between April and August in the Southern Hemisphere, and year round in the tropics. The vaccine available in the United States may not protect against new strains circulating in the Southern Hemisphere. Influenza vaccine is recommended for children at least 6 months of age; those younger than 9 years will need two doses of vaccine administered at least 4 weeks apart if they have received zero or one dose in prior seasons. The current vaccines are the trivalent or quadrivalent inactivated vaccine (IIV) given intramuscularly and the quadrivalent live attenuated vaccine (LAIV) given intranasally. It is preferable to be vaccinated at least 2 weeks prior to departure. The annual seasonal influenza vaccine may not be routinely available in the United States from the late spring to early fall, when it may be needed for travelers but may be available at some travel clinics. Revaccination is not recommended for those who will be traveling during April through September and were vaccinated the preceding fall.

Measles-Mumps-Rubella Vaccine

Measles remains endemic in many parts of the world, including Europe, Africa, and Asia, and outbreaks continue to occur worldwide. Susceptible travelers represent an important cause of outbreaks imported into the United States. Children as young as 6 months traveling outside the United States are recommended to receive the vaccine at least 2 weeks before departure, but any doses given prior to 12 months do not count toward an adequate two-dose series, as maternal antibodies may interfere with the immune response. These infants will still require one dose of measles-mumps-rubella (MMR) at 12–15 months of age and a second dose at 4–6 years of age. The second dose aims to protect those individuals (~ 5%) who did not respond the first time. If an accelerated schedule is required, two doses must be separated by a minimum of 4 weeks.

Meningococcal Vaccine

The highest risk for meningococcal disease is for travelers to the meningitis belt of Africa, (sub-Saharan region) especially during the dry season, and travelers on the Hajj or Umrah pilgrimage to Mecca. Notably, meningococcal disease is decreasing in this region due to vaccination against type A. Vaccination is recommended for those who live or travel to these areas with high rates of meningitis for children 2 months of age and older. The vaccine must be given at least 10 days before international travel. For children younger than 9 months, MenACWY-CRM should be used, and for those 9 months of age and older, either MenACWY or MenACWY-D can be used. Vaccination commencing at 2–6 months of age requires a four-dose series; children aged 7–23 months require a two-dose series at least 8 weeks apart, and those 2–55 years of age require one dose. The duration of protection is 3 years in children and 5 years in adults, and boosters are indicated for ongoing exposure and at-risk hosts.

Hib-MenCY-TT is approved for vaccination of children aged 6 weeks to 9 months. A combined Hib and *Neisseria meningitidis* serogroup C conjugate vaccine is licensed for infants younger than 6 weeks. These two vaccines should not be used for children traveling to the meningitis belt or the Hajj, as serogroup A is the predominant organism in these regions.

A previously vaccinated infant reaching the age of 9 months and traveling to endemic areas should be revaccinated with MCV4. MPSV4 should be used for persons older than 56 years. Meningococcal vaccination is required by the Saudi Arabian government for pilgrims undertaking the

Hajj or Umrah pilgrimage to Mecca and Medina, because of pilgrimage-related international outbreaks of *N meningitidis* A in 1987 and W-135 in 2000 and 2001. Further information concerning geographic areas recommended for meningococcal vaccination can be obtained from http://www.cdc.gov/travel.

Pneumococcal Vaccine

The indications for vaccination against *Streptococcus pneumoniae* in children traveling are the same as for routine vaccination. The 13-valent pneumococcal conjugate vaccine (PCV 13) is recommended for children aged 5 years or younger. For children aged 5 years or younger who have completed the PCV 7 series, a single additional dose of PCV 13 is recommended. The minimal interval is 4 weeks between the first three doses and 8 weeks between the third and fourth doses. In addition, the pneumococcal polysaccharide (PPSV23) is recommended for children and adults aged 2 years or older who have certain underlying medical conditions and for all adults aged 65 years or older.

Polio Vaccine

Transmission of wild-type polio still occurs in regions of Asia and Africa, and endemic transmission continues in Afghanistan and Pakistan; vaccine-derived polio is transmitted in other regions. Adequate immunization with inactivated polio vaccine (IPV) should be completed prior to travel to developing countries. The minimum age of administration is 6 weeks of age for IPV. The recommended interval between each dose is 4 weeks. One additional lifetime dose (a fifth dose) of the IPV should be given to caretakers who are traveling to areas with recent circulating polio.

Rotavirus Vaccine

Rotavirus is the most common cause of severe gastroenteritis in infants and young children worldwide, and vaccination with the complete series is recommended prior to travel if age-appropriate. The minimum and maximum age for the first dose is 4 weeks and 14 weeks, 6 days, respectively. There are insufficient data on the safety of older infants. The minimum interval between doses is 4 weeks.

Greenwood CS, Greenwood NP, Fischer PR: Immunization issues in pediatric travelers. Expert Rev Vaccines 2008 Jul;7(5): 651–661 [PMID: 18564019].

Myers AL, Christenson JC: Approach to immunization for the traveling child. Infect Dis Clin N Am 29 (2015) 745–757 [PMID: 26610424].

Rebaza A, Lee PJ: One more shot for the road: a review and update of vaccinations for pediatric international travelers. Pediatr Ann 2015 Apr;44(4):e89–e96 [PMID: 25875985].

VACCINATIONS—TRAVEL-SPECIFIC

Japanese Encephalitis Vaccine

Japanese encephalitis (JE) is caused by a flavivirus transmitted by the night-biting Culex mosquito. The risk of contracting severe JE is low, especially for travelers who will have a brief stay in an endemic area, as the infection rate in Culex mosquitoes is 3% or lower, and only 1 in 200 infections with JE leads to neuroinvasive disease. The symptoms of JE include seizures, paralysis, coma, and mental status changes; residual neurologic damage occurs in 50% of those with clinical disease (see Chapter 40). The case fatality rate is 30% in those with severe disease. Most symptomatic cases occur in children younger than 10 years and in the elderly. The areas at risk are within Asia, Eastern Russia, some areas of the Western Pacific, and the Torres Strait Islands of Australia. The peak season is between April and October, during and just after the rainy season. The JE vaccine licensed and available for use in the United States is Ixiaro, an inactivated Vero cell culture–derived vaccine. It was approved in May 2013 for use in children aged 2 months and older. The primary series is two doses administered 28 days apart. Each dose is 0.5 mL for adults and children aged 3 years and older, and 0.25 mL for children aged 2 months to 2 years. The JE vaccine is recommended for travelers who plan to spend at least 1 month in endemic areas during the JE transmission season. Vaccine should also be considered in the following scenarios: (1) short-term travelers to nonurban areas who will participate in outdoor activities; (2) travelers to an area with an ongoing JE outbreak; and (3) travelers to endemic areas who are uncertain of specific destinations, activities, or duration of travel.

Rabies Vaccine

Rabies is found worldwide and contracted through the bite or saliva-contaminated scratch of infected animals. Canine rabies is highly endemic in parts of Africa, Asia, and Central and South America (RabNet—www.who.int/rabies/rabnet/en/—provides country-specific animal and human data), where 40% of rabies occurs in children younger than 14 years. This increased risk is because children are attracted to animals, are more likely to be bitten, and may not report minor encounters with animals. Most cases of rabies in travelers occur through the bite of an infected dog, cat, or monkey (particularly those that live near temples in parts of Asia). Bats, mongooses, and foxes are other animals that can transmit disease.

Rabies vaccine is available for pre- and postexposure prophylaxis. It is recommended for travelers to areas in which rabies is endemic and for those who will have occupational or recreational exposure (such as cavers), especially if access to medical care will be limited when traveling. The risk of a bite from a potentially rabid animal is up to 2% for travelers to the developing world. The three types of inactivated virus vaccine available are administered prior to exposure in three doses at days 0, 7, and 21 or 28. Vaccination prior to exposure may not be completely protective; further doses are required if a high-risk bite occurs. The minimum age of administration is 1 year, and duration of protection is 2 years. Malaria chemoprophylaxis with mefloquine or chloroquine should begin 1 month after completing the rabies vaccine series to avoid interference with the immune response.

It is important to counsel travelers about animal avoidance, thorough cleansing of a bite wound with irrigation for at least 5 minutes. In the event of a bite in a nonvaccinated individual, rabies immunoglobulin and four doses of vaccine at days 0, 3, 7, and 14 are required, ideally within 24–48 hours after contact. In a fully vaccinated child exposed to rabies, two booster doses should be given on days 0 and 3 of exposure, and rabies immunoglobulin is not required.

Yellow Fever Vaccine

Yellow fever is a flavivirus transmitted by mosquitoes, found in urban and rural areas in sub-Saharan Africa and equatorial South America. Of those infected with the virus, 15% have moderate to severe infection. The licensed 17D strain live attenuated vaccine is highly effective. It must be administered 10 days before travel to an endemic region to allow for the development of protective antibodies. It is required by many countries for reentry after travel to an endemic area, and receipt of the vaccine should be documented in the International Certificate of Vaccination that became available in December 2007 (wwwnc.cdc.gov/travel/yellowbook provides an updated list of countries in which yellow fever vaccination is recommended). For this reason, it is administered only at certified clinics. The vaccine is given subcutaneously, and a single dose confers lifelong immunity. As of July 1, 2016, a completed International Certificate of Vaccination or Prophylaxis is valid for the entire lifetime of the vaccines, and countries cannot require proof of revaccination as a condition of entry, even if the last vaccination was more than 10 years prior. The recommended minimum age of administration is 9 months, and vaccine should not be administered to at-risk infants younger than 6 months, because of the increased risk of encephalitis (0.5–4 per 1000 vaccines). The risk of severe vaccine-related disease is also higher in adult caretakers older than 60 years. The decision to immunize infants who are 6–8 months of age must balance the infant's risk for exposure with the risk for vaccine-associated encephalitis. The vaccine is contraindicated in individuals with egg allergy or immunosuppression (including human immunodeficiency syndrome [HIV] with CD4 T-lymphocyte counts < 200 cells/mm^3 or a history of thymus disorder or thymectomy). A letter of medical exemption may be required for these travelers. In addition to age limitations, precautions to vaccination include asymptomatic HIV infection and CD4 T-lymphocyte count of 200–499 cells/mm^3, pregnancy, and breast-feeding. Adverse effects include encephalitis (15 per

million doses for those aged > 60 years) and multisystem disease (5 per million doses in older people). There is currently a shortage of US-manufactured yellow fever vaccine. A comparable alternative vaccine manufactured in France is available to certain travel clinics under an investigational new drug program. A list of clinics supplying yellow fever vaccine is available at the CDC's Traveler's Health Website (https://wwwnc.cdc.gov/travel/page/search-for-stamaril-clinics).

Cholera Vaccine

Cholera is an acute, watery diarrheal illness caused by *Vibrio cholerae* (O1 or O139 serogroups). Global pandemics continue to occur in developing countries. In 2016, the oral cholera vaccine was recommended for travelers 18 years or older to cholera-affected areas. The only cholera vaccine available in the United States is the CVD 103-HgR (Vaxchora), which is a live vaccine against serogroup O1. The vaccine is not indicated for use in children.

Typhoid Vaccine

The risk of typhoid fever in travelers is 1–10:100,000, depending on the destination. Areas at risk include South Asia, West and North Africa, South America, and Latin America. Travelers to the Indian subcontinent are at greatest risk. The vaccine is recommended for long-term travelers to an endemic area, those traveling off standard tourist routes, immunocompromised travelers, those of south Indian ancestry, and patients with cholelithiasis. There are two vaccines available: a capsular polysaccharide (ViCPS) and a live attenuated (Ty21a) vaccine. The ViCPS is given intramuscularly 2 weeks prior to travel. The minimum age of administration for this vaccine is 2 years; efficacy is 75% over 2 years. Fever, headache, and severe local pain and swelling are reported with the ViCPS more frequently than with other vaccines. The Ty21a is an oral vaccine in capsule form given every other day for four doses. The schedule needs to be completed more than 1 week prior to travel to be effective. The capsules should be refrigerated but not frozen and should not be taken with liquids warmer than 37°C. It is licensed for children older than 6 years; efficacy is 80% over 5 years. It is contraindicated in immunodeficient populations. Doses should be delayed for more than 72 hours after receipt of antibiotics, as they interfere with growth of the vaccine strain bacteria. Mefloquine, chloroquine, and prophylactic doses of atovaquone-proguanil can be given concurrently with the typhoid vaccine.

Tuberculosis

Tuberculosis risk is increased for travelers, especially when visiting Africa, Asia, Latin America, and the former Soviet Union. The risk is higher in long-term travelers to countries with a high incidence of tuberculosis and is highest among health care workers. Bacillus Calmette-Guérin (BCG) vaccination is given soon after birth in many countries, but not in the United States. It protects against miliary and meningeal tuberculosis, but not against pulmonary disease, with efficacy only established in children younger than 1 year. It may be considered in children younger than 5 years who will be in a high-risk area for a prolonged period and have a negative test for tuberculosis (tuberculin skin test [TST] or interferon-γ release assay [IGRA]). It should not be given to immunosuppressed individuals. BCG is not widely available in the United States but may be administered in the destination country. A preferred alternative is that travelers to high-prevalence areas have a test for tuberculosis prior to travel and 3 months after return. It should be noted that live virus vaccines can create an anergic state, in which tuberculosis testing can be falsely negative. Therefore, testing should be performed on the same day as any live vaccine administration or at least 28 days later.

Angelo KM et al: The rise in travel-associated measles infections—GeoSentinel, 2015–2019. J Travel Med 2019 Jun 20 [PMID: 31218359].

CDC Traveler's Health Yellow Book: https://wwwnc.cdc.gov/travel/yellowbook/2018/international-travel-with-infants-children/traveling-safely-with-infants-children.

Clemens JD, Nair GB, Ahmed T, Qadri F, Holmgren J: Cholera. Lancet 2017 Sep 23;390(10101):1539–1549 [PMID: 28302312].

Hatz CF, Kuenzli E, Funk M: Rabies: relevance, prevention, and management in travel medicine. Infect Dis Clin North Am 2012 Sep;26(3):739–753 [PMID: 22963781].

Hill DR et al: The practice of travel medicine: guidelines by the Infectious Diseases Society of America. Clin Infect Dis 2006 Dec 15;43(12):1499–1539 [PMID: 17109284].

TRAVELER'S DIARRHEA

Diarrhea is one of the most common illnesses in travelers to the developing world. Children are at highest risk, usually having more severe and prolonged illness than adults. Traveler's diarrhea is defined in adults as three or more loose stools in a 24-hour period, plus either fever, nausea, vomiting, or abdominal cramping. There is no strict definition in child travelers, as the pattern, consistency, and frequency of stools vary during childhood. A useful definition for traveling children is a change in normal stool pattern, with an increase in frequency (at least three stools per 24 hours) and a decrease in consistency to an unformed state. Most illnesses resolve over a 3- to 5-day period and occur in the first 2 weeks of travel. Enterotoxigenic *Escherichia coli* (ETEC) is the most common cause, accounting for up to one-third of cases. Other pathogens implicated are listed in Table 45–4. Counseling prior to travel includes education and caution with food handling and food and water consumption and provision for self-treatment in the event of illness.

▶ Prevention

Travelers should seek restaurants with a good safety reputation; eat hot, thoroughly cooked food; eat fruits and

Table 45–4. Pathogens causing traveler's diarrhea.

Bacterial
Enterotoxigenic *Escherichia coli* (ETEC)
Enteroaggregative *E coli*
Salmonella spp
Shigella spp
Campylobacter jejuni
Aeromonas spp
Plesiomonas spp
Vibrio cholera
Noncholerae *Vibrio* spp
Enterotoxigenic *Bacteroides fragilis*
Viral
Rotavirus
Noroviruses
Sapoviruses
Parasitic
Giardia lamblia
Cyclospora cayetanensis
Cryptosporidium hominis
Entamoeba histolytica

vegetables that can be peeled; and avoid tap water. They should also avoid ice cubes, fruit juices, fresh salads, unpasteurized dairy products, cold sauces and toppings, open buffets, undercooked foods, and food or beverages from street vendors. They should check the integrity of caps before buying bottled water to avoid bottles filled with tap water. It is also useful to remind travelers about hand washing after using the toilet and before eating. Families can consider using alcohol-containing hand sanitizers as an alternative to soap and water when access is limited during travel. Pasteurized or boiled milk is considered safe provided that it is stored at the appropriate temperature. It may be necessary to bring powdered milk to mix it with safe drinking water if the quality of milk is questionable. While these measures seem logical and should be recommended, there is little evidence that they prevent traveler's diarrhea, either in adults or in children.

Chemoprophylaxis & Treatment

The principles of treatment include adequate hydration and a short course of antibiotics when warranted; medical attention should be sought for severe or prolonged disease.

For mild disease, hydration may be all that is necessary, without any diet restriction. This can be achieved with oral rehydration therapy to supplement a regular diet. Packets of dry rehydration powder to be mixed with water are available from pharmacies, either prior to travel or at the destination. If this is not available, parents can be instructed on how to make oral rehydration solution (Table 45–5) or to use a sports drink such as Gatorade as a suitable alternative in older children and toddlers. The breast-fed infant should continue to breast-feed, in addition to receiving oral rehydration therapy.

Table 45–5. Recipe for oral rehydration solution.

- ¼ Teaspoon (1.25 cc) salt
- ¼ Teaspoon (1.25 cc) bicarbonate of soda[a]
- 2 Tablespoons (30 cc) sugar
- 1 L of water

[a]If bicarbonate of soda is not available, substitute an additional ¼ teaspoon (1.25 cc) of salt.

The vomiting child is at greater risk of dehydration, so aggressive rehydration is crucial. Parents should be reassured that some fluid will be absorbed even if vomiting is ongoing. This is best achieved with small amounts of fluid, given often to prevent further vomiting.

The antimotility agent loperamide, which is often used in adults to minimize symptom duration, is not advised for children because of the risk of adverse events such as toxic megacolon, ileus, extrapyramidal signs, hallucinations, and coma. Bismuth subsalicylate decreases the number of unformed stools in adults. Its routine use is not recommended in pediatrics, as aspirin is contraindicated in children younger than 18 years because of the risk of Reye syndrome, and dosing of bismuth has not been established for children.

For children with signs and symptoms of bacterial gastroenteritis, such as fever or blood in the stool, empiric antibiotic therapy should be considered. The drug of choice in children is azithromycin (10 mg/kg orally once a day for 3 days). It is available in a powdered form that can be reconstituted and stored without refrigeration. It is an ideal choice because of the growing resistance of many gastroenteritis-causing bacteria to ciprofloxacin. There are no pediatric trials of empiric azithromycin, so the dosing recommendations are based on pharmacokinetic data and studies involving the treatment of diarrhea in Africa and Thailand. Ciprofloxacin is currently not recommended for treatment of traveler's diarrhea in children, though it is used for treatment in adults.

Trimethoprim-sulfamethoxazole (TMP-SMX) has been used to treat traveler's diarrhea in children but is no longer recommended because of increasing antibiotic resistance. Rifaximin, a nonabsorbable derivative of rifamycin, is effective in treating ETEC and other noninvasive enteropathogens. Since it is not absorbed, high concentrations are achieved in the intestinal lumen and it has a good safety profile. It is licensed for patients 12 years and older at a treatment dose of 200 mg three times a day for 3 days.

The use of prophylactic antibiotics in children is not recommended because of the risk of adverse events to prevent a disease of limited morbidity, as well as the potential for emergence of antibiotic resistance. Rifaximin, based on adult studies, is a useful chemoprophylactic agent, but it is expensive and requires further study in pediatrics. Probiotics are of unproven benefit for the prevention of traveler's diarrhea, with a recent meta-analysis of five randomized controlled trials showing no benefit.

Ashkenazi S, Schwartz E, O'Ryan M: Travelers' diarrhea in children: what have we learnt? Pediatr Infect Dis J 2016 Jun;35(6): 698–700 [PMID: 26986771].

Giddings SL, Stevens AM, Leung DT: Traveler's diarrhea. Med Clin North Am 2016 Mar;100(2):317–330 [PMID: 26900116].

Kollaritsch H, Paulke-Korinek M, Wiedermann U: Traveler's diarrhea. Infect Dis Clin North Am 2012 Sep;26(3):691–706 [PMID: 22963778].

Steffen R, Hill DR, DuPont HL: Traveler's diarrhea: a clinical review. JAMA 2015 Jan 6;313(1):71–80 [PMID: 25562268].

MALARIA PROPHYLAXIS & PREVENTION (SEE ALSO CHAPTER 43)

Malaria is the most common preventable infectious cause of death among travelers, and a common cause of fever in the returned traveler. Children comprise 20% of imported cases of malaria. It is largely a preventable disease in travelers through personal protective measures and chemoprophylaxis. However, no method is 100% protective. The risk of acquiring malaria varies with the season, climate, altitude, number of mosquito bites, and destination, with the highest risk in Oceania, Africa, the Indian subcontinent, and the Amazon.

▶ Prevention of Mosquito Bites

Malaria is transmitted via the night-biting *Anopheles* mosquitoes. Mosquito bites are avoided by staying in well-screened and air-conditioned rooms from dusk until dawn, wearing clothing covering arms and legs, and avoiding scented soaps, shampoos, and perfumes. Mosquito nets are highly effective and can be used over beds, cribs, playpens, car seats, and strollers. Repellants containing 30% or less DEET are also recommended, as this concentration confers 5–8 hours of protection. When used appropriately, DEET is safe for infants and children older than 2 months. It should not be applied to children's hands, mouth, or near the eyes, and is best washed off upon returning indoors. There have been case reports of seizures and toxic encephalopathy with use of DEET, but these cases occurred with misapplication. Icaridin (also known as picaridin) is an alternative to DEET available in many countries. A concentration of 20% icaridin is as effective as DEET-containing products. It lacks the corrosiveness and greasy texture of DEET and is advised as safe for children by the American Academy of Pediatrics. However, because it is relatively new, it lacks the safety profile of DEET, especially for children. PMD is a plant-based repellant derived from lemon eucalyptus, and at a 30% concentration is equally effective as DEET. It may be used on children older than 6 months. It is considered safe if directions are followed and has been advocated for use by the Centers for Disease Control and Prevention. Clothing and bed nets may be sprayed with insecticides such as permethrin, which confers protection for 2–6 weeks, even with regular washing. Further studies are needed to establish its safety profile in children. The combination of DEET every 8–12 hours and permethrin on clothing is over 99% effective in preventing mosquito bites.

▶ Chemoprophylaxis

Prophylactic medications suppress malaria by killing asexual blood stages of the parasite before they cause disease, so protective levels of medication must be present in the blood before developing parasites are released from the liver. Therefore, it is necessary to start prophylaxis before the first possible exposure and to continue it for a sufficient period after return to a safe area.

The choice of antimalarial depends on the age of the child, resistance patterns, restrictions on the agent of choice, the child's ability to swallow tablets, the frequency of dosing, cost, availability of medication, and access to a compounding pharmacy for adequate dispensing of medication. For most children, once-weekly mefloquine is preferable and approved for children of any age. Atovaquone/proguanil is available in pediatric dosing, although only in tablet formulation. It is currently approved in most countries for children weighing greater than 5 kg. Doxycycline is another alternative but should be used only in children 8 years or older because of the risk of teeth staining. Chloroquine is the drug of choice in areas of chloroquine sensitivity (Mexico, Hispaniola, Central America, west and north of the Panama Canal, and parts of North Africa, the Middle East, and China). Pediatric and adult dosing, side effects, and other information about malaria chemoprophylaxis are in Table 45–6.

Antimalarial medications (with the exception of atovaquone/ proguanil) are bitter, so it may be necessary to grind the medication into a very sweet food, such as chocolate syrup or sweetened condensed milk. Infants may need to have their medication prepared by a compounding pharmacy, where the appropriate dose can be placed in a gelatin capsule, which can then be opened by the caregiver and mixed into food or liquid.

Genton B, D'Acremont V: Malaria prevention in travelers. Infect Dis Clin North Am 2012 Sep;26(3):637–654 [PMID: 22963775].

Kafai NM, Odom John AR: Malaria in children. Infect Dis Clin North Am 2018 Mar;32(1):189–200 [PMID: 29269188].

Lüthi B, Schlagenhauf P: Risk factors associated with malaria deaths in travellers: a literature review. Travel Med Infect Dis 2015 Jan–Feb;13(1):48–60 [PMID: 25022610].

Moore SJ, Mordue Luntz AJ, Logan JG: Insect bite prevention. Infect Dis Clin North Am 2012 Sep;26(3):655–673 [PMID: 22963776].

VISITS TO FRIENDS & RELATIVES (VFR) IN HIGH-RISK AREAS

Individuals who return to their home country are at the highest risk of travel-related infectious diseases. Sixty percent of malaria cases and over 75% of typhoid cases occur in these travelers, and VFR children are at highest risk of hepatitis A. The reasons for this include the following:

- Longer stays and increased likelihood of pregnancy or young age in the traveler
- Travel to remote rural areas
- Intimate contact with the local population
- Decreased likelihood of seeking (or following) pretravel advice because of familiarity with their home country
- Assumed immunity to infections
- Sociocultural barriers—for example, language barriers, belief systems of illness, prohibitive cost of vaccines and medications if lower socioeconomic status
- Eating and sleeping in local households, where hygiene may be suboptimal
- Use of high-risk forms of transportation

Thus, certain issues need to be emphasized when discussing travel for VFRs. Given the risk of waterborne infections, visiting families should boil water and milk if other safe drinking water is expensive; consume only piping hot foods and beverages; and follow proper hand-washing techniques at all times. Vaccination recommendations and malaria prophylaxis are of greater importance in VFRs, who have greater opportunities to contract vaccine-preventable diseases, such as typhoid, rabies, yellow fever, and meningococcal infection. VFRs have a higher risk of exposure to people with tuberculosis, so tuberculosis testing is recommended approximately 3 months after return from travel.

Feja KN, Tolan RW Jr: Infections related to international travel and adoption. Adv Pediatr 2013;60(1):107–139 [PMID: 24007842].

Hendel-Paterson B, Swanson SJ: Pediatric travelers visiting friends and relatives (VFR) abroad: illnesses, barriers and pre-travel recommendations. Travel Med Infect Dis 2011 Jul;9(4):192–203 [PMID: 21074496].

Leder K et al: Illness in travelers visiting friends and relatives: a review of the GeoSentinel Surveillance Network. Clin Infect Dis 2006;43(9):1185–1193 [PMID: 17029140].

HIV & SEXUALLY TRANSMITTED DISEASES (SEE ALSO CHAPTER 41)

Adolescent travelers might partake in high-risk activities while traveling, putting them at risk of human immunodeficiency virus (HIV) and other sexually transmitted diseases (STDs). The adolescent traveler should be counseled about the risks of STDs, safe sexual practices, and in particular, the importance of barrier contraception. Bringing a supply of latex condoms may be appropriate along with instruction on their proper use. They should be advised that HIV and STDs can also be contracted via oral sex and in nonsexual activities such as intravenous drug use, receiving tattoos, piercings, pedicures, and dental care while traveling. There may be a risk of HIV and other virus transmission through injections

Table 45–6. Malaria prophylaxis.

Drug	Usage	Adult Dose	Pediatric Dose	Directions	Comments
Atovaquone/proguanil	Prophylaxis in areas with chloroquine-resistant or mefloquine-resistant *Plasmodium falciparum*.	Adult tabs contain 250 mg atovaquone and 100 mg proguanil hydrochloride.	Pediatric tabs contain 62.5 mg atovaquone and 25 mg proguanil hydrochloride.	Begin 1–2 days before travel to malarious areas. Take daily at the same time each day while in the area and for 7 days after leaving such areas.	Contraindicated in persons with severe renal impairment (creatinine clearance < 30 mL/min). Atovaquone/proguanil should be taken with food or a milky drink.
		1 Adult tab orally, daily.	5–8 kg: 1/2 pediatric tablet daily > 8–10 kg: 3/4 pediatric tablet daily > 10–20 kg: 1 pediatric tablet daily > 20–30 kg: 2 pediatric tablets daily > 30–40 kg: 3 pediatric tablets daily > 40 kg: 1 adult tablet daily.		Not recommended for prophylaxis for children < 5 kg, pregnant women, and women breast-feeding infants weighing 5 kg, but consider if drug-resistant area (call CDC).
					Do not take with tetracycline, metoclopramide, rifampin, or rifabutin (all reduce atovaquone concentration).
Chloroquine phosphate	Prophylaxis only in areas with chloroquine-sensitive *P falciparum*.	150 and 300 mg base tabs (300 and 500 mg salt) orally, once per week (any age or size).	5 mg/kg base (8.3 mg/kg salt) orally, once per week, up to max adult dose. Tabs not scored.	Begin 1–2 wk before travel to malarious areas. Take weekly on the same day of the week while in the area and for 4 wk after leaving such areas.	Contraindicated in persons with prior retinal or visual field changes. May exacerbate psoriasis. Bitter taste. Interferes with rabies vaccine response. Not contraindicated in pregnancy.
Doxycycline	Prophylaxis in areas with chloroquine-resistant or mefloquine-resistant *P falciparum*.	100 mg orally, daily.	8 y of age: 2 mg/kg up to adult dose of 100 mg/day. Syrup available.	Begin 1–2 days before travel to malarious areas. Take daily at the same time each day while in the area and for 4 wk after leaving such areas.	Contraindicated in children < 8 y of age and pregnant women. May decrease oral contraceptive efficacy. Photosensitivity.
Hydroxychloroquine sulfate	An alternative to chloroquine in areas with chloroquine-sensitive *P falciparum*.	310 mg base (400 mg salt) orally, once per week.	5 mg/kg base (6.5 mg/kg salt) orally, once per week, up to max adult dose. Tabs not scored.	Begin 1–2 wk before travel to malarious areas. Take weekly on the same day of the week while in the area and for 4 wk after leaving such areas.	

Mefloquine	Prophylaxis in areas with chloroquine-resistant *P falciparum*.	228 mg base (250 mg salt) orally, once per week.	5–9 kg: 4.6 mg/kg base (5 mg/kg salt) orally, once per week. Tabs scored. 10–19 kg: ¼ tab once per week 20–30 kg: ½ tab once per week 31–45 kg: ¾ tab once per week: > 46 kg: 1 tab once per week.	Begin 1–2 wk before travel to malarious areas. Take weekly on the same day of the week while in the area and for 4 wk after leaving the area (start 2 wk prior if want to evaluate for side effects that may necessitate change).	Contraindicated in persons allergic to mefloquine or related compounds (eg, quinine and quinidine) and in persons with active depression, a recent history of depression, generalized anxiety disorder, psychosis, schizophrenia, other major psychiatric disorders, or seizures. Use with caution in persons with psychiatric disturbances. Not recommended for persons with cardiac conduction abnormalities. Not contraindicated in pregnancy. Bitter taste.
Primaquine (post-travel prophylaxis for long-term *Plasmodium vivax* and *Plasmodium ovale* exposure)	Used for presumptive antirelapse therapy (terminal prophylaxis) to decrease the risk of relapses of *P vivax* and *P ovale*.	30 mg base (52.6 mg salt) orally, once per day for 14 days after departure from the malarious area.	0.6 mg/kg base (1.0 mg/kg salt) up to adult dose orally, once per day for 14 days after departure from the malarious area.	Primaquine presumptive anti-relapse therapy is administered for 14 days after the traveler has left a malarious area. When chloroquine, doxycycline, or mefloquine is used for prophylaxis, primaquine is usually taken during the last 2 wk of postexposure prophylaxis, but may be taken immediately after those medications are completed. When atovaquone/proguanil is used for prophylaxis, primaquine may be taken either during the final 7 days of atovaquone/proguanil and then for an additional 7 days, or for 14 days after atovaquone/proguanil is completed.	Indicated for persons who have had prolonged exposure to *P vivax* and *P ovale* or both (eg, missionaries or peace corps volunteers). All persons who take primaquine should have a documented normal G6PD (glucose-6-phosphate dehydrogenase) level prior to starting this medication. Contraindicated in persons with G6PD1 deficiency. Also contraindicated during pregnancy and lactation unless the breast-fed infant has a documented normal G6PD level. Also an option for prophylaxis in special circumstances.

and blood transfusion, as many developing countries do not have adequate blood banking and transfusion protocols. In fact, 10%–20% of countries have inadequate screening.

Antiretroviral therapy is recommended if there is exposure to a known HIV-positive contact, and may be considered if the source is unknown but may be difficult to access in most countries (see Chapter 41).

Breuner CC: The adolescent traveler. Prim Care 2002 Dec;29(4): 983–1006 [PMID: 12687903].

Croughs M, Van den Ende JJ: Away from home: travel and sex. Lancet Infect Dis 2013 Mar;13(3):184–185 Epub 2012 Nov 22 [PMID: 23182930].

Mariano D, Smith DS: Safe travel preparation for HIV-infected patients. Curr Infect Dis Rep 2019 Mar 20;21(4):15 [PMID: 30895392].

MMWR: https://aidsinfo.nih.gov/contentfiles/NonOccupational ExposureGL.pdf.

FEVER IN THE RETURNED TRAVELER

More than one-half of travelers to the developing world experience a health-related travel problem during their trip; 8% require medical attention on return. The majority will develop common medical problems, such as upper respiratory tract infections, pneumonia, urinary tract infections, and otitis media, with the remainder developing travel-related infections. The most common travel-related diseases are malaria (21%), acute traveler's diarrhea (15%), dengue fever (6%), and typhoid/enteric fever (2%). Children who travel with caretakers visiting friends and relatives are at greatest risk. New pathogens and the changing epidemiology of some infectious diseases pose new risks to travelers—such as Ebola, avian influenza, multidrug-resistant TB, chikungunya virus, zika, and leishmaniasis.

Symptomatic returning travelers should be urgently and thoroughly evaluated for travel-related illness to prevent serious life-threatening disease and transmission to close contacts. The initial evaluation should include questions directed toward the travel itinerary, with dates of arrival and departure, specific activities, rural versus urban location, and accommodations. Specific information should be obtained regarding freshwater contact (eg, schistosomiasis, leptospirosis in some areas), sexual contacts, animal exposures, activities or hobbies, ill person contacts, and sources of food and water. A complete medication and vaccination history should be sought. Despite malaria chemoprophylaxis and protection against mosquitoes, no regimen is 100% protective. A thorough physical examination should include dermatologic examination, eye examination for scleral icterus, conjunctival injection or petechiae, and evaluation for hepatosplenomegaly or lymphadenopathy. Routine laboratory evaluation includes a complete blood count, erythrocyte sedimentation rate (ESR), C-reactive protein (CRP), serum chemistry, liver enzyme profile, and urinalysis. The laboratory evaluation

Table 45–7. Diagnostic evaluations to consider for fever in the returned traveler.

Routine
Hematologic
Complete blood count and differential
Thick and thin blood smear (ideally collect three at 12-h intervals)
Sedimentation rate
C-reactive protein
Electrolytes
Liver function tests
Blood culture
Urine
Urinalysis
Culture
Specific to presentation
Hematologic
Serologies for specific pathogens
Stool
Blood culture or polymerase chain reaction (PCR)
Fecal leucocytes
Giardia and *Cryptosporidium* antigen test
Clostridium difficile toxin (if antibiotic exposure)
Ova and parasite examination
Special studies (eg, stool for *Entamoeba histolytica* antigen, special stains)
Cerebrospinal fluid
Cell count with differential, protein, glucose, culture, freeze extra sample
Antibody and polymerase chain reaction tests as appropriate
Imaging studies
Chest radiography and abdominal ultrasound imaging as appropriate
Other specialized tests
Placement of PPD (purified protein derivative) or IGRA (interferon-γ release assay)
Morning gastric aspirates (culture) or sputum (culture or PCR) and AFB (acid-fast bacilli) stain
Bronchoscopy
Sigmoidoscopy, colonoscopy
Skin biopsy
Bone marrow aspirate
Skin snips (eg, for *Onchocerciasis*)

should also focus on diseases that are life threatening, with thick and thin smears for malaria (ideally three that are 12 hours apart), and blood cultures for typhoid fever. Specific testing should be done as directed by findings on history, physical examination, and preliminary laboratory test findings (Table 45–7). It may be necessary to seek the opinion of individuals with experience in international travel medicine, if available.

Fever is the most common complaint in a child who becomes ill after international travel. The most common travel-related infectious causes of fever are summarized in Table 45–8. A more detailed description of the symptoms,

Table 45–8. Illnesses in the returning traveler.

Disease	Etiology	Common Presenting Symptoms and Signs	Usual Incubation Period	Geographic Location	Mode of Transmission
Malaria	*Plasmodium falciparum*	Fever Headache Myalgias Chills Rigors	7–30 days	More prevalent in sub-Saharan Africa than in other regions of the world, also South East (SE) Asia, South America, Mexico	Bite from *Anopheles* mosquito
Malaria	*Plasmodium vivax*	As for *P falciparum*	10–17 days and up to 1 y	SE Asia, sub-Saharan Africa, South America, Central America	As for *P falciparum*
Malaria	*Plasmodium ovale*	As for *P falciparum*	16–18 days	West Africa, the Philippines, eastern Indonesia, and Papua New Guinea. It has been reported from Cambodia, India, Thailand, and Vietnam	As for *P falciparum*
Malaria	*Plasmodium malariae*	As for *P falciparum*	16–59 days	Sub-Saharan Africa, much of southeast Asia, Indonesia, on many of the islands of the western Pacific and in areas of the Amazon Basin of South America	As for *P falciparum*
Malaria	*Plasmodium knowlesi*	As for *P falciparum*	10–12 days	SE Asia	As for *P falciparum*
Dengue	Dengue virus	Fever Myalgias Maculopapular or petechial rash Arthralgias	2–7 days	Northern Australia, SE Asia, Mexico, Central America, South America, Puerto Rico, Florida Keys	Bite from *Aedes aegypti* mosquito
Typhoid fever	*Salmonella enterica* serovar *typhi*	Fever Malaise Anorexia Abdominal pain	10–14 days	South Asia, West and North Africa, South America, and Latin America	Ingestion of contaminated food/water
Paratyphoid fever	*S enterica* serovar *paratyphi*	Same as for typhoid fever	Same as for typhoid fever	Same as for typhoid fever	Same as for typhoid fever
Schistosomiasis	*Schistosoma mansoni*, *Schistosoma hematobium*, *Schistosoma japonicum*	Urticarial rash Fever Headache Myalgia Respiratory symptoms	23–70 days (average 1 mo)	*S mansoni*—South America, Caribbean *S hematobium*—Africa, Middle East *S japonicum*—Far East	Contaminated water containing freshwater snails
African tick typhus	*Rickettsia conorii*	Fever Headache Myalgia Maculopapular rash Malaise	5–7 days	Africa, Middle East, India, and Mediterranean Basin	Bite from hard ticks

(Continued)

Table 45–8. Illnesses in the returning traveler. (*Continued*)

Disease	Etiology	Common Presenting Symptoms and Signs	Usual Incubation Period	Geographic Location	Mode of Transmission
Scrub typhus	*Orientia tsutsugamushi*	Fever Headache Myalgia Possibly a maculopapular rash	10–12 days	"Tsutsugamushi triangle"—from northern Japan and Eastern Russia in the North, to Northern Australia in the South, to Pakistan and Afghanistan in the west	From chigger bites (the larval stage of the biculid mites)
Leptospirosis	*Leptospira* spp	Fever Headache Chills Myalgia Nausea Diarrhea Abdominal pain Uveitis Adenopathy Conjunctival suffusion	5–14 days (average 10 days)	Worldwide	Contact with urine from domestic and wild animals contaminating water and soil
Babesiosis	*Babesia microti, Babesia divergens, Babesia duncani*	Fevers Chills Symptoms similar to malaria	1–4 wk	Europe, United States, sporadic cases in Asia, Mexico, Africa	Bite of *Ixodes* ticks
Yellow fever	Yellow fever virus	Fever Chills Headache Jaundice Backache Myalgias Prostration Nausea Vomiting	3–6 days	Tropical and sub-Tropical Africa and South America, Caribbean (countries that lie within a band 15 degrees north to 10 degrees south of the Equator)	Bite of mosquitoes (*Aedes aegypti* and others)
Chikungunya	CHIK virus	Fever Joint pain Maculopapular rash Headache Nausea Vomiting Myalgias	2–12 days (usually 2–4 days)	Tropical Africa and Asia (SE Asia and India)	Bite from *Aedes* mosquitoes
Zika	Zika virus (ZIKV)	Fever Red eyes Joint pain Headache Maculopapular rash	3–12 days	Central, South America, Africa, Asia, South Pacific	Bite from *Aedes* mosquitoes
Amebiasis	*Entamoeba histolytica*	Fever Diarrhea Right upper quadrant pain	7–28 days	Worldwide, but higher incidence in developing countries	Contaminated food and water

signs, diagnosis, and treatment of these diseases that can occur in the returning traveler is presented in Chapters 40 to 43.

Centers for Disease Control and Prevention (CDC) Yellow Book: https://wwwnc.cdc.gov/travel/page/yellowbook-home. Accessed November 30, 2017.

Chen LH, Wilson ME: Dengue and chikungunya in travelers: recent updates. Curr Opin Infect Dis 2012 Oct;25(5):523–529 [PMID: 22825287].

Feja KN1, Tolan RW Jr: Infections related to international travel and adoption. Adv Pediatr 2013;60(1):107–139 [PMID: 24007842].

Kotlyar S, Rice BT: Fever in the returning traveler. Emerg Med Clin North Am 2013 Nov;31(4):927–944 [PMID: 24176472].

Thwaites GE, Day NPJ: Approach to fever in the returning traveler. New Engl J Med 2017;376(6):548–560 [PMID: 28467877].

REFERENCES

Web Resources

CDC traveler's health: http://www.cdc.gov/travel/destinat.htm.

CDCYellowBook:http://wwwnc.cdc.gov/travel/content/yellow-book/home-2010.aspx.

Centers for Disease Control and Prevention (CDC): http://www.cdc.gov/travel/index.htm.

GIDEON: http://www.cyinfo.com.

International Association for Medical Assistance to Travellers: http://www.iamat.org.

International Society of Travel Medicine: http://www.istm.org.

International SOS: http://www.internationalsos.com.

London School of Hygiene and Tropical Medicine: http://www.lshtm.ac.uk.

Malaria information specific to country: www.cdc.gov/malaria/risk_map.

ProMED: http://www.promedmail.org.

Rabies information specific to country: http://www.who.int/rabies/rabnet/en.

Royal Society of Tropical Medicine and Hygiene: http://www.rstmh.org.

The Malaria Foundation: http://www.malaria.org.

Travax Encompass: http://www.travax.com.

United States Department of State: http://www.travel.state.gov.

WHO for maps of vaccine preventable diseases: http://www.who.int.ith.

Yellow fever vaccine clinics: https://wwwnc.cdc.gov/travel/page/search-for-stamaril-clinics.

General References

Aung AK, Trubiano JA, Spelman DW: Travel risk assessment, advice and vaccinations in immunocompromised travellers (HIV, solid organ transplant and haematopoeitic stem cell transplant recipients): a review. Travel Med Infect Dis 2015 Jan–Feb;13(1):31–47 [PMID: 25593039].

Feja KN, Tolan RW Jr: Infections related to international travel and adoption. Adv Pediatr 2013;60(1):107–139 [PMID: 24007842].

Giddings SL, Stevens AM, Leung DT: Traveler's diarrhea. Med Clin North Am 2016 Mar;100(2):317–330 [PMID: 26900116].

Greenwood CS, Greenwood NP, Fischer PR: Immunization issues in pediatric travelers. Expert Rev Vaccines 2008 Jul;7(5): 651–661 [PMID: 18564019].

House HR, Ehlers JP: Travel-related infections. Emerg Med Clin North Am 2008 May;26(2):499–516 [PMID: 18406985].

Kohl SE, Barnett ED: What do we know about travel for children with special health care needs? A review of the literature. Travel Med Infect Dis 2019 Jun 21:101438 [PMID: 31233860].

Myers AL, Christenson JC: Approach to immunization for the traveling child. Infect Dis Clin North Am 2015 Dec;29(4): 745–757 [PMID: 26610424].

Rebaza A, Lee PJ: One more shot for the road: a review and update of vaccinations for pediatric international travelers. Pediatr Ann 2015 Apr;44(4):e89–e96 [PMID: 25875985].

Stauffer W, Christenson JC, Fischer PR: Preparing children for international travel. Travel Med Infect Dis 2008 May;6(3): 101–113 [PMID: 18486064].

Thwaites GE, Day NP: Approach to fever in the returning traveler. N Engl J Med 2017 Feb 9;376(6):548–560 [PMID: 28177860].

Trubiano JA, Johnson D, Sohail A, Torresi J: Travel vaccination recommendations and endemic infection risks in solid organ transplantation recipients. J Travel Med 2016 Sep 13;23(6) pii: taw058 [PMID: 27625399].

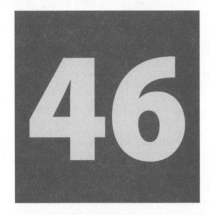

Chemistry & Hematology Reference Intervals

Melkon G. DomBourian, MD   Jordana E. Hoppe, MD

Aimee LeDoux, MT (ASCP)   Robert Snyder, MT (ASCP)

Laboratory tests provide valuable information necessary to evaluate a patient's condition and to monitor recommended treatment. Chemistry and hematology test results are compared with those of healthy individuals or those undergoing similar therapeutic treatment to determine clinical status and progress. In the past, the term *normal ranges* relayed some ambiguity because statistically; the term *normal* also implied a specific (Gaussian or normal) distribution, and epidemiologically it implied the state of the majority, which is not necessarily the desirable or targeted population. This is most apparent in cholesterol levels, where values greater than 200 mg/dL are common, but not desirable. Use of the term *reference range* or *reference interval* is therefore recommended by the International Federation of Clinical Chemistry (IFCC) and the Clinical and Laboratory Standards Institute (CLSI) to indicate that the values relate to a reference population and clinical condition.

Reference ranges are established for a specific age, sex, and sexual maturity; they are also defined for a specific pharmacologic status, dietary restrictions, and stimulation protocol. Similarly, diurnal variation is a factor as is degree of obesity. Some reference ranges are particularly meaningful when combined with other results (eg, parathyroid hormone and calcium), or when an entire set of analytes is evaluated.

Laboratory tests are becoming more specific and measure much lower concentrations than ever before. Therefore, reference ranges should reflect the analytical procedure as well as reagents and instrumentation used for a specific analysis. As test methodology continues to evolve, reference ranges are modified and updated.

CHALLENGES IN DETERMINING & INTERPRETING PEDIATRIC REFERENCE INTERVALS

The pediatric environment is particularly challenging for the determination of reference intervals since growth and developmental stages do not have a distinct and finite boundary by which test results can be tabulated. Furthermore, adult reference ranges are not always appropriate for pediatric patients. Reference ranges may overlap and, in many cases, complicate diagnosis and treatment. Collection and allocation of test results by age for the purpose of establishing a reference range is a convenient and manageable way to report them, but caution is needed in their interpretation and clinical correlation. Additionally, ethical concerns may exist related to blood draws in infants and young children to establish these reference ranges. Despite these challenges, there have been multicenter studies to improve the reference ranges for laboratory testing in pediatrics.

A particular difficulty lies in establishing reference ranges for analytes whose levels are changed under scheduled stimulation conditions. The common glucose tolerance test is such an example, but more complex endocrinology tests require skill and extensive experience to interpret. Reference ranges for these serial tests are established over a long period of time and are not easily transferable between test methodologies.

Adeli K: Special issue on laboratory reference intervals. eJIFCC. September 2008. http://www.ifcc.org/PDF/190201200801.pdf.

C28A3: *Defining, Establishing, and Verifying Reference Intervals in the Clinical Laboratory: Approved Guideline.* 3rd ed. http://www.clsi.org/source/orders.

Ozarda Y: Reference intervals: current status, recent developments and future considerations. Biochem Med 2016;26(1):5–16 [PMID: 26981015].

GUIDELINES FOR USE OF DATA IN A REFERENCE RANGE STUDY

The College of American Pathologists provides guidelines for the adoption of reference ranges used in hospitals and commercial clinical laboratories. It recognizes the enormous task of establishing a laboratory's own reference ranges and recommends alternatives to the process. A laboratory may acquire reference ranges by:

1. Conducting its own study to evaluate a statistically significant number of "healthy" volunteers. It is a monumental task for a laboratory to develop its own pediatric reference ranges due to the need for parental consent, approval by review boards, and the numerous age categories that need to be evaluated.

2. Adopting ranges established by the manufacturer of a particular analytical instrument. The laboratory must validate the data by analyzing a sample of 20 subjects representing that specific population to confirm that the adopted range is truly representative of that group.

3. Using reference data in the general medical literature and conferring with physicians to make sure the data agree with their clinical experience. A validation study is also recommended.

4. Analyzing hospital patient data. Laboratory test results from hospital patients have been used to compute reference ranges provided they fulfill stated clinical criteria. Patient records need to indicate that the patient's specific medical condition does not influence the analyte whose reference range is being determined. For example, a child undergoing surgery for bone fracture repair is expected to have normal electrolytes and thyroid function, whereas a child examined for precocious puberty should not be included in a reference range study for luteinizing hormone.

Statistically, the sample size of a hospital patient study should be considerably larger than that of a healthy group. A study from a healthy population may require 20 subjects to be statistically significant, whereas a hospital population should evaluate a minimum of 120 patients.

Biological Variation Database Reference List: http://www.westgard .com/biological-variation-database-reference-list.htm.
College of American Pathologists publication: http://www.cap .org/apps/docs/laboratory_accreditation/sample_checklist.pdf.
Schnabl K, Chan MK, Gong Y, Adeli K: Closing the gap on paediatric reference intervals: the CALIPER initiative. Clin Biochem Rev 2008 Aug;29(3):89–96 [PMID: 19107221].

STATISTICAL COMPUTATION OF REFERENCE INTERVALS

The establishment of reference intervals is based on a statistical distribution of test results obtained from a representative population. The CLSI recommendation for data collection and statistical analysis provides guidelines for managing the data. For clinicians, it is not important that they can reproduce the calculation. It is far more critical to understand the benefits and restrictions provided by the described statistical

approaches and to evaluate patient results with these limitations in mind.

The reference range includes 95% of all results obtained from a representative population. Note that 5% of that population will have "abnormal" results, when in fact they are "healthy" and an integral part of the reference group study. Similarly, an equivalent 5% of the "ill" population will have laboratory results within the reference range. These are inherent features of the statistical computation. Taking that analysis one step further, the probability of a healthy patient having a test result within a calculated reference range is

$$P = .95$$

When multiple tests or panels of tests are used, the combined probability of all the test results falling in their respective reference ranges drops dramatically. For example, the probability of all results from 10 tests in the complete metabolic panel being in the reference range is

$$P = (.95)^{10} = .60$$

Therefore, about one-third of healthy patients will have one test result in the panel that is outside the reference range. Clinical judgment is needed to determine the significance of test results falling outside the reference range.

A. Parametric Method of Computation

The parametric method of establishing reference intervals is simple, though not always representative, since it is based on the assumption that the data have a Gaussian distribution. A mean (x) and standard deviation (SD) are calculated; test results of 95% of that specific population will fall within the mean ±1.96 SD, as shown in Figure 46–1.

Where the distribution is not Gaussian, a mathematical manipulation of the values (eg, plotting the log of the value, instead of the value itself) may give a Gaussian distribution. The mean and SD are then converted back to give a usable reference range.

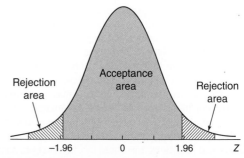

▲ **Figure 46–1.** Gaussian distribution and parametric calculation using $x \pm 1.96$ SD to define the range.

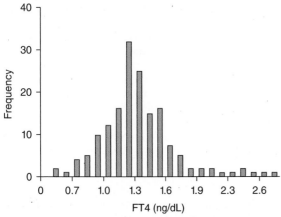

▲ **Figure 46–2.** Histogram of free thyroxine (FT₄) using clinic and hospital patients at Children's Hospital Colorado.

B. Nonparametric Method of Computation

The nonparametric method of establishing reference ranges is currently recommended by CLSI, since it defines outliers as those in the extreme 2.5 percentile of the upper and lower limits of data, respectively. The number of data points excluded at the limits depends on the skew of the curve, and so the computation accommodates a non-Gaussian distribution. A histogram depicting the non-Gaussian distribution of data from a free thyroxine reference range study conducted at Children's Hospital in Denver is shown in Figure 46–2.

Ichihara K, Boyd JC; IFCC Committee on Reference Intervals and Decision Limits (C-RIDL): An appraisal of statistical procedures used in derivation of reference intervals. Clin Chem Lab Med 2010 Nov;48(11):1537–1551 [PMID: 21062226].

WHY REFERENCE INTERVALS VARY

Recent modifications to reference ranges are due to the introduction of new and improved analytical procedures, advanced automated instrumentation, and standardization of reagents and reference materials. Reference ranges are also affected by preanalytical variations that can occur during sample collection, processing, and storage.

Preanalytical variations of biological origin can occur when specimens are drawn in the morning versus in the evening, or from hospitalized recumbent patients versus ambulatory outpatients. Variations also may be caused by metabolic and hemodynamic factors. Preanalytical factors may be a product of the socioeconomic environment or ethnic background (eg, genetic or dietary).

Analytical variations are caused by differences in analytical measurements and depend on the analytical tools as well as an inherent variability in obtaining a quantitative value.

Furthermore, new reagents, instruments, and improved testing procedures added to the clinical laboratory can result in an element of variability between tests.

1. **Antigen-antibody reactions** have revolutionized clinical chemistry but have also added a degree of variability because biologically derived reagents have different specificity and sensitivity. In addition to the targeted analyte, some of its metabolites are also measured, and these may or may not be biologically active.

2. **Reference materials** continue to be reviewed and evaluated by organizations such as the World Health Organization and the National Institute for Standards and Technology.

3. **Analytical instrumentation** with advanced electronics and robotics has improved the accuracy of results and increased throughput. However, they have added an element of variability between instruments from different manufacturers.

4. **Analytical detection methods** have also made big strides as they have expanded from simple ultraviolet-visible spectrophotometry to fluorescence, nephelometry, radioimmunoassay, and chemiluminescence.

Jung B, Adeli K: Clinical laboratory reference intervals in pediatrics: the CALIPER initiative. Clin Biochem 2009 Nov;42 (16–17):1589–1595. Epub 2009 Jul 7 [PMID: 19591815].

SENSITIVITY, SPECIFICITY, & PREDICITIVE VALUES

Despite its statistical derivation, a reference interval does not necessarily provide a finite and clear-cut guideline as to whether a patient has a condition. There will always be a segment of the population with test values that fall within the reference interval, but clinical manifestations that indicate disease is present. Similarly, a segment of the population will have test values outside the reference interval, but no clinical signs of disease. The ability of a test and corresponding reference interval to detect individuals with disease is defined by the diagnostic sensitivity of the test. Similarly, the ability of a test to detect individuals without disease is described by the diagnostic specificity. These characteristics are governed by the analytical quality of the test as well as the numerical parameters (reference interval) that define the presence of disease. The tolerance level for the desired sensitivity and specificity of a test requires significant input from clinicians.

Generally, specificity increases as sensitivity decreases. A typical distribution of test results, shown in Figure 46–3, provides information on individuals without disease (solid line) and individuals with the disease (dashed line). As with most tests, there is an overlap area. A patient with a test result of 1 is likely healthy, and the result indicates a true

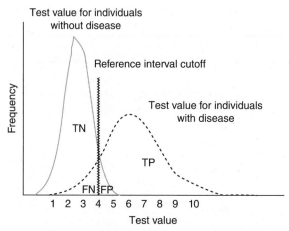

▲ **Figure 46–3.** Frequency distribution of test results for patients with and without disease. FN, false negative; FP, false positive; TN, true negative; TP, true positive.

negative (TN) for the presence of disease. A patient with a test result of 9 is likely to have the disease, and the test result is a true positive (TP). There is a small, but significant, population with a test result of 2–5 in whom the test is not 100% conclusive. A statistical analysis may determine the most likely cutoff for healthy individuals, but the clinically acceptable cutoff depends on the test as well as clinical correlation.

If cutoff values for the reference interval are such that a test result indicates that a healthy patient has the disease, the result is a false positive (FP). Conversely if a test result indicates that a patient is well when in fact he or she has the disease, the result is a false negative (FN). To define the ability of the test and reference interval to identify a disease state, the diagnostic sensitivity and specificity are measured.

$$\text{Diagnostic sensitivity} = TP/(TP + FN)$$

$$\text{Diagnostic specificity} = TN/(TN + FP)$$

In the example shown in Figure 46–3, a reference interval of 0.5–3 will provide more TN results and minimize FP results. Alternatively, a reference interval of 0.5–4 will increase the rate of FN. Thus, an increase in sensitivity leads to a decrease in specificity. A medical condition that requires aggressive treatment may necessitate a test and corresponding reference interval with a high sensitivity, which is a measure of the TP rate. This is accomplished at the expense of lowering specificity.

One must also consider that both diagnostic sensitivity and specificity as derived do not take into account disease prevalence. As shown in Figure 46–4, diagnostic sensitivity is calculated exclusively within a diseased population and the converse is true for diagnostic specificity. In a clinical setting, one is screening a population of individuals with and without disease. Therefore, positive predicative value (PPV) and negative predictive value (NPV) must also be used to better understand test screening performance and are defined as follows:

$$PPV = TP/(TP + FP)$$

$$NPV = TN/(FN + TN)$$

A reference interval is a statistical representation of test results from a finite population, but it is by no means inclusive of every member of the group. It is merely one component in the measure of a patient's status to be viewed in relation to a number of other testing factors.

PEDIATRIC REFERENCE INTERVALS

The establishment of reference ranges is a complex process. Assumptions are made in the management of data processes, regardless of the population used for the accumulation of test results. Analytical instrument manufacturers conduct large studies to identify reference intervals for each specific analyte, and pediatric values have always been the most challenging. Some of the manufacturers' recommended reference intervals are listed in Table 46–1 for general chemistry, Table 46–2 for endocrinology, and Table 46–3 for hematology. The interpretation of chemistry and hematology laboratory results is equally complex and forms a continuous challenge for physicians and the medical community at large.

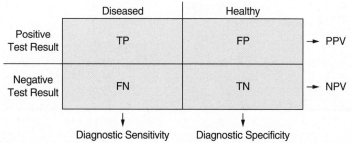

▲ **Figure 46–4.** Sensitivity, specificity, and predictive values of a test. FN, false negative; FP, false positive; NPV, negative predictive value; PPV, positive predictive value; TN, true negative; TP, true positive.

Table 46–1. General chemistry.

Analyte, Units Specimen Type	Age	Instrument	Male Range	Female Range
A$_{1C}$ hemoglobin (%) B	0 day–Adult	DCA Vantage	Normal: < 5.7% Prediabetes: 5.7%–6.5% Diabetes: > 6.5%	Normal: < 5.7% Prediabetes: 5.7%–6.5% Diabetes: > 6.5%
α-Fetoprotein (IU/mL) S, P	0–30 days 1–3 mo 4 mo–18 y > 18 y	Vitros 5600	50–100,000 40–1000 0–12 < 7.5	50–100,000 40–1000 0–12 < 7.5
α$_1$-Antitrypsin (mg/dL) S, P	0–1 mo 1–6 mo 6 mo–2 y 2–19 y > 19 y	Vitros 5600	79–223 71–190 60–161 70–179 88–183	79–223 71–190 60–161 70–179 88–183
Anti-streptolysin O (IU/mL) S, P	0–19 y > 19 y	Vitros 5600	< 241 < 200	< 241 < 200
Albumin (g/dL) S, P	0–7 days 8–30 days 1–2 mo 3–5 mo 6–12 mo 1–3 y 4–6 y 7–18 y ≥ 19 y	Vitros 5600	2.3–3.8 2.0–4.5 2.0–4.8 2.1–4.9 2.1–4.7 3.4–4.2 3.5–5.2 3.7–5.6 3.5–5.0	1.8–3.9 1.8–4.4 1.9–4.2 2.2–4.4 2.2–4.7 3.4–4.2 3.5–5.2 3.7–5.6 3.5–5.0
Allergens (KUA/L) S, P	0 day–Adult	Phadia ImmunoCAP	0–0.34	0–0.34
ALP (U/L) S, P	0–7 days 8–30 days 1–3 mo 4–6 mo 7–12 mo 1–3 y 4–6 y 7–9 y 10–11 y 12–13 y 14–15 y 16–18 y ≥ 19 y	Vitros 5600	77–265 91–375 60–360 55–325 60–300 129–291 134–346 156–386 120–488 178–455 116–483 58–237 38–126	65–270 65–365 80–425 80–345 60–330 129–291 134–346 156–386 116–515 93–386 62–209 45–116 38–126
ALT (U/L) S, P	0–3 y 4–13 y 14–18 y ≥ 19 y	Vitros 5600	12–45 10–41 11–26 < 50	14–45 11–28 10–35 5–34
Ammonia (μmol/L) P	0–1 days 1–13 y 14 d–17 y ≥ 18 y	Vitros 5600	64–107 56–92 21–50 9–33	64–107 56–92 21–50 9–33

(Continued)

Table 46–1. General chemistry. (*Continued*)

Analyte, Units Specimen Type	Age	Instrument	Male Range	Female Range
Amylase (U/L) S, P	0–2 mo	Vitros 5600	0–30	0–30
	3–5 mo		0–50	0–50
	6–11 mo		0–80	0–80
	1–18 y		30–100	30–100
	≥ 19 y		30–110	30–110
Anticardiolipin IGA (APL) S	0 day–Adult	Inova Bio-Flash	< 20	< 20
Anticardiolipin IGG (GPL) S	0 day–Adult	Inova Bio-Flash	< 20	< 20
Anticardiolipin IGM (MPL) S	0 day–Adult	Inova Bio-Flash	< 20	< 20
ASCA IGA (units) S	0 day–Adult	Inova DSX	< 20	< 20
ASCA IGG (units) S	0 day–Adult	Inova DSX	< 20	< 20
AST (U/L) S, P	0–7 days	Vitros 5600	30–100	24–95
	8–30 days		20–70	24–72
	1–3 mo		22–63	20–64
	4–6 mo		13–65	20–63
	7–12 mo		25–55	22–63
	1–3 y		20–60	20–60
	4–6 y		15–50	15–50
	7–9 y		15–40	15–40
	10–11 y		10–60	10–40
	12–15 y		15–40	10–30
	16–18 y		15–45	5–30
	≥ 19 y		17–59	14–36
Bilirubin direct (mg/dL) S, P	0–30 days	Vitros 5600	0–0.6	0–0.6
	> 1 mo		0–0.3	0–0.3
Bilirubin total (mg/dL) S, P	0–1 days	Vitros 5600	0.1–5.8	0.1–5.8
	1–2 days		0.1–8.5	0.1–8.5
	3–5 days		0.1–11.5	0.1–11.5
	6–30 days		< 11.5	< 11.5
	> 1 mo		0.2–1.2	0.2–1.2
Bilirubin indirect (mg/dL) S, P	0–30 days	Vitros 5600	0–0.6	0–0.6
	> 1 mo		0–0.3	0–0.3
BNP (ng/L) Whole blood (purple)	0 day–Adult	I-STAT	0–99	0–99
Pro-BNP (pg/mL) S, P	0 day–Adult	Vitros 5600	0–125	0–125
BUN (mg/dL) S, P	0–7 days	Vitros 5600	2–13	2–13
	8–30 days		2–16	2–15
	1–3 mo		2–12	2–14
	4–6 mo		1–14	1–13
	7–12 mo		2–14	1–13
	1–3 y		5–17	5–17
	4–13 y		7–17	7–17
	14–18 y		8–21	8–21
	≥ 19 y		9–20	7–17

(*Continued*)

Table 46–1. General chemistry. (*Continued*)

Analyte, Units Specimen Type	Age	Instrument	Male Range	Female Range
C3 (mg/dL) S, P	0–1 mo	Vitros 5600	55–129	55–129
	1–2 mo		61–155	61–155
	2–3 mo		67–136	67–136
	3–4 mo		64–182	64–182
	4–5 mo		67–174	67–174
	5–6 mo		77–178	77–178
	6–9 mo		78–173	78–173
	9–11 mo		76–187	76–187
	11–12 mo		87–181	87–181
	1–2 y		84–177	84–177
	2–3 y		80–178	80–178
	3–5 y		89–173	89–173
	5–8 y		92–161	92–161
	8–10 y		93–203	93–203
	10–19 y		86–184	86–184
	> 19 y		88–165	88–165
C4 (mg/dL) S, P	0–1 mo	Vitros 5600	9.2–33	9.2–33
	1–2 mo		9.7–37	9.7–37
	2–3 mo		11–35	11–35
	3–4 mo		11–50	11–50
	4–5 mo		9.3–47	9.3–47
	5–6 mo		11–55	11–55
	6–9 mo		12–48	12–48
	9–11 mo		16–51	16–51
	11–12 mo		16–52	16–52
	1–2 y		12–45	12–45
	2–3 y		13–47	13–47
	3–5 y		17–42	17–42
	5–8 y		16–42	16–42
	8–10 y		13–52	13–52
	10–19 y		10–40	10–40
	> 19 y		14–44	14–44
Ca (mg/dL) S, P	0–8 days	Vitros 5600	7.3–11.4	7.5–11.3
	8–30 days		8.6–11.7	8.4–11.9
	1–3 mo		8.5–11.3	8.0–11.1
	3–6 mo		8.3–11.4	7.7–11.5
	6–12 mo		7.7–11.0	7.8–11.1
	1–4 y		8.7–9.8	8.7–9.8
	4–10 y		8.8–10.1	8.8–10.1
	10–12 y		8.9–10.1	8.9–10.1
	12–14 y		8.8–10.6	8.8–10.6
	14–16 y		9.2–10.7	9.2–10.7
	16–19 y		8.9–10.7	8.9–10.7
	> 19 y		8.4–10.2	8.4–10.2
iCa (mmol/L) B	0–1 day	Radiometer ABL 90 flex	1.1–1.4	1.1–1.4
	1–3 days		1.1–1.5	1.1–1.5
	4–7 days		1.2–1.5	1.2–1.5
	8 days–1 mo		1.3–1.6	1.3–1.6
	1 mo–18 y		1.2–1.4	1.2–1.4
	> 18 y		1.2–1.3	1.2–1.3

(Continued)

Table 46–1. General chemistry. (*Continued*)

Analyte, Units Specimen Type	Age	Instrument	Male Range	Female Range
Chloride (mmol/L) S, P	0–8 days	Vitros 5600	96–111	96–111
	8 days–6 mo		96–110	96–110
	6–12 mo		96–108	96–108
	1–19 y		96–109	96–109
	> 19 y		98–107	98–107
Cholesterol (mg/dL) S, P	0 day–2 mo	Vitros 5600	45–177	63–198
	2–7 mo		60–197	66–218
	7–12 mo		89–208	74–218
	1–2 y		44–181	44–181
	2–18 y		< 170	< 170
	> 18 y		< 190	< 190
Creatine kinase (U/L) S, P	0–3 mo	Vitros 5600	28–300	42–470
	3–12 mo		24–170	26–240
	1–2 y		27–160	24–175
	2–11 y		30–150	24–175
	11–15 y		30–150	30–170
	15–19 y		33–145	27–140
Creatinine (mg/dL) S, P	0–3 days	Vitros 5600	0.33–1.08	0.33–1.08
	3–10 days		0.14–0.90	0.14–0.90
	10–17 days		0.14–0.61	0.14–0.61
	17 days–1 y		0.14–0.52	0.14–0.52
	1–11 y		0.23–0.61	0.23–0.61
	11–18 y		0.42–0.90	0.42–0.90
	> 18 y		0.71–1.18	0.52–0.99
Cystatin C (mg/L) S, P	0–3 mo	Vitros 5600	0.8–2.3	0.8–2.3
	4–12 mo		0.7–1.5	0.7–1.5
	> 1 y		0.5–1.3	0.5–1.3
Ferritin (ng/mL) S,P	0–6 wk	Vitros 5600	< 400	< 400
	7 wk–1 y		10–95	10–95
	1–10 y		10–60	10–60
	10–19 y		10–300	10–70
	19–50 y		n/a	6–137
	> 18 y		18–444	n/a
	> 50 y		n/a	11–264
Anti-deamidated gliadin peptide IgA	0 day–Adult	Bio-Flash	< 20	< 20
Anti-deamidated gliadin peptide IgG	0 day–Adult	Bio-Flash	< 20	< 20
GGT (U/L) S, P	0–8 days	Vitros 5600	25–148	19–131
	8–30 days		23–153	17–124
	1–4 mo		17–130	17–124
	4–7 mo		8–83	15–109
	7–12 mo		10–35	10–54
	1–4 y		5–16	5–16
	4–7 y		8–18	8–18
	7–10 y		11–21	11–21
	10–12 y		14–25	14–23
	12–14 y		14–37	12–21
	14–16 y		10–28	12–22
	16–19 y		9–29	9–23
	> 19 y		15–73	12–43

(*Continued*)

Table 46–1. General chemistry. (*Continued*)

Analyte, Units Specimen Type	Age	Instrument	Male Range	Female Range
Glucose (mg/dL) S, P	0–30 days > 1 mo	Vitros 5600	40–80 60–105	40–80 60–105
Glucose (2-h tolerance test) (mg/dL) S, P	0 day–Adult	Vitros 5600	< 200	< 200
Glucose–CSF (mg/dL) CSF	0 day–Adult	Vitros 5600	40–75	40–75
HDL (mg/dL) S, P	0 day–2 y 2 y–Adult	Vitros 5600	8–61 > 45	8–61 > 45
β_2-Glycoprotein 1-antibody, IgA (SAU) S	0 day–Adult	Inova Bio-Flash	0–20	0–20
β_2-Glycoprotein 1-antibody, IgG (SGU) S	0 day–Adult	Inova Bio-Flash	0–20	0–20
β_2-Glycoprotein 1-antibody, IgM (SMU) S	0 day–Adult	Inova Bio-Flash	0–20	0–20
IgA (mg/dL) S, P	0–30 days 1–6 mo 6–12 mo 1–4 y 4–7 y 7–10 y 10–13 y 13–16 y 16–19 y > 19 y	Vitros 5600	0–11 0–40 1–82 9–137 44–187 58–204 46–218 29–251 68–259 70–400	0–10 0–42 6–68 15–111 33–146 28–180 55–193 62–241 69–262 70–400
IgE (kU/L) S	0–12 mo 1–2 y 2–3 y 3–10 y 10 y–Adult	Phadia ImmunoCAP	0–29 0–49 0–45 0–52 0–87	0–29 0–49 0–45 0–52 0–87
IgG (mg/dL) S, P	0–30 days 1–6 mo 6–12 mo 1–4 y 4–7 y 7–10 y 10–13 y 13–16 y 16–19 y > 19 y	Vitros 5600	197–833 140–533 130–823 413–1112 468–1328 582–1441 685–1620 590–1600 522–1703 700–1600	136–872 311–664 325–647 421–1202 560–1319 485–1473 586–1609 749–1640 804–1817 700–1600

(Continued)

Table 46–1. General chemistry. (*Continued*)

Analyte, Units Specimen Type	Age	Instrument	Male Range	Female Range
IgM (mg/dL) S, P	0–30 days	Vitros 5600	0–65	0–57
	1–6 mo		0–84	0–127
	6–12 mo		15–117	0–130
	1–4 y		30–146	35–184
	4–7 y		31–151	42–184
	7–10 y		21–140	30–165
	10–13 y		27–151	42–211
	13–16 y		26–184	34–225
	16–19 y		28–179	42–224
	> 19 y		40–230	40–230
Iron (µg/dL) S, P	0–7 days	Vitros 5600	100–250	100–250
	7 d–1 y		40–100	40–100
	1–10 y		50–120	50–120
	> 10 y		49–181	37–170
Iron-binding capacity (mcg/dL) S	0 day–Adult	Vitros 5600	261–462	265–497
LDH (U/L) S, P	0–1 mo	Vitros 5600	550–2100	580–2000
	1–4 mo		480–1220	460–1150
	4–7 mo		400–1230	460–1150
	7–12 mo		380–1200	460–1060
	1–4 y		500–920	500–920
	4–7 y		470–900	470–900
	7–10 y		420–750	420–750
	10–12 y		432–700	380–700
	12–14 y		470–750	380–640
	14–16 y		360–730	390–580
	16–18 y		340–670	340–670
	> 18 y		313–618	313–618
LDL measured (mg/dL) S, P	0 day–Adult	Vitros 5600	< 100	< 100
Lead screen (mcg/dL) Whole blood-purple top	0 day–Adult	LeadCare	< 10	< 10
Magnesium (mg/dL) S, P	0–7 days	Vitros 5600	1.2–1.6	1.2–1.6
	7–30 days		1.6–2.4	1.6–2.4
	1 mo–2 y		1.6–2.6	1.6–2.6
	2–6 y		1.5–2.4	1.5–2.4
	6–10 y		1.6–2.3	1.6–2.3
	10–14 y		1.6–2.2	1.6–2.2
	> 14 y		1.5–2.3	1.5–2.3
iMg (mmol/L) B	0 day–Adult	Nova pHOx Ultra	0.45–0.60	0.45–0.60
Non-HDL cholesterol (mg/dL) S, P	2–18 y	Vitros 5600 (calculated)	< 120	< 120
	> 18 y		< 150	< 150
Potassium (mmol/L) S, P	0–7 days	Vitros 5600	3.7–5.9	3.7–5.9
	7 days–3 mo		4.1–5.3	4.1–5.3
	3 mo–18 y		3.4–4.7	3.4–4.7
	> 18 y		3.5–5.0	3.5–5.0

(*Continued*)

Table 46–1. General chemistry. (*Continued*)

Analyte, Units Specimen Type	Age	Instrument	Male Range	Female Range
Prealbumin (mg/dL) S, P	0–1 mo 1–6 mo 6 mo–4 y 4–6 y 6–14 y 14–19 y > 19 y	Vitros 5600	7–22 8–34 7–32 12–30 12–42 22–45 17–42	7–22 8–34 7–32 12–30 12–42 22–45 17–42
Phosphorus (mg/dL) S, P	0–15 days 15 days–1 y 1–5 y 5–13 y 13–16 y 16–19 y	Vitros 5600	5.85–10.9 5.05–8.76 4.52–7.09 4.37–6.25 3.41–5.82 3.19–5.29	5.85–10.9 5.05–8.76 4.52–7.09 4.37–6.25 3.78–6.47 3.19–5.29
Procalcitonin (ng/mL) P	0 day–Adult	Abbott Architect i1000	0–0.5	0–0.5
Prolactin (ng/mL) S, P	0 day–Adult	Vitros 5600	3.7–17.9	3.0–18.6
Sodium (mmol/L) S, P	0–8 days 8–30 days 1–6 mo 6–12 mo 1–19 y > 19 y	Vitros 5600	133–146 134–144 134–142 133–142 134–143 137–145	133–146 134–144 134–142 133–142 134–143 137–145
Anti–human tissue transglutaminase IgA	0 day–Adult	Bio-Flash	< 20	< 20
Anti–human tissue transglutaminase IgG	0 day–Adult	Bio-Flash	< 20	< 20
Troponin I (ng/mL) S, P	0 day–Adult	Vitros 5600	< 0.12	< 0.12
Total protein (g/dL) S, P	0–2 mo 2–6 mo 6–12 mo 1–4 y 4–7 y 7–10 y 10–20 y > 20 y	Vitros 5600	3.9–7.6 4.1–7.9 3.9–7.9 5.9–7.0 5.9–7.8 6.2–8.1 6.3–8.6 6.2–8.2	3.4–7.0 3.9–7.6 4.5–7.8 5.9–7.0 5.9–7.8 6.2–8.1 6.3–8.6 6.2–8.2
Triglycerides (mg/dL) S, P	0–9 y 10–18 y > 18 y	Vitros 5600	< 75 < 90 < 115	< 75 < 90 < 115
TCO_2-bicarb (mmol/L) S, P	0–7 days 7–30 days 1–6 mo 6–12 mo 1–19 y > 19	Vitros 5600	17–26 17–27 17–29 18–29 20–31 22–30	17–26 17–27 17–29 18–29 20–31 22–30

(Continued)

Table 46–1. General chemistry. (*Continued*)

Analyte, Units Specimen Type	Age	Instrument	Male Range	Female Range
Uric acid (mg/dL) S, P	0–30 days	Vitros 5600	2.0–5.2	2.0–5.2
	1–12 mo		2.5–9.0	2.5–9.0
	1–10 y		1.8–5.0	1.8–5.0
	10–12 y		2.3–5.4	3.0–4.7
	12–14 y		2.7–6.7	3.0–5.9
	14–16 y		2.4–7.8	3.0–5.9
	16–18 y		4.0–8.6	3.0–5.9
	> 18 y		3.5–8.5	2.5–7.5
Vitamin B$_{12}$ (pg/mL) S, P	0 day–Adult	Vitros 5600	163–949	163–949

ALP, alkaline phosphatase; ALT, alanine transaminase; ASCA, anti-*Saccharomyces cerevisiae* antibodies; AST, aspartate aminotransferase; B, whole blood; BNP, brain natriuretic peptide; BUN, blood urea nitrogen; Ca, calcium; CSF, cerebrospinal fluid; GGT, γ-glutamyl transpeptidase; HDL, high-density lipoprotein; iCa, ionized calcium; IgA, immunoglobulin A; IgE, immunoglobulin E; IgG, immunoglobulin G; IgM, immunoglobulin M; iMg, ionized magnesium; LDH, lactic dehydrogenase; P, plasma; S, serum; U, urine.
Data from Children's Hospital, Colorado, Chemistry Laboratory Procedure Manuals.

Table 46–2. Endocrine chemistry.

Analyte, Units, Specimen Type, Source	Age	Methodology	Male Range	Female Range
Cortisol (µg/dL) S, P	0 day–Adult (AM values) (PM values)	Vitros 5600	4.5–22.7 1.7–14.1	4.5–22.7 1.7–14.1
Estradiol (ng/mL) S	Prepuberty	HPLC/MS	< 1.5	< 1.5
	Tanner 1		0.5–1.1	0.5–2.0
	Tanner 2		0.5–1.6	1.0–2.4
	Tanner 3		0.5–2.5	0.7–6.0
	Tanner 4		1.0–3.6	2.1–8.5
	Tanner 5		1.0–3.6	3.4–17
FSH (mIU/mL) S, P	4 wk–11 mo	Siemens Immulite	0.16–4.1	0.24–14.2
	12 mo–8 y		0.26–3.0	1.0–4.2
	Tanner 1		0.26–3.0	1.0–4.2
	Tanner 2		1.8–3.2	1.0–10.8
	Tanner 3		1.2–5.8	1.5–12.8
	Tanner 4		2.0–9.2	1.5–11.7
	Tanner 5		2.6–11.0	1.0–9.2
	Adult		2.0–9.2	1.8–11.2
	Follicular			6–35
	Midcycle			1.8–11.2
	Luteal phase			
Growth hormone (ng/mL) S	0 day–Adult	Siemens Immulite	0–8	0–3

(*Continued*)

Table 46–2. Endocrine chemistry. (*Continued*)

Analyte, Units, Specimen Type, Source	Age	Methodology	Male Range	Female Range
IGF-BP3 (µg/mL) S, P	0–7 days	Siemens Immulite	0.1–0.7	0.1–0.7
	8–15 days		0.5–1.4	0.5–1.4
	16 days–1 y		0.7–3.6	0.7–3.6
	2 y		0.8–3.9	0.8–3.9
	3 y		0.9–4.3	0.9–4.3
	4 y		1.0–4.7	1.0–4.7
	5 y		1.1–5.2	1.1–5.2
	6 y		1.3–5.6	1.3–5.6
	7 y		1.4–6.1	1.4–6.1
	8 y		1.6–6.5	1.6–6.5
	9 y		1.8–7.1	1.8–7.1
	10 y		2.1–7.7	2.1–7.7
	11 y		2.4–8.4	2.4–8.4
	12 y		2.7–8.9	2.7–8.9
	13 y		3.1–9.5	3.1–9.5
	14 y		3.3–10.0	3.3–10.0
	15 y		3.5–10.0	3.5–10.0
	16 y		3.4–9.5	3.4–9.5
	17 y		3.2–8.7	3.2–8.7
	18 y		3.1–7.9	3.1–7.9
	19 y		2.9–7.3	2.9–7.3
	20 y		2.9–7.2	2.9–7.2
IGF-1 (ng/mL) S, P	0–3 y	Siemens Immulite	< 15.0–129.0	18.2–172.0
	4–6 y		22.0–208.0	35.4–232.0
	7–9 y		40.1–255.0	56.9–277.0
	10–11 y		68.7–316.0	118.0–448.0
	12–13 y		143.0–506.0	170.0–527.0
	14–15 y		177.0–507.0	191.0–496.0
	16–18 y		173.0–414.0	190.0–429.0
LH (mIU/mL) S, P	14 days–11 mo	Siemens Immulite	0.02–7.0	0.02–7.0
	12 mo–8 y		0.02–0.3	0.02–0.3
	Tanner 1		0.02–0.3	0.02–0.18
	Tanner 2		0.2–4.9	0.02–4.7
	Tanner 3		0.2–5.0	0.10–12.0
	Tanner 4		0.4–7.0	0.4–11.7
	Tanner 5		0.4–7.0	0.4–11.7
	Adult		1.5–9.0	2.0–9.0
	Follicular			18.0–49.0
	Midcycle			2.0–11.0
	Luteal			
T₃, total (ng/dL) S, P	0–3 days	Siemens Immulite	60–300	60–300
	4 days–1 y		90–260	90–260
	1–6 y		90–240	90–240
	7–11 y		90–230	90–230
	12–18 y		100–210	100–210
T₄ (µg/dL) S, P	0–3 days	Siemens Immulite	8–20	8–20
	3–30 days		5–15	5–15
	30 days–1 y		6–14	6–14
	1–6 y		4.5–12.5	4.5–12.5
	6–19 y		4.5–11.5	4.5–11.5
	> 19 y		4.5–11.5	5.5–11.5

(*Continued*)

Table 46–2. Endocrine chemistry. (*Continued*)

Analyte, Units, Specimen Type, Source	Age	Methodology	Male Range	Female Range
T₄ free (ng/dL) S	0–2 days	Siemens Immulite	2.0–5.0	2.0–5.0
	3–30 days		0.9–2.2	0.9–2.2
	1 mo–19 y		0.8–2.0	0.8–2.0
	> 19 y		0.78–2.19	0.78–2.19
TSH (μIU/mL) S, P	0–3 days	Vitros 5600	1.0–20.0	1.0–20.0
	3–30 days		0.5–8.0	0.5–8.0
	1–6 mo		0.5–6.0	0.5–6.0
	6 mo–5 y		0.5–6.0	0.5–6.0
	5–13 y		0.5–5.5	0.5–5.5
	> 13 y		0.5–5.0	0.5–5.0
Testosterone, total (ng/dL) S, P	Premature	Vitros 5600	37–198	5–22
	Newborn		75–400	20–64
	Prepubertal		1–10	1–10
	Tanner 1		1–10	1–10
	Tanner 2		18–150	7–28
	Tanner 3		100–320	15–35
	Tanner 4		200–620	13–32
	Tanner 5		350–970	20–38
Anti-thyroglobulin (IU/mL) S, P	0–Adult	Siemens Immulite	< 20	< 20
Thyroglobulin (ng/mL) S, P	0–Adult	Siemens Immulite	< 33	< 33

FSH, follicle-stimulating hormone; IGF-1, insulin-like growth factor 1; IGF-BP3, insulin-like growth factor–binding protein 3; LH, luteinizing hormone; T₃, triiodothyronine; T₄, thyroxine; TSH, thyroid-stimulating hormone.
Data from Children's Hospital, Colorado, Chemistry Laboratory Procedure Manuals.

Table 46–3. Hematology.

Analyte, Units, Specimen Type, Source	Age	Methodology	Male Range	Female Range
WBC (×10³/μL) EDTA whole blood	0–1 mo	Sysmex XN-Series	6.5–16.7	6.5–16.7
	1–24 mo		7.7–13.7	7.7–13.7
	2–12 y		5.7–10.5	5.7–10.5
	12–18 y		5.2–9.7	5.2–9.7
	> 18 y		5.8–10.3	5.8–10.3
RBC (×10⁶/μL) EDTA whole blood	0–14 days	Sysmex XN-Series	3.7–5.1	3.7–5.1
	15–30 days		3.25–4.62	3.25–4.62
	1–2 mo		3.0–4.3	3.0–4.3
	2–6 mo		3.3–4.7	3.3–4.7
	6 mo–6 y		3.75–4.9	3.75–4.9
	6–12 y		3.9–5.0	3.9–5.0
	12–18 y		4.1–5.4	3.9–5.0
	> 18 y		4.1–5.45	3.7–4.8

(Continued)

Table 46–3. Hematology. (*Continued*)

Analyte, Units, Specimen Type, Source	Age	Methodology	Male Range	Female Range
Hemoglobin (g/dL) EDTA whole blood	0–3 days	Sysmex XN-Series	12.8–18.1	12.8–18.1
	4–7 days		12.5–17.0	2.5–17.0
	8–14 days		11.9–16.3	11.9–16.3
	15–30 days		10.5–14.8	10.5–14.8
	1–6 mo		9.5–13.3	9.5–13.3
	6 mo–6 y		10.3–13.8	10.3–13.8
	6–12 y		11.1–14.5	11.1–14.5
	12–18 y		11.8–15.8	11.3–14.7
	> 18 y		11.8–16.4	11.2–14.3
HCT (%) EDTA whole blood	0–3 days	Sysmex XN-Series	36.5–51.4	36.5–51.4
	4–7 days		35.0–47.5	35.0–47.5
	8–14 days		33.6–45.0	33.6–45.0
	15–30 days		30.0–40.9	30.0–40.9
	1–6 mo		27.0–38.5	27.0–38.5
	6 mo–6 y		30.5–39.7	30.5–39.7
	6–12 y		32.9–41.5	32.9–41.5
	12–18 y		34.0–46.0	33.0–42.6
	> 18 y		34.0–48.0	33.0–42.6
MCV (fL) EDTA whole blood	0–3 days	Sysmex XN-Series	97.0–106.0	97.0–106.0
	4–7 days		90.0–101.0	90.0–101.0
	8–30 days		87.0–96.5	87.0–96.5
	1–2 mo		86.5–92.1	86.5–92.1
	2–6 mo		82.0–87.0	82.0–87.0
	6 mo–12 y		75.6–85.2	75.6–85.2
	12–18 y		80.8–87.7	80.8–87.7
	> 18 y		83.5–90.2	83.5–90.2
Polys (×10³/µL) (absolute) EDTA whole blood	0–3 days	Sysmex XN-Series	4.33–9.11	4.43–11.4
	4–30 days		3.33–9.42	3.18–9.43
	1 mo–2 y		1.5–6.0	1.5–6.0
	2–10 y		1.8–5.4	1.8–5.4
	10–18 y		2.0–5.8	2.0–5.8
	> 18 y		2.5–6.0	2.5–6.0
Bands (×10³/µL) (absolute) EDTA whole blood	0–1 mo	Sysmex XN-Series	0–3.5	0–3.5
	1 mo–Adult		0–1.0	0–1.0
Lymphs (×10³/µL) (absolute) EDTA whole blood	0–15 days	Sysmex XN-Series	1.35–4.09	1.35–4.09
	15–30 days		1.68–5.25	1.68–5.25
	1 mo–2 y		2.22–5.63	2.22–5.63
	2–6 y		1.33–3.47	1.33–3.47
	6–12 y		1.23–2.69	1.23–2.69
	> 12 y		1.03–2.18	1.03–2.18
Monos (×10³/µL) (absolute) EDTA whole blood	0–15 days	Sysmex XN-Series	0.52–1.77	0.52–1.77
	16 days–6 mo		0.28–1.38	0.28–1.38
	6 mo–2 y		0.25–1.15	0.25–1.15
	2 y–Adult		0.18–0.94	0.18–0.94
EOS (×10³/µL) (absolute) EDTA whole blood	0–1 mo	Sysmex XN-Series	0.03–0.51	0.03–0.51
	1 mo–Adult		0.01–0.42	0.01–0.42

(*Continued*)

Table 46–3. Hematology. (*Continued*)

Analyte, Units, Specimen Type, Source	Age	Methodology	Male Range	Female Range
Basos (×10³/μL) (absolute) EDTA whole blood	0–15 days 16 days–Adult	Sysmex XN-Series	0.02–0.11 0.01–0.07	0.02–0.11 0.01–0.07
Platelet (×10³/μL) EDTA whole blood	0 days–Adult	Sysmex XN-Series	150–500	150–500
MCH (pg) EDTA whole blood	0–3 days 4–60 days 2 mo–18 y > 18 y	Sysmex XN-Series	31.7–36.4 29.8–33.4 26.0–30.7 28.3–31.4	31.7–36.4 29.8–33.4 26.0–30.7 28.3–31.4
MCHC (g/dL) EDTA whole blood	0 day–Adult	Sysmex XN-Series	33.5–36.0	33.5–36.0

Data from Children's Hospital, Colorado, Hematology Laboratory Procedure Manual.

Index

Note: Page numbers followed by *f* and *t* indicate figures and tables.